YOUMANS
Neurological Surgery

YOUMANS
Neurological Surgery

Fifth Edition

H. Richard Winn, MD
Professor of Neurological Surgery
and Neuroscience
Mount Sinai School of Medicine
New York, New York

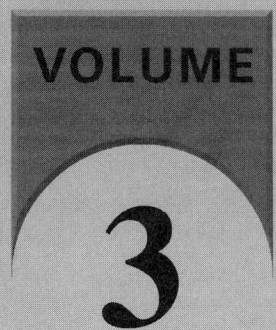
VOLUME
3

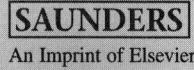
SAUNDERS
An Imprint of Elsevier

SAUNDERS
An Imprint of Elsevier

The Curtis Center
Independence Square West
Philadelphia, Pennsylvania 19106

YOUMANS NEUROLOGICAL SURGERY
Copyright 2004, Elsevier Inc. All rights reserved. ISBN 0-7216-8291-x.

Notice

Neurosurgery is an ever-changing field. Standard safety precautions must be followed, but as new research and clinical experience broaden our knowledge, changes in treatment and drug therapy become necessary or appropriate. Readers are advised to check the product information currently provided by the manufacturer of each drug to be administered to verify the recommended dose, the method and duration of administration, and the contraindications. It is the responsibility of the treating physician, relying on experience and knowledge of the patient, to determine dosage and the best treatment for each individual patient. Neither the publisher nor the editor assumes any responsibility for any injury and/or damage to persons or property arising from this publication.

The Publisher

First Edition 1973. Second Edition 1982. Third Edition 1990. Fourth Edition 1996.

Library of Congress Cataloging-in-Publication Data

Youmans neurological surgery / [edited by] H. Richard Winn.—5th ed.

   p. cm.

   Rev. ed. of: Neurological surgery / editor-in-chief, Julian R. Youmans; associate editors, Donald P. Becker . . . [et al.]. 4th ed. c1996.

   Includes bibliographical references and index.

   ISBN 0–7216–8291–X

   1. Nervous system—Surgery. I. Title: Neurological surgery. II. Winn, H. Richard. III. Youmans, Julian R., 1928–
   [DNLM: 1. Neurosurgical Procedures. 2. Nervous System Diseases—surgery. 3. Neurosurgery—methods. WL 368 Y671 2003]

   RE593 N4153 2003

   617.4′8—dc21
   2002017677

Vice President, Global Surgery: Richard Lampert

Developmental Editors: Anne Snyder, David Orzechowski

Project Manager: Jodi Kaye

Printed in the United States of America.

Last digit is the print number: 9 8 7 6 5 4 3 2 1

To my wife and family, and to my residents who have carried the message.

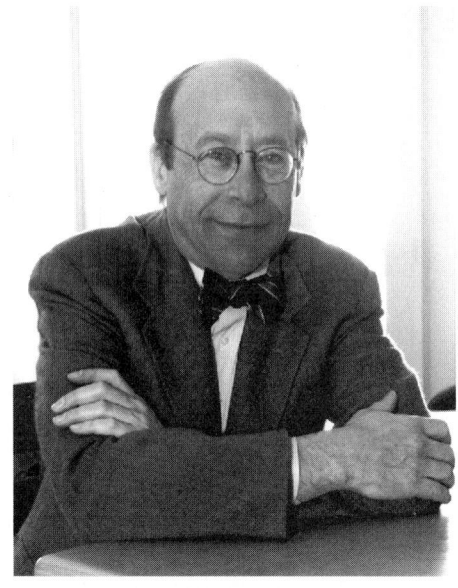

H. Richard Winn, MD
Professor of Neurological Surgery and
Neuroscience
Mount Sinai School of Medicine
New York, New York

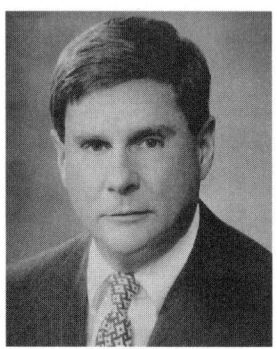

Ralph G. Dacey, Jr., MD
Henry G. and Edith R. Schwartz Professor and
Chairman
Department of Neurological Surgery
Washington University School of Medicine
St. Louis, Missouri

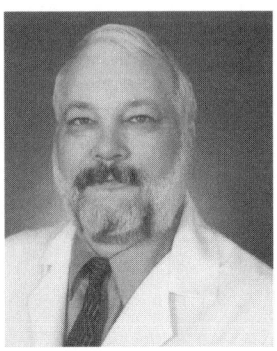

Roy A. E. Bakay, MD
Professor and Vice Chairman
Department of Neurosurgery
Rush Medical Center
Chicago, Illinois
Functional Neurosurgery, Volume 3

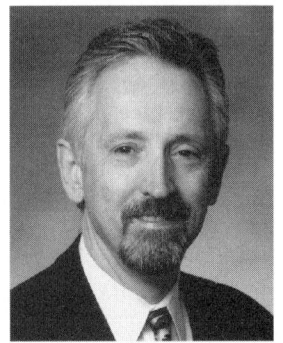

Kim J. Burchiel, MD
Professor and Chairman
Department of Neurological Surgery
Oregon Health & Science University
School of Medicine
Portland, Oregon
Functional Neurosurgery and Pain, Vol. 3

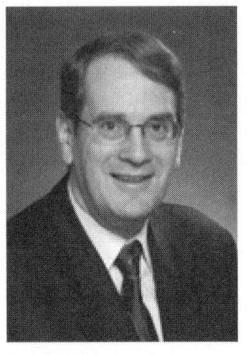

Henry Brem, MD
Harvey Cushing Professor of Neurosurgery,
Ophthalmology, and Oncology
Chairman, Department of Neurosurgery
Johns Hopkins University School of Medicine
Baltimore, Maryland
Oncology, Volume 1

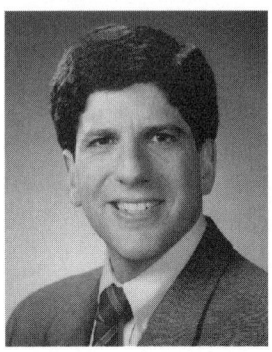

William A. Friedman, M.D.
Professor and Chair,
Department of Neurosurgery
University of Florida,
Gainesville, Florida
Radiation Therapy and Radiosurgery, Volume 4

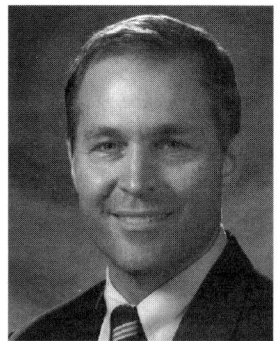

M. Sean Grady, MD

Charles Harrison Frazier Professor and Chair of the
Department of Neurosurgery
University of Pennsylvania School of Medicine
Philadelphia, Pennsylvania

Trauma, Volume 4

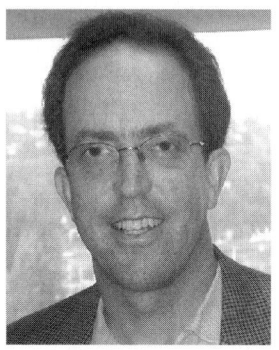

Michel Kliot, MD

Associate Professor of Neurosurgery
University of Washington School of Medicine
Seattle, Washington

*Introduction to Neurological Surgery, Volume 1; Peripheral
Nerve, Volume 4*

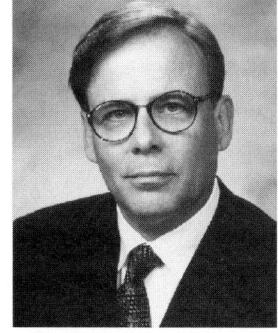

L. Dade Lunsford, MD

Lars Leksell Professor and Chairman of Neurological
Surgery, Radiology, and Radiology Oncology
University of Pittsburgh School of Medicine
University of Pittsburgh Medical Center
Pittsburgh, Pennsylvania

Radiation Therapy and Radiosurgery, Volume 4

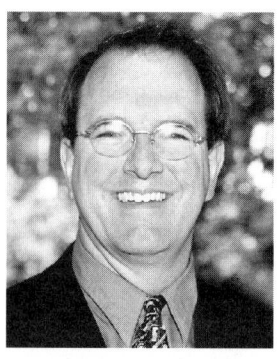

Joel D. MacDonald, MD

Assistant Professor of Neurosurgery
University of Utah Medical Center
Salt Lake City, Utah

Special Features

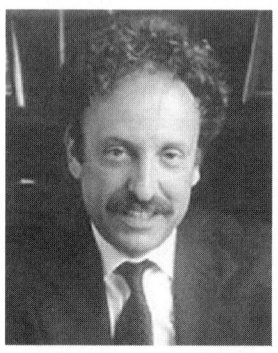

Lawrence F. Marshall, MD

Professor of Neurological Surgery
University of California, San Diego,
School of Medicine
San Diego, California

Trauma, Volume 4

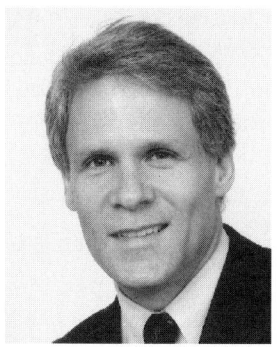

Marc R. Mayberg, MD

Chairman, Department of Neurosurgery
Cleveland Clinic Foundation
Cleveland, Ohio

Special Features

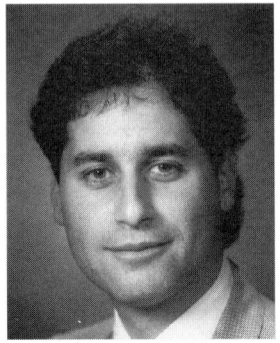

Fredric B. Meyer, MD
Professor of Neurosurgery
Mayo Medical School
Rochester, Minnesota
Vascular, Volume 2

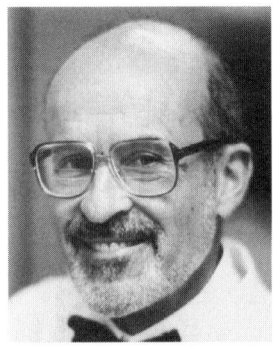

R. Michael Scott, MD
Professor of Neurological Surgery
Harvard Medical School
Boston, Massachusetts
Pediatric, Volume 3

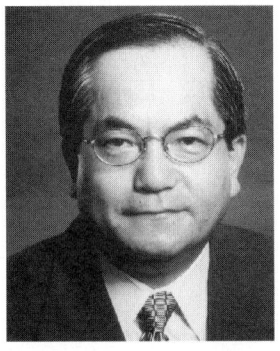

T. S. Park, MD
Shi H. Huang Professor of Neurosurgery and
Professor of Pediatrics and Anatomy and
Neurobiology
Washington University School of Medicine
St. Louis, Missouri
Pediatric, Volume 3

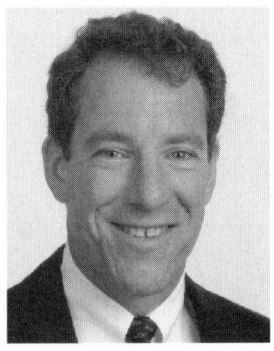

Daniel L. Silbergeld, MD
Associate Professor, Department of
Neurological Surgery
University of Washington School of Medicine
Seattle, Washington
Epilepsy, Volume 2

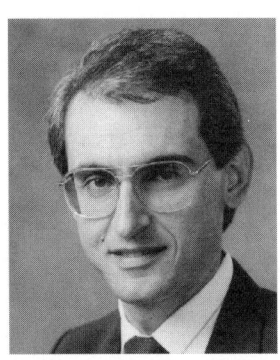

Raymond Sawaya, MD
Professor of Neurosurgery
University of Texas–Houston Medical School
Department of Neurosurgery
The University of Texas MD Anderson Cancer Center
Houston, Texas
Oncology, Volume 1

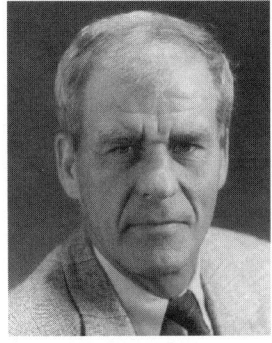

Volker K. H. Sonntag, MD
Clinical Professor of Neurosurgery
University of Arizona College of Medicine
Tucson, Arizona
Vice Chairman, Division of Neurological Surgery
Barrow Neurological Institute
Phoenix, Arizona
Spine, Volume 4

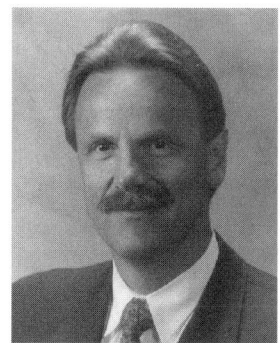

Robert F. Spetzler, MD
Professor, Department of Surgery,
Section of Neurosurgery
University of Arizona College of Medicine
Tucson, Arizona
Director and J. N. Harbor Chairman of
Neurological Surgery
Barrow Neurological Institute
Phoenix, Arizona
Vascular, Volume 2

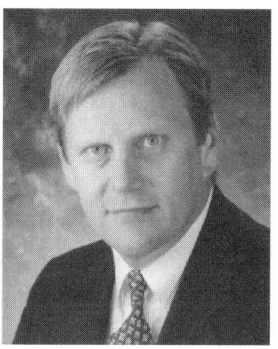

Dennis G. Vollmer, MD
Professor of Neurosurgery
University of Texas Health Science Center at Houston
Houston, Texas
Spine, Volume 4

CONTRIBUTORS

Khaled M. Abdel Aziz, MD, PhD

Resident, Department of Neurosurgery, University of Cincinnati College of Medicine and University Hospital, Cincinnati, Ohio
Dorsal Rhizotomy and Dorsal Root Ganglionectomy

Muwaffak M. Abdulhak, MD

Clinical Instructor, Department of Neurosurgery, Medical College of Wisconsin, Milwaukee, Wisconsin
Bone Metabolism as It Relates to Spinal Disease and Treatment

Saleem I. Abdulrauf, MD

Assistant Professor, Neurological Surgery and Director, Cerebrovascular and Skull Base Surgery Program, Saint Louis University School of Medicine; Director, Cerebrovascular and Skull Base Surgery Program, Saint Louis University Hospital, St. Louis, Missouri
Meningiomas

Dima Abi-Said, MD

Attending, Department of Neurosurgery, The University of Texas M.D. Anderson Cancer Center, Houston, Texas
Metastatic Brain Tumors

John R. Adler, Jr., MD

Professor, Department of Neurosurgery, Stanford University School of Medicine, Stanford, California
General and Historical Considerations of Radiotherapy and Radiosurgery

Robin Albert, MD, MPH

Research Coordinator, Center for Endovascular Surgery, Institute for Neurology and Neurosurgery, Beth Israel Medical Center, New York, New York
Endovascular Management of Brain Arteriovenous Malformations

A. Leland Albright, MD

Professor of Neurosurgery, University of Pittsburgh School of Medicine; Chief, Pediatric Neurosurgery, Childrens Hospital of Pittsburgh, Pittsburgh, Pennsylvania
Patient Selection in Movement Disorder Surgery; Brainstem Gliomas

Felipe C. Albuquerque, MD

Staff Neurosurgeon and Assistant Director, Endovascular Neurosurgery, Barrow Neurological Institute, Phoenix, Arizona
Carotid Angioplasty and Stenting: Interventional Treatment of Occlusive Vascular Disease; Basilar Trunk Aneurysms

Kenneth Aldape, MD

Assistant Professor, Department of Pathology, Neuropathology Unit, University of California, San Francisco, School of Medicine, San Francisco, California
Low-Grade Gliomas: Astrocytoma, Oligodendroglioma, and Mixed Gliomas

Eben Alexander III, MD

Associate Professor of Surgery, Department of Surgery, Division of Neurosurgery, University of Massachusetts Medical School; Attending Neurosurgeon, University of Massachusetts-Memorial Hospitals, Worcester, Massachusetts
Linac Radiosurgery

Michael J. Alexander, MD

Assistant Professor, Department of Surgery, Divisions of Neurosurgery and Interventional Neuroradiology, Duke University School of Medicine, Durham, North Carolina
Nonatherosclerotic Carotid Lesions

Mir Jafar Ali, MD

Resident, Department of Neurosurgery, University of Michigan Hospital, Ann Arbor, Michigan
Basilar Apex and Posterior Cerebral Artery Aneurysms

Ahmed Alkhani, MD

Fellow in Functional Neurosurgery, University of Toronto Faculty of Medicine and Toronto Western Hospital, Toronto, Ontario, Canada
Pallidotomy for Parkinson's Disease

Cargill H. Alleyne, Jr., MD

Co-Director, Neurosurgery Residency Program, University of Rochester School of Medicine and Dentistry; Chief, Division of Stroke and Cerebrovascular Surgery, Department of Surgery, Rochester General Hospital, Rochester, New York
Carotid Angioplasty and Stenting: Interventional Treatment of Occlusive Vascular Disease; Traumatic Carotid Injury

Ossama Al-Mefty, MD

Professor and Chairman, Department of
Neurosurgery, University of Arkansas for Medical
Sciences, Little Rock, Arkansas
Meningiomas

Mahmoud Al-Yamany, MD

Department of Neurosurgery, Riyadh Medical
Complex, King Saud University Affiliated Hospital,
Riyadh, Saudi Arabia
Intracranial Internal Carotid Artery Aneurysms

Arun Paul Amar, MD

Clinical Instructor, Department of Neurosurgery,
University of Southern California Keck School of
Medicine; Staff, Children's Hospital of Los Angeles,
Los Angeles, California
*Ventricular Tumors; Vagus Nerve Stimulation for
Intractable Epilepsy*

Christopher Ames, MD

Assistant Professor, Department of Neurological
Surgery, University of California, San Francisco,
School of Medicine, San Francisco, California
Differential Diagnosis of Altered States of Consciousness

Sepideh Amin-Hanjani, MD

Instructor in Surgery, Harvard Medical School;
Assistant Visiting Surgeon, Department of
Neurosurgery, Massachusetts General Hospital,
Boston, Massachusetts
Cerebral Lymphoma

Norberto Andaluz, MD

Clinical Fellow, Department of Neurosurgery,
University of Cincinnati College of Medicine,
Cincinnati, Ohio
Dorsal Rhizotomy and Dorsal Root Ganglionectomy

Peter Angevine, MD

Resident, Department of Neurological Surgery,
Columbia-Presbyterian Medical Center, New York,
New York
Anterior Lumbar Instrumentation

Ronald I. Apfelbaum, MD

Professor of Neurosurgery, University of Utah School
of Medicine; Attending, University of Utah Hospital
and Clinics, Salt Lake City, Utah
Treatment of Axis Fractures

Michael L. J. Apuzzo, MD

Edwin M. Todd/Treat M. Wells, Jr. Professor of
Neurological Surgery and Professor of Radiation
Oncology, Biology, and Physics, University of
Southern California Keck School of Medicine; Staff,
USC Care Medical Group, USC University Hospital,
and USC/Norris Cancer Hospital, Los Angeles,
California
*Ventricular Tumors; Vagus Nerve Stimulation for
Intractable Epilepsy*

Claire Ardouin, MA

Psychologist, Hôpital Albert Michallon, Grenoble,
France
Deep Brain Stimulation for Movement Disorders

E. Joy Arpin-Sypert, MD

Sypert Institute, Fort Myers, Florida
Evaluation and Management of the Failed Back Syndrome

James I. Ausman, MD

Professor of Neurosurgery, University of Illinois at
Chicago, Chicago, Illinois; Editor, *Surgical Neurology*
Extracranial Vertebral Artery Disease

Issam A. Awad, MD, MSc

Ogsbury-Kindt Professor and Chairman, Department
of Neurosurgery, and Professor of Neurosurgery,
Neurology, and Pathology, University of Colorado
School of Medicine, Denver, Colorado
*Surgical Management of Supratentorial Cavernous
Malformations*

Julian E. Bailes, MD

Professor and Chairman, Department of
Neurosurgery, West Virginia University School of
Medicine, Morgantown, West Virginia
Carotid Endarterectomy

Roy A. E. Bakay, MD

Professor and Vice Chairman, Director of Movement
Disorder Surgery, Rush-Presbyterian-St. Luke's
Medical Center, Chicago Institute of Neurosurgery
and Neuroresearch, Chicago, Illinois
*History of Functional Neurosurgery; Cellular
Transplantation in the Central Nervous System*

Perry A. Ball, MD

Attending Neurosurgeon, Section of Neurosurgery,
Dartmouth-Hitchcock Medical Center, Lebanon, New
Hampshire
Treatment of Disk Disease of the Lumbar Spine

Gordon H. Baltuch, MD, PhD

Assistant Professor, Department of Neurosurgery,
University of Pennsylvania School of Medicine;
Attending Neurosurgeon, Hospital of the University
of Pennsylvania, Pennsylvania Hospital, and
Philadelphia Veterans Administration Medical Center,
Philadelphia, Pennsylvania
Topectomy: Uses and Indications

Gene H. Barnett, MD

Professor of Surgery, Ohio State University College of
Medicine and Public Health, Columbus; Chairman,
Brain Tumor Institute, Cleveland Clinic Foundation,
Cleveland, Ohio
Surgical Navigation for Brain Tumors

Stanley L. Barnwell, MD, PhD

Associate Professor of Neurological Surgery, Oregon Health & Science University School of Medicine; Staff, Dotter Interventional Institute, Portland, Oregon
Cerebral Venous and Sinus Thrombosis

Jean-Claude Baron, MD

Professor of Stroke Medicine, Department of Neurology, University of Cambridge Faculty of Medicine; Neurology Consultant, Addenbrooke's Hospital, Cambridge, England
Positron Emission Tomography in Cerebrovascular Disease

Daniel L. Barrow, MD

MBNA-Bowman Professor and Chairman, Department of Neurological Surgery, Emory University School of Medicine; Chief, Neurological Service, and Co-Director, Emory Stroke Center, Emory University Hospital, Atlanta, Georgia
Treatment of Lateral-Sigmoid and Sagittal Sinus Dural Arteriovenous Malformations

Juan Bartolomei, MD

Assistant Professor, Department of Neurosurgery, Yale University School of Medicine, New Haven, Connecticut
Anterior Approach including Cervical Corpectomy (Degenerative)

Jonathan J. Baskin, MD

Attending Neurosurgeon, Atlantic Neurosurgical Specialists, Chatham, New Jersey
Carotid Angioplasty and Stenting; Interventional Treatment of Occlusive Vascular Disease; Anterior Cervical Instrumentation; Occipitocervical Fusion

H. Hunt Batjer, MD

Professor and Chair, Department of Neurological Surgery, Northwestern University Feinberg School of Medicine; Chairman, Department of Neurological Surgery, Northwestern Memorial Hospital, Chicago, Illinois
Basilar Apex and Posterior Cerebral Artery Aneurysms

Thomas K. Baumann, PhD

Associate Professor, Department of Neurological Surgery and Department of Physiology and Pharmacology, Oregon Health and Science University School of Medicine, Portland, Oregon
Physiologic Anatomy of Pain

Andrew Beaumont, MD

Neurosurgical Fellow, Virginia Commonwealth University School of Medicine, Richmond, Virginia
Physiology of the Cerebrospinal Fluid and Intracranial Pressure

Joshua Bederson, MD

Professor, Department of Neurosurgery, Mount Sinai School of Medicine; Vice Chairman, Department of Neurosurgery, Mount Sinai Medical Center, New York, New York
Infectious Intracranial Aneurysms

Ghassan K. Bejjani, MD

Clinical Assistant Professor, Department of Neurosurgery, University of Pittsburgh School of Medicine; Neurosurgeon, Presbyterian University Hospital, Pittsburgh, Pennsylvania
Orbital Tumors

J. Brad Bellotte, MD

Resident, Department of Neurosurgery, Allegheny General Hospital, Pittsburgh, Pennsylvania
Brain Death; Diagnosis and Management of Seventh and Eighth Cranial Nerve Injuries due to Temporal Bone Fractures

Alim L. Benabid, MD, PhD

Professor of Biophysics, University Joseph Fourier Medical School; Head, Neurosurgery, and Director, INSERM U.318 Research Laboratory of Preclinical Neurosciences, Hôpital Albert Michallon, Grenoble, France
Deep Brain Stimulation for Movement Disorders

Eduardo E. Benarroch, MD

Professor of Neurology, Mayo Medical School; Consultant in Neurology, Mayo Clinic, Rochester, Minnesota
Cerebral Blood Flow and Metabolism

Abdelhamid Benazzouz, PhD

Research Fellow, University of Bordeaux School of Medicine; Director of Research, Neurophysiology Laboratory, University Victor Segalan, Bordeaux, France
Deep Brain Stimulation for Movement Disorders

Bernard R. Bendok, MD

Assistant Professor, Department of Neurological Surgery, Northwestern University Feinberg School of Medicine, Chicago, Illinois
Basilar Apex and Posterior Cerebral Artery Aneurysms

Gregory J. Bennett, MD

Clinical Assistant Professor of Neurosurgery, University of Buffalo; Clinical Director of Neurosurgery, Erie County Medical Center, Buffalo, New York
Spondylolysis and Spondylolisthesis

Alejandro Berenstein, MD

Professor of Radiology, Neurosurgery, and Neurology, Albert Einstein College of Medicine of Yeshiva University, Bronx; Director, Center for Endovascular Surgery, and Director, Institute for Neurology and Neurosurgery, Beth Israel Medical Center, New York, New York

Endovascular Management of Brain Arteriovenous Malformations

Mitchel S. Berger, MD

Professor and Chair, Department of Neurological Surgery, University of California, San Francisco, School of Medicine, San Francisco, California

Low-Grade Gliomas: Astrocytoma, Oligodendroglioma, and Mixed Gliomas; Hemangioblastomas of the Central Nervous System; Interstitial and Intracavitary Irradiation of Brian Tumors

Matt A. Bernstein, PhD

Assistant Professor of Radiologic Physics, Mayo Medical School; Senior Associate Consultant in Radiology, Mayo Clinic, Rochester, Minnesota

Magnetic Resonance Angiography

José Biller, MD

Professor and Chairman, Department of Neurology, Indiana University School of Medicine, Indianapolis, Indiana

Carotid Occlusive Disease: Natural History and Medical Management

Jeffrey R. Binder, MD

Professor, Department of Neurology, Medical College of Wisconsin, Milwaukee, Wisconsin

Functional Magnetic Resonance Imaging in Epilepsy Surgery

Barry D. Birch, MD

Attending, Department of Neurosurgery, Mayo Clinic Scottsdale, Scottsdale, Arizona

Anterior Thoracic Instrumentation

Rolfe Birch, MChir

Visiting Professor, University College and Imperial College, London University, London; Orthopaedic Surgeon, Peripheral Nerve Injury Unit, Royal National Orthopaedic Hospital, Stanmore, England

Management of Acute Peripheral Nerve Injuries

Peter M. Black, MD, PhD

Franc D. Ingraham Professor of Neurosurgery, Harvard Medical School; Neurosurgeon-in-Chief, Brigham and Women's Hospital and Children's Hospital, and Chief, Neurosurgical Oncology, Dana-Farber Cancer Institute, Boston, Massachusetts

Craniopharyngioma in the Adult

Miroslav P. Bobek, MD

Attending Surgeon, Providence Medford Medical Center, Medford, Oregon

Brain Edema and Tumor-Host Interactions

Anne Boulin, MD

Neuroradiologist, Hôpital Foch, Suresnes, France

Osseous Tumors

Blaise F. D. Bourgeois, MD

Director, Division of Epilepsy and Clinical Neurophysiology, Department of Neurology, Children's Hospital, Boston, Massachusetts

Antiepileptic Medications: Principles of Clinical Use

Guy Bouvier, MD

Professor of Neurosurgery, University of Montreal Faculty of Medicine, Montreal; Neurosurgeon, Hôpital Notredame, Montreal; Medical Advisor to the Vice President, Western Region, Workers' Compensation Board of Appeal, St. Lambert, Quebec, Canada

Selective Peripheral Denervation for Spasmodic Torticollis

Frank J. Bova, PhD

Professor of Neurosurgery, University of Florida College of Medicine; Staff, Shand's Hospital, Gainesville, Florida

Fractionated and Stereotactic Radiation, Extracranial Stereotactic Radiation, Intensity Modulation, and Multileaf Collimation

Robin Bowman, MD

Assistant Professor of Neurosurgery, Northwestern University Feinberg School of Medicine; Attending Neurosurgeon, Children's Memorial Hospital, Chicago, Illinois

Birth Head Trauma

Adam Brant, MD

Staff Neurosurgeon, St. Agnes Medical Center, Fresno, California

Traumatic Cerebrospinal Fluid Fistulas

Henry Brem, MD

Harvey Cushing Professor of Neurosurgery, Ophthalmology, and Oncology and Chairman, Department of Neurosurgery, Johns Hopkins University School of Medicine; Director, Hunterian Neurosurgical Laboratory, and Neurosurgeon-in-Chief, Johns Hopkins Hospital, Baltimore, Maryland

Brain Tumors: General Considerations; Basic Principles of Cranial Surgery for Brain Tumors

Steven Brem, MD

Professor and Chief, Neurosurgery Service/Director, Neuro-oncology Research Laboratory/NABTT; and Investigator/Program Leader, Neuro-oncology Program, H. Lee Moffitt Cancer Center and Research Institute, Tampa, Florida

Angiogenesis and Brain Tumors

Gavin W. Britz, MD

Assistant Professor, Department of Neurological Surgery, University of Washington School of Medicine; Attending Neurosurgeon, Harborview Medical Center, Seattle, Washington

The Natural History of Unruptured Saccular Cerebral Aneurysms; Traumatic Cerebral Aneurysms Secondary to Penetrating Intracranial Injuries; Endovascular Treatment of Spinal Cord Arteriovenous Malformations; Magnetic Resonance Imaging for Peripheral Nerve Disorders

Carolyn D. Brockington, MD

Attending, Department of Neurology, Herbert and Nell Singer Division, Beth Israel Medical Center, New York, New York

Acute Medical Management of Ischemic Disease and Stroke

Jason A. Brodkey, MD

Staff, Michigan Brain & Spine Institute, Michigan Orthopedic Center, Ypsilanti, Michigan

Glomus Jugulare Tumors

Richard A. Bronen, MD

Associate Professor of Diagnostic Radiology and Neurosurgery, Yale University School of Medicine, New Haven, Connecticut

Preoperative Evaluation for Epilepsy Surgery: Computed Tomography and Magnetic Resonance Imaging

David J. Brooks, MD, DSc

Hartnett Professor of Neurology, Imperial College Faculty of Medicine; Consultant Neurologist, Hammersmith Hospital, London, England

Positron Emission Tomography in Movement Disorders

Jeffrey A. Brown, MD

Professor, Department of Neurosurgery, Wayne State University School of Medicine, Detroit, Michigan

Percutaneous Techniques (Trigeminal Neuralgia)

Robert D. Brown, Jr., MD

Associate Professor of Neurology, Mayo Medical School and Mayo Graduate School of Medicine; Chair, Division of Cerebrovascular Diseases, and Consultant, Department of Neurology, Mayo Clinic, Rochester, Minnesota

Natural History of Intracranial Vascular Malformations

Jeffrey N. Bruce, MD

Associate Professor of Neurological Surgery, Colombia University College of Physicians and Surgeons; Associate Attending in Neurological Surgery, New York Presbyterian Hospital, New York, New York

Pineal Tumors

John M. Buatti, MD

Professor and Head, Department of Radiation Oncology, University of Iowa Roy J. and Lucille A. Carver College of Medicine; Attending, University of Iowa Hospitals and Clinics, Iowa City, Iowa

Radiobiology; Radiotherapy for Benign Skull Base Tumors; Fractionated and Stereotactic Radiation, Extracranial Stereotactic Radiation, Intensity Modulation, and Multileaf Collimation

Robert J. Buchanan, MD

Assistant Professor, Department of Psychiatry, University of California, San Diego, School of Medicine; Chief Resident, Division of Neurosurgery, UCSD Medical Center, San Diego, California

Traumatic Cerebrospinal Fluid Fistulas

Dennis E. Bullard, MD

Associate Clinical Professor, Department of Surgery, Division of Neurosurgery, University of North Carolina at Chapel Hill School of Medicine, Chapel Hill; Chief, Division of Neurosurgery, Rex Hospital, Raleigh, North Carolina

Caudalis Nucleus Dorsal Root Entry Zone Procedure for the Treatment of Intractable Facial Pain

M. Ross Bullock, MD, PhD

Virginia Commonwealth University School of Medicine, Richmond, Virginia

Surgical Management of Traumatic Brain Injury

Kim J. Burchiel, MD

Professor and Chairman, Department of Neurological Surgery, Oregon Health & Science University School of Medicine, Portland, Oregon

Pain: General Historical Considerations; Alternative Surgical Treatments for Trigeminal Neuralgia

Matthew V. Burry, MD

Resident in Neurosurgery, University of Florida College of Medicine, Gainesville, Florida

Vein of Galen Malformations

Richard W. Byrne, MD

Assistant Professor of Neurosurgery, Rush Medical College of Rush University; Attending Neurosurgeon, Rush-Presbyterian-St. Luke's Medical Center, Chicago, Illinois

Multiple Subpial Transection

Jeffrey W. Campbell, MD

Assistant Professor of Neurosurgery, University of South Carolina College of Medicine; Director, Pediatric Neurosurgery, MUSC Children's Hospital, Charleston, South Carolina

Cerebellar Astrocytomas in Children

Martin B. Camins, MD

Clinical Professor of Neurological Surgery, Mount Sinai School of Medicine; Attending Neurosurgeon, Mount Sinai Hospital, New York, New York
Tumors of the Vertebral Axis: Benign, Primary Malignant, and Metastatic Tumors

Michael E. Carey, MD, MS

Professor of Neurosurgery, Louisiana State University School of Medicine in New Orleans, New Orleans, Louisiana
Bullet Wounds to the Brain among Civilians

Carlos Carlotti, MD

Neurosurgeon, Da Universidade de São Paulo, São Paulo, Brazil
Encephaloceles

Thomas Carlstedt, MD, DM

Associate Professor, Karolinska Institute, Stockholm, Sweden; Visiting Professor, Imperial College, London University, London, England; Consultant Orthopaedic Surgeon, Royal National Orthopaedic Hospital, Peripheral Nerve Injury Unit, Stanmore, England
Management of Acute Peripheral Nerve Injuries

Peter Carmel, MD, DMedSci

Professor and Chairman Department of Neurological Surgery, University of Medicine and Dentistry of New Jersey—New Jersey Medical School; Attending, University Hospital, Newark, New Jersey
Craniopharyngiomas; Brain Tumors of Disordered Embryogenesis

Andrew L. Carney, MD

Clinical Associate Professor of Neurosurgery, Radiology, and Orthopedics, University of Illinois at Chicago College of Medicine, Chicago, Illinois
Extracranial Vertebral Artery Disease

Benjamin S. Carson, Sr., MD

Professor of Neurosurgery, Oncology, Plastic Surgery, and Pediatrics, Johns Hopkins University School of Medicine; Director, Pediatric Neurosurgery, Johns Hopkins Hospital, Baltimore, Maryland
Ependymoma; Achondroplasia and Other Dwarfism

L. Philip Carter, MD

Clinical Professor of Neurosurgery, University of Arizona School of Medicine; Private Practice, Western Neurosurgery, Ltd., Tucson, Arizona
Historical Considerations [Vascular]

Kenneth F. Casey, MD

Associate Professor of Neurosurgery, Drexel University School of Medicine, Philadelphia; Attending, Department of Neurosurgery, Allegheny Hospital, Pittsburgh, Pennsylvania
Ablative Surgery for Spasticity

Mauricio Castillo, MD

Professor of Radiology and Chief and Program Director of Neuroradiology, University of North Carolina School of Medicine, Chapel Hill, North Carolina

Webster K. Cavenee, PhD

Professor of Medicine, Cancer Genetics Program, University of California, San Diego, School of Medicine; Director, Ludwig Institute for Cancer Research, La Jolla, California
Molecular and Cytogenetic Techniques

C. Michael Cawley, MD

Assistant Professor, Department of Neurological Surgery, Emory University School of Medicine, Atlanta, Georgia
Treatment of Lateral-Sigmoid, and Sagittal Sinus Dural Anteriovenous Malformations

Stephan Chabardès, MD

Assistant Neurosurgeon, Hôpital Albert Michallon, Grenoble, France
Deep Brain Stimulation for Movement Disorders

Marc C. Chamberlain, MD

Professor of Neurology and Neurosurgery, University of Southern California Keck School of Medicine; Co-Director, Neuro-oncology Program, Norris Comprehensive Cancer Center and Hospital, Los Angeles, California
Neoplastic Meningitis: Diagnosis and Treatment

Amitabha Chanda, MD, MCh

Staff, AMRI-Apollo Hospitals, Kolkata, West Bengal
Chordoma and Chondrosarcoma

Chandrasekar Kalavakonda, MD

Anna Nagar, Chennai, India
Chordoma and Chondrosarcoma

Eric L. Chang, MD

Staff, Department of Radiation Oncology, The University of Texas M.D. Anderson Cancer Center, Houston, Texas
Metastatic Brain Tumors

Steven D. Chang, MD

Assistant Professor, Department of Neurosurgery, Stanford University School of Medicine, Stanford, California
Surgical and Radiosurgical Management of Giant Arteriovenous Malformations; General and Historical Considerations of Radiotherapy and Radiosurgery

Tailoi Chan-Ling, MOptom, PhD

Associate Professor and National Health and Medical Research Council, Senior Research Fellow, Department of Anatomy, University of Sydney Faculty of Medicine, Sydney, New South Wales, Australia
Astrocytes

Paul H. Chapman, MD

Professor of Surgery (Neurosurgery), Harvard Medical School; Neurosurgical Director, Proton Radiosurgery Group, Massachusetts General Hospital, Boston, Massachusetts
Proton Radiosurgery

Ali Charara, PhD

Post-Doctoral Fellow, Department of Neuroscience, University of Pittsburgh School of Medicine, Pittsburgh, Pennsylvania
Anatomy and Synaptic Connectivity of the Basal Ganglia

Fady T. Charbel, MD

Professor and Head, Department of Neurosurgery, University of Illinois at Chicago College of Medicine, Chicago, Illinois
Extracranial Vertebral Artery Disease

Thomas C. Chen, MD, PhD

Assistant Professor of Clinical Surgery, University of Southern California University Hospital, Los Angeles, California
Intradiskal and Percutaneous Treatment of Lumbar Disk Disease

Gopal Chopra, MD

Neurosurgeon, Department of Neurosurgery, St. John Regional Hospital, Saint John, New Brunswick, Canada
Surgical Approaches for Anterior Circulation Aneurysms

Cindy Christian, MD

Assistant Professor of Pediatrics, University of Pennsylvania School of Medicine; Chair, Child Abuse and Neglect Prevention and Director, Child Abuse Program, Children's Hospital of Philadelphia, Philadelphia, Pennsylvania
Child Abuse

Richard C. Clatterbuck, MD, PhD

Assistant Professor, Department of Neurosurgery, Johns Hopkins University School of Medicine; Attending, Johns Hopkins Hospital, Baltimore, Maryland
Surgical Positioning and Exposures for Cranial Procedures; Sarcoidosis, Tuberculosis, and Xanthogranuloma

Elizabeth B. Claus, PhD, MD

Associate Professor, Department of Epidemiology and Public Health, Yale University School of Medicine, New Haven, Connecticut
Scalp Tumors; Shunt Infection

Charles S. Cobbs, MD

Associate Professor of Neurological Surgery, Department of Surgery, University of Alabama School of Medicine; Attending, Kirklin Clinic, UAB Medical Center, Birmingham, Alabama
Meningeal Hemangiopericytoma

Kimberly Peele Cockerham, MD

Assistant Professor, Drexel University School of Medicine, Philadelphia; Director, Neuro-ophthalmology, Orbital Disease and Reconstruction, Allegheny General Hospital, Pittsburgh, Pennsylvania
Orbital Tumors

P. H. Cogen, MD

Chairman, Department of Neurosurgery, Children's National Medical Center, Washington, DC
Occult Spinal Dysraphism and the Tethered Spinal Cord

Alan R. Cohen, MD

Professor of Neurological Surgery and Pediatrics, Case Western Reserve University School of Medicine; Chief, Pediatric Neurosurgery, Rainbow Babies and Children's Hospital, Cleveland, Ohio
Myelomeningocele and Myelocystocele; Intervertebral Disk Disease in Children

Wendy A. Cohen, MD

Professor of Radiology and Neurosurgery, University of Washington School of Medicine; Chief, Neuroradiology, Harborview Medical Center, Seattle, Washington
Radiology of the Spine

Domingos Coiteiro, MD

Staff, Dobelle Institute, Lisboa, Portugal
Revascularization Techniques for Complex Aneurysms and Skull Base Tumors

Antony Colantonio, MD

Pain Fellow, Department of Anesthesiology, Oregon Health & Science University, Portland, Oregon
Management of Pain by Anesthetic Techniques

Andrew J. Cole, MD

Associate Professor of Neurology, Harvard Medical School; Associate Neurologist, Massachusetts General Hospital, Boston, Massachusetts
Identification of Candidates for Epilepsy Surgery

John J. Collins, MD

Assistant Professor of Neurosurgery, Loma Linda University School of Medicine; Chief, Pediatric Neurosurgery, Loma Linda University Children's Medical Center and Loma Linda University Medical Center, Loma Linda, California
Nonsyndromic Craniosynostosis and Abnormalities of Head Shape

Edward S. Connolly, MD

Attending, Ochsner Clinic Foundation, New Orleans, Louisiana
Metabolic and Other Nondegenerative Causes of Low Back Pain

E. Sander Connolly, Jr., MD

Irving Assistant Professor, Department of Neurological Surgery, Columbia University College of Physicians and Surgeons; New York, New York
Techniques for Deep Hypothermic Circulatory Arrest

Stephen W. Coons, MD

Staff, Division of Neuropathology, Barrow Neurological Institute, Phoenix, Arizona
Proliferation Markers in the Evaluation of Gliomas

James J. Corbett, MD

McCarty Professor and Chairman, Department of Neurology, and Professor of Ophthalmology, University of Mississippi School of Medicine, Jackson, Mississippi; Lecturer in Ophthalmology, Harvard Medical School, Boston, Massachusetts
Neuro-ophthalmology

Daniel M. Corcos, PhD

Professor, Department of Kinesiology, College of Associated Health Professions, University of Illinois at Chicago; Director, Clinical Motor Control Laboratory, Department of Neurological Sciences, Rush-Presbyterian-St. Luke's Medical Center, Chicago, Illinois
Management of Spasticity by Central Nervous System Infusion Techniques

G. Rees Cosgrove, MD

Associate Professor of Surgery, Harvard Medical School; Associate Visiting Neurosurgeon, Massachusetts General Hospital, Boston, Massachusetts
Identification of Candidates for Epilepsy Surgery; Neurosurgery of Psychiatric Disorders

Neil R. Crawford, PhD

Coordinator, Spinal Biomechanics, Barrow Neurological Institute, Phoenix; Adjunct Assistant Professor, Department of Bioengineering, Arizona State University, Tempe, Arizona
Basic Principles of Spinal Internal Fixation

Kerry R. Crone, MD

Associate Professor of Neurosurgery, Director of Graduate Education in Pediatric Neurosurgery, University of Cincinnati College of Medicine; Director, Department of Pediatric Neurosurgery, Cincinnati Children's Hospital Medical Center, Cincinnati, Ohio
Neuroendoscopy

Raimondo D'Ambrosio, PhD

Associate Professor of Neurosurgery, University of Washington; Seattle, Washington
Basic Science of Post-traumatic Epilepsy

Carlos A. David, MD

Director, Cerebrovascular and Skull Base Surgery, Lahey Clinic, Burlington, Massachusetts
Intracranial Occlusion Disease and Moyamoya

Arthur L. Day, MD

Professor of Neurosurgery, Program Director, and Associate Chairman, Department of Neurosurgery, Harvard Medical School; Director, Cerebrovascular Center, Brigham and Women's Hospital, Boston, Massachusetts
Surgical Treatment of Intracavernous and Paraclinoid Internal Carotid Artery Aneurysms

J. Diaz Day, MD

Associate Professor of Neurosurgery, Drexel University School of Medicine, Philadelphia; Director, Center for Cerebrovascular Surgery and Stroke, Allegheny General Hospital, Pittsburgh, Pennsylvania
Basilar Trunk Aneurysms; Cavernous Carotid Fistulas

A. Lee Dellon, MD

Professor of Plastic Surgery, Johns Hopkins University School of Medicine and University of Maryland School of Medicine, Baltimore, Maryland; Professor of Plastic Surgery and Neurosurgery, University of Arizona College of Medicine, Tucson, Arizona; Private Practice, Institute for Peripheral Nerve Surgery, Baltimore, Maryland, and Institute for Peripheral Nerve Surgery: Southwest, Tucson, Arizona
History of Peripheral Nerve Surgery

Mahlon R. Delong, MD

Professor and Chairman, Department of Neurology, Emory University School of Medicine, Atlanta, Georgia
Rationale for Surgical Interventions in Movement Disorders

Franco Demonte, MD

Associate Professor, Department of Neurosurgery, University of Texas–Houston Medical School; Clinical Associate Professor, Department of Neurosurgery, Baylor College of Medicine; Attending, The University of Texas M.D. Anderson Cancer Center, Houston, Texas
Neoplasms of the Paranasal Sinuses

Robert J. Dempsey, MD

Professor and Chair, Department of Neurosurgery, University of Wisconsin Medical School; Attending, University of Wisconsin Hospitals and Clinics, Madison, Wisconsin
Recurrent Carotid Stenosis

Milind Deogaonkar, MD

Department of Neurosurgery, University of Arizona Health Sciences Center, Tucson, Arizona
Historical Considerations [Vascular]

Antonio A. F. De Salles, MD, PhD

Professor, Division of Neurosurgery, Department of Surgery, David Geffen School of Medicine at UCLA; Co-Director, Epilepsy Surgery Program, West LA Veterans Administration Medical Center, Los Angeles, California
Molecular Imaging of the Brain with Positron Emission Tomography; Sympathectomy for Pain

Nicolas De Tribolet, MD

Professor, University of Geneva Faculty of Medicine; Attending, Department of Neurosurgery, University Hospital, Geneva, Switzerland
Aspects of Immunology Applicable to Brain Tumor Pathogenesis and Treatment

Paul W. Detwiler, MD, PhD

Staff, Tyler Neurosurgical Group, Tyler, Texas
Infratentorial Cavernous Malformations; Classification of Spinal Cord Vascular Lesions

Harel Deutch, MD

Instructor, Department of Neurosurgery, Emory University School of Medicine; Spinal Surgery Fellow, Department of Neurosurgery, Emory University Hospital, Atlanta, Georgia
Complication Avoidance in Neurosurgery

Paul T. Diamond, MD

Associate Professor, Department of Physical Medicine and Rehabilitation, University of Virginia School of Medicine, Charlottesville, Virginia
Rehabilitation and Prognosis after Traumatic Brain Injury

Mark S. Dias, MD

Staff, Department of Neurosurgery, Section of Neurosurgery, Milton Hershey Medical Center, Pittsburgh, Pennsylvania
Normal and Abnormal Embryology of the Spinal Cord and Spine

Curtis A. Dickman, MD

Associate Chief, Spine Section, and Director, Spinal Research, Division of Neurological Surgery, Barrow Neurological Institute, Phoenix, Arizona
Basic Principles of Spinal Internal Fixation; Anterior Cervical Instrumentation; Occipitocervical Fusion; Thoracoscopic Approaches to the Spine

Pierre-Yves Dietrich, MD

Associate Professor, University of Geneva Faculty of Medicine; Head, Laboratory of Tumor Immunology, Division of Oncology, University Hospital, Geneva, Switzerland
Aspects of Immunology Applicable to Brain Tumor Pathogenesis and Treatment

Francesco DiMeco, MD

Faculty Member, Department of Neurosurgery, Istituto Nazionale Neurologico, Milan, Italy
Brain Tumors during Pregnancy

Jacques E. Dion, MD

Professor of Neuroradiology and Neurosurgery, Department of Radiology, Emory University School of Medicine; Director, Interventional Neuroradiology, Emory University Hospital, Atlanta, Georgia
Treatment of Lateral-Sigmoid and Sagittal Sinus Dural Arteriovenous Malformations

Carl B. Dodrill, PhD

Professor, Departments of Neurology, Neurological Surgery, and Psychiatry and Behavioral Sciences, University of Washington School of Medicine; Associate Director, Regional Epilepsy Center, Harborview Medical Center, Seattle, Washington
Neuropsychological Assessment of the Neurosurgical Patient; The Intracarotid Amobarbital Procedure or Wada Test

Aclan Dogan, MD

Fellow, Division of Neurosurgery, Louisiana State University Health Sciences Center, Shreveport, Louisiana
Recurrent Carotid Stenosis

Vinko V. Dolenc, MD, PhD

Professor of Neurosurgery, Medical School at Ljubljana University; Head, Neurosurgical Department, University Hospital Center, Ljubljana, Slovenia
Skull and Skull Base Tumors

Egon M. R. Doppenberg, MD

Resident, Department of Neurosurgery, Medical College of Virginia Hospitals, Richmond, Virginia
Pediatric Head Injury

Zeena Dorai, MD

Resident, Department of Neurosurgery, University of Texas Southwestern Medical Center at Dallas, Dallas, Texas
Posterior Fossa Arteriovenous Malformations

Stephen E. Doran, MD

Clinical Assistant Professor of Neurosurgery, Department of Surgery, University of Nebraska College of Medicine; Neurosurgeon, University Medical Associates and Midwest Neurosurgery, Omaha, Nebraska

Brain Tumors: Population-Based Epidemiology, Environmental Risk Factors, and Genetic and Hereditary Syndromes

Catherine J. Doty, MD

Clinical Assistant Professor in Pediatrics, Washington University School of Medicine; Attending, St. Louis Children's Hospital, St. Louis, Missouri

Cerebral Palsy: An Overview

James M. Drake, MBBCh, MSc

Associate Professor, Division of Neurosurgery, University of Toronto Faculty of Medicine; Neurosurgeon, The Hospital for Sick Children, Toronto, Ontario, Canada

Physiology of Cerebrospinal Fluid Shunt Devices

Ann-Christine Duhaime, MD

Professor of Neurosurgery, Dartmouth Medical School; Director, Pediatric Neurosurgery, Dartmouth-Hitchock Medical Center, Lebanon, New Hampshire

Child Abuse

Christopher M. Duma, MD

Medical Director, Hoag Gamma Knife Program, Hoag Memorial Hospital Presbyterian, Newport Beach, California

Functional Radiosurgery

Charles Duncan, MD

Professor and Head, Section of Pediatric Neurosurgery, Department of Neurosurgery, Yale University School of Medicine; Chief, Pediatric Neurosurgery, Yale–New Haven Hospital, New Haven, Connecticut

Shunt Infection

Marc E. Eichler, MD

Clinical Instructor, Harvard Medical School; Associate Surgeon, Department of Neurosurgery, Brigham and Women's Hospital and Boston Children's Hospital, Boston, Massachusetts

Cervical Spine Trauma

F. J. Eismont, MD

Vice Chairman, Department of Orthopedics and Rehabilitation, University of Miami School of Medicine; Orthopedic Surgeon, Jackson Memorial Hospital, Miami, Florida

Diagnosis and Management of Thoracic Spine Fractures

Elizabeth A. Eldredge, MD

Instructor in Anesthesia, Harvard Medical School; Staff Anesthesiologist, Children's Hospital, Boston, Massachusetts

Neuroanesthesia in Children

Hikmat El-Kadi, MD, PhD

Clinical Associate Professor of Neurosurgery, University of Pittsburgh School of Medicine, Pittsburgh Pennsylvania

Brain Death

Richard G. Ellenbogen, MD

Associate Professor, Department of Neurological Surgery, University of Washington School of Medicine; Chief and Theodore S. Roberts Endowed Chair, Division of Pediatric Neurological Surgery, Children's Hospital and Regional Medical Center, Seattle, Washington

Diagnosis and Management of Juvenile Angiofibroma; Choroid Plexus Tumors; Craniofacial Trauma

J. Paul Elliott, MD

Assistant Professor, Department of Neurosurgery, University of Colorado School of Medicine; Chief, Neurosurgery, Denver Health Medical Center, Denver, Colorado

Traumatic Cerebrovascular Injury

Syed A. Enam, MD, PhD

Staff Physician, Department of Neurosurgery, Henry Ford Hospital, Detroit, Michigan

Invasion in Malignant Glioma

Fred J. Epstein, MD

Professor of Neurosurgery, Albert Einstein School of Medicine of Yeshiva University, Bronx; Attending Physician, Institute for Neurology and Neurosurgery, Beth Israel Medical Center, New York, New York

Intraspinal Tumors in Infants and Children

Nancy E. Epstein, MD

Clinical Professor of Neurological Surgery, Albert Einstein College of Medicine of Yeshiva University, Bronx; Adjunct Clinical Associate Professor of Surgery/Neurosurgery, Cornell University, Joan and Sanford I. Weill Medical College, New York; Attending Neurosurgeon, North Shore–Long Island Jewish Health System, Manhasset and New Hyde Park, and Winthrop University Hospital, Mineola, New York

Lumbar Spinal Stenosis

Joseph Eskridge, MD

Professor, Departments of Radiology and Neurosurgery, University of Washington School of Medicine, Seattle, Washington

Endovascular Treatment of Spinal Cord Arteriovenous Malformations

Matthew G. Ewend, MD

Assistant Professor of Neurosurgery and Section Chief of Neuro-oncology Clinical Research, University of North Carolina Lineberger Comprehensive Cancer Center, University of North Carolina, Chapel Hill, North Carolina
Meningeal Sarcoma

Gary G. Ferguson, MD, PhD

Professor of Neurosurgery, Department of Clinical Neurological Sciences (Neurosurgery), University of Western Ontario Faculty of Medicine; Attending Neurosurgeon, London Health Sciences Centre, London, Ontario, Canada
Distal Anterior Cerebral Artery Aneurysms

Richard G. Fessler, MD, PhD

Professor of Neurosurgery, Department of Surgery, University of Chicago, Division of the Biological Sciences, Pritzker School of Medicine; Chief, Section of Neurosurgery, University of Chicago Hospital and Clinics, Chicago, Illinois
Benign Extradural Lesions of the Dorsal Spine; Posterior Lumbar Instrumentation

Matthew E. Fewel, MD

Instructor, Department of Neurosurgery, University of Michigan Medical School, Ann Arbor, Michigan
Skull Tumors

Paul E. Fewings, MBBS

Consultant Neurosurgeon, Hull Royal Infirmary, Hull, England
Medical Management of Chronic Pain

J. Max Findlay, MD, PhD

Clinical Professor, Division of Neurosurgery, University of Alberta Faculty of Medicine; Neurosurgeon, University of Alberta Hospital, Edmonton, Alberta, Canada
Cerebral Vasospasm

Andrew D. Fine, MD

Staff, Neurological Associates, PA, Sarasota, Florida
Benign Extradural Lesions of the Dorsal Spine

Howard A. Fine, MD

Branch Chief, Neuro-Oncology, National Cancer Institute, National Institute of Health, Bethesda, Maryland
Principles of Chemotherapy

Jill B. Firszt, PhD

Assistant Professor and Director, Koss Cochlear Implant Program, Department of Otolaryngology and Communication Sciences, Medical College of Wisconsin; Attending, Froedtert & Medical College Hospital and Children's Hospital of Wisconsin, Milwaukee, Wisconsin
Neuro-otology

Michael T. Fitch, MD, PhD

Resident in Emergency Medicine, Carolina Medical Center, Charlotte, North Carolina
Cellular and Molecular Mechanisms Mediating Injury and Recovery in the Nervous System

James D. Fleck, MD

Clinical Assistant Professor, Department of Neurology, Indiana University School of Medicine, Indianapolis, Indiana
Carotid Occlusive Disease: Natural History and Medical Management

Ian G. Fleetwood, MD

Chief Resident, Department of Neurosurgery, Foothills Medical Centre, Calgary, Alberta, Canada
Hemorrhagic Disease: Arteriovascular Malformations

Kelly D. Flemming, MD

Assistant Professor, Mayo Graduate School of Medicine; Consultant in Neurology, Mayo Clinic, Rochester, Minnesota
Natural History of Intracranial Vascular Malformations

Susan Fletcher, MB

Acting Assistant Professor of Anesthesiology, University of Washington School of Medicine; Attending Anesthesiologist, Harborview Medical Center, Seattle, Washington
Anesthesia: Preoperative Evaluation

John C. Flickinger, MD

Professor of Radiation Oncology and Neurological Surgery, University of Pittsburgh School of Medicine, Pittsburgh, Pennsylvania
Fractionated Radiotherapy for Pituitary Tumors

Nancy Foldvary, DO

Staff Neurologist, Cleveland Clinic, Cleveland, Ohio
[Surgical Treatment of Epilepsy in Children] Recognition of Surgical Candidates and the Presurgical Evaluation

Kenneth A. Follett, MD, PhD

Professor, Department of Neurosurgery, University of Iowa College of Medicine, Iowa City, Iowa
Neurosurgical Management of Intractable Pain

Kelly D. Foote, MD

Assistant Professor, Department of Neurosurgery, University of Florida School of Medicine, Gainesville, Florida
Radiosurgery for Arteriovenous Malformations

Daryl R. Fourney, MD

Assistant Professor, Division of Neurosurgery, University of Saskatchewan Faculty of Medicine; Attending, Royal University Hospital, Saskatoon, Saskatchewan, Canada
Neoplasms of the Paranasal Sinuses

Valerie Fraix, MD, PhD

Assistant Neurologist, Hôpital Albert Michallon, Grenoble, France
Deep Brain Stimulation for Movement Disorders

Paul C. Francel, MD, PhD

Associate Professor, Department of Neurosurgery, University of Oklahoma College of Medicine, Oklahoma City, Oklahoma
Mild Brain Injury in Children, including Skull Fractures and Growing Fractures

Itzhak Fried, MD, PhD

Associate Professor of Neurosurgery and Psychiatry and Biobehavioral Sciences, David Geffen School of Medicine at UCLA, Los Angeles, California; Associate Professor of Neurosurgery, Sackler School of Medicine, Tel-Aviv University, Tel-Aviv, Israel; Director, of Epilepsy Surgery, and Co-Director, UCLA Seizure Disorder Center, UCLA Medical Center, Los Angeles, California; Director, Functional Neurosurgery Unit, Tel-Aviv Medical Center, Tel-Aviv, Israel
Surgery for Extratemporal Lobe Epilepsy

Jonathan A. Friedman, MD

Chief Resident, Department of Neurologic Surgery, Mayo Clinic, Rochester, Minnesota
Middle Cerebral Artery Aneurysms

William A. Friedman, MD

Professor and Chair, Department of Neurosurgery, University of Florida; Attending, Shand's Hospital, Gainesville, Florida
Radiobiology; Radiosurgery for Arteriovenous Malformations; Fractionated and Stereotactic Radiation, Extracranial Stereotactic Radiation, Intensity Modulation, and Multileaf Collimation

David M. Frim, MD, PhD

Assistant Professor of Surgery and Pediatrics, University of Chicago, Division of the Biological Sciences, Pritzker School of Medicine; Chief, Pediatric Neurosurgery, University of Chicago Children's Hospital, Chicago, Illinois
Benign Tumors of the Vertebral Column in Children

Michael J. Fritsch, MD

Fellow in Neurological Surgery, University of Miami School of Medicine, Miami, Florida
Surgical Management of Supratentorial Arteriovenous Malformation

Herbert E. Fuchs, MD, PhD

Associate Professor, Department of Surgery, Division of Neurosurgery, Duke University School of Medicine, Durham, North Carolina
Benign Tumors of the Skull, including Fibrous Dysplasia

Gregory N. Fuller, MD, PhD

Professor of Pathology, University of Texas–Houston Medical School; Chief, Section of Neuropathology, The University of Texas M.D. Anderson Cancer Center, Houston, Texas
Brain Tumors: An Overview of Histopathologic Classification

Aurelie Funkiewiez, MA

Staff, Department of Neurology, Centre Hospitalier Universitaire de Grenoble, Grenoble, France
Deep Brain Stimulation for Movement Disorders

Michael R. Gallagher, MD

Clinical Assistant Professor, Department of Surgery, University of Tennessee, Chattanooga, College of Medicine; Staff Neurosurgeon, Baroness Erlanger Hospital and Memorial Hospital, Chattanooga, Tennessee
Spondyloarthropathies, including Ankylosing Spondylitis

Ira M. Garonzik, MD

Neurosurgery Fellow, Department of Neurosurgery, Johns Hopkins Hospital, Baltimore, Maryland
Thalamotomy for Tremor

Hugh Garton, MD, MHSc

Assistant Professor, Department of Neurosurgery, University of Michigan Medical School, Ann Arbor, Michigan
Neurosurgical Epidemiology and Outcomes Assessment

Marilyn L. Gates, MD

Assistant Professor, Uniformed Services University of the Health Sciences, Medicine; Assistant Director, Complex Spine Surgery, National Naval Medical Center Hospital, Bethesda, Maryland
Bone Metabolism as It Relates to Spinal Disease and Treatment

Stephen S. Gebarski, MD

Professor, Department of Radiology, Division of Neuroradiology, University of Michigan Medical School, Ann Arbor, Michigan
Skull Tumors

Christopher C. Getch, MD

Assistant Professor, Department of Neurological Surgery, Northwestern University Feinberg School of Medicine, Chicago, Illinois
Basilar Apex and Posterior Cerebral Artery Aneurysms

Sanjay Ghosh, MD

Staff, Senta Clinic, Division of Skull Base Surgery, San Diego, California
Ventricular Tumors; Cavernous Carotid Fistulas

Steven L. Giannotta, MD

Professor of Neurological Surgery, University of Southern California Keck School of Medicine; Chief, Neurosurgery, and Medical Director, USC University Hospital, Los Angeles, California
Basilar Trunk Aneurysms

Philip L. Gildenberg, MD, PhD

Clinical Professor of Neurosurgery and Radiation Oncology, Baylor College of Medicine; Clinical Professor of Psychiatry, University of Texas–Houston Medical School, Houston, Texas
Brainstem Procedures for Management of Pain

Howard J. Ginsberg, MD

Senior Resident, University of Toronto, Division of Neurosurgery, Toronto, Ontario, Canada
Physiology of Cerebrospinal Fluid Shunt Devices

Ziya L. Gokaslan, MD

Clinical Assistant Professor, Department of Neurosurgery, University of Texas–Houston Medical School; Attending, The University of Texas M.D. Anderson Cancer Center, Houston, Texas
Treatment of Disk and Ligamentous Diseases of the Cervical Spine

Joel Goldwein, MD

Professor of Radiation Oncology, University of Pennsylvania School of Medicine; Chief, Pediatric Radiation Oncology, Children's Hospital of Philadelphia, Philadelphia, Pennsylvania
Intracranial Ependymomas

Robert Goodkin, MD

Associate Professor, Department of Neurological Surgery, University of Washington School of Medicine; Chief, Neurosurgical Section, Veterans Administration Puget Sound Health Care System, Seattle, Washington
Legal Issues; General Principles of Operative Positioning; Magnetic Resonance Imaging for Peripheral Nerve Disorders

James Tait Goodrich, MD, PhD

Professor of Clinical Neurological Surgery, Pediatrics, and Plastic and Reconstructive Surgery, Leo Davidoff Department of Neurological Surgery, Albert Einstein College of Medicine of Yeshiva University; Director, Division of Pediatric Neurosurgery, Montefiore Medical Center, Bronx, New York
Neurological Surgery in Childhood: General and Historical Considerations

John P. Gorecki, MD

Clinical Assistant Professor, The University of Kansas Medical School, Wichita, Kansas
Dorsal Root Entry Zone and Brainstem Ablative Procedures

M. Sean Grady, MD

Charles Harrison Frazier Professor and Chair of the Department of Neurosurgery, University of Pennsylvania School of Medicine, Philadelphia, Pennsylvania
Cellular Basis of Injury and Recovery from Trauma; Initial Resuscitation and Patient Evaluation; Modern Neurotraumatology: A Brief Historical Review

Sylvie Grand, MD, PhD

Assistant Professor of Biophysics and Radiology, University Joseph Fourier; Staff Neuroradiologist, Hôpital Albert Michallon, Grenoble, France
Deep Brain Stimulation for Movement Disorders

Gerald A. Grant, MD

Acting Instructor, Department of Neurological Surgery, University of Washington School of Medicine; Attending, Children's Hospital and Regional Medical Center, Seattle, Washington
The Blood-Brain Barrier; Diagnosis and Management of Juvenile Angiofibroma; General Principles in Evaluating and Treating Peripheral Nerve Injuries; Magnetic Resonance Imaging for Peripheral Nerve Disorders

B. A. Green, MD

Professor and Chairman, Department of Neurosurgical Surgery, University of Miami School of Medicine; Chief, Department of Neurosurgery, Jackson Memorial Medical Center, Miami, Florida
Diagnosis and Management of Thoracic Spine Fractures

Michael W. Groff, MD

Director, Spinal Surgery, Indiana University Hospital, Indianapolis, Indiana
Concepts and Mechanisms of Biomechanics

Andreas Gruber, MD

Professor, Department of Neurosurgery, University of Vienna Medical School, Vienna, Austria
Embolization of Arteriovenous Malformations as a Primary Treatment Modality

Joseph S Gruss, MBBCh

Professor, Department of Surgery; Adjunct Professor, Department of Neurosurgery; and Marlys C. Larson Professor and Endowed Chair in Pediatric Craniofacial Surgery, University of Washington School of Medicine; Chief, Division of Craniofacial, Plastic and Reconstructive Surgery, Children's Hospital and Regional Medical Center; Attending Surgeon, Harborview Medical Center, Seattle, Washington
Craniofacial Trauma

Michael Guarnieri, PhD, MPH

Research Associate, Johns Hopkins University School of Medicine, Baltimore, Maryland
Ependymoma

James D. Guest, MD, PhD

Assistant Professor of Neurological Surgery, University of Miami School of Medicine; Scientific Faculty, The Miami Project to Cure Paralysis; Attending Neurosurgeon, University of Miami Hospital and Clinics and Miami Veterans Administration Medical Center, Miami, Florida
Biologic Strategies for Central Nervous System Repair

Abhijit Guha, MSc, MD

Associate Professor, Division of Neurosurgery, University of Toronto Faculty of Medicine; Attending Neurosurgeon, University Health Network; Co-Director, Arthur and Sonia Labatts Brain Tumor Center, The Hospital for Sick Children, Toronto, Ontario, Canada
Management of Peripheral Nerve Tumors

Mary Kay Gumerlock, MD

Professor of Neurosurgery, University of Oklahoma, College of Medicine, Oklahoma City, Oklahoma
Epidermoid, Dermoid, and Neurenteric Cysts

Murat Gunel, MD

Assistant Professor of Neurosurgery, Yale University School of Medicine, New Haven, Connecticut
Surgical Management of Supratentorial Cavernous Malformations

Kern H. Guppy, MD, PhD

Assistant Professor of Neurosurgery, University of Illinois at Chicago College of Medicine, Chicago, Illinois
Extracranial Vertebral Artery Disease

Nalin Gupta, MD, PhD

Assistant Professor, Department of Neurosurgery, University of California, San Francisco, School of Medicine, San Francisco, California
Benign Tumors of the Vertebral Column in Children

Lee R. Guterman, MD, PhD

Assistant Professor, Department of Neurosurgery and Co-Director Toshiba Stroke Research Center, University at Buffalo; Neurosurgeon, Kaleida Health, Buffalo, New York
Endovascular Treatment of Aneurysms

Barton L. Guthrie, MD

Associate Professor of Neurological Surgery, Department of Surgery, University of Alabama School of Medicine; Co-Director, Health South/UAB Gamma Knife Program, Health South Medical Center, Birmingham, Alabama
Meningeal Hemangiopericytoma

P. W. Gutin, MD

Chief, Department of Neurosurgery, Memorial Sloan-Kettering Cancer Center, New York, New York
Interstitial and Intracavitary Irradiation of Brain Tumors

Eldad Hadar, MD

Assistant Professor, Department of Surgery, Division of Neurosurgery, University of North Carolina at Chapel Hill School of Medicine, Chapel Hill, North Carolina
General and Historical Considerations of Epilepsy Surgery

Georges F. Haddad, MD

Clinical Assistant Professor, Department of Neurosurgery, American University of Beirut, Beirut, Lebanon

Regis W. Haid, MD

Associate Professor, Department of Neurological Surgery, Emory University School of Medicine, Atlanta, Georgia
Spondyloarthropathies, including Ankylosing Spondylitis

Stephen J. Haines, MD

Professor and Chair, Department of Neurological Surgery, Medical University of South Carolina College of Medicine, Charleston, South Carolina
Neurosurgical Epidemiology and Outcomes Assessment

H. Bruce Hamilton, MD

Private Practice, Neurosurgery, Waco, Texas
Metabolic and Other Nondegenerative Causes of Low Back Pain

Mark G. Hamilton, MDCM

Associate Professor of Neurosurgery, Department of Clinical Neurosciences, University of Calgary Faculty of Medicine; Director, Pediatric Neurosciences, Alberta Children's Hospital, Foothills Medical Centre, Calgary, Alberta, Canada
Hemorrhagic Disease: Arteriovascular Malformations

Thomas A. Hammeke, PhD

Professor, Department of Neurology (Neuropsychology), Medical College of Wisconsin, Milwaukee, Wisconsin
Functional Magnetic Resonance Imaging in Epilepsy Surgery

Patrick P. Han, MD

Chief Resident, Division of Neurological Surgery, Barrow Neurological Institute, Phoenix, Arizona
Epidemiology and Natural History of Cavernous Malformations

Russell W. Hardy, Jr., MD

Professor of Neurological Surgery, Department of Surgery, Case Western Reserve University School of Medicine; Co-Director, University Hospitals Spine Center, Cleveland, Ohio
Treatment of Disk Disease of the Lumbar Spine

Raymond I. Haroun, MD

Instructor, Department of Neurosurgery, Johns Hopkins University School of Medicine, Baltimore, Maryland
Anterior Communicating Artery and Anterior Cerebral Artery Aneurysms; Achondroplasia and Other Dwarfism

Mark R. Harrigan, MD

Lecturer, Department of Neurosurgery, University of Michigan Medical School, Ann Arbor, Michigan
Pregnancy and Treatment of Vascular Disease

Griffith R. Harsh IV, MD

Professor, of Neurosurgery, Stanford University School of Medicine; Director, Stanford Brain Tumor Center, Stanford, California
Cerebral Lymphoma

Jaimie M. Henderson, MD

Associate Staff, Department of Neurosurgery, Cleveland Clinic, Cleveland, Ohio
Medical Management of Chronic Pain

Jeffrey S. Henn, MD

Assistant Professor, Department of Neurological Surgery, University of Florida College of Medicine, Gainesville, Florida
Giant Aneurysms

Roberto C. Heros, MD

Professor, Department of Neurological Surgery, University of Miami School of Medicine; Attending Neurosurgeon, Jackson Memorial Hospital, Miami, Florida
Surgical Management of Supratentorial Arteriovenous Malformation

Karl Herrup, PhD

Professor of Neurosciences and Neurology, Case Western Reserve University School of Medicine; Director, University Memory and Aging Center, University Hospitals of Cleveland, Cleveland, Ohio
Neurons and Neuroglia

Jason Heth, MD

Chief Resident, Department of Neurosurgery, University of Iowa Hospitals and Clinics, Iowa City, Iowa
Tumors of the Craniovertebral Junction

Julian T. Hoff, MD

Professor and Chair, Department of Neurosurgery, University of Michigan Medical School, Ann Arbor, Michigan
Brain Edema and Tumor-Host Interactions; Skull Tumors; Treatment of Intractable Vertigo

Dominique Hoffmann, MD

Staff Neurosurgeon, Hôpital Albert Michallon, Grenoble, France
Deep Brain Stimulation for Movement Disorders

Brian L. Hoh, MD

Clinical Fellow in Surgery, Harvard Medical School; Resident, Neurosurgical Service, Massachusetts General Hospital, Boston, Massachusetts
Vertebral Artery, Posterior Inferior Cerebellar Artery, and Vertebrobasilar Junction Aneurysms

Anna Depold Hohler, MD

Chief, Neurology Clinic, Madigan Army Medical Center, Tacoma, Washington
Approach to Movement Disorders

Eric C. Holland, MD, PhD

Staff, Departments of Surgery (Neurosurgery), Neurology, and Cell Biology, Memorial Sloan-Kettering Cancer Center, New York, New York
Molecular Genetics and the Development of Targets for Glioma Therapy

James P. Hollowell, MD

Associate Professor of Neurosurgery, Medical College of Wisconsin; Staff, Neuroscience Research Laboratory and Veterans Affairs Medical Center, Milwaukee, Wisconsin
Concepts and Mechanisms of Biomechanics; Bone Metabolism as It Relates to Spinal Disease and Treatment

Mark D. Holmes, MD

Associate Professor of Neurology, University of Washington School of Medicine; Director of EEG, Regional Epilepsy Center, Harborview Medical Center, Seattle, Washington
Approaches to the Diagnosis and Classification of Epilepsy

John Honeycutt, MD

Assistant Professor, Department of Neurosurgery, University of Oklahoma College of Medicine, Oklahoma City, Oklahoma
Mild Brain Injury in Children, including Skull Fractures and Growing Fractures

L. Nelson Hopkins, MD

Professor and Chairman, Department of Neurosurgery, and Professor of Radiology, School of Medicine and Biomedical Sciences, State University of New York at Buffalo, Buffalo, New York
Endovascular Treatment of Aneurysms

Frank P. K. Hsu, MD, PhD

Assistant Professor of Neurosurgery, Department of Surgery, Loma Linda University School of Medicine, Loma Linda, California
Cerebral Venous and Sinus Thrombosis

Sherwin E. Hua, MD, PhD

Resident and Fellow, Department of Neurosurgery, Johns Hopkins Hospital, Baltimore, Maryland
Sarcoidosis, Tuberculosis, and Xanthogranuloma; Thalamotomy for Tremor

Alan R. Hudson, MBChB

Professor, Department of Surgery, University of Toronto Faculty of Medicine, Toronto, Ontario, Canada
Management of Peripheral Nerve Tumors

Robin P. Humphreys, MD

Emeritus Professor, Department of Surgery, University of Toronto Faculty of Medicine, Division of Neurosurgery, The Hospital for Sick Children, Toronto, Ontario, Canada
Arteriovenous Malformations and Intracranial Aneurysms in Children

John Huston III, MD

Assistant Professor of Radiology, Mayo Medical School; Consultant in Neurologic Radiology, Mayo Clinic, Rochester, Minnesota
Magnetic Resonance Angiography

Mark Iantosca, MD

Assistant Clinical Professor, Department of Neurosurgery, University of Connecticut School of Medicine; Director, Pediatric Neurosurgery, Connecticut Children's Medical Center, Farmington, Connecticut
Encephaloceles

Koji Ilhara, MD

Attending, Department of Neurosurgery, Toronto Western Hospital, University Health Network, Toronto, Ontario, Canada
Surgical Approaches for Anterior Circulation Aneurysms

Robert J. Jackson, MD

Department of Neurosurgery, Baylor College of Medicine; Attending, The University of Texas M.D. Anderson Cancer Center, Houston, Texas; Surgeon, Massoudi and Jackson Neurosurgical Medical Associates, Laguna Hills, California
Treatment of Disk and Ligamentous Diseases of the Cervical Spine

Deane B. Jacques, MD

Medical Director, The California Neuroscience Institute, Oxnard, California
Functional Radiosurgery

George I. Jallo, MD

Assistant Professor, Departments of Neurosurgery and Pediatrics, Albert Einstein School of Medicine of Yeshiva University, Bronx; Attending Physician, Institute for Neurology and Neurosurgery, Beth Israel Medical Center, New York, New York
Intraspinal Tumors in Infants and Children

C. David James, PhD

Professor of Laboratory Medicine, Mayo Medical School, Rochester, Minnesota
Molecular and Cytogenetic Techniques

John A. Jane, Sr., MD, PhD

Chairman, Department of Neurosurgery, University of Virginia School of Medicine, Charlottesville, Virginia
Esthesioneuroblastoma

Damir Janigro, PhD

Director, Cerebrovascular Center, Department of Neurosurgery, Cleveland Clinic, Cleveland, Ohio
The Blood-Brain Barrier; Electrophysiologic Properties of the Mammalian Nervous System

Peter J. Jannetta, MD

Professor of Neurosurgery, Drexel University College of Medicine, Philadelphia; Vice Chairman, Department of Neurosurgery, Allegheny General Hospital, Pittsburgh, Pennsylvania
Trigeminal Neuralgia: Microvascular Decompression of the Trigeminal Nerve for Tic Douloureux

Abel D. Jarell, MD

CPD Medical Corps, Department of the Army, Washington, DC
Growth Factors and Brain Tumors

Jeffrey G. Jarvik, MD, MPH

Associate Professor, Departments of Radiology and Neurosurgery, University of Washington School of Medicine; Adjunct Associate Professor, Department of Health Services, University of Washington School of Public Health; Director, Neuroradiology Fellowship, University of Washington Medical Center, Seattle, Washington
Radiology of the Spine; Magnetic Resonance Imaging for Peripheral Nerve Disorders

Kurt A. Jellinger, MD

Professor, University of Vienna Medical School, and Director, Ludwig Boltzmann Institute of Clinical Neurobiology, Vienna, Austria
Neuropathology of Movement Disorders

Arthur L. Jenkins III, MD, BA

Assistant Professor, Department of Neurosurgery, Mount Sinai School of Medicine, New York, New York

Complication Avoidance in Neurosurgery; Tumors of the Vertebral Axis: Benign, Primary Malignant, and Metastatic Tumors; Cervical Spine Trauma

Eric W. Johnson, MD

Chief, Molecular Genetics–Neurogenetics, Division of Neurology/Division of Neurosurgery, Barrow Neurological Institute, Phoenix, Arizona

The Genetics of Cerebral Cavernous Malformations

John Patrick Johnson, MD

Director, Cedars-Sinai Institute for Spinal Disorders, Los Angeles, California

Sympathectomy for Pain

Wayel Kaakaji, MD

Staff Neurosurgeon, Michigan Brain and Spinal Surgery Institute, Detroit, Michigan

Alternative Surgical Treatments for Trigeminal Neuralgia

Michael G. Kaiser, MD

Assistant Professor, Department of Neurological Surgery, Columbia University College of Physicians and Surgeons; Attending Neurosurgeon, New York Presbyterian Hospital, New York, New York

Anterior Thoracic Instrumentation; Anterior Lumbar Instrumentation

Iain H. Kalfas, MD

Head, Section of Spinal Surgery, Department of Neurosurgery, Cleveland Clinic, Cleveland, Ohio

Image-Guided Spinal Navigation

Paul M. Kanev, MD

Attending Neurosurgeon, Department of Surgery, Milton Hershey Medical Center, Hershey, Pennsylvania

Arachnoid Cysts

Yücel Kanpolat, MD

Professor and Chairman, Department of Neurosurgery, University of Ankara Faculty of Medicine; Ankara, Turkey

Cordotomy for Pain

Stuart S. Kaplan, MD

Assistant Professor of Neurosurgery, University of Cincinnati College of Medicine; Attending Neurosurgeon, Cincinnati Children's Hospital Medical Center, Cincinnati, Ohio

Birth Brachial Plexus Injury

Michael G. Kaplitt, MD, PhD

Assistant Professor, Department of Neurosurgery, Director, Center for Stereotactic and Functional Neurosurgery, Director, Laboratory of Molecular Neurosurgery, Cornell University Joan and Sanford I. Weill Medical College, New York, New York

Deep Brain Stimulation for Chronic Pain

Zvonimir S. Katusic, MD, PhD

Professor of Pharmacology, Mayo Medical School, Rochester, Minnesota

Cerebral Blood Flow and Metabolism

Bruce A. Kaufman, MD

Professor of Neurosurgery, Medical College of Wisconsin; Chief, Division of Pediatric Neurosurgery, Children's Hospital of Wisconsin, Milwaukee, Wisconsin

Medulloblastoma

Howard H. Kaufman, MD

Department of Neurosurgery, West Virginia University School of Medicine, Morgantown, West Virginia

Brain Death

Robert F. Keating

Associate Professor, Department of Neurosurgery, George Washington University School of Medicine; Chief, Children's National Medical Center, Washington; DC

Occult Spinal Dysraphism and the Tethered Spinal Cord

G. Evren Keles, MD

Assistant Professor, Department of Neurosurgery, University of California, San Francisco, School of Medicine; San Francisco, California

Low-Grade Gliomas: Astrocytoma, Oligodendroglioma, and Mixed Gliomas

John S. Kennerdell, MD

Professor of Ophthalmology, Drexel University Medical School, Philadelphia, and Adjunct Professor of Ophthalmology, University of Pittsburgh School of Medicine; Chairman, Department of Ophthalmology, Allegheny General Hospital, Pittsburgh, Pennsylvania

Orbital Tumors

Lawrence T. Khoo, MD

Department of Neurosurgery, University of Southern California Keck School of Medicine, Los Angeles, California

Intradiskal and Percutaneous Treatment of Lumbar Disk Disease

Vini G. Khurana, MD, PhD

Sundt Fellow, Departments of Neurologic Surgery and Molecular Pharmacology and Experimental Therapeutics, Mayo Clinic, Rochester, Minnesota

Cerebral Blood Flow and Metabolism

Monika Killer, MD

Attending, Christian Doppler Medical Center, Salzburg, Austria
Embolization of Arteriovenous Malformations as a Primary Treatment Modality

Jung Kim, MD

Professor, Department of Pathology, Yale University School of Medicine, New Haven, Connecticut
Unusual Gliomas

Thomas A. Kim, MD

Assistant Professor, Department of Radiology, University of Washington School of Medicine; Staff Neuroradiologist, Harborview Medical Center, University of Washington Medical Center, and Veterans Administration Puget Sound Medical Center, Seattle, Washington
Magnetic Resonance Imaging of Brain

Wesley A. King, MD

Associate Professor, Department of Neurosurgery, Mount Sinai School of Medicine; Attending Neurosurgeon, Mount Sinai Hospital, New York, New York
Neuro-otology

Gregory A. Kinney, PhD

Assistant Professor, University of Washington School of Medicine; Associate Director, Surgical Neuromonitoring University of Washington Medical Center and Harborview Medical Center, Seattle, Washington
Physiology of the Peripheral Nerve

Paul Klimo, MD

Resident, Department of Neurosurgery, University Hospital, Salt Lake City, Utah
Treatment of Axis Fractures

David G. Kline, MD

Boyd Professor and Chairman, Department of Neurosurgery, Louisiana State University School of Medicine at New Orleans; Visiting Staff, Medical Center of Louisiana at Charity Hospital and University Hospital; Academic Staff, Ochsner Foundation Hospital; Senior Staff, Touro Infirmary, S. Baptist and Mercy Hospitals; Consultant, Veterans Administration Hospital, New Orleans, Louisiana; and Keeslor AFB Hospital, Biloxi, Mississippi
Management of Peripheral Nerve Tumors

Michel Kliot, MD

Associate Professor of Neurosurgery, University of Washington School of Medicine; Attending Neurosurgeon, University of Washington Medical Center and Veterans Administration Puget Sound Health Care System, Seattle, Washington
Cellular and Molecular Mechanisms Mediating Injury and Recovery in the Nervous System; General Principles in Evaluating and Treating Peripheral Nerve Injuries; Magnetic Resonance Imaging for Peripheral Nerve Injuries; Carpal Tunnel Syndrome; Entrapment Syndromes of Peripheral Nerve Injuries

Douglas Kondziolka, MD, MSc

Professor of Neurological Surgery and Radiation Oncology, University of Pittsburgh School of Medicine, Pittsburgh, Pennsylvania
Patient Selection in Movement Disorder Surgery; Fractionated Radiotherapy for Pituitary Tumors; Gamma Knife Radiosurgery

Thomas A. Kopitnik, MD

Professor of Neurosurgery, University of Texas Southwestern Medical School; Director of Cerebrovascular Surgery, University of Texas Southwestern Medical Center at Dallas, Dallas, Texas
Posterior Fossa Arteriovenous Malformations

Oleg Kopyov, MD, PhD

Research Director, The California Neuroscience Institute, Oxnard, California
Functional Radiosurgery

Karl F. Kothbauer, MD

Assistant Professor, Department of Neurological Surgery, Albert Einstein College of Medicine of Yeshiva University, Bronx; Attending, Beth Israel Medical Center, New York, New York
Intraspinal Tumors in Infants and Children

Adnah Koudsié, MD

Staff Neurosurgeon, Hôpital Albert Michallon, Grenoble, France
Deep Brain Stimulation for Movement Disorders

Paul Krack, MD

Professor of Neurology, University Joseph Fourier Medical School; Staff Neurologist, Hôpital Albert Michallion, Grenoble, France
Deep Brain Stimulation for Movement Disorders

Michael A. Kraut, MD, PhD

Associate Professor of Radiology, Johns Hopkins University School of Medicine; Chief of Neuro–MRI, Johns Hopkins Hospital, Baltimore, Maryland
Radiologic Features of Central Nervous System Tumors

Lynda Kulawiak, RN

Research Associate, Department of Anesthesiology and Perioperative Medicine, Oregon Health & Science University, Portland, Oregon
Management of Pain by Anesthetic Techniques

V. G. R. Kumar, MBBS

Consultant Neurosurgeon, West Bank Hospital, Calcutta, West Bengal, India
Cervical Spondylotic Myelopathy

Lara J. Kunschner, MD

Assistant Professor, Department of Neurology, Drexel University College of Medicine, Philadelphia; Attending, Allegheny General Hospital, Allegheny Neurological Associates, Pittsburgh, Pennsylvania
Medulloblastoma

Charles Kuntz IV, MD

Assistant Professor of Neurosurgery, University of Cincinnati School of Medicine; Associate Director, Spine and Peripheral Nerve Surgery, The Maxfield Clinic and Spine Institute, and Director, Spine and Peripheral Nerve Research, Department of Neurological Surgery, The Neuroscience Institute, Cincinnati, Ohio
Approach to the Patient and Medical Management of Spinal Disorders

Inam Kureshi, MD

Department of Neurovascular Surgery, Hartford Hospital Stroke Center, Hartford, Connecticut
Revascularization Techniques for Complex Aneurysms and Skull Base Tumors

Arthur M. Lam, MD

Professor of Anesthesiology and Neurological Surgery, University of Washington School of Medicine; Head, Division of Neuroanesthesia, Harborview Medical Center, Seattle, Washington
Anesthesia: Preoperative Evaluation; Transcranial Doppler Ultrasonography

Lois A. Lampson, PhD

Associate Professor of Neurosurgery, Brigham and Women's Hospital, Harvard Medical School, Boston, Massachusetts
Basic Principles of Central Nervous System Immunology

Frederick F. Lang, Jr., MD

Attending, Department of Neurosurgery, The University of Texas M.D. Anderson Cancer Center, Houston, Texas
Medulloblastoma; Metastatic Brain Tumors

Guiseppe Lanzino, MD

Associate Professor, Department of Neurosurgery, University of Illinois College of Medicine at Peoria; Chief, Section of Cerebrovascular Surgery, Illinois Neurological Institute, Peoria, Illinois
Endovascular Treatment of Aneurysms

Donald Larsen, MD

Associate Professor, Department of Neurological Surgery, University of Southern California Keck School of Medicine; Director of Neuro-interventional Section, USC University Hospital, Los Angeles, California
Cavernous Carotid Fistulas

Sean D. Lavine, MD

Assistant Professor of Neurosurgery and Radiology, Columbia University, College of Physicians and Surgeons; Clinical Director, Endovascular Neurosurgery and Interventional Neuroradiology, Columbia-Presbyterian Medical Center, New York, New York
Basilar Trunk Aneurysms

Michael T. Lawton, MD

Tong-Po Kan Assistant Professor of Neurological Surgery, University of California, San Francisco, School of Medicine; Chief of Cerebrovascular Surgery, University of California, San Francisco Medical Center, San Francisco, California
Surgical Approaches for Posterior Circulation Aneurysms

Edward R. Laws, MD

Professor, Department of Neurosurgery, University of Virginia, Charlottesville, Virginia

Daniel A. Lazar, MD

Resident, Department of Neurological Surgery, University of Washington Hospitals, Seattle, Washington
Cellular and Molecular Mechanisms Mediating Injury and Recovery in the Nervous System

Jean F. Le Bas, MD, PhD

Professor of Biophysics and Radiology, University Joseph Fourier Medical School; Head, Division of Neuroradiology and MRI, and Director, Institut Federatif de Recherche eu IRM, Hôpital Albert Michallon, Grenoble, France
Deep Brain Stimulation for Movement Disorders

Chong C. Lee, MD, PhD

Resident, Department of Neurological Surgery, University of Washington, Seattle, Washington
Carpal Tunnel Syndrome; Entrapment Syndromes of Peripheral Nerve Injuries

Jang-Chul Lee, MD, PhD

Associate Professor, Department of Neurosurgery, Keimyung University School of Medicine, Taegu, Korea
Diagnostic Biopsy of Peripheral Nerves and Muscle

Jung-Il Lee, MD

Associate Professor, Department of Neurosurgery, Samsung Medical Center, Sungkyun Kwan University School of Medicine, Seoul, Korea
Thalamotomy for Tremor

Sunghoon Lee, MD

Administrative Chief Resident, Yale Neurosurgery Program, Yale–New Haven Medical Center, New Haven, Connecticut
Unusual Gliomas; Intracranial Monitoring

Elizabeth A. Leedom, JD

Lecturer, University of Washington School of Law, Seattle, Washington
Legal Issues

James W. Leiphart, MD, PhD

Resident in Neurosurgery, UCLA Medical Center, Los Angeles, California
Surgery for Extratemporal Lobe Epilepsy

G. Michael Lemole, Jr., MD

Private Practice, Huntingdon Valley, Pennsylvania
Giant Aneurysms

Frederick A. Lenz, MD

Professor of Neurosurgery, Johns Hopkins University School of Medicine; Attending Neurosurgeon, Johns Hopkins Hospital, Baltimore, Maryland
Thalamotomy for Tremor

Phillipp M. Lenzlinger, MD

Division of Trauma Surgery, Department of Surgery, University Hospital, Zuroch, Switzerland
Cellular Basis of Injury and Recovery from Trauma

Jeffrey R. Leonard, MD

Assistant Professor, Department of Neurosurgery, Washington University School of Medicine; Attending Neurosurgeon, St. Louis Children's Hospital, St. Louis, Missouri
Dandy-Walker Syndrome

Peter D. Le Roux, MB, ChB, MD

Associate Professor of Neurosurgery, University of Pennsylvania School of Medicine, Philadelphia, Pennsylvania
Surgical Decision Making for the Treatment of Cerebral Aneurysms

Allan D. O. Levi, MD, PhD

Assistant Professor, University of Miami School of Medicine; Chief, Section of Neurospinal Services, Jackson Memorial Hospital, Miami, Florida
Spine Trauma: Approach to the Patient and Diagnostic Evaluation

Elad I. Levy, MD

Neurosurgical Chief Resident, University of Pittsburgh Medical Center System, Pittsburgh, Pennsylvania
Trigeminal Neuralgia: Microvascular Decompression of the Trigeminal Nerve for Tic Douloureux

Michael L. Levy, MD, PhD

Associate Professor, Department of Neurosurgery, University of Southern California Keck School of Medicine, Los Angeles, California
Vagus Nerve Stimulation for Intractable Epilepsy

David H. Lewis, MD

Associate Professor of Radiology, University of Washington School of Medicine; Director, Division of Nuclear Medicine, Harborview Medical Center, Seattle, Washington
Single-Photon Emission Computed Tomography and Positron Emission Tomography

Patricia Limousin, MD, PhD

Senior Lecturer, Institute of Neurology, and Honorary Consultant Neurologist, National Hospital for Neurology and Neurosurgery, Queen's Square, London, England
Deep Brain Stimulation for Movement Disorders

E. Paul Lindell, MD

Attending Radiologist, Department of Radiology, Mayo Clinic, Rochester, Minnesota
Magnetic Resonance Imaging of Brain

Lawrence S. Liu, MD

Attending, Department of Neurosurgery, Kaiser-Permanente Los Angeles Medical Center, Los Angeles, California
Technical Aspects of Bone Graft Harvest and Spinal Fusion

Jay S. Loeffler, MD

Andreas Soriano Professor of Radiation Oncology, Harvard Medical School; Chair, Department of Radiation Oncology, Massachusetts General Hospital, Boston, Massachusetts
Proton Radiosurgery

Christopher Loftus, MD

Professor and Chairman, Department of Neurosurgery, University of Oklahoma College of Medicine, Oklahoma City, Oklahoma
Carotid Occlusive Disease: Natural History and Medical Management

William J. Logan, MD

Professor of Pediatrics and Medicine, University of Toronto Faculty of Medicine; Attending, Division of Neurology, The Hospital for Sick Children, Toronto, Ontario, Canada
Neurological Examination in Infancy and Childhood

Donlin M. Long, MD, PhD

Distinguished Service Professor of Neurosurgery, Johns Hopkins University School of Medicine; Active Staff, Johns Hopkins Hospital; Principal Staff, Applied Physics Laboratory, Johns Hopkins University, Baltimore, Maryland
Acoustic Neuroma

Luca Longhi, MD

Terapia Intensiva Neuroscienze, Padiglione Beretta Neuro II piano (Rianimazione), Ospedale Maggiore Policlinico IRCCS, Milano, Italy
Cellular Basis of Injury and Recovery from Trauma

James B. Lowe III, MD, MBA

Instructor in Surgery, Division of Plastic and Reconstructive Surgery, Washington University School of Medicine, St. Louis, Missouri
Ulnar Nerve Entrapment at the Elbow

Andres M. Lozano, MD, PhD

Professor of Neurosurgery and R. R. Tasker Chair in Functional Neurosurgery, University of Toronto Faculty of Medicine; Attending, Toronto Western Hospital, Toronto, Ontario, Canada
Pallidotomy for Parkinson's Disease; Deep Brain Stimulation for Chronic Pain

Mark Luciano, MD, PhD

Chief, Pediatric and Congenital Neurosurgery Section, and Director, Cleveland Clinic Hydrocephalus Project, Cleveland Clinic, Cleveland, Ohio
Infantile Posthemorrhagic Hydrocephalus

Jürgen Lüders, MD, PhD

Chairman, Department of Neurology, Cleveland Clinic Foundation, Cleveland, Ohio
General and Historical Considerations of Epilepsy Surgery

David Lundin, MD

Resident, Department of Neurological Surgery, University of Washington, Seattle, Washington
Spondylolisthesis

L. Dade Lunsford, MD

Lars Leksell Professor of Neurological Surgery, Radiology, and Radiology Oncology and Chairman, Department of Neurological Surgery, University of Pittsburgh School of Medicine; Director, Center for Image-Guided Neurosurgery, University of Pittsburgh Medical Center, Pittsburgh, Pennsylvania
Patient Selection in Movement Disorder Surgery; Radiosurgery of Tumors

W. David Lust, PhD

Professor of Neurological Surgery, Case Western Reserve University School of Medicine; Attending, Department of Neurological Surgery, and The Research Institute of University Hospitals of Cleveland, Cleveland, Ohio
Intraoperative Cerebral Protection

R. Loch MacDonald, MD, PhD

Professor, Department of Surgery, Division of the Biological Sciences, Pritzker School of Medicine University of Chicago; Attending Neurosurgeon, University of Chicago Medical Center, Chicago, Illinois
Perioperative Management of Subarachnoid Hemorrhage

Susan E. Mackinnon, MD

Shornberg Professor and Chief, Division of Plastic and Reconstructive Surgery, Department of Surgery, Washington University School of Medicine, St. Louis, Missouri
Ulnar Nerve Entrapment at the Elbow

Roger M. Macklis, MD

Professor of Radiology, Ohio State University College of Medicine and Public Health; Chairman, Department of Radiation Oncology, Cleveland Clinic, Cleveland, Ohio
Principles of Radiotherapy

Christopher Madden, MD

Clinical Assistant Professor, Ohio State University, Columbus, Ohio
Cervical Spondylotic Myelopathy

Parley W. Madsen III, MD, PhD

Staff, Department of Neurological Surgery, Conemaugh Memorial Medical Center, Johnstown, Pennsylvania
Diagnosis and Management of Thoracic Spine Fractures

Dennis J. Maiman, MD, PhD

Professor, Department of Neurosurgery, and Director, Spine Surgery Fellowship, Medical College of Wisconsin; Physical Medicine and Rehabilitation, Froedtert Hospital; Attending Neurosurgeon, Veterans Affairs Medical Center, Milwaukee, Wisconsin
Concepts and Mechanisms of Biomechanics

Allen Maniker, MD

Assistant Professor, Department of Neurological Surgery, University of Medicine and Dentistry of New Jersey, Newark; Attending Neurosurgeon, University Hospital, Newark, and Hackensack University Hospital, Hackensack, New Jersey
Peripheral Nerves

Scott C. Manning, MD

Professor, Department of Otolaryngology, University of Washington School of Medicine; Chief, Division of Pediatric Otolaryngology, Children's Hospital and Regional Medical Center, Seattle, Washington
Diagnosis and Management of Juvenile Angiofibroma

Timothy B. Mapstone, MD

Professor and Vice-Chairman, Department of Neurological Surgery, Emory University School of Medicine; Director, Pediatric Neurosurgery, Children's Health Care of Atlanta, Atlanta, Georgia
Intracranial Germ Cell Tumors

Kenneth Maravilla, MD

Professor of Radiology and Director of Neuroradiology, Department of Neurological Surgery, University of Washington School of Medicine; Research Affiliate, Center on Human Development and Disability, Seattle, Washington

Magnetic Resonance Imaging for Peripheral Nerve Disorders

Douglas A. Marchuk, PhD

Associate Professor, Department of Genetics, Duke University School of Medicine, Durham, North Carolina

The Genetics of Cerebral Cavernous Malformations

Paul J. Marcotte, MD

Associate Professor of Neurosurgery, University of Pennsylvania School of Medicine; Attending, Department of Neurosurgery, Hospital of the University of Pennsylvania, Philadelphia, Pennsylvania

Technical Aspects of Bone Graft Harvest and Spinal Fusion

Anthony Marmarou, PhD

Professor and Vice Chairman, Director of Research, Division of Neurosurgery, Virginia Commonwealth University School of Medicine, Richmond, Virginia

Physiology of the Cerebrospinal Fluid and Intracranial Pressure

Joseph C. Maroon, MD

Clinical Professor and Heindl Scholar, Department of Neurosurgery, University of Pittsburgh School of Medicine; Vice Chairman, Department of Neurosurgery, UPMC-Presbyterian Hospital, Pittsburgh, Pennsylvania

Orbital Tumors

Lawrence F. Marshall, MD

Professor of Neurological Surgery, University of California, San Diego, School of Medicine; Chief, Division of Neurosurgery, UCSD Medical Center, San Diego, California

Differential Diagnosis of Altered States of Consciousness; Modern Neurotraumatology: A Brief Historical Review; Traumatic Cerebrospinal Fluid Fistulas

Sharon B. Marshall

Director of Clinical Research, Department of Neurosurgery, University of California, San Diego, San Diego, California

Modern Neurotraumatology: A Brief Historical Review

Neil A. Martin, MD

Professor and Chair, Department of Neurosurgery, David Geffen School of Medicine at University of California, Los Angeles, Los Angeles, California

Revascularization Techniques for Complex Aneurysms and Skull Base Tumors

Timothy J. Martin, MD

Associate Professor of Surgical Sciences/ Ophthalmology, Department of Ophthalmology, Wake Forest University School of Medicine; Attending, Baptist Medical Center and Wake Forest University Eye Center, Winston-Salem, North Carolina

Neuro-ophthalmology

Robert E. Maxwell, MD, PhD

Professor and Chair, Department of Neurosurgery, University of Minnesota Medical School; Neurosurgery Clinical Service Chief, Fairview University Medical Center, Minneapolis, Minnesota

Standard Temporal Lobectomy and Transsylvian Amygdalohippocampectomy

Nina A. Mayr, MD

Professor and Director, Radiation Oncology, Oklahoma University Health Sciences Center, Oklahoma City, Oklahoma

Radiobiology

Kevin McCarthy, MD

Assistant Professor and Director, Department of Medicine, Nuclear Medicine Division, Louisiana State University School of Medicine in New Orleans, New Orleans, Louisiana

Intracranial Monitoring

Paul C. McCormick, MD, MPH

Professor of Clinical Neurosurgery, Department of Neurological Surgery, Columbia University College of Physicians and Surgeons; Attending Neurosurgeon, New York Presbyterian Hospital, New York, New York

Anterior Thoracic Instrumentation; Anterior Lumbar Instrumentation; Spinal Cord Tumors in Adults

M. W. McDermott, MD

Assistant Professor, Department of Neurological Surgery, University of California, San Francisco, School of Medicine, San Francisco, California

Interstitial and Intracavitary Irradiation of Brain Tumors

Cameron G. McDougall, MD, FRCS(C)

Director, Division of Endovascular Neurosurgery, Barrow Neurological Institute, Phoenix, Arizona

Carotid Angioplasty and Stenting: Interventional Treatment of Occlusive Vascular Disease

Tracy K. McIntosh, PhD

Professor of Neurosurgery, Pharmacology, and Bioengineering, Vice-Chair for Research and Director, University of Pennsylvania Head Injury Center, University of Pennsylvania, Philadelphia, Pennsylvania

Cellular Basis of Injury and Recovery from Trauma

Guy M. McKhann II, MD

Assistant Professor, Department of Neurological Surgery, Columbia University College of Physicians and Surgeons; Staff, The Neurological Institute, and Attending, New York Presbyterian Hospital, New York, New York
Electrophysiologic Properties of the Mammalian Central Nervous System

David G. McLone, MD, PhD

Staff, Department of Pediatric Neurosurgery, Children's Memorial Hospital, Chicago, Illinois
Normal and Abnormal Embryology of the Spinal Cord and Spine

Max B. Medary, MD

Director, Orlando Neurosurgical Foundation, Celebration, Florida
Carotid Endarterectomy

Sanford L. Meeks, PhD

Associate Professor of Radiology, University of Iowa Roy J. and Lucille A. Carver College of Medicine; Director of Medical Physics, Department of Radiation Oncology, University of Iowa Health Care, Iowa City, Iowa
Radiobiology; Radiotherapy for Benign Skull Base Tumors; Fractionated and Stereotactic Radiation, Extracranial Stereotactic Radiation, Intensity Modulation, and Multileaf Collimation

Minesh P. Mehta, MBChB

Associate Professor, Department of Human Oncology, University of Wisconsin—Madison Medical School, Madison, Wisconsin
Fractionated Radiation Therapy for Malignant Brain Tumors

Vivek Mehta, MD, MSc

Assistant Professor, Department of Neurosurgery, University of Alberta Faculty of Medicine; Attending, Walter MacKenzie Health Sciences Center, Edmonton, Alberta, Canada
Craniopharyngioma in the Adult

William P. Melega, PhD

Associate Professor, Department of Molecular and Medical Pharmacology, David Geffen School of Medicine at UCLA, Los Angeles, California
Molecular Imaging of the Brain with Positron Emission Tomography

Arnold H. Menezes, MD

Professor and Vice Chairman, Department of Neurosurgery, University of Iowa College of Medicine; Attending Neurosurgeon, University of Iowa Hospitals and Clinics, Iowa City, Iowa
Developmental Abnormalities of the Craniovertebral Junction; Acquired Abnormalities of the Craniocervical Junction; Tumors of the Craniovertebral Junction

Robert A. Mericle, MD

Assistant Professor, Department of Neurosurgery, University of Florida College of Medicine; Staff, McKnight Brain Institute, Gainesville, Florida
Vein of Galen Malformations

Glen S. Merry, MD

Professor of Neurosurgery, University of Queensland Faculty of Medicine; Consultant Neurosurgeon, Royal Brisbane Hospital, Brisbane Queensland, Australia
Mild Head Injury in Adults

Ali Mesiwala, MD

Resident, University of Washington Hospitals, Seattle, Washington
General Principles of Operative Positioning

Fredric B. Meyer, MD

Professor of Neurosurgery, Mayo Medical School; Staff, Departments of Diagnostic Radiology and Neurological Surgery, Mayo Clinic, Rochester, Minnesota
Cerebral Blood Flow and Metabolism; Multimodality Management of Complex Cerebrovascular Lesions

Jeff Michalski, MD

Associate Professor, Department of Radiation Oncology, Washington University School of Medicine; Clinical Director, Department of Radiation Oncology, Barnes-Jewish Hospital, St. Louis, Missouri
Radiotherapy of Tumors of the Spine

J. Parker Mickle, MD

Professor, Department of Neurosurgery, University of Florida College of Medicine; Staff, McKnight Brain Institute, Gainesville, Florida
Vein of Galen Malformations

Rajiv Midha, MD, MSc

Associate Professor, Department of Surgery, Division of Neurosurgery, University of Toronto Faculty of Medicine; Staff Neurosurgeon, Sunnybrook and Women's College Health Sciences Centre, Toronto, Ontario, Canada
Peripheral Nerve: Approach to the Patient

Tom Mikkelsen, MD

Co-Director, Hermelin Brain Tumor Center, and Attending, Henry Ford Hospital, Detroit, Michigan
Invasion in Malignant Glioma

Andrew N. Miles, MBBS

Consultant Neurosurgeon, Western Australian Comprehensive Epilepsy Service and Department of Neurosurgery, Royal Perth Hospital, Perth, Western Australia, Australia
Tailored Resections for Epilepsy

John W. Miller, MD, PhD

Professor of Neurology and Neurological Surgery, University of Washington School of Medicine; Director, Regional Epilepsy Center, University of Washington Medical Center, Seattle, Washington
Approaches to the Diagnosis and Classification of Epilepsy

Neil R. Miller, MD

Professor of Ophthalmology, Neurology, and Neurosurgery and Frank B. Walsh Professor of Neuro-Ophthalmology, Johns Hopkins University School of Medicine, Baltimore, Maryland
Pseudotumor Cerebri

Pedro Molina-Negro, MD, PhD

Professor of Surgery (Neurosurgery), University of Montreal Faculty of Medicine, Howick, Quebec, Canada
Selective Peripheral Denervation for Spasmodic Torticollis

Jacques J. Morcos, MD

Associate Professor, Department of Neurosurgery, University of Miami School of Medicine, Miami, Florida
Spontaneous Intracerebral Hemorrhage: Non–Arteriovenous Malformation, Nonaneurysm

Michael Kerin Morgan, MD

Professor of Neurosurgery, University of Sydney Faculty of Medicine, Sydney, New South Wales, Australia
Classification and Decision Making in Treatment and Perioperative Management, including Surgical and Radiosurgical Decision Making

Glenn Morrison, MD

Professor of Neurological Surgery, University of Miami School of Medicine; Chief, Division of Neurological Surgery, Miami Children's Hospital, Miami, Florida
Temporal and Extratemporal Lobe Resections for Childhood Intractable Epilepsy

Richard S. Morrison, PhD

Professor, Department of Neurological Surgery, University of Washington School of Medicine, Seattle, Washington
Growth Factors and Brain Tumors

Wade M. Mueller, MD

Associate Professor, Department of Neurosurgery, Medical College of Wisconsin, Milwaukee, Wisconsin
Functional Magnetic Resonance Imaging in Epilepsy Surgery

J. Paul Muizelaar, MD, PhD

Professor and Chair, Department of Neurological Surgery, University of California, Davis, School of Medicine, Davis; University of California, Davis, Medical Center, Sacramento, California
Clinical Pathophysiology of Traumatic Brain Injury

Jenny Multani, MD

Resident, Department of Neurosurgery, West Virginia University School of Medicine, Morgantown, West Virginia
Occult Spinal Dysraphism and the Tethered Spinal Cord

Karin M. Muraszko, MD

Associate Professor of Neurosurgery and Pediatric and Communicable Diseases, University of Michigan Medical School; Director, Pediatric Neurosurgery Program, C. S. Mott Children's Hospital, University of Michigan Hospital and Health Centers, Ann Arbor, Michigan
Primitive Neuroectodermal Tumors

Antonio C. M. Mussi, MD

Research Fellow, Department of Neurological Surgery, University of Florida College of Medicine, Gainesville, Florida
Surgical Anatomy of the Brain

Neal J. Naff, MD

Assistant Professor of Neurosurgery, Johns Hopkins University School of Medicine, Baltimore, and Uniformed Services University of Health Sciences, F. Edward Hébert School of Medicine, Bethesda; Chief of Neurosurgery, Sinai Hospital of Baltimore, Baltimore, Maryland
Endovascular Techniques for Brain Tumors

Blaine S. Nashold, MD

Professor Emeritus, Department of Surgery, Division of Neurosurgery, Duke University School of Medicine; Director, Neurosurgical Stereotactic Laboratory and Neuroprosthesis Laboratory, Duke University Medical Center, Durham, North Carolina
Caudalis Nucleus Dorsal Root Entry Zone Procedure for the Treatment of Intractable Facial Pain

Gary M. Nesbit, MD

Associate Professor, Department of Neurological Surgery, Diagnostic Radiology, and Neurology, Oregon Health & Science University School of Medicine and Dotter Interventional Institute; Chief, Neuroradiology and MRI, University Hospital, Portland, Oregon
Cerebral Venous and Sinus Thrombosis

David W. Newell, MD

Professor, Department of Neurological Surgery, University of Washington School of Medicine; Attending Neurosurgeon, Harborview Medical Center, University of Washington Medical Center, Children's Hospital Medical Center, and Veterans' Hospital Medical Center, Seattle, Washington

Transcranial Doppler Ultrasonography; Traumatic Cerebral Aneurysms Secondary to Penetrating Intracranial Injuries; Traumatic Cerebrovascular Injury

Douglas A. Nichols, MD

Associate Professor, Departments of Radiology and Neurosurgery, Mayo Medical School, Rochester, Minnesota

Multimodality Management of Complex Cerebrovascular Lesions

Ajay Niranjan, MBBS, MS, MCh

Assistant Professor, Department of Neurological Surgery, University of Pittsburgh School of Medicine; Director, Radiosurgery Research, University of Pittsburgh Medical Center System, Pittsburgh, Pennsylvania

Radiosurgery of Tumors

Russ P. Nockels, MD

Associate Professor and Vice Chair, Departments of Neurological Surgery and Orthopedic Surgery, Loyola University Stritch School of Medicine, Loyola University Medical Center, Maywood, Illinois

Diagnosis and Management of Thoracolumbar and Lumbar Spine Injuries

Michael J. Noetzel, MD

Professor of Neurology and Pediatrics, Washington University School of Medicine; Director, Clinical Services, Division of Pediatric Neurology, Washington University Medical Center; Medical Director, Clinical and Diagnostic Neuroscience Services, St. Louis Children's Hospital, St. Louis, Missouri

Acute Pediatric Neurorehabilitation

Patrick Noonen, MD

Department of Radiology, National Naval Medical Center, Bethesda, Maryland

Endovascular Techniques for Brain Tumors

Richard B. North, MD

Professor of Neurosurgery, Anesthesiology, and Critical Care Medicine, Johns Hopkins University School of Medicine, Baltimore, Maryland

Spinal Cord and Peripheral Nerve Stimulation for Chronic, Intractable Pain

Eric Nottmeier, MD

Chief Resident, Division of Neurosurgery, University of Missouri Hospitals and Clinics, Columbia, Missouri

Intracranial Occlusion Disease and Moyamoya

W. Jerry Oakes, MD

Professor of Neurosurgery and Pediatrics, University of Alabama School of Medicine; Chief, Pediatric Neurosurgery, University of Alabama Hospitals, Birmingham Alabama

Chiari Malformations

Maureen O'Donnell, MD, MSc

Assistant Professor and Head, Division of Developmental Pediatrics, Department of Pediatrics, University of British Columbia Faculty of Medicine; Medical Director, Child Development and Rehabilitation Program, Children's and Women's Health Centre of British Columbia, Vancouver, British Columbia, Canada

Intrathecal Baclofen Infusion

Christopher S. Ogilvy, MD

Associate Professor of Surgery, Harvard Medical School; Visiting Neurosurgeon, Massachusetts General Hospital, Boston, Massachusetts

Vertebral Artery, Posterior Inferior Cerebellar Artery, and Vertebrobasilar Junction Aneurysms

George A. Ojemann, MD

Professor of Neurological Surgery, University of Washington School of Medicine; Staff, University of Washington Regional Epilepsy Center, Seattle, Washington

Tailored Resections for Epilepsy

Jeffrey G. Ojemann, MD

Assistant Professor of Neurosurgery, Department of Neurological Surgery, and Assistant Professor of Pediatrics, Anatomy, Psychology, and Neurobiology, Washington University School of Medicine; Attending Neurosurgeon, St. Louis Children's Hospital, St. Louis, Missouri

Dandy-Walker Syndrome

Michael S. Okun, MD

Assistant Professor of Neurology, University of Florida College of Medicine; Co-Director, Movement Disorders Center, Department of Neurology, McKnight Brain Institute, Gainesville, Florida

Surgery for Dystonia

Edward H. Oldfield, MD

Chief, Surgical Neurology Branch, National Institute of Neurological Diseases and Stroke, National Institutes of Health, Bethesda, Maryland

Spinal Arteriovenous Malformations

Alessandro Olivi, MD

Professor of Neurosurgery, Johns Hopkins University School of Medicine, Baltimore, Maryland

Brain Tumors during Pregnancy

Stephen L. Ondra, MD

Assistant Professor of Neurosurgery, Northwestern University Feinberg School of Medicine, Chicago, Illinois
Adult Thoracolumbar Scoliosis

Michael Ostad, MD

Clinical Adjunct Assistant Professor of Urology, Cornell University, Joan and Sanford I. Weill College of Medicine; Attending Urologist, New York Presbyterian Hospital, New York, and North Shore University Hospital, Manhasset, New York
Neurourology

Renatta J. Osterdock, MD

Pediatric Neurosurgery Fellow, University of Tennessee, Memphis, College of Medicine and Semmes-Murphy Clinic, Memphis, Tennessee
Lipomyelomeningocele

Jeffrey H. Owen, PhD

President and Owner, Sentient Medical Systems, Cockeysville, Maryland
Intraoperative Electrophysiologic Monitoring of the Spinal Cord and Nerve Roots

Dachling Pang, MD

Professor of Clinical Neurosurgery, University of California, Davis, School of Medicine, Davis; Chief, Regional Center for Pediatric Neurosurgery, Kaiser Permanente Hospital, Oakland, California
Pediatric Vertebral Column and Spinal Cord Injuries

T. S. Park, MD

Shi H. Huang Professor of Neurosurgery and Professor of Pediatrics and Anatomy and Neurobiology, Washington University School of Medicine; Neurosurgeon-in-Chief, St. Louis Children's Hospital, St. Louis, Missouri
Birth Brachial Plexus Injury; Selective Dorsal Rhizotomy for Spastic Cerebral Palsy

Andrew T. Parsa, MD, PhD

Assistant Professor, Department of Neurological Surgery, University of California, San Francisco, School of Medicine, San Francisco, California
Anterior Thoracic Instrumentation; Anterior Lumbar Instrumentation

Michael Partington, MD

Neurosurgeon, Department of Pediatrics, Gillette Children's Specialty Healthcare, St. Paul, Minnesota
Normal and Abnormal Embryology of the Spinal Cord and Spine

Naresh P. Patel, MD

Assistant Professor of Neurosurgery, Mayo Medical School Scottsdale; Assistant Attending, Mayo Clinic Scottsdale, Scottsdale, Arizona
Complication Avoidance in Neurosurgery

Jogi V. Pattisapu, MD

Clinical Faculty, Department of Molecular Biology and Microbiology and Department of Nursing, College of Health Sciences, University of Central Florida; Medical Director, Pediatric Neurosurgery, Arnold Palmer Hospital for Women and Children, Florida Children's Hospital, Wade's Center for Hydrocephalus Research, HRI, Orlando, Florida
Infantile Posthemorrhagic Hydrocephalus

Richard D. Penn, MD

Professor of Neurosurgery, University of Chicago, Division of the Biological Sciences, Pritzker School of Medicine; Attending, Neuroscience Institute, Neurosurgery Division, Rush-Presbyterian-St. Luke's Medical Center, and University of Chicago Hospitals, Chicago, Illinois
Management of Spasticity by Central Nervous System Infusion Techniques; Intrathecal Drug Infusion for Pain

Noel I. Perin, MD

Clinical Associate Professor of Neurosurgery, Columbia University College of Physicians and Surgeons; Attending Physician, St. Luke's Roosevelt Beth-Israel Hospital, New-York, New York
Sacral Fractures

Richard G. Perrin, MD, MSc

Associate Professor of Neurological Surgery, Division of Neurosurgery, University of Toronto Faculty of Medicine; Staff, St. Michael's Hospital, Toronto, Ontario, Canada
Tumors of the Vertebral Axis: Benign, Primary Malignant, and Metastatic Tumors

Jonathan R. Perry, MD

Professor, Department of Radiology, University of Washington School of Medicine, Seattle, Washington
Radiology of the Spine

John A. Persing, MD

Professor, Department of Neurosurgery, Yale University School of Medicine; Chief, Section of Plastic Surgery, Yale–New Haven Hospital, New Haven, Connecticut
Scalp Tumors; Craniofacial Syndromes

Michael E. Phelps, PhD

Norton Simon Professor and Chair, Department of Molecular and Medical Pharmacology, David Geffen School of Medicine at UCLA; Director, Crump Institute for Molecular Imaging; Associate Director, Laboratory of Structural Biology and Molecular Medicine and Chief, Division of Nuclear Medicine, UCLA Medical Center, Los Angeles, California
Molecular Imaging of the Brain with Positron Emission Tomography

Loi K. Phuong, MD

Resident, Department of Neurology, Mayo Clinic, Rochester, Minnesota
Pediatric Cerebral Hemispheric Tumors

David G. Piepgras, MD

Professor of Neurologic Surgery, Mayo Medical School; Chairman, Department of Neurologic Surgery, Mayo Clinic, Rochester, Minnesota
Middle Cerebral Artery Aneurysms

Joseph Piepmeier, MD

Nixdorff-German Professor and Vice Chairman for Clinical Affairs, Department of Neurosurgery, Yale University School of Medicine; Director, Neuro-oncology Unit, Yale Comprehensive Cancer Center, New Haven, Connecticut
Unusual Gliomas

Webster H. Pilcher, MD, PhD

Professor and Chair, Department of Neurological Surgery, University of Rochester School of Medicine and Dentistry and School of Nursing; Staff, Eastman Dental Center and Strong Memorial Hospital, Rochester, New York
Epilepsy Surgery: Outcome and Complications

Frank A. Pintar, PhD

Professor, Department of Neurosurgery, Medical College of Wisconsin; Adjunct Professor of Biomedical Engineering, Marquette University; Director, Neuroscience Research Laboratories, and Principal Investigator/Biomedical Engineer, Veterans Administration Medical Center, Milwaukee, Wisconsin
Concepts and Mechanisms of Biomechanics

Joseph D. Pinter, MD

Assistant Professor of Neurology, University of California, Davis, School of Medicine, Davis; Attending, UC Davis Medical Center, Sacramento, California
Neuroembryology

Serge Pinto, PhD

Hôpital Albert Michallon, Service de Neurologie Grenoble and University Joseph Fourier, Grenoble, France
Deep Brain Stimulation for Movement Disorders

Farhad Pirouzmand, MD

Assistant Professor of Neurosurgery, University of Saskatchewan Faculty of Medicine; Program Director, Division of Neurosurgery, Royal University Hospital, Saskatoon, Saskatchewan, Canada
Arteriovenous Malformations and Intracranial Aneurysms in Children

Ian F. Pollack, MD

Professor of Neurosurgery, University of Pittsburgh School of Medicine; Co-Director, University of Pittsburgh Cancer Institute Brain Tumor Center, Children's Hospital of Pittsburgh, Pittsburgh, Pennsylvania
Brainstem Gliomas

Pierre Pollak, MD, PhD

Professor of Neurology, University Joseph Fourier Medical School; Head, Movement Disorders Unit, Hôpital Albert Michallon, Grenoble, France
Deep Brain Stimulation for Movement Disorders

Bruce E. Pollock, MD

Associate Professor, Department of Neurological Surgery, Mayo Medical School, Rochester, Minnesota
Multimodality Management of Complex Cerebrovascular Lesions

Randall W. Porter, MD

Chief, Interdisciplinary Skull Base Section, Barrow Neurological Institute, Phoenix, Arizona
Infratentorial Cavernous Malformations; Classification of Spinal Cord Vascular Lesions

Kalmon D. Post, MD

Professor and Chairman, Department of Neurosurgery, Mount Sinai School of Medicine; Chairman, Department of Neurosurgery, Mount Sinai Medical Center, New York, New York
Complication Avoidance in Neurosurgery; Trigeminal Schwannomas

Sujit S. Prabhu, MD

Director, Department of Neurosurgery, M.D. Anderson Cancer Center, Houston, Texas
Surgical Management of Traumatic Brain Injury

Charles J. Prestigiacomo, MD

Assistant Professor of Cerebrovascular/Endovascular Surgery, Departments of Neurological Surgery and Radiology, University of Medicine and Dentistry of New Jersey—New Jersey Medical School; Attending, Neurological Institute of New Jersey, University Hospital, Newark, New Jersey
Neurosonology

Robert Prost, PhD

Assistant Professor of Radiology, Medical College of Wisconsin; Attending, Froedtert & Memorial Lutheran Hospital, Milwaukee, Wisconsin
Magnetic Resonance Imaging of Brain

Chad J. Prusmack, MD

Resident, Department of Neurosurgery, University of Miami Hospital and Clinics, Miami, Florida
Spontaneous Intracerebral Hemorrhage: Non–Arteriovenous Malformation, Nonaneurysm

Donald O. Quest, MD

Professor, Department of Neurological Surgery, Columbia University College of Physicians and Surgeons; Attending, Department of Neurological Surgery, Neurological Institute of New York Presbyterian Hospital, and New York Presbyterian Medical Center, New York, New York
Neurosonology

Corey Raffel, MD, PhD

Professor of Neurosurgery, Mayo Medical School, Rochester, Minnesota
Pediatric Cerebral Hemispheric Tumors

Ramesh Raghupathi, PhD

Assistant Professor, Department of Neurobiology and Anatomy, Drexel University College of Medicine, Philadelphia, Pennsylvania
Cellular Basis of Injury and Recovery from Trauma

Frank A. Raila, MD

Professor Emeritus, Department of Radiology, University of Mississippi School of Medicine, Jackson, Mississippi
Radiology of the Skull

Zvi Ram, MD

Associate Professor of Surgery, Division of Neurosurgery, Tel Aviv University Sackler School of Medicine, Tel Aviv; Deputy Chairman, Department of Neurosurgery, Chaim Sheba Medical Center, Tel Hashomer, Israel
Principles of Gene Therapy

Bruce R. Ransom, MD, PhD

Professor and Chairman, Department of Neurology, University of Washington School of Medicine, Seattle, Washington
Astrocytes

Robert A. Ratcheson, MD

Professor of Neurological Surgery, Department of Neurological Surgery, Case Western Reserve University School of Medicine; Director, Department of Neurological Surgery, and the Research Institute, University Hospitals of Cleveland, Cleveland, Ohio
Intraoperative Cerebral Protection

Peter Raudzens, MD

Anesthesiologist, Department of Neuroanesthesia, Barrow Neurological Institute, Phoenix, Arizona
Anesthesia in Cerebrovascular Disease

Shlomo Raz, MD

Professor of Urology, Head of Reconstructive and Female Urology, David Geffen School of Medicine at UCLA, Los Angeles, California
Neurourology

Gary L. Rea, MD, PhD

Private Practice, University Orthopedic Physicians, Columbus, Ohio

Alyssa T. Reddy, MD

Assistant Professor of Pediatrics and Neurology, University of Alabama School of Medicine; Pediatric Neurologist, The Children's Hospital of Alabama, Birmingham, Alabama
Intracranial Germ Cell Tumors

Patrick M. Reilly, MD

Assistant Professor of Surgery, University of Pennsylvania School of Medicine, Philadelphia, Pennsylvania
Initial Resuscitation and Patient Evaluation

Harold L. Rekate, MD

Clinical Professor of Surgery, Division of Neurosurgery, University of Arizona College of Medicine, Tucson; Chairman, Section of Pediatric Neurosciences, and Director, Pediatric Neurosurgical Research Laboratory, Barrow Neurological Institute, Phoenix, Arizona
Hydrocephalus in Children

Ali R. Rezai, MD

Associate Professor and Head, Section for Stereotactic and Functional Neurosurgery, Department of Neurological Surgery, The Cleveland Clinic Foundation, Cleveland, Ohio
Deep Brain Stimulation for Chronic Pain

Laurence D. Rhines, MD

Assistant Professor of Neurosurgical Oncology, Department of Neurosurgery, University of Texas–Houston Medical School; Director, Spine Program, Department of Neurosurgery, The University of Texas M.D. Anderson Cancer Center, Houston, Texas
Brain Tumors during Pregnancy; Sarcoidosis, Tuberculosis, and Xanthogranuloma

Albert L. Rhoton, Jr., MD

R.D. Keene Family Professor, Chairman Emeritus, Department of Neurosurgery, University of Florida College of Medicine, Gainesville, Florida
Surgical Anatomy of the Brain

Teresa Ribalta, MD, PhD

Associate Professor of Pathology, University of Barcelona Medical School; Consultant, Department of Pathology, Hospital Clinic of Barcelona, Barcelona, Spain
Brain Tumors: An Overview of Histopathologic Classification

Bernd Richling, MD

Professor of Neurosurgery, Private Medical University of Salzburg, Salzburg Austria
Embolization of Arteriovenous Malformations as a Primary Treatment Modality

Charles J. Riedel, MD

Assistant Professor of Neurosurgery, Columbia University College of Physicians and Surgeons; Attending, Department of Neurological Surgery, Columbia-Presbyterian Medical Center, New York, New York
Surgical Exposures and Positioning for Spinal Surgery

Daniele Rigamonti, MD

Professor, Department of Neurosurgery, Johns Hopkins University School of Medicine; Director, Skeletal Dysplasias and Genetics, Johns Hopkins Hospital, Baltimore, Maryland
Anterior Communicating Artery and Anterior Cerebral Artery Aneurysms; Achondroplasia and Other Dwarfism

Howard A. Riina, MD

Assistant Professor of Neurological Surgery, Neurology, and Radiology, Cornell University Joan and Sanford I. Weill Medical College; Attending Neurosurgeon, New York Presbyterian Hospital, New York, New York
Giant Aneurysms; Classification of Spinal Cord Vascular Lesions

Michael E. C. Robbins, PhD

Professor, Department of Radiology, Wake Forest University School of Medicine; Head, Radiation Biology Section, Wake Forest Baptist Medical Center, Winston-Salem, North Carolina
Radiobiology

Claudia Robertson, MD

Professor, Department of Neurosurgery, Baylor College of Medicine; Medical Director, Neurosurgical Intensive Care Unit, Ben Taub General Hospital, Houston, Texas
Critical Care Management of Traumatic Brain Injury

Jon H. Robertson, MD

Chairman, Department of Neurosurgery, University of Tennessee, Memphis, College of Medicine, Memphis, Tennessee
Glomus Jugulare Tumors

Lawrence Robinson, MD

Professor and Chair, Department of Rehabilitation Medicine, University of Washington School of Medicine; Director, Electrodiagnostic Laboratory, Harborview Medical Center, Seattle, Washington
Electrodiagnostic Evaluation of Peripheral Nerves: Electromyography, Somatosensory Evoked Potentials, Nerve Action Potentials

Shenandoah Robinson, MD

Assistant Professor, Department of Neurological Surgery, Case Western Reserve University School of Medicine; Pediatric Neurosurgeon, Rainbow Babies and Children's Hospital, Cleveland, Ohio
Myelomeningocele and Myelocystocele; Intervertebral Disk Disease in Children

Mark A. Rockoff, MD

Professor of Anesthesia, Harvard Medical School; Vice-Chairman, Department of Anesthesia, Children's Hospital, Boston, Massachusetts
Neuroanesthesia in Children

Mark L. Rosenblum, MD

Chairman, Department of Neurosurgery, and Co-Director, Hermelin Brain Tumor Center, Henry Ford Hospital, Detroit, Michigan
Invasion in Malignant Glioma

Walter Royal III, MD

Associate Professor, Departments of Neurology, Morehouse School of Medicine, Atlanta, Georgia
Multiple Sclerosis

Ronald Ruff, PhD

Clinical Professor, Department of Psychiatry, University of California, San Francisco, School of Medicine, San Francisco, California
Sequelae of Traumatic Brain Injury

James T. Rutka, MD, PhD

Professor and Chairman, Division of Neurosurgery, University of Toranto Faculty of Medicine; Staff Neurosurgeon, The Hospital for Sick Children, Toronto, Ontario, Canada
Encephaloceles

Kathryn E. Saatman, MD

Associate Professor, Department of Neurosurgery, University of Pennsylvania School of Medicine, Philadelphia, Pennsylvania
Cellular Basis of Injury and Recovery from Trauma

Oren Sagher, MD

Associate Professor, Section of Neurosurgery, University of Michigan Medical College, Ann Arbor, Michigan
Diagnosis and Nonoperative Management [Trigeminal Neuralgia]

Sean A. Salehi, MD

Chief Resident, Department of Neurological Surgery, Northwestern Memorial Hospital, Chicago, Illinois
Adult Thoracolumbar Scoliosis

Ali Samii, MD

Assistant Professor of Neurology and Neurological Surgery, University of Washington School of Medicine, Seattle, Washington
Approach to Movement Disorders

Madjid Samii, MD

Professor and Chairman, Department of Neurosurgery, International Neuroscience Institute, Hanover, Germany
Basic Principles of Skull Base Surgery

Prakash Sampath, MD

Assistant Professor of Neurosurgery and Assistant Professor of Clinical Neurosciences, Brown University School of Medicine; Director, Neurosurgical Oncology, and Chief of Neurosurgery, Roger Williams Hospital, Providence, Rhode Island
Acoustic Neuroma; Sarcoidosis, Tuberculosis, and Xanthogranuloma

Duke Samson, MD

Professor and Chair, Department of Neurosurgery, University of Texas Southwestern Medical School, Dallas, Texas
Posterior Fossa Arteriovenous Malformations

Paul Santiago, MD

Resident, Department of Neurological Surgery, University of Washington Hospitals, Seattle, Washington
Malignant Gliomas: Anaplastic Astrocytoma, Glioblastoma Multiforme, Gliosarcoma, Malignant Oligodendroglioma; Benign Extradural Lesions of the Dorsal Spine

Harvey B. Sarnat, MD

Professor of Pediatrics (Neurology) and Pathology (Neuropathology), David Geffen School of Medicine at UCLA; Director, Division of Pediatric Neurology, and Neuropathologist, Cedars-Sinai Medical Center, Los Angeles, California
Neuroembryology

Raymond Sawaya, MD

Professor of Neurosurgery, University of Texas–Houston Medical School; Director, Brain Tumor Center, and Chairman, Department of Neurosurgery, The University of Texas M.D. Anderson Cancer Center, Houston, Texas
Brain Tumors: General Considerations; Metastatic Brain Tumors

Paul D. Sawin, MD

Private Practice, Orlando, Florida
Biology of Bone Grafting and Healing in Spinal Surgery; Posterior Cervical Stabilization and Fusion Techniques

Wouter I. Schievink, MD

Assistant Clinical Professor, Department of Neurological Surgery, University of California, Irvine, School of Medicine, Irvine; Attending Neurosurgeon, Cedars-Sinai Medical Center, and Co-Director, Neurovascular Surgery Program, Cedars-Sinai Neurosurgical Institute, Los Angeles, California
Genetics of Intracranial Aneurysms

Jay J. Schindler, MD, MS

Assistant Professor, Department of Neurologic Surgery, Mayo School of Medicine; Resident, Mayo Clinic, Rochester, Minnesota
Multimodality Management of Complex Cerebrovascular Lesions

James M. Schuster, MD, PhD

Assistant Professor of Neurosurgery, University of Pennsylvania School of Medicine; Attending, Department of Neurosurgery, Hospital of the University of Pennsylvania, Philadelphia, Pennsylvania
Growth Factors and Brain Tumors; Motor, Sensory, and Language Mapping and Monitoring for Cortical Resections; Posterior Thoracic Instrumentation

Theodore H. Schwartz, MD

Assistant Professor of Neurosurgery, Cornell University Joan and Sanford I. Weill Medical College; Assistant Attending in Neurosurgery, New York Presbyterian Hospital, New York, New York
Spinal Cord Tumors in Adults

R. Michael Scott, MD

Professor of Neurological Surgery, Harvard Medical School; Director, Clinical Pediatric Neurosurgery, The Children's Hospital and Medical Center, Boston, Massachusetts
Choroid Plexus Tumors; Cerebellar Astrocytomas in Children

Raymond Sekula, MD

Resident, Department of Neurosurgery, Allegheny General Hospital, Pittsburgh, Pennsylvania
Ablative Surgery for Spasticity

Laligam N. Sekhar, MD

Private Practice, Annandale, Virginia
Chordoma and Chondrosarcoma

Warren R. Selman, MD

Professor of Neurological Surgery, Department of Neurological Surgery, Case Western Reserve University School of Medicine; Vice Chairman, Department of Neurological Surgery, and The Research Institute, University Hospitals of Cleveland, Cleveland, Ohio
Intraoperative Cerebral Protection

Chandranath Sen, MD

Chairman, Department of Neurosurgery, and Co-Director, Center for Cranial Surgery, St. Luke's-Roosevelt Medical Center, New York, New York
Trigeminal Schwannomas

Joel L. Seres, MD

Clinical Professor, Department of Neurosurgery, Oregon Health Sciences University School of Medicine; Director, Northwest Occupational Medicine Center, Portland, Oregon
Approach to the Patient with Chronic Pain

Franco Servadei, MD

Professor of Neurotraumatology, Post-Graduate Medical School, University of Catania, Ancona; Director, WHO Neurotrauma Collaborating Center, Division of Neurosurgery, Hospital M. Bufalini, Cesena, Italy
Mild Head Injury in Adults

Avi Setton, MD

Attending, Center for Endovascular Surgery, Institute for Neurology and Neurosurgery, Beth Israel Medical Center, New York, New York
Endovascular Management of Brain Arteriovenous Malformations

Christopher I. Shaffrey, MD

Professor, Department of Neurological Surgery and Department of Orthopaedic Surgery, University of Virginia School of Medicine, Charlottesville, Virginia
Spondylolisthesis; Approach to the Patient and Medical Management of Spinal Disorders; Posterior Approach to Cervical Degenerative Disease

David Shafron, MD

Neurosurgeon, Phoenix Children's Hospital, Phoenix, Arizona
Benign Extradural Lesions of the Dorsal Spine

William R. Shapiro, MD

Professor of Neurology, University of Arizona College of Medicine, Tucson; Chief, Neuro-oncology, Division of Neurology, Barrow Neurological Institute, Phoenix, Arizona
Clinical Features: Neurology of Brain Tumor and Paraneoplastic Disorders

Michael Shea, MD

Attending, Department of Radiation Oncology, Hoag Memorial Hospital Presbyterian, Newport Beach, California
Functional Radiosurgery

Jonas M. Sheehan, MD

Chief, Division of Neuro-oncology and Cranial Base Surgery, Department of Neurosurgery, Pennsylvania State University Hospitals, Hershey, Pennsylvania
Esthesioneuroblastoma

Joseph H. Shin, MD

Assistant Professor of Surgery, Section of Plastic Surgery, Department of Surgery, Yale University School of Medicine; Director, Yale Craniofacial Center, Yale–New Haven Hospital, New Haven, Connecticut
Craniofacial Syndromes

Raj K. Shrivastava, MD

Chief Resident, Department of Neurosurgery, Mount Sinai Medical School,, New York, New York
Trigeminal Schwannomas

David Sibell, MD

Assistant Professor, Department of Anesthesiology and Perioperative Medicine, Oregon Health & Science University, Portland, Oregon
Management of Pain by Anesthetic Techniques

Bo K. Siesjö, Md, PhD

Professor, Center for the Study of Neurological Disease, The Queen's Neuroscience Institute, Honolulu, Hawaii
Cerebral Metabolism and the Pathophysiology of Ischemic Brain Damage

Peter Siesjö, MD, PhD

Assistant Professor, Department of Neurosurgery, University of Lund School of Medicine; Consultant, University Hospital, Lund, Sweden
Cerebral Metabolism and the Pathophysiology of Ischemic Brain Damage

Daniel L. Silbergeld, MD

Associate Professor, Department of Neurological Surgery, University of Washington School of Medicine, Seattle, Washington
Malignant Gliomas: Anaplastic Astrocytoma, Glioblastoma Multiforme, Gliosarcoma, Malignant Oligodendroglioma; Motor, Sensory, and Language Mapping and Monitoring for Cortical Resections

Jerry Silver, Ph.D.

Professor, Department of Neurosciences, Case Western Reserve University School of Medicine, Cleveland, Ohio
Cellular and Molecular Mechanisms Mediating Injury and Recovery in the Nervous System

Scott L. Simon, MD, MPH

Resident, Department of Neurosurgery, Hospital of the University of Pennsylvania, Philadelphia, Pennsylvania
Posterior Thoracic Instrumentation

Ran Vijai P. Singh, MBBS

Resident, Department of Neurosurgery, University of Miami Hospital and Clinics, Miami, Florida
Spontaneous Intracerebral Hemorrhage: Non–Arteriovenous Malformation, Nonaneurysm

Ash Singhal, MD

Senior Resident, Department of Neurosurgery, University of Toronto Faculty of Medicine, Toronto, Ontario, Canada
Tumors of the Vertebral Axis: Benign, Primary Malignant, and Metastatic Tumors

Grant Sinson, MD

Associate Professor of Neurosurgery, Medical College of Wisconsin, Milwaukee, Wisconsin
Initial Resuscitation and Patient Evaluation [Moderate and Severe Traumatic Brain Injury]

Stephen L. Skirboll, MD

Assistant Professor, Department of Neurosurgery, Stanford University; Staff, Palo Alto Veterans Affairs Medical Center, Palo Alto, California
Monitoring and Mapping of Vision in the Neurosurgical Patient

Jefferson Slimp, PhD

Associate Professor, Department of Rehabilitation Medicine, University of Washington School of Medicine; Director, Neurophysiological Monitoring, University of Washington Medical Center, Seattle, Washington
Electrodiagnostic Evaluation of Peripheral Nerves: Electromyography, Somatosensory Evoked Potentials, Nerve Action Potentials

Yoland Smith, PhD

Professor of Neurology, Emory University School of Medicine; Staff, Yerkes National Primate Research Center, Atlanta, Georgia
Anatomy and Synaptic Connectivity of the Basal Ganglia

P. K. Sneed, MD

Professor in Residence, Department of Radiation Oncology, University of California, San Francisco, San Francisco, California
Interstitial and Intracavitary Irradiation of Brain Tumors

Robert A. Solomon, MD

Byron Stookey Professor and Chairman, Department of Neurological Surgery, Columbia University College of Physicians and Surgeons, New York, New York
Techniques for Deep Hypothermic Circulatory Arrest

Volker K. H. Sonntag, MD

Clinical Professor of Surgery (Neurosurgery), University of Arizona College of Medicine, Tucson; Vice Chairman, Division of Neurological Surgery, Director, Residency Program, and Chairman, Spine Section, Barrow Neurological Institute, Phoenix, Arizona
Anterior Approach including Cervical Corpectomy; Anterior Cervical Instrumentation; Basic Principles of Spinal Internal Fixation; Occipitocervical Fusion; Overview and Historical Considerations [Spine];

Sulpicio G. Soriano, MD, MSEd

Associate Professor of Anesthesia, Harvard Medical School; Associate in Anesthesia, Children's Hospital, Boston, Massachussetts
Neuroanesthesia in Children

Dennis D. Spencer, MD

Professor, Department of Neurosurgery, Yale University School of Medicine, New Haven, Connecticut
Intracranial Monitoring

Robert F. Spetzler, MD

Professor, Department of Surgery, Section of Neurosurgery, University of Arizona College of Medicine, Tucson; Director and J. N. Harbor Chairman of Neurological Surgery, Barrow Neurological Institute, Phoenix, Arizona
Anesthesia in Cerebrovascular Disease; Traumatic Carotid Injury; Surgical Approaches for Posterior Circulation Aneurysms; Giant Aneurysms; Infratentorial Cavernous Malformations; Classification of Spinal Cord Vascular Lesions

Brett Stacey, MD

Associate Professor, Department of Anesthesiology and Perioperative Medicine, Oregon Health & Science University, Portland, Oregon
Management of Pain by Anesthetic Techniques

Gary K. Steinberg, MD, PhD

Lacroute-Hearst Professor and Chairman, Department of Neurosurgery, Stanford University School of Medicine, Stanford, California
Surgical and Radiosurgical Management of Giant Arteriovenous Malformations; General and Historical Considerations of Radiotherapy and Radiosurgery

Paul Steinbok, MBBS

Professor, Department of Surgery, University of British Columbia Faculty of Medicine; Head, Division of Pediatric Neurosurgery, Children's and Women's Health Centre, Vancouver, British Columbia, Canada
Intrathecal Baclofen Infusion

Barney J. Stern, MD

Professor and Executive Vice Chairman, Department of Neurology, Emory University School of Medicine, Atlanta, Georgia
Sarcoidosis, Tuberculosis, and Xanthogranuloma

David A. Steven, MD

Chief Resident, Department of Clinical Neurological Sciences (Neurosurgery), University of Western Ontario Faculty of Medicine, London, Ontario, Canada
Distal Anterior Cerebral Artery Aneurysms

Kimberly J. Stewart, PhD

Clinical Neuropsychologist, Hampton Roads Neuropsychology, Inc., Virginia Beach, Virginia
Rehabilitation and Prognosis after Traumatic Brain Injury

Charles B. Stillerman, MD

Clinical Professor, Department of Surgery, University of North Dakota School of Medicine, Grand Forks; Director, Department of Neurosurgery, Trinity Medical Center, Minot, North Dakota
Intradiskal and Percutaneous Treatment of Lumbar Disk Disease

John H. Suh, MD

Clinical Director, Department of Radiation Oncology, Cleveland Clinic, Cleveland, Ohio
Principles of Radiotherapy

Peter P. Sun, MD

Assistant Clinical Professor, Department of Neurological Surgery, University of California, San Francisco, School of Medicine, San Francisco; Chief, Division of Neurosurgery, Children's Hospital and Research Center at Oakland, Oakland, California
Pediatric Vertebral Column and Spinal Cord Injuries

Leslie N. Sutton, MD

Professor of Neurosurgery, University of Pennsylvania School of Medicine; Chief, Neurosurgery, Children's Hospital of Philadelphia, Philadelphia, Pennsylvania
Intracranial Ependymomas

Phillip D. Swanson, MD, PhD

Professor of Neurology, University of Washington School of Medicine, Seattle, Washington
History and Physical Examination [Introduction: Approach to the Patient]

Sara J. Swanson, PhD

Associate Professor, Department of Neurology, Medical College of Wisconsin, Milwaukee, Wisconsin
Functional Magnetic Resonance Imaging in Epilepsy Surgery

George W. Sypert, MD

Sypert Institute, Fort Myers, Florida
Evaluation and Management of the Failed Back Syndrome

Derek A. Taggard, MD

Chief Resident, Division of Neurosurgery, University of Iowa Hospitals and Clinics, Iowa City, Iowa
Treatment of Occipital C1 Injury

Jamal M. Taha, MD

Taha Neurosurgical Clinic Kettering; Ohio
Dorsal Rhizotomy and Dorsal Root Ganglionectomy

Rafael J. Tamargo, MD

Associate Professor, Department of Neurosurgery and Otolaryngology, Division of Head and Neck Surgery, Johns Hopkins University School of Medicine; Director, Division of Cerebrovascular Neurosurgery, Department of Neurosurgery, Johns Hopkins Hospital, Baltimore, Maryland
Surgical Positioning and Exposures for Cranial Procedures; Anterior Communicating Artery and Anterior Cerebral Artery Aneurysms

Nitin Tandon, MD

Chief Resident, Center for Neurosurgical Sciences, University of Texas Health Science Center; Chief Resident, University Hospital, Audie L Murphy VA Hospital, San Antonio, Texas
Infections of the Spine and Spinal Cord

Ronald Tasker, MD

Emeritus Professor, Division of Neurosurgery, Department of Surgery, University of Toronto Faculty of Medicine, Toronto, Ontario, Canada
Deep Brain Stimulation for Chronic Pain

Marcos Tatagiba, MD, PhD

Professor and Chairman, Department of Neurosurgery, University of Tuebingen, Tuebingen, Germany
Basic Principles of Skull Base Surgery

Christopher L. Taylor, MD

Resident, Department of Neurological Surgery, University Hospitals of Cleveland, Cleveland, Ohio
Intraoperative Cerebral Protection

Steven A. Telian, MD

John L. Kemink Professor of Neurotology, Department of Otolaryngology–Head and Neck Surgery, University of Michigan Medical School; Director, Division of Otology, Neurotology and Skull Base Surgery, and Medical Director, Cochlear Implant Program, University of Michigan Hospitals, Ann Arbor, Michigan
Treatment of Intractable Vertigo

Kamal Thapar, MD

Assistant Professor, Department of Neurosurgery, University of Toronto Faculty of Medicine, Toronto, Ontario, Canada

Nicholas Theodore, MD

Chief, Section of Neurosurgical Trauma, Division of Neurosurgery, Barrow Neurological Institute, Phoenix, Arizona
Anesthesia in Cerebrovascular Disease; Thoracoscopic Approaches to the Spine

Philip V. Theodosopoulos, MD

Assistant Professor, Department of Neurological Surgery, University of Cincinnati College of Medicine; Director, Skull Base Surgery, Mayfield Clinic, Cincinnati, Ohio

Ossification of the Posterior Longitudinal Ligament and Other Enthesopathies

B. Gregory Thompson, MD

Associate Professor, Department of Neurosurgery, University of Michigan Medical School; Director, Cerebrovascular and Skull Base Section, University of Michigan Hospitals, Ann Arbor, Michigan

Spinal Arteriovenous Malformations; Pregnancy and Treatment of Vascular Disease

Todd P. Thompson, MD

Chief of Neurosurgery, Straub Clinic and Hospital, Honolulu, Hawaii

Patient Selection in Movement Disorder Surgery

William E. Thorell, MD

Resident, Department of Neurosurgery, University of Nebraska Medical Center, Omaha, Nebraska

Brain Tumors: Population-Based Epidemiology, Environmental Risk Factors, and Genetic and Hereditary Syndromes

Robert Tiel, MD

Associate Professor, Department of Neurosurgery, Louisiana State University School of Medicine at New Orleans; Attending Neurosurgeon, Charity Hospital and Ochsner Hospital, New Orleans, Louisiana

Management of Peripheral Nerve Tumors

Suzie C. Tindall, MD

Professor, Department of Neurosurgery, Emory University School of Medicine, Atlanta, Georgia

Carpal Tunnel Syndrome; Entrapment Syndromes of Peripheral Nerve Injuries

Paul Tolentino, MD

Resident, Department of Neurosurgery, University of Florida College of Medicine, Gainesville, Florida

Posterior Lumbar Instrumentation

Tadanori Tomita, MD

Yeager Professor of Pediatric Neurosurgery, Northwestern University Feinberg Medical School; Chairman, Division of Neurosurgery, Children's Memorial Hospital, Chicago, Illinois

Birth Head Trauma

Steven A. Toms, MD, MPH

Assistant Professor, Department of Neurological Surgery, and Head, Section of Neurosurgical Oncology, Oregon Health & Science University School of Medicine; Chief, Section of Neurosurgery, Portland VA Medical Center, Portland, Oregon

Tumor Suppressor Genes and the Genesis of Brain Tumors

Kathleen R. Tozer, MD

Resident, Department of Neurosurgery, University of Washington, Seattle, Washington

Monitoring and Mapping of Vision in the Neurosurgical Patient

Bruce D. Trapp, PhD

Professor, Department of Neurosciences, Case Western Reserve University School of Medicine, Cleveland; Professor, Department of Cell Biology, Neurobiology, and Anatomy, Ohio State University, Cleveland; Professor Department of Chemistry, Cleveland State University, Cleveland; Professor Department of Cellular and Molecular Biology, Kent State University, Kent; Chairman, Department of Neurosciences, Lerner Research Institute, Cleveland Clinic Foundation, Cleveland, Ohio

Neurons and Neuroglia

Vincent C. Traynelis, MD

Professor of Neurosurgery, Department of Surgery, University of Iowa College of Medicine; Staff Neurosurgeon, University of Iowa Hospitals and Clinics, Iowa City, Iowa

Tumors of the Craniovertebral Junction; Treatment of Occipital C1 Injury

R. Shane Tubbs, MS, PA-C

Instructor in Anatomy, University of Alabama School of Medicine; Physician Assistant, Pediatric Neurosurgery Section, Children's Hospital, Birmingham, Alabama

Chiari Malformations

Ramachandra Tummala, MD

Resident, Department of Neurosurgery, University of Minnesota Medical School, Minneapolis, Minnesota

Standard Temporal Lobectomy and Transsylvian Amygdalohippocampectomy

Michael Tymianski, MD, PhD

Assistant Professor, Department of Surgery, University of Toronto Faculty of Medicine; Staff Neurosurgeon, Toronto Western Hospital, University Health Network, Toronto, Ontario, Canada

Surgical Approaches for Anterior Circulation Aneurysms

Atsushi Umemura, MD

Fellow in Stereotactic and Functional Neurosurgery, Department of Neurosurgery, University of Pennsylvania School of Medicine, Philadelphia, Pennsylvania
Topectomy: Uses and Indications

G. Edward Vates, MD, PhD

Staff, Department of Neurological Surgery, Brigham and Women's Hospital, Boston, Massachusetts
Hemangioblastomas of the Central Nervous System; Surgical Approaches for Posterior Circulation Aneurysms

A. Giancarlo Vishteh, MD

Co-Director, Neurotrauma, John C. Lincoln North Mountain Hospital, Phoenix, Arizona
Anesthesia in Cerebrovascular Disease; Traumatic Carotid Injury; Anterior Cervical Instrumentation;

André Visot, MD

Chief, Neurosurgical Service, Hôpital Foch, Suresnes, France
Osseous Tumors

Jerrold L. Vitek, MD, PhD

Professor, Department of Neurology, Emory University School of Medicine, Atlanta, Georgia
Surgery for Dystonia

Kenneth P. Vives, MD

Assistant Professor, Department of Neurosurgery, Yale University School of Medicine; Neurosurgeon, Yale Neurovascular Surgery Program, Neurovascular-Neuroscience Intensive Care Unit, Yale–New Haven Hospital, and Backus Hospital, New Haven, Connecticut
Unusual Gliomas; Surgical Management of Supratentorial Cavernous Malformations; Intracranial Monitoring

Dennis G. Vollmer, MD

Professor of Neurosurgery, University of Texas Health Science Center at Houston; Director, Comprehensive Center for Cerebrovascular Surgery, Memorial Hermann Hospital, Houston, Texas
Overview and Historical Considerations [Spine]; Infections of the Spine and Spinal Cord; Cervical Spine Trauma

Jennifer Vookles, MD

Assistant Professor, Department of Anesthesiology and Perioperative Medicine, Oregon Health & Science University, Portland, Oregon
Management of Pain by Anesthetic Techniques

Phillip A. Wackym, MD

John C. Koss Professor and Chairman, Department of Otolaryngology and Communication Sciences, Medical College of Wisconsin; Chief, Otolaryngology–Head and Neck Surgery, Froedtert & Medical College Hospital, and Children's Hospital of Wisconsin, Milwaukee, Wisconsin
Neuro-otology

Tom Wagner, PhD

Instructor, Department of Oncology, Mayo Graduate School of Medicine, Mayo Clinic; Therapeutic Radiological Physicist, St. Luke's Hospital, Jacksonville, Florida
Fractionated and Stereotactic Radiation, Extracranial Stereotactic Radiation, Intensity Modulation, and Multileaf Collimation

Gregory R. Wahle, MD

Clinical Associate Professor of Urology, Indiana University School of Medicine, Indianapolis, Indiana
Neurourology

Marion L. Walker, MD

Professor of Neurosurgery and Professor of Pediatrics, University of Utah School of Medicine; Chairman, Division of Pediatric Neurosurgery, Primary Children's Medical Center/University of Utah Medical Center, Salt Lake City, Utah
Nonsyndromic Craniosynostosis and Abnormalities of Head Shape

Paul R. Walker, PhD

Private Docent, University of Geneva, Faculty of Medicine; Biologist, University Hospital Geneva, Geneva, Switzerland
Aspects of Immunology Applicable to Brain Tumor Pathogenesis and Treatment

M. Christopher Wallace, MD

Chief, Division of Neurosurgery, University of Toronto Health Network, Toronto, Ontario, Canada
Intracranial Internal Carotid Artery Aneurysms

John W. Walsh, MD, PhD

Professor of Neurosurgery and Pediatrics, Tulane University Medical School; Chief, Section of Pediatric Neurosurgery, Tulane University Hospital and Clinic, New Orleans, Louisiana
Lipomyelomeningocele

Paul P. Wang, MD

Attending, Department of Neurological Surgery, Johns Hopkins Hospital, Baltimore, Maryland
Glomus Jugulare Tumors

John D. Ward, MD

Professor and Vice Chairman, Division of Neurosurgery, Department of Surgery, Virginia Commonwealth University School of Medicine, Richmond, Virginia
Pediatric Head Injury

Benjamin C. Warf, MD

Formerly Professor of Neurosurgery, University of Kentucky College of Medicine, Lexington, Kentucky
Tethered Spinal Cord

Ronald E. Warnick, MD

Professor of Neurosurgery, University of Cincinnati School of Medicine, Cincinnati, Ohio
Surgical Complications and Their Avoidance

Katherine E. Warren, MD

Tenure-Track Clinician, Pediatric Neuro-oncology, National Cancer Institute, National Institutes of Health, Bethesda, Maryland
Principles of Chemotherapy

W. Lee Warren, MD

Chief Resident, Department of Neurosurgery, Allegheny General Hospital, Pittsburgh, Pennsylvania
Diagnosis and Management of Seventh and Eighth Cranial Nerve Injuries due to Temporal Bone Fractures

Kyle D. Weaver, MD

Department of Neurosurgery, University of North Carolina at Chapel Hill School of Medicine, Chapel Hill, North Carolina

Jon Weingart, MD

Associate Professor of Neurosurgery and Oncology, Johns Hopkins University School of Medicine; Attending Neurosurgeon, Johns Hopkins Hospital, Baltimore, Maryland
Basic Principles of Cranial Surgery for Brain Tumors

Philip R. Weinstein, MD

Professor of Neurosurgery, University of California, San Francisco, School of Medicine, San Francisco, California
Ossification of the Posterior Longitudinal Ligament and Other Enthesopathies

Bryce Weir, MD

Interim Dean, Biological Sciences Division, University of Chicago Medical Center, Chicago, Illinois
Perioperative Management of Subarachnoid Hemorrhage

Hung Tzu Wen, MD

Courtesy Assistant Professor, Department of Neurological Surgery, University of Florida College of Medicine, Gainesville, Florida; Clinical Instructor, Division of Neurosurgery Hospital Das Clínicas—University of São Paulo; Clinical Associate, Hospital Samaritanod, São Paulo, Brazil
Surgical Anatomy of the Brain

G. Alexander West, PhD, MD

Associate Professor, Department of Neurological Surgery, Oregon Health & Science University Portland, Oregon
Traumatic Cerebral Aneurysms Secondary to Penetrating Intracranial Injuries

Michael F. Whelan, MD, DDS

Assistant Professor, Department of Surgery, Division of Craniofacial Plastic and Reconstructive Surgery, University of Washington School of Medicine; Attending Plastic and Craniofacial Surgeon, Children's Hospital and Regional Medical Center and Harborview Medical Center, Seattle, Washington
Craniofacial Trauma

Walter W. Whisler, MD

Professor and Chairman Emeritus, Department of Neurosurgery, Rush Medical College; Attending Neurosurgeon, Rush-Presbyterian-St. Luke's Medical Center, Chicago, Illinois
Multiple Subpial Transection

Jonathan White, MD

Assistant Professor of Neurosurgery, University of Texas Southwestern Medical School, Dallas, Texas
Posterior Fossa Arteriovenous Malformations

Thomas Wichmann, MD

Associate Professor of Neurology, Emory University School of Medicine, Atlanta, Georgia
Rationale for Surgical Interventions in Movement Disorders

Agadha Wickremesekera, MBChB (Ontario),

Consultant Neurosurgeon, Wakefield Hospital, Wellington, New Zealand
Infantile Posthemorrhagic Hydrocephalus

Gregory C. Wiggins, MD

Staff Neurosurgeon, David Grant Medical Center, Travis AFB, California
Posterior Approach to Cervical Degenerative Disease

James C. Wilberger, MD

Chair, Department of Neurosurgery, Allegheny General Hospital, Pittsburgh, Pennsylvania
Diagnosis and Management of Seventh and Eighth Cranial Nerve Injuries due to Temporal Bone Fractures

David M. Wildrick, PhD

Attending, Department of Neurosurgery, The University of Texas M.D. Anderson Cancer Center, Houston, Texas
Metastatic Brain Tumors

Lorna Sohn Williams, MD

Assistant Professor, Department of Radiology, University of Florida College of Medicine, Gainesville, Florida
Vein of Galen Malformations

H. Richard Winn, MD

Professor of Neurological Surgery and Neuroscience, Mount Sinai School of Medicine, New York, New York

The Natural History of Unruptured Saccular Cerebral Aneurysms; Surgical Decision Making for the Treatment of Cerebral Aneurysms; Traumatic Cerebral Aneurysms Secondary to Penetrating Intracranial Injuries; Monitoring and Mapping of Vision in the Neurosurgical Patient

Diana Barrett Wiseman, MD

Spine Fellow, Department of Neurological Surgery, University of Washington School of Medicine, Seattle, Washington

Spondylolisthesis

Jeffrey H. Wisoff, MD

Associate Professor of Neurosurgery and Pediatrics, New York University School of Medicine; Director, Division of Pediatric Neurosurgery, New York University Medical Center, New York, New York

Optic Pathway and Hypothalamic Gliomas in Children

Timothy F. Witham, MD

Department of Neurological Surgery, University of Pittsburgh School of Medicine, Pittsburgh, Pennsylvania

Gamma Knife Radiosurgery

W. Putnam Wolcott, MD

Department of Neurological Surgery, University of Virginia School of Medicine, Charlottesville, Virginia

Approach to the Patient and Medical Management, of Spinal Disorders

Donald C. Wright, MD

Surgeon, Washington Brain & Spine Institute, Bethesda, Maryland

Elaine Wyllie, MD

Head, Pediatric Epilepsy Program, Cleveland Clinic, Cleveland, Ohio

Recognition of Surgical Candidates and the Presurgical Evaluation

Kevin Yao, MD

Resident, Department of Neurosurgery, Mount Sinai Medical Center, New York, New York

Infectious Intracranial Aneurysms

Narayan Yoganandan, PhD

Professor and Chair, Department of Biomedical Engineering, and Professor, Department of Neurosurgery, Medical College of Wisconsin; Adjunct Professor of Biomedical Engineering, Marquette University, Milwaukee, Wisconsin

Concepts and Mechanisms of Biomechanics

Howard Yonas, MD

Peter J. Jannetta Professor of Neurological Surgery, University of Pittsburgh School of Medicine; Vice Chairman, Neurological Surgery, and Chief, Cerebrovascular Surgery, and Co-Director, University of Pittsburgh Medical Center Stroke Institute, University of Pittsburgh Medical Center-Presbyterian, Pittsburgh, Pennsylvania

Xenon Computed Tomography

Julie E. York, MD

Instructor, Department of Neurosurgery, Loyola University of Chicago Stritch School of Medicine, Maywood, Illinois

Treatment of Axis Fractures; Diagnosis and Management of Thoracolumbar and Lumbar Spine Injuries

Andrew S. Youkilis, MD

Chief Resident, Department of Neurosurgery, University Hospital, Ann Arbor, Michigan

Primitive Neuroectodermal Tumors; Diagnosis and Nonoperative Management [Trigeminal Neuralgia]

George P. H. Young, MD

Associate Professor of Clinical Urology, Cornell University Joan and Sanford I. Weill Medical College; Associate Attending Urologist and Director, Female Urology, Neurourology, Urodynamics, and Reconstructive Urology Unit, New York Presbyterian Hospital, New York, New York

Neurourology

David M. Yousem, MD

Professor of Radiology, Johns Hopkins University School of Medicine; Director, Division of Neuroradiology, Johns Hopkins Hospital, Baltimore, Maryland

Radiologic Features of Central Nervous System Tumors

Eric C. Yuen, MD

Associate Director of Clinical Research, Department of Clinical Neuroscience, Merck Research Laboratories, West Point, Pennsylvania

Peripheral Neuropathies; Electrodiagnostic Evaluation of Peripheral Nerves: Electromyography, Somatosensory Evoked Potentials, Nerve Action Potentials

Joseph M. Zabramski, MD

Chairman, Section of Cerebrovascular Surgery, Division of Neurological Surgery, Barrow Neurological Institute, Phoenix, Arizona

Epidemiology and Natural History of Cavernous Malformations; The Genetics of Cerebral Cavernous Malformations

Alois Zauner, MD

Clinical Instructor, Department of Radiology; University of California, Los Angeles, California

Surgical Management of Traumatic Brain Injury

Seth M. Zeidman, MD

Assistant Professor of Neurosurgery, University of Rochester School of Medicine and Dentistry; Chief, Division of Complex Neurological Surgery, Strong Memorial Hospital, and Attending Neurosurgeon, Highland Hospital, Park Ridge Hospital, and Rochester Memorial Hospital; Private Practice, Rochester Brain and Spine Neurosurgery, Rochester, New York

Hyperextension and Hyperflexion Injuries of the Cervical Spine

Gregory J. Zipfel, MD

Resident, Department of Neurological Surgery, University of Florida School of Medicine, Gainesville, Florida

Surgical Treatment of Intracavernous and Paraclinoid Internal Carotid Artery Aneurysms

Justin A. Zivin, MD, PhD

Professor of Neuroscience, University of California, San Diego, School of Medicine, La Jolla, California

Acute Medical Management of Ischemic Disease and Stroke

Geoffrey Zubay, MD

Chief Resident, Division of Neurological Surgery, Barrow Neurological Institute, Phoenix, Arizona

Basic Principles of Spinal Internal Fixation

Alexander Y. Zubkov, MD, PhD

Resident, Department of Neurology, University of Mississippi Medical Center, Jackson, Mississippi

Radiology of the Skull

Marike Zwienenberg-Lee, MD

Resident in Neurosurgery, Department of Neurological Surgery, University of California, Davis, Medical Center, Sacramento, California

Clinical Pathophysiology of Traumatic Brain Injury

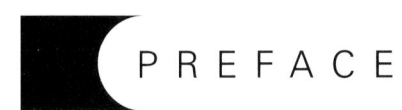

Neurological surgery is a dynamic field, but one that is built on and sustained by the broad shoulders of earlier scientific discoveries and clinical experiences. The fifth edition of *Neurological Surgery* reflects this ever-changing discipline and combines what is "new" with that which is not only "old," but enduring. Thus, this latest volume continues the original intent of the first[1] and subsequent texts edited by Julian Youmans. Reflecting the breadth and complexity of neurosurgery at the beginning of the 21st century, this new volume has had a long gestation period.

This edition has been radically restructured to reflect the ever-changing nature of our discipline. The initial section is focused on the key basic science areas and associated clinical disciplines, the knowledge of which is a necessity for the rational practice of neurosurgery. Subsequent sections reflect the mixture of time-tested information and new advances in the areas of oncology, vascular system, epilepsy, functional, pain, pediatrics, peripheral nerve, radiation therapy and radiosurgery, spine, and trauma. Each section begins with a consideration of general features and historical background that allows the reader to place in context the advances within each section. There then follow chapters dealing with basic scientific information and advances relevant to each area, whereas the subsequent topics within each section deal with clinical advances and surgical techniques. Thus, in all sections, we have added a wealth of new horizontally and vertically integrated information.

The overall aim of each section reflects the unifying goal of the entire book: to provide comprehensive knowledge of disorders and surgery of the nervous system to the student, whether that "student" is a junior resident or an experienced practitioner. Moreover, I hope that future physicians dealing with surgery of the nervous system, whether they are mechanical or biological surgeons,[2] will value the information contained in this text.

It is self-evident that these volumes represent the diligent work of many individuals. I enthusiastically express my appreciation to each of the Section Editors who contributed many long hours to the success of this effort: Roy Bakay (Functional), Henry Brem (Oncology), Kim Burchiel (Functional and Pain), Bill Friedman (Radiation Therapy and Radiosurgery), Sean Grady (Trauma), Michel Kliot (Introduction and Peripheral Nerve), Dade Lunsford (Radiation Therapy and Radiosurgery), Joel MacDonald (Special Features), Larry Marshall (Trauma), Marc Mayberg (Special Features), Fred Meyer (Vascular), T. S. Park (Pediatric), Ray Sawaya (Oncology), Michael Scott (Pediatric), Dan Silbergeld (Epilepsy), Volker Sonntag (Spine), Robert Spetzler (Vascular), and Dennis Vollmer (Spine). A special acknowledgement and thanks go to my long-time colleague, Ralph Dacey, Deputy Editor-in-Chief.

To bring to fruition a work of this magnitude requires a highly professional and disciplined editorial effort and for this I thank the members of the Saunders/Elsevier team: Publishing Directors, Richard Lampert and Richard Zorab (formerly); Developmental Editors, Anne Snyder and David Orzechowski (formerly); and Project Manager, Jodi Kaye. Most importantly, Margaret Connelly, my Editorial Assistant throughout this entire project, should be recognized for her vital and superb contributions.

A personal note of gratitude goes to my wife Debbie, our daughter Allison and her husband Adam, and our son Randy and his wife Tamara for their sustaining support and encouragement.

Lastly, matching the stellar quality of the Deputy Editor-in-Chief, the Section Editors, and the editorial team at Saunders/Elsevier, are the authors of the 335 chapters. With much enthusiasm, I thank them one and all. Their contributions are truly the broad shoulders upon which future care and advances in Neurosurgery will stand.

H. Richard Winn, MD
Editor-in-Chief
Professor of Neurological Surgery and Neuroscience
Mount Sinai School of Medicine New York, New York

1. Youmans JR: Neurological Surgery. Philadelphia, WB Saunders, 1973, pp xvii–xviii.
2. Winn HR, Howard MA: The next 100 years of neurosurgery. Lancet 354(Suppl):36, 1999.

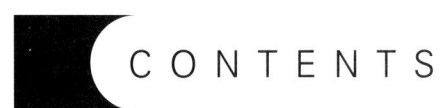

CONTENTS

VOLUME 1

VOLUME 2

VOLUME 3

VOLUME 4

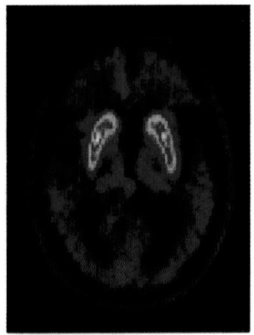 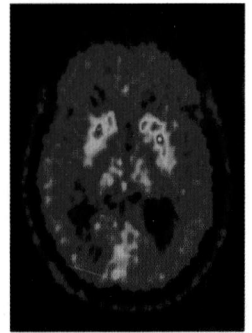 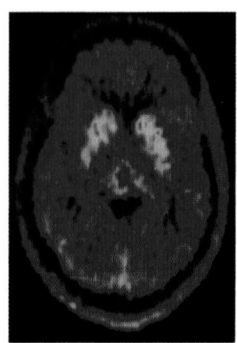

Normal subject   **Early Parkinson's disease**   **Advanced Parkinson's disease**

FIGURE 169-1. Positron emission tomographic images of striatal ¹⁸F-dopa uptake in early and advanced Parkinson's disease. The caudate is relatively spared compared with the putamen. (Courtesy of J. S. Rakshi, MRC Cyclotron Unit, Hammersmith Hospital, London, UK.)

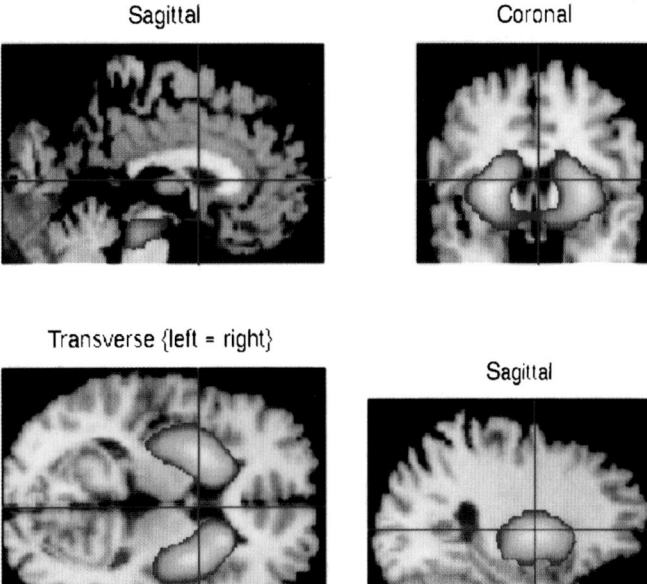

FIGURE 169-2. A statistical parametric map shows the location of significant reductions in ¹⁸F-dopa uptake for a group of seven patients with advanced Parkinson's disease compared with seven age-matched, normal controls ($P < .001$). The ¹⁸F-dopa uptake is reduced bilaterally in the putamen, caudate, and substantia nigra. (Courtesy of J. S. Rakshi, MRC Cyclotron Unit, Hammersmith Hospital, London, UK.)

Sagittal

Coronal

Transverse {left = right}

Sagittal

Pregraft   **8 Months**   **20 Months**

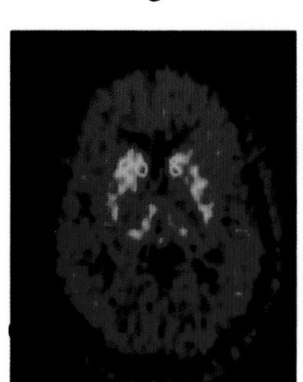 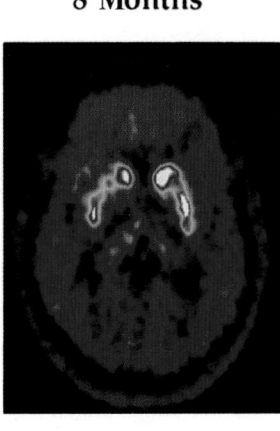 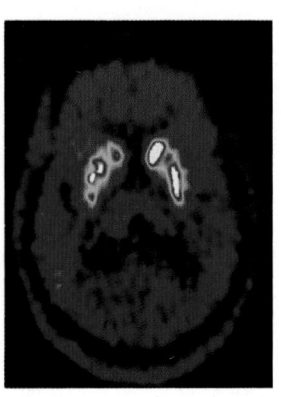

FIGURE 169-3. Positron emission tomographic images of striatal ¹⁸F-dopa uptake were collected 30 to 90 minutes after tracer administration for a patient with Parkinson's disease before, 8 months after, and 20 months after bilateral implantation of fetal mesencephalic tissue into the caudate and putamen. (Courtesy of P. Piccini, MRC Cyclotron Unit, Hammersmith Hospital, London, UK.)

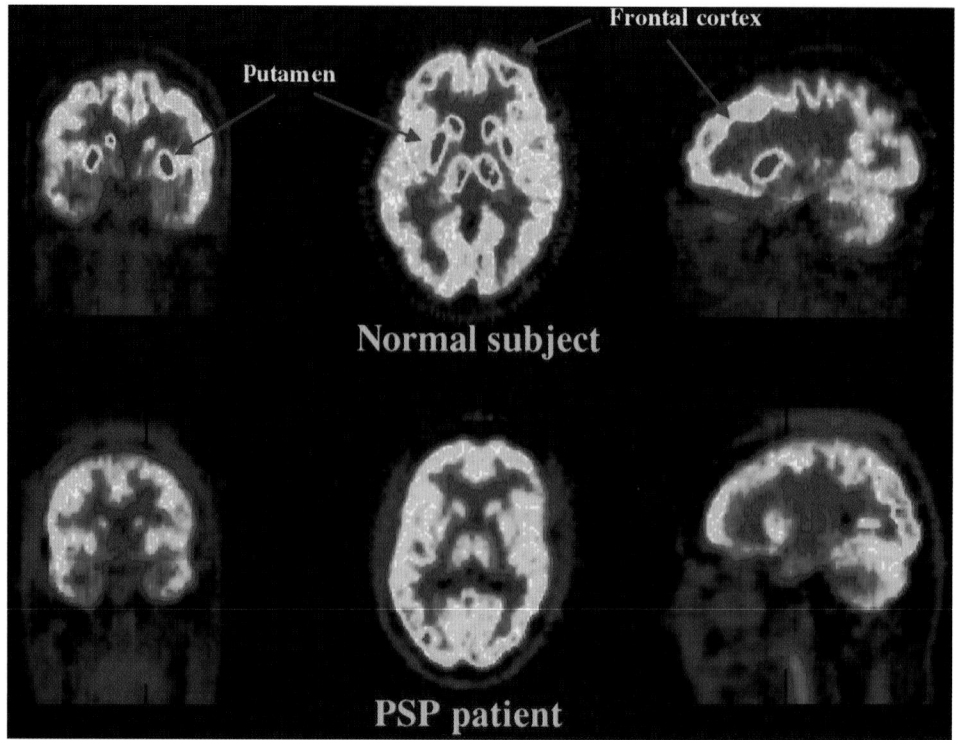

FIGURE 169-4. Fluorodeoxyglucose positron emission tomographic (^{18}FDG-PET) images of regional cerebral glucose metabolism for a normal person and a patient with progressive supranuclear palsy (PSP). The patient with PSP shows reduced frontal, striatal, and thalamic glucose use. (Courtesy of P. Piccini, MRC Cyclotron Unit, Hammersmith Hospital, London, UK.)

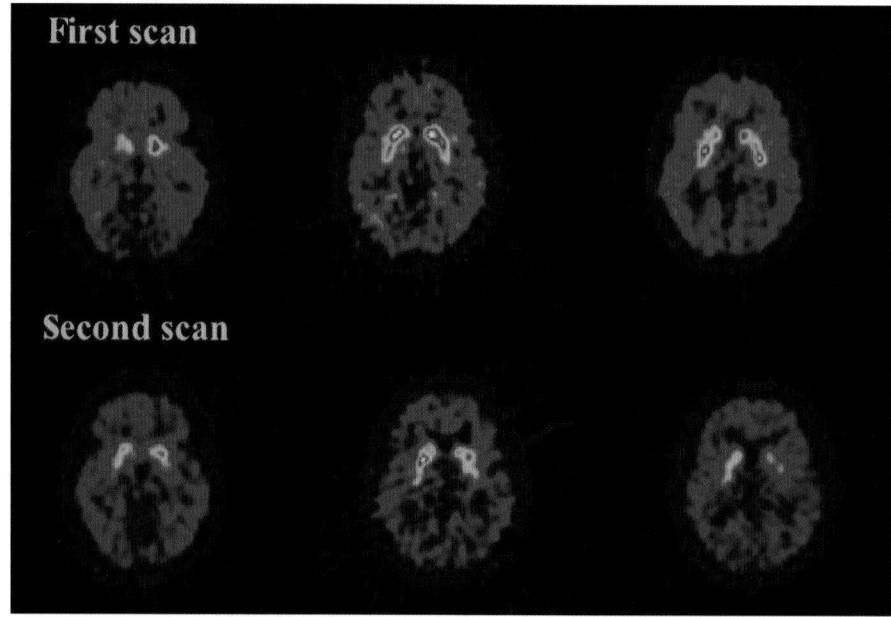

FIGURE 169-5. Positron emission tomographic images of serial striatal ^{11}C-SCH23390 uptake over 3 years for an adult who is an asymptomatic Huntington's disease gene carrier show progressive loss of striatal dopamine D1 binding. (Courtesy of T. Andrews, MRC Cyclotron Unit, Hammersmith Hospital, London, UK.)

Patient # 96

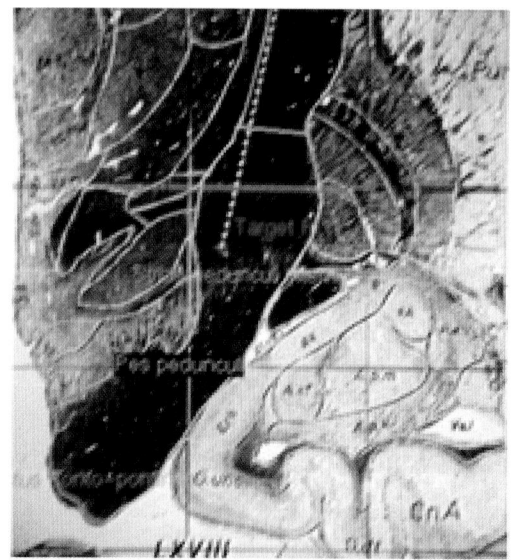

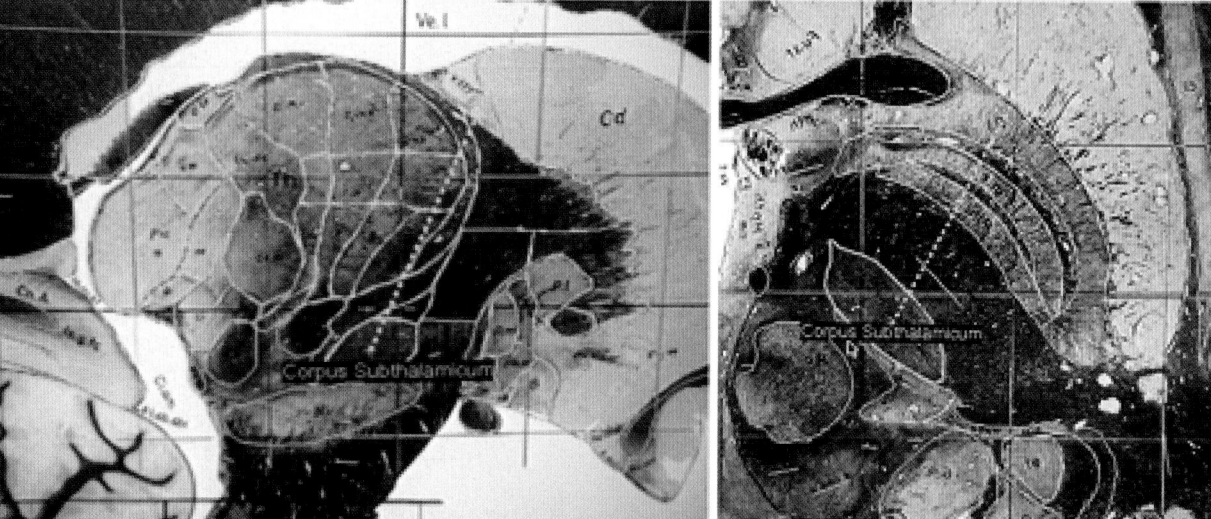

FIGURE 173-2. Demonstration of the mismatches in atlases. Shown is a target point using the Splan Radionics image-guidance software. It can be satisfactory on the sagittal and axial views, but it does not match with the coronal view, where the target representation is often in the peduncle. The three planes (axial, coronal, and sagittal) of the atlas were obtained in three different brains.

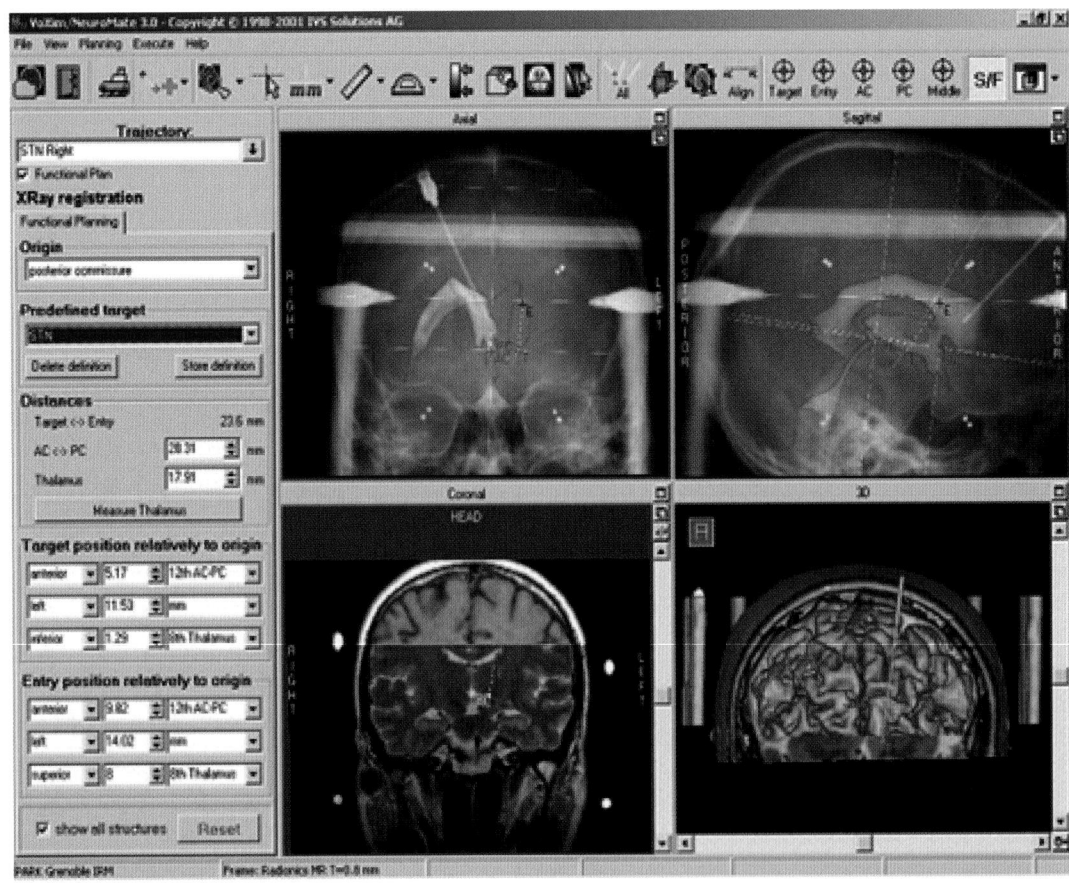

FIGURE 173-7. Computer screen display of the Voxim planning software of the Neuromate.

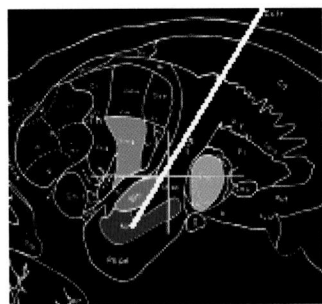

Silence in White Matter
Nucleus Signature
Nucleus Borders

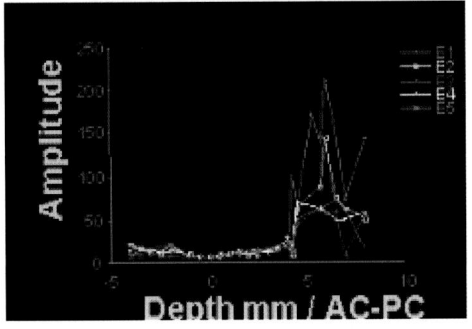

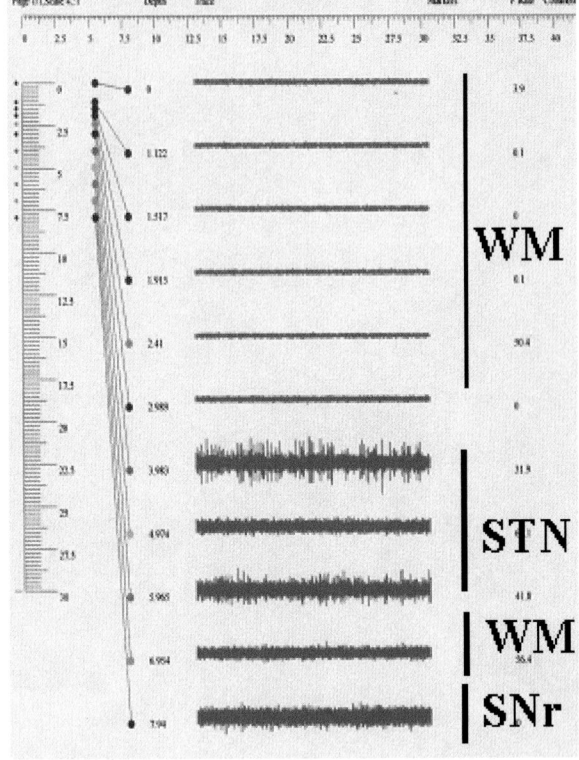

FIGURE 173-11. Electrophysiology using the Neurotrek system. Along the planned track through the basal ganglia, the electrophysiologic pattern changes from silence in the white matter of the internal capsule and between the subthalamic nucleus (STN) and substantia nigra pars reticularis (SNr) to typical neuronal firing in the nuclei. The plot of the signal amplitude clearly shows the entry and exit in and out of the STN.

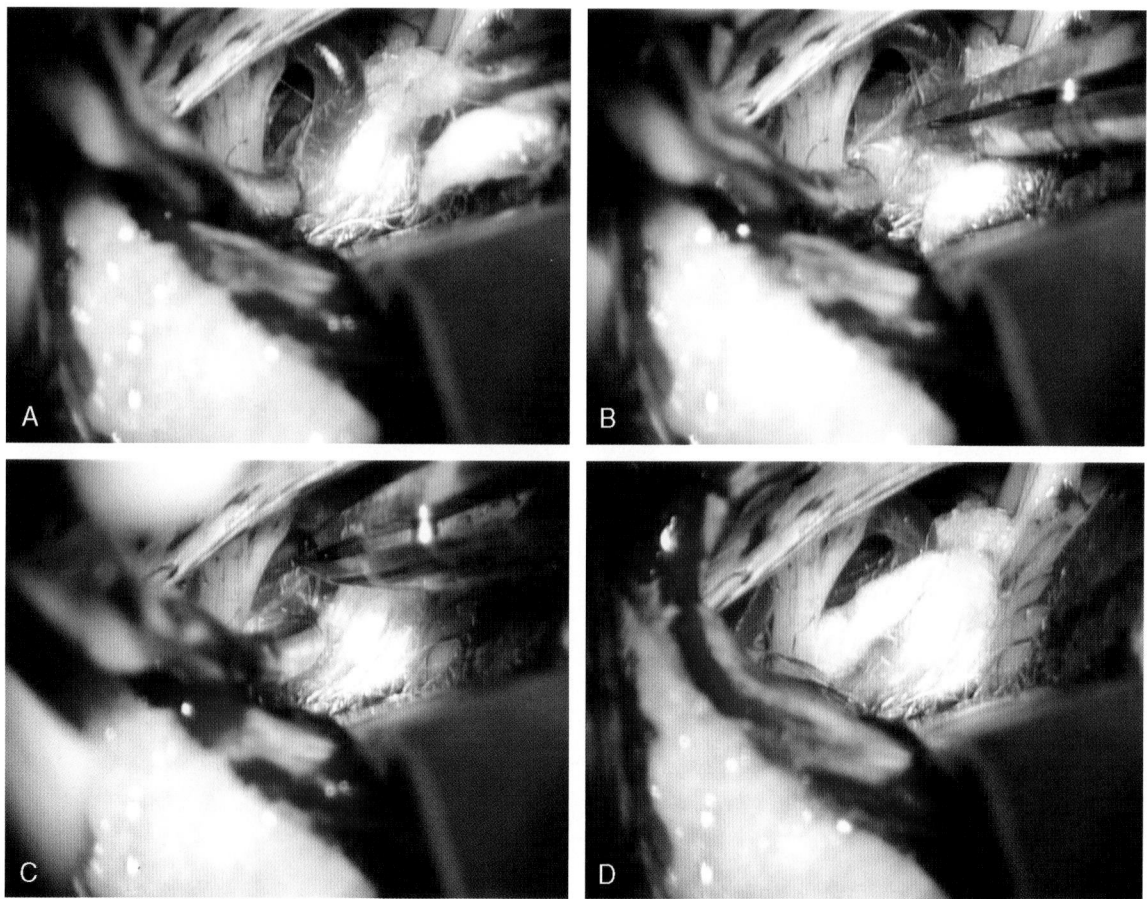

FIGURE 187-6. Intraoperative photograph of the superior cerebellar artery being lifted away with a suction device *(A)* and Teflon felt being placed in a proximal-to-distal fashion *(B, C)*, lifting the vessel *off* the root entry zone *(D)*. (From Burchiel KJ [ed]: Surgical Management of Pain. New York, Thieme, 2002.)

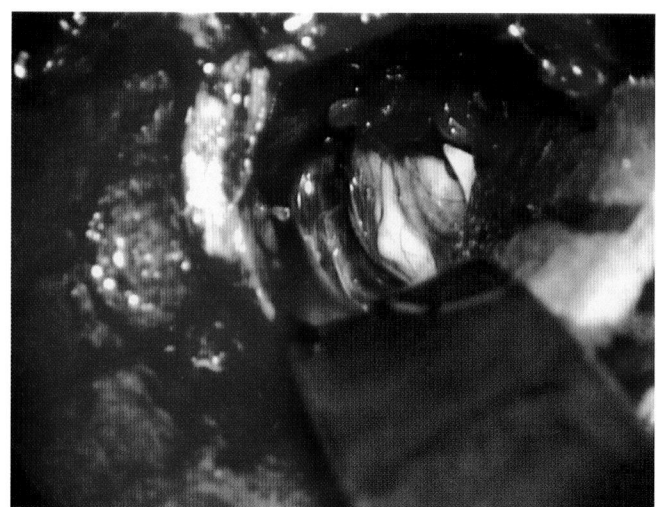

FIGURE 187-7. Intraoperative photograph demonstrating venous compression of the trigeminal nerve resulting in trigeminal neuralgia. (From Burchiel KJ [ed]: Surgical Management of Pain. New York, Thieme, 2002.)

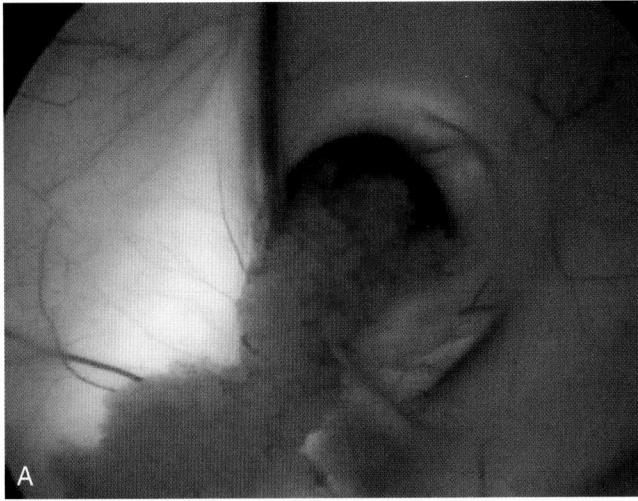
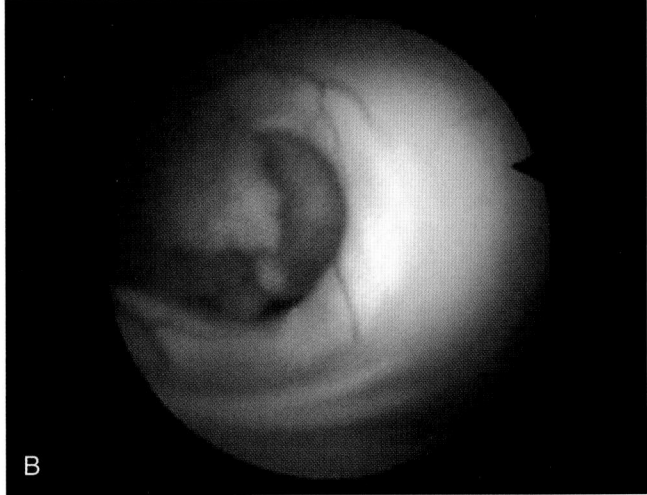

FIGURE 218-1. View of the foramen of Monro though the lateral ventricle using a rod-lens (rigid) endoscope *(A)* and a 4-mm steerable fiberscope *(B)*. (Courtesy of Mayfield Clinic, Cincinnati, OH.)

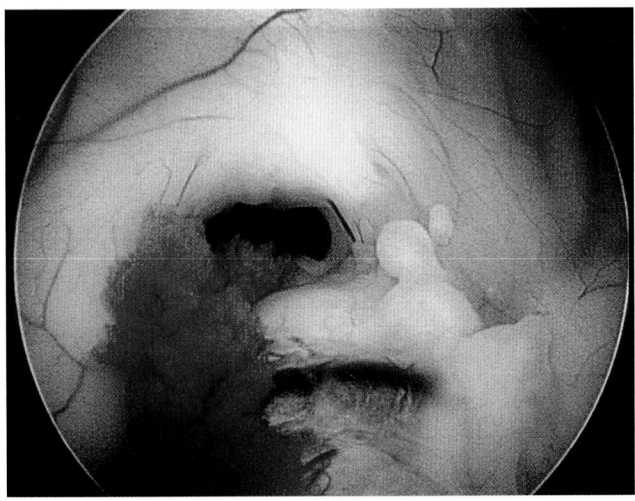

FIGURE 218-3. Endoscopic view of a thalamic tumor protruding through the ventricular wall at the time of shunt placement. The endoscopic biopsy determined it to be a low-grade glioma. (Courtesy of Mayfield Clinic, Cincinnati, OH.)

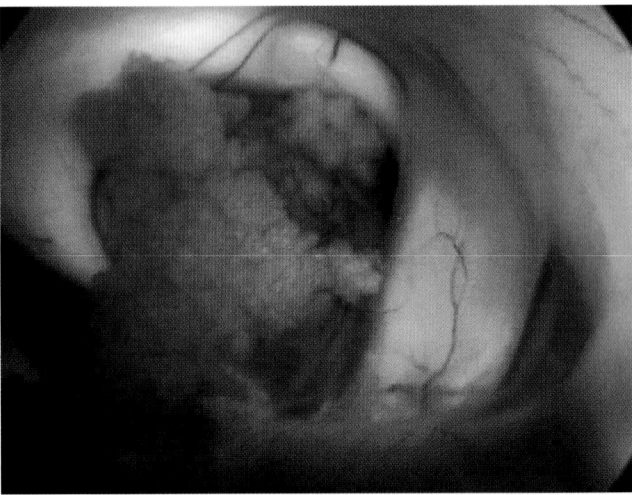

FIGURE 218-4. Endoscopic approach through the lateral ventricle to a third ventricular colloid cyst sitting just inside the foramen magnum, viewed through a rod-lens endoscope. (Courtesy of Mayfield Clinic, Cincinnati, OH.)

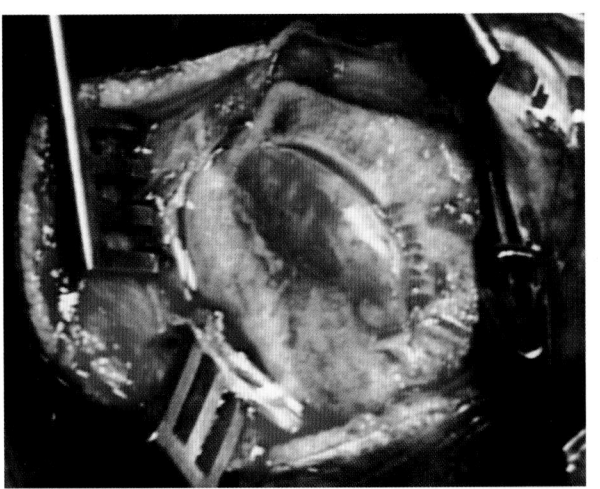

FIGURE 221-8. Operative exposure of a growing skull fracture. Notice the pulsatile mass located between scalloped bony edges. At surgery, the dural defect is always noted to be larger than the bony defect. The underlying brain is osseous and gliotic, with adhesions between the dura and the pia-arachnoid space. Brain that has extruded between the bony defects is potentially epileptogenic.

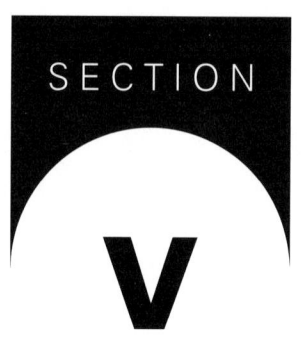

SECTION

V

Functional Neurosurgery

CHAPTER **163**

History of Functional Neurosurgery

ROY A. E. BAKAY

Functional neurosurgery is surgical intervention designed to alter the physiologic activity of the central nervous system (CNS). This surgical discipline has dramatically increased our knowledge about the mechanisms of many cortical functions such as memory, speech, somatomotor, somatosensory, vision, hearing, and affective behavior, as well as the function of subcortical structures that modulate these same functions. Recording, stimulation, ablation, and cellular and pharmacologic therapeutic procedures for the relief of functional neurological disorders have enabled neurosurgeons to become applied neurophysiologists in the study of regional and systematic neuroanatomy and electrophysiology of the human CNS. Functional neurosurgery is proving to be an indispensable subspecialty in neurosurgery and an important instrument for research on the functioning of the human brain. Functional neurosurgery has made significant contributions to neuroscience and promises to advance our understanding of the human brain even further.

The emergence of functional neurosurgery is also the result of the needs of neurologists, neuroradiologists, neurophysiologists, neuroanatomists, neuropathologists, and psychologists to provide more effective treatment of nervous system disorders. A variety of special talents have been recruited to these multidisciplinary teams, including electrophysiologists, molecular biologists, electronic engineers, and computer experts.

Neurosurgery began in prehistoric times, when trephinations were performed in many parts of the world. The reasons for these procedures are unknown, but they were presumably done for symptoms such as coma, convulsions, headache, and mental disorders. Many of these patients survived and occasionally could have benefited if hemorrhage or purulence was encountered. Trephinations became widely used by surgeons in Europe and the United States in the treatment of epilepsy during the 17th and 18th centuries. Even today, there are cults that believe in the beneficial "power" of trephination.

Rene Leriche[1, 2] used the term *functional surgery* to describe sympathetic neurectomies for pain and circulatory disturbances. Leriche removed the pejorative sense of the term *functional*, which was previously used to designate hysterical or conversion phenomena. He stated that this term should be used to denote physiologic function equally applied to normal and pathologic physiology. This was part of a growing philosophy that physiologic function is an important part of pathology and that it may precede or even create anatomic changes.

In 1956, Wertheimer, one of Leriche's disciples, for the first time assembled a book on functional neurosurgery, coining the name given to this division of neurosurgery.[3] Wertheimer's book includes the pathophysiology and treatment of movement disorders, epilepsy, pain, and mental illness. He recognized that the separation between functional and nonfunctional neurosurgery was artificial and included a chapter on the treatment of vascular pathology of the brain and a separate chapter on the treatment of brain edema and alternations of intracranial pressure. According to Wertheimer, functional neurosurgery would take advantage of the new neurophysiologic advances, and the neurosurgeons would perform interventions, guided by neurophysiologic information on the affected pathways.

Hughlings Jackson[4] stressed the importance of the correct use of the term *functional*. For him, *function* is a physiologic term: "Physiology deals with the dynamics of the organism—that is, with its function. I use the term 'function' with regards to nervous diseases in a strict sense, and never in the way it or its adjective (functional) is used when applied to the symptoms of a hysterical woman, or to minute or transitory changes of structure." Abnormal functions are to be distinguished from the pathologic changes that produced them.

General neurosurgery tends to concentrate on lesions, and functional neurosurgery tends to focus on the symptoms. Functional neurosurgery endeavors to correct abnormal function. The objective of functional neurosurgery is to treat, correct, or neutralize the functions of the brain that are altered by a pathologic state. Functional neurosurgery procedures often involve circuits or structures of the nervous system that may frequently be normal except for transient states of altered function. The circuits are not necessarily the same as those involved in the primary derangement of function. The cause of the functional abnormality may or may not require specific treatment because the lesion of origin often requires no treatment. Instead, emphasis is given to correction of the disordered function responsible for movement disorders, pain, epilepsy, or mental change and could include any symptom of the nervous system, even neuroendocrine disturbance.

ORIGINS OF FUNCTIONAL NEUROSURGERY

The early neurosurgical pioneers concentrated on the diagnosis and treatment of nervous system *lesions*. Significant exceptions were Sir Victor Horsley, Rene Leriche, and Otfrid Foerster, who concentrated on the study and treatment of epilepsy, pain, and movement disorders—*symptoms* of lesions that usually did not require treatment. Foremost among these was Sir Victor Horsley (Fig. 163–1), who can be considered the father of functional neurosurgery. Several of his operative procedures were forerunners of what gradually developed into the subspecialty of functional neurosurgery. The first of these was Horsley's introduction of the

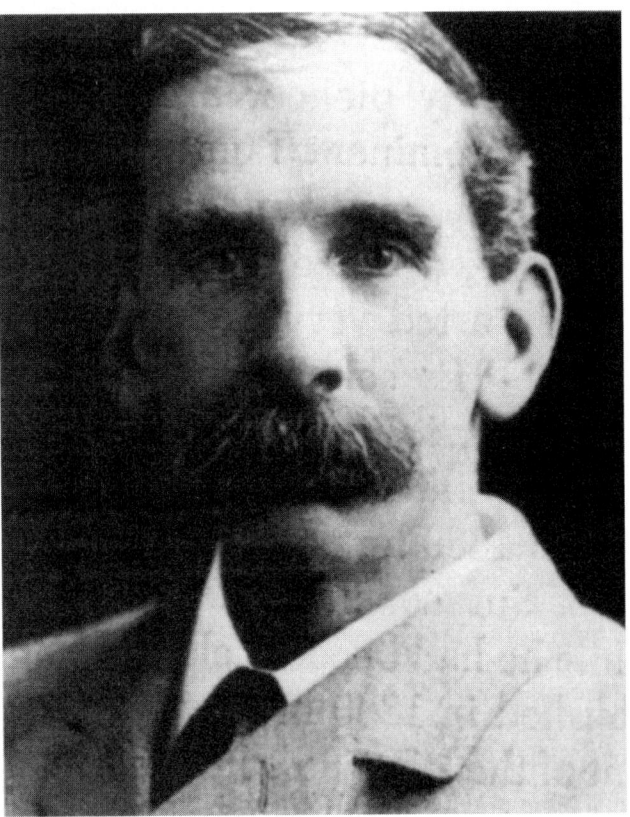

FIGURE 163–1. Sir Victor Horsley (1857–1916), father of stereotactic and functional neurosurgery.

excision of epileptogenic brain tissue for the treatment of focal epilepsy.[5] Knowledge of cortical localization arising from the perceptive studies of Jackson, Fritsch, Hitzig, and Ferrier, together with the advent of anesthesia, antisepsis, and asepsis, led to the development of more appropriate neurosurgical procedures for epilepsy by Foerster, Krause, Ballance, and other neurosurgical pioneers. It was Wilder Penfield's scholarly and progressive refinements of Foerster's cortical resection of epileptogenic cortex that gradually led to increasingly widespread acceptance of this surgical approach to epilepsy. The field of epilepsy surgery has expanded so extensively as to require its own chapter in this textbook (see Chap. 144).

The second precursor of functional neurosurgery was the introduction of gasserian ganglionectomy by Horsley.[6] Neurosurgical treatment of tic douloureux was later pioneered primarily by Krause, Frazier, and Dandy. Anterolateral cordotomy[7] for intractable extremity pain was performed after this pathway was discovered to conduct pain and further developed by Foerster and Frazier. Although neurotomies for pain have a long history in general surgery, it was these two procedures that produced the interest to develop modern functional neurosurgery, as exemplified by the comprehensive studies of pain by James White and William Sweet.[8, 9] Rapid advances in the understanding of neurophysiologic mechanisms of the central and peripheral nervous systems led to further expansion of the neurosurgical treatment of pain (see Chap. 180).

The third precursor forerunner of functional neurosurgery was Horsley's[10, 11] work in removing all or part of the motor cortex for treatment of movement disorders as early as 1890. One of the earliest reports of a systematic approach to movement disorders was that of Bucy and Buchanan.[12, 13] They extirpated the motor cortex for the treatment of athetosis in 1931, for the tremor of Parkinson's disease in 1932, and for cerebellar intention tremor in 1937. Although the patients' initial symptoms improved, they were frequently replaced by other major motor disabilities. In 1933, Putnam[14, 15] reported the first successful extrapyramidal system lesioning with alleviation of choreoathetosis by sectioning the spinal cord at C4-5, just below the exit of the respiratory fibers in the anterolateral quadrant and anterior to the pyramidal tract. However, it was ineffective against parkinsonian tremor.[16] In 1949, Oliver[17] reported that a longer incision helped the tremor, although at the expense of more severe motor deficit from damage to the corticospinal tract. Gillingham[18] went so far as to put lesions in the internal capsule. Until his death in 1992, Bucy insisted that improvement after surgery for Parkinson's disease was not entirely caused by interruption of the extrapyramidal system, but required the inclusion of injury to the pyramidal tract to get the best result. Bucy was wrong.

Moreover, Dandy[19] was convinced that lesioning of the basal ganglia would produce a disorder of consciousness, based on observations of patients with anterior cerebral artery infarcts. Dandy was wrong. However, he was so influential that the earliest surgical attempts to treat Parkinson's disease did not initially involve the basal ganglia. Russel Meyers[20–23] first attacked the basal ganglia directly in 1939, proving Dandy and Bucy wrong. He developed a number of surgical approaches, including a transventricular extirpation of the head of the caudate nucleus and adjacent structures in 1939 and sectioning of the ansa lenticularis by a subtemporal, interhemispheric, or transventricular approach in 1942. Meyers was forced to admit that the high morbidity and 15.7% mortality rates were prohibitive; however, this work was seminal in proving that it was possible to abolish involuntary movement disorders without impairing consciousness or imposing weakness or spasticity. This work set the stage for the development of stereotactic techniques.

Even after stereotactic techniques were introduced in 1947, many neurosurgeons were slow to embrace the stereotactic surgery, and open surgery continued to be more frequently used for treatment of movement disorders. In 1947, Browder[24, 25] revisited Meyer's surgery with extirpation of part of the head of the caudate nucleus and divided the anterior limb of the internal capsule, again with high morbidity and mortality, especially after bilateral surgery. These approaches did affect tremor and rigidity, but the postoperative deficits induced often were devastating to patients. In 1950, Fenelon[26] used a technical variation of open surgical ansotomy by manually inserting an electrode to interrupt the ansa lenticularis with electrical coagulation. In 1953, Guiot and Brion[27] used a similar freehand approach to coagulate the globus pallidus, even though accurate stereotactic guidance to that target had already been clearly demonstrated. During the same period, surgical excision of fiber bundles took aim at the corticospinal efferent pathways. These procedures induced less motor deficit, but they were also less effective. Walker[28] initially reported the use of mesencephalic tractotomy for the treatment of pain in 1942, but he later refined that procedure as a cerebral pedunculotomy with a subtemporal exposure, with the aim of interrupting the extrapyramidal tract and leaving the pyramidal tract intact for the treatment of hemiballismus.[29] Later, Guiot and Pecker[30] and Walker[31] reported the use of the same procedure for Parkinson's disease. Morbidity and mortality rates eventually ended open functional surgical procedures, because they could not compete with the 2.8% mortality rate of Spiegel and Wycis,[32] which was further decreased to less than 1% by Reichert.[33]

The treatment of spasticity and dystonia begins with Sir Victor Horsley. He noticed a transitory decrease in spasticity after cortical topectomy in the premotor area to control choreoathetotic movements.[11] Subsequently, to reduce spasticity, cortectomy and pyramidotomy were investigated in humans with the same results, yielding a flaccid palsy instead of spasticity.[34, 35]

This era was marked by empirical trial and error based on a rudimentary understanding of the neuroanatomy and pathophysiology. Progress was made through successes and failures. The latter is best exemplified by Irving Cooper. In 1951, while attempting a pedunculotomy, Cooper[36] tore the anterior choroidal artery, ligated it, and closed. Postoperatively, the patient was free of tremor and rigidity on the contralateral side. This surgical complication serendipitously demonstrated that ischemic lesioning of the pallidum could produce symptomatic relief of parkinsonian symptoms without corticospinal injury. Early claims of dramatic improvement with little or no morbidity damaged his reputation when deaths occurred after anterior choroidal ligations. The arterial supply to this region is quite variable and frequently includes the thalamus and internal capsule.[37] Given an unacceptable mortality rate of about 13%, Cooper directly targeted the pallidum for Parkinson's disease and dystonia through a pneumoencephalography-guided lateral transtemporal approach, into which he inserted a catheter to inject alcohol using a nonstereotactic guidance system.[38–40] The lesions were not always where expected. Upon autopsy, one of his more successful patients demonstrated a lesion in the lateral thalamus. This surgical complication of lesioning off target by several centimeters is frequently described as a second serendipitous finding that led to the discovery that the thalamus was a better target for tremor. The more scientific studies of Hassler and Riechert already had identified the ventrolateral thalamus as the better target for tremor.[41]

Cooper also advocated pulvinarotomy for spasticity[42] and stimulation of the anterior lobe of the cerebellum for epilepsy,[43] both of which proved useless when appropriately studied. Cooper never developed stereotactic techniques. His major contribution was a very large surgical experience. Superficial, nonstandardized, and unblinded clinical assessments and lack of confirmation of actual (rather than claimed) targets renders this and much of the data in this era suspect and unusable in any scientific attempt to determine precisely the relationships of lesion locations and response of clinical symptoms.

BIRTH OF STEREOTACTIC SURGERY

Multiple intracranial targets could be identified for functional neurosurgery, but a safe and effective way of operating was lacking. Before the development of a stereotactic frame, there were a number of aiming devices. The first experimental technique for the spatial localization of intracranial structures is credited to Dittmar,[44] who, in 1873, used a device to guide a knife in the performance of vasomotor physiologic studies in rat medulla oblongata. In 1897, a frame fixed on the skull of a patient was used to remove bullets that were localized with two perpendicular x-ray films. The only report of this procedure was given in the November 27, 1897, edition of a Parisian newspaper by Remy and Contremoulins (Le chercheur de projectiles, L'illustration). In 1889, Zernov[45] developed an encephalometer that helped localize surface areas of the brain, which was used clinically 2 years later by Altukhov.[46]

None of these techniques meets the criteria for a stereotactic device. A true stereotactic device requires a cartesian coordinate system that identifies a point in space by its mathematical relationship to three planes intersecting at right angles to each other and intersecting at a common point; this concept forms the basis for identifying a target in three-dimensional space.

Stereotactic surgery began with the use of cartesian principles by Sir Victor Horsley and Richard Clarke,[47] who described the first animal stereotactic apparatus in a landmark publication in 1908 (Fig. 163–2). Horsley was a neurophysiologist and neurosurgeon who looked for a technique to insert an electrode reliably into the dentate nucleus to study the cerebellum of the monkey. He collaborated with Clarke, a mathematician and inventor, to design a device that would accurately insert an electrode into any desired target. While recovering from pneumonia, Clarke conceptualized a device using geometric principles.[48] The resulting manuscript was divided into four parts. The first detailed the apparatus, the second illustrated the first stereotactic atlas of the monkey brain, the third described the lesions, and the fourth section discussed results of those lesions. The atlas sections were registered by a cartesian coordinate system to landmarks on the monkey's skull—the external auditory canals and the inferior orbital rim. These landmarks are still used today in monkey studies, but the use of imaging techniques to identify internal anatomy is replacing the use of atlases and external landmarks. The description of production of electrolytic lesions with direct current, a technique used in early clinical studies, is clear and precise. The physiologic observations of lesions made with the stereotactic apparatus are of minimal interest, but the

technology that allows them to be studied continues. Animal studies still use stereotactic frames to create lesions and to deliver drugs, cells, and electrical stimulation. These investigations have contributed greatly to our understanding of neuroanatomy and neuroelectrophysiology, and in some cases, they paved the way for new stereotactic procedures.

Horsley and Clarke called their technique *stereotaxic* from the Greek words *stereo* (three dimensional) and *taxic* (arrangement). Neurosurgeons later changed the name to *stereotactic* preferring the Latin *tactic* (to touch) as a more descriptive term for their technique. Although Clarke patented the idea for a human apparatus, the pair separated and did not develop that idea.[49] Clarke saw stereotactic surgery as a means to clinically treat tumor and pain, however Horsley did not. Horsley was wrong. It is ironic that the father of functional neurosurgery would invent the first stereotactic frame but never use it on a patient. In about 1918, Mussen, an engineer who had worked with the Horsley-Clarke stereotactic apparatus, designed a similar device for the human skull.[50] He could not persuade his neurosurgical colleagues to use it. Perhaps it was best that it was not used, because the variability between the human skull and the intracerebral structures is so great that it would have proved grossly inaccurate. He wrapped it in newspaper and stored it in his attic, where it was not discovered until after his death. The only evidence of its chronology was from the date of the newspaper, because he never reported the device in the literature.

Thirty years later, the concepts of human neurophysiology and imaging techniques had advanced enough to make the technique clinically useful. The key was to establish an accurate internal reference system for human stereotactic surgery. This problem was solved by Ernest Spiegel and Henry Wycis.[51] Spiegel was a professor of experimental neurology at Temple Medical School, and Wycis initially worked in Spiegel's laboratory as a medical student, after which he became a neurosurgeon and a collaborator. In 1947, they reported a human stereotactic apparatus that resembled the original Horsley-Clarke apparatus (Fig. 163–3). Anchored to the patient's head, it allowed orthogonal intraoperative pneumoencephalograms to be taken so that internal brain landmarks could be visualized and translated into three-dimensional space. Anatomic structures could be targeted by referring to a human stereotactic atlas, which they designed and later published.[52] They originally called this new science *stereo-encephalotomy* and called the frame Stereoencephalotome Model 1 (which is in the Smithsonian Institution). They continued to make improvements and to use Model V for all of their later work.

The timing was right for stereotactic surgery. The progress in clinical neuroanatomic and electrophysiologic understanding set the stage for the development of human stereotactic functional neurosurgery. Prefrontal lobotomy was a popular procedure in the period before adequate psychotropic medication.[53] Egas Moniz[54] applied observations by Fulton and Jacobsen[55] about frontal lobotomies in chimpanzees to patients

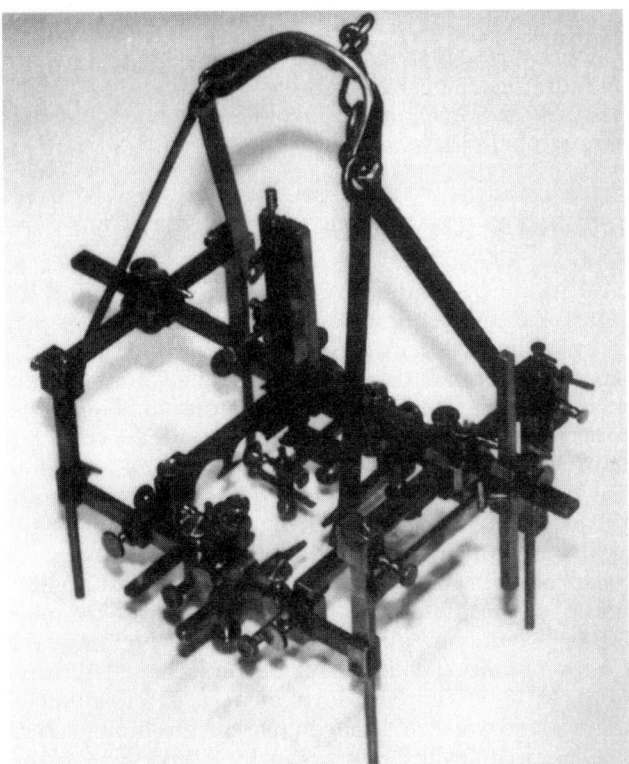

FIGURE 163–2. Horsley-Clarke frame as it might be assembled for use, showing ear bars, a mouth fixator, and a stand. (Courtesy of the Archives of the American Association of Neurological Surgeons, Rolling Meadows, IL.)

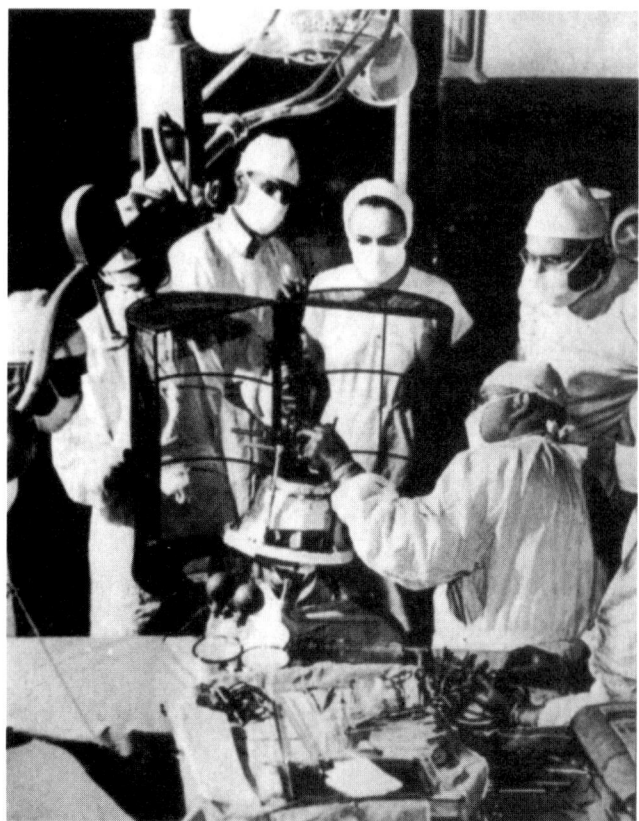

FIGURE 163–3. Spiegel and Wycis and their team during an early stereotactic procedure. (Courtesy of Time-Life Warner.)

with psychiatric disorders. The primary impetus for the development of stereotactic surgery was that Spiegel desired to refine the "ice pick" procedure to avoid its many complications. Spiegel wanted a device that could safely and effectively lesion the dorsomedial nuclei of the thalamus to interrupt the thalamofrontal circuits involved in affective disorders. However, after the technique was available, it was years before it was used for psychosurgery. Many surgical methods were used to interrupt pathways in the brain for the treatment of pain. The primary pain pathway as it ascended through the brainstem was understood, and the concept of the participation of the limbic system in pain perception was well developed.[56, 57] Modifications of these procedures involved surgical interruption of the pathways, approaches that are still in use today.[58, 59] The understanding of neurophysiology had advanced to the point where the concept of the extrapyramidal system and the pathways involved with movement disorders were defined,[60] to a large extent because of animal experimentation that involved stereotactic techniques.[61]

In 1946, Spiegel and Wycis performed the first stereotactic surgery on a patient with Huntington's chorea. They injected alcohol into the globus pallidus and medial thalamus in an attempt to spare the fibers *en passage*. They chose two separate targets: the pallidum to improve choreiform movement by interrupting the extrapyramidal circuit, and the dorsomedial nucleus of

the thalamus to lessen the emotional tone of the patient, because it was recognized that stress made the chorea worse.[62] Although the improvement was transient, the importance of the operation lay in the demonstration that pathways could be interrupted without a loss of neurological function and that targets deep within the brain could be selectively destroyed by minimally traumatic stereotactic techniques.

Spiegel and Wycis pioneered the scientific study of many of the targets for a variety of indications for stereotactic functional neurosurgery.[32, 63–66] Their philosophy was to perform a few well-done procedures on many neurological diseases. Every time an electrode was inserted into the human brain, it provided a unique research opportunity. Each operation involved physiologic confirmation of electrode position by neurophysiologic studies. Significant advances in our understanding of the human brain resulted from this careful evaluation of each patient, which led to additional indications and targets for stereotactic intervention. This philosophy should be the standard of contemporary stereotactic neurosurgeons. There is a need for patient service, but in a small, rapidly evolving subspecialty, we should learn something from each patient.

Neurosurgeons throughout the world entered the field of stereotactic neurosurgery during the 1950s. Talairach and Guiot in Paris; Hassler, Riechert, and Wolf in Germany; Gillingham in Great Britain; Leksell in Sweden; Krayenbuehl and Siegfried in Switzerland; Laitinen and Toivakka in Finland; Velasco-Suarez and Escobedo in Mexico; Obrador in Spain; Bechtereva and Kandel in Russia; Narabayashi in Japan; and others developed centers for functional stereotactic neurosurgery. In Canada, Bertrand and colleagues also incorporated stereotactic techniques into their treatment program for epilepsy. Within 20 years of its introduction, stereotactic surgery was practiced throughout the world. Spiegel estimated that more than 25,000 stereotactic cases had been done worldwide by 1965[67] and that 37,000 cases had been done by 1969,[66] with most performed for movement disorders.

EVOLUTION OF STEREOTACTIC SURGICAL TECHNOLOGY

Technologic innovation in stereotactic surgery came from improvements in the frame and imaging technique and from advancements in electrophysiology and pathophysiology. Progress in each of these areas would build on the other, but first, there was the problem of the frame. The first meeting of the International Society for Research and Stereoencephalotomy, which became the World Society for Stereotactic and Functional Neurosurgery in 1973, was held in Philadelphia in 1966. The meeting proceedings were published in *Confinia Neurologica* (or *Borderlands of Neurology*, which became Applied Neurophysiology in 1975 and Stereotactic and Functional Neurosurgery in 1988), which Spiegel edited.

Twenty years after the first human stereotactic procedure, the emphasis was on instrumentation. All major figures had their own instruments and instrumentation and were invited to bring their own apparatus to the meeting. More than 40 types of apparatus were presented, most of which were variations of the three basic designs: translational, arc centered, or ball and socket.[68] Almost all were custom made because there were few commercially available devices at that time. The Horsley-Clarke and Spiegel-Wycis frames were translational types of instruments (Fig. 163–4). The position of the electrode was changed by sliding the electrode carrier anteroposteriorly and mediolaterally

along a base plate, and a microdrive provided vertical positioning to set each of the three coordinates separately. This type of sliding base was later added to the arc-centered frame to optimize rectilinear translations. Angular settings were possible but required separate calculations.

The Leksell[69] and Riechert[70] frames and, later, the Todd-Wells frame[71] were arc-centered devices, and the three coordinates indicated the center of a semicircular arc along with a probe carrier when moved, always pointing the probe toward the isocenter. Because the target was always located at the center of the arc,

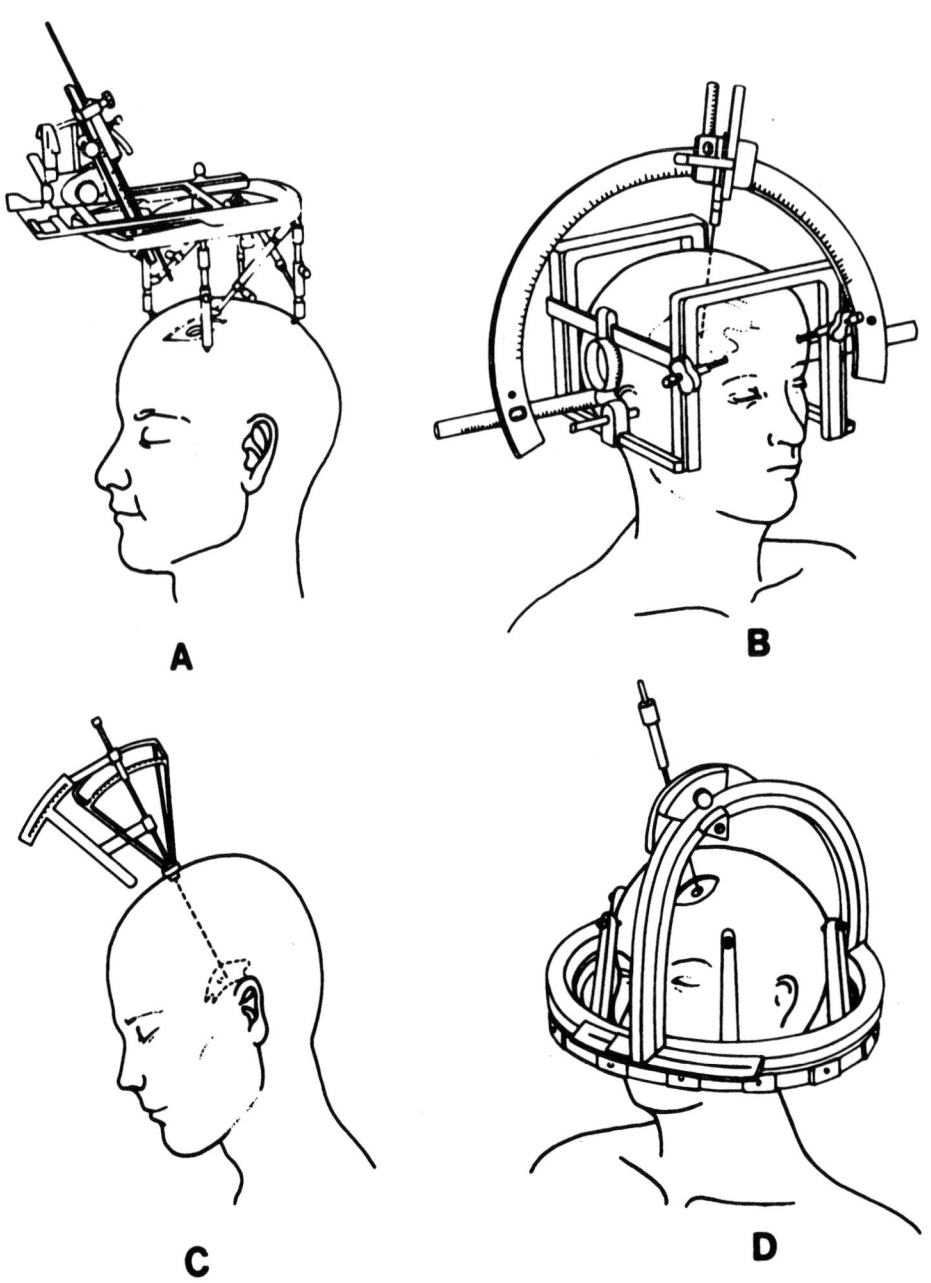

FIGURE 163–4. All frame-based stereotactic apparatus are of four basic designs: the translational system (Spiegel-Wycis model V) *(A)*, the arc-centered devices (Leksell, model B) *(B)*, a bur hole–mounted device *(C)*, and a system of interlocking arcs (Brown-Roberts-Wells frame) *(D)*. (From Gildenberg PL: Whatever happened to stereotactic surgery? Neurosurgery 20:983–987, 1987.)

insertion along any angle to the depth of the radius brought the probe to the target. The system was mounted in the bur holes and consisted of a multiple ball-and-socket probe to hold the probe and allow adjustments to direct the probe to the target and lock it into that trajectory. Many of these systems are aiming devices and not true stereotactic frames. Today, this type of system is primarily used for biopsies.[68] A fourth type of apparatus, introduced in 1980, is the Brown-Roberts-Wells frame, which is adjusted by a complicated system of interlocking arcs.[72] This system proved too difficult and counterintuitive and was abandoned. The Cosman-Roberts-Wells frame is an arc-based system that replaced it. During the 1960s and 1970s, the Todd-Wells system became the most popular in the United States, and the Leksell and Riechert-Mundinger systems became the most popular in Europe.[73, 74] The Brown-Roberts-Wells frame and, later, the Cosman-Roberts-Wells frame became standard in the United States for biopsy. The Leksell frame eventually became the most popular functional surgical frame worldwide. The Cosman-Roberts-Wells frame was modified; the functional Cosman-Roberts-Wells system has many of the desirable aspects of the Leksell frame and the ability to use a phantom to evaluate settings and angles preoperatively.

The second meeting of the International Society for Research and Stereoencephalotomy was held in Atlantic City in 1967. The emphasis at that meeting was on reviewing the large number of indications for stereotactic surgery and sharing clinical experiences. In their first case, Spiegel and colleagues[51] injected alcohol. Control of the lesion size and spread proved to be a source of variance and the technique would be abandoned. Many lesions were subsequently made with an electrolytic direct current, the same technique that Horsley and Clarke used 40 years earlier. Other techniques for making lesions, including mechanical disruption, ultrasonography, and irradiation, were soon developed but then abandoned because of the inability to control the lesion size. Cooper and Lee[75] developed a cryoprobe. Hassler and Riechert[41] introduced radiofrequency lesioning, which has evolved to become the standard. The heat lesioning technology proved superior because of the ability to produce highly reproducible lesions with much smaller probes.[76]

Advances in imaging were also pivotal to advancing stereotactic technology. Radiographic technology rapidly improved to eliminate distortion and evolved from air to positive contrast to allow greater detail in intraoperative films. The internal landmarks that Spiegel and Wycis first used were calcification in the pineal gland and the foramen of Monro as defined by pneumoencephalography.[51] Soon, the intercommissural line, as recommended by Talairach and coworkers[77] and by Hassler and Riechert,[41] was the state of the art. New stereotactic atlases were published, emphasizing the subnuclear structure of the thalamus[78] and later emphasizing neurophysiologic criteria.[79] These improvements meant that lesions were more precisely placed, lesions were smaller, and complication rates were lowered.

EARLY HISTORY OF FUNCTIONAL STEREOTACTIC SURGERY

The era before L-dopa was one of target exploration. Many different movement disorders were treated with functional and stereotactic surgery. Hassler's pathophysiologic concepts and Cooper's incidental observations about the anterior choroidal artery occlusion led many early neurosurgeons to lesion the pallidum. Lesions in the substantia nigra were used for treating hemiballismus[80, 81] and hypertonus.[82] Spiegel and Wycis were initially reluctant to make lesions in the globus pallidus in patients with Parkinson's disease because experimental pallidotomy produced hypokinesia in animals, and if this occurred clinically, it would make parkinsonian akinesia worse. They were wrong. After Hassler and Riechert[41] reported that they had successfully treated Parkinson's disease by ventrolateral thalamotomy (the target of the pallidofugal tract), Speigel and Wycis changed their thinking and made a lesion in the medial globus pallidus.[63] About the same time, Narabayashi[83] reported making a lesion with procaine oil injected into the pallidum. Improvements in rigidity and akinesia were good, but tremor was frequently not well treated.

In the late 1950s, after most neurosurgeons followed Hassler and Riechert's recommendation to lesion the thalamus, Spiegel and Wycis still preferred the pallidum as the target. In 1958, they commented that the lesion would be more effective against rigidity if it were placed more posteriorly than the tremor target to include the emerging ansa lenticularis fibers.[32] In 1959, Svennilson and colleagues[84] reviewed Leksell's cases and also advocated a lesion more ventral and posterior than that used by other surgeons. Ventral posterior pallidotomy has become the preferred target after L-dopa for treating parkinsonian rigidity, bradykinesia, and drug-induced dyskinesia.[85, 86]

By 1954, Hassler and Riechert[41] had defined their thalamic targets more precisely, with the ventral oral posterior (Vop) nucleus recommended for tremor and the ventral oral anterior (Voa) nucleus recommended for rigidity. Intention tremors were also treated with lesions in the ventrolateral nucleus,[87] as was hemiballismus.[88] Because the most dramatic effect of thalamotomy was the prompt and frequently complete abolition of tremor, this was felt to be the best target even though it did nothing to help the akinesia. For this reason, Gillingham tried pallidotomy first with thalamotomy as a second procedure if needed later.[18] The optimal target for tremor was eventually accepted to be the ventralis intermedius (Vim) nucleus of the thalamus,[89–92] and the pallidum eventually was abandoned as a target for Parkinson's disease in the mid-1960s.[93] There was still considerable disagreement, however, about where the ideal target was located.[94] Spiegel and Wycis moved their target to Forel's field, an area concentrating the pallidofugal fibers.[64, 65]

In 1962, microelectrode recording from the human brain was introduced as a surgical tool to confirm placement of the lesion in the ventralis intermedius.[95, 96]

The microelectrodes helped define the target and led to an understanding of the pathophysiology with identification of cells that burst in a tremor-synchronous manner.[97–99] The result was smaller, more effective lesions.[99–101] The science of microelectrode recording has advanced to the point where many consider it to be a routine technique in stereotactic functional neurosurgery.[102–106] A number of neurosurgeons use microelectrode recording to confirm placement of a lesion or deep brain stimulators in the globus pallidus internalis (GPi) and subthalamic nucleus (STN).[107–109]

Movement disorders are fascinating diseases to physicians but debilitating disorders for patients. Patients, desperate for treatment, have had lesions made in all parts of the central nervous system to relieve their symptoms. Serendipitous observations and trial and error were the hallmarks of surgery in this era. These early investigators were bold and innovative, although their studies were not scientific investigations but empirical trials. Those who succeeded became neurosurgical heroes, and those whose procedures were unsatisfactory went on to other things. The true heroes were the patients.

DECLINE AND REBIRTH OF STEREOTACTIC SURGERY

In 1968, L-dopa became generally available, and within a few months, the number of Parkinson's disease patients referred for surgery plummeted.[110] Only a few patients with primarily tremor came for stereotactic surgery during the next 2 decades, even though surgery was the most effective treatment for tremor. The number of neurosurgeons doing stereotactic surgery declined, and stereotactic surgery was practiced mainly by a few neurosurgeons in academic centers. Nevertheless, this became a time of refinement and greater sophistication in the development of stereotactic frames, intraoperative electrophysiologic technique (especially microelectrode recordings), imaging technique, and neuroanatomic and neurophysiologic understanding of the pathophysiology of multiple neurodegenerative disease, some never known to the first generation of functional neurosurgeons. It was not until the introduction of computed tomographic image–directed targeting that stereotactic surgery rebounded. However, functional neurosurgery was not the same as stereotactic neurosurgery, and progress in treating epilepsy and pain continued to flourish.

The stereotactic frame and stereotactic technique continued to be used in the development of stereotactic radiosurgery (see Chap. 261). Lars Leksell[111] coined the term *stereotactic radiosurgery*, and in 1951, he described its technical basis and many of the practical applications. Always an advocate of minimally invasive surgery, Leksell considered irradiation to be less invasive than the insertion of electrodes and decided to develop an instrument that would produce a lesion stereotactically with radiation. His first attempt was with an orthovoltage x-ray tube attached to his stereotactic frame so that radiation could be directed at the arc-centered target from many directions. The technology of radiotherapy of the day restricted the accuracy and application of this technique. In 1954, a report of charged particles focused with the use of stereotactic techniques for pituitary suppression[112] led to his second attempt and development of an apparatus that used a cyclotron to produce proton beams crossing at a target point.[113]

The cost and technical difficulties of cyclotron irradiation prompted Leksell to develop the gamma knife in 1967.[114] This was the first stereotactic radiosurgery device designed specifically to use radiation as a neurosurgical tool. In a repeat of history, the original intention was to use the system to interrupt pathways for functional stereotactic surgery, but the first patient treated had a craniopharyngioma. Treatment of other tumors and vascular malformations quickly followed. Leksell and others[115, 116] attempted functional stereotactic radiosurgery, but they abandoned it for lack of efficacy and safety. The second gamma knife, designed in 1975, allowed the indications for radiosurgery to be expanded.[117] More than 30 additional gamma knife units are in use worldwide.

During the same period, advancements in linear accelerator (LINAC) technology made it feasible for stereotactic radiosurgery. In 1972, Betti and Derechinsky[118] and Colombo and colleagues[119] reported modifications of LINACs to provide noncoplanar, isocentered administration of radiation for intracranial lesions. This technology was advanced further by the development of technology to quantify and calculate the dosimetry and ensure the accuracy of the system.[120, 121] The development of most commercially available systems was based on their concepts. Dosimetry-planning software became sophisticated, user-friendly, and efficient enough to be made commercially available.[122, 123] The development of LINAC-based stereotactic radiosurgery systems created competition for the gamma knife, because LINAC systems are more affordable, more widely available, and more versatile, with an ability to treat head and spinal diseases. In many cases, comparable results can be obtained, but LINAC systems have not been as rigorously studied as the gamma knife.[117]

Stereotactic and nonstereotactic psychosurgery has been performed and continues to be performed for depression and obsessive-compulsive disorder. The use of psychosurgery for drug addiction, violent behavior, and sexual dysfunction is no longer performed. In the 1960s, medical therapy was beginning to make progress in the management of the most aggressive or schizophrenic patients, and psychosurgery slowed but continued to be needed for medically refractory patients and was being re-evaluated with more refined targets. In 1972, the political campaign against psychosurgery reached Congress after a highly inflammatory article in the *New England Journal of Medicine*.[124] In a deliberate distortion, contemporary psychosurgery was equated with the type of lobotomy that had essentially been discontinued for more than a decade. False allegations were made that psychosurgery was being used primarily to subdue aggressive persons (especially minorities), always resulted in severe mental incapacity, and was of no psychological benefit. The National Commission for the Protection of Human Subjects was formed to study these allegations by retrospectively interviewing patients who had undergone cingulotomy.[125] They found that the procedure was generally safe and that patients functioned much better after surgery. Although the commission recommended that psychosurgery not be banned and should be considered safe and effective when properly performed, they recognized the need for additional safeguards and suggested increased research funding. Nevertheless, after several states banned psychosurgery, Congress made psychosurgery more difficult to perform, and no new money was set aside for research. Unfortunately, the ugly political upheaval that had been generated caused most neurosurgeons throughout the world to abandon the field. Psychosurgery never recovered. Today, few centers continue to be active, and only a few articles concerning the benefit of psychosurgery have been published. Advances in psychiatric medication and loss of interest in the field have all but vanquished this area of study. The development of deep brain stimulation (DBS) may reawaken the field because safe, effective, and reversible affective changes can be produced without permanent damage to the brain.[126]

Surgery for spasticity continued to evolve. Foerster[127] introduced dorsal rhizotomy for dystonia and spasticity, which was modified by Dandy, Bertrand, and others. Foerster's work was based on Sherrington's concept of the reflex arc, and the results he published were impressive. After the introduction of the stereotactic technique, destruction of the thalamus[128–130] in the neurosurgical treatment of spasticity was tried but abandoned because of the lack of clinical improvement in spasticity after ventrolateral thalamotomy and pulvinarotomy. Stereotactic dentatotomy may have some effect on spasticity, but the long-term follow-up results are rather disappointing.[131, 132] Thalamotomy and pallidotomy for dystonia proved beneficial,[98, 133, 134] and there has been a resurgence of interest in posterior ventral pallidotomy.[135, 136] The use of DBS may represent the greatest breakthrough in treatment of dystonia.[137] Interest in this destructive approach waned over the years because of the magnitude of the operation and the complications, which can include sensory loss and weakness. Improved surgical technique resulted in a resurgence of interest in treating the spasticity of cerebral palsy.[138–140] Electrostimulation of the spinal cord has produced modest improvements.[141] A new pharmacologic approach requiring implantation of a drug pump to deliver intrathecal baclofen has generated renewed enthusiasm for treating spasticity of spinal origin[142] or the injection of botulinum toxin for treatment to localize spastic dystonia.[143]

New areas of functional neurosurgery have evolved. In 1985, Backlund and associates[144] reported the first clinical stereotactic transplantation of autologous adrenal medullary tissue into the head of the caudate nucleus. Failure to produce clear improvement and the understanding from animal studies of the failure of adult tissue to survive without neurotrophic factors ended these pioneering trials. Two years later, Madrazo and colleagues[145] reported remarkable improvement in two patients. This and additional reports[146] stimulated great interest worldwide, and programs were begun at many institutions. Nevertheless, results were considered to be modest and of questionable duration[147, 148]; surgery to retrieve one adrenal gland was stressful to a fragile group of patients, resulting in frequent complications[149]; the adrenal gland was sometimes found to be atrophic[150]; and autopsy studies found few or no surviving cells.[151] Several complications resulted from the craniotomy by surgeons who placed the transplant tissue by open surgery, but very few complications resulted from surgery by those using stereotactic techniques.[149] By 1991, the procedure was essentially abandoned in the United States.

The short-lived interest in adrenal transplantation was a distraction from the transplantation of fetal nigral tissue. The experimental groundwork had already been done to a large extent in the late 1980s, first with parkinsonian rat models[152–154] and then in parkinsonian monkey models.[155–157] In 1989, the first two patients to receive fetal cell transplantation for the treatment of Parkinson's disease were reported,[158] and reports of others soon followed. Although research in this area continues, problems have been increasingly recognized, including difficulty in obtaining fetal tissue at the proper age and in the proper amounts, correct identification of the tissue, processing of the tissue, and coordination between obtaining the tissue and arranging for the implantation surgery.[148] There is a search for alternative tissues, especially among stem cells.[159, 160] The ultimate therapy, however, may be gene therapy for repair and eventual prevention.[161]

After years of drug trials, it became recognized that medical therapy was not the final answer to Parkinson's disease. As the disease progresses, symptoms become refractory to L-dopa, and side effects begin to appear. Response to medication eventually fluctuates, producing repeated on-off episodes during the course of the day, with dyskinesia alternating with freezing episodes. The introduction of multiple new drugs has not solved this problem. By the early 1980s, the increased safety and efficacy of stereotactic surgery was rewarded by patients with tremor being referred more frequently for thalamotomy. Stereotactic pallidotomy was revisited by Laitinen and colleagues.[94] Leksell reported more improvement in bradykinesia and rigidity than had been described by other investigators,[84] which Laitinen attributed to Leksell's placement of the lesion more ventrally and posteriorly than the target used by others. This area is the motor segment of the nucleus. In 1992, Laitinen[86] reported a significant improvement in rigidity, bradykinesia, tremor, and L-dopa–induced dyskinesia in Parkinson's disease patients who had become medically refractory and chronically disabled. Other investigators have confirmed these observations, including in blinded trials[162–164] and in open, long-term studies.[165–167]

Meanwhile, another promising field has emerged. Although it was known for sometime that intraoperative electrical stimulation of the thalamus could arrest tremor, Bechtereva[168] was the first to attempt therapeutic DBS. After implanting 20 to 40 electrodes, he stimulated for several weeks with some success. It was unclear whether improvement was caused by stimulation or by a lesion effect. Mundinger[169] and others[170–172] implanted stimulators for Parkinson's tremor and other movement disorders with only moderate success, in part because of an inability to generate high-frequency stimulation. In 1985, Siegfried[173] reported improvement in tremor in a Parkinson's disease patient who underwent deep brain implantation of an electrode capable of sustained high-frequency stimulation in the thalamus for treatment of pain. This observation encouraged Siegfried and Lippitz[174] and Benabid and coworkers[175] to implant high-frequency, chronically stimulating electrodes into the thalamus for the treatment of parkinsonian tremor and essential tremor (Fig. 163–5). Results are often dramatic, with prompt suppression of tremor when the stimulator is turned on, but with a rapid return of the tremor when the stimulator is turned off. Thalamic DBS has been just as effective as and safer than thalamotomy.[176] The use of chronic thalamic stimulation is preferred if patients are at high risk for complications, such as older patients or in cases of quadralateral procedure following a unilateral thalamotomy.[177] Later studies suggest that the globus pallidus[163, 173, 174, 178–180] or the STN [181–183] may be a better target for chronic stimulation to treat all the symptoms of Parkinson's disease.

The story behind STN DBS is hopefully the wave of the future for functional neurosurgery. Delong and colleagues[184] defined the electrophysiologic abnormalities in the basal ganglia of parkinsonian monkeys and determined that the increased excitatory output of the STN was in large part responsible for the symptoms of Parkinson's disease. They tested this hypothesis by lesioning the STN and reversed all symptoms in these monkeys.[185] This led Benabid and colleagues[186] to attempt the first electrical neuroinhibition in the STN. Cutting-edge neuroelectrophysiologic and neuroanatomic understanding led to bold therapeutic trials and opened frontiers in functional neurosurgery.[126]

After the introduction of computed tomography (CT) in 1973, there was a rapid development of new stereotactic techniques as image-based stereotactic surgery was born.[110] The breakthrough was the development of a fiducial system that contains all the information for three-dimensional targeting from a single two-dimensional image. Three sets of three rods, with each set in an N-shaped configuration (Z and V shapes were also introduced), allowed three coordinates for three points to be calculated, thereby defining the plane of the target. This system was first incorporated into the Brown-Roberts-Wells frame system,[72] but soon, similar technology was assimilated into other stereotactic systems.[187, 188] When magnetic resonance imaging (MRI) was introduced in the mid-1980s, it was rapidly incorporated into image-based stereotactic surgery, using techniques similar to those developed for functional neurosurgery with CT guidance. Functional stereotactic surgery for movement disorders is now performed with CT or MRI rather than with intraoperative ventriculography, although the latter is still occasionally used as an adjuvant intraoperative monitor. Introduc-

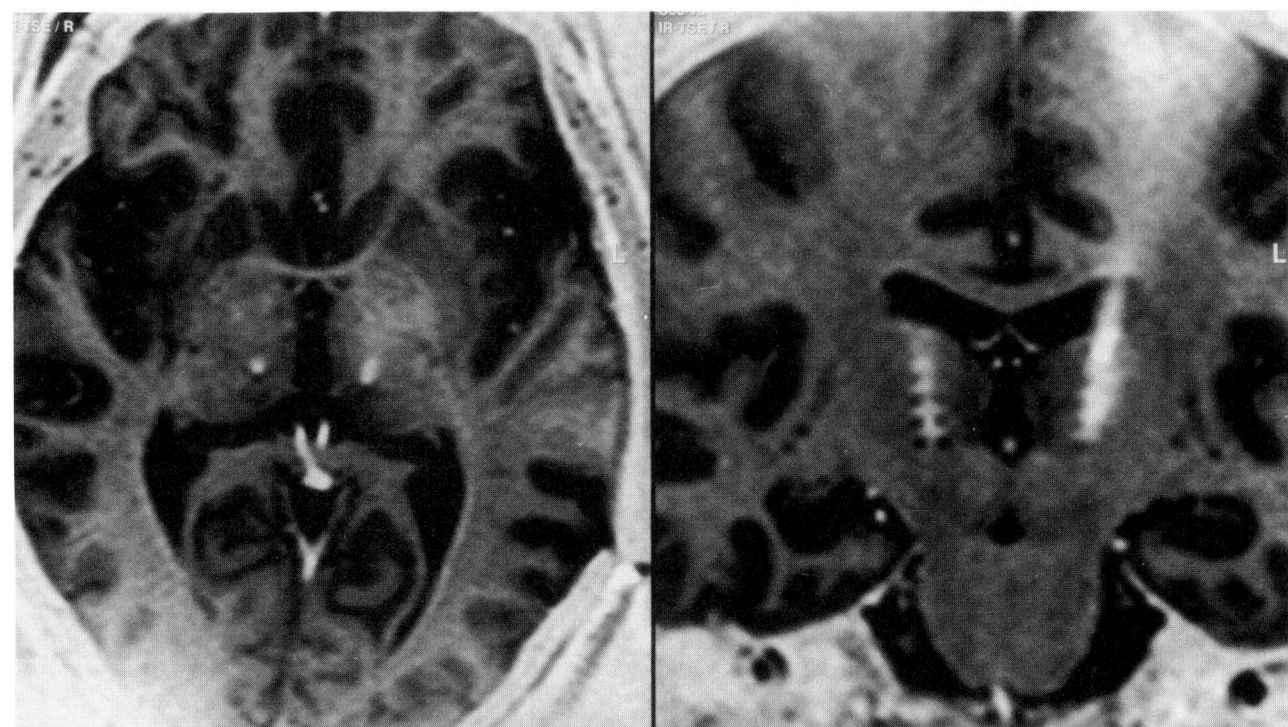

FIGURE 163–5. Magnetic resonance images of the axial *(left)* and coronal *(right)* locations of deep brain stimulators in the thalamus of a patient with essential tremor.

tion of computer workstations into stereotactic surgical planning allowed complex trajectories and target points to be calculated and visualized, and stereotactic atlases can to be superimposed and fitted to the anatomy on the scans of CT or MRI.[189–191] Anatomic targets can be reconstructed in three dimensions to facilitate functional stereotactic[192, 193] or epilepsy surgery.[194]

Although image-based neurosurgery for tumors or other mass lesions has advanced so rapidly that it now overshadows functional stereotactic surgery and will eventually be incorporated into the armamentarium of every general neurosurgeon,[195] functional stereotactic surgery remains a subspecialty for those knowledgeable in applied neurophysiology.[196] A group of stereotactic apparatuses were developed for use with computed tomographic scanning. Some depended on the calibrated movement of the scanner table between slices to define the vertical coordinate.[197–199] Laitinen developed a noninvasive device (i.e., no pin attachments) to be used with CT.[200] It was suggested that a computed tomographic scanner should incorporate a stereotactic head holder.[201] As an alternative, the scanner was installed in the operating room.[202]

Although MRI provides more information content than CT and its ability to display images in any plane is a significant advantage, magnetic resonance technology has introduced additional complexities. Because patients may not tolerate the length of time required to remain motionless in a claustrophobic environment, patients with movement disorders are particularly difficult to image. The magnetic field is subject to linear and nonlinear distortion, which can also cause errors of localization. There is an inherent distortion created just by placing the patient's head in the magnetic field. Any metal in the patient such as dental filling, plates, wires, and so on will distort the magnetic field. Add to that a stereotactic frame, even if nonferromagnetic, and there can be marked distortion of the field homogeneity.[190, 203] Ordinarily, the error produced is not enough to compromise the surgery, but large errors may not be recognized. This may not matter for a biopsy of a 1-cm tumor but could be a disaster for a target that requires an accuracy of millimeters. Techniques to fuse the images of MRI and CT may help correct linear MRI spatial distortions[123] but probably not nonlinear distortion.

The availability of image-based stereotactic surgery has enabled treatment of lesions that previously could be localized only indirectly and has drawn a large number of general neurosurgeons into the stereotactic

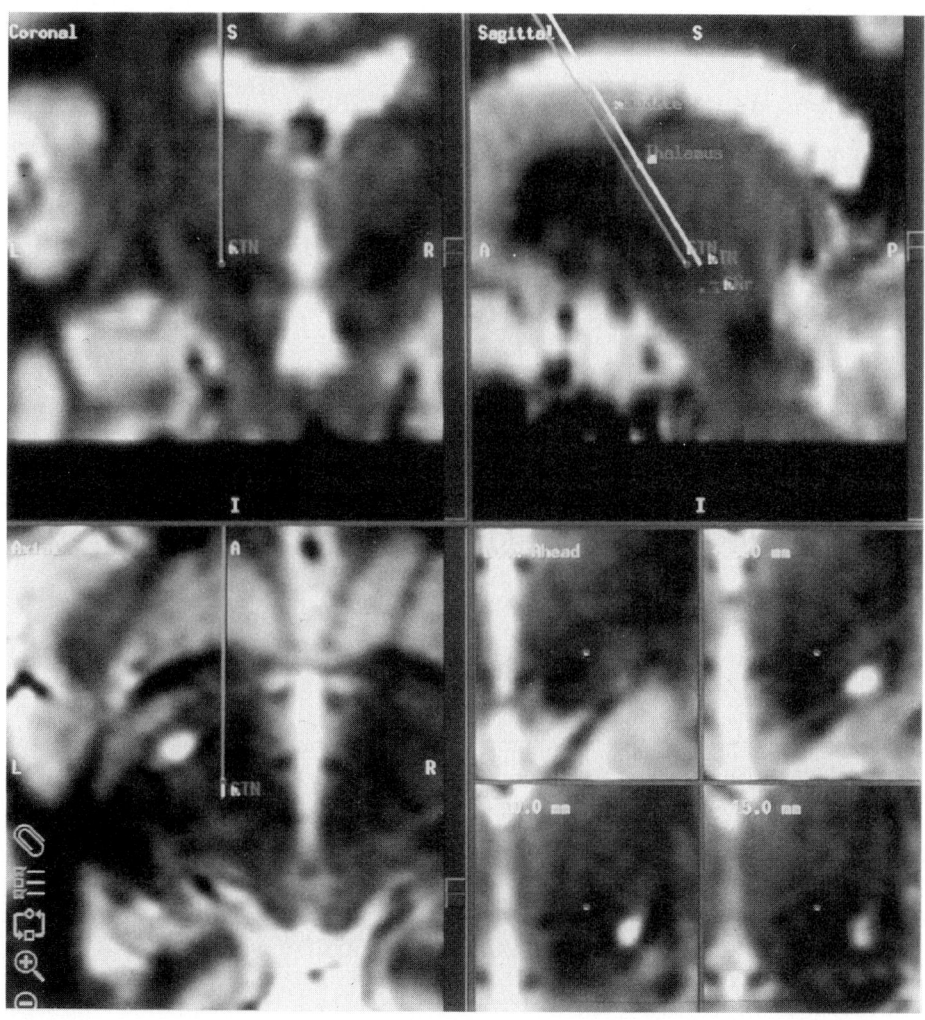

FIGURE 163–6. The StealthStation Treatment Guidance System (Medtronic Sofamor Danek, Memphis, TN) is used for magnetic resonance reconstructions, with stereotactic trajectories overlaid intraoperatively during microelectrode exploration of the subthalamic nucleus before placement of a deep brain stimulator.

field. During the past 15 years, the most common stereotactic procedure has been the biopsy.[74] Abscesses, hematomas, and cysts can be aspirated[204–208]; cannulas for brachytherapy[209] or isotope seeds[210] can be inserted into tumors; and endoscopy can be assisted by image guidance.[211] The approaches to and the boundaries of brain tumors can be defined before incision, and the stereotactic frame can be used to direct the surgeon to a target during craniotomy.[212]

Kelly[187, 213] developed the technology that made volumetric stereotactic guidance for tumor resection possible. The availability of three-dimensional data from computed tomographic scans enabled a target to be defined as a volume in space rather than a point in space. The volumetric image is displayed in the operating room to guide the surgical resection.[214] The stereotactic arc held a cylindrical retractor aimed at the center of rotation, which was used to direct the surgeon's view line along the same trajectory as the computer reconstruction. A heads-up display was added to the surgical microscope so that the surgeon could see the border of the tumor along the line of sight during resection.[214, 215] Similar techniques employ three-dimensional volumetric reconstruction to guide craniotomy, tumor resection, and endoscopy.[207, 216–218]

The introduction of computers brought another advance: development of frameless stereotactic systems. These systems allow coregistration of an instrument or a pointer relative to the patient's anatomy, as demonstrated by CT or MRI series (Fig. 163–6). Frameless systems generally are used to guide the surgeon during craniotomy and are not accurate enough to be employed for functional stereotactic neurosurgery. The first frameless system used the operating microscope to register in stereotactic space without the intervention of a frame by means of ultrasound triangulation and identified the view of the computed tomographic slices on a monitor in the operating room.[219] The first commercial frameless system was developed using a multiarticulated arm attached to the operating table or head holder.[220–222] A pointer is attached to the end of the arm. As the surgeon uses the pointer in the defined stereotactic space, the position of the pointer on the appropriate slice of the scan or three-dimensional display, or both, allows accurate determination of the relationship to the displayed structures.[223] Advances in frameless stereotactic surgery in this decade have been rapid, and newer systems no longer use multiarticulated arms but are freed by the use of ultrasonography,[224] light-emitting diodes,[225] or video "machine vision"[226] to localize hand-held pointers or instruments in stereotactic space. This powerful, rapidly expanding technology may soon add to the operative performance of all subspecialties of neurosurgery.

CONCLUSIONS

Functional neurosurgery has a long history and has evolved into many diverse disciplines. Stereotactic techniques have become a powerful tool for functional neurosurgical procedures. The stereotactic frame has become so linked to functional neurosurgery that the joint section of the American Association of Neurological Surgeons and the Congress of Neurological Surgeons combines them in the designation of *stereotactic and functional neurosurgery*. Stereotactic techniques have been so powerful that they have spread to other disciplines outside of functional neurosurgery as a means of neuronavigation, diagnosis, and treatment. Several functional disciplines, such as epilepsy and pain, have developed with minimal need of stereotactic techniques. Although epilepsy and pain are still considered functional issues, some investigators have attempted to develop them as independent disciplines. Other areas, such as movement disorders and psychosurgery, depend extensively on stereotaxis, and independence is nearly impossible.

The frame, however, may pass into history. The frame has been useful only as a means of registering a three-dimensional space. Imaging techniques are rapidly evolving so that four-dimensional space can easily be observed in real time and computer visualization can display rotations, scaling, translation, colorization, filtering, segmentation, and data manipulations to allow measurement enhancement of features, overlay of multidisciplinary data, and modeling of surfaces. Soon, holographic representations, heads-up displays, and virtual-reality technology will allow the surgeon to become completely integrated with the visualization of the target and the performance of the procedure. These improvements will allow greater precision, accuracy, and multiple interactions, even when the surgeon is earth bound and the operative field is in outer space.

Nevertheless, the basic driving elements of functional neurosurgery will remain the same. There will be a need to improve the quality of image acquisition and registration of the anatomy in stereotactic space. Moreover, such information would be useless unless we continue to expand our knowledge about the anatomy and physiology of disease and neurological injury such that accurate and precise interactions can be made to remedy abnormal function. In this regard, there will be decreasing use of lesioning and increasing use of stimulation. It is only natural that stimulation would be a useful technique in the central nervous system because it is an electrical organ.

The future of treatment may lie in cellular and gene therapy. There will always be a need for cellular replacement therapy to repair and restore lost function caused by disease or trauma. The ultimate goal is prevention, and as our understanding of the cellular and genetic basis of pathophysiology of disease and injury to the central nervous system develops, so shall our armamentarium of corrective and preventive therapies.

No matter how good the technology, the ultimate success of the discipline will reside in the performance of well-conducted clinical studies. Instead of accepting case reports, we should strive for a scientific approach. Even the great practitioners of functional neurosurgery were wrong sometimes, and because we all can be wrong about many things, the best way to test ideas is with rigorous, prospective, randomized studies employing standardized measures performed by experts blinded to the study paradigms.

REFERENCES

1. Leriche R: La Chirurgie de la Douleur. Paris, Masson, 1949.
2. Leriche R: La Philosophie de la Chirurgie. Paris, Flammarion, 1951.
3. Wertheimer P: Neurochirurgie Fonctionelle. Paris, Masson, 1956.
4. Taylor J (ed): Selected writings of John Hughlings. New York, Basic Books, 1958, pp 376–377.
5. Horsley SV: Brain-surgery. BMJ 2:670–675, 1886.
6. Horsley V, Taylor J, Colman W: Remarks on the various surgical procedures devised for the relief or cure of trigeminal neuralgia (tic douloureaux). BMJ 2:1139–1143, 1891.
7. Spiller W, Martin E: The treatment of persistent pain of organic origin in the lower part of the body by division of the anterolateral column of the spinal cord. JAMA 58:1489–1490, 1912.
8. White J, Sweet W: Pain: Its Mechanisms and Neurosurgical Control. Springfield, IL, Charles C Thomas, 1955.
9. White J, Sweet W: Pain and the Neurosurgeon. Springfield, IL, Charles C Thomas, 1969.
10. Horsley V: Remarks on the surgery of the central nervous system. BMJ, 1286–1292.
11. Horsley V: The Linacre Lecture of the function of the so-called motor area of the brain. BMJ 2:125–132, 1909.
12. Bucy P, Buchanan D: Athetosis. Brain 55:479–492, 1932.
13. Bucy P, Case T: Tremor. Physiologic mechanism and abolition by surgical means. Arch Neurol Psychiatry 41:721–746, 1939.
14. Putnam T: Treatment of athetosis and dystonia by section of the extrapyramidal motor tracts. Arch Neurol Psychiatry 29:504–521, 1933.
15. Putnam T: Results of treatment of athetosis by section of extrapyramidal tracts in the spinal cord. Arch Neurol Psychiatry 39:258–275, 1938.
16. Putnam T: Paralysis agitans and athetosis. Manifestations and methods of treatment. Arch Neurol Psychiatry 43:170–171, 1940.
17. Oliver L: Surgery in Parkinson's disease. Division of lateral pyramidal tract for tremor. Report on forty-eight operations. Lancet 1:910–913, 1949.
18. Gillingham F: Small localized lesions of the internal capsule in the treatment of dyskinesias. Confin Neurol 22:385–392, 1960.
19. Dandy W: Changes in our conceptions of localization of certain functions in the brain. Am J Physiol 93:643–647, 1930.
20. Meyers R: The modification of alternating tremors, rigidity and festination by surgery of the basal ganglia. Res Publ Assoc Res Nerv Ment Dis 21:602–665, 1942.
21. Meyers R: Surgical procedure for postencephalitic tremor, with notes on the physiology of premotor fibers. Arch Neurol Psychiatry 44:455–459, 1940.
22. Meyers R: Surgical experiments in the therapy of certain "extrapyramidal diseases." Acta Psychiatr Neurol 26:1–42, 1951.
23. Meyers R: Historical background and personal experiences in the surgical relief of hyperkinesia and hypertonus. In Fields W (ed): Pathogenesis and Treatment of Parkinsonism. Springfield, IL, Charles C Thomas, 1958.
24. Browder J: Parkinsonism—is it a surgical problem? N Y State Med J 47:2589–2592, 1947.
25. Browder J: Section of the fibers of the anterior limb of the internal capsule in parkinsonism. Am J Surg 72:264–268, 1948.
26. Fenelon F: Essais de traitement neurochirurgical du syndrom parkinsonien par intervention directe sur les voies extrapyramidales immediatement sousstriopallides (anse lenticulaire). Communication suivie de projection du dirm d'un des operes pris avant et apres l'intervention. Rev Neurol (Paris) 83:437–440, 1950.
27. Guiot G, Brion S, Fardeau M, et al: Dyskinesie volitionelle d'attitude supremee par la coagulation thalamo-capsulaire. Rev Neurol (Paris) 102:220–229, 1960.
28. Walker AE: Relief of pain by mesencephalic tractotomy. Arch Neurol Psychiatry 48:865–883, 1942.
29. Walker AE: Cerebral pedunculotomy for the relief of involuntary movements. I. Hemiballismus. Acta Psychiatr Neurol Scand 24:712–729, 1949.
30. Guiot G, Pecker J: Tractotomie mesencephalique anterieure pour tremblement parkinsonien. Rev Neurol (Paris) 81:387–388, 1949.
31. Walker AE: Cerebral pedunculotomy for the relief of involuntary movements: Parkinsonian tremor. J Nerv Ment Dis 116:766–775, 1952.
32. Spiegel EA, Wycis H, Baird HI: Long range effects of electropallido-ansotomy in extrapyramidal and convulsive disorders. Neurology 8:734–740, 1958.
33. Riechert T, Mundinger F: Indications, technique and results of the stereotactic operations upon the hypophysis using radioisotopes. J Nerv Ment Dis 13:1–9, 1960.
34. Bucy P: Cortical extirpation in the treatment of involuntary movements. Am J Surg 75:257–263, 1948.
35. Klemme R: Surgical treatment of dystonia, with report of one hundred cases. Assoc Res Nerv Ment Dis 21:596–601, 1942.
36. Cooper I: Ligation of the anterior choroidal artery for involuntary movements of parkinsonism. Psychiatr Q 27:317–319, 1953.
37. Rand R, Brown W, Stern W: Surgical occlusion of anterior choroidal arteries in parkinsonism: Clinical and neuropathologic findings. Neurology 6:390–401, 1956.
38. Cooper I: Chemopallidectomy. Science 121:217, 1955.
39. Cooper I: Chemopallidectomy and chemothalamectomy for parkinsonism and dystonia. Proc R Soc Med 52:47–60, 1959.
40. Cooper I, Bravo G, Riklan M, et al:, Chemopallidectomy and chemothalamectomy for parkinsonism. Geriatrics 13:127–147, 1958.
41. Hassler R, Reichert T: Indikation und Lokalisationsmethode der gezielten Hirnoperationen. Nervenarzt 25:441–447, 1954.
42. Cooper IS, et al: Clinical physiology of motor contribution of the pulvinar in man: A study of cryopulvinectomy. In Cooper IS, et al (eds): The Pulvinar-LP Complex. Springfield, IL, Charles C Thomas 1974, pp 220–232.
43. Cooper IS: Effect of chronic stimulation of anterior cerebellum on neurological disease. Lancet 1(7796):206, 1973.
44. Dittmar C: Ueber die Lage des sogenannten Gefaesszentrums in der Medulla oblongata. Bar Saech Ges Wiss Leipzig (Math Phys) 25:449–469, 1873.
45. Zernov D: Encephalometer. Device for estimation of parts of brain in human [in Russian]. Proc Soc Physiomed (Moscow) 2:70–80, 1889.
46. Altukhov NV: Encephalometric Investigations of the Brain Relative to the Sex, Age and Skull Indexes. Moscow, 1891.
47. Horsley V, Clarke R: The structure and functions of the cerebellum examined by a new method. Brain 31:45–124, 1908.
48. Fodstad H, Hariz M, Ljunggren B: History of Clarke's stereotactic instrument. Stereotact Funct Neurosurg 57:130–40, 1991.
49. Levy R: A Short History of Stereotactic Neurosurgery. Park Ridge, IL, American Association of Neurological Surgeons, 1992.
50. Olivier A, Bertrand G, Picard C: Discovery of the first human stereotactic instrument. Appl Neurophysiol 46:84–91, 1983.
51. Spiegel EA, Wycis H, Marks M, et al: Stereotaxic apparatus for operations on the human brain. Science 106:349–350, 1947.
52. Spiegel EA, Wycis H: Stereoencephalotomy. Part I. New York, Grune & Stratton, 1952.
53. Freeman W, Watts J: Psychosurgery: Intelligence, emotional and social behavior following prefrontal lobotomy for mental disorders. Springfield, IL, Charles C Thomas, 1942.
54. Moniz E: Tentatives operatoires dans le traitement de certaines psychoses. Paris: Mason & Cie, 1936, p 248.
55. Fulton JF, Jacobsen CF: The functions of the frontal lobes, a comparative study in monkeys, chimpanzees, and man. Presented at the Second International Neurological Congress, 1935, London.
56. Keele K: Anatomies of Pain. Baltimore, Williams & Wilkins, 1949.
57. Livingston W: Pain Mechanisms. New York, Macmillan, 1943.
58. Schwartz H, O'Leary J: Section of the spinothalamic tract in the medulla with observations on the pathways for pain. Surgery 9:183–193, 1941.
59. Dogliotti M: First surgical sections, in man, of the lemniscal lateralis (pain-temperature path) at the brain stem, for the treatment of diffuse rebellious pain. Anesth Analg 17:143–145, 1938.
60. Percheron G, Fenelon G, Leroux-Hugon V, Feve A: History of the basal ganglia system. Slow development of a major cerebral system [in French]. Rev Neurol (Paris) 150:543–554, 1994.

61. Abel-Fessard D, Arfel G, Guiot G, et al: Identification delimitation precise de certaines structures souscorticales de l'homme par l'electro-physiologie. C R Acad Sci III 243:2412–2414, 1961.

62. Spiegel EA, Wycis H: Pallido-thalamotomy in chorea. Arch Neurol Psychiatry 64:495–496, 1950.

63. Spiegel EA, Wycis H: Ansotomy in paralysis agitans. Arch Neurol Psychiatry 71:598–614, 1954.

64. Spiegel EA, Wycis H, Szekely E, et al: Campotomy in various extrapyramidal disorders. J Neurosurg 20:871–881, 1963.

65. Spiegel EA, Wycis H, Szekely E, et al: Stimulation of Forel's field during stereotaxic operations in the human brain. Electroencephalogr Clin Neurophysiol 16:537–548, 1964.

66. Spiegel EA: History of human stereotaxy (stereoencephalotomy). In Schaltenbrand G, Walker AAE (eds): Stereotaxy of the Human Brain: Anatomical, Physiological and Clinical Applications. Stuttgart, Georg Thieme Verlag, 1982, pp 3–10.

67. Spiegel EA: Methodological problems in stereoencephalotomy. Confin Neurol 26:125–132, 1965.

68. Gildenberg P, Tasker RR: Principles of stereotaxis and instruments. In DeSalles GS (ed): Stereotactic Surgery and Radiosurgery. Madison, WI, Medical Physics, 1993, pp 17–28.

69. Leksell L: A stereotaxic apparatus for intracerebral surgery. Acta Chir Scand 99:229–233, 1949.

70. Riechert T, Wolff M: Uber ein neues Zielgeraet zur intrakraniellen elektrischen Abteilung und Ausschaltung. Arch Psyhiatry Z Neurol 186:226–230, 1951.

71. Todd EM: Stereotaxic surgery of the basal ganglia. In Wells T (ed): Manual of Stereotaxic Procedures. Randolph, MA, Codman & Shurtleff, 1967.

72. Brown RA, Roberts TS, Osborn AG: Stereotaxic frame and computer software for CT-directed neurosurgical localization. Invest Radiol 15:308–312, 1980.

73. Gildenberg PL: Survey of stereotactic and functional neurosurgery in the United States and Canada. Appl Neurophysiol 38:31–37, 1975.

74. Gildenberg PL, Franklin P: Survey of CT-guided stereotactic surgery. Appl Neurophysiol 48:477–480, 1985.

75. Cooper I, Lee A: Cryostatic congelation. J Nerv Ment Dis 133:259–263, 1961.

76. Cosman ER, Nashold BS, Bedenbaugh P: Stereotactic radiofrequency lesion making. Appl Neurophysiol 46:160–166, 1983.

77. Talairach J, David M, Tournoux P, et al: Atals d'anatomie stereotaxique. Paris, Masson, 1957.

78. Schaltenbrand G, Bailey P: Introduction to Stereotaxis with an Atlas of the Human Brain. Stuttgart, Georg Thieme Verlag, 1959.

79. Tasker RR, Organ LW, Hawryishyn PA: The Thalamus and Midbrain of Man. A Physiological Atlas Using Electrical Stimulation. Springfield, IL, Charles C Thomas, 1982.

80. Spiegel EA, Wycis H: Stereoencephalotomy. Part II. Clinical and Physiological Applications. New York, Grune & Stratton, 1962.

81. Andy O: Diencephalic coagulation in the treatment of hemiballism. Confin Neurol 23:346–350, 1962.

82. Meyers R, Fry W, Fry F, et al: Early experiences with ultrasonic irradiation of the pallidofugal and nigra complexes in hyperkinetic and hypertonic disorders. J Neurosurg 16:32–54, 1959.

83. Narabayashi H, Okuma T: Procaine oil blocking of the globus pallidus for the treatment of rigidity and tremor of parkinsonism. Proc Japan Acad 29:310–318, 1953.

84. Svennilson E, Torvik A, Lowe R: Treatment of parkinsonism by stereotactic thermolesions in the pallidal region. A clinical evaluate of 81 cases. Acta Psychiatr Neurol Scand 35:358–377, 1960.

85. Laitinen LV, Bergenheim AT, Hariz MI: Leksell's posteroventral pallidotomy in the treatment of Parkinson's disease. J Neurosurg 76:53–61, 1992.

86. Laitinen LV, Bergenheim AT, Hariz MI: Ventroposterolateral pallidotomy can abolish all parkinsonian symptoms. Stereotact Funct Neurosurg 58:14–21, 1992.

87. Cooper I: Neurosurgical alleviation of intention tremor of multiple sclerosis and cerebellar disease. N Engl J Med 263:441–444, 1960.

88. Tsubokawa T, Moriyasu N: Lateral pallidotomy for relief of ballistic movement—its basic evidences and clinical application. Confin Neurol 37:10–15, 1975.

89. Tasker RR, Siqueira J, Hawrylyshyn P, Organ LW: What happened to VIM thalamotomy for Parkinson's disease? Appl Neurophysiol 46:68–83, 1983.

90. Kelly PJ, Ahlskog JE, Goerss SJ, et al: Computer-assisted stereotactic ventralis lateralis thalamotomy with microelectrode recording control in patients with Parkinson's disease. Mayo Clin Proc 62:655–664, 1987.

91. Reichert T: Long term follow-up of results of stereotaxic treatment of extrapyramidal disorders. Confin Neurol 22:356–363, 1962.

92. Mundinger F, Riechert T: Die stereotaktischen Hirnoperationen zur Behandlung extrapyramidaler Bewegungsstorungen (Parkinsonismus und Hyperkinesen) und ihre Resultate. Postoperative und Langzeitergebnisse der stereotakischen Hirnoperationen bei extrapyramidalmotorischen Bewedunasstrorungen. Teil B. Fortsch Neurol Psychiatry 31:69–120, 1963.

93. Levy A: Stereotaxic brain operations in Parkinson's syndrome and related motor disturbances. Comparison of lesions in the pallidum and thalamus with those in the internal capsule. Confin Neurol 29(Suppl):1–70, 1967.

94. Laitinen LV: Brain targets in surgery for Parkinson's disease: Results of a survey of neurosurgeons. J Neurosurg 62:349–351, 1985.

95. Guiot G, Hardy J, Albe-Fessard D: Delimitation precise des structures sous-corticales et identification de noyaux thalamiques chez l'homme par l'electrophysiologie stereotaxique. Neurochirurgie 5:1, 1962.

96. Guiot G, Arfel G, Derome P, Kahn A: Neurophysiologic control procedures for stereotaxic thalamotomy [in French]. Neurochirurgie 14:553–566, 1968.

97. Lenz FA, Tasker RR, Kwan HC, et al: Single unit analysis of the human ventral thalamic nuclear group: Correlation of thalamic "tremor cells" with the 3–6 Hz component of parkinsonian tremor. J Neurosci 8:754–764, 1988.

98. Tasker RR, Doorly T, Yamashiro K: Thalamotomy in generalized dystonia. Adv Neurol 50:615–631, 1988.

99. Ohye C, Maeda T, Narabayashi H: Physiologically defined VIM nucleus. Its special reference to control of tremor. Appl Neurophysiol 39:285–295, 1976.

100. Lenz FA, Normand SL, Kwan HC, et al: Statistical prediction of the optimal site for thalamotomy in parkinsonian tremor. Mov Disord 10:318–328, 1995.

101. Hirai T, Shibazaki T, Nakajima H, et al: Minimal effective lesion in the stereotactic treatment of tremor (proceedings). Appl Neurophysiol 42:307–308, 1979.

102. Ohye C, Hirai T, Miyazaki M, et al: Vim thalamotomy for the treatment of various kinds of tremor. Appl Neurophysiol 45:275–280, 1982.

103. Narabayashi H, Ohye C: Importance of microstereoencephalotomy for tremor alleviation. Appl Neurophysiol 43:222–227, 1980.

104. Narabayashi H, Gildenberg PL, Franklin PO: Proceedings of the meeting on the use of microphysiological recordings during stereotactic neurosurgery. Stereotact Funct Neurosurg 52:77–261, 1989.

105. Tasker RR, Dostrovsky JO: What goes on in the motor thalamus? Stereotact Funct Neurosurg 60:121–126, 1993.

106. Bertrand G, Jasper H: Microelectrode recording of unit activity in the human thalamus. Confin Neurol 26:205–208, 1965.

107. Hutchison WD, Lozano AM, Davis KD, et al: Differential neuronal activity in segments of globus pallidus in Parkinson's disease patients. Neuroreport 5:1533–1537, 1994.

108. Vitek JL, Bakay RA, Hashimoto T, et al: Microelectrode-guided pallidotomy: Technical approach and application for medically intractable Parkinson's disease. J Neurosurg 88:1027–1043, 1999.

109. Stereo D, Beric A, Dogali M, et al: Neurophysiological properties of pallidal neurons in Parkinson's disease. Ann Neurol 35:586–591, 1994.

110. Gildenberg PL: Whatever happened to stereotactic surgery? Neurosurgery 20:983–987, 1987.

111. Leksell L: The stereotaxic method and radiosurgery of the brain. Acta Chir Scand 102:316–319, 1951.

112. Tobias C, Lawrence J, Born J, et al: Pituitary irradiation with high-energy proton beams: A preliminary report. Cancer Res 18:121–134, 1958.

113. Larsson B, Leksell L, Rexed B: The high energy proton beam as a neurosurgical tool. Nature 82:1222–1223, 1958.

114. Leksell L: Stereotactic radiosurgery. J Neurol Neurosurg Psychiatry 46:797–803, 1983.

115. Steiner L, Forster D, Leksell L, et al: Gammathalamotomy in intractable pain. Acta Neurochir (Wien) 52:173–184, 1980.

116. Rand RW, Jacques DB, Melbye RW, et al: Gamma knife thalamotomy and pallidotomy in patients with movement disorders: Preliminary results. Stereotact Funct Neurosurg 61(Suppl 1):65–92, 1993.

117. Lunsford LD, Alexander E 3rd, Loeffler JS: General introduction: History of radiosurgery. In Alexander E 3rd, Loeffler JS, Lunsford LD (eds): Stereotactic Radiosurgery. New York, McGraw-Hill, 1993, pp 1–4.

118. Betti O, Derechinsky V: Hyperselective encephalic irradiation with a linear accelerator. Acta Neurochir Suppl (Wien) 33:385–390, 1984.

119. Colombo F, Benedetti A, Pozza F, et al: External stereotactic irradiation by linear accelerator. Neurosurgery 16:154–160, 1985.

120. Lutz W, Winston KR, Maleki N: A system for stereotactic radiosurgery with a linear accelerator. Int J Radiat Oncol Biol Phys 14:373–381, 1988.

121. Winston KR, Lutz W: Linear accelerator as a neurosurgical tool for stereotactic radiosurgery. Neurosurgery 22:454–464, 1988.

122. Friedman WA, Bova FJ: The University of Florida radiosurgery system. Surg Neurol 32:334–342, 1989.

123. Kooy HM, van Herk M, Barnes PD, et al: Image fusion for stereotactic radiotherapy and radiosurgery treatment planning. Int J Radiat Oncol Biol Phys 28:1229–1234, 1994.

124. Breggin P: The return of lobotomy and psychosurgery. Congressional Record 118:26–24, 1972.

125. National Commission for the Protection of Human Subjects of Biomedical and Behavioral Research: Report and Recommendations, Psychosurgery. Washington, DC, 1977.

126. Benabid AL, Koudsie A, Pollak P, et al: Future prospects of brain stimulation. Neurol Res 22:237–246, 2000.

127. Foerster O: On the indications and results of the excision of posterior spinal nerve roots in men. Surg Gynecol Obstet 16:463–474, 1913.

128. Ohye C: Role of thalamic nuclei in the hypertonia and tremor of Parkinson disease [in French]. Rev Neurol (Paris) 142:362–367, 1986.

129. Broggi G, Angelini L, Bono R, et al: Long term results of stereotactic thalamotomy for cerebral palsy. Neurosurgery 12:195–202, 1983.

130. Hassler R: Sagittal thalamotomy for relief of motor disorders in cases of double athetosis and cerebral palsy. Confin Neurol 34:18–28, 1972.

131. Siegfried J: Destructive stereotactic procedures for spasticity directed to the brain and the cerebellum. In Sindour M, Abbott R, Keravel Y (eds): Neurosurgery for Spasticity: A Multidisciplinary Approach. New York, Springer-Verlag, 1991, pp 187–190.

132. Siegfried J, Verdie JC: Long-term assessment of stereotactic dentatotomy for spasticity and other disorders. Acta Neurochir (Wien) 24(Suppl):41–48, 1977.

133. Cooper IS: 20-Year follow-up study of the neurosurgical treatment of dystonia musculorum deformans. Adv Neurol 14:423–452, 1976.

134. Hassler R: Stereotactic brain surgery for extrapyramidal motor disturbances. In Schaltenbrand G, Bailey P (eds): Introduction to Stereotaxis with an Atlas of the Human Brain. New York, Grune & Stratton, 1959.

135. Blount J, Kondoh T, Ebner TJ, et al: Pallidotomy for the treatment of dystonia. Presented at the American Association of Neurological Surgeons meeting, 1996, Minneapolis.

136. Vitek JL, Bakay RA: The role of pallidotomy in Parkinson's disease and dystonia. Curr Opin Neurol 10:332–339, 1997.

137. Blond S, Siegfried J: Thalamic stimulation for the treatment of tremor and other movement disorders. Acta Neurochir Suppl (Wien) 52:109–111, 1991.

138. Fasano VA, Broggi G, Barolat-Romana G, Sguazzi A: Surgical treatment of spasticity in cerebral palsy. Childs Brain 4:289–305, 1978.

139. Sindou M, Mertens P: Indications for surgery to treat adults with harmful spasticity. In Sindour M, Abbott R, Keravel Y (eds): Neurosurgery for Spasticity: A Multidisciplinary Approach. New York, Springer-Verlag, 1991, pp 211–213.

140. Park T, Phillips L, Peacock W: Management of Spasticity in Cerebral Palsy and Spinal Cord Injury. Philadelphia, Hanley & Belfus, 1989, p 506.

141. Cook AW, Weinstein SP: Chronic dorsal column stimulation in multiple sclerosis: Preliminary report. N Y State J Med 73:2868–2872, 1973.

142. Penn RD: Intrathecal baclofen for spasticity of spinal origin: Seven years of experience. J Neurosurg 77:236–240, 1992.

143. Benecke R: Botulinum toxin for spasms and spasticity in lower extremities. In Jankovic J, Hallett M (eds): Therapy with Botulinum Toxin. New York, Marcel Dekker, 1994, pp 557–565.

144. Backlund EO, Granberg PO, Hamberger B, et al: Transplantation of adrenal medullary tissue to striatum in parkinsonism. First clinical trials. J Neurosurg 62:169–173, 1985.

145. Madrazo I, Drucker-Colin R, Diaz V, et al: Open microsurgical autograft of adrenal medulla to the right caudate nucleus in two patients with intractable Parkinson's disease. N Engl J Med 316:831–834, 1987.

146. Drucker-Colin R, Madrazo I, Shkurovich M: Open microsurgical autograft of adrenal medulla to caudate nucleus of patients with Parkinson's disease. Presented at the Schmitt Neurological Sciences Symposium, 1987, Rochester, NY.

147. Goetz CG, De Long MR, Penn RD, Bakay RA: Neurosurgical horizons in Parkinson's disease. Neurology 43:1–7, 1993.

148. Bakay RA, Kordower JH, Starr PA: Restorative surgical therapies for Parkinson's disease. In Tuszynski MH, Kordower JH (eds): CNS Regeneration: Basic Science and Clinical Advances. New York, Academic Press, 1999, pp 389–417.

149. Bakay RA: Selection criteria for CNS grafting into Parkinson's disease patients. In Lindvall O, Bjorklund A, Widner H (eds): Intracerebral Transplantation in Movement Disorders: Experimental Basis and Clinical Experiences. New York, Elsevier Science, 1991, p 137.

150. Stoddard SL, Tyce GM, Ahlskog JE, et al: Decreased catecholamine content in parkinsonian adrenal medullae. Exp Neurol 104:22–27, 1989.

151. Kordower JH, Cochran E, Penn RD, Goetz CG: Putative chromaffin cell survival and enhanced host-derived TH-fiber innervation following a functional adrenal medulla autograft for Parkinson's disease. Ann Neurol 29:405–412, 1991.

152. Brundin P, Nilsson OG, Strecker RE, et al: Behavioural effects of human fetal dopamine neurons grafted in a rat model of Parkinson's disease. Exp Brain Res 65:235–240, 1986.

153. Dymecki J, Pucilowski O, Dyr W, et al: Effects of intracerebral transplantation of immature substantia nigra in rats with experimentally induced Parkinson's disease. III. Results of behavioural and biochemical investigations. Neuropatol Pol 23:287–295, 1985.

154. Bjorklund A, Stenevi U: Reconstruction of the nigrostriatal dopamine pathway by intracerebral nigral transplants. Brain Res 177:555–560, 1979.

155. Bakay RA, Fiandaca MS, Barrow DL, et al: Preliminary report on the use of fetal tissue transplantation to correct MPTP-induced Parkinson-like syndrome in primates. Appl Neurophysiol 48:358–361, 1985.

156. Redmond DE, Sladek JR Jr, Roth RH, et al: Fetal neuronal grafts in monkeys given methylphenyltetrahydropyridine. Lancet 1:1125–1127, 1986.

157. Bankiewicz KS, Plunkett RJ, Jacobowitz DM, et al: The effect of fetal mesencephalon implants on primate MPTP-induced parkinsonism. Histochemical and behavioral studies. J Neurosurg 72:231–244, 1990.

158. Lindvall O, Rehncrona S, Brundin P, et al: Human fetal dopamine neurons grafted into the striatum in two patients with severe Parkinson's disease. A detailed account of methodology and a 6-month follow-up. Arch Neurol 46:615–631, 1989.

159. Mezey E, Chandross KJ, Harta G, et al: Turning blood into brain: Cells bearing neuronal antigens generated in vivo from bone marrow. Science 290:1779–1782, 2000.

160. Bjornson CR, Rietze RL, Reynolds BA, et al: Turning brain into blood: A hematopoietic fate adopted by adult neural stem cells in vivo. Science 283:534–537, 1999.

161. Kordower JH, Emborg ME, Bloch J, et al: Neurodegeneration prevented by lentiviral vector delivery of GDNF in primate models of Parkinson's disease. Science 290:767–773, 2000.

162. Dogali M, Fazzini E, Kolodny E, et al: Stereotactic ventral pallidotomy for Parkinson's disease. Neurology 45:753–761, 1995.

163. Merello M, Nouzeilles MI, Kuzis G, et al: Unilateral radiofrequency lesion versus electrostimulation of posteroventral pallidum: A prospective randomized comparison. Mov Disord 14:50–56, 1999.

164. Lozano AM, Lang AE, Galvez-Jimenez N, et al: Effect of GPi pallidotomy on motor function in Parkinson's disease. Lancet 346:1383–1387, 1995.

165. Baron MS, Vitek JL, Bakay RA, et al: Treatment of advanced Parkinson's disease by unilateral posterior GPi pallidotomy: 4-year results of a pilot study. Mov Disord 15:230–237, 2000.

166. Fine J, Duff J, Chen R, et al: Long-term follow-up of unilateral pallidotomy in advanced Parkinson's disease. N Engl J Med 342:1708–1714, 2000.

167. Fazzini E, Dogali M, Sterio D, et al: Stereotactic pallidotomy for Parkinson's disease: A long-term follow-up of unilateral pallidotomy. Neurology 48:1273–1277, 1997.

168. Bechtereva NP, Bondartchuk AN, Smirnov VM, et al: Method of electrostimulation of the deep brain structures in treatment of some chronic diseases. Confin Neurol 37:136–140, 1975.

169. Mundinger F, Neumuller H: Programmed stimulation for control of chronic pain and motor diseases. Appl Neurophysiol 45:102–111, 1982.

170. Mazars G, Merienne L, Cioloca C: Control of dyskinesias due to sensory deafferentation by means of thalamic stimulation. Acta Neurochir Suppl (Wien) 30:239–243, 1980.

171. Brice J, McLellan L: Suppression of intention tremor by contingent deep-brain stimulation. Lancet 1:1221–1222, 1980.

172. Andy OJ: Thalamic stimulation for control of movement disorders. Appl Neurophysiol 46:107–111, 1983.

173. Siegfried J, Lippitz B: Chronic electrical stimulation of the VL-VPL complex and of the pallidum in the treatment of movement disorders: Personal experience since 1982. Stereotact Funct Neurosurg 62:71–75, 1994.

174. Siegfried J, Lippitz B: Bilateral chronic electrostimulation of ventroposterolateral pallidum: A new therapeutic approach for alleviating all parkinsonian symptoms. Neurosurgery 35:1126–1129, discussion 1129–1130, 1994.

175. Benabid AL, Pollak P, Gervason C, et al: Long-term suppression of tremor by chronic stimulation of the ventral intermediate thalamic nucleus. Lancet 337:403–406, 1991.

176. Schuurman PR, Bosch DA, Bossuyt PM, et al: A comparison of continuous thalamic stimulation and thalamotomy for suppression of severe tremor. N Engl J Med 342:461–468, 2000.

177. Benabid AL, Pollak P, Louveau A, et al: Combined (thalamotomy and stimulation) stereotactic surgery of the VIM thalamic nucleus for bilateral Parkinson disease. Appl Neurophysiol 50:344–346, 1987.

178. Burchiel KJ, Anderson VC, Favre J, et al: Comparison of pallidal and subthalamic nucleus deep brain stimulation for advanced Parkinson's disease: Results of a randomized, blinded pilot study. Neurosurgery 45:1375–1382, discussion 1382–1384, 1999.

179. Ghika J, Villemure JG, Fankhauser H, et al: Efficiency and safety of bilateral contemporaneous pallidal stimulation (deep brain stimulation) in levodopa-responsive patients with Parkinson's disease with severe motor fluctuations: A 2-year follow-up review. J Neurosurg 89:713–718, 1998.

180. Gross C, Rougier A, Guehl D, et al: High-frequency stimulation of the globus pallidus internalis in Parkinson's disease: A study of seven cases. J Neurosurg 87:491–498, 1997.

181. Benabid AL, Pollak P, Gross C, et al: Acute and long-term effects of subthalamic nucleus stimulation in Parkinson's disease. Stereotact Funct Neurosurg 62:76–84, 1994.

182. Molinuevo JL, Valldeoriola F, Tolosa E, et al: Levodopa withdrawal after bilateral subthalamic nucleus stimulation in advanced Parkinson disease. Arch Neurol 57:983–988, 2000.

183. Moro E, Scerrati M, Romito LM, et al: Chronic subthalamic nucleus stimulation reduces medication requirements in Parkinson's disease. Neurology 53:85–90, 1999.

184. DeLong MR: Primate models of movement disorders of basal ganglia origin. Trends Neurosci 13:281–285, 1990.

185. Bergman H, Wichmann T, DeLong MR: Reversal of experimental parkinsonism by lesions of the subthalamic nucleus. Science 249:1436–1438, 1990.

186. Limousin P, Pollak P, Benazzouz A, et al: Effect of parkinsonian signs and symptoms of bilateral subthalamic nucleus stimulation. Lancet 345:91–95, 1995.

187. Kelly PJ, Kall B, Goerss S, Alker GJ Jr: Precision resection of intra-axial CNS lesions by CT-based stereotactic craniotomy and computer monitored CO_2 laser. Acta Neurochir (Wien) 68:1–9, 1983.

188. Leksell L, Leksell D, Schwebel J: Stereotaxis and nuclear magnetic resonance. J Neurol Neurosurg Psychiatry 48:14–18, 1985.

189. Hardy TL: A method for MRI and CT mapping of diencephalic somatotopography. Stereotact Funct Neurosurg 52:242–249, 1989.

190. Gerdes JS, Hitchon PW, Neerangun W, Torner JC: Computed tomography versus magnetic resonance imaging in stereotactic localization. Stereotact Funct Neurosurg 63:124–129, 1994.

191. Peluso F, Gybels J: Computer calculation of the position of the side-protruding electrode tip during penetration in human brain. Confin Neurol 34:94–100, 1972.

192. Giorgi C, Garibotto G, Cerchiari U, et al: Neuroanatomical digital image processing in CT-guided stereotactic operations. Appl Neurophysiol 46:236–239, 1983.

193. Tasker RR, Organ LW, Hawrylyshyn P: Investigation of the surgical target for alleviation of involuntary movement disorders. Appl Neurophysiol 45:261–274, 1982.

194. Spenser D: Stereotactic methods in the management of epilepsy. In Heilbrun MP (ed): Stereotactic Neurosurgery. Baltimore, Williams & Wilkins, 1988, pp 161–178.

195. Lunsford LD, Coffey RJ, Cojocaru T, Leksell D: Image-guided stereotactic surgery: A 10-year evolutionary experience. Stereotact Funct Neurosurg 54–55:375–387, 1990.

196. Gildenberg PL: Where have we been? Where are we going? Stereotact Funct Neurosurg 68(Pt 1):1–9, 1997.

197. Barcia-Salorio JL, Broseta J, Hernandez G, et al: A new approach for direct CT localization in stereotaxis. Appl Neurophysiol 45:383–386, 1982.

198. Colombo F, Angrilli F, Zanardo A, et al: A new method for utilizing CT data in stereotactic surgery: Measurement and transformation technique. Acta Neurochir (Wien) 57:195–203, 1981.

199. Patil AA: Compute tomography-oriented stereotactic system. Neurosurgery 10:370–374, 1982.

200. Laitinen LV: Noninvasive multipurpose stereoadapter. Neurol Res 9:137–141, 1987.

201. Koslow M, Abele MG: A fully interfaced computerized tomographic–stereotactic surgical system. Appl Neurophysiol 43:174–175, 1980.

202. Lunsford LD: A dedicated CT system for the stereotactic operating room. Appl Neurophysiol 45:374–378, 1982.

203. Meuli RA, Verdun FR, Bochud FO, et al: Assessment of MR image deformation for stereotactic neurosurgery using a tagging sequence. AJNR Am J Neuroradiol 15:45–49, 1994.

204. Broggi G, Franzini A, Peluchetti D, Servello D: Treatment of deep brain abscesses by stereotactic implantation of an intracavitary device for evacuation and local application of antibiotics. Acta Neurochir (Wien) 76:94–98, 1985.

205. Backlund EO, von Holst H: Controlled subtotal evacuation of intracerebral haematomas by stereotactic technique. Surg Neurol 9:99–101, 1978.

206. Tanikawa T, Amano K, Kawamura H, et al: CT-guided stereotactic surgery for evacuation of hypertensive intracerebral hematoma. Appl Neurophysiol 48:431–439, 1985.

207. Zamorano L, Chavantes C, Dujovny M, et al: Stereotactic endoscopic interventions in cystic and intraventricular brain lesions. Acta Neurochir Suppl (Wien) 54:69–76, 1992.

208. Musolino A, Merckaert P, Munari C, et al: Stereotactic endocavitary treatment of cysts and pseudocysts of glioma. Preliminary report. J Neurosurg Sci 33:107–114, 1989.

209. Gutin PH, Hosobuchi Y, Phillips TL, Stupar TA: Stereotactic interstitial irradiation for the treatment of brain tumors. Cancer Treat Rep 65(Suppl 2):103–106, 1981.

210. Gildenberg PL, Pettigrew LC, Merrell R, et al: Transplantation of adrenal medullary tissue to caudate nucleus using stereotactic techniques. Stereotact Funct Neurosurg 54–55:268–271, 1990.

211. Shelden CH, McCann G, Jacques S, et al: Development of a computerized microstereotaxic method for localization and re-

moval of minute CNS lesions under direct 3-D vision. Technical report. J Neurosurg 52:21–27, 1980.

212. Whittle IR, Denholm SW, Elshunnar K: CT-guided stereotactic neurosurgery using the Brown-Roberts-Wells system: Experience with 125 procedures. Aust N Z J Surg 61:919–928, 1991.

213. Kelly PJ, Alker GJ Jr: A method for stereotactic laser microsurgery in the treatment of deep-seated CNS neoplasms. Appl Neurophysiol 43:210–215, 1980.

214. Kelly PJ, Kall BA, Goerss S: Transposition of volumetric information derived from computed tomography scanning into stereotactic space. Surg Neurol 21:465–471, 1984.

215. Kelly PJ: Tumor Stereotaxis. Philadelphia, WB Saunders, 1991.

216. Hardy TL, Brynildson L: Computerized atlas for functional stereotaxis, robotics, and radiosurgery. In Antonio A, DeSales J (eds): Stereotactic Surgery and Radiosurgery. Madison, WI, Medical Physics Publishing, 1993, pp 29–46.

217. Kelly PJ: Stereotactic technology in tumor surgery. Clin Neurosurg 35:215–253, 1989.

218. Gildenberg PL, Ledoux R, Cosman E, Labuz J: The exoscope—a frame-based video/graphics system for intraoperative guidance of surgical resection. Stereotact Funct Neurosurg 63:23–25, 1994.

219. Roberts DW, Strohbehn JW, Hatch JF, et al: A frameless stereotaxic integration of computerized tomographic imaging and the operating microscope. J Neurosurg 65:545–549, 1986.

220. Drake J, Rutka J, Hoffman H: ISG Viewing Wand system. Neurosurgery 34:1094–1097, 1994.

221. Watanabe E, Watanabe T, Manaka S, et al: Three-dimensional digitizer (neuronavigator): New equipment for computed tomography-guided stereotaxic surgery. Surg Neurol 27:543–547, 1987.

222. Guthrie B, Kaplan R, Kelly P: Neurosurgical stereotactic operating arm. Stereotact Funct Neurosurg 54:497–500, 1990.

223. Golfinos JG, Fitzpatrick BC, Smith LR, Spetzler RF: Clinical use of a frameless stereotactic arm: Results of 325 cases. J Neurosurg 83:197–205, 1995.

224. Roberts DW, Strohbehn JW, Friets EM, et al: The stereotactic operating microscope: Accuracy refinement and clinical experience. Acta Neurochir Suppl (Wien) 46:112–114, 1989.

225. Barnett GH, Kormos DW, Steiner CP, Weisenberger J: Use of a frameless, armless stereotactic wand for brain tumor localization with two-dimensional and three-dimensional neuroimaging. Neurosurgery 33:674–678, 1993.

226. Heilbrun MP, McDonald P, Wiker C, et al: Stereotactic localization and guidance using a machine vision technique. Stereotact Funct Neurosurg 58:94–98, 1992.

227. Spiegel EA, Wycis HT, Szekely E, et al: Role of the caudate nucleus in Parkinsonian bradykinesia. Confin Neurol 26:336–341, 1965.

228. Baird H, Wycis H, Spiegel EA: Treatment of convulsions by pallidoansotomy. Arch Neurol Psychiatr 75:446–447, 1956.

229. Heimburger RF: Putamenotomy as an aid to upper extremity control. Confin Neurol 37:16–23, 1975.

230. Spiegel EA, Wycis HT: The central mechanism of emotions. Am J Psychiatr 108:426–431, 1951.

231. Mundinger F: Stereotaxic interventions on the zona incerta area for treatment of extrapyramidal motor disturbances and their results. Confin Neurol 26:222–230, 1965.

232. Mundinger F, Riechert T, Disselhoff J: Long-term results of stereotactic treatment of spasmodic torticollis. Confin Neurol 34:41–50, 1972.

233. Jinnai D, Nishimoto A: Stereotaxic destruction of Forel H for treatment of epilepsy. Neurochirurgie 6:164–176, 1963.

234. Spiegel EA, Wycis H: Mesencephalotomy for relief of pain. In: Anniversary volume for O Poetzl. Vienna, 1948, p 438.

235. Hecaen H, Talairach T, David, et al: Memoires originaux. Coagulations limitees du thalamus dans les algies du syndrome thamique. Rev Neurol (Paris) 81:917–931, 1949.

236. Rand RW, Crandall PH, Adey WP, et al: Electrophysiologic investigations in Parkinson's disease and other dyskinesias in man. Neurology 12:754–770, 1962.

237. Andy OJ: Thalamotomy in hyperactive and aggressive behavior. Confin Neurol 32:322–325, 1970.

238. Jasper H, Bertrand G: Thalamic units involved in somatic sensation and voluntary and involuntary movements in man. In Purpura D, Yahr M (eds): The Thalamus. New York, Columbia University Press, 1966, pp 356–390.

239. Dieckmann G, Hassler R: Stereotaxic treatment of extrapyramidal myoclonus. Confin Neurol 34:57–63, 1972.

240. Mark VH, Ervin FR, Hackett TP: Clinical aspects of stereotactic thalamotomy in the human. Part I. Arch Neurol (Chicago) 3:17–32, 1960.

241. Hassler R, Dieckmann G: Stereotaxic treatment of compulsive and obsessive symptoms. Confin Neurol 29:153–158, 1967.

242. Kudo T, Yoshii N, Shimizu S, et al: Effects of stereotaxic thalamotomy on intractable pain and numbness: Preliminary report. Keio J Med 15:191–195, 1966.

243. Hassler R, Riechert T: Uber einen Fall von doppelseitiger Fornicotomies bei sogenannter temporaler epilepsie. Acta Neurochir 5:330–340, 1957.

244. Spiegel EA, Wycis HT, Szekely E, et al: Study of the mesencephalic tegmentum in paralysis agitans and Parkinsonism. Arch Neurol (Chicago) 2:46–54, 1960.

245. Spiegel EA, Wycis HT, Orchinik C: Thalamotomy and hypothalamotomy for the treatment of psychoses. Proc Assoc Res Nerv Ment Disord 31:379–391, 1953.

246. Sano K: Sedative neurosurgery with special reference to posteromedial hypothalamotomy. Neurol Med Chir 4:112, 1962.

247. Roeder FD: Stereotaxic lesion of the tubular cinereum in sexual deviation. Confin Neurol 27:162–163, 1966.

248. Nago T, Saito Y, et al: Stereotaxic amygdalotomy for behavior disorders. Arch Neurol (Chicago) 9:1–16, 1963.

249. Bouchard G, Kim YK, Umbach W: Stereotaxic methods in different forms of epilepsy. Confin Neurol 37:232–238, 1975.

250. Toth S: The effect of removal of the nucleus dentatus on the Parkinsonian syndrome. J Neurol Neurosurg Psychiatry 24:143–147, 1961.

251. Heimburger RF, Whitlock CC: Stereotaxic destruction of the human dentate nucleus. Confin Neurol 26:346–358, 1965.

252. Riechert T: Development of human stereotactic surgery. Confin Neurol 37:399–409, 1975.

253. Schaltenbrand G, Spuler H, Nadjmi M, et al: The stereotaxic treatment of epilepsy. Confin Neurol 27:111–113, 1966.

254. Gillingham F: Small localized lesions of the internale capsule in the treatment of the dyskinesias. Confin Neurol 22:385–392, 1962.

255. Dierssen G: Treatment of dystonic and athetoid symptoms by lesions in the sensory portio of the internal capsule. Confin Neurol 26:404–406, 1966.

256. Diemath HE, Heppner F, Enge S, Lechner H: Stereotactic anterior cingulotomy in therapy resistant generalized epilepsy. Confin Neurol 27:124–128, 1966.

257. Balasubramaniam V, Kanaka TS, Ramanujam PB: Stereotaxic cingulumotomy for drug addiction. Neurol India 21:63–66, 1973.

CHAPTER **164**

Rationale for Surgical Interventions in Movement Disorders

THOMAS WICHMANN ■ MAHLON R. DELONG

Neuroscience research over the past decade has led to major insights into the structure and function of the basal ganglia and the pathophysiologic basis of basal ganglia disorders, such as Parkinson's disease and Huntington's disease.[1–8] The renaissance of stereotactic surgery for Parkinson's disease and other movement disorders has provided valuable neuronal and imaging data from human subjects. This chapter examines pathophysiologic models of hypokinetic and hyperkinetic basal ganglia disorders, emphasizing the changes in neuronal activity in the basal ganglia–thalamocortical circuits that may underlie the different motor signs of these disorders.

ANATOMIC SUBSTRATE FOR CIRCUIT DYSFUNCTION IN MOVEMENT DISORDERS

Ultimately, an understanding of the pathophysiology of movement disorders must rest on a clear understanding of the relevant underlying anatomic and physiologic organization of the basal ganglia and related cortical, thalamic, and brainstem structures. These basic aspects are given attention first. A more detailed account may be found in Chapter 165 and in a discussion of the neurocircuitry of Parkinson's disease by Wichmann and DeLong.[9]

The basal ganglia are comprised of the neostriatum (i.e., caudate nucleus and putamen), the ventral striatum, the external (GPe) and internal segments (GPi) of the globus pallidus, the subthalamic nucleus (STN), and the substantia nigra with its pars reticulata (SNr) and pars compacta (SNc). The striatum and STN are the main entry points for cortical and thalamic inputs into the basal ganglia. From the input nuclei, information is conveyed over multiple pathways to the principal basal ganglia output nuclei, the GPi and SNr. Basal ganglia outflow from GPi and SNr is directed to frontal areas of the cerebral cortex (through the thalamus) and at various brainstem structures (e.g., superior colliculus, pedunculopontine nucleus, parvocellular reticular formation). The anatomy of the basal ganglia and related structures is shown schematically in Figure 164–1.

Input to the Basal Ganglia

The striatum and STN are the principal input structures of the basal ganglia. The more abundant corticostriatal projections are topographically organized.[10–12] In primates, projections from the somatosensory, motor, and premotor cortices terminate in the postcommissural putamen, whereas prefrontal cortical areas project to the caudate nucleus and the precommissural putamen, and projections from the limbic cortices, amygdala, and hippocampus terminate preferentially in the ventral striatum. Although the relationship between corticostriatal and corticospinal projection neurons is uncertain, it is clear that these projections arise from different groups of cortical neurons. Electrophysiologic experiments have shown that corticostriatal projection neurons have slower conduction velocities, have lower spontaneous discharge rates, and respond less frequently to somatosensory input than neighboring corticospinal neurons.[13, 14]

Projections from the frontal lobe to the STN are also topographically arranged.[15, 16] Afferents from the primary motor cortex reach the dorsolateral part of the STN, and afferents from premotor and supplementary motor areas innervate mainly the medial third of the

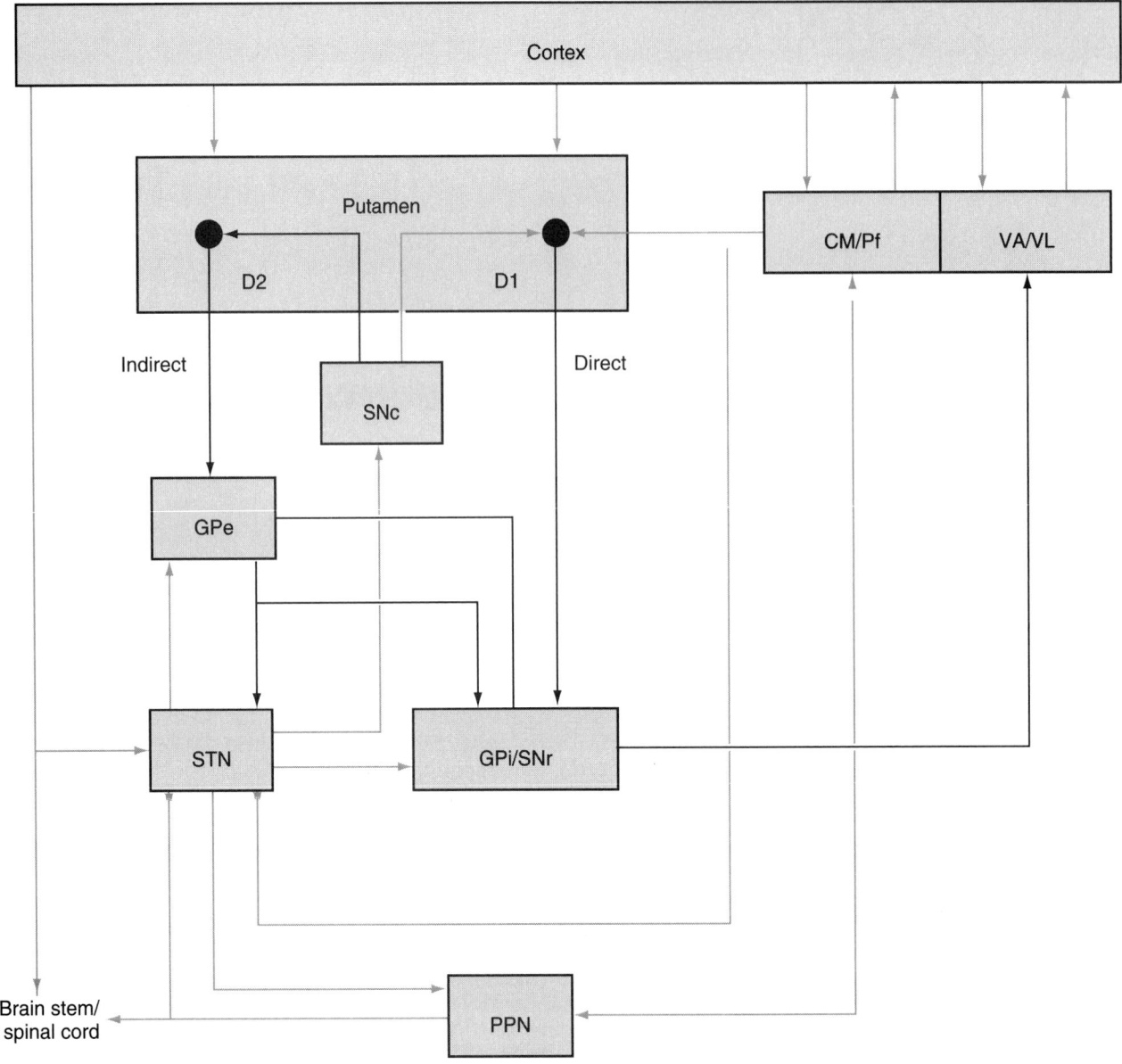

FIGURE 164–1. Schematic diagram of the basal ganglia–thalamocortical circuitry. Inhibitory connections are shown as filled arrows, excitatory connections as gray arrows. The principal input nuclei of the basal ganglia, the striatum and the STN are connected to the output nuclei, GPi and SNr. Basal ganglia output is directed at several thalamic nuclei (VA/VL and CM) and at brain stem nuclei (PPN and others). For abbreviations and further explanation of the model, see text.

nucleus.[17] The prefrontal or limbic cortices project to the ventral and most medial portions of the STN.

Topographically organized inputs to the striatum and STN also arise from the intralaminar nuclei of the thalamus, the centromedian and parafascicular nuclei. In primates, the centromedian nucleus projects to the motor portions of putamen and STN, whereas the parafascicular nucleus projects to associative and limbic territories.[18, 19]

Intrinsic Basal Ganglia Connections

The topography of the corticostriatal organization is maintained throughout the network of connections that link the striatum and the basal ganglia output structures, the GPi and SNr.[10] Although some striatofugal outputs collateralize to the GPe, GPi, and SNr,[20] most striatal projections to the other basal ganglia structures are organized into two distinct pathways, the so-called direct and indirect pathways.[3, 21]

The direct pathway arises from a discrete set of neurons that project monosynaptically to neurons in the GPi and SNr. The population of striatal neurons that gives rise to this pathway is further characterized by the presence of the neuropeptides substance P and dynorphin, by the preferential expression of the dopamine D_1 receptors, and by the fact that these neurons (and most striatal interneurons) appear to be the targets of thalamic inputs from the intralaminar nuclei of the thalamus.[22, 23]

The indirect pathway arises from a different set of striatal neurons that project to the GPe. These striatal neurons preferentially express enkephalin and dopamine D_2 receptors[24, 25] and may be a major target of cortical inputs.[22, 23] The indirect pathway is highly topographic.[26, 27] Populations of GPe neurons within the sensorimotor, cognitive, or limbic territory are reciprocally connected with populations of neurons in the same functional territories of the STN, and neurons in each of these regions innervate the same functional territory of the GPi.[26, 27]

The current model of the function of the basal ganglia–thalamocortical circuitry predicts that activation of striatal neurons that give rise to the direct pathway reduces inhibitory basal ganglia output from targeted neurons, with subsequent disinhibition of related thalamocortical neurons.[28] The net effect is increased activity in appropriate cortical neurons, resulting in facilitation of the movement. In contrast, activation of the striatal neurons that give rise to the indirect pathway leads to increased (inhibitory) basal ganglia output on thalamocortical neurons and to suppression of movement.

The segregation of D_1 and D_2 receptors between the direct and indirect pathways is probably not as strict as initially proposed,[25, 29] but it may still serve to explain the apparent differential action of dopamine on striatal output. Striatal dopamine appears to modulate the activity of the basal ganglia output neurons in GPi and SNr by facilitation of transmission over the direct pathway and inhibition of transmission over the indirect pathway.[30] The net effect of striatal dopamine release appears to be to reduce basal ganglia output to the thalamus and other targets. Dopamine may also more directly influence discharge patterns and rates in the STN and the pallidum through receptors located in these structures.

Output Projections of the Basal Ganglia

The caudoventral motor territory of the GPi projects almost exclusively to the posterior part of the ventrolateral nucleus, which sends projections toward the supplementary motor area (SMA),[31, 32] the primary motor cortex (M1), and premotor (PM) cortical areas.[33] The outflow from pallidal motor areas directed at cortical areas M1, PM, and SMA appears to arise from separate populations of pallidothalamic neurons.[33] The more rostromedial associative areas of the GPi project preferentially to the parvocellular part of the ventral anterior and the dorsal ventrolateral nucleus (VLc in macaques)[34, 35] and may be transmitted to prefrontal cortical areas[36, 37] and to motor and supplementary motor regions.[32, 38]

Other output projections from the GPi arise mostly as collaterals from the pallidothalamic projection. Prominent axon collaterals are sent in a segregated manner to the centromedian-parafascicular complex, projecting to the cortex and the striatum and constituting one of the many feedback circuits in the basal ganglia–thalamocortical circuitry.[34] Additional axon collaterals reach the noncholinergic portion of the pedunculopontine nucleus (PPN),[39, 40] which gives rise to ascending projections to the basal ganglia, thalamus, and basal forebrain and to descending projections to the pons, medulla, and spinal cord.[41]

Although the overlap between motor and nonmotor areas is probably greater in the SNr than the GPi,[42] the SNr can be broadly subdivided into a dorsolateral sensorimotor and a ventromedial associative territory.[43] Projections from the medial SNr to the thalamus terminate mostly in the medial magnocellular division of the ventral anterior nucleus (VAmc) and the mediodorsal nucleus (MDmc), which innervate anterior regions of the frontal lobe, including the principal sulcus and the orbital cortex in monkeys.[44] Neurons in the lateral SNr project preferentially to the lateral posterior region of VAmc and to parts of mediodorsal nucleus, which are predominately related to posterior regions of the frontal lobe, including the frontal eye field and areas of the premotor cortex.[44] The SNr also sends projections to the noncholinergic neurons of the pedunculopontine nucleus.[40, 45] Additional projections reach the parvicellular reticular formation, a region whose neurons are directly connected with orofacial motor nuclei,[46] and the superior colliculus, which plays a critical role in the control of saccades.[47]

PATHOPHYSIOLOGY OF MOVEMENT DISORDERS/PARKINSONISM

Pathologically, parkinsonism, the most common hypokinetic disorder, is characterized by progressive degeneration of the dopaminergic nigrostriatal projection, resulting clinically in the combination of akinesia, bradykinesia, rigidity, and tremor. The term *akinesia* is defined as poverty of movement, which is caused by impaired movement initiation, whereas *bradykinesia* refers to slowness of movement. Rigidity is characterized by an increased resistance to passive stretch, often associated with a rachety "cogwheel" sensation due to subclinical tremor. Parkinsonian tremor consists of low-frequency oscillations (4 to 6 Hz), mainly occurring at rest. The study of pathophysiologic changes in the basal ganglia that result from loss of dopaminergic transmission in the basal ganglia has been greatly facilitated by the discovery that primates treated with the neurotoxin l-methyl-4-phenyl-l,2,3,6-tetrahydropyridine (MPTP) develop behavioral and pathologic changes that closely mimic the features of Parkinson's disease in humans.[48, 49]

Changes in the activity over striatopallidal pathways were first suggested by studies in parkinsonian primates that indicated that metabolic activity (as measured with the 2-deoxy-glucose technique) is increased in both pallidal segments.[50, 51] This finding was interpreted as evidence for increased activity of the striatum-GPe connection and the STN-GPi pathway or, alternatively, as evidence for increased activity through the projections from the STN to both pallidal segments. Subsequent microelectrode recordings of neuronal activity in the primate MPTP model of parkinsonism showed directly that neuronal discharge is reduced in GPe and increased in STN and GPi compared with normal controls[52–54] (Fig. 164–2). In parkinsonian patients undergoing pallidotomy, it has similarly been shown that the discharge rates in the GPe are significantly lower than those in the GPi.[55–57] We have shown in the MPTP model of parkinsonism that the changes of neuronal activity in the second output nucleus of the basal ganglia, the SNr, are qualitatively similar to those occurring in the GPi.[58] The changes in discharge rates in the basal ganglia have been interpreted as indicating that striatal dopamine depletion leads to increased activity of striatal neurons of the indirect pathway, resulting in inhibition of the GPe and sub-

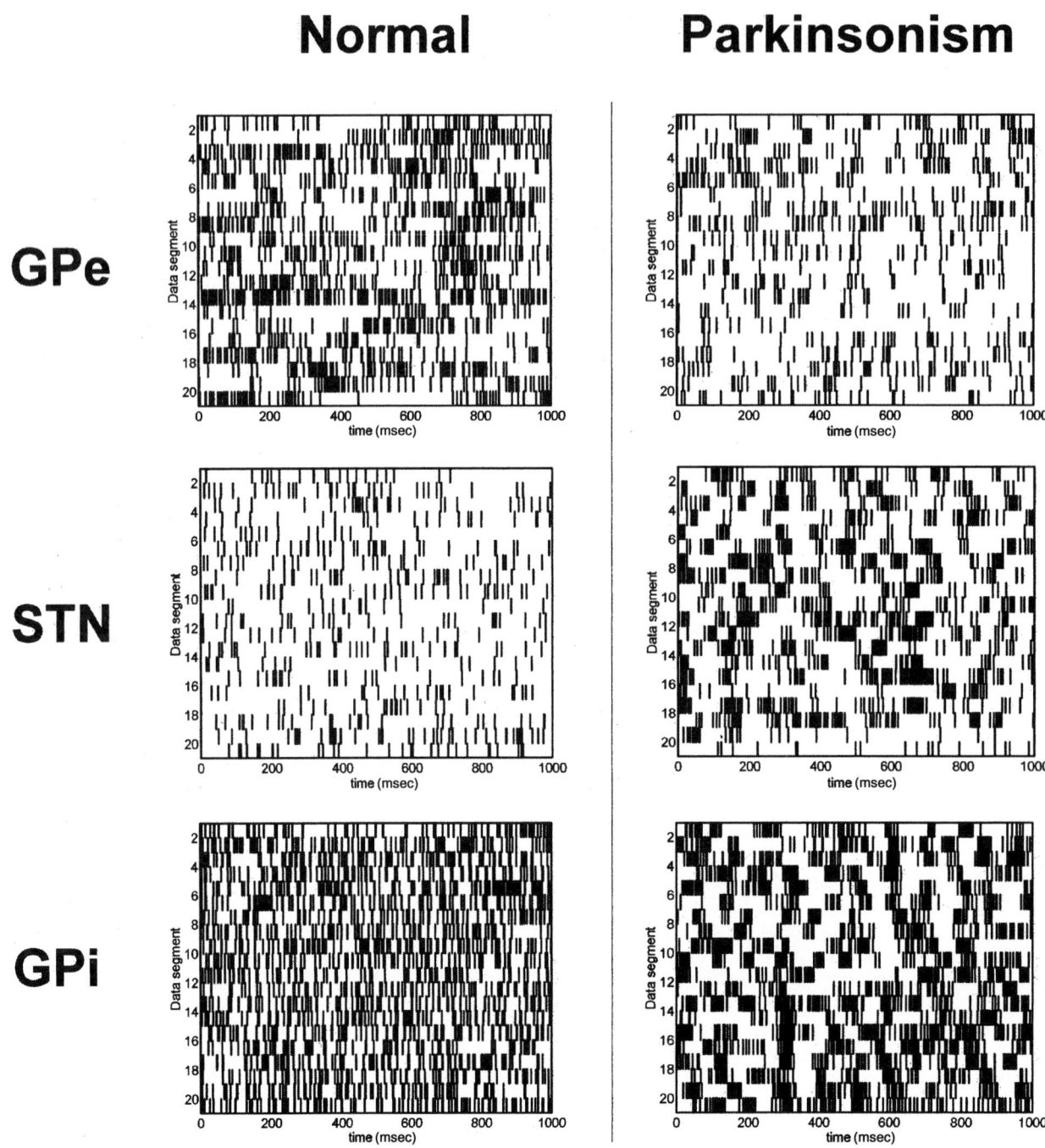

FIGURE 164–2. Raster displays of spontaneous neuronal activity recorded in the external and internal segments of the globus pallidus (GPe and GPi) in normal and parkinsonian primates. Each of the diagrams shows a 20-second segment of the spontaneous activity of a single neuron, which is displayed in 1-second intervals, with each tick representing a single action potential. In parkinsonism, the neuronal activity is reduced in the GPe and increased in the subthalamic nucleus (STN) and GPi. In addition to the rate changes, there are obvious changes in the firing patterns of neurons.

sequent disinhibition of the STN and GPi or SNr (Fig. 164–3). It is likely that other structures and feedback loops, such as those involving the pedunculopontine nucleus and the centromedian nucleus, aggravate or enhance the abnormalities of discharge in the basal ganglia output nuclei associated with Parkinson's disease. At the cortical level, studies of parkinsonian patients using positron-emission tomography (PET) have consistently shown reduced activation of motor and premotor areas.[59, 60]

Brainstem areas such as the pedunculopontine nucleus may also be directly (i.e., not through feedback interactions) involved in the development of parkinsonian signs. Lesions of this nucleus in normal monkeys can lead to akinesia, possibly by reducing stimulation of SNc neurons by input or by a direct influence on descending pathways.[61, 62]

The general pathophysiologic model outlined earlier is supported by the demonstration that lesions of the STN, GPi, or SNr in MPTP-treated primates reverse some or all signs of parkinsonism, presumably by reducing basal ganglia output.[63–65] During the past decade, these results have helped to rekindle interest in functional neurosurgical approaches to the treatment of medically intractable Parkinson's disease. This was first employed in the form of GPi lesions (i.e., pallidotomy)[66–69] and later in the form of STN lesions.[70] High-frequency deep brain stimulation (DBS) of the STN and GPi, whose mechanism of action is still uncertain, has been shown to reverse parkinsonian signs.[71, 72] PET studies in pallidotomy patients and in patients with DBS of the STN or GPi have shown a more normal pattern of activity after DBS in those frontal motor areas whose metabolic activity was reduced in the parkinsonian state.[67, 73]

The earlier rate-based circuit model of parkinsonism cannot explain many of the clinical and experimental features of the disease. Detailed studies of the results of lesions in human patients with parkinsonism have brought to light several findings that are incompatible with such models. For instance, lesions of the ventral anterior and ventrolateral nuclei of the thalamus (which completely remove thalamic output) do not lead to parkinsonism and are beneficial in the treatment of tremor and rigidity.[74, 75] Similarly, lesions of the GPi in the setting of parkinsonism improve all aspects of Parkinson's disease without producing dyskinesias or other obvious detrimental effects. In fact, they are highly effective in reducing drug-induced dyskinesias.[66, 67, 76] In contrast to the hypokinetic features of parkinsonism, dyskinesias appear to arise from pathologic reduction in basal ganglia outflow[77] and thus should not respond to, but should be made worse by further reduction of pallidal outflow.[78]

These seemingly paradoxical findings may be explained by the realization that parkinsonism may result from a combination of problems, including increased discharge rate, altered processing of proprioceptive input, and abnormal timing, patterning, and synchronization of discharge that introduces errors and nonspecific noise into the thalamocortical signal. Altered discharge patterns and synchronization between neighboring neurons have been extensively documented in parkinsonian monkeys and patients. For instance, neuronal responses to passive limb manipulations in the STN, GPi, and thalamus[52–54] have been shown to occur more often, to be more pronounced, and to have widened receptive fields after treatment with MPTP. There is also a marked change in the synchronization of discharge between neurons in the basal ganglia. In

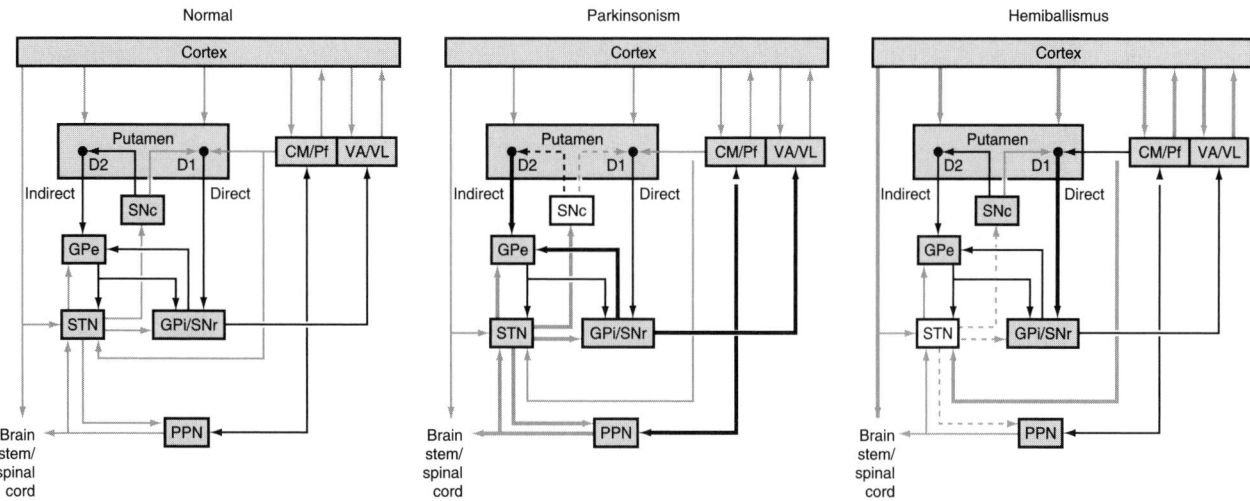

FIGURE 164–3. Changes in the neuronal activity of the basal ganglia–thalamocortical circuitry in movement disorders. The diagrams depict the changes encountered in parkinsonism *(center)*, a hypokinetic disorder, and in hemiballismus *(right)*, a hyperkinetic disorder. Inhibitory connections are shown as *filled arrows* and excitatory connections as *gray arrows*. Activity changes are indicated by the width of the respective arrows. In parkinsonism, the subthalamic nucleus (STN) drives the basal ganglia output structures. Hemiballismus is caused in most cases by a lesion of the STN, resulting in substantial reduction of activity in the internal segment of the globus pallidus (GPi) and the substantia nigra pars reticulata (SNr). For other abbreviations, please see text.

contrast to the virtual absence of synchronized discharge of such neurons in normal monkeys,[79] a substantial proportion of neighboring neurons in globus pallidus and STN discharge in unison in parkinsonian primates.[54] The proportion of cells in the STN, GPi, and SNr that discharge in oscillatory or nonoscillatory bursts is greatly increased in the parkinsonian state.[53, 54, 80] Oscillatory burst discharge patterns are often seen in conjunction with tremor, which may reflect tremor-related proprioceptive input or a more active participation of basal ganglia in the generation of tremor.

Conceivably, increased phasic activity in the basal ganglia may erroneously signal excessive movement or velocity to precentral motor areas, leading to slowing or premature arrest of ongoing movements and to greater reliance on external clues during movement. Alternatively, phasic alteration of discharge in the basal ganglia may introduce noise into thalamic output to the cortex that is detrimental to cortical operations. Parkinsonian patients have to compensate for the loss of basal ganglia contribution to movement and for the disruptive influence of the inappropriate basal ganglia output. The therapeutic benefits of GPi and STN lesions suggest that, in Parkinson's disease and other movement disorders, the total lack of basal ganglia output is more tolerable than disruptive abnormal output on brainstem and thalamocortical systems. Functional imaging studies have demonstrated that the surgical interventions do not necessarily normalize cortical motor mechanisms in parkinsonian subjects, but they may instead allow the intact portions of the thalamocortical and brainstem system to more effectively compensate for the loss of the basal ganglia contribution to movement.

Hyperkinetic Disorders

Hyperkinetic disorders encompass a spectrum of involuntary movements of different severity, ranging from mild restlessness to violent movements of entire limbs. The term *chorea* refers to discrete involuntary arrhythmic movements, and *ballismus* refers to proximal large-amplitude involuntary movements (likened to throwing motions). In chorea and ballism, purposeful movements can still be carried out, even in the presence of severe involuntary movements. The term *dystonia* refers to slower, more sustained movements and abnormal postures with prominent co-contraction of antagonist muscle groups and overflow of activation to inappropriate muscle groups, which is severely disruptive to the execution of intended movements.

Hyperkinetic disorders appear to have in common an overall reduction of basal ganglia output. This reduction is postulated to lead to disinhibition of thalamocortical neurons.[1, 3] Specific features of hyperkinetic disorders may be determined by abnormalities in the timing, patterning, and synchronization of basal ganglia output or by compensatory activity changes in subsequent stages of the thalamocortical circuitry.

HEMIBALLISM

Most cases of hemiballismus in humans and in animals result from lesions involving the STN. Studies in monkeys conducted in the 1940s and 1950s demonstrated that radiofrequency lesions of the STN that included at least 20% of the STN but spared pallidofugal fibers led to long-lasting, ballistic-appearing, choreiform movements, most commonly involving the leg.[81, 82] Similarly, small fiber–sparing lesions of the STN also result in dyskinesias of shorter duration.[83] A tight correlation between STN lesion and hemiballismus has also been described in humans. Magnetic resonance imaging (MRI) studies of patients with hemiballismus demonstrate in many cases discrete ischemic or hemorrhagic lesions of the STN.[84]

STN lesions interrupt the portion of the indirect pathway that traverses the STN (see Fig. 164–3). Metabolic and physiologic studies[85, 86] have demonstrated that STN lesions reduce neuronal activity in the GPe and GPi. In addition to the changes in discharge rate, the proportion of cells that respond to joint rotation with increases in discharge is greatly reduced in GPe and GPi under these conditions.[86] STN lesions in MPTP-treated animals also led to increases in discharge in thalamic areas that receive input from the basal ganglia, presumably because of lesion-induced reductions of (i.e., inhibitory) the GPi or SNr output to the thalamus (Yoshi Kaneoke and colleagues, unpublished observation, 1999). By virtue of feedback circuits, a reduction of basal ganglia output to the thalamus may further affect basal ganglia function. For instance, release of activity in the centromedian nucleus may lead to increased (i.e., excitatory) drive on striatal output neurons of the direct pathway, which would further reduce GPi output. This postulated positive feedback loop could contribute to the development of dyskinesias.

As is true for the other movement disorders, changes in overall basal ganglia output are probably not the only reason for the development of hemiballismus. Abnormally patterned activity may underlie the development of ballismus and other hyperkinetic disorders, and it may shape the specific features of the disorder in question.

HUNTINGTON'S DISEASE

Huntington's disease, a hereditary disorder resulting from pathologic expansion of CAG-trinucleotide repeat sequences in the Huntingtin gene on chromosome 4, is characterized by the gradual development of chorea and of cognitive and psychiatric abnormalities.[87] Pathologic studies[88, 89] have shown widespread neuronal degeneration, but striatal neurons appear to be a particularly affected group of cells.[90–93] Striatal degeneration first involves output neurons that project to the GPe.[93, 94] This may lead to reduced inhibition of neurons in GPe and subsequently to increased inhibition of STN neurons, resulting in decreased GPi output, the hallmark of hyperkinetic disorders. In later stages of the disease, inhibitory striatal output neurons to GPi begin to degenerate, which is postulated to result in disinhibition of GPi neurons. This may account for the late-stage reduction in chorea and the development of hypokinetic features.[93, 94]

Late stages of the disease are characterized by striatal degeneration that goes far beyond the motor portion of this structure. One of the most prominent anatomic and radiologic features of advanced Huntington's disease is caudate nucleus degeneration. Involvement of caudate associative and limbic circuits would affect nonmotor functions in particular and may contribute in part to the prominent psychiatric and cognitive abnormalities in this disease. Widespread neural degeneration in cortex, thalamus, and brainstem may also play a major role.

DRUG-INDUCED DYSKINESIA

After exposure to dopaminergic therapy for several years, a significant proportion of parkinsonian patients develop drug-induced dyskinesias. This has been attributed to transient shifts in the balance between the direct and the indirect pathway, with preponderance toward the direct pathway, resulting in decreased basal ganglia output. Dopamine receptor activation may result in activation of the direct pathway (through dopamine D_1 receptors), and inhibition of the putamen-GPe connection (part of the indirect pathway, through D_2 receptors). Both changes lead to reduced basal ganglia output and presumably to increased activity of thalamocortical neurons. It is questionable whether increased activity of the GPe, with resulting inhibition of STN and GPi, is the cause of drug-induced dyskinesias, because a study showed that excitotoxic lesions of GPe do not abolish L-dopa–induced dyskinesias in parkinsonian primates.[95] A more complex interaction between striatal dopamine D_1 and D_2 receptors[96] affecting the indirect and the direct pathway, or dopamine receptor activation at extrastriatal sites may play a role in drug-induced dyskinesias. It is also unclear why this phenomenon occurs predominantly after previous damage to the nigrostriatal system and exposure to L-dopa. Compensatory changes in dopamine receptor number or binding characteristics in response to dopamine depletion may be essential for this phenomenon.[30, 97, 98] In early parkinsonism, the "buffering capacity" of dopaminergic and other neurons for L-dopa may protect against the development of L-dopa–induced dyskinesias by preventing massive stimulation of postsynaptic dopaminergic receptors immediately after L-dopa administration. As more dopaminergic neurons are lost, this buffering capacity may be lost, leading to considerable oscillations in the level of dopaminergic stimulation in patients treated intermittently with L-dopa.[98]

Glutamatergic mechanisms may also play a significant role in the development of drug-induced dyskinesias. NMDA-receptor blockade can interrupt these drug-induced involuntary movements in experimental animals and in humans.[99] For example, the glutamate receptor antagonist amantadine has been shown to be effective in reducing drug-induced dyskinesias in patients and monkeys.[100, 101]

DYSTONIA

In patients with dystonia, normal movements are profoundly disrupted by co-contraction of agonist and antagonist muscles and by excessive activation of inappropriate musculature (i.e., overflow), leading to abnormal postures and slow involuntary movements. Dystonia may arise from a variety of disease processes, most of which involve the basal ganglia. Dystonia may occur in cases in which there is no clear cause identified (i.e., primary dystonias) and those with an underlying structural or biochemical defect (i.e., secondary dystonias). Secondary dystonia often develops after focal damage to the striatum (particularly the putamen), often occurring weeks or months after the inciting lesion. One of the main forms of primary dystonia is idiopathic torsion dystonia, which is caused by a genetic defect affecting chromosome 9.[102, 103] The gene (*DYT1*) codes for an ATP-binding protein, called torsinA,[104] which is found in particularly high concentrations in SNc neurons, suggesting a tie with dopamine function.

Dystonia is also frequently seen in patients with abnormalities of dopaminergic transmission. For instance, dystonia may develop in the context of parkinsonism, usually in patients who have been exposed to dopaminergic drugs, but it is also an early sign independent of antiparkinsonian medication. A group of patients with familial dystonia and parkinsonian features with onset at a young age respond dramatically to treatment with low-dose L-dopa (L-dopa–responsive dystonia[105, 106]), without the development of the troublesome, long-term motor side effects of this drug that are seen in patients with idiopathic Parkinson's disease. These patients suffer from a genetic defect of dopamine synthesis, caused by reduced GTP cyclohydrolase activity,[107–109] the rate-limiting enzyme in the biosynthesis of tetrahydrobiopterin a cofactor of the dopamine-synthesizing enzyme, tyrosine hydroxylase.

In cases in which dystonia results from lesions affecting the striatum or its dopaminergic supply,[110] such lesions may then affect the affinity or number of dopamine receptors in the unlesioned portion of the striatum or may lead to reorganization of striatal topography, resulting eventually in altered activity in the basal ganglia output structures. Metabolic studies in dystonic primates have suggested that dystonia may be associated with reduction of activity along the putamen-GPe connection and increased inhibition of the STN and GPi by GPe efferents.[111, 112] These activity changes in the indirect pathway are at odds with the results of PET studies and results of single-cell recordings in humans with dystonia that suggest activity changes in the direct pathway as well.

Unlike ballismus and chorea, in which involuntary movements occur independent of voluntary movements, the prominent dystonic features of co-contraction and "overflow" to inappropriate muscle groups are strongly tied to movement initiation and execution. The earliest manifestation of dystonia is often an "action dystonia," occurring only with attempted voluntary movement. This close dependence on movement initiation may be evidence that movement facilitation by the direct pathway of the basal ganglia may be affected more strongly in dystonia than in the other hyperkinetic movement disorders.

Pharmacologic studies suggest that abnormalities in the indirect and direct pathways are important in the development of dystonia. For instance, it has been shown that D_2-receptor antagonists have a substantial potential for inducing dystonia, presumably by increasing striatal outflow to the GPe through the indirect pathway, whereas D_1 receptor antagonists may be beneficial in this regard, presumably by reducing striatal outflow to the GPi along the direct pathway.[113, 114] By inference, these data suggest that a relative increase in the activity along the direct pathway (compared with that along the indirect pathway) may strongly contribute to dystonia. Supporting this concept, recording studies of patients undergoing pallidotomy as treatment for dystonia demonstrated lowered average discharge rates in both pallidal segments,[115] in contrast to parkinsonian patients in whom discharge rates in the GPi are increased.[56, 57, 116] The reduction of discharge in the GPe alone would lead to increased GPi discharge. The fact that discharge rates in GPi are reduced argues for additional overactivity of the direct (inhibitory) pathway. Increased activity along the direct pathway may be caused by activity changes in feedback loops that regulate GPi activity, such as the pathway through the centromedian nucleus (see Fig. 164–2). Cooper[117] reported that thalamic lesions were most effective against dystonia if they included the centromedian nucleus.

Phasic responsiveness of pallidal neurons to somatosensory stimuli in parkinsonism and dystonia is similar, with increased responses in both cases and with greater synchronicity between neighboring pallidal neurons. Increased phasic responses in the pallidum may result from increased STN input, because STN lesioning greatly reduces such responses in GPi neurons in normal animals.[86] The enhancement of phasic neuronal responses appears to differentiate dystonia from hemiballism physiologically.[86, 115]

Agonist-antagonist coactivation in dystonia may primarily reflect a defect in segregation of "channels" passing through the basal ganglia output nuclei (i.e., increased degree of synchronization). The development of dystonia would also depend on the presence of low overall discharge rates in the basal ganglia output nuclei, permitting excess movement. The degree of synchronization is probably determined for the most part by the presence or absence of dopamine in the striatum, but it could also be explained by extrastriatal dopamine loss, such as at the level of the STN. Given the differential effects of dopamine D_1- and D_2-receptor antagonists in the production of dystonia, the phenomenon of synchronization is likely to be primarily a function of abnormal discharge in the indirect pathway.

Lack of segregation may affect smaller channels within motor subcircuits or lead to synchronized activity between different subcircuits. The latter possibility has been favored by the results of PET studies of dystonic patients, which have demonstrated widespread changes in the activity of prefrontal areas.[118–121] The study by Karbe and colleagues[121] demonstrated reduced prefrontal activity (without further spatial subclassification), whereas later studies[118–120] demonstrated predominantly increased activity in SMA, anterior cingulate, and dorsolateral prefrontal motor areas. The differences between the studies may be explainable by the fact that focal and generalized dystonias of widely different causes were studied. Physiologic studies have also provided considerable evidence that dystonia is associated with increased excitability of motor areas (particularly the SMA), probably because of widespread decrease in cortical inhibition.[122–125]

These findings suggest that parkinsonism and dystonia may differ with regard to the level of activity in the direct pathway but that they have in common increased activity along the indirect pathway and increased phasic responsiveness and synchronization of pallidal discharge. From these considerations, it appears that the pathophysiology of dystonia may represent a combination of features of hyperkinetic and hypokinetic disorders.

CONCLUSIONS

Movement disorders are associated with increased and disordered discharge and with synchronization in motor areas of the basal ganglia–thalamocortical loops. Neuronal recording data and the observed effects of pallidal and thalamic lesions in these disorders suggest that the neuronal basis for the different basal ganglia movement disorders is not just changes in discharge rate, but also altered discharge patterns, abnormal and excessive synchronization of discharge, altered proprioceptive feedback, and the appearance of increased noise in the basal ganglia output signal. The effectiveness of ablative procedures and stimulation in treating hypokinetic and hyperkinetic disorders argues against a specific effect for these procedures on pathophysiologic processes. It is more likely that these interventions remove the abnormal signals directed to the thalamus, cortex, and brainstem, allowing the otherwise relatively intact systems to function undisturbed.

REFERENCES

1. DeLong MR: Primate models of movement disorders of basal ganglia origin. Trends Neurosci 13:281–285, 1990.
2. Wichmann T, DeLong MR: Functional and pathophysiological models of the basal ganglia. Curr Opin Neurobiol 6:751–758, 1996.
3. Albin RL, Young AB, Penney JB: The functional anatomy of basal ganglia disorders. Trends Neurosci 12:366–375, 1989.
4. Albin RL: The pathophysiology of chorea/ballism and parkinsonism. Parkinsonism Relat Disord 1:3–11, 1995.
5. Chesselet MF, Delfs JM: Basal ganglia and movement disorders: An update. Trends Neurosci 19:417–422, 1996.
6. Brooks DJ: The role of the basal ganglia in motor control: Contributions from PET. J Neurol Sci 128:1–13, 1995.
7. Graybiel AM: Basal ganglia: New therapeutic approaches to Parkinson's disease. Curr Biol 6:368–371, 1996.
8. Graybiel AM, Aosaki T, Flaherty AW, et al: The basal ganglia and adaptive motor control. Science 265:1826–1831, 1994.
9. Wichmann TM, DeLong R: Neurocircuitry of Parkinson's disease. In Davis KL, Charney D, Coyle JT, et al (eds): Neuropsychopharmacology: The Fifth Generation of Progress. New York, Lippincott Williams & Wilkins, 2002.

10. Alexander GE, DeLong MR, Strick PL: Parallel organization of functionally segregated circuits linking basal ganglia and cortex. Annu Rev Neurosci 9:357–381, 1986.
11. Parent A: Extrinsic connections of the basal ganglia. Trends Neurosci 13:254–258, 1990.
12. Haber SN, Kunishio K, Mizobuchi M, et al: The orbital and medial prefrontal circuit through the primate basal ganglia. J Neurosci 15:4851–4867, 1995.
13. Turner RS, DeLong MR: Corticostriatal activity in primary motor cortex of the macaque. J Neurosci 20:7096–7108, 2000.
14. Bauswein E, Fromm C, Preuss A: Corticostriatal cells in comparison with pyramidal tract neurons: Contrasting properties in the behaving monkey. Brain Res 493:198–203, 1989.
15. Monakow HK, Akert K, Kunzle H: Projections of the precentral motor cortex and other cortical areas of the frontal lobe to the subthalamic nucleus in the monkey. Exp Brain Res 33: 395–403, 1978.
16. Nambu A, Takada M, Inase M, et al: Dual somatopical representations in the primate subthalamic nucleus: Evidence for ordered but reversed body-map transformations from the primary motor cortex and the supplementary motor area. J Neurosci 16:2671–2683, 1996.
17. Takada M, Tokuno H, Hamada I, et al: Organization of cingulate motor areas inputs in primate basal ganglia. Eur J Neurosci 14: 1633–1650, 2001.
18. Smith Y, Parent A: Differential connections of caudate nucleus and putamen in the squirrel monkey (Saimiri sciureus). Neuroscience 18:347–371, 1986.
19. Sadikot AF, Parent A, Smith Y, et al: Efferent connections of the centromedian and parafascicular thalamic nuclei in the squirrel monkey: A light and electron microscopic study of the thalamostriatal projection in relation to striatal heterogeneity. J Comp Neurol 320:228–242, 1992.
20. Parent A, Charara A, Pinault D: Single striatofugal axons arborizing in both pallidal segments and in the substantia nigra in primates. Brain Res 698:280–284, 1995.
21. Alexander GE, Crutcher MD: Functional architecture of basal ganglia circuits: Neural substrates of parallel processing. Trends Neurosci 13:266–271, 1990.
22. Sidibe M, Smith Y: Differential synaptic innervation of striatofugal neurones projecting to the internal or external segments of the globus pallidus by thalamic afferents in the squirrel monkey. J Comp Neurol 365:445–465, 1996.
23. Parthasarathy HB, Graybiel AM: Cortically driven immediate-early gene expression reflects influence of sensorimotor cortex on identified striatal neurons in the squirrel. J Neurosci 17: 2477–2491, 1997.
24. Gerfen CR, Engber TM, Mahan LC, et al: D_1 and D_2 dopamine receptor-regulated gene expression of striatonigral and striatopallidal neurons. Science 250:1429–1432, 1990.
25. Surmeier DJ, Song WJ, Yan Z: Coordinated expression of dopamine receptors in neostriatal medium spiny neurons. J Neurosci 16:6579–6591, 1996.
26. Shink E, Bevan MD, Bolam JP, et al: The subthalamic nucleus and the external pallidum: Two tightly interconnected structures that control the output of the basal ganglia in the monkey. Neuroscience 73:335–357, 1996.
27. Smith Y, Bevan MD, Shink E, et al: Microcircuitry of the direct and indirect pathways of the basal ganglia. Neuroscience 86: 353–387, 1998.
28. Inase M, Buford JA, Anderson ME: Changes in the control of arm position, movement, and thalamic discharge during local inactivation in the globus pallidus of the monkey. J Neurophysiol 75:1087–1104, 1996.
29. Aizman O, Brismar H, Uhlen P, et al: Anatomical and physiological evidence for D_1 and D_2 dopamine receptor colocalization in neostriatal neurons. Nat Neurosci 3:226–230, 2000.
30. Gerfen CR: Dopamine receptor function in the basal ganglia. Clin Neuropharmacol 18(Suppl):S162–S177, 1995.
31. Schell GR, Strick PL: The origin of thalamic inputs to the arcuate premotor and supplementary motor areas. J Neurosci 4:539–560, 1984.
32. Inase M, Tanji J: Thalamic distribution of projection neurons to the primary motor cortex relative to afferent terminal fields from the globus pallidus in the macaque monkey. J Comp Neurol 353:415–426, 1995.

33. Hoover JE, Strick PL: Multiple output channels in the basal ganglia. Science 259:819–821, 1993.
34. Sidibe M, Bevan MD, Bolam JP. et al: Efferent connections of the internal globus pallidus in the squirrel monkey. I. Topography and synaptic organization of the pallidothalamic projection. J Comp Neurol 382:323–347, 1997.
35. DeVito JL, Anderson ME: An autoradiographic study of efferent connections of the globus pallidus in Macaca mulatta. Exp Brain Res 46:107–117, 1982.
36. Goldman-Rakic PS, Porrino LJ: The primate mediodorsal (MD) nucleus and its projection to the frontal lobe. J Comp Neurol 242:535–560, 1985.
37. Middleton FA, Strick PL: Anatomical evidence for cerebellar and basal ganglia involvement in higher cognitive function. Science 266:458–461, 1994.
38. Darian-Smith C, Darian-Smith I, Cheema SS: Thalamic projections to sensorimotor cortex in the macaque monkey: Use of multiple retrograde fluorescent tracers. J Comp Neurol 299: 17–46, 1990.
39. Harnois C, Filion M: Pallidofugal projections to thalamus and midbrain: A quantitative antidromic activation study in monkeys and cats. Exp Brain Res 47:277–285, 1982.
40. Rye DB, Lee HJ, Saper CB, et al: Medullary and spinal efferents of the pedunculopontine tegmental nucleus and adjacent mesopontine tegmentum in the rat. J Comp Neurol 269:315–341, 1988.
41. Inglis WL, Winn P: The pedunculopontine tegmental nucleus: Where the striatum meets the reticular formation. Prog Neurobiol 47:1–29, 1995.
42. Hedreen JC, DeLong MR: Organization of striatopallidal, striatonigral and nigrostriatal projections in the macaque. J Comp Neurol 304:569–595, 1991.
43. Deniau JM, Thierry AM: Anatomical segregation of information processing in the rat substantia nigra pars reticulata. Adv Neurol 74:83–96, 1997.
44. Ilinsky IA, Jouandet ML, Goldman-Rakic PS: Organization of the nigrothalamocortical system in the rhesus monkey. J Comp Neurol 236:315–330, 1985.
45. Steininger TL, Rye DB, Wainer BH: Afferent projections to the cholinergic pedunculopontine tegmental nucleus and adjacent midbrain extrapyramidal area in the albino rat. I. Retrograde tracing studies. J Comp Neurol 321:515–543, 1992.
46. von Krosigk M, Smith Y, Bolam JP, et al: Synaptic organization of GABAergic inputs from the striatum and the globus pallidus onto neurons in the substantia nigra and retrorubral field which project to the medullary reticular formation. Neuroscience 50: 531–549, 1993.
47. Wurtz RH, Hikosaka O: Role of the basal ganglia in the initiation of saccadic eye movements. Prog Brain Res 64:175–190, 1986.
48. Burns RS, Chiueh CC, Markey SP, et al: A primate model of parkinsonism: Selective destruction of dopaminergic neurons in the pars compacta of the substantia nigra by N-methyl-4-phenyl-1,2,3,6-tetrahydropyridine. Proc Natl Acad Sci U S A 80: 4546–4550, 1983.
49. Forno LS, DeLanney LE, Irwin I, et al: Similarities and differences between MPTP-induced parkinsonism and Parkinson's disease. Adv Neurol 60:600–608, 1993.
50. Crossman AR, Mitchell IJ, Sambrook MA: Regional brain uptake of 2-deoxyglucose in N-methyl-4-phenyl-1,2,3,6-tetrahydropyridine (MPTP)–induced parkinsonism in the macaque monkey. Neuropharmacology 24:587–591, 1985.
51. Schwartzman RJ, Alexander GM: Changes in the local cerebral metabolic rate for glucose in the 1-methyl-4-phenyl-1,2,3,6-tetrahydropyridine (MPTP) primate model of Parkinson's disease. Brain Res 358:137–143, 1985.
52. Filion M, Tremblay L, Bedard PJ: Abnormal influences of passive limb movement on the activity of globus pallidus neurons in parkinsonian monkeys. Brain Res 444:165–176, 1988.
53. Miller WC, DeLong MR: Altered tonic activity of neurons in the globus pallidus and subthalamic nucleus in the primate MPTP model of parkinsonism. In Carpenter MF, Jayaraman A (eds): The Basal Ganglia, II. New York, Plenum Press, 1987, pp 415–427.
54. Bergman H, Wichmann T, Karmon B, et al: The primate subthalamic nucleus. II. Neuronal activity in the MPTP model of parkinsonism. J Neurophysiol 72:507–520, 1994.

55. Dogali M, Beric A, Sterio D, et al: Anatomic and physiological considerations in pallidotomy for Parkinson's disease. Stereotact Funct Neurosurg 62:53–60, 1994.

56. Lozano A, Hutchison W, Kiss Z, et al: Methods for microelectrode-guided posteroventral pallidotomy. J Neurosurg 84:194–202, 1996.

57. Vitek JL, Kaneoke Y, Turner R, et al: Neuronal activity in the internal (GPi) and external (GPe) segments of the globus pallidus (GP) of parkinsonian patients is similar to that in the MPTP-treated primate model of parkinsonism. Soc Neurosci Abstr 19:1584, 1993.

58. Wichmann T, Bergman H, Starr PA, et al: Comparison of MPTP-induced changes in spontaneous neuronal discharge in the internal pallidal segment and in the substantia nigra pars reticulata in primates. Exp Brain Res 125:397–409, 1999.

59. Eidelberg D, Edwards C: Functional brain imaging of movement disorders. Neurol Res 22:305–312, 2000.

60. Ceballos-Baumann AO, Brooks DJ: Basal ganglia function and dysfunction revealed by PET activation studies. Adv Neurol 74:127–139, 1997.

61. Kojima J, Yamaji Y, Matsumura M, et al: Excitotoxic lesions of the pedunculopontine tegmental nucleus produce contralateral hemiparkinsonism in the monkey. Neurosci Lett 226:111–114, 1997.

62. Munro-Davies LE, Winter J, Aziz TZ, et al: The role of the pedunculopontine region in basal-ganglia mechanisms of akinesia. Exp Brain Res 129:511–517, 1999.

63. Bergman H, Wichmann T, DeLong MR: Reversal of experimental parkinsonism by lesions of the subthalamic nucleus. Science 249:1436–1438, 1990.

64. Wichmann T, Kliem MA, DeLong MR: Antiparkinsonian and behavioral effects of inactivation of the substantia nigra pars reticulata in hemiparkinsonian primates. Exp Neurol 167:410–424, 2001.

65. Lieberman DM, Corthesy ME, Cummins A, et al: Reversal of experimental parkinsonism by using selective chemical ablation of the medial globus pallidus. J Neurosurg 90:928–934, 1999.

66. Baron MS, Vitek JL, Bakay RAE, et al: Treatment of advanced Parkinson's disease by GPi pallidotomy: 1 year pilot-study results. Ann Neurol 40:355–366, 1996.

67. Dogali M, Fazzini E, Kolodny E, et al: Stereotactic ventral pallidotomy for Parkinson's disease. Neurology 45:753–761, 1995.

68. Laitinen LV, Bergenheim AT, Hariz MI: Leksell's posteroventral pallidotomy in the treatment of Parkinson's disease. J Neurosurg 76:53–61, 1992.

69. Lozano AM, Lang AE, Galvez-Jimenez N, et al: Effect of GPi pallidotomy on motor function in Parkinson's disease. Lancet 346:1383–1387, 1995.

70. Patel NK, Heywood P, O'Sullivan K, et al: Unilateral subthalamotomy in the treatment of Parkinson's disease. Brain 126:1136–1145, 2003.

71. Limousin-Dowsey P, Pollak P, van Blercom N, et al: Thalamic, subthalamic nucleus and internal pallidum stimulation in Parkinson's disease. J Neurol 246(Suppl 2):42–45, 1999.

72. Starr PA, Vitek JL, Bakay RA: Deep brain stimulation for movement disorders. Neurosurg Clin N Am 9:381–402, 1998.

73. Ceballos-Bauman AO, Obeso JA, Vitek JL, et al: Restoration of thalamocortical activity after posteroventrolateral pallidotomy in Parkinson's disease. Lancet 344:814, 1994.

74. Giller CA, Dewey RB, Ginsburg MI, et al: Stereotactic pallidotomy and thalamotomy using individual variations of anatomic landmarks for localization. Neurosurgery 42:56–62, 1998.

75. Tasker RR, Lang AE, Lozano AM: Pallidal and thalamic surgery for Parkinson's disease. Exp Neurol 144:35–40, 1997.

76. Rabey JM, Orlov E, Spiegelman R: Levodopa-induced dyskinesias are the main feature improved by contralateral pallidotomy in Parkinson's disease [abstract]. Neurology 45:A377, 1995.

77. Papa SM, Desimone R, Fiorani M, et al: Internal globus pallidus discharge is nearly suppressed during levodopa-induced dyskinesias. Ann Neurol 46:732–738, 1999.

78. Marsden CD, Obeso JA: The functions of the basal ganglia and the paradox of stereotaxic surgery in Parkinson's disease. Brain 117:877–897, 1994.

79. Wichmann T, Bergman H, DeLong MR: The primate subthalamic nucleus. I. Functional properties in intact animals. J Neurophysiol 72:494–506, 1994.

80. Filion M, Tremblay L: Abnormal spontaneous activity of globus pallidus neurons in monkeys with MPTP-induced parkinsonism. Brain Res 547:142–151, 1991.

81. Carpenter MB, Whittier JR, Mettler FA: Analysis of choreoid hyperkinesia in the rhesus monkey: Surgical and pharmacological analysis of hyperkinesia resulting from lesions in the subthalamic nucleus of Luys. J Comp Neurol 92:293–332, 1950.

82. Whittier JR, Mettler FA: Studies of the subthalamus of the rhesus monkey. II. Hyperkinesia and other physiologic effects of subthalamic lesions with special references to the subthalamic nucleus of Luys. J Comp Neurol 90:319–372, 1949.

83. Hamada I, DeLong MR: Excitotoxic acid lesions of the primate subthalamic nucleus result in transient dyskinesias of the contralateral limbs. J Neurophysiol 68:1850–1858, 1992.

84. Provenzale JM, Glass JP: Hemiballismus: CT and MR findings. J Comput Assist Tomogr 19:537–540, 1995.

85. Mitchell IJ, Sambrook MA, Crossman AR: Subcortical changes in the regional uptake of [³H]-2-deoxyglucose in the brain of the monkey during experimental choreiform dyskinesia elicited by injection of a gamma-aminobutyric acid antagonist into the subthalamic nucleus. Brain 108(Pt 2):405–422, 1985.

86. Hamada I, DeLong MR: Excitotoxic acid lesions of the primate subthalamic nucleus result in reduced pallidal neuronal activity during active holding. J Neurophysiol 68:1859–1866, 1992.

87. The Huntington's Disease Collaborative Research Group: A novel gene containing a trinucleotide repeat that is expanded and unstable on Huntington's disease chromosomes. Cell 72:971–983, 1993.

88. Mazurek MF, Garside S, Beal MF: Cortical peptide changes in Huntington's disease may be independent of striatal degeneration. Ann Neurol 41:540–547, 1997.

89. Heinsen H, Rub U, Gangnus D, et al: Nerve cell loss in the thalamic centromedian-parafascicular complex in patients with Huntington's disease. Acta Neuropathol 91:161–168, 1996.

90. Gutekunst CA, Levey AI, Heilman CJ, et al: Identification and localization of huntingtin in brain and human lymphoblastoid cell lines with anti-fusion protein antibodies. Proc Natl Acad Sci U S A 92:8710–8714, 1995.

91. Sapp E, Schwarz C, Chase K, et al: Huntingtin localization in brains of normal and Huntington's disease patients. Ann Neurol 42:604–612, 1997.

92. Furtado S, Suchowersky O: Huntington's disease: Recent advances in diagnosis and management. Can J Neurol Sci 22:5–12, 1995.

93. Albin RL, Reiner A, Anderson KD, et al: Striatal and nigral neuron subpopulations in rigid Huntington's disease: Implications for the functional anatomy of chorea and rigidity-akinesia. Ann Neurol 27:357–365, 1990.

94. Reiner A, Albin RL, Anderson KD, et al: Differential loss of striatal projection neurons in Huntington disease. Proc Natl Acad Sci U S A 85:5733–5737, 1988.

95. Blanchet PJ, Boucher R, Bedard PJ: Excitotoxic lateral pallidotomy does not relieve L-dopa–induced dyskinesia in MPTP parkinsonian monkeys. Brain Res 650:32–39, 1994.

96. Blanchet PJ, Grondin R, Bedard PJ: Dyskinesia and wearing-off following dopamine D₁ agonist treatment in drug-naive 1-methyl-4-phenyl-1,2,3,6-tetrahydropyridine–lesioned primates. Mov Disord 11:91–94, 1996.

97. Agid Y, Chase T, Marsden D: Adverse reactions to levodopa: Drug toxicity or progression of disease? Lancet 351:851–852, 1998.

98. Chase TN: The significance of continuous dopaminergic stimulation in the treatment of Parkinson's disease. Drugs 55(Suppl 1):1–9, 1998.

99. Blanchet PJ, Papa SM, Metman LV, et al: Modulation of levodopa-induced motor response complications by NMDA antagonists in Parkinson's disease. Neurosci Biobehav Rev 21(4):447–453, 1997.

100. Verhagen Metman L, Del Dotto P, van den Munckhof P, et al: Amantadine as treatment for dyskinesias and motor fluctuations in Parkinson's disease. Neurology 50:1323–1326, 1998; see comments.

101. Levesque D, Greenamyre JT: Amantadine suppresses dopamine agonist-induced dyskinesia in unilateral MPTP-treated monkey. Presented at the 6th Triennial Meeting of the International Basal Ganglia society, abstract volume 77, 1998.

102. Ozelius LJ, Hewett J, Kramer P, et al: Fine localization of the torsion dystonia gene (DYT1) on human chromosome 9q34: YAC map and linkage disequilibrium. Genome Res 7:483–494, 1997.

103. Risch N, deLeon D, Ozelius L, et al: Genetic analysis of idiopathic torsion dystonia in Ashkenazi Jews and their recent descent from a small founder population. Nat Genet 9:152–159, 1995.

104. Ozelius LJ, Hewett JW, Page CE, et al: The early-onset torsion dystonia gene (DYT1) encodes an ATP-binding protein. Nat Genet 17:40–48, 1997.

105. Nygaard TG: Dopa-responsive dystonia. Curr Opin Neurol 8:310–313, 1995.

106. Patel K, Roskrow T, Davis JS, et al: Dopa responsive dystonia. Arch Dis Child 73:256–257, 1995.

107. Ichinose H, Ohye T, Takayashi E, et al: Hereditary progressive dystonia with marked diurnal fluctuation caused by mutations in the GTP cyclohydrolase I gene. Nat Genet 8:236–242, 1994.

108. Nagatsu T, Ichinose H: GTP cyclohydrolase I gene, dystonia, juvenile parkinsonism, and Parkinson's disease. J Neural Transm Suppl 49:203–209, 1997.

109. Ichinose H, Nagatsu T: Molecular genetics of hereditary dystonia—mutations in the GTP cyclohydrolase I gene. Brain Res Bull 43:35–38, 1997.

110. Perlmutter JS, Tempel LW, Black LJ, et al: MPTP induces dystonia and parkinsonism. Clues to the pathophysiology of dystonia. Neurology 49:1432–1438, 1997.

111. Mitchell IJ, Luquin R, Boyce S, et al: Neural mechanisms of dystonia: Evidence from a 2-deoxyglucose uptake study in a primate model of dopamine agonist-induced dystonia. Mov Disord 5:49–54, 1990.

112. Hantraye P, Riche D, Maziere M, et al: A primate model of Huntington's disease: Behavioral and anatomical studies of unilateral excitotoxic lesions of the caudate-putamen in the baboon. Exp Neurol 108:91–104, 1990.

113. Gerlach J, Hansen L: Clozapine and D1/D2 antagonism in extrapyramidal functions. Br J Psychiatry 17(Suppl):34–37, 1997.

114. Casey DE: Dopamine D_1 (SCH23390) and D_2 (haloperidol) antagonists in drug-naive monkeys. Psychopharmacology 107:18–22, 1992.

115. Vitek JL, Zhang J, Evatt M, et al: GPi pallidotomy for dystonia: Clinical outcome and neuronal activity. In Fahn S, Marsden CD, DeLong MR (eds): Dystonia 3. Philadelphia, Lippincott-Raven, 1998, pp 211–220.

116. Sterio D, Beric A, Dogali M, et al: Neurophysiological properties of pallidal neurons in Parkinson's disease. Ann Neurol 35:586–591, 1994.

117. Cooper IS: Involuntary Movement Disorders. New York, Harper & Row, 1969, pp 160–161.

118. Eidelberg D, Moeller JR, Ishikawa T, et al: The metabolic topography of idiopathic torsion dystonia. Brain 118(Pt 6):1473–1484, 1995.

119. Galardi G, Perani D, Grassi F, et al: Basal ganglia and thalamocortical hypermetabolism in patients with spasmodic torticollis. Acta Neurol Scand 94:172–176, 1996.

120. Playford ED, Passingham RE, Marsden CD, et al: Increased activation of frontal areas during arm movement in idiopathic torsion dystonia. Mov Disord 13:309–318, 1998.

121. Karbe H, Holthoff VA, Rudolf J, et al: Positron emission tomography demonstrates frontal cortex and basal ganglia hypometabolism in dystonia. Neurology 42:1540–1544, 1992.

122. Hallett M, Toro C: Dystonia and the supplementary sensorimotor area. Adv Neurol 70:471–476, 1996.

123. Ikoma K, Samii A, Mercuri B, et al: Abnormal cortical motor excitability in dystonia. Neurology 46:1371–1376, 1996.

124. Hallett M: The neurophysiology of dystonia. Arch Neurol 55:601–603, 1998.

125. Berardelli A, Rothwell JC, Hallett M, et al: The pathophysiology of primary dystonia. Brain 121(Pt 7):1195–1212, 1998.

Anatomy and Synaptic Connectivity of the Basal Ganglia

YOLAND SMITH ■ ALI CHARARA

OVERALL ORGANIZATION OF THE BASAL GANGLIA

The basal ganglia are a group of subcortical nuclei of the mammalian brain that are intimately involved in motor control but also play complex roles in mediating cognitive and limbic functions. The basal ganglia traditionally include the striatum, which is composed of the caudate nucleus, the putamen, and the nucleus accumbens; the external globus pallidus (GPe; globus pallidus in nonprimates); the internal globus pallidus (GPi; entopeduncular nucleus in nonprimates); the substantia nigra, which includes the dopaminergic neurons in the substantia nigra pars compacta (SNc) and the γ-aminobutyric acid (GABAergic) neurons in the substantia nigra pars reticulata (SNr); and the subthalamic nucleus.

They are a complex and highly interconnected group of nuclei that have been the subject of intensive studies over many decades because of their clear involvement in neurological disorders that manifest as abnormal motor activities. The striatum and, to a lesser extent, the subthalamic nucleus are the main entrances of extrinsic information to the basal ganglia circuitry. The striatal architecture is divided into two compartments called *patches* (or striosomes) and *matrix,* which are characterized by differential expression of various neurotransmitters, receptors, and input-output connections.[1] The cerebral cortex and the intralaminar thalamic nuclei are the two major sources of excitatory glutamatergic afferents to the striatum and subthalamic nucleus. Dopaminergic inputs from the SNc and the ventral tegmental area, as well as serotonin inputs from the dorsal raphe, tightly interact with glutamatergic afferents to modulate striatal neuronal activity. After integration at the striatal level, the information is conveyed by medium-sized spiny projection neurons to the basal ganglia output nuclei (i.e., GPi and SNr) that forward basal ganglia outflow to frontal areas of the cerebral cortex through the ventrolateral thalamus or various brainstem structures (e.g., superior colliculus, lateral habenular nucleus, pedunculopontine nucleus, parvicellular reticular formation). Part of the informa-

tion flowing through the GPi returns to the striatum via connections with thalamostriatal neurons in the caudal intralaminar nuclei (Fig. 165–1).

Major aspects of the chemical anatomy and synaptic connectivity of the basal ganglia are reviewed in this chapter, and findings that have introduced novel concepts of basal ganglia organization are highlighted. A detailed account of the earlier literature is provided in several reviews published during the 1990s.[1–13]

AFFERENTS TO THE STRIATUM

Functional Organization of the Corticostriatal Projection

The entire cortical mantle provides a highly topographic input to the striatum. In primates, the somatosensory, motor, and premotor cortices project somatotopically to the postcommissural region of the putamen and the associative cortical areas project to the caudate nucleus and the precommissural putamen. The limbic cortices, the amygdala and the hippocampus, terminate preferentially in the ventral striatum, which includes the nucleus accumbens and the olfactory tubercle.[6, 7, 10, 12, 13]

Processing and integrating functionally related information within these striatal territories is probably very complex and governed by convergence and segregation of cortical inputs. For instance, projections from prefrontal oculomotor areas interconnected by corticocortical projections (i.e., frontal eye field and supplementary eye field) tightly overlap within the monkey striatum.[14] Conversely, Selemon and Goldman-Rakic[15] demonstrated that projections from connection-linked associative cortical areas in the frontal, parietal, and temporal lobes are completely segregated or interdigitated within a zone of overlap in the monkey striatum. The results of this study also introduced a novel concept of corticostriatal projection organization related to which associative cortices project to longitudinally extensive domains aligned along the mediolateral axis of the caudate nucleus in primates.[15] Complex patterns

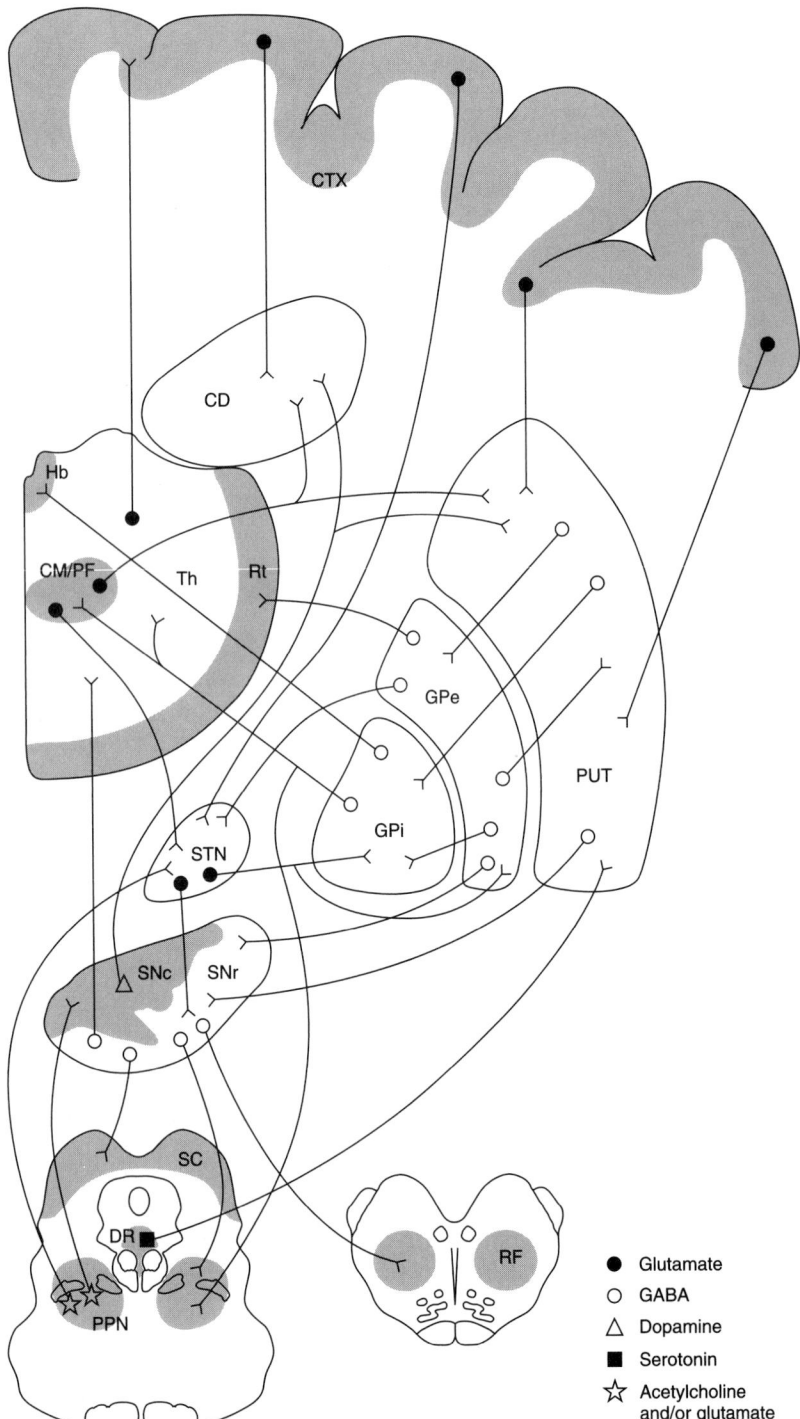

FIGURE 165–1. In the simplified schematic diagram of basal ganglia connectivity in primates, some connections have been omitted. The symbols used to label neuronal cell bodies indicate the main neurotransmitter used by these neurons. CD, caudate nucleus; CTX, cerebral cortex; CM/PF, center median/parafascicular nuclei; DR, dorsal raphe; GPe, globus pallidus, external segment; GPi, globus pallidus, internal segment; Hb, habenula; PUT, putamen; Rt, reticular nucleus; RF, reticular formation; SC, superior colliculus; SNc, substantia nigra, pars compacta; SNr, substantia nigra, pars reticulata; STN, subthalamic nucleus; Th, thalamus; PPN, pedunculopontine nucleus.

● Glutamate
○ GABA
△ Dopamine
■ Serotonin
☆ Acetylcholine and/or glutamate

of intrastriatal organization were also found for projections from sensorimotor cortical areas.[16, 17] For example, regions representing homologous body parts in different somatosensory cortical regions and primary motor cortex send projections that converge within the ipsilateral putamen, whereas contralateral projections from the primary motor cortex, except those from the face area, interdigitate with ipsilateral primary motor cortex and somatosensory cortical projection sites in squirrel monkeys.[17]

The striatum is composed of two main populations of neurons: the medium-sized GABAergic projection neurons, which have their dendrites densely covered with spines and account for more than 90% of the total neuronal population of the striatum, and the aspiny neurons, which are much less abundant and are generally considered to be interneurons.[3, 7, 10, 18] Dendritic spines of projection neurons are by far the main targets of corticostriatal afferents. Convergence of cortical and dopamine inputs at the level of individual spines was found to be a major feature of the synaptic connectivity of striatofugal neurons in rats and monkeys.[3, 12, 13] GABAergic interneurons also receive significant cortical inputs,[19] whereas cholinergic interneurons are almost completely devoid of cortical afferents except for sparse inputs on their distal dendrites.[20–21a] The projection neurons have extensive overlapping dendritic trees and emit axon collaterals that form symmetrical synapses with dendrites and spines of neighboring neurons in the striatum.[3, 7, 22] Although these intrastriatal connections have long been considered the main substrate for the mutual GABAergic inhibition between striatofugal neurons, electrophysiologic studies show that the inhibition among spiny neurons is rather weak.[23, 23a] This connection is powerful in terms of modulating the timing of action potentials generated by nearby spiny neurons.[23b] On the other hand, the feed-forward pathway through GABAergic interneurons is probably a better candidate for generating these inhibitory influences.[7, 8, 18, 24]

Three types of cortical neurons project to the striatum in rats.[7, 10] The most common type includes large cortical neurons located in deep layer V. These cells have extensive intracortical axon arborizations and emit fine collaterals, with only a few terminals in the ipsilateral striatum, which indicates that these cortical neurons innervate a limited population of striatal cells according to strict topographic organization. A less common type of pyramidal tract cell that contributes to the corticostriatal projection is medium sized and located in superficial layer V. These neurons have limited intracortical arborization but terminate profusely in the ipsilateral striatum. A third type of corticostriatal neuron is located in superficial layer V and the deep part of layer III. These neurons give rise to an extensive axonal arbor in the region of the parent perikaryon and form diffuse plexuses of axon terminals that occupy a large volume of the ipsilateral and contralateral striata. The region of the striatum innervated by these axons can be as large as 1 mm across, but within these regions, the density of axonal arborization is very sparse, leaving large areas not innervated. This pattern of arborization implies that individual cortical fibers cross the dendritic fields of many striatal neurons but form few synapses with any given cell.[8, 10] Conversely, striatal neurons can be expected to receive inputs from a large number of cortical fibers but not to receive many synapses from any one of them. The functional implications of such a pattern of organization are twofold. It suggests that striatal neurons may increase their firing rate only if there is activation of convergent input from many different cortical neurons and that nearby striatal neurons with totally overlapping dendritic volumes have few presynaptic cortical axons in common.[8, 10] These anatomic findings strongly support a high degree of specificity of the corticostriatal projection and explain the absence of redundancy in the responses of neurons near each other in the striatum.[7, 8]

Functional Organization of the Thalamostriatal Projection

In addition to the cerebral cortex, the intralaminar thalamic nuclei are a major source of excitatory afferents to the striatum. However, the influence of thalamic inputs on the activity of striatal neurons has received much less attention than corticostriatal projections. Anterograde tracing studies in rats and monkeys indicate that the thalamostriatal projection is massive, topographically organized, and highly specific.[6, 13, 25] In primates, the caudal intralaminar nuclear group (i.e., centromedian and parafascicular nuclei) provides massive inputs that largely terminate in different functional territories in the striatum.[6, 26, 27] Centromedian and parafascicular inputs terminate preferentially in the matrix compartment of the dorsal and ventral striatum.[26] The centromedian nucleus projects massively to the post-commissural sensorimotor part of the putamen, whereas the parafascicular nucleus innervates predominantly the caudate nucleus and, to a lesser extent, the ventral striatum.[26, 27] The striatal input from the parafascicular nucleus terminates in a patchlike manner that preferentially invades the matrix compartment in the caudate nucleus and the nucleus accumbens. The precommissural putamen receives inputs from the so-called dorsolateral parafascicular nucleus, a group of fusiform neurons that extends mediolaterally along the dorsal border of the centromedian.[28] In rats, thalamic inputs to the ventral striatum arise predominantly from midline and rostral intralaminar nuclei.[25] Specific relay nuclei also project to the striatum, although to a much lesser extent than intralaminar nuclei.[6, 13] As is the case for the motor and somatosensory cortical afferents, the centromedian nucleus input terminates in a bandlike fashion.[26, 27] Whether the thalamostriatal projection is somatotopic and overlaps with corticostriatal afferents is unknown.

The medium spiny neurons are the main targets of thalamic afferents, but in contrast to cortical terminals, which mostly terminate on the head of dendritic spines,[3] centromedian and parafascicular inputs preferentially innervate the dendritic shafts of striatal neurons.[13, 26, 27, 29] However, afferents from rostral intralaminar nuclei terminate almost exclusively on dendritic spines in rats.[30] In contrast to cortical and dopaminergic inputs, which often converge on common postsynaptic targets, centromedian and dopaminergic terminals largely innervate different striatal elements,[31] which suggests that dopaminergic afferents are located to subserve a more specific modulation of afferent cortical input than afferent thalamic input in the striatum. Striatal interneurons immunoreactive for choline acetyltransferase, parvalbumin, and somatostatin, but not those containing calretinin, receive inputs from the centromedian nucleus in monkeys.[32, 33] Centromedian inputs also display a high degree of specificity in their pattern of synaptic innervation of striatal projection neurons.

Together, these anatomic findings indicate that the thalamostriatal projections are more massive and much better organized than previously thought.[6, 13, 25–28, 31, 32] A major task for the coming years will be to elucidate the sources and better characterize the types of information transmitted by the different populations of thalamostriatal neurons. This will help to better understand the mechanisms by which thalamic and cortical inputs interact to control the activity of striatofugal neurons.

Some thalamic relay nuclei also project to the striatum in a highly specific and organized fashion.[34] Data demonstrate the convergence of interconnected cortical and ventral thalamic areas to specific regions of the sensorimotor striatum in monkeys.[35]

γ-Aminobutyric Acid and Glutamate Receptors in the Striatum

Although glutamate is the transmitter of cortical and thalamic afferents, highly specific actions on particular postsynaptic targets may be achieved through the different types of glutamate receptors. There are two categories of glutamate receptors: the ionotropic receptors, which mediate fast- and short-lasting excitatory effects, and the metabotropic receptors, which mediate slow- and long-lasting modulatory effects of glutamatergic transmission. Ionotropic glutamate receptors include *N*-methyl-D-aspartate (NMDA; NR1, NR2A-D), α-amino-3-hydroxyl-5-methyl-4-isoxazole-propionate (AMPA; GluR1 through GluR4), and kainate (GluR5 through GluR7, KA1, KA2) subtypes. Metabotropic receptors include eight subtypes pooled into three major groups: group I (mGluR1, mGluR5), group II (mGluR2, mGluR3), and group III (mGluR4, mGluR6, mGluR7, mGluR8). Study results indicate that various presynaptic and postsynaptic ionotropic and metabotropic glutamate receptors are involved in mediating and modulating excitatory effects in the striatum (Fig. 165–2).

Striatal projection neurons and interneurons express several NMDA, AMPA, and kainate receptor subunits.[36–40] AMPA and NMDA receptor subunits are found exclusively postsynaptically in the core of asymmetrical axodendritic and axospinous synapses in the rat striatum.[38, 41] Moreover, studies in the monkey striatum revealed that kainate receptors are found postsynaptically and presynaptically in cortical-like terminals making asymmetrical synapses.[42, 42a] In addition to ionotropic receptors, striatal neurons are enriched in metabotropic glutamate receptors. Group I and some of group III (mGluR4 and mGluR7) metabotropic glutamate receptors are expressed at a moderate to high level by most striatal neurons.[43, 44] Whereas strong immunoreactivity for group III mGluRs is found in glutamatergic corticostriatal terminals,[45, 46, 46a] group I mGluRs are found postsynaptically, perisynaptic to asymmetrical axospinous synapses, in the core of GABAergic synapses, and perisynaptic to dopaminergic synapses.[47, 48, 48a] The mGluR2 receptor is confined to striatal cholinergic interneurons, whereas mGluR3 is mostly expressed by glial cells.[43, 49, 50] A large population of corticostriatal terminals display mGluR2 and mGluR3 immunoreactivity.[51] These observations indicate that corticostriatal terminals are associated with presynaptic and postsynaptic glutamate receptors (see Fig. 165–2).

In addition to glutamatergic afferents, the striatum receives GABA-containing inputs from GABAergic interneurons, local collateral axons of medium-sized projection neurons, and from GPe cells. The inhibitory actions of GABA are mediated through two major groups of receptors: the ionotropic GABA$_A$ receptors, which are involved in fast synaptic inhibition and include 14 subunits (α_1 through α_6, β_1 through β_3, γ_1 through γ_3, δ, ϵ),[52, 53] and the metabotropic GABA$_B$ receptors, which mediate slow- and long-lasting inhibi-

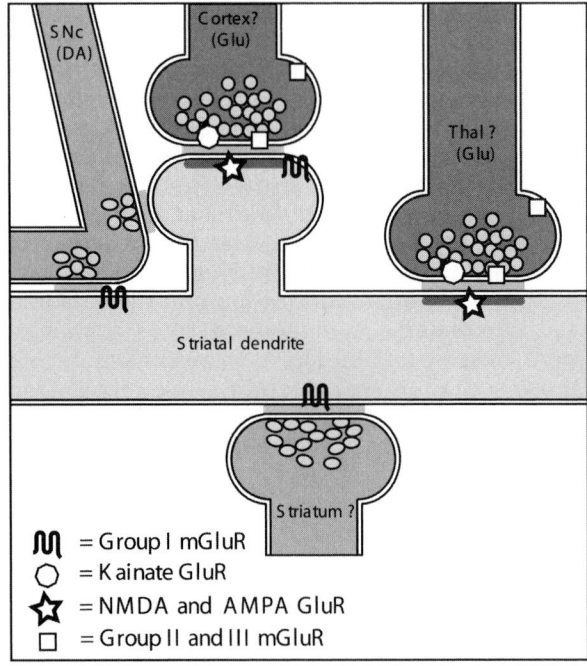
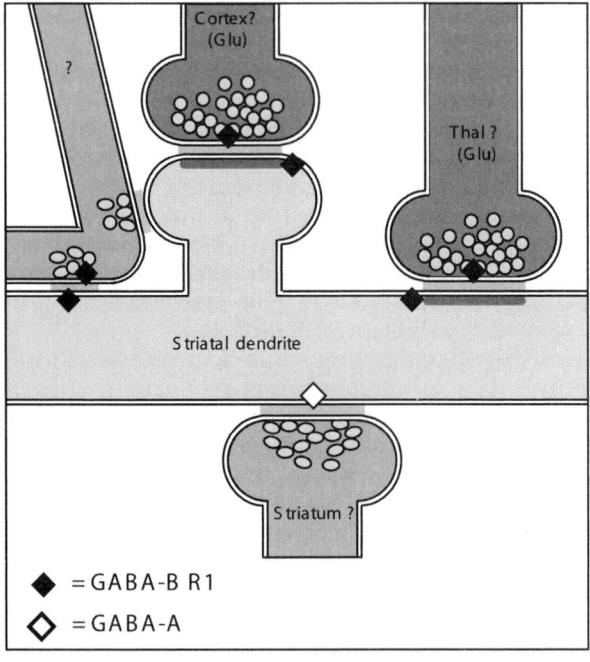

FIGURE 165–2. Schematic drawings of striatal dendrites show the pattern of subsynaptic distribution of glutamate and γ-aminobutyric acid (GABA) receptors in relation to the main striatal afferents in monkeys.

tion and include GABA$_B$-R1 and GABA$_B$-R2 subunits.[54-56] As expected, striatal neurons are enriched in GABA$_A$ and GABA$_B$ receptors.[53, 56-60] Whereas GABA$_B$ receptors are homogeneously distributed and found in medium-sized projection neurons and interneurons,[59] the GABA$_A$ receptor subunits display different patterns of distribution: the β_2 and β_3 subunits are confined to cholinergic neurons, whereas the α_1 subunit is abundant in the matrix compartment, where it is expressed in medium-sized aspiny neurons.[60] GABA$_A$ receptors are localized exclusively postsynaptically in the main bodies of symmetrical synapses.[60, 61] GABA$_B$ receptors are found postsynaptically in the main body of many symmetrical synapses and presynaptically in terminals making asymmetrical synapses (see Fig. 165–2).[48, 48a, 59] A small population of axons forming en passant type of symmetrical synapses also express GABA$_B$ receptors.[59] These data suggest that GABA can act postsynaptically through GABA$_A$ and GABA$_B$ receptors to modulate GABAergic transmission or presynaptically through GABA$_B$ receptors to modulate the activity of glutamatergic afferents in the striatum.

Other Afferents to the Striatum

The striatum is the target of many other afferents that are not discussed in detail in this chapter because of space limitations. These afferents include the massive projections from midbrain dopaminergic neurons in the SNc, ventral tegmental area, and retrorubral area[62, 63] as well as subthalamostriatal projections. In monkeys, subthalamic neurons that project to the caudate nucleus and putamen arise from two distinct neuronal populations; those that innervate the putamen are located in the sensorimotor-related dorsolateral two thirds of the subthalamic nucleus, and subthalamocaudate neurons are found ventromedially in the associative territory.[34, 64] Other minor inputs to the striatum arise from the tuberomamillary nucleus,[65] the brainstem pedunculopontine nucleus,[34, 66] the locus ceruleus,[34] the spinal nucleus of the trigeminal nerve,[67] the peripeduncular nucleus,[68] and the substantia innominata.[69]

DIRECT AND INDIRECT STRIATOFUGAL PROJECTIONS

The cortical inputs, together with the many other intrinsic and extrinsic afferents, are integrated by medium-sized projection neurons in the striatum. After processing at the striatal level, the cortical information is conveyed to the output nuclei of the basal ganglia (i.e., GPi and SNr) through two routes, the so-called direct and indirect striatofugal pathways.[10, 70-72] The *direct pathway* arises from a subpopulation of spiny neurons that project directly to the GPi or SNr, whereas the *indirect pathway* arises from a separate population of spiny neurons that project to the GPe. The GPe conveys the information to the subthalamic nucleus, which relays it to the output nuclei of the basal ganglia. The subpopulations of striatal output neurons that give

rise to the direct and indirect pathways are further distinguished by their expression of neuropeptides and dopamine receptor subtypes. Although all striatal spiny neurons use GABA as their main transmitter, the subpopulation that gives rise to the direct pathway is characterized by the presence of the neuropeptides substance P and dynorphin and by the preferential expression of the D$_1$ subtype of dopamine receptors. The subpopulation that gives rise to the indirect pathway expresses preferentially enkephalin and the D$_2$ subtype of dopamine receptors.[10] Imbalance in the activity of these two pathways underlies some of the motor deficits in Parkinson's disease.[10, 70, 72]

The model of direct and indirect pathways as originally introduced was by necessity a simplification and included only the major projections of subnuclei of the basal ganglia. Since its introduction, evolving knowledge about the anatomic and synaptic organization of the basal ganglia has led scientists to reconsider and update some aspects of the model. One of the most important new findings regarding the anatomic organization of the basal ganglia is the demonstration of multiple indirect pathways of information that flow through the basal ganglia. In addition to the classic indirect pathway through the GPe and the subthalamic nucleus, the GPe gives rise to GABAergic projections that terminate in basal ganglia output structures (i.e., GPi and SNr) and the reticular nucleus of the thalamus.[6, 12, 13] A projection from the GPe to the striatum, which in rats preferentially targets subpopulations of striatal interneurons,[73] has also been described.[6, 12, 13] Although the exact functions of these connections remain unknown, the circuitry of the basal ganglia as outlined in the original model of direct and indirect pathways is likely to be more complex than previously thought.[12]

Molecular and anatomic data challenge the organization of direct and indirect pathways. Reverse transcriptase polymerase chain reaction techniques show a higher level of colocalization of D$_1$ and D$_2$ receptors than that revealed by in situ hybridization methods in striatal neurons.[10] However, the relative abundance of the two receptor subtypes in direct and indirect striatofugal neurons is strikingly different, which is consistent with in situ hybridization data. Indirect striatofugal neurons that contain enkephalin express high levels of D$_2$ mRNA and low levels of D$_1$ mRNA, whereas direct striatofugal neurons that contain substance P express high levels of D$_1$ mRNA and low levels of D$_2$ mRNA. The only striatal projection neurons that coexpress high levels of D$_1$ and D$_2$ receptor subtypes are a small population of projection neurons that contain enkephalin and substance P. Another set of data that has led to the reconsideration of some aspects of the model was obtained in intracellular staining studies. These data showed that the segregation of striatofugal neurons into striatopallidal and striatonigral neurons is not as clear-cut as originally suggested based on differential peptide expression and retrograde double-labeling studies.[10] It appears that striatal projection neurons innervate the pallidal segments and the substantia nigra in rats and monkeys to some extent.[10] Kawaguchi and coworkers[22] divided striatofugal neurons into two major types based on their pattern of axonal arborization. The first type, referred to as *indirect* striatofugal neurons, has axons that arborize profusely and exclusively in the globus pallidus. The second type of neurons, referred to as *direct* striatofugal neurons, projects massively to the entopeduncular nucleus or the substantia nigra, or both, but also sends thin axon collaterals to the globus pallidus.[10] Although this does not rule out the concept of segregation of striatofugal neurons, these findings must be kept in mind while considering the functional significance of the direct and indirect striatofugal pathways.

Glutamate and γ-Aminobutyric Acid Receptors in the Globus Pallidus

GABA and glutamate are the two main transmitters that mediate activity along the direct and indirect pathways of the basal ganglia. Pallidal neurons receive massive axodendritic GABAergic inputs from the striatum and strong somatic innervation from local collaterals of GPe neurons. The glutamatergic terminals from the subthalamic nucleus, which account for less than 10% of the total population of boutons in contact with pallidal neurons, are homogeneously distributed among GABAergic terminals on neuronal cell bodies and dendrites (Fig. 165–3). The effects of GABA and

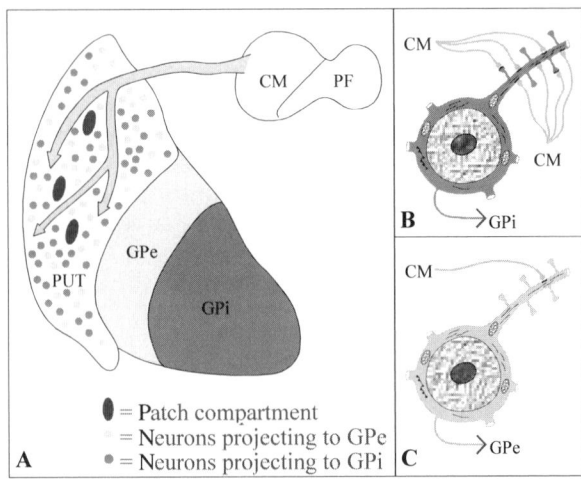

FIGURE 165–4. Compartmental *(A)* and synaptic *(B and C)* relationships between striatopallidal neurons and thalamic afferents from the centromedian (CM) nucleus in squirrel monkeys. These data were obtained after simultaneous injections of anterograde tracers in the CM nucleus and retrograde tracers in either segment of the globus pallidus. The thalamic inputs project mainly to the matrix striatal compartment *(A)* that contains neurons projecting to the external globus pallidus (GPe) *(light gray circles)* or internal globus pallidus (GPi) *(dark gray circles)*. The large ovoid black areas represent the patch compartment, which does not receive input from the CM. The thalamic terminals form asymmetrical synapses, frequently with striato-GPi neurons *(B)* but rarely with striato-GPe cells *(C)*. (Adapted from Sidibé M, Smith Y: Differential synaptic innervation of striatofugal neurons projecting to the internal or external segments of the globus pallidus by thalamic afferents in the squirrel monkey. J Comp Neurol 365:445–465, 1996.)

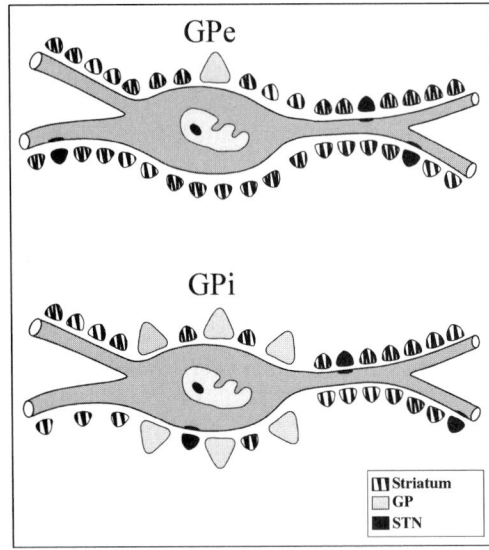

FIGURE 165–3. The pattern of innervation of neurons shown in both segments of the globus pallidus is based on data obtained in squirrel monkeys using anterograde tracing techniques and postembedding immunogold labeling for γ-aminobutyric acid (GABA) or glutamate. The relative size and proportion of each category of terminal are represented. The major difference between innervation of neurons of the two segments of the globus pallidus is that internal globus pallidus (GPi) neurons receive strong somatic inputs from the external globus pallidus (GPe), whereas striatal and subthalamic terminals are evenly distributed on GPe and GPi neurons. (Adapted from Smith Y, Bevan MD, Shink E, et al: Microcircuitry of the direct and indirect pathways of the basal ganglia. Neuroscience 86:353–387, 1998.)

glutamate on pallidal neurons depend on the subtype and subunit composition of the receptors expressed by the postsynaptic neurons and on their spatial relationships to glutamate and GABA release sites. In this respect, pallidal neurons express various NMDA and AMPA receptor subunits in the core of asymmetrical glutamatergic synapses in the rat pallidum.[41, 74] Pallidal neurons are also enriched in group I (mGluR1 and mGluR5) metabotropic glutamate receptors.[43] Surprisingly, both subtypes of group I mGluRs were found postsynaptically in the core of striatopallidal GABAergic synapses and perisynaptically at subthalamopallidal glutamatergic synapses in monkeys (Fig. 165–5).[47–48a, 75] However, pallidal neurons express low levels of group II mGluRs that abound in glial cells.[43, 49, 50] The group III mGluRs (mGluR4a and mGluR7a, b) are mostly expressed presynaptically in striatopallidal GABAergic terminals, where they may act as heteroreceptors to modulate GABA release from striatal terminals (see Fig. 165–5).[45–46a]

As expected, pallidal neurons express moderate to high levels of GABA$_A$ and GABA$_B$ receptors.[53, 58–60] The GABA$_A$ receptor subunits are mostly found postsynaptically in the core of symmetrical striatopallidal GABAergic synapses,[48a, 60, 76, 77] whereas the GABA$_B$ receptors are present on the postsynaptic membrane of striatopallidal synapses, perisynaptic to asymmetrical synapses, and presynaptic in subthalamic glutamatergic terminals (see Fig. 165–5).[48, 48a, 59] These data indicate that GABA_B receptors may act at various sites to modulate GABAergic and glutamatergic neurotransmission in the pallidal complex.

Differential Innervation of Direct and Indirect Striatofugal Neurons and Interneurons

Although all medium-sized spiny striatofugal neurons display a similar pattern of synaptic innervation, evidence indicates that some extrinsic afferents preferentially target direct or indirect striatal projection neurons (see Fig. 165–4). For instance, thalamic inputs from the centromedian nucleus form synapses much more frequently with direct than indirect striatofugal neurons in squirrel monkeys (see Fig. 165–4).[27] However, sensorimotor cortical inputs influence preferentially striato-GPe neurons in rats[78] and monkeys.[79] After microstimulation of physiologically corresponding sites in the primary motor cortex and somatosensory cortical region, 75% of the striatofugal neurons that displayed

FOS immunoreactivity (i.e., neurons that changed their activity) were enkephalin immunoreactive, indicating that they give rise to the indirect pathways. Whether those functional effects were mediated by a differential density of sensorimotor cortical terminals in contact with striato-GPe and striato-GPi neurons remains to be established. Such does not seem to be the case in rats, however, because inputs from the motor cortex form synapses more frequently with neurons of the direct pathway than those of the indirect pathways.[80]

This differential synaptic innervation was also found at the level of striatal interneurons. For example, cholinergic interneurons receive massive inputs from thalamic intralaminar nuclei but are much less innervated by cortical afferents.[20–21a, 81] However, calretinin-immunoreactive interneurons appear to be devoid of centromedian inputs, whereas parvalbumin- and somatostatin-containing neurons receive centromedian and cortical inputs in monkeys.[81] In rats, parvalbumin-containing neurons are preferentially innervated by cortical afferents.[33]

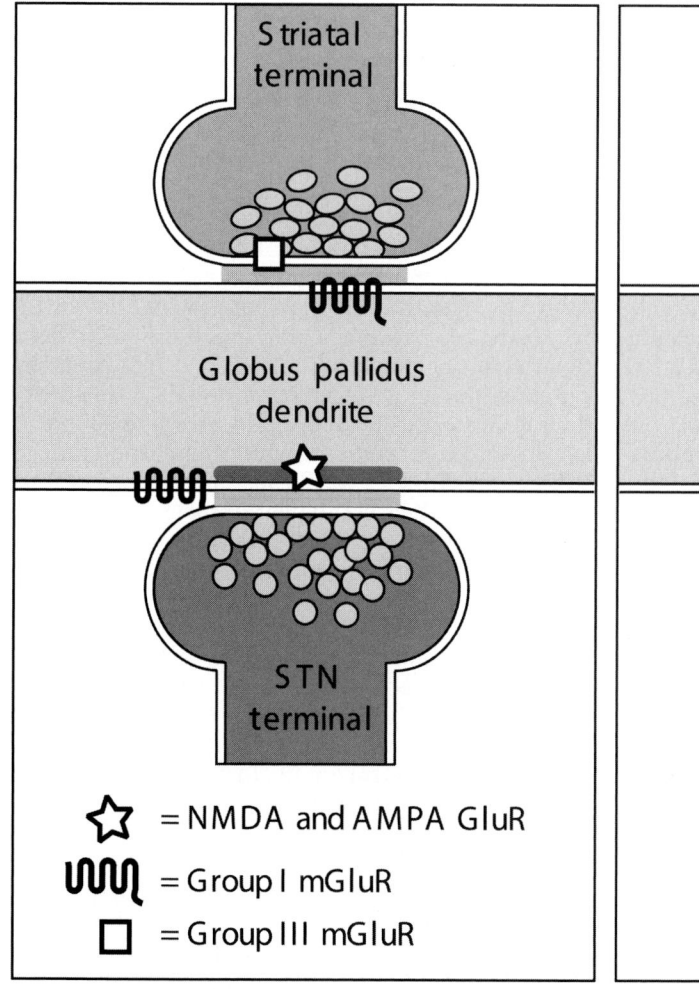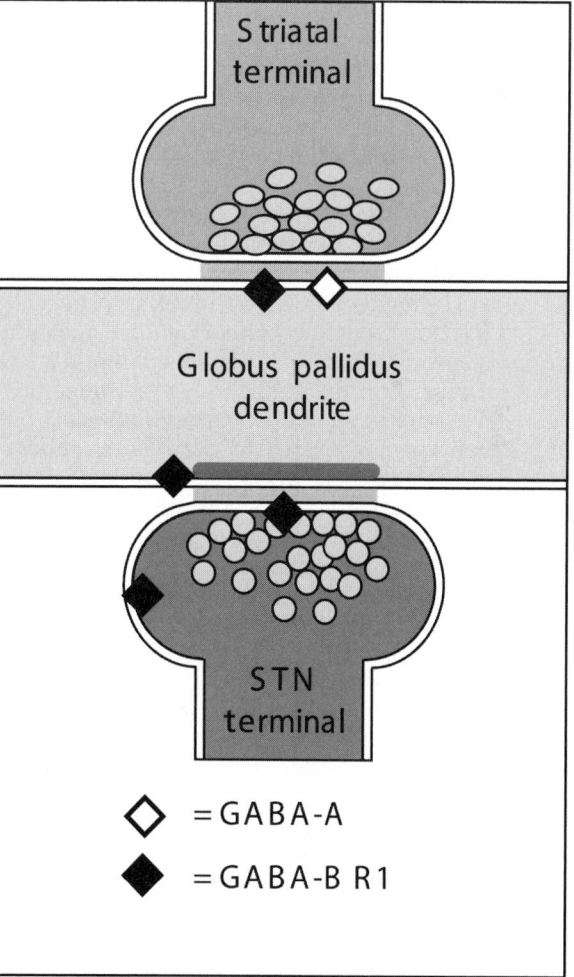

FIGURE 165–5. Schematic drawings of pallidal dendrites show the pattern of subsynaptic distribution of glutamate and γ-aminobutyric acid (GABA) receptors in relation to striatal and subthalamic afferents in monkeys.

CORTICOSUBTHALAMIC AND THALAMOSUBTHALAMIC PROJECTIONS: ADDITIONAL ENTRANCES TO THE BASAL GANGLIA CIRCUITRY

As is the case for the striatum, the subthalamic nucleus also receives excitatory glutamatergic projections from the cerebral cortex. In primates, anatomic evidence indicates that the corticosubthalamic projection is exclusively ipsilateral and arises mainly from the primary motor cortex (area 4), with a minor contribution of prefrontal and premotor cortices. Somatosensory and visual cortical areas do not project to the subthalamic nucleus, but they substantially innervate the striatum. Attempts to determine the exact origin of corticosubthalamic projections in the cat and monkey by retrograde transport have been inconclusive. In rats, however, the corticosubthalamic projection originates mainly from layer V neurons that, in some cases, send axons collateral to the striatum. In rats and monkeys, the corticosubthalamic projection is topographically organized so that afferents from the primary motor cortex are confined to the dorsolateral part of the subthalamic nucleus, whereas the premotor (areas 8, 9, and 6), supplementary motor, and presupplementary motor areas, as well as adjacent frontal cortical regions, innervate preferentially the medial third of the nucleus. Inputs from the prefrontal-limbic cortices are confined to the medial-most tip of subthalamic nucleus.[6, 12, 13] By virtue of its cortical inputs, the dorsolateral sector of the subthalamic nucleus is involved in the control of motor behaviors, whereas the ventromedial sector processes oculomotor, associative, and limbic information.[12, 13]

Like cortical afferents to the striatum, the corticosubthalamic projection from the primary motor cortex is somatotopically organized; the face area projects laterally, the arm area centrally, and the leg area medially. The arrangement of somatotopic representations from the supplementary motor area to the medial subthalamic nucleus is reversed from the ordering of the primary motor cortex to the lateral subthalamic nucleus in macaque monkeys.[82] The cerebral cortex imposes a specific functional segregation on the striatum and at the level of the subthalamic nucleus.[83] However, subthalamic nucleus neurons have long dendrites that may cross boundaries of functional territories imposed by cortical projections in rats.[84] This anatomic arrangement opens the possibility for some functionally segregated information at the level of the cerebral cortex to converge on individual subthalamic nucleus neurons in rodents.

As described for the striatum, another source of excitatory inputs to the subthalamic nucleus arises from the centromedian-parafascicular nuclear complex. No other thalamic nuclei are known to innervate the subthalamic nucleus. The thalamosubthalamic projection arborizes ipsilaterally in discrete portions of the subthalamic nucleus. This input respects the functional organization of the subthalamic nucleus (i.e., sensorimotor neurons in the centromedian terminate preferen-

tially in the dorsolateral part of the nucleus), whereas limbic- and associative-related neurons in the parafascicular nucleus project almost exclusively to the medial subthalamic nucleus. In rats, the thalamosubthalamic projection is excitatory and tonically drives the activity of subthalamic nucleus neurons. Although some parafascicular neurons that project to the striatum send axon collaterals to the subthalamic nucleus, the thalamosubthalamic and thalamostriatal projections largely arise from segregated populations of parafascicular neurons in rats.[85]

Even if cortical and thalamic inputs are relatively sparse and terminate on the distal dendrites and spines of subthalamic nucleus neurons, electrophysiologic experiments show that activation of these inputs results in very strong, short-latency, monosynaptic excitatory postsynaptic potentials in subthalamic nucleus neurons. The information flowing through the subthalamic nucleus reaches basal ganglia output structures much faster than information transmitted along the striatofugal pathways.[86–88a] These anatomic and electrophysiologic data suggest that the subthalamic nucleus is another main entrance of information to the basal ganglia circuitry.

γ-Aminobutyric Acid and Glutamate Receptors in the Subthalamic Nucleus

Subthalamic nucleus neurons display strong immunoreactivity for various GABA$_A$ receptor subunits,[48a, 77] which is consistent with electrophysiologic studies showing that the pallidal inhibition of subthalamic nucleus neurons is largely mediated by GABA$_A$ receptor activation. Subpopulations of subthalamic nucleus neurons display moderate immunoreactivity for GABA$_B$ receptors.[59] At the electron microscopic level, GABA$_B$ receptors are expressed postsynaptically on dendrites of subthalamic nucleus neurons and presynaptically in putative glutamatergic axon terminals.[59] Together, these data indicate that GABA$_A$ and GABA$_B$ receptors probably mediate postsynaptic inhibition from the GPe in subthalamic nucleus neurons. GABA$_B$ receptors also may control the activity of subthalamic nucleus neurons by presynaptic inhibition of neurotransmitter release from extrinsic or intrinsic, or both, glutamatergic terminals.

Subthalamic nucleus neurons express a high level of immunoreactivity for various NMDA and AMPA glutamatergic receptor subunits. Ultrastructural analysis reveals that both types of ionotropic glutamate receptors are expressed preferentially in the postsynaptic membrane of putative glutamatergic synapses, although AMPA receptor subunit immunoreactivity is also found at symmetrical GABAergic synapses in rats.[74] The synaptic localization of mGluRs has not been studied in great detail in the subthalamic nucleus, but preliminary data indicate that group I mGluRs are found postsynaptically at the edges of both asymmetrical glutamatergic synapses or symmetrical GABAergic synapses.[48a, 89] A particular feature that characterizes subthalamic nucleus neurons is their strong expression of group II (mGluR2) mGluR mRNAs relative to other populations of basal ganglia neurons.[43, 50] Consistent with this, group II mGluR agonists reduce subthalamic nucleus–mediated excitatory postsynaptic potentials in rat SNr neurons.[89a] These effects are probably mediated by activation of presynaptic mGluR2 receptors expressed on subthalamic nucleus axons and terminals in the SNr. Very low levels of group III mGluR mRNAs are found in subthalamic nucleus neurons.[43, 44]

THE MOTOR THALAMUS: A MAJOR TARGET OF BASAL GANGLIA AND CEREBELLAR OUTFLOW

The GPi and the SNr are the two output structures of the basal ganglia. They convey basal ganglia outflow to motor, cognitive, and intralaminar thalamic nuclei and to various brainstem structures (see Fig. 165–1). In this section, we discuss the organization of basal ganglia projections from GPi and SNr to the thalamus and compare the pattern of distribution of basal ganglia inputs with that of cerebellar afferents.

Nomenclature of Motor Thalamic Nuclei

The motor thalamus is composed of the ventral anterior and ventral lateral nuclear groups. Various nomenclatures have been introduced for the terminology of the subdivisions of motor thalamic nuclei in primates (Table 165–1). To facilitate the comparison of data obtained in different studies, it is important to understand the correspondence between these terminologies. Table 165–1 compares the nomenclature for the ventral anterior and ventral lateral subdivisions introduced by various groups to define motor thalamic nuclei in Old World[90–93] and New World[94] monkeys. Further details on the nomenclature of thalamic nuclei in humans and nonhuman primates are provided in an extensive review by Percheron and colleagues.[95]

Basal Ganglia and Cerebellar Inputs to Motor Thalamic Nuclei

Although the GPi and SNr project to the ventral anterior and ventral lateral nuclei, the nigral and pallidal afferents largely terminate in different subdivisions of this nuclear group,[96, 97] which were originally thought to be completely separate from cerebellar projection sites in the primate thalamus.[91, 96] However, investigations using multiple-labeling techniques have demonstrated that, even if cerebellar and pallidal projections mainly innervate different thalamic nuclei, a substantial level of convergence exists between these two major thalamic afferents.[98–101] These observations led to reconsideration of many aspects of basal ganglia thalamocortical relationships, taking into account that basal ganglia information is conveyed to premotor and supplementary motor cortical areas and the primary motor cortex. Conversely, the cerebellar outflow, which was thought to be conveyed exclusively to primary motor cortex, also reaches premotor and supplementary motor cortical regions.[98–102]

Another important concept that has been emphasized in the past few years is that cerebellar and basal ganglia thalamic projections terminate in motor thalamic territories and reach major associative and limbic regions of the primate thalamus.[102] Although the non-motor functions of basal ganglia and cerebellum have long been known, a series of anatomic data demonstrated the existence of various connections through which basal ganglia and cerebellar information can reach various cortical areas in the frontal, parietal, and temporal lobes known to be involved in cognitive functions.[102] The use of trans-synaptic, retrograde virus transport after injections in various cortical areas led Strick and associates[102] to propose that nigral, pallidal, and cerebellar outputs to the cerebral cortex flow through various channels that arise from segregated regions of basal ganglia output structures and deep cerebellar nuclei (Fig. 165–6).

NIGROTHALAMIC PROJECTION

The ventral anterior and mediodorsal thalamic nuclei are the main targets of nigrothalamic projections in primates.[6, 97] In an elegant anatomic study combining anterograde and retrograde labeling methods, Ilinsky and coworkers[97] came to some conclusions regarding the nigrothalamocortical projections in monkeys. First, inputs from the medial part of the SNr terminate mostly in the medial magnocellular divisions of the

T A B L E   1 6 5 – 1 ■ **Nomenclature of Subdivisions of the Ventral Anterior and Ventral Lateral Nucleus Nuclear Complex in New World and Old World Monkeys**

Olszewski[90]	VLo	VPLo	Area X	VLc (and VLps)	VLm	VApc	VAmc
Jones[91]	VLa	VLp	VLp	VLp	VMp	VA	VA
Ilinsky and Kultas-Ilinsky[92]	VAdc	VL	VL	VLd	VM	VApc	VAmc
Paxinos et al[93]	VAL (Vo)	VLL	VLM	VAL	VAM	VAL (Vo)	VAM
Stepniewska et al[94]	VLa	VLp	VLx	VLd	VM	VApc	VAmc

VA, ventral anterior nucleus; VAdc, ventral anterior nucleus, densocellular part; VAL, ventral anterior nucleus, lateral part; VAM, ventral anterior nucleus, medial part; VAmc, ventral anterior nucleus, magnocellular part; VApc, ventral anterior nucleus, parvocellular part; VL, ventral lateral nucleus; VLa, ventral lateral nucleus, anterior division; VLc, ventral lateral nucleus, pars caudalis; VLd, ventral lateral nucleus, dorsal division; VLL, ventral lateral nucleus, lateral part; VLM, ventral lateral nucleus, medial part; VLo, ventral lateral nucleus, pars oralis; VLp, ventral lateral nucleus, principal division; VLps, ventral lateral nucleus, pars posterma; VLx, ventral lateral nucleus, medial division; VM, ventral medial nucleus; VMp, ventral medial nucleus, principal division; Vo, ventralis oralis nucleus; VPLo, ventral posterior lateral nucleus, pars oralis.

PALLIDAL OUTPUT CHANNELS

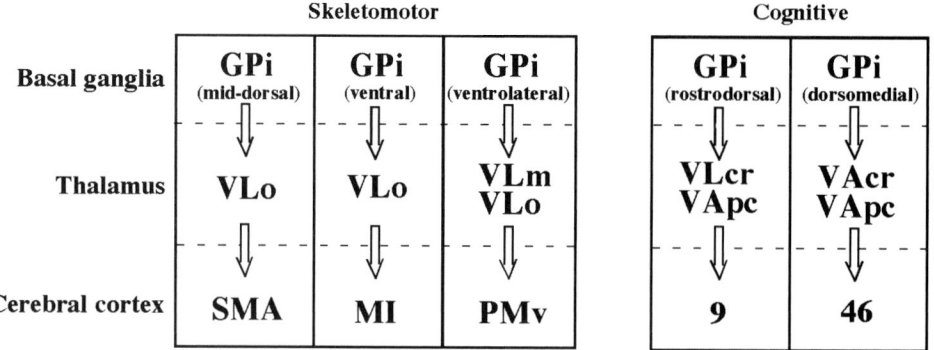

NIGRAL OUTPUT CHANNELS

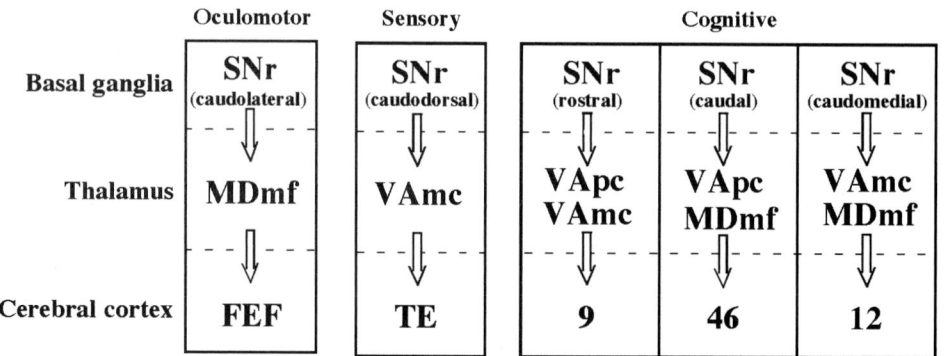

CEREBELLAR OUTPUT CHANNELS

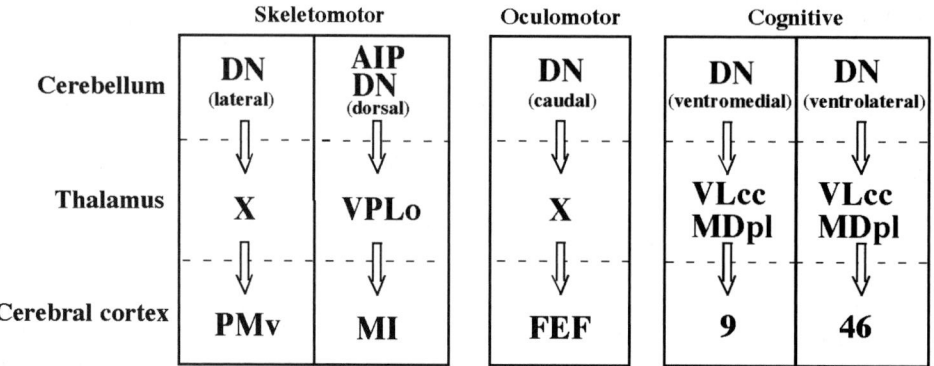

FIGURE 165–6. Motor and nonmotor connections between basal ganglia output structures or deep cerebellar nuclei and various functional regions of the monkey cerebral cortex. The internal globus pallidus (GPi), substantia nigra pars reticulata (SNr), and dentate cerebellar nucleus (DN) project to different subdivisions of the ventral anterior and ventral lateral (VA/VL) nuclei and the mediodorsal (MD) nucleus, which reach functionally segregated cortical areas involved in motor, cognitive, and sensory functions. The nomenclature of thalamic nuclei used in this diagram is that of Olszewski[90] (see Table 165–1). AIP, accessory interpositus nucleus; FEF, frontal eye field; MDmf, mediodorsal nucleus pars multiformis; MDpl, mediodorsal nucleus pars lateralis; TE, area of the inferotemporal cortex. (Adapted from Middleton FA, Strick PL: Basal ganglia and cerebellar loops: Motor and cognitive circuits. Brain Res Rev 31:236–250, 2000.)

ventral anterior nucleus (VAmc) and the mediodorsal nucleus (MDmc), which innervate anterior regions of the frontal lobe, including the principal sulcus (i.e., Walker's area 46) and the orbital cortex (i.e., Walker's area 11). Second, neurons in the lateral part of the SNr project preferentially to the lateral posterior region of the VAmc and to different parts of the mediodorsal nucleus mostly related to posterior regions of the frontal lobe, including the frontal eye field and areas of the premotor cortex. On the basis of retrograde transsynaptic viral tracing studies, Strick and associates[102] extended these findings and proposed that the nigral outputs to the thalamus flow along five separate channels that target various cortical areas involved in cognitive, sensory, and oculomotor functions (see Fig. 165–6). Another thalamic target of SNr neurons is the caudal intralaminar parafascicular nucleus.[94, 103] The organization of this projection is discussed in a separate section.

PALLIDOTHALAMIC PROJECTION

The main thalamic targets of GPi neurons are the ventral anterior and ventral lateral nuclei and caudal intralaminar thalamic nuclei.[6, 104] Efferents from the sensorimotor GPi remain largely segregated from the associative and limbic projections at the level of the thalamus, whereas, they partly overlap in the tegmental pedunculopontine nucleus (PPN).[104, 105] The limbic and associative pallidal projections innervate common nuclei in the thalamus and PPN.[104, 105] In squirrel monkeys, the sensorimotor GPi outputs are directed toward the posterior ventral lateral nucleus (VLp), whereas the associative and limbic GPi preferentially innervate the parvocellular ventral anterior nucleus (VApc) and the dorsal ventral lateral nucleus (VLd). The ventromedial nucleus receives inputs from the limbic GPi only.[104] These findings reveal that some associative and limbic cortical information, which is largely processed in segregated corticostriatopallidal channels, converge to common thalamic nuclei in monkeys.[104] After processing at the thalamic level, the basal ganglia influences are conveyed to the cerebral cortex through the ventral anterior and ventral lateral nuclei. Retrograde transneuronal virus studies showed that different populations of GPi neurons project to thalamocortical neurons directed toward the supplementary motor area, primary motor cortex, and premotor area,[102] each of which is involved in the control of various aspects of skeletomotor activity (see Fig. 165–6). The cognitive information from the dorsal part of GPi is transmitted to prefrontal cortical areas 9 and 46 and is involved in planning and spatial working memory through the VApc (see Fig. 165–6).[102] About 10% to 20% of pallidothalamic neurons in the monkey GPi project to the contralateral ventral anterior and ventral lateral nuclei.[106]

CEREBELLOTHALAMIC PROJECTION

Cerebellar afferents are partly segregated from nigral and pallidal projections in the primate thalamus. Although the cerebellum is commonly seen as a brain region involved in skeletomotor control, the importance of this structure in cognitive functions is well established.[101,107] In support of such nonmotor cerebellar functions, anatomic studies indicate that the dentate nucleus gives rise to at least two different channels of cognitive cerebellar-thalamic-cortical information in monkeys (see Fig. 165–6). These two circuits, which largely arise from the ventral part of the dentate nucleus, reach cortical areas 9 and 46 through relays in specific parts of the ventrolateral and mediodorsal nuclei (see Fig. 165–6). The skeletomotor-related outflow reaches premotor and primary motor cortical areas through relays in area X and VPLo, respectively. Cerebellar information related to eye movement arises from the caudal part of the dentate nucleus and reaches the frontal eye field cortical area through area X (see Fig. 165–6). Although cerebellar projections to the intralaminar thalamic nuclei have been described in nonprimates,[91, 108, 109] the existence of such connections still remains to be established in monkeys.

Basal Ganglia Inputs to Intralaminar Thalamic Nuclei

Most pallidal neurons that project to thalamic relay nuclei send axon collaterals to the caudal intralaminar nuclei, where they follow a highly specific pattern of distribution.[6, 104] Pallidal axons arising from the sensorimotor GPi terminate exclusively in the centromedian nucleus, where they form synapses with thalamostriatal neurons projecting back to the sensorimotor territory of the striatum (Fig. 165–7).[103, 104] In contrast, associative inputs from the caudate-receiving territory of the GPi terminate massively in a dorsolateral extension of the parafascicular nucleus (PFdL), which, surprisingly, does not project back to the caudate nucleus but rather innervates preferentially the precommissural region of the putamen (see Fig. 165–7).[103] The limbic GPi selectively innervates the rostrodorsal part of the parafascicular nucleus, which projects back to the nucleus accumbens. SNr projections are confined to the parafascicular nucleus, where they largely overlap with thalamostriatal neurons projecting to the caudate nucleus.[103] It appears that the centromedian-parafascicular complex is part of closed and open functional loops with the striatopallidal complex (see Fig. 165–7).

DESCENDING PALLIDAL AND NIGRAL PROJECTIONS TO THE TEGMENTAL PEDUNCULOPONTINE NUCLEUS

In monkeys, more than 80% of GPi neurons that project to the PPN send axon collaterals to the ventral thalamus.[6] In contrast to the ventral lateral nucleus, which largely conveys basal ganglia information to the cerebral cortex, the PPN gives rise to descending projections to the pons, medulla, and spinal cord as well as prominent ascending projections to the different structures of the basal ganglia, thalamus, and basal forebrain.[109–112] The pallidotegmental projection may be a

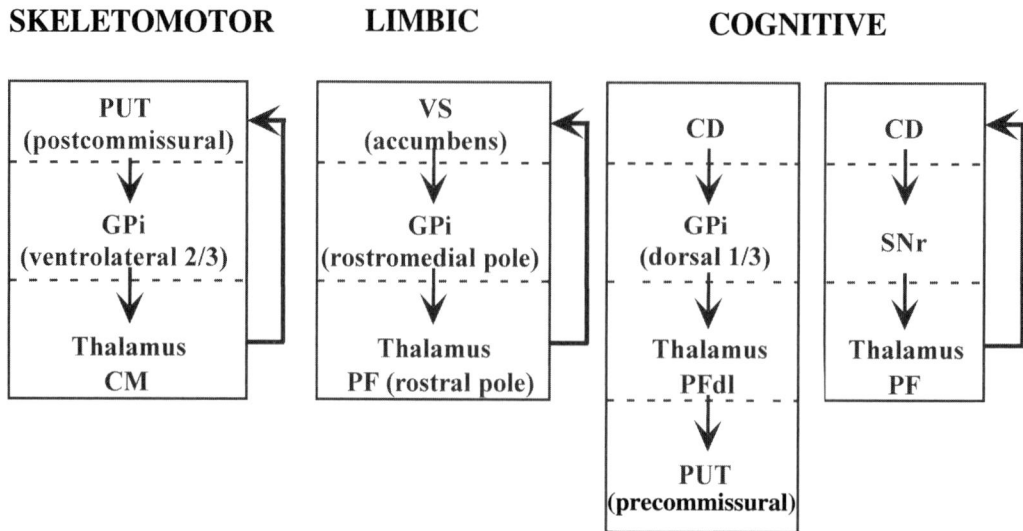

SKELETOMOTOR   **LIMBIC**   **COGNITIVE**

FIGURE 165–7. The functional interactions between the basal ganglia and thalamostriatal neurons in monkeys are shown schematically. These data were obtained after simultaneous injections of retrograde tracers in different functional territories of the striatum and anterograde tracers in the corresponding functional regions of internal globus pallidus (GPi) or substantia nigra pars reticulata (SNr) in squirrel monkeys. Notice that the caudal intralaminar thalamic nuclei (centromedian-parafascicular complex) and the basal ganglia are interconnected by closed and open functional loops. (Data from Sidibé M, Pare J-F, Smith Y: Nigral and pallidal inputs to functionally segregated thalamostriatal neurons in the centromedian/parafascicular intralaminar nuclear complex in monkey. J Comp Neurol 447:286–299, 2002; and Sidibé M, Bevan MD, Bolam JP, et al: Efferent connections of the internal globus pallidus in the squirrel monkey: I. Topography and synaptic organization of the pallidothalamic projection. J Comp Neurol 382:323–347, 1997.)

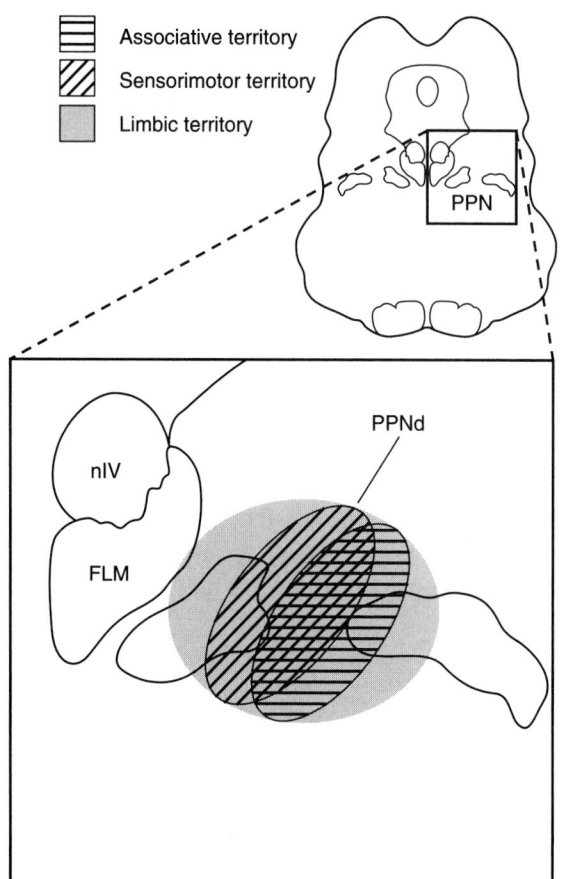

FIGURE 165–8. The location of anterogradely labeled fibers in the tegmental pedunculopontine nucleus (PPN) are shown schematically after injections of anterograde tracers in the associative, sensorimotor, and limbic territories of the internal globus pallidus (GPi) in squirrel monkeys. Notice that projections from the different functional territories of the GPi largely overlap in the pars diffusa of the PPN (PPNd). nIV, trochlear nucleus; FLM, medial longitudinal fasciculus; Sp, superior cerebellar peduncle. (Adapted from Shink E, Sidibé M, Smith Y: Efferent connections of the internal globus pallidus in the squirrel monkey: II. Topography and synaptic organization of the pallidal efferents to the pedunculopontine nucleus. J Comp Neurol 382:348–363, 1997.)

route by which information can escape from the basal ganglia–thalamocortical circuitry and reach lower motor and autonomic centers. Another possibility is that the PPN acts as an interface between different functional territories of the GPi and sends back the integrated information to the basal ganglia circuitry mainly through its massive projection to the dopaminergic neurons of the SNc.[6, 13] We investigated the pattern of distribution of functionally segregated pallidofugal information in the PPN of squirrel monkeys.[105] The results of this study are summarized in Figure 165–8. Injections of anterograde tracers in different functional territories of the GPi lead to anterograde labeling that largely converges to common regions of the so-called pars diffusa of the PPN (PPNd). The fields of fibers that arise from the associative and limbic territories of the GPi are more widely spread than the afferents from the sensorimotor territory of the GPi. Another major finding of this study is that pallidal fibers largely avoid cholinergic neurons in the pars compacta of the PPN. These anatomic data suggest that the noncholinergic neurons of the PPNd are potential targets for the integration of information arising from different functional territories of the GPi in primates. The PPNd is in a position to act as an interface for motivational, cognitive, and motor information transmitted along the pallidotegmental projection in primates (Fig. 165–8).

The SNr also provides substantial inputs to cholinergic and noncholinergic neurons of the PPN in rats.[113, 114] Although the existence of this projection has been shown in monkeys by means of retrograde labeling studies,[6] the exact targets of nigrotegmental projections remain to be established.

CONCLUSIONS

Our knowledge of the basal ganglia anatomy has increased tremendously over the past 10 years, mainly because of the introduction of highly sophisticated and sensitive tract-tracing and immunocytochemical methods suitable to light and electron microscopic analysis. Anatomic data led some to reconsider certain aspects of the functional circuitry of the basal ganglia. For instance, the thalamostriatal projection, which is largely neglected in functional models of basal ganglia connectivity, deserves attention. This projection is massive and follows a highly specific pattern of functional connectivity with the striatopallidal complex. The fact that thalamic inputs are directed preferentially toward specific populations of striatal projection neurons and interneurons strongly indicates that these inputs may play a major role in the basal ganglia circuitry.

An important concern has been raised during the past few years about the validity of the direct and indirect pathways of the basal ganglia. The evidence that subpopulations of striatofugal neurons express D_1 and D_2 dopamine receptors, combined with the fact that striatofugal neurons are more collateralized than previously thought, has challenged the concept of segregation of striatal projection neurons. Despite these anatomic refinements of the basal ganglia circuitry, it is clear that the functional concept of direct and indirect pathways still remains the basic working model for understanding changes in the basal ganglia circuitry in pathologic conditions and for developing more accurate surgical and pharmacologic therapies for basal ganglia diseases.

Another critical aspect of the basal ganglia circuitry, which should receive more attention, is the relative importance of the subthalamic nucleus and the striatum as major entrances of cortical information to the basal ganglia. Although the striatum receives a much more massive input from the cerebral cortex and thalamus than the subthalamic nucleus, the fact that the information flowing through the corticosubthalamic or thalamosubthalamic projections reaches the output structures of the basal ganglia (i.e., GPi and SNr) before the information traveling through the striatum deserves consideration. The long-held belief that the basal ganglia and cerebellum were solely involved in motor behaviors should be abandoned in light of various behavioral and clinical studies showing the clear implication of these brain regions in cognitive functions. The anatomic data presented in this chapter demonstrate that basal ganglia and cerebellar outflow have access to both motor-related cortical areas and invade large regions of the frontal, temporal, and parietal lobes devoted to various aspects of cognitive behaviors.

The large amount of neurotransmitters and neuropeptides involved in mediating synaptic communication between structures of the basal ganglia makes the chemical pedigree of basal ganglia structures extremely complex. Data showing that G protein–coupled glutamate and GABA receptors are largely expressed extrasynaptically or at synapses unrelated to the release site of their stimulating neurotransmitter further enhance this complexity and raise exciting issues about the functions and mechanisms of activation of metabotropic receptors in the basal ganglia.

ACKNOWLEDGMENTS

We thank Jean-François Paré and Jeremy Kieval for technical assistance, Frank Kiernan for photography, and Peggy Plant for clerical work. This work was supported by National Institutes of Health grants R01-37423, R01-37948, R01-42937, and RR 00165. Ali Charara held a fellowship from the Fonds Nature et Technologie of Quebec.

REFERENCES

1. Graybiel AM: Neurotransmitters and neuromodulators in the basal ganglia. Trends Neurosci 13:244–254, 1990.
2. Alexander GE, Crutcher MD: Functional architecture of basal ganglia circuits: Neural substrates of parallel processing. Trends Neurosci 13:266–271, 1990.
3. Smith AD, Bolam JP: The neural network of the basal ganglia as revealed by the study of synaptic connections of identified neurons. Trends Neurosci 13:259–265, 1990.
4. Joel D, Weiner I: The organization of the basal ganglia–thalamocortical circuits: Open interconnected rather than closed segregated. Neuroscience 63:363–379, 1994.
5. Joel D, Weiner I: The connections of the primate subthalamic nucleus: indirect pathways and the open-interconnected scheme

of basal ganglia-thalamocortical circuitry. Brain Res Rev 23: 62–78, 1997.

6. Parent A, Hazrati L-N: Functional anatomy of the basal ganglia. I. The cortico–basal ganglia–thalamo-cortical loop. Brain Res Rev 20:91–127, 1995.

7. Wilson CJ: Basal ganglia. In Shepherd GM (ed): The Synaptic Organization of the Brain. New York, Oxford University Press, 1998, pp 329–375.

8. Wilson CJ: The contribution of cortical neurons to the firing pattern of striatal spiny neurons. In Houk JC, Davis JL, Beiser DG (eds): Models of Information Processing in the Basal Ganglia. Cambridge, MA, MIT Press, 1995, pp 29–50.

9. Chesselet M-F, Delfs JM: Basal ganglia and movement disorders: An update. Trends Neurosci 19:417–422, 1996.

10. Gerfen CR, Wilson CJ: The basal ganglia. In Björklund A, Hökfelt T, Swanson L (eds): Handbook of Chemical Neuroanatomy: Integrated Systems of the CNS, Part III. Amsterdam, Elsevier, 1996, pp 369–466.

11. Levy R, Hazrati L-N, Herrero M-T, et al: Re-evaluation of the functional anatomy of the basal ganglia in normal and parkinsonian states. Neuroscience 76:335–343, 1997.

12. Smith Y, Bevan MD, Shink E, et al: Microcircuitry of the direct and indirect pathways of the basal ganglia. Neuroscience 86: 353–387, 1998.

13. Smith Y, Shink E, Sidibé M: Neuronal circuitry and synaptic connectivity of the basal ganglia. In Bakay AE (ed): Neurosurgery Clinics of North America. Philadelphia, WB Saunders, 1998, pp 203–222.

14. Parthasarathy HB, Schall JD, Graybiel AM: Distributed but convergent ordering of corticostriatal projections: Analysis of the frontal eye field and the supplementary eye field in the macaque monkey. J Neurosci 12:4468–4488, 1992.

15. Selemon LD, Goldman-Rakic PS: Longitudinal topography and interdigitation of corticostriatal projections in the rhesus monkey. J Neurosci 5:776–794, 1990.

16. Flaherty AW, Graybiel AM: Corticostriatal transformation in the primate somatosensory system: Projections from physiologically mapped body-part representations. J Neurophysiol 66:1249–1263, 1991.

17. Flaherty AW, Graybiel AM: Two input systems for body representations in the primate striatal matrix: Experimental evidence in the squirrel monkey. J Neurosci 13:1120–1137, 1993.

18. Kawaguchi Y, Wilson CJ, Augood SJ, et al: Striatal interneurons: Chemical, physiological and morphological characterization. Trends Neurosci 18:527–535, 1995.

19. Lapper SR, Smith Y, Sadikot AF, et al: Cortical input to parvalbumin-immunoreactive neurons in the putamen of the squirrel monkey. Brain Res 580:215–224, 1992.

20. Meredith GE, Wouterlood FG: Hippocampal and midline thalamic fibers and terminals in relation to the choline acetyltransferase–immunoreactive neurons in nucleus accumbens of the rat: A light and electron microscopic study. J Comp Neurol 296: 204–221, 1990.

21. Lapper SR, Bolam JP: Input from the frontal cortex and the parafascicular nucleus to cholinergic interneurons in the dorsal striatum of the rat. Neuroscience 51:533–545, 1992.

21a. Thomas TM, Smith Y, Levey AI, et al: Cortical inputs to m2-immunoreactive striatal interneurons in rat and monkey. Synapse 37:252–261, 2000.

22. Kawaguchi Y, Wilson CJ, Emson PC: Projection subtypes of rat neostriatal matrix cells revealed by intracellular injection of biocytin. J Neurosci 10:3421–3438, 1990.

23. Jaeger D, Kita H, Wilson CJ: Surround inhibition among projection neurons is weak or nonexistent in the rat neostriatum. J Neurophysiol 72:2555–2558, 1994.

23a. Stern EA, Jaeger D, Wilson CJ: Membrane potential synchrony of simultaneously recorded striatal spiny neurons *in vivo*. Nature 394:475–478.

23b. Oorschot DE, Tunstall MJ, Wickens JR: Local connectivity between striatal spiny projection neurons: A re-evaluation. In Nicholson LFB, Faull RLM (eds): The Basal Ganglia VII. New York, Plenum Press, 2002, pp 421–434.

24. Koos T, Tepper JM: Inhibitory control of neostriatal projection neurons by GABAergic interneurons. Nature Neurosci. 2:467–472.

25. Groenewegen HJ, Berendse HW: The specificity of the nonspecific midline and intralaminar thalamic nuclei. Trends Neurosci 17:52–57, 1994.

26. Sadikot AF, Parent A, Smith Y, et al: Efferent connections of the centromedian and parafascicular nuclei in the squirrel monkey: A light and electron microscopic study of the thalamostriatal projection in relation to striatal heterogeneity. J Comp Neurol 320:228–242, 1992.

27. Sidibé M, Smith Y: Differential synaptic innervation of striatofugal neurons projecting to the internal or external segments of the globus pallidus by thalamic afferents in the squirrel monkey. J Comp Neurol 365:445–465, 1996.

28. Sidibé M, Pare J-F, Raju D, Smith Y: Anatomical and functional relationships between intralaminar thalamic nuclei and basal ganglia in monkeys. In Nicholson LFB, Faull RLM (eds): The Basal Ganglia VII. New York, Plenum Press, 2002, pp 409–420.

29. Dubé L, Smith AD, Bolam JP: Identification of synaptic terminals of thalamic and cortical origin in contact with distinct medium-sized spiny neurons in the rat neostriatum. J Comp Neurol 267:455–471, 1988.

30. Xu ZC, Wilson CJ, Emson PC: Restoration of thalamostriatal projections in rat neostriatal grafts: An electron microscopic analysis. J Comp Neurol 303:22–34, 1991.

31. Smith Y, Bennett BD, Bolam JP, et al: Synaptic relationships between dopaminergic afferents and cortical or thalamic input to the sensorimotor territory of the striatum in monkey. J Comp Neurol 344:1–19, 1994.

32. Sidibé M, Smith Y: Thalamic inputs to striatal interneurons in monkeys: Synaptic organization and co-localization of calcium binding proteins. Neuroscience 89:1189–1208, 1999.

33. Rudkin TM, Sadikot AF: Thalamic input to parvalbumin-immunoreactive GABAergic interneurons: Organization in normal striatum and effect of neonatal decortication. Neuroscience 88: 1165–1175, 1999.

34. Smith Y, Parent A: Differential connections of caudate nucleus and putamen in the squirrel monkey (*Saimiri sciureus*). Neuroscience 18:347–371, 1986.

35. McFarland NR, Haber SN: Convergent inputs from thalamic motor nuclei and frontal cortical areas to the dorsal striatum in the primate. J Neurosci 20:3798–3813, 2000.

36. Standaert DG, Testa CM, Penney JB, et al: Organization of N-methyl-D-aspartate glutamate receptor gene expression in the basal ganglia of the rat. J Comp Neurol 343:1–16, 1994.

37. Kosinki CM, Standaert DG, Counihan TJ, et al: Expression of N-methyl-D-aspartate receptor subunit mRNAs in the human brain: Striatum and globus pallidus. J Comp Neurol 390:63–74, 1998.

38. Bernard V, Somogyi P, Bolam JP: Cellular, subcellular, and subsynaptic distribution of AMPA-type glutamate receptor subunits in the neostriatum of the rat. J Neurosci 17:819–833, 1997.

39. Bischoff S, Barhanin J, Bettler B, et al: Spatial distribution of kainate receptor subunit mRNA in the mouse basal ganglia and ventral mesencephalon. J Comp Neurol 379:541–562, 1997.

40. Wüllner U, Standaert DG, Testa CM, et al: Differential expression of kainate receptors in the basal ganglia of the developing and adult rat brain. Brain Res 768:215–223, 1997.

41. Bernard V, Bolam JP: Subcellular and subsynaptic distribution of NR1 subunit of the NMDA receptor in the neostriatum and globus pallidus of the rat: co-localization at synapses with the GluR2/3 subunit of the AMPA receptor. Eur J Neurosci 10: 3721–3736, 1998.

42. Charara A, Blankstein E, Smith Y: Presynaptic kainate receptor in the monkey striatum. Neuroscience 91:1195–1200, 1999.

42a. Kieval JZ, Hubert GW, Charara A, et al: Subcellular and subsynaptic localization of presynaptic and postsynaptic kainate receptor subunits in the monkey striatum. J Neurosci 21:8746–8757.

43. Testa CM, Standaert DG, Young, AB, et al: Metabotropic glutamate receptor mRNA expression in the basal ganglia of the rat. J Neurosci 14:3005–3018, 1994.

44. Ohishi H, Akazawa C, Shigemoto R, et al: Distribution of the mRNAs for L-2-amino-4-phosphonobutyrate-sensitive metabotropic glutamate receptors, mGluR4 and mGluR7, in the rat brain. J Comp Neurol 360:555–570, 1995.

45. Kinoshita A, Shigemoto R, Ohishi H, et al: Immunohistochemi-

cal localization of metabotropic glutamate receptors, mGluR7a and mGluR7b, in the central nervous system of the adult rat and mouse: A light and electron microscopic study. J Comp Neurol 393:332–352, 1998.

46. Bradley SR, Standaert DG, Rhodes KJ, et al: Immunohistochemical localization of subtype 4a metabotropic glutamate receptors in the rat and mouse basal ganglia. J Comp Neurol 407:33–46, 1999.

46a. Kosinski CM, Bradley SR, Conn PJ, et al: Localization of metabotropic glutamate receptor 7 mRNA and mGluR7a protein in the rat basal ganglia. J Comp Neurol 415:266–284.

47. Smith Y, Hubert GW, Paquet M, et al: Differential subcellular distribution of mGluR1a and mGluR5 in the primate basal ganglia. Neuropharmacology 43:309.

48. Smith Y, Charara A, Hanson JE, et al: GABAB and group I metabotropic glutamate receptors in the striatopallidal complex in primates. J Anat 196:555–576, 2000.

48a. Smith Y, Charara A, Paquet M, et al: Ionotropic and metabotropic GABA and glutamate receptors in primate basal ganglia. J Chem Neuroanat 22:13–42.

49. Ohishi H, Shigemoto R, Nakanishi S, et al: Distribution of the mRNA for a metabotropic glutamate receptor (mGluR3) in the rat brain: An in situ hybridization study. J Comp Neurol 335:252–266, 1993.

50. Ohishi H, Shigemoto R, Nakanishi S, et al: Distribution of the messenger RNA for a metabotropic glutamate receptor, mGluR2, in the central nervous system of the rat. Neuroscience 53:1009–1018, 1993.

51. Testa CM, Friberg IK, Weiss SW, et al: Immunohistochemical localization of metabotropic glutamate receptors mGluR1a and mGluR2/3 in the rat basal ganglia. J Comp Neurol 390:5–19, 1998.

52. Möhler H, Benke D, Benson J, et al: Diversity in structure, pharmacology, and regulation of GABAA receptors. In Enna SJ, Bowery NG (eds): The GABA Receptors. Totowa, NJ, Humana Press, 1997, pp 11–36.

53. Fritschy J-M, Mohler H: GABAA-receptor heterogeneity in the adult rat brain: Differential regional and cellular distribution of seven major subunits. J Comp Neurol 359:154–194, 1995.

54. Jones KA, Borowsky B, Tamm JA, et al: GABAB receptors function as heteromeric assembly of the subunits GABABR1 and GABABR2. Nature 396:674–679. 1998.

55. Kaupmann K, Malitschek B, Schuler V, et al: GABAB-receptor subtypes assemble into functional heteromeric complexes. Nature 396:683–687, 1998.

56. Kaupmann K, Huggel K, Heid J, et al: Expression cloning of GABAB receptors uncovers similarity to metabotropic glutamate receptors. Nature 396:239–246, 1997.

57. Fritschy J-M, Meskenaite V, Weinmann O, et al: GABAB-receptor splice variants GB1a and GB1b in rat brain: Developmental regulation, cellular distribution and extrasynaptic localization. Eur J Neurosci 11:761–768, 1999.

58. Margeta-Mitrovic M, Mitrovic I, Riley RC, et al: Immunocytochemical localization of GABAB receptors in the rat central nervous system. J Comp Neurol 405:299–321, 1999.

59. Charara A, Heilman TC, Levey AI: Pre- and post-synaptic localization of GABAB receptors in the basal ganglia in monkeys. Neuroscience 95:127–140, 2000.

60. Waldvogel HJ, Fritschy J-M, Mohler H: GABAA receptors in the primate basal ganglia: An autoradiographic and a light and electron microscopic immunohistochemical study of the α1 and β2/3 subunits in the baboon brain. J Comp Neurol 397:297–325, 1998.

61. Fujiyama F, Fritschy J-M, Stephenson FA, et al: Synaptic localization of GABA(A) receptor subunits in the striatum of the rat. J Comp Neurol 416:158–172, 2000.

62. Smith Y, Kieval JZ: Anatomy of the dopamine system in the basal ganglia. Trends Neurosci 23:28–33, 2000.

63. Joel D, Weiner I: The connections of the dopaminergic system with the striatum in rats and primates: An analysis with respect to the functional and compartmental organization of the striatum. Neuroscience 96:451–474, 2000.

64. Parent A, Smith Y: Organization of the efferent projections of the subthalamic nucleus in the squirrel monkey as revealed by retrograde labeling methods. Brain Res 436:296–310, 1987.

65. Steinbusch HWM, Sauren Y, Groenewegen HJ, et al: Histaminergic projections from the premammillary and posterior hypothalamic region to the caudate-putamen complex in the rat. Brain Res 368:389–393, 1986.

66. Jackson A, Crossman AR: Nucleus tegmenti pedunculopontinus: Efferent connections with special reference to the basal ganglia, studied in the rat by anterograde and retrograde transport of horseradish peroxidase. Neuroscience 10:725–765, 1983.

67. Yasui Y, Itoh K, Mizuno N: Direct projection from the caudal spinal trigeminal nucleus to the striatum in the cat. Brain Res 408:334–338, 1987.

68. Arnault P, Roger M: The connections of the peripeduncular area studied by retrograde and anterograde transport in the rat. J Comp Neurol 258:463–476, 1987.

69. Arikuni T, Kubota K: Substantia innominata projection to caudate nucleus in macaque monkeys. Brain Res 302:184–189, 1984.

70. Albin RL, Young AB, Penney JB: The functional anatomy of basal ganglia disorders. Trends Neurosci 12:366–375, 1989.

71. Alexander GE, Crutcher MD: Functional architecture of basal ganglia circuits: Neural substrates of parallel processing. Trends Neurosci 13:266–271, 1990.

72. Bergman H, Wichmann T, DeLong MR: Reversal of experimental parkinsonism by lesions of the subthalamic nucleus. Science 249:1436–1438, 1990.

73. Bevan MD, Booth PA, Eaton SA, et al: Selective innervation of neostriatal interneurons by a subclass of neurons in the globus pallidus of the rat. J Neurosci 18:9438–9452, 1998.

74. Clarke NP, Bolam JP: Distribution of glutamate receptor subunits at neurochemically characterized synapses in the entopeduncular nucleus and subthalamic nucleus of the rat. J Comp Neurol 397:403–420, 1998.

75. Hanson JE, Smith Y: Group I metabotropic glutamate receptors at GABAergic synapses in monkeys. J Neurosci 19:6488–6496, 1999.

76. Somogyi P, Fritschy J-M, Benke D, et al: The γ2 subunit of the GABAA receptor is concentrated in synaptic junctions containing the α1 and β2/3 subunits in hippocampus, cerebellum and globus pallidus. Neuropharmacology 35:1425–1444, 1996.

77. Charara A, Smith Y: Subsynaptic distribution of GABAA receptor subunits in the globus pallidus and subthalamic nucleus in monkeys. Soc Neurosci Abstr 24:1650, 1998.

78. Berretta S, Parthasarathy HB, Graybiel AM: Local release of GABAergic inhibition in the motor cortex induces immediate-early gene expression in indirect pathway neurons of the striatum. J Neurosci 17:4752–4763, 1997.

79. Parthasarathy HB, Graybiel AM: Cortically driven immediate-early gene expression reflects modular influence of sensorimotor cortex on identified striatal neurons in the squirrel monkey. J Neurosci 17:2477–2491, 1997.

80. Hersch SM, Ciliax BJ, Gutekunst C-A, et al: Electron microscopic analysis of D1 and D2 dopamine receptor proteins in the dorsal striatum and their synaptic relationships with motor corticostriatal afferents. J Neurosci 15:5222–5237, 1995.

81. Sidibé M, Smith Y: Thalamic inputs to striatal interneurons in monkeys: Synaptic organization and co-localization of calcium binding proteins. Neuroscience 89:1189–1208, 1999.

82. Nambu A, Takada M, Inase M, et al: Dual somatotopical representations of the primate subthalamic nucleus: Evidence for ordered but reversed body-map transformations from the primary motor cortex and the supplementary motor area. J Neurosci 16:2671–2683, 1996.

83. Wichmann T, Bergman H, DeLong MR: The primate subthalamic nucleus. I. Functional properties in intact animals. J Neurophysiol 72:494–506, 1994.

84. Bevan MD, Clarke NP, Bolam JP: Synaptic integration of functionally diverse pallidal information in the entopeduncular nucleus and subthalamic nucleus in the rat. J Neurosci 17:308–324, 1997.

85. Féger J, Hassani O-K, Mouroux M: The relationships between subthalamic nucleus, globus pallidus and thalamic parafascicular nucleus. In Ohye C, Kimura M, McKenzie JS (eds): The Basal Ganglia V. London, Plenum Press, 1995, pp 51–58.

86. Kita H: Physiology of two disynaptic pathways from the sensorimotor cortex to the basal ganglia output nuclei. In Percheron G, Mckenzie JS, Féger J (eds): The Basal Ganglia IV. New Ideas

and Data on Structure and Function. Advances in Behavioral Biology, vol 41. New York, Plenum Press, 1994, pp 263–276.

87. Maurice N, Deniau J-M, Menetrey A, et al: Prefrontal cortex-basal ganglia circuits in the rat: Involvement of ventral pallidum and subthalamic nucleus. Synapse 29:363–370, 1998.

88. Nambu A, Tokuno H, Hamada I, et al: Excitatory cortical inputs to pallidal neurons via the subthalamic nucleus in the monkey. J Neurophysiol 84:289–300, 2000.

88a. Nambu A, Tokuno H, Takada M: Functional significance of the cortico-subthalamo-pallidal "hyperdirect" pathway. Neurosci Res 43:111–117.

89. Smith Y, Paquet M, Hanson JE, et al: Subsynaptic localization of group I metabotropic glutamate receptors in the basal ganglia. In Graybiel AM, Kitai ST, DeLong MR (eds): The Basal Ganglia VI. New York, Plenum Press, 2003, pp 567–580.

89a. Bradley SR, Marino MJ, Wittman M, et al: Activation of group II metabotropic glutamate receptors inhibit synaptic excitation of the substantia nigra pars reticulata. J Neurosci 20:3085–3094.

90. Olszewski J: The Thalamus of the *Macaca mulatta*. An Atlas for Use with the Stereotaxic Instrument. Basel, Karger, 1952.

91. Jones EG: The Thalamus. New York, Plenum Press, 1985.

92. Ilinsky IA, Kultas-Ilinsky K: Sagittal cytoarchitectonic maps of the *Macaca mulatta* thalamus with a revised nomenclature of motor-related nuclei validated by observations on their connectivity. J Comp Neurol 262:331–364, 1987.

93. Paxinos G, Huang X-F, Toga AW: The rhesus monkey brain in stereotaxic coordinates. San Diego, CA, Academic Press, 2000.

94. Stepniewska I, Preuss TM, Kaas JH: Architectonic subdivisions of the motor thalamus of owl monkeys: Nissl, acetylcholinesterase, and cytochrome oxidase patterns. J Comp Neurol 349:536–556, 1994.

95. Percheron G, François C, Talbi B, et al: The primate motor thalamus. Brain Res Rev 22:93–181, 1996.

96. Srick PL: How do the basal ganglia and cerebellum gain access to the cortical motor areas? Behav Brain Res 18:107–123, 1985.

97. Ilinsky IA, Jouandet ML, Goldman-Rakic PS: Organization of the nigrothalamocortical system in the rhesus monkey. J Comp Neurol 236:315–330, 1985.

98. Rouillier E, Liang F, Babalian A, et al: Cerebellothalamocortical and pallidothalamocortical projections to the primary and supplementary motor cortical areas: A multiple tracing study in macaque monkeys. J Comp Neurol 345:185–213, 1994.

99. Sakai ST, Inase M, Tanji J: Comparison of cerebellothalamic and pallidothalamic projections in the monkey (*Macaca fuscata*): A double anterograde labeling study. J Comp Neurol 368:215–228, 1996.

100. Sakai ST, Inase M, Tanji J: Pallidal and cerebellar inputs to thalamocortical neurons projecting to the supplementary motor area in *Macaca fuscata*: A triple-labeling light microscopic study. Anat Embryol 199:9–19, 1999.

101. Sakai ST, Stepniewska I, Hui XQ, et al: Pallidal and cerebellar afferents to pre-supplementary motor area thalamocortical neurons in the owl monkey: A multiple labeling study. J Comp Neurol 417:164–180, 2000.

102. Middleton FA, Strick PL: Basal ganglia and cerebellar loops: Motor and cognitive circuits. Brain Res Rev 31:236–250, 2000.

103. Sidibé M, Pare J-F, Smith Y: Nigral and pallidal inputs to functionally segregated thalamostriatal neurons in the centromedian/parafascicular intralaminar nuclear complex in monkey. J Comp Neurol 447:286–299.

104. Sidibé M, Bevan MD, Bolam JP, et al: Efferent connections of the internal globus pallidus in the squirrel monkey: I. Topography and synaptic organization of the pallidothalamic projection. J Comp Neurol 382:323–347, 1997.

105. Shink E, Sidibé M, Smith Y: Efferent connections of the internal globus pallidus in the squirrel monkey: II. Topography and synaptic organization of the pallidal efferents to the pedunculopontine nucleus. J Comp Neurol 382:348–363, 1997.

106. Hazrati L-N, Parent A: Contralateral pallidothalamic and pallidotegmental projections in primates: An anterograde and retrograde labeling study. Brain Res 567:212–223, 1991.

107. Middleton FA, Strick PL: The cerebellum: An overview. Trends Neurosci 21:367–369, 1998.

108. Hendry SHC, Jones EG, Graham J: Thalamic relay nuclei for cerebellar and certain related fiber systems in the cat. J Comp Neurol 185:679–714, 1979.

109. Sakai ST, Patton K: Distribution of cerebellothalamic and nigrothalamic projections in the dog: A double anterograde tracing study. J Comp Neurol 330:183–194, 1993.

110. Inglis WL, Winn P: The pedunculopontine tegmental nucleus: Where the striatum meets the reticular formation. Prog Neurobiol 47:1–29, 1995.

111. Rye DB: Contributions of the pedunculopontine region to normal and altered REM sleep. Sleep 20:757–788, 1997.

112. Pahapill PA, Lozano AM: The pedunculopontine nucleus and Parkinson's disease. Brain 123:1767–1783, 2000.

113. Spann BM, Grofova I: Nigropedunculopontine projection in the rat: An anterograde tracing study with *Phaseolus vulgaris*-leucoagglutinin (PHA-L). J Comp Neurol 311:375–388, 1991.

114. Grofova I, Zhou M: Nigral innervation of cholinergic and glutamatergic cells in the rat mesopontine tegmentum: Light and electron microscopic anterograde tracing and immunohistochemical studies. J Comp Neurol 395:359–379, 1998.

Neuropathology of Movement Disorders

KURT A. JELLINGER

Movement disorders, according to their clinical phenotypes, can be divided into three main groups (Table 166–1); only the first two are discussed in this chapter. Most akinetic-rigid and hyperkinetic forms have their origin in basal ganglia dysfunction, and understanding of these movement disorders requires knowledge of the organization of basal ganglia and their anatomic and functional significance within the complex information circuits of the brain. Important insights into several movement disorders have come from a functional understanding of the basal ganglia. Their anatomy and functional circuits are reviewed.

ANATOMY AND FUNCTION OF BASAL GANGLIA

Anatomic Connections

The interconnections of the nuclei of the basal ganglia are shown schematically in Figure 166–1. The three main transmitter systems involved in the integration of basal ganglia function are glutamate, γ-aminobutyric acid (GABA), and dopamine. Normal movement is controlled by cortical–basal ganglia–thalamocortical circuits, in which the striatum receives glutamatergic input from the cerebral cortex and sends GABAergic output to substantia nigra pars compacta (SNc) and medial globus pallidus (GPi). These structures send GABAergic projections to specific thalamic nuclei, mainly to the medial and ventral thalamic nuclei and, to a lesser extent, to the deep layers of the superior colliculus and the mesencephalic reticular formation. These thalamic nuclei have an excitatory glutamatergic input to specific regions of the cerebral cortex involved in motor function. In this major circuit, the GABAergic output of the SNc and GPi diminishes the glutamatergic projections from the thalamus back to the cortex. Projections of the external globus pallidus (GPe), the dopaminergic SNc, and the subthalamic nucleus (STN) remain primarily within the realm of the basal ganglia, and these nuclei modulate the main flow of information through the basal ganglia.[1–3]

Basal Ganglia–Thalamocortical Circuits

Basal ganglia–thalamocortical circuits involve, in a sequential manner, specific parts of the prefrontal cortex, striatum, pallidal-nigral complex, medial or ventral thalamus, and the frontal (or prefrontal) cortical area of origin. Alexander and colleagues[4] tentatively defined five such basal ganglia–thalamocortical circuits: two loops involving motor (or premotor) cortical areas (i.e., motor circuit and an oculomotor circuit) and three loops involving different parts of the prefrontal association cortex (i.e., dorsolateral prefrontal circuit, lateral orbitofrontal circuit, and anterior cingulate or limbic circuit). These three main circuits include different frontal (or prefrontal) cortical areas as their starting focal point and involve different parts of the striatum, the pallidonigral complex, and the medial and ventral thalamus.[5]

Interactions between these circuits and the functional significance of such interactions are incompletely understood. There are, however, strong indications of a dominance in the flow of information from the limbic to the association circuit and subsequently to the motor circuit; the flow of information in the reverse direction is less prominent.[6] Two major loops modulate the cortical–basal ganglia–thalamocortical circuit (see Fig. 166–1), the balance between which appears to be crucial for the normal functioning of the basal ganglia.[3, 5, 7]

TABLE 166–1 ■ **Clinical Classification of Movement Disorders**

Akinetic-rigid forms
  Parkinsonism: Parkinson's disease; parkinsonian syndromes
  Stiff man syndrome
Hyperkinetic forms
  Chorea syndromes
  Dystonias
  Myoclonus
  Ballism
  Tics
Atactic movement disorders (not discussed)
  Cerebellar ataxias
  Spinocerebellar degeneration

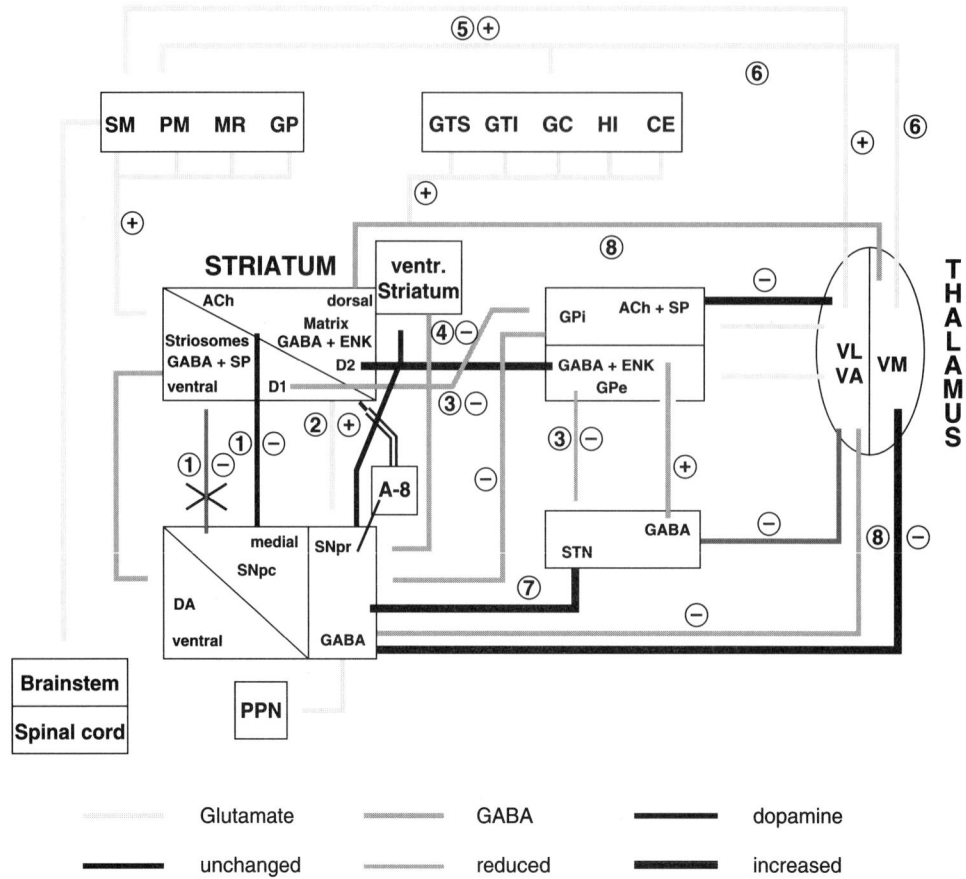

FIGURE 166–1. Schematic diagram of basal ganglia–thalamocortical circuitry under normal conditions and in Parkinson's disease. Several pathways are shown: 1, nigrostriatal dopaminergic pathway; 2, striatonigral pathway; 3, indirect loop; 4, direct loop; 5, motor or complex loop; 6, thalamocortical pathway; 7, pallidosubthalamic pathway. A-8, retrorubral field; ACh, acetylcholine; CE, entorhinal cortex; CS, superior colliculus; DA, dopamine; ENK, enkephalin; GC, gyrus cinguli; GP, postcentral gyrus; GPe, external globus pallidus; GPi, internal globus pallidus; HI, hippocampus; MPT, mesopontine tegmentum; MR, motor cortex; PM, premotor field; PPN, pedunculopontine nucleus; SM, supplementary motor field; SNpc, substantia nigra zona compacta; SNpr, substantia nigra reticulata; SP, substance P; STN subthalamic nucleus; VLM, ventrolateral/medial thalamus; VM, medioventral thalamus; +, excitatory; −, inhibitory. (Adapted from Jellinger KA: Neuropathology of movement disorders. Neurosurg Clin N Am 9:237–262, 1998.)

A nigrostriatal circuit, in which the SNc receives a GABAergic inhibitory projection from the striatum, feeds back to the striatum with a modulating dopaminergic input. Dopamine causes excitation of striatal neurons that project to the GPi or SNpr (by D_1 receptors) and thereby releases inhibition on the thalamic nuclei, maintaining normal speed and tone of movement. Dopamine also inhibits neurons that project to the GPe or STN (by D_2 receptors), keeping check on the normal negative effect on motor speed and tone associated with high output from the STN.

The GPe receives GABAergic input from the striatum and sends a GABAergic projection to the STN, which sends glutamatergic excitatory projections to the SNr and GPi. The STN "sets the throttle" on the activity of the cortical–basal ganglia–thalamocortical circuit, with a normal high output responsible for the SNr and GPi inhibiting thalamic excitation of the cortex. By inhibiting the basal ganglia output neurons in the GPi

and SNr, the thalamocortical system can be disinhibited, which leads to a higher output at the cortical level.

Activity of the output structures of the basal ganglia is controlled by two opposing striatal pathways, the direct and indirect pathways (see Fig. 166–1). The *direct pathway* consists of the striatal projections to the GPi and SNr. The medium-sized, densely spiny striatal projection neurons giving origin to this route contain GABA, substance P, and dynorphin as neurotransmitters and express mainly the dopamine D_1 receptor. Activation of these striatal neurons leads to inhibition of the tonically active pallidal and nigral neurons and consequently to a disinhibition of the basal ganglia target structures in the thalamus and midbrain. The direct pathway may be considered as facilitating thalamocortical activity and thereby facilitating motor and behavioral output.[3, 7]

The *indirect pathway* is sequentially composed of the striatal projections to the GPe, the GABAergic external pallidal projections to the STN, and the glutamatergic STN projections to the GPi and SNr. The striatopallidal projections are established by GABAergic, striatal, medium-sized spiny neurons that also contain enkephalin and that predominantly express the dopamine D_2 receptor. Activation of the striatal neurons in this pathway leads to inhibition of the tonically active neurons in GPe, which leads to a lesser inhibition at the level of the STN. A stronger activity of the excitatory, glutamatergic subthalamic outputs to the GPi and SNr leads to activation of these GABAergic output neurons and, ultimately, to a stronger inhibition of their thalamic and mesencephalic targets. The indirect pathway is thought to exert an inhibitory, modulating influence on the basal ganglia output structures in the thalamus and the midbrain, leading to suppression of motor and behavioral output.[3,7]

Balance between the direct and indirect pathways at the level of the pallidum and SN appears to be crucial for normal functioning of the basal ganglia–thalamocortical circuits. Dopamine has opposing ef-

fects on the two striatal output pathways: a stimulatory effect on the D_1 receptor–containing direct pathway and a suppressing effect on the D_2 receptor–containing indirect pathway. It facilitates the information flow through the direct pathway at the expense of the indirect pathway, which is suppressed by dopamine. Through enhanced inhibition of the basal ganglia output neurons, this leads to disinhibition of the thalamocortical system, facilitating expression of its motor, behavioral, and cognitive output. In contrast, dopamine depletion, as is the case in Parkinson's disease (PD), leads to a higher activity of neurons in the output structures and consequently to inhibition of their thalamic and midbrain targets (Fig. 166–2; see Fig. 166–1). Suppressing of the activity of the thalamocortical system may be, at least in part, an explanation for hypokinesia in PD. Hyperkinetic disorders, such as hemiballism (i.e., lesion of the STN) or Huntington's disease, can be explained by a lack of balance of the two striatal output pathways, leading to lower activity of neurons in the output structures of the basal ganglia

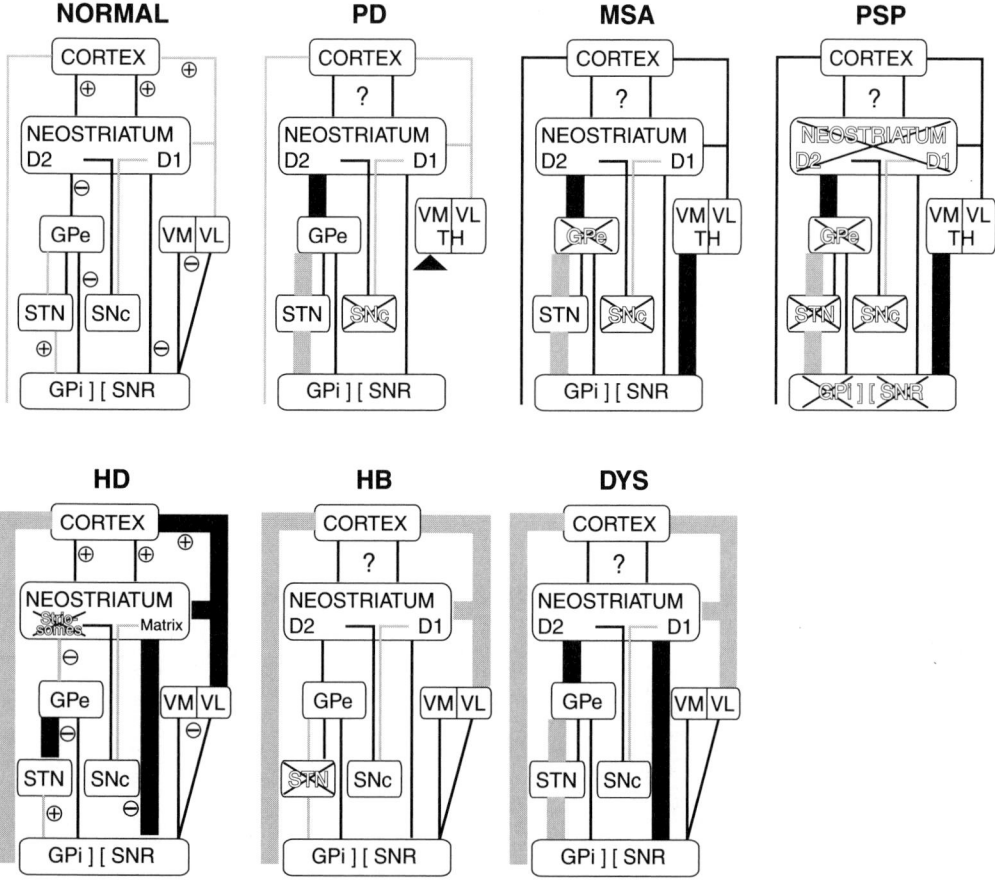

FIGURE 166–2. Schematic diagram of basal ganglia–thalamocortical circuitry under normal conditions and in hypokinetic and hyperkinetic movement disorders. The width of lines represents the relative change of activity compared with normal levels. *Disrupted lines* represent altered patterns with increase or decrease of neuronal activity; the *dashed arrow* indicates reduced activity; and the *solid arrow* indicates increased activity. D_1, dopamine type 1 receptor; D_2, dopamine type 2 receptor; DYS, dystonia; GPe, external segment of globus pallidus; GPi, internal segment of globus pallidus; HB, hemiballism; HD, Huntington's disease; MSA, multisystem atrophy; Normal, normal conditions; PD, Parkinson's disease; PSP, progressive supranuclear palsy; SNc, substantia nigra pars compacta; SNr, substantia nigra pars reticulata; STN subthalamic nucleus; TH, thalamus; VL, ventrolateral thalamic nuclei; VM, ventromedial thalamic nuclei.

T A B L E 1 6 6 – 2 ■ Ultrastructure, Immunohistochemistry, Biochemistry, and Distribution of Neuroglial Inclusions

TYPE OF INCLUSIONS	ULTRASTRUCTURES	IMMUNOHISTOCHEMISTRY								BIOCHEMISTRY	LESION PATTERN
		PHF	pNF	pTau	Ubi	ChrA	αBCrys	APP	αβTub		
Pick bodies	14–18 nm SF + 24 nm LPCT	++	+++	++	++	++	+	+	−	55–64 kDa 3-repeat tau doublet	Hippocampus, neocortex
Pick ballooned cells	Same	+	+++*	++	++	+	+	?	−	Same as above	Same as above
AD-NFT	22 nm PHF + 18 nm SF	+++	+++	+/+++	+/+++	−	−	+	−	PHF-tau (60, 64, 68 kDa triplet)	Hippocampus, cortex, amygdala
PEP-NFT	22 nm PHF	++	++	+/++	+	−	+	+	−	PHF-tau triplet	Brainstem, basal ganglia
PSP-NFT	14–15 nmST + 10 nm PHF	±	+/+++	+++	+	−	−	+	−	64, 69 kDa tau 4-repeat doublet	Basal ganglia, brainstem, cortex
PSP, ballooned cells	?	−	++	+	+	−	+	−	−	Same	Same
PSP, threads	14–15 nm SF	±/+	++	+	±/+	−	+	−	−	Same	Same
Lewy bodies, subcortical	7–20 nm (mean, 10 nm) SF	±/+	+++†	±‡	+++	+	+	−	+	α-synuclein + pNF + ubiquitin	Brainstem, nucleus basalis
"Pale" (pre-Lewy) bodies	10 nm SF	?	+	−	++	?	?	?	?	Same	Same
Lewy bodies, cortical	10, 12–18 nm SF	+	+*	−/±	++	+	?	+	?	α-synuclein + 68 kDa NF fragment	Cortex, amygdala
CBD inclusions (NFT-like)	26–28 nm PCT + 26 nm SF	+	+/+++	++§	±/−	−	−	?	?	64–69 kDa 4-repeat tau doublet	Cortex
CBD, ballooned cells	12–15 nm ST + 26 nm SF	−	+	±	−/+	−	++	−	?	Same	Basal ganglia, brainstem
MSA, neuronal inclusions	18–28 nm fibrils + 10 nm filam.	−	±	−	+++	−	?	?	−	α-synuclein	Cortex, basal ganglia
MSA, oligodendroglial incl.	21–30 nm tubules	+	−	++	++	−	−	?	++	α-synuclein + ubiquitin	White matter, cortex
MND; FTD and MND	13–25 nm SF	−	+	−	+++	?	−	−	−	?	Spinal cord neurons
FTD, ballooned cells		−	−	−	++	−	++	?	?	?	Cortex
Astrocytic inclusions: PSP,CBD, PiD	15–20 nm SF	−	+	++	±/+	−	−	?	?	64, 69 kDa tau doublet/triplet	Cortex, basal ganglia, brainstem, white matter
Oligodendroglia "coiled bodies," PSP, CBD, AD	13–15 nm SF¹, 15–20 nm SF + 26 nm LPCT	−	−	+	−	−	−	?	?	Tau doublet or triplet	White matter, cortex

*Persistent after phosphatase treatment.
†Nonpersistent after phosphatase treatment.
‡Also contain microtubule-associated protein 5 (MAP 5).
§Different from AD and PSP.

PHF, paired, helical filaments; pNF, phosphorylated neurofilament epitopes; pTau, phosphorylated tau protein; Ubi, ubiquitin; ChrA, chromogranin A; αBCrys, α-B crystallin; APP, amyloid precursor protein; αβTub, tubuline; SF, straight filaments; LPCT, long-period constricted tubules; LBD, Lewy body dementia; CBD, corticobasal degeneration; NF, neurofilaments; MND, motor neuron disease; FTD, frontotemporal dementia; PiD, Pick's disease.

and higher activity in the thalamocortical system (see Fig. 166–2).

CLASSIFICATION OF MOVEMENT DISORDERS

Most movement disorders related to basal ganglia dysfunction are neurodegenerative diseases that are morphologically characterized by neuronal degeneration and loss accompanied by astrocytosis in various, often disparate parts of the central nervous sytem (CNS) that may or may not be associated with cytoskeletal abnormalities (i.e., neuronal or glial inclusions) and representing important histologic signposts that, in some disorders, point to the diagnosis (Table 166–2). Nevertheless, clinical and morphologic overlaps between various phenotypes, lesion patterns, and cytopathologic hallmarks may impede the differential diagnosis. Because some movement disorders lack any such pathognomonic lesions, they are classified according to their morphologic lesion pattern or other criteria. Table 166–3 provides a morphologic classification of the major movement disorders related to basal ganglia dysfunction. For some of these disorders, consensus criteria for their clinical and neuropathologic diagnosis have been established,[8–17] although some criteria are still under discussion.

AKINETIC-RIGID MOVEMENT DISORDERS: PARKINSONISM

James Parkinson (1817) is credited with originally describing the disease that bears his name.[18] It is now recognized that there are many causes of shaking palsy or parkinsonism, with frequent clinical misclassification even if strict clinical diagnostic criteria are used. *Parkinsonism* describes the presence of extrapyramidal movement disturbance manifested by a combination of rigidity and bradykinesia, with or without resting tremor. Table 166–4 shows the main causes of parkinsonism.

According to the previously described morphologic-biochemical classification, akinetic-rigid movement disorders[1] include *synucleopathies*, which include Lewy body–associated disorders (e.g., PD, Lewy body dementia) and multiple system atrophy (MSA),[2] and *tauopathies*, all featuring neurofibrillary pathology.

Synucleopathies

α-Synuclein is a 140–amino acid protein normally present in presynaptic terminals in the human brain[19] that was initially discovered as a non-Aβ component of Alzheimer's disease (AD) amyloid.[20] Its gene, which is localized on chromosome 4, is mutated in rare familial forms of PD.[21] α-Synuclein was subsequently demonstrated in Lewy bodies and Lewy-related neuritic pathology in PD[22] and in neuronal and glial inclusions in MSA.[23] Given the fundamental nature of the α-synuclein–containing lesions in these disorders, Lewy body disease (LBD) and MSA are considered to be synucleinopathies.[13, 24]

TABLE 166–3 ■ Morphologic and Biochemical Classification of Degenerative Diseases with Movement Disorders

α-Synucleopathies

Parkinson's disease (brainstem type of Lewy body disease)
  Sporadic
  Familial with α-synuclein mutation
  Familial with other mutations
  Pure autonomic failure
  Lewy body dysphagia
Dementia with Lewy bodies; diffuse Lewy body disease
Multiple system atrophy (MSA)
  Striatonigral degeneration (MSA-P)
  Olivopontocerebellar atrophy
  Shy-Drager syndrome
Hallervorden-Spatz disease (specific forms)

Tauopathies

Progressive supranuclear palsy (PSP) (4-repeat tau doublet plus exon 19)
Corticobasal degeneration (CBD) (same)
Parkinson-dementia/ALS complex of Guam (3+4-repeat triplet)
Postencephalitic parkinsonism (3+4-repeat triplet)
Chromosome 17-linked familial dementia (frontotemporal dementia and parkinsonism) (FTDP-17) (tau doublet)
Pallido-ponto-nigral degeneration (PPND) (4-repeat tau)
Multiple system tauopathy with presenile dementia (MSTD)
Pick's disease (3-repeat tau doublet without exon 10)
Hallervorden-Spatz disease (with tangles)

Polyglutamine repeat (CAG) disorders

Huntington's disease
Choreoacanthocytosis (neuroacanthocytosis)
Machado-Joseph disease (SCA 3)
Dentatorubropallidoluysian atrophy (DRLPA)

Other heredodegenerative disorders

(Non)hereditary striatal degeneration
Pallidal degeneration and related variants
Hallervorden-Spatz disease (without α-synucleopathy)
Wilson's disease
Inherited dystonias

TABLE 166–4 ■ Causes of Parkinsonism

Common Causes of Parkinsonism

Idiopathic Parkinson's disease
Drug-induced parkinsonism
Multiple system atrophy
Progressive supranuclear palsy (i.e., Steele-Richardson-Olszewski syndrome)

Uncommon Causes of Parkinsonism

Vascular pseudoparkinsonism
Corticobasal degeneration
Alzheimer-type changes
Frontotemporal neurodegenerative disorders
Wilson's disease
Huntington's disease
Multisystem degenerations
Space-occupying lesions
Hydrocephalus
Toxin-induced parkinsonism
Boxer's encephalopathy (i.e., dementia pugilistica)

LEWY BODY–ASSOCIATED DISORDERS

The prominent cytoskeletal lesions are *Lewy bodies*, cytoplasmic inclusions occurring in many regions of the nervous system. They are morphologic hallmarks of PD (or brainstem LBD, and dementia with Lewy bodies [DLB]) and are also found in a variety of neurodegenerative disorders as an essential or coincidental feature.[13, 25]

Idiopathic Parkinson's Disease

Idiopathic PD is a progressive neurodegenerative disorder of advanced age, clinically characterized by motor symptoms such as bradykinesia, rigidity, tremor, and postural imbalance. Subtle cognitive dysfunctions and depression are often present early in the disease, whereas dementia is common in a later phase. Idiopathic PD is characterized by progressive degeneration of the dopaminergic nigrostriatal system and other cortical (or subcortical) neuronal networks associated with widespread occurrence of Lewy bodies and dystrophic neurites, leading to striatal dopamine deficiency and multiple other biochemical deficits that produce the variable clinical picture of this heterogeneous disorder. Accepted clinical criteria for the diagnosis of possible and probable PD[10] have a high sensitivity for detecting parkinsonism but have a specificity of only 75% for identifying idiopathic PD and to differentiate it from other Lewy body disorders, particularly DLB.[26] For the diagnosis of definite PD, histopathologic confirmation is required.[11, 13, 27–29] Several clinicopathologic studies have shown that LBD, including PD, represents 60% to 83% of cases, whereas other degenerative disorders masquerading as PD, such as DLB, MSA, and progressive supranuclear palsy (PSP), account for 15% to 30%. Other entities, referred to as *secondary parkinsonism*, are seen in 5% to 10% of patients (Table 166–5). Awareness of the high rate of misdiagnosis and refinements in

the clinical diagnostic criteria and approaches to early diagnosis of PD[30, 31, 31a] seem to have improved the accuracy of diagnosis to 85% (Table 166–6). Although data on the lesion pattern of the multisystem degeneration in PD have provided insights into the course and pathophysiology of its clinical subtypes,[28, 32, 33] the cause and pathogenesis of PD remain unclear.

Macroscopically, the brain is unremarkable or may show mild cortical atrophy and enlargement of the ventricular system. On cut surface, pallor of the SN and locus ceruleus (LC) is evident. PD is histopathologically characterized by the presence of Lewy bodies and Lewy neurites in association with variable neuron loss in the midbrain and other subcortical nuclei. In addition to degeneration of the dopamine-containing neurons in the SNc, other cell groups, including the LC and the basal nucleus of Meynert, are affected.[28, 29] According to the levels of calbindin in the midbrain, dopaminergic neurons of SNc have been divided into two major types with different vulnerabilities[34]: sparsely distributed neurons in a calbindin-rich matrix component and densely packed cells in five calbindin-poor nigrosomes. Melanized neurons (45% to 66%) and tyrosine hydroxylase–immunoreactive neurons (60% to 85%; mean, 75%) are severely depleted in the A9 group of SNc,[35, 36] particularly in the ventrolateral tier (area α, 91% to 97%), followed by the medioventral, dorsal, and lateral areas (Figs. 166–3 and 166–4). Cell loss in the nigrosomes ranges from 76% to 98% and is most severe in the initially involved main pocket I in the caudal and mediolateral part of SNc (98%), compared with 84% in the adjacent matrix. From here, cell depletion spreads to other nigrosomes, with pocket II being more affected (94% cell loss) than the medial matrix of the same level (77%), and finally to the matrix along a caudorostral, lateromedial, and ventrodorsal direction of progression (see Fig. 166–4*A* to *C*).[34] The temporospatial order is related to the somatotopic pattern of

T A B L E   1 6 6 – 5 ■ **Incidence of Different Types of Parkinsonism in Autopsy Series (Percentage)**

TYPE OF LESION	LITERATURE (MEAN)-JELLINGER[27]	HUGHES ET AL (1990–99)	JELLINGER (1957–70)	JELLINGER (1970–88)	JELLINGER (1989–2001)
Idiopathic Parkinson disease	44–94	50.0	15.3	17.0	57.6
Lewy body dementia	—	—	2.7	5.8	20.6
Lewy body disease (total)	(75)	50.0	78.0	82.8	78.0
Other degenerative Parkinsonism	0–30 (7)	33.0	10.0	8.9	13.2
Multiple system atrophy	?	22.0	4.6	2.3	3.5
Prog. supranuclear palsy	?	11.0	3.6		
Pick disease, corticobasal degen.	?		0.9	2.6	
Alzheimer disease	?	?	0.9	3.5	5.8
Secondary parkinsonism	0–50 (18)	17.0	12.0	8.3	8.4
Vascular (MIE, SAE, MIX)	0–15 (2)	?	2.0	4.2	
Postencephalitic	4–30 (13)	?	6.3		3.1
Sympt. (e.g., JCD, tumors)	?	?	—	0.3	0
Toxic/drug-induced	?	?	0.9	0.3	7.1
Posttraumatic/boxer dementia	?	?	0.9	0.3	1.1
Unclassified/no lesion	0–19 (2.6)	?	0.9	1.3	3.1
Total (n)	1400	143	110	400	260

† With substantia nigra lesion, 3.0.
* Figures within parentheses are percentages.
JCD, Creutzfeldt-Jakob disease; MIE, multiple infarct encephalopathy; MIX, mixed-type dementia (MIE + AI); SAE, subcortical arteriosclerotic encephalopathy.

TABLE 166-6 ■ **Misdiagnosis in Autopsy Series of Clinical Parkinson's Disease**

PATHOLOGY	HUGHES ET AL[30] (n = 100) %	HUGHES ET AL (n = 143) %	RAJPUT ET AL[133] (n = 41) %	JELLINGER[27] (1957–70) (n = 110) %	JELLINGER (1971–88) (n = 260) %	JELLINGER (1989–2000) (N = 145) %
Alzheimer's disease (AD)	6	?	2	0.9	2.6	1.8
Vascular encephalopathy (VaE)	0	?	2	4.6	3.5	0.8
Progressive supranuclear palsy	8	3.5	0	2.8	1.8	1.1
Multiple system atrophy	5	3.0	10	6.5	1.2	1.1
Nigral atrophy (unclassified)	2		2	3.6	0.5	0.6
MIX encephalopathy (AD+VaE)	0		0	1.5	0.5	0.6
Lewy body dementia	1		0	0.9	3.6	4.6
Pick's disease, corticobasal degen	0	8.7	0	2.8	0.2	—
Normal (essential tremor?)	1		0	0.0	0.3	0.8
Others (e.g., pallidonigral degen., toxic)	0		2	0.9	0.3	0.6
Postencephalitic parkinsonism	1		4	0.9	—	—
Total (%)	24	15.2	22	24.5	15.3	11.5

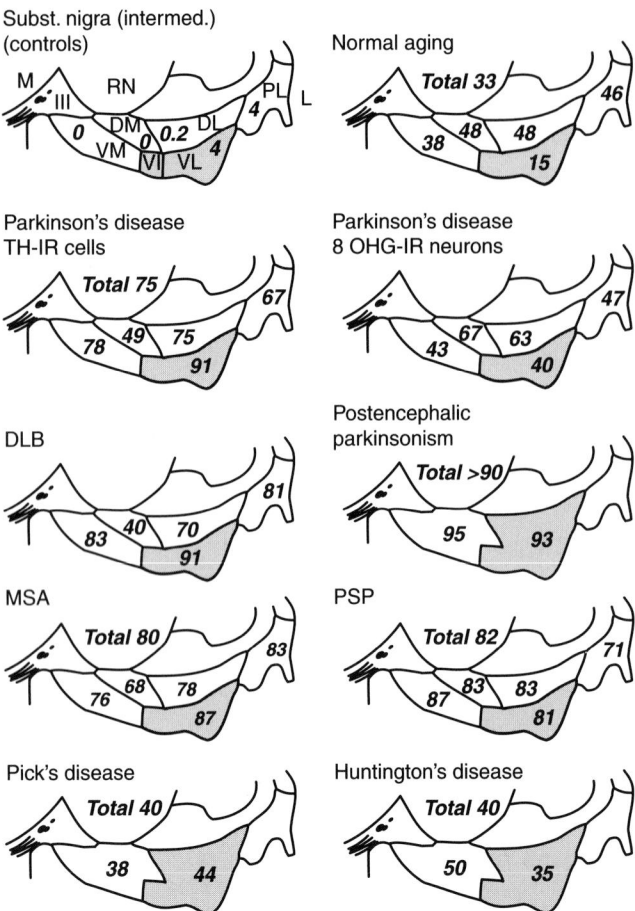

FIGURE 166–3. Drawings of coronal sections of the substantia nigra pars compacta (intermediate level) demonstrate 8-hydroxyguanidine–immunoreactive neurons in normal controls, as well as regional and total cell losses (%) in normal aging, Parkinson's disease, postencephalitic parkinsonism, dementia with Lewy bodies (DLB), multisystem atrophy (MSA-PI), progressive supranuclear palsy (PSP), Pick's disease, and Huntington's disease. Tyrosine hydroxylase–immunoreactive (TR-IR) cell loss in Parkinson's disease is also illustrated. DL, dorsolateral; M, medial group; RN, red nucleus; VL, ventrolateral thalamic nuclei; VM, ventromedial thalamic nuclei. (Adapted from Zhang J, Perry G, Smith MA, et al: Parkinson's disease is associated with oxidative damage to cytoplasmic DNA and RNA in substantia nigra neurons. Am J Pathol 154:1423–1429, 1999.)

dopaminergic terminal loss in striatum that is more severe in the dorsal and caudal putamen than in the caudate nucleus.[37] The degree of SNc cell loss shows close correlation to the duration and severity of motor dysfunction.[38, 39]

There is much less involvement of the A10 group (i.e., ventral tegmental area [VTA], nucleus parabrachialis, and nucleus parabrachialis pigmentosus) projecting to the cortical and limbic areas (i.e., mesocorticolimbic dopaminergic system). These nuclei suffer 40% to 50% cell loss,[40] whereas the periretrorubal A8 region, containing few tyrosine hydroxylase–immunoreactive but calbindin-rich neurons, and the central periventricular gray show no definite degeneration[40] or about 20% to 32% cell loss in A8 (see Fig. 166–4C and D).[34, 41] Cell loss in these nuclei shows no correlation to duration of disease.[34]

Showing an inverse pattern to the contents of calbindin and other calcium-binding proteins, SNc lesions in human PD are similar to those produced by the neurotoxin l-methyl-4-phenyl-l,2,3,6-tetrahydropyridine (MPTP), the most widely used model of PD.[11, 41] They differ from age-related lesions in the dorsal tier that is involved only in late stages of PD,[36, 42] and some studies show a 35% to 41% reduction in the total number of pigmented SN cells, with severe loss of dopamine transporter–immunoreactive neurons in older persons.[43] The estimated decrease in the total number of pigmented neurons and neuronal density in SNc is 9.8% and 7.4%, respectively, per decade, with a 4.4% decrease per decade in neuronal volume.[44] There is a similar distribution of reduced intensity of dopamine transporter messenger RNA in the remaining SNc neurons[45] and decreased α-synuclein mRNA expression in SN and cortex of PD brains,[46] with loss of the vesicular monoamine transporter VMAT2 (a dopaminergic neuronal marker) in striatum, orbitofrontal cortex, and amygdala in the early stages of PD but not in the SN.[47] Most mesotelencephalic dopamine neurons in A9 and A10 cell groups express high levels of dopamine transporter, whereas a smaller subpopulation of mesencephalic and all hypothalamic dopamine cell groups express little or no dopamine transporter.[48] PD shows an increase of 8-hydroxyguanidine, a common product of nucleic acid oxidation,[49] with similar cell loss but less production of 8-hydroxyguanidine in the SNc in the brains of patients with MSA and DLB (see Fig. 166–3). Whereas fibroblastic growth factor (FGF) immunoreactivity and its binding activity are retained in SNc neurons in PD,[50] brain-derived neurotrophic factor (BDNF) expression[51] and the number of neurons in SNc and VTA containing TRKB mRNA (a high-affinity BDNF receptor) are reduced in PD without a decrease of TRKB mRNA levels in the remaining neurons.[52, 53] These data suggest a selective vulnerability of neurons rich in neuromelanin with high expression of dopamine transporter mRNA,[54, 55] although not related to their intrinsic capacity of dopamine synthesis,[56] low content of calcium-binding proteins (protective role by preventing Ca^{2+} influx into cells),[34] and weaker neurotrophic support,[57] whereas BDNF protein expression appears not to protect melanized SNc cells from neurodegeneration.[53] This hypothesis is supported by preservation of the STN containing calcineurin and paralbumin (calcium-binding proteins)–immunoreactive neurons[58] and of nondopaminergic, GABAergic neurons in the SNr that are involved only in the terminal stages of PD with loss of paralbumin immunoreactivity.[36] However, there is selective involvement of the parabrachial nucleus of A10, which has neurons rich in tyrosine hydroxylase and GABA but poor in neuromelanin.[40] The severe decrease of caspase-3–positive, pigmented neurons in the SNc in PD (−76%) compared with controls suggests that distribution of this central effector enzyme of apoptosis[59] may contribute to regional vulnerability, whereas the regional increase of 8-hydroxyguanidine corresponding to the pattern of neurodegeneration in PD suggests increased oxidative damage to neuronal cytoplasm,[49] supporting the hy-

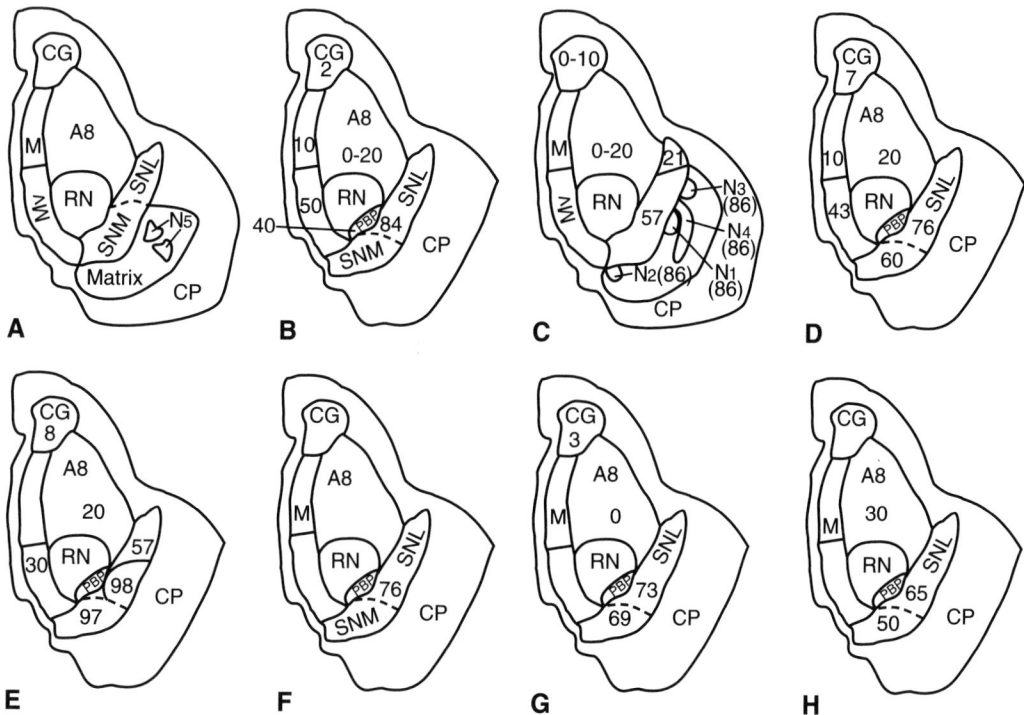

FIGURE 166–4. Neuronal loss in catecholaminergic nuclei of midbrain (intermediate level) in Parkinson's disease. *A,* Distribution of catecholaminergic nuclei. *B,* Distribution (%) of melanized, tyrosine hydroxylase–immunoreactive (TH-IR) neurons in normal controls. *C,* Average loss of TH-IR neurons in five cases of Parkinson's disease (PD) (duration of illness, 7 to 32 years). *D,* Percent average loss of TH-IR neurons in PD (no specific clinical type). *E,* Percent loss of TH-IR neurons in akinetic-rigid PD. *F,* Percent loss of caspase-3–positive, pigmented neurons in PD. *G,* Percent loss of TH-IR neurons in the tremor-dominant subtype of PD. *H,* Percent loss of calbindin-immunoreactive neurons in PD. A8, dopaminergic cell group A8; CG, central gray substance; CP, cerebral peduncle; M, medial group, Mv, medioventral group; N, nigrosome; PBP, parabrachial pigmented nucleus; RN, red nucleus; SNM, substantia nigra pars dorsalis; SNL, substantia nigra pars lateralis. (*A* and *C* from Damier P, Hirsch EC, Agid Y, et al: The substantia nigra of the human brain: II. Patterns of loss of dopamine-containing neurons in Parkinson's disease. Brain 122:1437–1448, 1999.)

pothesis that oxidative stress represents a major pathogenic factor in PD.[33, 60–65]

Symptom-Specific Lesion Pattern in Parkinson's Disease. Dopaminergic fibers, originating from different cell groups in the ventral mesencephalon (i.e., SNc [A9 cell group], VTA [A10], and the retrorubral area [A8]), strongly innervate the striatum and the cortex of the frontal lobe, including the prefrontal cortex and the motor and premotor areas.[66] Progressive degeneration of the dopaminergic system in PD affects functioning of the basal ganglia and cerebral cortex, particularly the frontal cortex. The major clinical subtypes of PD have specific morphologic lesion patterns of pathophysiologic relevance.[29, 33, 39]

In the *akinetic-rigid type,* the ventrolateral part of the SNc, which projects to the dorsal putamen, degenerates more severely than the medial part projecting to caudate nucleus and anterior putamen (see Fig. 166–4E), and there is a negative correlation between SNc neuron loss and the severity of akinesia-rigidity and dopamine loss in posterior putamen.[37, 38, 67] Damage to the nigrostriatal system caused by SN cell loss produces dopaminergic denervation of the striatum, whose efflux systems through the pallidum, SNr, and thalamus to the cortex and the parallel striatal-nigral-pallidal-cortical loop to premotor cortex remain intact in the early stages of PD. There is a ventromedial gradient loss of tyrosine hydroxylase– and dopamine transporter–immunoreactive fibers and endings (both frequently co-localized in synaptic vesicles and plasma membranes) progressing from dorsal to ventral putamen,[68] with predominant involvement of the met-enkephalin– and substance P–rich, acetylcholinesterase-poor striosomes of putamen projecting to the severely involved ventrolateral SNc. Preservation of the calbindin-positive, somatostatin-rich matrix, showing increased somatostatin mRNA expression[69] and projecting to GABA neurons of SNr and motor thalamus, and of periventricular islands of the caudate and nucleus accumbens suggests that the endings richest in dopamine transporter are most sensitive to degeneration.[70] Studies of caudate nucleus biopsies in PD patients have found reduced tyrosine hydroxylase immunostaining and revealed differences in substance P and met-enkephalin levels, with both being normal or variably reduced; low met-enkephalin immunostaining correlated with the severity of motor clinical symptoms.[71]

It has been estimated that the onset of clinical motor symptoms in PD occurs with loss of about 50% of SNc neurons, reduction of striatal dopamine uptake by 57% to 80%, and dopamine transporter loss of 56%.[67, 72, 73] Onset is preceded by a preclinical phase correlating with "incidental LBD,"[42] the duration and progression of which are still under discussion.[72, 74] Dopaminergic denervation of the striatum causes severe loss of dendrites on type I medium spiny neurons, the principal goal of dopaminergic input from SN[75] that, together with abundant α-synuclein pathology in strictures[76a] and ultrastructural findings in PD[76] and progressive loss of tyrosine hydroxylase– and dopamine transporter–immunoreactive nigrostriatal fibers, suggests trans-synaptic degeneration as a possible substrate for the severity of motor deficits and decreased efficacy of dopamine-mimetic treatment in late stages of PD.[77]

In PD, despite progressive dopaminergic denervation, the striatal matrix and the striatal efferents remain intact, but in MSA and PSP, loss of calcineurin-, calbindin-, methionine-, and substance P–immunoreactive neurons in the dorsolateral putamen, ventrolateral pallidum, and lateral SNc induce deafferentation of striatal efflux nuclei[77–79] and cause lesions of the striatal afferent and efferent projection systems (i.e., a motor loop). In the akinetic-rigid form of MSA, more severe atrophy in the lateral SNc (see Fig. 166–3) causes loss of calbindin-immunoreactive matrix cells in the caudal putamen with trans-synaptic degeneration of striatonigral efferents.[77, 79] Reduced dopaminergic input to the putamen but not the caudate causes increased activity of the GABAergic inhibitory "indirect" striatal efferent loop through SNr and GPi lesioning in PD,[78] leading to increased GABA output to the ventrolateral thalamus projecting to the cortex (i.e., thalamocortical motor loop) (see Fig. 166–2). The increased excitatory glutamatergic drive from STN and GPi/SNr leads, through reduced cortical activation by glutamate, to an akinetic-rigid syndrome.[7, 36] In MSA and PSP, there is additional severe damage to the GPi, SNr, and STN, causing dysfunction of these inhibitory nuclei projecting to the motor thalamus.[59, 78–80]

The *tremor-dominant type* of PD shows less severe total neuronal SNc loss (means, 52.8% versus 69%) and less severe depletion in the lateral than in the medial SNc,[39] but there is damage to the retrorubral A8 field (see Fig. 166–3G) that is usually preserved in akinetic-rigid PD.[34, 40] The A8 area, unlike A9 and A10, contains only few tyrosine hydroxylase– and dopamine transporter–immunoreactive and mainly contains calretinin-immunoreactive neurons.[81] A8 is largely independent of striatal influences and projects to the matrix of the dorsolateral striatum and ventromedial thalamus.[82, 83] The A8 and A10 areas directly influence the striatal efflux through the SNr to the thalamus and from there to the prefrontal cortex.[5, 84] Tremor-synchronous electric activity has been reported in the STN, GPi, and ventral intermedial thalamus (VIM),[85] and positron-emission tomographic studies suggest increased functional activity of ventral thalamic projections to cortical motor regions.[86, 87] Although autopsy cases of essential tremor show no pathologic changes—except for mild SN cell

loss[88]—in cases of essential and orthostatic tremor, bilateral overactivity of cerebellar connections has been reported.[89, 90] These data, differences in biopterin content of cerebrospinal fluid between akinetic-rigid and tremor-dominant PD, and the relation of dopa uptake between the caudate and putamen[91] suggest different pathophysiologic mechanisms for the two major clinical subtypes based on differential morphology, which has therapeutic implications, particularly for surgical treatment.

Because PD is a multisystem disorder, many other extranigral systems are involved[28, 29, 92]: noradrenergic LC, dorsal vagal nucleus, and adrenergic medullary nuclei; serotonergic dorsal raphe nuclei; nucleus of Meynert and other cholinergic brainstem nuclei (e.g., Westphal-Edinger nucleus, which controls pupillomotor functions and rapid eye movement sleep function); posterolateral hypothalamus, the center-median parafascicular thalamus, and parts of the limbic system, including the amygdaloid nucleus; hippocampal formation; anterior cingulate gyrus; limbic thalamic nucleus with prefrontal projection; other brainstem and entomeric systems; and other CNS regions. Most lesions are region specific, affecting not all neurons containing a specific transmitter or harboring Lewy bodies, and this may explain the complex patterns of morphologic, functional, biochemical, and clinical deficits of the disorder, including mental decline in idiopathic PD.[33, 93, 94] In incidental LB pathology, suggested to represent subclinical forms of PD, α-synuclein–immunoreactive LN and LB have been demonstrated in many reticular and raphe brainstem nuclei, the ceruleus–subceruleus and glossopharyngeus–vagus complexes, and olfactory bulb in the absence of nigral changes, suggesting early involvement of these systems with ascending progression.[41]

Lewy Bodies and Neuronal Cell Death. In PD and DLB, Lewy bodies occur in two forms: the classic brainstem type and the cortical type. Classic Lewy bodies are intraneuronal, cytoplasmic, spherical inclusions ranging from 8 to 30 μm in diameter with a hyaline eosinophilic core and a narrow, pale-stained halo. They are composed of radially arranged, 7- to 20-nm, intermediate filaments associated with a granular, electron-dense coating material and vesicular structures; the core contains densely packed filaments and dense granular material. Cortical Lewy bodies are eosinophilic, rounded, angular or reniform structures without an obvious halo. Ultrastructurally, they are composed of feltlike, arranged, intermediate filaments and granular material.[11, 13] Lewy bodies and pale bodies (their precursors[95]) are diagnostic hallmarks for PD and DLB, but they are not specific for these disorders; they have been described as secondary pathology in a variety of conditions, such as MSA, PSP, Lewy body dysphagia, corticobasal degeneration, motoneuron disease, Hallervorden-Spatz disease, ataxia-telangiectasia, sporadic and familial AD, Down syndrome, Meige syndrome, subacute sclerosing panencephalitis, and normal aging.[13, 25]

Lewy bodies are associated with coarse, dystrophic, neuritic changes—Lewy neurites, also decorated by ubiquitin and α-synuclein as inclusions in the axonal processes of neurons. They occur most frequently in the central and accessory cortical nuclei of the amygdala; in hippocampus, mainly the CA2 and CA3 subfields; in the periamygdaloid cortex; and in many brainstem nuclei, indicating involvement of multiple neuronal systems.[96–98] Absence of tyrosine hydroxylase immunoreactivity suggests that many of these neuritic processes are not derived from dopaminergic neurons.

The precise biochemical composition of Lewy bodies and Lewy neurites is unknown, but immunohistochemical studies have shown that major components are phosphorylated neurofilament proteins present in the core and periphery; ubiquitin, a heat shock protein targeting proteins for breakdown; enzymes associated with ubiquitin-mediated proteolysis and phosphorylation or dephosphorylation; cytosolic and microtubule-associated proteins, except for tau-protein; α − B-crystallin, probably mediating the aggregation of microfilaments; synaptophysin; synphylin, an α-synaptophysin–interacting protein, chromogranin A (suggesting that vesicular structures in Lewy bodies may represent degenerating nerve endings); enzymes, lipids, and the presynaptic nerve terminal protein α-synuclein.[22, 23, 99–101] α-Synuclein is one of the best markers for differentiating Lewy bodies and Lewy neurites from α-synuclein–negative neurofibrillary tangles (NFTs) or Pick bodies.[24]

Staining for α-synuclein will replace staining for ubiquitin as the preferred method for detecting Lewy bodies and Lewy neurites in the future.[13, 24, 25] Altered α-synuclein is incorporated into Lewy bodies, their precursors (i.e., pale bodies), and dystrophic Lewy neurites before ubiquitination[101]; it is aggregated and fibrillated in vitro, morphologically resembling Lewy body–like fibrils.[19] Cortical Lewy bodies show diffuse α-synuclein and ubiquitin labeling, while brainstem Lewy bodies exhibit a halo structure immunoreactive for α-synuclein and ubiquitin, probably representing later stages of LB formation. The fibrillar components in their central portion are suggested to undergo conformational changes revealing different epitopes in relation to Lewy body formation.[102] The mechanism of α-synuclein aggregation in vivo has not been elucidated. In cultured cells, aggregation of α-synuclein takes place under certain conditions, such as high temperature or low pH.[103] The wild type and mutant types of α-synuclein may undergo self-aggregation and form insoluble fibrillar aggregates with antiparallel β-sheet structure on incubation at physiologic temperature in vitro, which is accelerated for both known PD-linked point mutations.[104] Aggregation has been shown to be a nucleation-dependent process followed by fibril formation, and α-synuclein nucleation may be the rate-limiting step for the formation of the Lewy body α-synuclein fibril.[105]

Decreased α-synuclein mRNA in the SN and cortex of PD brain in the presence of preserved dopamine transporter and VMAT2 suggests that a decreased α-synuclein level is an early change in the process leading to neuron degeneration and preceding changes in tyrosine hydroxylase and dopaminergic markers. It may be considered a primary mediator of the disease process rather than a secondary change.[46] Studies have shown that abnormal aggregation and accumulation of synaptic proteins, such as α-synuclein, are also associated with plaque formation in AD and with Lewy body formation in DLB. This points to a potential role for this molecule in synaptic damage and neurotoxicity through amyloid-like fibril formation and mitochondrial dysfunction, linking α-synuclein to the pathogenesis of AD and DLB.[19] Lewy bodies and related cytoplasmic inclusions express CDK5, a proline-directed protein kinase involved in cell cycle regulation that probably catalyses in vivo phosphorylation of neurofilament proteins. The aberrant accumulation or ectopic expression of CDK5 and mitogen-activated protein kinase, normally not found in neurons and glia, may lead to the formation of pathologic cytoskeletal inclusions.[106] Studies on the development of α-synuclein–positive inclusions in brainstem suggest an initial intraneuronal appearance of fine, dustlike particles related to neuromelanin or lipofuscin, with aggregation of nondegradable material as small Lewy bodies and their shifting to processes of the involved neurons.[96, 107] The later, frequent extraneuronal deposition of Lewy bodies may be related to disappearance of the involved neurons.[11]

Lewy bodies are found in surviving neurons in the SN, LC, dorsal motor vagal nucleus, thalamus, hypothalamus, substantia innominata, mesocorticolimbic system, raphe nuclei, pedunculopontine and Westphal-Edinger nuclei, intermediolateral columns of the spinal cord, olfactory bulb, sympathetic and parasympathetic neurons, adrenal medulla, and enteric, cardiac, and pelvic nervous plexuses.[11, 13, 28, 33, 92]

α-Synuclein immunohistochemistry of cortical Lewy bodies is demonstrable in up to 100% of PD and DLB brains,[97, 101] particularly involving the cingulate gyrus, hippocampus, amygdala, and middle temporal gyrus.[14, 108] The importance of cortical Lewy bodies for mental dysfunction in PD is still a matter of discussion, because studies have demonstrated variable correlations between cognitive impairment and the numbers of cortical Lewy bodies[108–111] and the density of Lewy neurites in hippocampus that correlates significantly with that of Lewy bodies in all other brain areas. Regression analysis of PD cases with and without additional AD pathology indicates that the total number of cortical Lewy bodies is a strong predictor of cognitive impairment[109, 110] and appears to be correlated with the apolipoprotein E ε4 allele.[111] In contrast to AD, neocortical synapse density and synaptophysin concentration in PD and DLB patients (with and without dementia) do not significantly differ from control values and do not correlate with Lewy body density, whereas decreased cortical synaptophysin density,[112] a major substrate of dementia, is related to neuritic AD lesions.[110, 113] Recent studies in PD revealed significant correlation between cognitive impairment and neuritic AD pathology that caused significantly shorter survival (average 4.5 versus 10 years).[113a]

It is unknown whether Lewy bodies are cytotoxic or harmless by-products or markers of cell damage, although involvement of the ubiquitin proteolytic system suggests that they may be the structural manifestation of a cytoprotective response designed to eliminate damaged cellular elements. Deposits of insoluble proteinaceous fibrils may contribute to dysfunction or death of the involved cells.[114] However, the biologic significance of these cytoplasmic inclusions, especially the role they may play in neurodegeneration, is still enigmatic, because most SN neurons showing DNA fragmentation have no somal Lewy bodies,[115] suggesting that their presence does not predispose a neuron to undergo cell death. Lewy bodies, which are the sequelae of frustraneous proteolytic degradation of abnormal cytoskeletal elements, may represent—similar to other cellular inclusions such as NFTs in AD and Pick bodies—end products or reactions to unknown neuronal degeneration processes that are associated with disturbances of axonal protein transport and that lead to cell death.

SNc cell degeneration is preceded by loss of neurofilament proteins, neuronal tyrosine hydroxylase immunoreactivity; tyrosine hydroxylase, dopamine transporter, and neurofilament mRNA; tyrosine hydroxylase and dopamine transporter proteins; and cytochrome *c* oxidase, indicating functional neuronal damage.[33, 56, 116] It is accompanied by distribution of melanin with uptake into macrophages,[11] astroglial reaction, and proliferation of major histocompatibility complex class II–positive microglia, the latter by releasing cytokines, CD23, nitric oxide, and other substances mediating inflammatory reactions that may be inducing factors or sequelae of neuronal death.[65] Neurodegeneration in PD has been related to a cascade of multiple noxious factors, including formation of free radicals, lipid peroxidation, oxidative stress, melanin-iron interaction with increased iron content in the SN, mitochondrial dysfunction, disorders of calcium homeostasis, and inhibition or loss of neuroprotective mechanisms (Fig. 166–5).[33, 62–65, 117, 118]

Although the causes of neuronal death in PD and related neurodegenerative disorders are enigmatic, several mechanisms are being considered, including programmed versus passive cell death (i.e., apoptosis versus necrosis) and autophagy,[119–122] but the specific pattern of cell loss and the paucity of necrotic changes in the SN and other brainstem nuclei in PD have led to the suggestion that programmed cell death may be a major mechanism.[121] Studies demonstrating DNA fragmentation[118, 122] and an up-regulation of proapoptotic and cell death–regulating proteins and enzymes in programmed cell death[123] and in an MPTP mouse model[124] raise the question of whether apoptosis, a specific gene-directed form of programmed cell death, may represent a dominant pathway in the selective degeneration of specific neuronal populations.[64] Apoptosis, a morphologically and biochemically well-characterized form of programmed cell death to remove unnecessary or damaged cells in various situations, is characterized by nuclear fragmentation; condensation of nuclear chromatin with DNA fragmentation or laddering; breaking up of the cell into membrane-bound, ultrastructurally well-preserved fragments (i.e., apoptotic bodies), with preservation of intracellular organelles (mitochondria) and nuclear and cellular membranes; and lack of inflammatory reaction.[125]

Natural death of SN neurons with the apoptotic morphology occurs during normal development; its extent can be influenced by excitotoxic and hypoxic-ischemic injury in the striatum. Many of the noxious factors implicated in the pathogenesis of PD can bring about programmed cell death in other cell systems in vitro and in vivo and in SN neurons in experimental models of PD (e.g., 6-hydroxydopamine, MPTP), particularly in adult animals. In some of these reactions, active changes of apoptosis-related proteins have been observed.[120, 121]

DNA fragmentation and definite histologic features of apoptosis in nigral neurons in PD, DLB, and related disorders are rare (not detectable or less than 1%),[33, 64, 119, 122, 126–128] but they occur more frequently in glial cells. Some studies did not show convincing DNA fragmentation or apoptotic morphology in SN, LC, or cortical neurons with or without Lewy bodies, but variable numbers of terminal deoxynucleotidyl (TdT)–mediated dUTP-biotin nick-end labeling (TUNEL)-positive astrocytes, oligodendrocytes, and microglial cells were identified in the SN.[64, 126, 128] There were no significant differences in the expression of most apoptosis-related proteins in SN neurons among PD, DLB, and controls or between cortical and subcortical neurons with or without Lewy bodies. No expression of TP53, caspase-3, or stress proteins was seen in neurons, whereas reactive astroglia and microglia showed upregulation of several apoptosis-related proteins and caspase-3.[64] These and other data for AD[129] suggest that DNA fragmentation in neurodegenerative disorders indicates programmed cell death, only exceptionally following the classic pathways of apoptosis (i.e., its autophagic form), but rather reflecting the combined action of deficient DNA repair and accelerated DNA damage within susceptible neuron populations.[64, 130] Neurons in a proapoptotic environment may show increased vulnerability to metabolic disturbances related to the pathogenic factors suspected in these disorders (i.e., oxidative stress and mitochondrial impairment preceding DNA fragmentation), which may be early events in programmed cell death promoted by glutathione depletion or premortem factors (e.g., hypoxia pH changes), but a final trigger may occur during the terminal period of the patient's life.[127] Although Lewy bodies and other cytoskeletal inclusions, which are insoluble proteinaceous deposits, are thought to contribute to dysfunction of the involved cells,[114] in PD, AD, and Pick disease only a minority of cells with such inclusions display signs of programmed cell death,[115, 129, 131] and hippocampal neurons with NFTs in AD Parkinson-dementia complex (PDC) have been calculated to survive for years to decades.[132] Further elucidation of the basic mechanisms mediating cell degeneration in these disorders may lead to the development of novel approaches for their prevention and treatment.

Juvenile and Familial Parkinsonism

Parkinsonism with juvenile onset during the first 2 decades of life is uncommon, frequently autosomal

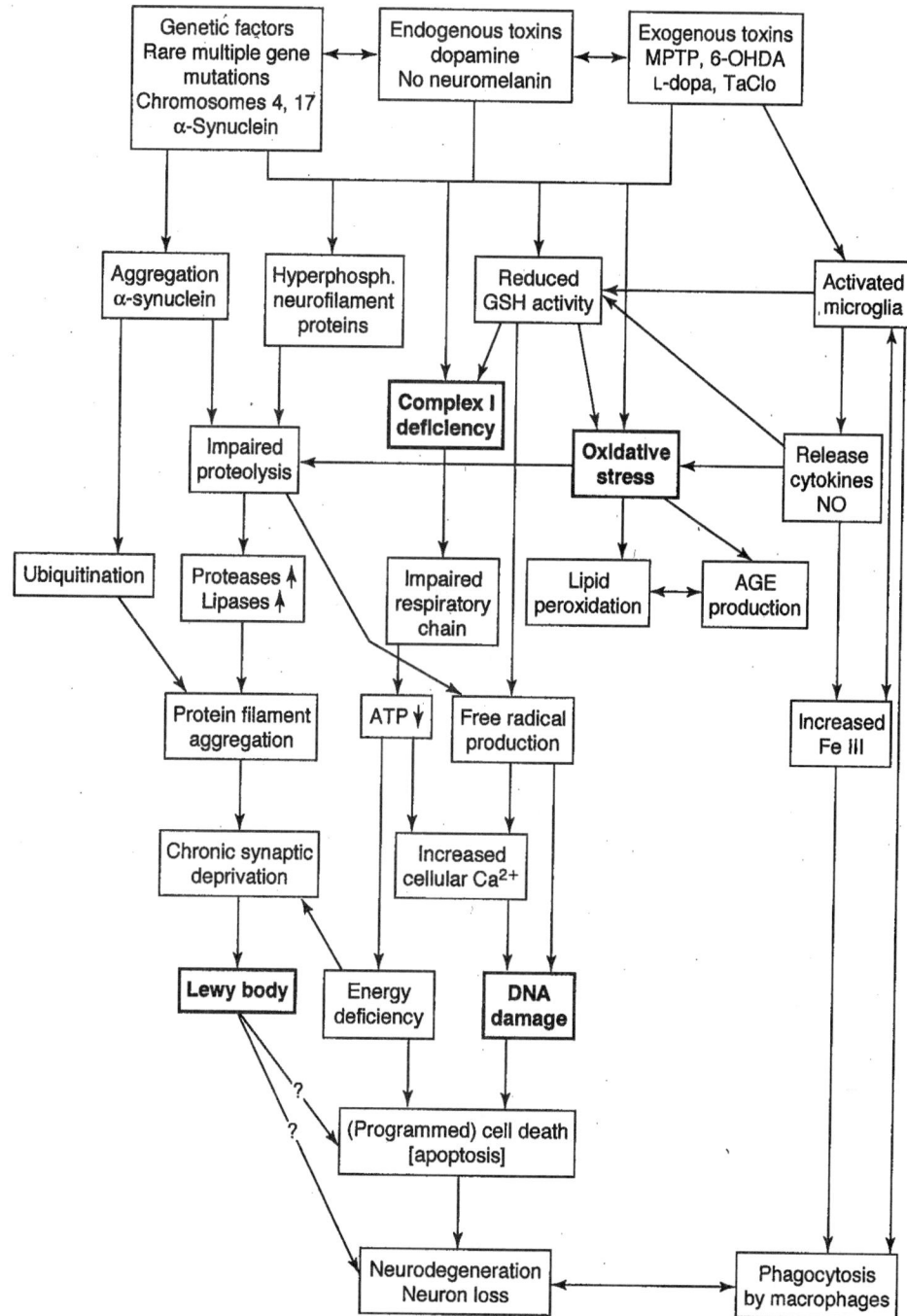

FIGURE 166–5: Hypothetical pathogenic cascade leading to neurodegeneration in Parkinson's disease.

dominant or autosomal recessive (AR-JP), and often associated with dystonia. There is clinical and pathologic overlap with dopa-responsive dystonia, showing normal or decreased numbers of neurons and tyrosine hydroxylase activity in the SN, no Lewy bodies, and no degenerative changes in the striatum,[133] although others show depigmentation of the SN and Lewy bodies.[134] Early onset, dopa-responsive parkinsonism with diurnal fluctuation (EPDF), mapped to a locus for AR-JP (mendelian inheritance in man 600116), is characterized by a benign course and relatively selective degen-

eration of SN neurons with no Lewy body formation.[135] Juvenile-onset parkinsonism has also been described with other types of pathology, including nuclear inclusions, neuroaxonal dystrophy, and multisystem degeneration.[135–139]

Most familial forms of PD associated with mutations of the α-synuclein gene *(SNCA)* at chromosome 4q21.3-q22 and the parkin gene *(PARK2)* at chromosome 6q25.2-q27 or with other known chromosomal loci (e.g., 2p12, 4p15.1, 4p14) are associated with early onset of PD without development of dementia.[117]

Autosomal-dominant familial parkinsonism with dementia, with or without dystonia, may pathologically resemble PD with neuronal loss in the SN and striatum, with or without subcortical and cortical Lewy bodies, amyloid plaques, and NFTs,[139–143] but it is different from that of idiopathic PD with a lack of Lewy bodies,[137] with neuronal loss in SNc and SNr, and hypopigmentation of SNc neurons with no or few Lewy bodies.[143]

Other familial disorders, including frontotemporal dementia with parkinsonism, multisystem degeneration referred to as pallidopontonigral degeneration,[140] and disinhibition-dementia-parkinsonism-amyotrophy complex, are clinically distinct conditions that are linked to intronic mutations of the tau gene located on chromosome 17q.[144]

Dementia with Lewy Bodies

DLB is distinguished from idiopathic PD or the pure brainstem type of LBD by clinical and morphologic features.[14, 17] DLB comprises a constellation of fluctuating, cognitive dysfunction; specific neuropsychiatric features; and motor impairments that combine to produce a severely disabling and sometimes very rapidly progressive clinical syndrome. A similar clinicopathologic picture may be seen in patients who initially present with the motor deficits of parkinsonism but later progress to an end stage of cognitive impairment and psychosis. Cognitive dysfunction in DLB has specific characteristics that aid in discrimination from AD. In autopsy series, DLB represented the second most frequent cause of dementia in the elderly, accounting for 7% to 30% (mean, 15% to 20%),[17] and represented 20% in our autopsy series of patients with parkinsonism (see Table 166–5). A community case register study in Camberwell, England, found 15% of elderly demented cases to have DLB at autopsy. The sensitivity of clinical diagnosis was low (0.22), but this may reflect the retrospective nature of the diagnostic procedures used.[145] Age at onset is 50 to 83 years, and the age at death is 68 to 92 years.[146] DLB is the preferred term[14] for such cases, which had received a variety of competing labels, including diffuse LBD,[147] the Lewy body variant of Alzheimer's disease,[148] and senile dementia of the Lewy body type.[109]

Pathologic analysis, in addition to diffuse brain atrophy, reveals numerous cortical Lewy bodies, particularly in the entorhinal cortex, cingulate cortex, hippocampus, inferior and middle temporal gyri, insula, and amygdala but less often in other isocortical areas.[113] Recommendations have been made about brain regions to be examined for Lewy bodies, and a simple semiquantitative scoring system has been devised.[14] This protocol has been simplified by excluding the frontal region because of the common finding of occasional Lewy bodies in this region in PD.[148a] The distribution of Lewy bodies in DLB does not follow the hierarchical spread of neurofibrillary tangles.[149] They are most commonly encountered in the pigmented midbrain and brainstem nuclei, the dorsal efferent vagal nucleus, the basal forebrain nuclei and limbic regions (amygdala,

entorhinal cortex, anterior cingulate gyrus), and the inferior temporal gyri and insula (less often in deep laminae of other isocortical areas), whereas they are rare in the occipital cortex.[17] The upper cerebral cortex frequently shows spongiform changes with loss of neurons and apical dendrites, but its cause remains undetermined. Positron emission tomography (PET) studies demonstrating hypometabolism in the primary and associated visual cortex in DLB, not present in AD, may be related to nonspecific white matter vacuolation in the occipital lobe.[149a] About 70% of DLB brains show severe nigral damage (see Fig. 166–3) with subcortical and cortical Lewy bodies and Lewy neurites in the C2 to C3 region of the hippocampus that is indistinguishable from idiopathic PD. They cause degeneration of the nigrostriatal projection, demonstrable by dopaminergic presynaptic ligand single-photon emission tomography (SPT) studies that distinguish AD DLB from AD.[149b] A minority of cases has only mild SN damage, comparable to that in AD. Pathologic features of AD are also commonly present in DLB, although with relative absence of neocortical neuritic AD pathology,[17, 148] preponderance of diffuse plaques with different proportions of plaques between DLB (less Aβ 1–40) and AD (more frequent Aβ 1–40 than 1–42 deposits),[150] and relative absence of AD-typical hyperphosphorylated tau protein or its restriction to the hippocampus.[17]

About 50% of DLB brains show neuritic AD changes restricted to the limbic system, with Braak[149] stages 3 and 4 corresponding to plaque-predominant AD[148] or isocortical AD stages meeting the CERAD (Consortium to Establish a Registry for Alzheimer's Disease) criteria of definite AD.[17, 93] In the former cases, referred to as diffuse LBD[17, 147] with or without dementia, neocortical synapse density and synapse proteins do not significantly differ from controls, whereas DLB cases with additional neuritic AD pathology show severe loss of synapse proteins, comparable to AD, and have been classified as Lewy body variant of AD (LBV/AD).[110] Irrespective of cortical AD pathology, DLB shows severe neuronal loss in the cholinergic magnocellular part of the nucleus of Meynert with neocortical cholinergic deficits and upregulation of cortical muscarinic receptors that correlate with dementia and abnormality of the nucleus of Meynert.[151–154] More severe depletion of presynaptic cholinergic neurons in DLB is associated with presynaptic and postsynaptic dopaminergic abnormalities in the striatum, which is not evident in AD.[155] There are no differences in Lewy body density in any brain area among DLB patients with cognitive changes or parkinsonism, no correlations of Lewy body density with Braak stage or frequency of neuritic plaques, and no correlations between Lewy bodies in the cortex and SN, suggesting that DLB should not be considered a severe form of idiopathic PD.[113] However, differences in the proportion of Aβ1–40 deposits, the distribution of neuritic AD pathology, tau proteins, and cholinergic biochemistry and genetic differences in ApoE ∈4 and ∈2 frequency[156] and absence in AD of the CP206 gene observed in PD and DLB[157] argue for a separation of DLB and AD. Whereas Lewy body densities, in general, cannot differentiate DLB from PD with dementia (PDD), temporal lobe Lewy bodies are usually rare in nondemented PD. The severity and duration of dementia appear to be related to both increasing parahippocampal Lewy body sensitivities and neuritic plaque grade. A simple screening algorithm has shown that semiquantitative Lewy body density thresholds in the parahippocampus can distinguish demented from nondemented DLB cases independent of other pathologies.[158]

In summary, there appear to be at least three recognizable anchor points along a spectrum of neurodegenerative disorders. Idiopathic PD is characterized by subcortical Lewy bodies and nigrostriatal degeneration. More extensively distributed Lewy bodies and significant senile plaque formation typifies DLB. Lewy bodies may also occur in AD, which is best defined by the presence of neocortical NFTs. The nosologic position of DLB within the spectrum of AD and LB disorders (including idiopathic PD) and the pathogenic relationship between cortical LB and AD diseases and their clinical implications await further elucidation. Cerebrovascular and systemic diseases frequently contribute to different pathologic and clinical profiles.[17]

MULTIPLE SYSTEM ATROPHY

MSA refers to a group of sporadic, rare, autosomal-dominant, progressive movement disorders with onset in middle age and with no known risk factors. Its prevalence is about 4.5 per 100,000. MSA is clinically characterized by various degrees of parkinsonism, cerebellar dysfunction, and autonomic dysfunction and accounts for 3% to 10% of autopsy cases with parkinsonian features.[15, 24]

Depending on the predominant lesion pattern of neurodegeneration, several clinical subtypes can be distinguished for which consensus criteria have been proposed.[9, 15, 159] MSA-P striatonigral degeneration is characterized by dopa-nonresponsive parkinsonism and may be difficult to differentiate from idiopathic PD or parkinsonism-plus syndromes, including DLB, corticobasal degeneration, and PSP. The clinical phenotype of MSA-C olivopontocerebellar atrophy is characterized by cerebellar ataxia and is only one of a heterogeneous group of spinocerebellar degenerations (i.e., spinocerebellar ataxia [SCA] 1, 2, 3, 6, and 7),[160] but the use of autonomic dysfunction, common to all forms of MSA and previously referred to as Shy-Drager syndrome, has been discouraged in the new consensus criteria.[9]

The brain shows mild cortical atrophy, atrophy and green-gray discoloration of the posterolateral putamen, and various degrees of atrophy of the cerebellum, cerebellar peduncles, and pons, occurring mainly in olivopontocerebellar atrophy. Histopathology reveals system-specific neuronal loss and gliosis in the posterolateral putamen, SN, cerebellum, pontine base, olivary nuclei, and intermediolateral cell column of spinal cord. In striatonigral degeneration, the severely damaged putamen reveals excessive accumulation of granular lipofuscin-iron pigment corresponding to hypointensity in the lateral putamen on magnetic resonance imaging (MRI) and differing from idiopathic

PD.[161] Degeneration of the SNc that is only rarely associated with Lewy bodies[15, 159] mainly involves the calbindin-positive cells in lateral parts (see Fig. 166–3), reflecting initial degeneration of the striatal matrix in the dorsal putamen with trans-synaptic degeneration of striatonigral efferents[77] that remain intact in idiopathic PD and PD-dementia complex of Guam. There is marked depletion of calcineurin-immunoreactive putaminal efferents in the posteroventral part of the GPi and GPe and in the ventrolateral portion of SNr topographically corresponding to the putaminal lesion,[162] with comparative preservation of the STN and thalamus. Based on semiquantitative assessment of neuronal loss, astrogliosis, and GCIs in striopallidum and substantia nigra in MSA-P, four degrees of severity can be distinguished, reflecting disease progression and dopa-responsibility.[16a] The degeneration affecting the direct and indirect striatal outflow pathways with variable activity of the STN and GPi may be responsible for parkinsonism (i.e., rigidity and bradykinesia) in patients with striatonigral degeneration (see Fig. 166–2).[162] These data and loss of striatal postsynaptic dopaminergic D_2 receptors, as in the late stages of idiopathic PD, are important reasons for the negative response to L-dopa substitution in some MSA patients.[77, 163] Striatonigral degeneration may be associated with olivopontocerebellar atrophy characterized by neuronal loss in the pontine nuclei and atrophy of inferior olives, lateral cerebellar cortex, and several other brainstem systems.[15, 159] Patients with Shy-Drager syndrome have widespread neuronal loss in the striatum, SN, cerebellar cortex, inferior olives, Westphal-Edinger nucleus, intermediolateral columns, and the Onufrowicz nucleus in the spinal cord. The degree of neuronal loss appears to be related to the duration of illness and the type of MSA.[15, 24, 162a] Selective involvement concerns neurochemically defined neuronal groups in the rostral and caudal ventrolateral medulla and locus ambiguus that contribute to autonomic disturbances.[163a] In addition to central neuropathology, peripheral nerve loss of small fibers has been observed.[164] Characteristic cytoskeletal changes in MSA are argyrophilic glial cytoplasmic inclusions in oligodendrocytes composed of 5- to 10-nm filaments coated with granular material and that are immunoreactive for α-synuclein, tau, ubiquitin, tubulin, αB-crystallin, and cyclin-dependent kinase.[15, 22–24, 107, 165] The anatomic distribution of the glial cytoplasmic inclusions follows that of neurodegeneration and shows only insignificant differences in the pattern and α-synuclein immunoreactivity between striatonigral degeneration and olivopontocerebellar atrophy. The argyrophilic glial cytoplasmic inclusions are diagnostic markers, even in atypical cases.[159] When in the basal ganglia, they contain iron pigment and induce widespread demyelination with the brunt of changes in affected white matter areas.[166] Neuronal cytoplasmic inclusions of similar composition are found in pontine and other brainstem nuclei, basal ganglia, hippocampus, and cerebral cortex, particularly in the anterior central gyrus and supplementary motor cortex, where they are associated with reduction of neuronal density.[15, 167] The latter changes may contribute to the cognitive deficits or dysexecutive striatofrontal syndrome resulting from deafferentation of the prefrontal cortex. Rare ubiquitin-positive neuronal nuclear or cytoplasmic inclusions resemble those in motoneuron diseases, whereas ubiquitin-positive neuritic degeneration resembling neurophil threads (NTs) but showing negative tau immunoreactivity is seen in affected areas in MSA.[15] In MSA, the inclusion bodies composed of insoluble α-synuclein filaments are more widespread in the brain than the obvious pathology, suggesting a fundamental molecular characteristic of the disorder.[168] The pathogenesis of MSA is obscure, but it is the only neurodegenerative disease in which oligodendroglial pathology is predominant. This suggests that the formation of GCIs is the primary lesion, which secondarily will affect nerve cells through the oligo-myelo-axon-neuron complex. The presumptive pathogenic mechanism in MSA is thus different from that proposed in other neurodegenerative disorders in which neurons rather than oligodendroglia play a pivotal role. The molecular mechanism of the fibrillogenesis of GCIs is unknown, but their occurrence suggests that the ectopic or aberrant expression of α-synuclein may cause abnormal phosphorylation of microtubular protein in the cytoplasm leading to GCI formation. However, abnormal α-synuclein is present not only in Lewy bodies but also in inclusions in MSA, which suggests a link between its selective and specific change and the development of degenerative changes.

Tauopathies

A series of neurodegenerative disorders referred to as tauopathies are morphologically characterized by widespread cellular aggregates of hyperphosphorylated microtubule-associated tau protein, previously known to be a key component of NFTs in AD. The characteristics of tau pathology that involves neurons and glia (i.e., astroglia and oligodendroglia) vary considerably among the different disorders.[169–171] In AD, postencephalitic parkinsonism, and Parkinson-dementia complex of Guam, all six tau isoforms with three and four microtubule-binding domains are hyperphosphorylated and detectable as a tau triplet (tau 55, 64, and 69); in corticobasal degeneration and PSP, only four-repeat tau isoforms as a doublet (tau 55 and 64) aggregate into randomly coiled filaments. In Pick's disease, which is rarely associated with extrapyramidal symptoms, another tau doublet (tau 55 and 64) of three-repeat isoforms aggregates into coiled filaments (see Table 166–2). In frontotemporal dementia with parkinsonism linked to chromosome 17, which has been related to mutations on the tau gene, the biochemical tau profile is similar to the tau triplet in AD, but a minor variant at 74 kDa is also found in some forms of postencephalitic parkinsonism and the PD-dementia complex of Guam.[171] These differences in tau isoforms may be related to degeneration of particular cell populations in a given disorder or aberrant cell trafficking of particular tau isoforms. The tauopathies exhibit specific patterns of CNS lesions but may also share clinical symptoms and histopathologic features, often obscuring the differential diagnosis.[13, 16, 172]

PROGRESSIVE SUPRANUCLEAR PALSY

PSP (i.e., Steele-Richardson-Olszewski syndrome) is the most common degenerative akinetic-rigid syndrome after PD, accounting for 3% to 6% of patients with parkinsonism (see Table 166–5). This sporadic, rarely familial, late-onset disorder is clinically characterized by rigidity, akinesia, postural instability, supranuclear vertical gaze palsy, and frontal lobe dementia.[173] Although the cause of the disease is unknown, some familial cases appear to be transmitted by mendelian inheritance.[174] Studies have shown overexpression of a four-repeat tau associated with a polymorphic tandem repeat allele, located in intron 9 of the tau gene, with prevalence of the tau genotype A0/A0,[175, 176] but no mutation in the tau gene similar to that in FTDP-17 was found in individuals with familial PSP.[177] Macroscopic changes include atrophy of the midbrain and pontine tegmentum, with pigment loss from the SN and LC and occasional frontal lobe atrophy. The major histologic features are multisystem neuronal loss and gliosis with widespread globose, non–flame-shaped tangles and NTs composed of 12- to 27-nm (mean, 15 nm), straight tubules with periodic constrictions at 80- to 120-nm intervals (see Table 166–2) composed of a 64-plus 69-kDa tau doublet with a sequence encoded by exon 10 (4-repeat tau isoforms) that differ from paired helical filaments in AD and from twisted filaments in corticobasal degeneration. The 13- to 15-nm, straight filaments are seen in PSP neurons, and "tufted" or thorn-shaped astrocytes immunoreactive for tau protein occur throughout the neuraxis.[13, 172, 178, 179] An increasingly recognized feature of PSP is the presence of swollen acromasic neurons in the cortex and basal ganglia that resemble those in corticobasal degeneration.[179] According to neuropathologic consensus criteria,[8] typical PSP confirming the original definition[173] is marked by variable neuronal loss and gliosis, with widespread NFTs and NTs in the basal ganglia, brainstem (including the SNc and SNr; see Fig. 166–3), LC, STN, pallidum, striatum, periaqueductal gray, red nucleus, raphe nuclei, oculomotor complex and trochlear nuclei, pontine tegmentum and basis, dentate and inferior olivary nuclei, and spinal gray matter.[8, 58, 180]

In PSP, extremely few tangle-bearing neurons but many glial cells, particularly tau-positive oligodendrocytes in brainstem tegmentum and pontine nuclei but not in SNc, show DNA fragmentation and may express ASPs (apoptosis-related proteins) or caspase-3.[64] Cortical involvement considerably differs from that in AD, with the highest density of tau pathology in prefrontal and angular gyri and decreasing density from frontal, cingulate, entorhinal, and hippocampal areas to superior temporal and occipital cortex. In PSP, NFTs and NTs are mainly located in the deepest cortical layers, in contrast to the bimodal distribution in AD, but entorhinal damage in both disorders is similar.[181]

Nigrostriatal dysfunction is a key feature of PSP, with 80% to 90% loss of dopamine, tyrosine hydroxylase, and postsynaptic D_2 receptors in the striatum, but the mesocorticolimbic system is relatively spared. Severe damage to the GPi, GPe, SNr, and STN causes considerable dysfunction of the striatal efflux to the motor thalamus accounting for akinesis-rigidity and its resistance to dopaminergic treatment (see Fig. 166–2). Cholinergic neurons are also lost in the striatum, the nucleus of Meynert, and various nuclei of the brainstem, along with loss of cholinergic innervation to the thalamus, which may play a role in motor, equilibrium, and cognitive dysfunction in PSP.[174, 182] Mental decline in PSP is often ascribed to subcortical pathology related to dysfunction of striatal-frontal (or prefrontal) circuits because of degeneration of basal ganglia and brainstem tegmental nuclei affecting hippocampal and prefrontal structures,[183, 184] but it has been shown to be related to neuroglial tau pathology ("tufted astrocytes") in neocortical, mainly prefrontal areas and in the limbic system.[185, 186] There is no difference in subcortical tau pathology between PSP cases with or without cognitive impairment. Atypical PSP includes histologic variants in which the severity or distribution of lesions, or both, deviate from the typical pattern due to less brainstem NFT involvement or more cortical changes.[8] The diagnosis of combined PSP is proposed in the presence of infarcts in brainstem and basal ganglia that could modify the clinical symptoms or other lesions, such as Lewy bodies or AD changes above age-associated levels.[8, 174]

CORTICOBASAL DEGENERATION

Corticobasal degeneration is a rare, sporadic, late-onset disorder manifesting with a rigid-akinetic syndrome with asymmetric limb apraxia, dystonia, action tremor and myoclonus, pseudobulbar palsy or supranuclear gaze palsy, and cognitive disturbance, and it may clinically resemble idiopathic PD or PSP.[187, 188] Several clinical features differentiate PSP from corticobasal degeneration.[16, 189] Whereas PSP patients often have severe postural instability at onset, symmetrical parkinsonism, vertical supranuclear gaze palsy, and speech and frontal lobe–type features, corticobasal degeneration manifests with lateralized motor (i.e., parkinsonism, dystonia, or myoclonus) and cognitive signs (i.e., ideomotoric apraxia, aphasia, or alien limb), but another phenotype of corticobasal degeneration in patients with early, severe frontal dementia, bilateral parkinsonism, and PSP without vertical gaze palsy is often misdiagnosed.

Corticobasal degeneration is associated with lobar frontal or parietal atrophy, severe neuronal loss and gliosis in the cortex, tau-positive ballooned neurons, NFT-like skein inclusions, widespread NTs, and tau-positive astrocytic plaques in the white matter.[13, 16, 172, 178, 190]

Basal ganglia and SN show severe degeneration and NFT-like neuronal tau aggregates that ultrastructurally differ from the paired helical filaments in AD but are almost identical to those in PSP, consisting of 15-nm, straight tubules and tubules with long, spaced constrictions[178, 190] and composed of 64- and 69-kDa tau doublets, lacking exon E3, which recognizes NFTs and NTs in PSP and AD.[172, 191] However, studies detecting tau isoforms with a sequence encoded by, but not without, exon 10 suggest that only four-repeat tau isoforms aggregate into filaments in corticobasal degeneration, as observed in PSP.[192] Although corticobasal degeneration may be difficult to distinguish from PSP and Pick's disease because of rare overlap between these disorders,[185, 187, 189, 193] and coexistent cortical AD pathology, biochemical tau profiles differ from those in AD, PSP, and Pick's disease.[171] Cortical inclusions in corticobasal degeneration, with the highest density in the prefrontal cortex and basal ganglia and in the thalamus and brainstem tegmentum, point to similarities with PSP,[194] whereas large numbers of thread-like processes and astroglial plaques distinguish corticobasal degeneration from PSP; the most striking difference is in the white matter, which shows more numerous and widespread threads and oligodendroglial inclusions in corticobasal degeneration than are found in PSP. Tau-positive astrocytes are more numerous in the deep gray matter in PSP than in corticobasal degeneration.[172] Mental decline with a dysexecutive syndrome, probably caused by degeneration of the basal ganglia and frontal cortex and asymmetric apraxia related to prefrontal and parietal lobe lesions, is caused by widespread tau cytopathology related to degeneration of cortical and subcortical areas.

POSTENCEPHALITIC PARKINSONISM

Postencephalitic parkinsonism is a rare, late sequela of encephalitis lethargica and other viral encephalitides. Sporadic cases have been reported.[195, 196] The intra vitam features are rather characteristic to enable diagnosis.[197] Despite epidemiologic evidence of a viral infection, even with modern molecular investigations, an infectious agent has not been identified.[197] Macroscopically, the brain may show mild generalized atrophy, with depigmentation of the SN and LC. Histologic analysis reveals severe, almost complete neuronal loss in the SNc (see Fig. 166–3), LC, and other parts of the rostral brainstem (e.g., midbrain raphe, pontine tegmentum), with diffuse gliosis and widespread occurrence of tau pathology in the form of NFTs and NTs that have morphologic and modular features identical to those in AD. The tangles and threads are composed of 22-nm, twisted tubules with occasional straight filaments containing the tau paired helical filament triplet and showing ubiquitin immunoreactivity, which is different from the NFTs in PSP and corticobasal degeneration (see Table 166–2). Tau-immunoreactive astroglia are seen in affected areas, whereas tufted astrocytes, oligodendroglial inclusions, and astrocytic plaques (typical features of PSP and corticobasal degeneration) and ballooned cells (typical of PSP or corticobasal degeneration) or Pick bodies are absent.[172] The distribution of subcortical NFTs and NTs resembles that in PSP, except for sparing or only mild involvement of several nuclei that are usually affected in PSP: striopallidal, thalamic, oculomotor complex, trochlear, vestibular nuclei, pontine basis, inferior olives, and dentate nucleus.

However, cholinergic subcortical supranuclear centers of gaze movement in some cases of postencephalitic parkinsonism may show lesions similar to those in PSP and causing similar gaze palsy and lid apraxia.[196] Cell loss in PSP and postencephalitic parkinsonism involves all parts of the SNc, with no predilection for the ventral tier specific for idiopathic PD (see Fig. 166–3). Cortical pathology is common in postencephalitic parkinsonism, with tangles found mainly in the hippocampus and entorhinal, temporal, frontal, and insular cortices and with relative preservation of the precentral, cingulate, and parietal regions; prominent involvement of layers II and III differs from that in AD.[198] There is no or only very little tau pathology in the white matter, which is consistently involved in PSP and corticobasal degeneration. Because of pathologic overlap, however, the differential diagnosis between postencephalitic parkinsonism and PSP may be difficult without clinical data.[197]

PARKINSON-DEMENTIA COMPLEX OF GUAM

The endemic combination of parkinsonism with dementia in the Chamorro population of Guam, on the Kii peninsula, and in West Guinea is characterized by cerebral and basal ganglia atrophy (rarely mimicking that of Huntington's disease) and prominent depigmentation of the SN and LC. Widespread neuronal loss and gliosis in the hippocampus, amygdala, nucleus of Meynert, striatum, pallidum, thalamus, hypothalamus, SN, brainstem tegmentum, and dentate nucleus are accompanied by abundant NFTs and by granulovacuolar degeneration and Hirano bodies in the hippocampus.[199] The ultrastructure, histochemistry, biochemistry, and distribution pattern of subcortical NFTs are similar to those in postencephalitic parkinsonism and AD,[195] but the distribution differs from that in AD. Severe atrophy of the frontal and temporal cortices, tegmentum, and base of the brainstem in the PD-dementia complex of Guam differs from brainstem lesions in PSP and AD. The loss of large neurons in the neostriatum and nucleus accumbens in the PD-dementia complex of Guam is more severe than in PSP, and the latter may be linked to marked degeneration of limbic areas.[200] The spinal cord shows degeneration of the lateral columns and neuronal loss and NFTs in the anterior horns.

Secondary Parkinsonism

About 10% of all patients with parkinsonism have secondary forms caused by certain drugs, toxins, metabolic disorders, viral infections, multiple infarcts, brain tumors, trauma, or hydrocephalus (see Table 166–4).

VASCULAR PARKINSONISM: ARTERIOSCLEROTIC PSEUDOPARKINSONISM

Vascular parkinsonism, or arteriosclerotic pseudoparkinsonism, is a rigid-akinetic syndrome usually manifesting as "lower body" parkinsonism with gait disorders, postural instability, and repeated falls. It is associated with lacunar infarcts in the basal ganglia and white matter or Binswanger's subcortical arteriosclerotic encephalopathy.[201–205] It may or may not be associated with infarction in the SN. The postmortem demonstration of Lewy bodies in about 13% of cases with multi-infarct encephalopathy, twice as common as in age-matched controls, suggests subclinical idiopathic PD.[206, 207] In large autopsy series of parkinsonism, purely cerebrovascular lesions without neurodegeneration are seen in less than 5% of patients (see Tables 166–5 and 166–6), but vascular lesions in the basal ganglia and white matter are observed in about 20% of all autopsy cases of idiopathic PD[206] and may be considered additional pathogenic factors in the movement disorder of such patients.

DRUG-RELATED AND TOXIC PARKINSONISM

Drug-induced parkinsonism, which can be clinically confused with akinetic-rigid idiopathic PD, is most often associated with neuroleptic drugs, calcium channel blocking agents, and other substances causing dopamine depletion or blockage of postsynaptic D_1 and D_2 receptors[208] or transient loss of tyrosine hydroxylase immunoreactivity of nigrostriatal neurons.[209] Incidental Lewy body disease is considered a preclinical phase of idiopathic PD, and age-related SNc cell loss occurring in about 10% of individuals older than 60 years of age may be unmasked by such substances and lead to parkinsonism related to reduced dopa uptake in the striatum.[31]

The pathology of parkinsonism resulting from carbon monoxide, carbon disulfide, and cyanide intoxication or postnarcotic encephalopathy shows anoxic lesions or necrosis of the pallidum and SN. Chronic lead intoxication causes SN damage, and manganese encephalopathy is characterized by widespread neuron loss and gliosis in the pallidum and striatum with little or no SN damage. Individuals who developed severe L-dopa–responsive parkinsonism after exposure to MPTP (1-methyl-4-phenyl-1,2,3,6-tetrahydropyridine), a synthetic heroin drug, have moderate to severe diffuse neuron loss and gliosis in the SNc, with extraneuronal melanin and activated microglia, without Lewy bodies or other neuronal inclusions, and with preservation of other brain regions.[210] Although the mechanism by which MPTP/MPP+ kills nigral neurons is unknown, data suggest that a single, time-limited insult to the nigrostriatal system can set in motion a self-perpetuating process of neurodegeneration, which has been experimentally reproduced in animals. MPTP and other piperidines cause rather selective damage (i.e., neuron loss and gliosis) of the dopaminergic area A9 (SNc), with relative sparing of other neuronal systems.[41] Eosinophilic inclusion bodies resembling Lewy bodies have been seen in the SN and LC of MPTP-treated, aged monkeys, but their ultrastructure differs from that of typical human Lewy bodies.[211]

OTHER LESIONS CAUSING PARKINSONISM

Parkinsonism has been observed in a wide variety of disorders involving the brainstem or SN, or both, and the dopaminergic projections, such as after head trauma causing direct destruction of the SN by bullet injury, direct traumatic impact, or herniation contusion of the upper brainstem or secondary damage to the midbrain resulting from vascular compression due to increased intracranial pressure. *Pugilistic encephalopathy,* or boxer's dementia, which often manifests with parkinsonian symptoms, is characterized by diffuse cortical atrophy; severe cell loss in the SN, LC, and striatum with widespread NFTs; and widely distributed β-amyloid deposits throughout the CNS. NFTs and β-A4 deposits are similar to those in AD.[212, 213] Parkinsonism has also been observed in rare cases of tuberculoma, tumors of the brainstem (e.g., lymphoma), solid tumors causing brainstem compression, calcification of the basal ganglia (i.e., Fahr's disease), viral encephalitis, subacute sclerosis panencephalitis, multiple sclerosis, and normal-pressure hydrocephalus (see Table 166–4).

HYPERKINETIC MOVEMENT DISORDERS

Several conditions are characterized by an excess of movement and may be grouped together as hyperkinetic disorders, in contrast to the poverty of movement seen in the akinetic-rigid movement disorders. The clinical disorders grouped in this section are chorea, myoclonus, ballism, dystonia, and tics (see Table 166–1).

Chorea

Chorea is characterized by nonrhythmic, rapid, involuntary movements. Causes may be divided into two main groups: hereditary and sporadic (Table 166–7).

HUNTINGTON'S DISEASE

Huntington's disease is an autosomal-dominant disorder characterized by chorea, involuntary movements,

T A B L E 1 6 6 – 7 ■ Causes of Chorea

Hereditary
Huntington's disease
Choreoacanthocytosis
Dentatorubropallidoluysian atrophy
Benign hereditary chorea
Paroxysmal choreoathetosis (i.e., paroxysmal dyskinesia)
Wilson's disease
Lesch-Nyhan syndrome
Hallervorden-Spatz disease
Pelizaeus-Merzbacher disease
Ataxia-telangiectasia

Sporadic
Sydenham's chorea
Chorea gravidarum
Systemic lupus erythematosus
Metabolic derangements
Drug-induced disease
Focal lesions

dystonia, intellectual impairment, and emotional disturbances.[214, 215] The gene for Huntington's disease, which is mutated in affected patients, has been mapped to chromosome 4p16.3. The mutation is an expanded polyglutamine repeat, $(CAG)_n$, within exon 1 of the gene. In the normal population, the number of CAG repeats ranges from 6 to 35, whereas in individuals affected by Huntington's disease, the repeat length ranges from 40 to 121. The age of onset is inversely related to CAG repeat length.[216-218] Macroscopically, the brain shows atrophy of the caudate nucleus and putamen, with enlarged ventricles and diffuse cortical atrophy and with sparing of the medial temporal lobe; striatal atrophy correlates with the severity of cortical atrophy, suggesting an associated disease process.[219] The neostriatum reveals severe loss of the medium, spiny, GABAergic type II neurons and gliosis progressing along posteroanterior, dorsoventral, and mediolateral directions. The severity of anatomic lesions correlates with clinical severity and has been classified into five grades, indicating no changes to severe striatal atrophy.[220] Grade 1 Huntington's disease is clinically manifested without macroscopic CNS changes but is characterized by a loss of GABAergic, enkephalin-containing striosome neurons and by gliosis in the neostriatum. The brain is macroscopically normal but microscopically reveals neuronal loss in the caudate tail and dorsal putamen involving the total striosomal system and extending to the ventral part of the nucleus accumbens. Grade 2 is associated with atrophy of the head of caudate. Grade 3 Huntington's disease exhibits severe atrophy of the head of the caudate and the putamen. In grade 4, severe atrophy of the total neostriatum (95% loss of caudate volume) and pallidum occurs with involvement of striosomes and matrix in a dorsoventral progression,[221] with relative sparing of the large cholinergic interneurons; the medium-sized, aspiny neurons; and the nitric oxide synthase–, and the nicotinamide adenine dinucleotide phosphate diaphorase–, somatostatin-, and neuropeptide Y–containing interneurons. Neostriatal pathology starts with the loss of spiny, enkephalin- and GABA-containing neurons[221, 222] that project to the GPe and correlate with the presence of chorea. This is consistent with current models of basal ganglia function in which hyperkinesia results from interruption of the indirect pathway involving the striatal GPe, STN, and GPi. This produces hyperactivity of the nigrostriatal pathway and of the thalamocortical feedback circuits due to reduced inhibitory effects of GPi and SNr, causing increased glutamatergic stimulation of the cortex (see Fig. 166–2). Recent studies provided evidence of distributed gray matter changes and progressive white matter atrophy with age before clinical onset of HD. In later stages, damage extends to the nucleus accumbens, pallidum, amygdala, ventrolateral thalamus, lateral tuberal nucleus of hypothalamus, STN, and SNc, with corticostriatal neurons disappearing from cortical layer V. These lesions and the loss of striatal GPi efferents (i.e., direct pathway) lead to decreased motor activity (i.e., bradykinesia) and rigidity in the later stages of Huntington's disease.[223] In juvenile cases corresponding to the early, severe rigidity in Westphal variants, striatal GPe and GPi efferents degenerate, suggesting that degeneration of the direct pathway is responsible for rigidity. Other lesions involve the pallidum, which shows loss of substance P and calcineurin-immunoreactive fibers and neurons, the ventrolateral thalamus, and the STN and SNc, with 40% to 50% cell loss[224] occurring more in medial than in lateral parts (see Fig. 166–3). The differences between rigid and choreiform Huntington's disease cases are not related to presynaptic SN damage, but to the involvement of striatal GABA–substance P neurons projecting to GPi that inhibit the increased dopaminergic activity of the neostriatum.[7] Functional neuroimaging studies have shown nonselective reductions in striatal D_1 and D_2 receptor binding, irrespective of clinical phenotype, although rigidity was associated with more severe loss of both receptors.[225] In asymptomatic gene carriers, putamen D_2 receptor binding is decreased by 6.3% per year.[226]

The coexistence of hyperkinetic and hypokinetic movement disorders in Huntington's disease patients may be explained by the involvement of direct and indirect pathways in the basal ganglia–thalamus–cortical motor circuit, as originally suggested by Thompson and colleagues.[227] Voluntary movement is slow and variable as a result of degeneration of the basal ganglia output (i.e., GPi) to supplementary motor areas concerned with initiation and maintenance of sequences of movement (see Fig. 166–2). Abnormalities of sensory function are also evident, but their clinical counterparts and the pathologic basis are poorly understood. Cortical somatosensory evoked potentials and long latency stretch reflexes in distal muscles of the upper limb are reduced. These findings may reflect a failure of thalamocortical relay of sensory information.[228] Extensive cortical cell loss in primary sensory and association areas, particularly in layers III, V, and IV[229]; in the corticostriatal neurons in frontal layer V, causing disorders of striatofrontal loops[167]; and in the deep entorhinal cortex[230] correlates with cognitive changes. Dystrophic ubiquitinated neurites resembling CA-2 or CA-3 and brainstem Lewy neurites in LBD are seen in many cortical areas and the SN. Their density does not correlate with the Vonsattel grade,[220] suggesting possible primary cortical pathology in Huntington's disease,[231, 232] and Jellinger[233] observed nonneuritic tau pathology in limbic areas and amyloid deposits in the neocortex of patients as young as 34 to 42 years of age. Although initial stages of AD-like lesions develop rather early in Huntington's disease patients, coexistence of Huntington's disease and AD is rare.

Other lesions involve the caudal central pontine nucleus and the rostral interstitial nucleus of the medial longitudinal fascicle, which are associated with saccade slowing[234] and cerebellar cortex, particularly in severe, early-onset cases. The extent of morphologic changes is closely related to the severity of the genetic defect, the age of onset, and the rate of progression of illness, which correlates with the expansion of a polymorphic trinucleotide repeat (i.e., the sequence CAG that codes for glutamine) to a length that exceeds 40 repeat units

in exon 1 of the gene for Huntington's disease. Coding for the huntingtin protein is normally localized in the cytoplasm, but the mutant protein is also found in the nucleus, suggesting that its translocation to this site is important for the pathogenesis of Huntington's disease.[235] In patients and in a transgenic mouse model of the disease, neuronal intranuclear inclusions, immunoreactive for huntingtin and ubiquitin, develop.[236, 237] Huntingtin interacts with several proteins and calmodulin, and mutant huntingtin that forms in vivo complexes with distinct context-dependent conformations of the polyglutamine segment is specifically cleaved by the proapoptotic enzyme caspase 3.[238] Various antibodies detect granular cytoplasmic deposits in cortical and striatal neurons that also contain intranuclear N-terminal huntingtin immunoreactivity. These data show a differential intracellular location of truncated huntingtin in the brains of patients with Huntington's disease. Cytoplasmic and nuclear aggregates of the protein fragments may be neurotoxic. The frequency of the cortical intranuclear inclusions correlates with the size of CAG expansion and is inversely related to the age at onset and the age at death. No such correlations were detected for the striatum, which most likely reflects a more advanced neuronal loss accrued by the time of death.[239] Findings about axonal transport of N-terminal huntingtin suggest that, in the earlier stages of Huntington's disease, its accumulation occurs in the cytoplasm together with dystrophic neurites and that it is associated with degeneration of the corticostriatal pathway.[240] The definite role of mutant huntingtin in neuronal degeneration has not been confirmed, and the pathogenic mechanisms are still unknown, but it is presumed that the mutant huntingtin has a toxic function that leads to cytoskeletal defects and results in the premature death of neurons. Evidence suggests that excitotoxicity, increased free radical production, elevated levels of oxidative damage products, early mitochondrial calcium defects, protein aggregation, impaired energy metabolism, and programmed cell death play pathologic roles.[241–244, 244a, 244b]

DENTATORUBROPALLIDOLUYSIAN ATROPHY

Dentatorubropallidoluysian atrophy is a rare, autosomal-dominant, neurodegenerative disorder that mainly occurs in Japan. It is caused by an unstable CAG trinucleotide repeat extension (more than 49 repeats) caused by a CTG-B37 mutation, which has been mapped to chromosome 12p13.31[245] and which encodes a protein called atrophin-1 that is present in many CNS areas.[246, 247] The clinical manifestation is diverse and includes cerebellar ataxia, epilepsy, myoclonus, choreoathetosis, and dementia with considerable intrafamilial variations.[245–248] Young-onset cases have the longest CAG repeats and manifest predominantly as progressive myoclonus epilepsy.[249] The neuropathology is characterized by MSA primarily involving the cerebellar dentate nucleus, red nucleus, external pallidum, and STN, with disruption of dentatorubral, pallidofugal, spinocerebellar, and motor systems. Milder changes involve the striatum, thalamus, SN, inferior olives, midbrain tegmentum, lateral cuneate nuclei, spinocerebellar tracts, and posterior spinal columns, often associated with neuroaxonal dystrophy.[245-248] Because dentatorubropallidoluysian atrophy has clinical and genetic similarities to Huntington's disease and spinocerebellar disorders (e.g., SCA1), differentiation from these and other multisystem degenerations may be difficult. Intranuclear inclusions immunoreactive for ubiquitin and huntingtin similar to those in Huntington's disease occur in dentatorubropallidoluysian atrophy. Their density correlates with the IT15 triplet repeat length, suggesting that these protein aggregates may be a common feature of the pathogenesis of glutamine repeat neurodegenerative disorders.[216-218, 250, 251]

MACHADO-JOSEPH DISEASE

Machado-Joseph disease is a rare, autosomal-dominant, progressive, ataxic disorder characterized by external ophthalmoplegia, facial fasciculations, and polyneuropathy. It has a worldwide distribution, and there are several clinical subtypes with pyramidal, cerebellar, and extrapyramidal signs, distal amyotrophies, and occasional dementia.[160, 218] The gene causing Machado-Joseph disease has been mapped to chromosome 14q24.3-q32 on the SCA3 locus, and it encodes the protein ataxin-3. Spinocerebellar ataxia type 3 (SCA3) and Machado-Joseph disease are caused by the same mutation in the *MJD* gene, with CAG repeat sizes of 61 to 84.[251, 252] Dentatonigrospinal degeneration occurs with lesions in the SN, dentate nucleus, pontine base nuclei, STN, many cranial nerve nuclei, spinal anterior horns, dorsal columns, and dorsale nuclei of Clarke, with variable neuronal loss occurring in the dorsal ganglia. The GPi is more affected than the GPe, an inverse pattern of that seen in dentatorubropallidoluysian atrophy, and the lesions of Clarke's column and dentate nuclei strongly resemble those in Friedreich's ataxia.[160, 218] Pathogenesis is related to the aggregation of ataxin-3, which causes neuron dysfunction and leads to selective cell loss.

NEUROACANTHOCYTOSIS

Neuroacanthocytosis is a rare, genetically heterogenous condition associated with acanthocytosis of the peripheral blood. It manifests clinically with chorea, dystonia, tics and vocalizations, amyotrophic mental deterioration, and later development of an akinetic-rigid parkinsonian syndrome.[253] The autosomal-recessive form is linked to a mutant sorting-associated protein on chromosome 9q21,[254, 254a] and the autosomal-dominant form overlaps with the X-linked McLeod syndrome, a distinct entity of acanthocytosis, weak expression of the Kell blood group system, and neurological abnormality. Patients have atrophy of the caudate nucleus and putamen with a loss of small and medium-sized neurons and later involvement of pallidonigral projections (i.e., neuron loss and gliosis in the pallidum). Less consistent is neuronal loss and gliosis in thalamus, SN, and ventral spinal horns. In contrast to Huntington's disease, the cerebral cortex, cerebellum, STN, and

brainstem nuclei are preserved; peripheral nerves may show chronic axonal neuropathy.[255]

HEREDITARY STRIATAL NECROSIS

Hereditary (holotopistic) striatal necrosis is a rare, autosomal-dominant or -recessive, progressive disorder. Patients have mental dystonia, rigidity, ataxia, and optic atrophy. The disorder is morphologically characterized by bilateral necrosis of the neostriatum and pallidum with vascular proliferation and is associated with similar lesions that variably involve the thalamus, SN, brainstem tegmentum, and rarely, the cerebral cortex. CNS pathology is similar to that in mitochondrial encephalomyelopathies and may be accompanied by Alzheimer type II astroglia in CNS gray matter and optic nerve atrophy.[256] The cause and genetics of hereditary striatal necrosis are unknown. Bilateral striatal lesions in childhood may occur in a variety of disorders.[257]

BENIGN HEREDITARY CHOREA

Benign hereditary chorea begins in childhood and persists into adult life. In contrast to Huntington's disease, there is no associated mental deterioration. Functional imaging studies have shown changes in basal ganglia similar to those of Huntington's disease.

SPORADIC CHOREA

The number of hereditary and nongenetic conditions in which chorea has been described is enormous (see Table 166-7). The following diagnoses should be considered: chorea gravidarum; Sydenham's chorea after streptococcal infection, often as part of classic rheumatic fever, or systemic lupus erythematosus with uncertain neuropathology[258]; polycythemia vera or vascular chorea due to small strokes in the striatum; and toxoplasma abscess in patients infected with the human immunodeficiency virus.[215, 259]

PROGRESSIVE PALLIDUM ATROPHY AND VARIANTS

A group of rare, autosomal-recessive or sporadic, neurodegenerative disorders manifesting with dystonia, choreoathetosis, rigid-akinesia, oculomotor and gait disorders, and pseudobulbar palsy is characterized anatomically by atrophy of various parts of the pallidoluysionigral system. The variants show much clinical and pathologic overlap.[29]

Pallidal degeneration is characterized by isolated bilateral atrophy of globus pallidus with gliosis and degeneration of efferent pallidal fibers. Patients with *pallidoluysian atrophy* have bilateral atrophy and gliosis of the GPe and STN.[260] *Pallidonigral degeneration* and *pallidonigroluysian degeneration*, which may be associated with pure L-dopa–resistant akinesia, are typified by involvement of the pallidum, STN, and SN with associated fiber systems, occasional involvement of the ventromedial thalamus, and iron deposition in the degenerated nuclei.[261, 262]

Pallidal degeneration with polyglucosan bodies has been described in single cases with progressive choreiform or dystonic disorder or nonprogressive cerebral palsy. Autopsy reveals symmetrical degeneration of the GPe or status marmoratus of the basal ganglia, associated with numerous polyglucosan bodies in neuronal perikarya, axons, and dendrites (i.e., Bielschowsky bodies).[263]

HALLERVORDEN-SPATZ DISEASE

Hallervorden-Spatz disease (i.e., pallidonigroluysian neuroaxonal dystrophy) is a rare, sporadic but often familial, autosomal-recessive, degenerative disorder of infantile, late infantile, juvenile, or adult onset. It is clinically characterized by progressive dystonia, choreoathetosis, rigidity or spasticity of the limbs, retinal degeneration, and mental deterioration.[264] It has been referred to as neurodegeneration with brain iron accumulation type 1 (NBIA1), pantothenate kinase–associated neurodegeneration (PKAN), or Hallervorden-Spatz syndrome.[266] It represents pantothenate kinase–associated neurodegeneration caused by the PNAK2 gene linked to chromosome 20p12.3-13.[265] Because an abnormality in ferritin strongly indicates a primary function for iron in the pathogenesis of this disorder, the term "ferritinopathy" has been proposed.[265a] Neuropathologic examination shows a rust-brown discoloration of the globus pallidus and SNr, a loss of neurons, gliosis, and iron-pigment deposits with an ultrastructure similar to that in striatonigral degeneration. Histologic markers are widespread axonal spheroids in the pallidum, SNr, and many other central and peripheral nervous system areas. Their ultrastructural identification enables in vivo diagnosis of Hallervorden-Spatz disease from peripheral nerve, conjunctival, skin, or rectal biopsies, which are now replaced by genetic studies to detect mutation in the pentothenate kinase gene.[266]

The disease is considered to be part of a wide spectrum of neuroaxonal dystrophy, which is subdivided into infantile neuroaxonal dystrophy; late infantile, juvenile, and adult-onset Hallervorden-Spatz disease; and presenile and senile (physiologic) neuroaxonal dystrophy.[267] The iron content of the basal ganglia is threefold higher than in controls, but no disturbance in iron metabolism has been found. On high-field MRI, decreased T2-weighted intensity in the pallidum and SN is related to increased iron content (i.e., tiger-eye phenomenon) and allows in vivo diagnosis of the disorder.[268] Although accumulation of cysteine acting as a chelating agent has been suggested as responsible for the accumulation of iron,[269] the cause and pathogenesis of the disorder are unknown. Lewy bodies have been found in cerebral cortex and brainstem of many patients, and studies revealed widespread occurrence of α-synuclein–immunoreactive inclusions in juvenile and adult-onset Hallervorden-Spatz disease,[270, 271] as well as extensive tau pathology with NFTs, often coexisting with Lewy bodies within the same neurons, the development of which could be related to disturbances of axonal transport caused by axonal spheroid formatin.[272] Axonal spheroids, the hallmark of NBIA1, contain immunoreactive neurofilament protein, ubiquitin, superoxide dismutase, amyloid precursor protein, and α-synuclein but are also variably immunoreactive for tau, ferritin, and iron II, suggesting that iron may also contribute to axonal damage.[272a] Additional lesions include GCIs, Lewy body–like intraneuronal inclusions, and dystrophic neurites. Ultrastructurally, the spheroids occurring in presynaptic terminals show accumulation of amorphous, granular, multilamellated, and dense bodies; mitochondria; and tubulovesicular structures in axoplasm but are different from those in infantile neuraxonal dystrophy (Seitelberger's disease).[267] Late infantile and adult cases show a three- to four-fold increase of iron in putamen and globus pallidus without signs of a generalized disorder of iron metabolism. However, the relationship between neuraxonal dystrophy and localized iron deposition in the brain to the defective PANK2 gene is unknown. Despite the demonstration of α-synuclein–positive inclusions in NBIA1 and extensive tau pathology with neurofibrillary tangles in some cases, the pathogenesis of this disorder is unknown.

Ballism and Hemiballismus

Ballism is a severe choreiform disorder characterized by involuntary, violent flinging movements of the limbs. When unilateral, it is called *hemiballismus*. In most cases, the cause is damage to the STN or its outflow tracts from vascular disease (i.e., infarcts or hemorrhages). Rarely, other focal lesions are caused by metastases, demyelination, toxoplasmosis, or tumors. Bilateral ballism is rare.[13, 263, 273] Histologic evaluation of experimental lesions in monkeys showed that more than 20% of the STN must be destroyed, while sparing surrounding white matter, to produce hemiballism. Lesions of the STN cause dysfunction in the inhibitory output from GPi and SNr, with reduced activity of the inhibitory GABAergic subthalamopallidal pathway to the thalamic nuclei. This increases glutamatergic cortical excitation, which may lead to the hyperkinetic disorder of ballism through increased synchronization of neuronal activity (see Fig. 166–2).[274]

Dystonia Syndromes

Dystonia has been defined as a syndrome of sustained muscle contractions, frequently causing twisting and repetitive movements or abnormal postures. The syndromes are classified by age of onset, severity, distribution of abnormal movements (e.g., focal, segmental, generalized, multifocal, unilateral), and cause, distinguishing primary dystonia, dystonia-plus, and secondary forms. Primary or idiopathic dystonia may be inherited or sporadic; dystonia-plus includes forms distinct from the hereditary and primary type. Secondary or symptomatic dystonia resulting from any insult to the brain can be associated with other neurological disorders, such as inherited neurological or neurometabolic disease, parkinsonism, and disorders with environmental causes.[275]

PRIMARY INHERITED DYSTONIAS

Primary torsion dystonia has an autosomal-dominant inheritance pattern. It generally starts in childhood or adolescence with abnormal movement of the neck or trunk and becomes rapidly generalized. The most frequent form is early-onset torsion or Oppenheim dystonia, an autosomal-dominant disorder associated with the *DYT1* locus on chromosome 9q34.1. Prevalent in Ashkenazi Jews, the causative mutation in most cases is deletion of a glutamate residue from the carboxyl terminus of tyrosine A, a 332–amino acid protein encoded by the *DYT1* gene.[276] The prominent expression of the *DYT1* gene within the SNc implicates a disturbance of dopaminergic functions in the pathophysiology of DYT1 dystonia. Other adult-onset familial forms of torticollis have been mapped to locus *DYT7* on chromosome 18p, to *DYT6* on chromosome 8p21.q22, or to other loci. Functional neuroimaging suggests inappropriate overactivity of the lentiform nucleus and promoter cortices.[277] Supported by neuronal recordings from the pallidum and thalamus at the time of stereotactic surgery in patients with primary dystonia, all evidence suggests that the dystonia results from a functional disturbance of the basal ganglia, particularly in the striatal control of the GPi and SNr, which causes altered thalamic control of cortical motor planning and executive areas and abnormal regulation of the brainstem and spinal cord inhibitory intraneuronal mechanisms (see Fig. 166–2).[276, 278] The limited studies of the neuropathology of these disorders report no abnormality or few NFTs in the brainstem nuclei and cell loss from the SN without Lewy bodies.[279, 279a] Cell loss and astrocytosis surrounding islands of preserved striatum in the caudate nucleus and putamen have been described in a male patient with severe generalized dystonia, although there was no family history of the disease, and extensive investigations during his life failed to reveal a cause for the dystonia.[280] The neuropathology of dopa-responsive dystonia seems to be independent of the genotype.[279a]

DYSTONIA-PLUS

The dystonia-plus category includes dystonia with parkinsonism and dystonia with myoclonus.[275] *Dystonia with parkinsonism* includes dopa-responsive dystonia, an autosomal-dominant dystonic disorder caused by mutation of the gene for guanosine triphosphate cyclohydrolyse-1, the key enzyme in tetrahydrobiopterin biosyntheses; the gene has been mapped to 14q22.1.[281] The mutation causes reduced activity of tyrosine hydroxylase and reduced dopamine synthesis. The pathologic investigation of dopa-responsive dystonia revealed no loss of neurons within the SNc, but these neurons were immature and had little neuromelanin. Neuromelanin synthesis requires dopamine (or other monoamines) as the initial precursor, and there is marked reduction of the dopamine concentration within the striatum.[282]

Rapid-onset dystonia-parkinsonism is an autosomal-dominant movement disorder characterized by sudden onset of persistent dystonia and parkinsonism. It usually manifests during adolescence, and patients have little or no response to L-dopa. The genetic mutation has been mapped to chromosome 19q13. Neuroimaging studies indicate no degeneration of dopaminergic nerve terminals, suggesting that the disorder, which is associated with decreased cerebrospinal fluid levels of the dopamine metabolite homovanillic acid, results from a functional deficit, as in dystonia, rather than neuronal loss or degeneration of dopaminergic striatal terminals, as in idiopathic PD.[283] No neuropathologic findings are available.

HEREDODEGENERATIVE DYSTONIAS

Heredodegenerative dystonias are a group of diseases in which heredodegenerations produce dystonia as a prominent feature and are associated with other neurological features (e.g., parkinsonism). An X-linked primary torsion dystonia, called *Lubac* or *X-linked dystonia-parkinsonism*, occurs on the island of Panay in the Philippines. The gene locus is within Xq12-q13.1. Positron-emission tomographic studies show decreased striatal metabolism with little or no decrease in dopa uptake, compatible with a mosaic pattern of gliosis and intact cell islands. The pathologic pattern is more severe in the putamen, with thinning of myelinated striatal fibers, than in the caudate nucleus.[284] A similar pattern of striatal gliosis was seen in progressive generalized dystonia.[285]

Craniofacial dystonia, or Meige's syndrome, is a segmental dystonia affecting the eyelids, face, and mouth. Pathologic examination has revealed no significant abnormalities or patchy neuronal loss and gliosis in the dorsal caudate nucleus and putamen[286] or identified Lewy body pathology and other structural lesions in the brainstem or diencephalon.[136]

SECONDARY DYSTONIA

Secondary or symptomatic dystonia, or hemidystonia, is associated with a wide range of structural pathologies in the basal ganglia, including infarcts, tumors, and the effects of head injury.[275]

Tic Disorders

Tics are involuntary, brief, stereotyped movements that can be suppressed at the expense of mounting inner tension. They may be subclassified as motor tics (i.e., brief movements), vocal tics (i.e., uttering brief sounds), and sensory tics (i.e., brief sensations). Tics may be simple or complex, and they may appear semi-purposeful (e.g., obscene gestures). Tics may be associated with several neurodegenerative diseases, may be a complication of drug therapy, or may occur with CNS infections.

The most common tic disorder is *Gilles de la Tourette syndrome*, clinically defined by the presence of motor and vocal tics. A genetic cause is indicated by high concordance of the condition in twin studies, but genetic heterogeneity seems likely,[287] and the idea of an autoimmune contribution to the cause is gaining in strength.[288] Neurochemical and functional imaging studies have revealed no consistent abnormalities,[289, 290] particularly no increased density of striatal presynaptic vesicles.[291] No specific anatomic CNS lesions have been observed, except for reduced dynorphin immunoreactivity in the GPe and SN in one case.[13]

Myoclonus

Myoclonus is a nonspecific sign of CNS disease, but it may point to a diagnosis. Prominent myoclonus and dementia are seen in many neurodegenerative disorders, including LBD, corticobasal degeneration,[292, 293] advanced AD, Creutzfeldt-Jakob disease, and dentatorubropallidoluysian atrophy. Myoclonus and epilepsy may be part of a defined epilepsy syndrome, but if associated with progressive neurological deficits, the sign may be caused by mitochondrial encephalopathies, Batten's or Lafora's disease, dentatorubropallidoluysian atrophy, or Baltic myoclonus.

Focal myoclonus is associated with lesions of the brainstem, such as palatal myoclonus with lesions of the central tegmental tract or dentate nucleus associated with hypertrophy of the inferior olives due to degenerative or other pathologies. *Segmental myoclonus* is associated with inflammatory, traumatic, or neoplastic diseases of the spinal cord. *Opsoclonus* (i.e., ocular myoclonus) is seen in children in association with neuroblastoma or in adults with CNS infections.[13, 294]

CONCLUSIONS

Despite some clinical and pathologic overlap, most types of movement disorders, particularly those of neurodegenerative origin, show characteristic pathologic patterns, with or without typical cytoskeletal signposts or distribution patterns of CNS lesions pointing to the correct diagnosis and to their pathophysiology (see Table 166–2). Because in vivo markers for these disorders, except for those with known molecular genetic backgrounds, are lacking, the diagnosis usually depends on clinicomorphologic features. Specific identification may be difficult because some of these disorders share morphologic features with other neurodegenerative diseases, and comprehensive morphologic studies using modern methods of neurobiology are needed for differentiating the different disease entities. Consensus data on clinical and neuropathologic criteria, together with molecular genetic and biochemical data, will aid correct classification and diagnosis of neurodegenerative disorders with extrapyramidal features and provide further insight into their pathophysiology and pathogenesis as a basis for future therapeutic strategies.

REFERENCES

1. Parent A, Hazrati L-N: Functional anatomy of the basal ganglia. I. The cortico-basal ganglia-thalamo-cortical loop. Brain Res Rev 20:91–127, 1995.
2. Parent A, Hazrati L-N: Functional anatomy of the basal ganglia. II. The place of subthalamic nucleus and external pallidum in basal ganglia circuitry. Brain Res Rev 20:128–154, 1995.
3. Gerfen CR, Wilson CJ: The basal ganglia. In Swanson LW, Björklund A, Hokfelt T (eds): Handbook of Chemical Neuroanatomy, vol 12. Integrated Systems of the CNS, part III. Amsterdam, Elsevier Science, 1996, pp 371–468.
4. Alexander GE, Crutcher MD, DeLong MR: Basal ganglia-thalamocortical circuits: Parallel substrates for motor, oculomotor, prefrontal and limbic functions. Prog Brain Res 85:119–146, 1990.
5. Groenewegen HJ: Cortical-subcortical relationships and the limbic forebrain. In Timble MR, Cummings JL (eds): Contemporary Behavioral Neurology. Boston, Butterworth-Heinemann, 1997, pp 29–48.
6. Heimer L, Zahm DS, Alheid GF: Basal ganglia. In Paxinos G (ed): The Rat Nervous System, 2nd ed. Sydney, Academic Press, 579–628, 1995.
7. Albin RL: The pathophysiology of chorea, ballism and parkinsonism. Parkinsonism Relat Disord 1:2–133, 1995.
8. Hauw JJ, Daniel S, Dickson D, et al: Preliminary NNDS neuropathologic criteria for Steele-Richardson-Olszewski syndrome (progressive supranuclear palsy). Neurology 44:2015–2019, 1994.
9. Gilman S, Low PA, Quinn N, et al: Consensus statement on the diagnosis of multiple system atrophy. J Neurol Sci 163:94–98, 1999.
10. Gelb DJ, Oliver E, Gilman S: Diagnostic criteria for Parkinson disease. Arch Neurol 56:33–39, 1999.
11. Forno LS: Neuropathology of Parkinson's disease. J Neuropathol Exp Neurol 55:259–272, 1996.
12. Litvan I, Hauw JJ, Bartko JJ, et al: Validity and reliability of the preliminary NINDS neuropathologic criteria for progressive supranuclear palsy and related disorders. J Neuropathol Exp Neurol 55:97–105, 1996.
13. Lowe J, Lennox G: Disorders of movement and system degenerations. In Graham D, Lantos PL (eds): Greenfield's Neuropathology, 7th ed. London, E Arnold, 2002, pp 325–430.
14. McKeith IG, Galasko D, Kosaka K, et al: Consensus guidelines for the clinical and pathological diagnosis of dementia with Lewy bodies (DLB): Report of the consortium on DLB International Workshop. Neurology 47:1113–1124, 1996.
15. Lantos PL: The definition of multiple system atrophy: A review of recent developments. J Neuropathol Exp Neurol 57:1099–1111, 1998.
16. Dickson DW, Bergeron C, Chin SS, et al: Office of Rare Diseases neuropathologic criteria for corticobasal degeneration. J Neuropathol Exp Neurol 61:935–946, 2002.
17. Ince PG, Perry EK, Morris AM: Dementia with Lewy bodies: A distinct non-Alzheimer dementia syndrome? Brain Pathol 8:299–324, 1998.
18. Parkinson J: An essay on the shaking palsy. London, Sherwood, Neely & Jones, 1817.
19. Hashimoto M, Masliah E: α-Synuclein in Lewy body disease and Alzheimer's disease. Brain Pathol 9:707–720, 1999.
20. Iwai A, Masliah E, Yoshimoto M, et al: The precursor protein of non-Aβ component of Alzheimer's disease amyloid is a presynaptic protein of the central nervous system. Neuron 14:467–475, 1995.
21. Polymeropoulos MHC, Leroy E, Die SE, et al: Mutation in the α-synuclein gene identified in families with Parkinson's disease. Science 276:2045–2047, 1997.
22. Spillantini MG, Crowther RA, Jakes R, et al: α-Synuclein in filamentous inclusions of Lewy bodies from Parkinson's disease and dementia with Lewy bodies. Proc Natl Acad Sci U S A 95:6469–6473, 1998.
23. Arima K, Uéda K, Sunohara N, et al: NACP/α-synuclein immunoreactivity in fibrillary components of neuronal and oligodendroglial cytoplasmic inclusions in the pontine nuclein in multiple system atrophy. Acta Neuropathol 96:439–444, 1998.
24. Galvin JE, Lee VM, Trojanowski JQ: Synucleinopathies: clinical and pathological implications. Arch Neurol 58:186–190, 2001.

25. Dickson DW: α-Synuclein and the Lewy body disorders. Curr Opin Neurol 14:423–432, 2001.
26. Litvan L, MacIntyre A, Goetz CG, et al: Accuracy of the clinical diagnoses of Lewy body disease, Parkinson disease, and dementia with Lewy bodies: A clinicopathologic study. Arch Neurol 55:969–978, 1998.
27. Jellinger K: Pathology of Parkinson's syndrome. In Calne DB (ed): Drugs for the treatment of Parkinson's disease. Berlin, Springer, 1989, pp 47–112.
28. Jellinger KA: Neuropathology of movement disorders. Neurosurg Clin N Am 9:237–262, 1998.
29. Jellinger KA: The pathology of Parkinson's disease. Adv Neurol 86:55–72, 2001.
30. Hughes AJ, Daniel SE, Kilford L, et al: Accuracy of clinical diagnosis of idiopathic Parkinson's disease: A clinico-pathological study of 100 cases. J Neurol Neurosurg Psychiatry 55:181–184, 1992.
31. Hughes AJ, Daniel SE, Lees AJ: Improved accuracy of clinical diagnosis of Lewy body Parkinson's disease. Neurology 57:1497–1499, 2001.
31a. Schrag A, Ben-Shlomo Y, Quinn N: How valid is the clinical diagnosis of Parkinson's disease in the community? J Neurol Neurosurg Psychiatry 73:529–534, 2002.
32. Graham JM, Sagar HJ: A data-driven approach to the study of heterogeneitiy in idiopathic Parkinson's disease: Identification of three distinct subgroups. Mov Disord 14:10–20, 1999.
33. Jellinger KA: Recent developments in the pathology of Parkinson disease. J Neural Transm 62(Suppl):347–376, 2002.
34. Damier P, Hirsch EC, Agid Y, et al: The substantia nigra of the human brain: II. Patterns of loss of dopamine-containing neurons in Parkinson's disease. Brain 122:1437–1448, 1999.
35. Ma SY, Rinne JO, Collan Y, et al: A quantitative morphometrical study of the neuron degeneration in the substantia nigra in patients with Parkinson's disease. J Neurol Sci 140:40–45, 1995.
36. Halliday GM, McRitchie DA, Cartwright HR, et al: Midbrain neuropathology in idiopathic Parkinson's disease and diffuse Lewy body disease. J Clin Neurosci 3:52–60, 1996.
37. Kish SJ, Shannak K, Hornykiewicz O, et al: Uneven pattern of dopamine loss in the striatum of patients with idiopathic Parkinson's disease: Pathophysiologic and clinical implications. N Engl J Med 318:876–880, 1988.
38. Ma SY, Röyttä M, Rinne JO, et al: Correlation between neuromorphometry in the substantia nigra and clinical features in Parkinson's disease using dissector counts. J Neurol Sci 151:83–87, 1997.
39. Paulus W, Jellinger K: The neuropathologic basis of different clinical subtypes of Parkinson's disease. J Neuropathol Exp Neurol 50:143–155, 1991.
40. McRitchie DA, Cartwright HR, Halliday GM: Specific A10 dopaminergic nuclei in the midbrain degenerate in Parkinson's disease. Exp Neurol 144:202–213, 1997.
41. Varastet M, Riche D, Maziere M, et al: Chronic MPTP treatment reproduces in baboons the differential vulnerability of mesencephalic dopaminergic neurons in Parkinson's disease. Neuroscience 63:47–56, 1994.
42. Fearnley JM, Lees AJ: Pathology of Parkinson's disease. In Calne DB (ed): Neurodegenerative Diseases. Philadelphia, WB Saunders, 1994, pp 545–554.
43. Ma SY, Ciliax BJ, Stebbins G, et al: Dopamine transporter-immunoreactive neurons decrease with age in the human substantia nigra. J Comp Neurol 409:25–37, 1999.
44. Ma SY, Röyttä M, Collan Y, et al: Unbiased morphometrical measurements show loss of pigmented nigral neurones with ageing. Neuropathol Appl Neurobiol 25:394–399, 1999.
45. Counihan TJ, Penney JB Jr: Regional dopamine transporter gene expression in the substantia nigra from control and Parkinson's diseased brains. J Neurol Neurosurg Psychiatry 65:164–169, 1998.
46. Neystat M, Lynch T, Przedborski S, et al: α-Synuclein expression in substantia nigra and cortex in Parkinson's disease. Mov Disord 14:417–422, 1999.
47. Ciliax BJ, Drash GW, Staley JK, et al: Immunocytochemical localization of the dopamine transporter in human brain. J Comp Neurol 409:38–56, 1999.
48. Miller GW, Erickson JD, Perez JT, et al: Immunochemical analy-
49. Zhang J, Perry G, Smith MA, et al: Parkinson's disease is associated with oxidative damage to cytoplasmic DNA and RNA in substantia nigra neurons. Am J Pathol 154:1423–1429, 1999.
50. Walker DG, Terai K, Matsuo A, et al: Immunohistochemical analyses of fibroblast growth factor receptor-1 in the human substantia nigra—comparison between normal and Parkinson's disease cases. Brain Res 794:181–187, 1998.
51. Mogi M, Togari A, Kondo T, et al: Brain-derived growth factor and nerve growth factor concentrations are decreased in the substantia nigra in Parkinson's disease. Neurosci Lett 270:45–48, 1999.
52. Benisty S, Boissiere F, Faucheux B, et al: TRKB messenger RNA expression in normal human brain and in the substantia nigra of parkinsonian patients—an in situ hybridization study. Neuroscience 86:813–826, 1998.
53. Parain K, Murer MG, Yan Q, et al: Reduced expression of brain-derived neurotrophic factor protein in Parkinson's disease substantia nigra. Neuroreport 10:557–561, 1999.
54. Joyce JN, Smutzer G, Whitty CJ, et al: Differential modification of dopamine transporter and tyrosine hydroxylase mRNAs in midbrain of subjects with Parkinson's, Alzheimer with parkinsonism, and Alzheimer's disease. Mov Disord 12:885–897, 1997.
55. Uhl GR: Hypothesis: The role of dopaminergic transporters in selective vulnerability of cells in Parkinson's disease. Ann Neurol 43:555–560, 1998.
56. Kingsbury AE, Marsden CD, Foster OJF: The vulnerability of nigral neurons to Parkinson's disease is unrelated to their intrinsic capacity for dopamine synthesis: An in situ hybridisation study. Mov Disord 14:206–219, 1999.
57. Nishio T, Furukawa S, Akiguchi I, et al: Medial nigral dopamine neurons have rich neurotrophin support. Neuroreport 9:2847–2851, 1998.
58. Hardman CD, Halliday GM, McRitchie DA, et al: The subthalamic nucleus in Parkinson's disease and progressive supranuclear palsy. J Neuropathol Exp Neurol 56:132–142, 1997.
59. Hartmann A, Hunot S, Michel FP, et al: Caspase-3: A vulnerability factor and final effector in apoptotic death or dopaminergic neurons in Parkinson's disease. J Neurosci 21:2247–2255, 2001.
60. Alam ZI, Jenner A, Daniel SE, et al: Oxidative DNA damage in the Parkinsonian brain: An apparent selective increase in 8-hydroxyguanine levels in substantia nigra. J Neurochem 69:1196–1203, 1997.
61. Floor E, Wetzel MG: Increased protein oxidation in human SNpc in comparison with basal ganglia and prefrontal cortex measured with an improved dinitrophenylhydrazine assay. J Neurochem 70:268–275, 1998.
62. Jenner P, Olanow CW: Understanding cell death in Parkinson's disease. Ann Neurol 44:S72–S84, 1998.
63. Jenner P: Oxidative mechanisms in nigral cell death in Parkinson's disease. Mov Disord 13:24–34, 1998.
64. Jellinger KA: Cell death mechanisms in Parkinson's disease. J Neural Transm 107:1–29, 2000.
65. Riederer P, Janetzky M, Gerlach M, et al: Parkinson's disease, iron, mitochondria, inflammatory responses, and oxidative stress: Prospectives for neuroprotection. Neurosci News 2:83–87, 1999.
66. Berger B, Gaspar P, Verney C: Dopaminergic innervation of the cerebral cortex: Unexpected differences between rodents and primates. Trends Neurosci 14:21–27, 1991.
67. Bernheimer H, Birkmayer W, Hornykiewicz O, et al: Brain dopamine and the syndromes of Parkinson and Huntington: Clinical, morphological and neurochemical correlations. J Neurol Sci 20:415–455, 1973.
68. Morrish PK, Sawle GV, Brooks DJ: Regional changes in [^{18}F]dopa metabolism in the striatum in Parkinson's disease. Brain 119:2097–2103, 1996.
69. Eve DJ, Nisbet AP, Kingsburg AE, et al: Selective increase in somatostatin mRNA expression in human basal ganglia in Parkinson's disease. Mol Brain Res 50:59–70, 1997.
70. Miller GW, Staley JK, Heilman CJ, et al: Immunochemical analysis of dopamine transporter protein in Parkinson's disease. Ann Neurol 41:530–539, 1997.
71. De Ceballos ML, Lopez-Lozano JJ: Subgroups of parkinsonian

patients differentiated by peptidergic immunostaining of caudate nucleus biopsies. Peptides 20:249–257, 1999.

72. Morrish PK, Rakshi JS, Bailey DL, et al: Measuring the rate of progression and estimating the preclinical period of Parkinson's disease with [18F]dopa PET. J Neurol Neurosurg Psychiatry 64:314–319, 1998.

73. Rinne JO, Nurmi E, Ruottinen HM, et al: [F-18]FDOPA and [F-18]CFT are both sensitive PET markers to detect presynaptic dopaminergic hypofunction in early Parkinson disease. Synapse 40:193–200, 2001.

74. Ito K, Morrish PK, Rakshi JS, et al: Statistical parametric mapping with 18F-dopa PET shows bilateral reduced striatal and nigral dopaminergic function in early Parkinson's disease. J Neurol Neurosurg Psychiatry 66:754–758, 1999.

75. Neill TH, Brown SA, Rafols JA, et al: Atrophy of medium spiny type I striatal dendrites in advanced Parkinson's disease. Brain Res 455:148–152, 1988.

76. Lach H, Grimes D, Benoit B, et al: Caudate nucleus pathology in Parkinson's disease: Ultrastructural and biochemical findings in biopsy material. Acta Neuropathol 83:352–360, 1992.

76a.Duda JE, Giasson BI, Mabon ME, et al: Novel antibodies to α-synuclein show abundant striatal pathology in Lewy body diseases. Ann Neurol 52:205–210, 2002.

77. Ito H, Kosaka H, Matsumoto S, et al: Striatal efferent involvement and its correlation to levodopa efficacy in patients with multiple system atrophy. Neurology 47:1291–1299, 1996.

78. Hardman CD, Halliday GM: The internal globus pallidus is affected in progressive supranuclear palsy and Parkinson's disease. Exp Neurol 158–142, 1999.

79. Hardman CD, Halliday GM: The external globus pallidus in patients with Parkinson's disease and progressive supranuclear palsy. Mov Disord 14:626–633, 1999.

80. Kume A, Takahashi A, Hashizume Y: Neuronal cell loss of the striatonigral system in multiple system atrophy. J Neurol Sci 117:33–40, 1993.

81. Mouatt-Prigent A, Agid Y, Hirsch EC: Does the calcium binding protein calretinin protect dopaminergic neurons against degeneration in Parkinson's disease? Brain Res 668:62–70, 1994.

82. Gerfen C: The neostriatal mosaic: Multiple levels of compartmental organization. Trends Neurosci 15:133–139, 1992.

83. Lynd-Balta E, Haber SN: Primate striatonigral projections: A comparison of the sensorimotor-related striatum and the ventral striatum. J Comp Neurol 345:562–578, 1994.

84. Percheron G, Francois C, Yelnik J, et al: The basal ganglia related system of primates: Definition, description and informational analysis. In Percheron G, McKensie JS, Féger J (eds): The Basal Ganglia, vol IV. New Ideas and Data on Structure and Function. New York, Plenum, 1994, pp 3–20.

85. Obeso JA, Guridi J, DeLong M: Surgery for Parkinson's disease. J Neurol Neurosurg Psychiatry 62:2–8, 1997.

86. Antonini A, Moeller JR, Nakamura T, et al: The metabolic anatomy of tremor in Parkinson's disease. Neurology 51:803–810, 1998.

87. Zirh TA, Lenz FA, Reich SG, et al: Patterns of bursting occurring in thalamic cells during parkinsonian tremor. Neuroscience 83:107–121, 1998.

88. Lee MS, Kim YD, Im JH, et al: 123I-IPT brain SPECT study in essential tremor and Parkinson's disease. Neurology 52:1422–1426, 1999.

89. Boecker H, Brooks DJ: Functional imaging of tremor. Mov Disord 13:64–72, 1998.

90. Lozza C, Marie RM, Baron JC: The metabolic substrates of bradykinesia and tremor in uncomplicated Parkinson's disease. Neuroimage 17:688–699, 2002.

91. Otsuka M, Ichiya Y, Kuwabara Y, et al: Differences in the reduced 18F-Dopa uptakes of the caudate and the putamen in Parkinson's disease: Correlation with the three main symptoms. J Neurol Sci 136:169–173, 1996.

92. Del Tredici K, Rub U, De Vos RA, et al: Where does Parkinson disease pathology begin in the brain? J Neuropathol Exp Neurol 61:413–426, 2002.

93. Jellinger KA: Neuropathological correlates of mental dysfunction in Parkinson's disease: An update. In Wolters EC, Scheltens P, Berendse HW (eds): Mental Dysfunction in Parkinson's Disease, II. Utrecht, Academic Pharmaceutical Productions, 1999, pp 82–105.

94. Wolters EC, Francot CMJE: The concept of mental dysfunction in Parkinson's disease. In Wolters EC, Scheltens P, Berendse HW (eds): Mental Dysfunction in Parkinson's Disease, II. Utrecht, Academic Pharmaceutical Productions, 1999, pp 35–48.

95. Dale GE, Probst A, Luthert P, et al: Relationship between Lewy bodies and pale bodies in Parkinson's disease. Acta Neuropathol 83:525–529, 1992.

96. Braak H, Sandmann-Keil D, Gai W, et al: Extensive axonal Lewy neurites in Parkinson's disease: A novel pathological feature revealed by α-synuclein immunocytochemistry. Neurosci Lett 265:67–69, 1999.

97. Braak H, Braak E: Pathoanatomy of Parkinson's disease. J Neurol 247(Suppl 2):II3–II10, 2000.

98. Gai WP, Blessing WW, Blumberg PC: Ubiquitin-positive degenerating neurites in the brainstem in Parkinson's disease. Brain 118:1447–1459., 1995.

99. Baba M, Nakajo S, Tu PH, et al: Aggregation of α-synuclein in Lewy bodies of sporadic Parkinson's disease and dementia with Lewy bodies. Am J Pathol 152:879–884, 1998.

100. Galvin JF, Lee VMY, Schmidt L, et al: Pathobiology of the Lewy body. Adv Neurol 80:313–324, 1999.

101. Irrizary MC, Growdon W, Gornez-Isla T, et al: Nigral and cortical Lewy bodies and dystrophic nigral neurites in Parkinson's disease and cortical Lewy body disease contain α-synuclein immunoreactivity. J Neuropathol Exp Neurol 57:334–337, 1998.

102. Sakamoto M, Uchihara T, Hayashi M, et al: Heterogeneity of nigral and cortical Lewy bodies differentiated by amplified triple-labeling for α-synuclein, ubiquitin, and thiazin red. Exp Neurol 177:88–94, 2002.

103. Hashimoto M, Hsu LJ, Sisk A, et al: Human recombinant NACP/α-synuclein is aggregated and fibrillated in vitro: Relevance for Lewy body disease. Brain Res 799:301–306, 1998.

104. Narhi L, Wood SJ, Steavenson S, et al: Both familial Parkinson's disease mutations accelerate α-synuclein aggregation. J Biol Chem 273:9843–9846, 1999.

105. Farrer M, Gwinn-Hardy K, Hutton M, Hardy J: The genetics of disorders with synuclein pathology and parkinsonism. Hum Molec Genet 8:1901–1905, 1999.

106. Nakamura S, Kawamoto Y, Nakano S, et al: Cyclin-dependent kinase 5 and mitogen-activated protein kinase in glial cytoplasmic inclusions in multiple system atrophy. J Neuropathol Exp Neurol 57:690–698, 1998.

107. Wakabayashi K, Hayashi S, Kakita A, et al: Accumulation of α-synuclein MACP is a cytopathological feature common to Lewy body disease and multiple system atrophy. Acta Neuropathol 96:445–452, 1998.

108. Samuel W, Galasko D, Masliah E, et al: Neocortical Lewy body counts correlate with dementia in the Lewy body variant of Alzheimer's disease. J Neuropathol Exp Neurol 55:44–52, 1996.

109. Hurtig HI, Trojanowski JQ, Galvin J, et al: α-Synuclein cortical Lewy bodies correlate with dementia in Parkinson's disease. Neurology 54:1916–1921, 2000.

109a.Haroutunian V, Serby M, Purohit DP, et al: Contribution of Lewy body inclusions to dementia in patients with and without Alzheimer disease neuropathological conditions. Arch Neurol 57:1145–1150, 2000.

110. Hansen LA, Daniel SE, Wilcock GK, et al: Frontal cortical synaptophysin in Lewy body diseases: Relation to Alzheimer's disease and dementia. J Neurol Neurosurg Psychiatry 64:653–656, 1998.

111. Wakabayashi K, Kakita A, Hayashi S, et al: Apolipoprotein E ε4 allele and progression of cortical Lewy body pathology in Parkinson's disease. Acta Neuropathol 95:450–454, 1998.

112. Brown DF, Risser RC, Bigio EH: Lewy body density does not correlate with neocortical synapse density in the Lewy body variant of Alzheimer disease. J Neuropathol Exp Neurol 57:515, 1998.

113. Gómez-Tortosa E, Newell K, Irizarry MC, et al: Clinical and quantitative pathologic correlates of dementia with Lewy bodies. Neurology 53:1284–1291, 1999.

113a.Jellinger KA, Seppi K, Wenning GK, Poewe W: Impact of coexistent Alzheimer pathology on the natural history of Parkinson's disease. J Neural Transm 109:329–339, 2002.

114. Trojanowski JQ, Lee VMY: Aggregation of neurofilament and α-synuclein proteins in Lewy bodies. Implications for the patho-

genesis of Parkinson's disease and Lewy body dementia. Arch Neurol 55:151–152, 1998.

115. Tompkins MM, Hill WD: Contribution of somal Lewy bodies to neuronal death. Brain Res 775:24–29, 1997.

116. Itoh K, Weis S, Mehraein P, et al: Defects of cytochrome *c* oxidase in the substantia nigra of Parkinson's disease: An immunohistochemical and morphometric study. Mov Disord 12:9–16, 1997.

117. Mizuno Y, Hattori N, Kitada T, et al: Genetic aspects in Parkinson's disease. In Wolters EC, Scheltens P, Berendse HW (eds): Mental Dysfunction in Parkinson's Disease, II. Utrecht, Academic Pharmaceutical Productions, 1999, pp 49–61.

118. Olanow CW, Tatton WG: Etiology and pathogenesis of Parkinson's disease. Annu Rev Neurosci 22:123–144, 1999.

119. Anglade P, Vyas S, Javoy-Agid F, et al: Apoptosis and autophagy in nigral neurons of patients with Parkinson's disease. Histol Histopathol 12:25–31, 1997.

120. Burke RE, Kholodilov NG: Programmed cell death: Does it play a role in Parkinson's disease? Ann Neurol 44(Suppl 1):S126–S133, 1998.

121. Tatton WG, Olanow CW: Apoptosis in neurodegenerative diseases: The role of mitochondria. Biochem Biophys Acta 1410:195–214, 1999.

122. Tompkins MM, Basgall EJ, Zamrini E, et al: Apoptotic-like changes in Lewy body–associated disorders and normal aging in substantia nigral neurons. Am J Pathol 150:119–131, 1997.

123. Marshall KA, Daniel SE, Cairns N, et al: Upregulation of the anti-apoptotic protein Bcl-2 may be early event in neurodegeneration: Studies on Parkinson's incidental Lewy body disease. Biochem Biophys Res Commun 240:84–87, 1997.

124. Duan W, Zhang Z, Gash DM, et al: Participation of prostate apoptosis response-4 in degeneration of dopaminergic neurons in models of Parkinson's disease. Ann Neurol 46:587–597, 1999.

125. Bredesen DE: Neural apoptosis. Ann Neurol 38:839–851, 1995.

126. Banati RB, Daniel SE, Path MRC, et al: Glial pathology but absence of apoptotic nigral neurons in long-standing Parkinson's disease. Mov Disord 13:221–227, 1998.

127. Kingsbury AE, Mardsen CD, Foster OJF: DNA fragmentation in human substantia nigra: Apoptosis or perimortem effect? Mov Disord 13:877–884, 1998.

128. Wüllner U, Kornhuber J, Weller M, et al: Cell death and apoptosis regulating proteins in Parkinson's disease—a cautionary note. Acta Neuropathol 97:408–412, 1999.

129. Stadelmann C, Brück W, Bancher C, et al: Alzheimer disease: DNA fragmentation indicates increased neuronal vulnerability, but not apoptosis. J Neuropathol Exp Neurol 57:456–464, 1998.

130. Graeber MB, Grasbon-Frodl E, Abell-Aleff P, et al: Nigral neurons are likely to die of a mechanism other than classical apoptosis in Parkinson's disease. Parkinsonism Relat Disord 5:187–192, 1999.

131. Gleckman AM, Jiang Z, Liu Y, et al: DNA fragmentation in neurons and glial cells indicates cellular injury but not apoptosis in Pick's disease. Acta Neuropathol 99:55–61, 1999.

132. Morsch R, Simon W, Coleman PD: Neurons may live for decades with neurofibrillary tangles. J Neuropathol Exp Neurol 58:188–197, 1999.

133. Rajput AH, Rozdilsky B, Rajput A: Accuracy of clinical diagnosis in parkinsonism: A prospective study. Can J Neurol Sci 18:275–278, 1991.

134. Olsson JE, Brunk U, Lindvall B, et al: Dopa-responsive dystonia with depigmentation of the substantia nigra and formation of Lewy bodies. J Neurol Sci 112:90–95, 1992.

135. Matsumine H, Yamamura Y, Kobayashi T, et al: Early onset parkinsonism with diurnal fluctuation maps to a locus for juvenile parkinsonism. Neurology 50:1340–1345, 1998.

136. Mark MH, Sage JI, Dickson DW, et al: Meige syndrome in the spectrum of Lewy body disease. Neurology 44:1432–1436, 1994.

137. Takahashi H, Ohama E, Suzuki S, et al: Familial juvenile parkinsonism: Clinical and pathologic study in a family. Neurology 44:437–441, 1994.

138. Yoshimura N, Yoshimura I, Asada M, et al: Juvenile Parkinson's disease with widespread Lewy bodies in the brain. Acta Neuropathol 77:213–218, 1988.

139. Denson MA, Wszolek ZK, Pfeiffer RF, et al: Familial parkinsonism, dementia and Lewy body disease: Study of family G. Ann Neurol 42:638–643, 1997.

140. Muenter MD, Forno LS, Hornykiewicz O, et al: Hereditary form of parkinsonism-dementia. Ann Neurol 43:768–781, 1998.

141. Bhatia KP, Daniel SE, Marsden CD: Familial parkinsonism with depression: A clinicopathological study. Ann Neurol 34:842–847, 1993.

142. Golbe LI, Lazzarini AM, Schwarz KO, et al: Autosomal dominant parkinsonism with benign course and typical Lewy-body pathology. Neurology 43:2222–2227, 1993.

143. Dwork AJ, Balmaceda C, Fazzini EA, et al: Dominantly inherited early-onset parkinsonism: Neuropathology of a new form. Neurology 43:69–74, 1993.

144. Foster NL, Wilhelmsen K, Sima AAF, et al: Frontotemporal dementia and parkinsonism linked to chromosome 17—a consensus conference. Ann Neurol 41:706–715, 1997.

145. Holmes C, Cairns N, Lantos P, et al: Validity of current clinical criteria for Alzheimer's disease, vascular dementia and dementia with Lewy bodies. Br J Psychiatry 174:45–50, 1999.

146. Papka M, Rubio A, Schiffer RB: A review of Lewy body disease, an emerging concept of cortical dementia. J Neuropsychiatry Clin Neurosci 10:267–279, 1998.

147. Kosaka K, Yoshimura M, Ikeda K, et al: Diffuse type of Lewy body disease: Progressive dementia with abundant cortical Lewy bodies and senile changes of varying degree—a new disease? Clin Neuropathol 3:185–192, 1984.

148. Hansen LA, Masliah E, Galasko D, et al: Plaque-only Alzheimer disease is usually the Lewy body variant and vice versa. J Neuropathol Exp Neurol 52:648–654, 1993.

148a. Harding AJ, Halliday GM: Simplified neuropathological diagnosis of dementia with Lewy bodies. Neuropathol Appl Neurobiol 24:195–201, 1998.

149. Bruak H, Braak E: Neuropathological staging of Alzheimer-related changes. Acta Neuropathol 82:239–259, 1991.

149a. Higuchi M, Tashiro M, Arai H, et al: Glucose hypometabolism and neuropathological correlates in brains of dementia with Lewy bodies. Exp Neurol 162:247–256, 2000.

149b. Walker Z, Costa DC, Walker RW, et al: Differentiation of dementia with Lewy bodies from Alzheimer's disease using a dopaminergic presynaptic ligand. J Neurol Neurosurg Psychiatry 73:134–140, 2002.

150. Lippa CF, Ozawa K, Mann DMA, et al: Deposition of β-amyloid subtypes 40 and 42 differentiates dementia with Lewy bodies from Alzheimer disease. Arch Neurol 56:1111–1118, 1999.

151. Samuel W, Alford M, Hofstetter CR, et al: Dementia with Lewy bodies versus pure Alzheimer's disease: Differences in cognition, neuropathology, cholinergic dysfunction, and synaptic density. J Neuropathol Exp Neurol 56:499–508, 1997.

152. Perry E, Court J, Goodchild R: Clinical neurochemistry: Developments in dementia research based on brain bank material. J Neural Transm 105:915–934, 1998.

153. Lippa CF, Smith TW, Perry E: Dementia with Lewy bodies: Choline acetyltransferase parallels nucleus basalis pathology. J Neural Transm 106:525–535, 1999.

154. Shiozaki K, Iseki E, Uchiyama H, et al: Alterations of muscarinic acetylcholine receptor subtypes in diffuse Lewy body disease: Relation to Alzheimer's disease. J Neurol Neurosurg Psychiatry 67:209–213, 1999.

155. Piggot MA, Perry EK, Marshall EF, et al: Nigrostriatal dopaminergic activites in dementia with Lewy bodies in relation to neuroleptic sensitivity: Comparison with Parkinson's disease. Biol Psychiatry 44:765–774, 1998.

156. Martinoli MG, Trojanowski JQ, Schmidt ML, et al: Association of apolipoprotein ε4 allele and neuropathological findings in patients with dementia. Acta Neuropathol 90:239–243, 1995.

157. Tanaka S, Chen X, Xia Y, et al: Association of CYP2D microsatellite polymorphism with Lewy body variant of Alzheimer's disease. Neurology 50:1556–1562, 1998.

158. Harding AJ, Halliday GM: Cortical Lewy body pathology in the diagnosis of dementia. Acta Neuropathol 102:355–363, 2001.

159. Wenning GK, Tison F, Ben Shlomo Y, et al: Multiple system atrophy: A review of 203 pathologically proven cases. Mov Disord 2:133–147, 1997.

160. Koeppen AH: The hereditary ataxias. J Neuropathol Exp Neurol 57:531–543, 1998.

161. Kraft E, Schwarz J, Trenkwalder C, et al: The combination of hypointense and hyperintense signal changes of T-1 weighted

magnetic resonance imaging sequences: a specific marker of multiple system atrophy? Arch Neurol 56:225–228, 1999.

162. Goto S, Matsumoto S, Ushio Y, et al: Subregional loss of putaminal efferents to the basal ganglia output nuclei may cause parkinsonism in striatonigral degeneration. Neurology 47:1032–1036, 1996.

162a. Wenning GK, Seppi K, Tison F, Jellinger K: A novel grading scale for striatonigral degeneration (multiple system atrophy). J Neural Transm 109:307–320, 2002.

163. Tison F, Wenning GK, Daniel SE, et al: The pathophysiology of parkinsonism in multiple system atrophy. Eur J Neurol 2:435–444, 1995.

163a. Benarroch EE: New findings on the neuropathology of multiple system atrophy. Auton Neurosci 96:59–62, 2002.

164. Toghi H, Tabuchi M, Tomonaga M, et al: Selective loss of small myelinated and unmyelinated fibers in Shy-Drager syndrome. Acta Neuropathol 57:282–286, 1982.

165. Tu P-H, Galvin JE, Baba M, et al: Glial cytoplasmic inclusions in white matter oligodendrocytes of multiple system atrophy brains contain insoluble α-synuclein. Ann Neurol 44:415–422, 1998.

166. Gai WP, Powert JHT, Blumberge PC, et al: Alpha-synuclein immunoisolation of glial inclusions from multiple system atrophy brain tissue reveals multiprotein components. J Neurochem 73:2093–2100, 1999.

167. Matsuo A, Akiguchi I, Lee GC, et al: Myelin degeneration in multiple system atrophy detected by unique antibodies. Am J Pathol 153:735–744, 1998.

168. Dickson DW, Liu WK, Hardy J, et al: Widespread alterations of alpha-synuclein in multiple system atrophy. Am J Pathol 155:1241–1251, 1999.

169. Morris HR, Lees AJ, Wood NW: Neurofibrillary tangle parkinsonian disorders—tau pathology and tau genetics. Mov Disord 14:731–736, 1999.

170. Jellinger KA: Movement disorders with tau protein cytoskeletal pathology. Adv Neurol 80:303–311, 1999.

171. Buée L, Delacourte A: Comparative biochemistry of tau in progressive supranuclear palsy, cortico-basal degeneration, FTDP-17 and Pick's disease. Brain Pathol 9:681–693, 1999.

172. Feany MB, Mattiace LA, Dickson DW: Neuropathologic overlap of progressive supranuclear palsy, Pick's disease, and cortico-basal degeneration. J Neuropathol Exp Neurol 55:53–67, 1996.

173. Steele JC, Richardson JC, Olszewski J: Progressive supranuclear palsy. Arch Neurol 10:333–359, 1964.

174. Litvan I: Progressive supranuclear palsy revisited. Acta Neurol Scand 98:73–84, 1998.

175. Baker M, Litvan I, Houlden H, et al: Association of an extended haplotype in the tau gene with progressive supranuclear palsy. Hum Mol Genet 8:711–715, 1999.

176. Chambers CB, Lee JM, Troncoso JC, et al: Overexpression of four-repeat tau mRNA isoforms in progressive supranuclear palsy but not in Alzheimer's disease. Ann Neurol 46:325–332, 1999.

177. Hoenicka J, Perez M, Perez-Tur J, et al: The tau gene A9 allele and progressive supranuclear palsy. Neurology 53:1219–1225, 1999.

178. Komori T: Tau-positive glial inclusions in progressive supranuclear palsy, cortico-basal degeneration and Pick's disease. Brain Pathol 9:663–679, 1999.

179. Mackenzie I, Hudson L: Achromatic neurons in the cortex of progressive supranuclear palsy. Acta Neuropathol 90:615–619, 1995.

180. Hardman CD, Halliday GM, McRitchie DA, et al: Progressive supranuclear palsy affects both the substantia nigra pars compacta and reticulata. Exp Neurol 144:183–192, 1997.

181. Verny M, Duyckaerts C, Agid Y, Hauw J: The significance of cortical pathology in progressive supranuclear palsy. Clinicopathological data in 10 cases. Brain 119:1123–1136, 1996.

182. Shinotoh H, Namba H, Yamaguchi M, et al: Positron emission tomographic measurement of acetylcholinesterase activity reveals differential loss of ascending cholinergic systems in Parkinson's disease and progressive supranuclear palsy. Ann Neurol 46:62–69, 1999.

183. Litvan I, Paulsen JS, Mega MS, et al: Neuropsychiatric assessment of patients with hyperkinetic and hypokinetic movement disorders. Arch Neurol 55:1313–1319, 1998.

184. Pillon B, Gouider-Khouja N, Deweer B, et al: Neuropsychological pattern of striatonigral degeneration: Comparison with Parkinson's disease and progressive supranuclear palsy. J Neurol Neurosurg Psychiatry 58:174–179, 1995.

185. Bergeron C, Davis A, Lang AE: Cortico-basal ganglionic degeneration and progressive supranuclear palsy presenting with cognitive decline. Brain Pathol 8:355–365, 1998.

186. Bigio EH, Brown DF, White CL III: Progressive supranuclear palsy with dementia: Cortical pathology. J Neuropathol Exp Neurol 58:359–364, 1999.

187. Dickson DW: Progressive supranuclear palsy and corticobasal degeneration., In Hof PR, Mobbs CV (eds): Functional Neurobiology of Aging. New York, Academic Press, 2001, pp. 155–171.

188. Boeve BF, Maraganore DM, Parisi JE, et al: Pathologic heterogeneity in clinically diagnosed cortico-basal degeneration. Neurology 53:795–800, 1999.

189. Litvan I, Agid Y, Goetz C, et al: Accuracy of the clinical diagnosis of cortico-basal degeneration: A clinicopathologic study. Neurology 48:119–125, 1997.

190. Takahashi T, Amano N, Hanihara T, et al: Cortico-basal degeneration: Widespread argentophilic threads and glia in addition to neurofibrillary tangles. Similarities of cytoskeletal abnormalities in cortico-basal degeneration and progressive supranuclear palsy. J Neurol Sci 138:66–77, 1996.

191. Ksiezak-Reding H, Tracz E, Yang L-S, et al: Ultrastructural instability of paired helical filaments from cortico-basal degeneration as examined by scanning transmission electron microscopy. Am J Pathol 149:639–651, 1996.

192. Sergeant N, Wattez A, Delacourte A: Neurofibrillary degeneration in progressive supranuclear palsy and cortico-basal degeneration: Tau pathologies with exclusively "exon 10" isoforms. J Neurochem 72:1243–1249, 1999.

193. Jendroska K, Rossor MN, Mathias CJ, et al: Morphological overlap between cortico-basal degeneration and Pick's disease: A clinicopathological report. Mov Disord 10:111–114, 1995.

194. Matsumoto S, Udaka F, Kameyama M, et al: Subcortical neurofibrillary tangles, neuropil threads, and argentophilic glial inclusions in cortico-basal degeneration. Clin Neuropathol 15:209–214, 1996.

195. Geddes JF, Hughes AJ, Lees AJ, et al: Pathological overlap in cases of parkinsonism associated with neurofibrillary tangles. A study of recent cases of postencephalitic parkinsonism and comparison with progressive supranuclear palsy and Guamanian parkinson-dementia complex. Brain 116:281–302, 1993.

196. Wenning GK, Jellinger K, Litvan I: Supranuclear gaze palsy and eye lid apraxia in postencephalitic parkinsonism. J Neural Transm 104:845–865, 1997.

197. Litvan I, Jankovic J, Goetz CG, et al: Accuracy of the clinical diagnosis of postencephalitic parkinsonism: A clinicopathologic study. Eur J Neurol 5:451–457, 1998.

197a. McCall S, Henry JM, Reid AH, Taubenberger JK: Influenza RNA not detected in archival brain tissue from acute encephalitic lethargica cases of postencephalitic parkinsonism. J Neuropathol Exp Neurol 60:606–704, 2001.

198. Hof PR, Perl DP, Loerzel AJ, et al: Amyotrophic lateral sclerosis and parkinsonism-dementia from Guam: Differences in neurofibrillary tangle distribution and density in the hippocampal formation and neocortex. Brain Res 650:107–116, 1994.

199. Perl DP: Amyotrophic lateral sclerosis/parkinsonism-dementia complex of Guam. In Esiri MM, Morris JH (eds): The Neuropathology of Dementia. Cambridge, Cambridge University Press, 1997, pp 184–203.

200. Oyanagi K, Wada M: Neuropathology of parkinsonism-dementia complex and amyotrophic lateral sclerosis of Guam: an update. J Neurol 246(Suppl 2):19–27, 1999.

201. Chang CM, Yu YL, Ng KH, et al: Vascular pseudoparkinsonism. Acta Neurol Scand 85:588–592, 1992.

202. Fénelon G, Gray F, Wallys C, et al: Parkinsonism and dilatation of perivascular spaces (état criblé) of the striatum: A clinical, magnetic resonance imaging, and pathological study. Mov Disord 10:754–760, 1995.

203. Horner S, Niederkorn K, Ni SK, et al: Evaluation vaskulärer Risikofaktoren bei Patienten mit Parkinson-Syndrom. Nervenarzt 68:967–971, 1997.

204. Mark MH, Sage JI, Walters AS, et al: Binswanger's disease

presenting as levodopa-responsive parkinsonism: Clinicopathologic study of three cases. Mov Disord 10:450–454, 1995.

205. Van Zagten M, Lodder J, Kessels F: Gait disorder and parkinsonian signs in patients with stroke related to small deep infarcts and white matter lesions. Mov Disord 13:89–95, 1998.

206. Winikates J, Jankovic J: Clinical correlates of vascular parkinsonism. Arch Neurol 56:98–102, 1999.

207. Jellinger K: Evaluation vaskulärer Risikofaktoren bei Parkinson-Syndrom. Nervenarzt 69:929–930, 1998.

208. Llau ME, Nguyen L, Senard JM, et al: Drug induced parkinsonism. Rev Neurol 150:757–762, 1994.

209. Veitch K, Hue L: Flunarizine and cinnarizine inhibit mitochondrial complexes I and II. Possible implication for parkinsonism. Mol Pharmacol 45:156–163, 1994.

210. Langston JW, Forno LS, Tetrud J, et al: Evidence of active nerve cell degeneration in the substantia nigra of humans years after 1-methyl-4-phenyl-1,2,3,6-tetrahydropyridine exposure. Ann Neurol 46:598–605, 1999.

211. Forno LS, DeLanney LE, Irwin I, et al: Electron microscopy of Lewy bodies in the amygdala-parahippocampal region. Comparison with inclusion bodies in the MPTP-treated squirrel monkey. Adv Neurol 69:217–224, 1996.

212. Allsop D, Haga S, Bruton C, et al: Neurofibrillary tangles in some cases of dementia pugilistica share antigens with amyloid β-protein in Alzheimer's disease. Am J Pathol 136:255–260, 1990.

213. Hof PF, Bouras C, Buée L, et al: Differential distribution of neurofibrillary tangles in the cerebral cortex of dementia pugilistica and Alzheimer's disease cases. Acta Neuropathol 85: 23–30, 1992.

214. Kremer B, Weber B, Hayden MR: New insights into the clinical features, pathogenesis and molecular genetics of Huntington's disease. Brain Pathol 2:321–335, 1992.

215. Quinn N, Schrag A: Huntington's disease and other choreas. J Neurol 245:709–716, 1998.

216. Ross CA, Becher HW, Colomer V, et al: Huntington's disease and dentatorubral-pallidoluysian atrophy: Proteins, pathogenesis and pathology. Brain Pathol 7:1003–1018, 1997.

217. Ross CA, Margolis RL, Rosenblatt A, et al: Huntington disease and the related disorder, dentatorubral-pallidoluysian atrophy (DRPLA). Rev Mol Med 76:305–338, 1997.

218. Robitaille A, Lopes-Cendes I, Becher M, et al: The neuropathology of CAG repeat diseases: Review and update of pathogenetic and molecular features. Brain Pathol 7:901–926, 1997.

219. Halliday GM, McRitchie DA, Macdonald Y, et al: Regional specificity of brain atrophy in Huntington's disease. Exp Neurol 154:663–672, 1998.

220. Vonsattel JP, Myers RH, Stevens TJ, et al: Neuropathological classification of Huntington's disease. J Neuropathol Exp Neurol 44:559–577, 1985.

221. Hedreen JC, Folstein SE: Early loss of neostriatal striosome neurons in Huntington's disease. J Neuropathol Exp Neurol 54: 105–120, 1995.

222. Ferrante RJ, Kowall NW, Beal MF, et al: Morphologic and histochemical characteristics of a spared subset of striatal neurons in Huntington's disease. J Neuropath Exp Neurol 46:12–27, 1987.

222a. Thieben MJ, Duggins AJ, Good CD, et al: The distribution of structural neuropathology in pre-clinical Huntington's disease. Brain 125:1815–1828, 2002.

223. Storey E, Beal MF: Neurochemical substrates of rigidity and chorea in Huntington's disease. Brain 116:1201–1222, 1993.

224. Oyanagi K, Takeda S, Takahashi H: A quantitative investigation of the substantia nigra in Huntington's disease. Ann Neurol 26: 13–19, 1989.

225. Turjanski N, Weeks R, Dolan R, et al: Striatal D1 and D2 receptor binding in patients with Huntington's disease and other choreas: PET study. Brain 118:689–696, 1995.

226. Antonini A, Leenders KL, Spiegel R, et al: Striatal glucose metabolism in asymptomatic gene carriers and patients with Huntington's disease. Brain 119:2085–2095, 1996.

227. Thompson PD, Berardelli A, Rothwell JC, et al: The coexistence of bradykinesia and chorea in Huntington's disease and its implications for theories of basal ganglia control of movement. Brain 111:223–244, 1988.

228. Berardelli A, Noth J, Thompson PD, et al: Pathophysiology of chorea and bradykinesia in Huntington's disease. Mov Disord 14:398–403, 1999.

229. Heinsen H, Strik M, Bauer M, et al: Cortical and striatal neurone number in Huntington's disease. Acta Neuropathol 88:320–333, 1994.

230. Braak H, Braak E: The human entorhinal cortex: Normal morphology and lamina-specific pathology in various diseases. Neurosci Res 15:6–31, 1992.

231. Jackson M, Gentleman S, Lennox S, et al: The cortical neuritic pathology of Huntington's disease. Neuropathol Appl Neurobiol 21:18–26, 1995.

232. Jones AL, Wood JD, Harper PS: Huntington's disease—advances in molecular and cell biology. J Inherit Metab Dis 20:125–138, 1997.

233. Jellinger KA: Alzheimer-type lesions in Huntington's disease. J Neural Transm 105:787–799, 1998.

234. Koeppen AH: The nucleus pontis centralis caudalis in Huntington's disease. J Neurol Sci 91:129–141, 1989.

235. Boutell JM, Thomas P, Neal JW, et al: Aberrant interactions of transcriptional repressor proteins with the Huntington's disease gene product, huntingtin. Hum Mol Genet 8:1647–1655, 1999.

236. DiFiglia M, Sapp E, Chase KO, et al: Aggregation of huntingtin in neuronal intranuclear inclusions and dystrophic neurites in brain. Science 277:1990–1993, 1997.

237. Maat-Schieman MLC, Dorsman JC, Smoor MA, et al: Distribution of inclusions in neuronal nuclei and dystrophic neurites in Huntington disease brain. J Neuropathol Exp Neurol 58: 129–137, 1999.

238. Persichetti F, Trettel F, Huang CC, et al: Mutant huntingtin forms in vivo complexes with distinct context-dependent comformations of the polyglutamine segment. Neurobiol Dis 6: 364–375, 1999.

239. Sieradzan KA, Merchan AO, Jones L, et al: Huntington's disease intranuclear inclusions contain truncated ubiquitinated huntingtin protein. Exp Neurol 156:92–99, 1999.

240. Sapp E, Penney J, Young A, et al: Axonal transport of N-terminal huntingtin suggests early pathology of corticostriatal projections in Huntington disease. J Neuropathol Exp Neurol 58:165–173, 1999.

241. Petersen Å, Mani K, Brundin P: Recent advances on the pathogenesis of Huntington's disease. Exp Neurol 157:1–18, 1999.

242. Browne SE, Ferrante RJ, Beal MF: Oxidative stress in Huntington's disease. Brain Pathol 9:147–163, 1999.

243. Reddy PH, Williams M, Tagle DA: Recent advances in understanding the pathogenesis of Huntington's disease. Trends Neurosci 22:248–255, 1999.

244. Tabrizi SJ, Cleeter MWJ, Xuereb J, et al: Biochemical abnormalities and excitotoxicity in Huntington's disease brain. Ann Neurol 45:25–32, 1999.

244a. Ho LW, Carmichael J, Swartz J, et al: The molecular biology of Huntington's disease. Psychol Med 31:3–14, 2001.

244b. Panov AV, Gutekunst CA, Leavitt BR, et al: Early mitochondrial calcium defects in Huntington's disease are a direct effect of polyglutamines. Nat Neurosci 5:731–736, 2002.

245. Becher MW, Rubinsztein DC, Leggo J, et al: Dentatorubral and pallidoluysian atrophy (DRPLA). Clinical and neuropathological findings in genetically confirmed North American and European pedigrees. Mov Disord 12:519–530, 1997.

246. Ikeuchi T, Koide R, Tanaka H, et al: Dentatorubral-pallidoluysian atrophy: Clinical features are closely related to unstable expansions of trinucleotide (CAG) repeat. Ann Neurol 37:769–775, 1995.

247. Koide R, Onodera O, Ikeuchi T: Atrophy of the cerebellum and brainstem in dentatorubral pallidoluysian atrophy: Influence of CAG repeat size on MRI findings. Neurology 49:1605–1612, 1997.

248. Komure O, Sano A, Shino N, et al: DNA analysis in hereditary dentatorubral-pallidoluysian atrophy. Neurology 45:143–149, 1995.

249. Warner TT, Williams LD, Walker RWH, et al: A clinical and molecular genetic study of dentatorubropallidoluysian atrophy in four European families. Ann Neurol 37:452–459, 1995.

250. Becher MW, Kotzuk JA, Sharp AH, et al: Intranuclear neuronal inclusions in Huntington's disease and dentatorubral and pallidoluysian atrophy: Correlation between the density of inclu-

sions and IT15 CAG triplet length. Neurobiol Dis 4:387–397, 1998.

251. Koshy BT, Zoghbi HY: The CAG/polyglutamine tract diseases: Gene products and molecular pathogenesis. Brain Pathol 7:927–942, 1997.

252. Watanabe M, Abe K, Aoki M, et al: Analysis of CAG trinucleotide expansion associated with Machado-Joseph disease. J Neurol Sci 136:101–107, 1996.

253. Hardie RJ, Pullon HWS, Harding AE, et al: Neuroacanthocytosis: A clinical, haematological and pathological study of 19 cases. Brain 114:13–49, 1991.

254. Rubio JP, Danek A, Stone C, et al: Chorea-acanthocytosis: genetic linkage of chromosome 9q21. Am J Hum Genet 61:899–908, 1997.

254a. Rampoldi L, Dobson-Stone C, Rubio JP, et al: A conserved sorting-associated protein is mutant in chorea-acanthocytosis. Nat Genet 28:119–120, 2001.

255. Rinne JQ, Daniel SE, Scaravilli F, et al: The neuropathological features of neuroacanthocytosis. Mov Disord 9:297–304, 1994.

256. Bruyn GW, Bots GTAM, Went LN, et al: Hereditary spastic dystonia with Leber's hereditary optic atrophy: Neuropathological findings. J Neurol Sci 103:195–202, 1992.

257. Roig M, Calopa M, Rovira A, et al: Bilateral striatal lesions in childhood. Pediatr Neurol 9:349–358, 1993.

258. Cardoso F, Vargas AP, Oliveira LD, et al: Persistent Sydenham's chorea. Mov Disord 14:805–807, 1999.

259. Janavs JI, Aminoff MJ: Dystonia and chorea in acquired systemic disorders. J Neurol Neurosurg Psychiatry 65:436–445, 1998.

260. Wooten GF, Lopes MBS, Harris WO, et al: Pallidoluysian atrophy: Dystonia and basal ganglia functional anatomy. Neurology 43:1764–1768, 1993.

261. Kawai J, Sasahara M, Hazawa F, et al: Pallidonigroluysian degeneration with iron deposition: A study of three autopsy cases. Acta Neuropathol 86:609–616, 1993.

262. Katayama S, Watanabe C, Khoriyama T, et al: Slowly progressive L-dopa nonresponsive pure akinesia due to nigropallidal degeneration: A clinicopathological case study. J Neurol Sci 161:169–172, 1998.

263. Jellinger KA: Neurodegenerative disorders with extrapyramidal features: A neuropathological overview. J Neural Transm Suppl 46:33–56, 1995.

264. Hallervorden J, Spatz H: Eigenartige Erkrankung im extrapyramidalen System mit besonderer Beteiligung des Globus pallidus und der Substantia nigra. Ein Beitrag zu den Beziehungen zwischen diesen beiden Zentren. Zentralbl Gesamte Neurol 79:254–302, 1922.

265. Zhou B, Westaway SK, Levinson B, et al: A novel pantothenate kinase gene (PANK2) is defective in Hallervorden-Spatz syndrome. Nat Genet 28:345–349, 2001.

265a. Curtis AR, Fey C, Morris CM, et al: Mutation in the gene encoding ferritin light polypeptide causes dominant adult-onset basal ganglia disease. Nat Genet 28:350–354, 2001.

266. Hyflick SJ, Westaway SK, Levinson B, et al: Genetic, clinical and radiographic delineation of Hallervorden-Spatz syndrome. N Engl J Med 348:33–40, 2003.

267. Seitelberger F: Neuroaxonal dystrophy: Its relation to aging and neurological diseases. In Vinken PJ, Bruyn GW, Klawans HL (eds): Handbook of Clinical Neurology, vol 5. Amsterdam, Elsevier Science, 1986, 391–415.

268. Savoiardo M, Haliday WC, Nardocci N, et al: Hallervorden-Spatz disease: MR and pathologic findings. AJNR Am J Neuroradiol 14:155–162, 1993.

269. Perry TL, Norman MG, Yong VW, et al: Hallervorden-Spatz disease: Cysteine accumulation and cysteine dioxygenase deficiency in the globus pallidus. Ann Neurol 18:482, 1985.

270. Arawaka S, Saito Y, Murayama S, Mori H: Lewy body in neurodegeneration with brain iron accumulation type 1 is immunoreactive for α-synuclein. Neurology 51:887–889, 1998.

271. Wakabayashi K, Yoshimura M, Fukushima T, et al: Widespread occurrence of α-synuclein/NACP-immunoreactive neuronal inclusions in juvenile and adult-onset Hallervorden-Spatz disease

with Lewy bodies. Neuropathol Appl Neurobiol 25:363–368, 1999.

272. Saito Y, Kawai M, Inoue K, et al: Widespread expression of α-synuclein and tau immunoreactivity in Hallervorden-Spatz syndrome with protracted clinical course. J Neurol Sci 177:48–59, 2000.

272a. Neumann M, Adler S, Schluter O, et al: α-Synuclein accumulation in a case of neurodegeneration with brain iron accumulation type 1 (NBIA-1, formerly Hallervorden-Spatz syndrome) with widespread cortical and brainstem-type Lewy bodies. Acta Neuropathol 100:568–574, 2000.

273. Krauss JK, Pohle T, Borreman JJ: Hemichorea and hemiballism associated with contralateral hemiparesis and ipsilateral basal ganglia lesions. Mov Disord 14:497–501, 1999.

274. Vitek JL, Chockkan V, Zhang J-Y, et al: Neuronal activity in the basal ganglia in patients with generalized dystonia and hemiballismus. Ann Neurol 46:22–33, 1999.

275. Fahn S, Bressman SB, Marsden CD: Classification of dystonia. Adv Neurol 78:1–10, 1998.

276. Augood SJ, Penney JB, Friberg IK, et al: Expression of the early-onset torsion dystonia gene (DYT1) in human brain. Ann Neurol 43:669–673, 1998.

277. Eidelberg D, Moeller JR, Ishikawa T, et al: The metabolic topography of idiopathic torsion dystonia. Brain 118:1473–1484, 1995.

278. Berardelli A, Rothwell JC, Hallett M, et al: The pathophysiology of primary dystonia. Brain 121:1195–1212, 1998.

279. Zweig RM, Hedreen JC: Brainstem pathology in cranial dystonia. Adv Neurol 49:395–407, 1988.

279a. Grotzsch H, Pizzolato GP, Ghika J, et al: Neuropathology of a case of dopa-responsive dystonia associated with a new genetic locus, DYT14. Neurology 58:1839–1842, 2002.

280. Factor SA, Barron KD: Mosaic pattern of gliosis in the neostriatum of a North American man with craniocervical dystonia and parkinsonism. Mov Disord 12:783–789, 1997.

281. Nygaard TG, Wilhelmsen KC, Risch NJ, et al: Linkage mapping of dopa-responsive dystonia (DRD) to chromosome 14q. Nat Genet 5:386–391, 1993.

282. Rajput AH, Gibb WRG, Zhong XH, et al: DOPA-responsive dystonia: Pathological and biochemical observations in a case. Ann Neurol 35:396–402, 1994.

283. Kramer PL, Mineta M, Klein C, et al: Rapid-onset dystonia-parkinsonism: Linkage to chromosome 19q13. Ann Neurol 46:176–182, 1999.

284. Waters CH, Faust PL, Powers J, et al: Neuropathology of Lubag (X-linked dystonia-parkinsonism). Mov Disord 8:387–390, 1993.

285. Gibb WRG, Kilford L, Marsden CD: Severe generalized dystonia with a mosaic pattern of striatal gliosis. Mov Disord 7:217–223, 1992.

286. Altrocchi PH, Forno LS: Spontaneous oro-facial dyskinesias: Neuropathology of a case. Neurology 33:802–805, 1983.

287. Nemeth AH, Mills KR, Elston JS, et al: Do the same genes predispose to Gilles de la Tourette syndrome and dystonia? Report of a new family and review of the literature. Mov Disord 14:826–831, 1999.

288. Robertson MM, Stern JS: Tic disorders: New developments in Tourette syndrome and related disorders. Curr Opin Neurol 11:373–380, 1998.

289. Eidelberg D, Moeller JR, Antonini A, et al: The metabolic anatomy of Tourette's syndrome. Neurology 48:927–934, 1997.

290. Peterson BS, Skudlarski P, Anderson AW, et al: A functional magnetic resonance imaging study of tic suppression in Tourette syndrome. Arch Gen Psychiatry 54:326–333, 1998.

291. Meyer P, Bohnen NI, Minshima S, et al: Striatal presynaptic monoaminergic vesicles are not increased in Tourette's syndrome. Neurology 53:371–374, 1999.

292. Carella F, Ciano C, Panzica F, et al: Myoclonus in cortico-basal degeneration. Mov Disord 12:598–603, 1997.

293. Thompson PD, Day BL, Rothwell JC, et al: The myoclonus in cortico-basal degeneration: Evidence for two forms of cortical reflex myoclonus. Brain 117:1197–1207, 1995.

294. Young CA, Mac KJ, Chadwick DW, et al: Opsoclonus-myoclonus syndrome: An autopsy study of three cases. Eur J Med 2:239–241, 1993.

CHAPTER **167**

Approach to Movement Disorders

ANNA DEPOLD HOHLER ■ ALI SAMII

In this chapter we provide an overview of movement disorders. We begin with a review of nomenclature used to describe movement disorders, followed by a discussion of the basal ganglia circuitry. Individual movement disorder syndromes are then addressed, as well as treatment options, including, when applicable, neurosurgical treatment.

TERMINOLOGY

The term *movement disorder* is used in two contexts: (1) as a physical sign of involuntary movement or abnormal movement, and (2) to describe a syndrome that causes involuntary movement.[1] Before discussing the different movement disorder syndromes, it is imperative to define the types of movement that exist to ensure a common language among practitioners.

Tremor is defined as a rhythmic oscillation of a body part by alternating or synchronous contraction of agonist and antagonist muscles.[2] It may be seen at rest or with action. It commonly affects the hands but may also involve the head, jaw, voice, tongue, or lower limbs. *Resting tremor* occurs while the limb is not active. The typical resting tremor is the finger and wrist tremor in Parkinson's disease, seen while the hand is resting on the patient's lap. *Action tremor* can be postural (seen during sustained posture, such as hands in the outstretched position), intention (seen during trajectory movement, such as finger-nose-finger), or task specific (seen while performing a specific activity, for example, only when writing).

Dystonia is an abnormal sustained muscle contraction causing twisting or turning around one or multiple joints. It may be present in a variety of locations, including the neck (cervical dystonia, or *torticollis*), eyelids (*blepharospasm*), or vocal cords (*spasmodic dysphonia*). Dystonia can be focal, segmental, or generalized.

An example of focal limb dystonia is writer's cramp. In segmental dystonia, an entire limb or trunk is involved. Generalized dystonia is multifocal, involving several body parts.

Myoclonus is defined as a sudden, brief, shocklike involuntary muscle contraction or inhibition. Positive myoclonus occurs with active muscle contraction, and negative myoclonus causes inhibition of the activated muscle. An example of negative myoclonus is asterixis (brief interruption of muscle contraction in the extended arm and wrist). Myoclonus is classified by the body part involved (focal or multifocal) and in relation to its cause (e.g., postanoxic) or site of origin (cortical or subcortical).[3] Some types of myoclonus are stimulus sensitive or action induced.

Chorea is derived from the Greek word meaning "dance." Chorea consists of complex involuntary movements resembling exaggerated fidgetiness. The movements are usually generalized, purposeless, and absent during sleep. *Choreoathetosis* is the term used when the movements are slow and writhing. In mild cases, the choreic movements can be blended into natural movements and appear more purposeful.

Ballismus is characterized by large-amplitude, proximal chorea. At times, it can be quite violent. The onset is often sudden and is typically related to an infarct in the contralateral subthalamic nucleus. It usually occurs on one side of the body, hence the term *hemiballismus*. Hemiballismus usually evolves into the less violent hemichorea over time.

Tics are temporarily suppressible movements seen in Tourette's syndrome. The frequency and severity of tics are exacerbated after voluntary suppression; this is a rebound effect. Tics can be motor or vocal in nature. Simple motor tics are isolated, brief, sudden movements involving one body part. Complex motor tics may involve more than one body part and may have a component of dystonia or tremor. Complex motor tics may take the form of purposeful movements. A complex motor tic that is an obscene gesture is termed *copropraxia*. A simple vocal tic may be a grunt or throat clearing. Complex vocal tics may be more elaborate vocalizations, words, or phrases. When the words include profanity, the term *coprolalia* is used.

Bradykinesia literally means slowness of movement. It is used to describe slow voluntary movements such as those seen in Parkinson's disease. The amplitude of fine movements is typically decreased. When there is a lack of movement, the term *akinesia* is used. *Akinesia* and *bradykinesia* are frequently used interchangeably.

Freezing is an arrest of gait and is usually associated with bradykinesia. It may occur during gait initiation, when approaching an obstacle, or when attempting to turn. Freezing is a specific gait phenomenon that is often seen with Parkinson's disease.

Dyskinesia means abnormal involuntary movement. It is frequently seen in patients with Parkinson's disease receiving dopaminergic therapy and usually takes the form of chorea or dystonia. *Tardive dyskinesia* refers to late-onset dyskinesia secondary to the long-term use of medications. Neuroleptic and antiemetic medications are the usual culprits in those with tardive dyskinesia.

Akathisia is defined as motor activity that is the result of a voluntary effort to relieve an uncomfortable sensation of inner restlessness. It is often manifested by an inability to remain seated, a shifting of weight, or pacing. Akathisia usually occurs following the administration of neuroleptic medications. It may occur shortly after exposure (acute akathisia) or as a late complication of treatment (tardive akathisia).[4]

Hyperekplexia is an exaggerated startle response to a sudden, unexpected stimulus. An individual may experience loss of postural control without loss of consciousness. It may be symptomatic or can be inherited as an autosomal-dominant condition. The latter has been defined as a mutation in the $\alpha 1$ subunit of the glycine receptor.[5]

BASAL GANGLIA ANATOMY AND CONNECTIONS

There has been a significant amount of research on the mechanisms by which movements, and hence movement disorders, occur. Here we briefly describe the current understanding of the function of the basal ganglia. It must be emphasized that the model of the basal ganglia circuitry presented here is simplistic (Fig. 167–1). Much work is needed to better elucidate the inconsistencies of this model.[6–8]

The basal ganglia are composed of the striatum (caudate nucleus and putamen), globus pallidus (internal and external), substantia nigra (pars compacta and pars reticularis), and subthalamic nucleus. The pedunculopontine nucleus is not traditionally included as part of the basal ganglia, though there are significant connections between them.

The corpus striatum is composed of the caudate, the putamen, and the globus pallidus. The striatum is made up of the putamen and the caudate nucleus. The lentiform nucleus is made up of the putamen and both segments of the globus pallidus.

The striatum, particularly the putamen, receives excitatory glutamatergic input from the primary and secondary sensorimotor cortices. Medium spiny neurons

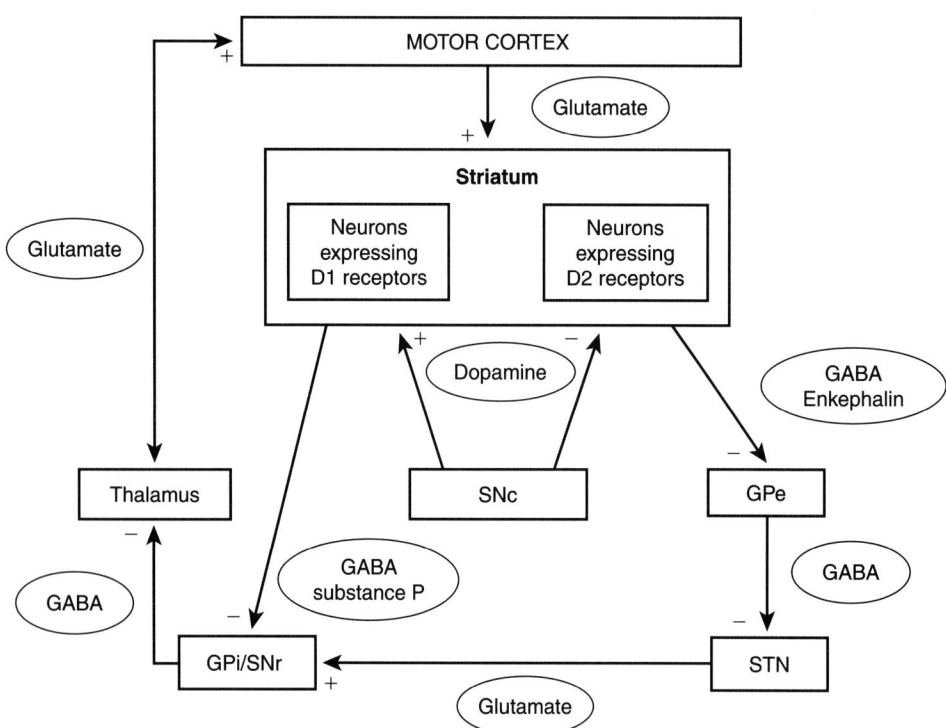

FIGURE 167–1. The basal ganglia circuitry.

(MSNs) make up 75% of the neurons in the striatum. Two major pathways, direct and indirect, arise from the MSNs. The population of MSNs rich in D_1 dopamine receptors form the direct pathway and project to the internal globus pallidus (GPi) and substantia nigra pars reticularis (SNr). These neurons coexpress γ-aminobutyric acid (GABA) and substance P. The population of MSNs rich in D_2 dopamine receptors form the indirect pathway and project to the external globus pallidus (GPe). These neurons coexpress GABA and enkephalin.

The GPi and SNr are the sensorimotor output nuclei of the basal ganglia. They have GABAergic projections to ventrolateral, ventral-anterior, and centromedian nuclei of the thalamus. GPi and SNr neurons have high spontaneous discharge rates (60 to 80 Hz)

The GPe is part of the indirect pathway. It receives input from the striatal MSNs that coexpress GABA and enkephalin. The GPe has GABAergic projections mainly to the subthalamic nucleus (STN) and receives glutamatergic feedback from it. It also has GABAergic projections directly to the GPi and SNr.

The STN is part of the indirect pathway. It receives inhibitory input from the GPe and excitatory input from cortex. It has glutamatergic excitatory projections to the GPi and SNr.

The substantia nigra pars compacta is the origin of the dopaminergic nigrostriatal pathway. Dopamine acts differently on the direct and indirect pathways. Activation of striatal MSNs that project to the GPi and SNr (direct pathway) is achieved by activation of D_1 receptors in the striatum. Suppression of striatal MSNs that project to the GPe (indirect pathway) occurs by activation of D_2 receptors in the striatum. The overall effect of dopamine release in the striatum is a reduction of GPi and SNr inhibition of thalamus, which leads to increased activity of excitatory thalamocortical projections. The pars compacta also sends projections to the STN, GPi, and SNr.

The pedunculopontine nucleus receives mostly inhibitory collaterals from the GPi and SNr as they project to the thalamus. It sends excitatory projections back to the GPi and SNr. The pedunculopontine nucleus also has connections to the STN, brainstem, and spinal cord.

The basal ganglia and their connections are responsible for the orderly control of normal movements. As disease processes develop, different components of these circuits are affected. With an understanding of these abnormal circuits, the neurosurgeon can better conceptualize the mechanism behind the surgical interventions now available for the treatment of certain movement disorders.

MOVEMENT DISORDER SYNDROMES

Essential Tremor

Essential tremor is the most common movement disorder.[9] The tremor is present during action and absent at rest. (It may be postural, trajectory, or occur while performing a task.) The pathophysiologic mechanism of tremor is not well understood. Mechanical, reflex

oscillators and central neuronal pacemakers or circuits (e.g., olivar-cerebellar-thalamic circuit) have all been implicated in various types of tremor.[2] Essential tremor has been correlated to cortical activity, particularly in the sensorimotor area.[10]

Essential tremor is more symmetrical than the tremor of Parkinson's disease, and rigidity and bradykinesia are not seen. The tremor often involves the upper extremities, head, and voice. Unlike Parkinson's disease, there is no significant response to anti-Parkinson medications.[11] A family history is positive in one half of patients. In patients with hereditary essential tremor, there is autosomal-dominant inheritance. Men and woman are affected equally. Head tremor is invariably mild, and 75% is of a "no-no" type. Relatives of patients with essential tremor are five times as likely to develop symptoms of the disorder.[12]

Medical therapy for essential tremor may start with either primidone or propranolol. The starting dose of primidone is 25 to 50 mg at bedtime, with gradually increasing doses up to 500 or 750 mg daily. Propranolol may be started at 10 mg daily and titrated as tolerated to 300 mg daily. Primidone and propranolol can be administered together. Phenobarbital, gabapentin, topiramate, and benzodiazepines may also help relieve symptoms.[13–15] Botulinum toxin may improve tremor severity, but it is usually limited to the treatment of dystonic tremor.[16]

There are a number of surgical options for the treatment of tremor. With isolated tremor, the target of either ablative surgery or deep brain stimulation (DBS) is the ventrointermediate nucleus of the thalamus. Unilateral thalamotomy improves contralateral tremor.[17] Bilateral thalamotomy is rarely performed because it can cause cognitive and gait disturbances.[18]

In contrast to ablative surgery, DBS is reversible and potentially adjustable. The goal of DBS is to render a target nonfunctional by stimulating it at high frequency. Unilateral thalamic DBS improves contralateral hand tremor. It is used mainly for essential tremor.[19, 20] Bilateral thalamic DBS can improve tremor in both hands and in the head. Side effects may include serious cognitive and gait disturbances. The stimulation-related adverse effects of bilateral thalamic DBS may be more reversible than the adverse effects of bilateral thalamotomies.

Parkinson's Disease

James Parkinson originally described Parkinson's disease (PD) as "shaking palsy" in 1817.[21] For 4 decades, very little was added to the original description.[22] In the 1860s, Charcot began to elucidate the clinical features of this entity.[23] The four cardinal features of PD are tremor, bradykinesia, rigidity, and postural instability.[24] *Parkinsonism* is a nonspecific term used to describe a constellation of signs on physical examination similar to those seen in PD. PD is defined as asymmetrical parkinsonism with no known cause, characterized by most of the four cardinal features and responsive to anti-Parkinson medications. The diagnostic criteria for

PD have become more rigorous with gradations of diagnostic certainty[25] (Table 167–1).

The mean age of onset is in the mid-50s.[26] Young-onset PD begins between 21 and 40 years, and juvenile-onset PD starts before age 20.[27] Individuals with young-onset PD constitute 5% to 10% of patients at referral centers.[28] PD is believed to become clinically manifest once a threshold of injury in the nigrostriatal pathway has occurred. Clinical signs of PD appear when 80% of striatal dopamine and 50% of nigral neurons are lost.[29]

The etiopathogenesis of PD is unknown, but it is probably a complex trait with a multifactorial cause.[30] Aging, environmental factors, and genetic predisposition all play a role in whether a person will develop PD.[31] Epidemiologic studies have linked PD to pesticides, well water drinking, rural living, and infectious agents.[32–34] For unclear reasons, there is an inverse relationship between cigarette smoking and the development of PD.[35] The only environmental agent that has been directly linked to the development of levodopa-responsive parkinsonism indistinguishable from PD is 1-methyl-4-phenyl-1,2,3,6-tetrahydropyridine (MPTP).[36] MPTP was a contaminant analog of meperidine that caused parkinsonism in a small number of illicit narcotic drug users. MPTP has been used to develop a primate model of PD.[37]

A family history of PD in a first-degree relative exists in approximately 15% of patients.[38, 39] A positive family history does not necessarily imply a genetic predisposition, however, because it could be explained by common environmental exposure.[40] Genetic abnormalities have been identified in the alpha-synuclein gene[41] and the parkin gene.[42] The former is seen in a few families worldwide, and the latter is seen in some cases of young- and juvenile-onset PD.[43] Mutations in these genes are present in only an extremely small number of PD patients. A large twin study points away from genetic influences in patients with disease onset after age 50.[44] Genomic screening suggests involvement of multiple susceptibility genes,[45] supporting the idea that the pathogenesis of PD involves interactions between genetic predisposition and environmental exposure.

TABLE 167–1 ■ Diagnostic Criteria for Parkinson's Disease

Clinically Possible PD

Any one of the following: resting tremor, rigidity, or bradykinesia

Clinically Probable PD

Any two of the four cardinal signs*
Alternatively, any one of the following: asymmetrical resting tremor, asymmetrical rigidity, or asymmetrical bradykinesia

Clinically Definite PD

Any combination of three of the cardinal signs*
Alternatively, two cardinal signs* with asymmetry and response to antiparkinsonian medications

* The four cardinal signs are tremor, bradykinesia, rigidity, and postural instability.
PD, Parkinson's disease.

Tremor is the first symptom in 70% of PD patients.[46] The mechanisms underlying Parkinson's tremor are not well understood.[47] The tremor may result from dopamine loss unmasking pacemaker properties in the basal ganglia. The tremor is 3 to 5 Hz, with varying amplitude; it has been described as "pill rolling" and is seen at rest. Initially, it is distal more than proximal and may be intermittent. It is almost always asymmetrical. It worsens with anxiety, contralateral motor tasks, and during ambulation.

Bradykinesia and rigidity are believed to be due to the overactivity of the GPi and SNr. This leads to excessive inhibition of the thalamus. The same symptoms may occur with overactivity of the STN. There is reduced activation of cortical areas by excitatory thalamocortical projections. In PD, there is a loss of dopaminergic input to the striatum. This leads to increased activation of the indirect pathway and decreased activation of the direct pathway. Bradykinesia is usually proportional to rigidity in a given limb. Limb bradykinesia may be tested by finger tapping, alternating forearm movements, foot tapping, and opening and closing fists, as outlined in the Unified Parkinson Disease Rating Scale.[48] Timed motor tasks such as the Purdue pegboard test may also be used. Bradykinesia has the best correlation with disease severity. This has been evaluated by functional imaging (positron emission tomography or single photon emission computed tomography) of the nigrostriatal pathway.[49, 50] Rigidity is defined as an increased resistance to passive movement of joints. It may have a "lead pipe" or "cogwheel" quality, and it is also asymmetrical.

Postural instability and gait abnormalities are the least specific cardinal features of PD. There is often loss of arm swing on one or both sides, neck and trunk flexion, and shortened stride length. Gait is described as shuffling, and there is an inability to turn quickly. Freezing may be seen in more advanced disease. Patients have an impaired ability to recover when pulled from behind.

Exclusion criteria for PD include exposure to drugs known to cause parkinsonism such as neuroleptics and some antiemetic medications. Cerebellar deficits, corticospinal tract signs, and oculomotor deficits other than slight limitation of upward gaze are also exclusion criteria. Finally, autonomic impairment independent of anti-Parkinson medications, early moderate to severe postural instability, and early dementia also suggest an alternative diagnosis.[25, 51]

MEDICAL THERAPY

Medical therapy for PD is extensive.[52] The first medication shown to be effective in the treatment of PD was levodopa. It has been used as a mainstay of medical therapy ever since its development in the 1960s.[53] Levodopa is combined with carbidopa or benserazide in formulation to prevent peripheral conversion to dopamine by dopa-decarboxylase. Patients may have mild nausea and vomiting with treatment. Side effects are reduced by starting at a low dose and titrating to a goal of four times a day over a period of days to weeks. Lightheadedness and vivid dreams are also early reported side effects. Although motor symptoms may improve dramatically on this therapy, the underlying degeneration of dopamine-containing neurons is not arrested.

Late complications of levodopa therapy are motor fluctuations and dyskinesias. The motor fluctuations result in distinct "on" and "off" periods, representing times when the patient is responding or not responding to the medication. After patients have been on levodopa therapy for 4 to 6 years, 40% of them experience motor fluctuations. The same percentage is afflicted with dyskinesias.[54, 55]

In an attempt to slow the progression of PD, a variety of medications have been tested, including vitamin E and selegiline (a monoamine oxidase-B inhibitor). Vitamin E was not found to be beneficial in a large multicenter trial of patients with early PD.[56] After multiple studies, it is still unclear whether selegiline has a neuroprotective effect. The efficacy of selegiline in delaying the initiation of levodopa is likely due to symptomatic relief of motor symptoms rather than neuroprotection.[57, 58]

Dopamine agonists have also been used in the treatment of PD. The agonists available in the United States include bromocriptine, pergolide, pramipexole, and ropinirole. Patients taking dopamine agonists have fewer dyskinesias than their counterparts on levodopa.[59, 60] When using dopamine agonist therapy instead of levodopa, PD symptoms are less effectively treated, and there is an increased risk of developing somnolence, hallucinations, and edema. Most patients on dopamine agonist monotherapy require the addition of levodopa after approximately 3 to 5 years of therapy.[59, 60]

Patients with onset of PD before 40 years of age are at greater risk of developing motor fluctuations and dyskinesias. As many as 90% of such patients may have these complications.[61] There has been considerable debate about whether these patients should be initiated on dopamine agonist monotherapy versus low-dose combination therapy. Recent studies suggest that dopamine agonist monotherapy is associated with a slower rate of nigrostriatal neuronal loss compared with levodopa monotherapy.[62]

With prolonged levodopa use, motor fluctuations invariably occur, including end-of-dose wearing off. If this occurs, the physician must ensure that the patient is not taking the medication in conjunction with a high-protein meal, which can decrease absorption and limit the medication's ability to cross the blood-brain barrier.[63] There are a variety of techniques for decreasing "off" periods. For a patient on levodopa monotherapy, the overall daily intake of levodopa may be increased by increasing the individual doses or by adding additional doses. Alternatively, a dopamine agonist may be added. Entacapone, a catechol-O-methyltransferase (COMT) inhibitor, may relieve end-of-dose wearing off because it enhances the duration of action of levodopa. Inhibition of COMT results in a prolonged half-life of circulating levodopa. Tolcapone, another COMT inhibi-

tor, has been shown to cause fatal liver failure and is rarely used.[64] COMT inhibitors can exacerbate all levodopa-induced adverse effects; therefore, the levodopa dose may need to be reduced. In addition, diarrhea is a common side effect of COMT inhibitors.

Dyskinesias can be treated by adding a dopamine agonist and reducing the dose of levodopa. COMT inhibitors do not provide relief of dyskinesias and may actually exacerbate them. Other agents such as amantadine may help reduce dyskinesias.[65] Surgical therapy has also been advocated in patients with severe dyskinesias.

SURGICAL OPTIONS

There are several surgical options for the treatment of PD. Ablative surgical procedures or DBS targeting the thalamus, globus pallidus, or STN are currently available. Transplantation surgery for PD remains investigational. Thalamotomy is typically reserved for patients with isolated tremor, because this procedure has less impact on the rigidity and dyskinesias seen with PD.[18]

Pallidotomy and subthalamotomy decrease the tremor, rigidity, and dyskinesias seen with PD. The target for pallidotomy is the posteroventrolateral portion of the globus pallidus. Unilateral pallidotomy improves mainly contralateral tremor and dyskinesia.[66] These results were sustained in 4-year follow-up studies.[67, 68] These results are seen only in patients who are levodopa responders, however. As with all surgical interventions, there are risks. Surgical side effects include hemorrhage, infarct, aphonia, and cognitive and gait disturbances. Because side effects are greater for bilateral pallidotomies, they are not typically recommended.[69–71]

Subthalamotomy improves most of the contralateral motor symptoms of PD. Bilateral subthalamotomy also helps reduce the need for anti-Parkinson medications. Rare but significant side effects of this surgery are irreversible ballismus and chorea. This procedure is not done in the United States because of these potentially dangerous side effects.

DBS has several advantages over ablative surgery. It causes less brain trauma, is reversible, and can be modified in terms of which of the four stimulation sites is active. Adjustments to the intensity, duration, and frequency of the stimulation can be made, and the procedure can be performed bilaterally. Side effects of the surgical procedure include brain hemorrhage, infarct, seizures, and death. Disadvantages of DBS include the hours required to adjust the settings, lead damage or failure, the need to replace batteries after 3 to 5 years, the potential for infection, and erosion of the device through the skin. Worsening dyskinesia (in cases of STN stimulation), paresthesias, and subtle cognitive and mood changes have also been reported. Some of these side effects may be reversible by adjusting stimulation parameters, but hardware failure requires removal or replacement of parts or of the entire device.

Thalamic DBS, much like thalamotomy, is effective in reducing contralateral PD tremor.[72] As with thalamotomy, the dyskinesias seen with late-stage PD are not significantly improved. For this reason, PD patients are now typically recommended for globus pallidus or subthalamic surgical intervention. Unilateral thalamic DBS can also be performed on a patient who has already had a contralateral thalamotomy.

Similar to ablative surgery, the target for pallidal DBS is the GPi. However, the surgery is done bilaterally, which is an advantage over pallidotomy. With DBS, there are fewer adverse effects than with bilateral pallidotomies. Bilateral GPi stimulation improves tremor, rigidity, and dyskinesia. The benefit in terms of tremor and bradykinesia is seen in the levodopa "off" state. There has been a trend toward improvement in the levodopa "on" state as well, mostly with a reduction in dyskinesia.[73, 74] Bilateral GPi stimulation usually does not allow a reduction in the overall dosages of anti-Parkinson medications. Unilateral pallidal DBS has been performed after contralateral pallidotomy in a few PD patients, with positive results.[75]

DBS of the STN is usually performed bilaterally and has shown a 40% to 60% improvement in levodopa "off" states.[76–80] Another advantage is that anti-Parkinson medications can often be reduced after the procedure. Some patients are even able to discontinue levodopa altogether.[76, 80] The effects of the procedure appear to be present at 2-year follow-up assessment. Most of the motor symptoms of PD are improved by bilateral STN stimulation. Levodopa nonresponders do not appear to respond to this procedure. Reported side effects include cognitive, speech, and language deficits; eyelid opening apraxia; confusion; and hallucinations. Bilateral STN stimulation may be superior to bilateral GPi stimulation in PD patients,[81] but the debate about the optimal stimulation target continues. A large, randomized, multicenter study comparing bilateral STN and bilateral GPi stimulation is currently under way.

Various combinations of different stereotactic neurosurgical procedures for advanced PD have been reported. Merello reported on the lack of efficacy of unilateral STN stimulation contralateral to a previous pallidotomy.[82] Moro and coworkers reported a patient who benefited from bilateral STN stimulation after unilateral pallidotomy and unilateral thalamotomy.[83] Houeto and colleagues reported on two patients in whom bilateral GPi stimulation failed to provide long-term improvement.[84] The GPi electrodes were then removed, and bilateral STN electrodes were implanted; the subsequent improvement was superior to that achieved with bilateral GPi stimulation. Several patients have undergone bilateral STN stimulation after unilateral pallidotomy.[85] One patient underwent bilateral STN stimulation after bilateral pallidotomies, with no added benefit from DBS.[86] In summary, the efficacy of DBS after ablative surgery must be studied further.

Appropriate patient selection is extremely important for achieving a positive outcome from stereotactic surgery. Strict inclusion and exclusion criteria must be used. A recent large multicenter study used specific criteria that included "a good response to levodopa."[87] Table 167–2 summarizes basic guidelines for inclusion

TABLE 167–2 ■ Inclusion and Exclusion Criteria for Patient Selection for Stereotactic Surgery in Parkinson's Disease

Inclusion Criteria

Clinically definite Parkinson's disease (see Table 167–1 for diagnostic criteria)

Hoehn and Yahr stage 2–4 (patient should be independently ambulatory)

Levodopa responsive with clearly defined "on" periods (i.e., symptoms improve at least partially with levodopa administration)

Persistent disabling symptoms (e.g., dyskinesias, motor fluctuations, disabling "off" periods several hours per day) despite optimal medication therapy

Age 20–80 yr

Exclusion Criteria

"Parkinson's plus" syndromes, atypical parkinsonism, or secondary parkinsonism (e.g., progressive supranuclear palsy, striatonigral degeneration, multiple system atrophy, vascular parkinsonism, drug-induced parkinsonism)

Medical contraindications to surgery or stimulation (e.g., serious comorbid medical conditions, chronic anticoagulation, pregnancy)

Contraindication to magnetic resonance imaging (e.g., indwelling metal fragments or implants)

Dementia or other active neuropsychiatric dysfunction (e.g., untreated depression, psychosis)

Intracranial abnormalities that contraindicate surgery (e.g., stroke, tumor, vascular abnormality affecting the target area)

---

and exclusion criteria. Each patient must be considered individually.

The goal of transplantation is to replace neuronal tissue lost to the neurodegenerative process of PD. Initial trials involved transplantation of the adrenal medulla.[88] The initial positive results were short-lived,[89] and this procedure was abandoned. Dopaminergic transplantation, in the form of fetal mesencephalic tissue, has also been used. It is thought that neurotropic factors secreted by the implanted cells may contribute to the benefits seen with transplantation.[90] Moderate or marked improvement was reported in these patients, though none had resolution of PD symptoms. Few patients were able to discontinue levodopa therapy.[91–93] Graft survival is evident on positron emission tomography scanning and on autopsy.[91–95] A side effect of the transplant seen in 15% of patients is severe and disabling dyskinesias.[96] In a randomized, sham surgery–controlled study, there was some improvement in the medication-off state in younger patients, but disabling dyskinesia was again problematic.[97] Additional research is ongoing. Stem cell transplantation is currently an area of great interest. It is hoped that eventually cells from a patient can be dedifferentiated into stem cells and then redifferentiated into dopamine-producing cells to be implanted in PD patients.

DIFFERENTIAL DIAGNOSIS

The differential diagnosis of PD includes normal aging, essential tremor, drug-induced parkinsonism, vascular parkinsonism, progressive supranuclear palsy, corticobasal degeneration, multiple system atrophy, and diffuse Lewy body disease.[98] Less common entities with parkinsonism include dopa-responsive dystonia, normal-pressure hydrocephalus, prion diseases, pallidopontonigral degeneration, disinhibition-dementia-parkinsonism-amyotrophy complex, and neuromanganism.

Normal Aging. It is difficult to define normal aging of the nervous system.[99, 100] Slowness of movement, stooped posture, and gait instability are not uncommon in the elderly population. Pathologically, aging is associated with loss of pigmented neurons in the substantia nigra,[101] and functional imaging has shown an age-related attrition of striatal dopamine.[102] If signs of PD are present in an elderly patient, a trial of levodopa therapy should help determine medication responsiveness and hence establish the diagnosis.

Drug-Induced Parkinsonism. Drug-induced parkinsonism is often seen after exposure to neuroleptics.[103] Antiemetics, pro-motility agents, reserpine, and tetrabenazine can also cause parkinsonism. The symptoms are symmetrical, and there is resolution of parkinsonian symptoms when the offending medications are discontinued. It may take months for complete resolution.

Vascular Parkinsonism. Vascular parkinsonism is often due to multiple infarcts in the basal ganglia or their connecting fibers.[104] Symptoms are more prominent in the legs. Typically, there is absence of tremor. Brain imaging reveals extensive small vessel disease. Dementia and pseudobulbar and pyramidal signs are seen. There is a lack of significant therapeutic response to dopaminergic therapy.

Progressive Supranuclear Palsy. Progressive supranuclear palsy is characterized by parkinsonism with progressive gaze disturbance.[105] There is a symmetrical onset, early postural instability, severe axial rigidity, and absence of tremor. Supranuclear gaze palsy, especially of down-gaze, is characteristic. Blepharospasm, eyelid opening apraxia, early dementia, and lack of significant therapeutic response to dopaminergic therapy are also seen. Trazodone may help with sleep disturbance, and botulinum toxin injections may be used for blepharospasm. Gaze paresis may be helped with prisms.

Corticobasal Degeneration. Corticobasal degeneration manifests with asymmetrical parkinsonism and cortical signs.[106–110] The patient exhibits marked asymmetry, tremor, limb dystonia, limb apraxia, and corticospinal tract signs. Cortical myoclonus, early oculomotor and eyelid abnormalities, and cortical sensory signs are often seen. The alien limb phenomenon and lack of response to dopaminergic medications help confirm the diagnosis. In the alien limb, the sensory systems are impaired. The patient describes the limb as not belonging to him or her.[111] This sensation is combined with involuntary movements of the limb. For example, the limb may pick at buttons, grasp objects, or even choke the patient. The tremor and myoclonus of corticobasal degeneration can be partially controlled with clonazepam. Baclofen may help reduce rigidity. Botulinum toxin injections may help reduce the pain from dystonia, but they do not improve mobility.

Multiple System Atrophy. Multiple system atrophy (MSA) is divided into three clinically distinct categories.[112, 113] MSA-A, or Shy-Drager syndrome, is characterized by an autonomic predominance with parkinsonism. MSA-P, or striatonigral degeneration, has a parkinsonian predominance. MSA-C, or olivopontocerebellar atrophy, has cerebellar signs with parkinsonism. MSA-A manifests with orthostatic hypotension, urinary incontinence, bowel dysfunction, and impairment of temperature regulation and sweating. Symptoms are more symmetrical than in PD, and severe hypotension occurs with treatment with anti-Parkinson medications. MSA-P most resembles PD. However, it is more symmetrical, with early and pronounced postural instability, dysarthria, and dysphonia. There is no resting tremor, and progression of symptoms is more rapid than in PD. Corticospinal tract signs and respiratory stridor are also seen. There is a poor response to anti-Parkinson medications. MSA-C shows progressive cerebellar ataxia and parkinsonism. Sustained nystagmus, ocular dysmetria, oculomotor instability, and impaired smooth pursuits are noted. In addition, gait and limb ataxia, early dysarthria and dysphagia, corticospinal tract signs, peripheral neuropathy, and retinal degeneration occur.

Diffuse Lewy Body Disease. This disease is characterized by progressive parkinsonism and dementia.[114] There is minimal or no resting tremor. Early cognitive dysfunction, psychiatric features, and depression are noted. Hallucinations, paranoid delusions, rapid eye movement sleep disorders, and psychotic symptoms may be present before the administration of anti-Parkinson medication and are exacerbated by even small doses of these medications. These patients typically have dramatic fluctuations in their symptoms from hour to hour or day to day. Cognitive function may improve with central cholinesterase inhibitors.[115]

OTHER MOVEMENT DISORDERS

Wilson's Disease

Wilson's disease is an autosomal-recessive disorder of copper metabolism resulting from the absence or dysfunction of a copper-transporting P-type adenosine triphosphatase encoded on chromosome 13.[116] The term *hepatolenticular degeneration* is also used, because the disease affects the liver and causes movement disorders related to changes in the basal ganglia. The primary problem is a defect in copper metabolism, causing its buildup in the liver, brain, and eye. Numerous cognitive, psychiatric, and movement disorders may be seen with this disease. The neurological manifestations include tremor (typically a proximal or "wing beating" tremor), dystonia, dysmetria, dysrhythmia, ataxia, and dysarthria.[117] Testing for Wilson's disease involves assessment of liver function, ceruloplasmin, and serum and urine copper. Liver function abnormalities in the face of low ceruloplasmin and high urinary copper levels should prompt a diagnosis. Slit-lamp examination may reveal Kayser-Fleischer rings, and magnetic resonance imaging (MRI) often shows abnormal T2 signal in the basal ganglia.

It is important to recognize this syndrome, because treatment is available. The typical patient presents in early or middle adulthood with hepatic, psychiatric, or neurological symptoms. The psychiatric and neurological symptoms may rarely precede the diagnosis of hepatic dysfunction. Medical therapies include reducing copper in the diet and treating with zinc, penicillamine, or trientine.[118, 119] Liver transplantation also provides symptomatic benefit. Thalamotomy has been used in these patients, but because of the progressive nature of the disease and the availability of medical options, it is rarely performed.[120]

Huntington's Disease

Huntington's disease (HD) is an autosomal-dominant inherited disorder localized to the short arm of chromosome 4. It is characterized by a CAG trinucleotide repeat. Children of affected individuals who also express the gene show *anticipation*, which is an expansion of the trinucleotide repeat resulting in an earlier onset and more severe symptoms. HD typically manifests in the third to fourth decade and is characterized by movement disorders and cognitive decline.[121] Depression and high rates of suicide are also noted. The movement disorders can be varied, although most patients manifest with chorea.[122]

The chorea seen in HD is thought to result from the loss of striatal projection neurons to the GPe. In early stages of the disease, there is reduced inhibition of the GPe and increased inhibition of the STN, as well as reduced inhibitory output from the GPi and SNr to the thalamus. In more advanced stages, striatal projections to the GPi also degenerate, causing reduced chorea and development of bradykinesia.

Juvenile-onset HD presents by age 20 years and is characterized by an akinetic-rigid state. More rapid progression is seen, and seizures are more prominent in juvenile HD.[123, 124] Diagnosis is based on clinical presentation and imaging studies and confirmed by genetic testing. Imaging studies reveal atrophy of the caudate and putamen.

Medical treatment of the chorea includes dopamine antagonist therapy with haloperidol, phenothiazines, or atypical neuroleptics such as olanzapine. Benzodiazepines may also be helpful in suppressing the choreiform movements when they become disabling. Tetrabenazine is also used to suppress chorea. Unfortunately, none of these treatments is very effective.

Pallidotomy has been attempted in HD patients with dystonia.[125] Although there was some symptomatic improvement, the background of dementia and the underlying progression of the disease make this a short-term solution. Surgical treatment with neural transplantation has been studied in a small number of patients.[126] Motor and cognitive functions were im-

proved in three of five patients who underwent bilateral fetal neuroblast transplantation in the striatum. Further work is needed in this area.

Other Disorders Causing Chorea

Chorea can be seen with a variety of movement disorders in addition to HD. Neuroacanthocytosis; benign hereditary chorea; and infectious, autoimmune-mediated, drug-induced, metabolic, and vascular causes have been described.

Neuroacanthocytosis is a disorder of red blood cell morphology that is autosomal recessive and linked to chromosome 9.[127] It manifests in early adulthood with a variety of movement disorders, including chorea, tics, and dystonia. A kinetic-rigid variant has also been described.[128] Reflexes are almost always diminished or absent, suggesting peripheral involvement. Electromyography reveals axonal neuropathy and amyotrophy. Imaging studies often reveal caudate atrophy. Treatment of the movement component involves the use of neuroleptic medications. This is a progressive disorder, with death occurring approximately 9 years after the onset of symptoms.

Benign hereditary chorea typically presents in girls younger than 5 years. The chorea is independent of dementia, and the symptoms do not progress. Genetic investigation in these cases has not revealed a trinucleotide expansion.[129, 130]

Sydenham's chorea is the most common postinfectious chorea described.[131] It is seen after infection with group A β-hemolytic streptococci in 20% to 30% of cases. The chorea is commonly generalized, although hemichorea may be seen. The chorea usually remits in days to weeks; however, it may recur in 20% of patients. Young girls are affected most frequently, and treatment consists of anticonvulsants or neuroleptics. Sydenham's chorea may recur during pregnancy (chorea gravidarum).[132] Again, treatment is with neuroleptic agents or tetrabenazine; however, because of the self-limited nature of the disease, treatment is not warranted in all individuals.

Systemic lupus erythematosus is associated with chorea in 1% of cases.[133] Chorea may precede the diagnosis of lupus in some cases. It is important to assess for lupus as an underlying diagnosis, because steroid therapy often improves symptoms. Dopamine antagonists can also improve the choreic symptoms. Chorea is also associated with the antiphospholipid antibody syndrome.[134]

A variety of medications have been shown to produce chorea. Levodopa, anticonvulsants, stimulants, and antidepressants have all been implicated.[135, 136] Oral contraceptive agents have also been associated with chorea, typically in patients with a history of Sydenham's chorea. Symptoms often develop within weeks of exposure to these medications. Once the medication has been stopped, symptoms resolve over several weeks to months.

Hyperthyroidism, electrolyte derangements, and central pontine myelinolysis have all been associated with chorea.[137–139] Hyperthyroidism may be associated with chorea in up 2% of cases.[139] The chorea is usually generalized and persistent; rarely, a paroxysmal chorea has been described. The striatal dopamine receptors are thought to have enhanced sensitivity. Correction of the thyroid imbalance leads to resolution of the chorea.

Vascular causes of chorea have been reported.[140] Chorea can result from lesions to the midbrain as well as the basal ganglia. Hemiballismus, a severe form of chorea, results from a lesion in the contralateral STN.[141] With hemiballismus, there is interruption of the indirect pathway and unopposed activity of the direct pathway. There is loss of the excitatory drive from the STN to the GPi and SNr, along with reduced inhibitory output from the GPi and SNr to the thalamus. Treatment includes dopamine antagonist therapy and benzodiazepines.

Dystonia

Dystonia is a symptom of a variety of disorders. Dystonic contractions are often aggravated by purposeful actions, may be task specific, and are often worsened by stress. Dystonia can be classified according to age of onset, distribution, or cause. With the recent discovery of certain genes linked to types of dystonia, the classification is occasionally based on genetics.[142, 143] Here we focus on the cause-based classification, which divides dystonia into primary, dystonia plus, secondary, and heredodegenerative.[144]

In primary dystonia, dystonia is the most pronounced symptom, and no underlying injury or disease can be identified. The sporadic and many of the genetic dystonias fall into this category. In dystonia plus, patients have other symptoms such as tremor, myoclonus, or parkinsonism associated with the dystonia. The disorders of dopamine synthesis are in this category, but not the neurodegenerative diseases. Secondary dystonia includes dystonia caused by a wide variety of insults to the central nervous system, including stroke and trauma to the brain, neck,[145] or limbs. In heredodegenerative dystonia, the dystonia occurs in conjunction with a progressive neurological disorder such as PD, MSA, Wilson's disease, or mitochondrial disorders.

Primary dystonia can be further divided into sporadic and genetic types. The sporadic primary type is the most common form of dystonia and includes the common focal dystonias.[146] Torticollis, blepharospasm, isolated hand and foot dystonias, and task-specific dystonias fall into this category. This is a diagnosis of exclusion. There are numerous genetically localized dystonia syndromes that are subclassified into dystonia-torsion (DYT) categories. The most common cause of early-onset generalized dystonia is DYT1 dystonia, localized to chromosome 9.[147–151] The pattern of inheritance is autosomal dominant with reduced penetrance. The average age of onset is 12 years. The dystonia generally begins in one limb and then generalizes. DYT7, or adult-onset focal dystonia, is another well-described genetic dystonia. It is localized to chromosome 18 and is also an autosomal-dominant form.[152, 153]

The average age of symptom onset is 43 years. Symptoms have been focal or multifocal in all cases.

Dystonia plus can be divided into dopa-responsive dystonia, dystonia-parkinsonism, myoclonus-dystonia, and paroxysmal dystonia. Dopa-responsive dystonia, labeled DYT5, is characterized clinically as childhood-onset dystonia with a dramatic and sustained response to relatively low doses of levodopa. Dystonia is often the presenting feature, but patients then progress to parkinsonian features.[154, 155] An autosomal-dominant form is localized to chromosome 14, and an autosomal-recessive subtype is localized to chromosome 11. The dystonia may become worse during the day and improve after napping.[156] A dystonia-parkinsonism syndrome is seen in patients with a tyrosine hydroxylase defect.[157–159] Treatment with levodopa bypasses the defect and results in symptomatic benefit.

DYT11 is a myoclonus-dystonia syndrome with onset in childhood or adolescence.[160] In most cases, there is an autosomal-dominant pattern of inheritance, and some patients have been linked to an abnormality on chromosome 7.[161] The symptoms are not progressive and respond well to small doses of alcohol.[162]

In paroxysmal kinesigenic (triggered by voluntary movement) and nonkinesigenic dystonia syndromes, the neurological examination is normal between events. Epilepsy must be excluded in these patients. Paroxysmal nonkinesigenic dystonia (DYT8) has been linked to chromosome 2.[163–165] The inheritance is autosomal dominant with variable penetrance, and the onset is in childhood or adolescence. The dystonia lasts from 2 minutes to 4 hours, and the frequency varies from daily to only a few times a year. In DYT9, the dystonia is associated with episodic ataxia, dysarthria, paresthesias, and double vision. Several patients also displayed spastic paraplegia during and between attacks. The gene for this disorder has been mapped to chromosome 1.[166]

Secondary dystonia can be related to a number of cerebral or peripheral insults. In evaluating a patient with dystonia, it is important to identify any possible underlying abnormalities, particularly ones that may be treatable. Secondary dystonias are related to perinatal cerebral injuries, congenital malformations, central and peripheral nervous system insults or injuries, infections, inflammatory processes, paraneoplastic syndromes, drug or toxin exposures, and metabolic disorders. Tardive dystonia results from exposure to neuroleptics. It can best be avoided by using low doses and slowly increasing these medications as needed.

There are a number of treatments available for dystonia. Patients with a primary dystonia or a dystonia-parkinsonism syndrome should have a trial of levodopa. These dystonias are typically generalized and often present in childhood. Pharmacologic interventions for generalized dystonia include discontinuation of the offending agent (e.g., neuroleptic) and the use of anticholinergic agents, benzodiazepines, muscle relaxants, anticonvulsants, and clozapine.[167–171] Other medical options for the treatment of severe generalized dystonia include intrathecal baclofen[172] and tetrabenazine.[173] Pallidotomy is superior to thalamotomy in relieving dystonia.[174] Now, bilateral pallidal DBS is being performed for severe cases of generalized dystonia, especially those associated with the *DYT1* gene abnormality.[175]

Focal dystonias can be treated with the same medications used in generalized dystonia. However, botulinum toxin injections are the first line of therapy for focal dystonias, allowing for specifically localized treatment.[176–178] The primary effect of botulinum is to reduce muscle contractions of the injected skeletal muscles by blocking neuromuscular signal transmission. Electromyography is useful to localize the specific muscles that are contracting. Side effects of the injections include local bruising or infection, muscle atrophy, and dysphagia or ptosis (if the injection leaches to adjacent areas). Antibodies to botulinum toxin may develop, but if this occurs, it is usually a late consequence of the treatment. It can be avoided by giving injections only once every 3 or 4 months. With the newer formulation of botulinum toxin, antibody formation to the toxin and subsequent lack of efficacy are rare.

Myoclonus

Myoclonus can be classified according to its site of origin. It is also useful to subdivide myoclonus according to its cause.[179] Physiologic myoclonus occurs in normal subjects and includes sleep jerks and anxiety- or exercise-induced myoclonus. Essential myoclonus has no known cause, and there are no other gross neurological deficits; there is a hereditary form[180] and a sporadic form. In epileptic myoclonus, seizures dominate, and initially there is no encephalopathy. The myoclonus can be related to fragments of epilepsy,[181] or it can manifest as childhood myoclonic epilepsy[182] or benign familial myoclonic epilepsy.[183] Finally, in symptomatic myoclonus, a progressive or static encephalopathy dominates. Symptomatic forms of myoclonus may have vascular, infectious, traumatic, autoimmune-related, metabolic, toxin-related, or paraneoplastic causes, as well as being a component of hereditary mitochondrial and storage diseases.[184]

Cortical, subcortical, and spinal (including propriospinal) types of myoclonus have been described. In cortical myoclonus, the abnormal activity originates in the sensorimotor cortex and is transmitted down the spinal cord via the pyramidal tract.[185] Cortical myoclonus is thus a fragment of epilepsy.

Treatment of myoclonus is based on reversing the underlying pathology, as appropriate, and on localizing the myoclonus. If the myoclonus is related to an epileptic syndrome, anticonvulsant therapy is used. Valproic acid, clonazepam, and primidone are often used in combination. The use of several anticonvulsants acting on different sites has also been advocated.[186] Piracetam[187] and levetiracetam[188] suppress myoclonus as well. Negative myoclonus (asterixis) does not appear to respond to medical therapy. Stereotactic thalamotomy has been used in the past to treat myoclonus,[189] and more recently, thalamic stimulation has been successful in treating hereditary myoclonus.[190] Neurosurgical treatment of myoclonus has not been well studied.

AUTOSOMAL-RECESSIVE ATAXIAS

Friedreich's Ataxia

Friedreich's ataxia is the most common genetic ataxia. It affects males and females equally. The disorder is due to a GAA trinucleotide repeat and is localized to chromosome 9.[191] Criteria for classification include onset before age 10 years, gait ataxia, dysarthria, dorsal column signs, weakness, and lack of deep tendon reflexes. Hearing loss, visual loss, and sphincter dysfunction occur late and are not universal. There is an atypical form of Friedreich's ataxia with retained deep tendon reflexes and a later onset. Imaging studies reveal spinal cord atrophy with relative preservation of the cerebellum. More than half of patients die of cardiac causes. Genetic testing is available for Friedreich's ataxia.

Ataxia-Telangiectasia

Ataxia-telangiectasia is a disease that begins with postural instability and ataxia within 12 to 14 months of birth.[192] Later, the ataxia is associated with hypotonia, bradykinesia, choreoathetosis, areflexia, and proprioceptive deficits. The disorder is localized to chromosome 11. Patients have an inability to initiate saccades. Telangiectasias develop between 3 and 6 years of age and spread in a symmetrical fashion. Patients are often chair-bound by the second decade, and death occurs in the fourth to fifth decade due to pulmonary infection or malignancy. Alpha fetoprotein levels are elevated in these patients. Nerve conduction studies show abnormal sensory nerve action potentials, and MRI shows atrophy of the cerebellum.

Ataxia with Selective Vitamin E Deficiency

Ataxia with vitamin E deficiency is due to a mutation in the gene coding for alpha-tocopherol transfer protein, located on the long arm of chromosome 8.[193, 194] It is characterized by the onset in childhood of ataxia, dysarthria, areflexia, proprioceptive deficits, extensor plantar responses, and skeletal deformities. It is important to screen for this disorder, because early treatment with vitamin E may slow or reverse symptoms.

Ataxia with Oculomotor Apraxia

Ataxia with oculomotor apraxia is an autosomal-recessive disorder consisting of ataxia, oculomotor apraxia, choreoathetosis, and mild mental retardation.[195] The disease is linked to chromosome 9.[196] Late in the disease, some individuals develop hypoalbuminemia and hypercholesterolemia.[197]

AUTOSOMAL-DOMINANT ATAXIAS

The trinucleotide repeat disorders typically demonstrate anticipation, meaning that subsequent generations of affected individuals tend to have a larger number of repeats and therefore earlier and more severe symptoms. Spinocerebellar ataxia (SCA) type 6 does not demonstrate this phenomenon. Anticipation occurs most often with paternal inheritance, except for SCA 8, in which anticipation occurs more often with maternal inheritance.[198] There is a significant amount of clinical overlap in the SCAs. It is difficult to diagnose a patient based purely on the clinical manifestations. All the SCAs are associated with cerebellar features, all are inherited, and all show some degree of abnormality on imaging studies.[199]

Spinocerebellar Ataxia Type 1

SCA 1 is due to a CAG trinucleotide repeat on chromosome 6p.[200] Onset is in the third or fourth decade. Patients present with ataxia, dysarthria, and brisk deep tendon reflexes. Sensory neuropathy, dysphagia, spasticity, dystonia, and chorea may occur later in the disease. MRI reveals pontocerebellar disease, and pathologic examination reveals severe loss of Purkinje cells, olivary neurons, and pontine neurons that project to the cerebellum.

Spinocerebellar Ataxia Type 2

SCA 2 presents with gait and limb ataxia, diminished deep tendon reflexes, and dysarthria.[201] Extreme slowing of saccades is observed in most patients. Sensory impairment, postural tremor, and cognitive problems are often seen. Rarely, patients may complain of muscle cramps, fasciculations, and sphincter disturbances. SCA 2 is due to a CAG trinucleotide repeat on chromosome 12q. Nerve conduction studies show a predominantly sensory neuropathy, and MRI shows pontocerebellar or isolated cerebellar atrophy. Pathologic studies show severe loss of Purkinje cells, mild loss of granule cells, and brainstem loss of inferior olivary neurons and pontocerebellar neurons. The substantia nigra shows severe loss of cells, and the spinal cord shows loss of myelin in the posterior columns and loss of cells in the anterior horn.

Spinocerebellar Ataxia Type 3

SCA 3, also known as Machado-Joseph disease, is due to a CAG trinucleotide repeat on chromosome 14q.[202] Patients develop ataxia, hyperreflexia, nystagmus, and dysarthria early in the disease. Oculomotor signs include gaze-evoked nystagmus and ophthalmoparesis leading to diplopia, which is frequently disabling. Facial and tongue atrophy, perioral fasciculations, and peripheral nerve disease appear with muscle atrophy and sensory loss. Patients with early-onset disease may also have spasticity, rigidity, dystonia, bradykinesia, and tremor responsive to levodopa. Electrodiagnostic studies show evidence of a sensory neuropathy as well as involvement of the anterior horn cells. MRI shows pontocerebellar and spinal cord atrophy. Pathologic studies demonstrate cell loss in the pontine basis, substantia nigra, and anterior horn cells. There is relative sparing of the Purkinje cells.

Spinocerebellar Ataxia Type 4

SCA 4 is localized to chromosome 16q. It is rare and has been described in a single family from Utah. Onset of symptoms is in the third or fourth decade with progressive ataxia, profound sensory loss, areflexia, and distal wasting.[203]

Spinocerebellar Ataxia Type 5

SCA 5, localized to chromosome 11, occurs in family members who are descendants of the grandparents of Abraham Lincoln.[204] It is a syndrome of pure cerebellar ataxia. Progression of the disease is slow.

Spinocerebellar Ataxia Type 6

SCA 6 is a CAG trinucleotide repeat disorder located on chromosome 19p13.[205] The protein involved is an α1A voltage-dependent calcium channel. SCA 6 manifests with mostly cerebellar symptoms, such as cerebellar ataxia, nystagmus, and mild sensory loss. Progression of the disease is slow. MRI studies reveal atrophy of the cerebellum, with relative sparing of the pons. Pathologic studies reveal cerebello-olivary atrophy, with no involvement of the pons.

Spinocerebellar Ataxia Type 7

In SCA 7, the age of onset is bimodal, with peaks in childhood (younger than 10 years) and again in adulthood (between 30 and 39 years). It is localized to chromosome 3p.[206] Ataxia, hyperreflexia, visual loss, and slow saccades characterize adult-onset disease. The childhood version is more severe and combines visual loss, ataxia, upper motoneuron signs, seizures, myoclonus, and dementia. Children typically die within 5 years of onset.

Spinocerebellar Ataxia Type 8

SCA 8 is a CTG trinucleotide repeat disorder localized to chromosome 13.[207] It is a slowly progressive ataxia with pronounced cerebellar atrophy, brisk reflexes, decreased vibratory sense, and a normal life span.[208] Cognitive impairment has been noted in at least one family.

Spinocerebellar Ataxia Type 10

SCA 10 has an ATTCT repeat on chromosome 22.[209] It may be associated with seizures.

Episodic Ataxia

Two forms of episodic ataxia (EA) have been described. They are caused by ion channel mutations—EA 1 by mutations in a potassium channel gene,[210] and EA 2 by mutations in a voltage-dependent calcium channel.[211] EA 2, SCA 6, and one type of familial hemiplegic migraine all represent allelic mutations of the same calcium channel gene on chromosome 19.[212] EA 1 typically manifests during the first decade and often attenuates after 20 years. Myokymia is present, and attacks last seconds to minutes. The symptoms are induced by startling or exercise. EA 2 has a lifelong duration. Nystagmus is common, and symptoms last minutes to hours. Vertigo may be present, and patients later have permanent ataxia. EA 2 patients may get some symptomatic relief from acetazolamide.

Dentatorubral-Pallidoluysian Atrophy

Dentatorubral-pallidoluysian atrophy is the most commonly reported ataxia in Japan. It is a CAG trinucleotide repeat localized to chromosome 12p. There are childhood- and adult-onset types. The childhood-onset type is characterized by myoclonic epilepsy, dementia, ataxia, and chorea. In the adult-onset type, ataxia, chorea, and dementia are often misdiagnosed as HD. Other signs include psychosis, slow saccades, dyskinesias, rigidity, bradykinesia, and hyperreflexia.[213] MRI shows pontocerebellar atrophy, with hyperintensity in the periventricular white matter. Pathologic study reveals cell loss in the dentate, red nucleus, globus pallidus, and STN.

Diagnosis

The diagnosis of hereditary ataxia is based on clinical findings, family history, clinical testing, and DNA-based testing. Clinical testing for ataxia-telangiectasia and for vitamin E deficiency involves measurements of alpha fetoprotein and vitamin E levels, respectively. Genetic counseling is recommended in patients suspected of having any inherited disorder. Genetic testing is available for SCAs 1, 2, 3, 6, 7, 8, and 10 and for dentatorubral-pallidoluysian atrophy.[214]

ACKNOWLEDGMENT

We would like to thank Mrs. Yalda Danesh Farnia for careful editing and preparing Figure 167–1.

REFERENCES

1. Kishore A, Calne DB: Approach to the patient with a movement disorder and overview of movement disorders. In Watts RL, Koller W (eds): Movement Disorders: Neurologic Principles and Practice. New York, McGraw-Hill, 1997, pp 3–14.
2. Deuschl G, Lindemann M, Krack P: The pathophysiology of tremor. Muscle Nerve 24:716–735, 2001.
3. Hallett M, Marsden CD: Cortical reflex myoclonus. Neurology 29:1107–1125. 1979.
4. Chung WS: Drug-induced akathisia revisited. Br J Clin Pract 50: 270–278, 1996.
5. Vergouwe MN, Peters AC, Wielaard R, Frants RR: Hyperekplexia phenotype due to compound heterozygosity for GLRA1 gene mutations. Ann Neurol 46:634–638, 1999.
6. Brown P, Marsden CD: What do the basal ganglia do? Lancet 351:1801–1804, 1998.
7. Parent A, Cicchetti F: The current model of basal ganglia organization under scrutiny. Mov Disord 13:199–202, 1998.
8. Wichman T, DeLong M: Functional and pathophysiological models of the basal ganglia. Curr Opin Neurobiol 6:751–758, 1996.
9. Jankovic J: Essential tremor: Clinical characteristics. Neurology 54(Suppl 4):S21–S25, 2000.
10. Hellwig B, Schelter B, Lauk M, et al: Tremor-correlated cortical activity in essential tremor. Lancet 357:519–523, 2001.
11. Brin MF, Koller W: Epidemiology and genetics of essential tremor. Mov Disord 13(Suppl 3):55–63, 1998.
12. Louis ED, Ford B, Frucht S, et al: Risk of tremor and impairments from tremor in relatives of patients with essential tremor: Community-based family study. Ann Neurol 49:761–769, 2001.
13. Koller WC, Busenbark K: Essential tremor. In Watts RL, Koller W (eds): Movement Disorders: Neurologic Priciples and Practice. New York, McGraw-Hill, 1997, pp 365–385.
14. Gironell A, Kulisevesky J, Barbanoj M, et al: A randomized placebo-controlled comparative trial of gabapentin and propranolol in essential tremor. Arch Neurol 56:475–480, 1999.
15. Galvez-Jimenez N, Hargreave M: Topiramate and essential tremor. Ann Neurol 47:837–838, 2000.
16. Jankovic J, Schwartz K, Clemence W, et al: A randomized, double-blind, placebo-controlled study to evaluate botulinum toxin type A in essential hand tremor. Mov Disord 11:250–256, 1996.
17. Goldman MS, Kelly PJ: Stereotactic thalamotomy for medically intractable essential tremor. Stereotact Funct Neurosurg 58:22–25, 1992.
18. Tasker RR: Thalamotomy for Parkinson's disease and other types of tremor. In Tasker R, Gildenberg PL (eds): Textbook of Stereotactic and Functional Neurosurgery. New York, McGraw-Hill, 1998, pp 1179–1198.
19. Koller W, Pahwa R, Busenbark K, et al: High-frequency unilateral thalamic stimulation in the treatment of essential and parkinsonian tremor. Ann Neurol 42:292–299, 1997.
20. Benabid AL, Pollak P, Seigneuret E, et al: Chronic VIM thalamic stimulation in Parkinson's disease, essential tremor and extrapyramidal dyskinesias. Acta Neurochir Suppl (Wien) 53:39–44, 1993.
21. Parkinson J: An Essay on the Shaking Palsy. London, Sherwood, Neely, & Jones, 1817.
22. Louis ED: The shaking palsy, the first forty-five years: A journey through the British literature. Mov Disord 12:1068–1072, 1997.
23. Bonduelle M: Charcot. Dates. Legend and reality. Hist Sci Med 28:289–295, 1994.
24. Pal PK, Samii A, Calne DB: Cardinal features of early Parkinson's disease. In Factor SA, Weiner WJ (eds): Parkinson's Disease: Diagnosis and Clinical Management. New York, Demos Medical, 2002, pp 41–56.
25. Calne DB, Snow B, Lee C: Criteria for diagnosing Parkinson's disease. Ann Neurol 32(Suppl S1):25–27, 1992.
26. Hoehn MM, Yahr MD: Parkinsonism: Onset, progression and mortality. Neurology 17:427–442, 1967.
27. Muthane UB, Swamy H, Satishchandra P, et al: Early onset Parkinson's disease: Are juvenile- and young-onset different? Mov Disord 9:539–544, 1994.
28. Golbe LI: Young-onset Parkinson's disease: A clinical review. Neurology 41:168–173, 1991.
29. Fearnley JM, Lees A: Aging and Parkinson's disease: Substantia nigra regional selectivity. Brain 114:2283–2301, 1991.
30. Lander ES, Schor N: Genetic dissection of complex traits. Science 265:2037–2048, 1994.
31. Samii A, Calne DB: Research into the etiology of Parkinson's disease. In Oertel W, LeWitt P (eds): Parkinson's Disease: The Treatment Options. London, Martin Dunitz, 1999, pp 229–243.
32. Hubble JP, Cao T, Hassanein RE, et al: Risk factors for Parkinson's disease. Neurology 3:1693–1697, 1993.
33. Priyadarshi A, Khuder SA, Schaub EA, Priyadarshi SS: Environmental risk factors and Parkinson's disease: A metaanalysis. Environ Res 86:122–127, 2001.
34. Tsui JK, Calne DB, Wang Y, et al: Occupational risk factors in Parkinson's disease. Can J Public Health 90:334–337, 1999.
35. Hernan MA, Zhang SM, Rueda-deCastro AM, et al: Cigarette smoking and the incidence of Parkinson's disease in two prospective studies. Ann Neurol 50:780–786, 2001.
36. Langston JW, Ballard P, Tetrud JW, Irwin I: Chronic parkinsonism in humans due to a product of meperidine-analog synthesis. Science 219:979–980, 1983.
37. Burns RS, Chiueh CC, Markey SP, et al: A primate model of parkinsonism: Selective destruction of dopaminergic neurons in the pars compacta of the substantia nigra by N-methyl-4-phe-

nyl-1,2,3,6-tetrahydropyridine. Proc Natl Acad Sci U S A 80: 4546–4550, 1983.

38. Maraganore DM, Harding AE, Marsden CD: A clinical and genetic study of familial Parkinson's disease. Mov Disord 6: 205–211, 1991.

39. Payami H, Larsden K, Bernard S, Nutt J: Increased risk of Parkinson's disease in parents and siblings of patients. Ann Neurol 36:659–661, 1994.

40. Calne S, Schoenberg B, Martin W, et al: Familial Parkinson's disease: Possible role of environmental factors. Can J Neurol Sci 14:303–305, 1987.

41. Polymeropoulos MH, Lavedan C, Leroy E, et al: Mutation in the alpha-synuclein gene identified in families with Parkinson's disease. Science 276:2045–2047, 1997.

42. Kitada T, Asakawa S, Hatorri N, et al: Mutations in the parkin gene cause autosomal recessive juvenile parkinsonism. Nature 392:605–608, 1998.

43. Mizuno Y, Hattori N, Kitada T, et al: Familial Parkinson's disease: Alpha-synuclein and parkin. Adv Neurol 86:13–21, 2001.

44. Tanner CM, Ottoman R, Goldman SM, et al: Parkinson disease in twins: An etiologic study. JAMA 281:341–346, 1999.

45. Scott WK, Nance MA, Watts RL, et al: Complete genomic screen in Parkinson disease: Evidence for multiple genes. JAMA 286: 2239–2244, 2001.

46. Calne DB, Stoessl AJ: Early parkinsonism. Clin Neuropharmacol 9(Suppl 2):S3–S8, 1986.

47. Deuschl G, Raethjen J, Baron R, et al: The pathophysiology of parkinsonian tremor: A review. J Neurol 247(Suppl 5):V33–V48, 2000.

48. Martinez-Martin P, Gil-Nagel A, Gracia LM, et al: Unified Parkinson's Disease Rating Scale characteristics and structure: The Cooperative Multicenter Group. Mov Disord 9:76–83, 1994.

49. Vingerhoets FJ, Schulzer M, Calne DB, Snow BJ: Which clinical sign of Parkinson's disease best reflects the nigrostriatal lesion? Ann Neurol 41:58–64, 1997.

50. Shonitoh H, Uchida Y, Ito H, Harrori T: Relationship between striatal (123I)beta-CIT binding and four major clinical signs in Parkinson's disease. Ann Nucl Med 14:199–203, 2000.

51. Gelb DJ, Oliver E, Gilman S: Diagnostic criteria for Parkinson disease. Arch Neurol 56:33–39, 1999.

52. Samii A, Letwin S, Calne DB: Prospects for new drug treatment in idiopathic parkinsonism. Drug Discov Today 3:131–140, 1998.

53. Yahr MD, Duvoisin RC, Schear MJ, et al: Treatment of parkinsonism with levodopa. Arch Neurol 21:343–354, 1969.

54. Ahlskog JE, Muenter M: Frequency of levodopa-related dyskinesias and motor fluctuations as estimated from the cumulative literature. Mov Disord 16:448–458, 2001.

55. Ahlskog JE: Parkinson's disease: Medical and surgical treatment. Neurol Clin 19:579–605, 2001.

56. Parkinson Study Group: Effects of tocopherol and deprenyl on the progression of disability in early Parkinson's disease. N Engl J Med 328:176–183, 1993.

57. Schulzer M, Mak E, Calne DB: The antiparkinson efficacy of deprenyl derives from transient improvement that is likely to be symptomatic. Ann Neurol 32:795–798, 1992.

58. Vingerhoets FJ, Uitti RJ, Calne DB: Deprenyl and the issue of neuroprotection. Eur Neurol 34:1–3, 1994.

59. Rascol O, Brooks DJ, Korczyn AD, et al: A five-year study of the incidence of dyskinesia in patients with early Parkinson's disease who were treated with ropinirole or levodopa. 056 Study Group. N Engl J Med 342:1484–1491, 2000.

60. Parkinson Study Group: Pramipexole vs levodopa as initial treatment for Parkinson disease. JAMA 284:1931–1938, 2000.

61. Quinn N: Young onset Parkinson's disease. Mov Disord 2:73–91, 1987.

62. Marek K, Seibyl J, Shoulson I, et al: Parkinson Study Group: Dopamine transporter brain imaging to assess the effects of pramipexole vs levodopa on Parkinson disease progression. JAMA 287:1653–1661, 2002.

63. Nutt JG, Woodward WR, Hammerstad JP, et al: The "on-off" phenomenon in Parkinson's disease: Relation to levodopa absorption and transport. N Engl J Med 310:483–488, 1984.

64. Assal F, Spahr L, Hadengue A, et al: Tolcapone and fulminant hepatitis. Lancet 352:958, 1998.

65. Verhagen Metman L, Del Dotto P, van den Munckhof P, et al: Amantadine as treatment of dyskinesias and motor fluctuations in Parkinson's disease. Neurology 50:1323–1326, 1998.

66. Samii A, Turnbull IM, Kishore A, et al: Reassessment of unilateral pallidotomy in the treatment of Parkinson's disease: A two year follow-up study. Brain 122:417–425, 1999.

67. Baron MS, Vitek JL, Bakay RA, et al: Treatment of advanced Parkinson's disease by unilateral posterior Gpi pallidotomy: 4-year results of a pilot study. Mov Disord 15:230–237, 2000.

68. Fine J, Duff J, Chen RM: Long-term follow-up of unilateral pallidotomy in advanced Parkinson's disease. N Engl J Med 342:1708–1714, 2000.

69. Ghika J, Ghika-Schmid F, Fankhauser H, et al: Bilateral contemporaneous posteroventral pallidotomy for the treatment of Parkinson's disease: Neuropsychological and neurological side effects. Report of four cases and review of the literature. J Neurosurg 91:313–321, 1999.

70. Hallett M, Litvan I: Scientific position paper of the Movement Disorder Society evaluation of surgery for Parkinson's disease. Task Force on Surgery for Parkinson's Disease of the American Academy of Neurology Therapeutic and Technology Assessment Committee. Mov Disord 15:436–438, 2000.

71. Lang AE: A surgery for Parkinson's disease: A critical evaluation of the state of the art. Arch Neurol 57:1118–1125, 1995.

72. Schuurman PR, Bosch DA, Bossuyt PM, et al: A comparison of continuous thalamic stimulation and thalamotomy for suppression of severe tremor. N Engl J Med 342:461–468, 2000.

73. Volkmann J, Sturm V, Weiss P, et al: Bilateral high-frequency stimulation of the internal globus pallidus in advanced Parkinson's disease. Ann Neurol 44:953–961, 1998.

74. Burchiel KJ, Anderson VC, Favre J, Hammerstad JP: Comparison of pallidal and subthalamic nucleus deep brain stimulation for advanced Parkinson's disease: Results of a randomized, blinded pilot study. Neurosurgery 45:1375–1382, 1999.

75. Galvez-Jimenez N, Lozano A, Tasker R, et al: Pallidal stimulation in Parkinson's disease patients with a prior unilateral pallidotomy. Can J Neurol Sci 25:300–305, 1998.

76. Moro E, Scerrati M, Romito LM, et al: Chronic subthalamic nucleus stimulation reduces medication requirements in Parkinson's disease. Neurology 53:85–90, 1999.

77. Kumar R, Lozano A, Kim YJ, et al: Double-blind evaluation of subthalamic nucleus deep brain stimulation in advanced Parkinson's disease. Neurology 51:850–855, 1998.

78. Limousin P, Krack P, Pollak P, et al: Electrical stimulation of the subthalamic nucleus in advanced Parkinson's disease. N Engl J Med 339:1105–1111, 1998.

79. Ardouin C, Pillon B, Peiffer E: Bilateral subthalamic or pallidal stimulation for Parkinson's disease affects neither memory nor executive functions: A consecutive series of 62 patients. Ann Neurol 46:217–223, 1999.

80. Molinuevo JL, Valldeoriola F, Tolosa E, et al: Levodopa withdrawal after bilateral subthalamic nucleus stimulation in advanced Parkinson's disease. Arch Neurol 57:983–988, 2000.

81. Krack P, Pollak P, Limousin P: Subthalamic nucleus or internal pallidal stimulation in young onset Parkinson's disease. Brain 121:451–457, 1998.

82. Merello M: Subthalamic stimulation contralateral to a previous pallidotomy: An erroneous indication? Mov Disord 14:890, 1999.

83. Moro E, Esselink RA, Van Blercom N, et al: Bilateral subthalamic nucleus stimulation in a parkinsonian patient with previous unilateral pallidotomy and thalamotomy. Mov Disord 15:753–755, 2000.

84. Houeto JL, Bejjani PB, Damier P, et al: Failure of long-term pallidal stimulation corrected by subthalamic stimulation in PD. Neurology 55:728–730, 2000.

85. Mogilner AY, Sterio D, Rezai AR, et al: Subthalamic nucleus stimulation in patients with a prior pallidotomy. J Neurosurg 96:660–665, 2002.

86. Samii A, Giroux ML, Slimp JC, Goodkin R: Bilateral subthalamic nucleus stimulation after bilateral pallidotomies in a patient with advanced Parkinson's disease. Parkinsonism Relat Disord 9:159–162, 2003.

87. The Deep-Brain Stimulation for Parkinson's Disease Study Group: Deep-brain stimulation of the subthalamic nucleus or the pars interna of the globus pallidus in Parkinson's disease. N Engl J Med 345:956–963, 2001.

88. Madrazo I, Drucker-Colin R, Diaz V, et al: Open microsurgical autograft of adrenal medulla to the right caudate nucleus in two patients with intractable Parkinson's disease. N Engl J Med 316:831–834, 1987.

89. Olanow CW, Koller W, Goetz CG, et al: Autologous transplantation of adrenal medulla in Parkinson's disease: 18-month results. Arch Neurol 47:1286–1289, 1990.

90. Ahlskog JE: Cerebral transplantation for Parkinson's disease: Current progress and future prospects. Mayo Clin Proc 68:578–591, 1993.

91. Freeman TB, Olanow CW, Hauser RA: Bilateral fetal nigral transplantation in the postcommissural putamen in Parkinson's disease. Ann Neurol 38:379–388, 1995.

92. Hauser RA, Freeman T, Snow BJ, et al: Long-term evaluation of bilateral fetal nigral transplantation in Parkinson's disease. Arch Neurol 5:179–187, 1999.

93. Lindvall O: Update on fetal transplantation: The Swedish experience. Mov Disord 13:83–87, 1998.

94. Freed CR, Breeze RE, Rosenberg NL, et al: Survival of implanted fetal dopamine cells and neurologic improvement 12 to 46 months after transplantation for Parkinson's disease. N Engl J Med 327:1549–1555, 1992.

95. Kordower JH, Freeman TB, Snow BJ, et al: Neuropathological evidence of graft survival and striatal reinnervation after the transplantation of fetal mesencephalic tissue in a patient with Parkinson's disease. N Engl J Med 332:1118–1124, 1995.

96. Greene PE, Fahn S, Tsai WY: Severe spontaneous dyskinesias: A disabling complication of embryonic dopaminergic tissue implants in a subset of transplanted patients with advanced Parkinson's disease. Mov Disord 14:904–910, 1999.

97. Freed CR, Greene PE, Breeze RE, et al: Transplantation of embryonic dopamine neurons for severe Parkinson's disease. N Engl J Med 344:710–719, 2001.

98. Stoessl AJ, Rivest J: Differential diagnosis of parkinsonism. Can J Neurol Sci 26(Suppl 2):S1–S4, 1999.

99. Rowe JW, Kahn RL: Human aging: Usual and successful. Science 237:143–149, 1987.

100. Calne DB, Eisen A, Meneilly G: Normal aging of the nervous system. Ann Neurol 30:206–207, 1991.

101. McGeer PL, McGreer EG, Suzuki JS: Aging and extrapyramidal function. Arch Neurol 34:33–35, 1977.

102. Cordes M, Snow BJ, Cooper S, et al: Age-dependent decline of nigrostriatal dopaminergic function: A positron emission tomographic study of grandparents and their grandchildren. Ann Neurol 36:667–670, 1994.

103. Jimenez-Jimenez FJ, Garcia-Ruiz PJ, Molina JA: Drug induced movement disorders. Drug Saf 16:180–204, 1997.

104. Foltynie T, Barker R, Brayne C: Vascular parkinsonism: A review of the precision and frequency of the diagnosis. Neuroepidemiology 21:1–7, 2002.

105. Rajput A, Rajput AH: Progressive supranuclear palsy: Clinical features, pathophysiology and management. Drugs Aging 18:913–925, 2001.

106. Rinne JO, Lee MS, Thompson PD, Marsden CD: Corticobasal degeneration; a clinical study of 36 cases. Brain 117:1183–1196, 1994.

107. Riley DE, Lang AE, Lewis MB: Corticobasal ganglionic degeneration. Neurology 40:1203–1212, 1990.

108. Leiguarda R, Merello M, Balej J: Apraxia in corticobasal degeneration. In Goetz G, Litvan I, Lang A (eds): Corticobasal Degeneration. Philadelphia, Lippincott Williams & Wilkins, 2000, pp 103–121.

109. Stover NP, Watts RL: Corticobasal degeneration. Semin Neurol 21:49–58, 2001.

110. Vanek ZF, Jankovic J: Dystonia in corticobasal degeneration. In Goetz G, Litvan I, Lang A (eds): Corticobasal Degeneration. Philadelphia, Lippincott Williams & Wilkins, 2000, pp 61–67.

111. Hanna PA, Doody RS: Alien limb sign. In Goetz G, Litvan I, Lang A (eds): Corticobasal Degeneration. Philadelphia, Lippincott Williams & Wilkins, 2000, pp 135–145.

112. Hanna PA, Jankovic J, Kilpatrick JB: Multiple system atrophy, the putative causative role of environmental toxins. Arch Neurol 56:90–94, 1999.

113. Gilman S, Low PA, Quinn N: Consensus statement on the diagnosis of multiple system atrophy. J Neurol Sci 163:94–98, 1999.

114. Kosaka K: Diffuse Lewy body disease. Neuropathology 20(Suppl):S73–S78, 2000.

115. McKeith I, Del Ser T, Spano P, et al: Efficacy of rivastigmine in dementia with Lewy bodies: A randomised, double-blind, placebo-controlled international study. Lancet 356:2031–2036, 2000.

116. Loudianos G, Gitlin JD: Wilson's disease. Semin Liver Dis 20:353–364, 2000.

117. Robertson WM: Wilson's disease. Arch Neurol 57:276–277, 2000.

118. Brewer GJ: Treatment of Wilson's disease with zinc. J Lab Clin Med 134:322–324, 1999.

119. Schilsky ML: Diagnosis and treatment of Wilson's disease. Pediatr Transplant 6:15–19, 2002.

120. Laitinen LV, Hariz MI: Movement disorders. In Winn RH (ed): Youman's Neurological Surgery, 4th ed. Philadelphia, WB Saunders, 1996, pp 3575–3609.

121. Harper PS: The epidemiology of Huntington's disease. Hum Genet 89:365–376, 1992.

122. Feifin A, Kieburtz K, Shoulson I: Treatment of Huntington's disease and other choreic disorders. In Kurlan R (ed): Treatment of Movement Disorders. Philadelphia, JB Lippincott, 1995, pp 337–364.

123. Bittenbender JB, Quadfasel FA: Rigid and akinetic forms of Huntington's chorea. Arch Neurol 7:37–50, 1962.

124. Foroud T, Gray J, Ivashina J, Conneally PM: Differences in duration of Huntington's disease based on age of onset. J Neurol Neurosurg Psychiatry 66:52–56, 1999.

125. Cubo E, Shannon KM, Penn RD, Kroin JS: Internal globus pallidotomy in dystonia secondary to Huntington's disease. Mov Disord 15:1248–1251, 2000.

126. Bachoud-Levi AC, Remy P, Nguyen JP, et al: Motor and cognitive improvements in patients with Huntington's disease after neural transplantation. Lancet 356:1975–1979, 2000.

127. Rubio JP, Danek A, Stone C, et al: Chorea-acanthocytosis: Genetic linkage to chromosome 9q21. Am J Hum Genet 61:899–908, 1997.

128. Mark MH: Other choreatic disorders. In Watts RL, Koller WC (eds): Movement Disorders. New York, McGraw-Hill, 1997, pp 527–541.

129. Hageman G, Ippel PF, van Hout MS, Rozeboom AR: A Dutch family with benign hereditary chorea of early onset: Differentiation from Huntington's disease. Clin Neurol Neurosurg 98:165–170, 1996.

130. Freidrich RL: Benign hereditary chorea improved on stimulant therapy. Pediatr Neurol 14:326–327, 1996.

131. Genel F, Arslanoglu S, Uran N, Saylan B: Sydenham's chorea: Clinical findings and comparison of the efficacies of sodium valproate and carbamazepine regimens. Brain Dev 24:73–76, 2002.

132. Cardoso F: Chorea gravidarum. Arch Neurol 59:868–870, 2002.

133. Kaell AT, Shetty M, Lee BC, Lockshin MD: The diversity of neurologic events in systemic lupus erythematosus: Prospective clinical and computed tomographic classification of 82 events in 71 patients. Arch Neurol 43:273–276, 1986.

134. Levine SR, Welch KM: Antiphospholipid antibodies. Ann Neurol 26:386–389, 1989.

135. Fahn S: The spectrum of levodopa-induced dyskinesias. Ann Neurol 47:S2–S11, 2000.

136. Shoulson I: On chorea. Clin Neuropharmacol 9(Suppl 2):S85–S99, 1986.

137. Tison FX, Ferrer X, Julien J: Delayed onset movement disorders as a complication of central pontine myelinolysis. Mov Disord 6:171–173, 1991.

138. Tsutada T, Hayashi H, Kitano S, et al: A case report of central pontine myelinolysis and extrapontine myelinolysis which occurred during pregnancy and was accompanied by choreic movement. Clin Neurol 29:1294–1297, 1989.

139. Yen DJ, Shan DE, Lu S: Hyperthyroidism presenting as recurrent short paroxysmal kinesigenic dyskinesia. Mov Disord 13:361–363, 1998.

140. Ghika-Schmid F, Ghika J, Regli F, Bogousslavsky J: Hyperkinetic movement disorders during and after acute stroke: The Lausanne Stroke Registry. J Neurol Sci 146:109–116, 1997.

141. Gioino GG, Dierssen G, Cooper IS: The effect of subcortical lesions on production and alleviation of hemiballistic or hemichoreic movements. J Neurol Sci 3:10, 1966.

142. Klein C, Breakefield XO, Ozelius LJ: Genetics of primary dystonia. Semin Neurol 19:271, 1999.

143. Nemeth AH: The genetics of primary dystonias and related disorders. Brain 125:695–721, 2002.

144. Fahn S: Concept and classification of dystonia. Adv Neurol 50:1–8, 1988.

145. Samii A, Pal PK, Schulzer M, et al: Post-traumatic cervical dystonia: A distinct entity? Can J Neurol Sci 27:55–59, 2000.

146. Nutt JG, Muenter M, Aronson A, et al: Epidemiology of focal and generalized dystonia in Rochester, Minnesota. Mov Disord 3:188, 1988.

147. Ozelius LJ, Kramer PL, de Leon D, et al: Strong allelic association between the torsion dystonia gene (DYT1) and loci on chromosome 9q34 in Ashkenazi Jews. Am J Hum Genet 50:619, 1992.

148. Ozelius LJ, Hewett JW, Page CE, et al: The early-onset torsion dystonia gene (DYT1) encodes an ATP-binding protein. Nat Genet 17:40, 1997.

149. Warner TT, Fletcher NA, Davis MB, et al: Linkage analysis in British and French families with idiopathic torsion dystonia. Brain 116:739, 1993.

150. Bressman SB, de Leon D, Kramer PL, et al: Dystonia in Ashkenazi Jews: Clinical characterization of a founder mutation. Ann Neurol 36:771, 1994.

151. Bressman SB, de Leon D, Raymond D, et al: Clinical-genetic spectrum of primary dystonia. Adv Neurol 78:79, 1998.

152. Leube B, Rudicki D, Ratzlaff T, et al: Idiopathic torsion dystonia: Assignment of a gene to chromosome 18p in a German family with adult onset, autosomal dominant inheritance and purely focal distribution. Hum Mol Genet 5:1673, 1996.

153. Leube B, Hendgen T, Kessler KR, et al: Sporadic focal dystonia in northwest Germany: Molecular basis on chromosome 18p. Ann Neurol 42:111, 1997.

154. Nygaard TG: Dopa-responsive dystonia: Delineation of the clinical syndrome and clues to pathogenesis. Adv Neurol 60:577, 1993.

155. Segawa M, Nomura Y: Hereditary progressive dystonia with marked diurnal fluctuation: Pathophysiological importance of the age of onset. Adv Neurol 60:568–76, 1993.

156. Segawa M, Hosaka A, Miyagawa F, et al: Hereditary progressive dystonia with marked diurnal fluctuations. Adv Neurol 14:215, 1976.

157. Bartholome K, Ludecke B: Mutations in the tyrosine hydroxylase gene cause various forms of L-dopa-responsive dysonia. Adv Pharmacol 42:48, 1998.

158. Ludecke B, Dworniczak B, Bartholome K, et al: A point mutation in the tyrosine hydroxylase gene associated with Segawa's syndrome. Hum Genet 95:123, 1995.

159. Ludecke B, Knappskog P, Clayton PT: Recessively inherited L-dopa-responsive parkinsonism in infancy caused by a point mutation (L205P) in the tyrosine hydroxylase gene. Hum Mol Genet 5:1023–1028, 1996.

160. Gasser T: Inherited myoclonus-dystonia syndrome. Adv Neurol 78:325, 1998.

161. Klein C, Schilling K, Saunders-Pullman RJ, et al: A major locus for myoclonus-dystonia maps to chromosome 7q in eight families. Am J Hum Genet 67:1314, 2000.

162. Quinn NP: Essential myoclonus and myoclonic dystonia. Mov Disord 11:19, 1996.

163. Fink JK, Rainer S, Wilkowski J, et al: Paroxysmal dystonic choreoathetosis: Tight linkage to chromosome 2q. Am J Hum Genet 59:140–145, 1996.

164. Fouad GT, Servidei S, Durcan S, et al: A gene for familial paroxysmal dyskinesia (FPD1) maps to chromosome 2q. Am J Hum Genet 59:135–139, 1996.

165. Raskind WH, Brolin T, Wolff J, et al: Further localization of a gene for paroxysmal dystonic choreoathetosis to a 5-cM region on chromosome 2q34. Hum Genet 102:93–97, 1998.

166. Auburger G, Ratzlaff T, Lunkes A, et al: A gene for autosomal dominant paroxysmal choreoathetosis/spasticity (CSE) maps to the vicinity of a potassium channel gene cluster on chromosome 1p, probably within 2 cM between D1S443 and D1S197. Genomics 31:90–94. 1996.

167. Karp BI, Goldstein SR, Chen R, et al: An open trial of clozapine for dystonia. Mov Disord 14:652–657, 1999.

168. Marsalek M: Tardive drug-induced extrapyramidal syndromes. Pharmacopsychiatry 33(Suppl 1):14–33, 2000.

169. Simpson GM: The treatment of tardive dyskinesia and tardive dystonia. J Clin Psychiatry 61(Suppl 4):39–44, 2000.

170. Wirshing WC: Movement disorders associated with neuroleptic treatment. J Clin Psychiatry 62(Suppl 21):15–18, 2001.

171. Misbahuddin A, Warner TT: Dystonia: An update on genetics and treatment. Curr Opin Neurol 14:471–475, 2001.

172. Albright AL, Barry MJ, Shafton DH, Ferson SS: Intrathecal baclofen for generalized dystonia. Dev Med Child Neurol 43:652–657, 2001.

173. Jankovic J, Orman J: Tetrabenazine therapy of dystonia, chorea, tics, and other dyskinesias. Neurology 38:391–394, 1988.

174. Yoshor D, Hamilton WJ, Ondo W, et al: Comparison of thalamotomy and pallidotomy for the treatment of dystonia. Neurosurgery 48:818–826, 2001.

175. Krack P, Vercueil L: Review of the functional surgical treatment of dystonia. Eur J Neurol 8:389–399, 2001.

176. Jankovic J, Brin MF: Therapeutic uses of botulinum toxin. N Engl J Med 324:1186–1194, 1991.

177. Clarke CE: Therapeutic potential of botulinum toxin in neurological disorders. Q J Med 82:197–205, 1992.

178. Bentivoglio AR, Albanese A: Botulinum toxin in motor disorders. Curr Opin Neurol 12:447–456, 1999.

179. Blindauer K: Myoclonus and its disorders. Neurol Clin 19:723–734, 2001.

180. Fahn S, Sjaastad O: Hereditary essential myoclonus in a large Norwegian family. Mov Disord 6:237–247, 1991.

181. Niedermeyer E, Fineyre F, Riley T, Bird B: Myoclonus and the electroencephalogram, a review. Clin Electroencephalogr 10:75–95, 1979.

182. Oguni H, Hayashi K, Awaya Y, et al: Severe myoclonic epilepsy in infants: Review based on the Tokyo Women's Medical University series of 84 cases. Brain Dev 23:736–748, 2001.

183. Plaster NM, Uyama E, Uchino M, et al: Genetic localization of the familial adult myoclonic epilepsy (FAME) gene to chromosome 8q24. Neurology 53:1180–1183, 1999.

184. Caviness JN: Myoclonus. Mayo Clin Proc 71:679–688, 1996.

185. Mima T, Nagamine T, Nishitani N, et al: Cortical myoclonus: Sensorimotor hyperexcitability. Neurology 50:933–942, 1998.

186. Obeso JA: Therapy of myoclonus. Clin Neurosci 3:253–257, 1995.

187. Brown P, Steiger MJ, Tompson PD, et al: Effectiveness of piracetam in cortical myoclonus. Mov Disord 6:73–75, 1993.

188. Schauer R, Singer M, Saltuari L, Kofler M: Suppression of cortical myoclonus by levetiracetam. Mov Disord 17:411–415, 2002.

189. Laitinen L: Thalamotomy in progressive myoclonus epilepsy. Acta Neurol Scand 43(Suppl 31):170, 1967.

190. Kupsch A, Trottenberg T, Meissner W, Funk T: Neurostimulation of the ventral intermediate thalamic nucleus alleviates hereditary essential myoclonus. J Neurol Neurosurg Psychiatry 67:415–416, 1999.

191. Durr A, Cossee M, Agid Y, et al: Clinical and genetic abnormalities in patients with Friedreich's ataxia. N Engl J Med 335:1169–1175, 1996.

192. Spacey SD, Gatti RA, Bebb G: The molecular basis and clinical management of ataxia telangiectasia. Can J Neurol Sci 27:184–191, 2000.

193. Cavalier L, Ouahchi K, Kayden H, et al: Ataxia with isolated vitamin E deficiency: Heterogeneity of mutations and phenotypic variability in a large number of families. Am J Hum Genet 62:301–310, 1998.

194. Yokota T, Shiojiri T, Gotoda T, et al: Friedreich-like ataxia with retinitis pigmentosa caused by the His101Gln mutation of the alpha-tocopherol transfer gene protein gene. Ann Neurol 41:826–832, 1997.

195. do Ceu Moreira M, Barbot C, Tachi N, et al: Homozygosity mapping of Portuguese and Japanese forms of ataxia-oculomotor apraxia to 9q13, and evidence for genetic heterogeneity. Am J Hum Genet 68:501–508, 2001.

196. Nemeth AH, Bochukova E, Dunne E, et al: Autosomal recessive cerebellar ataxia with oculomotor apraxia (ataxia-telangiectasia-like syndrome) is linked to chromosome 9q34. Am J Hum Genet 67:1320–1326, 2000.

197. Date H, Onodera O, Tanaka H, et al: Early-onset ataxia with ocular motor apraxia and hypoalbuminemia is caused by muta-

tions in a new HIT superfamily gene. Nat Genet 29:184–188, 2001.

198. Koob MD, Moseley M, Schut LJ, et al: An untranslated CTG expansion causes a novel form of spinocerebellar ataxia. Nat Genet 21:379–384, 1999.

199. Nance MA: Clinical aspects of CAG repeat diseases. Brain Pathol 7:881–900, 1997.

200. Orr HT, Zoghbi HY: SCA1 molecular genetics: A history of a 13 year collaboration against glutamines. Hum Mol Genet 10:2307–2311, 2001.

201. Wadia N, Pang J, Desai J, et al: A clinicogenetic analysis of six Indian spinocerebellar ataxia (SCA2) pedigrees: The significance of slow saccades in diagnosis. Brain 121(Pt 12):2341–2355, 1998.

202. Cemal CK, Huxley C, Chamberlain S: Insertion of expanded CAG trinucleotide repeat motifs into a yeast artificial chromosome containing the human Machado-Joseph disease gene. Gene 236:53–61, 1999.

203. Nagaoka U, Takashima M, Ishikawa K, et al: A gene on SCA4 locus causes dominantly inherited pure cerebellar ataxia. Neurology 54:1971–1975, 2000.

204. Ranum LP, Schut LJ, Lundgren JK, et al: Spinocerebellar ataxia type 5 in a family descended from the grandparents of President Lincoln maps to chromosome 11. Nat Genet 8:280–284, 1994.

205. Watanabe H, Tanaka F, Matsumoto M, et al: Frequency analysis of autosomal dominant cerebellar ataxias in Japanese patients and clinical characteristics of spinocerebellar ataxia type 6. Clin Genet 53:13–19, 1998.

206. Michalik A, Del-Favero J, Mauger C, et al: Genomic organisation of the spinocerebellar ataxia type 7 (SCA7) gene responsible for autosomal dominant cerebellar ataxia with retinal degeneration. Hum Genet 105:410–417, 1999.

207. Day JW, Schut LK, Moselry ML, et al: Spinocerebellar ataxia type 8: Clinical features in a large family. Neurology 55:649–657, 2000.

208. Juvonen V, Hietala M, Paivarinta M, et al: Clinical and genetic findings in Finnish ataxia patients with the spinocerebellar ataxia 8 repeat expansion. Ann Neurol 48:354–361, 2000.

209. Matsuura T, Yamagata T, Burgess DL: Large expansion of the ATTCT pentanucleotide repeat in spinocerebellar ataxia type 10. Nat Genet 26:191–194, 2000.

210. Browne DL, Gancher ST, Nutt JG, et al: Episodic ataxia/myokymia syndrome is associated with point mutations in the human potassium channel gene, KCNA1. Nat Genet 8:136–140, 1994.

211. Ophoff RA, Terwindt G, Vergouwe MN, et al: Familial hemiplegic migraine and episodic ataxia type 2 are caused by mutations in the Ca^{2+} channel gene CACNL1A4. Cell 87:543–552, 1996.

212. Elliott MA: Familial hemiplegic migraine. Adv Clin Neurosci 7:197–214, 1997.

213. Ikeuchi T, Koide R, Tanaka H, et al: Dentatorubral-pallidoluysian atrophy: Clinical features are closely related to unstable expansions of trinucleotide (CAG) repeat. Ann Neurol 37:769–775, 1995.

214. Potter NT: Genetic testing for ataxia in North America. Mol Diagn 52:91–99, 2002.

CHAPTER 168

Patient Selection in Movement Disorder Surgery

TODD P. THOMPSON ■ L. DADE LUNSFORD ■
DOUGLAS KONDZIOLKA ■ A. LELAND ALBRIGHT

The surgical treatment of patients with movement disorders continues to evolve. A greater understanding of relevant anatomy, improved imaging, advanced stereotactic systems, and new implantable devices has allowed neurosurgeons to improve the lives of patients. Successful surgical treatment of movement disorders requires proper diagnosis, understanding of the unique pathophysiology, and careful patient selection.

In this chapter, we review the distinguishing clinical characteristics of the movement disorders that are currently treated with surgical intervention, the relevant diagnostic tests, and the differential diagnosis. As their diagnostic skills improve and the therapeutic armamentarium grows, neurosurgeons will likely treat an increased number of movement disorders. The current medical philosophy considers surgical treatment of movement disorders when standard medical therapies have been exhausted. With improved understanding of such disorders, some diseases may be arrested or even reversed with early surgical intervention. We believe that successful patient selection is achieved through the multidisciplinary collaboration of neurosurgeons, neurologists, psychiatrists, physiatrists, and orthopedic surgeons (when there are associated tendon contractures).

HISTORY

As Osler professed years ago, listening to the patient will most often yield the correct diagnosis. Understanding the patients' complaints is essential to accurately diagnosing movement disorders. Although a patient may have a well-labeled and characterized disorder, the primary cause of disability may be unique to the patient's situation. For example, a patient with marked tremor caused by Parkinson's disease (PD) may not have much functional disability due to the tremor. The patient's activity may be most affected by periods of freezing or dyskinesias. Additionally, a patient's expectations of surgical interventions must be understood. A patient with PD who expects that a pallidotomy will eliminate a flat affect, improve gait, and reduce the need for continued medication is certain to be disappointed. Important characteristics of the history include the age at and rapidity of onset, the family history, environmental exposure, the temporal characteristics, the presence or absence of abnormal movements during sleep, exacerbating or alleviating factors and concurrent medical conditions, and previous interventions.

A review of the patient's current medicines is essential. Medications, particularly neuroleptics, can cause a number of confounding movement disorders. The neuroleptics can induce acute dystonic reactions, parkinsonism, and neuroleptic malignant syndrome. In addition, tardive tremor, chorea, akathisia, myoclonus, and parkinsonism can occur with chronic use.

EXAMINATION

The physical examination of a patient with a movement disorder is of critical importance because many disorders are defined solely by their physical manifestations. Movement disorders are characterized according to the involvement of the axial versus appendicular musculature. The axial disorders are divided into those affecting the head and neck and those affecting the trunk. Extremity movements are described in terms of their occurrence with intentional movements, with sustained postural movements, or at rest. Disorders may be focal, affecting one extremity; lateralized, affecting one side of the body; or generalized. Disorders may also be characterized as isokinetic or hyperkinetic. Isokinetic disorders such as spasticity and ataxia have a normal amount of movement, but the movement itself is abnormal. Hyperkinetic disorders such as dystonia or tremor have increased amounts of movement. The frequency, rate, rhythm, and magnitude of abnormal movements are significant components. The examination should include a thorough evaluation of the cranial nerves, muscle strength, tone, reflexes, fine motor movement, balance, and coordination. Provocative testing can include walking, turning, rising from the sitting position, and task performance with stress-inducing or distracting maneuvers.

PARKINSON'S DISEASE

Parkinson's disease is the most prevalent movement disorder. Although the incidence of PD is estimated at 15 per 100,000, its prevalence is much greater.[1] The diagnosis of PD is clinical, based on the presence of at least two of the triad of clinical hallmarks of PD (tremor, bradykinesia, and rigidity) and a favorable response to dopaminergic therapy. There is a spectrum of clinical signs and symptoms as well as a long differential list of possible confounding diagnoses that have a different clinical course and response to therapy. The hallmarks of PD include a resting tremor, muscular rigidity, gait and postural disturbances, and bradykinesia. Bradykinetic symptoms include slow initiation of movement, freezing, short steps, festinating gait, reduced spontaneous movements, micrographia, difficulty arising from a chair, postural instability, dysphonia, dysarthria, and dysphagia. The initial symptoms of PD, mild unilateral tremor or decreased arm motion with ambulation, are often missed until the patient develops additional symptoms. With progressive bradykinesia and rigidity, patients may suffer respiratory distress. Gait and postural instability are usually late symptoms. If observed early in the disease, caution should be taken as to the correctness of the diagnosis.

Patients without significant tremor are often more difficult to recognize. Early signs may include complaints of fatigue, slightly increased muscle rigidity, failure to swing the arm with ambulation, and extinction of the blink reflex with tapping on the bridge of the nose (Myerson's sign). PD may include psychological symptoms such as anxiety, depression, hallucinations, and poor memory and concentration.

PD presenting in the adult population is most often the result of the loss of dopaminergic neurons in the substantia nigra. Children or young adults with parkinsonian features should be suspected to have hepatolenticular degeneration and evaluated for liver disease and Kayser-Fleischer rings (corneal pigmentation), serum ceruloplasmin, and urinary copper excretion.

Tests for evaluating PD include clinical rating scales, timed motor tests, a trial of L-dopa therapy, and positron emission tomography (PET) studies.[2, 3] The Unified Parkinson's Disease Rating Scale (UPDRS) is a detailed scoring system that evaluates patients' cognition, activities of daily living, motor skills, complications of medical therapy, and overall impairment of function[4-6] (Table 168–1). The Hoehn and Yahr staging scale defines the extent of patients' disability. These two scales are components of the Core Assessment Program for Intracerebral Transplantation (CAPIT) that has been instituted to allow consistent evaluation of surgical interventions.[7, 8] Other components of the CAPIT protocol are timed motor tests, an L-dopa test, video analysis, and, when available, PET (Table 168–2).

The differential diagnosis of PD includes the Parkinson's plus syndromes (or multiple system atrophy disease). These degenerative disorders need to be recognized because they respond poorly to current ablative or stimulation techniques. Such conditions include Shy-Drager syndrome, striatonigral degeneration, progressive supranuclear palsy, olivopontocerebellar degeneration, and the "multiple system atrophy" disorders. Clinically, signs of autonomic dysfunction, long tract signs, cerebellar deficits, extraocular movement abnormalities, increased axial tone, and a lack of response to L-dopa therapy are indicators that a Parkinson's plus disorder exists. In addition to thorough neurological assessment,

TABLE 168–1 ■ Unified Parkinson's Disease Rating Scale

I.	Mentation, Behavior, and Mood	0–16 points
	1 Intellectual impairment	
	2 Thought disorder	
	3 Depression	
	4 Motivation/initiative	
II.	Activities of Daily Living	0–52 points
	2 Speech	
	3 Salivation	
	4 Swallowing	
	5 Handwriting	
	6 Cutting food and handling utensils	
	7 Dressing	
	8 Hygiene	
	9 Turning in bed and adjusting bedclothes	
	10 Falling, unrelated to freezing	
	11 Freezing when walking	
	12 Walking	
	13 Tremor	
	14 Sensory complaints related to parkinsonism	
III.	Motor Examination	0–108 points
	15 Speech	
	16 Facial expression	
	17 Tremor at rest	
	18 Action or postural tremor of hands	
	19 Rigidity	
	20 Finger taps	
	21 Hand movements	
	22 Rapid alternating movements of the hands	
	23 Leg agility	
	24 Rising from chair	
	25 Posture	
	26 Gait	
	27 Postural stability	
	28 Body bradykinesia and hypokinesia	
IV.	Complications of Therapy (in the past week)	0–23 points
	29 Duration of dyskinesia	
	30 Disability from dyskinesia	
	31 Pain from dyskinesia	
	32 Early morning dystonia	
	33 Predictable off periods	
	34 Unpredictable off periods	
	35 Sudden-onset off periods	
	36 Proportion of day spent in the off state	
	37 Anorexia, nausea, vomiting	
	38 Sleep disturbance	
	39 Symptomatic orthostasis	
Total Points		0–199 points

The UPDRS gives 0–4 points for each item, with higher scores reflecting greater disability. Normal function is scored '0'. In section IV, items 32, 33, 34, and 39 are scored 0–4. The others are scored as 0 = no, 1 = yes. Section V (not shown) evaluates the activities of daily living with eight categories, each scored 0–5. This section of the UPDRS is similar to the Hoehn and Yahr staging scale. Section VI (not shown) gives a percentage of normal function score to patients, with normal function considered 100%.

TABLE 168–2 ■ Hoehn and Yahr Staging

STAGE	DEFINITION
1	Unilateral involvement only
1.5	Unilateral and axial involvement
2	Bilateral involvement without impairment of balance
2.5	Mild bilateral involvement with recovery on retropulsion test
3	Mild to moderate bilateral involvement, some postural instability, physically independent
4	Severe disability, able to stand and walk unassisted
5	Wheelchair-bound or bedridden except when assisted

preoperative computed tomography (CT) and magnetic resonance imaging (MRI) are important to exclude multi-infarct dementia. PET has been shown to be useful in helping distinguish progressive supranuclear palsy and corticobasal degeneration from PD.[9]

Even with the proper diagnosis, it remains challenging to choose the best surgical procedure for a given set of clinical problems. Our current practice is to perform a pallidotomy for those patients who are most disabled by dopa-induced dyskinesias, with or without tremor. The consistent efficacy of pallidotomy to treat tremor has not been fully established. PD patients affected primarily by tremor are advised to have a thalamotomy or placement of a thalamic stimulator. Only patients with multiple medical problems or contraindications to open surgery are considered for stereotactic radiosurgical thalamotomy. It has been suggested that stimulation of the subthalamic nucleus (STN) relieves akinesia, L-dopa–induced dyskinesias, tremor, and rigidity.[10, 11] Many of the same results can be achieved with stimulation of the internal segment of the globus pallidus (GPi). It has also been suggested that bilateral STN stimulation may alter the progression of the disease. STN stimulation can be performed bilaterally with an acceptable rate of complications. At this time, a definitive long-term experience with either STN or GPi stimulation is not available.

CHOREA AND ATHETOSIS

Chorea (from the Greek, meaning "dance") describes brief irregular involuntary muscle contractions that are rapid, rhythmic, and unpatterned, with variable timing, generally affecting the upper extremities more than the lower extremities. Choreiform movements may appear purposeful but disordered. They interfere with intentional efforts, contributing to an ataxic appearance,[12] but there is no true ataxia or incoordination. Athetosis describes a slow writhing distal movement, often masked with semi-purposeful gestures. Chorea and athetosis often do overlap. Like chorea, athetosis is more prominent in the distal musculature and in the upper extremities. Unilateral chorea is sometimes considered hemiballismus, particularly when it involves the proximal musculature. Ballistic (from the Greek, meaning "jump") movements are forceful, vio-

lent movements that are most evident when present in the proximal musculature. In reality, there is a continuum of chorea and hemiballismus.

Chorea is associated with a number of degenerative diseases that affect the basal ganglia, such as Huntington's disease, ataxia-telangiectasia, and Wilson's disease. Chorea may exist with cerebral palsy. Chorea can also be a secondary symptom of infection or autoimmune disease (Sydenham's chorea due to rheumatic fever, systemic lupus erythematosus), drug side effects (L-dopa, anticholinergics, antipsychotics), metabolic disorders (hyperthyroidism, oral contraceptives, pregnancy), or vascular lesions or be idiopathic.[13] In each of these syndromes the corticospinal system is intact.

There is no effective medical therapy for chorea. Prior to 1960, both pallidotomy and thalamotomy were tried for patients with chorea and athetosis but with poor results.[14] Spiegel and Wycis found improvements in three of nine chorea patients treated by pallidotomy and one of three patients treated with medial thalamotomy.[15, 16] Narabayashi and Okuma effectively treated two chorea patients by chemopallidotomy.[17, 18] Although the literature does not encourage the surgical treatment of chorea, re-evaluation with modern techniques should be explored. Figure 168–1 illustrates two children with chorea (in one the disorder was caused by cerebral palsy and in the other by a thalamic hemorrhage) treated with thalamic stimulators. Both children had disabling unilateral chorea that was most pronounced in the upper extremity. Thalamic stimulation improved the functional ability of both children.

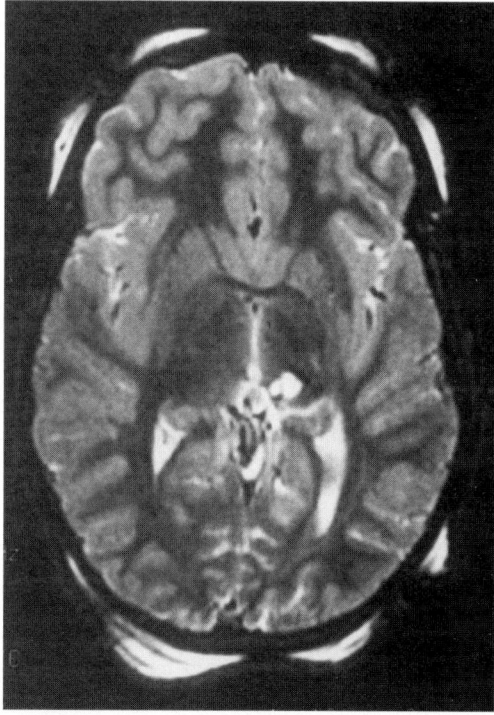

FIGURE 168–1. Magnetic resonance imaging in a 10-year-old girl who developed a progressive choreiform movement disorder 4 years after an intracerebral hemorrhage. The patient was treated with a left thalamic stimulator that resulted in improved function of the right upper extremity.

DYSTONIA

Dystonia is an extreme variant of athetosis, with co-contraction of agonist and antagonist muscles resulting in an abnormal posture.[19] Dystonic movements are most often slow, enduring, forceful contractions of either axial or appendicular musculature. They may also be repetitive phasic movements that can be differentiated from tremor by the irregular movement intervals. Dystonia is categorized as focal, segmental, hemidystonia, or generalized, describing the affected body region, and by the age at onset and etiology (secondary or idiopathic). Primary dystonia was previously called dystonia musculorum deformans.

Dystonia is augmented with patient activity or excitement and diminished with sleep. Patients are often thin, owing to the energy expended through dystonic movements. In cerebral palsy (CP), dystonia may progress from 3 to 15 years of age. The initial absence of dystonia with CP may be related to the initial hypomyelination of the corticospinal system. The clinical diagnosis of dystonia may be supported by radiographic imaging. Whereas primary dystonia patients will have normal MRI, with PET overactive prefrontal and underactive motor cortical areas are demonstrated.[20] Patients with secondary dystonias may have detectable abnormalities in the basal ganglia on MRI.[21-23]

CP is the most common cause of dystonia, which generally manifests as a generalized disorder. Dystonia also may be caused by a number of degenerative diseases, including trauma, kernicterus, Hallervorden-Spatz disease, Huntington's chorea, Wilson's disease, PD, lipid storage diseases, basal ganglia calcifications, and Leigh's disease and by drugs such as the phenothiazines, butyrophenones (haloperidol), and metoclopromide.[23] Dystonia must be distinguished from spasticity, with which it is often mistaken, and choreoathetosis. Dystonic CP must be distinguished from dopa-responsive dystonia (DRD or Segawa's disease).[24] DRD begins in childhood, often with gait difficulties or with dystonia in a foot, often has diurnal variations and a family history, and may have associated parkinsonian features or spasticity.[23] A trial of L-dopa is useful in clarifying the presence of DRD in dystonic CP when there is not a clear history of CP or radiographic correlation.

Oral medications are successful in less than half of the affected patients and may have significant side effects. Commonly used medicines include baclofen, trihexyphenidyl (Artane), diazepam, clonazepam, carbamazepine, L-dopa, propranolol, and haloperidol. Among the medical options, baclofen and trihexyphenidyl are the most successful. Patients who are unresponsive to medical therapy, including baclofen, may respond well to intrathecal baclofen (ITB) therapy (Fig. 168–2).[25, 26]

Patient selection for ITB therapy is facilitated by a trial of continuous ITB infusion because dystonia often does not respond to intermittent bolus by lumbar puncture.[26] The protocol at Children's Hospital of Pittsburgh delivers 200 μg/day through an intrathecal catheter with the tip positioned at C5–T2. The dose is increased

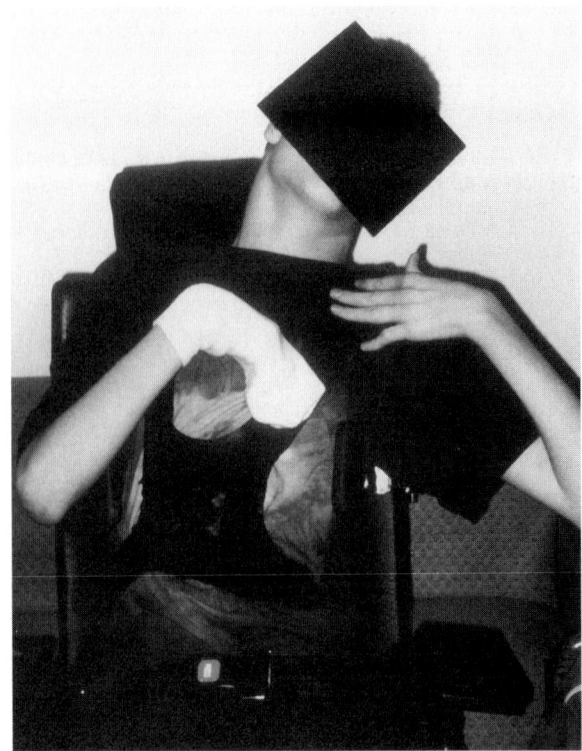

FIGURE 168–2. Patient with generalized dystonia secondary to cerebral palsy affecting the neck, trunk, and upper and lower extremities. This patient achieved improved function and comfort with intrathecal therapy with baclofen.

by 50 μg every 12 hours until a beneficial effect is achieved, side effects limit greater doses, or a maximum of 900 μg/day is reached. Responses typically occur with 400 to 600 μg/day. The response to baclofen is assessed with the Barry-Albright Dystonia Scale, a modified Fahn-Marsden scale that does not include an assessment of functional abilities because many patients with dystonia are not able to care for themselves (Table 168–3).[25, 27] (The Fahn-Marsden scale evaluates patients according to provoking and severity factors, based primarily on function.[28]) In addition to the quantitative evaluation, patients are assessed for subjective gains in general comfort, sleeping, and ease of positioning. In our 7-year experience with ITB for generalized dystonia, approximately 90% of individuals responded to the screening infusion with a 25% or greater decrease in the Barry-Albright Dystonia Scale scores. Of those implanted with a pump for chronic ITB infusion, approximately 90% have sustained improvement with their dystonia.

There is a long history of surgery for dystonia.[14] Success with thalamotomy can be achieved, but this procedure is infrequently performed because of the relatively low long-term success rate and need in most cases to perform bilateral procedures. The use of pallidotomy and GPi stimulation for dystonia is being studied.

TREMOR

Tremor is the most common type of involuntary movement and has many clinical manifestations, a few of

TABLE 168-3 ■ **Barry-Albright Dystonia Scale**

Patient's Name: _____   **Date:** _____

Directions. Assess the patient for dystonia in each of the following regions: eyes, mouth, neck, trunk, and each upper and lower extremity (8 body regions). Write the scores on the lines provided. Rate severity based only on dystonia as evidenced by abnormal movements or postures. When assessing functional limitations, do not score dystonia based on other factors, such as weakness, lack of motor control, cognitive deficits, primitive reflexes, and/or other movement disorders as defined below:

Dystonia: Sustained muscle contractions causing twisting and repetitive movements or abnormal postures
Spasticity: Velocity-dependent resistance to passive stretch
Athetosis: Distal writhing or contorting movements
Chorea: Brief, rapid, unsustained, irregular movements
Ataxia: Incoordination of movement characterized by wide-based unsteady gait, flailing movements

Eyes. Signs of dystonia of the eyes include prolonged eyelid spasms, forced eye deviations, or both.
0   Absence of eye dystonia
1   Slight: Dystonia less than 10% of the time and does not interfere with tracking
2   Mild: Frequent blinking without prolonged spasms of eye closure, and/or eye movements less than 50% of the time
3   Moderate: Prolonged spasms of eyelid closure, but eyes open most of the time, and/or eye movements more than 50% of the time that interfere with tracking, but able to resume tracking
4   Severe: Prolonged spasms of eyelid closure, with eyes closed at least 30% of the time, and/or eye movements more than 50% of the time that prevent tracking
*   Unable to assess eye movements
Eyes: _____

Mouth. Signs of dystonia of the mouth include grimacing, clenched or deviated jaw, forced open mouth, forceful tongue thrusting, or any combination thereof.
0   Absence of mouth dystonia
1   Slight: Dystonia less than 10% of the time and does not interfere with speech and/or feeding
2   Mild: Dystonia less than 50% of the time and does not interfere with speech and/or feeding
3   Moderate: Dystonia more than 50% of the time, and/or dystonia that interferes with speech and/or feeding
4   Severe: Dystonia more than 50% of the time, and/or dystonia that prevents speech and/or feeding
*   Unable to assess mouth movements
Mouth: _____

Neck. Signs of dystonia of the neck include pulling of the neck into any plane of motion: extension, flexion, lateral flexion, or rotation.
0   Absence of neck dystonia
1   Slight: Pulling less than 10% of the time and does not interfere with lying, sitting, standing, and/or walking
2   Mild: Pulling less than 50% of the time and does not interfere with lying, sitting, standing, and/or walking
3   Moderate: Pulling more than 50% of the time and/or dystonia that interferes with lying, sitting, standing, and/or walking
4   Severe: Pulling more than 50% of the time and/or dystonia that prevents sitting in standard wheelchair, standing, and/or walking (e.g., requires more than standard headrest for seating)
*   Unable to assess neck movements
Neck: _____

Trunk. Signs of dystonia of the trunk include pulling of the trunk into any plane of motion: extension, flexion, lateral flexion, or rotation.
0   Absence of trunk dystonia
1   Slight: Pulling less than 10% of the time and does not interfere with lying, sitting, standing, and/or walking
2   Mild: Pulling less than 50% of the time and does not interfere with lying, sitting, standing, and/or walking
3   Moderate: Pulling more than 50% of the time and/or dystonia that interferes with lying, sitting, standing, and/or walking
4   Severe: Pulling more than 50% of the time and/or dystonia that prevents positioning in standard wheelchair, standing, and/or walking (e.g., requires adapted seating system to control posturing, such as ASIS bar)
*   Unable to assess eye movements
Trunk: _____

Upper extremities. Signs of dystonia of the upper extremities include sustained muscle contractions causing abnormal posturing of the upper extremities.
0   Absence of upper extremity dystonia
1   Slight: Dystonia less than 10% of the time and does not interfere with normal positioning and/or functional activities
2   Mild: Dystonia less than 50% of the time and does not interfere with normal positioning and/or functional activities
3   Moderate: Dystonia more than 50% of the time and/or dystonia that interferes with normal positioning and/or upper extremity function
4   Severe: Dystonia more than 50% of the time and/or dystonia that prevents normal positioning and/or upper extremity function (e.g., arms restrained in wheelchair to prevent injury)
*   Unable to assess upper extremity movements
Left upper extremity: _____
Right upper extremity: _____

Lower extremities. Signs of dystonia of the lower extremities include sustained muscle contractions causing abnormal posturing of the lower extremities.
0   Absence of lower extremity dystonia
1   Slight: Dystonia less than 10% of the time and does not interfere with normal positioning and/or functional activities
2   Mild: Dystonia less than 50% of the time and does not interfere with normal positioning and/or functional activities
3   Moderate: Dystonia more than 50% of the time and/or dystonia that interferes with normal positioning and/or lower extremity weight bearing or function
4   Severe: Dystonia more than 50% of the time and/or dystonia that prevents normal positioning and/or lower extremity weight bearing and/or function (e.g., cannot maintain standing due to severe dystonia at ankles)
*   Unable to assess eye movements
Left lower extremity: _____
Right lower extremity: _____

Total Score: _____   Rater's initials:

TABLE 168-4 ■ **Differential Diagnosis of Tremor**

Age
Alcohol use
Hepatocellular degeneration
Hyperthyroidism
Hysteric
Intention/ataxic
Peripheral neuropathy
Intention
Orthostatic
Palatal
Physiologic
Postural/action
Parkinson's disease
Essential tremor

which are currently treated by the neurosurgeon (Table 168–4). Tremor is a rhythmic movement that is classified as resting, intentional/kinetic, action, or postural/essential. Tremor can be described by its location, rate, and presence or absence with sleep. Exacerbating and alleviating factors are important, as are the functional implications of the tremor. Not all tremors fit clearly into these categories. Tremors can be associated with dystonia, myoclonus, asterixis, and orthostasis. As always, the history is important. In particular, family history, medical history, and environmental exposures are significant in diagnosing tremor.

Environmental exposures associated with a postural tremor include beta-agonists, dopamine agonists, amphetamines, lithium, tricyclic antidepressants, neuroleptics, theophylline, caffeine, valproic acid, alcohol, mercury, lead, arsenic, and other heavy metals. Heavy metals can also precipitate intentional tremors. Degenerative diseases associated with resting tremors include PD and Wilson's disease. Physiologic tremors can occur with emotional stress, extreme fatigue, or use of sympathomimetic medication. Tremors may also be psychogenic, but this is certainly a diagnosis of exclusion.[29]

The most common tremor and most common movement disorder is a 4- to 8-Hz "essential" or "benign" tremor that affects 415 of 100,000 adults older than the age of 40.[30] Familial autosomal dominant and sporadic variants exist. When this tremor presents late in life, it is referred to as a senile tremor. By definition, there are no other neurological symptoms or diseases. Classically, the essential tremor is postural and/or an action tremor of 4 to 11 Hz. Only in the most severe forms does it occur at rest. The tremor often presents in early adulthood. The term "benign" is inaccurate, because the amplitude can increase with age, severely limiting functional activity. Essential tremor preferentially affects the hands and upper extremities, but it can affect the oropharyngeal muscles and lower extremities. With thalamic stimulation, even voice tremor can be improved in three fourths of the patients.[31]

Parkinson's tremor occurs at rest, is exacerbated by anxiety, and disappears with activity and sleep. The tremor, often described as "pill rolling," owing to the flexion-extension movements of the fingers and wrist,

has a typical frequency of 3 to 5 Hz with variable amplitude. The "resting tremor" will disappear when the extremity is completely supported and without tone. Because a patient's extremities usually have some degree of muscular contraction, the tremor is usually present when the patient is awake and without volitional movement. Stress will augment the tremor. Parkinsonian tremor may affect the leg, jaw, lips, eyelids, and tongue. In advanced PD, postural and/or action tremor may also be present.

Intention tremor or kinetic tremor, the current preferred name, occurs with movement, is an involuntary, rhythmic 2- to 4-Hz oscillation, and often is present bilaterally. The hallmark of the kinetic tremor is the occurrence with precise movements. The tremor is absent at rest and during the initial portions of a movement but increases in amplitude as the movement progresses to fine motor control.[19] This tremor may also be referred to as an ataxic, cerebellar, or rubral tremor. The physiology of kinetic tremor is attributed to injury of the cerebellum and its corresponding tracts or the pathways between the motor cortex and the cerebellum. The etiology is variable, including postviral encephalitic syndromes, trauma, multiple sclerosis, or Wilson's disease.

Patients with bilateral tremor can be considered for thalamic stimulation on at least one side to minimize the risk of complications due to bilateral thalamotomy. If bilateral procedures are performed, the second procedure is often performed 6 to 12 months after the first. For PD patients, even those with tremor predominance, STN or GPi stimulators have been used to treat the tremor and present or future PD symptoms.

SPASTICITY

Spasticity defines the velocity-dependent increase in resistance to passive muscle movements that occurs with injury to the corticospinal tract or motor cortex. Spasticity is associated with weakness, hyperactive deep tendon reflexes, and clonus. The most common causes of spasticity include cerebral palsy, stroke, multiple sclerosis, and traumatic brain or spinal cord injuries. Pathologically, alpha motoneurons receive less inhibition. The alpha motoneurons develop an uninhibited reflex arc with the Ia afferents from muscle spindles. Spasticity must be distinguished from the conditions that often coexist: dystonia, rigidity, athetosis, ataxia, dyskinesia, and chorea.[32]

Selective dorsal rhizotomy (SDR) has been a common treatment of lower extremity spasticity since the mid-1980s. SDR may provide improved upper extremity spasticity in half the patients. An alternative nondestructive therapy for spasticity is the infusion of ITB by a subcutaneous pump. The clinical guidelines and physical size of the subcutaneous pump limit the implantation to those older than 4 years of age. However, size is the main consideration. We have implanted a pump into a 20-lb, 1-year-old child. Before either procedure is performed, patients should be clinically stable, at least 1 year beyond an inciting injury.[32] The only

TABLE 168–5 ■ Ashworth Score

1	No increase in tone
2	Slight increase in tone, a catch with passive flexion or extension
3	More prominent increase in tone
4	Marked increase in tone
5	Affected muscle group rigid with flexion or extension

From Ashworth B: Preliminary trial of carisoprodol in multiple sclerosis. Practitioner 192:540–542, 1964.

contraindications for ITB therapy are active infection or allergy to baclofen. Relative contraindications include hypotonia of the head and neck, a seizure disorder, renal failure, autonomic dysreflexia, psychotic disorders, age younger than 4 years, and pregnancy/lactation.

Patients' spasticity, motor strength, and functional ability need to be evaluated together. The Ashworth rating scale measures spasticity on a five-point scale that is reproducible[33] (Table 168–5). Spasticity is routinely measured in the quadriceps, abductors, hamstrings, and gastrocnemius. An average score is calculated, based on the number of muscle groups evaluated. Patients with mild spasticity are probably not candidates for surgical intervention, because mild spasticity is often a useful compensatory reaction to weakness. Patients with predominant lower extremity spasticity, without weakness, may benefit from either SDR or ITB. Patients with significant lower extremity spasticity and weakness may benefit most from ITB, because there is less risk of significant weakness from ITB than SDR.[34] Patients with upper and lower extremity spasticity are candidates for ITB. This option allows greater relief of the upper extremity symptoms than is possible with a dorsal rhizotomy, especially if the catheter tip is at the T4-6 level. In general, younger patients are better candidates for SDR, because they have a greater ability to acquire skills and develop strength (Fig. 168–3).

Before implantation of an ITB pump, patients undergo a trial of ITB. This may be done with escalating doses of baclofen delivered by sequential lumbar punctures (50, 75, and 100 μg of baclofen) or with continu-

ous infusion of ITB. A significant response to baclofen (a one- to two-point decrease in the Ashworth score) predicts a good clinical response to ITB therapy. Patients with excessive loss of tone during the trial are not excluded from ITB therapy because the implanted pump allows gradual titration of the dose. The primary risk of an indwelling intrathecal catheter is meningitis.[34]

Spasticity is a common clinical manifestation of CP and often coexists with other clinical conditions such as tendon contractures and learning disabilities. To best delineate the functional limitations of patients with spasticity and select the most appropriate clinical intervention, all new spasticity patients are evaluated in a multidisciplinary clinic that includes neurosurgery, physical therapy, orthopedic surgery, and social services. Each member of the team meets with the patient and family to make an independent assessment of the patient's abilities and disabilities, possible therapeutic interventions, and the patient's goals. The collaborative team then meets to discuss the patient's disorder and develop a consensus treatment plan. At the end of the clinic, the patient meets with a member of the treatment team to review the suggested therapeutic options and answer questions. Common treatment goals include improving function (e.g., gait), facilitating care, and delaying or preventing the development of contractures.

The multidisciplinary clinic facilitates the clinical evaluation of the patient, allowing him or her to see several clinicians on the same morning. It also allows members of the team to methodically organize the treatment plan. Orthopedic procedures may be delayed until the inciting spasticity is reduced. Physical therapy precedes neurosurgical procedures for patients at risk for greater weakness from neurosurgical procedures.

MYOCLONUS

Myoclonus is a sudden brief involuntary movement that is usually arrhythmic and irregular. Positive myoclonus describes the active contraction of muscles. Negative myoclonus describes the inhibition of ongoing muscle activity. An example of the latter is asterixis. Benign myoclonus most commonly occurs at the onset of sleep. Pathologic myoclonus is also associated with seizure disorders. Medical therapy with serotonin precursors, sodium valproate, and clonazepam can improve symptoms.[35] No surgical treatment for myoclonus exists.

HEMIFACIAL SPASM

Hemifacial spasm is a unique focal movement disorder often caused by vascular compression of the seventh cranial nerve, typically at the dorsal root exit zone. Hemifacial spasm typically begins around the eye and progresses caudad, to envelop the entire facial musculature and platysma. When present for a long time, tonus phenomenon, a sustained muscular contraction, is common. The standard therapy is microvascular de-

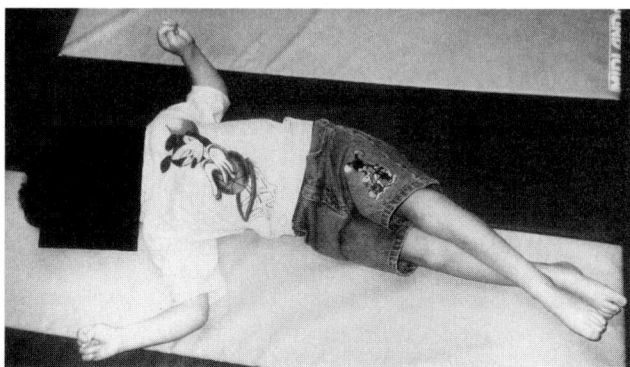

FIGURE 168–3. Patient with spastic cerebral palsy and scissoring of the lower extremities caused by spasticity.

compression via a retromastoid craniectomy. The differential diagnosis of hemifacial spasm includes essential blepharospasm (involuntary, bilateral repetitive and symmetric blinking), facial myokymia (continuous facial spasm often associated with a lesion of the brainstem), "habit" spasm (volitional), focal motor seizures, synkinesis after nerve injury, tardive dyskinesia, and Meige's syndrome (oromandibular dystonia and blepharospasm).[36-38] There is no evidence that these diseases will respond to microvascular decompression.

CONTRAINDICATIONS TO SURGERY

Relative contraindications to intracranial stereotactic procedures include coagulopathy, use of antiplatelet agents, and poorly controlled hypertension. These must be controlled before considering surgery. All aspirin-type products are discontinued 1 week before surgery. Intraoperatively, it is essential to monitor the patient's systolic blood pressure, because hypertension will significantly increase the risk of an intracerebral hemorrhage. We do not perforate the dura or lesion the brain until the systolic blood pressure is controlled, below 160 mm Hg.

These same conditions should be considered absolute contraindications for implantation of mechanical devices. There are several relative contraindications that apply to both implantable infusion pumps and deep brain stimulators that should be considered. Patients and families must understand that pumps and stimulators require ongoing maintenance. Poor access to facilities and staff who can maintain and adjust these devices should be considered before surgery. Furthermore, patients who are unreliable, demented, or psychologically impaired should not be offered this form of therapy.

ABLATION VERSUS STIMULATION

Whereas stereotactic ablative procedures may often achieve the same results as deep brain stimulation, the patient's unique situation must also be considered. In general, there is a trend toward deep brain stimulation in younger patients, with the belief that it avoids a permanent lesion, allows adjustment of the "physiologic lesion" as the disease progresses, and reserves the potential for future restorative procedures as they become available. The positive aspects must be balanced with the higher cost of deep brain stimulation, the need for frequent initial adjustments, and the need to replace the power source periodically. Deep brain stimulation is also preferred for bilateral procedures, to minimize the risk associated with bilateral lesion procedures.

CONCLUSION

The treatment of movement disorders is a challenging but rewarding area for neurosurgeons. The proper selection of surgical candidates is critical to achieving positive outcomes. Both the selection of patients and

TABLE 168-6 ■ **International Classification of Diseases, Tenth Revision: Neurological Adaptation (ICD-10 NA)**

Primary, Idiopathic

Classical type
Akinetic type
Tremor type
Postural instability—gait difficulty type
Hemiparkinsonism

Secondary Parkinsonism

Malignant neuroleptic syndrome
Other drug-induced secondary parkinsonism (neuroleptics, antiemetics, reserpine, lithium, diltiazem)
Secondary parkinsonism due to external agents (carbon monoxide, cyanide, methanol, MPTP)

Postencephalitic Parkinsonism (Encephalitis Lethargica, Slow Virus Infections)

Parkinsonism in Diseases Classified Elsewhere

Sporadic degenerative diseases
Familial degenerative and metabolic disorders (Huntington's disease, Leigh's disease, Wilson's disease)
Infectious diseases (AIDS, Creutzfeldt-Jakob disease, syphilis)
Parkinsonism in brain tumors, cerebrovascular disease, hydrocephalus, paraneoplastic syndromes and psychosomatic

Other Degenerative Diseases of the Basal Ganglia

Hallervorden-Spatz disease
Progressive supranuclear palsy
Striatonigral degeneration
Hemiparkinsonism-hemiatrophy syndrome
Corticobasal gangionic degeneration
Pallido-pyramidal-dentato-luysian degeneration
Dentato-rubral-pallido-lysian atrophy
Guamanian-type parkinsonism
Parkinsonism associated with calcification of the basal ganglia (Fahr's disease, hypoparathyroidism, pseudopoparathroidism, familial basal ganglia calcifications)

Dystonia

Drug-induced (acute and tardive dystonia and dyskinesia) tremor
Idiopathic familial dystonia
Idiopathic nonfamilial dystonia
Spasmotic torticollis
Idiopathic orofacial dystonia
Blepharospasm

Other Extrapyramidal and Movement Disorders

Essential tremor
Drug-induced tremor
Myoclonus
Drug-induced chorea
Other chorea
Drug-induced tics

From Jankovic J: International Classification of Diseases Tenth Revision: Neurological Adaptation (ICD-10 NA): Extrapyramidal and movement disorders. Mov Disord 10:533–540, 1995.

the follow-up evaluation can be facilitated with the use of standardized evaluation scales. Through multidisciplinary collaboration, neurosurgeons are able to improve the lives of patients who have a variety of movement disorders (Table 168-6).[39]

REFERENCES

1. Bennett DA, Beckett L, Murray A, et al: Prevalence of parkinsonian signs and associated mortality in a community population of older people. N Engl J Med 334:71–76, 1996.

2. Brooks DJ, Salmon EP, Mathias CJ, et al: The relationship between locomotor disability, autonomic dysfunction, and the integrity of the striatal dopaminergic system in patients with multiple system atrophy, pure autonomic failure, and Parkinson's disease, studied with PET. Brain 113:1539–1552, 1990.

3. Takikawa S, Dhawan V, Chaly T, et al: Input functions for 6-[fluorine-18] fluorodopa quantitation in parkinsonism: Comparative studies and clinical correlations. J Nucl Med 35:955–963, 1994.

4. Fahn S, Elton RI, Members of the UPDRS Development Committee: Unified Parkinson's disease rating scale. In Fahn S, Marsden CD, Calne DB, et al (eds): Recent Developments in Parkinson's Disease. Park Ridge, NJ, Parthenon, 1992, pp 89–112.

5. Goetz CG, Stebbins GT, Shale HM, et al: Utility of an objective dyskinesia rating scale for Parkinson's disease: Inter- and intrarater reliability assessment. Mov Disord 9:390–394, 1986.

6. Richards M, Marder K, Cote L, Mayeux R: Interrater reliability of the Unified Parkinson's Disease Rating Scale motor examination. Mov Disord 9:89–91, 1994.

7. Lang AE, Benabid AI, Koller WC, et al: The core assessment program for intracerebral transplantation. Mov Disord 10:527–528, 1995.

8. Langston JW, Widner H, Goetz CG, et al: Core assessment program for intracerebral transplantations (CAPIT). Mov Disord 7:2–13, 1992.

9. Brooks DJ: Positron emission tomography studies in movement disorders. Neurosurg Clin 9:263–281, 1998.

10. Broggi G: Chronic deep brain stimulation: Clinical results. In Germano IM (ed): Neurosurgical Treatment of Movement Disorders. Park Ridge, IL, American Association of Neurological Surgeons, 1998, pp 159–168.

11. Limousin P, Krack P, Pollak P, et al: Electrical stimulation of the subthalamic nucleus in advanced Parkinson's disease. N Engl J Med 339:1105–1111, 1998.

12. Bannister R: Extrapyramidal syndromes. In Bannister R (ed): Brain's Clinical Neurology, 6th ed. Frome, England, Butler & Tanner, 1987.

13. Jankovic J: The extrapyramidal disorders. In Wyngaarden JB, Smith LH, Bennett JC (eds): Cecil Textbook of Medicine, 19th ed. Philadelphia, WB Saunders, 1992, pp 2135–2136.

14. Tasker RR: Surgical treatment of the dystonias. In Gildengerg PL, Tasker RR (eds): Textbook of Stereotactic and Functional Neurosurgery. New York, McGraw-Hill, 1998.

15. Spiegel EA, Wycis HT: Effect of thalamic and pallidal lesions upon involuntary movements in choreoathetosis. Trans Am Neurol Assoc 75:234–236, 1950.

16. Spiegel EA, Wycis HT: Pallidothalamotomy in chorea. Arch Neurol Psychiatry 64:295–296, 1950.

17. Narabayashi H, Okuma T: Procaine-oil blocking of the globus pallidus for the treatment of rigidity and tremor of parkinsonism. Proc Jpn Acad 29:134–137, 1953.

18. Narabayashi H, Okuma T: Procaine-oil blocking of the globus pallidus. Arch Neurol 75:36–48, 1956.

19. Adams RD: Disorders of motility. In Adams RD (ed): Principles of Neurology, 4th ed. New York, McGraw-Hill, 1989.

20. Ceballos-Baumann AO, Passingham R, Warner T, et al: Overactive prefrontal and underactive motor cortical areas in idiopathic dystonia. Ann Neurol 37:363–372, 1995.

21. Marsden CD, Obeso JA, Zarranz JJ, Lang AE: The anatomical basis of symptomatic hemidystonia. Brain 108:463–483, 1985.

22. Nardocci N, Zorzi G, Grisoli M, et al: Acquired hemidystonia in childhood: A clinical and neuroradiological study of thirteen patients. Pediatr Neurol 15:108–113, 1996.

23. Albright AL: Spasticity and movement disorders. In Albright AL, Pollack I, Adelson PD (eds): Principles and Practice of Pediatric Neurosurgery. New York, Thieme, 1999.

24. Boyd K, Patterson V: Dopa responsive dystonia: A treatable condition misdiagnosed as cerebral palsy. BMJ 298:1019–1020, 1989.

25. Albright AL, Barry MJ, Painter MJ, Shultz B: Infusion of intrathecal baclofen for generalized dystonia in cerebral palsy. J Neurosurg 88:73–76, 1998.

26. Albright AL, Barry MJ, Fasick P, et al: Continuous intrathecal baclofen infusion for symptomatic generalized dystonia. Neurosurgery 38:934–939, 1996.

27. Barry MJ, Van Swearingen JM, Albright AL: Reliability and responsiveness of the Barry-Albright Dystonia Scale. Dev Med Child Neurol 41:404–411, 1999.

28. Fahn S, Marsden CD, Calne DB: Classification and investigation of dystonia. In Marsden CD, Fahn S (eds): Movement Disorders 2. London, Butterworth, 1987, pp 332–358.

29. Jankovic J, Lang AE: Classification of movement disorders. In Germano IM (ed): Neurosurgical Treatment of Movement Disorders. Park Ridge, Ill, American Association of Neurological Surgeons, 1998.

30. Haerer AF, Anderson DW, Schoenberg BS: Prevalence of essential tremor. Arch Neurol 39:750, 1982.

31. Osenbach RK, Burchiel KJ: Thalamotomy: Indications, techniques, and results. In Germano IM (ed): Neurosurgical Treatment of Movement Disorders. Park Ridge, Ill, American Association of Neurological Surgeons, 1998.

32. Albright AL: Spastic cerebral palsy: Approaches to drug treatment. CNS Drugs 4:17–27, 1995.

33. Ashworth B: Preliminary trial of carisoprodol in multiple sclerosis. Practitioner 192:540–542, 1964.

34. Albright AL: Baclofen in the treatment of cerebral palsy. J Child Neurol 11:77–83, 1996.

35. Bannister R: The dyskinesias. In Bannister R (ed): Brain's Clinical Neurology, 6th ed. Frome, England, Butler & Tanner, 1987.

36. Blair RL, Berry H: Spontaneous facial movement. J Otolaryngol 10:459–462, 1981.

37. Wilkins RH: Hemifacial spasm: A review. Surg Neurol 36:251–277, 1991.

38. Jannetta PJ, McLaughlin MR: Operative treatment of hemifacial spasm. In Germano IM (ed): Neurosurgical Treament of Movement Disorders. Park Ridge, Ill, American Association of Neurological Surgeons, 1998.

39. Jankovic J: International Classification of Diseases, Tenth Revision: Neurological Adaptation (ICD-10 NA): Extrapyramidal and movement disorders. Mov Disord 10:533–540, 1995.

Positron Emission Tomography in Movement Disorders

DAVID J. BROOKS

Positron emission tomography (PET) provides a sensitive means of detecting and characterizing the regional changes in brain metabolism and receptor binding associated with movement disorders. It can have diagnostic value and help to throw light on the pathophysiology underlying parkinsonian syndromes and involuntary movement disorders. PET also provides a means of detecting subclinical disease in the subcortical degenerations and of objectively following the progression of Parkinson's disease (PD) and Huntington's disease (HD).

PET cameras can detect 10^{-12} molar concentrations of radiotracers and have a resolution of 3 to 5 mm. They allow quantitative, in vivo examination of regional cerebral blood fow (rCBF); glucose, oxygen, and dopa metabolism; and brain neuroreceptor binding. The PET radiotracers commonly used for studying movement disorders are provided in Table 169–1.

The changes in regional cerebral function that characterize different movement disorders can be examined in two main ways. First, focal changes in resting levels of regional cerebral metabolism, blood flow, and neuroreceptor binding can be measured. Second, abnormal patterns of brain activation can be detected when patients with movement disorders perform motor and cognitive tasks.

PARKINSON'S DISEASE

The pathologic hallmark of PD is degeneration of pigmented and other brainstem nuclei in association with the formation of neuronal Lewy inclusion bodies. Loss of cells from the substantia nigra in PD results in profound dopamine depletion in the striatum, with lateral nigral projections to posterior putamen being most affected. The pathology of PD targets subcortical nuclei, but the cortex is also involved. It remains uncertain whether Lewy body dementia and PD represent ends of a spectrum.

Presynaptic Dopaminergic System

The function of the presynaptic dopaminergic system in PD can be examined in vivo with PET in three ways:

by measuring terminal dopa decarboxylase (DDC) activity by uptake of ^{18}F-dopa; by assessing the availability of dopamine transporters with ^{11}C-nomifensine or the tropane-based tracers ^{11}C-CFT, ^{18}F-CFT, and ^{11}C-RTI-32; and by estimating dopamine vesicle transporter density with ^{11}C-dihydrotetrabenazine (DHTBZ).

After intravenous administration, ^{18}F-dopa is taken up by the terminals of dopaminergic projections, where it is converted to ^{18}F-dopamine and stored in vesicles. In early hemiparkinsonism, ^{18}F-dopa PET shows preserved caudate but bilaterally reduced putamen tracer uptake and indicates depressed activity in the putamen contralateral to the affected limbs.[1] Subclinical disease can be detected by PET in early PD as evidenced by involvement of the "asymptomatic" putamen contralateral to clinically unaffected limbs. Cases of early PD (i.e., Hoehn and Yahr stage 1) show a 30% to 40% loss of ^{18}F-dopa uptake in the putamen contralateral to the affected limbs, suggesting that this loss of DDC activity is the threshold for the onset of symptoms (Fig. 169–1). On average, PD patients have a 50% loss of specific putamen ^{18}F-dopa uptake, compared with a 60% to 80% loss of ventrolateral nigra compacta cells at postmortem.[2] As putamen dopamine levels are reduced by more than 90% in end-stage PD, striatal uptake of ^{18}F-dopa reflects dopamine terminal density rather than striatal levels of endogenous dopamine.

Initially, PET data sets of regional brain tracer uptake were collected in two-dimensional mode, that is, only recorded activity emitted within a given transaxial slice is recorded. PET data are now acquired in three-dimensional mode, which simultaneously detects all the activity in the three-dimensional brain volume. Although this leads to increased levels of scatter, the advantage is a sixfold increase in the signal-to-noise ratio and increased spatial resolution, allowing regions with low ^{18}F-dopa uptake to be sampled more sensitively. The increased signal allows scans to be converted from raw images of ^{18}F-dopa uptake to parametric influx constant (K_i) maps representing dopa decarboxylase activity on a voxel-by-voxel basis.

The advantage of generating K_i images is that significant changes in dopaminergic function associated

TABLE 169–1 ■ **PET Tracers Used for Studying Movement Disorders**

BIOLOGIC APPLICATION	TRACER
Blood flow	$H_2^{15}O$
Oxygen metabolism	$^{15}O_2$
Glucose metabolism	^{18}F-2-fluoro-2-deoxyglucose (^{18}FDG)
Dopamine storage	^{18}F-6-fluorodopa (^{18}F-dopa)
Dopamine vesicle transporters	^{11}C-dihydrotetrabenazine (DHTBZ)
Dopamine transporters	^{11}C-CFT, ^{18}F-CFT, ^{11}C-RTI-32, ^{11}C-methylphenidate (^{11}C-MP)
Dopamine D_1 sites	^{11}C-SCH 23390
Dopamine $D_{2/3}$ sites	^{11}C-raclopride, ^{11}C-methylspiperone ^{76}Br-bromospiperone, ^{18}F-spiperone
MAOB activity	^{11}C-deprenyl
Opioid binding sites	^{11}C-diprenorphine
Central benzodiazepine	^{11}C-flumazenil
Peripheral benzodiazepine	^{11}C-PK11195
Muscarinic	^{11}C-NMPB
Acetylcholine esterase	^{11}C-physostigmine

MAOB, monoamine oxidase B.

with PD can be localized throughout the whole brain volume using statistical parametric mapping. First, parametric images of ^{18}F-dopa influx constants (K_i) on a voxel-by-voxel basis are transformed into standard stereotactic space. Images of mean tracer K_i with associated standard deviations are then generated for the separate groups of controls and PD patients and used to compare ^{18}F-dopa storage on a voxel-by-voxel basis. The locations of volumes of significantly altered K_i values at a preassigned threshold (at least $P < .001$ to minimize spurious changes arising from the multiple comparisons performed) are then displayed, and the magnitudes of the changes are measured by sampling the transformed or untransformed data sets. This statistical parametric mapping approach is advantageous because it can detect changes in regional dopaminergic function in brain areas that might not have been predicted.

There is a strong dopaminergic projection from the midbrain tegmentum to prefrontal areas, and the substantia nigra is also rich in dopamine terminals. Three-dimensional ^{18}F-dopa PET coupled with statistical parametric mapping has been used to demonstrate bilateral K_i reductions in the caudate, putamen, midbrain, and anterior cingulate with disease progression, and individual K_i values correlate with the severity of disability on the Unified Parkinson's Disease Rating Scale (UPDRS) (Fig. 169–2).[3,4] It is severity of bradykinesia and rigidity, rather than tremor, that correlates with dopamine terminal function in PD.[5]

The PET dopamine transporter ligands ^{11}C-nomifensine, ^{11}C-CFT, ^{18}F-CFT, and ^{11}C-RTI-32 and the vesicle transporter tracer ^{11}C-DHTBZ also provide a sensitive means of differentiating PD patients from normal subjects.[6–10] Putamen uptake inversely correlates with locomotor disability. A direct comparison of putamen ^{18}F-dopa, ^{11}C-DHTBZ, and ^{11}C-methylphenidate uptake in PD has suggested that ^{18}F-dopa may overestimate and dopamine transporter tracers underestimate dopamine terminal function relative to ^{11}C-DHTBZ.[11]

Detection of Preclinical Disease

^{18}F-dopa PET has been used to study asymptomatic adult relatives in kindreds with familial PD.[12] Affected individuals from such kindreds show the typical pattern of striatal ^{18}F-dopa storage reduction associated with sporadic PD; putamen tracer uptake is more severely reduced than caudate uptake. Twenty-five percent of asymptomatic adult relatives scanned have shown significantly reduced levels of putamen ^{18}F-dopa uptake, and one third of these subclinical cases have gone on to develop clinical parkinsonism during 5 years of follow-up.

^{18}F-dopa PET findings have also been reported for 18 monozygotic and 16 dizygotic asymptomatic co-

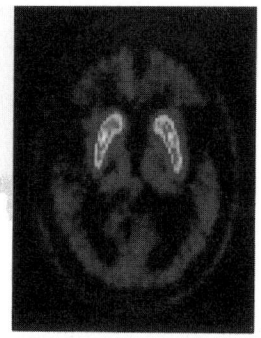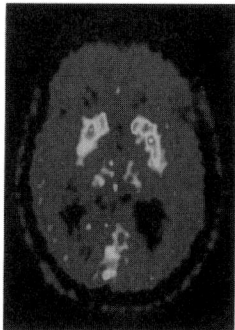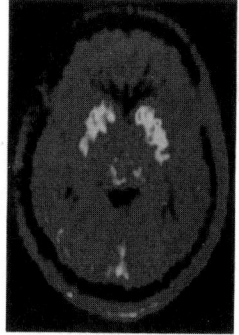

Normal subject **Early Parkinson's disease** **Advanced Parkinson's disease**

FIGURE 169–1. Positron emission tomographic images of striatal ^{18}F-dopa uptake in early and advanced Parkinson's disease. The caudate is relatively spared compared with the putamen (see color section in this volume). (Courtesy of J. S. Rakshi, MRC Cyclotron Unit, Hammersmith Hospital, London, UK.)

Saggital

Coronal

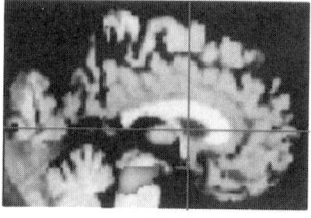

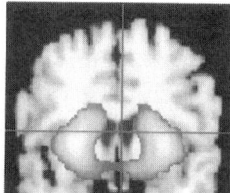

Transverse {left = right}

Saggital

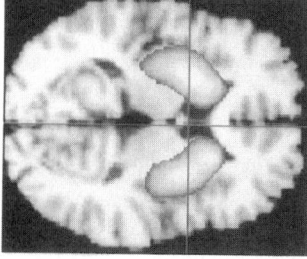

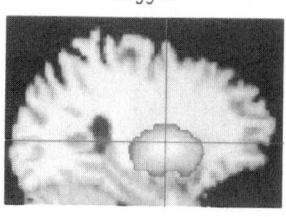

FIGURE 169–2. A statistical parametric map shows the location of significant reductions in ^{18}F-dopa uptake for a group of seven patients with advanced Parkinson's disease compared with seven age-matched, normal controls ($P < .001$). The ^{18}F-dopa uptake is reduced bilaterally in the putamen, caudate, and substantia nigra (see color section in this volume). (Courtesy of J. S. Rakshi, MRC Cyclotron Unit, Hammersmith Hospital, London, UK.)

twins of PD patients with sporadic disease.[13] Both twin groups had a mean age close to 60 years. Ten of the 18 monozygotic and two of the 16 dizygotic co-twins had reduced levels of putamen ^{18}F-dopa uptake, yielding significantly different 56% and 12% concordances for dopaminergic dysfunction ($P < .03$). Over 5 years, the monozygotic co-twin cohort showed further mean reductions in putamen ^{18}F-dopa uptake (4.5% per year), whereas the dizygotic co-twin group showed no significant change (1.3% per year). Two of the monozygotic co-twins developed clinical signs of parkinsonism. These findings strongly support a role of inheritance in apparently sporadic PD.

Measuring Progression of Parkinson's Disease

Vingerhoets and coworkers[14] were the first to demonstrate that loss of striatal ^{18}F-dopa uptake occurs more rapidly in PD than in age-matched controls. One difficulty with this study, however, was that whole striatal regions of interest were employed to analyze disease progression, whereas the pathologic process of PD targets dopamine levels in the dorsal putamen. Such an approach, therefore, inevitably underestimates disease progression.

Morrish and coworkers[15] directly measured dorsal putamen ^{18}F-dopa influx constants and found a mean 12% annual decline in baseline putamen K_i values for a group of 17 PD patients with a baseline clinical disease duration of 40 months when scanned serially a mean period of 18 months apart. Ten controls showed

no significant change in putamen ^{18}F-dopa uptake over 3 years. These workers subsequently extended their data set to a cohort of 32 PD patients and reported mean 9% and 3% annual declines of putamen and caudate ^{18}F-dopa K_i values, respectively.[16] When the duration of clinical disease was less than 2 years, patients appeared to be losing dopaminergic function most rapidly (18% versus 2% per year). Extrapolation of levels of putamen ^{18}F-dopa uptake suggested a preclinical disease window of 6 ± 3 years and symptom onset after a 30% fall in putamen ^{18}F-dopa uptake from normal mean levels.

These ^{18}F-dopa PET findings are strikingly similar to those reported in a cross-sectional study in which postmortem nigral cell counts were correlated with estimated clinical disease duration.[17] This study suggested that nigral cell loss occurs at 10 times the rate of loss associated with natural aging (4.5% versus 0.47% per year) and estimated a mean preclinical disease period in PD of 4.7 years and symptom onset after a 30% loss of nigral dopamine neurons due to the disease process.

A subsequent ^{18}F-dopa PET study from Finland reported a 9% per year loss of dopamine terminal function in PD patients and a mean 2-year duration of clinical symptoms.[18] Such PET studies open the way to objectively test the efficacy of putative neuroprotective agents for this disorder. A tracer, ^{11}C-PK11195, has been developed as a marker of neuroinflammation.[19] This ligand binds to peripheral benzodiazepine sites expressed by the mitochondria of activated microglia in the brain. It is possible to demonstrate the presence of such binding in the brainstem and basal ganglia of PD patients.[20] This opens the intriguing possibility of being able to monitor the inflammatory component of this degenerative disorder and possibly detect beneficial effects of anti-inflammatory agents.

Fetal Graft Function in Parkinson's Disease

As well as providing a means of following natural disease progression, ^{18}F-dopa PET provides a means of examining the function of restorative therapies in PD, such as striatal implants of fetal mesencephalic tissue. The Lund group[21] reported serial clinical and ^{18}F-dopa PET findings over 6 years for two PD patients after fetal engraftment into the putamen contralateral to their more affected limbs. Both patients have maintained significant clinical improvement, particularly in time spent "on" and in dexterity of the limbs contralateral to the putamen engrafted. One of the two received bilateral putamen implants after 5 years, and the other was satisfied with his situation and did not want further surgery.

Another four unilaterally transplanted PD patients showed ^{18}F-dopa PET evidence of graft function 1 year after surgery, and all had a second graft into the opposite putamen.[21] Three of these four responded well to transplantation, but the fourth deteriorated and is showing signs suggestive of atypical disease. Another series of five PD patients transplanted bilaterally into the putamen and caudate is also showing a good clini-

Pregraft   8 Months   20 Months

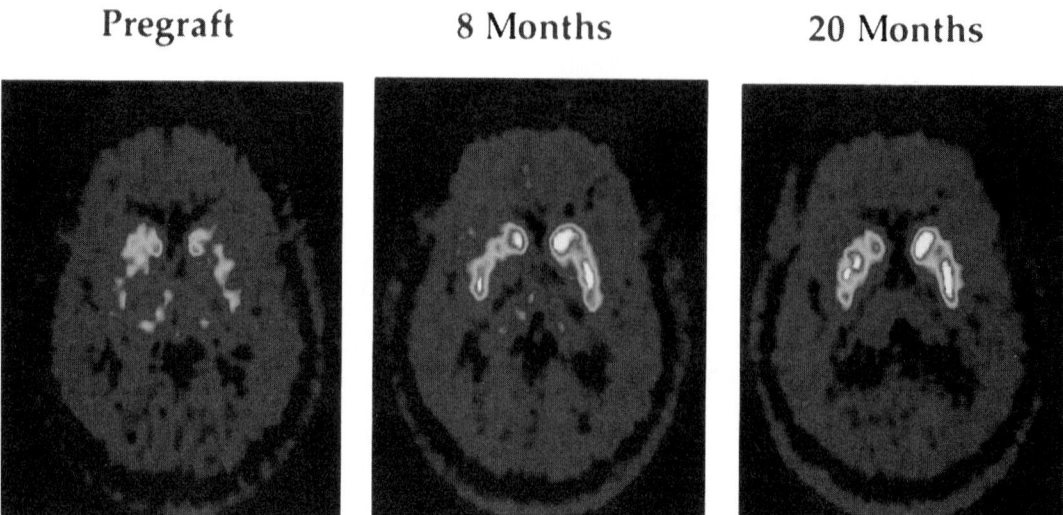

FIGURE 169–3. Positron emission tomographic images of striatal ^{18}F-dopa uptake were collected 30 to 90 minutes after tracer administration for a patient with Parkinson's disease before, 8 months after, and 20 months after bilateral implantation of fetal mesencephalic tissue into the caudate and putamen (see color section in this volume). (Courtesy of P. Piccini, MRC Cyclotron Unit, Hammersmith Hospital, London, UK.)

cal response (Fig. 169–3).[22] Putamen and caudate ^{18}F-dopa uptake increased by 61% and 24%, respectively, over 2 years, and the UPDRS motor score improved by 54%. L-dopa medication could be withdrawn in one of these five cases.

Clinically successful transplantation of fetal tissue with corroborative serial ^{18}F-dopa PET findings has also been reported for five PD patients in a 2-year follow-up French study and for four PD patients in a series from Tampa, Florida.[24] In the French study, grafted putamen K_i values were shown to correlate well with the percentage of time spent in the "on" state during the day and measures of finger dexterity while in the "off" state. One of the transplanted PD patients in the Florida series subsequently died of an unrelated cause, and at postmortem, viable tyrosine hydroxylase–staining graft tissue forming connections with host neurons was seen.[25] This finding confirms that ^{18}F-dopa PET is measuring graft function rather than simply reflecting a host reaction to foreign tissue or the presence of blood-brain barrier breakdown. As a consequence of these pilot data, two major studies on the efficacy of implantation of fetal cells in PD have been sponsored by the National Institutes of Health in the United States.

Postsynaptic Dopamine System and Dyskinesias

^{11}C-SCH23390 PET studies suggest that striatal dopamine D_1 site binding is normal in untreated PD, whereas patients who have been exposed to L-dopa show mild reductions.[26–28] Levels of striatal D_1 binding appear to be similar in PD patients who have sustained or have fluctuating or dyskinetic responses to treatment, provided they are matched for clinical disease duration. This suggests that onset of treatment complications is not primarily related to changes in striatal D_1 receptor availability.

Several PET ligands have been used to study striatal D_2 receptor binding in PD. Striatal uptake of ^{11}C-methylspiperone is normal in de novo PD patients,[29] whereas ^{11}C-raclopride PET studies show 10% to 20% increases in putamen D_2 binding in de novo hemiparkinsonism contralateral to the more affected limbs.[27, 30] Striatal ^{11}C-methylspiperone binding is not influenced by levels of endogenous dopamine, but ^{11}C-raclopride competes with dopamine for D_2 sites. These findings suggest that overall D_2 receptor density may be normal in de novo PD but that availability of these sites to ^{11}C-raclopride becomes increased because of the low levels of endogenous dopamine present.

Striatal D_2 binding in treated PD cases has been reported to be normal or mildly decreased.[27, 31] Serial ^{11}C-raclopride PET studies suggest that the initially increased putamen D_2 binding in de novo PD patients normalizes after several months of exposure to L-dopa.[32] Long-term–treated PD cases continue to show normal levels of putamen but develop reduced caudate D_2 binding. Levels of putamen and caudate D_2 binding appear to be similar in treated PD patients, regardless of whether they have sustained or have fluctuating or dyskinetic responses to treatment, provided they are matched for clinical disease duration. It seems likely that development of dyskinetic responses to L-dopa involves changes in function of postsynaptic, nondopaminergic pathways rather than dopaminergic pathways. Animal models of PD suggest that dyskinesias may be associated with abnormal rises in basal ganglia enkephalin and dynorphin levels. PET evidence of reduced opioid receptor availability to ^{11}C-diprenorphine in the striatum and cingulate of dyskinetic PD patients has been reported in support of this hypothesis.[33]

Resting Brain Metabolism

PET studies have shown relatively raised levels of resting oxygen and glucose metabolism in the contralateral lentiform nucleus of hemiparkinsonian patients with early disease, whereas PD patients with established bilateral involvement have normal levels of lentiform metabolism.[34, 35] Principal component analysis applied to [18]fluorodeoxyglucose positron emission tomography ([18]FDG-PET) findings, however, reveals an abnormal metabolic pattern in all PD cases, with relatively raised resting lentiform nucleus and lowered frontal metabolism in these patients.[36] The degree of expression of this component has been reported to correlate with disease severity.[37]

Initially, nondemented PD patients were thought to have normal cortical metabolism, but this view is changing. [18]FDG-PET data from our unit has shown reduced absolute parietotemporal glucose metabolism in one third of such patients.[38] Principal component analysis applied to [18]FDG-PET findings has revealed a component with relative parietal hypofunction, expression of which correlates with performance on tests of verbal memory and visual perception.[39] The [18]FDG-PET scans of frankly demented patients show an Alzheimer pattern of impaired brain glucose use, with the posterior parietal and temporal association areas being most affected and with lesser involvement of the prefrontal cortex.[40] It is unclear whether this pattern of glucose hypometabolism in demented PD patients reflects coincidental Alzheimer's disease (AD), cortical Lewy body disease (LBD), loss of cholinergic projections, or some other degenerative process. PET studies have shown that frontal muscarinic binding is elevated in demented PD patients from the loss of acetylcholine.[41] One clinicopathologic series suggested that AD and LBD are associated with similar cortical patterns of metabolic dysfunction but that LBD cases have greater occipital involvement.

Pallidotomy is effective therapy for PD. Current theories on basal ganglia connectivity argue that loss of striatal dopamine in PD is associated with increased excitation of the internal globus pallidus (GPi) by the striatum, resulting in excessive inhibitory pallidal output to the ventral thalamus and cortex. By lesioning the motor GPi, it was argued that the excessive inhibition would be removed, facilitating volitional movements in PD patients. It is now established that pallidotomy leads to moderate improvements in rigidity and bradykinesia, but paradoxically, its main effect appears to be to abolish L-dopa–induced dyskinesias.

One [18]FDG-PET study reported the functional effects of medial pallidotomy in PD on regional resting glucose metabolism.[42] Postoperatively, pallidotomy was found to have increased the resting metabolism of primary motor cortex, lateral premotor cortex (LPMC), and dorsolateral prefrontal cortex (DLPFC). Preoperative levels of lentiform nucleus metabolism correlated with postoperative clinical outcome. Principal component analysis showed that the PD patient group preoperatively expressed the usual abnormal pattern of relatively increased lentiform and reduced premotor resting metabolism. Medial pallidotomy resulted in relative declines in resting lentiform and thalamic glucose metabolism and increases in supplementary motor area (SMA) metabolism, normalizing this pattern. The degree of change in this pattern of covariance postoperatively correlated with improvement of clinical disability. Perhaps surprisingly, postoperative clinical outcome and resting metabolic changes did not correlate with the size of the pallidotomy lesion as measured volumetrically with magnetic resonance imaging (MRI).

Activation Studies

Studies of resting cerebral blood flow and metabolism provide insight into the pathophysiology of the cerebral dysfunction underlying movement disorders. A more sensitive way of elucidating the nature of the functional disturbance underlying the bradykinesia of PD is to challenge the system by asking patients to perform motor or cognitive tasks. Associated changes in regional cerebral blood flow (rCBF) can then be measured with $H_2^{15}O$ PET.

When normal subjects make paced movements of a joystick in freely selected directions with their right hands, there are associated rCBF increases in contralateral sensorimotor cortex (SMC) and lentiform nucleus and bilaterally in anterior cingulate cortex, SMA, LPMC, and DLPFC.[43] Self-paced extensions of the index finger result in a similar pattern of activation.[44] When PD patients, scanned after stopping their medication for 12 hours, perform the same motor tasks, normal levels of activation of SMC, PMC, and lateral parietal association areas are seen. However, there is selectively impaired activation of the contralateral lentiform nucleus and the anterior cingulate, SMA, and DLPFC in cortical areas that receive a major input from the basal ganglia.

It is thought that the DLPFC plays a crucial role in motor decision making and that the SMA prepares and optimizes volitional motor programs, once selected. In contrast, the LPMC is believed to have a primary role in facilitating motor responses to external visual and auditory stimuli. An inability to activate SMA and DLPFC during freely selected movements could explain the difficulty that PD patients experience in initiating such movements. In contrast, their ability to activate the LPMC normally allows them to respond effectively to visual and auditory cues. This may explain why stepping over lines on the floor aids their walking. It has been shown that, during performance of sequential finger movements, PD patients overactivate lateral parietal and premotor areas[45] and the cerebellum.[46]

If akinesia in PD results from a failure to activate the basal ganglia–SMA and DLPFC projections because of a loss of dopamine, replacement therapy should restore activation of this system. When apomorphine, a combined D_1 plus D_2 agonist, is given subcutaneously to PD patients, resolution of their akinesia is associated with selective increases in SMA and DLPFC blood flow, providing further evidence for the role of these structures in the generation of motor programs.[47, 48]

Two centers have reported the functional effects of pallidotomy on cerebral activation in PD. Grafton and coworkers[49] examined the regional cerebral activation in six PD patients associated with reaching out to grasp lighted targets every 3 seconds while off medication. Despite an absence of change in patient performance, this patient group showed significantly increased SMA and lateral premotor activation after pallidotomy. This externally cued motor task was not designed to activate prefrontal areas. Subsequently, we demonstrated significantly increased activation of the SMA, LPMC, and DLPFC in PD patients after pallidotomy when making joystick movements in freely selected directions while off medication.[50] The findings of these activation studies therefore lend support to the hypothesis that pallidotomy results in removal of excess pallidal inhibitory drive to frontal association areas in PD patients.

There have been three PET reports on the effects of high-frequency electrical pallidal stimulation on regional brain function. In one study, levels of resting rCBF were measured with the stimulator switched off, switched on at a subeffective intensity, and switched on at an effective intensity.[51] Effective GPi stimulation improved contralateral bradykinesia and rigidity in eight of the nine PD patients when they were assessed off medication, and this was associated with increased resting SMA and putamen or external pallidal rCBF. Stimulation of the GPi at a lower intensity did not lead to clinical improvement or increase SMA rCBF. The investigators concluded that decreased akinesia in PD after pallidal stimulation resulted from increased SMA activation, although this study was not strictly an activation study. The investigators thought that the increased levels of putamen or external pallidal rCBF reflected antidromic stimulation.

In two $H_2^{15}O$ PET studies, changes in regional brain activation associated with moving a joystick in freely chosen directions or with reaching to touch a visual target were measured during pallidal stimulation. In the first report, six PD patients were studied while off medication with the GPi stimulator switched off and then with the stimulator switched on.[52] In this study, clinically effective GPi stimulation did not lead to any significant changes in levels of SMA or DLPFC activation during free choice joystick movements. In the second study, clinically effective GPi stimulation led to increased lateral premotor and anterior cingulate activation during the reaching task.[53]

Taken together, the findings of these PET studies lend support to the hypothesis that a reduction in internal pallidal output by lesioning or high-frequency stimulation results in removal of excess inhibitory drive to premotor and prefrontal areas in PD, improving fluency of movement.

Although the excessive inhibitory output of the GPi can be reduced by medial pallidotomy, an alternative approach is to reduce the excitatory input to GPi from the subthalamic nucleus (STN) by means of high-frequency electrical stimulation. This approach has resulted in dramatic relief of bradykinesia and rigidity, although it may be less effective than pallidotomy in relieving dyskinesias.

There have been two reports of $H_2^{15}O$ PET activation findings in PD patients before and after STN stimulation. In both studies, levels of rCBF were measured in patients with PD when off medication during performance of paced joystick movements in freely selected directions. The first study reported relative increases in activation of rostral SMA, lateral premotor, LPMC, and DLPFC during movement when the STN stimulator was switched on. These findings were similar to those reported after pallidotomy. In contrast to pallidotomy, STN stimulation was also associated with reduced motor cortex activation and led to increases in resting thalamic and decreases in resting motor cortex and caudal SMA rCBF.[52] The second study also found that STN stimulation in their six PD patients led to increased SMA and DLPFC activation and decreased motor cortex activation.[54] The mechanism causing the decreased motor cortex activation remains unclear, although antidromic stimulation of direct projections to STN may be a possibility.

Pallidotomy, pallidal stimulation, and subthalamic stimulation all appear to increase levels of premotor and dorsal prefrontal activation in PD along with resolution of bradykinesia, adding further support to the suggestion that these areas play a primary role in planning and preparing actions.

Dopaminergic Function and Tremor

^{18}F-dopa PET studies on patients with postural, rest, and rubral tremors have been reported. One study involved 31 patients with isolated tremor, including 20 with predominantly postural tremor (8 familial and 12 sporadic) and 11 with predominantly parkinsonian rest tremor.[55] Striatal ^{18}F-dopa uptake fell in the normal range for all eight familial essential tremor cases. However, 2 of 12 patients with sporadic postural tremor had subnormal putamen ^{18}F-dopa K_i values, with one falling in the PD range for a patient who later became akinetic as disease progressed. These findings argue against dopaminergic dysfunction being associated with most essential tremors but confirm that postural tremor occasionally can be a presenting feature of PD.

In contrast, all 11 patients with resting tremor showed reduced putamen but preserved caudate ^{18}F-dopa uptake, a pattern of loss similar to that found in patients fulfilling the UK Brain Bank criteria for PD. Remy and coworkers[56] also reported that six patients with midbrain tremors associated with peduncular lesions had reduced putamen ^{18}F-dopa uptake. Playford and colleagues[57] performed ^{18}F-dopa PET on three essential tremor patients who developed a transient parkinsonian rest tremor during neuroleptic exposure. Striatal ^{18}F-dopa uptake was entirely normal in these patients. Combined, these ^{18}F-dopa PET findings support Lamarre's hypothesis that a postural "essential" tremor arises from overactivity of olivorubrocerebellar connections, whereas a parkinsonian rest tremor requires additional interruption of dopaminergic connections structurally or through dopamine receptor blockade.[58]

ATYPICAL PARKINSONIAN SYNDROMES

Multiple System Atrophy

Multiple system atrophy (MSA) includes striatonigral degeneration (SND), olivopontocerebellar atrophy (OPCA), and progressive autonomic failure (PAF) within its spectrum. [18]FDG-PET studies of patients with probable SND have reported reduced levels of striatal glucose metabolism, in contrast to PD, in which striatal metabolism is preserved.[59] In one series, 8 of 10 L-dopa–nonresponsive, akinetic-rigid patients were reported to have reduced striatal metabolism. L-dopa–responsive patients had a normal or raised striatal metabolism.[60] This study also reported that akinetic-rigid patients with low levels of striatal glucose metabolism, regardless of L-dopa response, showed little improvement after pallidotomy.[61] When patients have the full syndrome of MSA with parkinsonism, autonomic failure, and cerebellar ataxia, cerebellar metabolism is also reduced.[62] [18]FDG-PET therefore provides a sensitive means of detecting the presence of striatal and cerebellar dysfunction when atypical parkinsonism is suspected.

In patients with probable SND, function of the presynaptic and postsynaptic dopaminergic systems is impaired. As in PD, specific putamen ^{18}F-dopa and ^{11}C-nomifensine uptake is reduced to about 50% of normal levels in established SND, and individual levels of putamen ^{18}F-dopa uptake correlate with locomotor status.[2] In patients with the full syndrome of MSA, caudate uptake of ^{18}F-dopa and ^{11}C-nomifensine is significantly more depressed than in PD patients.[59, 63] This finding suggests that the nigra is more uniformly involved by the pathology of SND than PD, and pathologic studies confirm this. The pattern of caudate and putamen ^{18}F-dopa uptake, however, only discriminates SND from PD with 70% specificity,[64] and [18]FDG-PET appears to provide a more sensitive tool than ^{18}F-dopa PET for this purpose.[65]

Striatal dopamine D_1 and D_2 binding has been studied with PET in SND. Mild but significant reductions in mean putamen ^{11}C-SCH23390 and ^{11}C-raclopride uptake have been reported, although an overlap of the SND, normal, and PD ranges is evident.[28, 66, 67] Striatal D_1 and D_2 binding does not appear to provide sensitive differentiation of possible SND from PD, although it characterizes the full syndrome of MSA. Because a significant number of parkinsonian patients who respond poorly to L-dopa retain normal levels of striatal D_2 binding, it seems likely that degeneration of downstream brainstem and pallidal, rather than striatal, projections is responsible for their poor response to L-dopa. The basal ganglia are rich in opioid peptides and their binding sites, and they are differentially affected in SND and PD. ^{11}C-diprenorphine is a nonspecific opioid antagonist binding with equal affinity for μ, κ, and δ sites. In nondyskinetic PD patients, caudate and putamen uptake of ^{11}C-diprenorphine is preserved, whereas putamen uptake is reduced in 50% of patients thought to have SND.[68]

Progressive Supranuclear Palsy

Progressive supranuclear palsy (PSP) usually refers to Steele-Richardson-Olszewski syndrome. It is characterized pathologically by neurofibrillary tangle formation and neuronal loss in the basal ganglia, superior colliculi, brainstem nuclei, and the periaqueductal grey matter. There have been a number of studies of regional cerebral glucose and oxygen metabolism in patients with probable PSP, several of whom have later had the diagnosis confirmed at autopsy. Cortical metabolism is globally depressed in this condition, and frontal areas are particularly targeted, with levels of metabolism correlating with disease duration and performance on psychometric tests of frontal function.[69–72] Hypofrontality, however, is not specific for PSP; it can be seen in PD, SND, Pick's disease, HD, and depression. Basal ganglia, cerebellar, and thalamic glucose metabolism are also depressed in PSP, distinguishing it from PD, in which metabolism is preserved (Fig. 169–4). Although [18]FDG-PET reliably distinguishes PSP from PD, it is not able to discriminate PSP from SND, because striatal and frontal hypometabolism can occur in both disorders.

Because the pathologic process of PSP targets nigrostriatal dopaminergic projections, striatal ^{18}F-dopa uptake in PSP is significantly reduced, and levels correlate with disease duration.[2, 73, 74] Unlike PD, however, putamen and caudate ^{18}F-dopa uptake appear to be equally affected in PSP, suggesting that the nigra is uniformly involved by the pathology, which is in line with pathologic reports. One report suggests that this is also the case for uptake of the dopamine transporter ligand ^{11}C-CFT.[75] In practice, 90% of PSP patients can be discriminated from PD cases with ^{18}F-dopa PET on the basis of uniform caudate and putamen involvement.[64] There appears to be little correlation between levels of striatal ^{18}F-dopa uptake in PSP and the degree of disability. Unlike PD and SND, in which locomotor impairment appears to principally result from loss of dopaminergic fibers, loss of mobility in PSP is probably determined by degeneration of other basal ganglia and brainstem projections. An ^{11}C-physostigmine PET study reported reduced striatal acetylcholine esterase activity in PSP but not in PD.[76] Reductions in striatal ^{11}C-physostigmine uptake correlated with locomotor disability in PSP, and striatal cholinergic function may play a role in determining the mobility of these patients.

Caudate and putamen D_2 binding in PSP has also been extensively studied with PET. Although mean binding is invariably reduced, only 50% to 70% of PSP patients have significant receptor loss.[66, 77] It is likely that, as in SND, degeneration of downstream pallidal and brainstem projections is also in part responsible for the poor L-dopa response of PSP patients. One study has examined striatal opioid binding in PSP.[68] Striatal ^{11}C-diprenorphine was reduced in all six cases studied, and in contrast to SND in which caudate function was spared, caudate and putamen were equally affected in PSP.

Corticobasal Degeneration

Corticobasal degeneration (CBD) is also known as corticobasal ganglionic degeneration, corticodentatonigral

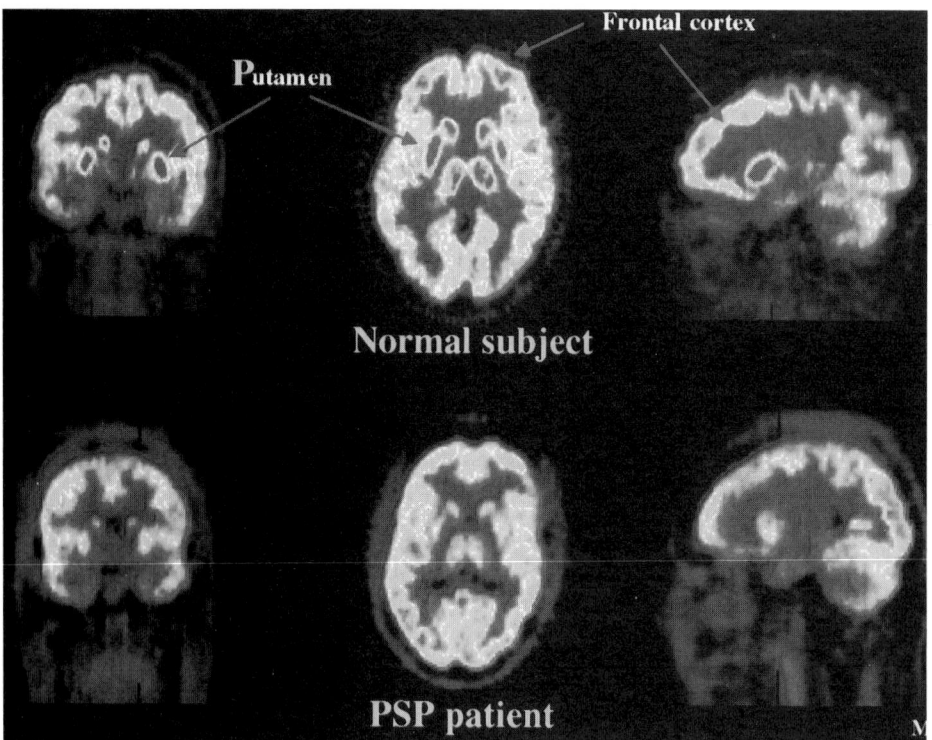

FIGURE 169–4. Fluorodeoxyglucose positron-emission tomographic (¹⁸FDG-PET) images of regional cerebral glucose metabolism for a normal person and a patient with progressive supranuclear palsy (PSP). The patient with PSP shows reduced frontal, striatal, and thalamic glucose use (see color section in this volume). (Courtesy of P. Piccini, MRC Cyclotron Unit, Hammersmith Hospital, London, UK.)

degeneration, and neuronal achromasia. Patients present with an akinetic-rigid, apraxic limb that may exhibit alien behavior. Cortical sensory loss, dysphasia, myoclonus, supranuclear gaze problems, and bulbar dysfunction are also features, but intellect is spared until late in the course of disease. Eventually, all four limbs become involved, and the condition is invariably poorly responsive to L-dopa. The pathology consists of collections of swollen, achromatic, tau-positive–staining Pick cells in the absence of argyrophilic Pick bodies, which target the posterior frontal, inferior parietal, and superior temporal lobes; the substantia nigra; and the cerebellar dentate nuclei.

PET studies of patients with the clinical syndrome of CBD have shown the greatest reductions in resting cortical oxygen and glucose metabolism in posterior frontal, inferior parietal, and superior temporal regions.[78–80] The thalamus and striatum are also involved, and the metabolic reductions are strikingly asymmetrical; they are most severe contralateral to the more affected limbs. This pattern contrasts with that seen in nondemented PD patients, who generally show preserved and symmetrical levels of regional cerebral glucose metabolism.

Striatal ¹⁸F-dopa uptake is reduced in CBD in an asymmetrical fashion and is most depressed contralateral to the more affected limbs.[78] In contrast to PD but similar to PSP, caudate and putamen tracer uptake are equally depressed in CBD. These PET findings help to differentiate CBD from Pick's disease, in which inferior frontal hypometabolism predominates; from PD, in which cortex striatal and glucose metabolism is preserved and caudate ¹⁸F-dopa uptake is spared; and from PSP, in which frontal and striatal metabolism

are more symmetrically involved and inferior parietal metabolism is often spared.[81]

INVOLUNTARY MOVEMENT DISORDERS

Huntington's Disease and Other Choreas

HD is an autosomal-dominant disorder associated with an excess (>38) of CAG triplet repeats in the *IT15* gene on chromosome 4. The function of this gene is still uncertain, but the pathology of HD targets medium-sized spiny projection neurons in the striatum. Patients with predominant chorea show a selective loss of striatolateral pallidal projections, which express γ-aminobutyric acid (GABA) and enkephalin, whereas those with a predominant akinetic-rigid syndrome show additional severe loss of striatomedial pallidal fibers containing GABA and dynorphin. Several other degenerative disorders can lead to chorea with background rigidity, including neuroacanthocytosis, dentatorubropallidoluysian atrophy, and benign familial chorea.

Inflammatory diseases such as systemic lupus erythematosus and Sydenham's chorea can be associated with chorea, as can tardive dyskinesia. The mechanism underlying tardive dyskinesia is uncertain; postmortem studies have reported low levels of subthalamic and pallidal glutamate decarboxylase activity, and neurochemical studies on a primate tardive dyskinesia model have reported severe depletion of subthalamic and pallidal GABA. These findings suggest that tardive dyskinesia, like HD, may be associated with deranged basal ganglia GABA transmission.

Clinically affected HD gene carriers show severely reduced levels of glucose and oxygen metabolism of the caudate and lentiform nuclei.[82–84] Levels of resting putamen metabolism correlate with locomotor function and caudate metabolism with performance on tests sensitive to frontal lobe function.[85, 86] In early HD, cortical metabolism is preserved, but as the disease progresses and dementia becomes prominent, it also declines, with the frontal cortex being targeted.[87] Caudate hypometabolism is not specific to HD. It is also seen in neuroacanthocytosis, dentatorubropallidoluysian atrophy, and some cases of benign familial chorea.[88, 89] In contrast, striatal glucose metabolism has been reported to be normal or elevated in chorea resulting from systemic lupus erythematosus, Sydenham's chorea, and tardive dyskinesia.[90–92]

Two $H_2^{15}O$ PET studies have examined patterns of cerebral activation in HD. Weeks and colleagues[93] found that HD patients showed impaired activation of contralateral putamen, sensorimotor cortex, caudal SMA and anterior cingulate, bilateral dorsal prefrontal and orbitofrontal cortex, and bilateral posterior parietal cortex when moving a joystick with the right arm in freely chosen directions. Insular activation was increased bilaterally. Weindl and associates[94] had their HD patients perform a paced finger opposition task and found impaired striatal, cingulate, SMA, and LPMC activation. Activation was bilaterally increased in inferolateral parietal area 40. The results from these two series are in reasonable agreement, both suggesting that the striatum and its frontal projection areas are underactive in HD during limb movement. This pattern is reminiscent of that seen in PD, although motor cortex and LPMC are underactive rather than overactive. This may well explain why choreic HD patients are also bradykinetic and have difficulties with neurobehavioral tests of frontal function.

The medium-sized spiny striatal neurons that degenerate in HD express D_1, D_2, opioid, and benzodiazepine receptors. PET studies have reported that striatal D_1 and D_2 binding is reduced in parallel, with at least a 30% loss in clinically affected HD gene carriers and with rigid cases being most severely affected.[31, 95, 96] Striatal opioid and benzodiazepine binding also are reduced in clinically affected HD patients.[97, 98] Reductions are relatively small (20%) compared with the mean 60% loss of dopamine receptor binding.

The finding of reduced striatal dopamine receptor binding in patients with HD is not specific; a mean 70% reduction of striatal ^{11}C-raclopride binding has been reported in neuroacanthocytosis.[99] In contrast, normal striatal D_2 binding has been reported in systemic lupus erythematosus chorea and tardive dyskinesia.[100, 101] This finding argues against the hypothesis that tardive dyskinesia results from striatal D_2 receptor supersensitivity after prolonged exposure to neurolepsis and suggests that the finding of downstream reductions in pallidal and subthalamic GABA levels may be of greater relevance.

DETECTION OF PRECLINICAL DISEASE

Clinically affected HD patients show at least a 30% loss of striatal glucose metabolism and dopamine receptor binding, suggesting that ^{18}FDG, ^{11}C-SCH23390, and ^{11}C-raclopride PET should all be capable of detecting subclinical dysfunction when present in asymptomatic HD gene carriers. Reduced striatal glucose metabolism and reduced D_1 and D_2 binding have been reported in 30% to 50% of asymptomatic adult gene carriers (Fig. 169–5).[102, 103] One study compared expression of abnormal metabolic patterns of regional brain glucose metabolism, detected with ^{18}FDG-PET and principal component analysis, and striatal dopamine receptor binding in asymptomatic and clinically affected HD gene carriers.[104] The study found that some asymptomatic HD

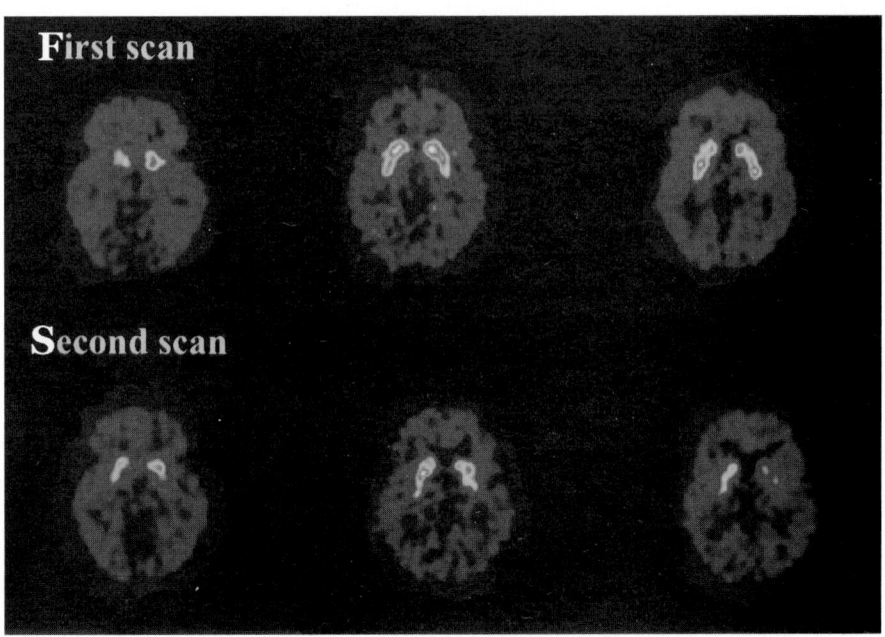

FIGURE 169–5. Positron emission tomographic images of serial striatal ^{11}C-SCH23390 uptake over 3 years for an adult who is an asymptomatic Huntington's disease gene carrier show progressive loss of striatal dopamine D_1 binding (see color section in this volume). (Courtesy of T. Andrews, MRC Cyclotron Unit, Hammersmith Hospital, London, UK.)

gene carriers expressed an abnormal pattern of relatively reduced striatal and mesial temporal glucose metabolism even in the presence of intact striatal D_2 binding.

MEASURING PROGRESSION OF HUNTINGTON'S DISEASE

With the advent of putative neuroprotective agents and therapeutic trials of striatal implants of fetal striatal cells in HD, the use of functional imaging as a surrogate marker of disease progression has become highly relevant. Using [18]FDG-PET, the caudate glucose metabolism was found to decline annually by 3% in early HD patients.[105, 106] Striatal D_1 and D_2 binding appears to be lost faster, falling at a mean annual rate of 4% to 6% in HD gene carriers with early clinical or subclinical disease.[106, 107] These findings suggest that PET provides an objective means of following HD progression. If future studies want to follow the function of implants of fetal striatal cells or the action of neurotrophic factors in HD, monitoring striatal dopamine receptor binding has an advantage over monitoring glucose metabolism. Regeneration of dopamine receptors should be a clear indication of cell regeneration, whereas increased glucose metabolism may reflect increased glial activity or an inflammatory process. Regeneration of striatal dopamine receptors after implantation with fetal striatal tissue has been demonstrated with PET in a rodent model of HD.[108]

Dystonia

Idiopathic torsion dystonia (ITD) is a dominantly inherited condition with a 40% penetrance and variable phenotype characterized by involuntary posturing and muscle spasms. The *DYT1* gene, which codes for the ATP-binding protein torsinA, has been localized to chromosome 9q34. Most Caucasian and Jewish kindreds with young-onset disease have a GAG deletion in the *DYT1* gene. TorsinA is expressed in the nigra and other brain areas, but pathologic studies have failed to identify consistent structural or neurotransmitter abnormalities in ITD. Patients with acquired hemidystonia often have associated structural lesions of the lentiform nucleus or posterior thalamus. Based on this observation, it has been suggested that ITD arises primary from basal ganglia dysfunction, reduced inhibitory output from the pallidum to ventral thalamus, and frontal association areas, causing them to become inappropriately overactive.

There have been a number of [18]FDG-PET studies on resting levels of regional cerebral glucose metabolism in dystonia. A problem in interpreting the findings of early studies arises from the heterogeneity of the patient groups recruited; familial, sporadic, and acquired dystonia have all been considered together, and patients with focal or hemidystonia have been favored to allow side-to-side comparisons of basal ganglia function. As a consequence, the relevance of some PET findings for familial ITD is uncertain. Some patients, supposedly at rest, were experiencing active muscular

spasms during scanning. Resting lentiform nucleus metabolism in dystonia has been variously reported to be increased,[109, 110] normal,[111–113] and decreased.[114]

Principal component analysis has been applied to [18]FDG-PET data obtained for symptomatic and clinically unaffected *DYT1* gene carriers.[115] Symptomatic carriers have also been studied when awake with dystonic spasms and again after drug-induced sleep when spasm free. This has allowed movement-free and related abnormal patterns of resting regional cerebral glucose metabolism to be identified in *DYT1* gene carriers. The movement-free pattern was characterized by a relatively raised resting metabolism in the striatum, cerebellum, and SMA. The movement-related pattern was characterized by midbrain, cerebellum, and thalamic hypermetabolism.

Cerebral activation studies of dystonia have been conducted. When ITD patients perform paced joystick movements with their right hands in freely selected directions, they show significantly increased levels of contralateral putamen, rostral SMA, LPMC, and DLPFC activation.[116, 117] In contrast, activation of contralateral sensorimotor cortex and caudal SMA, cortical executive areas that send direct pyramidal tract projections to the spinal cord, is impaired. Using a vibrotactile stimulator, Tempel and Perlmutter[118] also reported impairment of sensorimotor cortex and caudal SMA activation during sensory stimulation in ITD. The pattern of activation in dystonia therefore differs from the pattern associated with PD, in which the primary motor cortex activates normally, whereas striatal, SMA, and prefrontal areas underfunction.

Resting and activation PET studies suggest that dystonic limb movements in ITD are associated with inappropriate overactivity of basal ganglia–frontal association area projections. Patients with acquired hemidystonia or focal dystonia due to basal ganglia and thalamic lesions also show increased levels of mesial and LPMC and DLPFC activation during arm movement.[119] In contrast to ITD patients, however, acquired dystonia patients show raised rather than reduced primary motor cortex activation. This finding suggests that the pathology of ITD may have a direct inhibitory effect on primary motor cortex function.

ITD patients and normal subjects activate the DLPFC and rostral SMA equivalently when imagining rather than performing joystick movements in freely chosen directions.[120] This implies that the primary functional deficit in idiopathic dystonia must lie at an executive rather than a planning level. Whether the frontal association area overactivity results from primary basal ganglia overactivity or represents an adaptive phenomenon in a conscious attempt to suppress the syndrome remains unclear. To investigate further, writer's cramp patients have been scanned while writing before and after successful treatment with botulinum toxin.[121] These patients demonstrated premotor overactivity and sensorimotor underactivity while writing continuously, but this pattern did not reverse after relief of the associated forearm cramp with botulinum toxin. This suggests that the frontal overactivity seen in dystonics is part of the pathophysiology of the syndrome and not simply an adaptive phenomenon to the presence of involuntary muscle spasms.

PET reports on dopaminergic function in dystonia have suffered from inclusion of heterogeneous groups of patients; reduced and elevated putamen ^{18}F-dopa uptake values have been reported.[112, 122] The only study to assess striatal ^{18}F-dopa uptake in purely familial ITD found that 8 of 11 ITD patients had normal striatal tracer uptake, but 3 patients with severe disease taking high doses of anticholinergics showed mild impairment of putamen ^{18}F-dopa uptake.[123] The investigators concluded that dopamine terminal function was normal in most ITD cases.

Striatal D_2 binding has also been studied in dystonia. An ^{18}F-spiperone PET study reported reduced mean putamen D_2 binding in a group of nine patients with Meige syndrome and seven patients with writer's cramp. Because there was an extensive overlap with the normal binding range, the physiologic significance of this finding is unclear.[124] The investigators suggested that their data supported dystonia being associated with underactivity of the indirect striatopallidal pathway.

Dopa-Responsive Dystonia and Dystonia-Parkinsonism

Dopa-responsive dystonia (DRD) is related to GTP-cyclohydrolase-1 deficiency in most cases. DRD is dominantly inherited, and the genetic defect is located on chromosome 14. GTP-cyclohydrolase-1 constitutes part of the tetrahydrobiopterin synthetic pathway, the cofactor for tyrosine hydroxylase. Patients are unable to manufacture L-dopa, and hence dopamine, from endogenous tyrosine but can still convert exogenous L-dopa to dopamine. DRD generally manifests in childhood with diurnally fluctuating dystonia and later with background parkinsonism. Occasionally, the condition manifests later as pure parkinsonism.

18F-dopa PET findings are normal in most cases of DRD, which distinguishes this condition from early-onset dystonia-parkinsonism, which is characterized by severely reduced putamen ^{18}F-dopa storage.[125, 126] ^{11}C-raclopride PET studies show raised striatal D_2 binding in dopa-naive DRD cases in response to the chronically low levels of striatal dopamine present, whereas L-dopa–treated DRD cases show normal levels of striatal D_2 binding.[127]

CONCLUSIONS

PET can demonstrate and distinguish the characteristic patterns of derangement of regional resting cerebral metabolism and neuropharmacology in typical and atypical parkinsonian syndromes, HD and other choreas, and dystonic syndromes. PET provides a means of detecting subclinical dysfunction in at-risk PD relatives and in HD and dystonia gene carriers. It has provided strong support for a role of inheritance in apparently sporadic PD.

PET allows PD and HD progression to be objectively monitored. In the future, it will play an important role in evaluating the efficacy of putative neuroprotective agents, neurotrophic factors, and neurotransplantation. PET activation studies have established that the akinesia of PD is associated with selective underfunctioning of the SMA and dorsal prefrontal cortex and that inappropriate overactivity of these areas is associated with dystonia.

REFERENCES

1. Morrish PK, Sawle GV, Brooks DJ: Regional changes in [18F]dopa metabolism in the striatum in Parkinson's disease. Brain 119: 2097–2103, 1996.
2. Brooks DJ, Ibañez V, Sawle GV, et al: Differing patterns of striatal ^{18}F-dopa uptake in Parkinson's disease, multiple system atrophy and progressive supranuclear palsy. Ann Neurol 28: 547–555, 1990.
3. Ito K, Morrish PK, Rakshi JS, et al: Statistical parametric mapping with ^{18}F-dopa PET demonstrates bilaterally reduced striatal and nigral dopaminergic function in early Parkinson's disease. J Neurol Neurosurg Psychiatry 66:754–758, 1999.
4. Rakshi JS, Uema T, Ito K, et al: Frontal, striatal, and midbrain dopaminergic function in early and advanced Parkinson's disease: A 3D ^{18}F-dopa PET study. Brain 122:1637–1650, 1999.
5. Otsuka M, Ichiya Y, Kuwabara Y, et al: Differences in the reduced ^{18}F-dopa uptakes of the caudate and the putamen in Parkinson's disease: Correlations with the three main symptoms. J Neurol Sci 136:169–173, 1996.
6. Salmon EP, Brooks DJ, Leenders KL, et al: A two-compartment description and kinetic procedure for measuring regional cerebral ^{11}C]nomifensine uptake using positron emission tomography. J Cereb Blood Flow Metab 10:307–316, 1990.
7. Frost JJ, Rosier AJ, Reich SG, et al: Positron emission tomographic imaging of the dopamine transporter with ^{11}C-WIN 35,428 reveals marked declines in mild Parkinson's disease. Ann Neurol 34:423–431, 1993.
8. Rinne JO, Bergman J, Ruotinnen H, et al: Striatal uptake of a novel PET ligand, ^{18}F] β-CFT, is reduced in early Parkinson's disease. Synapse 31:119–124, 1999.
9. Guttman M, Burkholder J, Kish SJ, et al: [11]C]RTI-32 PET studies of the dopamine transporter in early dopa-naive Parkinson's disease: Implications for the symptomatic threshold. Neurology 48:1578–1583, 1997.
10. Frey KA, Koeppe RA, Kilbourn MR, et al: Pre-synaptic monoaminergic vesicles in Parkinson's disease and normal aging. Ann Neurol 40:873–884, 1996.
11. Lee CS, Samii A, Sossi V, et al: Effect of striatal dopaminergic denervation on [18F]Dopa-, [11C]DTBZ, and [11C]MP-PET scans: A comparative study in patients with Parkinson's disease. Neurology 52(Suppl 2):A175, 1999.
12. Piccini P, Morrish PK, Turjanski N, et al: Dopaminergic function in familial Parkinson's disease: A clinical and ^{18}F-dopa PET study. Ann Neurol 41:222–229, 1997.
13. Piccini P, Burn DJ, Ceravalo R, et al: The role of inheritance in sporadic Parkinson's disease: Evidence from a longitudinal study of dopaminergic function in twins. Ann Neurol 45:577–582, 1999.
14. Vingerhoets FJG, Snow BJ, Lee CS, et al: Longitudinal fluorodopa positron emission tomographic studies of the evolution of idiopathic parkinsonism. Ann Neurol 36:759–764, 1994.
15. Morrish PK, Sawle GV, Brooks DJ: An [18F]dopa PET and clinical study of the rate of progression in Parkinson's disease. Brain 119:585–591, 1996.
16. Morrish PK, Rakshi JS, Sawle GV, Brooks DJ: Measuring the rate of progression and estimating the preclinical period of Parkinson's disease with [18F]dopa PET. J Neurol Neurosurg Psychiatry 64:314–319, 1998.
17. Fearnley JM, Lees AJ: Ageing and Parkinson's disease: Substantia nigra regional selectivity. Brain 114:2283–2301, 1991.
18. Nurmi EM, Ruottinen HM, Bergman J, et al: The rate of progression in Parkinson's disease: A [18F]Dopa PET study. Neurology 52(Suppl 2): A91, 1999.

19. Banati RB, Goerres G, Perkin D, et al: Imaging microglial activation in vivo. J Cereb Blood Flow Metab 17(Suppl 1):S435–S436, 1997.

20. Banati R, Cagnin A, Myers R, et al: In vivo detection of activated microglia by [¹¹C]PK11195-PET indicates involvement of the globus pallidum in idiopathic Parkinson's disease. Parkinsonism Relat Disord 5:S56, 1999.

21. Hagell P, Schrag AE, Piccini P, et al: Sequential bilateral transplantation in Parkinson's disease: Effects of the second graft. Brain 122:1121–1132, 1999.

22. Piccini P, Ceravalo R, Hagell P, et al: Task related cortical function in Parkinson's disease after bilateral dopaminergic grafts. Mov Disord 13(Suppl 2):128–130, 1998.

23. Remy P, Samson Y, Hantraye P, et al: Clinical correlates of [¹⁸F]fluorodopa uptake in five grafted parkinsonian patients. Ann Neurol 38:580–588, 1995.

24. Freeman TB, Olanow CW, Hauser RA, et al: Bilateral fetal nigral transplantation into the post-commissural putamen as a treatment for Parkinson's disease: Six months follow-up. Ann Neurol 38:379–388, 1995.

25. Kordower JH, Freeman TB, Snow BJ, et al: Neuropathological evidence of graft survival and striatal reinnervation after the transplantation of fetal mesencephalic tissue in a patient with Parkinson's disease. N Engl J Med 332:1118–1124, 1995.

26. Rinne JO, Laihinen A, Nagren K, et al: PET demonstrates different behaviour of striatal dopamine D1 and D2 receptors in early Parkinson's disease. J Neurosc Res 27:494–499, 1990.

27. Turjanski N, Lees AJ, Brooks DJ: PET studies on striatal dopaminergic receptor binding in drug naive and L-dopa treated Parkinson's disease patients with and without dyskinesia. Neurology 49:717–723, 1997.

28. Shinotoh H, Inoue O, Hirayama K, et al: Dopamine D₁ receptors in Parkinson's disease and striatonigral degeneration: A positron emission tomography study. J Neurol Neurosurg Psychiatr 56:467–472, 1993.

29. Leenders KL, Herold S, Palmer AJ, et al: Human cerebral dopamine system measured in vivo using PET. J Cereb Blood Flow Metab 5(Suppl 1):S157–S158, 1985.

30. Antonini A, Schwarz J, Oertel WH, et al: [¹¹C]raclopride and positron emission tomography in previously untreated patients with Parkinson's disease: Influence of L-dopa and lisuride therapy on striatal dopamine D₂-receptors. Neurology 44:1325–1329, 1994.

31. Antonini A, Leenders KL, Vontobel P, et al: Complementary PET studies of striatal neuronal function in the differential diagnosis between multiple system atrophy and Parkinson's disease. Brain 120:2187–2195, 1997.

32. Rinne JO, Laihinen A, Rinne UK, et al: PET study on striatal dopamine D₂ receptor changes during the progression of early Parkinson's disease. Mov Disord 8:134–138, 1993.

33. Piccini P, Weeks RA, Brooks DJ: Opioid receptor binding in Parkinson's patients with and without levodopa-induced dyskinesias. Ann Neurol 42:720–726, 1997.

34. Miletich RS, Chan T, Gillespie M, et al: Contralateral basal ganglia metabolism is abnormal in hemiparkinsonian patients. An FDG-PET study. Neurology 38:S260, 1988.

35. Wolfson LI, Leenders KL, Brown LL, Jones T: Alterations of regional cerebral blood flow and oxygen metabolism in Parkinson's disease. Neurology 35:1399–1405, 1985.

36. Eidelberg D, Moeller JR, Dhawan V, et al: The metabolic topography of parkinsonism. J Cereb Blood Flow Metab 14:783–801, 1994.

37. Eidelberg D, Moeller JR, Ishikawa T, et al: Assessment of disease severity in Parkinsonism with fluorine-18-fluorodeoxyglucose and PET. J Nucl Med 36:378–383, 1995.

38. Hu M, Taylor-Robinson SD, Chaudhuri KR, et al: Evidence for cortical dysfunction in non-demented Parkinson's disease patients: A proton MR spectroscopy study. J Neurol Neurosurg Psychiatry 67:20–26, 1999.

39. Mentis M, Edwards C, Krch D, et al: Metabolic abnormalities associated with cognitive dysfunction in Parkinson's disease. Neurology 52(Suppl 2):A221, 1999.

40. Vander-Borght T, Minoshima S, Giordani B, et al: Cerebral metabolic differences in Parkinson's and Alzheimer's disease matched for dementia severity. J Nucl Med 38:797–802, 1997.

41. Asahina M, Suhara T, Shinotoh H, et al: Brain muscarinic receptors in progressive supranuclear palsy and Parkinson's disease: A positron emission tomographic study. J Neurol Neurosurg Psychiatry 65:155–163, 1998.

42. Eidelberg D, Moeller JR, Ishikawa T, et al: Regional metabolic correlates of surgical outcome following unilateral pallidotomy for Parkinson's disease. Ann Neurol 39:450–459, 1996.

43. Playford ED, Jenkins IH, Passingham RE, et al: Impaired mesial frontal and putamen activation in Parkinson's disease: A PET study. Ann Neurol 32:151–161, 1992.

44. Jahanshahi M, Jenkins IH, Brown RG, et al: Self-initiated versus externally triggered movements: Measurements of regional cerebral blood flow and movement-related potentials in normals and Parkinson's disease. Brain 118:913–933, 1995.

45. Samuel M, Ceballos-Baumann AO, Blin J, et al: Evidence for lateral premotor and parietal overactivity in Parkinson's disease during sequential and bimanual movements: A PET study. Brain 120:963–976, 1997.

46. Rascol O, Sabatini U, Fabre N, Brefel C, et al: The ipsilateral cerebellar hemisphere is overactive during hand movements in akinetic parkinsonian patients. Brain 120:103–110, 1997.

47. Jenkins IH, Fernandez W, Playford ED, et al: Impaired activation of the supplementary motor area in Parkinson's disease is reversed when akinesia is treated with apomorphine. Ann Neurol 32:749–757, 1992.

48. Brooks DJ, Jenkins IH, Passingham RE: Positron emission tomography studies on regional cerebral control of voluntary movement. In Mano N, Hamada I, DeLong MR (eds): Role of the cerebellum and basal ganglia in voluntary movement. New York, Excerpta Medical, 1993, pp 267–274.

49. Grafton ST, Waters C, Sutton J, et al: Pallidotomy increases activity of motor association cortex in Parkinson's disease—a positron emission tomographic study. Ann Neurol 37:776–783, 1995.

50. Samuel M, Ceballos-Baumann AO, Turjanski N, et al: Pallidotomy in Parkinson's disease increases SMA and prefrontal activation during performance of volitional movements: An H₂¹⁵O PET study. Brain 120:1301–1313, 1997.

51. Davis KD, Taub E, Houle S, et al: Globus pallidus stimulation activates the cortical motor system during alleviation of parkinsonian symptoms. Nat Med 3:671–674, 1997.

52. Limousin P, Greene J, Polak P, et al: Changes in cerebral activity pattern due to subthalamic nucleus or internal pallidum stimulation in Parkinson's disease. Ann Neurol 42:283–291, 1997.

53. Eidelberg D, Nakamura T, Mentis M, et al: Brain activation responses with internal pallidal stimulation in Parkinson's disease. Neurology 52(Suppl 2):A176, 1999.

54. Ceballos-Baumann AO, Bartenstein P, Von Falkenhayn I, et al: Parkinson's disease ON and OFF subthalamic nucleus stimulation: A PET activation study. Neurology 48(Suppl 2):A250, 1997.

55. Brooks DJ, Playford ED, Ibanez V, et al: Isolated tremor and disruption of the nigrostriatal dopaminergic system: An ¹⁸F-dopa PET study. Neurology 42:1554–1560, 1992.

56. Remy P, De Recondo A, Defer G, et al: Peduncular "rubral" tremor and dopaminergic denervation: A PET study. Neurology 45:472–477, 1995.

57. Playford ED, Britton TC, Thompson PD, et al: Exacerbation of postural tremor with emergence of parkinsonism following neuroleptic administration. J Neurol Neurosurg Psychiatry 58:487–489, 1995.

58. Lamarre Y: Animal models of tremor. In Findley LJ, Capildeo R (eds): Movement Disorders: Tremor. London, Macmillan, 1984, pp 183–194.

59. Otsuka M, Ichiya Y, Hosokawa S, et al: Striatal blood flow, glucose metabolism, and ¹⁸F-dopa uptake: Difference in Parkinson's disease and atypical parkinsonism. J Neurol Neurosurg Psychiatry 54:898–904, 1991.

60. Eidelberg D, Takikawa S, Moeller JR, et al: Striatal hypometabolism distinguishes striatonigral degeneration from Parkinson's disease. Ann Neurol 33:518–527, 1993.

61. Eidelberg D, Moeller JR, Kazumata K, et al: Metabolic correlates of pallidal neuronal activity in Parkinson's disease. Brain 120:1315–1324, 1997.

62. De Volder AG, Francard J, Laterre C, et al: Decreased glucose utilisation in the striatum and frontal lobe in probable striatonigral degeneration. Ann Neurol 26:239–247, 1989.

63. Brooks DJ, Salmon EP, Mathias CJ, et al: The relationship between locomotor disability, autonomic dysfunction, and the integrity of the striatal dopaminergic system, in patients with multiple system atrophy, pure autonomic failure, and Parkinson's disease, studied with PET. Brain 113:1539–1552, 1990.

64. Burn DJ, Sawle GV, Brooks DJ: The differential diagnosis of Parkinson's disease, multiple system atrophy, and Steele-Richardson-Olszewski syndrome: Discriminant analysis of striatal ^{18}F-dopa PET data. J Neurol Neurosurg Psychiatry 57:278–284, 1994.

65. Antonini A, Kazumata K, Feigin A, et al: Differential diagnosis of parkinsonism with [^{18}F]Fluorodeoxyglucose and PET. Mov Disord 13:268–274, 1998.

66. Brooks DJ, Ibanez V, Sawle GV, et al: Striatal D$_2$ receptor status in Parkinson's disease, striatonigral degeneration, and progressive supranuclear palsy, measured with ^{11}C-raclopride and PET. Ann Neurol 31:184–192, 1992.

67. Shinotoh H, Aotsuka A, Yonezawa H, et al: Striatal dopamine D$_2$ receptors in Parkinson's disease and striato-nigral degeneration determined by positron emission tomography. In Nagatsu T, Fisher A, Yoshida M (eds): Basic, Clinical, and Therapeutic Advances of Alzheimer's and Parkinson's disease, Vol 2. New York, Plenum Press, 1990, pp 107–110.

68. Burn DJ, Rinne JO, Quinn NP, et al: Striatal opioid receptor binding in Parkinson's disease, striatonigral degeneration, and Steele-Richardson-Olszewski syndrome: An ^{11}C-diprenorphine PET study. Brain 118:951–958, 1995.

69. Foster NL, Gilman S, Berent S, et al: Cerebral hypometabolism in progressive supranuclear palsy studied with positron emission tomography. Ann Neurol 24:399–406, 1988.

70. Blin J, Baron JC, Dubois P, et al: Positron emission tomography study in progressive supranuclear palsy. Arch Neurol 47:747–752, 1990.

71. Goffinet A, DeVolder AG, Gillain C, et al: Positron tomography demonstrates frontal lobe hypometabolism in progressive supranuclear palsy. Ann Neurol 25:131–139, 1989.

72. Otsuka M, Ichiya Y, Kuwabara Y, et al: Cerebral blood flow, oxygen and glucose metabolism with PET in progressive supranuclear palsy. Ann Nuc Med 3:111–118, 1989.

73. Leenders KL, Frackowiak RS, Lees AI: Steele-Richardson-Olszewski syndrome: Brain energy metabolism, blood flow and fluorodopa uptake measured by positron emission tomography. Brain 111:615–630, 1988.

74. Bhatt MH, Snow BJ, Martin WRW, et al: Positron emission tomography in progressive supranuclear palsy. Arch Neurol 48:389–391, 1991.

75. Ilgin N, Zubieta J, Reich SG, et al: PET imaging of the dopamine transporter in progressive supranuclear palsy and Parkinson's disease. Neurology 52:1221–1226, 1999.

76. Pappata S, Traykov L, Tavitian B, et al: Striatal reduction of acetylcholinesterase in patients with progressive supranuclear palsy (PSP) as measured in vivo by PET and ^{11}C-physostigmine (^{11}C-PHY). J Cereb Blood Flow Metab 17(Suppl 1):S687, 1997.

77. Baron JC, Maziere B, Loc'h C, et al: Loss of striatal (^{76}Br)bromospiperone binding sites demonstrated by positron tomography in progressive supranuclear palsy. J Cereb Blood Flow Metab 6:131–136, 1986.

78. Sawle GV, Brooks DJ, Marsden CD, Frackowiak RSJ: Corticobasal degeneration: A unique pattern of regional cortical oxygen metabolism and striatal fluorodopa uptake demonstrated by positron emission tomography. Brain 114:541–556, 1991.

79. Eidelberg D, Dhawan V, Moeller JR, et al: The metabolic landscape of corticobasal ganglionic degeneration: Regional asymmetries studied with positron emission tomography. J Neurol Neurosurg Psychiatr 54:856–862, 1991.

80. Blin J, Vidhailhet M-I, Pillon B, et al: Corticobasal degeneration: Decreased and asymmetrical glucose consumption as studied by PET. Movement Disorders 7:348–354, 1992.

81. Nagahama Y, Fukuyama H, Turjanski N, et al: Cerebral glucose metabolism in corticobasal degeneration: Comparison with progressive supranuclear palsy and normal controls. Mov Disord 12:691–696, 1997.

82. Kuhl DE, Phelps ME, Markham CH, et al: Cerebral metabolism and atrophy in Huntington's disease determined by ^{18}FDG and computed tomographic scans. Ann Neurol 12:425–434, 1982.

83. Leenders KL, Frackowiak RSJ, Quinn N, Marsden CD: Brain energy metabolism and dopaminergic function in Huntington's disease measured in vivo using positron emission tomography. Mov Disord 1:69–77, 1986.

84. Hayden MR, Martin WRW, Stoessl AJ, et al: Positron emission tomography in the early diagnosis of Huntington's disease. Neurology 36:888–894, 1986.

85. Young AB, Penney JB, Starosta-Rubinstein S, et al: PET scan investigations of Huntington's disease: Cerebral metabolic correlates of neurological features and functional decline. Ann Neurol 20:296–303, 1986.

86. Berent S, Giordani B, Lehtinen S, et al: Positron emission tomographic scan investigations of Huntington's disease—cerebral metabolic correlates of cognitive function. Ann Neurol 23:541–546, 1988.

87. Kuwert T, Lange HW, Langen KJ, et al: Cortical and subcortical glucose consumption measured by PET in patients with Huntington's disease. Brain 113:1405–1423, 1990.

88. Dubinsky RM, Hallett M, Levey R, Di Chiro G: Regional brain glucose metabolism in neuroacanthocytosis. Neurology 39:1253–1255, 1989.

89. Hosokawa S, Ichiya Y, Kuwabara Y, et al: Positron emission tomography in cases of chorea with different underlying diseases. J Neurol Neurosurg Psychiatry 50:1284–1287, 1987.

90. Guttman M, Lang AE, Garnett ES, et al: Regional cerebral glucose metabolism in SLE chorea: Further evidence that striatal hypometabolism is not a correlate of chorea. Mov Disord 2:201–210, 1987.

91. Weindl A, Kuwert T, Leenders KL, et al: Increased striatal glucose consumption in Sydenham chorea. Movement Disorders 8:437–444, 1993.

92. Pahl JJ, Mazziotta JC, Cummings J, et al: Positron emission tomography in tardive dyskinesia and Huntington's disease. J Cereb Blood Flow Metab 7:1253–1255, 1987.

93. Weeks RA, Ceballos-Baumann AO, Boecker H, et al: Cortical control of movement in Huntington's disease: A PET activation study. Brain 120:1569–1578, 1997.

94. Weindl A, Bartenstein P, Boecker H, et al: PET investigations on central motor processing in Huntington's disease. Neurology 48(Suppl 2):A120, 1997.

95. Hagglund J, Aquilonius SM, Eckernas SA, et al: Dopamine receptor properties in Parkinson's disease and Huntington's chorea evaluated by positron emission tomography using ^{11}C-N-methyl-spiperone. Acta Neurol Scand 75:87–94, 1987.

96. Turjanski N, Weeks R, Dolan R, et al: Striatal D$_1$ and D$_2$ receptor binding in patients with Huntington's disease and other choreas: A PET study. Brain 118:689–696, 1995.

97. Weeks RA, Cunningham VJ, Piccini P, et al: ^{11}C-diprenorphine binding in Huntington's disease: A comparison of region of interest analysis and statistical parametric mapping. J Cereb Blood Flow Metab 17:943–949, 1997.

98. Holthoff VA, Young AB, Koeppe RA, et al: Benzodiazepine changes in Huntington's disease. J Cereb Blood Flow Metab 11(Suppl 2):S810, 1991.

99. Brooks DJ, Ibanez V, Playford ED, et al: Presynaptic and postsynaptic striatal dopaminergic function in neuroacanthocytosis: A positron emission tomographic study. Ann Neurol 30:166–171, 1991.

100. Turjanski N, Burn DJ, Lammertsma AA, et al: PET studies on D$_1$ and D$_2$ receptor status in chorea. Neurology 43(Suppl 2):A333, 1993.

101. Blin J, Baron JC, Cambon H, et al: Striatal dopamine D$_2$ receptors in tardive dyskinesia: PET study. J Neurol Neurosurg Psychiatr 52:1248–1252, 1989.

102. Weeks RA, Piccini P, Harding AE, Brooks DJ: Striatal D$_1$ and D$_2$ dopamine receptor loss in asymptomatic mutation carriers of Huntington's disease. Ann Neurol 40:49–54, 1996.

103. Antonini A, Leenders KL, Spiegel R, et al: Striatal glucose metabolism and dopamine D-2 receptor binding in asymptomatic gene carriers and patients with Huntington's disease. Brain 119:2085–2095, 1996.

104. Feigin A, Moeller JR, Messimer J, et al: Metabolic brain networks and dopamine D$_2$ receptor binding in presymptomatic and symptomatic Huntington's disease. Neurology 52(Suppl 2):A377, 1999.

105. Grafton ST, Mazziotta JC, Pahl JJ, et al: Serial changes of cerebral glucose metabolism and caudate size in persons at risk for Huntington's disease. Arch Neurol 49:1161–1167, 1992.
106. Antonini A, Leenders KL, Feigin A, et al: PET studies of Huntington's disease rate of progression. Neurology 48(Suppl 2): A120, 1997.
107. Andrews TC, Weeks RA, Brooks DJ: [11C]raclopride and [11C]SCH23390 PET and the Unified Huntington's Disease Rating Scale can be used to monitor disease progression in asymptomatic Huntington's disease gene carriers. Soc Neurosci Abstracts 23:741.17–741.10, 1997.
108. Torres EM, Fricker RA, Hume SP, et al: Assessment of striatal graft viability in the rat *in vivo* using a small diameter PET scanner. Neuroreport 6:2017–2021, 1995.
109. Chase T, Tamminga CA, Burrows H: Positron emission studies of regional cerebral glucose metabolism in idiopathic dystonia. Adv Neurol 50:237–241, 1988.
110. Eidelberg D, Dhawan V, Cedarbaum J, et al: Contralateral basal ganglia hypermetabolism in primary unilateral limb dystonia. Neurology 40(Supp 1):399, 1990.
111. Gilman S, Junck L, Young AB, et al: Cerebral metabolic activity in idiopathic dystonia studied with positron emission tomography. Adv Neurol 50:231–236, 1988.
112. Otsuka M, Ichiya Y, Shima F, et al: Increased striatal ^{18}F-Dopa uptake and normal glucose metabolism in idiopathic dystonia syndrome. J Neurol Sci 111:195–199, 1992.
113. Stoessl AJ, Martin WRW, Clark C, et al: PET studies of cerebral glucose metabolism in idiopathic torticollis. Neurology 36:653–657, 1986.
114. Karbe H, Holthoff VA, Rudolf J, et al: Positron emission tomography in dystonia: Frontal cortex and basal ganglia hypometabolism. Mov Disord 7(Suppl 1):144, 1992.
115. Eidelberg D, Moeller JR, Antonini A, et al: Functional brain networks in DYT1 dystonia. Ann Neurol 44:303–312, 1998.
116. Ceballos-Baumann AO, Passingham RE, Warner T, et al: Overactivity of rostral and underactivity of caudal frontal areas in idiopathic torsion dystonia: A PET activation study. Ann Neurol 37:363–372, 1995.
117. Playford ED, Passingham RE, Marsden CD, Brooks DJ: Increased activation of frontal areas during arm movement in idiopathic torsion dystonia. Movement Disorders 13:309–318, 1998.
118. Tempel LW, Perlmutter JS: Abnormal cortical responses in patients with writer's cramp. Neurology 43:2252–2257, 1993.
119. Ceballos-Baumann AO, Passingham RE, Marsden CD, et al: Overactivity of primary and accessory motor areas after motor reorganisation in acquired hemi-dystonia: A PET activation study. Ann Neurol 37:746–757, 1995.
120. Ceballos-Baumann AO, Marsden CD, Passingham RE, et al: Cerebral activation with performing and imagining movement in idiopathic torsion dystonia (ITD): A PET study. Neurology 44(Suppl 2):A338, 1994.
121. Ceballos-Baumann AO, Sheean G, Marsden CD, et al: Botulinum toxin does not reverse the cortical dysfunction associated with writer's cramp. Brain 120:571–582, 1997.
122. Martin WRW, Stoessl AJ, Palmer M, et al: PET scanning in dystonia. Adv Neurol 50:223–229, 1988.
123. Playford ED, Fletcher NA, Sawle GV, et al: Integrity of the nigro-striatal dopaminergic system in familial dystonia: An ^{18}F-dopa PET study. Brain 116:1191–1199, 1993.
124. Perlmutter JS, Stambuk MK, Markham J, et al: Decreased [F-18] spiperone binding in putamen in idiopathic focal dystonia. J Neurosci 17:843–850, 1997.
125. Sawle GV, Leenders KL, Brooks DJ, et al: Dopa-responsive dystonia: [^{18}F]dopa positron emission tomography. Ann Neurol 30: 24–30, 1991.
126. Snow BJ, Nygaard TG, Takahashi H, Calne DB: Positron emission tomography studies of dopa-responsive dystonia and early-onset idiopathic parkinsonism. Ann Neurol 34:733–738, 1993.
127. Kunig G, Leenders KL, Antonini A, et al: D$_2$ receptor binding in dopa-responsive dystonia. Ann Neurol 44:758–762, 1998.

CHAPTER **170**

Thalamotomy for Tremor

SHERWIN E. HUA ■ IRA M. GARONZIK ■ JUNG-IL LEE ■ FREDERICK A. LENZ

The pallidum was an early stereotactic target for the treatment of Parkinson's disease.[1, 2] In 1951, Hassler and Riechert[3] applied stereotactic techniques to functional surgery of the thalamus. Hassler reasoned that the thalamic termination of pallidal efferents might be a more effective site for a lesion to relieve parkinsonian symptoms than was the pallidum. Indeed, the effect of thalamotomy on tremor was greater than that of pallidotomy, and rigidity was also improved. For the next 2 decades, surgery for Parkinson's disease was dominated by thalamotomy (see Chapter 163).[4]

In the modern era, thalamic lesions for the treatment of movement disorders have been made in the ventral nuclear group of the thalamus. According to Hassler's classification,[5] the nuclei in the ventral nuclear group, from anterior to posterior, are the pallidal relay nucleus (ventral oral [Vo]), the cerebellar relay nucleus (ventral intermediate [Vim]), and the principal somatic sensory nucleus (ventral caudal [Vc]).[6, 7] On the basis of surgical experience, Hassler proposed that the anterior portion of Vo, the nucleus ventralis oralis anterior (Voa), was a better target for rigidity, whereas the nucleus ventralis oralis posterior (Vop) was better for the relief of tremor. With the aid of microelectrode recordings, an area posterior to Vop was later found to have rhythmic bursting activity close to the frequency of tremor.[8] The nucleus in this location, Vim, became the target of choice for tremor of all types. This chapter presents the technique of thalamotomy for tremor. The mechanism of tremor and the indications and results of thalamotomy are discussed separately for parkinsonian, essential, and cerebellar (intention) tremor.

Some of the studies described in this chapter were supported by grants to Dr. Lenz from the National Institutes of Health (NS28598, K08-NS1384, P01 NS32386-Proj. 1, NS38493).

STEREOTACTIC SURGICAL TECHNIQUE

Many techniques can be used to carry out functional stereotactic procedures within the standard of care. The goal of thalamotomy is to lesion a population of cells within Vim that is involved in the mechanism of tremor. Radiologic and physiologic landmarks provide the most accurate localization of the target. At our institution, we have localized the anterior commissure (AC), the posterior commissure (PC), and the border between the capsule and thalamus radiologically by using both computed tomography (CT) and magnetic resonance imaging (MRI). We refine the radiologic estimate of location by microelectrode physiologic localization[9] and then carry out radiofrequency lesioning. Alternative approaches are to localize radiologically by ventriculography or CT-MRI fusion techniques; to localize physiologically by semi-microelectrode recording or macrostimulation, or both; and to lesion by radiosurgery. The relative efficacy and safety of these different techniques have not been examined systematically.

Radiologic Localization

Radiologic targeting can be used to determine the location of the AC and PC by ventriculography, MRI, or CT. AC and PC predict the locations of the different thalamic nuclei in stereotactic space. At our institution, the sagittal sections of the Schaltenbrand and Bailey atlas[10] are transformed to match the AC-PC line in the patient.[11] In this way, the nuclear locations predicted radiographically in that patient are displayed in the coordinates of the Leksell frame. The laterality of the target is determined from a fast-inversion-recovery MRI sequence. This sequence is used to determine the position of the capsule and the medial dorsal nucleus (MD) as a large dorsal, periventricular, thalamic, high-intensity T2 signal (Lenz, Eckell, Bryant, unpublished observations). Because the MD forms the medial boundary of Vim and Vop, the center of Vim is midway between the lateral border of MD and the medial border of the capsule.[10] This central plane is matched to the closest sagittal section of the atlas. The first microelectrode trajectories target Vc in this plane; physiologic observations are recorded, with pen and paper, on the atlas map. Alternative approaches to targeting Vim from the AC-PC line include the geometric construction for approximating nuclear location as described by Guiot.[12, 13]

Ventriculography as a means of locating the AC-PC line has largely been replaced by CT and MRI. CT is as accurate as ventriculography[14] and does not carry the risks of ventricular puncture and instillation of air or contrast medium into the ventricles. MRI is slightly less accurate than CT, with errors of approximately 2 mm on average and 4 mm at maximum.[15–17] These errors are due to artifacts related to inhomogeneities in the magnetic field and nonlinearities in the gradient field—the position-dependent variation in the magnetic field.[18] These artifacts can be induced by metal or magnetic susceptibility artifacts—produced at the interface between materials (e.g., air and bone) that have different tendencies to affect the magnetic field in a region.

Attempts to decrease errors in MRI scans due to these artifacts include software modifications and overlapping (fusion) of the MRI database with the CT database, which is not prone to these types of artifacts.[19] Targeting in thalamotomy can then be accomplished by computer programs that relate atlas maps of anatomy to the radiologic anatomy. These programs display atlas maps transformed to match either the AC-PC line in isolation[20] or the AC-PC line and other structures, such as the margins of the third ventricle or the internal capsule.[21]

Physiologic Localization

Radiologic targeting can be further refined by identifying the different thalamic nuclei, including Vim, Vop, and Vc, on the basis of their electrophysiologic properties. These properties are defined in terms of spontaneous activity, neuronal response to passive and active movements, and sensory responses to natural or electrical stimulation. Physiologic localization has been carried out by stimulation with a macroelectrode (impedance <1000 ohm) or by stimulation and recording with a semi-microelectrode (impedance <100 kohm) or a microelectrode (impedance >500 kohm).

MICROELECTRODE LOCALIZATION

Microelectrodes for physiologic monitoring and recording are designed to isolate single action potentials.[22–24] In addition, the electrode must be durable enough to withstand microstimulation, which degrades the insulation. Typically these characteristics are

achieved by constructing electrodes from a platinum-iridium alloy or from tungsten, producing a tapered tip, and insulating with glass.[22, 24–28] The electrode impedance is usually greater than 500 kohm.[22, 23, 29] A high-impedance microelectrode is required to isolate single units.[22] Passing current through the electrode during microstimulation degrades insulation and lowers impedance, which makes it harder to isolate single units (Fig. 170–1).

The assembled electrode is attached to a hydraulic microdrive and mounted on the stereotactic frame. Some microdrive systems incorporate a coarse drive so that overlying structures can be traversed quickly. The tip is then retracted into a protective cylindrical housing while the whole assembly is advanced to a new depth.[29] The microdrive may then be used from this new depth for detailed exploration of deeper structures. Another option is to use the microdrive throughout the trajectory by advancing it each time it reaches the end of its traverse.[22]

The signal from the microelectrode is amplified and filtered. Multiple neuronal discharges of various sizes may be seen on an oscilloscope and heard by use of an audio monitor. The "all or none" principle of neuronal discharge provides that an action potential signal of constant shape and amplitude will be produced from

A

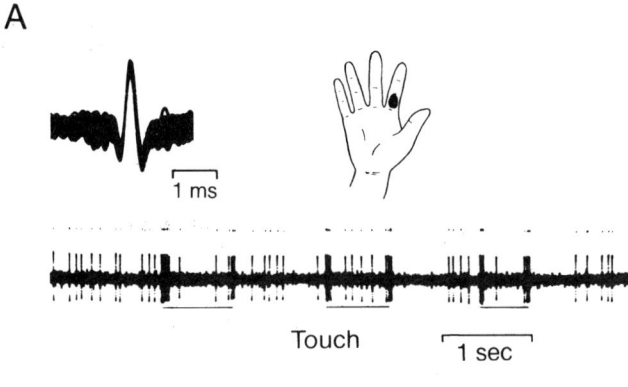

B

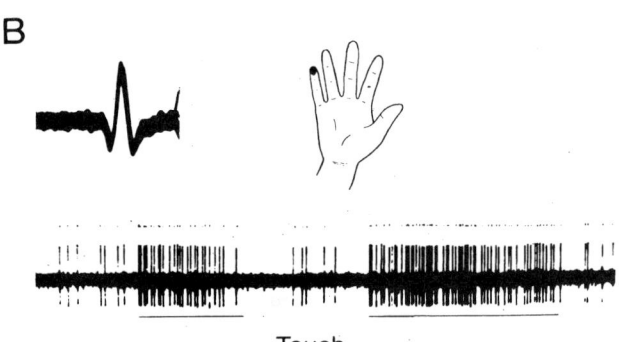

FIGURE 170–1. *A* and *B*, Examples of two thalamic cells with sensory receptive fields. The lower oscilloscope tracing in each part shows single-unit activity evoked during sensory testing. The approximate duration of somatosensory stimulation is indicated by the horizontal bars below the spike train. The approximate receptive field is indicated in the upper right of each part. (Adapted from Lenz FA, Dostrovsky JO, Tasker RR, et al: Single-unit analysis of the human ventral thalamic nuclear group: Somatosensory responses. J Neurophysiol 59:299–316, 1988.)

any one neuron. Therefore, a window discriminator may be used to isolate individual neuronal firing activity. The analog signal may be stored for later analysis.

In addition to recording, microstimulation of subcortical structures through the microelectrode may be employed in physiologic localization. Current can be delivered through the same electrode used for recording by disconnecting it from the preamplifier and connecting it to the output of a current-isolation stimulator. To minimize damage to the electrode tip, microstimulation is delivered in biphasic, square-wave pulse trains of 0.1 to 0.3 msec for up to 10 seconds at a frequency of 300 Hz.[30] The current used in stimulation determines the amount of local current spread. Stimulation in Vc evokes somatic sensations,[31] whereas stimulation in Vim may alter the ongoing tremor (see Chapter 173) or dystonia (Fig. 170–2).[32]

Cells responding to sensory stimulation in small, well-defined, receptive fields are found in Vc (see Fig. 170–1).[33] Some have described a mediolateral somatotopy within Vc[23, 33] proceeding from representation of oral structures medially to leg laterally. Anterior to Vc, in Vim and Vop, Raeva has shown thalamic neuronal firing that was correlated with movement in response to commands, the active phase of movement, and to a state of maximal muscle contraction.[34] A large percentage of neuronal activity demonstrated statistical changes in rate of firing related to active movement (voluntary cells).[35, 36] The movement-related activity of most cells in Vim and Vop is preferentially related to execution of particular movements, with a somatotopy parallel to that of the sensory thalamus.[35] As shown in Figure 170–2, some neurons respond both to active movement and to somatosensory stimulation (combined cells).[35, 37] Combined cells fire in response to passive movements of a joint and during active movements of the same joint. The sensory cells are found in Vc and thus are located posterior to the cells with responses during active movement, as shown in Figure 170–3.

Cells in Vc, Vim, and Vop often exhibit activity at about the frequency of tremor. Correlations between thalamic neuronal activity and tremor have been suggested previously by visual or auditory inspection.[23, 38–40] Quantitative analysis techniques have allowed clearer demonstration of correlation between thalamic neuronal firing and electromyographic (EMG) activity during tremor,[41–43] as shown in Figure 170–4.

LOCALIZATION WITH MACROSTIMULATION OR SEMI-MICROELECTRODE

Semi-microelectrode recordings are carried out using microelectrodes with impedances of less than 100 kohm. The semi-microelectrode signal is often amplified against a concentric ring electrode located on a radius of 0.4 mm around the microelectrode.[13, 44, 45] Bipolar stimulation has been used through a concentric

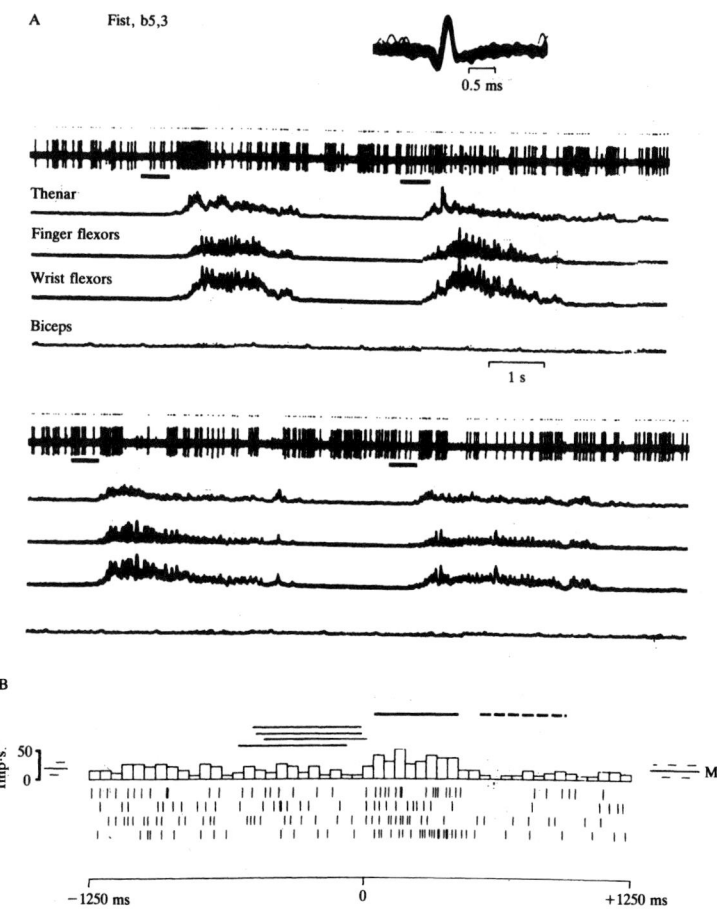

FIGURE 170–2. Example of a thalamic cell with movement-related activity. *A,* The spike train with electromyographic (EMG) signals of four contralateral muscles is shown. The lower panel in *A* is a continuation of the upper panel. The bar underneath the spike train indicates the verbal cue to begin a fist-making movement. *B,* Raster and histogram of the neuronal activity shown in *A,* but time-locked to the onset of EMG activity. The stacked lines above the histogram indicate the verbal cue to move. (From Lenz FA, Kwan H, Dostrovsky JO, et al: Single unit analysis of the human ventral thalamic nuclear group: Activity correlated with movement. Brain 113:1795–1821, 1990.)

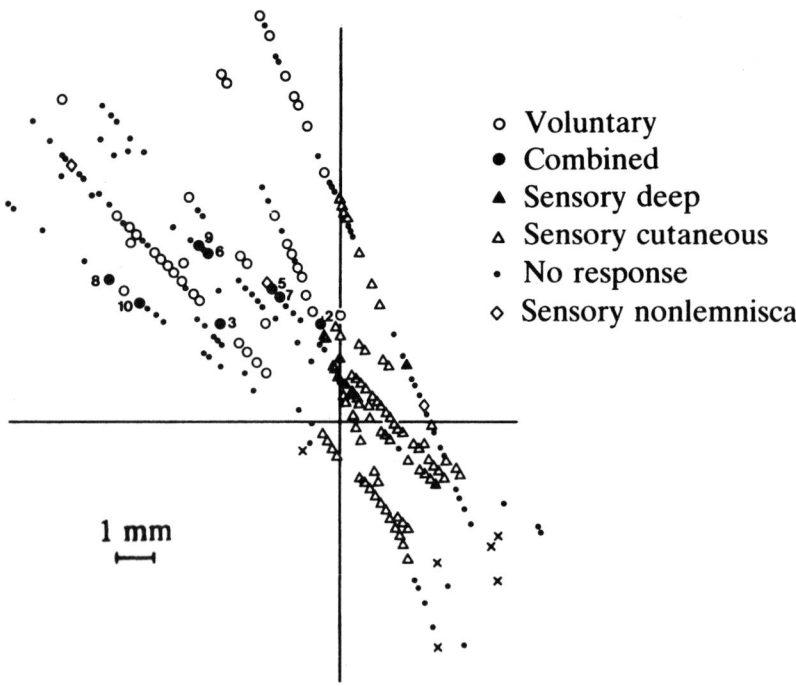

○ Voluntary
● Combined
▲ Sensory deep
△ Sensory cutaneous
· No response
◇ Sensory nonlemniscal

1 mm

FIGURE 170–3. Relative locations of cells identified by functional category from microelectrode studies during thalamotomy for tremor. The results have been pooled from planes in several patients where the majority of cells had activity related to hand and wrist movements. The horizontal line represents the anterior commissure–posterior commissure line. The vertical line represents the anterior-posterior position of the most anterior cell responding to sensory stimulation. Therefore, the principal sensory nucleus (ventral caudal [Vc]) is to the right of the vertical line, and the cerebellar relay (ventral intermediate [Vim]) is to the left. Numbers apply to combined cells. Each x marks the site where the last somatic action potential was recorded along that trajectory. (Adapted from Lenz FA, Kwan H, Dostrovsky JO, et al: Single unit analysis of the human ventral thalamic nuclear group: Activity correlated with movement. Brain 113:1795–1821, 1990.)

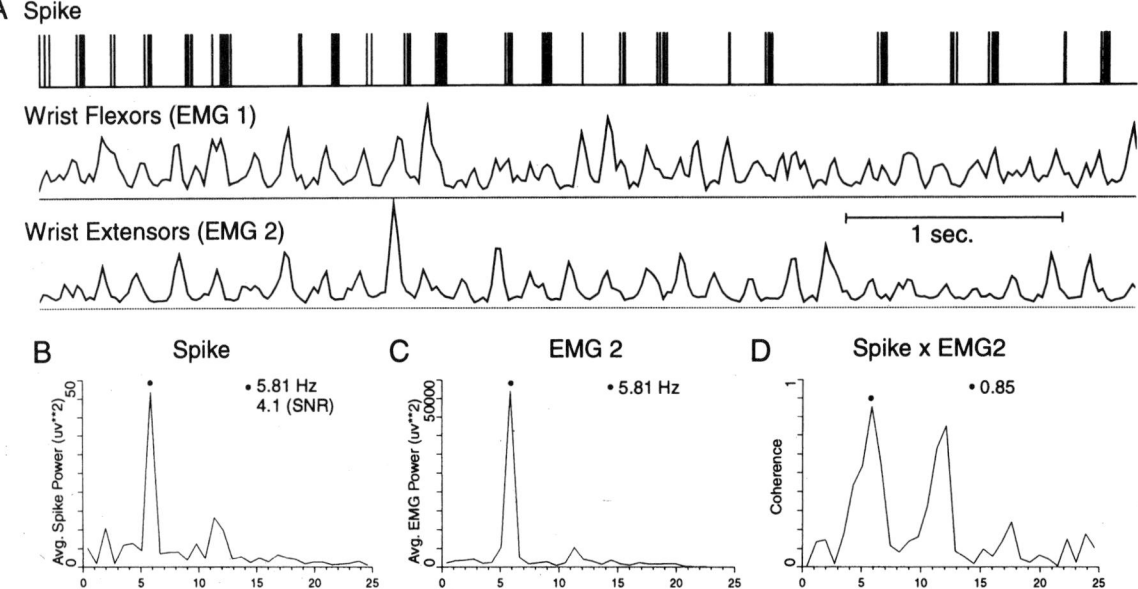

FIGURE 170–4. Simultaneous recording of thalamic single-neuron activity and peripheral electromyographic (EMG) activity during tremor in a patient with essential tremor. *A,* Digitized spike train (upper trace) and EMG channels (lower two traces). *B,* Autopower spectrum of the spike train illustrated in *A. C,* Autopower spectrum for EMG 2. *D,* Coherence spectrum of the spike × EMG 2 function.[41, 42] The autopower spectrum measures power or the intensity of the signal as a function of frequency. The coherence is a statistical function used to estimate the probability that two signals are correlated at a given frequency. As computed by this method, a coherence greater than 0.42 indicates significant probability ($P < 0.05$) of a linear relationship between the two signals.[41] (Adapted from Hua S, Lenz FA, Zirh TA, et al: Thalamic activity correlated with essential tremor. J Neurol Neurosurg Psychiatry 64:273–276, 1998.)

ring electrode alone or in combination with recording through a semi-microelectrode or recording of a scalp electroencephalogram.[46–48]

Macrostimulation through a low-impedance electrode (impedance often <1000 kohm) can reliably identify the capsule by stimulation-evoked tetanic contraction of skeletal muscle at a low threshold.[46, 47] Stimulation of intralaminar nuclei, medial to Vc or Vim, may evoke the recruiting response—long latency, high voltage, negative waves occurring over much of the cortex at the frequency of stimulation (usually <10 Hz).[6, 49] A recruiting response localized over the precentral cortex has been described in response to stimulation of Vim.[50] The target area in Vim can be identified by a stimulation-evoked increase or decrease in the amplitude of tremor.[47] Although macrostimulation in Vc evokes paresthesias, similar sensations can be evoked by stimulation in Vim.[47] Therefore, recording of responses to tactile stimulation localizes Vc more accurately.[46] Currently, macrostimulation is commonly used in conjunction with semi-microelectrode recordings.

Semi-microelectrode recordings[13, 27, 45, 51] reveal patterns of neuronal activity parallel to those of microelectrode recordings. Vc can be identified by a high level of neural activity and by responses to tactile stimulation. As with the microelectrode, recording responses are usually evoked from stimulation of lips and fingers with a medial lateral somatotopy, as described earlier.[51–54] Median or tibial nerve evoked potentials are characterized by a large positive deflection[48, 55]; these are maximal in Vc, although such evoked potentials can be recorded for a distance around Vc.[56, 57]

Vim, and perhaps Vop, can be identified by the presence of responses to stimulation of deep structures (e.g., squeezing tendons) or movement of joints.[25, 38, 40] Phasic tremor frequency activity can also be recorded in Vim and, to a lesser extent, in Vop.[58–64] Vim may also be identified by median or tibial nerve evoked potentials, which are characterized by an initial negative deflection that inverts as the electrode traverses posteriorly into Vc (see earlier).[13, 48, 56, 65] It has been reported that Vop may also be identified by spindles, an electroencephalographic pattern characterized by a 7- to 10-per-second rhythm, with increases and decreases in amplitude that occur over many seconds.[13] Semi-microelectrode recordings are simpler and less time consuming than microelectrode recordings, but they do not provide the spatial resolution of single-cell recordings.

Stereotactic Lesioning

RADIOFREQUENCY

In our technique, coordinates are taken from both radiographic studies and physiologic observations to predict the best target to lesion those neurons involved in tremor. One study suggests that the optimal target for treating parkinsonian tremor is the site of cells with activity related to tremor,[66] that is, 2 mm anterior to Vc and 3 mm above the AC-PC line. Other approaches

have been applied to define the optimal site for thalamotomy. Targets have been placed anterior to the site at which evoked potentials can be recorded in response to cutaneous stimulation of the fingers.[51, 53, 67] Lesions have been made in the region where electrical stimulation produces effects on tremor and anterior to the region where electrical stimulation evokes sensations.[47] Lesions have also been made in the region where cells respond to somatosensory stimulation of muscle, joint, and tendon.[68]

One or two lesions are made at the target defined by the previously mentioned algorithms. Radiofrequency coagulation is performed with an electrode with a 1.1-mm outer diameter and a 3-mm exposed tip and a thermistor at the tip of the electrode (TM electrode; Radionics Inc., Burlington, MA). Temperature is held constant at 60°C over a 1-minute interval. The temperature is increased in increments of 5°C to 10°C during subsequent 1-minute intervals to a level of approximately 80°C. Because temperature is increased in steps of about 10°C, the time to make the lesion is 4 minutes. Neurological examination stressing lemniscal sensory function, pyramidal function, cerebellar function, and speech should be carried out before, during, and after each stage of lesion making. The coagulum of each separate lesion made by this technique is approximated by a cylinder with a diameter of 3 mm and a length of 5 mm.[66, 69, 70]

RADIOSURGERY

The use of MRI to provide radiologic localization has led to the development of stereotactic radiosurgical thalamotomy without physiologic confirmation. Gamma knife thalamotomy is carried out with 4-mm collimators, sometimes located on a secondary collimator helmet[71] and sometimes on the standard 201-cobalt source helmet. Maximal doses of 120 to 160 Gy are delivered. Lesions with a volume of approximately 250 mm^3 are created.[71, 72] The lesion placement is estimated from the usual location of Vim in relation to the anterior and posterior commissures and the internal capsule.[71, 72]

In the largest of these series, MRI-guided gamma knife procedures were carried out in 34 patients at high risk for standard stereotactic procedures.[72] Patients rated their own outcomes using the Unified Parkinson's Disease Rating Scale (UPDRS). A good to excellent result was reported in 78%, which was less than the success rate with standard stereotactic procedures. Another series of MRI-guided gamma knife radiosurgery reported complete to nearly complete relief of tremor in 88% of cases ($n = 27$).[71] In an older series of patients with intention, parkinsonian, and undefined tremor, MRI-guided gamma knife thalamotomy resulted in good outcomes in 66% of cases ($n = 9$).[73] No neurological complications were reported in any of these series, but neurological injury and death have been reported in abstracts. The conclusion of most of these reports,[71, 72] as well as a recent review,[74] is that radiosurgical thalamotomy may have a role in the treatment of tremor in patients with significant medical contraindications for microelectrode-guided thalamotomy.

TREMOR OF PARKINSON'S DISEASE

Parkinson's disease affects approximately 1% of the population older than 65 years,[75] or approximately 1 million patients in North America. The three cardinal signs of Parkinson's disease are resting tremor, cogwheel rigidity, and bradykinesia. The 3- to 5-Hz resting, pill-rolling tremor is sometimes the first manifestation of the disease and may be the only symptom for years before the development of clinically significant bradykinesia and rigidity. The tremor is typified by alternating contraction of extensor and flexor antagonists when the arm is at rest. As the tremor progresses, it may involve posture and active movement and become a significant source of disability. Parkinsonian tremor often does not respond to medication,[76, 77] so some of these patients may be candidates for thalamic surgical procedures.[78, 79]

Mechanisms of Tremor

Two mechanisms have been proposed as the basis for the tremor of Parkinson's disease.[80–83] The central oscillator hypothesis proposes that tremor is caused by pacemaker cells located in the basal ganglia or thalamus. Alternatively, the peripheral hypothesis suggests that parkinsonian tremor results from peripheral feedback loops that have become unstable and oscillate.

CENTRAL OSCILLATOR HYPOTHESIS

The thalamus could be the site of a central oscillator that drives tremor. Thalamic neurons function in at least two modes: the transfer mode and the oscillatory mode. The transfer mode occurs during wakefulness and is associated with neuronal depolarization and a constant firing rate.[84] The oscillatory mode occurs during drowsiness and slow-wave sleep and is associated with neuronal hyperpolarization with a burst firing pattern. Recordings of thalamic neurons during the oscillatory mode show a prolonged decrease in firing rate, followed by a high-frequency burst of action potentials—a spike associated with a calcium burst. This burst is thought to result from a somatic calcium spike that occurs during the recovery from hyperpolarization. Because hyperpolarization follows the burst, periodic burst firing occurs during this mode. This type of burst is characterized by progressively lengthening interspike intervals.[85–87] The central oscillator hypothesis for parkinsonian tremor predicts that overactivity in the internal segment of the globus pallidus (GPi) causes a relative hyperpolarization of cells in Vop, a pallidal relay nucleus. When hyperpolarized, thalamic cells display calcium spike–related bursting activity, which could form the basis for thalamic tremor-related activity.[88–91]

In recordings from Vim and Vop in parkinsonian patients undergoing thalamotomy, the calcium spike–associated pattern of firing was found in only 1 of 118 cells.[92, 93] This cell had tremor-related activity[41] but was located in Vim, not in Vop, as predicted by the model. Alternatively, transmission of bursting activity from GPi to cells in Vop, which are in the transfer mode (i.e., slightly depolarized), could be a central generator of thalamic tremor-related activity. This hypothesis suggests that activity correlated with tremor should be maximal in the pallidal relay nucleus of the thalamus. However, the incidence of tremor-related activity was equal in Vim (25%) and in Vop (21%).[37, 94] Further, GPi activity at tremor frequency is rarely correlated with tremor in Parkinson's disease[95] (compare reference 96) or in monkey models of parkinsonism.[97] Therefore, the activity of cells in the thalamus and pallidum is not consistent with a pallidal generator for parkinsonian tremor.

PERIPHERAL FEEDBACK HYPOTHESIS

The other major hypothesis of the generation of parkinsonian tremor involves abnormal sensory feedback to the central nervous system. According to this hypothesis, stretch reflex arcs traverse the motor cortex in much the same way that tendon tap reflexes traverse the spinal cord.[98–100] The increased gain of these reflexes may cause tremor in Parkinson's disease similar to the way that increased tendon tap reflexes cause clonus in spasticity.[99–101] This hypothesis has been studied by comparing the activity of thalamic relay cells with sensory inputs to that of relay cells without sensory inputs.[35, 37, 102, 103] Tremor-related activity of sensory cells in the sensory relay nucleus Vc lags behind parkinsonian tremor.[37] This result is easily understood, because tremor causes somatosensory input, which is transmitted to the thalamus after a conduction delay. Combined cells are those cells activated in response to passive movement and in advance of active movement, so they can be distinguished from sensory cells.[35] Combined cell activity is correlated with and leads to tremor, which suggests that activity of these cells may be involved in the generation of parkinsonian tremor by a feedback mechanism.[37] Systems analysis demonstrates feedback mechanisms in the transfer function relating thalamic activity to tremor for greater than 90% of cells in Vim and Vop.[104, 105] Thus, peripheral feedback loops appear to play an important role in the mechanism of tremor. This feedback may be involved in an unstable reflex loop or may modulate the activity of a central oscillator.

INSIGHTS THROUGH FUNCTIONAL NEUROIMAGING

Positron emission tomography (PET) scanning produces an image of brain function by measuring regional cerebral blood flow, glucose metabolism, or oxygen metabolism. PET technology has been used to study parkinsonian tremor after reversible suppression by Vim stimulation. Deiber and coworkers[106] showed that effective suppression of parkinsonian tremor by Vim stimulation is associated with a decreased level of activity bilaterally in the medial and paramedial cerebellum. Stimulation at a frequency that is inadequate to alleviate tremor is not associated with a decrease in cerebellar activity, although such inadequate stimulation results in a decrease in the ipsilateral cerebral cortex similar to that seen during adequate stimulation. Other studies have shown that adequate thalamic stimulation is associated with cerebellar vermis and deep nuclear reductions in regional cerebral blood flow.[107] Other investigators[108] have confirmed a decrease in cerebellar blood flow with Vim stimulation, but only in the hemisphere ipsilateral to the tremor. This evidence supports the idea that parkinsonian tremor is mediated through a cerebellothalamocortical circuit; however, the exact role of the cerebellum in tremor has been debated. Cerebellar blood flow reductions after tremor alleviation could be an epiphenomenon if the cerebellum were either mediating proprioceptive feedback or somehow involved in stabilizing tremor during movement.[109] Nevertheless, the interruption of the cerebellothalamocortical pathway by thalamotomy[66] abolishes parkinsonian tremor, which suggests that abnormal cerebellar or thalamic function produces tremor.

Indications for Thalamotomy

Medical therapy is the mainstay of treatment for parkinsonian tremor, with L-dopa–carbidopa and anticholinergics being the most effective agents.[77] After an adequate trial of medical therapy, parkinsonian patients with significant tremor and minimal other parkinsonian symptoms may be candidates for unilateral thalamotomy. Such patients should satisfy the following criteria[110, 111]: (1) Parkinson's disease (idiopathic, juvenile, or postencephalitic)[112] with disabling unilateral or asymmetrical tremor or drug-induced dyskinesias and (2) poor response to or intolerance of optimal medical management. Contraindications include Parkinson's plus syndromes (e.g., Shy-Drager, multisystem degeneration), significant dementia, and significant medical illness. Bilateral procedures are now relatively contraindicated because of the high incidence of dysarthria following the second lesion.[111] Therefore, deep brain stimulation (DBS) may be a viable option for treatment of tremor on the second side. DBS in Vim involves implantation of a stimulator to block both neuronal activity and tremor transiently during stimulation.[113–115] Side effects complicating Vim-DBS, such as dysesthesia or dysarthria, may be reversible by altering stimulation.[79]

Results

Vim thalamotomies have been performed for more than 5 decades, and improved technology during this period has enhanced the accuracy and safety of this operation. CT and MRI, as well as microelectrode recording, have advanced the technical standards of thalamotomy. Tasker reported that for surgeries performed before 1967, thalamotomy achieved good results in 45% of cases, compared with 86% to 96% for surgeries carried out during the 1970s.[116] Reports of thalamotomies performed from 1980 to 1990 reveal good results in 86% to 94% of cases.[110, 117]

Jankovic and coworkers[110] reviewed the results of Vim thalamotomy performed between 1982 and 1994 in 42 patients with severe, asymmetrical, medically intractable parkinsonian tremor. Thalamotomies were guided by CT or ventriculographic localization and microelectrode recording. A neurologist or the surgeon assessed outcome using the UPDRS and a global tremor rating scale. Tremor was completely abolished in 74% of cases (31 of 42), and an additional 14% (6 of 42) showed significant improvement in tremor and functional ability. None of the patients had worsening of tremor contralateral to the thalamotomy, and 84% of patients reported that they would undergo the procedure again.

Similar efficacy rates were reported by Fox and coworkers.[117] In their study, 37 thalamotomies were performed between 1984 and 1989 for medically refractory parkinsonian tremor. CT localization and microelectrode guidance were used, and the lesions targeted Vim. At the time of discharge, complete abolition of contralateral tremor was seen in 94% of cases (34 of 36 patients). At 3 months, 31 of 36 patients had no tremor, and at 3 years, 13 of 16 patients remained tremor free. When tremor recurred, it was always within 3 months of surgery.

At our institution, the effectiveness of thalamotomy in 20 patients (3 operated on bilaterally) for medically intractable parkinsonian tremor of the upper extremity was assessed by use of a blinded measure of outcome.[118] Function, tremor amplitude, and handwriting/drawing were rated before surgery and 12 months afterward. The handwriting/drawing score was rated by a neurologist blinded to patient identity, laterality of surgery, and operative status. Compared with baseline, all three scores improved significantly after surgery.

The long-term success of thalamotomy has been hard to assess because of the difficulty of follow-up in these patients and the slow progression of the disease. One blinded long-term assessment of the efficacy of thalamotomy compared tremor in the arm contralateral to thalamotomy with that in the ipsilateral arm.[119] Thalamotomies were performed between 1976 and 1985, and patients were followed for a mean of 10 years. A significant concordance for the UPDRS was demonstrated among blinded raters, and tremor severity scores were consistently better contralateral to surgery. These results suggest that the effect of thalamotomy may last for up to 10 years.

Tasker[112] has also reported that the effect of thalamotomy on tremor is long lasting. In his experience, tremor that was completely abolished contralateral to a thalamic lesion for 3 months never recurred. Such results have prompted some authors to propose that thalamotomy may actually alter the course of Parkinson's disease.[120] An investigation into this issue has revealed three subgroups of Parkinson's disease in which the disease progresses so slowly that elimination of the major symptoms may appear to alter the progression of the disease. Patients with young-onset Parkinson's disease or the postencephalitis type and a subset of patients with idiopathic parkinsonism all seem to have very slow progression of their parkinsonian symptoms.[112] Thus, elimination of tremor in these patients might give the appearance of a long-term "cure."

In addition to the reduction of tremor symptoms, several studies have shown that patients require less or no L-dopa after thalamotomy.[110, 117] This decreased requirement for L-dopa helps reduce the drug-related side effects (e.g., dyskinesias). Independent of this reduction in the need for L-dopa, thalamotomy has been shown to reduce L-dopa–induced dyskinesias.[110] Narabayashi and colleagues[121] reported that although L-dopa dyskinesias are ameliorated by Vim thalamotomy, the optimal site for a lesion to relieve dyskinesias may be Vop, just anterior to Vim. This reduction of dyskinesia and increased tolerance of L-dopa are important for patients who have other parkinsonian symptoms, such as bradykinesia and rigidity, in addition to tremor.[77] In these patients, thalamotomy not only reduces tremor but also allows them to tolerate higher doses of L-dopa for management of their other symptoms.

Summary

Thalamotomy is a safe and effective procedure for the treatment of asymmetrical, severe, and medically intractable parkinsonian tremor.[118, 122–126] Recent experience has confirmed the early observation that thalamotomy is not effective for the treatment of bradykinesia, micrographia, or difficulty with gait or speech caused by Parkinson's disease.[78] Noninvasive computerized imaging provides optimal radiologic localization, and microelectrode recording provides optimal physiologic localization.[111]

Patients with tremor-predominant Parkinson's disease often develop other symptoms that do not respond to thalamic procedures. Thus, neurosurgeons are reluctant to make lesions that might make future interventions ineffective. Such interventions include DBS in Vim, GPi, or the subthalamus.[113, 114, 127] The latter two procedures may be considered later in the course of the disease for symptoms that develop after tremor. For these reasons, Vim stimulation may be preferable to thalamotomy for the treatment of parkinsonian tremor.[79, 111] In turn, DBS in GPi or the subthalamus can be effective against many symptoms of Parkinson's disease in addition to tremor,[113, 114] so these procedures may replace thalamic procedures for the treatment of Parkinson's tremor.

ESSENTIAL TREMOR

Essential tremor is the most common adult movement disorder, with a prevalence estimated at 4.1 to 39.2 cases per 1000 persons.[128] It is defined as a bilateral, largely symmetrical, postural or action tremor that occurs in the absence of any condition or drug known to cause enhanced physiologic tremor, in the absence of cerebellar signs and symptoms, and in the absence of Parkinson's disease, dystonia, hyperthyroidism, chronic alcoholism, peripheral neuropathy, or an anxiety state.[129, 130] It has a frequency range of 4 to 11 Hz.[129] The tremor preferentially affects both upper extremities and the head; the lower extremities are affected to a lesser extent.

Mechanism of Tremor

A familial form of essential tremor is transmitted in an autosomal-dominant pattern with high penetrance.[129, 131] The cause of this condition is poorly understood, however, despite investigations into the neurophysiologic mechanisms. Animals treated with β-carboline drugs such as harmaline develop a tremor similar to essential tremor.[132, 133] Harmaline tremor has been shown to originate in the inferior olive and to be expressed through the cerebellobulbospinal pathways.

In essential tremor, PET scans have shown that the cerebellum, contralateral red nucleus, thalamus, and sensorimotor cortex display overactivity.[134] Thalamic single neuron activity recorded during thalamotomy has been compared with forearm EMG activity (see Fig. 170–4). These studies indicate that thalamic cells have tremor frequency firing patterns that are linearly related to forearm EMG signals during essential tremor (tremor-related activity). One third of cells with tremor-related activity responded to sensory stimulation. Three models could account for this correlation: thalamic activity drives EMG activity, thalamic activity is driven by sensory input generated by tremor movement (for one third of cells), or an oscillator outside the thalamus drives both thalamic and EMG activity. Surgical lesions in the thalamus abolish essential tremor.[110, 123, 135] Therefore, it seems likely that thalamic mechanisms are involved in essential tremor, perhaps by transmission of cerebellar tremor-related activity to the periphery via the cortex.[42]

Indications for Thalamotomy

Surgery is an option for patients with disabling essential tremor who are unresponsive to or intolerant of optimal medical management and who do not have significant medical illness.[110, 123, 135] Approximately two thirds of patients are satisfactorily controlled with first-line therapy consisting of beta-blockers and primidone or with clonazepam.[130] The average functional status of patients with essential tremor undergoing stereotactic thalamotomy in our institution is outlined in Table 170–1.[135] The functional measure was obtained by grading speech, hygiene, eating, drinking, dressing, writing, and work separately, on a scale of 0 to 4. A score of 0 indicates that the patient's function is normal, and a score of 4 indicates that the patient requires assistance to complete the activity. Therefore, a score of 28 indicates that a patient is completely dependent. The mean disability score of 13 (see Table 170–1) indicated that most patients were moderately disabled preoperatively. Both writing and drawing (spiral and straight line) tests were administered and graded by a blinded asses-

T A B L E 1 7 0 – 1 ■ Total Functional, Blinded Handwriting/Drawing, and Amplitude (Action and Posture) Scores for Patients with Essential Tremor

TIME OF EVALUATION	AVERAGE SCORE—MEAN (SD)			
	Functional	Blinded Handwriting/ Drawing	Postural Tremor Amplitude	Action Tremor Amplitude
Preoperative	13.4 (1.8)	6.3 (0.7)	3.0 (0.3)	3.5 (0.2)
Postoperative 3 mo	4.7 (1.5)	2.8 (0.4)	0.7 (0.4)	0.6 (0.4)
Postoperative 1 yr	4.5 (1.3)	2.9 (0.3)	0.9 (0.4)	0.6 (0.4)
Significance				
Preoperative vs 3 mo	$P < 0.001$	$P < 0.001$	$P < 0.05$	$P < 0.05$
Preoperative vs 1 yr	$P < 0.001$	$P < 0.001$	$P < 0.05$	$P < 0.05$

From Zirh AT, Reich SG, Dougherty PM, Lenz FA: Stereotactic thalamotomy in the treatment of essential tumor of the upper extremity. J Neurol Neurosurg Psychiatry 66:772–775, 1999.

sor on a scale of 0 to 4 (Fig. 170–5), with 4 indicating an inability to complete the task. The three scores were added to obtain the composite writing score, out of a possible 12. The mean preoperative score of 6 indicated that the patients' writing and drawing were disrupted by tremor. Postural tremor amplitude and action tremor amplitude were rated by the surgeon, with 0 indicating no tremor and 4 indicating tremor with a greater than 2 cm amplitude.

Results

The results of several large clinical series of thalamotomies for essential tremor have been published. Al-

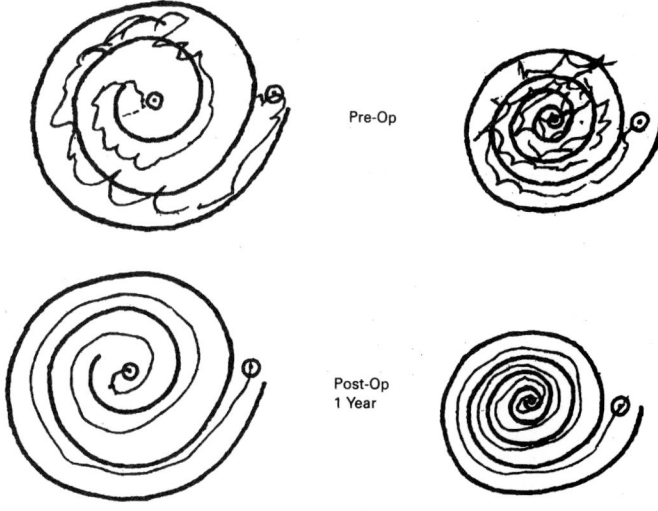

WRITE (with dominant hand only) "TODAY IS A NICE DAY IN BALTIMORE," SIGN YOUR NAME AND WRITE THE DATE JULY 4, 1776.

Pre-Op

Post-Op 1 Year

CONNECT THE DOTS ON EACH FIGURE WITH THE RIGHT HAND:

Pre-Op

Post-Op 1 Year

FIGURE 170–5. Example of the handwriting/drawing component of the standard rating scale of tremor in a patient with essential tremor. The preoperative sample is shown above in each case, and the 1-year postoperative sample is shown below. Both writing and spiral drawing were scored at 3 (with 4 being the worst score) preoperatively. Postoperatively, writing was scored at 0, and the spiral drawing task was scored at 1. (From Zirh AT, Reich SG, Dougherty PM, Lenz FA: Stereotactic thalamotomy in the treatment of essential tremor of the upper extremity: Re-assessment including a blinded measure of outcome. J Neurol Neurosurg Psychiatry 66:772–775, 1999.)

though these studies were conducted using different operative techniques, each demonstrated that the majority of patients undergoing the procedure had a significant reduction in tremor. This tremor control was maintained for extended periods (10 years or more). Nagaseki and colleagues[136] reported the outcome for 43 patients undergoing stereotactic lesioning of Vim between August 1975 and April 1982. Of these patients, 16 had essential tremor, and the remainder had Parkinson's disease. Of the 16 patients with essential tremor, complete abolition of tremor by thalamotomy was reported in 11 patients; a significant reduction of tremor was reported in the remaining 5. One patient subsequently underwent the procedure on the contralateral side, and one patient had a recurrence leading to a second procedure on the ipsilateral side. Fifteen of 16 patients returned to work, and 11 patients were able to discontinue their pharmacologic therapy. The mean follow-up period for this series was 6.25 years.

Mohadjer and associates[125] reported on 105 patients with essential tremor operated on between 1964 and 1984. Their anatomic target was the zona incerta either alone or in combination with other target points. They reported a 93.7% improvement in tremor control in the immediate postoperative period. A follow-up questionnaire was sent to all 105 patients, with a mean follow-up period of 8.6 years. Of the 65 patients who responded, 68.7% felt that they were still enjoying significant benefits from the surgery.

In a series of 60 patients undergoing Vim thalamotomy for tremor, Jankovic and coworkers[110] reported on 6 patients with essential tremor. Outcome was based on a global scale measuring improvement in tremor and functional status (scores ranged from 0, no effect, to 4, marked improvement in movement disorder and function). The mean outcome for essential tremor patients was 3.3, corresponding to a moderate improvement in tremor and functional status, with a mean follow-up of 59.2 months. Overall, 83% of patients (five of six) experienced improvement in their tremor.

Eight patients were treated surgically for essential tremor at the Mayo Clinic between 1984 and 1991.[123] Pre- and postoperative assessments were made for each patient with regard to disability in handwriting, speaking, feeding, hygiene, dressing, and working. Maximal disability represented a score of 28, and minimal disability was scored 0. The mean follow-up was 17.3 months postoperatively. All eight patients had improvement postoperatively. The mean disability score was reduced from 21.1 preoperatively to 3.9 postoperatively. Further, voice tremor was abolished or significantly improved in 71.4% of patients.

In another study, a disability scale, a blinded handwriting/drawing scale (see Fig. 170–5), and a tremor amplitude scale[137] were applied to assess the outcome of thalamotomy in 21 essential tremor patients.[135] Overall, the average patient was moderately disabled by tremor, with a mean functional disability score of 13.4 preoperatively; this score was reduced to 4.5 at 1 year postoperatively. Patients had significant improvements in all three scales. Figure 170–5 shows an example of the handwriting and spiral drawing tasks with pre- and postoperative samples.

Summary

Essential tremor is the ideal indication for thalamotomy because, unlike with Parkinson's disease, other symptoms do not develop over time. The benefit is long lasting, so no further procedures are required for this monosymptomatic condition. The alternative to thalamotomy for essential tremor is Vim-DBS; however, thalamotomy produces good, long-lasting control for essential tremor without the need for maintenance of the device, battery changes, and so forth. Unlike the radiofrequency lesion of thalamotomy, which is permanent, DBS can be adapted to treat the patient's symptoms and decrease the side effects.[79, 138] By reducing, modifying, or stopping stimulation, some side effects can be reduced or eliminated. This is particularly advantageous for bilateral procedures, in which the incidence of dysarthria approaches 30% to 60% of patients after bilateral thalamotomy.[110, 123, 135] The decision to carry out thalamotomy or Vim-DBS (see later) is based on the patient's acceptance of a somewhat higher risk (thalamotomy) versus the lifelong maintenance of an implanted device (Vim-DBS).[127]

CEREBELLAR TREMOR

Cerebellar tremor is characterized by tremor with intention—the increase in tremor amplitude as the target is approached during visually guided movements to a target. Specifically, cerebellar tremor is defined as a unilateral or bilateral intention tremor with a frequency usually below 5 Hz; postural tremor may be present, but not rest tremor.[129] Cerebellar tremor may occur from multiple causes, including inherited, traumatic, inflammatory, neoplastic, and vascular disorders that affect the cerebellum.

Mechanism of Tremor

The mechanism of intention tremor after lesions of the cerebellum or cerebellar pathways (cerebellar tremor) is still uncertain, although numerous mechanisms have been proposed. Cerebellar tremor may arise from alternating transcortical stretch reflex activity in antagonist muscle pairs.[139, 140] Alternatively, cerebellar tremor may result from voluntary corrections for errors in following a movement trajectory.[141–144] Finally, tremor may be related to interruption of cerebellar feed-forward control of the motor cortex responsible for the antagonist muscle activity that brakes movement.[145] In the absence of cerebellar feed-forward control of antagonists, sensory (feedback) control may take precedence so that cortical activity related to antagonists lags behind rather than leads movement. In monkeys with cerebellar tremor produced by cooling of the deep cerebellar nuclei, delayed antagonist activation correlates with delayed motor cortical activity related to antagonists.[145] Thus, cerebellar tremor is the result of a delay in the control signal to antagonist muscles during movement.[146, 147] This pathologic delay should be reflected in thalamic activity, because cerebellar efferents project to the motor cortex[148–152] via the thalamus.[153–155]

Thalamic recordings in patients with cerebellar tremor provide support for the third model. In patients with cerebellar tremor, neurons in Vim have significantly lower firing rates than do those in patients operated on for the treatment of pain (controls).[156] The degree of correlation between the thalamic and neuronal activities during tremor was not significantly different between neurons in Vim and neurons in Vop. Cellular activity lagged behind EMG activity more often in Vim than in Vop. The phase lag in Vim of cerebellar tremor patients is in contrast to the results of studies in normal monkeys carrying out active wrist oscillations. In these monkeys, the activity of cells in VPLo, corresponding to human Vim,[7] was correlated with and led wrist oscillations.[157] This suggests that cerebellar feedback to motor cortex is delayed by cerebellar lesions, leading to tremor during movement. Sensory cells had maximal activity at the frequency of tremor, and sensory cell activity was significantly correlated with movement more commonly than was the activity of nonsensory cells. These results suggest that delay in cerebellar input to the thalamus may explain cerebellar tremor.

Indications for Thalamotomy

As with other types of tremor, surgery is an option for patients with disabling cerebellar tremor who are unresponsive to or intolerant of optimal medical management and who do not have significant medical contraindications to surgery. Concomitant ataxic components in the limb are contraindications. The optimal medical management of this condition is less well defined than that for the other types of tremor, so the end point of medical management is less clear.[158]

Results

A study of 11 patients with multiple sclerosis treated with thalamotomy reported a good effect on tremor in 8 cases (73%) and moderate improvement in 2 (18%).[159] Significant improvement in arm function was noted in six cases (54%), and moderate improvement in two (18%). In another study, moderate or good improvement in activities of daily living was noted in 44% of patients (four of nine) with multiple sclerosis undergoing thalamotomy for pronounced, coarse intention tremor.[126]

Goldman and Kelly[123] reported complete abolition or marked reduction in 82% of 14 patients with intention tremor caused by head injury, multiple sclerosis, or stroke. As measured by a standard scale of tremor disability,[137] a significant decrease in median disability score was noted. In another study, eight patients with intention tremor (kinetic, eight of eight patients) with or without postural tremor (seven of eight patients) after severe head injury underwent thalamotomy.[160] Seven of eight had marked improvement, and the

eighth had 50% improvement. Two of the eight had gradual improvement in function over several weeks after the procedure. Intention tremor of multiple causes (not including multiple sclerosis) responded to lesions of less than 300 mm³ in 15 of 18 cases reported by Hirai and coworkers.[124]

In our experience, a statistically significant improvement in functional scores was found in intention tremor patients (*n* = 11) undergoing Vim thalamotomy.[118] The mean change in writing/drawing scores, determined by a blinded assessor, was not significant. A within-patient analysis demonstrated a significant improvement in the majority of patients (6 of 11).

Summary

Comparisons of the results of thalamotomy make it clear that thalamotomy is less effective for cerebellar tremor than for parkinsonian or essential tremor. Patients with cerebellar tremor are more disabled, however, because their tremor occurs with action and thus interferes directly with voluntary movement. A good result in these patients, although less common than with other tremors, is particularly satisfying for everyone involved. DBS is not approved in the United States for these patients, although it can be of some benefit.[79, 161] Thus, thalamotomy is still the procedure of choice for the treatment of disabling, medically intractable cerebellar tremor.

COMPLICATIONS

Complications from Vim thalamotomy fall into two categories: those that result from neural injury related to lesion making and those considered to be general risks of stereotactic surgery. Neither type of complication is directly related to the indication for thalamotomy, so we discuss the complications of thalamotomy for parkinsonian, essential, and cerebellar tremors together.

Complications from stereotactic surgery can arise from infection or intracranial hemorrhage. Infection of pin sites and meningitis have been reported in about 1% of stereotactic surgeries.[162] Hemorrhages account for a significant percentage of operative mortality in stereotactic surgery, with rates reported from 1% to 6%.[163] Hemorrhages may occur at the lesion site or at cortical sites, resulting in intracerebral or subdural hematomas. In four large series of thalamotomies (*n* = 242 patients), no hemorrhages were reported.[110, 117, 125, 136] In the same series, mortality after thalamotomy was a single death from a pulmonary embolus. Two deaths were reported in small series of patients (*n* = 53) operated on for cerebellar tremor.[122, 123, 126, 159, 160]

Functional deficits account for the majority of postoperative complications in thalamotomy. Functional deficits can be explained by lesion-induced disruption of the cerebellothalamocortical pathway or damage to thalamic nuclei and nearby structures. Large or incorrectly placed lesions are often responsible for deficits.

Lesions made posterior to Vim (in Vc) may cause sensory deficits (dysesthesia or paresthesia). A laterally placed lesion may injure internal capsule fibers, leading to weakness. Inferiorly placed lesions may cause hemiballismus by damage to the subthalamic nucleus. Additionally, left-sided or dominant hemispheric thalamic lesions may be associated with postoperative dysarthria and verbal memory impairment.[164]

In a series of 60 patients with essential, parkinsonian, or cerebellar tremor, functional deficits in the immediate postoperative period were reported in 58% of patients.[110] These transient deficits included weakness (34%), dysarthria (29%), ataxia (8%), dystonia (5%), and sensory deficits (3%). Cognitive deficits included disorientation and somnolence, as well as speech and language deficits and hypophonia. Transient deficits may have occurred from edema surrounding the acute lesion site.[165] Functional deficits persisted in 23% of patients but were generally mild and did not increase disability.[110] In a series of 105 patients with essential tremor, Mohadjer and coworkers[125] reported that 9 patients had persistent side effects, 5 had contralateral weakness, 1 had verbal dysarthria, and 3 showed signs of cerebellar dysfunction. Nagaseki and colleagues[136] reported that among 43 patients undergoing Vim thalamotomy for essential or parkinsonian tremor, there was one case each of meningitis and limb weakness.

In a series of 34 patients operated on for parkinsonian tremor, 14% (5) had permanent complications, including apraxia (1), dysarthria (2), dysphasia (1), and abulia (1).[117] Transient complications in 61% included cognitive decline (5), central facial (10) or hand (7) weakness, and hand numbness (2). Half the transient deficits resolved by 1 week, and most were absent at the 3-month follow-up visit. Thus, the rate of permanent, functionally significant postoperative deficits is low.

THALAMOTOMY VERSUS THALAMIC DEEP BRAIN STIMULATION

The primary alternative to Vim thalamotomy for essential tremor has been DBS through electrodes implanted in Vim (Vim-DBS). Although thalamotomy produces good tremor control for this condition, it was postulated that using stimulation rather than thermal coagulation would reduce the frequency of long-term side effects from these procedures. Unlike the radiofrequency lesion of thalamotomy, which is permanent, Vim-DBS can tailor the stimulation patterns to match the patient's symptoms.[79, 138] By reducing, modifying, or stopping stimulation, unpleasant or disabling side effects can be reduced or eliminated. This is particularly advantageous for bilateral procedures, where the postoperative incidence of dysarthria ranges from 30% to 60%.[110, 123, 135]

Tasker and coworkers[166] retrospectively reviewed their case series of Vim-DBS implants and thalamotomies for both Parkinson's disease and essential tremor. Because of the small number of patients with essential

tremor, the results were pooled with those for the parkinsonian patients for evaluation. The authors reported complete abolition of tremor in 42% of both groups and near abolition in 79% of DBS patients and 69% of thalamotomy patients. Tremors recurred in 5% of Vim-DBS patients and in 15% of thalamotomy patients. Ataxia, dysarthria, and gait disturbance occurred in 42% of the thalamotomy patients and 26% of the Vim-DBS patients: 15% of patients required a repeat thalamotomy, but none required a second Vim-DBS procedure. On the basis of these results, the authors concluded that Vim-DBS and thalamotomy produce equivalent degrees of tremor control, but that Vim-DBS produces these results with less morbidity. Of note, this study was neither prospective nor randomized, and several authors have reported a lower complication rate for thalamotomy than the 42% mentioned by Tasker.[166] A recent randomized, prospective study confirmed that Vim-DBS and thalamotomy are equally effective for tremor control.[169]

Additionally, implantation of a stimulating electrode involves the long-term maintenance of the stimulator. The burden of this maintenance can be estimated from large single-institution studies of DBS (141 patients followed over 20 years)[167] and spinal cord stimulation for the treatment of chronic pain (249 patients followed over 14 years).[168] The accumulated complications in these studies included infection, erosion, foreign body reaction, lead fracture, and stimulator failure. The morbidity rate from these complications in the two studies was 17% and 36%, respectively. In their most recent review (117 patients followed over 8 years), Benabid and associates[79] noted complications of this type in 7% of cases. This lower figure may result from technical refinements or may reflect the shorter follow-up in the latter study. Finally, DBS requires the cost and inconvenience of readjusting the stimulator periodically and of changing the battery at 3- to 5-year intervals. DBS has the obvious advantage of being reversible and adjustable, allowing the option of reversing some functional deficits. These advantages make bilateral procedures safer and more practical. The balance of the cost and inconvenience of lifelong maintenance of the device versus the lower complication rate of DBS can best be sorted out by a large, randomized outcome trial of Vim-DBS versus thalamotomy.

REFERENCES

1. Spiegel EA, Wycis HT: Ansotomy in paralysis agitans. Arch Neurol Psychiatry 71:598–614, 1954.
2. Narabayashi H, Okuma T: Procaine oil blocking of the globus pallidus for the treatment of rigidity and tremor of parkinsonism. Proc Jpn Acad 29:310–318, 1953.
3. Hassler R, Riechert T: Indikationen und Lokalisations-methode der gezielten Hirnoperationen. Nervenarzt 25:441–447, 1954.
4. Gildenberg PL: The present role of stereotactic surgery in the management of Parkinson's disease. Adv Neurol 40:447–453, 1984.
5. Hassler R: Architectonic organization of the thalamic nuclei. In Schaltenbrand G, Walker AE (eds): Stereotaxy of the Human Brain. Stuttgart, Germany, Thieme, 1982, pp 140–180.
6. Jones EG: The Thalamus. New York, Plenum, 1985.
7. Hirai T, Jones EG: A new parcellation of the human thalamus on the basis of histochemical staining. Brain Res Rev 14:1–34, 1989.

8. Guiot G, Hardy J, Albe-Fessard DG: Delimitation precis des structures sous-corticales et identification de noyaux thalamiques chez l'homme par l'electrophysiologie stereotactic. Neurochirurgia 5:1–18, 1962.

9. Mandir AS, Rowland LH, Dougherty PM, Lenz FA: Microelectrode recording and stimulation techniques during stereotactic procedures in the thalamus and pallidum. Adv Neurol 74:159–168, 1997.

10. Schaltenbrand G, Bailey P: Introduction to Stereotaxis with an Atlas of the Human Brain. Stuttgart, Germany, Thieme, 1959.

11. Hawrylyshyn P, Rowe IH, Tasker RR, Organ LW: A computer system for stereotaxic neurosurgery. Comput Biol Med 6:87–97, 1976.

12. Guiot G, Derome P: The principle of stereotaxic thalamotomy. In Kahn EA, Crosby EC, Schneider RC, Taren J (eds): Correlative Neurosurgery. Springfield, Ill, Charles C Thomas, 1969, pp 376–401.

13. Burchiel KJ: Thalamotomy for movement disorders. In Gildenberg PL (ed): Neurosurgery Clinics of North America. Philadelphia, WB Saunders, 1995, pp 55–71.

14. Tasker RR, Dostrovsky JO, Dolan EJ: Computerized tomography (CT) is just as accurate as ventriculography for functional stereotactic thalamotomy. Stereotact Funct Neurosurg 57:157–166, 1991.

15. Kondziolka D, Dempsey PK, Lunsford LD, et al: A comparison between magnetic resonance imaging and computed tomography for stereotactic coordinate determination. Neurosurgery 30:402–407, 1992.

16. Gerdes JS, Hitchon PW, Neerangun W, Torner JC: Computed tomography versus magnetic resonance imaging in stereotactic localization. Stereotact Funct Neurosurg 63:124–129, 1994.

17. Holtzheimer PE III, Roberts DW, Darcey TM: Magnetic resonance imaging versus computed tomography for target localization in functional stereotactic neurosurgery. Neurosurgery 45:290–298, 1999.

18. Hardy PA, Barnett GH: Spatial distortion in magnetic resonance imaging: Impact on stereotactic localization. In Gildenberg PL, Tasker RR (eds): Textbook of Stereotactic and Functional Neurosurgery. New York, McGraw-Hill, 1998, pp 271–280.

19. Alexander E, Kooy HM, van Herk M, et al: Magnetic resonance image–directed stereotactic neurosurgery: Use of image fusion with computerized tomography to enhance spatial accuracy. J Neurosurg 83:271–276, 1995.

20. Dostrovsky JO: The use of inexpensive personal computers for map generation and data analysis. In Gildenberg PL, Tasker RR (eds): Textbook of Stereotactic and Functional Neurosurgery. New York, McGraw-Hill, 1998, pp 2031–2036.

21. Cooper IS, Bergmann LL, Caracalos A: Anatomic verification of the lesion which abolishes parkinsonian tremor and rigidity. Neurology 13:779–787, 1963.

22. Lenz FA, Dostrovsky JO, Kwan HC, et al: Methods for microstimulation and recording of single neurons and evoked potentials in the human central nervous system. J Neurosurg 68:630–634, 1988.

23. Jasper HH, Bertrand G: Thalamic units involved in somatic sensation and voluntary and involuntary movements in man. In Purpura DP, Yahr MD (eds): The Thalamus. New York, Columbia University Press, 1966, pp 365–390.

24. Hubel DH: Tungsten microelectrode for recording from single units. Science 125:549–550, 1957.

25. Umbach W, Ehrhardt KJ: Micro-electrode recording in the basal ganglia during stereotaxic operations. Confinia Neurol 26:315–317, 1965.

26. Albe-Fessard DG: Electrophysiological methods for the identification of thalamic nuclei. Z Neurol 205:15–28, 1973.

27. Ohye C: Depth microelectrode studies. In Schaltenbrand G, Walker AE (eds): Stereotaxy of the Human Brain: Anatomical, Physiological and Clinical Applications. Stuttgart, Germany, Thieme, 1982, pp 372–389.

28. Wolbarsht ML, MacNichol EF Jr, Wagner HG: Glass insulated platinum microelectrode. Science 132:1309–1310, 1960.

29. Vitek JL, Bakay RAE, Hashimoto T, et al: Microelectrode-guided pallidotomy: Technical approach and application for treatment of medically intractable Parkinson's disease. J Neurosurg 88:1027–1043, 1998.

30. Ranck JB: Which elements are excited in electrical stimulation of mammalian central nervous system? A review. Brain Res 98:417–440, 1975.

31. Lenz FA, Seike M, Lin YC, et al: Thermal and pain sensations evoked by microstimulation in the area of the human ventrocaudal nucleus (Vc). J Neurophysiol 70:200–212, 1993.

32. Lenz FA, Seike MS, Jaeger CJ, et al: Thalamic single neuron activity in patients with dystonia: Dystonia-related activity and somatic sensory reorganization. J Neurophysiol 82:2372–2392, 1999.

33. Lenz FA, Dostrovsky JO, Tasker RR, et al: Single-unit analysis of the human ventral thalamic nuclear group: Somatosensory responses. J Neurophysiol 59:299–316, 1988.

34. Raeva SN: Localization in human thalamus of units triggered during "verbal commands," voluntary movements and tremor. Electroencephalogr Clin Neurophysiol 63:160–173, 1986.

35. Lenz FA, Kwan H, Dostrovsky JO, et al: Single unit analysis of the human ventral thalamic nuclear group: Activity correlated with movement. Brain 113:1795–1821, 1990.

36. Crowell RM, Perret E, Siegfried J: "Movement units" and "tremor phasic units" in the human thalamus. Brain Res 11:481–488, 1968.

37. Lenz FA, Kwan HC, Martin RL, et al: Single neuron analysis of the human ventral thalamic nuclear group: Tremor-related activity in functionally identified cells. Brain 117:531–543, 1994.

38. Raeva SN: Unit activity of some deep nuclear structures of the human brain during voluntary movements. In Somjen G (ed): Neurophysiology Studied in Man. Amsterdam, Excerpta Med, 1972, pp 64–78.

39. Bertrand C, Martinez SN, Hardy J, et al: Stereotactic surgery for parkinsonism: Microelectrode recording, stimulation, and oriented sections with a leucotome. In Krayenbuhl H, Maspes PE, Sweet WH (eds): Progress in Neurological Surgery. Basel, Karger, 1973, pp 79–112.

40. Hongell A, Wallin G, Hagbarth KE: Unit activity connected with movement initiation and arousal situations recorded from the ventrolateral nucleus of the human thalamus. Acta Neurol Scand 49:681–698, 1973.

41. Lenz FA, Tasker RR, Kwan HC, et al: Single unit analysis of the human ventral thalamic nuclear group: Correlation of thalamic "tremor cells" with the 3–6 Hz component of parkinsonian tremor. J Neurosci 8:754–764, 1988.

42. Hua S, Lenz FA, Zirh TA, et al: Thalamic activity correlated with essential tremor. J Neurol Neurosurg Psychiatry 64:273–276, 1998.

43. Lenz FA, Tasker RR, Kwan HC, et al: Cross-correlation analysis of thalamic neurons and EMG activity in parkinsonian tremor. Appl Neurophysiol 48:305–308, 1985.

44. Taren J, Guiot G, Derome P, Trigo JC: Hazards of stereotactic thalamectomy. J Neurosurg 29:173–182, 1968.

45. Ohye C: Neural noise recording in functional neurosurgery. In Gildenberg PL, Tasker RR (eds): Textbook of Stereotactic and Functional Neurosurgery. New York, McGraw-Hill, 1998, pp 941–948.

46. Ojemann GA, Ward AA Jr: Abnormal movement disorders. In Youmans JR (ed): Neurological Surgery, 2nd ed. Philadelphia, WB Saunders, 1982, pp 3821–3857.

47. Tasker RR, Organ LW, Hawrylyshyn P: The Thalamus and Midbrain in Man: A Physiologic Atlas Using Electrical Stimulation. Springfield, Ill, Charles C Thomas, 1982.

48. Laitinen LV, Hariz MI: Movement disorders. In Youmans JR (ed): Neurological Surgery, 4th ed. Philadelphia, WB Saunders, 1996, pp 3575–3609.

49. Fisher RS, Uematsu S, Krauss GL, et al: Placebo-controlled pilot study of centromedian thalamic stimulation in treatment of intractable seizures. Epilepsia 33:841–851, 1992.

50. Housepian EM, Purpura DP: Electrophysiological studies of subcortical-cortical relations in man. Electroencephalogr Clin Neurophysiol 15:20–28, 1963.

51. Kelly PJ, Ahlskog JE, Goerss SJ, et al: Computer-assisted stereotactic ventralis lateralis thalamotomy with microelectrode recording control in patients with Parkinson's disease. Mayo Clin Proc 62:655–664, 1987.

52. Bates JAV: Electrical recording from the thalamus in human subjects. In Iggo A (ed): Handbook of Sensory Physiology:

Somatosensory System. Berlin, Springer Verlag, 1972, pp 561–578.

53. Guiot G, Derome P, Arfel G, Walter SG: Electrophysiological recordings in stereotaxic thalamotomy for parkinsonism. In Krayenbuehl H, Maspes PE, Sweet WH (eds): Progress in Neurological Surgery. Basel, Karger, 1973, pp 189–221.

54. McComas AJ, Wilson P, Martin-Rodriguez J, et al: Properties of somatosensory neurons in the human thalamus. J Neurol Neurosurg Psychiatry 33:716–717, 1970.

55. Shima F, Morioka T, Tobimatsu S, et al: Localization of stereotactic targets by microrecording of thalamic somatosensory evoked potentials. Neurosurgery 28:223–230, 1991.

56. Albe-Fessard D: Electrophysiological recording in functional neurosurgery. Part I. Use of thalamic evoked potentials to improve the stereotactic localization of electrodes in the human brain. In Gildenberg PL, Tasker RR (eds): Textbook of Stereotactic and Functional Neurosurgery. New York, McGraw-Hill, 1998, pp 911–924.

57. Larson SJ, Sances A Jr: Averaged evoked potentials in stereotactic surgery. J Neurosurg 28:227–232, 1968.

58. Velasco F, Molina-Negro P: Electrophysiologic topography of the human diencephalon. J Neurosurg 38:204–214, 1973.

59. Li CL, van Buren JM: Microelectrode recordings in the brain of man with particular reference to epilepsy and dyskinesia. In Somjen G (ed): Neurophysiology Studied in Man. Amsterdam, Excerpta Med, 1972, pp 49–63.

60. Donaldson IML: The properties of some human thalamic units. Brain 96:419–440, 1973.

61. Fukamachi A, Ohye C, Narabayashi H: Delineation of the thalamic nuclei with a microelectrode in stereotaxic surgery for parkinsonism and cerebral palsy. J Neurosurg 39:214–225, 1973.

62. Alberts WW, Libet B, Wright EW, Feinstein B: Physiological mechanisms of tremor and rigidity in parkinsonism. Confinia Neurol 26:318–327, 1965.

63. Albe-Fessard DG, Arfel G, Guiot G, et al: Thalamic unit activity in man. Electroencephalogr Clin Neurophysiol 25:132–143, 1967.

64. Lucking CH, Struppler A, Erbel F, Reiss W: Stereotactic recording from human subthalamic structures. In Somjen G (ed): Neurophysiology Studied in Man. Amsterdam, Excerpta Med, 1972, pp 95–99.

65. Birk P, Riescher H, Struppler A, Keidel M: Somatosensory evoked potentials in the ventrolateral thalamus. Appl Neurophysiol 49:327–335, 1986.

66. Lenz FA, Normand SL, Kwan HC, et al: Statistical prediction of the optimal lesion site for thalamotomy in parkinsonian tremor. Mov Disord 10:318–328, 1995.

67. Kelly PJ, Derome P, Guiot G: Thalamic spatial variability and the surgical results of lesions placed with neurophysiologic control. Surg Neurol 9:307–315, 1976.

68. Ohye CH, Narabayashi H: Physiological study of presumed ventralis intermedius neurons in the human thalamus. J Neurosurg 50:290–297, 1979.

69. Tasker RR, Yamashiro K, Lenz FA, Dostrovsky JO: Thalamotomy in Parkinson's disease: Microelectrode techniques. In Lundsford D (ed): Modern Stereotactic Surgery. Norwell, Mass, Academic Press, 1988, pp 297–313.

70. Cosman ER, Cosman BJ: Methods of making nervous system lesions. In Wilkins RH, Rengachary SS (eds): Neurosurgery. New York, McGraw-Hill, 1985, pp 2490–2499.

71. Young RF, Shumway-Cook A, Vermeulen SS, et al: Gamma knife radiosurgery as a lesioning technique in movement disorder surgery. J Neurosurg 89:183–193, 1998.

72. Duma CM, Jacques DB, Kopyov OV, et al: Gamma knife radiosurgery for thalamotomy in parkinsonian tremor: A five year experience. J Neurosurg 88:1044–1049, 1998.

73. Rand RW, Jacques DB, Melbye RW, et al: Gamma knife thalamotomy and pallidotomy in patients with movement disorders: Preliminary results. Stereotact Funct Neurosurg 61 (Suppl 1): 65–92, 1992.

74. Kondziolka D, Lunsford LD: Functional radiosurgery using the gamma knife: Current and future applications. In Gildenberg PL, Tasker RR (eds): Textbook of Stereotactic and Functional Neurosurgery. New York, McGraw-Hill, 1998, pp 871–880.

75. Adams RD, Victor M, Ropper AH: Principles of Neurology. New York, McGraw-Hill, 1996.

76. Paulson HL, Stern MB: Clinical manifestations of Parkinson's disease. In Watts RL, Koller WC (eds): Movement Disorders. New York, McGraw-Hill, 1997, pp 183–199.

77. Poewe W, Granata R: Pharmacologic treatment of Parkinson's disease. In Watts RL, Koller WC (eds): Movement Disorders. New York, McGraw-Hill, 1997, pp 201–220.

78. Tasker RR, Siqueira J, Hawrylyshyn PA, Organ LW: What happened to VIM thalamotomy for Parkinson's disease? Appl Neurophysiol 46:68–83, 1983.

79. Benabid AL, Pollak P, Gao D, et al: Chronic electrical stimulation of the ventralis intermedius nucleus of the thalamus as treatment of movement disorders. J Neurosurg 84:203–214, 1996.

80. Elble RJ, Koller W: Tremor. Baltimore, Johns Hopkins University Press, 1990.

81. Lamarre Y, Joffroy AJ: Experimental tremor in monkey: Activity of thalamic and precentral cortical neurons in the absence of peripheral feedback. Adv Neurol 24:109–122, 1979.

82. Marsden CD: Origins of normal and pathological tremor. In Findley LJ, Capildeo R (eds): Movement Disorders: Tremor. London, Macmillan, 1984, pp 37–85.

83. Stein RB, Lee RG: Tremor and clonus. In Brooks VB (ed): Handbook of Physiology, sec 1, vol 2. Bethesda, Md, American Physiological Society, 1981, pp 325–343.

84. Steriade M, Deschenes M: The thalamus as a neuronal oscillator. Brain Res Rev 8:1–63, 1984.

85. Roy JP, Clercq M, Steriade M, Deschenes M: Electrophysiology of neurons of lateral thalamic nuclei in cat: Mechanisms of long-lasting hyperpolarizations. J Neurophysiol 51:1220–1235, 1984.

86. Domich L, Oakson G, Steriade M: Thalamic burst patterns in the naturally sleeping cat: A comparison between cortically-projecting and reticularis neurones. J Physiol (Lond) 379:429–449, 1986.

87. Jahnsen H, Llinas R: Ionic basis for the electroresponsiveness and oscillatory properties of guinea-pig thalamic neurones in vitro. J Physiol (Lond) 349:247–349, 1984.

88. Alexander GE, DeLong MR, Strick PL: Parallel organization of functionally segregated circuits linking basal ganglia and cortex. Annu Rev Neurosci 9:357–381, 1986.

89. Filion M, Tremblay L, Bedard PJ: Abnormal influences of passive limb movement on the activity of globus pallidus neurons in parkinsonian monkeys. Brain Res 444:165–176, 1988.

90. Pare D, Curro Dossi R, Steriade M: Neuronal basis of the parkinsonian resting tremor: A hypothesis and its implications for treatment. Neuroscience 35:217–226, 1990.

91. Buzsaki G, Smith A, Berger S, et al: Petit mal epilepsy and parkinsonian tremor: Hypothesis of a common pacemaker. Neuroscience 36:1–14, 1990.

92. Zirh AT, Lenz FA, Reich SG, Dougherty PM: Patterns of bursting occurring in thalamic cells during parkinsonian tremor. Neuroscience 83:107–121, 1997.

93. Lenz FA, Vitek JL, DeLong MR: Role of the thalamus in parkinsonian tremor: Evidence from studies in patients and primate models. Stereotact Funct Neurosurg 60:94–103, 1993.

94. Hua S, Reich SG, Zirh AT, et al: The role of the thalamus and basal ganglia in parkinsonian tremor. Mov Disord 13(Suppl 3): 40–42, 1998.

95. Lemstra AW, Verhagen Metman L, Lee J-I, et al: Tremor-frequency (3–6 Hz) activity in the sensorimotor arm representation of the internal segment of the globus pallidus in patients with Parkinson's disease. Neurosci Lett 267:129–132, 1999.

96. Hutchinson WD, Benko R, Dostrovsky JO, et al: Coherent relation of rest tremor to pallidal tremor cells in Parkinson's disease patients. Mov Disord 13(Suppl 2):204, 1998.

97. Raz A, Fiengold A, Vaadia E, et al: Neuronal oscillations in the globus pallidus of tremulous MPTP-treated monkeys—are they synchronized? Mov Disord 13(Suppl 2):184, 1998.

98. Lenz FA, Tatton WG, Tasker RR: Electromyographic response to displacement of different forelimb joints in the squirrel monkey. J Neurosci 3:783–794, 1983.

99. Lenz FA, Tatton WG, Tasker RR: The effect of cortical lesions on the electromyographic response to joint displacement in the squirrel monkey forelimb. J Neurosci 3:795–805, 1983.

100. Desmedt JE: Progress in Clinical Neurophysiology. Cerebral Motor Control in Man: Long Loop Mechanisms. Basel, Karger, 1978.

101. Lenz FA, Tasker RR, Tatton WG, Halliday W: Long-latency reflex activity in squirrel monkeys with occlusion of the middle cerebral artery. Electroencephalogr Clin Neurophysiol 67:238–246, 1987.

102. Vitek JL, Ashe J, DeLong MR, Alexander GE: Physiologic properties and somatotopic organization of the primate motor thalamus. J Neurophysiol 71:1498–1513, 1994.

103. Strick PL: Activity of ventrolateral thalamic neurons during arm movement. J Neurophysiol 39:1032–1044, 1976.

104. Schnider SM, Kwong RH, Lenz FA, Kwan HC: Detection of feedback in the central nervous system using system identification techniques. Biol Cybern 60:203–212, 1989.

105. Lenz FA, Schnider S, Tasker RR, et al: The role of feedback in the tremor frequency activity of tremor cells in the ventral nuclear group of human thalamus. Acta Neurochir (Wien) 39:54–56, 1987.

106. Deiber M-P, Pollak P, Passingham RE, et al: Thalamic stimulation and suppression of parkinsonian tremor: Evidence of cerebellar deactivation using positron emission tomography. Brain 116:267–279, 1993.

107. Parker F, Tzourio N, Blond S, et al: Evidence for a common network of brain structures involved in parkinsonian tremor and voluntary repetitive movement. Brain Res 584:11–27, 1992.

108. Davis KD, Taub E, Houle S, et al: Globus pallidus stimulation activates the cortical motor system during alleviation of parkinsonian symptoms. Nat Med 3:671–674, 1997.

109. Deuschl G, Wilms H, Krack P, et al: Function of the cerebellum in parkinsonian rest tremor and Holmes' tremor. Ann Neurol 46:126–128, 1999.

110. Jankovic J, Cardoso F, Grossman RG, Hamilton WJ: Outcome after stereotactic thalamotomy for parkinsonian, essential and other types of tremor. Neurosurgery 37:680–687, 1995.

111. Hallett M, Litvan I, members of the Task Force on Surgery for Parkinson's Disease of the American Academy of Neurology Therapeutic and Technology Assessment Committee: Evaluation of surgery for Parkinson's disease. Neurology 53:1910–1921, 1999.

112. Tasker RR: Ablative therapy for movement disorders: Does thalamotomy alter the course of Parkinson's disease? Neurosurg Clin N Am 9:375–380, 1998.

113. Limousin P, Krack P, Pollak P, et al: Electrical stimulation of the subthalamic nucleus in advanced Parkinson's disease. N Engl J Med 339:1105–1111, 1998.

114. Siegfried J, Lippitz B: Bilateral chronic electrostimulation of the ventroposterolateral pallidum: A new therapeutic approach for alleviating all parkinsonian symptoms. Neurosurgery 35:1126–1130, 1994.

115. Kumar R, Lozano AM, Kim YJ, et al: Double blind evaluation of subthalamic nucleus deep brain stimulation in advanced Parkinson's disease. Neurology 51:850–855, 1998.

116. Tasker RR: Thalamotomy. Neurosurg Clin N Am 1:841–864, 1990.

117. Fox MW, Ahlskog EJ, Kelly PJ: Stereotactic ventrolateralis thalamotomy for medically refractory tremor in post-levodopa era Parkinson's disease patients. J Neurosurg 75:723–730, 1991.

118. Lenz FA, Dougherty PM, Reich SG: The effectiveness of thalamotomy for treatment of tremor and dystonia. Mov Disord 11:18, 1996.

119. Diederich N, Goetz CG, Stebbins GT, et al: Blinded evaluation confirms long-term asymmetric effect of unilateral thalamotomy or subthalamotomy on tremor in Parkinson's disease. Neurology 42:1311–1314, 1992.

120. Matsumoto K, Schichijo F, Fukami T: Long-term follow-up review of cases of Parkinson's disease after unilateral or bilateral thalamotomy. J Neurosurg 53:332–337, 1984.

121. Narabayashi H, Yokochi F, Nakajima Y: Levodopa-induced dyskinesia and thalamotomy. J Neurol Neurosurg Psychiatry 47:831–839, 1984.

122. Perry VL, Lenz FA: Ablative surgery for treatment of movement disorders: Thalamotomy for Parkinson's disease. Neurosurg Clin N Am 9:317–324, 1998.

123. Goldman MS, Kelly PJ: Symptomatic and functional outcome of stereotactic ventralis lateralis thalamotomy for intention tremor. J Neurosurg 77:223–229, 1992.

124. Hirai T, Miyazaki M, Nakajima H, et al: The correlation between tremor characteristics and the predicted volume of effective lesions in stereotaxic nucleus ventralis intermedius thalamotomy. Brain 106:1001–1018, 1983.

125. Mohadjer M, Goerke H, Milios E, et al: Long term results of stereotaxy in the treatment of essential tremor. Stereotact Funct Neurosurg 54–55:125–129, 1990.

126. Wester K, Hauglie-Hanssen E: Stereotactic thalamotomy—experiences from the levodopa era. J Neurol Neurosurg Psychiatry 53:427–430, 1990.

127. Clatterbuck R, Lee J-I, Lenz FA: Lesions versus stimulation for the neurosurgical treatment of movement disorders. In Lozano A (ed): Progress in Neurological Surgery, vol 15. New York, Karger, 2000.

128. Louis ED, Ottman R, Hauser WA: How common is the most common adult movement disorder? Estimates of the prevalence of essential tremor throughout the world. Mov Disord 13:5–10, 1998.

129. Deuschl G, Bain PB, Brin MF, et al: Consensus statement of the Movement Disorder Society on tremor. Mov Disord Suppl 3:2–23, 1998.

130. Koller WC, Busenbark KL: Essential tremor. In Koller WC, Watts RL (eds): Movement Disorders. New York, McGraw-Hill, 1997, pp 365–386.

131. Brin MF, Koller W: Epidemiology and genetics of essential tremor. Mov Disord 13:55–63, 1998.

132. Lamarre Y: Central mechanisms of experimental tremor and their clinical relevance. In Findley LJ, Capildeo R (eds): Handbook of Tremor Disorders. New York, Marcel Dekker, 1995, pp 103–118.

133. Elble RG: The pathophysiology of tremor. In Watts RL, Koller WC (eds): Movement Disorders. New York, McGraw-Hill, 1997, pp 405–417.

134. Jenkins IH, Bain PB, Colebatch JG, et al: A positron emission tomography study of essential tremor: Evidence of overactivity of cerebellar connections. Ann Neurol 34:82–90, 1993.

135. Zirh AT, Reich SG, Dougherty PM, Lenz FA: Stereotactic thalamotomy in the treatment of essential tremor of the upper extremity: Re-assessment including a blinded measure of outcome. J Neurol Neurosurg Psychiatry 66:772–775, 1999.

136. Nagaseki Y, Shibazaki T, Hirai T, et al: Long-term follow-up results of selective VIM-thalamotomy. J Neurosurg 65:296–302, 1986.

137. Fahn S, Tolosa E, Marin C: Clinical rating scale for tremor. In Jankovic J, Tolosa E (eds): Parkinson's Disease and Movement Disorders. Baltimore, Urban & Schwartzenberg, 1988, pp 225–234.

138. Koller W, Pahwa R, Busenbark K, et al: High frequency unilateral thalamic stimulation in the treatment of essential and parkinsonian tremor. Ann Neurol 42:292–299, 1997.

139. Flament D, Hore J: Comparison of cerebellar intention tremor under isotonic and isometric conditions. Brain Res 439:179–186, 1988.

140. Diener HC, Dichgans J: Pathophysiology of cerebellar ataxia. Mov Disord 7:95–109, 1992.

141. Growdon JH, Chambers WW, Liu CN: An experimental study of cerebellar dyskinesia in the rhesus monkey. Brain 90:603–632, 1967.

142. Holmes G: The Croonian lectures on the clinical symptoms of cerebellar disease. Lancet 100:1177–1182, 1922.

143. Holmes G: The Croonian lectures on the clinical symptoms of cerebellar disease. Lancet 100:111–115, 1922.

144. Goldberger ME, Growdon JH: Pattern of recovery following cerebellar deep nuclear lesions in monkeys. Exp Neurol 39:307–322, 1973.

145. Hore J, Flament D: Changes in motor cortex neural discharge associated with the development of cerebellar limb ataxia. J Neurophysiol 60:1285–1302, 1988.

146. Vilis T, Hore J: Central neural mechanisms contributing to cerebellar tremor produced by limb perturbations. J Neurophysiol 43:279–291, 1980.

147. Vilis T, Hore J: Effects of changes in mechanical state of limb on cerebellar intention tremor. J Neurophysiol 40:1214–1224, 1977.

148. Jones EG, Wise SP, Coulter JD: Differential thalamic relationships of sensory-motor and parietal cortical fields in monkeys. J Comp Neurol 183:833–882, 1979.

149. Kievit J, Kuypers HGJM: Organization of the thalamo-cortical connections to the frontal lobe in the rhesus monkey. Exp Brain Res 29:299–322, 1977.
150. Mehler WR: Idea of a new anatomy of the thalamus. J Psychiatr Res 8:203–217, 1971.
151. Strick PL: Anatomical analysis of ventrolateral thalamic input to primate motor cortex. J Neurophysiol 39:1020–1031, 1976.
152. Walker AE: The Primate Thalamus. Chicago, University of Chicago Press, 1938.
153. Chan-Palay V: Cerebellar Dentate Nucleus: Organization, Cytology and Transmitters. New York, Springer, 1977.
154. Kalil K: Projections of the cerebellar and dorsal column nuclei upon the thalamus of the rhesus monkey. J Comp Neurol 195:25–50, 1981.
155. Tracey DJ, Asanuma C, Jones EG, Porter R: Thalamic relay to motor cortex: Afferent pathways from brain stem, cerebellum, and spinal cord in monkeys. J Neurophysiol 44:532–554, 1980.
156. Jaeger CJ, Lenz FA, Seike M, et al: Single unit analysis of thalamus in patients with cerebellar tremor. Mov Disord 9(Suppl 1):22, 1994.
157. Butler EG, Horne MK, Churchward PR: A frequency analysis of neuronal activity in monkey thalamus, motor cortex and electromyograms in wrist oscillations. J Physiol (Lond) 445:49–68, 1992.
158. Gilman S: Clinical features and treatment of cerebellar disorders. In Watts RL, Koller WC (eds): Movement Disorders. New York, McGraw-Hill, 1999, pp 577–585.
159. Speelman JD, Van Manen J: Stereotactic thalamotomy for the relief of intention tremor of multiple sclerosis. J Neurol Neurosurg Psychiatry 47:596–599, 1984.
160. Andrew J, Fowler CJ, Harrison MGH: Tremor after head injury and its treatment by stereotaxic surgery. J Neurol Neurosurg Psychiatry 45:815–819, 1982.
161. Geny C, Nguyen J-P, Pollin B, et al: Treatment of severe postural cerebellar tremor in multiple sclerosis by chronic thalamic stimulation. Mov Disord 11:489–494, 1996.
162. Hood TW, Yap JC: A survey of infections in stereotactic surgery. Appl Neurophysiol 44:314–319, 1981.
163. Louw DF, Burchiel KJ: Ablative therapy for movement disorders: Complications in the treatment of movement disorders. Neurosurg Clin N Am 9:367–373, 1999.
164. Ojemann GA, Hoyenga KB, Ward AA: Prediction of short-term verbal memory disturbance after ventrolateral thalamotomy. J Neurosurg 35:203–210, 1971.
165. Tomlinson FH, Jack CR Jr, Kelly PJ: Sequential magnetic resonance imaging following stereotactic radiofrequency ventralis lateralis thalamotomy. J Neurosurg 74:579–584, 1991.
166. Tasker RR, Munz M, Junn FSCK, et al: Deep brain stimulation and thalamotomy for tremor compared. Acta Neurochir Suppl (Wien) 68:49–53, 1997.
167. Levy RM, Lamb S, Adams JE: Treatment of chronic pain by deep brain stimulation: Long term follow-up and review of the literature. Neurosurgery 21:885–893, 1987.
168. North RB, Kidd DH, Zahurak M, et al: Spinal cord stimulation for chronic intractable pain: Experience over two decades. J Neurosurg 32:384–395, 1993.
169. Schuurman PR, Bosch DA, Bossuyt PM, et al: A comparison of continuous thalamic stimulation and thalamotomy for suppression of severe tremor. N Engl J Med 342:461–468, 2000.

Pallidotomy for Parkinson's Disease

ANDRES M. LOZANO ■ AHMED ALKHANI

The burden of disability produced by Parkinson's disease (PD) is augmenting with the increasing age of the population. Current figures estimate the overall incidence at 0.3%, increasing to 3% in persons older than 65 years of age.[1] Although medical therapy can be effective in many patients, particularly early in the disease, there continues to be a large number of patients with PD who continue to have profound motor disability or have significant drug-related adverse effects. Thus, alternate treatment strategies and a reexamination of surgical procedures in the treatment of PD are important.

Surgical treatment for PD and other movement disorders is not new; indeed, there is nearly a century-long history of these procedures.[2] Whereas surgery was initially the mainstay of treatment, the discovery of the dopamine deficiency in the striatum in PD changed the landscape. With the introduction of L-dopa in the 1960s and the realization of its striking clinical benefit, surgical procedures ground to a standstill. With time and increasing experience with the use of L-dopa and other medications, the shortcomings of pharmacotherapy have become problematic for many patients. The long-term use of antiparkinsonian drugs is associated with loss of therapeutic efficacy and with motor and non-motor complications, including fluctuations in motor performance with sometimes disabling drug-induced involuntary movements (dyskinesias) and gastrointestinal, cognitive, and psychiatric adverse effects. It is in the context of the failure of contemporary medical therapy that a reappraisal of surgical procedures is taking place. This re-evaluation has been encouraged by significant developments in surgical techniques and by important advances in the understanding of the pathophysiology of parkinsonism, which for the first time provide a sound scientific rationale for surgical interventions in various components of the basal ganglia. These developments and the initial reports of striking benefits with contemporary surgical interventions are responsible for spearheading the renaissance of surgical procedures in the treatment of PD and movement disorders in general and for the large recent increase in the use of pallidotomy (Fig. 171–1).

PATHOPHYSIOLOGY OF PARKINSON'S DISEASE AND PALLIDOTOMY

The human substantia nigra contains approximately 450,000 dopaminergic neurons.[3] Although other neu-

ronal populations such as those in the cholinergic, serotonergic, and catecholaminergic system are also affected, the most striking loss is that of pigmented neural melanin-laden dopaminergic neurons of the pars compacta of the substantia nigra (SNc).[4] The cause of this degeneration remains largely unknown, although important genetic and environmental factors are being identified.[4-6] Signs and symptoms of PD appear when approximately half of this neuronal population is lost. The most striking consequence of this neuronal loss is a severe dopamine deficiency in the striatum, in particular the dorsal putamen.[7]

Significant advances in our understanding of the pathophysiology of parkinsonian signs and symptoms have come about through the establishment of animal models. The administration of the neurotoxin 1-methyl-4-phenyl-1,2,3,6-tetrahydropyridine (MPTP) to nonhuman primates results in severe degeneration of dopaminergic neurons and a clinical picture characterized by akinesia, bradykinesia, and tremor remarkably similar to that encountered in patients with PD.[8] The development of this animal model has allowed neurophysiologists to obtain direct measures of cellular activity in the basal ganglia of parkinsonian animals and discover the pathophysiologic correlates of the motor abnormalities. The most striking finding in the parkinsonian state is the hyperactivity of neurons in the internal segment of the globus pallidus (GPi).[9, 10] This comes about by a combination of two mechanisms: first, decreased inhibition from the diminished activity in an inhibitory direct striatopallidal projection; and, second, through enhanced driving from an overactive glutaminergic excitatory subthalamic nucleus projection.[11] Because the globus pallidus and its related structure, the substantia nigra pars reticulata (SNpr), constitute the entire output from the basal ganglia, they are in a pivotal position and exert a powerful influence on thalamocortical and brainstem motor areas to which they project. The final consequence of the dopamine deficiency state is thus a heightened and excessively inhibitory outflow from the globus pallidus that disrupts thalamocortical and brainstem motor function, leading to the poverty of movement and unregulated movement encountered in parkinsonism. Consistent with this mechanism is the observation that the impaired activation of the supplementary motor cortex in PD is reversed when the akinesia is treated with

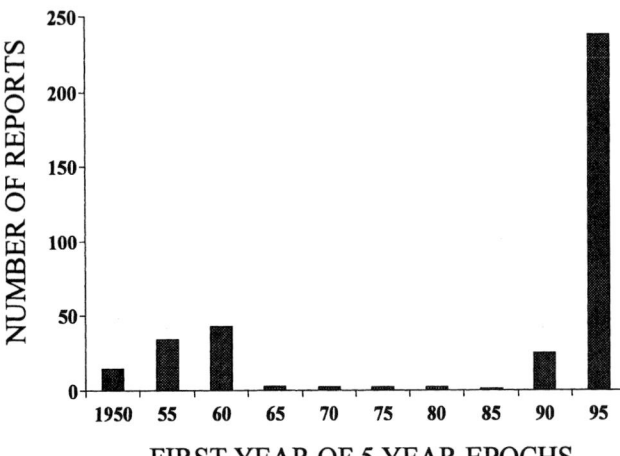

FIGURE 171–1. The number of reports in the literature on pallidotomy in 5-year epochs as a measure of the use of pallidotomy. Reports from 1966 to 1999 were obtained by using a PubMed literature search using the word "pallidotomy" as a key word. Before 1966, the number of reports on pallidotomy was estimated by counting publications listed in a bibliography on Parkinson's disease published by the National Institutes of Health. (Data from Parkinson's Disease and Related Disorders. Cumulative bibliography: 1800–1970. Bethesda, MD, National Institutes of Health, 1971.)

dopaminergic agents.[12] The surgical strategy is to remove this abnormal output from the globus pallidus to the thalamus and downstream cortex as well as the brainstem, to restore their function, and to reverse the motor abnormalities.

Although there is no direct evidence that GPi is overactive in humans, there are several lines of evidence that support this. First, hyperactivity in the internal segment of the globus pallidus can be demonstrated using 18-fluorodeoxyglucose positron emission tomography in PD patients.[13] Second, animal experiments have confirmed hyperactivity in the GPi in the MPTP parkinsonian state.[14] Third, although no control values are available, GPi neurons in PD patients have high rates of discharge, on the order of 80 to 100 Hz, and these rates fall dramatically with the administration of dopaminergic agents.[15] These observations suggest that GPi is hyperactive in the parkinsonian state, that dopaminergic drugs may act by reducing GPi overactivity, and that reducing GPi activity is important for improvement in motor function.

PATIENT SELECTION

Indications for Pallidotomy

Pallidotomy is used for patients with PD who continue to have significant motor disability despite the best medical management. The best candidates are patients with idiopathic PD who respond to L-dopa and who are disabled by motor fluctuations, dyskinesias, tremor, bradykinesia, and rigidity. Patients with asymmetric disease stand to benefit most from unilateral pallidotomy. Patients with prominent gait disturbances can

also benefit, but this symptom may be less responsive to unilateral pallidotomy. It is controversial whether patients who are non–L-dopa responsive or who have one of the so-called Parkinson's plus syndromes, such as multiple system atrophy or progressive supranuclear palsy, respond to pallidotomy and should undergo the operation. Preliminary reports suggest that these patients do not obtain substantial benefit from this procedure. Pallidotomy is also being used for primary dystonia and dystonia-like syndromes, with several centers reporting sometimes striking benefit.[16, 17]

Because the benefits of pallidotomy are predominantly contralateral, patients with asymmetric disease are particularly good candidates for the procedure. The ipsilateral benefits of unilateral pallidotomy are small in magnitude and often dissipate after a few months. In patients with bilateral symptoms, surgery should be performed contralateral to the most affected side. If both sides are equally affected, then surgery should be directed to improve the dominant side of the body. Although certain patients do show benefit with pallidotomy, in general, patients with prominent axial, postural abnormalities and speech impairments are not ideal candidates because these features are less responsive to pallidotomy. Furthermore, cognitive and psychiatric disturbances, autonomic disturbances, and speech and swallowing disturbances cannot only fail to improve but may also worsen after pallidotomy.

Diagnostic Evaluation

It is essential that a thorough neurological evaluation be completed to confirm the diagnosis of PD and its responsiveness to dopaminergic drugs and rule out some of the many other causes of parkinsonism. In 20% to 25% of patients diagnosed with PD by consultant neurologists a different disorder is found at autopsy.[18] Brain imaging can be useful in revealing structural causes of parkinsonism, including ischemic white matter disease, hydrocephalus, and space-occupying lesions, and in identifying some of the Parkinson's plus syndromes, such as striatonigral degeneration, which are associated with characteristic magnetic resonance imaging (MRI) signal changes in the striatum. Significant coexisting medical conditions, psychiatric disease, or focal abnormalities on brain imaging are relative contraindications.

The age of the patient is not a primary concern, although several reports suggest that younger patients derive more benefit from surgery.[19, 20] The procedure should not be offered to patients whose disorder is well controlled with medications or who have minimal disability that does not significantly interfere with their work or lifestyle. As a general rule, patients who have significant cognitive impairment are not good candidates for the procedure. Cognitive disturbance is common, with an estimated approximately 30% of PD patients having dementia.[21] Patients with cognitive impairments are sometimes uncooperative in the operating room, and the motor benefits they receive from the procedure can have sometimes only minor impact in the context of a significant cognitive disability. In addition, these patients are at risk for worsening of cognitive function after pallidotomy. As an office screening test, patients scoring less than 25 of 30 in the Mini-Mental State evaluation[22] should raise concern and may merit further neuropsychological assessment.

TREATMENT

Surgical Techniques

The surgical technique is divided into three stages: imaging, physiologic mapping, and lesioning. Modern imaging has had an important impact on the resurgence of pallidotomy. There has been a steady transition from ventriculography to computed tomography (CT) and MRI to help localize the targets. In a survey of the literature, we found that the majority of centers employ MRI (45%), with approximately 10% of centers using only CT and 2.5% of centers using only ventriculography. The rest of the centers use a combination of these procedures.[23] There are two approaches to deriving the pallidotomy target. It can be estimated as a function of its relationship to the anterior and posterior commissure, or it can be targeted directly from MRI. Laitinen and colleagues have popularized a pallidotomy target of 2 to 3 mm anterior to the midcommissural point, 3 to 6 mm below the intercommissural line, and 18 to 21 mm to the midline.[24] Although these coordinates are an approximation of the pallidotomy target, they do not take into account anatomic variations in the size and position of the pallidal complex nor the width of the third ventricle.[25] In part to address these issues there has been a move toward direct visualization of the globus pallidus and targeting from MR images.[26] There are advocates of both CT and MRI techniques for localization. CT has a greater spatial resolution and accuracy, but MRI provides better anatomic definition. It is clear that if MRI is used, particular attention has to be placed on how the images are acquired and on quality control for the intrinsic distortions, which may occur with MRI. To overcome some of these difficulties, certain centers are fusing CT and MRI images.

MAPPING

The purpose of mapping is to confirm the anatomic data obtained from imaging, to identify the optimal surgical target for clinical improvement, and to diminish the possibility of adverse effects. The goals of physiologic mapping in the globus pallidus are to identify the sensorimotor portion of the globus pallidus, the optic tract, and the internal capsule.

Two forms of physiologic mapping are possible: macroelectrode stimulation and microelectrode recording stimulation. With macroelectrode stimulation three types of information can be obtained. First and most reliably, the induction of contractions related to current spread to the internal capsule can be elicited with stimulation at the various frequencies; commonly, 2 or 100 Hz is used. The current threshold required to

elicit this response is a function of the distance separating the electrode to the internal capsule. An estimate of the proximity of the optic tract can also be obtained by stimulating at high frequencies and asking the patient to report the occurrence of visual perceptions or phosphenes in the contralateral visual field. This is completely dependent on the patient's subjective response and has been found on some occasions (in approximately 10% of cases) to be unreliable. The false-negative reports of visual perceptions may be responsible for the cases of visual field deficits after pallidotomy. To avoid this difficulty, recording light flash–induced volleys of action potentials or evoked potentials from optic tract axons using microelectrodes can unambiguously identify the optic tract (Fig. 171–2). This technique offers the advantage that it does not rely on the patient's subjective report and that the optic tract can be identified even under general anesthesia. There is also some indication that, in some patients, acute intraoperative stimulation of the globus pallidus can lead to clinical improvement. This is not universally seen but is potentially a promising indication of an appropriate location for lesioning.

The main advantage of microelectrode recordings is that they permit the acquisition of direct measures of cellular activity of the pallidal complex (see Fig. 171–2) and provide unambiguous definition of axonal and neuronal territories.[27, 28] The internal capsule and optic tract are devoid of large somatodendritic action potentials and are characterized by relative electrical silence in recordings. In contrast, nuclear structures feature a high density of units that generate large action potentials. Furthermore, the white matter laminae that separate the external from the internal segments of the globus pallidus and indeed that subcompartmentalize the internal segment into external and internal compartments can also be identified (Fig. 171–3). The identification of neurons whose spontaneous rate of discharge changes in response to active or passive movements of limbs or body parts identifies the sensorimotor territory of GPi. It is this region of GPi that occupies the posterior ventral one third of GPi and that is distinct from the associative and limbic regions of GPi, which is believed to be the optimal surgical target for the alleviation of parkinsonian symptoms. The technical details of microelectrode recording techniques have been covered elsewhere.[28, 29] The number of microelectrode recording trajectories required to identify the optic tract, internal capsule, and sensorimotor GPi varies from two to four per case. On average, each recording tract takes 30 minutes to 1 hour if one stops to examine each neuron and determine its movement-related receptive field. Examples of microelectrode recording trajectories and findings are shown in Figures 171–2 and 171–3. Once the sensorimotor GPi, the internal capsule, and the optic tract have been identified, surgery progresses to lesion making.

LESION MAKING

Two alternate strategies are commonly used: either a single lesion or multiple smaller contiguous or stacked

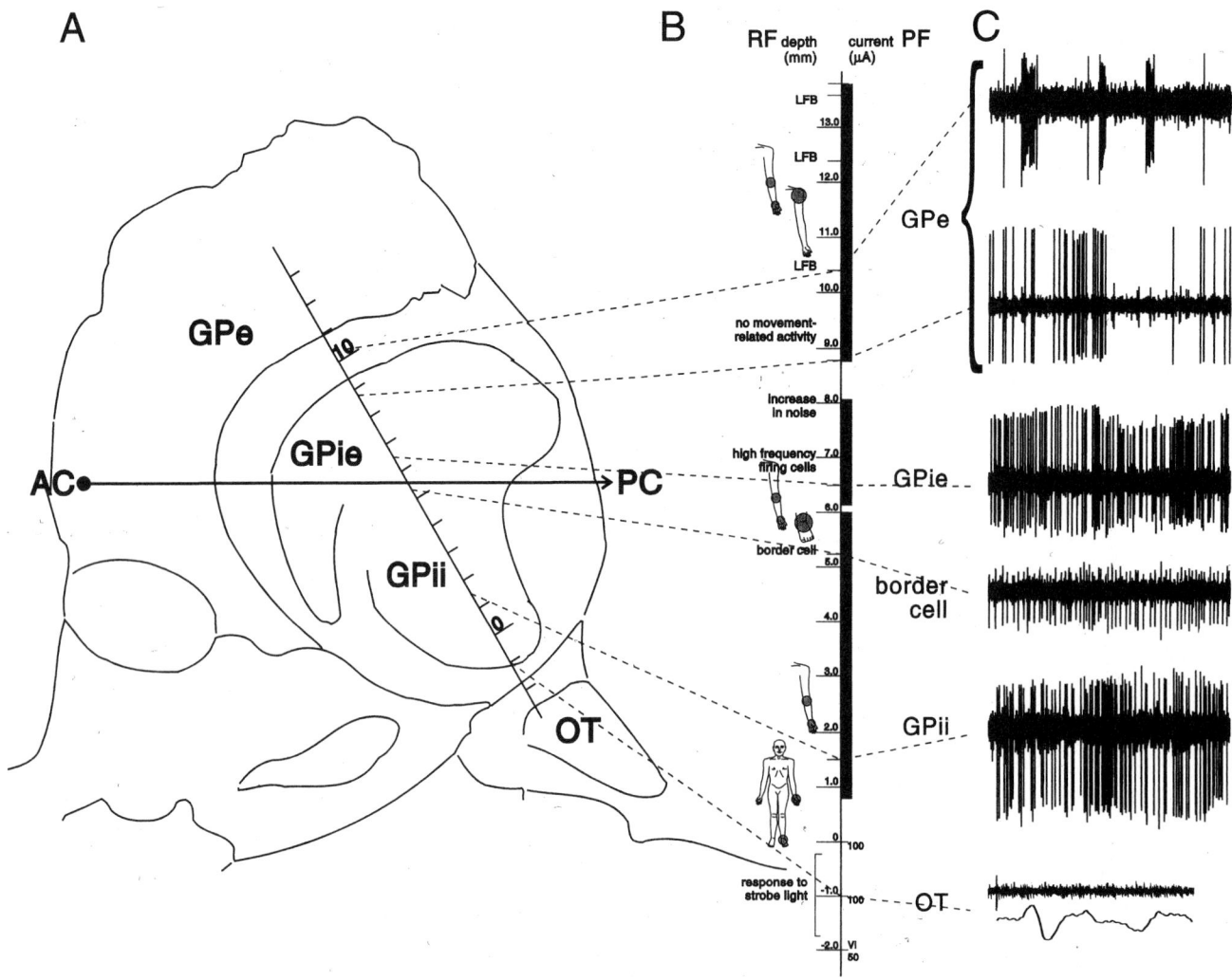

FIGURE 171–2. Physiologic data obtained from one trajectory through the globus pallidus and optic tract, plotted on the 20-mm sagittal map from the Schaltenbrand and Wahren stereotactic atlas *(A)*. *B,* The locations of neurons and their responses as well as intraoperative observations of the characteristics of recordings. *C,* Oscilloscope traces of representative examples of the neuronal types described in text. At the bottom is shown a single sweep of the filtered trace where the optic tract field potential to visual stimuli was heard but not readily seen. With appropriate filter settings for visual evoked potential measurement from the optic tract (OT), the visual evoked potential (VEP) can be seen, as illustrated below (the smooth trace). GPe, external, and GPi, internal, segments; AC, PC, anterior and posterior commissures; LFB, low-frequency burst neuron. (From Lozano A, Hutchison W, Kiss Z, et al: Methods for microelectrode-guided posteroventral pallidotomy. J Neurosurg 84: 194–201, 1996.)

radiofrequency lesions. The relative merits of each of these strategies are largely unknown. In general, radio-frequency lesions are made with electrodes with exposed tips from 1 to 3 mm long and between 1 and 1.8 mm in diameter. Lesions are made sequentially for periods of up to 1 minute at 45°C, 60°C, 70°C, and 80°C up to 90°C. Using a lesioning electrode with a 3-mm exposed tip at 90°C for 60 seconds produces a lesion approximately 6 mm in diameter (Fig. 171–4). Patients are operated on in the "off" drug condition to accentuate the signs and symptoms of PD and to provide immediate feedback of the effects of incremental lesions. There should be immediate improvements in bradykinesia and rigidity with lesioning. Tremor improvements are often delayed, and the improvements

in gait and postural instability are not practically tested in the operating room. Improvements in L-dopa dyskinesias in the operating room are also difficult to assess. It has been suggested that the acute onset of dyskinesias with lesioning may prove to be a good prognostic sign for a beneficial effect on parkinsonian symptoms.

Complications

Pallidotomy is a relatively safe procedure. However, adverse effects are not uncommon. A compilation of reported adverse effects of pallidotomy is presented in Table 171–1. Mortality is estimated to be on the order of 0.3% and mostly related to cerebral hemorrhage. The most significant morbidities include hemorrhage,

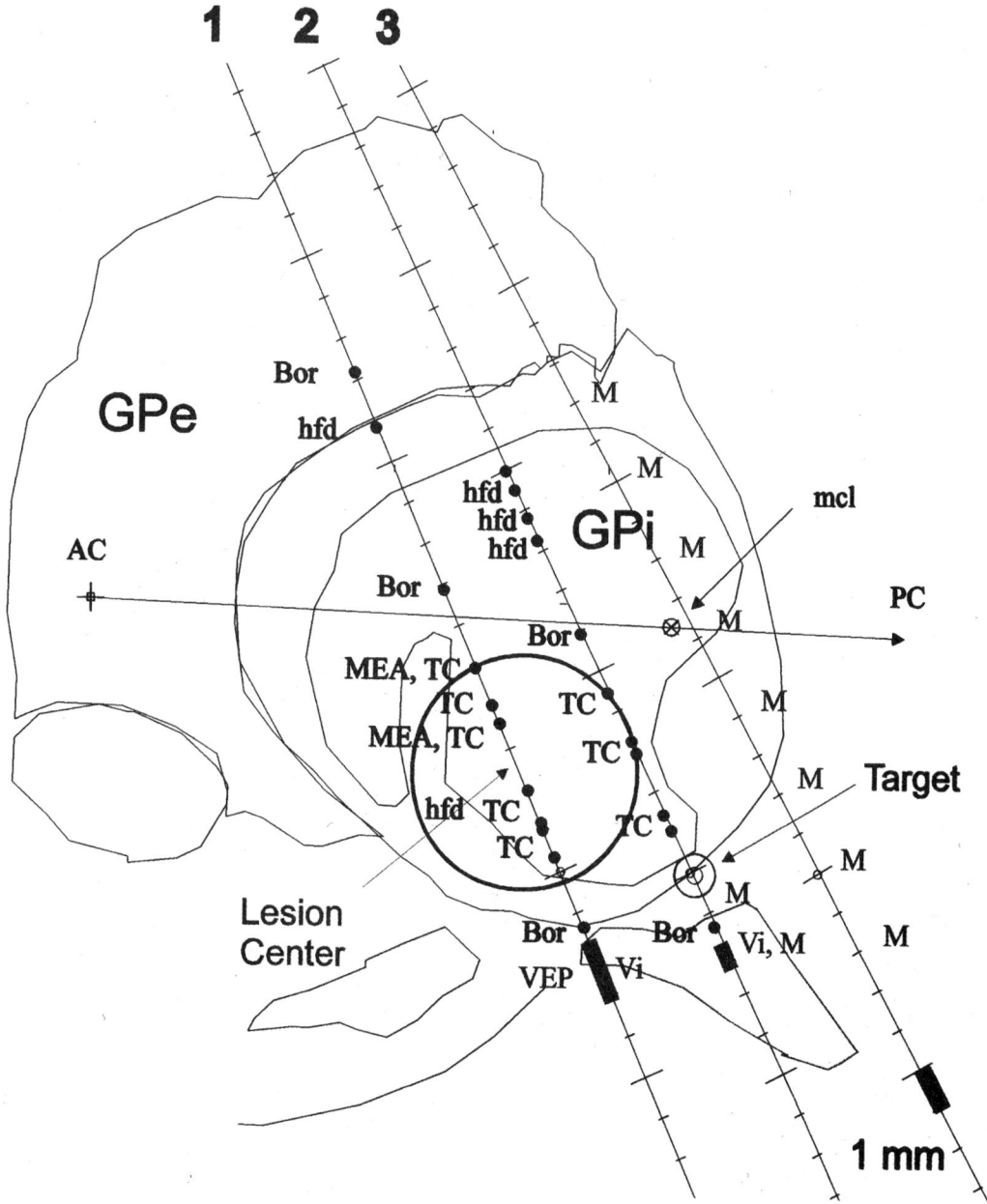

FIGURE 171–3. Final physiologic map for one case consisting of three sequential electrode trajectories showing the major findings, superimposed on a sagittal map of the globus pallidus 20 mm lateral to the midline. The map outline used is the same as in Figure 171–2. Note that in this case the recommended target site determined by anatomic localization methods was too close to both the internal capsule and the optic tract. Based on the physiologic findings, the final lesion site was modified an additional 3 mm anterior and 3 mm superior to the original target. Microrecording results are shown left of the track and microstimulation results on the right. Bor, border cell; hfd, high-frequency discharge cell; mcl, midcommissural line; MEA, movement-evoked activity; TC, tremor cell. The optic tract, located ventral to GPi was found by recording visual-evoked potentials (VEP) and patient's reports of visual responses (Vi) to microstimulation (<100 mA). The internal capsule (posterior to GPi) was located by observation of motor (M) responses to microstimulation. *Large circle* shows the estimated final lesion size. (From Lozano AM, Hutchison WD: Microelectrode guided pallidotomy. In Rengachary S, Wilkins RH (eds): Neurosurgical Operative Atlas, vol 7. American Association of Neurological Surgeons, 1997, pp 27–33.)

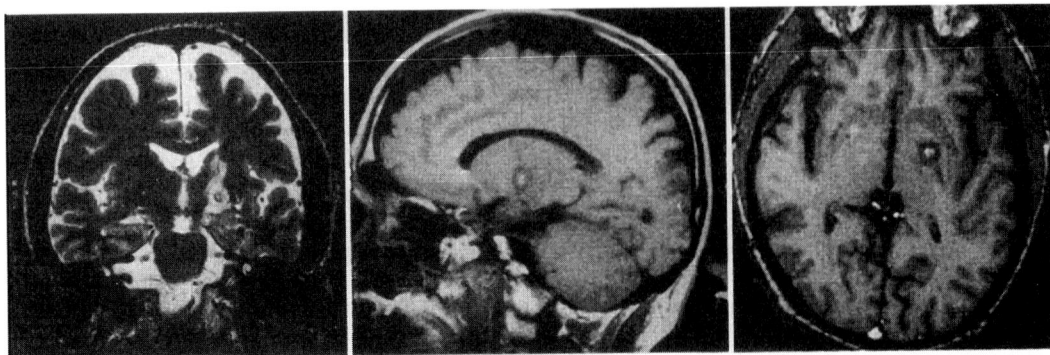

FIGURE 171–4. Location of the globus pallidus lesion in a patient with idiopathic Parkinson's disease shown on magnetic resonance images of the brain in *(from left to right)* coronal, sagittal, and horizontal planes. (From Lozano A, Hutchison W, Kiss Z, et al: Methods for microelectrode-guided posteroventral pallidotomy. J Neurosurg 84:194–201, 1996.)

visual field defect, contralateral weakness, dysarthria, dysphagia, hypophonia, and cognitive changes. Cerebral hemorrhages are said to occur in 1% to 2% of cases. This includes only symptomatic hemorrhages and does not take into account small asymptomatic

TABLE 171–1 ■ Reported Complications of Pallidotomy*

MORBIDITIES	TOTAL NO. PATIENTS	RATE (%)
Cerebral hemorrhage†	26	1.7
Postoperative psychosis	8	0.5
Hypersalivation (sialorrhea)	9	0.6
Postoperative seizure	8	0.5
Hypophonia	20	1.3
Visual field (total)	30	2.0
Visual field (persistent)	23	1.5
Depression	13	0.9
Acute postoperative confusion	40‡	2.6
Facial weakness		
Total	56‡	3.7
Persistent	19	1.3
Dysarthria		
Total	48	3.2
Persistent	24	1.6
Dysphagia		
Total	18	1.2
Persistent	8	0.5
Impaired memory		
Total	19	1.3
Persistent	14	0.9
Limb weakness		
Total	24	1.6
Persistent	14	0.9
Other complications	30	2.0
Total patients with complications	349/1510	23.1
Total patients with persistent complications	216/1510	14

*The values listed are derived from a review of 85 published studies from 1992 to 1999 on pallidotomy describing nearly 2000 patients. Data on complications were available on 1510 patients who underwent pallidotomy.
†Not including mortality cases.
‡Not including one study that reported "several" transient deficits in 15 patients.[20]
From Alkhani A, Lozano AM: Pallidotomy for Parkinson's disease: A review of the contemporary literature. J Neurosurg 94:43–49, 2001.

hemorrhages that occur along the electrode trajectories. Visual field deficits have been reported to complicate approximately 2% of pallidotomy cases, although the incidence varies largely from 0% to 40%. The reasons for this large variability in incidence of this complication have to do with series size and the degree to which visual field deficits have been ascertained. Experience also plays a role in preventing such complications, with initial series often reporting a higher incidence than subsequent reports from the same center. Contralateral weakness in the limbs or face may occur after pallidotomy, with an incidence of 4% being reported in the literature. Other complications, including persistent dysarthria, dysphagia, and hypophonia, also have an incidence of approximately 4%. Acute postoperative confusion is not uncommon after pallidotomy. Several series have reported the occurrence of this adverse effect in approximately 10% and up to 40% of patients. There are several reports of mild cognitive disturbances that occur with pallidotomy; however, in all but a few exceptions the authors report that the motor improvements obtained outweigh the mild cognitive deficits.

Clinical Outcome

A summary of clinical outcomes in pallidotomy is presented in Table 171–2. The clinical feature that responds best to pallidotomy is the cessation of the contralateral drug-induced involuntary movements. Several studies have documented improvements in the contralateral dyskinesia score of 80% to 90%. This effect is seen within days of the surgery and lasts for at least 2 years,[30] with indications that it may last 5 years or longer (Lang and Lozano, unpublished results). The improvements in "off" period contralateral rigidity are 50% to 60%. These benefits are immediate and last for several years. Improvements in activities of daily living and the bradykinesia scores in the "off" period are on the order of 30%. These benefits last at least 5 years. The gait and postural instability scores after pallidotomy improve 20% to 30%; however, the beneficial effects to gait appear to be short-lived, with much of the initial benefit being lost after 6 months. There is an

TABLE 171–2 ■ **Effects of Pallidotomy on Major Motor Manifestations of Parkinson's Disease***

ASSESSMENT SCALE	6-MONTHS' FOLLOW-UP DATA				12-MONTHS' FOLLOW-UP DATA			
	No. Patients	Preop. Mean	Postop. Mean	Improvement (%)	No. Patients	Preop. Mean	Postop. Mean	Improvement (%)
UPDRS (II & III) during "off"	142	74,2	48.8	34.2	99	75.3	48.4	35.7
Motor UPDRS during "off"	256	45.8	27.2	40.6	161	43.9	23.6	45.3
Schwab & England ADL "off"	87	47.2	61.8	31.1	86	44.8	63.3	41.3
Contralateral dyskinesias "on"	94	2.26	0.60	73.5	71	2.35	0.32	86.4

*The values listed are derived for a review of 85 published studies from 1992 to 1999 on pallidotomy.
ADL, activities of daily living; UPDRS, Unified Parkinson's Disease Rating Scale part II (ADL) and part III (motor examination); "on" and "off" refer to practically defined on and off states.
  From Alkhani A, Lozano AM: Pallidotomy for Parkinson's disease: A review of the contemporary literature. J Neurosurg 94:43–49, 2001.

ipsilateral improvement of dyskinesias on the order of 30% that wanes after approximately 6 months.[30] In addition, pallidotomy unequivocally increases patient function and can restore some independence.[30, 31]

It is clear that other than patient selection, the size and location of the pallidotomy lesion may also have a profound influence on clinical benefit. Gross and associates have used postoperative MRI to localize the site of pallidotomy lesions within the internal segment of the globus pallidus.[25, 32] Some clear-cut differences have been seen in outcome as a function of lesion location (Fig. 171–5). These researchers have also shown that anterior medial lesions in GPi benefit rigidity and drug-induced involuntary movements whereas central lesions most benefit bradykinesia and tremor as well as rigidity and drug-induced involuntary movements and that the most posterior lesions are especially beneficial for tremor. These types of observations may explain in part the discrepancies among various surgical series.

Most reported series state that drug dosages are uninfluenced or only slightly reduced by pallidotomy. In some cases because of the elimination of drug-induced involuntary movements, drugs have actually been increased after pallidotomy, resulting in a better and longer duration of the "on" period.

CONCLUSION

Pallidotomy is useful for patients with advanced PD with significant bradykinesia, rigidity, tremor, motor fluctuations, and drug-induced involuntary movements (dyskinesias). Improvement after unilateral pallidotomy appears to be greatest for drug-induced dyskinesias and least for gait and postural disturbances. Improvements in contralateral dyskinesias, tremor, rigidity, and bradykinesia last at least 5 years. Symptoms that persist in the "on" state (e.g., freezing, falls, dysarthria) are less responsive to pallidotomy. Because benefits are predominantly contralateral, asymmetric patients stand to improve the most with pallidotomy. There are insufficient reliable data on the indications, safety, or benefits of bilateral pallidotomy. The available data, however, suggest that bilateral pallidotomy may be associated with a higher incidence of neurological adverse effects, particularly speech complications.[33] Nevertheless, small bilateral lesions have been pro-

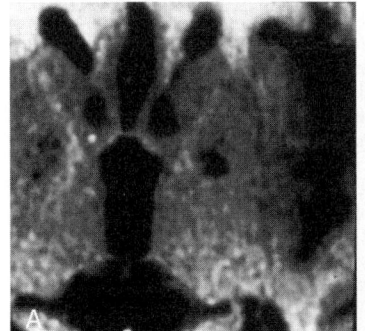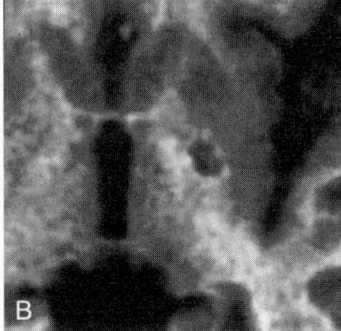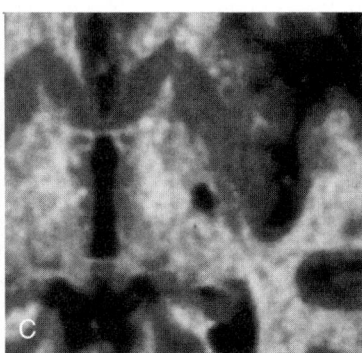

FIGURE 171–5. Clinical correlates of lesion location. Lesions within different regions of GPi have differential effects on parkinsonian symptoms. Anteromedial lesions *(A)* are most effective for relieving drug-induced dyskinesias and rigidity. Central lesions *(B)* are most effective for akinesia. Posterolateral GPi lesions *(C)* are especially effective for tremor. (From Gross RE, Lombardi WJ, Lang AE, et al: Relationship of lesion location to clinical outcome following microelectrode-guided pallidotomy for Parkinson's disease. Brain 22(Pt 3):405–416, 1999.)

duced with good clinical benefit and few adverse effects.[34] The optimal lesion size, location, duration of benefit, and incidence of adverse effects with bilateral pallidotomy are unresolved.

Emerging Alternatives to Pallidotomy: Gamma-Knife Pallidotomy, Subthalamic Nucleus Lesions, Chronic Brain Stimulation

There are a small number of studies using image-guided radiosurgical pallidotomy.[35–42] Based on the available reports of limited benefits and substantial complications, the radiosurgical, nonphysiologically guided approach cannot be recommended at the present time.

An alternative lesioning target is the subthalamic nucleus. Preliminary reports suggest that substantial improvement in parkinsonism can be achieved with radiofrequency lesions of the subthalamic nucleus and that the risk of producing hemiballism is minimal.[43] Further studies and longer term follow-up are required.

Deep brain stimulation (DBS) is also emerging as a surgical alternative. The advantage of stimulation versus lesioning is its safety, reversibility, and adaptability. DBS also provides the possibility of adjustment of stimulation parameters as the clinical features change over time. DBS is therefore becoming attractive for patients who require bilateral procedures or as a contralateral procedure in a patient who has had a pallidotomy.

Several reports on bilateral GPi stimulation for PD[44–51] and dystonia[52] have appeared. Bilateral GPi DBS for PD has produced improvements in bradykinesia, gait, tremor, and drug-induced dyskinesias. The clinical effects are dependent on which parts of the pallidum are stimulated and which stimulating parameters are used.[46, 53] Recent functional imaging data[54] suggest that GPi stimulation, like pallidotomy,[55] improves parkinsonian features by activating supplementary motor cortical areas whose underactivity in PD is thought to underlie major clinical signs and symptoms. This finding suggests that pallidal stimulation blocks GPi overactivity to disinhibit the downstream thalamus and thalamocortical system. Recent work shows that pallidotomy can be combined with contralateral pallidal DBS[47] to provide clinical benefit with the advantage of the reversibility of DBS. Similar striking improvements in parkinsonism are being seen with subthalamic nucleus stimulation.[56–58] Among the important unresolved issues in movement disorder surgery are the relative merits of lesioning versus stimulation and the relative attributes of the GPi and the subthalamic nucleus as targets for the treatment of PD.

Acknowledgments

The authors thank Drs. Lang, Hutchison, Dostrovsky, and Tasker for their ongoing collaboration. Dr. Lozano is a Medical Research Council of Canada Clinician-Scientist. This work is supported by the Parkinson's Foundation of Canada.

REFERENCES

1. Moghal S, Rajput AH, D'Arcy C, Rajput R: Prevalence of movement disorders in elderly community residents. Neuroepidemiology 13:175–178, 1994.
2. Guridi J, Lozano AM: A brief history of pallidotomy. Neurosurgery 41:1169–1180; discussion 1180–1183, 1997.
3. German DC, Schlusselberg DS, Woodward DJ: Three-dimensional computer reconstruction of midbrain dopaminergic neuronal populations: From mouse to man. J Neural Transm 57:243–254, 1983.
4. Lang AE, Lozano AM: Parkinson's disease: First of two parts. N Engl J Med 339:1044–1053, 1998.
5. Polymeropoulos MH, Lavedan C, Leroy E, et al: Mutation in the alpha-synuclein gene identified in families with Parkinson's disease. Science 276:2045–2047, 1997.
6. Kitada T, Asakawa S, Hattori N, et al: Mutations in the parkin gene cause autosomal recessive juvenile parkinsonism [see comments]. Nature 392:605–608, 1998.
7. Kish SJ, Shannak K, Hornykiewicz O: Uneven pattern of dopamine loss in the striatum of patients with idiopathic Parkinson's disease. N Engl J Med 318:876–880, 1988.
8. Langston JW, Forno LS, Rebert CS, Irwin I: Selective nigral toxicity after systemic administration of 1-methyl-4-phenyl-1,2,5,6-tetrahydropyrine (MPTP) in the squirrel monkey. Brain Res 292:390–394, 1984.
9. Filion M, Boucher R, Bedard P: Globus pallidus unit activity in the monkey during the induction of parkinsonism by 1-methyl-4-phenyl-1,2,3,6-tetrahydropyridine (MPTP). Brain Res 11:1160, 1985.
10. Miller WC, DeLong MR: Altered tonic activity of neurons in the globus pallidus and subthalamic nucleus in the primate MPTP model of parkinsonism. In Carpenter MB, Jayaraman A (eds): The Basal Ganglia II. New York, Plenum, 1987.
11. DeLong MR: Primate models of movement disorders of basal ganglia origin. Trends Neurosci 13:281–285, 1990.
12. Jenkins IH, Fernandez W, Playford ED, et al: Impaired activation of the supplementary motor area in Parkinson's disease is reversed when akinesia is treated with apomorphine. Ann Neurol 32:749–757, 1992.
13. Eidelberg D, Moeller JR, Kazumata K, et al: Metabolic correlates of pallidal neuronal activity in Parkinson's disease. Brain 120:1315–1324, 1997.
14. Crossman AR, Mitchell IJ, Sambrook MA: Regional brain uptake of 2-deoxyglucose in N-methyl-4-phenyl-1,2,3,6-tetrahydropyridine (MPTP)-induced parkinsonism in the macaque monkey. Neuropharmacology 24:587–591, 1985.
15. Hutchison WD, Levy R, Dostrovsky JO, et al: Effects of apomorphine on globus pallidus neurons in parkinsonian patients. Ann Neurol 42:767–775, 1997.
16. Lozano AM, Kumar R, Gross RE, et al: Globus pallidus internus pallidotomy for generalized dystonia [see comments]. Mov Disord 12:865–870, 1997.
17. Ondo WG, Desaloms JM, Jankovic J, Grossman RG: Pallidotomy for generalized dystonia. Mov Disord 13:693–698, 1998.
18. Hughes AJ, Daniel SE, Kilford L, Lees AJ: Accuracy of clinical diagnosis of idiopathic Parkinson's disease: A clinico-pathological study of 100 cases [see comments]. J Neurol Neurosurg Psychiatry 55:181–184, 1992.
19. Lang AE, Lozano AM, Montgomery E, et al: Posteroventral medial pallidotomy in advanced Parkinson's disease [see comments]. N Engl J Med 337:1036–1042, 1997.
20. Baron MS, Vitek JL, Bakay RA, et al: Treatment of advanced Parkinson's disease by posterior GPi pallidotomy: 1-year results of a pilot study [see comments]. Ann Neurol 40:355–366, 1996.
21. Aarsland D, Tandberg E, Larsen JP, Cummings JL: Frequency of dementia in Parkinson disease. Arch Neurol 53:538–542, 1996.
22. Folstein MF, Folstein SE, McHugh PR: Mini-mental state: A practical method for grading the cognitive state of patients for the clinician. J Psychiatr Res 12:189–198, 1975.
23. Alkhani A, Lozano AM: Pallidotomy for Parkinson's disease: A review of the contemporary literature. J Neurosurg 94:43–49, 2001.
24. Laitinen LV, Bergenheim AT, Hariz MI: Leksell's posteroventral pallidotomy in the treatment of Parkinson's disease. J Neurosurg 76:53–61, 1992.

25. Gross RE, Lombardi WJ, Hutchison WD, et al: Variability in lesion location after microelectrode-guided pallidotomy for Parkinson's disease: Anatomical, physiological, and technical factors that determine lesion distribution. J Neurosurg 90:468–477, 1999.

26. Starr PA, Vitek JL, DeLong M, Bakay RA: Magnetic resonance imaging-based stereotactic localization of the globus pallidus and subthalamic nucleus. Neurosurgery 44:303–313; discussion 313–314, 1999.

27. Lozano AM, Hutchison WD, Kiss ZHT, et al: Methods for microelectrode-guided posteroventral pallidotomy. J Neurosurg 84:194–202, 1996.

28. Vitek JL, Bakay RA, DeLong MR: Microelectrode-guided pallidotomy for medically intractable Parkinson's disease. Adv Neurol 74:183–198, 1997.

29. Lozano A, Hutchison W, Kiss Z, et al: Methods for microelectrode-guided posteroventral pallidotomy. J Neurosurg 84:194–202, 1996.

30. Lang AE, Lozano AM, Montgomery E, et al: Posteroventral medial pallidotomy in advanced Parkinson's disease. N Engl J Med 337:1036–1042, 1997.

31. de Bie RM, de Haan RJ, Nijssen PC, et al: Unilateral pallidotomy in Parkinson's disease: A randomised, single-blind, multicentre trial [In Process Citation]. Lancet 354:1665–1669, 1999.

32. Gross RE, Lombardi WJ, Lang AE, et al: Relationship of lesion location to clinical outcome following microelectrode-guided pallidotomy for Parkinson's disease [see comments]. Brain 122:405–416, 1999.

33. Taha J, Favre J, Burchiel KJ: Bilateral pallidotomy for the treatment of Parkinson's disease. In Krauss J, Grossman R, Jankovic J (eds): Pallidal Surgery for Movement Disorders. Philadelphia, Lippincott-Raven, 1998, pp 173–178.

34. Scott R, Gregory R, Hines N, et al: Neuropsychological, neurological and functional outcome following pallidotomy for Parkinson's disease: A consecutive series of eight simultaneous bilateral and twelve unilateral procedures. Brain 121:659–675, 1998.

35. Hirai T, Ryu H, Nagaseki Y, et al: Image-guided electrophysiologically controlled posteroventral pallidotomy for the treatment of Parkinson's disease: A 28-case analysis. Adv Neurol 80:585–591, 1999.

36. Friedman DP, Goldman HW, Flanders AE, et al: Stereotactic radiosurgical pallidotomy and thalamotomy with the gamma knife: MR imaging findings with clinical correlation—preliminary experience. Radiology 212:143–150, 1999.

37. Young RF, Vermeulen S, Posewitz A, Shumway-Cook A: Pallidotomy with the gamma knife: A positive experience. Stereotact Funct Neurosurg 70(Suppl 1):218–228, 1998.

38. Young RF, Shumway-Cook A, Vermeulen SS, et al: Gamma knife radiosurgery as a lesioning technique in movement disorder surgery. J Neurosurg 89:183–193, 1998.

39. Bonnen JG, Iacono RP, Lulu B, et al: Gamma knife pallidotomy: Case report. Acta Neurochir 139:442–445, 1997.

40. Friedman JH, Epstein M, Sanes JN, et al: Gamma knife pallidotomy in advanced Parkinson's disease. Ann Neurol 39:535–538, 1996.

41. Young RF: Functional neurosurgery with the Leksell Gamma knife. Stereotact Funct Neurosurg 66:19–23, 1996.

42. Rand RW, Jacques DB, Melbye RW, et al: Gamma knife thalamotomy and pallidotomy in patients with movement disorders: Preliminary results. Stereotact Funct Neurosurg 61:65–92, 1993.

43. Gill SS, Heywood P: Bilateral dorsolateral subthalamotomy for advanced Parkinson's disease. Lancet 350:1224, 1997.

44. Gross C, Rougier A, Guehl D, et al: High-frequency stimulation of the globus pallidus internalis in Parkinson's disease: A study of seven cases. J Neurosurg 87:491–498, 1997.

45. Ardouin C, Pillon B, Peiffer E, et al: Bilateral subthalamic or pallidal stimulation for Parkinson's disease affects neither memory nor executive functions: A consecutive series of 62 patients [In Process Citation]. Ann Neurol 46:217–223, 1999.

46. Bejjani B, Damier P, Arnulf I, et al: Pallidal stimulation for Parkinson's disease: Two targets? Neurology 49:1564–1569, 1997.

47. Galvez-Jimenez N, Lozano A, Tasker R, et al: Pallidal stimulation in Parkinson's disease patients with a prior unilateral pallidotomy. Can J Neurol Sci 25:300–305, 1998.

48. Ghika J, Villemure JG, Fankhauser H, et al: Efficiency and safety of bilateral contemporaneous pallidal stimulation (deep brain stimulation) in levodopa-responsive patients with Parkinson's disease with severe motor fluctuations: A 2-year follow-up review. J Neurosurg 89:713–718, 1998.

49. Tronnier VM, Fogel W, Kronenbuerger M, Steinvorth S: Pallidal stimulation: An alternative to pallidotomy? J Neurosurg 87:700–705, 1997.

50. Vingerhoets G, van der Linden C, Lannoo E, et al: Cognitive outcome after unilateral pallidal stimulation in Parkinson's disease. J Neurol Neurosurg Psychiatry 66:297–304, 1999.

51. Volkmann J, Sturm V, Weiss P, et al: Bilateral high-frequency stimulation of the internal globus pallidus in advanced Parkinson's disease. Ann Neurol 44:953–961, 1998.

52. Kumar R, Dagher A, Hutchison WD, et al: Globus pallidus deep brain stimulation for generalized dystonia: Clinical and PET investigation. Neurology 53:871–874, 1999.

53. Krack P, Pollak P, Limousin P, et al: Opposite motor effects of pallidal stimulation in Parkinson's disease. Ann Neurol 43:180–192, 1998.

54. Davis KD, Taub E, Houle S, et al: Globus pallidus stimulation activates the cortical motor system during alleviation of parkinsonian symptoms [see comments]. Nat Med 3:671–674, 1997.

55. Ceballos-Baumann AO, Obeso JA, Vitek JL, et al: Restoration of thalamocortical activity after posteroventral pallidotomy in Parkinson's disease. Lancet 344:814, 1994.

56. Kumar R, Lozano AM, Sime E, et al: Comparative effects of unilateral and bilateral subthalamic nucleus deep brain stimulation. Neurology 53:561–566, 1999.

57. Limousin P, Krack P, Pollak P, et al: Electrical stimulation of the subthalamic nucleus in advanced Parkinson's disease. N Engl J Med 339:1105–1111, 1998.

58. Kumar R, Lozano AM, Kim YJ, et al: Double-blind evaluation of subthalamic nucleus deep brain stimulation in advanced Parkinson's disease. Neurology 51:850–855, 1998.

CHAPTER 172

Surgery for Dystonia

MICHAEL S. OKUN ■ JERROLD L. VITEK

Dystonia is a movement disorder characterized by sustained muscle contractions, twisting and repetitive movements, and abnormal postures.[1-3] Dystonia can be classified by cause or by body region. Dystonia without a defined cause is referred to as *primary* or *idiopathic dystonia*. Dystonia with a cause, such as trauma, metabolic alterations, degenerative disease, drugs, or stroke, is classified as *secondary dystonia*. Primary dystonia may have a known genetic linkage, such as *DYT1*,[4] or it may occur sporadically without an associated or identifiable gene location.[4-6] Many genetic loci have been identified in dystonia patients, but those with genetic causes still represent the minority of patients with this disease. Dystonia also may be described in terms of the affected body regions, such as focal dystonia, segmental dystonia, hemidystonia, or generalized dystonia.[3]

Although there is no specific medical therapy for dystonia, observation and limited studies have resulted in trials of different drugs, including anticholinergic medications, muscle relaxants, and benzodiazepines.[2, 7-9] Most drugs used to treat dystonia have limited efficacy at low doses and intolerable side effects at high doses. In light of the failure of medical therapy in most patients, considerable effort has been invested in developing alternative treatment strategies. These strategies have included a variety of surgical approaches, including peripheral nerve denervation,[10, 11] dorsal column stimulation,[12] pallidotomy,[13] thalamotomy,[14-16] and pallidal[17-22] and thalamic deep brain stimulation (DBS).[23-26]

Before the 1990s, the largest experience in dystonia surgery was with thalamotomy, with only a few poorly detailed cases of pallidotomy reported in the literature.[13, 14, 27-31] Although pallidotomy[13, 32] and thalamotomy[15, 16, 28, 31, 33, 34] were effective in improving motor function in some patients, others did not benefit, or they worsened. Many patients undergoing bilateral thalamotomy and pallidotomy experienced bulbar complications including dysarthria and dysphagia. Because of the inconsistent benefit of these procedures and their associated complications, they were largely abandoned and only recently revived. The resurgence of surgical therapy resulted from a better understanding of the functional organization of the basal ganglia and improved comprehension of the pathophysiologic basis of movement disorders.

BASAL GANGLIA: FUNCTIONAL ORGANIZATION AND ROLE IN DYSTONIA

The basal ganglia are viewed as components of segregated circuits, including motor, oculomotor, associative, and limbic circuits. The motor circuit is implicated in the pathophysiology of hyperkinetic disorders (e.g., dystonia, drug-induced dyskinesias) and hypokinetic disorders (e.g., Parkinson's disease [PD]). The basal ganglia–thalamocortical motor circuit originates from precentral and postcentral sensorimotor fields and engages specific portions of the putamen, the external (GPe) and internal (GPi) segments of the globus pallidus, the substantia nigra pars reticulata (SNr), the subthalamic nucleus (STN) and portions of the motor thalamus (i.e., ventralis lateralis pars oralis [VLo; VOP or VOA in humans], ventralis anterior [VA]), and returns to the same precentral motor fields from which it took origin. The striatum, the major input structure of the basal ganglia, influences GPi, the major output structure, through two routes arising from separate subpopulations of inhibitory neurons: a direct pathway and an indirect pathway involving the GPe and STN. All the intrinsic connections of the basal ganglia are inhibitory, except for the STN to GPi or SNr pathway, which is glutamatergic and excitatory.

The dopaminergic nigrostriatal pathway (from the substantia nigra pars compacta [SNc]) appears to modulate the activity of the two striatopallidal pathways differentially by activation of different dopamine receptors (Fig. 172-1). Dopamine appears to facilitate transmission in the direct pathway through D_1 receptors and inhibit transmission in the indirect pathway through D_2 receptors.[35, 36] According to this model, depletion of dopamine in the striatum, as occurs in PD, causes increased activity in the GPi, which results in excessive inhibition of the pallidal receiving areas of the thalamus, VLo and VA. It has been postulated that the resulting increased level of inhibition in the thalamus leads to the hypokinetic features of PD.[35] In contrast to excessively increased GPi output in hypokinetic disorders, hyperkinetic disorders are thought to result from abnormally lowered GPi output, leading to disinhibition and increased activity of thalamocortical

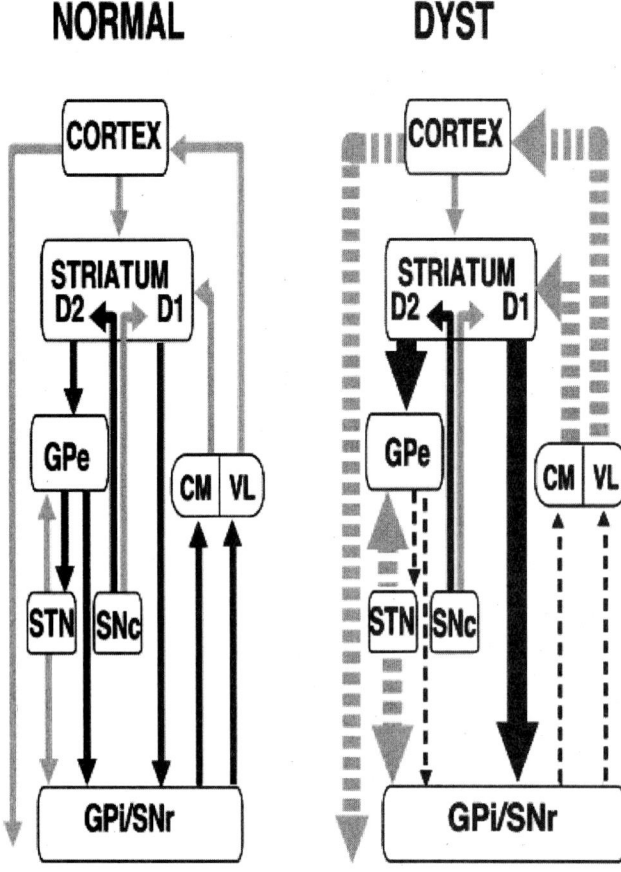

NORMAL   **DYST**

FIGURE 172–1. Model of dystonia based on observations of altered patterns of neuronal activity that interrupt thalamocortical and corticocortical activity leading to altered cortical output. CM, projections from center median thalamic nuclei; D1, dopamine 1 receptor; D2, dopamine 2 receptor; DYST, dystonia; GPe, external segment of the globus pallidus; GPi, internal segment of the globus pallidus; NORMAL, normal conditions; SNc, substantia nigra pars compacta; SNr, substantia nigra pars reticulata; STN, subthalamic nucleus; VL, projections from ventral lateral thalamic nuclei.

neurons. Consistent with this hypothesis, metabolic mapping studies have suggested that activity in the direct pathway is increased in dyskinetic parkinsonian monkeys.[37–39] Recordings of neuronal activity in humans with idiopathic PD and in l-methyl-4-phenyl-l,2,3,6-tetrahydropyridine (MPTP)–treated parkinsonian monkeys with dyskinesia have shown a decreased mean discharge rate of neurons in the GPi.[40] Similar reductions in mean discharge rates in the GPi have also been reported in humans with dystonia, hemiballismus, and drug-induced dyskinesia.[41–43] The precise pathophysiologic differences between the different types of hyperkinetic disorders (e.g., chorea, drug-induced dyskinesia, dystonia) is uncertain, but they may occur in part as the result of differences in the balance between the direct and indirect pathways.[35, 36, 44–46] For example, chorea and drug-induced dyskinesias may occur because of excessive activity in the GPe, leading to a reduction of excitatory drive from the STN to the GPi, whereas dystonia may result from increased

activity in the direct pathway, leading to excessive inhibition of the GPi from the putamen.[43]

TREATMENT

Medical Therapy

Before considering surgical approaches for patients with dystonia, a trial of medical therapy should be undertaken. The mainstay of medical therapy has been anticholinergic drugs (i.e., trihexyphenidyl and ethopropazine), which are often used in conjunction with benzodiazepines (i.e., diazepam, lorazepam, and clonazepam), dopamine-depleting drugs (i.e., tetrabenazine), and anticonvulsants and muscle relaxants (i.e., carbamazepine and baclofen). Trihexyphenidyl is the most efficacious oral agent in the treatment of dystonia.[8, 9] Trihexyphenidyl is frequently useful in treatment of dystonias that are etiologically different. It is hypothesized to work through a central muscarinic effect, but the mechanism may be different at higher doses. Doses should be titrated until clinical benefit is maximized or side effects are intolerable. Peripheral side effects such as dry mouth, blurred vision, constipation, and difficulties with urination can be treated with appropriate adjunctive drug therapies. Central side effects of confusion, memory problems, and hallucinations should prompt the practitioner to decrease the dose or discontinue therapy. Special care should be exercised with the elderly, who may be particularly susceptible to drowsiness or confusion. The combination of an anticholinergic, muscle relaxant, and benzodiazepine is often used to provide the optimal benefit for symptom control.

Many neurologists prefer the use of botulinum toxin over drug therapy for treating focal dystonias. The most efficacious treatment for torticollis is botulinum toxin, which exerts its effects by a paralytic action. After endocytosis, the toxin undergoes disulfide cleavage. The remaining light chain enters the cytosol and blocks normal binding of vesicles to the axon's presynaptic terminal membrane. By strongly binding to presynaptic neuromuscular cholinergic receptors, the toxin decreases the frequency of acetylcholine release. Patients typically require injections every 3 to 6 months. Dysphagia is the most common worrisome side effect, and it is caused primarily by spread of toxin to pharyngeal muscles.

Patients with dystonia without a satisfactory response to medication or botulinum toxin should be considered for surgical intervention.

Surgery

SELECTION CRITERIA FOR DYSTONIA SURGERY

Although no specific selection criteria for dystonia surgery have been published, the experience of many neurologists and neurosurgeons and the emerging literature have begun to address this important question. The best candidates have primary dystonia, particularly those with the *DYT1* gene.[47, 48] Patients with secondary dystonia respond much less consistently and to a lesser degree, with the exception of tardive dystonia, for which preliminary data have shown a response to surgery similar to that of primary dystonia (Vitek, unpublished observations).[49–51] Independent of cause, other characteristics need to be taken into account when evaluating a patient for surgery, including the patient's cognitive status, psychiatric state, and whether or not the dystonic abnormalities are fixed or phasic. Patients who are younger (i.e., physiologic age of less than 70 years), have mobile dystonia,[47] and have normal cognition are better candidates than those who are older, or have abnormal cognition or active psychiatric problems. To define the best candidates for dystonia surgery, additional studies are needed to characterize the pertinent clinical variables and determine their effects on clinical outcome.

PERIPHERAL DENERVATION SURGERY, DORSAL COLUMN STIMULATION, AND CEREBELLAR STIMULATION

Peripheral surgical denervation, although not considered useful for segmental, hemidystonia, or generalized dystonia because of the multiple muscle groups involved in these syndromes, may still have a role in the treatment of cervical dystonia refractory to medical treatment. Although effective in some cases, results may be unpredictable and can be associated with severe weakness, dysphagia, sensory disorders, and in a few cases, trauma to the vertebral artery.[52] There have been no prospective, randomized trials of this therapy, and with the introduction of botulinum toxin therapy and DBS, its role in the treatment of cervical dystonia seems to be diminishing. Dorsal column and cerebellar stimulation as well as ablation of various portions of the cerebellum have all met with mixed success in the treatment of dystonia and are no longer in wide clinical use.[53]

LESIONS: THALAMOTOMY AND PALLIDOTOMY

Historically, thalamotomy has been the most widely used surgical procedure for the treatment of dystonia. The studies range from a single case report[54] to those with long-term follow-up of multiple patients.[15, 16, 31, 55] There are four major studies of thalamotomy for dystonia.[15, 16, 31, 55] All studies reported that it was effective in alleviating primary and secondary dystonia; however, the benefits to individual patients varied from none to marked, with approximately one third showing marked benefit, one third with mild to moderate benefit, and one third with little or no benefit.[56] Many patients who experienced initial improvement after surgery gradually lost benefit over the ensuing months. These patients were often reoperated, and the lesion was gradually expanded with the hope of regaining lost benefit. An average of two operations per patient was reported by Cooper[31] in his seminal work published in 1976, although it is worth noting that some patients underwent as many as seven operations. This variable outcome and gradual loss of benefit reported

in patients may have stemmed in part from a lack of a common target. Surgeons performing operations before the 1990s targeted various combinations of thalamic subnuclei, including the ventralis intermedius, ventralis posterior, ventralis anterior, center median, ventralis caudalis, centromedian, and pulvinar nucleus.[15, 31, 55, 56]

The published complication rate for thalamotomy in dystonia ranges from 2% to 56%.[13, 15, 16, 31, 52, 57] The side effect profile includes dysarthria, hemiparesis, dysphonia, dysphagia, dysphasia, worsening gait, and ataxia. Some of the side effects associated with thalamotomy resulted from encroachment of lesions into adjacent areas, such as the internal capsule and the thalamic subnuclei subserving language function, memory, attention, and sensation. Given the complicated, onion-skin somatotopy of the motor thalamus, in which distal to proximal portions of the limb are represented in different concentric layers,[58–60] a large lesion usually is needed to involve the proximal portions of the body. These types of lesions are more likely to be associated with a greater risk of complication as a result of encroachment on adjacent thalamic subnuclei.

Pallidotomy may offer an advantage over thalamotomy as a surgical target for dystonia, because lesions of the pallidal target (i.e., sensorimotor portion of GPi) are relatively free of the complications often associated with thalamotomy. Compared with thalamotomy, however, pallidotomy for dystonia was performed infrequently until the mid-1990s.[41, 61–64] Although good results were sometimes observed after pallidotomy, results were mostly inconsistent and often disappointing. The signs of dystonia frequently were improved after surgery, similar to results after thalamotomy, but many patients had regression or worsening of signs over the ensuing weeks to months. The underlying basis for these variable results remain speculative because there is little histologic or radiographic evidence of the lesion site, and rigorous and comprehensive preoperative and postoperative evaluations of motor, cognitive, and emotional changes were not done. It is likely, however, that the reasons for this variability in patient outcome stemmed from a combination of differences in patient selection and from problems with target localization and lesioning techniques. In some of the cases in which little or no benefit was achieved, lesions may have been placed in the more rostral-medial "associative" territory of GPi, the site commonly targeted by surgeons at that time.

Lesion location in dystonia surgery is a critical factor in patient outcome, and it probably accounts for much of the variability in clinical outcome reported in earlier surgical series. The lesson of pallidotomy for PD was that the outcome appeared to depend critically on the site of the lesion.[65–68] In our experience, lesions involving the caudal "sensorimotor" portions of GPi have been more effective in alleviating parkinsonian motor signs than more rostrally placed lesions. Lesions only a few millimeters apart may have vastly different long-term results.[65–68] Marked improvement in patients with primary dystonia with lesions in the posterolateral, sensorimotor portion of the GPi, confirmed using high-resolution magnetic resonance imaging (MRI), suggests that lesions in this region of the pallidum can be highly effective in the alleviation of this disorder.[61–64, 69, 70] Overall improvement of 20% to 60% has been reported with unilateral pallidotomy, and 50% to 80% improvement has been reported with bilateral procedures (i.e., unilateral pallidotomy plus contralateral DBS or bilateral pallidotomy).[43, 62, 63, 71]

Previous studies of pallidotomy or thalamotomy, as well as recent observations by us and others, suggest that patients with neck, trunk, or other axial symptoms require bilateral procedures.[19, 72] Although the incidence of complications associated with bilateral pallidotomy for patients with dystonia is considered to be low,[63, 73, 74] only a handful of patients have been reported in the literature. In the largest series of pallidotomy for dystonia reported by Ondo,[63, 73, 74] five patients with generalized dystonia underwent bilateral pallidotomy. The length of follow-up was 4 months. The mean scores for the Fahn-Marsden Dystonia Rating Scale (FMDRS) improved 61%, and scores for the Unified Dystonia Rating Scale (UDRS) improved 66%. Complications were transient or mild and consisted of postoperative lethargy in one patient and transient weakness in another. No cognitive or bulbar compromise was reported. Although these observations suggest that bilateral pallidotomy may be a safe procedure, before these results can be generalized, we need careful documentation in a greater number of patients followed for a longer period.

DEEP BRAIN STIMULATION

Concerns about the development of permanent side effects related to lesioning and the high incidence of side effects associated with bilateral ablative procedures have led investigators to consider alternative forms of surgery for the treatment of dystonia and other movement disorders. With the development of DBS, a procedure in which the surgeon can adjust stimulation parameters to obtain the optimal alleviation of motor symptoms while minimizing associated side effects, patients have an alternative to lesioning. Although the application of chronic stimulation is new, the concept is not. Hassler and associates[14, 28] described suppression of dystonic movements in patients with torsion dystonia after high-frequency (>25 Hz) electrical stimulation used before ablation of the GPi. At that time, there were no methods available to provide patients with a means for chronic DBS, and ablations were continued. As a result of the development of chronic stimulation for DBS and the reversibility of its side effects, many patients now choose DBS over ablative therapy.

We and others have successfully used GPi DBS for the treatment of primary dystonia.[19–21, 72] The largest reported series of patients with DBS for dystonia is that of Coubes.[21] Seven patients with DYT1-positive generalized dystonia underwent bilateral GPi DBS. Improvement as determined using the FMDRS varied from 60% to 100%. Patients were followed for 1 year without signs of regression, and only one patient experienced a complication. This complication was related to a scalp infection, requiring the lead to be removed. It was subsequently replaced 6 months later with return of benefit. Another report of bilateral GPi DBS for a case of generalized dystonia supports these findings, reporting an improvement of 67% in the FMDRS.[20] Our data have demonstrated a marked improvement (50% to 80%) in trunk, neck, and limb dystonia after GPi DBS, but similar to previous observations, optimal improvement in axial symptoms did not occur without bilateral procedures.[71] Similar to our observations of improvement in neck dystonia after a second procedure on the unoperated hemisphere in a patient with axial dystonia (i.e., GPi DBS on the side contralateral to a previous pallidotomy), Krauss and associates[75] reported significant improvement in cervical dystonia for three patients after bilateral GPi DBS, and Bereznai and colleagues[76] saw improvement in five patients with focal or cervical dystonia. Taken together, these studies suggest that GPi DBS can be an effective therapy for patients with generalized or focal dystonia. Although results vary across studies, the benefit of GPi DBS provides hope for patients with primary dystonia in whom all previous therapies have failed. Results for secondary dystonia, although favorable in many cases, have been less consistent, and the benefits have been smaller in magnitude.[75, 77–80] Although the reasons for this have not been delineated, it probably reflects the variable causes and resultant differences in the pathophysiologic mechanism underlying the development of dystonia in these cases.

In addition to the advantages offered by DBS, there are also disadvantages. These include the risk of infection, the need for frequent visits to adjust stimulation parameters, mechanical breakdown, and cost.[81, 82] The voltage requirements for patients with dystonia are considerably higher than those for patients with PD or tremor. Replacement of the internal pulse generator (IPG) may be required as often as every 8 to 12 months, resulting in considerable cost to the patient. For younger patients, the costs associated with bilateral procedures may be prohibitive if IPGs require replacement every year. Younger patients will continue to grow and may need to have adjustments made to the device to allow for this growth. Younger patients may benefit the most from a reversible procedure that leaves them free to explore potentially curative therapies if they become available in the future. Newer-generation IPGs will be rechargeable and allow minor modifications in stimulation parameters by the patient. Depending on the relative risk of side effects for ablation versus stimulation, the risk of mechanical failure, and the cost for replacement of the IPG, the choice of procedures may depend on whether there is a significant difference in the clinical benefit between GPi and thalamic DBS. This remains to be determined, because there are no randomized trials comparing the relative efficacy of these two procedures.

TECHNIQUES FOR DYSTONIA SURGERY AND MICROELECTRODE RECORDING

Many approaches can be used for target localization when performing an ablative or DBS procedure. Most approaches include some combination of imaging (e.g., pneumoencephalography, MRI, computed tomography [CT], MR-CT fusion), electrophysiologic recording, and macrostimulation. The surgical procedure for the thalamic and pallidal targets has been addressed in several papers[42, 65, 83–91] and is therefore not discussed here, other than to point out that not all groups use the microelectrode in the same fashion.[42, 65, 83–89, 91] Some groups use only one microelectrode pass, but others use multiple passes to identify the target, define its borders, and identify nearby critical structures. The danger of the single pass approach is that a single pass can fit on multiple planes and different anteroposterior sites of the same plane. Although a single pass may ensure that the target has been identified, it does not allow accurate determination of the location within the target structure.

CONCLUSION

Many therapies, including medications, botulinum toxin, and surgery, are available for patients with focal and generalized dystonia. Medications such as anticholinergics, muscle relaxants, and benzodiazepines are of limited use for most patients. Botulinum toxin is a safe and effective therapy for many focal dystonias, but it is not generally helpful for patients with segmental, hemidystonia, or generalized dystonia. Surgical therapies in the form of cerebellar stimulation and dorsal column stimulation are rarely used. Peripheral denervation may be effective in some patients with cervical dystonia, but most centers use ablative therapy and DBS targeting the pallidum or thalamus. Although the thalamus was targeted almost exclusively in previous years, most centers now target the internal segment of the pallidum. Both sites are effective. There have been no direct comparisons of the site (pallidum versus thalamus) or the surgical method (lesioning versus stimulation). More consistent and greater improvement has been reported for primary than for secondary dystonia. Further studies will be needed to determine the optimal target for patients with different kinds of dystonia (primary versus secondary) and to determine whether stimulation, lesioning, or a combination of stimulation and lesioning provides the best clinical result.

REFERENCES

1. Bressman SB: Dystonia. Curr Opin Neurol 11:363–372, 1998.
2. Bressman SB: Dystonia update. Clin Neuropharmacol 23:239–251, 2000.
3. Fahn S, Bressman SB, Marsden CD: Classification of dystonia. Adv Neurol 78:1–10, 1998.
4. Bressman SB, Sabatti C, Raymond D, et al: The DYT1 phenotype and guidelines for diagnostic testing. Neurology 54:1746–1752, 2000.
5. Ozelius LJ, Hewett JW, Page CE, et al: The gene (DYT1) for early-onset torsion dystonia encodes a novel protein related to the Clp protease/heat shock family. Adv Neurol 78:93–105, 1998.
6. Ozelius LJ, Page CE, Klein C, et al: The TOR1A (DYT1) gene family and its role in early onset torsion dystonia. Genomics 62:377–384, 1999.
7. Burke RE: The relative selectivity of anticholinergic drugs for the M1 and M2 muscarinic receptor subtypes. Mov Disord 1:135–144, 1986.
8. Burke RE, Fahn S: Pharmacokinetics of trihexyphenidyl after short-term and long-term administration to dystonic patients. Ann Neurol 18:35–40, 1985.
9. Burke RE, Fahn A: Serum trihexyphenidyl levels in the treatment of torsion dystonia. Neurology 35:1066–1069, 1985.
10. Freckmann N, Hagenah R: Relationship between the spinal accessory nerve and the posterior root of the first cervical nerve in spasmodic torticollis and common autopsy cases. Zentralbl Neurochir 47:134–138, 1986.
11. Freckmann N, Hagenah R, Herrmann HD, Muller D: Bilateral microsurgical lysis of the spinal accessory nerve roots for treatment of spasmodic torticollis. Follow up of 33 cases. Acta Neurochir 83:47–53, 1986.
12. Gildenberg PL: Treatment of spasmodic torticollis with dorsal column stimulation. Acta Neurochir Suppl (Wien) 24(Suppl):65–66, 1977.
13. Gros C, Frerebeau P, Perez-Dominguez E, et al: Long term results of stereotaxic surgery for infantile dystonia and dyskinesia. Neurochirurgia 19:171–178, 1976.
14. Hassler R, Dieckmann G: Stereotactic treatment of different kinds of spasmodic torticollis. Confin Neurol 32:135–143, 1970.
15. Andrew J, Fowler CJ, Harrison MJG: Stereotaxic thalamotomy in 55 cases of dystonia. Brain 106:981–1000, 1983.
16. Tasker RR, Doorly T, Yamashiro K: Thalamotomy in generalized dystonia. In Fahn C, Marsden C, Calne D (eds): Advances in Neurology: Dystonia 2. New York, Raven Press, 1988, pp 615–631.
17. Vitek J: Surgery for dystonia. In Bakay R (ed): Neurosurgery Clinics of North America. Philadelphia, WB Saunders, 1998, pp 345–366.
18. Vitek J, Bakay R: The role of pallidotomy in Parkinson's disease and dystonia. Curr Opin Neurol 10:332–339, 1997.
19. Vitek J, et al: Pallidotomy and deep brain stimulation as a treatment for dystonia. Neurology 52(Suppl 2):S46.006, 1999.
20. Kumar R, Dagher A, Hutchison WD, et al: Globus pallidus deep brain stimulation for generalized dystonia: Clinical and PET investigation. Neurology 53:871–874, 1999.
21. Coubes P, Roubertie A, Vayssiere N, et al: Treatment of DYT1-generalised dystonia by stimulation of the internal globus pallidus [letter]. Lancet 355:2220–2221, 2000.
22. Krauss JK, Pohle T, Weber S, et al: Bilateral stimulation of globus pallidus internus for treatment of cervical dystonia. Lancet 354:837–838, 1999.
23. Benabid AL, Pollak P, Gao D, et al: Chronic electrical stimulation of the ventralis intermedius nucleus of the thalamus as a treatment of movement disorders. J Neurosurg 84:203–214, 1996; see comments.
24. Sellal F, Hirsch E, Barth P, et al: A case of symptomatic hemidystonia improved by ventroposterolateral thalamic electrostimulation. Mov Disord 8:515–518, 1993.
25. Benabid AL, Koudsie A, Pollak P, et al: Future prospects of brain stimulation. Neurol Res 22:237–246, 2000.
26. Vercueil L, Koudsie A, Benazzouz A, et al: Deep brain stimulation in the treatment of severe dystonia. J Neurol 248:695–700, 2001.
27. Hassler R: Anatomy of the thalamus. In Schaltenbrand G, Bailey P (eds): Introduction to Stereotaxis with an Atlas of the Human Brain. Stuttgart, Thieme, 1959, pp 230–290.
28. Hassler R, Dieckmann G: Locomotor movements in opposite directions induced by stimulation of pallidum of putamen. J Neurol Sci 8:189–195, 1968.
29. Hassler R, Mundinger F, Riechert T: Correlations between clinical and autopsic findings in stereotactic operations of parkinsonism. Confin Neurol 26:282–290, 1965.
30. Benabid AL, Pollak P, Seigneuret E, et al: Chronic VIM thalamic stimulation in Parkinson's disease, essential tremor and extrapyramidal dyskinesias. Acta Neurochir Suppl (Wien) 58:39–44, 1993.
31. Cooper IS: 20-Year followup study of the neurosurgical treatment of dystonia musculorum deformans. In Eldridge R, Fahn S (eds): Advances in Neurology. New York, Raven Press, 1976, pp 423–452.
32. Burzaco J: Stereotactic pallidotomy in extrapyramidal disorders. Appl Neurophysiol 48:283–287, 1985.

33. Hassler R, et al: Physiological observations in stereotaxic operations in extrapyramidal motor disturbances. Brain 83:337–350, 1960.

34. Andrew J, Edwards JM, Rudolf NDM: The placement of stereotaxic lesions for involuntary movements other than in Parkinson's disease. Acta Neurochir (Wien) 21(Suppl):39–47, 1974.

35. DeLong MR: Primate models of movement disorders of basal ganglia origin. Trends Neurosci 13:281–285, 1990.

36. DeLong MR, Alexander GE: Organization of basal ganglia. In Asbury AK, McKhann GM, McDonald WI (eds): Disease of the Nervous System. London, William Heinemann Medical Books, 1986, pp 379–393.

37. Crossman AR: A hypothesis on the pathophysiological mechanisms that underlie levodopa- or dopamine agonist-induced dyskinesia in Parkinson's disease: Implications for future strategies in treatment. Mov Disord 5:100–108, 1990.

38. Crossman AR, Clarke CE, Boyce S, et al: MPTP-induced parkinsonism in the monkey: Neurochemical pathology, complications of treatment and pathophysiological mechanisms. Can J Neurol Sci 14(Suppl):428–435, 1987.

39. Crossman AR, Mitchell IJ, Sambrook MA: Regional brain uptake of 2-deoxyglucose in N-methyl-4-phenyl-1,2,3,6-tetrahydropyridine (MPTP)–induced parkinsonism in the macaque monkey. Neuropharmacology 24:587–591, 1985.

40. Papa SM, Desimone R, Fiorani M, Oldfield EH: Internal globus pallidus discharge is nearly suppressed during levodopa-induced dyskinesias. Ann Neurol 46:732–738, 1999.

41. Lozano A, Kumar R, Gross RE, et al: Globus pallidus internus pallidotomy for generalized dystonia. Mov Disord 12:865–870, 1997.

42. Vitek J, et al: Neuronal activity in the pallidum in patients with medically intractable dystonia [abstract]. Mov Disord 12:9, 1997.

43. Vitek JL, Chockkan V, Zhang JY, et al: Neuronal activity in the basal ganglia in patients with generalized dystonia and hemiballismus. Ann Neurol 46:22–35, 1999.

44. DeLong MR, et al: Anatomical and functional aspects of basal ganglia-thalamocortical circuits. In Winslow W (ed): Studies in Neuroscience. Manchester, UK, Manchester University Press, 1989.

45. Alexander GE, Crutcher MD, DeLong MR: Basal ganglia-thalamocortical circuits: Parallel substrates for motor oculomotor, "prefrontal" and "limbic" functions. Prog Brain Res 85:119–146, 1990.

46. Albin RL, Young AB, Penney JB: The functional anatomy of basal ganglia disorders. Trends Neurosci 12:366–375, 1989.

47. Krack P, Vercueil L: Review of the functional surgical treatment of dystonia. Eur J Neurol 8:389–399, 2001.

48. Vesper J, Klostermann F, Funk T, et al: Deep brain stimulation of the globus pallidus internus (GPI) for torsion dystonia—a report of two cases. Acta Neurochir Suppl 79:83–88, 2002.

49. Weetman J, Anderson IM, Gregory RP, Gill SS: Bilateral posteroventral pallidotomy for severe antipsychotic induced tardive dyskinesia and dystonia. J Neurol Neurosurg Psychiatry 63:554–556, 1997.

50. Wang Y, Turnbull I, Calne S, et al: Pallidotomy for tardive dyskinesia. Lancet 349:777–778, 1997.

51. Hillier CE, Wiles CM, Simpson BA: Thalamotomy for severe antipsychotic induced tardive dyskinesia and dystonia. J Neurol Neurosurg Psychiatry 66:250–251, 1999.

52. Kandel E: Functional and Stereotactic Neurosurgery. New York, Plenum Publishing, 1989, p 606.

53. Tasker R: Surgical treatment of the dystonias. In Gildenberg P, Tasker R (eds): Textbook of Stereotactic and Functional Neurosurgery. New York, McGraw-Hill, 1996, pp 1015–1032.

54. Spiegel E, Wycis H, Freed H: Stereoencephalotomy: Thalamotomy and related procedures. JAMA 148:446–451, 1952.

55. Cardoso F, Jankovic J, Grossman RG, Hamilton WJ: Outcome after stereotactic thalamotomy for dystonia and hemiballismus. Neurosurgery 36:501–508, 1995.

56. Tasker RR, et al: Thalamotomy in Parkinson's disease: Microelectrode techniques. In Lundsford D (ed): Modern Stereotactic Surgery. Norwell, MA, Academic Press, 1988, pp 297–313.

57. Laitinen LV, Bergenheim AT, Hariz MI: Leksell's posteroventral pallidotomy in the treatment of Parkinson's disease. J Neurosurg 76:53–61, 1992.

58. Jones EG, Leavitt RY: Retrograde axonal transport and the dem-

59. Jones EG, Friedman DP: Projection pattern of functional components of thalamic ventrobasal complex on monkey somatosensory cortex. J Neurophysiol 48:521–543, 1982.

60. Vitek J, et al: Functional organization of the motor thalamus in the nonhuman primate: Application to functional neurosurgery. Presented at the Satellite Symposium on Stereotactic Neurosurgery, Abstract, 1993.

61. Lin JJ, Lin SZ, Lin GY, et al: Treatment of intractable generalized dystonia by bilateral posteroventral pallidotomy—one-year results. Zhonghua Yi Xue Za Zhi (Taipei) 64:231–238, 2001.

62. Ondo W, Desaloms JM, Jankovic J, Grossman RG: Pallidotomy for generalized dystonia. Mov Disord 13:693–698, 1998.

63. Ondo W, et al: Pallidotomy for dystonia [abstract]. Ann Neurol 42:446, 1997.

64. Vitek J, et al: Pallidotomy as a treatment for medically intractable dystonia. Ann Neurol 42:409, 1997.

65. Vitek J, Bakay R, DeLong M: Microelectrode-guided pallidotomy for medically intractable Parkinson's disease. In Obeso J (ed): Advances in Neurology. Philadelphia, Lippincott-Raven, 1997, pp 183–198.

66. Gross RE, Lombardi WJ, Lang AE, et al: Relationship of lesion location to clinical outcome following microelectrode-guided pallidotomy for Parkinson's disease. Brain 122(Pt 3):405–416, 1999; see comments.

67. Eskandar EN, Cosgrove GR, Shinobu LA, Penney JB Jr: The importance of accurate lesion placement in posteroventral pallidotomy. Report of two cases. J Neurosurg 89:630–634, 1998.

68. Bronte-Stewart H, et al: Lesion location predicts clinical outcome of pallidotomy. Mov Disord 13:300, 1998.

69. Lozano AM, Kumar R, Gross RE, et al: Globus pallidus internus pallidotomy for generalized dystonia. Mov Disord 12:865–870, 1997.

70. Vitek JL, Zhang J, Evatt M, et al: GPi pallidotomy for dystonia: Clinical outcome and neuronal activity. Adv Neurol 78:211–219, 1998.

71. Vitek JL, Evatt M, Zhang J, et al: Pallidotomy and deep brain stimulation as a treatment for dystonia. Neurology 52(Suppl 2):S46.006, 1999.

72. Vitek JL: Surgery for dystonia. Neurosurg Clin N Am 9:345–366, 1998.

73. Ondo W, Jankovic J, Schwartz K, et al: Unilateral thalamic deep brain stimulation for refractory essential tremor and Parkinson's disease tremor. Neurology 51:1063–1069, 1998.

74. Ondo WG, Desaloms JM, Jankovic J, Grossman RG: Pallidotomy for generalized dystonia. Mov Disord 13:693–698, 1998; see comments.

75. Krauss JK, Loher TJ, Pohle T, et al: Pallidal deep brain stimulation in patients with cervical dystonia and severe cervical dyskinesias with cervical myelopathy. J Neurol Neurosurg Psychiatry 72:249–256, 2002.

76. Bereznai B, Steude U, Seelos K, Botzel K: Chronic high-frequency globus pallidus internus stimulation in different types of dystonia: A clinical, video, and MRI report of six patients presenting with segmental, cervical, and generalized dystonia. Mov Disord 17:138–144, 2002.

77. Volkmann J, Benecke R: Deep brain stimulation for dystonia: Patient selection and evaluation. Mov Disord 17(Suppl 3):S112–S115, 2002.

78. Vercueil L, Krack P, Pollak P: Results of deep brain stimulation for dystonia: A critical reappraisal. Mov Disord 17(Suppl 3):S89–S93, 2002.

79. Muta D, Goto S, Nishikawa S, et al: Bilateral pallidal stimulation for idiopathic segmental axial dystonia advanced from Meige syndrome refractory to bilateral thalamotomy. Mov Disord 16:774–777, 2001.

80. Parkin S, Aziz T, Gregory R, Bain P: Bilateral internal globus pallidus stimulation for the treatment of spasmodic torticollis. Mov Disord 16:489–493, 2001.

81. Koller WC, Lyons KE, Wilkinson SB, et al: Long-term safety and efficacy of unilateral deep brain stimulation of the thalamus in essential tremor. Mov Disord 16:464–468, 2001.

82. Lyons KE, Koller WC, Wilkinson SB, Pahwa R: Long term safety and efficacy of unilateral deep brain stimulation of the thalamus

for parkinsonian tremor. J Neurol Neurosurg Psychiatry 71:682–684, 2001.

83. Bakay R, et al: Use of microelectrode recordings to characterize optimal target localization for posteroventral pallidotomy [abstract]. Congress of Neurological Surgeons, 1993.

84. Bakay RA, Starr PA, Vitek JL, DeLong MR: Posterior ventral pallidotomy: Techniques and theoretical considerations. Clin Neurosurg 44:197–210, 1997.

85. Bakay RAE, Vitek JL, DeLong MR: Thalamotomy for tremor. In Rengachary S, Wilkins R (eds): Neurosurgical Operative Atlas. Baltimore, Williams & Wilkins, 1992, pp 299–312.

86. Lenz FA, Jaeger CJ, Seike MS, et al: Thalamic single neuron activity in patients with dystonia: Dystonia-related activity and somatic sensory reorganization. J Neurophysiol 82:2372–2392, 1999.

87. Lenz FA, Kwan HC, Martin RL, et al: Single unit analysis of the human ventral thalamic nuclear group: Tremor-related activity in functionally identified cells. Brain 117:531–543, 1994.

88. Lenz FA, Suarez JI, Metman LV, et al: Pallidal activity during dystonia: Somatosensory reorganisation and changes with severity. J Neurol Neurosurg Psychiatry 65:767–770, 1998.

89. Vitek JL, Bakay RA, Hashimoto T, et al: Microelectrode-guided pallidotomy: Technical approach and its application in medically intractable Parkinson's disease. J Neurosurg 88:1027–1043, 1998; see comments.

90. Lozano AM, et al: Methods for microelectrode-guided posteroventral pallidotomy. J Neurosurg 84:194–202, 1996.

91. Lozano AM, Hutchison WD, Tasker RR, et al: Microelectrode recordings define the ventral posteromedial pallidotomy target. Stereotact Funct Neurosurg 71:153–163, 1998.

Deep Brain Stimulation for Movement Disorders

ALIM L. BENABID ■ JEAN F. LEBAS ■ SYLVIE GRAND ■ ABDELHAMID BENAZZOUZ ■
PIERRE POLLACK ■ PAUL KRACK ■ ADNAN KOUDSIÉ ■ STEPHAN CHABARDÈS ■
VALÉRIE FRAIX ■ PATRICIA LIMOUSIN ■ SERGE PINTO ■ DOMINIQUE HOFFMANN ■
CLAIRE ARDOUIN ■ AURÉTIE FUNKIEWIEZ

NEUROSURGERY FOR MOVEMENT DISORDERS

Movement disorders, pain, epilepsy, spasticity, and mental disorders have constituted the field of functional neurosurgery for several decades. Movement disorders deserve special consideration because of the importance of the patient's deficit, which necessitates a cure. Knowledge of the physiology and pharmacology of the basal ganglia provides an understanding of the mechanism of disease and helps establish the basis of the therapeutic approach. Before the discovery of dopamine, this approach was based primarily on an empirical process, from serendipitous findings to audacious human experiments, suggested by experiments in small animals and by theoretical assumptions based on mostly anatomic considerations.[1]

This led neurosurgeons to consider the ventral intermedius nucleus (Vim) as a target. Its destruction was highly effective in alleviating tremor, the most spectacular but not the most disabling symptom of Parkinson's disease. Use of this procedure extended rapidly, and it was the major focus of functional neurosurgery for decades, until the 1960s. This surgical experience improved the understanding of the pathophysiology of the disease and the physiology of motility. The parallel progress of neurophysiology and the rapid development of neuropharmacology, initially as a tool for neurophysiologists and secondarily as fertile ground for the drug industry, yielded the discovery of dopamine and its effects, which soon led to its clinical application. Because of the spectacular effect of L-dopa and its absence of immediate permanent side effects (versus the complications of surgery, which could be disabling and permanent), neurosurgery for the treatment of parkinsonian tremor fell out of favor. Neurosurgery was restricted to the treatment of essential tremor, which is not sensitive to drugs. L-Dopa had a "honeymoon" period with both patients and doctors, but after 5 to 10 years of medication, dyskinesias developed that were as disabling as the disease itself, although patients generally preferred to be hyperactive rather than feeling that they were buried alive.

DEEP BRAIN STIMULATION

These complications revived the need for surgery—in fact, for a new surgery. It had to alleviate the symptoms and at the same time allow diminished drug doses while producing fewer side effects and fewer permanent motor, sensory, or cognitive deficits. During the attempt to develop a less invasive procedure for thalamotomies, investigators observed that tremor was influenced by stimulation performed to identify the neural structures traversed by the stereotactic probe. This influence was frequency dependent; that is, low frequencies ($\leqq 30$ Hz) usually increased the intensity of the tremor, very low frequencies (around 5 Hz) drove the tremor, and high frequencies (100 to 2500 Hz) stopped the tremor totally and reversibly. Deep brain stimulation (DBS) had been used since the 1950s for various indications, mainly for the treatment of pain. Thus, the technology was available to be applied to movement disorders, and it was developed as an alternative to ablative methods and insufficient medical treatment. Since 1987, DBS has proved to be a safe, efficient, and stable method of producing neural inhibition in the thalamus and the pallidum, as well as locations that were considered dangerous, such as the subthalamic nucleus (STN) or corpus luysi.[2–5]

SUBTHALAMIC NUCLEUS: THE MAIN TARGET IN PARKINSON'S DISEASE

The role of the various basal ganglia nuclei in controlling motility has long been known to involve the thalamus, the pallidum, and the STN, as well as other structures such as the centromedian-parafascicularis complex (CM-Pf) and the substantia nigra pars reticularis (SNr). Currently, there are three surgical targets for Parkinson's disease, which can be represented on Guiot's scheme based on the posterior and anterior commissures, the height of the thalamus, and the width of the third ventricle at the midline.

- The thalamic target is the Vim, and additionally the CM-Pf.[6]
- The globus pallidus internalis (GPi) is the second target, which was reintroduced by Laitinen and coworkers[7] after being initiated by Leksell.[8]
- The STN is our preferred target for advanced stages of Parkinson's disease.

Although highly efficient for tremor, thalamic Vim stimulation did not result in any significant improvement of other parkinsonian symptoms, essentially rigidity and akinesia, which was already known about thalamotomy.[9–25] Therefore, the evolution of the disease in these patients from tremulous to akinetic-rigid made Vim stimulation useless.[26] There was no treatment for these highly disabling symptoms in advanced stages, except for pallidotomy or, more recently, brain grafting, which is still experimental.[27] DBS permitted the performance of bilateral implantation of the GPi, decreased the incidence of complications, and lowered the possibility of neuropsychological complications from bilateral pallidotomies. There is still controversy about the respective efficiencies of stimulating the GPi and the STN. The main difference is the possibility of significantly decreasing, or even eliminating, the need for dopaminergic treatment in STN-stimulated patients, which might play a role in the occurrence of postoperative depression. Introduction of the STN as a target was based on data obtained by neurophysiologists in rodents and monkeys, showing that the STN plays a key role in the organization of basal ganglia[28–34] and allowing its use as a human therapeutic target.[35–38]

From a neurosurgical point of view, the method is fairly uniform. Its variations in Parkinson's disease as well as in other diseases (e.g., epilepsy, neuropsychiatric disorders, endocrinologic disturbances) are a matter of targets, which in neurosurgical terms are a matter of coordinates.

METHODS

General Principles

DBS must be performed stereotactically. Precise placement of the electrode is the most important criterion of efficacy. Variations and innovations in methodology should be compared on the basis of the quality of the clinical results obtained. The exact method used depends on the skill, experience, technical expertise, and habits of the surgical team, and all variations are acceptable as long as the results are satisfactory.

The basic approach of targeting the basal ganglia is the same for most nuclei; any differences are primarily in the coordinates. For this reason, STN, GPi, and Vim targets can be considered simultaneously. However, specific features are used to distinguish them and to accurately determine their limits to ensure precise placement of the electrode in the main core of one nucleus, considered the target. There is now sufficient evidence that the quality of the functional results, in terms of alleviation of symptoms, is closely related to the precision of the implantation. Ideally, targeting consists of gathering all data about a target to ensure the highest probability of putting the final electrode in the correct site. It should be within a statistical range of coordinates, and the neuronal firing should fit a given pattern, such as responses to external stimuli, particularly to proprioceptive inputs, in a somatotopically organized manner. Moreover, this placement should provide the best clinical improvement of symptoms using stimulation parameters based on the chronic situation. The latter criterion is by far the most reliable and important, because it actually mimics the functional benefit for the patient, which is the ultimate purpose of the surgery.

Radiologic data are of great interest, but each modality has drawbacks. Ventriculography is the most precise method, and it is safe when performed according to strict technical procedures; however, it provides more indirect targeting and is more invasive than magnetic resonance imaging (MRI). MRI is the best method for visualizing the STN and, to some extent, for discerning the Vim, but it is plagued by unpredictable and irreproducible deformations that induce systematic distortion. Without doubt, these flaws will be corrected in the near future, which will help in placement of the electrode.

General Strategy

To ensure the most precise localization of the ideal target and to avoid a lengthy procedure for the patient, we have divided the surgery for thalamic implantation of electrodes into five steps (three surgical sessions and two MRI sessions) on different days:

Step 1: Ventriculography and implantation of titanium skull screws for repositioning.
Step 2: Targeting MRI.
Step 3: Implantation of electrodes into the target.
Step 4: Postimplantation control MRI.
Step 5: Implantation of the programmable stimulator.[26]

We base our method on ventriculography, which is still (in our opinion) the gold standard, and we use it to build a diagram that allows pretargeting for most of the targets (Fig. 173–1) on the lateral and anteroposterior (AP) views. MRI is also used, but computerized image guidance is not sufficient, because atlases can be misleading when targeting one nucleus; for instance, MRI can be satisfactory on the sagittal and axial views, but frequently it does not match with the coronal view, where the target representation is often in another

FIGURE 173–1. Schematic drawings for determining the ventral intermedius nucleus (Vim), subthalamic nucleus (STN), and globus pallidus internalis (GPi) deep brain stimulation targets based on third ventricle anatomic landmarks. The upper graph represents the antero-posterior (AP) view; the width is in millimeters, and the vertical axis is based on one eighth the height of the thalamus. The lower graph represents the lateral view; the horizontal axis represents the distance from the posterior commissure (PC) based on one twelfth of the anterior commissure–posterior commisure (AC-PC) length, and the vertical axis is based on one eighth the height of the thalamus. The STN target extends over the middle third of the AC-PC, below the line. On the AP view, the average laterality is 12 mm, and the STN extends from 11 to 13 mm. Projected on this view are the image of the average target *(black and gray square)* and the limits of the standard deviations around the average target *(rectangle)*. The lateral view shows the trajectory; the theoretical angle of the track with the AC-PC is 63.57 ± 2.34 degrees on the basis of Guiot's scheme, and in actuality, it is 63.11 ± 3.87 degrees on the right side and 62.81 ± 4.59 degrees on the left side. The GPi target is situated in the anterior third of the AC-PC, from one eighth of the height of the thalamus to two eighths below the AC-PC plane. The laterality extends 15 to 22 mm from the midline. Vim is 14 mm from the midline and is about two twelfths to three twelfths of the AC-PC distance, ahead of the PC.

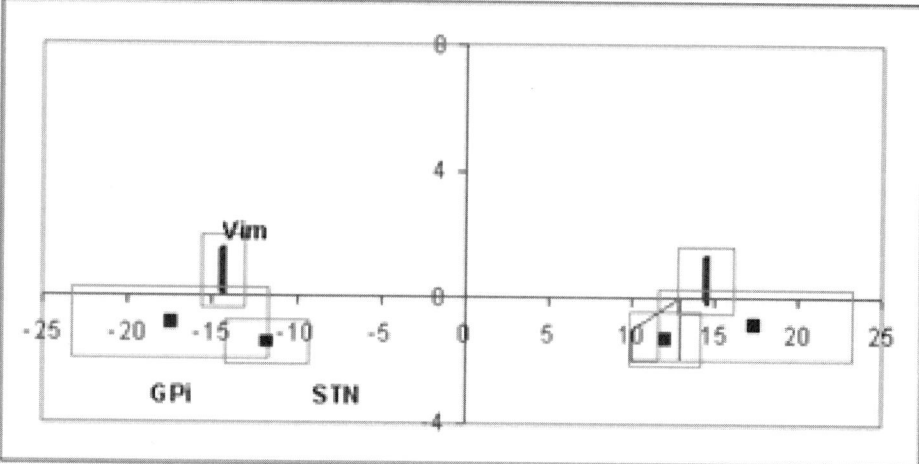

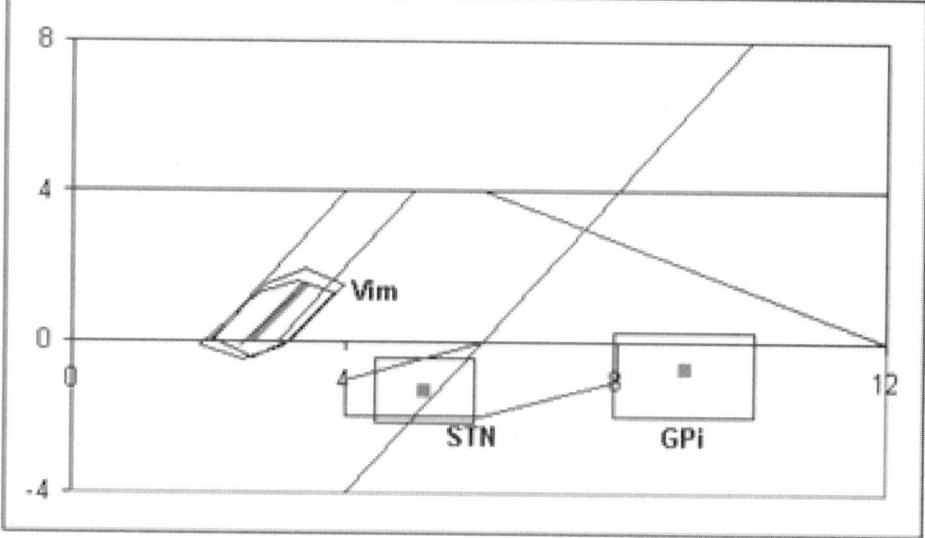

structure (Fig. 173–2; see color section in this volume). Therefore, we still use electrophysiology during surgery to ensure that we are in the right location.[39–41] In this chapter, we describe our procedure, with enough details to make it reproducible.

Localization of Targets

VENTRICULOGRAPHY

Anesthesia and Preparation. The patient is placed in the horizontal position; general anesthesia, orotracheal intubation, and assisted ventilation are used for step 1. Additional local anesthesia is used to decrease bleeding at the skin incisions.

Frame and Screws. Bone screws (Stevis, SOFAMOR) are implanted into the skull and will remain in place for several days after the completion of steps 2, 3, and 4. The patient is placed in the stereotactic frame, the pins are inserted into the screw holes, and the numerical values of their positions are recorded to allow painless repositioning during the next steps.

X-Ray Setup. X-ray films are taken under teleradiologic conditions (3.5 m between the x-ray tube and the film, with an average magnification coefficient of 1.05) in the supine and prone positions.

Ventricular Puncture. Positive contrast ventriculography is performed by direct puncture of the frontal horn of the lateral ventricle (90 mm from the nasion; 25 mm from the midline) with a 65-mm-long Cushing cannula. Placement is confirmed by control radiographs after injection of a 5-mL air bubble. Using these landmarks and the air bubble test, we have never observed any of the reported complications (hemorrhages in the thalamus and in the brainstem)[42, 43]; in our opinion, these are not potential risks of ventriculography but only the expected results of technical errors.

Contrast Enhancement and Reconstitution of the Ventriculogram. Injection of 6.5 mL of Iopamiron 200 (Schering) is performed. AP and lateral radiographs are taken in the supine and ventral positions to visualize the posterior commissure (PC) and anterior commissure (AC). This necessitates turning the patient up-

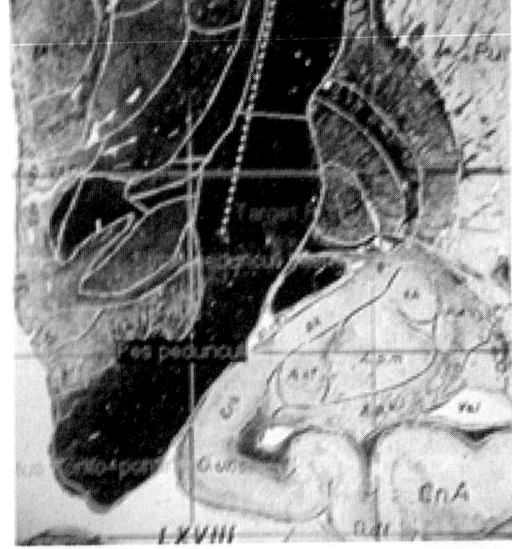

● Patient # 96

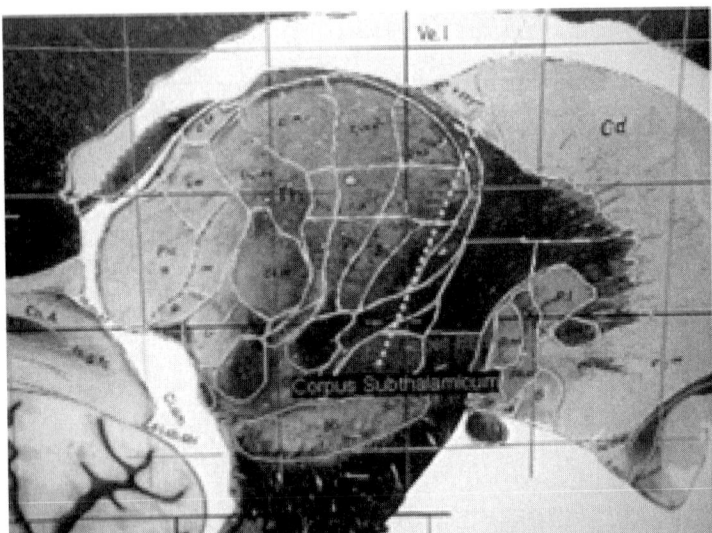

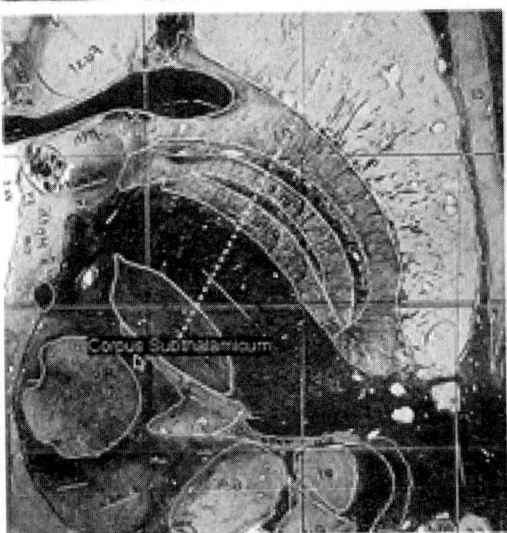

FIGURE 173–2. Demonstration of the mismatches in atlases. Shown is a target point using the Splan Radionics image-guidance software. It can be satisfactory on the sagittal and axial views, but it does not match with the coronal view, where the target representation is often in the peduncle. The three planes (axial, coronal, and sagittal) of the atlas were obtained in three different brains (see color section in this volume).

side down using the frame, which allows a 360-degree rotation of the patient along its own axis. The radiologic images provide a precise delineation of the midline of the third ventricle and of the AC and PC. This information is obtained by drawing from a superimposition of the AP and lateral radiographs in the supine and prone positions, which are used as a coordinate system to calculate a statistical estimation of the coordinates of the targets. Additionally, these data are used to build Guiot's scheme,[44] which will be used as the template for final targeting. These coordinates were initially derived from the stereotactic atlases of Schaltenbrand and Wahren[45] and Talairach and coworkers[22, 46] and then further validated by correlation with the clinical results. The average dimensions of the third ventricle are as follows: AC-PC length, 24.63 ± 1.64 mm (N = 153; range, 21.21 to 27.59 mm); height of thalamus (HT), 16.62 ± 1.47 mm (N = 153; range,

12.57 to 19.95 mm); width, 5.22 ± 1.64 mm (N = 153; range, 1.52 to 19.46 mm).

Talairach System and the Guiot Diagram. On the lateral view, a rectangle is constructed with the AC-PC line as its base; the ends rise perpendicular to the AC-PC line, one at the inner border of the AC and the other at the inner border of the PC. The top is a line parallel to the AC-PC line, tangential to the top of the thalamus. A third line, parallel to the AC-PC line, is drawn at the midheight of the thalamus. The AC-PC line is divided into 12 parts, and the height of the thalamus is divided into 8 parts (see Fig. 173–1). On the AP view, the vertical coordinates are also expressed as one eighth of the height of the thalamus. However, the width is expressed in millimeters from the midline, as there is no good normalization method for this axis of coordinates. Based on Guiot's scheme, the various targets have different ventriculographic characteristics.[13, 44, 46] The coordinates of the various nuclei are given later.

MAGNETIC RESONANCE IMAGING

Sequences. Stereotactic MRI is performed as step 2 (between steps 1 [ventriculography] and 3 [electrode implantation]), to help determine the target site for STN and GPi but not for Vim stimulation, and as step 4 (between steps 3 [electrode implantation] and 5 [pulse generator implantation]), to check the position of the electrodes. Precise calibration of MRI gradients ensures minimal distortion of the images in the central part of the brain, including the basal ganglia. The patient is placed in a modified MRI-compatible (Fischer-Leibinger, Leksell, or CRW Radionics) stereotactic frame capable of reproducible repositioning, using the implanted screws. This frame is equipped with copper sulfate–filled MRI fiducial tubes. The titanium screws make repositioning fast, easy, and painless (local anesthesia is not required). MRI examination is performed in a 1.5-tesla Philips Gyroscan. T1-weighted images are made in the sagittal and coronal (perpendicular to the AC-PC line) planes and allow direct visualization of the thalamus and the pallidum and indirect visualization of the thalamus. T2-weighted coronal sections are taken in planes perpendicular to the AC-PC line to show the STN. These images can be enlarged to the same degree of magnification as the x-ray images obtained by ventriculography, thereby allowing accurate matching of the two sets of morphologic data by simple superimposition or with image guidance software. Stereotactic MRI slices taken in the plane of the trajectory show the position of the pyramidal tract and can help in positioning the electrode in an oblique trajectory parallel to the internal capsule. It also shows the cortical sulci, between the superior and middle frontal gyri (F1-F2), which should be avoided because of the bleeding risk.

Target Visibility. Stereotactic MRI is the key investigation for STN localization. T2-weighted images clearly show the STN as a small, almond-shaped structure situated 1 to 2 mm anterior to the red nucleus, 2 to 3 mm superior and slightly lateral to the SNr, externally limited by the internal capsule, and posterior to the mamillary bodies (Fig. 173–3), allowing precise determination of the coordinates of the center of this small nucleus.

In contrast, the Vim is not visible on MRI. However, on axial T1-weighted images, one can recognize the external limit of the thalamus, which corresponds to the lateral border of the Vim, at one fourth the AC-PC line, anterior to the PC, in the AC-PC horizontal plane. The mesial limit of the Vim might be recognized as the slight change in density that marks the intralaminar nuclei. Similar observations are made on coronal sections. On sagittal sections, the somatosensory thalamus is visible, limited in front by the oblique hypersignal of the internal capsule and posteriorly by the hyposignal of the pulvinar.

The GPi is visible on T1- and T2-weighted images as a strong hyposignal, although the putamen has an even stronger signal than the pallidum on T1-weighted images, where it marks the external limit of the pallidum; this is important posteriorly, where the target is situated. The GPi is clearly separated from the globus pallidus externalis (Gpe), and its division into mesial

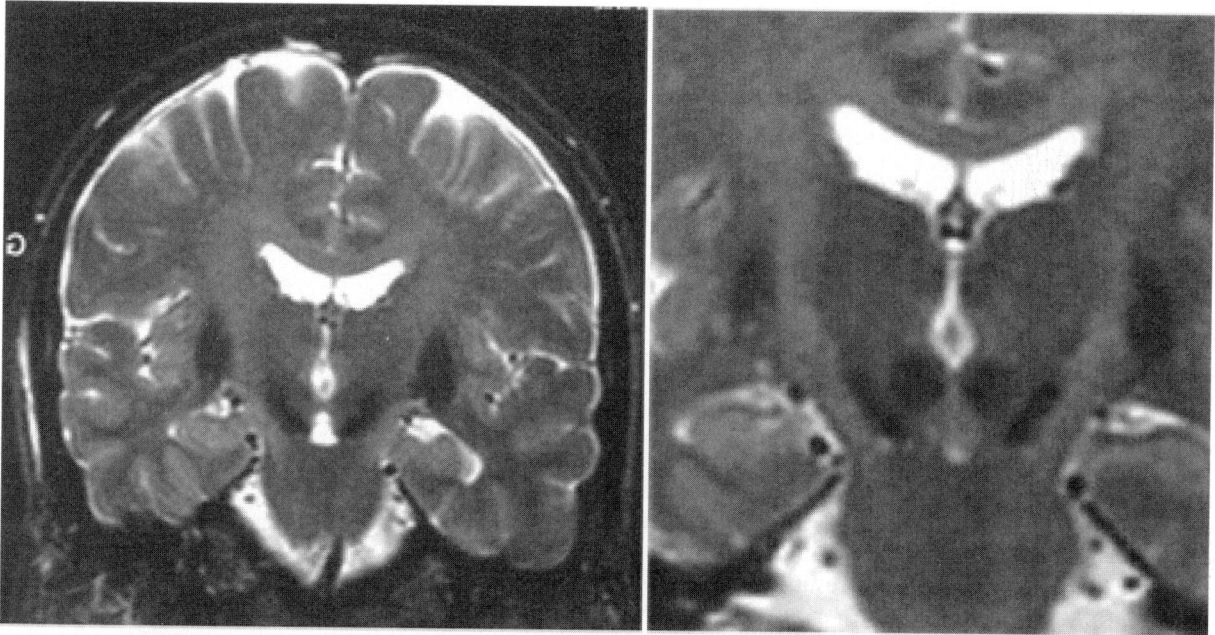

FIGURE 173–3. Magnetic resonance images of the functional targets on coronal T2-weighted sections. The striatum, pallidum, subthalamic nucleus, and substantia nigra, as well as the red nucleus, are visible as strong hyposignals. The thalamic complex is outlined by the oblique relative hypersignal of the internal capsule.

and lateral parts is often visible. The internal capsule and optic tract are also visible on coronal and sagittal T1- and T2-weighted images.

Computed Tomography. Although computed tomography (CT) has made tremendous progress in both spatial and density resolution, and although it provides good three-dimensional reconstructed images, this modality does not match the quality of MRI. CT is not used in our institution as a primary mode of target determination, although AC and PC reconstructed images from high-resolution helicoid CT might be acceptable for targeting based on the AC-PC and midline system of target coordinates. In theory, the data from CT are reconstructed without spatial deformation, whereas those from MRI may be distorted for several reasons: inhomogeneity of the primary magnetic field due to improper tuning of the shim gradients, which tend to achieve a homogeneity of at least 10^{-5}, or due to changes in the magnetic susceptibility of the patient, even though he or she might not have metallic (e.g., dental) implants. As a result, the spatial data, which are dependent on a frequency coding of the space by a linear magnetic gradient, provide erroneous data, which are translated into a wrong position of the corresponding point on the final MRI scan. The extent of these errors depends on the direction in which one looks at the values (coaxial or orthogonal to the main magnetic field) as well as on the sequences of the MRI acquisition protocol. They are larger at a greater distance from the axis of the main magnet and are therefore smaller close to the midline of the patient; they are smaller for STN than for Vim or even Gpi. They can be minimized by careful tuning of the machines, requiring close cooperation from the MRI unit personnel.

Fusion of MRI and CT data might in theory circumvent these errors, provided that the fusion process reformats the MRI data in the nondeformed space represented by the CT image. Currently, the available software does not achieve this reformatting. It matches the two sets of data, with a precision depending on the algorithm used (usually using a least squares method), meaning that the process superimposes the two sets of data in such a way that the average value of the distance of two corresponding points is minimized. Even if this average value is reduced to zero, this does not mean that for a given point its position has been corrected.

Precision of Magnetic Resonance Imaging. This theoretical error may or may not be negligible, but this is not usually known at the time of measurement. A simple way to assess this potential error is to use the software of the image guidance system to measure the AC-PC length on MRI as well as on the ventriculogram (V). Figure 173–4 shows how these data compare in a series of 18 patients after proper tuning of the MRI parameters. On average, the data look similar: AC-PC length (MRI)/AC-PC length (V) = 0.99 ± 0.04 mm (range, 0.92 to 1.08 mm; or an error of ± 8%). The distortion is maximum in the Z (vertical) direction, where the average ratio of Z MRI/V is 0.13 ± 1.27

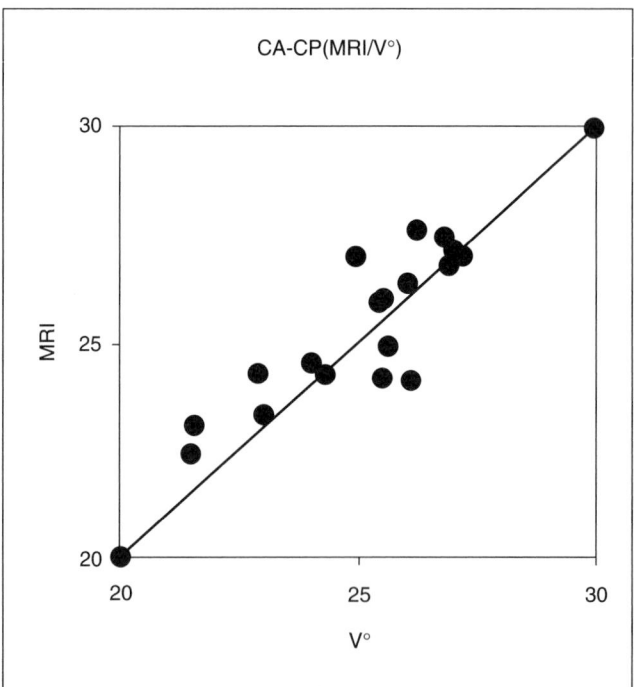

FIGURE 173–4. Distortion on magnetic resonance imaging (MRI). Plot of the anterior commissure–posterior commissure line length as measured on MRI versus ventriculography.

mm, but the true error varies between −3.2 and +3.6 mm, which corresponds to the length of about four contacts of the series 3389 reduced-space electrode.

Postoperative Magnetic Resonance Imaging and Security Issues. A control stereotactic MRI is performed using titanium screws a few days after electrode implantation. The safety of this procedure has been shown, provided some precautions are observed.[47, 48] The Medtronic tetrapolar electrodes, series 3387 and 3389, are MRI compatible and provide images in which the four contacts can be located precisely by the small magnetic artifact surrounding an area devoid of signal. The former monopolar electrode SP.5535, now called series 3388, was used mainly for Vim due to its particular metallic composition; it had a larger magnetic artifact that prevented good localization of the electrode tip.

ATLASES AND TARGETS

Atlases[49–63] can be misleading when targeting one nucleus, because matching of the three planes is rarely achieved; for instance, the STN target representation can be satisfactory on the sagittal and axial views, but frequently it does not match with the coronal view, where the target is often projected in the peduncle (see Fig. 173–2). This is understandable, because usually the three planes (axial, coronal, and sagittal) of an atlas have been obtained in three different brains; we will have to wait for electronically reconstructed atlases to avoid this drawback. All atlases have been drawn from anatomic postmortem examinations of a limited number of brains. Their statistical value is low, and artifacts

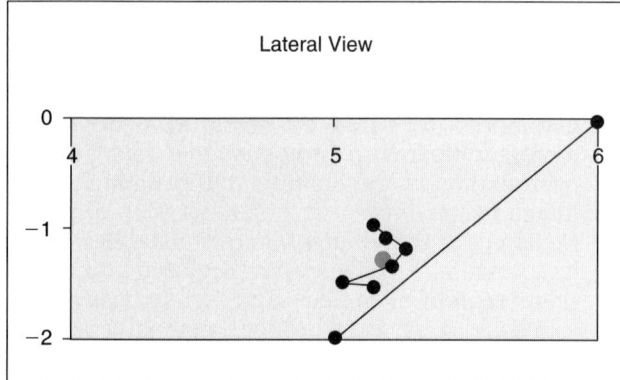

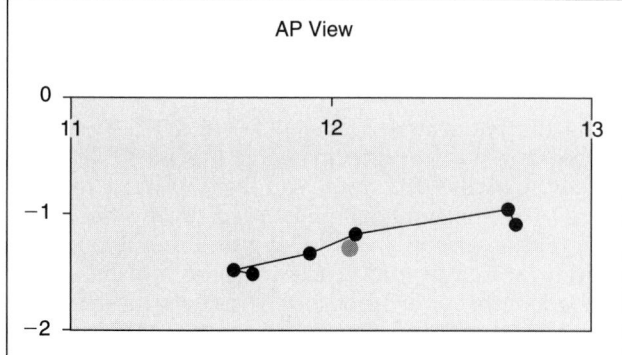

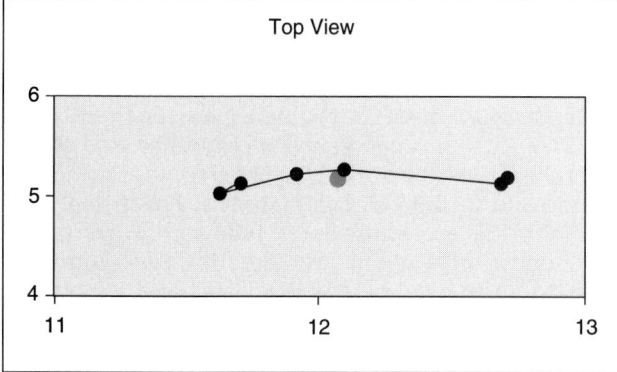

FIGURE 173–5. Evolution of the clinically validated coordinates of the subthalamic nucleus "theoretic" target in consecutive groups of 50 patients, plotted on lateral, anteroposterior, and top views using Guiot's coordinates.

due to fixation and sections are difficult to assess and correct. Adaptations for the specific dimensions of the patient have to be made, using either the proportional grid system of Talairach or the newly designed computerized methods. However, due to the high topologic stability of the brain, atlases are valuable for pretargeting of the basal ganglia, provided that the coordinates of the target are referred to anatomic landmarks visible on the neuroradiologic images (ventriculography, CT, or MRI).

Final Coordinates of the Theoretic Target. Each of the three targets currently used can be defined by the conjunction of data based on (1) geometric landmarks

obtained from ventriculography (which provides a preliminary statistical estimation of the target position), using the modified proportional geometric scheme of Guiot based on the AC-PC line (see Fig. 173–1), and (2) MRI data (which shows neighboring structures of the Vim, clearly visualizes the GPi and STN, and may help in adjusting the coordinates for each patient, particularly for width, which is the only target not normalized). On this basis, the stereotactic parameters (x, y, and z coordinates) of the target point and the entry point are calculated manually or using image-guided neuronavigation software, which guides the trajectories aiming at the target point with microelectrodes for recording and stimulation. The final site for implantation of the chronic tetrapolar electrodes is determined on the basis of the data obtained during this electrophysiology session. The clinical data observed by the clinician in the postoperative period identify the contacts responsible for the best improvement of symptoms. Their coordinates provide the data to calculate the average values of the coordinates of the "clinically validated targets."

Justification of Clinically Validated Targets. The coordinates of the targets are drawn on the ventriculogram, according to the values determined for the whole series of patients, in correlation with the clinical results of stimulation of each contact in all patients. The coordinates obtained are actually adjusted for each new patient and may change if the targeting is incorrect. In fact, if the initial targeting is too posterior, for instance, the electrophysiologic study tends to provide better data on the more anterior electrodes. Their coordinates therefore influence the average value of the AP coordinate toward values closer to the AC. This principle works in all three cartesian dimensions. Figure 173–5 shows the evolution of the "theoretic" target in our experience in groups of 50 patients.

Numerical Values for Coordinates and Third Ventricle Features

Subthalamic Nucleus. On the sagittal view, the STN is situated in the middle third of the AC-PC distance, 0 to 6 mm below this plane and 10 to 14 mm from the midline. The coordinates are as follows: AP, 5.28 ± 0.58 mm × 1/12 of AC-PC length (range, 2.88 to 7.08 mm); vertical, −1.22 ± 0.65 mm × 1/8 of HT (range, −3.29 ± 0.19 mm); width, 12.14 ± 2.05 mm from midline (range, 9 to 15.2 mm) (see Fig. 173–1; Tables 173–1 and 173–2).

Ventral Intermedius Nucleus. The Vim is situated in the posterior fourth of the AC-PC distance, at the level of the AC-PC and about 15 mm from the midline. The coordinates are as follows: AP, 3.53 ± 0.91 mm × 1/12 of AC-PC length (range, 1.43 to 5.98 mm); vertical, 1.15 ± 1.18 mm × 1/8 of HT (range, −2.37 ± 4.26 mm); width, 15.36 ± 1.61 mm from midline (range, 12.27 to 19.22 mm). To take into account changes in the width of the third ventricle (which directly affect the position of the Vim, which is lateral to the third ventricle, but not of the STN, which is below it), one can use

TABLE 173-1 ■ **Statistical Values of Third Ventricle Dimensions***

ALL TARGETS (N = 197)	WIDTH OF V3 (mm)	AC-PC LENGTH (mm)	HEIGHT OF THALAMUS (mm)
Mean	6.25	24.82	16.53
Standard deviation	2.31	1.44	1.57
Minimum	2.21	20.97	10.48
Maximum	14.63	30.48	20.82

* These dimensions were measured on the ventriculogram and divided by the magnification coefficient (1.05).
AC-PC, anterior commissure–posterior commissure; V3, third ventricle.

the "rule of Tasker," where the width of Vim is 11.5 mm + (third ventricle width)/2.

Globus Pallidus Internalis. The GPi target is situated at a distance of two thirds of AC-PC length in front of PC, at the level of the AC-PC, and about 20 mm from the midline. The coordinates are as follows: AP, 8.4 ± 1.2 mm $\times$ 1/12 of AC-PC length (range, 6.6 to 9.9 mm); vertical, -0.7 ± 0.8 mm $\times$ 1/8 of HT (range, -1.7 to 0.3 mm); width, 19.1 ± 2.9 mm from midline (range, 16.0 to 23.2 mm).

Software. Surgery is done on a stereotactic frame, which is used mainly to hold the head of the patient. The frame accessories (goniometer, probe holder) are replaced by a robotized arm (ISS Neuromate), which is driven by either Radionics Splan software or ISS Voxim software. Both types of neuronavigational software can drive the robot on the basis of either MRI or ventriculogram data, or a combination of both. Built-in atlases allow comparison of the position of the electrode during surgery with theoretic anatomic landmarks and structures.[64]

Every frame has its own software, which consists of the following:

- Importation of MRI and CT images, usually in the DICOM 3 format, through an ethernet connection between the operating room and the MRI and radiology facilities or through the transfer of data by magnetic tape.
- Acquisition of x-ray images through digitized subtraction angiography for angiography or ventriculography, or through a scanner to digitize the conventional radiographs.

- Recognition of the fiducials of the specific localizers (angiography, CT, MRI), schematically made of a set of opaque beads or N-shaped tubes containing contrast (iodine for CT and x-ray films, gadolinium for MRI), the section of which on the tomographic images provides three dots, allowing computation of the altitude and inclination of the image plane.
- Matching of the different image modalities, which is automatic when they are acquired during the same session with the same set of frames and localizers. This must be done manually when at least one of the various modalities has not been acquired stereotactically.

Implantation of Electrodes

AIMING AT THE TARGET

Using the Neuromate (Figs. 173–6 and 173–7), repositioning is easy to perform using the screw holes, in which the pins of the frame can dock, and the readings of the verniers, previously recorded during the ventriculographic session and allowing millimetric precision. As in most image-guided software, the coordinates can be loaded through numerical windows in which the values are typed or obtained from the MRI scans by pointing at the anatomic structures considered the target or at the point drawn on the ventriculogram using Guiot's scheme and the geometric determination of the targets, according to the clinically validated theoretic targets.

Determination of Coordinates on the Ventriculogram. We currently use ventriculography-based coordinates (Fig. 173–8), primarily in the STN for Parkinson's disease and in the GPi for dystonias. For instance, for the STN, the procedure is as follows: On the lateral view, one draws a line through the midcommissure point and a point situated at the level of the top of the thalamus, at ten twelfths of the AC-PC distance ahead of the vertical to the PC. This line intersects the floor of the third ventricle at a point whose coordinates are AP = 11.02 ± 0.90 mm (or 5.03 ± 0.61 mm $\times$ 1/12 AC-PC distance) and vertical = -3.36 ± 0.59 mm (or -1.54 ± 0.34 mm $\times$ 1/8 HT), which is at an average distance of 0.74 ± 0.55 mm from the theoretic target, whose coordinates are AP = 5.28 ± 0.58 mm $\times$ 1/12 AC-PC distance, vertical = -1.22 ± 0.65 mm $\times$ 1/8 HT. This simple graphic method provides an easy way

TABLE 173-2 ■ **Statistical Values of Coordinates of All Targets***

	VIM (mm)	STN (mm)	GPi (mm)	
AC-PC/PC	2.87 ± 0.37	5.16 ± 0.73	8.99 ± 1.04	$^1/_{12}$ AC-PC length
Width	13.77 ± 1.65	11.52 ± 2.11	16.65 ± 5.53	mm (corrected)
Height/AC-PC	0.65 ± 0.71	-1.30 ± 0.84	-0.85 ± 1.13	$^1/_8$ thalamus height

* These dimensions were measured on the ventriculogram and normalized to AC-PC length for anteroposterior coordinates, to the height of the thalamus for the vertical coordinate, and divided by the magnification coefficient (1.05) for the width.
AC-PC, anterior commissure–posterior commissure; GPi, globus pallidus internalis; STN, subthalamic nucleus; Vim, ventral intermedius nucleus.

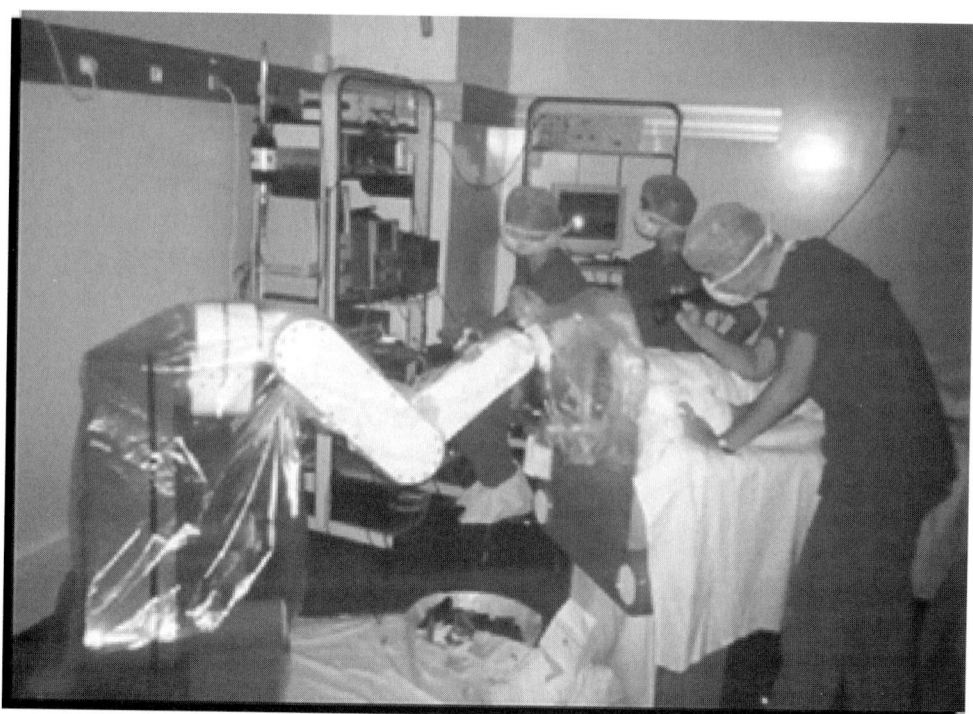

FIGURE 173–6. Robotic arm Neuromate.

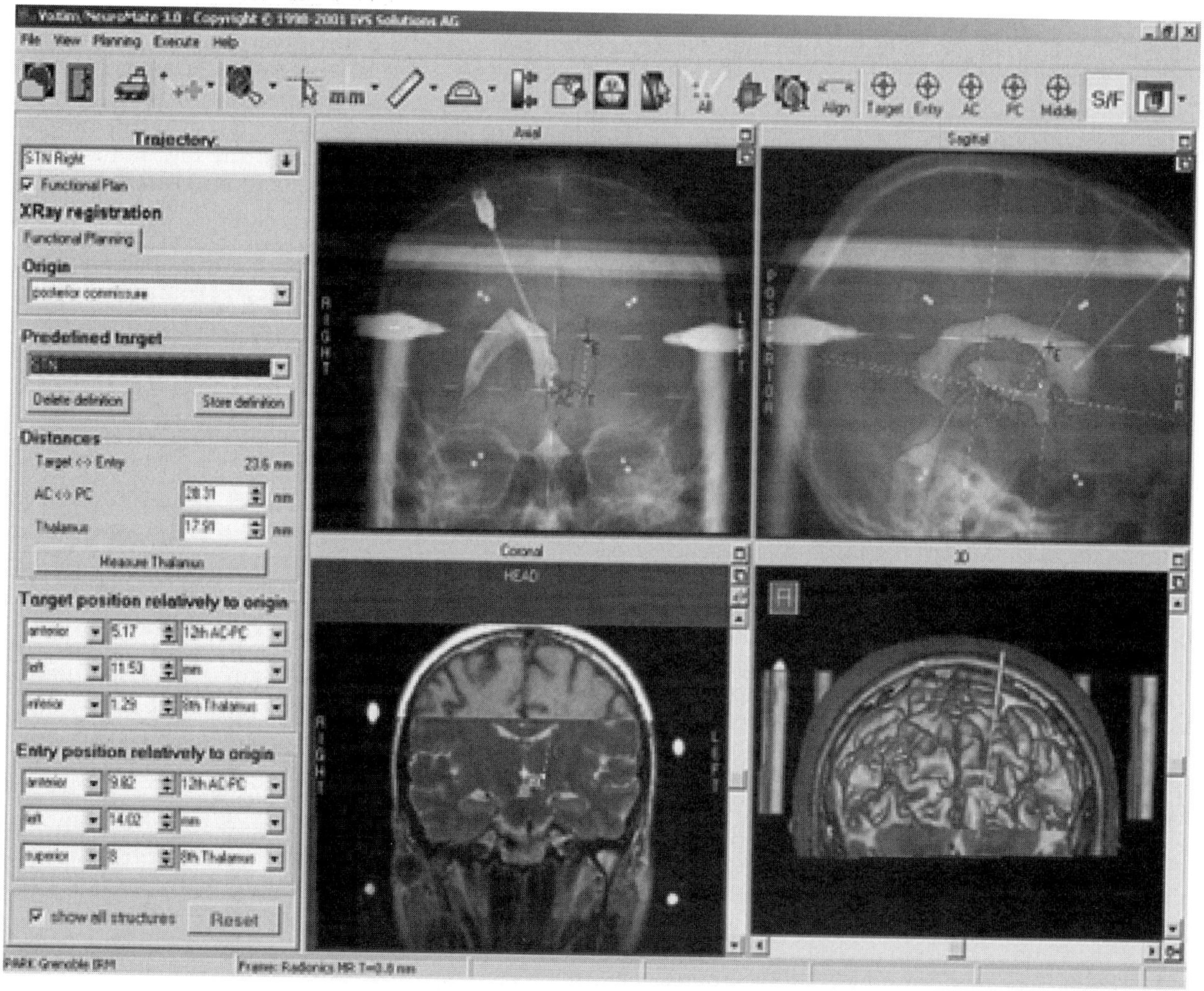

FIGURE 173–7. Computer screen display of the Voxim planning software of the Neuromate.

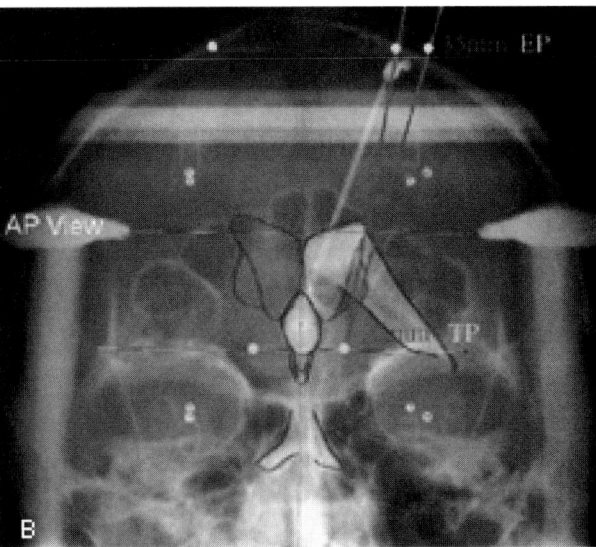

FIGURE 173–8. *A* and *B*, Ventriculographic determination of target coordinates. AC, anterior commissure; EP, entry point; HT, height of thalamus; PC, posterior commissure; TP, target point.

of drawing the target. Then the altitudes of the intersection of the track with the floor of the third ventricle and with the inner table of the skull to the reference line between the screws. These values are reported on the AP x-ray view. From the midline of the third ventricle, the lateral point of the STN target is set at 12.14 mm, and the lateral extent of the entry point is set at between 25 and 35 mm. This point is then adjusted on the MRI scans loaded in the image-guidance software.

The Vim and GPi are consistently implanted parallel to the midline plane. Our first 50 STN patients were also implanted parallel to the midline plane, but the risk of hitting a vessel, such as a branch of the pericallosal artery, was too high and was actually responsible for a supraventricular hematoma. The theoretic STN target is currently approached in double obliquity and parallel to the anterior border of Vim (average coronal angle, 13.1 ± 7.4 degrees; average sagittal angle on the AC-PC plane: theoretic from Guiot's scheme, 63.6 ± 2.4 degrees; actual, 59.5 ± 17.4 degrees). This difference is due to adjustment of the entry point on MRI, using image-guidance software, to avoid cortical veins, the F1-F2 sulcus, and, if possible, the lateral ventricle.

Description and Use of the Five-Channel Guide System: "Ben Gun." Since 1994, we have treated 220 patients (36 Vim, 172 STN, 12 GPi) with a new system designed to allow simultaneous introduction of a set of five parallel recording-stimulating electrodes (four electrodes concentrically placed around a central one at 2-mm distance; tungsten microelectrodes, 1-μm tip, 10 Mohm, protruding from the guide tube by 15 mm to avoid lesion of the target by the guide tubes) aimed directly at the theoretic location of the target. A 6-mm bur hole is made in the skull, without opening the dura, and a five-channel barrel is inserted into it. The dura is pierced with a sharp stylet, 1.3-mm external diameter guide tubes are introduced, and progression into the brain parenchyma is achieved using a blunt

stylet to avoid vascular damage. When the tips of the tubes are 25 mm from the intended target, the stylets are withdrawn and replaced by the microelectrodes. During this exploration, electrophysiologic procedures are performed. The track that provides the best functional results is chosen for final implantation of the DBS electrode, which is inserted in place of the test electrode. The corresponding guide tube and microelectrode are withdrawn, and the four remaining electrodes are left in place to avoid brain shift. The chronic electrode is precisely guided and inserted exactly where the best results were observed. The four remaining tubes and microelectrodes are then withdrawn, the five-channel barrel is withdrawn by 3 cm while the DBS electrode is kept at the same depth, and the electrode is secured by a nylon ligature secured to the skull through a thin, oblique hole drilled in the rim of the 6-mm bur hole. Pieces of Surgicel dipped in liquid dental cement are packed in the hole, occluding it and at the same time embedding the electrode. When the cement is fully polymerized, the inner stylet of the DBS electrode is withdrawn, the system is dismantled, and the electrode is bent over the external table of the skull under the galea, where it will stay until it is connected to the cable of the generator. On the one hand, the risk of hitting a blood vessel is theoretically five times higher with this method than with the previous one, but this was not confirmed in our series. On the other hand, because a larger area is probed, the probability of finding the best electrode location is increased.

We aim at the target with a set of five microelectrodes, and microstimulation and microrecording are performed all along the track. At the end of exploration, the multidisciplinary team compiles the information that will be required during surgery, including microrecordings and recognition of typical neuronal firing patterns, beneficial effects of microstimulation on the clinical symptoms, and side effects, to predict the long-term therapeutic result. Finally, based on this brainstorming session, the best electrode (the one yielding the best positive effects and the fewest side effects) is withdrawn and replaced by the chronic electrode (DBS 3389, Medtronic, Minneapolis, MN; four contacts, 1.27-mm diameter, 1.5-mm long, 0.5-mm spacing), which is secured to the skull.

Electrode number 1, or the central one aimed at the estimated target, is chosen in only 41.6% of cases; in the remaining cases, the electrode choice is almost equally distributed among the other four tracks (18% lateral, 17% anterior, 12% mesial, and 11% posterior), which are just 2 mm apart. When electrode number 1 is not chosen as the best target, its efficiency would still be acceptable in 26.3% of cases. This means that if electrode number 1 were used as the sole electrode aimed at the target on the basis of anatomic and radiologic data only, this would lead to a clinically acceptable result in about 70% of cases and to an unacceptable outcome in about 30%. These failures warrant the use of intraoperative electrophysiologic assessment, at least by stimulation. The positioning of the contralateral electrode is asymmetrical in 63.7% of cases, emphasizing how important it is to assess the functional location of the target during surgery on both sides, even if the anatomic positioning looks correct. The placement was symmetrical in 12.4% of cases for the central electrode, 7.82% for the anterior, 5.25% for the lateral, 1.7% for the posterior, and 0% for the mesial in 57 consecutive patients bilaterally implanted with 114 electrodes.

MICRORECORDING AND MICROSTIMULATION

Electrophysiology (stimulation and recording) provides the functional signature of the target (Fig. 173–9). Owing to individual variations, the target is identified during the procedure by the electrophysiologic study, including recording with microelectrodes of the specific neuronal activity of the target neurons and stimulation at high frequency, the clinical effects of which (alleviation of symptoms and production of side effects) are observed with the cooperation of a neurologist. The final target may be significantly different from the theoretic target (based on atlases, ventriculography, and MRI), when the electrophysiologic data gathered along the five tracks are taken into account (e.g., specific spontaneous and evoked neuronal firing patterns, positive and negative effects of stimulation). Investigations are performed all along the last 10 to 15 mm before the theoretic target is reached.

Microrecording

Spontaneous as well as evoked multiunit and single-unit neuronal activities are considered the signature of the explored structure. For our first 130 patients, neuronal patterns were recorded at various sites along the trajectory using conventional preamplifiers (WPI DAM-5A), AC-DC amplifiers (Neurolog NL106), filters (Neurolog NL125), and spike triggers (Neurolog NL201) and processed through a MacLab 4 WPI system

and a MacIntosh II CX computer. The development of this branch of functional neurosurgery has motivated manufacturers to design systems that can assist neurosurgical teams in performing electrophysiologic investigations in the operating room. For our last 60 patients, we used the AlphaOmega integrated system Neurotrek (Fig. 173–10), which allows simultaneous recording from five electrodes and data processing (frequency analysis, interspike histogram, dot raster display, spike sorting, cross- and autocorrelograms, and storage and stimulation). It is equipped with a microdrive controlled from the computer keyboard. The LeadPoint Medtronic system also has the capability of recording simultaneously on four channels. The recorded pattern depends on the nucleus investigated and the type of electrode used. With a semi-macroelectrode, only multiunit activity can be recorded; the amplitude of the spikes, described as "neural noise,"[65, 66] varies along the track and can provide information about the boundaries of the different nuclei. White matter bundles are usually silent and recognizable by their low neural noise. This neural noise is high in the Vim and diminishes markedly when the electrode enters the internal capsule. Similar patterns are observed in the STN and GPi.[67] With a microelectrode (FHC Brunswick), single units are recorded in all three nuclei. The exact position of each stimulating or recording site is checked by x-ray films and mapped onto the final operating diagram.

Ventral Intermedius Nucleus. Neuronal activity can be recorded along the track in both the Vim and the VPL. In the Vim, cells fire in bursts of 5 to 10 large spikes. Some cells have spontaneous bursting activity independent of any peripheral stimulation or muscular activity. Others fire synchronously with the tremor and also respond to passive movements of the limbs. Similarly, evoked activities are easily recorded in VPL in response to superficial stimulation of the skin (touch, pressure). As has already been shown, neurons firing in bursts synchronous with the tremor are recorded in the Vim, and thalamotomy at this site provides good results,[41, 44, 68] as does, in our experience, stimulation at high frequency.

Globus Pallidus Internalis. The GPi is a larger structure than the Vim or STN, but we do not have clear data about functional spatial distribution within this nucleus, which makes electrode placement difficult. Depending on the obliquity of the exploration track, electrophysiologic recording provides characteristic firing patterns, originally described by Hutchinson and coworkers,[67] which allows one to recognize the GPe, where two types of cells are recorded (low-frequency discharge-burst neurons [10.6 ± 8.9 Hz] and higher-frequency neurons [60 ± 36 Hz] with an irregular pattern and pauses in activity), and the GPi, where neurons are firing at a high rate with a very irregular firing pattern (55 ± 27 Hz in the external part, and 82 ± 32 Hz in the medial part). These three subnuclei are also separated by border cells with a regular firing pattern of about 30 Hz. Below the GPi, the adjacent structure that runs obliquely parallel to the main axis

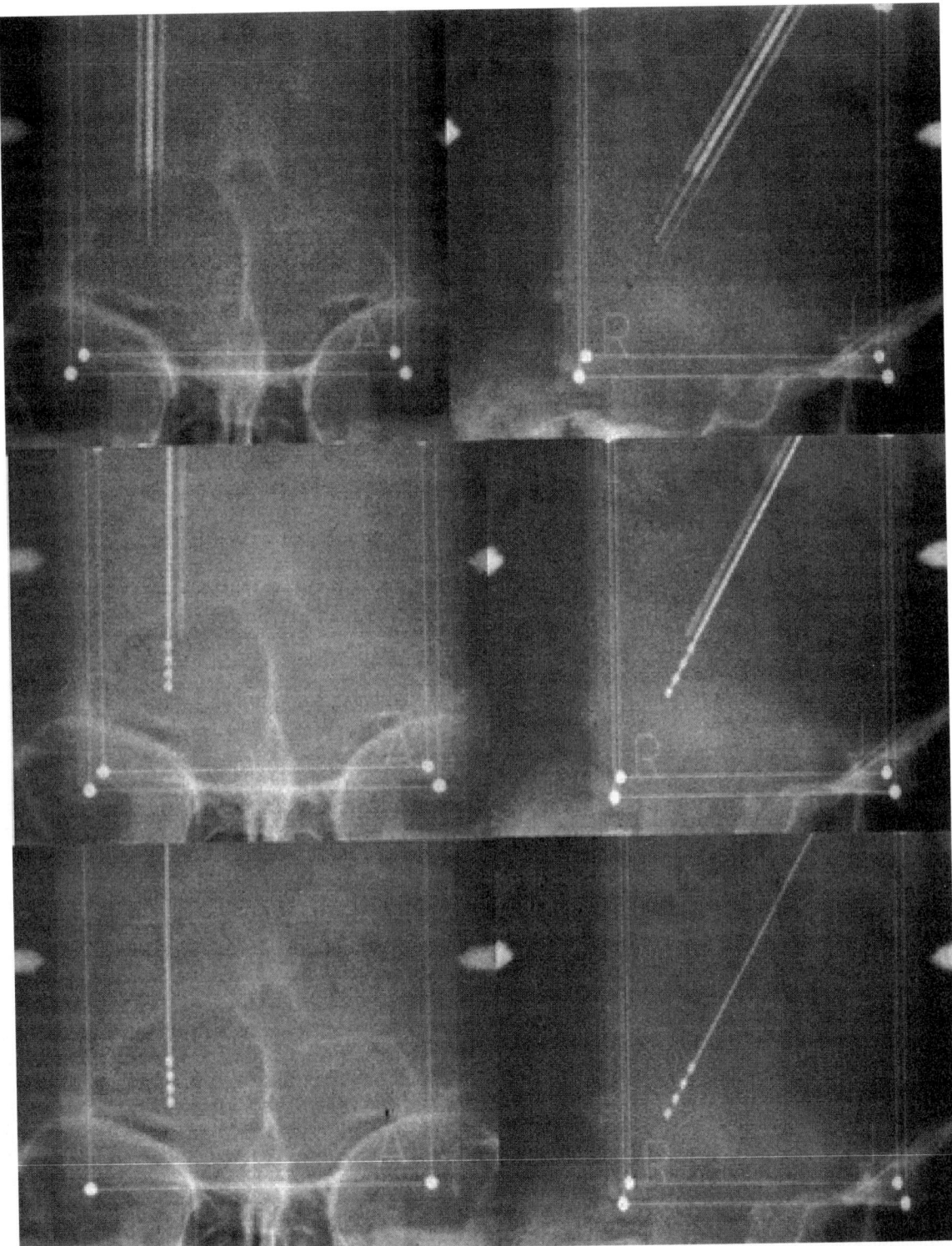

FIGURE 173–9. Five-channel guide. Anteroposterior and lateral x-ray views of the different steps: introduction of the guide tubes with microelectrodes, replacement of the best microelectrode by the chronic deep brain stimulating electrode, and final control of the electrode as it is secured to the skull.

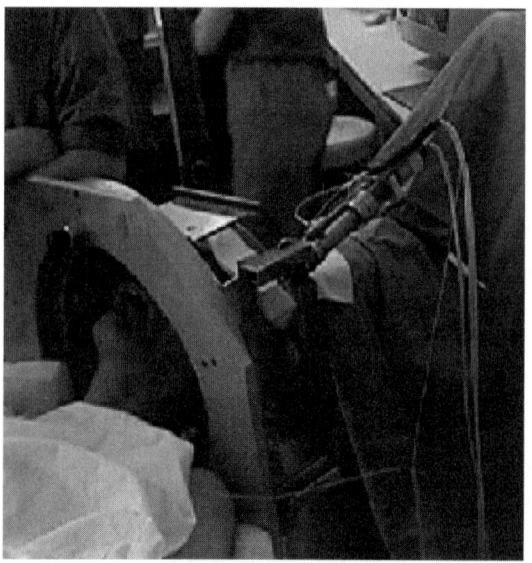 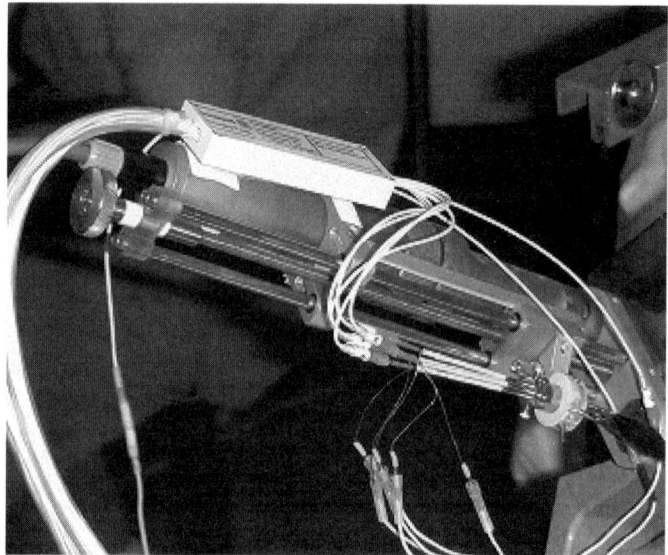

FIGURE 173–10. Microguide setup. *Left*, General assembly of the frame on the rotating stand and of the microguide system on the frame. *Right*, Detail of the microguide showing the microelectrode and the motorized drive.

of GPi is the optic tract, where light flashes induce evoked potentials and stimulation induces phosphene perception.

Subthalamic Nucleus. Electrophysiology enables precise identification of the STN. At the site of the STN as located by MRI, and at the place where the best effects on rigidity and akinesia were obtained, recordings showed an increase in the neuronal firing rate in the STN compared with the surrounding area. The majority of STN cells produce large, asymmetrical spikes with a high-frequency (35.2 ± 8.8 Hz) firing rate and biphasic spikes at a lower rate (11.1 ± 2.3 Hz) responsive to passive movements and to tremor. Below the STN level, even larger, very symmetrical spikes can be recorded with a lower, irregular firing rate and unresponsive to all kinds of stimuli in the SNr. Farther below this area, neuronal silence is characteristic of the internal capsule and provides the inferior limit for electrode positioning (Fig. 173–11; see color section in this volume).

Microstimulation

Even though MRI visualization of the STN and GPi evidently helps pinpoint the track, shifts of several millimeters between the theoretic (MRI or ventriculography based) and the corrected (electrophysiology based) targets may be observed, confirming the necessity of electrophysiologic studies for target localization, although this is still a matter of controversy.[69] However, these shifts are rather small, and the first localization of the target by the ventriculographic approach is nearly always correct (average distance from the active contact to the theoretic target is 2.1 ± 0.9 mm for the STN). These data support the ability of ventriculography to define the target, whether or not an electrophysiologic study is performed, although the utility of ventriculog-

raphy is also a matter of controversy.[70] Stimulation may identify surrounding structures and essentially provides the functional criteria of effectiveness by showing directly, during surgery, to what extent tremor or other symptoms are suppressed by stimulation and where this can be achieved. Contrary to common belief, efficient microstimulation can be routinely and safely performed, with currents up to 10 mA through 0.1- to 0.3-Mohm microelectrodes, provided that trains of stimulation are kept shorter than 10 seconds. This has the advantage of allowing the comparison of recorded data and the effects of stimulation at the same site. The exact position of each stimulating or recording site is checked by radiographs and mapped onto the final operating diagram. This provides a set of data with which the exact location of the chosen nucleus can be mapped, providing a corrected target into which the chronic DBS electrode will be implanted (Fig. 173–12). A constant-current stimulator (WPI Accupulser A310) with an isolation unit (WPI A365R) was used in the past to stimulate structures during the electrode placement procedure at various sites along the trajectory, but this has been replaced by the stimulation unit included into the AlphaOmega Neurotrek. Test stimulation was done with a 60-msec pulse width, a 130-Hz frequency, and a current intensity that varied from 0.1 to 10 mA. The electrode is always used as a cathode, and the positive electrode is a large conducting rubber electrode (4 by 5 cm) glued with conductive gel on the subclavicular area.

Ventral Intermedius Nucleus. The effect of stimulation on tremor was quantified using an accelerometer attached to the patient's finger. The effect of stimulation (130 Hz, 60-msec pulse width) on Vim tremor suppression with the lowest (0.2 to 2 mA) current strength is the major criterion in choosing the final placement. For instance, as the electrode approaches

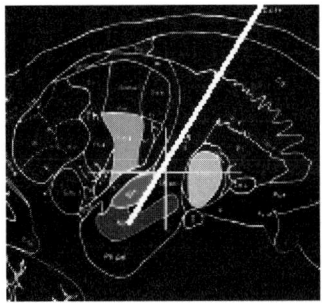

Silence in White Matter
Nucleus Signature
Nucleus Borders

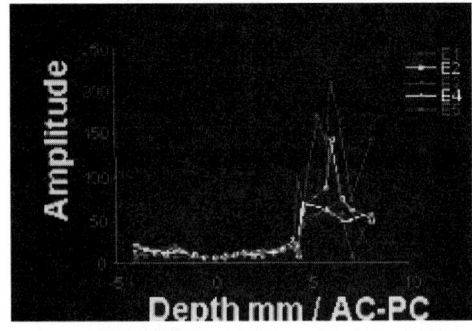

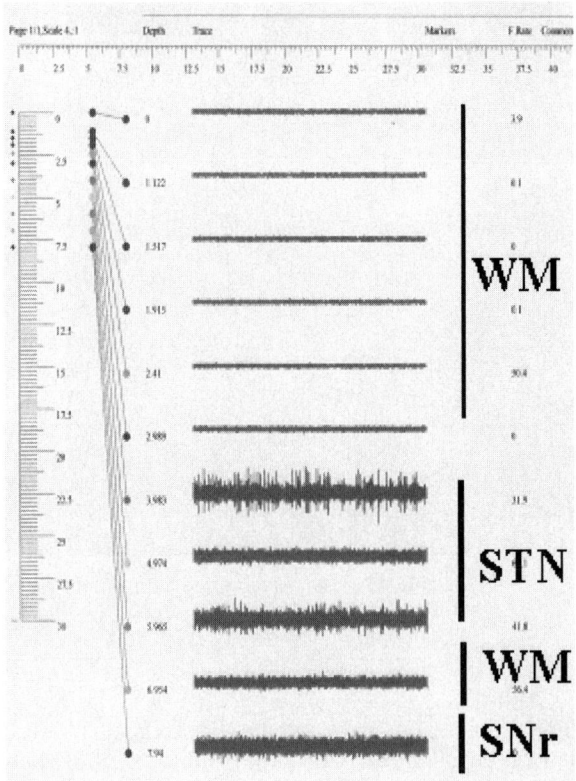

FIGURE 173–11. Electrophysiology using the Neurotrek system. Along the planned track through the basal ganglia, the electrophysiologic pattern changes from silence in the white matter of the internal capsule and between the subthalamic nucleus (STN) and substantia nigra pars reticularis (SNr) to typical neuronal firing in the nuclei. The plot of the signal amplitude clearly shows the entry and exit in and out of the STN (see color section in this volume).

the Vim target, the current intensity threshold necessary to obtain total arrest of the tremor decreases, from more than 10 mA at 20 mm from PC to between 0.1 and 1 mA at the level of the Vim area as determined by Guiot's scheme, which is reached at about 8 mm from PC. The lowest value of this threshold is used to

determine the site of maximal effectiveness into which the DBS electrode is finally implanted. For each track, comparison between motor and sensory thresholds helps determine the optimal electrode placement. Progression of the electrode farther than this point usually leads to the need for greater current values to suppress

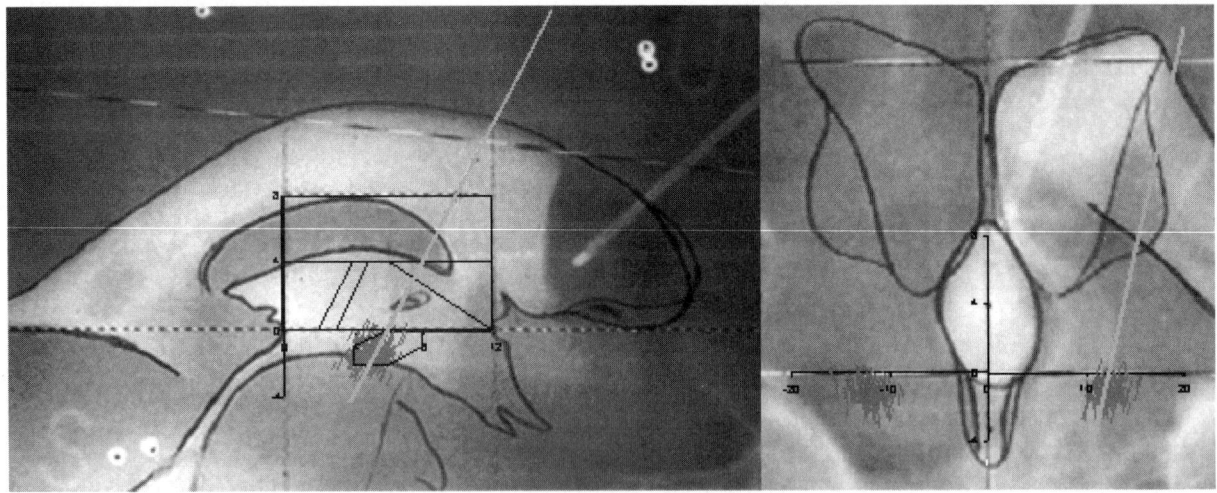

FIGURE 173–12. Distribution of all subthalamic nucleus electrodes, represented on the ventriculogram.

tremor, and permanent paresthesias caused by stimulation of the VPL are progressively and increasingly induced. In the Vim area, stimulation with currents as low as 0.2 mA induces immediate suppression of the tremor in an intensity-dependent manner. With sufficient current values, the tremor disappears at the onset of the current, with no more than 1 or 2 seconds of delay, and recurs almost as quickly when the current is turned off. When an aftereffect is observed, it lasts no more than 10 to 20 seconds. The effect is polarity sensitive, as the stimulating electrode is negative. When the polarity is reversed, the effect disappears or is at least strongly decreased. Brief paresthesias, which disappear within 10 seconds, are often described by the patient at the onset of stimulation. Stimulation-induced paresthesias in the commissure of the first two fingers are indicative of correct lateral position for tremor suppression in the upper limb. Paresthesias elicited in the face indicate that the track is too medial, whereas paresthesias in the fifth finger or even in the leg mean that the track is too lateral. During progression of the electrode toward the final target, a decrease in spontaneous tremor intensity is often observed, together with increased stimulation aftereffects and difficulty in reinducing the tremor. This is considered a minor equivalent of the thalamotomy-like effect that is classically observed when entering the thalamotomy target with a larger electrode.

Globus Pallidus Internalis. Stimulation of the GPi can produce a clear decrease in rigidity or even in akinesia and tremor. This is used to guide correct electrode placement. However, L-dopa–induced dyskinesias or abnormal involuntary movements cannot be easily tested in the operating room during the electrophysiologic session, except if the apomorphine test is performed. The GPi is a larger structure than the Vim or STN, but we do not have clear data about functional spatial distribution within this nucleus, which makes electrode placement difficult.

Subthalamic Nucleus. During STN stimulation, continuous monitoring by the neurologist of passive rigidity of the patient's wrist reveals changes related to efficient stimulation. The STN target is located where the best effects on rigidity and akinesia are obtained. STN stimulation induces a recovery of limb akinesia when the patient is "frozen." Motor performance rates are significantly increased, although this type of assessment's reproducibility is limited, owing to patient fatigue. A significant decrease in wrist rigidity is actually the most reliable intraoperative test. When the symptoms (tremor or bradykinesia) are bilateral, the contralateral side is implanted during the same session.

Introduction and Fixation of the Chronic Deep Brain Stimulating Electrode

As of this writing, a total of 545 electrodes have been implanted in 305 patients: 121 in Vim (64 bilateral), 12 in Gpi (8 bilateral), and 172 in STN (4 unilateral). A total of 340 STN tetrapolar electrodes have been implanted in 172 patients, parallel to the midsagittal plane in 54 patients (99 electrodes) and in double obliquity in the other 241. The first 108 electrodes were monopolar (Medtronic SP.5535; currently, DBS series 3388) with an insulated tip, 1.27-mm diameter, and 3.5 mm long. The remaining 437 were tetrapolar (Medtronic series 3387 or 3389) with four contacts, 1.27-mm diameter, and 1.5 mm long, separated by 1.5 or 0.5 mm. When control radiographs confirm the correct final placement, the electrode is fixed to the skull by a suture anchored in the skull through a short drilled hole intersecting the track hole in a Y-shaped pattern. The bur hole is filled with hemostatic sponge (Surgicel) dipped in semiliquid dental cement, and the knot in the suture is embedded using dental cement (methyl methacrylate). Because the dura is not opened and has only five punctures, there is no leakage of cement or solvent into the subdural space. We never used the bur hole cap provided with the series 3387 or 3389 kits. The extra length of wire is folded under the pericranium, which is carefully closed, as is the skin. All incisions are closed by nonresorbant sutures after local irrigation with an antibiotic (rifamycin). When the symptoms (tremor or bradykinesia) are bilateral, the contralateral side is implanted during the same session, using the same procedure.

IMPLANTATION OF THE PROGRAMMABLE GENERATOR

Timing and Procedure. Internalization of the stimulator can be done after implantation of the electrodes. In our institution, this is done within a week after electrode implantation under general anesthesia. This delay may allow preliminary testing, recovery of the patient from the implantation step, and MRI control of the position of the electrodes, which we do not perform when the implantable programmable generator (IPG) is internalized, although it has been shown that this can be done safely.[71] The distal part of the DBS electrode is introduced into the connector of the extension. This connector has to be secured with silicon glue to achieve correct insulation and to avoid disconnection. It also must be placed under the galea to avoid skin erosion and exteriorization of the material, which could lead to infection and require ablation. It also has to be placed above the level of the mastoid, ideally at the level of the convexity, to prevent any movement at the level of the lead, which is the fragile part; its fracture would have critical consequences and require electrode reimplantation. The extension between the electrodes and the IPG must be performed by subcutaneous tunnelization, as for ventriculoperitoneal or atrial shunts; the depth has to be carefully controlled and must not be too superficial, to avoid subdermal fibrosis and adhesion of the extension to the superficial layers of the skin, which is painful. The programmable stimulus generator (Medtronic Itrel I in the first 23 patients, and Itrel II in the last 169 patients) is placed in a subcutaneous pocket in the subclavicular area and connected to the distal tip of the electrode via an extension passed subcutaneously up the neck to the cephalic area (Fig. 173–13). This allows independent selection of each of-

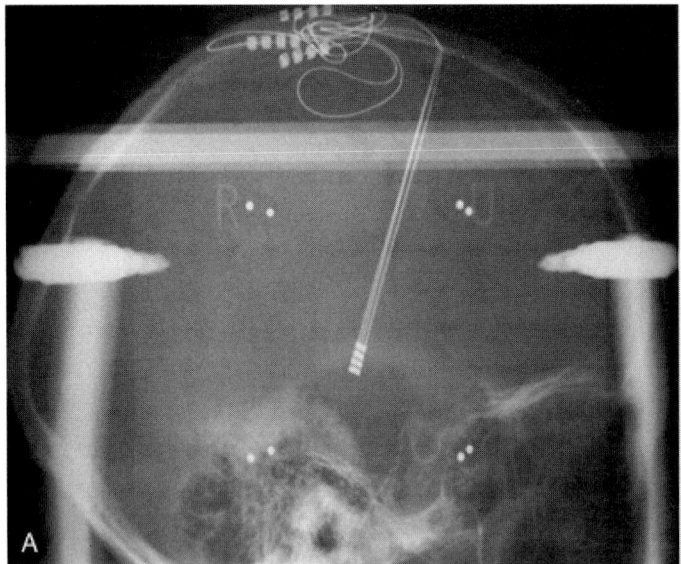
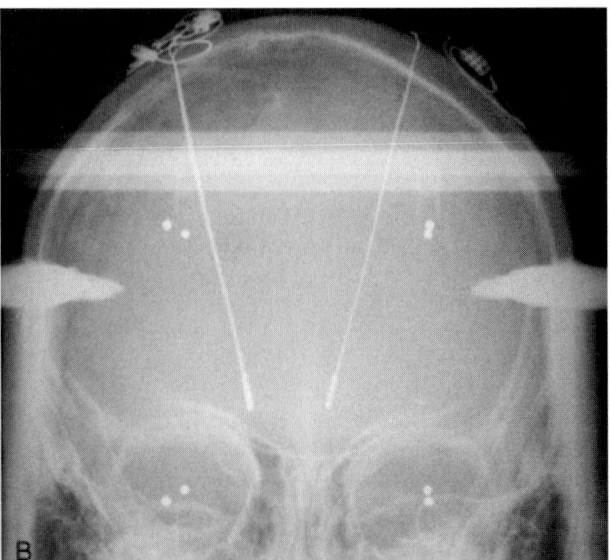
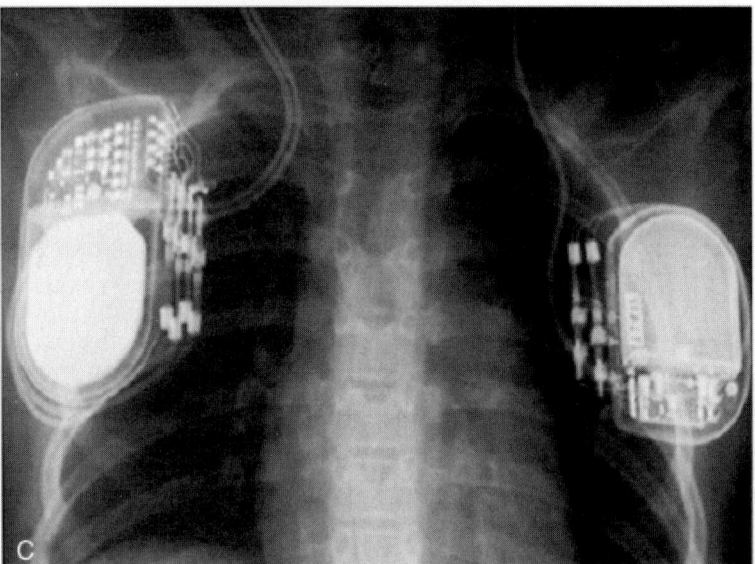

FIGURE 173–13. Final x-ray control of electrodes and implanted generator. In this case, two electrodes were implanted in the right subthalamic nucleus, connected to a Kinetra generator; one was implanted on the left side, connected to an Itrel II generator.

the four contacts of the series 3389 electrode. A double-channel IPG Kinetra, allowing independent programming of each of the two electrodes, one for each side, has been used since January 1999. This makes the implantation step unilateral and easier, and only one system has to be replaced when the battery is exhausted. Local instillation of antibiotics (rifamycin) is done at the level of every surgical wound.

Tuning of Parameters. After implantation of the Itrel (replaced by Soletra) or Kinetra stimulators, patients are kept in the hospital for at least a week for evaluation of the effects of stimulation and other symptoms and fine-tuning of the stimulator parameters. All quantitative tests performed in the preoperative period are performed again. In particular, the effects of Vim DBS on tremor are assessed clinically using a 5-point scale:

4, complete disappearance of tremor in all circumstances; 3, reappearance of slight tremor on rare occasions (e.g., under stress, mental calculation, motor activation); 2, moderate benefit; 1, slight but definite benefit without any real improvement in daily living; and 0, no benefit. Clinical assessment of rigidity and bradykinesia are based on the Unified Parkinson's Disease Rating Scale (UPDRS) part II, Hoehn and Yahr scales, Schwab and England scores, and neuropsychological evaluation (Mattis, Beck scales).

Setting up the parameters of the IPGs can be done rather quickly after some experience. Initial settings are 130-Hz frequency, 60-μsec pulse width, and 0.5 to 4 V, depending on the target and on the clinical effects. If necessary, the frequency range of the Itrel II can be extended to 185 Hz. Each of the four contacts are then successively tested as the amplitude is progressively increased and the patient is examined for alleviation of symptoms and induction of side effects (e.g., paresthesias; contractions of the limb, face, or ocular muscles; flashing lights; strange feelings). The contact that provides the best benefit–to–side effects ratio is selected for chronic stimulation. These parameters are adjusted according to the needs of each patient during the follow-up period; adjustments in voltage amplitude are usually required. These fine-tunings must not be considered drawbacks of the method, as they correspond to drug dosage adjustments in medical therapy. They also allow adaptations to postoperative healing after ablative surgery or to evolution of the disease.

AVAILABLE TARGETS

Data gathered over the last 2 decades from animal experiments and pathologic findings in cases of movement disorders have led to the current concept of the parallel processing model, which, if not accurate, has the immense value of being didactic and providing a practical basis for reasoning. As in every model, the precise mechanisms are probably far more complicated, but so far, most of the clinical and experimental observations fit rather closely to its predictions, indicating that the general structure of the model is reasonably close to reality. According to this current concept,[28, 29, 33] degeneration of the dopaminergic neurons of the substantia nigra pars compacta deafferentates the striatum (putamen and caudate nucleus) from the regulatory neurotransmitter dopamine. The D1 and D2 receptors of the striatum are then deprived and undergo a process of deafferentation supersensitivity, and the two output GABAergic pathways originating from them become unbalanced. The direct pathway impinges on the GPi and SNr, and the indirect pathway connects to the GPe, which in turn exerts its GABAergic influence on the STN. The STN is a glutamatergic nucleus that sends excitatory axons to the complex SNr-GPi. In this concept, the SNr and GPi are placed in the same functional "black box," which sends a globally inhibitory GABAergic output to the motor thalamic nuclei. This is supposed to be the basis of the akinesia of Parkinson's disease. Obviously, the model is too simple: it does not explain tremor or the effect on tremor of destroying or inhibiting the STN, GPi, Vim, and CM-Pf. The STN receives GABAergic input from the GPe, but also glutamatergic input from the cortex and the CM-Pf. The SNr does not have the same therapeutic properties as the GPi when stimulated in Parkinson's disease, contrary to what the model suggests. It is obvious that the data gathered in patients stimulated at high frequency in the Vim, STN, and GPi under various pathologic circumstances will provide new insight into the mechanisms of both normal and abnormal motility. According to this concept, the decrease in striatal dopamine levels induces hyperactivity in the STN as well as in the GPi and SNr, while neuronal firing in the ventrolateral motor thalamus and the cortex is reduced. Accordingly, one might expect that destruction of the STN or GPi would improve symptoms by erasing the abnormal neuronal activity in these two nuclei, which is coherent with clinical observations following subthalamotomy and pallidotomy or neuroinhibition of these structures by high-frequency stimulation.

Substantia Nigra Pars Reticularis

According to the current concept of the organization of the basal ganglia, the GPi and SNr are supposed to have equivalent properties and share common features and roles in the control of motility. Therefore, the SNr should have the same properties as the GPi and could be considered a functional target. Its position just below the STN makes it easy to explore as well as to stimulate with the lower contacts of the electrode used for STN stimulation. Unfortunately, as could have been predicted from the different electrophysiologic properties of the SNr, the neuronal firing does not change in response to any stimulus. Stimulation of the SNr has no effect on parkinsonian symptoms, independent of the frequency. Further studies are needed to evaluate the effects, or absence of effects, of SNr stimulation on ocular motility, taking into account the projection of the SNr onto the superior colliculus. This connection might be useful in treating epilepsy.[72–74]

Globus Pallidus Externalis

In theory, the GPe is a potent GABAergic structure that should exert a strong inhibitory action on both the STN and the GPi. However, this has never been observed, although there has been no definite attempt to explore its properties.

Cortex

Motor cortex stimulation is being investigated and seems to be effective in relieving some forms of intractable pain. It has been reported that intraoperative cortex stimulation might stop parkinsonian tremor and that chronic stimulation could alleviate action tremor.[75, 76]

Pedunculopontine Nucleus

From animal experiments and basic neurophysiology, there is evidence that the pedunculopontine nucleus might play an important role in the control of motility. However, the pedunculopontine nucleus is subject to degeneration in Parkinson's disease, and results of the first attempts to lesion or stimulate it in animal models have been ambiguous.[77] The pedunculopontine nucleus seems to be difficult to access safely and might not be a practical target in human patients.

INDICATIONS AND PATIENT SELECTION

Surgical treatment is not a treatment per se. It has to be part of a strategy and is used only when medical treatment fails. Our primary selection criterion is severe disability with conserved response to a L-dopa treatment, and the patient must not be demented.

Patients were selected for treatment on the basis of the existence of on-off periods, involuntary abnormal movements, and periods of severe akinesia despite high daily doses of L-dopa. Implantation was always performed bilaterally in the STN for bradykinesia and unilaterally for predominant tremor (four cases). In one case, STN implantation was contralateral to GPi implantation.

In all cases, DBS is proposed to patients when:

- Medical treatment has been inefficient in achieving a satisfactory functional result and cannot be improved on.
- Medical treatment is efficient but is not tolerated (e.g., because of disabling abnormal involuntary movements) at the doses required for a satisfactory functional result.
- Remaining disability is great enough to significantly disturb the patient's activities of daily living.
- There are no general contraindications for surgery.
- There is no significant alteration of mental functions.
- There is no psychiatric or severe depressive state.

Parkinson's Disease

Parkinson's disease is by far the best indication for high-frequency stimulation of deep brain targets. Schematically, tremor is controlled by Vim DBS, L-dopa–induced dyskinesias by GPi DBS, and akinesia and rigidity by STN DBS. In fact, GPi DBS is also efficient in tremor and akinesia and rigidity, as previously reported for pallidotomies. When the electrode placement is correct, STN DBS is able to completely control tremor, akinesia, and rigidity and allows a significant decrease in drug dosage, which in turn suppresses the L-dopa–induced dyskinesias. The consistently positive results obtained with STN DBS have led us to choose it as the primary target in Parkinson's patients. The response to the L-dopa test is a good predictive index, and the effect of STN DBS is close to the best clinical improvement under L-dopa. Multiple systemic atrophy and other atypical parkinsonian syndromes are not considered for DBS procedures.

Essential Tremor

So far, Vim is the only target that has been able to alleviate essential tremor, as was true for thalamotomies.[10] However, cases of tolerance of DBS, with loss of functional benefit, in patients with essential tremor may reflect a similar problem described with thalamotomy.[68]

Dyskinesias

L-Dopa–induced dyskinesias are poorly controlled by Vim DBS, electively suppressed by GPi DBS, and indirectly suppressed by STN DBS through the decreased drug dosage allowed by the striking improvement of akinesia and rigidity.

Dystonias

Generalized primary dystonia is variably improved by Vim DBS (four cases) and more recently by GPi DBS (five cases). The general experience is still limited, and although there is no doubt that improvement occurs, the precise target must be clearly identified. The severity of this disease, the number of candidate patients, and the absence of any efficient treatment are determining factors in favor of the use of DBS for these indications, and even limited improvement has a considerable impact on the daily lives of these patients and their families.

Although there are no published series on this issue, there appears to be preliminary consensus on the following ranking of indications, as far as outcome is concerned: primary generalized dystonias are most improved (especially those related to mutation of the *DYT1* gene); nonprimary generalized dystonias (anoxic, toxic, allergic, anesthetic, Hallervorden-Spatz disease) are next most improved; and the unilateral dystonias are more improved than the focal dystonias (see Chapter 172). Recent preliminary results report the improvement of spasmodic torticollis by bilateral GPi stimulation (or lesions).

Other Movement Disorders

Tremor of multiple sclerosis is a good indication for Vim DBS when it is postural, and even more so when it is distal. However, the evolution of the disease usually erases the tremor suppression and induces new symptoms, making the initial benefit temporary. Other types of movement disorders may respond, but the proper targets remain to be discovered.

RESULTS

Specific Effects of Targets

So far, the thalamic target Vim is the only efficient structure for DBS. It was considered the best target for essential tremor during the thalamotomy era but seems to be less useful for DBS, owing to the occurrence of tolerance in about 20% of cases.

THALAMUS

Vim DBS is effective on tremor, particularly parkinsonian rest tremor.[5] There was almost no change in bradykinesia or any other symptom of Parkinson's disease. Unilateral pain, which accompanies severe tremor and rigidity in many cases, was greatly reduced. The effect on tremor was scored independently by the neurologist on a 5-point scale. Immediately after surgery, a microthalamotomy-like effect was responsible for transitory tremor suppression for a few days (22 of 107 patients [20.5%], 23 of 153 electrodes [15%]). A very good result (scores 3 and 4) was obtained in 71% of the operated sides (88% of patients with Parkinson's disease, 68% of those with essential tremor, and 18% of cases related to other causes). In these last cases, the effect was often complete during the first postoperative month, but an action component recurred later. Resting tremor was better controlled than action tremor, distal limb tremor better than proximal or axial tremor, and upper limb tremor better than lower limb tremor. In all cases, the effect was strictly coincident with the stimulation, without significant delay at the onset or cessation of stimulation. The L-dopa dosage was decreased by 20% at 3 months' follow-up in 39 of 80 Parkinson's patients (48.7%). There were only 12 patients (15%) available at the last follow-up, owing to progression of the disease. Caparros-Lefebvre and colleagues[6] reported much better results in five patients with L-dopa–induced choreic and ballistic dyskinesias, which were clearly improved by thalamic stimulation.

Thalamic stimulation was applied in four cases of idiopathic generalized dystonia. Out of seven stimulated thalami, a moderate long-term benefit was achieved for contralateral limb dystonia in four cases. In two cases of familial dystonia, the effect of Vim DBS consisted mainly of a decrease in limb rigidity and an increased facility in nursing care; reduction in hip, knee, and elbow flexed positions; and decrease in saliva inhalation, all leading to a global improvement in general status. In these disabling dystonias, the benefit of Vim stimulation is appreciated mainly by family members and caregivers rather than being reflected by the current dystonia scales, because it affects essentially the patient's general status and daily life activities. Establishment of the effect was delayed, and the pulse width was 450 msec.

Essential tremor is also significantly improved by Vim stimulation. In some cases, a tolerance effect may result in total loss of efficacy. This may relate to the mechanism of action, which is still unknown. During the initial postoperative period on a tremor rating scale from 0 (no tremor) to 4 (no effect on patient's tremor), scores of 3 or 4 were obtained in the upper limbs in 27 of the 36 operated sides (75%), and the remaining 25% had scores of 2 or 1. At the last follow-up, these scores remained similar. Global scores for the four limbs were 4 or 3 in 69% at 3 months and in 59% at the last follow-up.

GLOBUS PALLIDUS

Pallidal DBS is a safe and effective procedure for treatment of advanced Parkinson's disease. Compared with pallidotomy, the advantages of pallidal DBS are its reversibility and the option of performing bilateral surgery in one session. Bilateral DBS results in an approximately 34% reduction in the activities of daily living score during the off period and 35% to 40% improvement in the motor score during the off period. In addition, there are significant improvements in patients' symptoms during the on period and in on-off motor fluctuations. Compared with STN stimulation, the L-dopa–induced dyskinesias are directly diminished even when the drug dosage is not decreased. Actually, GPi stimulation does not allow a significant decrease in drug dosage (+10% at 6 months, −15% at 36 months).

SUBTHALAMUS

Dyskinesias. Improvement of L-dopa–induced dyskinesias following STN stimulation is due to the improvement of akinesia and rigidity,[78, 79] which allows the drug dosage to be decreased by about 55%, thus eliminating the drug-induced dyskinesias. About 10% of our patients are now drug free. Actually, by overstimulating the patient beyond the level needed to control the parkinsonian symptoms, one can induce ballismus or choreoballic dyskinesias. It is interesting to note that because of this decrease in L-dopa doses and the continuous stimulation, there is a tendency for these patients not to react so strongly to L-dopa challenges that had previously induced dyskinesia. Similarly, the tendency to develop abnormal movements under STN stimulation vanishes with time, which raises the question of postsynaptic desensitization, which is also observed during long-term apomorphine administration. The improvement is visible in midline symptoms as well: gait, rising, and stability are improved; speech is also improved to a lesser extent. One of the most spectacular symptoms, off-dystonia, was much improved in 16 of 20 patients. When the stimulator was turned on, dystonia disappeared within seconds, and when the stimulator was turned off again, it reappeared just as quickly, as well as the akinesia and rigidity.

Hypophonia. Hypophonia must not be considered a complication of surgery, and it may respond to increased doses of L-dopa or even to stimulation. However, the reduction in voice volume may be disabling, rendering the patient barely understandable. The current hypothesis to explain this phenomenon is that it might be due to a somatotopic organization of the STN. The current functional method of targeting is actually based on rigidity as assessed by passive mobilization of the wrist, which is a good indicator for the limbs but probably not for orofacial activity. If the midline functions, such as the voice, are located in a different part of the STN, we might consistently miss it according to the method employed. Therefore, during chronic stimulation, the patient is much improved as far as rigidity and akinesia of the limbs are concerned and is consequently deprived of L-dopa, which is no longer useful and may cause dyskinesias. As a result, as far as the hypophonia is concerned, the patient is not being medically treated because of the significant reduction in drug doses and is not being surgically treated because the electrode in the STN is not located in an area corresponding to voice control. This must be confirmed, but it points out the need to develop intraoperative methods of voice exploration that would allow us to better target this symptom.

Cognitive Function and Quality of Life. Overstimulation may be responsible for spreading the current to immediately adjacent structures and for inducing side effects related to these structures. This could result in depressive states or, conversely, irrepressible laughter, as we observed in one patient. Neuropsychological testing has not shown any change after long-term stimulation in the STN.

At 12 months' follow-up, bilateral STN stimulation greatly improved motor symptoms (UPDRS III, 55%) and activities of daily living (UPDRS II, 45%; Schwab and England scale, +142%) in the off-drug condition as well as dyskinesias in the on-drug condition (−90%). Dopaminergic treatment (L-dopa equivalent dose) was decreased by 50%. Patients were only mildly depressed before surgery (Beck Depression Inventory, 10.45 ± 6.6), and there was a very mild but significant improvement of mood after surgery (Beck Depression Inventory, 8.5 ± 4.1). No significant differences were found in the on-drug condition for motor score, activities of daily living, or mentation and behavior as assessed by UPDRS I.

The Parkinson's disease quality of life (PDQL) total score improved from 90.3 to 129 (maximum 185), parkinsonian symptoms improved from 33.2 to 49.1 (maximum 70), systemic symptoms from 17.3 to 23.1 (maximum 35), emotional functioning from 24.2 to 31.2 (maximum 45), and social functioning from 15.7 to 25.6 (maximum 35).

Improvement in the UPDRS III score was significantly correlated with improvement in the total PDQL score. We found an improvement in health-related quality of life with bilateral STN stimulation. Bilateral STN stimulation improved all aspects of health-related quality of life in Parkinson's disease, including emotional and social functioning. Although quality of life improved, it did not normalize; rather, it improved to the level of a large population of Parkinson's patients with less advanced disease. This finding is not surprising, as bilateral STN stimulation improves only motor symptoms in the off-drug condition and only dyskinesias in the on-drug condition. On-period symptoms as well as cognitive symptoms show little or no improvement. Decreasing the social isolation of Parkinson's patients is the real success of STN stimulation. Therefore, in selected, highly L-dopa–sensitive patients suffering from motor complications of dopaminergic treatment and without severe depression, the motor complications seem to be the main determinant of quality of life.

Side effects related to surgery, stimulation, or changes in medication are likely to influence quality of life. However, the overall study tended to confirm that the benefit of motor improvement largely overshadowed the impact of side effects on quality of life. Thus, it is worth taking the relatively small risk and operating on patients before their quality of life has reached a low level.

Rigidity, Akinesia, and Tremor. The clinical changes, as well improvement in quantitative testing, were strongly evident when stimulation was turned on and off.[35-37, 80] Moreover, surface electromyographic recording of agonist and antagonist muscles of the forearm during passive wrist manipulation showed that reflex hyperactivity of the stretched antagonist muscle, which is typical of extrapyramidal rigidity, was almost completely suppressed during STN stimulation, similar to that observed after apomorphine injection or L-dopa administration. The continuous follow-up of these patients[35] showed that all symptoms were improved by about 60% (evaluated on the corresponding scales) with a 30% to 100% (mean, 50%) decrease in drug dosage, which was responsible for the disappearance of L-dopa–induced dyskinesias. Patients who had preoperative L-dopa–induced involuntary movements may exhibit similar dyskinesias with STN stimulation while on their regular drug regimen. This attenuation continues as long as drug dosages are progressively decreased.[17] Tremor is abolished by STN DBS in a way comparable to Vim DBS. As a general rule, it may be said that STN DBS provides patients with a permanent level of improvement equal to their best status during on-periods and that all L-dopa–sensitive parkinsonian symptoms are similarly improved.

COMPLICATIONS

Some side effects are not related to the target and happen as a consequence of the procedure and the general condition of the patient. Observation of complications in patients treated in the Vim or GPi in our center may help define the specific morbidity of STN implantation versus the nonspecific complications of DBS. In more than 197 patients undergoing operation on 316 sides, all three targets included, we observed 1 large supraventricular hematoma (0.5% of patients, 0.3% of operated sides); 3 microhematomas with transient or minor permanent symptoms (1.7% of patients, 0.95% of operated sides); 3 asymptomatic microhematomas (1.7% of patients, 0.95% of operated sides); 2 subdural hemorrhages (1.01% of patients, 0.6% of operated sides; one was surgically explored); 3 MRI hypersignals along the electrode tracks (1.7% of patients, 0.95% of operated sides); 3 asymptomatic presence of blood in the ventricles, related to the transventricular approach of the target (1.7% of patients, 0.95% of operated sides); 7 local late infection, erosion, or granuloma of the external leads (3.5% of patients, 2.2% of operated sides); 1 local hematoma in the stimulator subcutaneous pocket (0.5% of patients, 0.3% of operated sides); 4 ruptures of the external extension, needing replacement (2% of patients, 1.3% of operated sides); 3 repositioning of the stimulators because of patient discomfort (1.7% of patients, 0.95% of operated sides); 3 cases of thrombophlebitis with 2 pulmonary embolisms, with good resolution (1.7% of patients, 0.95% of operated sides); and 17 cases of postoperative confusion, often related to the general status of the patient (8.6% of patients, 5.4% of operated sides). Apraxia of eyelid opening was observed in 11 of 51 STN patients (21.6% of patients, 11.6% of operated sides); 6 of these patients needed botulinum toxin injection, and in 3 of them, the problem lasted more than 6 months. Apraxia of eyelid opening was also observed in 1 GPi patient. Four patients who had previous demented states were not improved and had permanently impaired mental status. There were five transient psychiatric complications (one mania, one paranoia, and three depressions, including one suicide and two suicide attempts). These complications can also be analyzed for each target.

According to the Target

THALAMUS

With Vim stimulation (134 patients, 202 implanted sides),[5] four intracranial microhematomas induced a long-term thalamotomy-like effect or slight motor neglect, which resolved over several weeks. Three others were detected only on routine postoperative CT. In this series, no epileptic seizures were induced by thalamic kindling. Five patients were confused and disoriented for a few days. There were no complications related to ventriculography. Any adverse effects of stimulation (contralateral paresthesias [9%], limb dystonia [9%], dysequilibrium [7.6%], and dysarthria) were mild, were well tolerated by the patients, and disappeared immediately when stimulation was decreased or stopped. Dysarthria occurred more often in patients who had had previous contralateral thalamotomy (12 of 23 patients [51.7%]) than in those who were bilaterally stimulated (10 of 66 patients [15%]), suggesting that the morbidity rate from dysarthria for Vim stimulation is lower than that for thalamotomy. Switching the stimulator off induced transient rebound tremor in about half the patients, without clinical implications. However, in some patients (7 of 20), mainly those with action tremor, continuous stimulation induced a tolerance phenomenon, causing a progressive loss of stimulation efficacy.

GLOBUS PALLIDUS

Our experience with GPi is too limited to be significant. The current literature tends to show a relatively low rate of complication during GPi stimulation. However, in one case, we had to withdraw by 2 mm an electrode whose tip was against the optic tract and induced visual flashes, which disappeared thereafter.

SUBTHALAMUS

Complications and side effects have been infrequent. We had two hematomas in 100 patients—one in the supraventricular area from a pericallosal branch injured by the exploratory electrode (the patient died 3 years later), and one in the thalamus. We had three asymptomatic hemorrhages along the tracks of the electrode. Five patients had postoperative or late infections. On postoperative MRI, three patients showed the asymptomatic presence of blood in the ventricular system, due to the transventricular approach. One patient had a secondary scalp ulceration in front of the electrode-to-extension connection. Permanent hemiballismus was never observed during clinical follow-up. However, acute and transient hemiballismus (resolved within 24 hours) was observed in one case at the moment of insertion of the permanent series 3389 electrode. In several cases, advancement of recording electrodes, and in five cases, final insertion of chronic electrodes, induced various degrees of peripheral limb dyskinesias and involuntary movements, which we considered symptoms of STN penetration. In three cases, a lesioning direct-current leak from a defective test generator was responsible for transient hemiballismus, but one patient, at 6 months after surgery, still experiences a major resolution of the parkinsonian symptoms with no deficit, making stimulation unnecessary so far. Seven patients were confused and disoriented for a few days to 3 months; this temporary mental confusion is related to the patient's clinical state and age, with younger patients being better off. Such confusion has never left any permanent sequelae. We observed eyelid apraxia in about 20% of cases; of 11 patients with transient eyelid opening apraxia, 4 needed botulinum toxin injection. Eyelid opening apraxia is known to occur in Parkinson's patients, but the pathophysiology is unknown. It could be related to the proximity of the SNr, which projects onto the superior colliculus; this is related to vertical ocular motility, including extrinsic motility of the eyelids. Hypophonia (discussed earlier) was observed in about 20% of patients. Worsening of motor performance is extremely rare, and it is possible to abnormally induce dyskinesias similar to L-dopa–induced involuntary movements. Most patients had weight gain related to recovery of normal behavior and loss of dyskinesias; it is not related to hypothalamic-like hormonal disturbances, because it is also observed after pallidotomy.[81]

The follow-up was 87.4 ± 13.9 months (minimum, 61; maximum, 123).

Mortality. There was no operative mortality. One patient died suddenly on the 11th postoperative day from pulmonary embolism due to previously existing cardiovascular insufficiency. Seven others died from various non-neurological diseases at 3, 6, 7, 10, 11, 23, and 116 months. Owing to the long-distance referral of most of these patients, postmortem pathologic examination was not possible.

Immediate Postoperative Morbidity. Immediate postoperative morbidity has been observed to be higher in STN patients than in Vim patients. This might be related to differences in the patient populations. Although STN-implanted patients are not older (56.6 ± 7.6 years; $N = 60$) than Vim bilaterally implanted patients (59.3 ± 11.4 years; $N = 118$), they are in a more severe stage of their disease. The difference in morbidity could also be attributable to the target itself and to localization of the stereotactic approach. The target itself does not seem to be responsible for the observed side effects, as these were not always present. The track, however, was closer to the midline, and at the upper level it might have involved the white matter of the supplementary motor area or the thalamocortical frontal projections.

According to the Steps of the Method

We carefully reviewed complications of all types in a total of 166 patients operated on in the STN. Eighty-eight patients (54%) were complication free, and 75 patients (46%) had at least one complication: 11 (6.7%) after the initial ventriculographic step, 52 (31.9%) after electrode implantation, and 12 (7.4%) after the IPG implant.

Side Effects of Stimulation

Chronic use of DBS was associated with 6 cases of hypophonia, 22 blepharospasms (12 needed botulinum toxin injections), and 26 psychic manifestations. In the immediate postoperative period and at 12 months, the incidence of apathy was 2% and 11%, respectively; it was 11% and 7% for depression and 6% and 8% for apathy associated with depression. One patient committed suicide, and three patients attempted it. The causes of depression and suicide are multifactorial, involving primarily the withdrawal or significant decrease of L-dopa doses and the important changes in the social and familial context for these patients, who had been dependent for 10 to 15 years. This stresses the importance of a careful preoperative neuropsychological evaluation and postoperative psychological support, associated with a cautious and slow withdrawal of L-dopa or agonists.

COMPARISON WITH OTHER METHODS

Ablative Methods

The present data are significant enough to demonstrate that STN DBS relieves parkinsonian tremor, rigidity, akinesia, and dyskinesias; has no unavoidable complications, such as hemiballismus; and has no specific side effects. Ventroposterolateral pallidotomy[71, 81–85] has recently been reintroduced and is under investigation in several centers. The results reported are similar to those of STN DBS, and it has been claimed that pallidotomy relieves all the motor symptoms of Parkinson's disease, especially dyskinesia. However, bilateral procedures have been reported to produce cognitive dysfunction and increased complication rates. Moreover, the growing experience acquired by several teams using pallidal DBS[80, 86, 87] suggests that pallidal inhibitions can be done by DBS rather than by destruction, and bilateral procedures have less morbidity using DBS methods. We compared the merits of STN DBS and GPi DBS in two matched series of young-onset Parkinson's patients. Our conclusions favored STN DBS, which has become our primary therapeutic intervention for akinetic-rigid as well as tremulous Parkinson's disease.[78, 79, 86] We showed[78, 86] that STN improves all the UPDRS items by more than 60%, whereas they are improved by less than 60% in GPi-stimulated patients, in the off-medication situation. When patients are on medication, GPi stimulation appears to cause a loss of sensitivity to L-dopa treatment, and the dosage has to be increased.[81, 88]

Neural Grafts

In our opinion, the indications for STN DBS are the same as those for neural grafts. Considering the ethical and technical problems raised by neural grafts that have yet to be resolved, and the only moderate improvement reported so far,[27] STN DBS can be offered as a proven alternative.

TRENDS AND FUTURE APPLICATIONS

Technical Developments

Triggered Generators. Although the effects of DBS are in general immediately reversible, at least as far as tremor is concerned, intermittent stimulation triggered by specific events might be useful.

Shielded Generators. MRI examinations are the most advanced form of imaging and the most frequently used modality of diagnostic investigation, morphologic as well as functional. When they are composed of nonferromagnetic alloys, electrodes are compatible with MRI, with limited magnetic artifacts and no side effects, as confirmed by our 11-year experience.

More casually, the magnetic switch of the IPG may be activated in various situations of daily life. For example, refrigerator doors have built-in magnets that may turn the IPG on and off when the door is open and shut if it is too close to the patient's chest. Similarly, domestic tools with rotors and magnets must be handled with care. Security gates may be based on various methodologies that could affect the IPG, and they should be avoided, as for patients with cardiac pacers. Exposure of these devices to radiofrequency irradiation has to be carefully evaluated to identify potential hazards, such as diathermia and cardioversion.[89, 90]

Waveforms. Rectangular pulses are the easiest to produce but may not be the most physiologically suited in terms of safety and efficiency. Other waveforms must be tried. Balanced bipolar pulses are supposed to avoid electrical charge accumulation.

New Targets

Basic research will suggest new targets where the network could be modulated. The reversibility and low morbidity of high-frequency stimulation by DBS will allow these new solutions to be investigated with reasonable safety for patients.

Understanding the Role of Basal Ganglia in Motor Control

Observations made during surgery may provide insight into the functional model of motor control by the basal ganglia. For instance, the SNr, which fits into the same functional box as the GPi, does not behave like the GPi. When electrodes enter the SNr area at the bottom of the STN, they do not record any evoked activity or proprioceptive activity in the SNr, in contrast to what is observed in the STN and GPi. The activity of the SNr cells, whose neuronal firing patterns are clearly distinguishable from those of STN neurons, does not respond to the classic maneuvers we use to monitor patients, and the stimulation has none of the beneficial effect usually observed in the STN and even in the GPi. Thus, the role of the SNr seems to be different from that suggested by the currently accepted model.

COSTS

DBS is more expensive than thalamotomy. In addition to the stereotactic procedure, which is almost the same in both methods, stimulation requires electrodes, extension leads, and impulse generators. Due to the high frequency at which the Itrel II is used (130 to 185 Hz), the battery life is relatively short; the lifetime of the 90 Itrel IIs implanted in the STN averages 87 months. Itrel I stimulators have already been replaced in 18 of 20 patients after 38.7 ± 23.5 months (range, 17 to 109 months). However, the significant decrease in drug dosage observed in STN patients reduces overall costs, which may make this procedure competitive with medical treatment.

CONCLUSION

Because of its total and immediate reversibility, Vim DBS has been attempted in patients presenting with parkinsonian tremor or essential tremor. Other targets have been selected based on their potential effect on extrapyramidal symptoms without the consequences of lesions. Stimulation of the STN to treat hypertonia with or without bradykinesia and, more recently, stimulation of the GPi to treat dyskinesia have been tried with significant results. Owing to the low morbidity of the procedure, bilateral implantation of one of these three nuclei can be performed in the same session, without inducing the classic side effects of bilateral thalamotomies or STN lesions, such as hemiballismus. The excellent results obtained by DBS justify its use as first-line surgical treatment for parkinsonian symptoms. Because electrical stimulation is reversible and its effects on symptoms are more easily observable, this method may lead to a better understanding of the underlying mechanisms of tremor and other movement disorders.

It is important to note that the effects of high-frequency stimulation of the STN are stable in patients operated on 6 years ago, and some of them are almost drug free. The advantages of this type of treatment are its reversibility (particularly in the case of misplacement of the electrode, which can be changed or replaced); adaptability of the parameters to fit the patient's clinical status and even follow the evolution of the disease; ability to perform bilateral implantation in

one session without significant permanent neuropsychological side effects; reduction of L-dopa doses, which decreases dyskinesias; and potential neuroprotective effect. STN high-frequency stimulation is a remarkable therapeutic agent for all symptoms of Parkinson's disease and can be proposed as a first alternative when evolution of the disease and failure of medical treatment to provide an acceptable quality of life call for a surgical approach. Moreover, this procedure does not exclude patients from receiving other types of treatment, such as fetal neural tissue transplants, in the future. Finally, because of its reversibility and adaptability, STN DBS provides the opportunity to study and understand the mechanisms of Parkinson's disease as well as normal motor control in humans.

REFERENCES

1. Benabid AL, Benazzouz A, Hoffmann D, et al: Long term electrical inhibition of deep brain targets in movement disorders. Mov Disord 13:119–125, 1998.
2. Albe-Fessard D, Arfel G, Guiot G, et al: Dérivations d'activités spontanées et évoquées dans les structures cérébrales profondes de l'homme. Rev Neurol (Paris) 106:89–105, 1962.
3. Benabid AL, Pollak P, Louveau A, et al: Combined (thalamotomy and stimulation) stereotactic surgery of the Vim thalamic nucleus for bilateral Parkinson disease. Appl Neurophysiol 50:344–346, 1987.
4. Benabid AL, Pollak P, Gervason C, et al: Long-term suppression of tremor by chronic stimulation of the ventral intermediate thalamic nucleus. Lancet 337:403–406, 1991.
5. Benabid AL, Pollak P, Gao DM, et al: Long-term suppression of tremor by chronic electrical stimulation of the ventralis intermedius nucleus of the thalamus as a treatment of movement disorders. J Neurosurg 84:203–214, 1996.
6. Caparros-Lefebvre D, Blond S, Feltin MP, et al: Improvement of levodopa induced dyskinesias by thalamic deep brain stimulation is related to slight variation in electrode placement: Possible involvement of the centro-median and parafascicularis complex. J Neurol Neurosurg Psychiatry 67:306–314, 1999.
7. Laitinen L, Bergenheim AT, Hariz MI: Leksell's posteroventral pallidotomy in the treatment of Parkinson's disease. J Neurosurg 76:53–61, 1992.
8. Svennilson E, Torvik A, Lowe R, Leksell L: Treatment of parkinsonism by stereotactic thermolesions in the pallidal region: A clinical evaluation of 81 cases. Acta Psychiatr Neurol Scand 35: 358–377, 1960.
9. Derôme PJ, Jedynak CP, Visot A, Delalande O: Traitement des mouvements anormaux par lésions thalamiques. Rev Neurol (Paris) 142:391–397, 1986.
10. Fox MW, Ahlskog JE, Kelly PJ: Stereotactic ventrolateralis thalamotomy for medically refractory tremor in post-levodopa era Parkinson's disease patients. J Neurosurg 75:723–730, 1991.
11. Goldman MS, Ahlskog JE, Kelly PJ: The symptomatic and functional outcome of stereotactic thalamotomy for medically intractable essential tremor. J Neurosurg 76:924–928, 1992.
12. Hirai T, Miyazaki M, Nakajima H, et al: The correlation between tremor characteristics and the predicted volume of effective lesions in stereotaxic nucleus ventralis intermedius thalamotomy. Brain 106:1001–1018, 1983.
13. Kelly P, Derome P, Guiot G: Thalamic spatial variability and the surgical results of lesions placed with neurophysiological control. Surg Neurol 9:307–315, 1978.
14. Matsumoto K, Asano T, Baba T, et al: Long-term follow-up review of cases of Parkinson's disease after unilateral or bilateral thalamotomy. Appl Neurophysiol 39:257–260, 1976–1977.
15. Matsumoto K, Shichijo F, Fukami T: Long-term follow-up review of cases of Parkinson's disease after unilateral or bilateral thalamotomy. J Neurosurg 60:1033–1044, 1984.
16. Nagaseki Y, Shibazaki T, Hirai T, et al: Long term follow-up of selective Vim-thalamotomy. J Neurosurg 65:296–302, 1986.

17. Narabayashi H: Stereotaxic Vim thalamotomy for treatment of tremor. Eur Neurol 29:29–32, 1989.
18. Ohye C, Maeda T, Narabayashi H: Physiologically defined Vim nucleus: Its special reference to control of tremor. Appl Neurophysiol 39:285–295, 1977.
19. Ohye C, Hirai T, Miyazaki M, et al: VIM thalamotomy for the treatment of various kinds of tremor. Appl Neurophysiol 45:275–280, 1982.
20. Ohye C: Rôle des noyaux thalamiques dans l'hypertonie et le tremblement de la maladie de Parkinson. Rev Neurol (Paris) 142:362–367, 1986.
21. Stellar S, Cooper IS: Mortality and morbidity in cryothalamectomy for Parkinson's disease: A statistical study of 2868 consecutive operations. J Neurosurg 28:459–467, 1968.
22. Talairach J, Hecaen H, David M, et al: Recherches sur la coagulation thérapeutique des structures sous-corticales chez l'homme. Rev Neurol (Paris) 81:4–24, 1949.
23. Taren J, Guiot G, Derome P, Trigo JC: Hazards of stereotaxic thalamotomy: Added safety factors in corroborating x-ray target localization with neurophysiological methods. J Neurosurg 29:173–182, 1968.
24. Tasker RR, Organ LW, Hawrylyshyn PA: Investigation of the surgical target for alleviation of involuntary movement disorders. Appl Neurophysiol 45:261–274, 1982.
25. Tasker RR, Siquiera J, Hawrylyshyn P, Organ LW: What happened to Vim thalamotomy for Parkinson's disease? Appl Neurophysiol 46:68–83, 1983.
26. Benabid AL, Benazzouz A, Hoffmann D, et al: Chronic electrical stimulation of the ventralis intermedius nucleus of the thalamus and of other nuclei as a treatment for Parkinson's disease. Tech Neurosurg 5:5–30, 1999.
27. Kordower JH, Freeman TB, Chen EY, et al: Fetal nigral grafts survive and mediate clinical benefit in a patient with Parkinson's disease. Mov Disord 13:383–393, 1998.
28. Albin RL, Young AB, Penney JB: The functional anatomy of basal ganglia disorders. Trends Neurosci 12:365–375, 1989.
29. Alexander GE, Crutcher MD: Functional architecture of basal ganglia circuits: Neural substrates of parallel processing. Trends Neurosci 13:266–271, 1990.
30. Aziz TZ, Peggs D, Sambrook MA, Crossman AR: Lesion of the subthalamic nucleus for the alleviation of 1-methyl-4-phenyl-1,2,3,6-tetrahydro-pyridine (MPTP)–induced parkinsonism in the primate. Mov Disord 6:288–292, 1991.
31. Benazzouz A, Gross C, Feger J, et al: Reversal of rigidity and improvement in motor performance by subthalamic high-frequency stimulation in MPTP-treated monkeys. Eur J Neurosci 5:382–389, 1993.
32. Bergman H, Wichmann T, DeLong MR: Reversal of experimental parkinsonism by lesions of the subthalamic nucleus. Science 249:1346–1348, 1990.
33. DeLong M: Primate models of movement disorders of basal ganglia origin. Trends Neurosci 13:281–285, 1990.
34. Feger J, Robledo P: The effects of activation or inhibition of the subthalamic nucleus on the metabolic and electrophysiological activities within the pallidal complex and substantia nigra in the rat. J Neurosci 3:947–952, 1991.
35. Limousin P, Pollak P, Benazzouz A, et al: Effect on parkinsonian signs and symptoms of bilateral subthalamic nucleus stimulation. Lancet 345:91–95, 1995.
36. Limousin P, Pollak P, Benazzouz A, et al: Bilateral subthalamic nucleus stimulation for severe Parkinson's disease. Mov Disord 10:672–674, 1995.
37. Limousin P, Krack P, Pollak P, et al: Electrical stimulation of the subthalamic nucleus in advanced Parkinson's disease. N Engl J Med 339:1105–1111, 1998.
38. Pollak P, Benabid AL, Gross C, et al: Effets de la stimulation du noyau sous-thalamique dans la maladie de Parkinson. Rev Neurol (Paris) 149:175–176, 1993.
39. Albe-Fessard D, Arfel G, Guiot G, et al: Identification et délimitation précise de certaines structures sous-corticales de l'homme par l'électrophysiologie. Son interêt dans la chirurgie stéréotaxique des dyskinesies. C R Acad Sci Paris 253:2412–2414, 1961.
40. Albe-Fessard D, Arfel G, Guiot G: Activités électriques caractéristiques de quelques structures cérébrales chez l'homme. Ann Chir 17:1185–1214, 1963.
41. Guiot G, Derome P, Arfel G, Walter S: Electrophysiological recordings in stereotaxic thalamotomy for parkinsonism. Prog Neurol Surg 5:189–221, 1973.
42. Cheshire WP, Ehle AL: Hemi-parkinsonism as a complication of an Ommaya reservoir. J Neurosurg 73:774–776, 1990.
43. Marks PV, Wild AM, Gleave JRW: Long-term abolition of parkinsonian tremor following attempted ventriculography. Br J Neurosurg 5:505–508, 1991.
44. Guiot G, Arfel G, Derôme P: La chirurgie stéréotaxique des tremblements de repos et d'attitude. Gaz Méd France 75:4029–4056, 1968.
45. Schaltenbrand G, Wahren W: Atlas for Stereotaxy of the Human Brain, 2nd ed. Stuttgart, Georg Thieme Verlag, 1977.
46. Talairach J, David M, Tournoux P, et al: Atlas d'anatomie stéréotaxique des noyaux gris centraux. Paris, Masson, 1957.
47. Rezai AR, Lozano AM, Crawley AP, et al: Thalamic stimulation and functional magnetic resonance imaging: Localization of cortical and subcortical activation with implanted electrodes. Technical note. J Neurosurg 90:583–590, 1999.
48. Rezai AR, Finelli D, Nyenhuis JA, et al: Neurostimulation systems for deep brain stimulation: In vitro evaluation of magnetic resonance imaging-related heating at 1.5 tesla. J Magn Reson Imaging 15:241–250, 2002.
49. Alesch F, Koos WT: Computer-assisted multidimensional atlas for functional stereotaxy. Acta Neurochir (Wien) 133:153–156, 1995.
50. Benabid AL, Hoffmann D, Ashraf A, et al: [The robotization of neurosurgery: State of the art and future outlook.] Bull Acad Natl Med 181:1625–1635, discussion 1635–1636, 1997.
51. Berks G, Pohl G, Keyserlingk DG: 3D-VIEWER: An atlas-based system for individual and statistical investigations of the human brain. Methods Inf Med 40:170–177, 2001.
52. Gybels J, Suetens P: [Image-guided surgery.] Verh K Acad Geneeskd Belg 59:35–57, 1997.
53. Hardy TL, Smith JR, Brynildson LR, et al: Magnetic resonance imaging and anatomic atlas mapping for thalamotomy. Stereotact Funct Neurosurg 58:30–32, 1992.
54. Nowinski WL, Fang A, Nguyen BT, et al: Multiple brain atlas database and atlas-based neuroimaging system. Comput Aided Surg 2:42–66, 1997.
55. Nowinski WL, Yeo TT, Thirunavuukarasuu A: Microelectrode-guided functional neurosurgery assisted by Electronic Clinical Brain Atlas CD-ROM. Comput Aided Surg 3:115–122, 1998.
56. Nowinski WL, Yang GL, Yeo TT: Computer-aided stereotactic functional neurosurgery enhanced by the use of the multiple brain atlas database. IEEE Trans Med Imaging 19:62–69, 2000.
57. diPierro CG, Francel PC, Jackson TR, et al: Optimizing accuracy in magnetic resonance imaging–guided stereotaxis: A technique with validation based on the anterior commissure–posterior commissure line. J Neurosurg 90:94–100, 1999.
58. Serra L, Nowinski WL, Poston T, et al: The Brain Bench: Virtual tools for stereotactic frame neurosurgery. Med Image Anal 1:317–329, 1997.
59. Shabalov VA, Kazarnovskaya MI, Borodkin SM, et al: Functional neurosurgery using 3-D computer stereotactic atlas. Acta Neurochir Suppl (Wien) 58:65–67, 1993.
60. Vannier MW, Marsh JL: Three-dimensional imaging, surgical planning, and image-guided therapy. Radiol Clin North Am 34:545–563, 1996.
61. Vayssiere N, Hemm S, Cif L, et al: Comparison of atlas- and magnetic resonance imaging–based stereotactic targeting of the globus pallidus internus in the performance of deep brain stimulation for treatment of dystonia. J Neurosurg 96:673–679, 2002.
62. Yeo TT, Nowinski WL: Functional neurosurgery aided by use of an electronic brain atlas. Acta Neurochir Suppl (Wien) 68:93–99, 1997.
63. Zincone A, Landi A, Piolti R, et al: Physiologic study of the subthalamic volume. Neurol Sci 22:111–112, 2001.
64. Benabid AL, Hoffmann D, Ashraf A, et al: Robotic guidance in advanced imaging environments. In Alexander GE, Maciunas RJ (eds): Advanced Neurosurgical Navigation. New York, Thieme Medical Publishers, 1999, pp 571–583.
65. Ohye C, Narabayashi H: Physiological study of presumed ventralis intermedius neurons in the human thalamus. J Neurosurg 50:290–297, 1979.

66. Ohye C, Shibazaki T, Hirai T, et al: Further physiological observations on the ventralis intermedius neurons in the human thalamus. J Neurophysiol 61:488–500, 1989.

67. Hutchinson WD, Lozano AM, Davis KD, et al: Differential neuronal activity in segments of globus pallidus in Parkinson's disease patients. Neuroreport 5:1533–1537, 1994.

68. Guiot G, Derome P, Trigo JC: Le tremblement d'attitude. Indication la meilleure de la chirurgie stéréotaxique. Presse Med 75: 2513–2518, 1967.

69. Hariz MI, Fodstad H: Do microelectrode techniques increase accuracy or decrease risks in pallidotomy and deep brain stimulation? A critical review of the literature. Stereotact Funct Neurosurg 72:157–169, 1999.

70. Alterman RL, Kall BA, Cohen H, Kelly PJ: Stereotactic ventrolateral thalamotomy: Is ventriculography necessary? Neurosurgery 37:717–721, discussion 721–722, 1995.

71. Tronnier VM, Fogel W, Kronenbuerger M, Steinvorth S: Pallidal stimulation: An alternative to pallidotomy? J Neurosurg 87:700–705, 1997.

72. Benabid AL, Minotti L, Koudsie A, et al: Antiepileptic effect of high-frequency stimulation of the subthalamic nucleus (corpus luysi) in a case of medically intractable epilepsy caused by focal dysplasia: A 30-month follow-up: Technical case report. Neurosurgery 50:1385–1392, 2002.

73. Depaulis A: The inhibitory control of the substantia nigra over generalized non-convulsive seizures in the rat. J Neural Transm Suppl 35:125–139, 1992.

74. Iadarola MJ, Gale K: Substantia nigra: Site of anticonvulsant activity mediated by gamma-aminobutyric acid. Science 218: 1237–1240, 1982.

75. Nguyen JP, Pollin B, Feve A, et al: Improvement of action tremor by chronic cortical stimulation. Mov Disord 13:84–88, 1998.

76. Woolsey CN, Erickson TC, Gilson WE: Localization in somatic sensory and motor areas of human cerebral cortex as determined by direct recording of evoked potentials and electrical stimulation. J Neurosurg 51:476–506, 1979.

77. Nandi D, Liu X, Winter JL, et al: Deep brain stimulation of the pedunculopontine region in the normal non-human primate. J Clin Neurosci 9:170–174, 2002.

78. Krack P, Limousin P, Benabid AL, Pollak P: Chronic stimulation of the subthalamic nucleus improves levodopa-induced dyskinesias in Parkinson's disease. Lancet 350:1676, 1997.

79. Krack P, Pollak P, Limousin P, et al: From off-period dystonia to peak-dose chorea: The clinical spectrum of varying subthalamic nucleus activity. Brain 122:1133–1146, 1999.

80. Lozano AM, Lang AM, Galvez-Jimenez N, et al: Effect of GPi pallidotomy on motor function in Parkinson's disease. Lancet 346:1383–1387, 1995.

81. Lang AE, Lozano A, Tasker R, et al: Neuropsychological and behavioral changes and weight gain after medial pallidotomy. Ann Neurol 41:834–836, 1997.

82. Baron MS, Vitek JL, Bakay RA, et al: Treatment of advanced Parkinson's disease by posterior GPi pallidotomy: 1-year results of a pilot study. Ann Neurol 40:355–366, 1996.

83. Dogali M, Fazzini E, Kolodny E, et al: Stereotactic ventral pallidotomy for Parkinson's disease. Neurology 45:753–761, 1995.

84. Eskandar EN, Cosgrove GR, Shinobu LA, Penney JB: The importance of accurate lesion placement in posteroventral pallidotomy. J Neurosurg 89:630–634, 1998.

85. Lang AE, Lozano AM, Montgomery E, et al: Posteroventral medial pallidotomy in advanced Parkinson's disease. N Engl J Med 337:1036–1042, 1997.

86. Krack P, Pollak P, Limousin P, et al: Opposite effects of pallidal stimulation in Parkinson's disease. Ann Neurol 43:180–192, 1998.

87. Siegfried J, Lippitz B: Bilateral chronic electrostimulation of ventroposterolateral pallidum: A new therapeutic approach for alleviating all parkinsonian symptoms. J Neurosurg 35:1126–1130, 1994.

88. Verhagen L, Mouradian M, Chase T: Altered levodopa dose-response profile after pallidotomy [abstract]. Neurology 46:A416–A417, 1996.

89. Nutt JG, Anderson VC, Peacock JH, et al: DBS and diathermy interaction induces severe CNS damage. Neurology 56:1384–1386, 2001.

90. Yamamoto T, Katayama Y, Fukaya C, et al: Thalamotomy caused by cardioversion in a patient treated with deep brain stimulation. Stereotact Funct Neurosurg 74:73–82, 2000.

CHAPTER 174

Cellular Transplantation in the Central Nervous System

ROY A. E. BAKAY

Transplantation is the process of removing a live organ or tissue and transferring it to a host (self or nonself) with the objective of restoring lost function. The word *transplant* is properly used to refer to an entire organ or a very large part of an organ that is transplanted into a host. A *graft* refers to the insertion of a small piece or pieces of tissue into the host (Table 174–1). The insertion process may be described as *transplantation* or *grafting*. This process is distinct from *regeneration,* in which the host generates its own tissue to restore function.

Like their theoretical understanding of the atom, the ancient Greeks understood the concepts of regeneration and transplantation. However, they also understood an even older concept—that once the central nervous system (CNS) was severely injured, the injury was permanent, and restoration of function would not occur. This pessimism is first recorded in the Smith papyrus, in which the ancient Egyptian physicians indicated that severe head injuries were in the category of "I do not treat."

The ability to graft a patient's own skin (i.e., autograft) was developed to a very high degree of sophistication in India more than 2600 years ago. Blood transfusions representing the first transplantation from one human to another (i.e., allograft) occurred approximately 100 years ago. The first solid organ (i.e., kidney) transplantation occurred approximately 50 years ago between identical twins (i.e., isograft), and even more recently, grafting between genetically different individuals (i.e., allografts) was achieved. The first approach to grafting of tissue between another species and humans (i.e., xenograft) was performed more than 40 years ago. Against this backdrop, attempts at CNS transplantation have occurred only during the past 2 decades.

There is great resistance to the concept of CNS transplantation, and many people remain skeptical such procedures have ever been successful. The first fully accepted, successful, and well-documented survival of grafted neural tissue was performed by Elizabeth Dunn at the University of Chicago.[1] In a series of experiments from 1907 to 1917, she clearly demonstrated the ability of fetal tissue to successfully graft to mature neural tissue and to form structures that could survive over a long period. Despite publication in a major neurological journal of these remarkable findings by a reputable scientist in a highly respected academic center, little interest developed in the field of CNS transplantation. The next major contribution came from Medawar, who demonstrated the remarkable ability of graft tissue to survive in the CNS compared with other locations in the body, which led to the concept of the brain as an *immunologically privileged site.* Despite these and other reports of successful grafting into the CNS, the potential for clinical use was not anticipated because these anatomic studies did not demonstrate restored function.[2]

There was a sudden and dramatic change in the appreciation of CNS transplantation when investigations by Lars Olson and colleagues[3, 4] at the Karolinska demonstrated anatomic and electrophysiologic interactions between grafts and host in the anterior eye chamber model (another immunologically privileged site). In 1979, the Olson laboratory[5] and Bjorklund and colleagues[6] demonstrated for the first time quantified behavioral improvement as a result of fetal mesencephalic transplantation in a rat parkinsonian model compared with controls. The demonstration that isolated adrenal medullary tissue could produce large quantities of dopamine and quantitatively reverse behavioral deficits in a rat parkinsonian model occurred very shortly thereafter.[7] All the basic principles have been proved.[8–10]

The field of CNS transplantation has developed rapidly, with advances in molecular biology pushing the field forward and expanding understanding at an exponential rate. It is important for the neurosurgeon to understand developments in this field and contribute to the application of these techniques. The stereotactic neurosurgeon especially will remain an essential part of the delivery system for this technology. Stereotactic techniques are still the best means to place specific tissues, particles, or drugs into predetermined sites within the CNS. We have entered the age of CNS repair and restoration.

T A B L E   1 7 4 – 1 ■ **Terminology**

Transplantation	Process of removing an organ or part of an organ and transferring it to a host that can be the same or another subject
Transplant	Usually refers to the whole or a substantial part of an organ that has been inserted into a host; a brain transplant refers to the whole brain from one animal that has been transferred into another
Graft	Usually refers to a small part of an organ that has been transferred to a host; a brain graft refers to small pieces of tissue placed into the host brain
Autograft	Graft from one part of an individual's body to another part (i.e., adrenal to brain grafts in the same patient)
Isograft	Graft between two individuals who are genetically identical (i.e., identical twins)
Allograft	Graft from a donor to a recipient of the same species but genetically different (i.e., human-to-human fetal grafts)
Xenograft	A graft between animals of different species

BACKGROUND

CNS transplantation holds great potential as a means of repairing and restoring function to degenerative and injured brain or spinal cord.[8, 9, 11, 12] The main focus of this chapter is an examination of transplantation for Parkinson's disease (PD). Patients with PD are ideal candidates for CNS transplantation because the disease is associated with a well-characterized and specific neuronal degeneration, dopamine replacement therapy provides dramatic clinical benefit, dopamine neurons serve a modulatory function and under physiologic conditions provide tonic stimulation of target receptors, and there are well-defined target areas for neural transplantation.

PD is a progressive neurodegenerative disorder characterized by a loss of melanized neurons in the pars compacta of the substantia nigra, a reduction in striatal dopamine, and the presence of intracytoplasmic inclusions or Lewy bodies. It affects approximately 1% of the population older than 50 years of age. Estimates indicate that up to 1 million people may be affected in the United States, and this number will increase as the elderly population of the country increases. The cardinal symptoms are resting tremor, rigidity, akinesia, and gait disturbance.[13] The resting tremor is the most dramatic symptom, but the slowness of movement (i.e., bradykinesia) and the difficulty in initiating movement (i.e., akinesia) represent the patient's most severe debilitating symptoms and the ones that are the most difficult to treat. Dopamine replacement strategies that use L-dopa or dopamine agonists have provided substantial reductions in morbidity and mortality but are associated with adverse side effects, including dyskinesias and fluctuations in motor performance.[14]

The problem of patients with severe PD is not that they are unable to synthesize dopamine, but rather that they cannot store and release it when needed. Wide fluctuations in levels of L-dopa produce the on-off syndrome.[15, 16] Alternation in motor function between complete immobility and uncontrollable dyskinetic movement leaves these patients extremely disabled and shortens their life expectancy. Parkinsonian disability continues to progress and is ultimately associated with clinical features that do not respond to L-dopa replacement therapy. Efforts to provide neuroprotective treatment with deprenyl can delay the need for L-dopa therapy but have not been conclusively demonstrated to influence the natural history of PD.[17] This has led to a search for alternative treatments designed to restore function and halt disease progression.

Several investigators have demonstrated that fetal mesencephalic tissue grafted into the denervated striatum can reduce the parkinsonian symptoms in rats with lesions produced by 6-hydroxydopamine.[18, 19] The behavioral improvements follow the grafting of solid pieces or of cell suspensions.[5, 6, 20–22] Fetal mesencephalic grafts can form synaptic connections with host neurons and reinnervate up to two thirds of the denervated rat striatum in an organotypic pattern.[21–23] The presumed mechanism of restoration of function is by synaptic reinnervation, but other mechanisms are possible (Fig. 174–1). Mature dopaminergic grafts exhibit electrical discharge patterns similar to those of the normal substantia nigra, and they have the ability for synthesis and release of dopamine.[24, 25] After fetal mesencephalic grafting in rodents, functional recovery, as characterized by the amelioration of motor dysfunction, can persist for the life of the rodents.[26] The restoration of function appears to depend on the continued presence of donor dopaminergic cells and is lost immediately after their removal or destruction.[18, 27, 28] Fetal mesencephalic tissue grafted into the dorsal striatum ameliorates rotational asymmetries, whereas those grafted into the ventrolateral striatum ameliorate sensorimotor deficits.[20, 29] Neither intrastriatal grafts of nondopaminergic tissue (e.g., mesencephalic raphe) nor dopaminergic implants placed into nonstriatal regions improve motor asymmetries, which attests to the neurochemical and structural specificity of this phenomenon.[27] Despite the fact that these are allografts, rejection is rarely a problem.[12, 30] The functional recovery observed after transplantation correlates with the site of implantation and the type of tissue used.

Similar results have been observed in primate models using N-methyl-4-pheny-1,2,3,6-tetrahydropyridine (MPTP), in which fetal ventral mesencephalic allografts have been shown to survive transplantation, partially reinnervate host striatum, and improve hypokinesia, rigidity, and other parkinsonian symptoms.[31–38] Such effects can also be achieved with human fetal tissue grafted into immunocompromised rats.[28, 39–42] Although neurite outgrowth and functional recovery occur over a more protracted time course, consistent with the maturation of human fetal tissue, the xenografts more com-

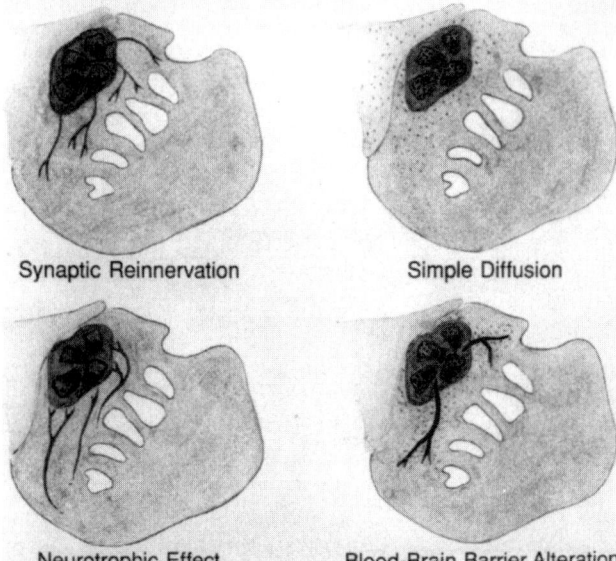

Synaptic Reinnervation

Simple Diffusion

Neurotrophic Effect

Blood-Brain Barrier Alteration

FIGURE 174–1. The most commonly proposed mechanism by which successful graft-host interaction can occur is synaptic reinnervation. In this instance, the graft reinnervates the host, providing the appropriate neurotransmitter to the appropriate receptor sites. This mechanism alone cannot explain bilateral effects, nor can it explain why a very small area of innervation can have such a dramatic effect on behavior. Simple diffusion of the appropriate neurotransmitter substances from the graft into the host is another mechanism by which graft-host interaction can occur. Difficulties with this hypothesis rest with the facts that diffusion can occur for only a very short distance and that, although it may be effective in the rat brain, this type of mechanism seems unlikely in the human brain, which is 400 times larger. As a result of the grafting procedures, neurotrophic factors are released. The graft may also release neurotrophic factors that further stimulate reinnervation through a host sprouting mechanism. Whether persistence of the graft is required for reinnervation of the host remains to be determined. The neurotrophic effects from brain injuries can result in elevated levels of neurotrophic factors bilaterally and may explain the bilateral changes observed. The magnitude of the effect is relatively small, and to be effective, this mechanism requires the host to have a significant reserve of dopaminergic neurons. Revascularization of the graft can result in alteration of the blood-brain barrier, which may serve as a mechanism for graft-host interaction. A variety of substances that normally cannot cross the blood-brain barrier become free to enter the host and may have significant effects on the local neurotransmitter receptors. This mechanism still relies on diffusion over a large enough area—even with alteration of the blood-brain barrier—having a significant neurotransmitter effect or an effect that is bilateral. (Adapted from Bakay RA: Neural transplantation—what are the real possibilities? Clin Neurosurg 37:179–192, 1991.)

pletely reinnervate the host striatum. These studies demonstrate the robust capacity of fetal grafts to provide functional restoration in models of dopamine deficiency and suggest that CNS grafting is a logical and appropriate therapeutic application for PD. However, ethical issues regarding the use of aborted human fetal tissue and practical issues regarding graft tissue availability have led to a search for alterative sources of dopamine-producing cells. Graft of sympathetic ganglia, carotid body glomus cells, PC12 cells (i.e., pheochromocytoma), and neuroblastoma cells have been tested and do not produce significant, long-lasting functional recovery in animal models.[35, 43–46]

The most studied paraneural source of catecholamines is the chromaffin cells of the adrenal medulla. These cells normally produce a small amount of dopamine, but dopamine levels can be substantially increased if these cells are removed from glucocorticoid inhibition by means of their separation from the overlying adrenal cortex. Grafts of adrenal medulla tissue placed into the denervated striatum or lateral ventricle of 6-hydroxydopamine–lesioned rats[7, 39, 47] or primates with MPTP-induced parkinsonism provide only limited behavioral improvements.[7, 39, 47–51] The magnitude or duration of these effects is not as great as those observed with fetal nigral grafts.

In 1982, Backlund and colleagues[52] performed the initial human trials. Adrenal medullary tissue was stereotactically transplanted into the striatum of seriously affected patients and did not demonstrate significant clinical benefit. In 1987, Madrazo and coworkers reported "dramatic amelioration of symptoms" in two patients after autologous adrenal medullary transplantation into the caudate with an open microsurgical procedure.[53] However, investigators using similar techniques failed to replicate these dramatic effects.[54, 55] The most consistent finding was a reduction in percent of off time and a modest improvement in motor function during off periods. However, benefits were largely transient, and the procedure was associated with significant morbidity and mortality.[56] It is now thought that the resultant benefits observed do not justify the surgical risk, and the procedure has been abandoned.

The lack of a more dramatic benefit may reflect the fact that adult chromaffin cells survive poorly after intrastriatal transplantation in primate models and in clinical series.[15, 49, 50, 57–63] Despite poor survival, host dopaminergic sprouting responses have been observed.[54, 57–68] Enhanced chromaffin cell viability and behavioral improvement can be obtained with the infusion of neurotrophic growth factor–secreting cells.[39, 69, 70] Clinical trials with neurotrophic growth factor infusion[71] and Schwann cell (i.e., neurotrophic growth factor–secreting cells) co-grafts were successful, but long-term benefits are not comparable with those observed after fetal tissue transplantation.[72–74] Fetal tissue transplantation also obviates the need for an additional harvesting operation and is associated with less surgical morbidity and mortality. It is likely that, compared with adrenal tissue grafting, transplantation of fetal mesencephalic cells offers patients with PD a better chance of obtaining a good clinical response with the least morbidity and mortality.

The focus of clinical activity has shifted to the use of fetal tissue.[75] Although the procedures remain investigational, reports of human fetal mesencephalic tissue implantation into the caudate nucleus and putamen of idiopathic parkinsonian or MPTP-induced parkinsonian patients have indicated that this technique seems to be a step toward the successful relief of the symptoms in advanced parkinsonism. However, because this technology is still evolving, no universally accepted standard technique is available. Many of the basic methodologic issues, including the age of the donor tissue, the method of tissue preparation and storage, the amount of tissue needed, the implantation technique, the location for placement of the graft, and the use of immunosuppression, have been addressed in preclinical studies, and general guidelines are available.

PATIENT SELECTION

In light of the experimental nature and potential risks of transplantation of fetal tissue, patients considered for this procedure should have moderate or severe parkinsonian symptoms (i.e., Hoehn and Yahr stage 3 or 4 in an off period). They should still be responsive to L-dopa but have a clinically unsatisfactory, fluctuating motor response. In general, the selection criteria include a clearly established diagnosis of PD, with persistent responsiveness to L-dopa therapy (despite the occurrence of motor fluctuations); good general health; no neurologic disease other than parkinsonism; and mental competence. Exclusion criteria include significant volume loss within the striatum as observed on magnetic resonance imaging (MRI); failure to show clinical deterioration on a drug holiday or the absence of on-off phenomenon; MRI evidence for nonidiopathic PD or additional neurological conditions; age older than 70 years (most investigators consider physiologic age rather than chronologic age, but with lack of response in patients older than 60 years,[76] more restricted age limits should be used); history of myocardial infarction within 6 months or of other significant medical, neoplastic, or infectious conditions; dementia; and prior surgery for PD.

The rationales for these criteria are in part derived from analysis of prior CNS transplantation experiences.[56] Patients must be fully informed of the design of the study, and an Institutional Review Board should approve any study. Randomization and use of surgical shams for phase II/III studies is controversial,[77, 78] but it has become the Federal Drug and Alcohol standard.

PATIENT ASSESSMENT

The severity of the disability associated with PD can be difficult to assess, and a neurologist or group of neurologists with specific expertise in movement disorders can add credibility to the transplant team's assessment of patients with this disease preoperatively and postoperatively. All patients must be thoroughly examined for confirmation of the diagnosis. PD in patients who are young (<40 years), have a short duration of symptoms, and have an atypical response to therapy should suggest the possibility of an erroneous diagnosis.

Use of the Core Assessment Program for Intracerebral Transplantation (CAPIT) is recommended for diagnosis and evaluation to provide a standardized basis for assessing patients preoperatively and postoperatively.[79] Clinical evaluations provide scores of disability and motor function during on and off states, as well as a determination of the percent of on time with and without dyskinesias. The CAPIT uses the United Parkinson's Disease Rating Scale (UPDRS), modified Hoehn and Yahr staging, a dyskinetic rating scale, and a self-reporting diary (Table 174–2). Time testing and pharmacologic studies are also useful. Because of the fluctuations that may be observed during examination, the preoperative clinical evaluation should span at least 3 months. During this time, medications are kept constant, and a minimum of two to three separate core assessment program examinations are performed in on and off conditions. Postoperatively, these same parameters should be evaluated in an identical setting. These examinations should be considered a minimal evaluation; most centers perform their own measures of quantitative behavioral improvement.

Preoperative MRI should be performed to exclude

TABLE 174–2 ■ **Core Assessment Program for Intracerebral Transplantation**

Clinical Rating Scales
1. The Unified Parkinson's Disease Rating Scale
2. Hoehn and Yahr staging
3. Dyskinesia rating scale
4. Self-Assessment Diary collected for the week before each visit, quantifying the hours spent in *on*, partial *on*, *on* without dyskinesias, *off*, and asleep

Timed Motor Testing
1. Pronation-supination test: time in seconds to perform 20 cycles of alternating tapping of the knee with the palm and dorsal surface of the hand
2. Hand/arm movement between two points: time in seconds to perform 10 cycles of tapping of the index finger between two points spaced 30 cm (12 in) apart horizontally
3. Finger dexterity: time in seconds to perform 10 cycles of tapping of the thumb with each finger in rapid succession
4. Stand-walk-sit test: time in seconds to stand from a chair, walk 7 m (23 ft), turn, walk back to chair, and sit

Levodopa Test
After a 12-hour rest, the Unified Parkinson's Disease Rating, Hoehn and Yahr staging, dyskinesias rating, and time tests are performed immediately before and then every 20 minutes after the patient has received the standard early morning dose of levodopa or carbidopa. Record best on score and stop. If the patient fails to respond by 120 minutes, repeat the procedure in 1 week with 1.5 times the normal morning dose. If still no response by 120 minutes, repeat 1 week later with 2 times the normal morning dose. If still no response, exclude patient from study.

any underlying disease and to provide a baseline for postoperative studies. Positron-emission tomography (PET) scanning with fluorodopa (^{18}F-dopa) is an increasingly important part of the preoperative and postoperative evaluation.[80, 81] It helps confirm the diagnosis, documents postoperative changes, and facilitates the planning of graft placement.

PREPARATION OF DONOR TISSUE

Although it is generally agreed that the elective abortion of fetuses provides the optimal donor tissue, the ethics of this approach are complex.[40, 41, 77, 82, 83] Each institution must develop its own protocols in accordance with the guidelines of the National Institutes of Health and with federal, state, and local laws (Table 174–3). The issue of tissue donation should not be raised until after the decision to abort a fetus has been made. After permission to use the fetal tissue has been obtained, the tissue must be considered an anonymous gift; with this approach, the possibility of any monetary gain is precluded, and the mother remains unaware of whether the tissue was used and who reviewed the tissue. This anonymity is similar to that for other transplant donations and prevents a woman from becoming pregnant to donate specifically to a relative or for monetary gain. Because only one in four fetuses (or fewer) is usable, anonymity can be achieved.

There must be no change in the indications for abortions or alteration of clinical care given on the basis of the acceptance or refusal to participate in the research program. During the 30-year history of fetal tissue research, no evidence indicates that participation in this type of research has had any influence on the

demographics of voluntary therapeutic abortions in the United States.

Although spontaneously aborted fetuses have been used, such fetuses are far less satisfactory sources of tissue than those electively aborted.[84] Spontaneous, first-trimester abortions frequently have chromosomal aberrations and are more likely to be infected with bacteria, viruses, or protozoa.[85, 86] Even under optimal conditions, it is not known how long a fetus has been dead, and with fetal death preceding spontaneous abortion in 50% of cases, the viability of the tissue would remain in doubt.

The optimal donor age for graft survival is thought to be from the time that dopaminergic cells first appear (i.e., final mitosis) to the time that they differentiate and extend neuritic processes.[21] After neuritic processes are formed, cells are less likely to survive transplantation, probably because they are axotomized during preparation. Study of the ontogeny of dopamine-producing cells indicates that dopamine neurons first appear in the ventricular floor at postconception week 5.5 and are rare by week 10. Neurite processes are first observed in postconception week 8 and reach the striatum by week 9. These observations suggest that the ideal donor age for transplantation of human embryonic mesencephalic dopamine cells is probably through 8 weeks after conception (Fig. 174–2). Human-to-rodent nigral xenografts confirm that optimal survival of suspension grafts is up to 8 weeks after conception and that of solid grafts is up to 9 weeks after conception.[40, 41, 83, 87, 88]

Ideally, preoperative ultrasonography would be performed before abortion for estimation of the crown-rump length and Carnegie staging.[89–95] In general, optimal human mesencephalic tissue is obtained with a crown-rump length between 14 mm (Carnegie stage 17 or 18) and 30 mm (Carnegie stage 23). Staging can be performed on examination of the products of abortion, but its accuracy is decreased, and the difficulties associated with properly identifying tissue for staging are increased. If ultrasonography is not used, the degree of development of the extremities (especially the hand), hand width, foot length, and ocular pigmentation can be used to stage the embryo or fetus (Table 174–4). The use of the last menstrual period alone for staging is inadequate. The postconception and postovulation age usually vary by only 1 day and have been used interchangeably. The postconception period generally starts 2 weeks after the last menstrual period. Crown-rump length and the morphologic characteristics of the hands and feet are used to correct postconception estimations and are best expressed with Carnegie staging.[90, 92, 93] At Carnegie stage 23, hand width is 4.0 to 4.5 mm and foot length is 4 to 6 mm. Postconception week 9 (crown-rump length, 50 mm) begins the fetal stage; at this time, hand width is 5.0 to 5.5 mm, and foot length is 7 to 8 mm. By postconception week 10 (crown-rump length, 60 mm), the face is very developed, hair begins to appear, and foot length is 8 to 10 mm.

The tissue is obtained during routine suction abortion procedure. For ethical reasons, the abortion procedure can be modified only if the modification does not

TABLE 174–3 ■ Guidelines for Performing Abortions

1. All decisions regarding abortion are made by the patient and the physician performing the abortion.
2. The timing or the indication for abortion is not altered.
3. The abortion is performed by a physician who is not involved in the transplantation process.
4. No investigator encourages or counsels women to have an abortion.

To ensure that women do not have an abortion for the purpose of providing tissue for transplantation, the following guidelines apply:

1. Consent for the use of cadaver fetuses are requested after surgical consent for abortion has been signed.
2. No monetary or other inducement is provided to the mother for tissue donation.
3. No monetary or other inducement is provided to the physician or center performing the abortion, with the exception of reimbursement of direct costs.
4. There is no advertising for donors.
5. Patients undergoing abortion are not to be denied medical care for refusal to donate tissue for transplantation.
6. The confidentiality of donor and recipient is maintained.
7. The donation of embryonic tissue is made without restriction as to the individual who may be the transplant recipient.
8. No assurance is provided that donated tissue will be employed for clinical transplantation.

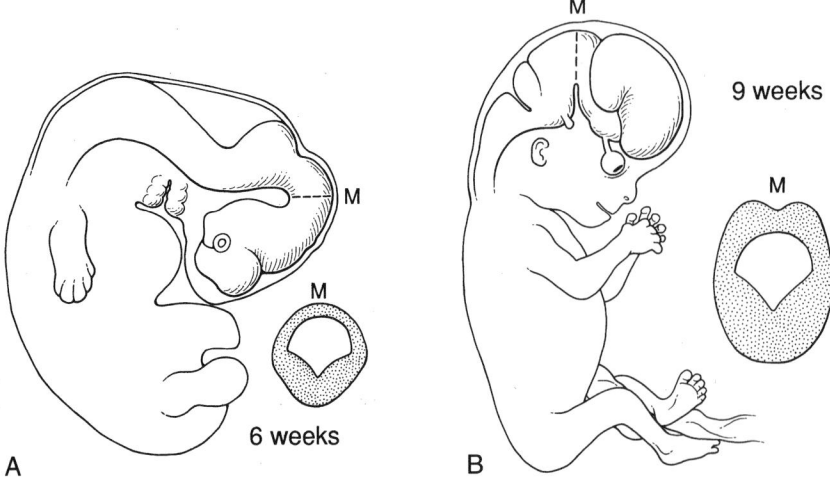

FIGURE 174–2. Line drawings demonstrate fetal systemic and central nervous system development from 6 to 9 weeks' gestation. *A,* At 6 weeks, the eye is pigmented but very poorly developed. Finger rays are evident, but the foot remains a plate. Remnants of the pharyngeal arches are evident, as are maxillary and mandibular processes, but the midface structures have not yet merged. The brain makes three distinct flexures: the cervical flexure at the junction of the spinal cord and brain (1), the pontine flexure in the hindbrain at the level of the enlarged fourth ventricle (2), and the mesencephalic flexure at the level of the midbrain (3). *B,* Considerable development has occurred by 9 weeks. A temporal pole has emerged and begins to cover the insula. Eye, ear, and facial development are advanced. The flexures have been grossly collapsed but are clearly evident. The cerebellum is still relatively small compared with the mesencephalon. Cranial nerves are readily visible. Sections through the mesencephalon designated by the *dotted line,* and the letter *M* demonstrates the development of the tectum and tegmentum, with increasing bulk to the tegmentum as the crus cerebri begins to develop during the initial fetal stage. The aqueduct is still relatively large in relation to the tissues of the mesencephalon.

TABLE 174–4 ■ Staging

WEEKS POSTCONCEPTION	CARNEGIE STAGE	POSTOVULATION AGE (D)	GREATEST LENGTH (MM)	APPENDAGE		MORPHOLOGIC CHARACTERIZATION AND ULTRASOUND FINDINGS
				Hand	Foot	
5 wk	16	37	8–11			Retina has pigment Upper and lower limbs are only buds
	17	41	11–14			Head with large fourth ventricle visible Finger rays appear Embryonic movement can be detected by ultrasonography
6 wk	18	44	13–17			Toe rays begin to appear
	19	48	16–18			Pharyngeal arches gone Toe rays clearly present
7 wk	20	51	18–22			Superficial vascular plexus first appears in frontal temporal area Fourth ventricle no longer seen Upper limbs bent at elbows
	21	52	22–24			Superficial vascular plexus over halfway up from ears to vertex Hands and feet approach each other in the midline as observed on ultrasound
8 wk	22	54	23–28			Eyelids and auricles well formed Hands and fingers may overlap in the midline as observed on ultrasonography
	23	57	27–31			Head more round Ultrasonographic measurement of umbilical vesicle diameter is 5.5 mm

increase the risk to the mother or adversely affect the successful completion of the abortion procedure. Techniques already available and in clinical application include the use of slightly larger bore instruments or low-pressure aspiration techniques. The uterine contents are sterile, but the approach through the vagina can introduce a variety of infective organisms. The physician can reduce the risk of infection by swabbing the vagina and cervical orifice with antiseptics and by using a single instrument passage to obtain the fetal material. Because maternal blood is an additional contaminant, blood samples must be tested for the presence of human immunodeficiency virus, hepatitis A, hepatitis B, hepatitis C, cytomegalovirus, herpes simplex, and syphilis. Once obtained, the fetal tissue must be rinsed multiple times with sterile saline and cultured to ensure sterility. Inclusion of an infectious disease specialist on the transplantation team is recommended.

Identification and separation of the appropriate mesencephalic tissue is a delicate and arduous task. The technique must be practiced on multiple occasions before clinical studies. Absolute sterility and skillful dissection under the microscope are required. Sterile, calcium-free Hank's solution buffered at pH 7.4 is used to sustain the tissue and protect it from calcium-mediated injury during preparation. The addition of antibiotics such as gentamicin sulfate (50 mg/L) helps ensure

sterility. Microdissection is performed in a Petri dish against a dark background, which contrasts with the white embryonic tissue. During examination of the tissue, the brainstem is often fractured at some point above the spinal cord. Frequently, the fracture occurs at the mesencephalic juncture, but it can occur at the pontine flexure or cervical flexure. The tectal or cerebellar primordial constitute landmarks for orienting the brainstem in the rostral-caudal direction.

Mesencephalic dopaminergic tissue lies on either side of the mesencephalic flexure (Fig. 174–3). A 2- to 8-mm³ segment can be obtained. After this tissue is dissected free, it is essential to remove only meningeal attachments. The blood vessels outline the meninges, and with the use of two fine Dumont watchmaker forceps, gentle removal of this tissue is possible. In younger tissue, these attachments are extremely difficult to remove, because the pia mater and the dura are not well defined until Carnegie stage 19. Even at stage 23, the arachnoid is still difficult to define.

Under optimal conditions, the fetal tissue is implanted within 4 to 6 hours of harvesting. This situation is possible in Sweden, where the laws allow for advanced screening and investigators know far in advance when tissue will be harvested. In most other situations, however, a significant delay is incurred while the mother and fetus are screened for viruses. Most centers also evaluate the tissue for bacterial con-

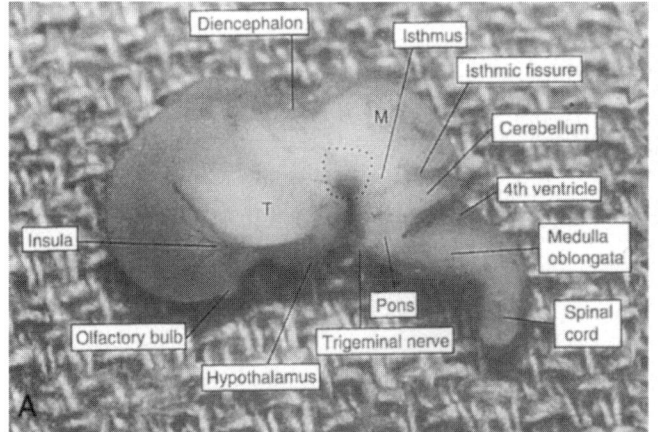

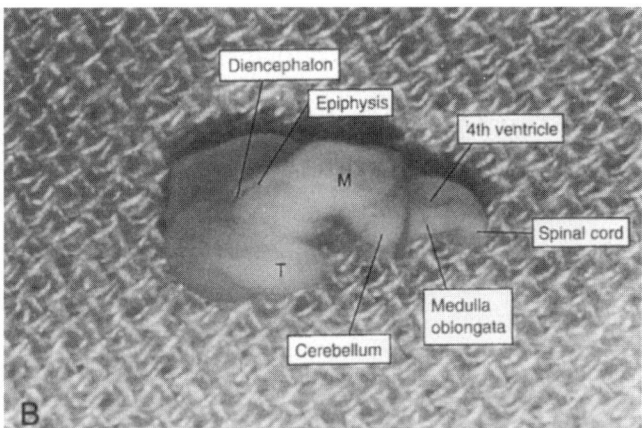

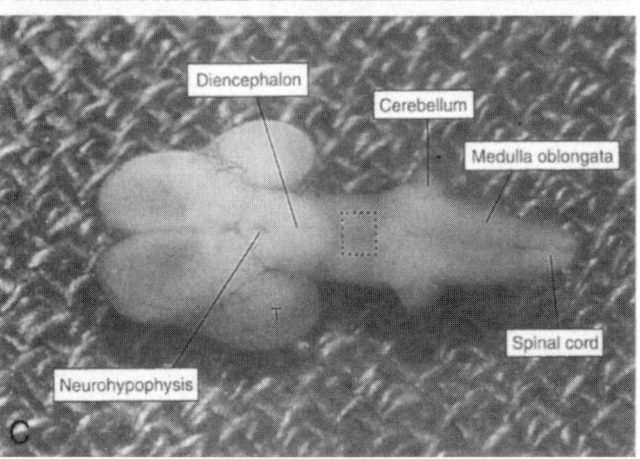

FIGURE 174–3, *A* to *C,* Multiple views of a Carnegie stage 23 rhesus monkey obtained during hysterectomy are labeled to help identify its anatomy. The area of interest is identified by the *dotted line.* Human specimens are usually torn into multiple fragments, but identification of key elements of the anatomy, especially the mesencephalic flexure, allows the harvesting of tissue containing dopaminergic neurons. M, tectal aspect of the mesencephalon; T, developing temporal lobe.

tamination by performing Gram's staining and by attempting to grow any potential contaminating organisms on culture media. To prepare tissue for transplantation, Swedish investigators prefer enzymatic and mechanical disruption of the tissue to form single-cell and cell-aggregate suspensions.[96–99] Investigators at the University of Colorado extrude tissue through glass pipettes to form several "cores" (200 mm in diameter), which are placed in F12 medium supplemented with 5% human placental serum.[100] This configuration allows the tissue to be conserved in a less traumatic manner than is the case with cell suspension while it is still easily transported and distributed throughout the host striatum. Maintaining the tissue in culture allows monitoring of dopamine metabolite production and provides time for performing chromosomal studies, bacterial cultures, immunologic screening for viruses, and tissue typing. Contaminated tissue or tissue that fails to produce adequate amounts of dopamine is discarded. Fetal tissue can be left in culture at 37°C for only 2 to 3 days; however, it can be left in hibernation media for 7 to 10 days without having its viability adversely affected.[101, 102] Alternatively, investigators at Yale University have used cryoprotected and frozen tissue, although this technique appears to be less successful, as demonstrated in animal and human studies on the storage of dopamine cells.[102–107] In vitro survival of cells maintained in freeze-storage does not predict the potential for in vivo survival.

Cell viability is frequently tested with the use of small aliquots of the cell suspension and dye extrusion procedures. Trypan blue exclusion is the simplest procedure. More sensitive is the use of acridine orange and ethidium bromide for staining live and dying cells, respectively, to provide the best possible evaluation of graft viability.[108] Assessment of the portion of tyrosine hydroxylase–immunoreactive neurons on a smear also provides an estimate of success but sacrifices tissue for grafting. Other investigators prefer to evaluate dopamine production using the culture media.

Approximately 5% to 10% of dopamine neurons survive the transplantation process; the remainder are destroyed as a result of mechanical disruption, ischemia, and apoptosis.[41] Behavioral improvement can be observed after transplantation of a human fetal ventral mesencephalon into a lesioned rat striatum; however, the human striatum is several orders of magnitude larger than that of the rat, and it is estimated that mesencephalic tissue from at least three donors is necessary for complete restoration of dopaminergic innervation to a single human putamen.[97] The larger the area planned for reinnervation, the greater number of fetuses required. This is reflected in the results of a number of clinical studies in which the number of fetuses used was progressively increased in the effort to obtain greater behavioral improvement. The use of more tissue and increases in the area of distribution are one answer to the problem of reinnervation of the striatum, but improvement of neuronal survival and axonal extension is the ultimate solution.

SURGERY

Surgical Techniques

The rationale behind fetal mesencephalic grafting is that the dopaminergic cells lost in PD can be replaced with grafted dopaminergic cells. For effective replacement to occur, cells of the appropriate age must be grafted into the appropriate target. Immature cells may not have undergone the differentiation necessary for them to mature and form dopaminergic cells, and cells harvested too late in development do not survive the trauma of axotomy associated with the grafting process in sufficient numbers to effect behavioral change. The cells must be of the appropriate age and must be implanted in the correct target site (i.e., the area of denervation). Transplanted human fetal mesencephalic cells send out axonal processes for only 2 to 7 mm.[109] Tracts 5 to 7 mm operant should provide confluence, but in the best autopsy data, only about 50% of the postcommissural putamen is reinnervated. It remains to be determined whether reconstructive methods that allow these cells to be placed in their proper anatomic location can be developed. Transplantation into the substantia nigra has been shown to improve symptoms in MPTP-treated primates,[110] and at least one clinical trial has included this location with striatal implants.[111]

The key target is the putamen,[112] where dopamine depletion is most dramatic in idiopathic PD.[113, 114] The loss is bilateral, and bilateral distribution of transplant tissue over wide areas is recommended. Rodent and primate experiments have demonstrated that functional recovery after dopamine neuronal grafting is site specific.[27, 29, 38] In patients with PD, the posterior putamen (i.e., postcommissural area) should be considered as the primary site for grafting, because autopsy and PET studies demonstrate greater dopamine depletion within the posterior putamen than in the anterior putamen or caudate nucleus.[113, 115–118] Degeneration of the substantia nigra in PD preferentially occurs in regions that project to the putamen. In primates, the postcommissural putamen receives input from the precentral motor fields, and microstimulation studies within the putamen evoke discrete movements of contralateral body parts.[119–121] The caudate nucleus and the anterior putamen are less related to primary motor circuitry and receive extensive innervation from the prefrontal cortex and frontal eyefields.[122] Although the rodent does not have a distinctly separate caudate nucleus and putamen, the dorsal striatum is believed to be homologous with the putamen. Grafts placed into the dorsal striatum of rats with 6-hydroxydopamine–induced lesions ameliorate sensorimotor attention deficits.[27, 29] Experiments in primates similarly demonstrate that dopamine grafts placed into the putamen can induce significant improvement of motor function.[35, 38]

However, other evidence indicates that the caudate nucleus may be an important target for transplantation. Hemiparkinsonism can be induced by the injection of MPTP into the caudate nucleus, and fetal mesencephalic grafts placed into the caudate nucleus of monkeys treated with the same drugs can produce significant functional recovery.[32, 37] The pattern of behavioral improvement in these primates differs after fetal mesencephalic grafting into the caudate nucleus compared with the putamen.[38] Clinical benefits also have been reported after grafting of dopaminergic tissues into the caudate nucleus of PD patients, although the underlying mechanism remains uncertain.[84, 98, 106, 107, 123–127] Fetal mesencephalic grafts placed into the caudate nucleus may alter the clinical outcome associated with or independent of neural tissue grafting into the putamen.

After unilateral transplantation, improvement in PD patients has occurred primarily on the side contralateral to that receiving the graft.[84, 100, 105–107, 123–128] Several groups have used PET to follow survival of fetal transplants in the striatum.[98–100, 112, 129, 130] PET-monitored ^{18}F-dopa uptake increased in successful grafting,[99] and uptake has been observed in autopsy-proven cases with dopamine cell survival.[109, 131, 132] Remy and colleagues[133] correlated increased ^{18}F-dopa uptake with clinical improvement, and Wenning and colleagues[130] observed decreased ^{18}F-dopa uptake in the contralateral, nongrafted side, where the disease continued to progress. In the patients followed for the longest time, there is PET evidence for graft survival at 6 years.[99, 130] Freed[76] suggested that ^{18}F-dopa PET might not be the best surrogate marker for clinical improvement.

These observations suggest that better results may be obtained with bilateral implants. Potential risks from host injury are associated with bilateral procedures, but these can be minimized by staging the two procedures at an interval of 4 weeks or more. Immunosuppressants are administered throughout this period to address the potential for graft rejection. The best results were obtained by a Swedish group, which used this technique to distribute fetal tissue bilaterally into the caudate nucleus and putamen.[98] It is unclear whether the results from Sweden were excellent because additional tissue was placed into the caudate nucleus (i.e., a more uniform innervation of the striatum), because multiple fetuses were used (i.e., increased number of dopaminergic cells in the area of distribution), or because they studied patients with MPTP-induced PD (a potentially more treatable disease entity) and not those with idiopathic parkinsonism. In England, Hitchcock and colleagues[123, 124] systematically grafted tissue into the caudate nucleus or the putamen unilaterally and later used either target bilaterally. Because of suboptimal fetal age and preparation of tissue, they have been unable to ascertain which target or targets are optimal.

Another important technical point concerns the outer diameter of the insertion device. The use of large needles appears to interfere with transplantation success. Lindvall and coworkers[134] initially used a cannula with a 2.5-mm outer diameter in their 1987 transplantation experiment. Patient status worsened for about 2 months after surgery but then recovered back to baseline and showed some improvement over baseline status. Lindvall and colleagues[97] subsequently obtained better results by using a 1.5-mm guide cannula and a cannula with a 1.0-mm outer diameter to penetrate the

caudate nucleus and putamen. Most investigators who apply stereotactic incision techniques use a gradually tapering cannula with a final outer diameter of 1 mm. This instrument has the rigidity necessary to traverse the pathway to the target and causes minimal tissue injury at the target site. The best clinical results have been reported with the use of an insertion cannula with an outer diameter of 1 mm. Surgeons at the University of Colorado have further refined the needle size and use cannulas with outer diameters that range from 0.46 to 0.64 mm.[97–100, 123, 124]

The importance of understanding the basic principles of transplantation before clinical application is illustrated in an autopsy case. Folkerth and Durso[135] documented the presence of bone, mature hyaline cartilages, hair shafts, and squamous epithelium with keratinous debris after placement of fetal tissue into the ventricular system of a patient with PD. The patient had tissue from fetuses grafted into the right caudate nucleus and left putamen; then a suspension from a third embryo was injected into the ventricular system. The patient died 23 months later from ventricular obstruction from growth of the suspension graft in the fourth ventricle. There were serious flaws in the choice of transplantation techniques: incorrect fetal age (too old); tissue obtained from wrong region (not strictly ventral mesencephalon); poor dissection (included non-CNS tissue); and inappropriate grafting technique (intraventricular suspension grafts).[136] At autopsy 23 months postoperatively, no dopamine cells were present. The clinical and PET data on this patient cannot be interpreted because of the lack of baseline data. The clinical data are based on patient and family reports and did not include standardized UPDRS rating scales. The observations were confounded by manipulations of antiparkinsonian medications. This report documents what can occur when neural transplantation is performed in an unscientific fashion. The key point is the failure to take advantage of preclinical information, to perform precise transplantation technique based on established preclinical data, and failure to conduct rigorous clinical studies. It is because of this type of cases that the U.S. Food and Drug Administration has proposed regulating fetal tissue transplantation.[137]

Postoperative Management

The need for immunosuppressant drugs in patients who receive allogenic fetal tissue implants in the CNS remains controversial.[8, 138] Although immune response to allographic fetal donor tissue is a concern,[30] rejection has not been demonstrated in any clinical study. Moreover, cyclosporine has a mild neurotrophic effect that may confound clinical studies.[139] Using stereotactic techniques, immunologic response to fetal CNS allografts in monkeys may be restricted to a local inflammatory reaction.[138, 140–142] Evidence from primate models suggests that CNS allografts do not evoke donor-specific lymphocytotoxic sensitization.[140, 141] The several CNS-grafted human patients studied also lack humoral or cellular systemic sensitization.[138] Autopsy data also fail to show rejection, but microglia and peripheral immune cells were observed in healthy grafts.[109, 131, 136, 143] A similar infiltrate response is observed in fetal cell–grafted, MPTP-induced primates without evidence of host sensitization and sham-operated monkeys in response to CNS trauma.[140] Freed and colleagues[100] initially used immunosuppression on every other patient, and graft rejection was not observed. This group no longer uses immunosuppression and has had clinical improvement and graft survival.[76] Nevertheless, most investigators begin immunosuppression preoperatively to ensure maximum protection and by which time the blood-brain barrier is closed, and inflammation resolved after 6 months. The use of multiple fetuses and staggered grafting times may increase the risk of rejection.

Patients in most studies perioperatively received prophylactic anticonvulsants and antibiotics. Parkinsonian medications are initially kept at preoperative levels and adjusted as needed. Most patients can be discharged within 72 hours of surgery.

Surgical Results

Stereotactic grafting techniques appear to be safe and effective. Among the reported cases, no major intraoperative complications have occurred. Open operative techniques are not as safe as stereotactic methods.[106, 126] All reports indicate that improvements are delayed and gradual, with the greatest benefits occurring in patients with MPTP-induced parkinsonism who received bilateral caudate and putamen grafts into the right side of the caudate nucleus. However, the marked variations in technique, patient selection, and potential viability in evaluation do not allow firm conclusions to be made. The improvements probably do not result from nonspecific placebo effects[77] or nonspecific host responses.[132]

Fetal tissue transplantation started in 1989.[134] The Swedish experience in the use of fetal grafting reported by Lindvall and colleagues in their first two PD patients was disappointing. A stereotactic technique was used to graft a cell aggregate suspension from four fetuses at a postconception age of 6 to 8 weeks unilaterally into the caudate nucleus or putamen of each patient. During the 6-month postoperative observation period, patients exhibited a small but significant improvement in motor performance during off periods. However, no change was seen in the duration of response to a single dose of L-dopa. PET studies did not demonstrate a significant increase in ^{18}F-dopa uptake at the graft site at 6 months; however, at 12 months, the first patient demonstrated an increase in uptake in the caudate nucleus, and both patients demonstrated increased uptake in the putamen on the side receiving the grafts. Follow-up at 2 years showed no major change in one patient and gradual loss of postoperative improvement in the other starting at 10 months postoperatively.

Subsequently, two additional PD patients underwent transplantation procedures to receive mesencephalic tissue derived from four fetuses at a postconception age of 6 to 8 weeks into the putamen only; a small-gauge implantation needle was used in these two patients.[97] After initial worsening, the patients experienced gradual and significant improvement of parkinsonian features, beginning 6 to 12 weeks after transplantation and lasting throughout the 1-year observation period. Improvement in bradykinesia and rigidity was observed bilaterally but was more pronounced on the side contralateral to the surgical procedure. Motor performance during off episodes progressively improved, and the percent of off time and the number of daily off periods significantly decreased. PET studies with ^{18}F-dopa performed at approximately 6, 12, and 36 months after surgery showed a progressive increase in tracer uptake within the grafted putamen that was consistent with graft survival coupled with a decline in tracer uptake on the side not operated on, which was presumed to result from disease progression.[80, 97, 99] At 3 years postoperatively, the third patient continued to have reduced off periods and increased motor functions in the contralateral limbs during both on and off periods but demonstrated increasing bradykinesia, rigidity, and loss of tone in the ipsilateral limbs.[99] The fourth patient continued to experience a reduction in rigidity and an increase in the speed of motion on the side contralateral to that receiving the grafts, despite withdrawal of L-dopa treatment at 32 months postoperatively.

More impressive are the results of fetal mesencephalic tissue grafting in two patients with MPTP-induced parkinsonism. They received bilateral grafts into the caudate nucleus and putamen from 3 to 4 embryos at a postconception age of 6 to 8 weeks per side.[98] They experienced progressive improvement in motor function, beginning at 3 to 4 months after the transplantation procedure. Striatal ^{18}F-dopa uptake on PET was markedly increased bilaterally at 12 and 24 months. These patients achieved a greater improvement than had been observed after fetal tissue grafting in patients with PD. This finding may be related to the bilateral implantation of nucleus and putamen. Alternatively, fetal tissue grafting into patients with parkinsonism induced by MPTP, who have a relatively static and more purely nigral lesion, may not be the same as grafting into patients with PD who have progressive neuronal degeneration.

In a study at Yale University,[107] four patients diagnosed as having severe PD underwent stereotactic implantation into the right side of the caudate nucleus of fragments of cryopreserved mesencephalic tissue obtained from embryos at postconception ages of 7 to 11 weeks. The courses of these patients were compared with those of three randomized PD patients who did not undergo operation. Eighteen months after surgery, transplant recipients showed statistically significant improvement in their activities of daily living (ADLs) and Schwab-England scores when these were compared with their preoperative findings; however, they did not show improvement compared with controls. Although the magnitude of clinical improvement was greater in transplant patients, control patients also experienced improvement; differences between the groups were not statistically significant. Transplant patients received significantly less L-dopa than controls received. Autopsy of one patient who died 4 months after surgery revealed striatonigral degeneration rather than PD, and no dopamine neurons were present in the graft.[105] This study underscores the importance of maintaining a control group, the need for accurate clinical diagnosis, and the necessity to fully test tissue processing techniques in preclinical studies before clinical use.

A group of seven patients from the University of Colorado received unilateral grafts into the caudate nucleus and putamen on the side opposite that of the maximal clinical deficit (n = 2) or bilateral putamen grafts (n = 5).[100, 128] One patient received fetal tissue from a single embryo at a postconception age of 8 to 9 weeks. At 12 months, statistically significant improvement in the ADL subscale of the UPDRS was observed in the on and off states; the scores for facial expression, postural control, gait, and bradykinesia were also improved. L-dopa doses were reduced by an average of 39%. This was followed by a double-blind, randomized trial with 40 patients assigned to receive fetal neural transplants or undergo sham surgery.[144] The primary outcome measure was a subjective global rating of the change in the severity of disease, as scored by the patients, 1 year after surgery. The transplantation procedure included collection of mesencephalic tissue from four embryos, which were maintained in culture for extended periods while their ability to produce dopamine was evaluated before implantation into the putamen. The grafts were placed bilaterally, using an anterior-to-posterior trajectory through the dorsal and ventral lengths of the nucleus. The global rating scale scores failed to demonstrate significant differences between the transplanted-treated and sham-treated groups, demonstrating a powerful placebo effect. In an evaluation of secondary end points, it was observed that younger patients (≤60 years) demonstrated significant improvement when evaluated using the UPDRS ($P = .01$) and the Schwab and England Disability Score ($P = .006$). There was no significant improvement among older patients, despite increased ^{18}F-dopa uptake on PET scans. The conclusion was that "human embryonic dopamine-neuron transplants survive in patients with severe PD and result in some clinical benefit in younger but not older patients."[144] Although viewed by many as disappointing, the analysis by others, in light of prior studies and the fact it may take 3 or more years to reach optimal benefits, is more optimistic.[145]

The key concern is that 5 (15%) of the 33 patients who ultimately received fetal transplants developed dystonia and dyskinesia that persisted even after reduction or elimination of dopaminergic agonist therapy. This was not a major problem with respect to frequency or magnitude in any of the previously reported open studies.[3] The group of patients with these symptoms is interesting. All patients were in the younger treatment group, they all exhibited very good 1-year improvements in their parkinsonian symptoms, and they had histories of dyskinesia before surgery. They began developing these symptoms approximately

2 years after transplantation. This finding demands further study.[146]

Hitchcock and associates[123, 124] have been examining in a systematic way the optimal site for implantation. Each of six series consisted of 12 patients. In series I (i.e., pilot study), implantation was made only into the right side of the caudate nucleus at a single site. Series II and III included randomized patient populations; the series II patients received implants in the left putamen, and series III patients acted as the control for 1 year. Series III patients then received implants in the right caudate. Series IV patients received right caudate and putamen implants. Modest to moderate improvement was observed in series I through III. Because of Hitchcock's death, the study with series V patients, who were to receive bilateral caudate implants, and with series VI patients, who were to receive bilateral caudate implants with co-grafts of mesencephalic and striatal tissue, was never completed. No immunosuppression was used for any patient. However, the major criticism was that tissue for grafting was harvested at postconception weeks 11 through 19, at which time axon extension to the striatum should have occurred; the resultant axotomy would result in minimal cell survival. Autopsy studies of five of the patients have confirmed no dopamine cells in two and very few in three.[143] Similar to the Yale group that used fetal tissue that was too old, the presence of neuromelanin, which is abnormal for tissue this age, was observed.

The University of South Florida reported results for four patients who, at 6-month follow-up, had a 22-point increase in the total UPDRS score in off and a reduction in off time and a corresponding increase in on time without dyskinesias. Two patients died 18 months after grafting from causes unrelated to transplantation.[109, 131, 132] Both patients had received bilateral grafts into the putamen of tissue from six to seven fetuses (postconception ages of 6.4 to 9 weeks). The patients had been immunosuppressed for 6 months after transplantation. Many dopamine cells (up to 49,336 per graft) were observed in the grafts. Clusters of dopamine cells within the grafts displayed classic organotypic organization, appearing morphologically identical to the substantia nigra pars compacta. There was dense reinnervation within the graft and many fibers that crossed the graft-host interface. These fibers reinnervated the adjacent striatum in a patch-matrix pattern and extended neuronal processes up to 7 mm into the surrounding normal brain. The graft fibers formed synaptic contacts with the host neurons.[143] There was no evidence of host-derived dopamine sprouting, and in nongrafted regions, innervation was negligible. These studies demonstrated that human fetal neural allografts can survive and robustly reinnervate host tissue, and they suggested that long-term immunosuppression (>6 months after transplantation) might not be needed for survival of the allografts, even if multiple donors are used. The investigators are performing a second randomized, sham-controlled National Institutes of Health study.

Fetal grafting has been conducted in several other institutions in the United States (Table 174–5) and the

TABLE 174–5 ■ Current Experience of Fetal Transplantation for Parkinson's Disease in Humans: USA Experience

REFERENCES	TECHNIQUE	NO. OF PATIENTS TREATED		NO. OF IMPLANTS		FETAL TISSUE		USE OF IMMUNO-SUPPRESSION	LENGTH OF FOLLOW-UP (MO)	FUNCTION RATINGS SCALES	REPORTED OUTCOME
		Unilateral	Bilateral	Caudate	Putamen	No. of Donors Patients	Post gestational Age (wk)				
Freed et al, 1992 (Colorado)	Stereotactic	2 —	— 5	4 —	6 12–16	1 1–2	5–6 5–6	Every other patient	12–46	UPDRS HY	Mild to moderate motor improvement ↓ L-Dopa need ↓ Off time
Spencer et al, 1992 (Connecticut)	Stereotactic	4	—	2–4	—	1	5–9	Yes	4–18	UPDRS HY	Mild motor improvement ↓ L-Dopa need
Iacono et al, 1992 (Arizona)	Delayed stereotactic	—	5	—	—	2–3	?	Yes	2–22	HY	Improved motor ↓ L-Dopa need On-off
Freeman et al, 1995 (Florida)	Stereotactic	—	4	—	6–8	6–8	6.5–9	Yes	6	UPDRS CAPIT	Moderate motor improvement Improved UPDRS ↓ Off time
Kopyov et al, 1996 (California)	Stereotactic	9	13	Mixed patterns	—	1–3	6–10	Yes	6–24	UPDRS CAPIT	Mild to moderate motor improvement ↓ L-Dopa need Improved UPDRS
Freed, 2001 (Colorado)	Stereotactic	—	20	—	2*	4	5–6	No	12	UPDRS CAPIT	Moderate motor improvement Improved UPDRS ↓ Off time

↓, Decreased; UPDRS, United Parkinson's Disease Rating Scale; HY, Hoehn Yahr staging system; SEADL, Schwab-England Activities of Daily Living Scale; WRS, Webster Rating Scale; NUDS, Northwestern University Disability Scale; CAPIT, Core Assessment Program for Intracerebral Transplantation.
*Vertical rather than horizontal.
†Substantia nigra also implanted bilaterally.
Adapted from Boyer and Bakay. Neurosurg Clin N Am 6:113–135, 1995.

world (Tables 174–6 and 174–7), but the data from these institutions are insufficient for a proper analysis. Several centers in Eastern Europe, Russia, China, Mexico, Cuba, and South America have not published results in refereed journals or have basic medical delivery systems that are different enough to make comparison of their results with those of the aforementioned studies difficult. Even the studies described in this chapter are difficult to evaluate because of marked differences in patient demographics, entry criteria, surgical techniques, tissue preparation, outcome measures, adjustment of antiparkinsonian medications in the postoperative period, and expertise of the evaluators. Complications have been relatively few. There were several transient psychiatric complications, including hallucinations,[129, 147, 148] panic attacks,[107] and obsessive-compulsive disorders.[129] Major complications reported include an infection,[99, 148] seizures,[107, 112] off-period dyskinesias,[76, 148] and cerebral hemorrhage.[112, 148] There were several complications of immunosuppressive therapy requiring its cessation.[149] Two deaths can be attributed to late complications of grafting.[135, 150]

RESEARCH GOALS

Alternative Tissue Sources

Multiple technical problems must be solved before CNS transplantation can become widely accepted as standard treatment for PD.[151, 152] A source of tissue other than human fetuses must be found. In the most successful human fetal transplant protocols, less than 10% of implanted dopaminergic cells survive, and reinnervation of host structures occurs only over a few millimeters. Attempts to increase survival by lazaroids (21-aminosteroids)[153] and neurotrophic factors[111] have been tried but with apparently limited success. The most successful clinical transplantation protocols have been those implanting the most tissue, often requiring six to eight fetuses per procedure.[8, 9, 154] Because each fetus must be obtained from an elective abortion taking place 6 to 9 weeks after conception and only one of four fetuses can be used, harvesting enough appropriately aged tissue for a single therapeutic PD transplantation program is logistically difficult. There is not enough fetal tissue available to meet the needs of large-scale PD treatment programs, and in the future, there will be even fewer fetuses available. With ethical concerns presenting problems for many physicians and patients,[75, 155] the abortion rate decreasing, and the availability of RU384, alternative tissue sources are being explored. Xenografts, stem cells, and genetically engineered cells are the most actively researched areas for CNS transplantation.

The use of porcine xenografts for dopaminergic neuronal cell transplantation has been actively investigated. Immune-mediated rejection of xenografts is more vigorous than that of allografts.[156] This could limit the clinical utility of xenografts. However, in immunosuppressed rats, porcine fetal mesencephalon cells can survive, extend processes, and integrate into surrounding brain tissue.[157, 158] Phase I clinical trials with porcine xenografts in PD patients have been performed as an alternative to human fetal allografts.[159, 160] One autopsy study has been published on a PD patient who died (pulmonary embolus) 7 months after intrastriatal transplantation of porcine fetal mesencephalon.[161] The patient had been immunosuppressed with cyclosporine. There was evidence of graft survival and extension of processes into the host brain, although cell survival and growth were not nearly as robust as in the best human fetal mesencephalon allograft transplantation. This autopsy suggested the need for more cells to be implanted in more sites. A phase II/III, randomized, sham-operated–controlled trial was completed, but it failed to show statistically significant differences (unpublished data). Porcine retroviral activation or mutation to produce a cross-species pathogen has not been observed. Porcine embryos contain microglia and endothelial cells that express alpha-galactosyl, which increases rejection by CD4-positive T cells and, when the cells are pretreated to eliminate these cells, the immunogenicity of porcine tissue in xenotransplants.[162]

Another source of dopaminergic cells is the retinal-pigmented epithelial cells, which can be harvested from eye banks and grown in culture to standardize the quality of the tissue. Results in MPTP-treated monkeys[163] and open-labeled clinical studies are promising.[164] An alternative strategy is to sequester xenografts from the host immune system by encapsulating the tissue within a synthetic, biologically compatible polymer coating that allows diffusion of small xenograft-produced molecules out but prevents immune attack of the xenograft.[165, 166] In hemiparkinsonian, MPTP-treated monkeys, implantation of polymer-encapsulated PC12 cells, a dopamine-secreting cell line derived from a rat pheochromocytoma, is effective in ameliorating parkinsonian symptoms.[165] A disadvantage of implanting encapsulated tissue is that it prevents most graft-host interactions, which may be an important mechanism of behavioral recovery. With time, the cells die, and the capsule must be replaced. This technology remains unexplored.

The ability to have a stable and readily available dopaminergic cell line would be ideal for CNS grafting into PD patients.[167] Human fetal brain progenitor cell lines have been produced but not for dopaminergic or other useful neuronal cell types. Attempts to develop an immortalized cell line do increase the potential for tumor genesis after intracerebral grafting. The use of neural cultures suffers from the same problem of potentially uncontrolled mitotic activity. These tissues would have to be allografts and subject to potential immune rejection.

The future awaits the introduction of neural precursor stem cells. Stem cells are characterized by a capacity for self-renewal and a capacity for differentiation into multiple cells lineages. Not all stem cells are the same. The totipotent stem cells occur only in the zygote, pluripotent stem cells occur in embryonic tissue, and adult stem cells are multipotent (hemopoietic) or partially committed cell-lineage progenitor cells. Tech-

TABLE 174–6 ■ **Current Experience of Fetal Transplantation for Parkinson's Disease in Humans: Non-USA Experience**

REFERENCES	TECHNIQUE	NO. OF PATIENTS TREATED		NO. OF IMPLANTS		FETAL TISSUE		USE OF IMMUNO-SUPPRESSION	LENGTH OF FOLLOW-UP (MO)	FUNCTION RATINGS SCALES	REPORTED OUTCOME
		Unilateral	Bilateral	Caudate	Putamen	No. of Donors Patients	Post gestational Age (wk)				
Lindvall et al, 1990, 1994, Widner et al, 1992 (Sweden)	Stereotactic	2 2 —	— — 2†	1 — 0–1	2 3 3	4 4 6–8	8–10 6–8 7–9	Yes Yes Yes	15 12–24	SEADL UPDRS	Modest Moderate motor improvement Marked
Subrt et al, 1991 (Prague)	Stereotactic	3	—	1	—	1	7–8	No	6–12	HY	Mild motor improvement ↓L-Dopa need
Wu et al, 1994* (China)	Stereotactic	4 1	— —	1–2 Many	— —	1 1	12–14	Yes Yes	14–23	UPDRS	Moderate motor improvement
Molina et al, 1994 (Cuba)	Stereotactic	7	9	1	2	1	8–13	Yes	3–18	UPDRS	Moderate motor improvement L-Dopa Off phase
Hitchcock et al, 1994, 1995 (UK)	Stereotactic	24 12 —	— — 12	1 — 1	— 1 1	1 1 1	12–19 12–19 12–19	No No No	>12	WRS NUDS	Mild to moderate motor improvement No change L-Dopa
Defer et al, 1996 (France)	Stereotactic	4 1	— —	1 —	3 3	1–3	6–9	Yes	12–24	UPDRS CAPIT	Improved UPDRS Moderate motor improvement ↓L-Dopa need
Mendez et al, 2002	Stereotactic	—	3	—	4+	6	6–9	No	12	UPDRS CAPIT	Moderate motor improvement Improved UPDRS ↓Off time

*One patient grafted with fetal adrenal and FM tissue; all had VIM thalamotomy.
SEADL, Schwab-England Activities of Daily Living Scale; HY, Hoehn Yahr staging system; WRS, Webster Rating Scale; NUDS, Northwestern University Disability Scale; UPDRS, United Parkinson's Disease Rating Scale; CAPIT, .

nology exists to turn blood cells into brain cells[168] and brain cells into blood cells.[169] Bjorklund and colleagues[170] transplanted partially differentiated mouse embryonic stem cells into a rat model of PD and found some cells did become dopaminergic in the grafts of 56% of animals but in none of 24%, and 20% had lethal teratomas. The techniques for differentiation of the stem cells before implantation, inhibition of mitotic activity, the high rate of successful survival after grafting, projection of axons throughout the target, and phenotypical behavior of a substantia nigra dopaminergic neuron (not just a dopamine neuron) remain to be developed.

Hematopoietic stem cells from the patients' bone marrow could avoid the ethical issue of fetal stem cells as well as immune issues and still provide the source for neurons and glia for transplantation. Use of adult neural progenitor cells removes many ethical concerns, but it remains to be proved that specific neuronal phenotypes can be generated efficiently and safely. Partially differentiated and lineage-restricted progenitor cells eliminate the concern about teratomas and can generate large numbers of dopaminergic neurons.[171–173] The problems of poor survival after grafting and migration throughout the CNS remain unsolved. Several select populations of neurons and glia precursors continue to proliferate into adulthood.[174] Capable of self-renewal, these multipotential cells could be an inexhaustible clonal source of replacement cells. Three neurogenesis sites have been identified: subventricular zone of the lateral ventricle, subgranular layers of the dentate gyrus, and subgranular layers of the cerebellar cortex. The key will be the manipulation and purification of select phenotypes before transplantation. Whether these stem cells can be induced to replicate and differentiate into the desired neurons is being explored in a limited number of laboratories, but the potential for the future is tremendous.[175]

Intracerebral Delivery of Neurotrophins

Intracerebral transplantation of dopamine-secreting cells can correct the symptomatic dopamine depletion in host tissue, but it does not address the fundamental pathology of PD. There has been interest in identifying a neurotrophic factor, which could halt or reverse the loss of dopaminergic neurons. Such a factor could provide a more direct and effective treatment for PD and could be particularly useful for early PD, before the extreme loss of dopaminergic cells. It is possible that transplanted cells are subject to the same degenerative process as host dopaminergic cells. These same neurotrophic factors could prove useful for transplantation studies.[8, 73, 176, 177] Interest in neurotrophic factors includes neuronal rescue, stimulation of axonal growth, and metabolic maintenance.

Many neurotrophic factors affect dopaminergic neurons.[178–180] The two best studied are brain-derived neurotrophic factor (BDNF) and glial cell line–derived neurotrophic factor (GDNF). Both enhance the survival of mesencephalic dopaminergic neurons in tissue culture and rescue dopaminergic neurons from the effects

TABLE 174–7 ■ Fetal Transplantation for Parkinson's Disease in Humans: Non-USA Experience

REFERENCES	TECHNIQUE	NO. OF PATIENTS TREATED Unilateral	Bilateral	NO. OF IMPLANTS Caudate	Putamen	FETAL TISSUE No. of Donors Patients	Post gestational Age (wk)	USE OF IMMUNO-SUPPRESSION	LENGTH OF FOLLOW-UP (MO)	FUNCTION RATINGS SCALES	REPORTED OUTCOME
Madrazo et al, 1990 (Mexico)	Craniotomy Microsurgery	7	—	1	—	1	12–14	Yes	6–19	HY UPDRS SEADL	Motor improvement ↓L-Dopa need
Molina et al, 1994 (Cuba)	Craniotomy Microsurgery	30	—	1	—	1	6–12	Yes	39–60	CAPIT	Moderate motor improvement L-Dopa Off phase
Zhang et al, 1994 (Poland)	Craniotomy Microsurgery	3	—	1	—	1	11–12	Yes	30	HY	Motor improvement No change L-Dopa Off phase
Lopez-Lorenzo et al, 1995, 1997 (Spain)	Craniotomy	10	—	1	—	1	6–8	Yes	60	UPDRS NUDS	Motor improvement Improved UPDRS ↓L-Dopa need

↓, Decreased; UPDRS, United Parkinson's Disease Rating Scale; SEADL, Schwab-England Activities of Daily Living Scale; CAPIT, Core Assessment Program for Intracerebral Transplantation; NUDS, Northwestern University Disability Scale.

of axotomy or neurotoxins.[73, 181] Of these factors, GDNF has been shown to be the most potent and the most specific for dopaminergic neurons.[182] GDNF is a member of the transforming growth factor-β superfamily. It was isolated in 1993 on the basis of its ability to support the survival and differentiation of embryonic midbrain dopaminergic neurons in culture.[183] Intraniagral injections of GDNF produces long-term enhancement of dopaminergic function.[178] Intracerebral injection of GDNF has been shown to protect adult rodent midbrain dopaminergic neurons from death after axotomy.[184] GDNF enhances survival of substantia nigra dopaminergic neurons and ameliorates motor abnormalities in rodent models of PD.[181, 185, 186] Fetal dopaminergic graft survival is increased after incubation with GDNF[187, 188] or by implants of polymer-encapsulated cells genetically modified to produce GDNF.[189] In the MPTP-treated primate model of PD, intracerebral administration of GDNF improves tremor, rigidity, and bradykinesia and increases the size of dopaminergic neurons within the lesioned nigra.[190] Striatal dopamine concentration remained depleted after GDNF treatment, supporting the possibility that amelioration of parkinsonian motor signs may not depend strictly on restoration of striatal dopamine.

A clinical trial of intraventricular administration of GDNF in PD patients began in 1996.[73] Unfortunately, the trial was terminated because of side effects and lack of efficiency, probably because of failure to deliver GDNF to the target.[191] The critical lesson is the need to restrict the delivery to a specific target region. Intraparenchymal infusion has shown promise but life-long drug delivery is needed, and chronic infusion has risks, including tissue necrosis, infection, and cyst formation. An exciting alternative is lentivirus *GDNF* gene therapy,[192] which may provide therapeutic and preventive effects.

The Future of Transplantation

CNS transplantation for PD must develop techniques to increase the survival of dopamine grafted cells and degree of reinnervation of the striatum for PD. Neurotrophic factors are the key to expanding the effectiveness of CNS grafts, but they are only part of the molecular biology that must be mastered. If the environment is hostile to axonal extension, the extracellular matrix substance may need to be modified to allow neuronal axonal growth columns to find their appropriate targets.

The study of PD remains the model for the development of transplantation techniques because of its comparatively simple pathophysiology. Although clinical trials have already begun for the study of Huntington's disease and Alzheimer's disease, true improvement cannot come until we have effective systematic treatment that can be replicated in the transplantation technology. These diseases may have to wait for a better understanding of the underlying pathophysiology. Fetal cells are the current gold standard but remain an interim type of cells until stem cells can be perfected. Ultimately, the tissue of choice may be that which comes from the patient. Genetic engineering of host cells may provide a readily available tissue source unhindered by immunologic or ethical concerns.[193] The protein products are similar to conventional protein replacement therapy, such as insulin for diabetes mellitus. Gene therapy may be the ultimate form of pharmacotherapeutics.

The future depends on the development of molecular biologic techniques for understanding the disease pathophysiology, providing therapy through gene transfer, and developing animal models. Advances in molecular biology have allowed us to understand the genetic basis for disease, and a logical extension is combining the genetic modification of cells with transplantation techniques. In 1994, there were more than 100 clinical gene therapy studies involving more than 600 patients in the United States. All such clinical studies must have the approval of the National Institutes of Health, the U.S. Food and Drug Administration, and the Recombinant DNA Advisory Committee of the National Institutes of Health. Most gene therapy trials are phase I evaluations of the safety of gene transfer in humans. The primary focus has been on gene therapy for somatic disease with the same type of risk-benefit ratio evaluation as conducted in conventional therapy. Most of the work is directed at alleviating systemic, single-gene deficiencies, but there is at least one attempt to devise a novel basis for treatment of cancer.[194] Success in correcting X-linked severe combined immunodeficiency for more than 2 years has demonstrated the therapeutic potential of gene therapy.[195] Unfortunately, the death of an 18-year-old patient in 1999 in a gene therapy trial for a nonlethal disease has slowed progress in this field.[196] Gene transfer to human embryos to alter the genome is not considered ethically justifiable.

The first step in any such therapy is isolation of the required gene and demonstration of authenticity by protein expression in cultured cells. Second, the delivery system for this gene must be demonstrated to be capable of augmenting or replacing single-gene proteins within the CNS. Third, the delivery system for this gene must be demonstrated to be safe and efficacious. Genetically engineered cells that can produce neural-specific enzymes have been shown to be capable of augmenting or replacing single-gene proteins within the CNS.[147, 197] Findings of the Human Genome Project and discernment of the molecular pathophysiology of neurological diseases will stimulate the potential for gene therapy to unprecedented levels. It is predicted that genes will be created for the production of neurotransmitters, growth factors, receptors, cell matrix, and any imaginable genetic replacement alleles. Although there is good reason to be optimistic about the ultimate success of gene therapy, there is still too much to be learned to expect quick cures.

The general exclusion criteria for a donor population are that the cells should not elicit an inflammatory response, migrate through the host CNS, or generate uncontrolled growth.[198] The specific criteria for choosing a donor cell population for transduction include accessibility of the donor cell population, stability of the population in culture, and cell division in culture, so that the transgenes can be incorporated into the donor cell genome with resultant long-term survival but without injury to the host after grafting. To completely circumvent the immunologic complexity of xenotransplantation or allotransplantation, a patient's own tissues could be removed, genetically engineered to adopt a useful phenotype, and then reimplanted into the host brain.[198, 199] Most primary non-neuronal cells have the advantages of being easily obtainable from the host for ex vivo genetic manipulation or an autograph, and they are unlikely to be tumorigenic. Genetically engineered fibroblasts have already been demonstrated to express the transgene and produce L-dopa that can restore behavior in the rodent model of PD.[200] Improvement started to decline after 2 weeks, and the fibroblasts showed some signs of neoplasms.[147] Tyrosine hydroxylase expression was observed in genetically engineered fibroblasts in MPTP-treated primates.[201–203] Fibroblasts were initially favored for experimental purposes because of the ease of harvesting this tissue from skin biopsy, the efficiency of transfection due to rapid cell division in culture, the ability to survive in the CNS, and the long-term potential expression of the transgenes that result in a high rate of synthesis and secretion of transgene product.

Most of this experimental work has been done with retroviral vectors. The disadvantage of this tissue is that the rate of proliferation is much slower in adults, and there is less efficient gene transfer and expression. Concerns about collagen production over the long term are not resolved. Schwann cells are also candidates for ex vivo gene therapy. Although the source of Schwann cells is limited, this tissue should be a much more appealing population for autograft cell lines. These cells appear to be capable of living in the CNS without producing adverse products, and they release neurotrophic factors that may be of value to the reparative process. The use of plasmid-transfected primary cultured muscle cells in the same experimental paradigm resulted in more stable behavioral amelioration, with evidence of continued L-dopa secretion, up to 6 months after transplantation. A disadvantage of using genetically engineered non-neuronal tissues is that it is not possible for such tissues to form functional synapses with host tissue, and they therefore cannot reform circuits. Although apparently unimportant for some substances (e.g., dopamine), for others (e.g., nerve growth factor), unregulated, inappropriate, excessive, or ectopic release may be harmful to the host.

CNS-derived tissue may provide endogenous neurotrophic substances or cell-cell interactions essential to host response. Future developments in gene delivery to the brain for some diseases may emphasize the use of neurons or neural progenitors for ex vivo genetic manipulation and refinement of techniques for the direct injection of therapeutic genes into neurons in vivo.[204, 205] A promising technique is use of retroviral vectors to genetically modify fetal neurons so that they continue to divide in culture (at 30°C) and are immortalized, but at higher temperatures (38°C to 39°C), they are rendered permanently amitotic.[206] When transfected to produce tyrosine hydroxylase, these cells have been shown in rat and monkey hemiparkinsonian models to reverse behavioral deficits without evidence of tumor formation.[161]

Gene therapy may make xenografts safer. Transgenic fetal pig tissue with human complement genes escapes the first phase of immune rejection and has been transplanted into PD patients. In the future, neuronal progenitor cells combined with gene therapy may be a powerful technique for repair and restoration of neurological function.[207] However, long-term transgene expression using viral promoters is difficult to achieve with current gene transfer methods. In the long term, any graft propensity for continued growth is a concern because of a mass effect.

Successful gene therapy depends on highly efficient transfection. Calcium phosphate transfection, lipofection, and electroporation are simple methods for gene transfer that typically exploit normal mechanisms for cellular uptake and transport of macromolecules. Although these methods are of value in systemic disorders, in the CNS, they are limited by the low efficiency of stable gene expression in the target cells, with less than 1% of treated cells incorporating a functional transgene. High-efficiency gene transfer is desirable in primary cells that grow slowly in vitro. However, primary cell culture time may be limited, and the ability to induce genetic material into the genome of a wide variety of target cells with high efficiency currently requires a viral vector. Successful vectors include retrovirus, adenovirus, adeno-associated virus, and herpesvirus (Table 174–8).

Replication-deficient recombinant retroviruses have been used extensively as a gene delivery system, and their success rates have been well established. Retroviruses are RNA viruses with a single-stranded RNA genome that is converted to DNA by reverse transcriptase carried in the viral particle. Replication-defec-

TABLE 174–8 ■

VECTOR FAMILY	NUCLEIC ACID TYPE	GENETIC INSERT	NUCLEUS INTEGRATION
Rentovirus	RNA	10 kb	Yes
Adenovirus	DNA	8 kb*–30 kb†	No
Adeno-associated virus	DNA	4–5 kb	Yes
Herpes	DNA	20–30 kb	Yes and No

*Standard adenovirus.
† "Gutless."
kb = kilobases

tive retroviruses are the most commonly used vector for in vitro gene therapy, and they have been used in more than 70% of clinical trials. The major advantages of the retrovirus vectors are the high efficiency of nuclear integration; stable expression of induced gene products, even after multiple cell divisions, and host cells that do not express viral proteins. The disadvantages of the retrovirus vector is the poor infection of nonreplicating cells, the limited amount of genetic material that can be introduced, and the potential toxicity from chronic overexpression or insertional mutagenesis. Specific retroviruses can infect rodent and primate cells with high efficiency. Integration of the retrovirus into the CNS appears to require at least one cell division; once incorporated, the transgene is part of the target cell genome and is replicated with each cell division. Because oncogenesis is possible, use in the adult CNS may be limited to transfection of glia. Attachment to the cell surface requires a receptor for the retrovirus membrane, which then results in fusion and release of the viral particle content into the cytoplasm of the cell. Once inside, the RNA genome undergoes reverse transcription into DNA, which is then transported to the nucleus of the target cell. A significant advance in retroviral vectors has been the development of lentivirus particles.[208] Lentiviruses are capable of integrating into dividing and nondividing cells. Expression is preferentially in neurons.

The second most popular viral vector is the adenovirus. Replication-defective adenoviruses have been developed to introduce double-stranded DNA into the target cells. The amount of genetic material transferred is about the same as with retroviruses. The advantages are that transfection can occur in any type of tissue in dividing and nondividing cells and that the organism can be grown in very high titers. The disadvantages are that the DNA is not incorporated into the target cell genome, the adenovirus vectors evoke nonspecific inflammation and antivectoral cellular immunity responses, and the expression of the genetic material appears to be transient. Because the "free" DNA is gradually degraded, repeat administration may be required to maintain expression. This may not be possible because of immune responses resulting in host injury. There is less concern about oncogenesis. This vector continues to express viral proteins that can cause inflammatory responses and rejection of transfected cells. A major advance is the development of "gutless" vectors that retain the advantages of the adenovirus packaging but eliminate all of the viral genes.[209] These constructs need further testing to determine whether they are safe and effective.[210, 211]

Because of these differences, additional viruses have also been explored, including adeno-associated[212] and herpes simplex viruses.[213] The adeno-associated viruses (e.g., parvovirus) are small, single-stranded, DNA viruses that can efficiently integrate into a specific site on chromosome 19. The major advantages are that they do not produce an immunologic response, they can infect many cell types, and they are a ubiquitous nonpathogen. The major disadvantages are the small amount of DNA packaged, the reliability of vector expression in this particular family of viruses, the difficulty in producing high titers, and potential "helper" adenovirus contamination. Herpes simplex viruses are neurotrophic viruses and can persist in the nervous system for long periods—suggesting distinct advantages for the CNS. However, replication-defective herpes simplex virus vectors have a toxic effect on transfected cells and are therefore unlikely to be used extensively, except for treating CNS tumors. Designing a vector that removes the lytic destructive genes has improved their utility, but because they are nonintegrating, long-term expression is uncertain. However, short-term expression may have advantages in CNS host repair, through short-term growth factor to support graft survival, or in cancer treatment to limit toxicity. Most vectors are broad spectrum, and the strategy of the future is to increase specificity.

The main lessons from clinical studies is that continued expression is a problem.[194] There has not been unequivocal evidence of therapeutic benefit, and there is only one phase III trial. Undoubtedly, a novel system for gene delivery remains to be discovered. Once introduced, regulation of transgene expression becomes the next major goal. We can be confident that rapidly advancing molecular technology will provide the means to precisely and efficiently integrate and regulate a multitude of genes into target cells, allowing optimal therapeutic intervention. Increasing the specificity of the vector may enable a specific population of cells to have one gene and another population to have a complementary gene, allowing greater control over expression and production of the transgene proteins.

In vitro techniques provide the optimal conditions for genetic transfer. Growth in culture and multiple diversions are required for optimal gene transfer. The environment in culture can be well controlled, and introduction of multiple growth factors and genetic manipulation for differentiation or differentiation can enhance transgenic incorporation and stimulate the desired transformation of the genetically engineered cell population. Increasingly, the same process is being performed in vivo.[113, 214] Long-term in vivo expression by an adenovirus has been observed.[215] In vivo transfection of a *GDNF* transgene into substantia nigra cells in rodent models is protective,[216] and expression in primates is being explored.[217] Lentiviral transfection of *GDNF* prevents the loss of axotomized substantia nigra neurons.[218] Long-term expression of lentivirus[109] and adeno-associated virus[203, 219] transgene products has been observed in primates. Oncogenic studies are under way in settings in which transfection occurs in vivo. Direct modification of cells in vivo may avoid many of the problems with cellular transplantation.[193] It may be possible that direct intracellular grafting is not required and that viral capsules could be developed that would be capable of targeting a specific cell population.

CONCLUSIONS

The clinical experience supports the concept of CNS transplantation as a means of treating patients with

PD, but the procedure remains experimental. Clinical observations of patients who have received fetal mesencephalic grafts indicate that the grafts may be able to reverse the symptoms of rigidity, akinesia, and bradykinesia, as well as L-dopa–related side effects of on and off phenomena. However, it has not been clearly established that grafting effects positive changes in gait abnormalities, postural instability, tremor, or the dyskinesias induced by L-dopa therapy. Symptomatic relief should be anticipated for the factors directly related to dopaminergic deficiency. Idiopathic PD patients are also affected by noradrenergic, serotonergic, and cholinergic dysfunction, which can lead to autonomic disturbances, depression, and dementia, and it is therefore unlikely that the use of fetal mesencephalic grafts will ever cure PD.

Although CNS grafting technology is in its second stage, the initial experience with the adrenal medullary grafts should not be forgotten. Improvements in off time of 30% to 50% and improvements in rating scale scores of 20% to 30% with statistically significant improvement in the motor component have been observed in some of the better adrenal medullary transplantation studies. Whether further study is needed to define the best possible technique before a randomized, controlled study is performed and whether current techniques should be used for proving that fetal grafting has an advantage over other treatments are unresolved issues, but the answers to each of these questions should be *yes.* Improvement can come through experimentation with the grafting technique. Although improvements in stereotactic technique are important, the major breakthroughs will come through an increased understanding of the biology of the graft tissue, the graft-host interaction, and the host response to the grafting procedure. Methods to increase cell survival and to reinnervate greater volumes of striatum with grafted dopaminergic neurons need to be developed so that the transplantation techniques will depend less on widespread distribution of tissue from multiple fetuses. The goal must be complete reinnervation of the striatum bilaterally to maximize recovery. Advancements in molecular biology are likely to be the main source of increased effectiveness, and it is important to clearly document the degree to which they are effective, regardless of the mechanism of action. These techniques must be more powerful than the placebo effect, and they must eventually compete with other surgical therapies and with new medications.

Implantation of fetal tissue grafts is the gold standard, but the opportunities for using alterative tissues are rapidly expanding. Development of neuronal progenitor stem cell lines that are more readily available for large-scale surgical studies and that do not carry the same ethical concerns as fetal tissue is being actively pursued. Nevertheless, problems of poor graft survival and limited striatal innervation must be resolved, regardless of the cell source. Although no evidence indicates immunologic rejection, rejection remains a concern throughout the life of the patient. Genetic engineering of the patient's own cells in vitro or in situ may offer the best alterative to the use of fetal tissue.

REFERENCES

1. Dunn E: Primary and secondary findings in a series of attempts to transplant cerebral cortex in albino rat. J Comp Neurol 27: 565–582, 1917.
2. Medawar P: Immunity of homologous grafted skin. III. The fate of skin homografts transplanted to the brain, to subcutaneous tissue and to the anterior chamber of the eye. Br J Exp Pathol 29:58–69, 1948.
3. Olson L, Malmfors T: Growth characteristics of adrenergic nerves in the adult rat. Fluorescence histochemical and ^{3}H-noradrenaline uptake studies using tissue transplantations to the anterior chamber of the eye. Acta Physiol Scand Suppl 348: 1–112, 1970.
4. Olson L, Seiger A: Brain tissue transplanted to the anterior chamber of the eye. 1. Fluorescence histochemistry of immature catecholamine and 5-hydroxytryptamine neurons reinnervating the rat iris. Z Zellforsch Mikrosk Anat 135:175–194, 1972.
5. Perlow MF, Freed WF, Hoffer BJ, et al: Brain grafts reduce motor abnormalities produced by destruction of nigrostriatal dopamine system. Science 204:643–647, 1979.
6. Bjorklund A, Stenevi U: Reconstruction of the nigrostriatal dopamine pathway by intracerebral nigral transplants. Brain Res 177:555–560, 1979.
7. Freed WJ, Morihisa JM, Spoor E, et al: Transplanted adrenal chromaffin cells in rat brain reduce lesion-induced rotational behaviour. Nature 292:351–352, 1981.
8. Lindvall O: Neural transplantation: A hope for patients with Parkinson's disease. Neuroreport 8:iii–x, 1997.
9. Bakay RA, Kordower JH, Starr PA: Restorative surgical therapies for Parkinson's disease. In Tuszynski MH, Kordower JH (eds): CNS Regeneration: Basic Science and Clinical Advances. New York, Academic Press, 1999.
10. Dunnett S, Bjorklund A: Mechanisms of function of neural grafts in the injured brain. In Dunnett S, Bjorklund A (eds): Functional Neural Transplantation. New York, Raven Press, 1994, pp 531–567.
11. Sladek JR Jr, Gash DM: Nerve-cell grafting in Parkinson's disease. J Neurosurg 68:337–351, 1988.
12. Oyesiku N, Bakay RA: Central nervous system transplantation. In Crockard A, Hayward R, Hoff J (eds): Neurosurgery. Oxford, Blackwell Scientific, 1992, pp 448–469.
13. Miller WC, DeLong MR: Parkinsonian symptomatology: An anatomical and physiological analysis. Ann N Y Acad Sci 515: 287–302, 1988.
14. Caline D: Treatment of Parkinson's disease. N Engl J Med 329: 1021–1027, 1993.
15. Hoehn MM, Crowley TJ, Rutledge CO: Dopamine correlates of neurological and psychological status in untreated Parkinsonism. J Neurol Neurosurg Psychiatry 39:941–951, 1976.
16. Marsden CD, Parkes JD: Success and problems of long-term levodopa therapy in Parkinson's disease. Lancet 1:345–349, 1977.
17. Group PSS: Effects of tocopherol and deprenyl on the progression of disability in early Parkinson's disease. N Engl J Med 328:176–183, 1993.
18. Freed W: Substantia nigra grafts and Parkinson's disease: From animal experiments to human therapeutic trials. Restor Neurol Neurosci 3:109–134, 1991.
19. Bjorklund A: Dopaminergic transplants in experimental parkinsonism: Cellular mechanisms of graft-induced functional recovery. Curr Opin Neurobiol 2:683–689, 1992.
20. Dunnett S, Bjorklund A, Stenevi U, et al: Behavioral recovery following transplantation of substantia nigra in rats subjected to 6-OHDA lesions of the nigrostriatal pathway: I. Unilateral lesions. Brain Res 215:147–161,1981.
21. Bjorklund A, Stenevi U, Schmidt RH, et al: Intracerebral grafting of neuronal cell suspensions. II. Survival and growth of nigral cell suspensions implanted in different brain sites. Acta Physiol Scand Suppl 522:9–18, 1983.
22. Brundin P, Bjorklund A: Survival, growth and function of dopaminergic neurons grafted to the brain. Prog Brain Res 71:293–308, 1987.
23. Mahalik TJ, Finger TE, Stromberg I, et al: Substantia nigra transplants into denervated striatum of the rat: Ultrastructure of graft and host interconnections. J Comp Neurol 240:60–70, 1985.

24. Wuerthele SM, Freed WJ, Olson L, et al: Effect of dopamine agonists and antagonists on the electrical activity of substantia nigra neurons transplanted into the lateral ventricle of the rat. Exp Brain Res 44:1–10, 1981.

25. Schmidt RH, Ingvar M, Lindvall O, et al: Functional activity of substantia nigra grafts reinnervating the striatum: Neurotransmitter metabolism and (^{14}C)2-deoxy-D-glucose autoradiography. J Neurochem 38:737–748, 1982.

26. Freed WJ, Perlow MJ, Karoum F, et al: Restoration of dopaminergic function by grafting of fetal rat substantia nigra to the caudate nucleus: Long-term behavioral, biochemical, and histochemical studies. Ann Neurol 8:510–519, 1980.

27. Dunnett SB, Hernandez TD, Summerfield A, et al: Graft-derived recovery from 6-OHDA lesions: Specificity of ventral mesencephalic graft tissues. Exp Brain Res 71:411–424, 1988.

28. Brundin P, Widner H, Nilsson OG, et al: Intracerebral xenografts of dopamine neurons: The role of immunosuppression and the blood-brain barrier. Exp Brain Res 75:195–207, 1989.

29. Dunnett SB, Bjorklund A, Schmidt RH, et al: Intracerebral grafting of neuronal cell suspension: IV. Behavioral recovery in rats with unilateral 6-OHDA lesions following implantation of nigral cells suspensions in different forebrain sites. Acta Physiol Scand Suppl 522:29–37, 1983.

30. Widner H, Brundin P: Immunological aspects of grafting in the mammalian central nervous system: A review and speculative synthesis. Brain Res Rev 13:287–324, 1988.

31. Bakay RA, Fiandaca MS, Barrow DL, et al: Preliminary report on the use of fetal tissue transplantation to correct MPTP-induced Parkinson-like syndrome in primates. Appl Neurophysiol 48:358–361, 1985.

32. Redmond DE, Sladek JR Jr, Roth RH, et al: Fetal neuronal grafts in monkeys given methylphenyltetrahydropyridine. Lancet 1:1125–1127, 1986.

33. Sladek JR Jr, Collier TJ, Haber SN, et al: Survival and growth of fetal catecholamine neurons transplanted into primate brain. Brain Res Bull 17:809–818, 1986.

34. Bakay RA, Barrow DL, Fiandaca MS, et al: Biochemical and behavioral correction of MPTP Parkinson-like syndrome by fetal cell transplantation. Ann N Y Acad Sci 495:623–640, 1987.

35. Fine A, Hunt S, Gertel W, et al: Transplantation of embryonic marmoset dopaminergic neurons to the corpus striatum of marmosets rendered parkinsonian by 1-methyl-4-phenyl-1,2,3,6-tetrahydropyridine. Prog Brain Res 78:479–489, 1988.

36. Freed CR, Richards JB, Sabol KE, et al: Fetal substantia nigra transplants lead to dopamine cell replacement and behavioral improvement in Bonnet monkeys with MPTP-induced parkinsonism. In Beart P, Woodruff G, Jackson D (eds): Pharmacological and Functional Regulation of Dopaminergic Neurons. New York, Macmillan, 1988, pp 353–360.

37. Bankiewicz KS, Plunkett RJ, Jacobowitz DM, et al: The effect of fetal mesencephalon implants on primate MPTP-induced parkinsonism. Histochemical and behavioral studies. J Neurosurg 72:231–244, 1990.

38. Dunnett SB, Annett LE: Nigral transplants in primate models of parkinsonism. In Lindvall O, Bjorklund A, Widner H (eds): Intracerebral Transplantation in Movement Disorders. New York, Elsevier Science, 1991, pp 27–50.

39. Stromberg I, Herrera-Marschitz M, Ungerstedt U, et al: Chronic implants of chromaffin tissue into the dopamine-denervated striatum. Effects of NGF on graft survival, fiber growth and rotational behavior. Exp Brain Res 60:335–349, 1985.

40. Brundin P, Nilsson OG, Strecker RE, et al: Behavioural effects of human fetal dopamine neurons grafted in a rat model of Parkinson's disease. Exp Brain Res 65:235–240, 1986.

41. Brundin P, Strecker RE, Widner H, et al: Human fetal dopamine neurons grafted in a rat model of Parkinson's disease: Immunological aspects, spontaneous and drug-induced behaviour, and dopamine release. Exp Brain Res 70:192–208, 1988.

42. van Horne CG, Mahalik T, Hoffer B, et al: Behavioral and electrophysiological correlates of human mesencephalic dopaminergic xenograft function in the rat striatum. Brain Res Bull 25:325–334, 1990.

43. Hefti F, Hartikka J, Schlumpf M: Implantation of PC12 cells into the corpus striatum of rats with lesions of the dopaminergic nigrostriatal neurons. Brain Res 348:283–288, 1985.

44. Jaeger CB: Morphological and immunocytochemical characteristics of PC12 cell grafts in rat brain. Ann N Y Acad Sci 495:334–350, 1987.

45. Itakura T, Kamei I, Nakai K, et al: Autotransplantation of the superior cervical ganglion into the brain. A possible therapy for Parkinson's disease. J Neurosurg 68:955–959, 1988.

46. Pasik P, Martinez JF, Yahr MD, et al: Grafting of human sympathetic ganglia into the brain of MPTP-treated monkeys [abstract]. Soc Neurosci Abstr 14:4, 1988.

47. Freed WJ: Functional brain tissue transplantation: Reversal of lesion-induced rotation by intraventricular substantia nigra and adrenal medulla grafts, with a note on intracranial retinal grafts. Biol Psychiatry 18:1205–1267, 1983.

48. Bankiewicz KS, Plunkett RJ, Kophin IJ, et al: Transient behavioral recovery in hemiparkinsonian primates after adrenal medullary allografts. Prog Brain Res 78:543–549, 1988.

49. Yong VW, Guttman M, Kim SU, et al: Transplantation of human sympathetic neurons and adrenal chromaffin cells into parkinsonian monkeys: No reversal of clinical symptoms. J Neurol Sci 94:51–67, 1989.

50. Plunkett RJ, Bankiewicz KS, Cummins AC, et al: Long-term evaluation of hemiparkinsonian monkeys after adrenal autografting or cavitation alone. J Neurosurg 73:918–926, 1990.

51. Watts RL, Bakay RA, Herring CJ, et al: Preliminary report on adrenal medullary grafting and cografting with sural nerve in the treatment of hemiparkinson monkeys. Prog Brain Res 82:581–591, 1990.

52. Backlund EO, Granberg PO, Hamberger B, et al: Transplantation of adrenal medullary tissue to striatum in parkinsonism. First clinical trials. J Neurosurg 62:169–173, 1985.

53. Madrazo I, Drucker-Colin R, Diaz V, et al: Open microsurgical autograft of adrenal medulla to the right caudate nucleus in two patients with intractable Parkinson's disease. N Engl J Med 316:831–834 1987.

54. Bakay RA, Allen GS, Apuzzo M, et al: Preliminary report on adrenal medullary grafting from the American Association of Neurological Surgeons Graft Project. Prog Brain Res 82:603–610, 1990.

55. Goetz CG, Stebbins GT: Effects of head trauma from motor vehicle accidents on Parkinson's disease. Ann Neurol 29:191–193, 1991.

56. Bakay RAE: Selection criteria for CNS grafting into Parkinson's disease patients. In Lindvall O, Bjorklund A, Widner H (eds): Intracerebral Transplantation in Movement Disorders. New York, Elsevier Science, 1991, p 137.

57. Dohan FC, Robertson JT, Feler C, et al: Autopsy findings in a Parkinson's disease patient treated with adrenal medullary to caudate nucleus transplant [abstract]. Soc Neurosci Abstr 14:8, 1988.

58. Dubach M, German DC: Extensive survival of chromaffin cells in adrenal medulla "ribbon" grafts in the monkey neostriatum. Exp Neurol 110:167–180 1990.

59. Fiandaca MS, Kordower JH, Hansen JT, et al: Adrenal medullary autografts into the basal ganglia of Cebus monkeys: Injury-induced regeneration. Exp Neurol 102:76–91, 1988.

60. Hansen JT, Kordower JH, Fiandaca MS, et al: Adrenal medullary autografts into the basal ganglia of Cebus monkeys: Graft viability and fine structure. Exp Neurol 102:65–75, 1988.

61. Morihisa JM, Nakamura RK, Freed WJ, et al: Adrenal medulla grafts survive and exhibit catecholamine-specific fluorescence in the primate brain. Exp Neurol 84:643–653, 1984.

62. Peterson DI, Price ML, Small CS: Autopsy findings in a patient who had an adrenal-to-brain transplant for Parkinson's disease. Neurology 39:235–238, 1989.

63. Walters AM, Clarke DJ, Bradford HF, Stern GM: The properties of cultured fetal human and rat brain tissue and its use as grafts for the relief of the parkinsonian syndrome. Neurochem Res 17:893–900, 1992.

64. Goetz CG, Stebbins GT 3rd, Klawans HL, et al: United Parkinson Foundation Neurotransplantation Registry on adrenal medullary transplants: Presurgical, and 1- and 2-year follow-up. Neurology 41:1719–1722, 1991.

65. Hirsch EC, Duyckaerts C, Javoy-Agid F, et al: Does adrenal graft enhance recovery of dopaminergic neurons in Parkinson's disease? Ann Neurol 27:676–682, 1990.

66. Hurtig H, Joyce J, Sladek JR Jr, Trojanowski JQ: Postmortem analysis of adrenal-medulla-to-caudate autograft in a patient with Parkinson's disease. Ann Neurol 25:607–614, 1989.

67. Jankovic J, Grossman R, Goodman C, et al: Clinical, biochemical, and neuropathologic findings following transplantation of adrenal medulla to the caudate nucleus for treatment of Parkinson's disease. Neurology 39:1227–1234, 1989.

68. Kordower JH, Notter MF, Gash DM: Neuroblastoma cells in neural transplants: A neuroanatomical and behavioral analysis. Brain Res 417:85–98, 1987.

69. Kordower JH, Fiandaca MS, Notter MF, et al: NGF-like trophic support from peripheral nerve for grafted rhesus adrenal chromaffin cells. J Neurosurg 73:418–428, 1990.

70. Cunningham LA, Hansen JT, Short MP, Bohn MC: The use of genetically altered astrocytes to provide nerve growth factor to adrenal chromaffin cells grafted into the striatum. Brain Res 561:192–202, 1991.

71. Olson L, Backlund EO, Ebendal T, et al: Intraputaminal infusion of nerve growth factor to support adrenal medullary autografts in Parkinson's disease. One-year follow-up of first clinical trial. Arch Neurol 48:373–381, 1991.

72. Pate BD, Kawamata T, Yamada T, et al: Correlation of striatal fluorodopa uptake in the MPTP monkey with dopaminergic indices. Ann Neurol 34:331–338, 1993.

73. Lindsay RM: Neuron saving schemes. Nature 373:289–290, 1995.

74. Date I, Ohmoto T, Imaoka T, et al: Chromaffin cell survival and host dopaminergic fiber recovery in a patient with Parkinson's disease treated by cografts of adrenal medulla and pretransected peripheral nerve: Case report. J Neurosurg 84:685–689, 1996.

75. Bakay RA, Sladek JR Jr: Fetal tissue grafting into the central nervous system: Yesterday, today, and tomorrow. Neurosurgery 33:645–647, 1993.

76. Freed CR, Greene PE, Breeze RE, et al: Transplantation of embryonic dopamine neurons for severe Parkinson's disease. N Engl J Med 344:710–719, 2001.

77. Freeman TB, Vawter DE, Leaverton PE, et al: Use of placebo surgery in controlled trials of a cellular-based therapy for Parkinson's disease. N Engl J Med 341:988–992, 1999.

78. Dekkers W, Boer G: Sham neurosurgery in patients with Parkinson's disease: Is it morally acceptable? J Med Ethics 27:151–156, 2001.

79. Langston JW, Widner H, Goetz CG, et al: Core assessment program for intracerebral transplantations (CAPIT). Mov Disord 7:2–13, 1992.

80. Sawle GV, Bloomfield PM, Bjorklund A, et al: Transplantation of fetal dopamine neurons in Parkinson's disease: PET (^{18}F)6-L-fluorodopa studies in two patients with putaminal implants. Ann Neurol 31:166–173, 1992.

81. Brooks DJ: Positron emission tomography studies in movement disorders. Neurosurg Clin N Am 9:263–282, 1998.

82. Health At.t.D.o.t.N.I.o: Report of the human fetal tissue transplantation research. Bethesda, National Institutes of Health, 1988, p 2-E1.

83. Freeman RB, Kordower JR: Human cadaver embryonic substantia nigra grafts: Effects of ontogeny, preoperative graft preparation, and tissue storage. In Lindvall O, Bjorklund A, Widner H (eds): Intracerebral Transplantation in Movement Disorders. New York, Elsevier Science, 1991, pp 163–169.

84. Madrazo I, Franco-Bourland R, Ostrosky-Solis F, et al: Fetal homotransplants (ventral mesencephalon and adrenal tissue) to the striatum of parkinsonian subjects. Arch Neurol 47:1281–1285, 1990.

85. Sever JL: Infectious causes of human reproductive loss. In Porter IH, Hood B (eds): Human Embryonic and Fetal Death. Orlando, Academic Press, 1980, pp 169–175.

86. Warburton D, Stein Z, Klein J, et al: Chromosome abnormalities in spontaneous abortion. In Porter IH, Hood B (eds): Human Embryonic and Fetal Death. Orlando, Academic Press, 1980, pp 281–287.

87. Freeman TB, Spence MS, Boss BD, et al: Development of dopaminergic neurons in the human substantia nigra. Exp Neurol 113:344–353, 1991.

88. Freeman TB, Sanberg PR, Nauert GM, et al: The influence of donor age on the survival of solid and suspension intraparen-

chymal human embryonic nigral grafts. Cell Transplant 4:141–154, 1995.

89. Streeter GL: Weight, sitting height, head size, foot length, and menstrual age of the human embryo. Contrib Embryol Carnegie Inst 11:143–170, 1920.

90. O'Rahilly R, Gardner E: The timing and sequence of events in the development of the limbs in the human embryo. Anat Embryol (Berl) 148:1–23, 1975.

91. Drumm JE, O'Rahilly R: The assessment of prenatal age from the crown-rump length determined ultrasonically. Am J Anat 148:555–560, 1977.

92. Hern WM: Correlation of fetal age and measurements between 10 and 26 weeks of gestation. Obstet Gynecol 63:26–32, 1984.

93. O'Rahilly R, Muller F: Developmental stages in human embryos, including a revision of Streeter's "horizons" and a survey of the Carnegie collection. In The Carnegie Institution of Washington. Meriden, Meriden-Stinehour Press, 1987.

94. Muller F, O'Rahilly R: The human brain at stages 21–23, with particular reference to the cerebral cortical plate and to the development of the cerebellum. Anat Embryol (Berl) 182:375–400, 1990.

95. O'Rahilly R, Muller F: Human Embryology and Teratology. New York, Wiley-Liss, 1994.

96. Lindvall O: Transplantation into the human brain: Present status and future possibilities. J Neurol Neurosurg Psychiatry xx (Suppl):39–54, 1989.

97. Lindvall O, Brundin P, Widner H, et al: Grafts of fetal dopamine neurons survive and improve motor function in Parkinson's disease. Science 247:574–577, 1990.

98. Widner H, Tetrud J, Rehncrona S, et al: Bilateral fetal mesencephalic grafting in two patients with parkinsonism induced by 1-methyl-4-phenyl-1,2,3,6-tetrahydropyridine (MPTP). N Engl J Med 327:1556–1563, 1992.

99. Lindvall O, Sawle G, Widner H, et al: Evidence for long-term survival and function of dopaminergic grafts in progressive Parkinson's disease. Ann Neurol 35:172–180, 1994.

100. Freed CR, Breeze RE, Rosenberg NL, et al: Survival of implanted fetal dopamine cells and neurologic improvement 12 to 46 months after transplantation for Parkinson's disease. N Engl J Med 327:1549–1555, 1992.

101. Sauer H, Brundin P: Effects of cool storage on survival and function of intrastriatal ventral mesencephalic grafts. Restor Neurol Neurosci 2:123–135, 1991.

102. Dong JF, Detta A, Hitchcock ER: Susceptibility of human foetal brain tissue to cool- and freeze-storage. Brain Res 621:242–248, 1993.

103. Jensen S, Sorensen T, Moller AG, Zimmer J: Intraocular grafts of fresh and freeze-stored rat hippocampal tissue: A comparison of survivability and histological and connective organization. J Comp Neurol 227:559–568, 1984.

104. Chanaud CM, Das GD: Growth of neural transplants in rats: Effects of initial volume, growth potential, and fresh vs frozen tissues. Neurosci Lett 80:127–133, 1987.

105. Redmond DE Jr, Leranth C, Spencer DD, et al: Fetal neural graft survival. Lancet 336:820–822, 1990.

106. Madrazo I, Franco-Bourland R, Aguilera M, et al: Can an analogy be drawn between the clinical evolution of Parkinson's patients who undergo autoimplantation of adrenal medulla and those of fetal ventral mesencephalon transplant recipients? In Lindvall O, Bjorklund A, Widner H (eds): Intracerebral Transplantation in Movement Disorders. New York, Elsevier Science, 1991, pp 123–130.

107. Spencer DD, Robbins RJ, Naftolin F, et al: Unilateral transplantation of human fetal mesencephalic tissue into the caudate nucleus of patients with Parkinson's disease. N Engl J Med 327:1541–1548, 1992.

108. Brundin P, Isacson O, Bjorklund A: Monitoring of cell viability in suspensions of embryonic CNS tissue and its use as a criterion for intracerebral graft survival. Brain Res 331:251–259, 1985.

109. Kordower JH, Freeman TB, Snow BJ, et al: Neuropathological evidence of graft survival and striatal reinnervation after the transplantation of fetal mesencephalic tissue in a patient with Parkinson's disease. N Engl J Med 332:1118–1124, 1995.

110. Starr PA, Wichmann T, van Horne C, Bakay RA: Intranigral transplantation of fetal substantia nigra allograft in the hemiparkinsonian rhesus monkey. Cell Transplant 8:37–45, 1999.

111. Mendez I, Dagher A, Hong M, et al: Simultaneous intrastriatal and intranigral fetal dopaminergic grafts in patients with Parkinson disease: A pilot study. Report of three cases. J Neurosurg 96:589–596, 2002.

112. Freeman TB, Olanow CW, Hauser RA, et al: Bilateral fetal nigral transplantation into the postcommissural putamen in Parkinson's disease. Ann Neurol 38:379–388, 1995.

113. Bernheimer H, Birkmayer W, Hornykiewicz O, et al: Brain dopamine and the syndromes of Parkinson and Huntington. Clinical, morphological and neurochemical correlations. J Neurol Sci 20:415–455, 1973.

114. Fearnley JM, Lees AJ: Ageing and Parkinson's disease: Substantia nigra regional selectivity. Brain 114(Pt 5):2283–2301, 1991.

115. Brooks DJ, Ibanez V, Sawle GV, et al: Striatal D2 receptor status in patients with Parkinson's disease, striatonigral degeneration, and progressive supranuclear palsy, measured with 11C-raclopride and positron emission tomography. Ann Neurol 31:184–192, 1992.

116. Kish SJ, Shannak K, Hornykiewicz O: Uneven pattern of dopamine loss in the striatum of patients with idiopathic Parkinson's disease: Pathophysiologic and clinical implications. N Engl J Med 318:876–880, 1988.

117. Leenders KL, Salmon EP, Tyrrell P, et al: The nigrostriatal dopaminergic system assessed in vivo by positron emission tomography in healthy volunteer subjects and patients with Parkinson's disease. Arch Neurol 47:1290–1298, 1990.

118. Nyberg P, Nordberg A, Webster P: Dopaminergic deficiency is more pronounced in putamen than in nucleus caudatus in Parkinson's disease. Neurochem Pathol 1:193–202, 1983.

119. Alexander GE, DeLong MR: Microstimulation of the primate neostriatum. II. Somatotopic organization of striatal microexcitable zones and their relation to neuronal response properties. J Neurophysiol 53:1417–1430, 1985.

120. Kunzle H: Bilateral projections from precentral motor cortex to the putamen and other parts of the basal ganglia. An autoradiographic study in Macaca fascicularis. Brain Res 88:195–209, 1975.

121. Szabo J: Organization of the ascending striatal afferents in monkeys. J Comp Neurol 189:307–321, 1980.

122. Kunzle H: An autoradiographic analysis of the efferent connections from premotor and adjacent prefrontal regions (areas 6 and 9) in *Macaca fascicularis*. Brain Behav Evol 15:185–234, 1978.

123. Hitchcock E, Henderson B, Hughes R, et al: United Kingdom experience with neural transplantation for advanced Parkinson's disease. Restor Neurol Neurosci 4:230–231, 1992.

124. Hitchcock E, Henderson B, Kenny B: Stereotactic implantation of fetal mesencephalon. In Lindvall O, Bjorklund A, Widner H (eds): Intracerebral Transplantation in Movement Disorders. New York, Elsevier Science, 1991, pp 79–86.

125. Lopez-Lozano JJ, Bravo G, Brera B, et al: Can an analogy be drawn between the clinical evaluation of Parkinson's patients who undergo autoimplantation of adrenal medulla and those of fetal ventral mesencephalon transplant recipients? In Lindvall O, Bjorklund A, Widner H (eds): Intracerebral Transplantation in Movement Disorders. New York, Elsevier Science, 1991, pp 87–98.

126. Molina H, Quinones R, Alvarez L, et al: Transplantation of human fetal mesencephalic tissue in caudate nucleus as treatment for PD: The Cuban experience. In Lindvall O, Bjorklund A, Widner H (eds): Intracerebral Transplantation in Movement Disorders. New York, Elsevier Science, 1991, pp 99–105.

127. Molina H, Quinones R, Alvarez L, et al: Stereotactic transplantation of fetal ventral mesencephalic cells: Cuban experience from five patients with idiopathic Parkinson's disease. J Neurol Transplant Plast 3:338–339, 1992.

128. Freed CR, Breeze RE, Rosenberg NL, et al: Transplantation of human fetal dopamine cells for Parkinson's disease: Results at 1 year. Arch Neurol 47:505–512, 1990.

129. Peschanski M, Defer G, N'Guyen JP, et al: Bilateral motor improvement and alteration of L-dopa effect in two patients with Parkinson's disease following intrastriatal transplantation of foetal ventral mesencephalon. Brain 117(Pt 3):487–499, 1994.

130. Wenning GK, Odin P, Morrish P, et al: Short- and long-term survival and function of unilateral intrastriatal dopaminergic grafts in Parkinson's disease. Ann Neurol 42:95–107, 1997.

131. Kordower JH, Rosenstein JM, Collier TJ, et al: Functional fetal nigral grafts in a patient with Parkinson's disease: Chemoanatomic, ultrastructural, and metabolic studies. J Comp Neurol 370:203–230, 1996.

132. Kordower JH, Freeman TB, Chen EY, et al: Fetal nigral grafts survive and mediate clinical benefit in a patient with Parkinson's disease. Mov Disord 13:383–393, 1998.

133. Remy P, Samson Y, Hantraye P, et al: Clinical correlates of (^{18}F)fluorodopa uptake in five grafted parkinsonian patients. Ann Neurol 38:580–588, 1995.

134. Lindvall O, Rehncrona S, Brundin P, et al: Human fetal dopamine neurons grafted into the striatum in two patients with severe Parkinson's disease. A detailed account of methodology and a 6-month follow-up. Arch Neurol 46:615–631, 1989.

135. Folkerth RD, Durso R: Survival and proliferation of nonneural tissues, with obstruction of cerebral ventricles, in a parkinsonian patient treated with fetal allografts. Neurology 46:1219–1225, 1996.

136. Kordower JH, Styren S, Clarke M, et al: Fetal grafting for Parkinson's disease: Expression of immune markers in two patients with functional fetal nigral implants. Cell Transplant 6:213–219, 1997.

137. Food and Drug Administration: Proposed approach to regulation of cellular and tissue-based products. J Hematother 6:195–212, 1997.

138. Freed CR, et al: Fetal neural transplantation for Parkinson's disease. In Rich RR (ed): Clinical Immunology: Principles and Practice. New York, Mosby, 1995, pp 1677–1687.

139. Borlongan CV, et al: Cyclosporine-A increases spontaneous and dopamine agonist-induced locomotor behavior in normal rats. Cell Transplant 4:65–73, 1995.

140. Bakay RA, Boyer KL, Freed CR, Ansari AA: Immunological responses to injury and grafting in the central nervous system of nonhuman primates. Cell Transplant 7:109–120, 1998.

141. Fiandaca MS, Bakay RA, Sweeney KM, Chan WC: Immunologic response to intracerebral fetal neural allografts in the rhesus monkey. Prog Brain Res 78:287–296, 1988.

142. Howel LL, Byrd LD, McDonough AM, et al: Behavioral evaluation of hemiparkinsonian MPTP monkeys following dopamine pharmacological manipulation and adrenal co-graft transplantation. Cell Transplant 9:609–622, 2000.

143. Kordower JH, Hanbury R, Bankiewicz KS: Neuropathology of dopaminergic transplants in patients with Parkinson's disease. 1998.

144. Freed CR, Green PE, Breeze RE, et al: Embryonic dopamine cell transplantation for advanced Parkinson's disease—a double blinded neurological study. ,2000.

145. Isacson O, Bjorklund L, Pernaute RS: Parkinson's disease: Interpretations of transplantation study are erroneous. Nat Neurosci 4:553, 2001.

146. Bakay RA: Is transplantation to treat Parkinson's disease dead? Neurosurgery 49:576–580, 2001.

147. Fisher LJ, Jinnah HA, Kale LC, et al: Survival and function of intrastriatally grafted primary fibroblasts genetically modified to produce L-dopa. Neuron 6:371–380, 1991.

148. Cesaro P, Peschanski M, N'Guyen JP: Treatment of Parkinson's disease by cell transplantation. Funct Neurol 16:21–27, 2001.

149. Lopez-Lozano JJ, Bravo G, Brera B, et al: Long-term improvement in patients with severe Parkinson's disease after implantation of fetal ventral mesencephalic tissue in a cavity of the caudate nucleus: 5-year follow up in 10 patients. Clinica Puerta de Hierro Neural Transplantation Group. J Neurosurg 86:931–942, 1997.

150. Mamelak AN, Eggerding FA, Oh DS, et al: Fatal cyst formation after fetal mesencephalic allograft transplant for Parkinson's disease. J Neurosurg 89:592–598, 1998.

151. Hauser RA, Freeman TB, Snow BJ, et al: Long-term evaluation of bilateral fetal nigral transplantation in Parkinson disease. Arch Neurol 56:179–187, 1999.

152. Fischbach GD, McKhann GM: Cell therapy for Parkinson's disease. N Engl J Med 344:763–765, 2001.

153. Widner H: The Lund transplant program for Parkinson's disease and patients with MPTP-induced parkinsonism. In Freeman TB, Widner H (eds): Cell Transplantation for Neurological Disorders: Toward Reconstruction of the Human Central Nervous System. Totowa, NJ, Human Press, 1998, pp 1–17.

154. Bakay RA: Transplantation into the central nervous system: A therapy of the future. Neurosurg Clin N Am 1:881–895, 1990.

155. Vawter D, Gervais K, Caplan A: Risks of fetal tissue donation to women. J Neural Transplant Plast 3:322, 1992.

156. Emerich DF, et al: A novel approach to neural transplantation in Parkinson's disease: Use of polymer-encapsulated cell therapy. Neurosci Biobehav Rev 16:437–437 1992.

157. Deacon TW, Pakzaban P, Burns LH, et al: Cytoarchitectonic development, axon-glia relationships, and long distance axon growth of porcine striatal xenografts in rats. Exp Neurol 130: 151–167, 1994.

158. Isacson O, Deacon TW, Pakzaban P, et al: Transplanted xenogeneic neural cells in neurodegenerative disease models exhibit remarkable axonal target specificity and distinct growth patterns of glial and axonal fibres. Nat Med 1:1189–1194, 1995.

159. Deacon T, Schumacher J, Dinsmore J, et al: Histological evidence of fetal pig neural cell survival after transplantation into a patient with Parkinson's disease. Nat Med 3:350–353, 1997.

160. Edge A, Dinsmore J: Xenotransplantation in the central nervous system. Xeno 5:23–25, 1997.

161. Bredesen DE, Manaster JS, Rayner SEA: Functional improvement in parkinsonism following transplantation of temperature-sensitive immortalized neural cells. Neurology 41:325, 1991.

162. Brevig T, Meyer M, Kristensen T, et al: Xenotransplantation for brain repair: Reduction of porcine donor tissue immunogenicity by treatment with anti-Gal antibodies and complement. Transplantation 72:190–196, 2001.

163. Subramanian T, Bakay RAE, Cornfeldt ME, et al: Blinded placebo-controlled trial to assess the effects of striatal transplantation of human retinal pigmented epithelial cells attached to microcarriers (hRPE-M) in parkinsonian monkeys. Parkinsonism Relat Disord 5:S111, 1999.

164. Watts RL, Raiser CD, Stover NP, et al. AAN. Paper presented at the 54th Annual Meeting of the American Academy of Neurology, 2002, Denver, CO.

165. Aebischer P, Goddard M, Signore AP, Timpson RL: Functional recovery in hemiparkinsonian primates transplanted with polymer-encapsulated PC12 cells. Exp Neurol 126:151–158, 1994.

166. Aebischer P, Tresco PA, Winn SR, et al: Long-term cross-species brain transplantation of a polymer-encapsulated dopamine-secreting cell line. Exp Neurol 111:269–275, 1991.

167. Fisher LJ: Neural precursor cells: Applications for the study and repair of the central nervous system. Neurobiol Dis 4:1–22, 1997.

168. Mezey E, Chandross KJ, Harta G, et al: Turning blood into brain: Cells bearing neuronal antigens generated in vivo from bone marrow. Science 290:1779–1782, 2000.

169. Bjornson CR, Rietze RL, Reynolds BA, et al: Turning brain into blood: A hematopoietic fate adopted by adult neural stem cells in vivo. Science 283:534–537, 1999.

170. Bjorklund LM, Sanchez-Pernaute R, Chung S, et al: Embryonic stem cells develop into functional dopaminergic neurons after transplantation in a Parkinson rat model. Proc Natl Acad Sci U S A 99:2344–2349, 2002.

171. Potter ED, Ling ZD, Carvey PM: Cytokine-induced conversion of mesencephalic-derived progenitor cells into dopamine neurons. Cell Tissue Res 296:235–246, 1999.

172. Studer L, Tabar V, McKay RD: Transplantation of expanded mesencephalic precursors leads to recovery in parkinsonian rats. Nat Neurosci 1:290–295, 1998.

173. Ling ZD, Potter ED, Lipton JW, Carvey PM: Differentiation of mesencephalic progenitor cells into dopaminergic neurons by cytokines. Exp Neurol 149:411–423, 1998.

174. Gage FH: Mammalian stem cells. Science 287:1433–1439, 1999.

175. McKay R: Immortal mammalian neuronal stem cells differentiate after implantation into the developing brain. In Gage FH, Christen Y (eds): Gene Transfer and Therapy in the Nervous System. Berlin, Springer-Verlag, 1997, pp 76–85.

176. Kromer LF, Cornbrooks CJ: Identification of trophic factors and transplanted cellular environments that promote CNS axonal regeneration. In Azmitia EC, Bjorklund A (eds): Cell and Tissue Transplantation into the Adult Brain. New York, Academy of Sciences, 1987, pp 207–225.

177. Yurek DM, Lu W, Hipkens S, Wiegand SJ: BDNF enhances the functional reinnervation of the striatum by grafted fetal dopamine neurons. Exp Neurol 137:105–118, 1996.

178. Bjorklund A, Rosenblad C, Winkler C, Kirik D: Studies on neuroprotective and regenerative effects of GDNF in a partial lesion model of Parkinson's disease. Neurobiol Dis 4:186–200, 1997.

179. Bohn MC, Choi-Lundberg DL, Davidson BL, et al: Adenoviral-mediated gene expression in the nonhuman primate brain. Hum Gene Ther 10:1175–1184, 1999.

180. Collier TJ, Sortwell CE: Therapeutic potential of nerve growth factors in Parkinson's disease. Drugs Aging 14:261–287, 1999.

181. Kearns CM, Gash DM: GDNF protects nigral dopamine neurons against 6-hydroxydopamine in vivo. Brain Res 672:104–111, 1995.

182. Gash DM, Zhang Z, Gerhardt G: Neuroprotective and neurorestorative properties of GDNF. Ann Neurol 44(Suppl 1):S121–S125, 1998.

183. Lin LF, Doherty DH, Lile JD, et al: GDNF: A glial cell line–derived neurotrophic factor for midbrain dopaminergic neurons. Science 260:1130–1132, 1993.

184. Beck KD, Valverde J, Alexi T, et al: Mesencephalic dopaminergic neurons protected by GDNF from axotomy-induced degeneration in the adult brain. Nature 373:339–341, 1995.

185. Hoffer BJ, Hoffman A, Bowenkamp K, et al: Glial cell line–derived neurotrophic factor reverses toxin-induced injury to midbrain dopaminergic neurons in vivo. Neurosci Lett 182: 107–111, 1994.

186. Tomac A, Lindqvist E, Lin LF, et al: Protection and repair of the nigrostriatal dopaminergic system by GDNF in vivo. Nature 373:335–339, 1995.

187. Granholm AC, et al: Glial cell line-derived neurotrophic factor improves survival of ventral mesencephalic grafts to the 6-hydroxydopamine lesioned striatum. Exp Brain Res 116:29–38, 1997.

188. Rosenblad C, Martinez-Serrano A, Bjorklund A: Glial cell line–derived neurotrophic factor increases survival, growth and function of intrastriatal fetal nigral grafts. Neuroscience 75:979–985, 1996.

189. Sautter J, Tseng JL, Braguglia D, et al: Implants of polymer-encapsulated genetically modified cells releasing glial cell line–derived neurotrophic factor improve survival, growth, and function of fetal dopaminergic grafts. Exp Neurol 149:230–236, 1998.

190. Gash DM, Zhang Z, Ovadia A, et al: Functional recovery in parkinsonian monkeys treated with GDNF. Nature 380:252–255, 1996.

191. Kordower JH, Palfi S, Chen EY, et al: Clinico-pathological findings following intraventricular GDNF treatment in a patient with Parkinson's disease. Ann Neurol 46:419–424, 1999.

192. Kordower JH, Sortwell CE: Neuropathology of fetal nigra transplants for Parkinson's disease. Prog Brain Res 127:333–344, 2000.

193. Horellou P, Mallet J: Gene therapy for Parkinson's disease. Mol Neurobiol 15:241–256, 1997.

194. Blau HM, Springer ML: Gene therapy—a novel form of drug delivery. N Engl J Med 333:1204–1207, 1995.

195. Hacein-Bey-Abina S, Le Deist F, Carlier F, et al: Sustained correction of X-linked severe combined immunodeficiency by ex vivo gene therapy. N Engl J Med 346:1185–1193, 2002.

196. Halim N: Aftermath of tragedy. Scientist Jan 10:6, 2000.

197. Gage FH, Friedmann T, Fisher L, et al: Genetically modified cells: Potential therapeutic application to Parkinson's disease. In Lindvall O, Bjorklund A, Widner H (eds): Intracerebral Transplantation in Movement Disorders. New York, Elsevier Science, 1991, pp 259–266.

198. Tuszynski MH, Gage FH: Somatic gene therapy for nervous system disease. Ciba Found Symp 196:85–94, 1996, discussion 94–97.

199. Wolff JA, Lederberg J: A history of gene transfer and therapy. In Wolff J (ed): Gene Therapeutics: Methods and Application of Direct Gene Transfer. Boston, Birkhauser, 1994, pp 3–25.

200. Wolff JA, Fisher LJ, Xu L, et al: Grafting fibroblasts genetically modified to produce L-dopa in a rat model of Parkinson disease. Proc Natl Acad Sci U S A 86:9011–9014, 1989.

201. Bankiewicz KS, Bringas JR, McLaughlin W, et al: Application of gene therapy for Parkinson's disease: Nonhuman primate experience. Adv Pharmacol 42:801–806, 1998.

202. Bankiewicz KS, Emborg ME, McLaughlin W, et al: Utilization

of a non-human model of Parkinson's disease for therapeutic applications of gene therapy. Exp Neurol 145:S15, 1997.

203. Bankiewicz KS, Snyder R, Zhou S, et al: Adeno-associated (AAV) viral vector-mediated gene delivery in non-human primates [abstract]. Soc Neurosci Abstr 22:768, 1996.

204. Snyder EY: Grafting immortalized neurons to the CNS. Curr Opin Neurobiol 4:742–751, 1994.

205. Tuszynski MH, Gage FH: Somatic gene therapy for nervous system disease. In Symposium CF (ed): Growth Factors as Drugs for Neurological and Sensory Disorders. Chichester, UK, Wiley, 1996, pp 85–97.

206. Anton R, Kordower JH, Maidment NT, et al: Neural-targeted gene therapy for rodent and primate hemiparkinsonism. Exp Neurol 127:207–218, 1994.

207. Snyder EY: Retroviral vectors for the study of neuroembryology: Immortalization of neural cells. In Kaplit MG, Lowey AD (eds): Viral Vectors: Tools for Analysis and Genetic Manipulation of the Nervous System. New York, Academic Press, 1995, pp 435–475.

208. Naldini L, Blomer U, Gallay P, et al: In vivo gene delivery and stable transduction of nondividing cells by a lentiviral vector. Science 272:263–267, 1996.

209. Kochanek S, Clemens PR, Mitani K, et al: A new adenoviral vector: Replacement of all viral coding sequences with 28 kb of DNA independently expressing both full-length dystrophin and beta-galactosidase. Proc Natl Acad Sci U S A 93:5731–5736, 1996.

210. Horellou P, Bilang-Bleuel A, Mallet J: In vivo adenovirus-mediated gene transfer for Parkinson's disease. Neurobiol Dis 4:280–287, 1997.

211. Smith GM: Adenovirus-mediated gene transfer to treat neurologic disease. Arch Neurol 55:1061–1064, 1998.

212. Xiao X, Li J, McCown TJ, Samulski RJ: Gene transfer by adeno-associated virus vectors into the central nervous system. Exp Neurol 144:113–124, 1997.

213. Lachmann RH, Efstathiou S: Utilization of the herpes simplex virus type 1 latency–associated regulatory region to drive stable reporter gene expression in the nervous system. J Virol 71:3197–3207, 1997.

214. Bing GY, Notter MF, Hansen JT, Gash DM: Comparison of adrenal medullary, carotid body and PC12 cell grafts in 6-OHDA lesioned rats. Brain Res Bull 20:399–406, 1988.

215. Goodman JC, Trask TW, Chen SH, et al: Adenoviral-mediated thymidine kinase gene transfer into the primate brain followed by systemic ganciclovir: Pathologic, radiologic, and molecular studies. Hum Gene Ther 7:1241–1250, 1996.

216. Bohn MC: A commentary on glial cell line-derived neurotrophic factor (GDNF). From a glial secreted molecule to gene therapy. Biochem Pharmacol 57:135–142, 1999.

217. Bohn MC, Choi-Lundberg DL, Davidson BL, et al: Adenovirus-mediated transgene expression in nonhuman primate brain. Hum Gene Ther 10:1175–1184, 1999.

218. Deglon NJ, Tseng L, Bensadoun J-C, et al: Protection of dopaminergic neurons from axotomy-induced degeneration with a GDNF-expressing lentiviral vector [abstract]. Soc Neurosci Abstr 24:1008, 1998.

219. Bankiewicz KS, Leff SE, Nagy D, et al: AAV-mediated gene expression in the striatum of hemiparkinsonian monkeys [abstract]. Presented at the 5th International Neurotransplantation Meeting, 1997, San Diego, CA.

CHAPTER 175

Neurosurgery of Psychiatric Disorders

G. REES COSGROVE

For most patients with significant psychiatric illness, the accepted therapeutic approach consists of a combination of well-supervised pharmacologic, behavioral, and in some instances, electroconvulsive therapies. However, not all patients respond to these modern treatment methods, and many remain severely disabled. It is reasonable to consider that some of these patients may be appropriate candidates for surgical treatment if the overall result and level of functioning could be improved.

Surgery for intractable neuropsychiatric illness and behavioral disorders has been performed for many years and has generated considerable controversy for a variety of scientific, social, and philosophical reasons. In this chapter, I review the historical issues underlying this debate and discuss the anatomic and physiologic basis for surgical intervention. Guidelines for the appropriate selection of surgical candidates are presented, and the four most common psychosurgical procedures are described. The indications, results, complications, and overall experience for each procedure are reviewed and compared.

HISTORICAL PERSPECTIVE

Surgical intervention for neuropsychiatric disease was first reported by Burckhardt[1] in 1891, when he performed bilateral cortical excision in six demented and aggressive patients with mixed results. In 1935, Fulton and Jacobsen[2] presented their experience with primate behavior after ablation of the frontal cortices and observed less "experimental neurosis" in the lobectomized animals. These observations prompted Egas Moniz[3] to perform prefrontal leukotomies by injection of absolute alcohol into the frontal lobes of a small group of severely ill, institutionalized patients. Moniz[3] reported that 14 of 20 patients showed "worthwhile" improvement and coined the term *psychosurgery* to describe his interventions. Moniz[3] later described his experience with larger numbers of patients after more specific and restricted frontal lobe lesions were created using a leukotome. At the time, few satisfactory treatment options existed, and the asylums for the insane were overflowing with the chronic mentally ill. Despite

the lack of objective data and long-term follow-up, an enthusiastic response was obtained from the medical and lay communities, which resulted in Moniz receiving the Nobel Prize in Medicine in 1949.

One of the most enthusiastic proponents of the procedure was Walter Freeman, a psychiatrist, who performed the first prefrontal lobotomy in the United States with James Watts, a neurosurgeon.[4] The Freeman-Watts prefrontal lobotomy was performed through bilateral bur holes placed in the inferior frontal region with a specially designed, calibrated instrument that was inserted blindly to the midline and swept back and forth to interrupt the white matter tracts in the frontal lobes. In reporting their results on the first 200 patients in 1942, Freeman and Watts[5] were favorably impressed, although they did admit to a significant complication rate, including frontal lobe syndrome, seizures, apathy, decreased attention, and inappropriate behavior. Despite these side effects, prefrontal lobotomy became widely performed throughout the United States, largely because of the lack of satisfactory therapeutic alternatives and the promotional zeal of Freeman himself.

Over time, Watts gradually became disillusioned with Freeman and terminated his collaboration. Freeman subsequently developed a novel technique of "transorbital leucotomy," which involved inserting a small, sharp instrument under the eyelids and pushing it through the bony orbit with a sweeping motion to sever the frontal-thalamic radiations in the posterior frontal orbital cortex.[6] This so-called ice pick procedure was performed quickly and with minimal anesthesia, often in the immediate postictal phase after an induced electroshock treatment. Outcomes were generally favorable, although the procedure was associated with significant morbidity. The broad and somewhat indiscriminate application of this particular technique by Freeman probably contributed to the subsequent decline of psychosurgery in later years.

Tooth and Newton[7] reviewed 10,365 standard prefrontal lobotomy operations performed between 1943 and 1954 and confirmed that the rate of "improvement" was about 70%, but they also reported a 6% mortality rate, 1% epilepsy rate, and 1.5% rate of marked disinhibition. These complications prompted

Fulton and others to call for a less radical and more selective approach to the surgery. By the late 1940s, more precise open surgical procedures were described, including bilateral inferior leukotomy, bimedial frontal leukotomy, orbital gyrus undercutting, cerebral topectomies, and anterior cingulectomies.[8–12] During the same period, human stereotaxy was introduced. It allowed accurate and reproducible placement of lesions in specific target sites. The results of stereotactic anterior cingulotomy were first reported by Foltz and White[13] in 1962, and results of subcaudate tractotomy were reported by Knight[14] in 1964. Lars Leksell[15] described his experience with anterior capsulotomy in 1972, and Kelly[16] reported limbic leukotomy (i.e., subcaudate tractotomy and cingulotomy combined) in 1973. Isolated reports of hypothalamotomy, bilateral amygdalotomy, and thalamotomy can also be found in the literature during this same period.[17–19]

Despite generally favorable results, criticism and concerns about surgery for psychiatric illness and allegations of abuse prompted calls for a careful review of the issues. In the United States, the report of the National Commission for the Protection of Human Subjects of Biomedical and Behavioral Research indicated that psychosurgery was efficacious in more than one half of the 400 operations performed annually between 1971 and 1973 and that no psychologic deficits could be attributed to the procedures.[20] Preoperative and postoperative studies by independent observers of smaller groups of patients undergoing cingulotomy demonstrated a marked improvement in psychiatric symptoms in most, along with a significant improvement in full-scale, verbal, and performance IQ.[21] Fears that psychosurgery was being used on minority and disadvantaged populations for social control were unsubstantiated. The commission's conclusions argued against the public perception that psychosurgery was dangerous, ineffective, and experimental, but opposition remained despite its formal acceptance in position statements by organized psychiatry in many countries around the world.

With the introduction of chlorpromazine in 1954 and the additional psychotropic agents that followed, satisfactory medical management of psychiatric illness led to a rapid decline in surgery for mental illness. However, despite the vast array of specific psychotropic medications available today, many patients are refractory to treatment and may be considered appropriate candidates for surgery. Although it has been estimated that fewer than 25 patients were operated on annually in the United States and Great Britain,[22] there is a resurgence of interest in surgical options, perhaps because of the favorable emerging data on ablative procedures and excitement about the prospect of deep brain stimulation (DBS).

Over the past 2 decades, significant progress has been made in understanding the neurobiologic basis of psychiatric illness and in its diagnosis and treatment. The availability of precise neurosurgical techniques along with sophisticated clinical and neuroimaging assessment strategies promises better data to help guide researchers and clinicians in the refinement of these interventions. Increasingly, prospective outcome studies in psychiatric surgery using clinically validated rating scales are being reported in an ongoing attempt to provide relief in a scientific and ethical manner.

ANATOMIC AND PHYSIOLOGIC BASES FOR SURGERY

In 1937, a year after Moniz reported his initial experience with prefrontal lobotomy, Papez[23] postulated that a reverberating circuit in the human brain might be responsible for emotion, anxiety, and memory. The components of this rudimentary limbic system included the hypothalamus, septal nuclei, hippocampi, mamillary bodies, anterior thalamic nuclei, cingulate gyri, and their interconnections. It was subsequently expanded by McLean[24] in 1952 to incorporate paralimbic structures, including orbital frontal, insular, and anterior temporal cortices; the amygdala; and dorsomedial thalamic nuclei. Neurosurgical interventions for psychiatric disorders have always been directed at various targets within this system, and some have proposed the term *limbic system surgery* as an alternative to psychosurgery.

Although the exact mechanisms are unknown, there is mounting evidence that the limbic system and its interconnections with the cortical-striatal-thalamic circuits play a central role in the pathophysiology of major affective illness, obsessive-compulsive disorder (OCD), and other anxiety disorders. Electrical stimulation of specific areas within the limbic system (i.e., anterior cingulum and subcaudate region) has been shown in humans to alter autonomic responses and anxiety levels.[25] Stimulation of the hypothalamus in animals produces autonomic, endocrine, and complex motor effects, which suggest that the hypothalamus integrates and coordinates the behavioral expression of emotional states.[26] The Papez circuit has direct input to the hypothalamus and is influenced by the paralimbic structures as well as the medial orbitofrontal cortex, forming a link between neocortex and the limbic system proper. The limbic system appears strategically located to mediate and interconnect somatic and visceral stimuli with higher cortical functions. It is likely that certain psychiatric disorders (i.e., depression, OCD, and other anxiety disorders) may reflect a final common pathway of limbic system dysregulation.

Data from clinical and neuroimaging studies have converged to implicate the cortical-striatal-thalamic circuits in the pathophysiology of OCD.[27, 28] The frontal-striatal-pallidal-thalamic-frontal loop, which has been so well characterized for its control of motor function in Parkinson's disease, may also explain some features of OCD. From a clinical perspective, rare neurological movement disorders such as von Economo's encephalitis and Sydenham's chorea are known to affect the basal ganglia and have been associated with obsessive and compulsive symptoms.[29, 30] Many patients with Tourette's syndrome, another disorder of the basal ganglia characterized by coprolalia and motor tics, have significant OCD symptoms throughout their lives. This close association has led some observers to the hypothesis that Tourette's syndrome and OCD may be different phenotypic manifestations of similar basal ganglia pathology.[31] Orbitofrontal cortex has also been implicated in OCD because the cognitive and behavioral features associated with lesions in this area, such as decreased response inhibition, inflexibility, and overattention to irrelevant details, are reminiscent of OCD symptoms.

Magnetic resonance imaging (MRI) has demonstrated specific brain lesions in the frontal, temporal, and cingulate areas in some cases of new-onset OCD.[32] Detailed morphometric analysis of MRI scans in OCD patients has also suggested focal abnormalities in striatal areas with subtle volumetric abnormalities involving caudate nuclei.[33] Positron emission tomography (PET) has provided perhaps the most compelling evidence implicating orbitofrontal cortex and basal ganglia dysfunction in OCD. Studies of children and adults using ^{18}F-fluorodeoxyglucose PET (FDG-PET) have consistently reported significant elevation of absolute glucose metabolic rates for the cerebral hemispheres and orbital gyri and somewhat less consistently for the caudate nucleus in OCD patients compared with normal controls.[34-36] In one study of clomipramine treatment in childhood-onset OCD, 6 patients who failed to respond had significantly higher right anterior cingulate and right orbital metabolism than did 11 drug-responsive patients.[37] Two reports have found regional decreases in metabolic activity correlating with a decrease in the severity of OCD symptoms as measured by the Yale-Brown Obsessive-Compulsive Scale (YBOCS) after successful pharmacologic or behavioral treatment; one reported decreased caudate activity, and the other decreased right orbitofrontal metabolism.[35, 38]

These findings prompted several investigators to propose a model of OCD based on abnormal activity in the frontal-striatal-pallidal-thalamic-frontal loop.[31, 39] Neuroanatomic evidence supports the existence of functional circuits linking cortical, striatal, and thalamic nuclei in a series of topographically defined feedforward loops.[40] These circuits separately influence motor activity, eye movement, cognition, and emotion, each by corresponding basal ganglia–thalamocortical pathways. The loop underlying emotion and psychiatric symptoms has two components: an orbitofrontal-thalamic interconnection (i.e., direct loop) and an orbitofrontal-striatal-thalamic interconnection (i.e., indirect loop), and each is mediated by various neurotransmitters. Just as with Parkinson's disease, it is hypothesized that one pathway modulates the activity of the other. According to this model, overactivity in the orbitofrontal-thalamic interconnection gives rise to obsessive thoughts and consequently increases anxiety. In the normal state, the orbitofrontal area would at the same time stimulate the caudate, which would modulate overactivity of the orbitofrontal-thalamic interconnection by means of pallidal-thalamic output. OCD symptoms may arise from overactivity in the orbitothalamic pathway or dysfunction in the modulating effect of the frontal-caudate-pallidal-thalamic interconnection. Either situation would result in an overactive frontothalamic circuit associated with obsessive and anxiety symptoms. In this model, compulsions are hypothesized to be ritualized activities that recruit the striatum in a compensatory attempt to regulate frontothalamic overactivity. Theoretically, lesions placed in these circuits may reduce overactivity or reroute compensatory strategies more efficiently.

It is possible to speculate about how disruption of different pathways affects the direct or indirect frontal-striatal-thalamic pathways so as to normalize activity, leading to symptom improvement. In humans, it has been shown that lesions in the substantia innominata after subcaudate tractotomy cause extensive degeneration in the ventral portion of the internal capsule.[41] The fiber tract degeneration can be traced back to the dorsomedial nucleus of the thalamus, which has extensive interconnections with various parts of the limbic system.[42] Rauch and associates[43] reported atrophy in the caudate body in subjects who had undergone one or more cingulotomies approximately 6 months before the morphometric studies. Such investigations are beginning to demonstrate the functional connectivity of the cortical and subcortical brain regions. Lesions in one region may affect the integrity and function of other brain regions. Preliminary evidence suggests that patients with OCD or major depressive disorder do not improve immediately after psychosurgery and that several weeks to months are required for positive clinical effects to be fully manifested. It is likely that secondary nerve degeneration or metabolic alterations in brain areas other than the region where the lesions are actually made are involved in the therapeutic effect.

Although the exact neuroanatomic and neurochemical mechanisms underlying depression, OCD, and other anxiety states remain unclear, it is known that the basal ganglia, limbic system, and frontal cortex play a principal role in the pathophysiology of these diseases. Similarly, lesions that affect these target areas can be expected to modulate neuropsychiatric dysfunction.

PATIENT SELECTION

Only patients with severe, chronic, disabling, and treatment-refractory psychiatric illness should be considered for surgical intervention. Chronicity in this context refers to the enduring nature of the illness without extended periods of symptomatic relief and may be less important than the severity of the illness. The severity of the patient's illness is manifested in terms of subjective distress and a decrement in psychosocial functioning. The illness must prove to be refractory to systematic trials of pharmacologic, psychologic, and when appropriate, electroconvulsive therapy before considering neurosurgical intervention. As in all medical decisions, the potential benefit from such an intervention must be balanced against the risks imposed by surgery.

Thoughtful assessment of psychosurgical candidacy requires that criteria for severity, chronicity, disability, and treatment refractoriness be operationalized to form guidelines. In this regard, chronicity would require at least 1 year of enduring symptoms without significant remission, although practically, confirmation of treatment refractoriness usually requires more than 5 years of illness before surgery. Severity is usually measured using validated clinical research instruments corresponding to specific indicators, such as a YBOCS score greater than 20 for OCD or a Beck Depression Inventory (BDI) score greater than 30. Disability may be reflected, for instance, by a Global Assessment of Function (GAF) score of less than 50.

The major psychiatric diagnostic groups, as defined by the revised third edition of the *Diagnostic and Statistical Manual of Mental Disorders* (DSM-III-R), that might benefit from surgical intervention include OCD and major affective disorder (i.e., unipolar major depression or bipolar disorder).[44] In many instances, patients present with mixed disorders combining symptoms of anxiety, depression, and OCD, and these patients remain candidates for surgery. Schizophrenia is not considered an indication for surgery. A history of personality disorder, substance abuse, or other significant axis II symptomatology is often a relative contraindication to surgery. In rare instances, patients with severe violent outbursts and the potential for serious injury or self-mutilation may be considered for bilateral amygdalotomy, limbic leukotomy, or hypothalamotomy.

To determine that their psychiatric illness is refractory to treatment despite appropriate care, all patients must be referred for surgical intervention by their treating psychiatrists. The referring psychiatrist must demonstrate an ongoing commitment to the patient and the evaluation process and must also agree to be responsible for postoperative management. Detailed questionnaires that document the extent and severity of the illness as well as a thorough account of the diagnostic and therapeutic history must be provided by the psychiatrist. The specifics of pharmacologic trials should include the agents used, dose, duration, response, and the reason for discontinuation for any suboptimal trial. Adequate trials of electroconvulsive therapy or behavioral therapy, when clinically appropriate, must also be demonstrated.

The patient and family must agree to participate completely in the evaluation process and in the postoperative psychiatric treatment program. In general, only adult patients (older than 18 years) who are able to render informed consent and who express a genuine desire and commitment to proceed with surgery are accepted. Surgery should be performed only to help a sick patient and never for social or political reasons.

After meeting these criteria, a patient at my institution undergoes a more detailed presurgical screening evaluation by an experienced, multidisciplinary group of psychiatrists, neurosurgeons, and neurologists (i.e., Cingulotomy Assessment Committee). Thorough review of the medical record is carried out to ensure that the illness is refractory to an exhaustive array of conventional therapies. The Massachusetts General Hospital (MGH) evaluation also includes brain MRI, neuropsychologic testing, and independently conducted clinical examinations by a psychiatrist, neurologist, and neurosurgeon in the outpatient setting. An electrocardiogram and appropriate blood tests are obtained to assess medical risks and to exclude organic causes for mental status abnormalities. Validated clinical research instruments (e.g., YBOCS, BDI, Minnesota Multiphasic Personality Inventory [MMPI]) are employed to quantify psychiatric symptom severity and outcomes. There must be unanimous agreement that the patient satisfies selection criteria, that the surgery is indicated, and that the requirements for informed consent are fulfilled. A family member or close relative must also understand the evaluation process, including the indications for, risks of, and alternatives to surgery, and agree to be available to provide emotional support for the patient during the hospitalization.

SURGICAL APPROACHES

Although many methods have been used in the neurosurgical treatment of psychiatric disease, four procedures have evolved as the safest and most effective: anterior cingulotomy, subcaudate tractotomy, limbic leukotomy, and anterior capsulotomy. They are all performed bilaterally and under stereotactic conditions to ensure precise lesioning of target structures. Each procedure has different indications, techniques, results, and complications.

DBS has been tried in a handful of cases as an alternative to lesioning.[45] The reversibility of DBS has theoretical and philosophical advantages, but significant practical and scientific issues remain. Most experience has been in stimulation of the anterior capsule, but the number of patients in whom this procedure has been performed is too small for any meaningful conclusions.

Anterior Cingulotomy

Fulton was the first to suggest that the anterior cingulum would be an appropriate target for psychosurgical intervention, and cingulotomy was initially carried out as an open procedure.[46, 47] Foltz and White[13] reported their experience with stereotactic cingulotomy for intractable pain and noticed that the best results were in patients with concurrent anxiety-depressive states. Ballantine and Giriunas[48] subsequently demonstrated the safety and effectiveness of cingulotomy in a large number of patients, and it has been the surgical procedure of choice in North America during the past 30 years. Current surgical indications are for treatment-refractory major affective disorder and chronic anxiety states, including OCD. The procedure is still performed occasionally for some patients with severe, chronic pain.

Initially, these procedures were carried out with ventriculography, but over the past decade, this has been replaced by MRI-guided stereotactic techniques.[49] Target coordinates are calculated for a point in the cingulum 7 mm from the midline and 20 to 25 mm posterior to the tip of the frontal horns. Lesions are created by heating the 10-mm exposed tip of a thermocoagulation electrode to 85°C for 90 seconds. Intraoperative stimulation is not performed routinely. On the day after surgery, a postoperative MRI scan is obtained to document the placement and extent of the lesions (Fig. 175–1).

Although the patient may experience an immediate reduction in anxiety, there is generally a delay to the onset of beneficial effect on depression and OCD. This latency may be as long as 6 to 12 weeks and must be clearly explained to the patient and referring psychiatrist. If there has been no response to the initial cingulotomy after 3 to 6 months, reoperation and enlargement of the cingulotomy lesion or conversion to limbic leukotomy is considered.

The results of bilateral cingulotomy in 198 patients suffering from a variety of psychiatric disorders were reported retrospectively by Ballantine and coworkers[50] in 1987. With a mean follow-up of 8.6 years, 62% of patients with severe affective disorder were found to have had worthwhile improvement. Similarly, approximately 56% of patients with OCD had worthwhile improvement. Of 14 patients suffering from nonobsessive anxiety disorders, 50% were found to be functionally well, and 29% showed marked improvement. Another retrospective study evaluating cingulotomy in 33 patients with refractory OCD using strict outcome criteria and independent observers demonstrated that at least 25% to 30% of patients benefited substantially from the procedure.[51]

In a prospective, long-term follow-up study of 18 patients who underwent cingulotomy for intractable OCD, 5 patients met very conservative criteria as treatment responders (i.e., more than 35% improvement in

YBOCS scores), and 2 others were considered possible responders for an overall response rate of 28% to 40%.[52] The average duration of follow-up was more than 2 years. Overall, the entire group improved significantly in terms of functional status, and no serious adverse effects were found. This was the first study to demonstrate in a prospective way that cingulotomy was effective in treating OCD as measured by standardized psychiatric rating scales and independent observers. Another prospective, long-term follow-up study by the same group of investigators using the same strict outcome criteria reported similar findings for 44 treatment-refractory OCD patients.[53] Between 32% and 45% of patients were judged to be responders, with a mean follow-up of almost 3 years.

In more than 800 cingulotomies performed at the MGH since 1962, there have been no deaths and only two infections. Early in the series, two acute subdural hematomas resulted from laceration of a cortical artery at the time of introduction of ventricular needles, but only one patient suffered permanent neurological impairment. An independent analysis of 34 patients who underwent cingulotomy demonstrated no significant behavioral or intellectual deficits as a result of the cingulate lesions themselves.[21] Subsequent evaluation of 57 patients before and after cingulotomy found no evidence of lasting neurological or behavioral deficits after surgery.[54] A comparison of preoperative and postoperative Wechsler IQ scores demonstrated significant gains postoperatively. This improvement was greatest in patients with chronic pain and depression but negligible in those with the diagnosis of schizophrenia.

Subcaudate Tractotomy

Subcaudate tractotomy was introduced by Knight[14] in Great Britain in 1964. It was one of the first attempts to restrict the size of the surgical lesion and therefore minimize the side effects seen with standard prefrontal lobotomy. The aim was to interrupt white matter tracts between orbital cortex and subcortical structures by placing a lesion in the region of the substantia innominata, just below the head of the caudate nucleus. Surgical indications included major depressive illness, OCD, and anxiety states, as well as a variety of other psychiatric diagnoses.

The surgical procedure was performed with stereotactic technique using bony landmarks and a ventricular outline. Target coordinates were calculated as 15 mm from the midline and approximately 10 to 11 mm above the planum sphenoidale at the most anterior part of the sella turcica. Intraoperative stimulation was performed looking for autonomic responsivity (e.g., alterations in heart rate, respiration, blood pressure), and targets were typically moved more posteriorly until such responses were obtained. Lesions were originally created using rows of implantable radioactive yttrium-90 seeds, which yielded large lesional volumes of approximately 2000 mm². Smaller lesions are now created by thermocoagulation with MRI stereotactic guidance (Fig. 175–2).

Total improvement or improvement with minimal

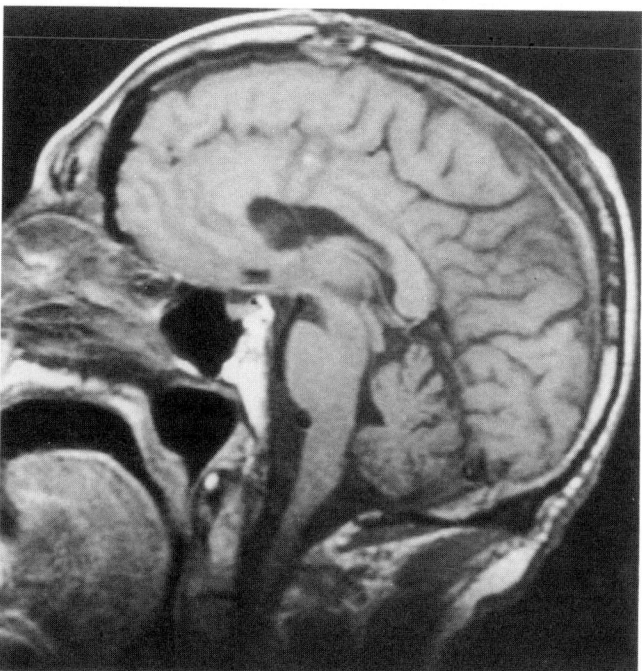

FIGURE 175–1. Sagittal T1-weighted magnetic resonance scan after cingulotomy. Notice the lesions coalesce to ablate approximately 1.0 cm of the anterior cingulate cortex.

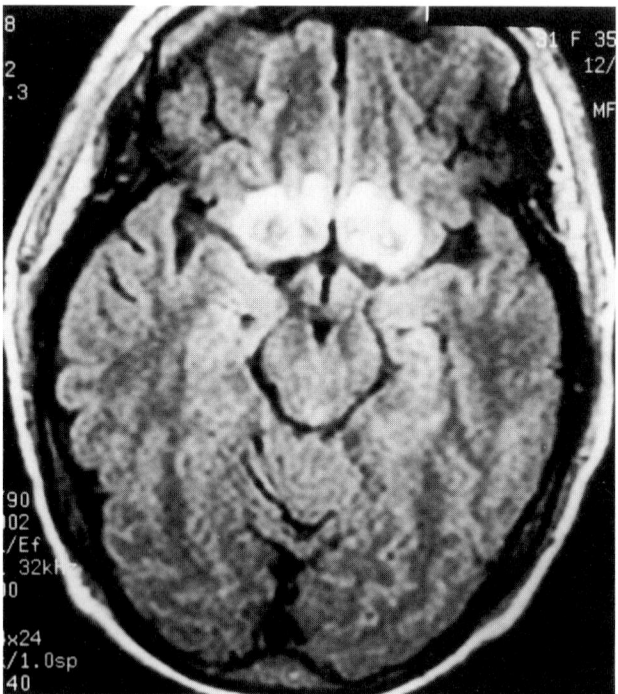

FIGURE 175–2. This axial, T2-weighted magnetic resonance scan was obtained 48 hours after subcaudate tractotomy for bilateral lesions measuring approximately 15 mm in diameter.

symptoms was clinically observed in two thirds of patients with depression and OCD. The best review of the surgical results for subcaudate tractotomy was presented by Goktepe and colleagues[55] in 1975. Using a five-point global scale and rating scales for depression and anxiety, they reviewed 208 patients after a mean follow-up period of 2.5 years. Of the 134 patients available for structured interview, good results were seen in 68% of those suffering from depression, 62.5% of patients with anxiety states, and 50% of patients with obsessive neurosis. Patients with schizophrenia, personality disorder, drug abuse, or alcohol abuse did poorly. Some patients who had only temporary benefit from the initial lesion had second lesions created lateral to the first, with good results seen in about one half.

The incidence of complications was small but included postoperative seizures in 2.2% and undesirable personality traits in 6.7%. Transient disinhibition was common. Of the 25 patients who had died at the time of review, 3 patients had committed suicide. One patient died of inadvertent destruction of the hypothalamus when an yttrium seed migrated off target.

Limbic Leucotomy

Limbic leukotomy was introduced by Kelly and co-workers[56] in 1973. It combines subcaudate tractotomy with anterior cingulotomy. This procedure was designed to disconnect orbital-frontal-thalamic pathways with the former lesion and interrupt an important portion of Papez's circuit with the latter. Kelly and associates[56] reasoned that these two lesions might lead to a

better result for the symptoms of OCD than either lesion alone. Indications for surgical intervention included obsessional neurosis, anxiety states, depression, and a variety of other psychiatric diagnoses.[57]

This procedure was carried out stereotactically, and three 6-mm-diameter lesions were placed in the lower medial quadrant of each frontal lobe, and two lesions were placed in each cingulate gyrus. Intraoperative stimulation was carried out, and if pronounced autonomic responses were observed, this approach was thought to provide physiologic proof of correct location. Lesions were created using a cryoprobe or by thermocoagulation (Fig. 175–3).

Using the same five-point scale described in the study of Goktepe, 66 patients were assessed preoperatively and postoperatively (mean, 16 months). Among patients with obsessional neurosis, 89% were clinically improved; 66% of those with chronic anxiety were improved; 78% of those with depression were improved; and in a small number of schizophrenics, more than 80% were improved. Kelly[57] later reported, for 49 patients with OCD, that 84% were improved 20 months after surgery. They also noticed that postoperative symptom improvement was not immediate; instead a fluctuating but progressive reduction of symptoms occurred over the first postoperative year. Although many patients complained of lethargy, confusion, and a lack of sphincter control in the early postoperative period, persistent complications were rare. No patients developed seizures postoperatively, one patient suffered severe memory loss due to improper lesion placement, and 12% of patients complained of persistent lethargy. Measurements of IQ showed slight improvement postoperatively.[58]

Results were reported for 21 patients in a later series of MRI-guided stereotactic limbic leukotomies.[59] Mean follow-up was more than 2 years, and 35% to 50% of patients were considered to be treatment responders

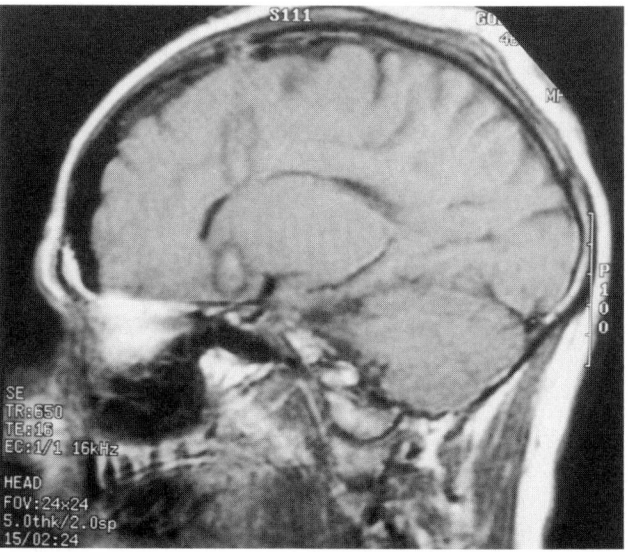

FIGURE 175–3. A sagittal, T1-weighted magnetic resonance scan demonstrates the limbic leukotomy, consisting of anterior cingulotomy combined with subcaudate tractotomy.

using clinically validated rating scales. Transient side effects were more common than after cingulotomy alone, with permanent minor memory loss or urinary difficulties observed in approximately 10% of patients. Limbic leukotomy has also been used successfully in a small number of patients with severe, self-injurious behavior.[60]

Anterior Capsulotomy

Although Talairach and associates[61] were the first to describe anterior capsulotomy, Leksell popularized the procedure for patients with a variety of psychiatric disorders.[15] The aim was to interrupt presumed fronto-thalamic connections in the anterior limb of the internal capsule, where they pass between the head of the caudate nucleus and the putamen. Clinical indications for capsulotomy initially included schizophrenia, depression, chronic anxiety states, and obsessional neurosis, but current indications are almost entirely limited to OCD.

The exact target coordinates as described by Leksell are in the anterior one third of the anterior limb of the internal capsule, 5 mm behind the tip of the frontal horns and 20 mm lateral to the midline at the level of the intercommissural plane. Intraoperative electrical stimulation has not been helpful in terms of determining optimal placement of lesions within the capsule. Lesions were created by thermocoagulation using a bipolar electrode system and were typically about 15 mm high and 4 to 5 mm in diameter (Fig. 175–4). Lesions can also be created using the gamma knife.

In the first 116 patients operated on by Leksell, 50% with obsessional neurosis and 48% with depression had a satisfactory response.[15] Only 20% of patients with anxiety neurosis and 14% of patients with schizophrenia were improved. In this classification system, only patients who were free of symptoms or markedly improved were judged as having a satisfactory response. Of the patients who were rated as worse after capsulotomy, nine had schizophrenia, four had depression, and three had obsessive symptoms. In another series of 35 patients with OCD who underwent capsulotomy and were followed prospectively by independent psychiatrists, 16 were rated as free of symptoms, and 9 were much improved, for an overall satisfactory result of 70%.[62] In a review of all cases of capsulotomy previously reported in the literature, Mindus and colleagues[63] found sufficient data to categorize the outcomes of 213 of the 362 patients. Of these, 137 (64%) were deemed to have a satisfactory result.

Mindus and associates[64] followed 24 patients prospectively with standardized rating scales. Complications of the surgery included transient episodes of confusion during the first week in 19 of 22 patients available for follow-up and occasional nocturnal incontinence. One patient had an intracranial hemorrhage without neurological sequelae, and one patient had seizures. One patient committed suicide in the postoperative phase, and eight patients suffered from depression requiring treatment. Excessive fatigue was a complaint of seven patients, and four had poor memory.

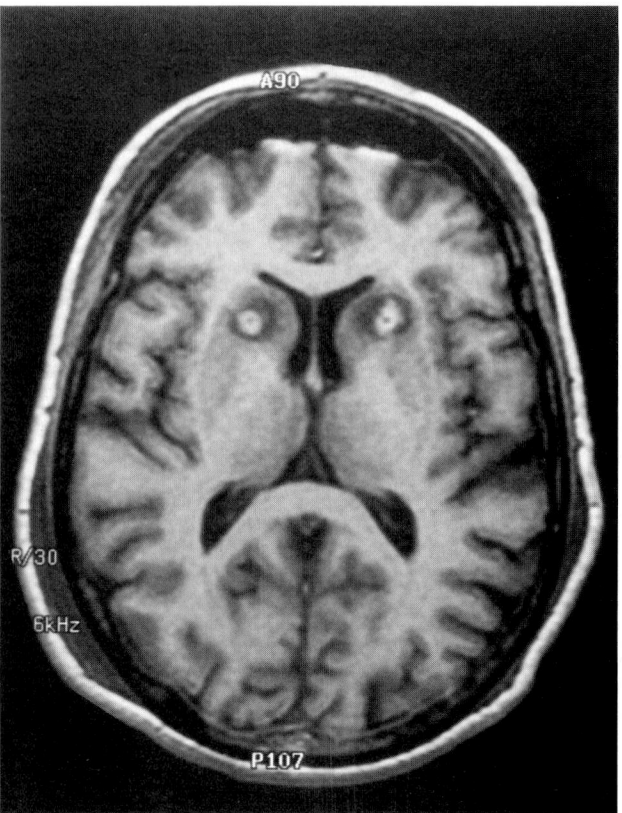

FIGURE 175–4. This axial, T1-weighted magnetic resonance scan was obtained 48 hours after anterior capsulotomy.

Two patients showed slovenliness. Weight gain is also common after capsulotomy, with an overall mean weight gain of about 10% in all patients. Reoperation was required in two patients who did not achieve a satisfactory result, and only one improved after the second operation. Burzaco[65] subjected 17 of his 85 patients to a second procedure, at which time the lesions were enlarged, and one half of these reoperations yielded satisfactory results.

Capsulotomy using the gamma knife has yielded insights into the importance of lesion placement. Initial treatment with a single lesion in the ventral to middle third of the anterior capsule produced a satisfactory clinical result in only 1 of 15 patients with severe treatment-refractory OCD. Reoperation with enlargement of the lesion inferiorly in 13 patients who had failed the initial surgery yielded satisfactory results in 6 patients, for an overall response rate of 36% at 2 years and 58% at 3 years of follow-up. Similar results were obtained for an additional 20 patients who had the two lesions placed at the initial gamma knife surgery. Two important observations arise from this experience. The effective portion of the lesion appears to be in the ventral portion of the capsule close to the subcaudate tractotomy lesion, and the results appear to improve over time.[66]

USE OF PSYCHOSURGERY

Much of the controversy surrounding the use of psychosurgery may be attributed to its rather indiscriminate application and the high incidence of side effects seen with the early procedures. Stereotactic techniques have minimized side effects, but the issue of case selection remains a major consideration. Although initially any patient with a severe psychiatric illness was considered a candidate for surgical intervention, the current indications for psychosurgery are more restrictive. There is general agreement among treatment centers that patients with major affective disorder, chronic anxiety states, and OCD are the best candidates for surgery. Schizophrenia is not an indication for psychosurgery, although patients with concomitant psychotic disorders and depression may still be helped with surgery and should not be excluded. Personality disorders or psychoactive substance use disorder are also significant relative contraindications to surgery. Appropriate selection of patients for surgery remains a major issue and the responsibility of the psychiatrist, guided by the informed and expert opinions of the other members of the psychosurgical team. Advanced neuroimaging data may ultimately aid in optimal patient selection, and preliminary PET studies of patients with OCD indicate that preoperative cerebral metabolic rates within a territory of posterior cingulate cortex predict subsequent outcome after cingulotomy.[67]

With the available data, it is impossible to determine whether there is one optimal surgical technique or strategy. All procedures seem to be generally well tolerated and have few side effects or complications when applied with modern stereotactic techniques. No matter which structure in the limbic system is chosen for ablation, the overall clinical outcome appears quite similar. Obstacles that prevent a direct comparison of results across centers include diagnostic inaccuracies, nonstandardized presurgical evaluation tools, center bias, and varied outcome assessment scales. However, in virtually all published reports, some modification of the Clinical Global Improvement (CGI) scale or equivalent has been used to determine clinical outcome.[68] The CGI rates outcome in seven categories:

1. Very much improved
2. Much improved
3. Slightly improved
4. Unchanged
5. Slightly worse
6. Much worse
7. Very much worse

Although comparisons are imperfect, these scales do appear to have some clinical validity. If category 1 and 2 are considered a satisfactory outcome or favorable response, cingulotomy was effective in 56% of patients with OCD, subcaudate tractotomy in 50%, limbic leukotomy in 61%, and capsulotomy in 67%. In patients with major affective disorder, cingulotomy was effective in 56%, subcaudate tractotomy in 50%, limbic leukotomy in 61%, and capsulotomy in 67%.[69]

In 1977, Kullberg[70] attempted to compare cingulotomy and capsulotomy in the treatment of 26 patients in a randomized fashion. Six of 13 capsulotomy patients and 3 of 13 cingulotomy patients were better,

but transient deterioration in mental status was much worse after capsulotomy than after cingulotomy.

One of the major difficulties in evaluating surgery for neuropsychiatric illness is that many centers report their results using subjective rating scales. Only when centers report their experience using validated, objective rating scales (e.g., YBOCS, BDI) will comparisons be possible. Based on current methods of comparison, the clinical superiority of any one procedure is not convincing. Although many centers claim advantages for their specific surgical intervention, it is not possible to determine whether one of the four major psychosurgical procedures is superior to the others. Cingulotomy is more commonly performed in the United States, whereas in Europe, capsulotomy and limbic leukotomy are more prevalent. They all appear roughly equivalent from a therapeutic point of view, but in terms of unwanted side effects, cingulotomy appears to be the safest of all procedures performed. Cingulotomy also appears to be especially effective for major depression.

At first glance, it would appear that cingulotomy, anterior capsulotomy, subcaudate tractotomy, and limbic leukotomy are distinct surgical procedures with unique anatomic targets. However, remarkable similarities exist, especially between anterior capsulotomy and subcaudate tractotomy. It is apparent that the effective portion of the anterior capsulotomy lesion is the inferior or ventral part of the lesion below the intercommissural plane. This is the same area encompassed by the superior or dorsal portion of the subcaudate tractotomy lesion, and it contains the ventral striatum or nucleus accumbens, an area of the brain implicated in many human behavioral studies. In retrospect, this area was also the target of many of the early psychosurgical interventions.

Not all surgical interventions are performed in a similar fashion from one center to another. For any given procedure, there may be significant differences in lesion location, volume, and extent, and it is therefore critical to define lesion characteristics with postoperative MRI.

Regardless of the choice of procedure, surgical failures should be investigated, and if the lesion size or location is suboptimal, consideration should be given to another procedure. The rate of repeat surgery in capsulotomy patients has been reported as 20%. In 5 of the 24 patients in the Mindus series,[64] a significant correlation was found between neuroradiologic ranking of a target site and the psychiatric outcome, suggesting that the site and extent of lesion may be important factors influencing outcome. At least 45% of patients undergoing cingulotomy require repeat operations, with good results being salvaged in one half.[49] The exact size or volume of tissue required for an effective outcome at each of the target sites has yet to be determined.

The method used for creating the lesion itself does not appear to influence results. There is considerable interest in the use of external radiosurgical techniques for psychosurgery, but this remains controversial. Although radiosurgery does not require introduction of a subcortical electrode, it remains a surgical procedure with a small but significant complication rate.[71] Little is known about the exact dosimetry required for satisfactory lesions, and the latency to onset of beneficial effect as radionecrosis develops may not be reasonable for patients with a grave psychiatric condition. There is considerable variability in terms of the lesion volume between individuals for the same radiation dose.[72] In view of the proliferation of radiosurgical centers and the inexperience of these same groups with psychosurgery, the potential for misapplication of this technique is great.

Although controversy exists regarding the exact choice of surgical procedure to be employed, there is unanimous agreement that the presurgical evaluation be performed by committed multidisciplinary teams with expertise and experience in the surgical treatment of psychiatric illness. Diagnosis based on the DSM-III-R classification scheme is encouraged, and although it is impossible to mandate uniformly across all centers, prospective trials employing standardized clinical instruments with long-term follow-up are needed. Comparisons of preoperative and postoperative functional status remain an important parameter in addition to target psychiatric symptoms in characterizing outcomes. All centers with experience emphasize the importance of rehabilitation postoperatively and the need for ongoing psychiatric follow-up. The operation is not a panacea and should be considered as only one aspect in the overall management of these patients. Despite the advent of new and effective psychopharmacologic agents, it is generally thought that the procedure is underused by centers employing this form of psychosurgery. Caution must be urged, however, regarding the surgical treatment of psychiatric disease to ensure that the indiscriminate application of this form of therapy never recurs.

CONCLUSIONS

The surgical treatment of psychiatric disease can be helpful in certain patients with severe, disabling, and treatment-refractory major affective disorders, OCD, and chronic anxiety states. Psychosurgical treatment should be carried out only by an expert multidisciplinary team with experience in these disorders. Surgery should be considered as one part of an entire treatment plan and must be followed by an appropriate psychiatric rehabilitation program. Many patients are greatly improved after surgery, and the complications or side effects are few. Surgical intervention remains an important therapeutic option for disabling psychiatric disease and is probably underused.

REFERENCES

1. Burckhardt G: Uber Rindenexcisionen, als Beitrag zur operativen Therapie der Psychosen. Z Psychiatr 47:463–548, 1891.
2. Fulton JF, Jacobsen CF: Fonctions des lobes frontaux; etude comparee chez l'homme et les singes chimpanzes. In Proceedings of the International Neurological Congress. London, 1935, pp 70–71 (abstract).
3. Moniz E: Prefrontal leucotomy in the treatment of mental disorders. Am J Psychiatry 93:1379–1385, 1937.
4. Freeman W, Watts JW: Prefrontal lobotomy in the treatment of mental disorders. South Med J 30:23–31, 1937.
5. Freeman W, Watts JW: Psychosurgery: Intelligence, emotion and social behavior following prefrontal lobotomy for mental disorders. Springfield, IL, Thomas, 1942.
6. Freeman W: Transorbital leucotomy. Lancet 2:371–373, 1948.
7. Tooth JC, Newton MP: Leucotomy in England and Wales 1942–1954. Reports on public health and medical subjects No. 104. London, Her Majesty's Stationary Office, 1961.
8. Pool JL: Topectomy: A surgical procedure for the treatment of mental illness. J Nerv Ment Dis 110:164–173, 1949.
9. Poppen JL: Technique of prefrontal lobotomy. J Neurosurg 5:514–520, 1948.
10. Scoville W: Selective cortical undercutting. J Neurosurg 6:65, 1949.
11. Whitty CWM, Duffield JE, Tow PM, et al: Anterior cingulectomy in the treatment of mental disease. Lancet 1:475–481, 1952.
12. Falconer MA, Schurr PH: Surgical treatment of mental illness: Recent progress in psychiatry, vol 3. London, J&A Churchill, 1959, pp 352–367.
13. Foltz EL, White LE Jr: Pain relief by frontal cingulotomy. J Neurosurg 19:89–94, 1962.
14. Knight GC: The orbital cortex as an objective in the surgical treatment of mental illness. The development of the stereotactic approach. Br J Surg 51:114–124, 1964.
15. Herner T: Treatment of mental disorders with frontal stereotactic thermal lesions: A follow-up study of 116 cases. Acta Psychiatr Neurol Scand 158:36, 1961 (abstract).
16. Kelly D, Richardson A, Mitchell-Heggs N: Stereotactic limbic leucotomy: Neurophysiologic aspects and operative technique. Br J Psychiatry 123:133–140, 1973.
17. Narabayashi H, Nagao T, Saito Y, et al: Stereotactic amygdalotomy for behavior disorders. Arch Neurol 9:1–16, 1963.
18. Hassler R, Dieckmann NG: Relief of obsessive compulsive disorders, phobias and tics by stereotactic coagulation of the rostral intralaminar and medial thalamic nuclei. In Laitinen LV, Livingston KV (eds): Surgical Approaches in Psychiatry. Proceedings of the Third International Congress of Psychosurgery. Baltimore, University Park Press, 1973, pp 206–212.
19. Dieckmann NG, Hassler R: Treatment of sexual violence by stereotactic hypothalamotomy. In Sweet WH, Obrador S, Martin-Rodriguez JG (eds): Neurosurgical Treatment in Psychiatry, Pain and Epilepsy. Baltimore, University Park Press, 1977, pp 451–462.
20. National Commission for the Protection of Human Subjects of Biomedical and Behavioral Research: Report and Recommendations: Psychosurgery. Department of Health and Human Services, publication number (OS) 77-002. Washington, DC: US Government Printing Office, 1979.
21. Corkin S, Twitchell TE, Sullivan EV: Safety and efficacy of cingulotomy for pain and psychiatric disorders. In Hitchcock ER, Ballantine HT, Myerson BA (eds): Modern Concepts in Psychiatric Surgery. Amsterdam, Elsevier, 1979, pp 253–272.
22. Hay P, Sachdev P, Cumming S, et al: Treatment of obsessive-compulsive disorder by psychosurgery. Acta Psychiatr Scand 87:197–207, 1993.
23. Papez JW: A proposed mechanism of emotion. Arch Neurol Psychiatry 38:725–743, 1937.
24. McLean PD: Some psychiatric implications of physiologic studies on the frontotemporal portion of limbic system. Electroencephalogr Clin Neurophysiol 4:407–418, 1952.
25. Laitinen LV: Emotional responses to subcortical electrical stimulation in psychiatric patients. Clin Neurol Neurosurg 81:148–157, 1979.
26. Ranson SW: The hypothalamus: Its significance for visceral innervation and emotional expression. Trans Coll Physicians Phila (Series IV) 2:222–242, 1934.
27. Rauch SL, Jenike MA: Neurobiological models of obsessive compulsive disorder. Psychosomatics 34:20–32, 1993.
28. Insel TR: Toward a neuroanatomy of obsessive-compulsive disorder. Arch Gen Psychiatry 49:739–744, 1992.
29. Weilburg JB, Mesulam MM, Weintraub S, et al: Focal striatal abnormalities in a patient with obsessive compulsive disorder. Arch Neurol 46:233–236, 1989.

30. LaPlane E, Levasseur M, Pillon B, et al: Obsessions-compulsions and behavioral changes with bilateral basal ganglia lesions: A neuropsychological, magnetic resonance imaging and positron tomography study. Brain 112:699–725, 1989.

31. Baxter LR, Schwartz JM, Guze BH, et al: Neuroimaging in obsessive compulsive disorder: Seeking the mediating neuroanatomy. In Jenike MA, Baer L, Minichiello WE (eds): Obsessive Compulsive Disorder: Theory and Management, 2nd ed. Chicago, Year Book Medical Publishers, 1990, pp 167–188.

32. Berthier ML, Kulisevsky J, Gironell A, et al: Obsessive-compulsive disorder associated with brain lesions: Clinical phenomenology, cognitive function, and anatomic correlates. Neurology 47: 353–361, 1996.

33. Jenike MA, Breiter HCR, Baer L, et al: Cerebral structural abnormalities in patients with obsessive-compulsive disorder: A quantitative morphometric magnetic resonance imaging study. Arch Gen Psychiatry 53:625–632, 1996.

34. Saxena S, Brody AL, Maidment KM, et al: Localized orbitofrontal and subcortical metabolic changes and predictors of response to paroxetine treatment in obsessive-compulsive disorder. Neuropsychopharmacology 21:683–693, 1999.

35. Baxter LR Jr, Schwartz JM, Bergman KS, et al: Caudate glucose metabolic rate changes with both drug and behavior therapy for obsessive compulsive disorder. Arch Gen Psychiatry 49:681–689, 1992.

36. Nordahl TE, Benkelfat C, Semple WE, et al: Cerebral glucose metabolic rates in obsessive-compulsive disorder. Neuropsychopharmacology 2:23–28, 1989.

37. Swedo SE, Schapiro MB, Grady CL, et al: Cerebral glucose metabolism in childhood-onset obsessive-compulsive disorder. Arch Gen Psychiatry 46:518–523, 1989.

38. Swedo SE, Pietrii P, Leonard HL, et al: Cerebral glucose metabolism in childhood-onset obsessive-compulsive disorder: Revisualization during pharmacotherapy. Arch Gen Psychiatry 49:690–694, 1992.

39. Modell J, Mountz J, Curtis G, et al: Neurophysiologic dysfunction in basal ganglia/limbic striatal and thalamocortical circuits as a pathogenetic mechanism of obsessive compulsive disorder. J Neuropsychiatry 1:27–36, 1989.

40. Alexander GE, Crutcher MD, DeLong MR: Basal ganglia-thalamocortical circuits: Parallel substrates for motor, oculomotor, "prefrontal" and "limbic" functions. Prog Brain Res 85:119–146, 1990.

41. Strom-Olsen R, Carlisle S: Bi-frontal stereotactic tractotomy: A follow-up study of its effects on 210 patients. Br J Psychiatry 118: 141–154, 1971.

42. Mesulam M-M: Patterns in behavioral neuroanatomy: Association areas, the limbic system, and hemispheric specialization. In Mesulam M-M (ed): Principles of Behavioral Neurology. Philadelphia, FA Davis, 1985, pp 1–70.

43. Rauch SL, Kim H, Makris N, et al: Volumetric reduction in caudate nucleus following stereotactic lesions of anterior cingulate cortex in humans: A morphometric magnetic resonance imaging study. J Neurosurg 93:1019–1025, 2000.

44. American Psychiatric Association: Diagnostic and Statistical Manual of Mental Disorders, 3rd ed., revised. Washington, DC, American Psychiatric Association, 1987.

45. Nuttin B, Gabriels L, Cosyns P, et al: Electrical stimulation of the brain for psychiatric disorders. CNS Spectrums 5:35–39, 2000.

46. Fulton JE: Frontal Lobotomy and Affective Behavior: A Neurophysiological Analysis. New York, WW Norton, 1951.

47. Le Beau J: Anterior cingulectomy in man. J Neurosurg 11:268–276, 1954.

48. Ballantine HT, Giriunas IE: Treatment of intractable psychiatric illness and chronic pain by stereotactic cingulotomy. In Schmidek HH, Sweet WH (eds): Operative Neurosurgical Techniques. New York, Grune & Stratton, 1982, pp 1069–1075.

49. Spangler W, Cosgrove GR, Ballantine HT, et al: MR-guided stereotactic cingulotomy for intractable psychiatric disease. Neurosurgery 38:1071–1078, 1996.

50. Ballantine HT, Bouckoms AJ, Thomas EK, et al: Treatment of psychiatric illness by stereotactic cingulotomy. Biol Psychiatry 22:807–819, 1987.

51. Jenike MA, Baer L, Ballantine HT, et al: Cingulotomy for refractory obsessive compulsive disorder: A long term follow-up of 33 patients. Arch Gen Psychiatry 48:548–555, 1991.

52. Baer L, Rauch SL, Ballantine HT, et al: Cingulotomy for treatment of refractory obsessive-compulsive disorder: Prospective long-term follow-up of 18 patients. Arch Gen Psychiatry 52:384–392, 1995.

53. Dougherty DD, Baer L, Cosgrove GR, et al: Update on cingulotomy for intractable obsessive-compulsive disorder: Prospective long-term follow-up of 44 patients. Am J Psychiatry 159: 269–275, 2002.

54. Corkin S: A prospective study of cingulotomy. In Valenstein ES (ed): The psychosurgery debate. San Francisco, WH Freeman, 1980, p 264.

55. Goktepe EO, Young LB, Bridges PK: A further review of the results of stereotactic subcaudate tractotomy. Br J Psychiatry 126: 270–280, 1975.

56. Kelly D, Richardson A, Mitchell-Heggs N: Technique and assessment of limbic leucotomy. In Laitinen LV, Livingston KE (eds): Surgical Approaches in Psychiatry. Baltimore, University Park Press, 1973, pp 165–173.

57. Kelly D: The Limbic System. Sex, Anxiety and Emotions: Physiologic Basis and Treatment. Springfield, IL, Charles C Thomas, 1980, pp 197–300.

58. Mitchell-Heggs N, Kelly D, Richardson A: Stereotactic limbic leucotomy—a follow-up at 16 months. Br J Psychiatry 128:226–240, 1976.

59. Montoya A, Weiss AP, Price BH, et al: Magnetic resonance image-guided stereotactic limbic leucotomy for intractable psychiatric disease. Neurosurgery 50:1043–1052, 2002.

60. Price BH, Baral I, Cosgrove GR, et al: Improvement in severe self-mutilation following limbic leucotomy: A series of 5 consecutive cases. J Clin Psychiatry 62:925–932, 2001.

61. Talairach J, Hecaen H, David M: Lobotomie prefrontale limitee par electrocoagulation des fibres thalamo-frontalis leur emergence du bras anterior de la capsule interne. In Proceedings of the 4th Congress Neurologique Internationale. Paris, Masson, 1949, p 141.

62. Mindus P: Capsulotomy in anxiety disorders: A multidisciplinary study [thesis]. Stockholm, Karolinska Institute, 1991.

63. Mindus P, Rasmussen SA, Lindquist C: Neurosurgical treatment for refractory obsessive-compulsive disorder: Implications for understanding frontal lobe function. J Neuropsychiatry 6:467–477, 1994.

64. Mindus P, Edman G, Andreewitch S: A prospective, long-term study of personality traits in patients with intractable obsessional illness treated by capsulotomy. Acta Psychiatr Scand 99:40–50, 1999.

65. Burzaco J: Stereotactic surgery in the treatment of obsessive compulsive neurosis. In Perris C, Struwe G, Janssen B (eds): Biological Psychiatry. Amsterdam, Elsevier, 1981, pp 1108–1109.

66. Rasmussen S, Greenberg B, Mindus P, et al: Neurosurgical approaches to intractable obsessive-compulsive disorder. CNS Spectrums 5:23–34, 2000.

67. Rauch SL, Dougherty DD, Cosgrove GR, et al: Cerebral metabolic correlates as potential predictors of response to anterior cingulotomy for obsessive compulsive disorder. Biol Psychiatry 50: 659–667, 2001.

68. Pippard J: Rostral leucotomy: A report on 240 cases personally followed up after one and one half to five years. J Mental Sci 101:756–773, 1955.

69. Cosgrove GR, Rauch SL: Psychosurgery. In Gildenberg PH (ed): Neurosurgical Clinics of North America. Philadelphia, WB Saunders, 1995.

70. Kullberg G: Differences in effect of capsulotomy and cingulotomy. In Sweet WH, Obrador S, Martin-Rodriguez JG (eds): Neurosurgical Treatment in Psychiatry, Pain and Epilepsy. Baltimore, University Park Press, 1977, pp 301–308.

71. Leksell L, Backlund EO: Stereotactic gamma capsulotomy. In Hitchcock ER, Ballantine HT Jr, Meyerson BA (eds): Modern Concepts in Psychiatric Surgery. Amsterdam, Elsevier/North Holland Biomedical Press, 1979, p 213.

72. Lindquist C, Hindmarsh T, Kihlstrom L, et al: MRI and CT studies of radionecrosis development in the normal human brain. In Steiner L (ed): Radiosurgery Baseline and Trends. New York, Raven Press, 1992, pp 245–256.

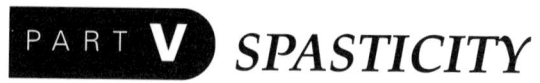

Ablative Surgery for Spasticity

KENNETH F. CASEY ■ RAYMOND SEKULA

HISTORY OF SPASTICITY

The history of spasticity in some respects mirrors the history of neurology and neurosurgery. Just over a century ago, Sherrington[1] demonstrated that sectioning a cat's brainstem just above the vestibular nuclei produced an animal with increased stretch reflex and increased tone in the extensor muscles. The cat retained the ability to stand on all four extremities with rigid legs.[1] This has been called *decerebrate rigidity.* Further research demonstrated that rigidity was influenced by certain supratentorial influences through the spinal cord and that normal movement might be said to represent a pattern of facilitated disinhibition. In a case in 1908, Sir Victor Horsley dramatically relieved spasmodic movements of the left upper extremity in a 14-year-old boy by resection of the precentral gyrus. Cortical resections for treatment of movement disorders, tremor, and spasticity followed through the 1930s. In 1946, Magoun and Rhines[2] regarded spasticity and rigidity as an uncontrolled and augmented stretch reflex, which they thought was produced by loss of the inhibitory pathways from the cortex. They postulated that these pathways arose from area 4, area 4S, and perhaps area 6. In 1940, Tauer[3] stated that a pure cortical lesion in a monkey only caused flaccid paralysis. In 1943, Fulton[4] observed that ablation of area 6 in the brain caused spasticity but that it was accompanied by other symptoms related to the cortical lesion. However, when Magoun and Rhines[2] referred to the loss of inhibitory pathways from area 4S, located between areas 4 and 6, they regarded this as a suppression zone that used the pathways of the reticulospinal system to influence the cord.

In 1939, the efforts of Meyers[5] produced some of the current concepts of the operative treatment of movement disorders, including spasticity and dyskinesia. Meyers examined the role of the basal ganglia in the production of movement disorders and the interruption of these structures as treatment. Putnam[6] had opted for interruption of the descending motor fibers at the level of the cervical cord, and Walker[7] had sectioned them to the level of the cerebral peduncles. These surgeons' efforts directed at the pyramidal motor system were effective in relieving involuntary movements of spasticity but produced hemiparesis. The work of Meyers on the basal ganglia produced relief of rigidity and tremor, especially when the target was the medial globus pallidus. This led him to conclude that interruption of the pallidal-fugal pathway through the transventricular approach with secondary interruption of the ansa lenticularis was the most effective way to relieve tremor rigidity.[5]

Ablative operations for spasticity built on this understanding that rigidity and spasticity result from the natural imbalance or interruption of pathways from the cortex to the basal ganglia and back. Interruption or facilitation of the feedback loop can address spasticity and rigidity (Fig. 176–1). Sherrington[1] was able

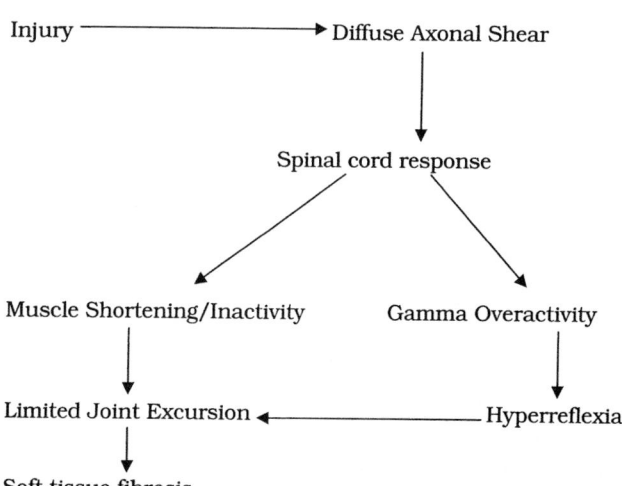

FIGURE 176–1. The pathologic process leads to muscle shortening, hyperreflexia, and the secondary effects of spasticity.

to eliminate the rigidity in the cat preparation by cutting some of the dorsal roots directly. This set the stage for the ablative and neuro-augmentative procedures for spasticity.

OUTCOME MEASURES FOR SPASTICITY MANAGEMENT

As we deal with patients with spasticity, it becomes obvious that there is a need to assess the treatment we are rendering to the patient. Treatment and assessment of outcomes occurs on four levels: assessing the technical outcome, functional outcome, cost-effectiveness of the treatment, and patient satisfaction. The need for assessment has been increasing in the past several years, driven by third-party payers and clinicians who recognize the need to reproducibly evaluate and compare the effects of different treatments as we strive to find what is best for our patients. In the past, assessment tools have been difficult to apply universally for patients with spasticity. Several issues have caused this problem, particularly the time of day, positional issues, drugs and coincident use, concurrent illnesses, emotional states, and training effects, all of which directly affect the degree of spasticity and underlying tone.[8] Some knowledge of these different effects can be applied in such a way that testing occurs at a reasonably relevant interval and allows reproducibility day by day. Unfortunately, the effects of training and the emotional states, for example, are difficult to factor in, and this suggests the need for the surgeon to be aware of multiple avenues of assessment.

The ideal test would have a well-defined scoring system, be easy to administer, and require a relatively short time frame so that it could be used daily. Very few clinical spasticity tests meet these criteria, and they are difficult to address to different patient populations in view of language skills, clinical requirements, and local versus global effects of a procedure. When looking at the issue of spasticity, even for technical outcomes, a test is needed that looks beyond the limb or side in question, taking into account the global effects of spasticity and the potential changes if spasticity decreases. A common example is the use of a test dose of intrathecal baclofen, with which the reduction in tone is quite appropriate, but a great deal of function is lost because the patient had been using some of the spasticity previously present to support gait, turning, or other activities. For focal spasticity in a single limb or several limbs in sequence, different electrodiagnostic tests have been used with some reliability. Electromyography can demonstrate the activity of the muscles at rest, patterns of overactivity and underactivity, incomplete recruitment, and patterns of co-contraction during simple movement.[8] Pretreatment and post-treatment recordings, especially after local blocks, can be quite useful.

Objective technical measures of spasticity have traditionally been aimed at a single joint or a group of joints such as angled torque measurements, the H-reflex, and the vibratory inhibitory reflex.[9] Although

TABLE 176–1 ■ **Modified Ashworth Scale**

SCORE	TONE*
1	Minimal resistance at elbow
2	Moderate resistance at elbow
3	Difficult to flex/extend at elbow
4	Cannot flex/extend at elbow

*The modified Ashworth scale, which provides a reproducible, ordinal scale of tone, is defined only at the elbow, although it has been widely applied to other joints.

these are precise measurements, they are clinically not useful because of their limitations of expense and lack of portability. Katz and colleagues[10] described a relationship between the clinical assessment of spasticity as included in the Ashworth scale[11] (Table 176–1) and these biomechanical measurements, including the H-reflex and pendulum test.[10, 11] They also assessed the Fugl-Meyer scale, which is a measurement of motor impairment. In the upper extremity, the Ashworth and Fugl-Meyer scores correlated well. In the lower extremity, the Ashworth scale did not correlate well with Fugl-Meyer score but did with the pendulum test.[10]

Overall, a simple preassessment test for the surgeon is the Ashworth scale (recognizing its limitations) used with a joint angle measurement test using a goniometer; x-ray studies and torque angles can be useful as well. Unfortunately, no ideal test exists to measure the technical aspects of spasticity care. For functional independence, the Functional Independence Measure and the Barthel Index are examples of multidimensional scales in which performance on many items is rated individually; the scores are added, and an overall score is reached.[12] These types of scales are different in that the intervals are not assumed to be equal; the difference between 1 and 2 may not be equal in severity to the interval between 6 and 7. The noninterval scaling is nonparametric, and probabilistic measurements, including the Rasch analysis, must be used. This mathematical procedure uses a total of scores that represent some interval data, usually in ordinals, and that is divided in a manner that equalizes the data. Although this is useful for interventional testing or study, it is quite limited for day-to-day use.[13, 14]

Quality-of-life indexes are measures that have received increasing attention in the literature. They include the Sickness Impact Profile and the 36-item Short Form Health Survey (SF-36), which are in widespread use and are easily applied. Scoring can be accomplished after a short interval of assessment (see Appendix). These indexes, however, do not have stroke or spasticity specific questions and are global assessment tests. The Canadian Occupational Performance Measure computes individualized areas, including self-care, productivity, and leisure. This involves a patient interview. Goals are defined and then weighted, and the assessment after therapy is repeated and compared with the pretreatment status.[15]

Spasticity defined as loss of independent muscle contraction is only part of the triad of dysfunction that these patients have.[16] Muscle shortening that starts shortly after the injury to the brain is typically accompanied by overactivity, especially in the spinal cord at the level of the alpha motoneuron. This has classically been thought to be related to the removal of suprasegmental inhibitory influences.[17] Any treatments, in conceptualization of the treatment and the assessment of their outcome, should focus on reduction of spasticity as a marker for the degree of muscle overactivity, but ablative therapy must also be combined with muscle lengthening to allow more effective joint motion and produce patient satisfaction.

All therapies, whether they are chemically ablative, surgically ablative, or chemically or electrically neuroaugmentive, aim to improve the degree of muscle stretch (i.e., lengthening the muscle) and therefore reduce pain and improve activity. Muscle lengthening is best achieved with continuous application of stretching devices. This includes rigid or semi-rigid splints, dynamic splints, serial casting, and some automated devices.[17, 18] Muscle relaxation then can be achieved with chemical means orally, locally, or regionally or by ablated neural input to the muscle.

ABLATIVE PHARMACOLOGIC TREATMENTS FOR SPASTICITY

In this section, we review the pathophysiology, purported local pharmacology, and risks and benefits associated with local anesthetics, any alcohol, and cold in the ablative treatment of spasticity (Table 176–2).

Local anesthetics are ionic channel-blocking agents that alter the time of sodium conductance in the tissue to which they are applied. Their action is reversible, and in appropriate concentrations, there is no structural damage to the nerve fibers or muscle cells injected. They act on peripheral nerve tissue and can have central action when administered intravenously.[19] Gasser and Erlinger[20] described the various sizes of nerve fibers, and Erlanger reported that the small nerve fibers are more readily affected than large nerve fibers. Franz and Perry[21] suggested that the shorter internodal distance and small axons were responsible for the more rapid onset and slower recovery from the block. Some ionic channel blockers can have differential effects on the types of fibers despite their similar size. Etidocaine has a prolonged effect on motor fibers compared with sensory fibers of the same size.

Each anesthetic has a pharmacologic profile that addresses the onset of action (range, 3 to 15 minutes), the duration of action (20 to 45 minutes), and the toxic dose (3 to 7 mg/kg). The duration of the effect can be altered by the amount of drug given. Up to the limit of toxicity, however, local efforts to isolate the drug in a limb, including the concomitant use of epinephrine, the local application of cold, and isolation of the limb with a tourniquet (e.g., lidocaine regional block), are all examples of this concept. Systemic toxicity is also affected by the degree of absorption into the circulation, and this is an additional reason to use local vasoconstrictors in areas of high blood flow. The toxic effects of local anesthetics in common use (e.g., lidocaine, etidocaine, bupivacaine) involve the cardiovascular system and the central nervous system. In the cardiovascular system, blood pressure may be affected by dilatation of the arterial tree, and cardiac collapse and changes in the myocardium may occur with alterations in excitability and conduction time. In the central nervous system, restlessness and seizures may occur, and when local anesthetics are used, intravenous access should be readily available for this reason.

When selecting local anesthetics, the duration of action can aid in the evaluation of the patient. For diagnostic evaluations, lidocaine, which has the shortest time to onset and the shortest duration, can be used for sampling of several different muscle groups in a given day. The lidocaine dose is typically between 0.5% and 2.0% up to 7 mg/kg. Etidocaine and bupivacaine have a greater time to onset of action, typically 15 to 30 minutes, and a prolonged duration (4 to 6 hours in the case of bupivacaine). The standard dose of bupivacaine involves solutions of 0.25% to 0.75%, and the toxic dose is thought to be 3 mg/kg. Bupivacaine allows the clinician to evaluate the effect of muscle lengthening while the longer-lasting block is sustained, but etidocaine has a greater propensity to block autofibers and somatic fibers and can be quite useful in that regard. Etidocaine can be used in 0.5% to 1.0% solutions, and the dose is up to 6 mg/kg without epinephrine. A local anesthetic treatment can allow the clinician and the patient to determine which of the triad (i.e., spasticity, muscle contraction, and overactivity of co-contractile muscles) is most operative in a particular patient. This allows the clinician to select the type of block and more precisely identify the site of an ablative procedure.

These blocks can be performed intramuscularly near the motor end points and within the muscle itself with the use of larger volumes to allow diffusion throughout the muscle. In nerve block techniques, the mixed peripheral nerve is identified, and the agent is placed in proximity, with the understanding that the distance away from the nerve and diffusion into the nerve can take a variable amount of time. The literature suggests that the duration of the block is greatest in the central fibers of any nerve because of the uptake profile across the epineurium into the core fibers. Technical adjuncts to intramuscular or peripheral nerve blocks can involve the use of hollow-core Teflon needles through which low-grade stimulation and recording can be performed. In the case of a mixed nerve block, the needle is placed as close as possible to the nerve by identifying the lowest current required to produce nerve activity or achieve a threshold of sensation. In the case of motor point blocks, the needle is positioned until minimal stimulation is required to produce a small twitch, and the technique involves the use of short pulse width and very low milliamperage.

Chemical neurolysis can be achieved with phenol or alcohol and is effective for children and adults.[22, 23] Awad[24] carefully investigated phenol blocks for muscle spasticity and found that peripheral neurolysis could be quite effective for up to 12 months.[25] Phenol has

TABLE 176–2 ■ **Spasticity Treatment**

TREATMENT	ROUTE	WHERE DONE	MECHANISM	ADVANTAGES (BENEFIT)	DISADVANTAGES (COSTS)	DURATION OF EFFECT
Biofeedback	Training	IH	Patient learns how to inhibit spasms	No medication	Requires concentration; may not be sufficient	Long term
Wheelchair positioning		IH	Inhibits spasticity	6–12 h per day	Expensive; skin risk if improperly placed	As long as in wheelchair plus long term
Physical and occupational therapy	Active and passive ROM	IH	Stretches tissues, inhibits spasticity	No meds: professional staff can customize treatment and monitor	Subject to staffing, transport	1–7 days
Continuous passive motion (CPM)		IH	Maintains ROM, inhibits spasticity	Does not need therapist; gentle; as much as necessary	Needs daily setup; less customized; skin risk; not yet covered	As much as needed
Baclofen oral (Lioresal)	Oral medication	IH	Blocks nerve transmission selectively	Rare side effects or toxicity; selectively inhibits spastic muscle	Cannot increase or decrease suddenly; must take several times per day	Approx. 6 hours
Diazepam (Valium)	Oral medication	IH	Blocks nerve transmission selectively	Selectively inhibits spastic muscle	Dependency; sedation; must take several times per day	6–12 hours
Dantrium	Oral medication	IH	Blocks muscle transmission nonselectively	Always works	Affects good and bad muscles—causes some weakness; liver toxicity—blood every month; must take for rest of life	6–12 hours
Lidocaine or bupivacaine	Injection of nerve or motor point	IH	Temporarily blocks nerve and muscle	Reversible	Must be followed by permanent injection, which may have different effect	4–6 hours
Phenol	Injection of nerve or motor point	IH	Damages nerve along its path	Always works to some degree; oral meds not needed; can be done at IH	Partly permanent; can cause pain	6–52 weeks
Alcohol	Injection	IH	Damages nerve along its path	Same as phenol	Same as phenol	Months to years
Botox	Injection of motor point	Hospital and surgery	Blocks transmission of nerve to muscle	No oral meds; reversible	Only one muscle at a time; must be repeated; may become ineffective; not yet covered by some insurance	3–6 months
Baclofen pump	Neurosurgery	Hospital and surgery	Blocks nerve transmission in spinal cord	Minimal oral meds; adjustable	Pump must be filled periodically; risk of pump failure; not covered by some insurance	Months to years
Dorsal column stimulator	Neurosurgery	Hospital and surgery	Sends alternate message to pain fibers	Relatively benign	Often not effective	None to years
Radiofrequency neurolysis	Neurosurgery	Hospital and surgery	Damages nerve	Permanent; one time	Irreversible; requires hospitalization and anesthesia	Months to years
Dorsal rhizotomy	Neurosurgery	Hospital, inpatient	Cuts nerves	Permanent	Spasticity may recur or move elsewhere	Months to years
Myelotomy	Neurosurgery	Hospital, inpatient	Cuts tracts of spinal cord	One time	Variable effectiveness	Months to years
Flap surgery (skin or skin plus muscle)	Plastic surgery	Hospital, inpatient	Moves good skin and/or muscle to cover open wound	Quicker healing than non-flap	Requires clean wound; permanent risk of recurrence; not all wounds can be flapped	Months to years
Tenotomy	Orthopedic surgery	Hospital, inpatient	Cuts tendons	Permanent	May redevelop contractures in same or opposite side of joint	Months to years

ROM, range of motion.

been used percutaneously in peripheral nerves and motor end-point blocks by open injection into motor branches of peripheral nerves during muscle-lengthening procedures, and perineurally at a distance from target muscles that are technically more inaccessible, including the deep muscles of the back and pelvis. The latter procedure is used because peripheral nerves commonly contain motor and sensory fibers. Phenol can reduce sensation and produce chemical neuritis and secondary dysesthesia. Surgically exposing the motor branch of the nerve allows selective injection. This typically is not done as an isolated procedure but can be done in the context of other procedures. The painful dysesthesia, typically occurring in 1% to 35% of patients, tends to diminish through the first month.[26]

Contraindications to long-term blocks include a known coagulopathy or an induced coagulopathy (e.g., coumadin, Plavix), localized cellulitis or active skin breakdown in proximity to the intended injection site, and the presence of a systemic infection or ongoing fever.

Phenol is the most commonly used agent. It is used in concentrations of 2% to 5%. At 2%, it tends to have less of a lytic effect and more of a local, reversible effect. Phenol is benzoyl alcohol, and it denatures protein and causes tissue breakdown. Some surgeons have suggested that the effect is greater than that from alcohol, but that has not diminished the overall use. The effect is nonselective; it crosses all fiber sizes and is long lasting. Although wallerian degeneration occurs in affected neural tissue and necrosis and scarring occur in affected muscle tissue, the time of regeneration is predictably months to years, as discussed by Burkel and McPhee.[27] Phenol was previously placed epidurally or in the subarachnoid space with good histopathologic effects; however, spinal cord injury and an inability to control the spread of the phenol has led to avoidance of that route. When the concentration exceeds 3% to 6% of phenol, the effect on the muscles is nearly immediate, and within 2 days, the clinical effect on the nerve and muscle is nearly complete. As in the case of the extended lidocaine blocks, it is possible to determine the effect of co-contraction of antagonist muscles and apply additional treatments for muscle lengthening.

Typically, injection of phenol is somewhat more painful, with patients reporting a burning sensation during injection, and chronic dysesthesia has occurred but is usually short term. Skin slough and some local edema have been reported. The lethal dose of phenol is 8.5 g, and overdose can cause central nervous system collapse and cardiovascular collapse.[25, 28]

The use of phenol has become popular because of the clinical observation that phenol treatment has a differential effect on reflexes. Voluntary strength appears to be preserved at a more functional level than that of the reflexes relative to stretch. Several investigators, including Carpenter,[23] have reported that, when alcohol is combined with phenol and the phenol is placed on a peripheral nerve, the amount of soft tissue damage and surrounding damage is diminished. In this case, when all fibers in the nerve are affected

equally, with the core fibers equally affected by phenol (unlike the situation with lidocaine), a reduction in some of the reflex loops relative to spasticity, including the gamma motoneurons and the afferents from the muscle spindle, may be enough to reduce the spasticity reflex arc, but the concomitant reduction in a number of alpha motoneurons is less clinically evident because of their greater number. The duration of the effect appears to be partly dose related, with several researchers reporting that 2% to 3% phenol did not have as long-lasting or as widespread an effect as a 5% block.[26, 28] The effect lasts 10 to 840 days, which is consistent with Petrillo's report[29] of a duration up to 22 months with a higher concentration. It appears that the intensity of effect initially and the long-term duration are dose related. However, some degree of local damage occurs, and efficacy is affected by muscle necrosis and fibrosis, neural changes, denaturation of the protein locally, the degree and extent of wallerian degeneration, and subsequent efforts at repair by the nerve. In clinical practice, alcohol and phenol injections may be superior to botulinum toxin because of their rapid onset and enhanced duration of effect. They also have a somewhat higher degree of selectivity given the neural effects. Although pain and local muscle dysfunction can occur as a consequence of the blocks, their low cost, ease of administration, and reproducibility may favor their use in selected spasticity.

Some patients, however, require a more global approach, such as the use of botulinum toxin intrathecally or the use of oral antispasticity agents. Many oral medications have been incompletely studied for spasticity of cerebral origin, and they fall into four categories: baclofen, which is an example of a gamma analog agonist; diazepam, which is a centrally acting lytic agent; dantrolene sodium, which is a direct muscle implant agent; and tizanidine, which is an α_2-adrenergic agonist.

The most common use of baclofen is in patients with multiple sclerosis or asbestos-related spinal cord pathology. It has its greatest effect in reduction of flexor spasms in cases of spinal cord injury. Baclofen can be sedating, and patients may develop tolerance. It is not absorbed directly. The usual starting dose is 20 mg three times per day, and as much as 200 mg per day has been used.[30]

Diazepam is the oldest antispasticity medicine and is still quite useful, especially for multiple sclerosis and spinal cord injury. It has also been studied to some degree in stroke patients. It binds the brainstem reticulospinal neurons, and the effect is dose dependent. Unfortunately, it has a marked sedating effect at higher doses and is associated with early tolerance. The standard initial dose is 5 mg taken once or twice each day, with 2-mg supplements as needed.

Dantrolene sodium has been thought to be the most effective agent for treating spasticity of cerebral origin.[31] It affects ion flux in the muscles and appears to directly affect calcium release in skeletal muscle. There is virtually no effect on smooth muscle and cardiac muscle, but dantrolene can reduce voluntary muscle power and spastic power. Dantrolene is mildly sedating but has a lower incidence of cognitive changes compared with diazepam or middle to higher doses of baclofen. Typically, the drug is started at 25 mg per day, increasing to 100 mg per day.

Tizanidine has been approved to treat spasticity of spinal cord origin in adults. Sedation is the most common side effect. The α_2-adrenergic receptor binds intracranial and spinal sites and acts to reduce excitatory amino acids. Tizanidine has been proffered as having an anti-nociceptive effect because of its interaction with the release of glycine. Doses of 6 to 36 mg per day have been used in studies comparing it with baclofen.[32] Tizanidine has a greater effect in patients who are still ambulatory at the time of initiation of use. It improves walking and positioning in preference to stretch reflexes at rest.

SURGICAL PROCEDURES

Spinal Cord Procedures

Percutaneous interventional procedures that are ablative include cryorhizotomy. In a study on rabbits, Zhou and collegues[33] demonstrated that application of cold in the perineural region resulted in alteration of the somatosensory potentials for up to 180 to 200 days with no disruption of the histologic structure of the nerve. Their findings were particularly significant because of the amount of cold required to produce these changes. They demonstrated that $-180°C$ to $-200°C$ was the ideal temperature for the most long-lasting effect.[33] This study was then conducted in humans with facet arthropathy (15 patients) and spasticity (12 patients). In this study, patients received two lesions directly to the offending nerve root in a foraminal location. Lesioning at $-180°C$ was applied for 1 minute. We used a double-nitrogen technique, with rapid rewarming to avoid cellular dehydration and subsequent cell injury (BioLife Solutions, Binghamton, NY). The lesions overlapped by 1 mm, given the standard size in vivo of the cold cone (Figs. 176–2 to 176–4). The second lesion was placed 3 mm distally. The result was an immediate reduction in spasticity, with less than a 5% reduction in voluntary motor strength as assessed by independent, blinded examiners. These effects persisted up to 3 months. No complications were encountered. This small study suggested the potential for cryoneurolysis with appropriate lesioning parameters.

Radiofrequency rhizotomy has been advocated, first by Uematsu[34] for pain and then extended to treating spasticity by several investigators. Herz and colleagues[35] reported that 32 of 77 patients required an additional procedure. These patients exhibited "generalized spasticity" rather than focal problems. Most were treated for lower extremity symptoms. With the two procedures (i.e., radiofrequency foraminal rhizotomies and radiofrequency sciatic neurolysis), 66 of 77 were judged to be "completely relieved." Recurrences were common (61%) but yielded to a repeat procedure.[35] Complications were minimal and transient.

Selective peripheral neurectomies constitute a direct

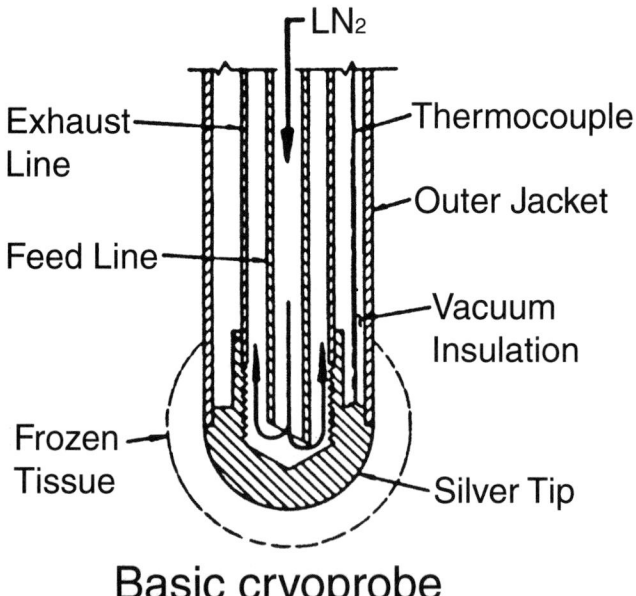

FIGURE 176–2. A diagram of the cryoprobe shows the dual-line liquid nitrogen technology that provides rapid cooling and rewarming. Notice the thermocouple. (Courtesy of BioLife Solutions, Binghamton, NY.)

approach to focal spasticity. Most often indicated for lower extremity problems, the potential surgical lesion can be simulated with the use of an anesthetic block. The open neurectomy is supplemented by a soft tissue release (muscle or tendon) to correct the deformity. This allows postoperative splinting and therapy a chance to maintain the therapeutic result. Intraoperative stimulation techniques can help with identification

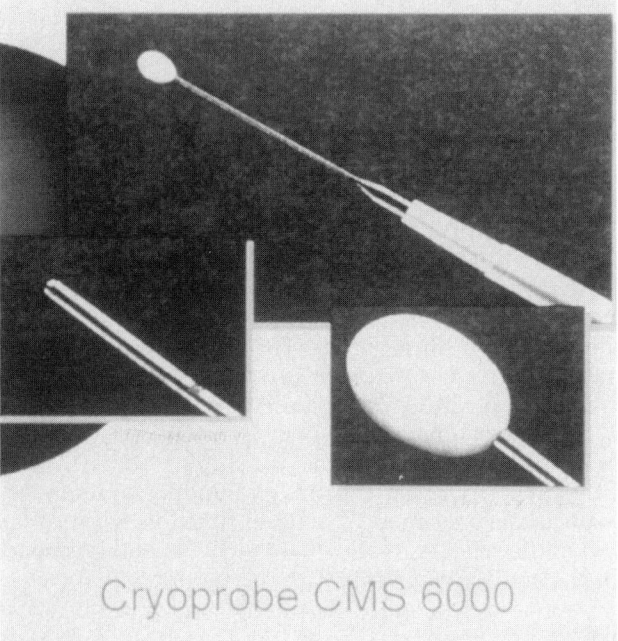

FIGURE 176–3. The dimensions of the cooling cone at -180°C. (Courtesy of BioLife Solutions, Binghamton, NY.)

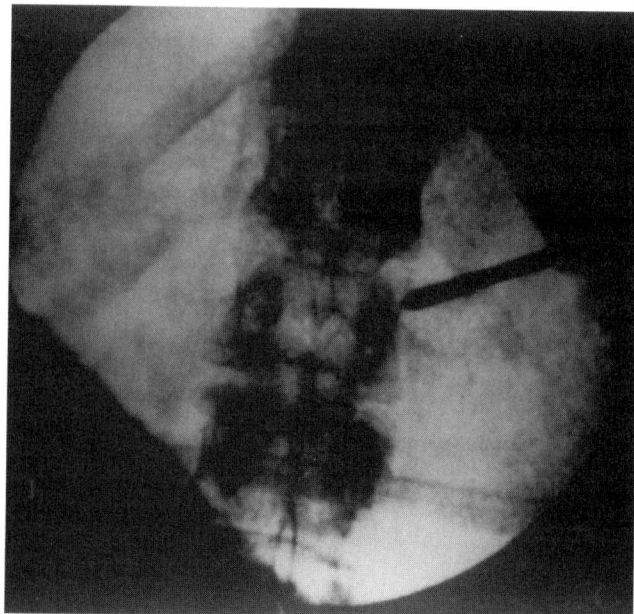

FIGURE 176–4. The cryoprobe is placed at the level of the mammillo-accessory ligament to access the medial dorsal ramus of the nerve.

of distal branches and their function. The goal is to minimize loss of voluntary control, when present.[36] Selective tibial neurectomy can improve foot deformity, ankle motion, and gait. This is a less debilitating procedure for patients with preserved gait.[37]

POSTERIOR RHIZOTOMY

In 1898, Sherrington[1] conducted a classic series of experiments in a decerebrate cat model. He performed dorsal rhizotomies to reduce hypertonus in individual limbs. Somewhat later, Abbe and Dana[38] performed dorsal rhizotomies in patients with pain. In 1908, it was Forster,[39] although he credited Munro with performing similar work in 1904, who first reported the utility of posterior rhizotomy for patients with spasticity. He emphasized that patient selection was critical. Spasticity must be differentiated from conditions such as rigidity and dystonia, which may respond better to other therapeutic modalities. In a large series of 158 patients, he performed an L2-S2 laminectomy with complete division of the posterior roots, sparing only the L4 root to preserve knee extension for standing.[39] He outlined the tenets of surgery for spasticity, which largely hold true today. He also recognized what Sindou later called *harmful and helpful spasticity*. He withheld the operation from those who depended on spasticity for antigravity control because any procedure to reduce spasticity might exaggerate weakness. He is also credited with first using intraoperative electrical stimulation to discern posterior from anterior roots. Because of a high incidence of differentiation problems, the procedure was overlooked until used by Gros and coworkers[40] in the 1960s.

POSTERIOR LUMBOSACRAL RHIZOTOMY

Recognizing the difficulties associated with whole sectioning of posterior roots, Gros and associates[40] proposed sectioning four fifths of each rootlet in an effort to spare sensation and strength. The group[40] further refined the procedure with the addition of intraoperative electromyography to preserve muscle groups with useful function while identifying the rootlets presumably involved with spasticity. In the 1970s, Fasano and colleagues[41] postulated that "abnormal" rootlets could be identified by their abnormal response to intraoperative electrical stimulation. The rootlets with abnormal responses are presumed to have synapses with hyperactive motoneurons in the anterior motor horns, which may lead to clonus or hyperactive responses with or without spread. Numerous protocols have been devised to discern which rootlets are most responsible for spasticity. Despite numerous researchers' conclusions that intraoperative stimulation is superior to random partial sectioning, no good prospective studies are available to support partial selective sectioning versus random partial sectioning. Mittal and coworkers[42] and Fukuhara and colleagues[43] reported the value of intraoperative electrophysiologic monitoring in selective posterior rhizotomy. Peacock and Arens[44] were concerned about the potential effects on the sphincters and proposed the surgical site be in the lumbosacral canal to aid root identification.

Surgical Technique

With the help of a short-acting muscle paralyzing agent, general endotracheal anesthesia is administered, and no relaxants are used after initial induction. The patient is placed in the prone position on a Kambin frame, but a similar radiolucent frame can be used to assist in visualization. A system that allows the abdominal wall to move freely is essential to minimize venous epidural bleeding. A laminectomy (or laminoplasty) is performed from L1 to S1. The dura is opened, and the nerve root exit points are visualized. X-ray studies or fluoroscopy is used to identify level in cases of anatomic irregularity. Bladder and bowel sphincters are monitored along with muscle responses. Dorsal roots are separated from ventral roots and stimulated. Generally, 60% of the dorsal rootlets are sectioned. The number at each level is determined by the electrophysiologic results. It is not unusual for most rootlets to respond abnormally at a single level. Various surgeons section 50% to 100% of the rootlets in that setting.[45–49] If more than 50% of the rootlets are sectioned at a given level, Abbott and associates[49] report that they limit the procedure to two successive levels. The adjacent levels are restricted to sectioning of less than 50%.

Most reports concern children, and the range of success is 45% to 80%. The functional parameters used vary widely, making comparisons difficult. Complications are incompletely reported, but in two pediatric populations, intraoperative pulmonary events were seen in 2% to 6%, dysesthesias in 9% to 25%, and bladder problems in 10%.[50–55] Late scoliosis is mentioned, but no documentation is offered. Late back pain occurred in 10% of patients.[48, 49]

POSTERIOR CERVICAL RHIZOTOMY

A long-standing tenet of surgery for spasticity has been that improvement is seen in those with lower extremity rather than upper extremity spasticity.[56] In 1970, Kottke[57] challenged this notion when he performed rhizotomies of the whole posterior nerve roots from C1 to C3. In 1973, Heimberger[50] followed with a series of 15 patients treated with posterior cervical rhizotomies. He showed improvement in upper extremity spasticity in 13 patients but functional improvement in only 11. Although others reported similar results, the procedure had largely fallen out of favor until recently. In 2000, Bertelli and coworkers[56] reported on 13 patients treated with cervical dorsal rhizotomy. They proposed dorsal rhizotomy from C5 to C7 in those with spastic shoulder and elbow. If the hand is involved, C8 should be added. If only the hand and wrist are involved, C7 and C8 rhizotomies are recommended. Relief of spasticity and functional improvement in arm/hand was seen in all patients, with a mean follow-up period of 15.6 months. The surgeons reported preservation of hand sensation despite sectioning of the whole dorsal roots from C5 to C8. They postulated that light touch and pain sensation in the hand might be conducted along other afferent pathways, such as adjacent cervical and thoracic dorsal roots or the brachial plexus ventral root.

ANTERIOR RHIZOTOMY

Anterior rhizotomy was proposed by Munro.[58] This procedure involved a laminectomy from T9 to L1. The dentate ligaments were sectioned and the conus rotated to bring the ventral rootlets into view. Sectioning produced paraplegia and did eliminate spasticity. The major complications included bladder and bowel problems and decubitus ulcers resulting from muscle atrophy.

Central Ablative Approaches

CORDECTOMY

Theoretically, the excitatory input to the motor horn may be interrupted at the level of the spinal cord. In 1949, McCarty and Kiefer[59] described such a procedure, the cordectomy. This radical procedure produced complete motor and sensory loss and bladder disturbances.

MYELOTOMY

In 1951, Bischof[60] described an elegant procedure in which the sensory fibers within the spinal cord and adjacent to nearby motor tracts were severed with the hope of reducing spasticity. Because of the risk of damaging uninvolved nearby tracts and high recurrence of spasticity, this procedure has largely been abandoned. Its importance, however, is certain in that it provided the basis for the modern dorsal root entry zone (DREZ) procedure.

DORSAL ROOT ENTRY ZONE PROCEDURE

In the 1960s, Sindou[61] reported neuroanatomic findings showing that the posterior roots demonstrated a grouping of fibers relative to their anatomic position in the posterior root. He concluded that this grouping was in preparation for the fiber types to enter the cord and move to their appropriate sites. In his initial series of patients, pain relief was the major target of the surgery, and the lesion was ventral to the DREZ, severing the deep fibers and maintaining the anterior rootlets.

The microsurgical DREZ procedure is a refinement of Sindou's original procedure. The DREZ procedure is designed to destroy the nociceptive and myotactic fibers, allowing preservation of the lemniscal fibers with resultant interruption of reflex and nociceptive pathways. It involves lesioning the afferent fibers as they enter the posterolateral sulcus of the spinal cord. A 3-mm-deep microsurgical incision directed at a 45-degree angle is made in the posterolateral sulcus with bipolar coagulation at the level of the rootlets into the dorsal sulcus. It is still thought to be more successful for pain relief than for spasticity. Mertens and Sindou[62] described 121 patients who underwent the procedure, with spasticity being the overriding consideration in all patients, pain in 75 patients, and hyperactive bladder responses in 38. The overall success rates for spasticity, spasm, and pain were 78%, 88%, and 82%, respectively. Complications were reported in 32 patients, and 5 patients died. The report emphasizes the severe preoperative impairment and poor preoperative medical condition of some of the patients to explain the high morbidity and mortality rates.

Stereotactic neurosurgical procedures were tried in the 1950s. Targets included the thalamus (VIM), the globus pallidus, and the dentate nucleus in the cerebellum. The dystonias are characterized by abnormal muscle tone, co-contraction of agonist and antagonist muscle pairs, and minimal hyperreflexia. Interruption of basal ganglia targets gave moderate relief to this group. The results were more variable with spasticity. Current investigations are centered on identifying a suitable target for high-frequency stimulation to address spasticity. Cooper and associates[63] introduced chronic cerebellar stimulation. Initially, electrodes were applied to the cerebellar surface; later, the cerebellar peduncle was selected with good results. Russman and Gahm[64] performed a double-blind study for the cerebellar cortex site and could not find a significant improvement in spasticity. They did not evaluate the superior peduncle site, as performed by Galanda and Hovath.[65] Zervas[66] commented on the potential role for dentatectomy after a thalamotomy.

CONCLUSIONS

The ablative approaches for spasticity have revealed much information about how the process evolves. As with many ablative procedures, we need to understand what compensatory pathways are activated after ablation. We also need to gauge the effects of these pathways on the primary problem of spasticity. Early efforts with neuro-augmentative procedures hold promise for timed, limited incursions into the central nervous system. The ideal approach may combine limited ablation followed by neuroaugmentation to maintain the result. This approach allows patients to tailor the outcomes to meet their daily requirements for positioning and movement. This has been the promise in other areas of minimally incisional, maximally effective neurosurgery. The ideal operation for spasticity does not exist. Selective dorsal rhizotomy enjoys the most popularity among pediatric practitioners. For most adults, the origin of their spasticity partly directs the selection of operative technique, but the microsurgical DREZ approach seems to be slightly less destructive and leaves room for redress, which is often needed. Future approaches need to address the overactivity with the loss of suprasegmental inhibition. The promise for neuroaugmentation is to simulate that control in the remaining descending pathways.

REFERENCES

1. Sherrington CS: Decerebrate rigidity and reflex coordination of movements. J Physiol 22:319–322, 1898.
2. Magoun HW, Rhines R: An inhibitory mechanism in the bulbar reticular formation. J Neurophysiol 9:165–171, 1946.
3. Duce PC: Surgical relief of tremor at rest. Ann Surg 122:933–941, 1945.
4. Klemme RM: Surgical treatment of distilla, paralysis agitans and athetosis. Arch Neurol Psychiatry 44:926–928, 1940.
5. Meyers R: Surgical interruptions of the palatal fugal fibers. N Y State J Med 42:317–325, 1942.
6. Putnam TJ: Relief from unilateral paralysis agitans by section of thermal trac. Arch Neurol Psychiatry 40:1049–1050, 1938.
7. Walker A: Cerebral pedunculotomy for the relief of involuntary movements. J Nerv Ment Dis 116:766–775, 1952.
8. Goldberg MJ: Measuring outcomes in cerebral palsy. J Pediatr Orthop 11:682–685, 1991.
9. Mayer NH: Functional management in spasticity after head injury. J Neurol Rehabil 5:1–11, 1991.
10. Katz RT, Rovai GP, Brait C, Rymer WZ: Objective quantification of spastic hypertonia: Correlation with clinical findings. Arch Phys Med Rehabil 73:339–347, 1992.
11. Ashworth B, Walsh EG: Scope and limitation to the manual assessment of muscle tone. Spinal Cord 35:64, 1997.
12. Mahoney F, Barthel D: Functional evaluation: The Barthel Index. Md State Med J 14:61–65, 1965.
13. Fisher WP, Fisher AG: Applications of the Rasch analysis to studies in occupational therapy. Phys Med Rehabil Clin N Am 4:493–526, 1993.
14. Fugl-Meyer AR, Jaasko L, Layman I, et al: The post-stroke hemiplegic patient: A method for evaluation of physical performance. Scand J Rehabil Med 7:13–31, 1975.
15. Pollock N, Baptiste S, Law M, et al: Occupational performance measures: A review based on the guidelines for client-centered practice of occupational therapy. Can J Occup Ther 57:77–81, 1990.
16. Lance JW: Symposium synopsis. In Feldman RG, Young RR, Koella WP (eds): Spasticity: Disordered Motor Control. Chicago, Yearbook Medical, 1980.
17. Odwyer NJ, Ada L, Neilson PD: Spasticity in muscle contracture following stroke. Brain 119:1737–1749, 1966.
18. Feldmen PA: Upper extremity casting and shunting. In Glen MB, Whyte J (eds): Practical Management of Spasticity in Children and Adults. Philadelphia, Lea & Febiger, 1990.
19. Bonica JJ: History, current status and future of regional anesthesia. Ann Chir Gynecol 73:108–117, 1984.
20. Gasser HS, Erlinger J: The role of fiber size in the establishment in a nerve block by pressure or cocaine. Am J Physiol 88:581–591, 1929.
21. Franz DN, Perry RS: Mechanisms for differential blocks among single myelinated and non-myelinated axons by procaine. J Physiology (Lond) 236:193–210, 1974.
22. Helweg-Larsen J, Jacobsen E: Treatment of spasticity in cerebral palsy by means of phenol nerve block of peripheral nerves. Dan Med Bull 16:20–25, 1969.
23. Carpenter EB, Seitz DG: Intramuscular alcohol as an aid in the management of spastic cerebral palsy. Dev Med Child Neurol 22:497–501, 1980.
24. Awad EA: Intramuscular neurolyses for stroke. Minn Med 8:711–713, 1972.
25. Glen M: Nerve blocks. In Glen M, Whyte J (eds): Practical Management of Spasticity in Children and Adults. Philadelphia, Lea & Febiger, 1990.
26. Khalili AA: Physiatric management of spasticity by phenol nerve and motor point block. In Ruskin AP (ed): Current Therapy and Physiatry. Philadelphia, WB Saunders, 1984.
27. Burkel WE, McPhee M: Effective phenol injection into peripheral nerve of rat: Electron microscope studies. Arch Phys Med Rehabil 51:391–397, 1970.
28. Halpern D: Histologic studies in animals after intramuscular neurolyses with phenol. Arch Phys Med Rehabil 58:438–443, 1978.
29. Petrillo CR, Chuds, Davis SW: Phenol block of the tibial nerve in the hemiplegic patient. Orthopedics 3:871–874, 1980.
30. Gracies J-M, Elovic E, McGuire J, Simpson DM: Traditional pharmacologic treatments for spasticity: Local treatments. Muscle Nerve Suppl 20(Suppl 6):S61–S91, 1997.
31. Nogen AG: Medical treatment for spasticity in children with cerebral palsy. Childs Brain 2:304–308, 1976.
32. Haslam RAJ, Walcher JR, Lietman PS, et al: Dantrolene sodium in children with spasticity. Arch Phys Med Rehabil 55:384–388, 1974.
33. Zhou L, Kambin P, Casey K, et. al: Mechanism research of cryoanalgesia. Neurol Res 17:307–311, 1995.
34. Uematsu S, Udvarhelyi GB, Benson DW, Siebens AA: Percutaneous radiofrequency rhizotomy. Surg Neurol 2:319–325, 1974.
35. Herz DA, Looman JE, Tiberio A, et al: The management of paralytic spasticity. Neurosurgery 26:300–306, 1990.
36. Decq PH, Cuny E, Filipetti P, et al: Peripheral neurotomy in the treatment of spasticity: Indications, techniques and results to the lower extremities. Neurochirurgie 44:175–182, 1988.
37. Caillet F, Mertens P, Rabaseda S, Boisson D: The study of the evolution of walking in the hemiplegic patients after selective tibial neurotomy. Neurochirurgie 44:183–191, 1998.
38. Abbe R: Resection of posterior roots of spinal nerves to relieve pain, pain reflex, athetosis, and spastic paralysis—Dana's operation. Med Rec 79:377–381, 1911.
39. Forster O: On the indications and results of the excision of the posterior spinal roots in men. Surg Gynecol Obstet 16:463–475, 1913.
40. Gros C, Frerebeau PH, Kuhner A, Perez-Dominguez E: Technical modification in the Forster operation. Selective posterior root section: The results of 18 years of practice. Paper presented at the Fifth International Congress of Neurosurgery, 1973, Tokyo, Japan.
41. Fasano VA, Baralott G, Zeme S, et al: Electrophysiologic assessment of spinal circuits in spasticity by direct dorsal root stimulation. Neurosurgery 4:146–151, 1979.
42. Mittal S, Farmer JP, Poulin C, et al: Reliability of intraoperative electrophysiological monitoring in selective posterior rhizotomy. J Neurosurg 95:67–75, 2001.
43. Fukuhara T, Najm IM, Levin KH, et al: Nerve rootlets to be sectioned for spasticity resolution in selective dorsal rhizotomy. Surg Neurol 54:126–132, 2000.
44. Peacock WJ, Arens LJ: Selective posterior rhizotomy for the treatment of spasticity in cerebral palsy. S Afr Med J 62:119–124, 1982.
45. Boop FA, Woo R, Maria BL: Consensus statement on the surgical management of spasticity related to cerebral palsy. J Child Neurol 16:68–69, 2001.
46. Engsberg JR, Olree KS, Ross SA, et al: Spasticity and strength changes as a function of selective dorsal rhizotomy. J Neurosurg 88:1020–1026, 1998.
47. Fukuhara T, Najm IM, Levin KH, et al: Nerve rootlets to be sectioned for spasticity resolution in selective dorsal rhizotomy. Surg Neurol 54:126–132, discussion 133, 2000.

48. Steinbok P, Schrag C: Complications after selective posterior rhizotomy for spasticity in children with cerebral palsy. Pediatr Neurosurg 28:300–313, 1998.

49. Abbott R, Foram SL, Johann M: Selective posterior rhizotomy for the treatment of spasticity: A review. Childs Nerv Syst 5: 337–346, 1989.

50. Heim RC, Park TS, Vogler GP, et al: Changes in hip migration after selective dorsal rhizotomy for spastic quadriplegia in cerebral palsy. J Neurosurg 82:567–571, 1995.

51. Lazorthes Y, Sol JC, Sallerin B, et al: The surgical management of spasticity. Eur J Neurol 9(Suppl 1):35–41, 2002.

52. Mittal S, Farmer JP, Poulin C, et al: Reliability of intraoperative electrophysiological monitoring in selective posterior rhizotomy. J Neurosurg 95:67–75, 2001.

53. Ojemann JG, Park TS, Komanetsky R, et al: Lack of specificity in electrophysiological identification of lower sacral roots during selective dorsal rhizotomy. J Neurosurg 86:28–33, 1997.

54. Smyth MD, Peacock WJ: The surgical treatment of spasticity. Muscle Nerve 23:153–163, 2000.

55. Steinbok P, Keyes R, Langill L, et al: The validity of electrophysiological criteria used in selective functional posterior rhizotomy for treatment of spastic cerebral palsy. J Neurosurg 81:354–361, 1994.

56. Bertelli JA, Ghizoni MF, Michels A: Brachial plexus dorsal rhizotomy in the treatment of upper-limb spasticity. J Neurosurg 93: 26–32, 2000.

57. Kottke FJ: Modification of athetosis by denervation of the tonic neck reflex. Dev Med Child Neurol 12:236–237, 1970.

58. Munro D: The rehabilitation of patients totally paralyzed below the waist: With special reference to making them ambulatory and capable of earning their living: Anterior rhizotomy for spastic paraplegia. N Engl J Med 233:453–461, 1945.

59. Durward QJ, Rice GP, Ball MJ, et al: Selective spinal cordectomy: clinicopathological correlation. J Neurosurg 56:359–367, 1982.

60. Bischof W: Die longitudinale Myelotomie. Zentralbl Neurochir 2: 79–88, 1951.

61. Sindou M, Jeanmonod D, Merten P: Ablative neurosurgical procedures for the treatment of chronic pain. Neurophysiol Clin 20: 399–423, 1990.

62. Mertens P, Sindou M: The microsurgical DREZ-otomy in the treatment of spasticity of the lower extremities. Neurchirurgie 44:209–128, 1998.

63. Cooper IS, Upton AR, Amin I: Chronic cerebellar stimulation (CCS) and deep brain stimulation (DBS) in involuntary movement disorders. Appl Neurophysiol 45:209–217, 1982.

64. Russman DS, Gahm NH: Spasticity in cerebral palsy in the selective posterior rhizotomy procedure. J Child Neurol 6:277–278, 1991.

65. Galanda M, Hovath S: Different effect of chronic electrical stimulation of the region of superior cerebellar peduncle in the nucleus ventralis intermedius of the thalamus and the treatment of movement disorders. Stereotact Funct Neurosurg 69(Part 2):116–120, 1997.

66. Zervas N: Long-term review of dentatectomy and dystonia musculorum deformans in cerebral palsy. Acta Neurochir (Wein) (Suppl 24):49–51, 1977.

67. Bergner M, Bobbitt RA, Carter WB, Gilson BS: The Sickness Impact Profile: Final revision of a health status measure. Med Care 19:787–805, 1981.

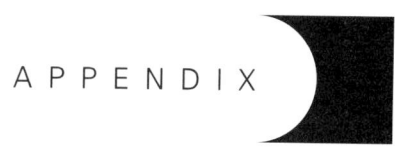

FUNCTIONAL SCALES

SICKNESS IMPACT PROFILE

The Sickness Impact Profile[67] is an interval scale, referring to the weighted scoring for items in 12 subsections. The patient or caregiver can complete it with an interviewer. The global rating scale is widely applicable but is not disease specific. The subscales can be applied individually. Reproducibility is good among different care settings. It requires 30 minutes to apply in its full form.

SF-36 HEALTH SURVEY

The SF-36 Health Survey is a patient report of 36 items that relate to the perception of current health and the limitations and burdens imposed by a disease process. It may underestimate severe states because of patient reporting. Easily administered, it can be used in the 36-item or 12-item (SF-12) formats for daily use.

The SF-36 Health Survey can be obtained by writing to Medical Outcome Trust, 20 Park Plaza, Suite 1014, Boston, MA 02116.

Management of Spasticity by Central Nervous System Infusion Techniques

RICHARD D. PENN ■ DANIEL M. CORCOS

Chronic intrathecal infusion of baclofen has been extremely successful for the treatment of spasticity.[1] Because baclofen does not cure spasticity, most treated patients need to be maintained on intrathecal baclofen for the rest of their lives. This long-term commitment to treatment is similar to maintaining shunt function in hydrocephalics and may be equally rewarding or frustrating. To make proper use of this powerful tool, neurosurgeons need to understand the pharmacology and distribution of intrathecal baclofen and how pumps are employed to infuse the drug. Proper selection of patients requires an understanding of the physiology of spasticity and its clinical manifestations. Other neurosurgical methods for reducing spasticity are considered elsewhere; in particular, dorsal rhizotomy for spastic cerebral palsy in children is discussed in Chapter 243. Other forms of pharmacotherapy are discussed by Noth.[2]

DEFINITION OF SPASTICITY

Spasticity is a term that can refer to a wide variety of motor problems and has numerous associated definitions.[3] It has been used to connote difficulty with coordinated movements, spasms, rigidity, abnormal primitive reflexes, and hyperactive reflexes. Researchers studying spasticity tend to stress definitions that emphasize abnormal reflex responses, whereas clinicians tend to stress more global definitions, primarily related to movement impairment. To further complicate the issue, many clinical syndromes associated with spasticity are caused by injuries in a multiplicity of sites in the neuraxis, and the pathologic mechanisms producing motor dysfunction are equally varied.

For the sake of clarity, a narrow physiologic definition is used in this chapter, with note made when more general meanings arise in clinical situations. Following the definition of Lance, spasticity, is "a motor disorder characterized by a velocity-dependent increase in tonic stretch reflexes (i.e., muscle tone) with exaggerated tendon jerks, resulting from hyperexcitability of the stretch reflex, as one component of the upper motoneuron syndrome."[4] The important point to stress about this definition is that spasticity is a velocity-dependent phenomenon. This velocity dependence differentiates spasticity from other, non–velocity-dependent forms of rigidity that can be caused by contractures, dystonias, or Parkinson's disease. In addition to hyperactive reflexes, spasticity can be associated with various symptoms that can be viewed in terms of positive and negative categories.[5] Positive signs are produced by overactivity (i.e., disinhibition) of certain pathways as a result of injury to a specific part of the motor system; negative symptoms are caused by lack of function of the injured area. In spasticity, an increase in deep tendon reflexes and resistance to passive stretch of the limb are positive signs. Negative symptoms are weakness and loss of dexterity. It is the negative symptoms that usually create the clinically significant problems that are disabling for the patient. Occasionally, muscle rigidity, clonus, and hyperactive reflexes can interfere with initiation and smooth completion of a movement. Spasms, although often associated with hyperactive reflexes, are not a necessary concomitant of hyperreflexia and should be considered separately.

The relation between physiologic abnormalities and motor function disabilities is a major area of investigation and of more than academic interest. It is uncertain how or to what extent the velocity-dependent increase in stretch reflexes interferes with movements.[6] Therapies that reduce reflex excitability may not necessarily improve the symptoms of spasticity.[3, 7] To evaluate and treat patients with spasticity, the physician must have a basic understanding of the pathophysiology of spasticity and knowledge about scales of measurement and modes of treatment.

PHYSIOLOGIC BASIS OF SPASTICITY

The final common pathway to the muscle is the alpha motoneuron. Many mechanisms influence the output of the alpha motoneuron and may therefore exaggerate this neuron's response to stretch. The muscles contain receptors called *spindles*, which are diagrammed in the

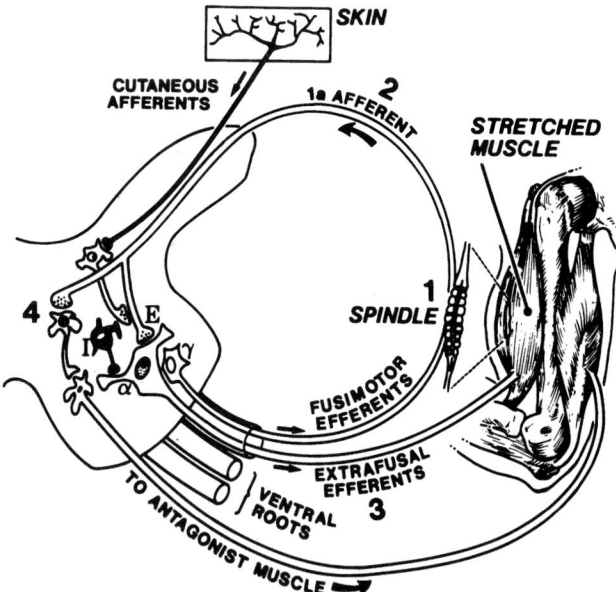

FIGURE 177–1. Structures involved in the control of movement at the spinal and peripheral levels. The text describes the sequence of events (1 through 4) that occur in the stretch reflex arc. α, alpha motoneuron; γ, gamma motoneuron; E, excitatory presynaptic ending; I, inhibitory interneuron.

center portion of Figure 177–1. The spindle is made up of intrafusal fibers, attached to which are primary sensory endings. The primary sensory endings, which are extensions of the large, myelinated Ia afferents, attach at the noncontractile equatorial region of the intrafusal fibers. The spindle organs are attached at both ends of the muscle mass, which is composed of extrafusal fibers. Because the spindles are attached in this way, they undergo the same changes in length as the overall muscle and monitor changes in muscle length. The spindles themselves are under the control of fusimotor efferents (i.e., gamma system).

If the stretch reflex operated only in conjunction with the alpha motoneuron, voluntary movements would be difficult to make, because a change in alpha activity would cause contraction of the extrafusal fibers, which would shorten the muscle. As the muscle shortened, the intrafusal fibers of the muscle would slacken and would not monitor length changes. Gamma innervation prevents this and assists in controlling movement by indirectly increasing alpha motoneuron activation through Ia feedback. Gamma innervation also serves to increase reciprocal inhibition of the antagonist muscle.

When a muscle is stretched, it contracts to try to regain its original length. This response can be broken down into five events, four of which are diagrammed in Figure 177–1:

1. Sensory impulses are generated as a result of stretching of muscle spindles.

2. The afferent volley ascends to the spinal cord.

3. It excites discharge of the alpha motoneuron of the same muscle.

4. It inhibits the motoneuron pools of antagonistic muscles through a disynaptic pathway.

5. It facilitates, probably monosynaptically, the motoneurons of synergistic pools (not shown in Fig. 177–1).[8]

Mechanisms Underlying Reflex Function

To understand how changes in these mechanisms lead to spasticity, we must trace the events that occur when a muscle is stretched. In a closed-loop system, it is impossible to identify the beginning and end of a sequence of events. For simplicity of presentation, the various mechanisms are discussed in the following order: Ia monosynaptic connection, Ia excitatory polysynaptic pathways, reciprocal Ia inhibition, group II pathways, decreased recurrent inhibition, alpha motoneuron hyperexcitability, gamma motoneuron hyperactivity, and group Ib inhibition. A detailed discussion of these mechanisms has been presented by Pierrot-Deseilligny,[9, 10] Deseilligny and Mazieres,[11] and Sehgal and McGuire.[12] Sehgal and McGuire[12] also provide a detailed explanation of the different electrophysiologic testing procedures that are used to deduce which mechanisms underlie spasticity.

Ia MONOSYNAPTIC CONNECTION

When a muscle is stretched, the Ia afferent neuron transmits excitatory messages from its receptor, the muscle spindle, to the alpha motoneuron of the same muscle by means of a monosynaptic connection. It has been suggested that the Ia discharge is normally reduced by presynaptic inhibition and that reduced levels of presynaptic inhibition could lead to an increased stretch reflex.[11] For example, Calancie and colleagues[13] argued that presynaptic inhibition is elevated in patients in the acute stage of spinal cord injury but is reduced in the chronic stage of spinal cord injury. This reduction in presynaptic inhibition could give rise to an increased reflex response. There is also evidence that there is a decrease in presynaptic inhibition in paraplegic patients but not in hemiplegic patients.[14]

Ia EXCITATORY POLYSYNAPTIC PATHWAYS

The alpha motoneuron can also be affected by the Ia excitatory polysynaptic pathway (Fig. 177–2).[15] The tonic vibration reflex is defined as vibration-induced activity in group Ia fibers that produces a tonic contraction of the vibrated muscle through Ia excitatory polysynaptic pathways; it can sometimes increase and sometimes decrease in spastic patients.[16] Facilitation of this pathway can lead to an increased stretch reflex.

RECIPROCAL Ia INHIBITION

When a muscle is stretched, the reflex evoked in that muscle is normally accompanied by inhibition of the opposing muscle. This finding of reciprocal inhibition has had a pervasive influence on our understanding of movement control.[17] It has been assumed that, as a

Descending pathways

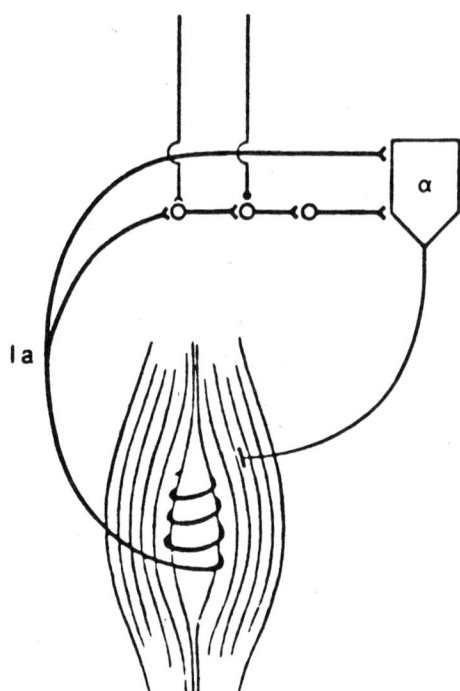

FIGURE 177–2. In addition to monosynaptic Ia excitatory pathways, there are polysynaptic pathways converging on the alpha motoneuron. Interneurons interposed in these pathways *(open circles)* are controlled by descending pathways. Excitatory synapses are represented as *angular* and inhibitory synapses as a *dot.* (From Pierrot-Deseilligny E: Pathophysiology of spasticity. Triangle 22:165–174, 1983.)

movement is made, stretch-related activation in the antagonist muscle is suppressed by reciprocal inhibition. A lack of reciprocal inhibition can lead to unwanted activation of the antagonist muscle and impede movement. The Ia inhibitory interneuron receives excitatory synaptic inputs from numerous descending pathways, including the corticospinal tract.[18] The input from the descending tracts is combined with the output from the Ia afferent of the contracting agonist muscle.[19] If the Ia interneuron does not receive input from the corticospinal tract, reciprocal inhibition may become ineffective, a phenomenon observed in some spastic patients.[20]

GROUP II PATHWAYS

Group II endings (i.e., secondary endings), like Ia endings, are located on intrafusal muscle fibers and are most sensitive to dynamic stretch. Their role in spasticity is not well understood.

DECREASED RECURRENT INHIBITION

Recurrent inhibition refers to the phenomenon whereby motor axons give off recurrent collaterals that activate Renshaw cells, which inhibit alpha motoneurons.[9] Renshaw cells are influenced by supraspinal control, which can facilitate and inhibit them. At rest, a

complicated picture emerges with respect to recurrent inhibition.[21] In about 40% of patients tested, there is no evidence for abnormal recurrent inhibition at rest. In patients with hemiplegia (most often from stroke) and in patients with spinal cord injury (most often from trauma), recurrent inhibition increases. In patients with progressive paraparesis, especially in the case of hereditary spastic paraparesis or amyotrophic lateral sclerosis, recurrent inhibition is reduced.

In the case of active movements in spastic patients, an increased reflex response may be caused by lack of inhibition of Renshaw cells. In healthy subjects, there is inhibition of Renshaw cells, which inhibits the Ia inhibitory interneuron directed to the antagonist motoneuron. This prevents decreased inhibition of the Ia inhibitory interneuron by the Renshaw cells and allows reciprocal inhibition to function to suppress a stretch reflex in the antagonist muscles.[22] Lack of descending control of the Renshaw cells can lead to impaired voluntary movements and prevent modulation of control of the antagonist muscle, as has been shown by Katz and Pierrot-Deseilligny.[23]

ALPHA MOTONEURON HYPEREXCITABILITY

The alpha motoneuron receives excitatory input from segmental and descending pathways. Lesions at numerous levels of the central nervous system may upset the delicate balance between excitatory and inhibitory inputs influencing the alpha motoneuron. There also may be a change in the intrinsic properties of motoneurons.[10] However, the influence of alpha hyperexcitability is impossible to assess in humans because it involves knowing the firing level of motoneurons deprived of any sensory input.[9] There is no evidence for or against the involvement of alpha hyperexcitability in spasticity, although Noth[2] has argued that it does play a role.

GAMMA MOTONEURON HYPERACTIVITY

The gamma system modulates the length of the intrafusal fibers and therefore is responsible for establishing the thresholds for Ia and group II neurons (Fig. 177–3). Incorrect setting of the thresholds for the afferent neurons can lead to a hyperactive response. Evidence to support gamma hyperactivity is derived from analogy with the decerebrate cat, from selective blockade of the fusimotor system using local anesthetics, from the Jendrassik maneuver, and from comparison of the tendon jerk and the H-reflex. The selective blockade of the fusimotor system is the most important experimental manipulation, and this procedure has been used clinically for spastic patients. Injection of dilute procaine into the motor points of spastic and rigid muscles of human patients was found to decrease muscle tone.[24] This result seems to support the view that spasticity is related to an imbalanced fusimotor system, because stretch reflexes were abolished as a result of lack of gamma influence on the spindle, but voluntary muscle power remained because the larger alpha motoneurons were unaffected. However, the use of intrathecal and

Descending pathways

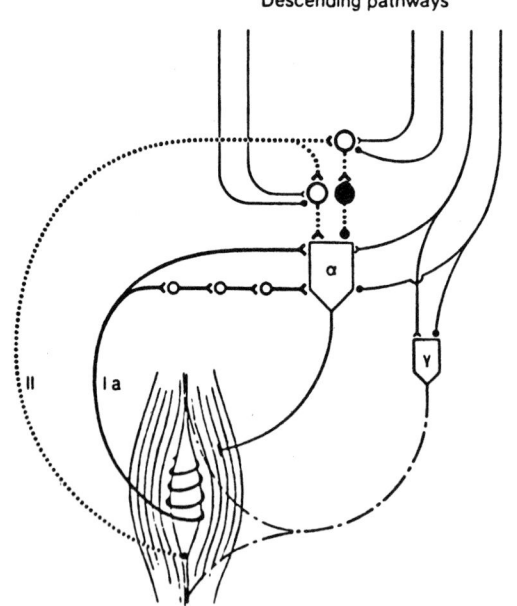

FIGURE 177–3. Muscle spindle afferents and fusimotor innervation. Ia pathways are described in Figure 177–2. Two pathways from group II afferents *(dotted line)* to homonymous motoneurons are represented: excitatory (synapses represented as *angular*, interneurons as *open circles*) and inhibitory (synapses represented as *filled circles*, interneurons as *solid circles*). Notice that α and γ motoneurons are controlled by descending pathways. (From Pierrot-Deseilligny E: Pathophysiology of spasticity. Triangle 22:165–174, 1983.)

epidural injections of local anesthetics has established no link between increased fusimotor activity and spasticity.[25] Additional evidence against the gamma hyperactivity hypothesis comes from the finding that the discharge rate of primary spindle endings is the same in spastic and normal individuals.[26] Increased gamma activity should lead to an increased sensitivity in the discharge rate of primary spindle endings in spastic patients. Although the gamma hyperactivity hypothesis has been influential, the evidence to support it is indirect, inconclusive, and circumstantial.[27]

DECREASED Ib INHIBITION

Golgi tendon organs are very sensitive to stretch because they lie in series with the muscle. On muscle stretch, impulses from Ib fibers are transmitted to homonymous motoneuron pools and heteronymous pools acting synergistically to inhibit stretch.[28] Lack of inhibition can result in an increased response to stretch and thereby contribute to spasticity. This has been demonstrated by Delwaide and Oliver,[29] who showed that Ib inhibition was markedly reduced in spastic patients.

SUMMARY OF MECHANISMS

Contributions of the different spinal mechanisms to hyperreflexia are summarized in Table 177–1. The information in this table should be treated with caution, because there is considerable variability in the tests

used to draw conclusions and in the types of patients who were evaluated in the different studies. Under the Mechanism column, we have listed the putative mechanism by which hyperreflexia could occur. The evidence is strong that decreased presynaptic inhibition, decreased inhibition from supraspinal centers, and decreased Golgi tendon organ inhibition can each play a role in hyperreflexia. However, each mechanism does not necessarily play a role in hyperreflexia of all causes. The research that has been conducted over the past 10 years makes it strikingly clear that different causes of spasticity can have opposite effects on the patterns of inhibition and excitation observed in different spinal pathways.

Why Do Spinal Circuits Malfunction?

There are two reasons why the spinal circuits can malfunction: abnormal descending control and local changes at the spinal level.

ABNORMAL DESCENDING CONTROL

One way to consider the diminished motor control in patients with spasticity is from a developmental perspective.[30, 31] It is well known that babies demonstrate a mass of uncontrolled reflexes. Before a baby can stand, the flexor reflexes in the lower limbs must be inhibited and the extensor reflexes enhanced to brace the limbs against gravity, a function of vestibulospinal and facilitatory reticulospinal tracts. After the child has learned how to stand, the next step is walking. For the child to walk, the extensor pattern of reflex standing in the lower limbs must be inhibited, and the flexor synergy of the lower limbs must be integrated into a walking pattern. This requires the involvement of the motor cortex to inhibit extensor activity and facilitate flexors.

As maturity is reached, the pyramidal tract exerts control over the direct connections to the anterior horn cells and, in conjunction with the basal ganglia and cerebellum, the brainstem. If the motor cortex or its projections are damaged, the brainstem exerts control. If the brainstem assumes complete control, individuals develop decorticate posture, with flexion of the upper limbs and extension of the lower limbs. In cerebral spasticity, there is enhancement of stretch reflexes in upper limb flexors and lower limb extensors. If the spinal cord is damaged, even brainstem control is interfered with, so that flexor reflexes and stretch reflexes are released. This can lead to any or all of the following physical signs[31]:

1. Disinhibition of the stretch reflex
   a. Increased muscle tone
   b. Exaggerated tendon jerks (i.e., phasic stretch reflexes)
   c. Radiation of phasic stretch reflexes in response to percussion
   d. Clonus
2. Disinhibition of flexor reflexes (in lower limbs)
   a. Clasp-knife phenomenon

T A B L E 1 7 7 – 1 ■ **Spinal Mechanisms of Hyperreflexia**

NEURONS	MECHANISM	INCREASE/ DECREASE	INVOLVEMENT IN HYPERREFLEXIA	REFERENCE
1a Monosynaptic connection	Presynaptic inhibition	Decrease Increase No change Decrease	Yes (chronic spinal cord injury) No (acute spinal cord injury) No (hemiplegics) No (paraplegics)	Calancie et al, 1993[13] Calancie et al, 1993[13] Faist et al, 1994[14] Faist et al, 1994[14]
1a Excitatory polysynaptic pathways	Excitation	Increase	Possibly	Hagbarth, 1973[16]
1a Reciprocal inhibitory	Inhibition Inhibition Inhibition	Decreased Increased (Released)	Possibly (multiple sclerosis) Possibly (spinal cord injury) Possibly (capsular hemiplegia) (During voluntary movement)	Crone et al, 1994[94] Ashby and Wiens, 1989[95] Yanagisawa et al, 1976[20]
Group II	Inhibition (decreased)		No evidence	
Renshaw cells	Recurrent inhibition (at rest)	Increased Increased Decreased Decreased	No (hemiplegia) No (spinal cord injury, trauma) Possibly (hereditary spastic paraparesis) Possibly (amyotrophic lateral sclerosis)	Katz and Pierrot-Deseilligny, 1982[23] Shefner et al, 1992[96] Mazzocchio and Rossi, 1997[97] Raynor and Shefner, 1994[98]
	Recurrent inhibition (movement) (Decrease of supraspinal control)		Yes	Katz and Pierrot-Deseilligny, 1982[23]
Alpha motoneuron	Hyperexcitability		Possibly; no evidence	See Katz and Rymer, 1989, for discussion[99]
Gamma motoneuron GTO 1b inhibition	Gamma hyperactivity Inhibition	(Released)	No evidence Yes (hemiplegia from stroke)	Burke, 1983[27] Delwaide and Oliver, 1988[29]

 b. Flexor spasms
 c. Extensor plantar response (i.e., Babinski's phenomenon)
3. Withdrawal of pyramidal facilitation
 a. Weakness of extensor and abductor muscles in upper limbs
 b. Weakness of flexor muscles in lower limbs

Lack of descending control is the initial impetus for the hyperexcitability of the stretch reflex, which is the cardinal sign of spasticity. Any lesion that affects upper motoneurons can cause spasticity. However, there are numerous factors to consider in trying to establish the effect of such a lesion (e.g., age, precise location of the lesion, time since lesion, cause of lesion). These lesions upset the delicate balance between excitation and inhibition in the spinal cord.

The transection of the spinal cord results in spinal shock, abolition of reflexes, and muscle flaccidity.[32] After different periods, muscle tone and reflex activity reappear and then become excessive. These increases may be caused by loss of descending control, but this loss cannot explain the reflex exaggeration as time proceeds. It is best explained by reorganization of spinal cord circuitry and alterations in levels of presynaptic inhibition.[13] A detailed review of the neurophysiology of spinal spasticity has been provided by Ashby and McCrea.[33]

LOCAL CHANGES AT THE SPINAL LEVEL

Most evidence for plastic changes at the spinal level is based on experience with spinal hemisection.[34, 35]

Changes in the spinal cord may be structural or functional, or both. Collateral sprouting of peripheral afferents has been shown to occur. In the hemisected spinal cord, a greater number of dorsal root fibers are eventually found on the hemisected side than on the intact side. This suggests that the Ia fibers may eventually constitute 10% of the synapses on motoneurons instead of the normal 1%, which may account for the exaggerated tendon reflexes.[32]

There is evidence that changes can occur in the spinal circuitry of humans who have suffered perinatal injuries to the immature nervous system.[36–38] In adults who suffered birth-onset injuries, rapid stretch of the soleus muscle elicits a reflex in the soleus and the tibialis anterior muscles. This phenomenon of reciprocal excitation is in marked contrast to the normal occurrence of reciprocal inhibition in the nonstretched muscle, suggesting that some disorders (e.g., cerebral palsy) may be characterized by abnormal spinal cord circuitry and brain damage.

CHANGES IN MUSCLE FIBER AND CONNECTIVE TISSUE

In the previous discussion in this chapter, the mechanisms underlying spasticity have been postulated to be neural. However, alterations in the functioning of these neural mechanisms can lead to numerous changes in muscle that may be partially responsible for the symptoms of spasticity. The mechanical properties of muscles and joints in spastic limbs can change in several ways.[39] The degree of abnormality of the muscles of children with cerebral palsy depends on which muscle groups are involved.[40] Examples have been found of atrophy, hypertrophy, and myopathy. During long-term spastic hemiplegia in human patients, some motor units develop increased fatigability and prolonged twitch-contraction times, causing changes in the dynamic properties of muscle.[41] Several studies on locomotion and interlimb coordination have suggested that, because hypertonia is present without concomitant changes on electromyography, it must be caused by muscle properties.[42–48] For example, histochemistry and morphometry of the spastic muscle of four individuals revealed increased atrophy of muscle fibers (especially type II) and a predominance of type I fibers if spasticity was established.[49]

In some patients, another likely explanation for spastic hypertonia is that some muscle fibers are replaced by connective tissue. In the more severely atrophic muscles, an increase in the amount of perimysial-endomysial connective tissue and interstitial tissue and an increase in the number of internal nuclei have been found.[40]

MEASUREMENT OF SPASTICITY

Methods for evaluating and measuring spasticity can be divided into three categories: clinical evaluation, whereby limbs are manipulated by a clinician and patients are observed making movements; passive quantifiable evaluation, whereby limbs are mechanically moved or different components of the reflex pathway are electrically stimulated; and active quantifiable evaluation, whereby movements are generated by the patient.

Clinical Evaluation

Clinically, spasticity is rarely graded in any way but qualitatively. Muscle response to stretch is judged by deep tendon reflexes elicited by a reflex hammer and by the spread of the response to other muscle groups. This is demonstrated in Figure 177–4, which illustrates the overreaction that can occur to a very light stimulus.[50] The stimulus was a tap to the right quadriceps tendon while the patient was performing Jendrassik's maneuver.

Asymmetry of response is more important than the strength of the response, and even a few beats of clonus in both ankles may be normal. Resistance to passive stretch can be a gauge of spasticity but often reflects other problems, such as contractures or ankylosis of the joint being tested. Spasticity may vary because of factors such as fatigue and emotional state. Normal individuals may even have sustained clonus under these conditions.[51] Position (i.e., vestibular input) dramatically changes spasticity. For example, patients with partial cord injuries, when tested in the upright position or in a wheelchair, may demonstrate much less resistance than when supine. Voluntary movement is assessed by analysis of gait and the ability to generate rapid successive movements.

To provide a simple grading system that would be useful for repeated clinical examinations, Ashworth devised the scale shown in Table 177–2.[52] A graded scale is appropriate because the response of a muscle

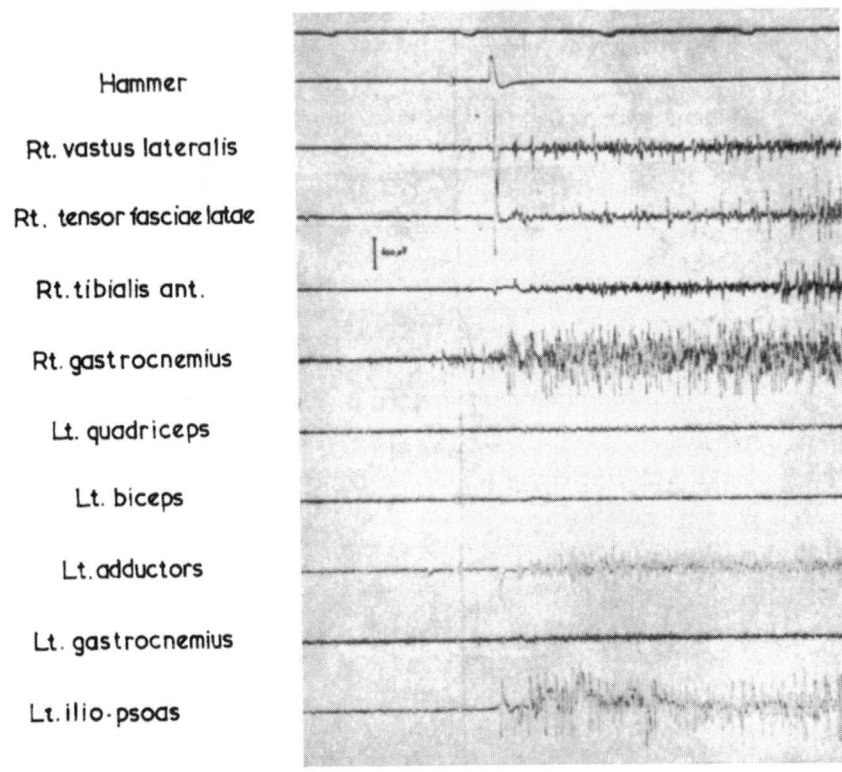

FIGURE 177–4. Electromyography of a knee jerk in a patient with severe spasticity. A tap on the right quadriceps tendon causes spreading activity in muscles of both lower limbs. (From Dimitrijevic M, Nathan P: Studies of spasticity in man. II. Analysis of stretch reflexes in spasticity. Brain 90:333–358, 1967.)

TABLE 177-2 ■ **Assessment of Spasticity: The Ashworth Scale**

SCORE*	CHARACTERISTIC
1	No increase in tone
2	Slight increase in tone, giving a "catch" when the affected part is moved in flexion and extension
3	More marked increase in tone but affected parts easily flexed
4	Considerable increase in tone—passive movement difficult
5	Affected parts rigid in flexion or extension

* The original Ashworth scale was scored on a scale of 1 to 4.

to stretch can vary considerably for a normal individual, and the spastic patient's increased response represents the higher end of a continuum. In general, the categories are distinct enough that changes in spasticity can be judged accurately during repeated examinations. However, one problem with the scale is that the scores of many patients cluster in the middle. Thus, it is worth considering the modified Ashworth scale, which tries to account for this problem by adding an extra scoring category.[53] Another problem with the scale is that the factors that affect the response of a muscle to stretch are not differentiated (i.e., reflex abnormalities versus contractures). Numerous other outcome measures can be used to facilitate the effective management of spasticity, and they are summarized by Pierson.[54]

It is desirable to use objective tests whenever possible, as is obvious from the suggestion that up to 50% of patients tested claim a favorable response to an inert substance if told that it is a new form of treatment for spasticity.[55]

Passive Quantifiable Tests

The normal limb can be passively extended or flexed without encountering resistance. This is not the case, however, for a spastic limb. After movement of a spastic limb has been initiated, the following characteristics can be recognized: resistance that increases gradually through the movement; resistance that may suddenly subside as the limits of range of motion are reached (i.e., clasp-knife phenomenon); resistance that is proportional to the velocity of stretch; and a stretch reflex that is position dependent.[56]

Any quantitative measures must record the velocity of the stretch, the resistance to stretch, and if possible, the electromyographic response of the stretched muscle. Several such tests have been developed.[57–60] One of the simplest evaluations appropriate for clinical use is a drop test.[61] To do this, the patient is placed on his or her back. The patient's leg is lifted to a horizontal position and then allowed to fall freely as the knee angle and the quadriceps response are recorded. Figure 177–5 shows how different degrees of spasticity are manifested in the knee goniogram and quadriceps electromyogram.

A wide variety of electrophysiologic tests can be used to explore the neurophysiologic mechanisms that

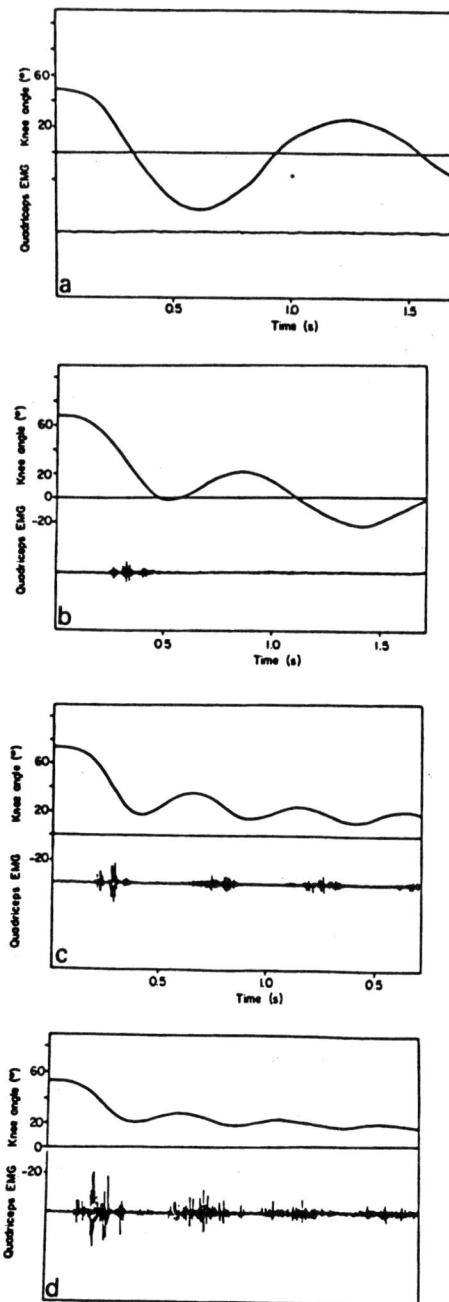

FIGURE 177–5. Degrees of spasticity: Absent *(A)*, slight *(B)*, moderate *(C)*, and severe *(D)*. (Adapted from Bajd T, Bowman B: Testing and modeling of spasticity. J Biomed Eng 4:90–97, 1982.)

underlie spasticity. A comprehensive explanation of these tests is provided by Sehgal and McGuire.[12]

Reflexes are more easily measurable than activities of daily living but are less representative of changes in general motor performance.[62] It is important to bridge this gap by the use of isokinetic measurements, gait studies, and studies of general movements.

Active Tests of Movement

Perhaps the most interesting question concerning the signs of spasticity is whether they have any relation to the paucity of movement experienced by many patients with this disorder. It is possible for the signs of spasticity to interfere with voluntary movement in a direct or an indirect way.

DIRECT INTERFERENCE IN MOVEMENT CAPABILITY

Deficits in the ability to generate movements can be tested and analyzed in numerous ways. The most common methods have been studies of unidirectional or reciprocal movements, use of ergometers, and evaluation of gait.[44, 63–65] The definition of spasticity used at the beginning of this chapter suggests that a reflex can be elicited in the muscle antagonistic to a movement. The evidence for this assertion, however, is contradictory. It has been suggested that there is no relationship between hyperactive reflexes and movement deficits,[65] but it has also been shown that reflexes in patients with mild spasticity are suppressed during voluntary movement.[66] It has been suggested that abolition of hyperactive stretch reflexes does not necessarily improve motor performance.[3, 7, 25] However, direct evidence showing the effect of reflex involvement in movement impairment has also been observed.[50, 64, 67, 68] Boorman and colleagues[69] found a loss of supraspinal control over spinal inhibitory mechanisms during cycling movements in patients with spinal cord injury.

Studies that have investigated gait have described the abnormal features of locomotion by the use of force plate recordings, accelerometry, and photography, alone or in conjunction with electromyography. The findings emphasize large interindividual variations in underlying mechanisms. For instance, the same diagnosis (e.g., footdrop) can be caused by diverse mechanisms.[70] Often, the observed paralysis of the foot is caused by the pull of the hypertonic triceps surae muscle.

INDIRECT INTERFERENCE IN MOVEMENT CAPABILITY

For patients with spasticity associated with paraplegia, even though a full range of movements is available in the upper limbs, spasms and contractures in the lower limbs can make such movements very unpleasant or impossible. The spasms and contractures also can severely limit the ability of these individuals to bend or stretch in everyday reaching movements, such as tying their shoelaces. The movements of the upper limbs indirectly stretch the muscles of the lower limbs and trigger the spasms or contractures. Any treatment that can effectively reduce the frequency or severity of these occurrences indirectly influences the individual's ability to move.

Measurement of Spasms

Lesions of the central nervous system often produce spasms and spasticity. The lesions are frequently in the spinal cord and cause a release of inhibition that results in the exaggeration of the flexor reflex. Spasms are often associated with pain, can compromise standing and sitting, and may facilitate the development of contractures. One of the few objective methods for documenting spasms involves placing electrodes over the ankle flexors and using a rectifier circuit to create an envelope of electromyograph activity that is easy to count visually or electronically.[71] Patients can then be tested during sleep (approximately 6 to 9 hours).

TREATMENT OF SPASTICITY

The goal of therapy is to improve neurological function by decreasing the effects of spasticity. However, because the disability that results from the hyperexcitability of the motoneuron can have numerous causes, disability varies from patient to patient and from lesion to lesion. In some patients, limb rigidity leads to poorly coordinated walking, and clonus may limit the speed of movement. In other patients, neither of these aspects of spasticity may be significant, and only associated spasms or motor weakness may cause problems.

Consideration of the pathophysiology also makes it clear that a wide variety of measures can be taken to reduce motoneuron hyperexcitability. Alterations to one or more of the pathways and connections of the reflex arc have been postulated to play an instrumental role in spasticity. However, studies that selectively reduce spasticity by allegedly influencing a single mechanism should be viewed with caution because that mechanism may not be responsible for the spasticity.[10] Reduction of excitatory input from suprasegmental levels, spinal circuits, or dorsal roots reduces motoneuron drive, as does activation of inhibitory pathways. Even if a particular input is not the primary cause of motoneuron excitation, reducing it or eliminating it may have the desired therapeutic effect. The success of therapy directed at one mechanism influencing the motoneuron pool does not imply that the cause of the spasticity is understood. It is rare that a drug or operative treatment has a simple physiologic effect. Therapy is empirical, and results must be interpreted with care because responses among patients can be significantly different.

Intrathecal Baclofen

The rationale for using baclofen intrathecally is analogous to that for using intrathecal morphine. In both cases, the drug acts on receptors in the dorsal gray matter of the spinal cord, and the direct infusion into the cerebral spinal fluid concentrates the drug where it is needed for its therapeutic effect. Systemic delivery could produce the same concentrations in the spinal cord, but the medication would be distributed equally to the entire brain, and the result would be somnolence or even coma. The use of an implanted drug pump with a catheter in the lumbar subarachnoid space not only concentrates the drug regionally but also provides a means of achieving constant levels. The rate of infusion can be adjusted to allow drug titration for a precise therapeutic effect.

PHYSIOLOGIC EFFECTS OF BACLOFEN

Baclofen was designed to be a lipophilic γ-aminobutyric acid (GABA) agonist that could pass through the blood-brain barrier.[72] However, it only partially permeates from blood to brain and does not fully resemble gamma-aminobutyric acid in its physiologic actions.[73] Two types of receptors for gamma-aminobutyric acid are found in the brain and spinal cord, and baclofen affects only the B type. This receptor has recently been identified and sequenced.[74] It is a transmembrane protein that affects calcium and potassium channels. Immunohistologic staining of the spinal cord has shown a high concentration of $GABA_B$ receptors in layer II of the dorsal gray matter.[75] Physiologic experiments on isolated perfused spinal cords have demonstrated that baclofen produces a profound reduction in monosynaptic and polysynaptic spinal reflexes.[76] This effect is caused by activation of the $GABA_B$ receptors, which reduce the influx of calcium in presynaptic terminals of afferent fibers, the result being a reduction of the release of excitatory transmitters. Baclofen can also affect the postsynaptic membrane by increasing potassium influx, thereby stabilizing or increasing the membrane potential and causing inhibition of the neuron firing.[77,78]

The sum of these presynaptic and postsynaptic effects is to decrease drive on the motoneurons. Diazepam, the other centrally active antispastic medication, works differently. It binds to the presynaptic membrane and facilitates GABA–mediated presynaptic inhibition. Unlike baclofen, which directly activates the receptor, diazepam works only when GABA is released, increasing the response to that acid (Fig. 177–6).[79]

The physiologic effects of baclofen have been studied most frequently in the normal spinal cord. After spinal cord injury, spasticity develops slowly and is related to the plastic changes in the spinal cord circuitry. The physiology of the damaged spinal cord is significantly changed and so is its response to medications. Tests have shown that, after a cervical injury, the rat lumbar cord increases the number of its $GABA_B$ receptors by 30%.[80] Other experiments in rats and cats have demonstrated that bladder reflexes change after cord injury and that the modified reflexes are inhibited by morphine and baclofen.[81] These animal findings are paralleled by clinical observations. Intrathecal baclofen given to normal patients does not interfere with movement or decrease strength, but the same dose given to a spastic patient markedly decreases spasticity and muscle tone. Ninety-six percent or more of patients with spasticity from multiple sclerosis or spinal cord injury have responded to intrathecal baclofen in double-blind studies.[82] The reason baclofen is so effective in reducing spasticity is that the same changes in the spinal cord that produce spasticity increase sensitivity to baclofen.

KINETICS AND DISTRIBUTION OF INTRATHECAL BACLOFEN

Baclofen, like morphine, is primarily water soluble. This means that only a small amount crosses the blood-

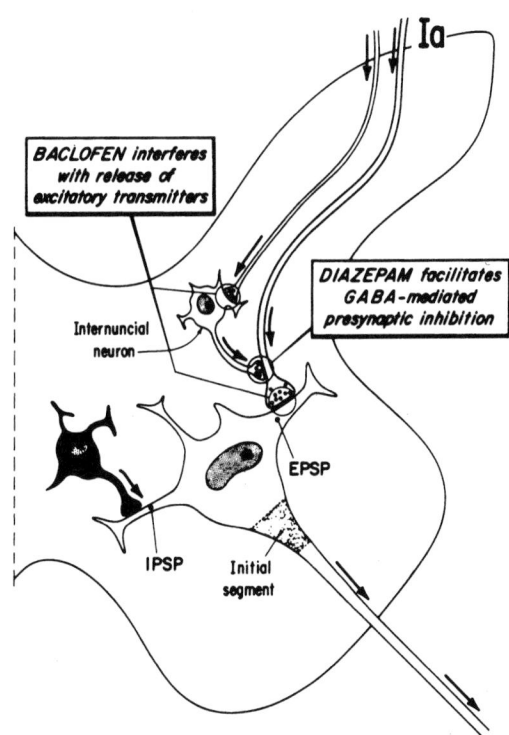

FIGURE 177–6. Enlargement of the left half of Figure 177–1. Synaptic mechanisms at the spinal level are responsible for excitation (EPSP) and two types of inhibition: postsynaptic (IPSP) and presynaptic. The sites of action are schematically illustrated. GABA, γ-aminobutyric acid. (From Young RR, Delwaide PJ: Drug therapy: Spasticity. Part 2. N Engl J Med 304:96–99, 1981.)

brain barrier.[73] Similarly, little of the drug introduced into the cerebrospinal fluid is lost by movement across membranes into the systemic circulation. Flow of cerebrospinal fluid is therefore the only source for distribution of intrathecal baclofen to the spinal cord. If a bolus dose is given by lumbar puncture, it mixes rapidly in the lumbar subarachnoid space and then is gradually carried upward along the spinal cord.[83] In 3 to 6 hours, it reaches the brainstem and then goes over the convexities and is eliminated into the systemic circulation at the arachnoid granulations. Bolus administration leads to transient but very high drug levels at the spinal cord and, later, at the brainstem. The half-life for a bolus of baclofen in the cerebrospinal fluid is about 90 minutes.[84] It is stable in the cerebrospinal fluid and does not become metabolized by tissue.

If baclofen is given by slow infusion, a different distribution is reached. The concentration gradually reaches the steady-state situation, in which the same amount of baclofen is being removed from the cerebrospinal fluid as is being infused; this occurs at about 12 to 18 hours (i.e., seven times the half-life). As has been measured in patients, the final steady-state concentration is directly proportional to the drug infusion rate.[85] Doubling the rate doubles the concentration (Fig. 177–7). Other measurements in patients have demonstrated that, at the steady state, the concentration of baclofen is decreased to one fourth from the lumbar area to the high cervical region. The manner in which the

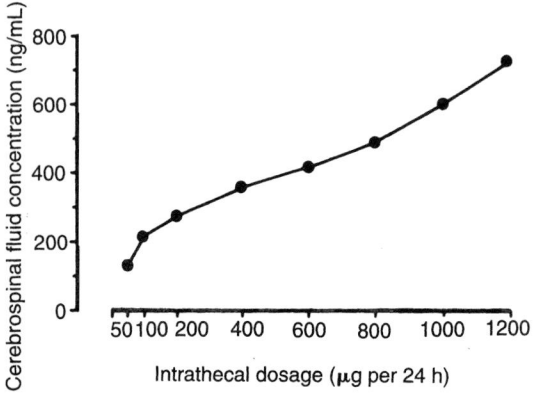

FIGURE 177–7. Lumbar cerebrospinal fluid concentration of baclofen in relation to a continuously infused intrathecal dosage. Concentrations are presented for eight patients receiving different daily doses of baclofen infusion. (Adapted from Müller H, Zierski J, Penn R: Local-Spinal Therapy of Spasticity. Berlin, Springer-Verlag, 1988.)

concentration varies along the spinal cord is indicated by indium-111 flow studies of cerebrospinal dynamics in patients with implanted pumps.[83] These tests indicate that the decrease in concentration is gradual and almost linear along the cord (Fig. 177–8).

Results of these kinetic and distribution studies have practical consequences:

1. Bolus administration produces immediate and extremely high, transient levels in the spinal cord, and several hours later, baclofen reaches the brainstem, causing side effects such as lightheadedness and drowsiness.

2. Slow, constant delivery with a drug pump produces levels of drug proportional to the delivery rate.

3. A change in delivery rate takes at least 12 hours to reach a constant level in the cerebrospinal fluid. Rates should not be adjusted more than twice each day.

4. A constant infusion into the lumbar space distributes baclofen along the cord so that the concentration decreases directly with distance and is about one fourth as high at the brainstem as it is at the point of infusion. Fewer brainstem effects are likely to occur if a constant infusion is employed and infusion is in the lumbar intrathecal space.

Another point of considerable clinical significance is that, to have its physiologic effect, baclofen must get from the cerebrospinal fluid to the spinal cord receptors, a distance of 2 to 5 mm through cord tissue. Diffusion is a very slow process. This accounts for the 45- to 60-minute delay from the time a bolus dose is injected until spasticity is reduced. After the receptors have been reached, diffusion back to the cerebrospinal fluid is equally slow. A single bolus dose may reduce spasticity for 4 to 12 hours; its maximum effect occurs when the level in cerebrospinal fluid has decreased almost to zero.[86] This slow diffusion from tissue also means that a large, single overdose causes a long-lasting respiratory depression and coma, even after cerebrospinal fluid levels have come down. In giving medication intrathecally, the physician must always be aware that the clinical effects are slow to appear and equally slow to clear, because the drug requires time for diffusion into the spinal cord and the cord tissue acts as a reservoir after it is loaded.

EFFICACY OF INTRATHECAL BACLOFEN FOR SPINAL SPASTICITY

The most effective use of oral baclofen has been in the treatment of spasticity caused by spinal cord injury or multiple sclerosis. The initial intrathecal studies were done on these patient groups after oral medications proved unsuccessful or had unacceptable side effects such as drowsiness. In this well-defined patient population, a bolus of 50 to 100 µg of intrathecal baclofen

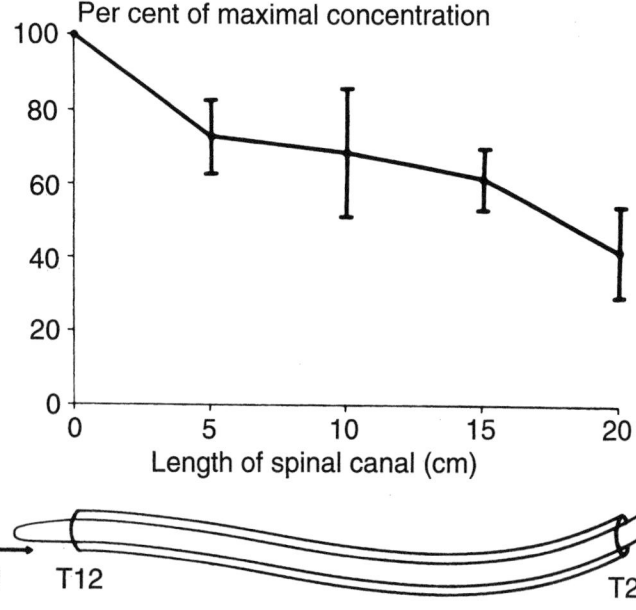

FIGURE 177–8. Decline of ^{111}In-diethylenetriamine pentaacetic acid concentration as the compound ascends the thoracic spinal column after slow intrathecal infusion. The 0-cm point is at the T12 vertebra, and the 20-cm point is at the T2 vertebra. The percentage of maximum concentration is the ratio of counts at points along the spinal canal to the level measured at T12. Data are presented as means ± standard deviations for four patients. (Adapted from Kroin J, Ali A, York M, et al: The distribution of medication along the spinal canal after chronic intrathecal administration. Neurosurgery 33:226–230, 1993.)

TABLE 177-3 ■ **Studies of Intrathecal Baclofen for Spinal Spasticity**

REFERENCE	COUNTRY	NO. OF PATIENTS	TYPE OF STUDY	RESULTS
Penn et al, 1989[100]	United States	20	Double-blind	Excellent
Penn, 1992[82]	United States	62	Prospective	Excellent
Ochs et al, 1989[101]	Germany/Sweden, Belgium/ Holland, United Kingdom	28	Prospective, multicenter	Excellent
Lazorthes et al, 1990[102]	France	38 ports 18 pumps	Prospective	Excellent
Müller, 1991[103]	Germany	211	Prospective, multicenter	Excellent
Loubser et al, 1991[104]	United States	9	Prospective	Excellent
Coffey et al, 1993[105]	United States	75	Double-blind	Excellent

reduced abnormal muscle tone two or more points on the Ashworth scale for almost all patients. If patients had spasms, they were also significantly reduced. The short-term effect could be maintained with constant delivery. Individual and multicenter studies in the United States and Europe have demonstrated that the control of spasticity and spasms can be achieved over years using implanted drug pumps to deliver baclofen (Table 177–3 and Fig. 177–9).

The efficacy of chronic intrathecal baclofen is clear and unequivocal, but several questions need to be answered. What are the drug's side effects? How difficult is it to maintain long-term baclofen treatment? What other patient groups can benefit from this treatment?

DRUG SIDE EFFECTS

The side effects from intrathecal baclofen are similar to those of oral baclofen and are dose related. Although some protection from central side effects is afforded by the fact that the baclofen concentration is higher in the lumbar region than at the brainstem, increasing dosage can lead to adverse effects. Common problems from high dosage include drowsiness, mental confusion,

lightheadedness, and ataxia. Weakness can be induced in some patients, as can loss of function because of reduction in spasticity. This is not a true side effect, because baclofen is intended to reduce muscle tone. A 10% to 20% reduction in dosage usually eliminates these symptoms. Bolus administration, used for testing before implantation of a pump, is more frequently associated with these same side effects and occasionally produces hypotension, nausea, and respiratory depression. A large overdose, in the range of 1 to 20 mg, results in coma, flaccidity, hypotension, and respiratory depression.[87] If an overdose occurs, the patient must be followed with apnea monitoring and, if necessary, ventilatory support. No deaths from overdose have been reported, but the intrathecal route of drug administration can result in potent and serious side effects. Treatment of a moderate overdose with physostigmine (0.5 to 2 mg) often reverses the somnolence and respiratory effects.[88] This treatment does not work for large overdoses and should not be given to patients with heart conduction defects. The central effects of an overdose should clear in 24 to 48 hours.

Tolerance to baclofen develops in most patients. Over the first 6 to 12 months, the dose of baclofen

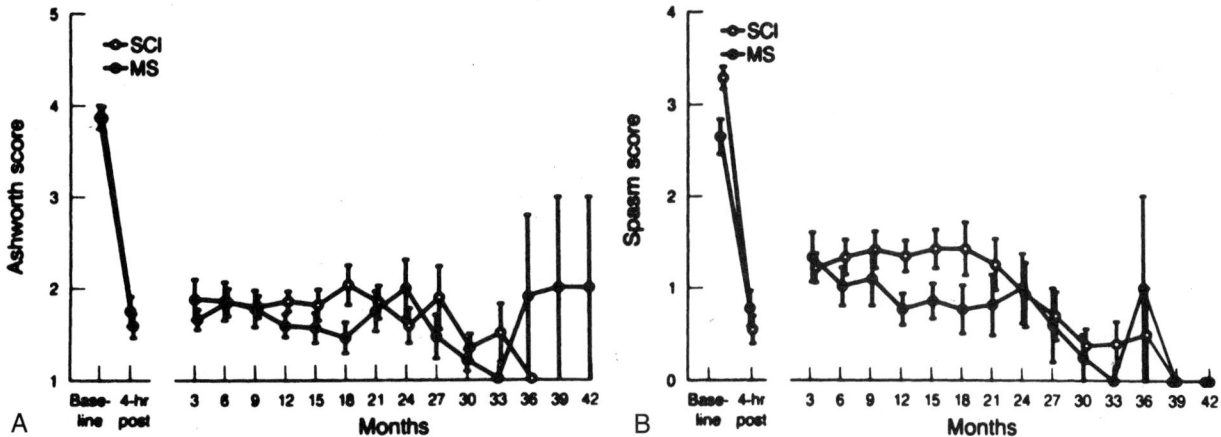

FIGURE 177–9. Effects of chronic intrathecal baclofen administration in 47 patients with spinal cord injury (SCI) and in 27 patients with multiple sclerosis (MS). Values are expressed as means ± standard deviations. *A,* Ashworth scale scores over time since pump implantation. *B,* Spasm frequency scores over time since pump implantation. (Adapted from Coffey JR, Cahill D, Steers W, et al: Intrathecal baclofen for intractable spasticity of spinal origin: Results of a long-term multicenter study. J Neurosurg 78:226–232, 1993.)

required to achieve a given clinical effect usually doubles and then eventually stabilizes.[82] In a few patients, tolerance has been a significant problem, necessitating "drug holidays" for several weeks or a switch to intrathecal morphine, which has some of the antispastic effects of baclofen. Most often, the need for increasing dosage after the first year is related to a problem with drug delivery through the catheter rather than true tolerance.

Seizures and hallucinations can occur if baclofen is suddenly withdrawn. After intrathecal treatment has been initiated, oral baclofen should be withdrawn gradually over several weeks. Baclofen may change the seizure threshold in some patients and has been associated with the onset of seizures in a few patients. It may make prior seizures more difficult to control. Sudden withdrawal of intrathecal baclofen produces a rebound phenomenon of spasticity and spasms that is worse than those that occurred before baclofen was started. This increased spasticity gradually dissipates over several days. It also frequently causes a tickling and dysesthetic skin sensation.

Recently a rare life-threatening baclofen withdrawal syndrome has been described of high fever, altered mental states, and profound muscular rigidity that can lead to fatal rhabdomyolysis. The most effective treatment is rapid reinstating of intrathecal baclofen. Oral and intravenous medicines including high-dose benzodiazepines and supportive care are useful.[88a]

DELIVERY SYSTEMS

Intrathecal baclofen therapy depends completely on the proper function of the pump and catheter system used to deliver the drug. Pump designs, catheter systems, and implantation procedures have been discussed for morphine delivery and are the same as for baclofen. The incidence of pump failure is low, approximately 0.5% per year, and the only common failures are stalling or stopping. Overdosing is rare, except for iatrogenic causes such as misprogramming.

The major cause of disruption of drug delivery is that catheters are thin walled and small in caliber so that they can easily be passed into the subarachnoid space without causing injury to the nerve roots.[82] Despite anchoring devices, they can pull out of position because of movement. Catheters also can tear, disconnect, or occlude. Often, the problem can be diagnosed by plain radiography. If the cause is not obvious, indium 111 can be placed in the pump, and the patient can be scanned at 24 and 48 hours to check catheter patency.[89] The indium-111 study has the advantage of showing the flow of cerebrospinal fluid, and it can demonstrate a subarachnoid block caused by arachnoiditis or fibrosis around the catheter tip. Sometimes, a pinhole leak in a catheter cannot be seen on any study, and the cause is found only when the catheter is replaced.

As with any implanted device, infection is a potential problem. The bacteriostatic filter on the pump blocks any contamination in the pump reservoir from reaching the cerebrospinal fluid. However, localized infection around the pump or meningitis from the catheter in the cerebrospinal fluid has occurred in a few patients (<3%). Infection usually requires removal of the hardware. Intrathecal antibiotics delivered by pump can sometimes successfully treat an infection of the cerebrospinal fluid.

Long-term management of patients requires regular pump refills, dose adjustments, and diagnosis and treatment of complications.[90] Despite these requirements, the dropout rate of implanted patients is quite low. In a 7-year study, no patients were lost because of medication side effects, and although more than 30% had pump or catheter problems requiring operative repair, only 10% decided not to continue long-term treatment.[82] Key to management is a well-trained nurse-practitioner who can help with patient education, pump refills, and dose adjustments.

PATIENT SELECTION

The U.S. Food and Drug Administration first approved pump implantation and intrathecal baclofen treatment for spasticity caused by multiple sclerosis or spinal cord injury on the basis of several double-blind, multicenter studies. Approval has been extended to patients with cerebral spasticity and those with cerebral palsy. These and other conditions in which spasticity may be reduced with baclofen are provided in Table 177–4. In general, if a patient has the classic signs of spasticity, baclofen can decrease them. Athetosis and generalized dystonia do not usually improve, although exceptions are found.[90, 91] Focal, painful, lower limb dystonias may be helped considerably.[92] Stiff-man syndrome, in which spinal GABA-producing neurons are thought to be lost and the patient suffers from episodes of severe axial and limb spasms and rigidity, is markedly improved.[93]

Because a prediction cannot be always made about

TABLE 177–4 ■ **Conditions Responding to Intrathecal Baclofen**

SPASTICITY-ASSOCIATED CONDITION	REFERENCE
Spinal cord injury	
Cerebral palsy	Albright et al, 1993[106]
	Albright et al, 1991[107]
Hydromyelia	Case reports
Spondylosis	
Progressive lateral sclerosis	Case reports
Traumatic brain injury	Meythaler et al, 1999[108]
	Meythaler et al, 1997[109]
	Becker et al, 1997[110]
	Rifici et al, 1994[111]
	Saltuari et al, 1992[112]
Dystonias	
Axial	Ford et al, 1996[91]
Cerebral palsy	Albright et al, 1993[106]
	Albright et al, 1991[107]
Distal extremity – foot	Meythaler et al, 1999[113]
Miscellaneous	
Stiff-man syndrome	Penn et al, 1993[93]
Painful leg moving—toes	Penn et al, 1995[92]

response to intrathecal baclofen, a trial dose of 50 to 100 μg should be tried. This easy test, done under observation in the hospital, has few side effects and provides the physician and the patient a good chance to understand what baclofen can accomplish in their particular situation. The only caveat is that a bolus frequently reduces spasticity so much that motor function may be lost if some rigidity is required. Patients must be warned about this possibility. For most patients, careful dosage adjustment after implantation allows titration to a level that improves spasticity without significantly interfering with motor function.

The indications for intrathecal treatment of spasticity are straightforward for most patients: spasticity that has not responded to oral antispastic medications and a successful trial of intrathecal baclofen (50 to 100 μg). The drug should be used in patients whose spasticity is severe enough to cause significant disability, difficulties in self-care, or pain from spasms. The use of destructive neurolytic or neurosurgical procedures should be limited to the few patients who cannot be maintained on intrathecal baclofen or who have no useful motor function. The most difficult decisions are for patients for whom it is unclear whether reduction in spasticity will improve motor function and for those in whom baclofen treatment decreases functionally useful rigidity. This group includes many patients with spastic cerebral palsy. The results of dorsal rhizotomy are difficult to compare with intrathecal baclofen because rhizotomy is usually performed on young children and pumps are implanted in older children who weigh more than 50 pounds. Both procedures reduce spasticity. A pump requires continuous treatment and many dose adjustments; on the positive side, it is reversible, and the amount of spasticity reduction can be titrated to meet the patient's needs. Rhizotomy is irreversible and requires a long recovery period. In many cerebral palsy patients, regardless of the method used to reduce spasticity, motor function improves only slightly because of the widespread damage to the nervous system, but care becomes much easier.

REFERENCES

1. Campbell S, Almeida G, Penn R, et al: The effects of intrathecally administered baclofen on function in patients with spasticity. Phys Ther 75:21–31, 1995.
2. Noth J: Trends in the pathophysiology and pharmacotherapy of spasticity. J Neurol 238:131–139, 1991.
3. Landau W: Spasticity: The fable of the neurological demon and the emperor's new therapy. Arch Neurol 31:217–219, 1974.
4. Lance J: Symposium synopsis. In Feldman R, Young R, Koella W (eds): Spasticity: Disordered Motor Control. Chicago, Year Book Medical Publishers, 1980, pp 485–494.
5. Jackson J: On the comparative study of diseases of the nervous system. In Taylor J (ed): Selected Writings of John Hughlings Jackson. New York, Basic Books, 1958, pp 393–410.
6. Dietz V: Spasticity: Exaggerated reflexes or movement disorder? In Forssberg H, Hirschfeld H (eds): Movement Disorders in Children. Medicine and Sports Science Series, vol 36. Basel, Karger, 1992, pp 225–233.
7. Landau W: Spasticity: What is it? What is it not? In Feldman R, Young R, Koella W (eds): Spasticity: Disordered Motor Control. Chicago, Year Book Medical Publishers, 1980, pp 17–24.
8. Rushworth G: Some pathophysiological aspects of spasticity and the search for rational and successful therapy. Int Rehab Med 2:460–465, 1977.
9. Pierrot-Deseilligny E: Pathophysiology of spasticity. Triangle 22:165–174, 1983.
10. Pierrot-Deseilligny E: Electrophysiological assessment of the spinal mechanisms underlying spasticity. Electroencephalogr Clin Neurophysiol Suppl 41:264–273, 1990.
11. Pierrot-Deseilligny E, Mazieres L: Spinal mechanisms underlying spasticity. In Delwaide P, Young R (eds): Clinical Neurophysiology in Spasticity. Amsterdam, Elsevier, 1985, pp 63–76.
12. Sehgal N, McGuire J: Beyond Ashworth. Electrophysiological Quantification of Spasticity. Phys Med Rehabil Clin N Am 9:949–979, 1998.
13. Calancie B, Broton J, Klose K, et al: Evidence that alterations in presynaptic inhibition contribute to segmental hypo- and hyperexcitability after spinal cord injury in man. Electroencephalogr Clin Neurophysiol 89:177–186, 1993.
14. Faist M, Mazevet D, Dietz V, et al: A quantitative assessment of presynaptic inhibition of Ia afferents in spastics: Differences in hemiplegics and paraplegics. Brain 117:1449–1455, 1994.
15. Hultborn H, Wigstrom H: Motor response with long latency and maintained duration evoked by activity in Ia afferents. In Desmedt J (ed): Spinal and Supraspinal Mechanisms of Voluntary Control and Locomotion: Progress in Clinical Neurophysiology. Basel, Karger, 1980, pp 99–116.
16. Hagbarth K: The effect of muscle vibration in normal man and in patients with motor disorders. In Desmedt J (ed): New Developments in Electromyography and Clinical Neurophysiology. Basel, Karger, 1973, pp 428–443.
17. Sherrington C: The Integrative Action of the Nervous System. New Haven, Yale University Press, 1906.
18. Hultborn H: Transmission in the pathway of reciprocal Ia inhibition to motoneurons and its control during the tonic stretch reflex. In Homma S (ed): Understanding the Stretch Reflex: Progress in Brain Research. Amsterdam, Elsevier, 1976, pp 235–255.
19. Tanaka R: Reciprocal Ia inhibition during voluntary movements in man. Exp Brain Res 21:529–540, 1974.
20. Yanagisawa N, Tanaka R, Ito Z: Reciprocal Ia inhibition in spastic hemiplegia of man. Brain 99:555–574, 1976.
21. Katz R, Pierrot-Deseilligny E: Recurrent inhibition in humans. Prog Neurobiol 57:325–355, 1999.
22. Hultborn H, Pierrot-Deseilligny E: Changes in recurrent inhibition during voluntary soleus contractions in man studied by an H-reflex technique. J Physiol 297:229–251, 1979.
23. Katz R, Pierrot-Deseilligny E: Recurrent inhibition of motoneurons with upper motor lesions. Brain 105:103–124, 1982.
24. Rushworth G: Spasticity and rigidity: An experimental study and review. J Neurol Neurosurg Psychiatry 23:99–118, 1960.
25. Landau W, Weaver R, Hornbein T: Fusimotor nerve function in man: Differential nerve block studies in normal subjects and in spasticity and rigidity. Arch Neurol 3:10–23, 1960.
26. Hagbarth K, Wallin G, Lofstedt L: Muscle spindle responses to stretch in normal and spastic subjects. Scand J Rehab Med 5:156–159, 1973.
27. Burke D: Critical examination of the case for or against fusimotor involvement in disorders of muscle tone. In Desmedt J (ed): Motor Control Mechanisms in Health and Disease. Advances in Neurology, vol 39. New York, Raven Press, 1983, pp 133–150.
28. Eccles J, Eccles R, Lundberg A: Synaptic actions on motoneurons caused by impulses in Golgi tendon organ afferents. J Physiol (Lond) 138:227–252, 1957.
29. Delwaide P, Oliver E: Short-latency, autogenic inhibition (IB inhibition) in human spasticity. J Neurol Neurosurg Psychiatry 51:1546–1550, 1988.
30. Lance J: The control of muscle tone, reflexes, and movement: Robert Wartenberg Lecture. Neurology 30:1303–1313, 1980.
31. Lance J: Pathophysiology of spasticity and clinical experience with baclofen. In Feldman R, Young R, Koella W (eds): Spasticity: Disordered Motor Control. Chicago, Year Book Medical Publishers, 1980, pp 185–203.
32. Woolsey R: Symposium on spasticity and spasms. J Am Paraplegia Soc 5:3–9, 1982.
33. Ashby P, McCrea D: Neurophysiology of spinal spasticity. In Davidoff R (ed): Handbook of the Spinal Cord. New York, Marcel Decker, 1987, pp 119–143.

34. Malmsten J: Time course of segmental reflex changes after chronic spinal cord hemisection in the rat. Acta Physiol Scand 119:435–443, 1983.

35. McCouch G, Austin G, Liu C, et al: Sprouting as a cause of spasticity. J Neurophysiol 21:205–216, 1958.

36. Gottlieb G, Myklebust B, Penn R, et al: Reciprocal excitation of muscle antagonists by the primary afferent pathway. Exp Brain Res 46:454–465, 1982.

37. Myklebust B, Gottlieb, G, Penn R, et al: Reciprocal excitation of antagonistic muscles as a differentiating feature in spasticity. Ann Neurol 12:367–374, 1982.

38. Corcos D, Pfann K, Penn R: The control of movement in Parkinson's disease and spasticity: Role of inhibition and excitation. In Crockard A, Hoff R, Hoff J (eds): Neurosurgery: The Scientific Basis of Clinical Practice. Boston, Blackwell Scientific Publications, 2000.

39. Lowenthal M, Tobis J: Contractures in chronic neurologic disease. Arch Phys Med Rehabil 38:640–645, 1957.

40. Castle M, Reyman T, Schneider M: Pathology of spastic muscle in cerebral palsy. Clin Orthop 142:223–233, 1979.

41. Young J, Mayer R: Physiological alterations of motor units in hemiplegia. J Neurol Sci 54:401–412, 1982.

42. Ahlqvist G, Landin S, Wrobblewski R: Ultrastructure of skeletal muscle in patients with Parkinson's disease and upper motor lesions. Lab Invest 32:673–679, 1975.

43. Berger W, Horstmann G, Dietz V: Tension development and muscle activation in the leg during gait in spastic hemiparesis: Independence of muscle hypertonia and exaggerated stretch reflexes. J Neurol Neurosurg Psychiatry 47:1029–1033, 1984.

44. Dietz V, Berger W: Normal and impaired regulation of muscle stiffness in gait: A hypothesis about muscle hypertonia. Exp Neurol 79:680–687, 1983.

45. Dietz V, Berger W: Interlimb coordination of posture in patients with spastic paresis. Brain 107:965–978, 1984.

46. Dietz V, Quintern J, Berger W: Electrophysiological studies of gait in spasticity, and rigidity: Evidence that altered mechanical properties of muscle contribute to hypertonia. Brain 104:431–499, 1981.

47. Edstrom L: Selective changes in the sizes of red and white muscle fibers in upper motor neuron lesions and Parkinsonism. J Neurol Sci 11:537–550, 1970.

48. Hufschmidt A, Mauritz K: Chronic transformation of muscle in spasticity: A peripheral contribution to increased tone. J Neurol Neurosurg Psychiatry 48:676–685, 1985.

49. Dietz V, Ketelsen U, Berger W, et al: Motor unit involvement in spastic paresis: Relationship between leg muscle activation and histochemistry. J Neurol Sci 75:89–103, 1986.

50. Dimitrijevic M, Nathan P: Studies of spasticity in man. II. Analysis of stretch reflexes in spasticity. Brain 90:333–358, 1967.

51. Gottlieb G, Agarwal G: Physiological clonus in man. Exp Neurol 54:616–621, 1977.

52. Ashworth B: Preliminary trial of carisoprodol in multiple sclerosis. Practitioner 192:540–542, 1964.

53. Bohannon R, Smith M: Interrater reliability of a modified Ashworth scale of muscle spasticity. Phys Ther 67:206–207, 1987.

54. Pierson S: Outcome measures in spasticity management. Muscle Nerve Suppl 6:S36–60, 1997.

55. Burry H: Objective measurement of spasticity. Dev Med Child Neurol 14:508–510, 1972.

56. Bishop B: Spasticity: Its physiology and management. Phys Ther 57:371–401, 1977.

57. Burke D, Gillies J, Lance J: The quadriceps stretch reflex in human spasticity. J Neurol Neurosurg Psychiatry 33:216–223, 1970.

58. Burke D, Gillies J, Lance J: Hamstring stretch reflex in human spasticity. J Neurol Neurosurg Psychiatry 34:231–235, 1971.

59. Gottlieb G, Agarwal G, Penn R: Sinusoidal oscillation of the ankle as a means of evaluating the spastic patient. J Neurol Neurosurg Psychiatry 41:32–39, 1978.

60. Lehmann J, Price R, deLateur B, et al: Spasticity: Quantitative measurements as a basis for assessing effectiveness of therapeutic intervention. Arch Phys Med Rehabil 70:6–15, 1989.

61. Bajd T, Bowman B: Testing and modeling of spasticity. J Biomed Eng 4:90–97, 1982.

62. Pederson E: Evaluation of antispastic therapy. In Delwaide P,

Young R (eds): Restorative Neurology: Clinical Neurophysiology in Spasticity, vol 1. Amsterdam, Elsevier, 1985, pp 221–223.

63. Benecke R, Conrad B, Meinck H, et al: Electromyographic analysis of bicycling on an ergometer for evaluation of spasticity of lower limbs in man. In Desmedt J (ed): Advances in Neurology, vol 39. Motor Control Mechanisms in Health and Disease. New York, Raven Press, 1983, pp 1035–1046.

64. Mizrahi E, Angel R: Impairment of voluntary movement by spasticity. Ann Neurol 5:594–595, 1979.

65. Sahrmann S, Norton B: The relationship of voluntary movement to spasticity in the upper motor syndrome. Ann Neurol 2:460–465, 1977.

66. McLellan D: Co-contraction and stretch reflexes in spasticity during treatment with baclofen. J Neurol Neurosurg Psychiatry 1:30–38, 1977.

67. Corcos D, Gottlieb G, Penn R, et al: Movement deficits caused by hyperexcitable stretch reflexes in spastic humans. Brain 109:1043–1058, 1986.

68. Knuttson E, Martensson A: Dynamic motor capacity in spastic paresis and its relation to prime mover dysfunction, spastic reflexes and antagonistic coactivation. Scand J Rehab Med 12:93–106, 1980.

69. Boorman G, Becker W, Morrice B, et al: Modulation of the soleus H-reflex during pedalling in normal humans and in patients with spasticity. J Neurol Neurosurg Psychiatry 55:1150–1156, 1992.

70. Dimitrijevic M, Faganel J, Sherwood A, et al: Activation of paralyzed leg flexors and extensors during gait in patients after stroke. Scand J Rehab Med 13:109–115, 1981.

71. Pederson E, Klemar B, Torring J: Counting of flexor spasms. Acta Neurol Scand 60:164–169, 1979.

72. Faigle J, Keberle H, Degen P: Chemistry and pharmacokinetics of baclofen. In Feldman R, Young R, Koella W (eds): Spasticity: Disordered Motor Control. Miami, Symposia Specialists, 1980.

73. Knutsson E, Lindbloom U, Martensson A: Plasma and cerebrospinal fluid levels of baclofen (Lioresal) at optimal therapeutic responses in spastic paresis. J Neurol Sci 23:473–484, 1974.

74. Kaupmann K, Huggel K, Heid J, et al: Expression cloning of GABA$_B$ receptors uncovers similarity to metabotropic glutamate receptors. Nature 386:239–246, 1997.

75. Price G, Wilkin G, Turnbull M, et al: Are baclofen-sensitive GABA-B receptors present on primary afferent terminals of the spinal cord? Nature 307:71–74, 1984.

76. Ault B, Evans R: The depressant action of baclofen on the isolated spinal cord of the neonatal rat. Eur J Pharmacol 71:357–364, 1981.

77. Azouvi P, Roby-Brami A, Biraben A, et al: Effect of intrathecal baclofen on the monosynaptic reflex in humans: Evidence for a postsynaptic action. J Neurol Neurosurg Psychiatry 56:515–519, 1993.

78. Zieglglansberger W, Howe J, Sutor B: The neuropharmacology of baclofen. In Muller H, Zierski J, Penn R (eds): Local Spinal Therapy of Spasticity. Berlin, Springer-Verlag, 1988, pp 37–49.

79. Young R, Delwaide P: Drug therapy: Spasticity. Part 2. N Engl J Med 304:96–99, 1981.

80. Kroin J, Bianchi G, Penn R: Intrathecal baclofen downregulates GABA B receptors in the rat substantia gelatinosa. J Neurosurg 79:544–549, 1993.

81. DeGroat W: Nervous control of the urinary bladder of the cat. Brain Res 87:201–211, 1975.

82. Penn R: Intrathecal baclofen for spasticity of spinal origin: Seven years of experience. J Neurosurg 77:236–240, 1992.

83. Kroin J, Ali A, York M, et al: The distribution of medication along the spinal canal after chronic intrathecal administration. Neurosurgery 33:226–230, 1993.

84. Kroin J: Which drugs? What space? In Penn R (ed): Neurological Applications of Implanted Drug Pumps. New York, New York Academy of Sciences, 1988, pp 40–47.

85. Muller H, Zierski J, Penn R: Local-Spinal Therapy of Spasticity. Berlin, Springer-Verlag, 1988.

86. Penn R, Kroin J: Intrathecal baclofen alleviates spinal cord spasticity. Lancet 1:1078, 1984.

87. Delhaas E, Brouwers J: Intrathecal baclofen overdose: Report of 7 events in 5 patients and review of the literature. Int J Clin Pharmacol Ther Toxicol 29:274–280, 1991.

88. Muller-Schwepe G, Penn R: Physostigmine in the treatment of intrathecal baclofen overdose: Reports of three cases. J Neurosurg 71:273–275, 1989.

88a. Coffey RJ, Edgar TS, Francisco GE, et al: Abrupt withdrawal from intrathecal baclofen: Recognition and management of a potentially life-threatening syndrome. Arch Phys Med Rehabil 83:735–741, 2002.

89. Rosenson A, Ali A, Fordham E, et al: Indium-111 DPTA flow study to evaluate surgically implanted drug delivery system. Clin Nuclear Med 15:154–156, 1990.

90. Naravan R, Loubser P, Jankovic J, et al: Intrathecal baclofen for intractable axial dystonia. Neurology 41:1141–1142, 1991.

91. Ford B, Greene P, Louis E, et al: Use of intrathecal baclofen in the treatment of patients with dystonia. Arch Neurol 53: 1241–1246, 1996.

92. Penn R, Gianino J, York M: Intrathecal baclofen for motor disorders. Mov Disord 10:675–677, 1995.

93. Penn R, Mangieri E: Stiff-man syndrome treated with intrathecal baclofen. Neurology 43:2412, 1993.

94. Crone C, Nielsen J, Petersen N, Ballegaard M, et al: Disynaptic reciprocal inhibition of ankle extensors in spastic patients. Brain 117:1161–1168, 1994.

95. Ashby P, Wiens M: Reciprocal inhibition following lesions of the spinal cord in man. J Physiol (Lond) 414:145–157, 1989.

96. Shefner J, Berman S, Sarkarati M, et al: Recurrent inhibition is increased in patients with spinal cord injury. Neurology 42: 2162–2168, 1992.

97. Mazzocchio R, Rossi A: Involvement of spinal recurrent inhibition in spasticity: Further insight into the regulation of Renshaw activity. Brain 120:991–1003, 1997.

98. Raynor E, Shefner J: Recurrent inhibition is decreased in patients with amyotrophic lateral sclerosis. Neurology 44:2148–2153, 1994.

99. Katz R, Rymer W: Spastic hypertonia: Mechanisms and measurement. Arch Phys Med Rehabil 70:144–155, 1989.

100. Penn R, Savoy S, Corcos D, et al: Intrathecal baclofen for severe spinal spasticity: A double-blind crossover study. N Engl J Med 320:1517–1521, 1989.

101. Ochs G, Struppler A, Meyerson B, et al: Intrathecal baclofen for long-term treatment of spasticity: A multi-centre study. J Neurol Neurosurg Psychiatry 52:933–939, 1989.

102. Lazorthes Y, Sallerin-Caute B, Verdie J, et al: Chronic intrathecal baclofen administration for control of severe spasticity. J Neurosurg 72:393–402, 1990.

103. Müller H: Treatment of severe spasticity: Results of a multicenter trial conducted in Germany involving the intrathecal infusion of baclofen by an implantable drug delivery system. Rev Eur Technol Biomed 13:184–186, 1991.

104. Loubser P, Narayan P, Sandin K, et al: Continuous infusion of intrathecal baclofen: Long-term effects on spasticity in spinal cord injury. Paraplegia 29:48–64, 1991.

105. Coffey JR, Cahill D, Steers W, et al: Intrathecal baclofen for intractable spasticity of spinal origin: Results of a long-term multicenter study. J Neurosurg 78:226–232, 1993.

106. Albright AL, Barron W, Fasick M, et al: Continuous intrathecal baclofen infusion for spasticity of cerebral origin. JAMA 270: 2475–2477, 1993.

107. Albright AL, Cervi A, Singletary J: Intrathecal baclofen for spasticity in cerebral palsy. JAMA 265:1418–1422, 1991.

108. Meythaler JM, Guin-Renfroe SG, Grabb P, et al: Long-term continuously infused intrathecal baclofen for spastic-dystonic hypertonia in traumatic brain injury: 1-year experience. Arch Phys Med Rehabil 80:13–19, 1999.

109. Meythaler JM, Hadley M, McCary A: Prospective study on the use of continuously infused intrathecal baclofen for spasticity due to acquired brain injury: A preliminary report. J Neurosurg 87:415–419, 1997.

110. Becker R, Alberti O, Bauer BL: Continuous intrathecal baclofen infusion in severe spasticity after traumatic or hypoxic brain injury. J Neurol 244:160–166, 1997.

111. Rifici C, Kofler M, Kronenberg M, et al: Intrathecal baclofen application in patients with supraspinal spasticity secondary to severe traumatic brain injury. Funct Neurol 9:29–34, 1994.

112. Saltuari L, Kronenberg M, Marosi MJ, et al: Long-term intrathecal baclofen in supraspinal spasticity. Acta Neurol 14:195–207, 1992.

113. Meythaler JM, Guin-Renfroe SG, Hadley MN: Continuously infused intrathecal baclofen for spastic-dystonic hemiplegia: A preliminary report. Am J Phys Med Rehabil 78:247–254, 1999.

Selective Peripheral Denervation for Spasmodic Torticollis

GUY BOUVIER ■ PEDRO MOLINA-NEGRO

Spasmodic torticollis is a manifestation of dystonia. Dystonia may be segmentary or generalized. Regardless of whether it is segmentary or generalized, most patients carry a genetic predisposition for dystonia.[3] In a few patients, the dystonia may result from a lesion involving the basal ganglia and their connections.[2] The objective of selective peripheral denervation is to correct the abnormal posture and abolish the abnormal movements of the head while preserving the function of muscles not involved in dystonic movement.

This chapter is intended to help physicians recognize the various forms of spasmodic torticollis, better understand the role of specific muscles, and ultimately determine which muscles should be denervated and which ones should be preserved. A historical review of various surgical techniques for the treatment of spasmodic torticollis has been provided by Bertrand and colleagues.[3] The same group described the normal anatomy of the cervical muscles in relation to the various types of movements and their respective innervation.

PHYSIOPATHOLOGY

Movements of the head are made essentially on three cartesian axes:

> Horizontal axis: rotatory movements (i.e., toward the right or the left)
> Sagittal axis: movements of flexion or extension
> Frontal axis: movements of lateral inclination (i.e., right and left)

In spasmodic torticollis, simple movements occur on one of the cartesian axes, or more frequently, complex movements occur on various axes.

The main muscle responsible for a specific movement is called an *agonist*. A muscle that has an action contrary to the agonist is called an *antagonist*. Agonist and antagonist actions are reinforced by one or more *synergistic muscles*.

In simple movements, it is possible to distinguish between an agonist, a synergist, and an antagonist muscle. However, in complex movements, it is sometimes difficult to establish which muscle is the agonist and which is the antagonist or the synergist.

The law of reciprocal innervation stipulates that the contraction of an agonist is followed by a reflex inhibition of the antagonist. For example, in a left rotatory movement, there is a contraction of the main agonist (i.e., right sternocleidomastoid muscle) and a reflex inhibition of the antagonist (i.e., left sternocleidomastoid muscle).

In dystonia, the reciprocal innervation law is broken. For example, if a patient with a left rotatory torticollis tries to turn the head to the right, there is a paradoxical inhibition of the agonist of this movement, the left sternocleidomastoid muscle. Simultaneously, the antagonist to the movement of rotation to the right, the right sternocleidomastoid muscle, remains contracted in a paradoxical manner.

CLINICAL FORMS OF TORTICOLLIS

Because spasmodic torticollis is an exaggeration of normal, simple or complex movements, we can describe the different types of movements of the head in relation to the cartesian axes. Simple movements refer to rotation, lateral tilting, extension, and flexion. A complex movement may contain a combination of more than one movement, with some being predominant and others relatively secondary. In such instances, contributions of the agonist and the synergist vary. The description of a complex movement must clearly identify which movement is predominant (e.g., rotation, lateral tilting, flexion). In this example, rotation is dominant, and flexion is less dominant; the agonist is the muscle responsible for rotation, and the synergist is the muscle responsible for flexion, or a complex movement may be seen, with flexion, lateral tilting, and rotation. In the former example, the muscle responsible for flexion was the synergist, and in the latter example, the same muscle (synergist) becomes the agonist.

To simplify the classification, we define a single combination of complex movements, even if there could be some type in which some movement would be predominant. The academic interest of defining the main agonist and synergist has no impact on the proposed surgical procedure.

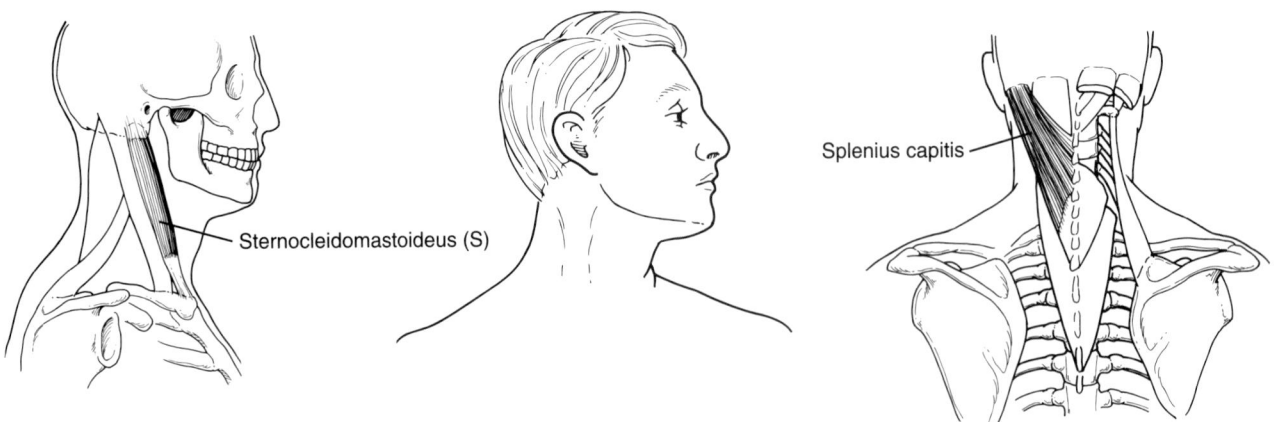

FIGURE 178–1. Rotatory torticollis. SCM (C), cleidal portion of the sternocleidomastoid muscle.

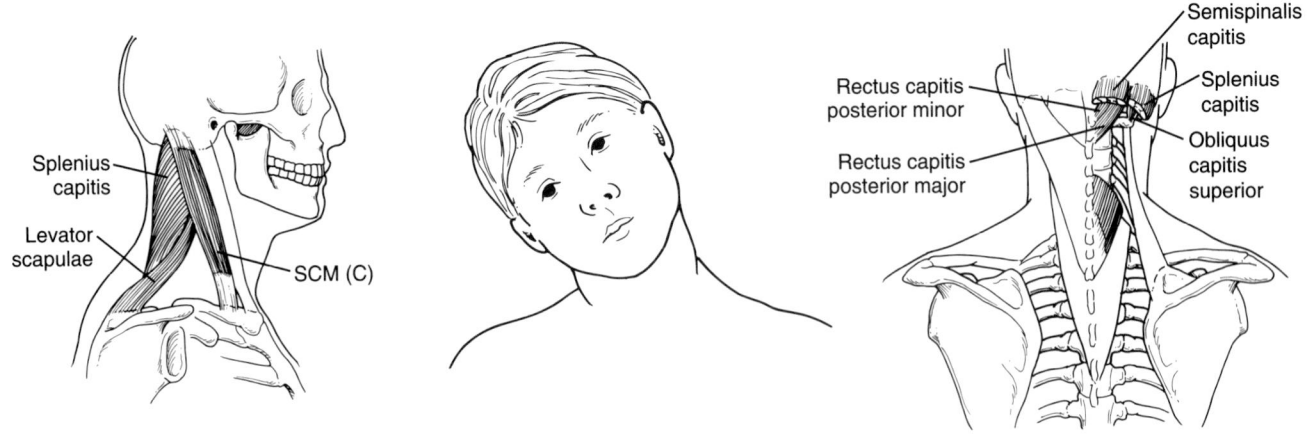

FIGURE 178–2. Laterocollis.

I. SIMPLE MOVEMENTS
  A. Rotation
    The main agonists are the sternocleidomastoid muscle opposite to the rotation and the posterior muscles on the side of the rotation.
    Clinical type: rotatory torticollis (Fig. 178–1)
  B. Lateral tilting
    The main agonist is the levator scapulae, and the synergists are the posterior muscles on the same side.
    Clinical type: laterocollis (Fig. 178–2)
  C. Extension
    Simultaneous contraction of the recti and obliqui muscles occurs with the synergistic action of the splenius capitis and semispinalis capitis muscles.

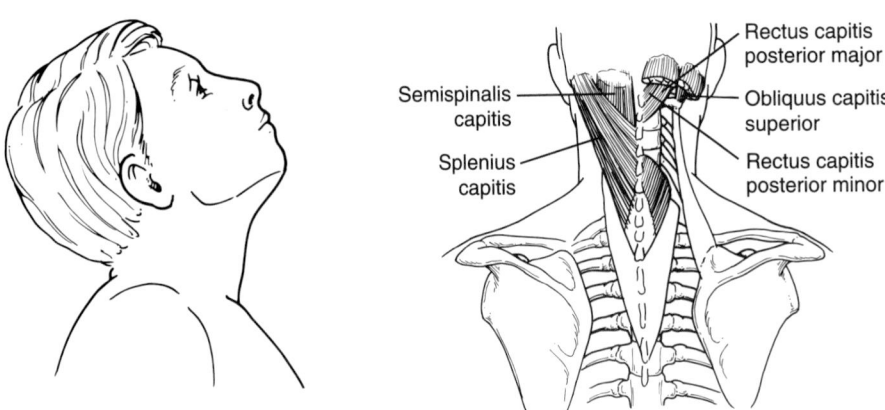

FIGURE 178–3. Superior retrocollis.

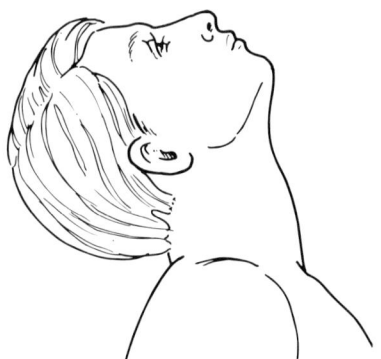

FIGURE 178–4. Inferior retrocollis.

Clinical type: superior retrocollis (Fig. 178–3)
   This "chin-up" movement should be distinguished from the extension of the cervical and dorsal spine (inferior retrocollis) (Fig. 178–4) associated with abnormal contraction of the lower cervical and upper dorsal muscles.
D. Flexion
   Simultaneous contraction of both sternocleidomastoid muscles occurs with the synergistic action of the longus capitis and longus colli muscles.
   Clinical type: antecollis
II. COMPLEX MOVEMENTS
   A. Rotation
      1. Rotation and lateral tilting
         Agonist: sternal portion of the sternocleidomastoid muscle, opposite to the rotation; posterior group on the side of the rotation
         Synergist: levator scapulae on the side of the tilting
         Clinical type: rotatory laterocollis (Fig. 178–5)
      2. Rotation plus extension
         Agonist: contraction of the sternocleidomastoid muscle on the side opposite to the rotation and contraction of the posterior muscles on the side of the rotation
         Synergist: obliquus superior and semispinalis capitis on the side opposite to the rotation
         Clinical type: rotatory retrocollis (Fig. 178–6)
      3. Rotation and flexion
         Agonist: contraction of the sternocleidomastoid to the side opposite to the rotation; contraction of the cleidal part of the sternocleidomastoid on the side of the flexion

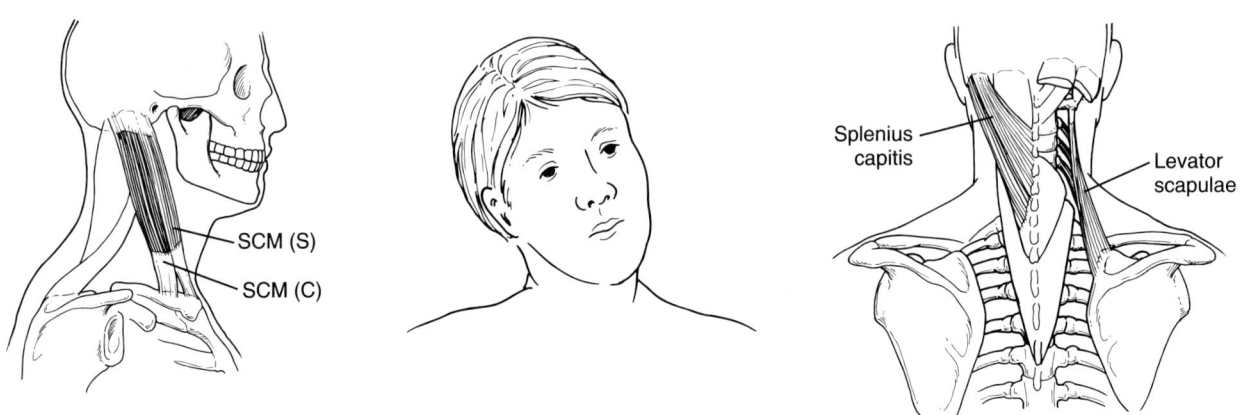

FIGURE 178–5. Rotation and contralateral tilting. SCM (S), sternal portion of the sternocleidomastoid muscle.

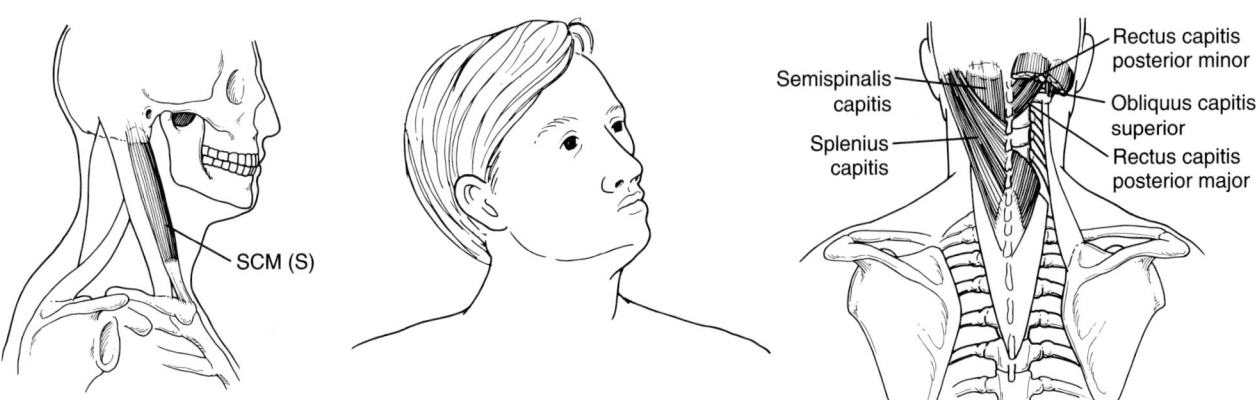

FIGURE 178–6. Rotation and retrocollis.

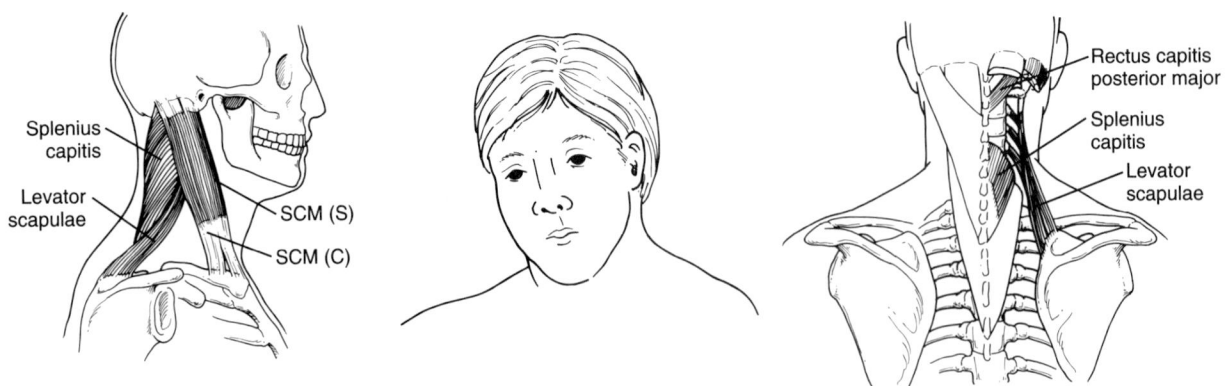

FIGURE 178–7. Rotation and ipsilateral tilting.

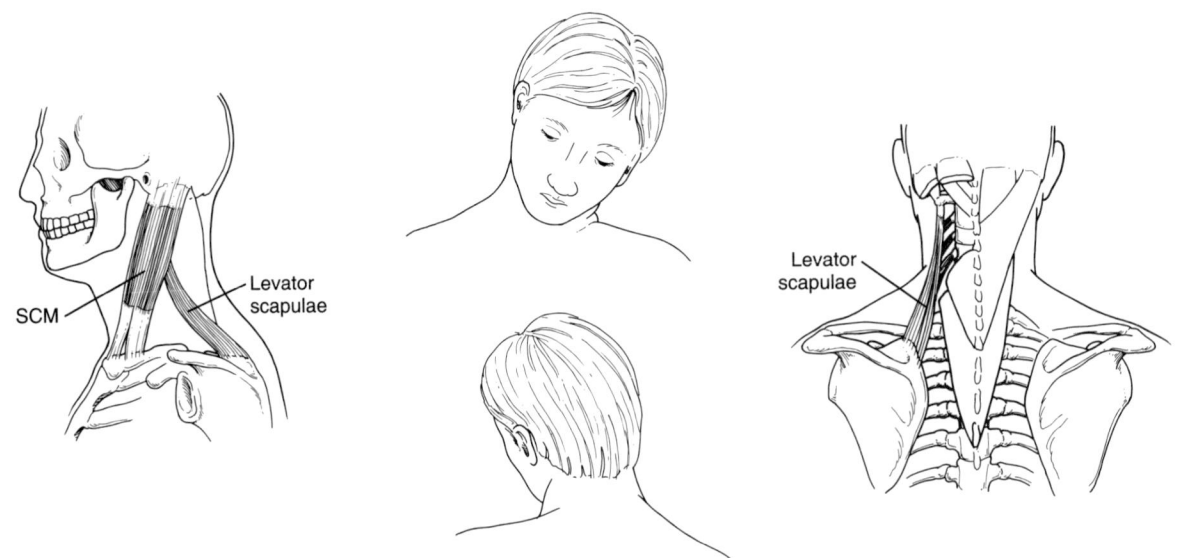

FIGURE 178–8. Laterocollis and antecollis.

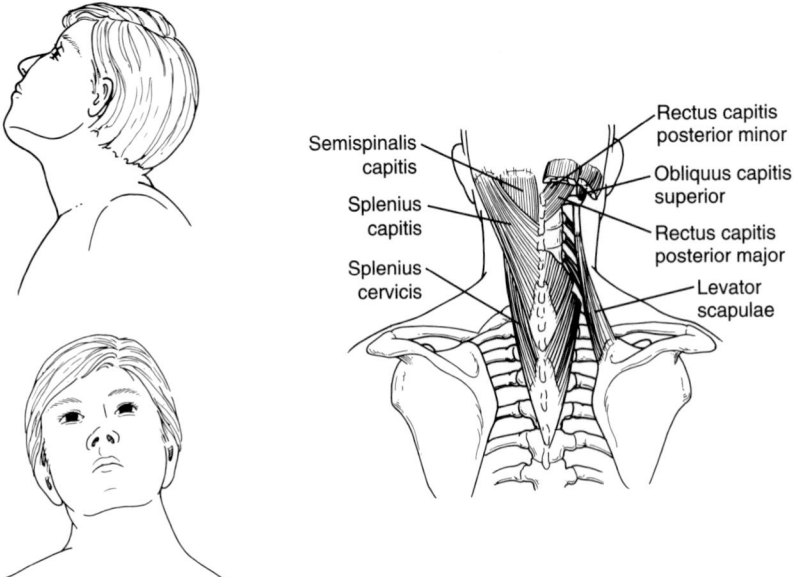

FIGURE 178–9. Laterocollis and retrocollis.

Synergist: posterior muscles on the side of
the rotation
Clinical type: rotatory antecollis (Fig. 178–7)
4. Rotation, lateral tilting, and flexion
Agonist: sternal portion of the sternocleidomastoid on the side opposite to the rotation;
cleidal portion of the sternocleidomastoid
on the side of the tilting; levator scapulae
on the side of the tilting
Synergist: muscles of the posterior group on
the side of the rotation
5. Rotation, lateral tilting, and extension
Agonist: sternal portion of the sternocleidomastoid muscle on the side opposite to the
rotation; levator scapulae on the side of the
tilting; posterior muscles on the side of the
tilting
Synergist: semispinalis capitis on the side opposite to the rotation
B. Lateral tilting
1. Lateral tilting and flexion
Agonist: main agonists are the levator scapulae and the cleidal portion of the sternocleidomastoid muscle on the side of the tilting
Synergist: posterior muscles on the side of
the tilting
Clinical type: lateroantecollis (Fig. 178–8)
2. Lateral tilting and extension
Agonist: levator scapulae as the main agonist
Synergist: posterior muscles on the same side
Clinical type: lateroretrocollis (Fig. 178–9)
C. Extension
D. Flexion
Complex movements involving extension or
flexion have been described previously (A2.
through B2.) (Table 178–1).

ELECTROMYOGRAPHY

The clinical evaluation is completed by electromyographic analysis of spontaneous and induced movements. After the clinical evaluation, the hypotheses
on the agonists and synergists must be validated by
electromyography, a procedure used for recording the
activity in at least four muscles, to establish the pri-
mum movens of each movement. Proper knowledge of
the anatomy and function of each muscle is essential.
The activity recorded during spontaneous movements
is compared with the activity recorded at the time of
movements executed on command with or without
resistance. This allows definition of the phenomenon
of paradoxical contraction or inhibition.

Postoperative electromyographic analysis can confirm that the denervation has been completed, define
muscles that have been spared at the time of the first
operation, and identify the muscles responsible for the
abnormal residual movements. To verify the contribution of a specific muscle in complex movements, blocks
using a local anesthetic agent under electromyographic
control may be useful.

INDICATIONS FOR SELECTIVE PERIPHERAL DENERVATION

The main criterion in determining whether surgery is
indicated is the clinical identification, confirmed by
electromyographic analysis, of the agonist and synergist muscles responsible for the abnormal posture and
movements. The torticollis must be present for at least
3 years and stable for 1 year. A positive therapeutic
result from a temporary, selective denervation using
botulinum toxin (Botox) indicates a good surgical result
with selective peripheral denervation.

For a simple movement, selective peripheral denervation is performed in one step, which consists of
denervation of the agonists and synergists. For complex movements, the surgeon must decide which muscles have to be denervated; some surgeons prefer to
denervate all muscles involved in one surgical procedure, but we prefer to proceed step by step. For example, in the case of a patient with a combination of left
rotation and extension, we start by correction of the
rotation, and according to the results, we treat the
extension if necessary. The first procedure consists of
denervation of the right sternocleidomastoid muscle
associated with a left posterior ramisectomy from C1
to C6. If a second procedure is performed, it consists
of a right superior ramisectomy from C1 to C4.

Patients with generalized dystonia should be carefully evaluated to establish the appropriateness of surgical treatment. In most patients with generalized dystonia, selective peripheral denervation is not indicated,
because it is rarely possible to define a particular pattern from clinical and electromyographic evidence that
would allow the possibility of this surgical approach.
In these cases, there is also a possibility of a flare-up
of the dystonia after surgery. Although aggravation of
the clinical picture is usually temporary, we had two
patients with permanent aggravation of the dystonia.
It can be argued that such aggravation would eventually have taken place, even if the patient has not been
subjected to surgery, but the patient should be made
aware of this possible complication.

Selective peripheral denervation may be indicated
in cases of generalized dystonia under the following
conditions:

1. There is a definite pattern from the clinical and
electromyographic evidence that makes it possible to
define a particular form of torticollis.
2. This particular abnormal movement is for the
patient a major handicap that prevents her or him from
enjoying a normal life.

Since the previous edition of this textbook, we had
the opportunity to operate on three patients with severe, generalized dystonia in which a specific form of
torticollis was clearly identified. In all three cases, the
result was at least as good as in the pure form of
segmental dystonia. Generalized dystonia is not an
absolute contraindication for selective peripheral denervation.

T A B L E 1 7 8 – 1 ■ **Surgical Techniques for Clinical Forms of Spasmodic Torticollis**

		PROPOSED SURGICAL PROCEDURE*					
MOVEMENT	**TYPE OF TORTICOLLIS**	**DM Right SCM Muscle**	**DM Left SCM Muscle**	**RPR Right C1–6**	**LPR Left C1–6**	**DM Right Levator Scapulae**	**DM Left Levator Scapulae**
Simple Movements							
Rotation	Left rotatory torticollis	√			√		
	Right rotatory torticollis		√	√			
Lateral tilting	Left laterocollis						√
	Right laterocollis					√	
Extension	Superior retrocollis			√	√		
	Inferior retrocollis						
Flexion	Superior antecollis	√	√				
	Inferior antecollis						
Complex Movements							
Rotation							
Rotation and lateral tilting	Left rotatory torticollis, left laterocollis	√			√		√
	Left rotatory torticollis, right laterocollis	√			√	√	
	Right rotatory torticollis, right laterocollis		√	√		√	
	Right rotatory torticollis, left laterocollis		√	√†			√
Rotation and extension	Left rotatory torticollis, right retrocollis	√			√		
	Right rotatory torticollis, left retrocollis		√	√	√†		
	Left rotatory torticollis, bilateral retrocollis	√		√	√		
	Right rotatory torticollis, bilateral retrocollis		√	√	√		
Rotation and flexion	Left rotatory torticollis, right flexion	√			√		
	Left rotatory torticollis, left flexion	√	√		√		
	Right rotatory torticollis, left flexion	√	√	√			
	Right rotatory torticollis, right flexion	√	√	√			
Rotation, lateral tilting and flexion	Right rotatory torticollis, right laterocollis, right flexion	√	√	√		√	
	Left rotatory torticollis, left laterocollis, left flexion	√	√		√		√
Rotation, lateral tilting and extension	Right rotatory torticollis, right laterocollis, right retrocollis		√	√		√	
	Right rotatory torticollis, right laterocollis, left retrocollis		√	√	√†	√	
	Left rotatory torticollis, left laterocollis, left retrocollis	√			√		√
	Left rotatory torticollis, left laterocollis, right retrocollis	√	√†		√		√
Lateral tilting							
Lateral tilting and flexion	Right lateral tilting, right flexion	√				√	
	Left lateral tilting, left flexion		√				√
Lateral tilting and extension	Right lateral tilting, right extension			√†		√	
	Left lateral tilting, left extension				√†		√

* Each patient deserves an individual approach because of the protean forms characteristic of spasmodic torticollis.
† Left or right superior ramisectomy, C1-4.
DM, denervation and myectomy; LPR, left posterior ramisectomy; RPR, right posterior ramisectomy; SCM, sternocleidomastoid.

SURGICAL TECHNIQUE

The general principles of the surgical technique were described by Bertrand and coworkers.[3] Since then, the technique has evolved and has been simplified. The procedure is performed under light general anesthesia, without curarization but with invasive and noninvasive monitoring.

Selective peripheral denervation cannot be performed without proper stimulation during the entire surgical procedure. Stimulation is mandatory for proper identification of the spinal accessory nerve and its rootlets to the sternocleidomastoid muscle and the trapezius and for identification of the anterior rami for the cleidal portion of the sternocleidomastoid muscle. Stimulation is also essential for identification of all the posterior rami from C1 to C6 and especially the anterior branches of C1 and C2, which contribute to deglutition. Stimulation is also useful in the identification of the anterior rami that innervate the levator scapulae.

Some muscles have different innervation sources. For example, the trapezius receives innervation from the spinal accessory nerve and from the anterior rami at C2 and C3. While denervating the levator scapulae, we expect the contraction to be limited to the levator scapulae. The anterior rami at C3 and C4 may innervate the trapezius, the deltoid, or the diaphragm. The surgeon must remember the principle of sparing the innervation of nondystonic muscles, maintaining a good function, and avoiding a neurological deficit.

Position

The procedure can be accomplished in various positions, including the dorsal decubitus position with rotation of the head contralateral to the denervation of the sternocleidomastoid muscle and, if posterior ramisectomy has to be done, repositioning the patient in the lateral or prone position for the posterior ramisectomy. Some may prefer the prone position with an initial rotation of the head to allow denervation of the sternocleidomastoid muscle and a return to the neutral position for the posterior ramisectomy.

We prefer the sitting position, with the head slightly flexed and maintained with the Gardner headrest, unless there is a congenital cardiac abnormality (e.g., patent foramen ovale). This position allows direct and easy access to the sternocleidomastoid muscle and the posterior rami in one operative field. The position is comfortable for the patient and ergonomic for the surgeon. Even if magnification is unnecessary, the use of the microscope for teaching purposes is compatible with this type of positioning. In the sitting position, the operative field remains dry, permitting safe and easy access to the posterior arches of C1 and C2, the vertebral artery, and the articular facets down to T1. The only disadvantage of this position is the possibility of air embolism, which can be controlled by proper monitoring and by meticulous technique with control of venous bleeding.

Posterior Ramisectomy

A midline incision is carried out from the external protuberance down to T1. Sharp and blunt dissections are carefully performed over the midline, avoiding unnecessary bleeding until the posterior tubercle of C1 and the spinous processes of C2 through C6 are exposed.

Sectioning is performed at the superior nuchal line of the skull, leaving a fringe of 1 cm to suture the semispinalis capitis, splenius capitis, and trapezius muscles. This permits good exposure of the suboccipital bone and the posterior arches of C1 and C2 as laterally as possible on the side of the ramisectomy.

There is a plane of cleavage between the anterior surface of the splenius capitis and splenius cervicis muscles and the posterior surface of the semispinalis capitis. This plane is followed laterally and leads directly to the articular facets at C2-3, C3-4, C4-5, and C5-6. We then proceed to the identification of the suboccipital triangle, which is formed by the rectus capitis major (medially), the superior oblique muscle of the head (superiorly), and the inferior oblique (inferiorly).

At the center of the triangle and above the posterior arch of C1, the surgeon can see the vertebral artery and, ventrally and laterally, the posterior ramus of C1. Proper stimulation is done to identify the anterior branch of C1 and spare this branch to avoid swallowing problems.

The posterior ramus of C2 is found underneath the inferior oblique muscle at its external edge. Stimulation is used to identify the anterior branch, and sectioning is performed laterally to this branch for the same reason.

Because it is extremely important to identify the anterior branch at C1 and C2 (in some circumstances) when the obliqui and the rectus capitis are hypertrophied, a myectomy of these muscles is recommended to have a better approach to C1 and C2 and their anterior branches.

The posterior rami are found at the level of each articular facet. They run over and across the deep muscles and over the posterior aspect of the longissimus capitis muscle. This muscle is cut progressively and retracted laterally to identify deeper branches. Dissection is pursued anteriorly until the four attachments of the levator scapulae are visualized. These bundles are anchored on the posterior tubercle of the transverse processes of C1, C2, C3, and C4. Each facet joint is exposed and denuded to ensure there are no rootlets remaining from the posterior rami.

Denervation of the Levator Scapulae

Until recently, denervation and myectomy of the levator scapulae was performed through a posterior approach. The procedure is relatively simple when denervation and myectomy had to be performed on the side of the posterior ramisectomy. The four attachments of the levator scapulae were already exposed, and each was cut. Stimulation was then used to identify the anterior ramus at C3 and C4. Unless there were isolated contractions of the levator scapulae, the anterior rami were left intact. The posterior approach is much more complex when performed on the side opposite to the posterior ramisectomy. Because it was usually difficult to perform proper denervation of the levator scapulae, we adopted a direct lateral approach and abandoned the posterior approach.

The incision follows the posterior border of the sternocleidomastoid muscle. The bulk of the levator scapulae is found between the posterior part of the sternocleidomastoid muscle and the anterior part of the trapezius; superiorly and posteriorly, there is the splenius capitis, and anteriorly and inferiorly, there are the scalene muscles (i.e., posterior, medial, and anterior). After cutting the platysma, the surgeon encounters the cervical fascia, through which travel the external jugular vein, the lesser occipital nerve, and the greater auricular nerve. Next is the levator scapulae. Stimulation is necessary to identify the branches of C3 and C4 ending in the muscle. Denervation is performed when there are isolated contractions in the levator scapulae. After the denervation, the myectomy of the levator scapulae completes the procedure.

Denervation of the Sternocleidomastoid Muscle

The technique used for denervation of the sternocleidomastoid muscle is identical to the one described by Bertrand and colleagues.[3] We therefore reproduce in full the description given by Bertrand:

> *The incision starts at the mastoid process and curves slightly backward as it is continued downward along the posterior limit of the sternocleidomastoid muscle to finish near the point of penetration of the spinal accessory nerve into the trapezius muscle, at the junction of the vertical and horizontal portions of the trapezius. Care is taken to identify and spare the greater auricular nerve to avoid numbness around the ear. Selective stimulation is used to identify the spinal accessory nerve. Its dissection is carried out upward to the level of the styloid process. The surgeon should be wary of a kink along the course of the nerve, before or as it divides into branches going to the sternocleidomastoid muscle. Because the spinal accessory nerve is exposed along its entire length, any traction or compression of the nerve must be carefully avoided to protect the innervation of the trapezius. All the branches that emerge from the spinal accessory nerve are dissected and stimulated. If stimulation produces isolated contraction of the sternocleidomastoid, the branch is clipped and sectioned peripheral to the clip. There are usually four to six branches going to the sternocleidomastoid, and occasionally a branch is found at the level of the styloid*

> *process. At the end, only the main trunk remains, with one or two branches to the trapezius. During dissection of the spinal accessory nerve, the surgeon must keep in mind the possibility of anatomical variations.*

Extensive myectomy of the sternocleidomastoid muscle should be performed to prevent reattachment of both ends of the muscle. When there is an associated movement of anteflexion, the main agonist appears to be the cleidal portion of the sternocleidomastoid muscle. This portion is innervated by anterior rami from C3 and C4. To avoid incomplete denervation or reinnervation, selective anterior ramisectomy should be performed.

Because there is a large cavity from the myectomy, a drain may be placed in the cavity and exteriorized with a contraincision. Proper hemostasis is required. The aponeurosis is sutured, and metallic clips are applied to the skin.

LONG-TERM RESULTS OF SELECTIVE PERIPHERAL DENERVATION

Abnormal movements may recur within a short time after surgery. The results of denervation are considered stable after a period of 6 months. For a long time, the presence of residual abnormal movements after selective peripheral denervation was related to a poor denervation or to reinnervation. Assuming that the denervation is complete, the surgeon must be sure that identification of all involved muscles has been accomplished. Some muscles have more than one source of innervation, and different muscles may share some sources of innervation. For example, the sternocleidomastoid muscle and the trapezius are innervated by the spinal accessory nerve. Occasionally, the cleidal part of the sternocleidomastoid muscle is innervated by an anterior ramus from C3 or C4. The semispinalis capitis, which is usually innervated by the posterior rami, may receive innervation from anterior rami at C3 through C5. Reoperation to complete selective peripheral denervation by denervation of the anterior rami has eliminated residual abnormal movements in most cases.

Because dystonia evolves, surgery never cures the progressive disorder. After several years, new abnormal movements may appear. Two patients, who were operated on 8 and 11 years earlier for rotatory torticollis with no abnormal movements, sought medical con-

T A B L E   1 7 8 – 2 ■ **Patient and Surgeon Degree of Satisfaction after Surgery**

DEGREE OF SATISFACTION	PATIENT AFTER SURGERY	PATIENT AT REVIEW	SURGEON AT LAST VISIT
Very satisfied	29 (37.7%)	22 (28.6%)	29 (37.7%)
Satisfied	37 (48.1%)	36 (46.8%)	24 (31.2%)
Moderately satisfied	3 (3.9%)	6 (7.8%)	6 (7.8%)
Unsatisfied	8 (10.4%)	13 (16.9%)	2 (2.6%)
Total	77 (100%)	77 (100%)	61*

* We lack medical follow-up in 16 (20.8%) cases.

T A B L E 1 7 8 – 3 ■ Cumulative Degree of Satisfaction after Surgery

DEGREE OF SATISFACTION	PATIENT AFTER SURGERY	PATIENT AT REVIEW	SURGEON AT LAST VISIT
Satisfied	66 (85.8%)	58 (75%)	53 (68.9%)
Unsatisfied	11 (14.2%)	19 (25%)	8 (10.4%)

sultations again because of the appearance of rotatory torticollis toward the opposite side. Both patients had selective peripheral denervation that corrected these new abnormal movements.

In a review of our long-term surgical results at Notre-Dame Hospital (De Soultrait and Dulou, unpublished observations, 2002),[4] the follow-up period varied between 3 and 16 years. A questionnaire was mailed to our patients, and 77 provided sufficient data to complete a statistical analysis. Subjective evaluations made immediately postoperatively and at the time of the survey were compared with our own degree of satisfaction at the time of each patient's last visit (Table 178–2). Cumulative values of satisfied and unsatisfied responses were also tabulated (Table 178–3). Long-term results declined from 85% satisfied initially to 75% satisfied in the long term. Overall subjective improvement compared favorably with our own evaluation.

Persistence of pain after surgery was the most common reason for reported lack of satisfaction, followed by disappointment regarding head and neck posture compared with the patient's preoperative expectations. Reduction of satisfaction by 10% of patients after prolonged follow-up may be explained by the progressive nature of dystonia.

CONCLUSIONS

Selective peripheral denervation is the only surgical technique used at Notre-Dame Hospital for the surgical treatment of spasmodic torticollis since it was proposed and developed by Claude Bertrand with the collabora-

tion of Pedro Molina-Negro. This technique has developed progressively during the last 25 years. Preoperative and postoperative clinical and electromyographic evaluations have allowed us to better understand the physiopathology of dystonic movements in spasmodic torticollis. It is now possible to define more precisely the particular characteristics of innervation of different muscles and to establish which surgical technique is appropriate for the different clinical forms.

Selective peripheral denervation is true to its name because it allows adjustment of the surgical technique to each particular clinical form. Improved knowledge of the anatomy and the innervation of the cervical muscles has enabled us to avoid side effects such as decreased range of motion of the neck, dysphagia, and weakness of the shoulder. The encouraging long-term results strongly support selective peripheral denervation as the best technique for the surgical treatment of spasmodic torticollis.

REFERENCES

1. Ozelius L, Kramer PL, Moscowitz CB, et al: Human gene for torsion dystonia located on chromosome 9q32-q34. Neuron 2: 1427–1434, 1989.
2. Molina-Negro P: Neurology of brain functional disorders. In Rassmussen T, Marino R Jr (eds): Functional Neurosurgery. New York, Raven Press, 1979, pp 25–44.
3. Bertrand C, Molina-Negro P, Bouvier G, et al: Surgical treatment of spasmodic torticollis. In Youmans JR (ed): Neurological Surgery, 4th ed. Philadelphia, WB Saunders, 1996.
4. Molina-Negro P, Bouvier G: Surgical treatment of spasmodic torticollis by peripheral denervation. In Tarsi D, Vitek JL, Lozano AM (eds): Surgical Treatment of Parkinson's Disease and Other Movement Disorders. Totowa, NJ, Humana Press, 2003, pp 275–286.

CHAPTER 179

Treatment of Intractable Vertigo

STEVEN A. TELIAN ■ JULIAN T. HOFF

Vestibular symptoms may result from a variety of inner ear, cerebellopontine angle, and central nervous system (CNS) lesions. Labyrinthine symptoms accompany a wide variety of otologic disorders, including Ménière's disease, vestibular neuritis, chronic otitis media, labyrinthine injury, and the effects of ototoxic drugs. These symptoms are frequently of great concern to the patient and may cause occupational and social disability. Physical discomfort due to nausea, vomiting, and diarrhea may accompany the attacks. Central nervous system disease, including tumors, vascular insufficiency, demyelinating diseases, and vascular compression syndromes, may also cause dizziness. Lesions of the peripheral or central vestibular system are identified, beginning with the history and physical examination, followed by appropriate audiometric, vestibular, and radiographic studies. Unstable lesions of the peripheral vestibular system are often amenable to surgical treatment if the offending labyrinth can be identified with certainty.

CLASSIFICATION

Vestibular symptoms may be caused by peripheral or central vestibular disorders.[1] Generally, peripheral vestibular disorders are associated with a fairly intense sensation of motion (i.e., vertigo or pulsion) and with somatic vegetative symptoms, especially pallor, nausea, and vomiting. Central vestibular disorders other than those associated with devastating acute pontine infarction or hemorrhage are usually characterized by a more chronic dysequilibrium and may be associated with other neurological abnormalities. Although the classic clinical characteristics of peripheral and central vestibular disorders are well described, disease variability and the individual patient's description of the symptoms may obscure the correct diagnosis.

Central Vestibular Disorders

The differential diagnosis of vertigo includes diseases affecting the brainstem and those that are focused more peripherally. Although peripheral disorders are more common, the following central vestibular disorders should be considered in the patient with vertigo.

VERTEBROBASILAR ISCHEMIA

Reduced blood flow in the vertebrobasilar system may cause dizziness of any form. Transient symptoms may accompany arterial hypotension from a variety of causes, including cardiac arrhythmias and orthostatic hypotension induced by medications or postural changes. The same symptoms may develop from focal ischemia in the brainstem caused by small-vessel thrombosis. The advent of magnetic resonance imaging (MRI) has assisted in documenting this phenomenon. Acute vertigo caused by central ischemia or hemorrhage is usually associated with nystagmus and occasionally with hearing loss and tinnitus. If these signs and symptoms are related to posterior fossa ischemia rather than an acute labyrinthine event, they are usually accompanied by other brainstem or cerebellar symptoms such as diplopia, ataxia, dysarthria, and dysphagia. The diagnosis of posterior fossa syndromes related to ischemia is essentially a clinical one. Transcranial Doppler studies have been used to help document chronic vascular insufficiency.[2] Other studies, including angiography, may or may not be definitive.

Vertigo may be the initial symptom of spontaneous cerebellar hemorrhage or infarction. Rapidly progressive cerebellar and, later, brainstem signs suggest the diagnosis. Sometimes, the lesion may be relatively silent neurologically and imitate a classic peripheral lesion such as vestibular neuritis.[3] MRI or computed tomography (CT) should be obtained when potentially serious vascular insults are suspected.

MIGRAINE

Patients who suffer from classic migraine sometimes have vertigo before or during a typical headache because of vascular changes within the vestibular nucleus.[4, 5] Some may have a migraine equivalent that causes vertigo without headache. This diagnosis may be suspected when there is a significant family or personal history of migraine. This condition may lead to diagnostic confusion because the vertigo spells are very similar to those of Ménière's disease. They may be distinguished from Ménière's attacks because hearing loss and other auditory symptoms rarely or never accompany migraine-associated vertigo. Confirmation of the diagnosis comes only with successful administration of a therapeutic trial of migraine prophylaxis. Abortive therapy at the onset of symptoms may also prove effective.

CONGENITAL ANOMALIES

Skull base and posterior fossa CNS anomalies may be associated with vertigo. The Arnold-Chiari malformation and platybasia causing brainstem distortion are examples of potentially symptomatic congenital deformities. Generally, these disorders manifest with vague symptoms and central abnormalities identified on oculomotor testing. A combination of routine skull radiographs, CT, and MRI substantiate the clinical diagnosis.

DEMYELINATING DISEASE

Vertigo or dizziness is the initial symptom in up to 25% of patients with multiple sclerosis. Nearly 75% of patients with this disease experience vertigo at some time during the course of the illness. Vertigo may be transient or sustained, and it is usually accompanied by nystagmus. Other focal neurological signs, separated by time and location, suggest a demyelinating disease. Although the diagnosis depends primarily on clinical interpretation, vestibular testing, cerebrospinal fluid studies, MRI, and evoked potential studies are helpful for confirmation.

EPILEPSY

Temporal lobe seizures may be heralded by a vertiginous aura. Loss of consciousness usually follows, although motor or sensory phenomena sometimes develop without altered consciousness. Electroencephalography and imaging studies establish the diagnosis.

PARANEOPLASTIC SYNDROME

Crippling vestibular symptoms may result from anti-Purkinje cell antibodies associated with a remote neoplasm.[6] The tumors are most often adenocarcinomas and are frequently occult when the patient presents. Such patients have rapidly deteriorating vestibulocerebellar function, are almost always bedridden, and usually have a dismal prognosis. This diagnosis may be confirmed by lumbar puncture if the disease is suspected.

Peripheral Vestibular Disorders

MÉNIÈRE'S DISEASE

Ménière's disease, or endolymphatic hydrops, is a symptom complex consisting of fluctuating sensorineural hearing loss, episodic vertigo, tinnitus, and aural fullness. This has been attributed to an imbalance in the fluid compartments within the inner ear. By definition, Ménière's disease is idiopathic in origin, although an inherited susceptibility and a variety of triggering in-

sults may play a role.[7] The same symptom complex may result years after an injury to the inner ear from a temporal bone fracture, an otologic surgical procedure, or chronic suppurative otitis media. This condition is sometimes designated *Ménière's syndrome*. A more descriptive term that has gained wide acceptance for describing this subset of patients is *delayed endolymphatic hydrops*.

Classically, Ménière's disease begins with discrete episodes of aural fullness and tinnitus, followed by sensorineural hearing loss and episodic vertigo. Initially, episodes last up to several hours, with clearing of all symptoms between acute spells. As time progresses, a permanent sensorineural hearing loss develops because of accumulated damage within the cochlea, but the hearing acuity continues to fluctuate from the new baseline with subsequent episodes. Long-standing Ménière's disease may produce a mild, chronic unsteadiness that continues between spells. The vertigo spells commonly become more sudden in onset and shorter in duration in the late stages of the disease. Sometimes, they occur with no warning, because the auditory function has deteriorated to the point that it can no longer fluctuate with spells. The onset of drop attacks (i.e., otolithic crises of Tumarkin) is a serious complication that may occur later in the disease process. These attacks result from a sudden loss of limb extensor tone because of sudden changes in neural input to the vestibular nuclei from the otolithic organs in the involved ear. Such spells often necessitate destruction of the labyrinth to prevent severe patient injury from falls.

Two subclasses of idiopathic endolymphatic hydrops exist. Cochlear hydrops is characterized as fluctuating sensorineural hearing loss, tinnitus, and aural fullness without vertigo. Conversely, vestibular hydrops causes episodic vertigo and aural fullness without auditory changes. As expected, the latter form is very difficult to distinguish from migraine equivalent vertigo unless auditory symptoms eventually emerge. Ménière's disease becomes bilateral in 10% to 40% of patients. Although the disease may occur in any age group, it most commonly affects those between the ages of 30 and 50 years, and it almost never develops before the late teenage years.

Although the clinical history is generally sufficient to make the diagnosis, supporting audiologic and vestibular studies are helpful. Classically, the patient has low-frequency sensorineural hearing loss, and serial audiograms may document fluctuation of the hearing level in the involved ear (Fig. 179–1). The electronystagmographic examination is typically normal early in the disease, but a unilaterally reduced vestibular response frequently develops over time. Results of auditory brainstem response testing and imaging studies are normal.

VESTIBULAR NEURITIS

Vestibular neuritis is characterized by the sudden onset of vertigo that is not associated with auditory symptoms such as sensorineural hearing loss, tinnitus, or

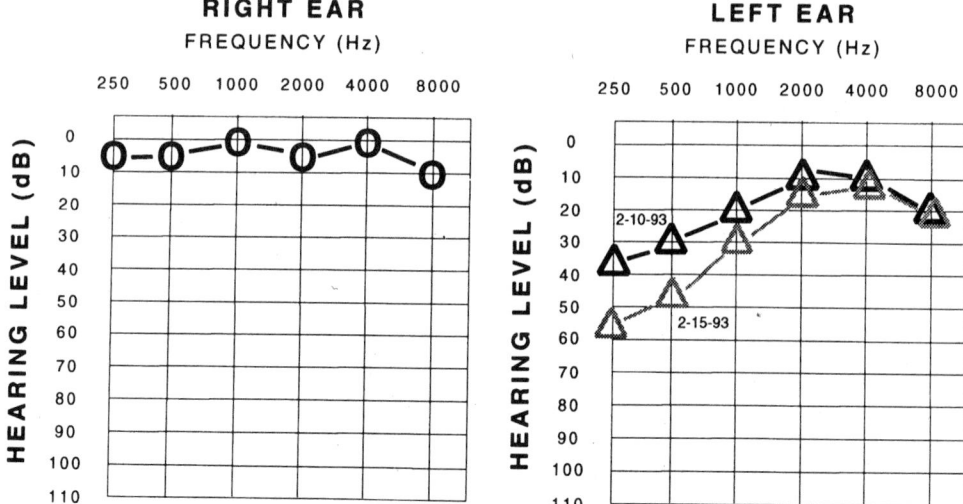

FIGURE 179–1. The typical audiometric findings in unilateral Ménière's disease involve a low-frequency sensorineural hearing loss with frequent fluctuations in auditory acuity, often preceding attacks of vertigo.

aural fullness. The etiologic factor is generally believed to be a viral infection, although other causes, including vascular occlusion, have been proposed. The acute vertigo is quite intense and usually debilitating. The intensity decreases over 24 to 72 hours as the acute phase of vestibular compensation rectifies neural activity in the vestibular nuclei. Residual dysequilibrium or positional vertigo may persist for months until the chronic phase of vestibular compensation is complete. In most patients, symptoms resolve completely without specific treatment. In some patients, motion-provoked vertigo or a degree of dysequilibrium may persist long term. This condition is known as *uncompensated vestibular neuritis*, a diagnosis that encompasses a large number of patients with chronic vestibular complaints. The condition usually is not responsive to surgical treatment.

The classic clinical history is usually diagnostic of vestibular neuritis, but other otologic diseases should be excluded by otoscopic and audiometric examination, auditory brainstem response testing, and appropriate radiologic studies. Electronystagmographic testing demonstrates spontaneous nystagmus unless compensation is complete. A reduced vestibular response to caloric irrigations is anticipated but not universally documented. Rotational chair studies usually show an increase in the phase lead and may also demonstrate an asymmetrical vestibulo-ocular reflex response to rightward versus leftward acceleration. When present, the caloric weakness and rotational chair asymmetry allow for identification of the pathologic side. Results of auditory brainstem responses and imaging studies are normal.

LABYRINTHITIS

Inflammatory conditions of the inner ear may result from viral, bacterial, or syphilitic infections. There may also be immune-mediated or vasculitic involvement of the membranous labyrinth. The unifying feature of these diagnoses is the presence of a sensorineural hearing loss accompanying the vertigo. Test results are similar to those seen in vestibular neuritis, except that the audiogram is abnormal.

BENIGN PAROXYSMAL POSITIONAL VERTIGO

Benign paroxysmal positional vertigo (BPPV) is characterized by bursts of short-duration vertigo associated with specific head positions or movements. There may also be a continuous but not disabling unsteadiness. BPPV is thought to result from otoconia that have dislodged from the utricular macula, settling into one of the semicircular canals and rendering it gravity sensitive. The posterior semicircular canal is the most commonly affected, but variations of this disease involving the horizontal or superior semicircular canal have also been documented. In one form of this disease, called *canalithiasis*, the otoconia are floating freely in the endolymph of the canal. The spell lasts up to 30 seconds, unless returning to a nonprovocative head position interrupts it. Usually, the onset is delayed (i.e., latent form) for 2 to 5 seconds after assuming the position, after which the intensity of the associated nystagmus crescendos over a few seconds and then decrescendos. The response fatigues if the stimulating head position is assumed repeatedly. The ear that is dependent when the symptoms are produced is almost always the pathologic ear. Another less common form of BPPV, called *cupulolithiasis*, develops when the otoconia become adherent to the cupula of a semicircular canal. This results in a continuous nystagmus and vertigo lasting as long as the position is maintained. Both conditions are self-limited, typically resolving without treatment within 2 months, but recurrences are common.

PERILYMPH FISTULA

Perilymph fistula is a controversial diagnosis that centers on the phenomenon of inner ear fluid (i.e., perilymph) leaking into the middle ear through the oval window, round window, or other fibrous clefts in the bony otic capsule that may be abnormally patent. The fistulas may develop after stapedectomy surgery, penetrating middle ear trauma, head trauma, barotrauma, or possibly spontaneously. Uncertainty regarding the clinical criteria for the diagnosis and the inability to document the presence of a microfistula at surgery contribute to the problematic nature of this condition.

OSCILLOPSIA

Complete absence of peripheral vestibular function (i.e., Dandy's syndrome) results in oscillopsia, the sensation of bobbing of the visual surroundings with head motion. Patients with this disorder have constant dysequilibrium but do not have vertigo. Partial accommodation to these symptoms does occur because of the use of visual and proprioceptive inputs, allowing most patients to ambulate unassisted under ideal conditions. However, they are at considerable risk in darkness, on uneven surfaces, and especially in the relatively weightless underwater environment because of the lack of labyrinthine inputs to the balance system. Affected individuals may be unable to drive because of the disturbing motion of the horizon associated with bumps in the road, and almost all are unable to read street signs without dramatically slowing or stopping the car.

Certain individuals are highly susceptible to this complication because of a mitochondrial DNA mutation that interferes with the intracellular metabolism of aminoglycosides. The diagnosis should be suspected in patients developing symptoms after treatment of a serious infection using aminoglycoside antibiotics, even if drug levels were never above the therapeutic range. It is confirmed when vestibular testing documents a severe bilateral reduction of the caloric responses and the vestibulo-ocular reflex gain.

OTHER VESTIBULAR ABNORMALITIES

Vestibular symptoms may result from other disturbances of the inner ear, such as idiopathic or immune-mediated progressive sensorineural hearing loss, temporal bone fracture, acute or chronic otitis media, temporal bone lesions, and cerebellopontine angle tumors. Each of these conditions may be associated with dysequilibrium or episodic vertigo and can be identified by careful otologic consultation.

DIAGNOSIS

Clinical Features

The history and physical examination is paramount in determining the nature of vestibular system dysfunction. Important indicators of peripheral (i.e., labyrinthine or cranial nerve VIII) disease include a history of sudden onset, episodic rotational sensation, nausea, vomiting, and exacerbation by head motion. The initial onset of symptoms provides an important clue to the disease process. A history of sudden onset of vertigo with associated auditory symptoms is helpful in identifying peripheral labyrinthine disease. The presence of asymmetrical or fluctuating unilateral sensorineural hearing loss in a patient with vertigo is the single strongest indicator of the involved labyrinth. A history of previous temporal bone trauma, ear infection, or otologic surgery is important. Certain characteristics of balance disturbances, such as vague dysequilibrium, floating sensations, gradual onset, and unremitting symptoms, are more indicative of central or nonspecific conditions, such as anxiety disorders. The major exception to this principle is when the patient has a remote but definite history of a severe peripheral labyrinthine crisis. In such cases, the diagnosis is more likely to be an uncompensated peripheral vestibular syndrome. All patients should be asked to recount the very first episode of dizziness they experienced.

Although results of the physical examination of the ear are frequently normal for patients with dizziness, otoscopic examination may identify underlying chronic ear disease. A positive fistula test result (i.e., nystagmus with the application of positive or negative external auditory canal pressure) suggests sensitivity of the inner ear to middle ear pressure variations. This may be associated with perilymph fistula, internal traumatic disruption of inner ear membranes, labyrinthine erosion by cholesteatoma, syphilis, or Ménière's disease. Neurological examination assesses the presence of other cranial nerve deficits, cerebellar dysfunction, or brainstem signs. Facial nerve dysfunction associated with vertigo suggests an intratemporal mass lesion. The presence of lower cranial nerve deficits strongly suggests a posterior fossa or skull base lesion.

Audiometry

Audiometry evaluates auditory sensitivity to identify a conductive or sensorineural hearing loss. A complete audiogram evaluates pure tone thresholds and speech discrimination ability. Unexpectedly poor speech discrimination scores suggest a retrocochlear process, such as acoustic neuroma. Serial audiograms may show progression or fluctuation of sensorineural hearing loss, documenting inner ear dysfunction. The presence of an asymmetrical sensorineural hearing loss is a strong lateralizing sign of labyrinthine pathology. In the absence of a conflicting clinical history, the vestibular periphery responsible for the vertigo is almost invariably the side with the sensorineural hearing loss.

Auditory brainstem response testing may be used to identify a lesion of cranial nerve VIII or to confirm the true hearing sensitivity when behavioral audiometric results are suspect. Auditory brainstem response testing is quite effective in screening for cerebellopontine angle tumors, although the sensitivity for detecting the smallest tumors is reduced. This study has also been used to help identify demyelination and vascular loop compression syndromes of cranial nerve VIII.

Vestibular Testing

Clinical vestibular testing extends beyond conventional electronystagmography (ENG) to include rotational chair testing (i.e., sinusoidal harmonic acceleration) and a functional measure of balance capabilities known as dynamic posturography. These study findings can help to guide the diagnosis and treatment of dizziness. Although discussed here briefly, a complete investigation of vestibular physiology and the various testing modalities is beyond the scope of this chapter, but more complete examinations of the topics can be found elsewhere.[8, 9]

ENG includes a battery of tests that assesses oculomotor control of voluntary and involuntary eye movements, identifies pathologic eye movements such as spontaneous or positional nystagmus, and evaluates the individual responsiveness of each labyrinthine organ. The oculomotor battery includes measurement of saccade latencies and velocities, smooth pursuit ability, gaze stability, and nystagmus evoked by optokinetic stimuli. If all results are normal, any spontaneous or positional nystagmus is almost certainly of peripheral origin. The examination also includes caloric testing, which measures the intensity of the nystagmus generated by the instillation of cool and warm water into the ear canals. These results allow calculation of two important parameters: unilateral weakness, which is the relative strength of each labyrinth, and directional preponderance, which is the tendency of the system to permit right-beating versus left-beating nystagmus. Evidence of unilateral weakness of the vestibular response is particularly helpful in the presence of accompanying ipsilateral auditory symptoms or audiometric abnormalities. Unfortunately, the test evaluates only the function of the horizontal semicircular canal and the related portion of the superior vestibular nerve. No available test can independently assess the function of the posterior and superior semicircular canals or the otolithic organs. It is possible to have a normal ENG result even when a significant disorder such as vestibular neuritis or acoustic neuroma is present. Between spells, findings in cases of Ménière's disease may be normal as well.

Generally, peripheral vestibular lesions are paretic in nature and produce spontaneous nystagmus with the fast-phase beating away from the offending ear. However, the examiner should be cautious about implicating the pathologic ear by the direction of spontaneous nystagmus alone because "irritative" nystagmus may occur in some conditions, causing the fast phase of the nystagmus to beat toward the affected ear. Rapid positioning tests such as the Dix-Hallpike maneuver may be helpful in determining the involved labyrinth in BPPV. The most common and classic form of BPPV is caused by canalithiasis of the posterior semicircular canal. The downward ear that produces a positive Dix-Hallpike response contains the offending labyrinth in this form of BPPV. It is associated with rotary nystagmus that beats toward the downward ear when observing the eyes directly. When the nystagmus is recorded with electro-oculography, the nystagmus may paradox-

ically seem to be reversed. The examiner should not be confused by this phenomenon, which results from the difficulty of recording torsional nystagmus accurately. There are many other, less common forms of BPPV. The characteristics of the nystagmus observed during positional testing and rapid positioning maneuvers allow the clinician to distinguish canalithiasis from cupulolithiasis and to identify which semicircular canal is involved.[10] It is important to make such distinctions on clinical grounds because the treatment paradigms depend on an accurate diagnosis of the involved canal.

Rotational chair testing may provide supportive evidence for peripheral labyrinthine disease, but it is not independently reliable for identifying the pathologic labyrinth. This modality is most useful in the assessment of patients with bilateral vestibular lesions and those who cannot cooperate with conventional ENG, such as young children or the mentally handicapped. It is also helpful in the determination of central compensation status after vestibular injuries. Dynamic posturography is helpful in quantifying the functional result of vestibular disorders that affect postural control, for monitoring response to treatment, and for identifying malingerers.

Radiology

Radiologic evaluation of the temporal bone and posterior cranial fossa is indicated for individuals with asymmetrical sensorineural hearing loss or significant ENG abnormalities. A variety of temporal bone lesions (e.g., congenital and acquired cholesteatomas, glomus tumors, metastatic tumors, cholesterol cysts) and posterior fossa lesions (e.g., acoustic neuromas, meningiomas, brainstem lesions) may manifest clinically with vertigo. MRI with gadolinium enhancement is exquisitely sensitive for detection of mass lesions of the internal auditory canal and cerebellopontine angle, as well as for ischemic or demyelinating disease of the brainstem. High-resolution CT is preferred for the assessment of bony anatomy when intrinsic lesions of the temporal bone are suspected.

TREATMENT

Medical Management

Many patients with vertigo suffer from ineffective management instituted after an incorrect diagnosis. The history and results of diagnostic testing must be used to establish the appropriate diagnosis. Specifically, any tendency to apply the diagnosis of Ménière's disease too broadly should be avoided in light of the plethora of therapeutic options propagated through the lay press and Internet resources.

VESTIBULAR SUPPRESSION

Vestibular suppressants may be beneficial in the management of patients with vertigo, particularly during the acute phase of their symptoms.[11] Unfortunately, all vestibular suppressants act through CNS depression and may delay the natural processes of central vestibular compensation. Some patients have dysequilibrium and positional vertigo long after the acute insult because complete compensation has been prevented by inactivity and continued use of centrally acting medications. Tachyphylaxis is nearly universal when these drugs are taken regularly, rendering them ineffective when severe spells do occur. It is wise to avoid long-term, regular use of vestibular suppressants.

Although patient response to different medications is quite unpredictable, diazepam is generally the single most potent drug for the suppression of severe, disabling attacks of vertigo. Other milder but frequently effective vestibular suppressants include meclizine and dimenhydrinate. None of these medications prevents spells of vertigo from beginning, but they may provide a margin of relief after a spell occurs. The physician may consider the use of promethazine or phenothiazine antiemetics when nausea or vomiting is prominent among the symptoms. Transdermal scopolamine or propantheline may be helpful in controlling chronic symptoms that are not otherwise treatable, but use of these drugs is limited by the side effects of dry mouth and blurred vision. Dermatologic sensitivity to the transdermal patch may occur, although local skin reactions can be avoided by moving the patch to a different location with each application. The rare patient may notice subjective beneficial effects from vasodilators such as niacin, isoxsuprine, and cyclandelate.

TREATMENT OF MÉNIÈRE'S DISEASE

The diagnosis of Ménière's disease is based on the history of typical symptoms and the results of appropriate diagnostic testing. This classification must be accurate because the management of Ménière's disease involves several unique medical and operative treatments not appropriate for other syndromes. A very strict low-sodium diet (1500 to 2000 mg/day) is the hallmark of treatment, which generally requires patients to prepare meals using fresh ingredients without adding salt. Although these low-sodium diets are very restrictive, many patients recognize this stringent reduction of salt as essential for controlling their symptoms. Some patients notice that the intake of caffeine or nicotine exacerbates their symptoms.

Medications used to control the symptoms of Ménière's disease can be divided into two categories: those that may affect the underlying endolymphatic hydrops (usually diuretics) and those that provide symptomatic relief by suppressing vestibular responses. Control of vertigo by salt restriction and diuretic use may be accompanied by stabilization of hearing and decrease in the amount of tinnitus and aural fullness.

AMINOGLYCOSIDE ADMINISTRATION

Complete therapeutic ablation of peripheral vestibular function using intramuscular streptomycin sulfate was first reported by Schuknecht in 1956.[12] This method

reliably relieves vertigo but is complicated by oscillopsia (i.e., Dandy's syndrome). In an attempt to avoid oscillopsia, subtotal ablation has been advocated using titration methods of administering intramuscular streptomycin therapy. These continue to be appropriate in bilateral Ménière's disease or when the actively symptomatic ear is the only one with residual, useful hearing.[13] Administration of streptomycin is monitored by audiometric and caloric testing. Rotational chair protocols can identify the dosage level at which the first measurable reduction of vestibular function occurs and have helped to further refine this treatment modality. The total streptomycin dose required may be 10 to 50 g, administered as 1 g twice daily.

Intratympanic administration of ototoxic antibiotics, usually gentamicin, into the middle ear on the affected side to control unilateral Ménière's disease has gained widespread acceptance.[14] This has the theoretical advantage of leaving the opposite ear unaffected, avoiding any possibility of oscillopsia. However, the dosage administered to the inner ear is uncertain because of variable retention of the injected liquid in the middle ear and unpredictable absorption through the round window membrane. These variables may lead to widely disparate therapeutic responses, ranging from no response after numerous injections to a profound chemical labyrinthectomy after the first injection. In the latter group, there is often an associated profound loss of residual hearing in the involved ear.

In light of the relative simplicity and safety of this treatment option, many patients prefer intratympanic gentamicin injections to surgical intervention, knowing that surgery can be pursued later if the spells are not controlled by the injection protocol. Although results have been promising, the ideal protocol for this technique remains undefined, and there seems to be a significant risk to hearing, even when using conservative dosing schedules.[15]

Vestibular Rehabilitation

Motion-provoked vertigo or chronic dysequilibrium, or both, may persist because of poor CNS compensation after an acute peripheral injury, even if labyrinthine function is stable. Some patients adopt maladaptive postural control strategies in the setting of vestibular dysfunction that may be destabilizing in certain environments. These patients often benefit from a customized outpatient program of vestibular rehabilitation therapy, supervised by an appropriately trained physical therapist.[16] The program typically consists of a combination of habituation exercises designed to facilitate compensation by extinguishing pathologic responses to head motion, postural control exercises, and a general conditioning program. The benefits of such programs are widely accepted. Although the treatment is not always curative, most patients with stable but uncompensated lesions improve considerably. Similar treatment protocols are appropriate after any operation undertaken to ablate unilateral vestibular function.

Specific particle-repositioning maneuvers have been developed to treat BPPV caused by canalithiasis. These maneuvers may successfully reposition offending oto-lithic particles within the inner ear and eliminate the symptoms after one treatment. Success depends on the correct identification of the offending canal. Additional physical therapy techniques are widely available to treat cupulolithiasis or canalithiasis syndromes that are refractory to particle-positioning techniques. Conventional habituation protocols are also effective in treating BPPV. These measures should always be attempted before resorting to other medical or surgical interventions for BPPV.

Operative Management

RATIONALE FOR SURGERY IN VESTIBULAR DISORDERS

When vertigo results from acute disturbances of the peripheral labyrinth or vestibular nerve, the patient initially experiences intense symptoms that gradually subside. If the lesion is self-limited and stable (e.g., acute viral labyrinthitis), it does not produce fluctuating or progressive dysfunction of the system. In this setting, the process of central vestibular compensation reliably relieves dizziness in most cases by adjusting to the altered sensory inputs from the periphery. This is true unless some adverse factor prevents compensation or causes decompensation at a later date. Similarly, ongoing vestibular compensation can minimize symptoms of vestibular loss from lesions that produce an insidious progressive deterioration, such as vestibular schwannoma. However, if the lesion is unstable from day to day or rapidly progressive in nature, central compensation is not possible unless the ear can be stabilized by medical or surgical treatment. Ménière's disease is the prototypical disorder in this category, in which the ear fluctuates between allowing normal labyrinthine function and causing dramatic cochleovestibular symptoms. Vestibular system surgery is most likely to succeed when it is undertaken to stabilize an unstable inner ear by correcting an underlying defect or by ablating vestibular function in the pathologic ear. It is less likely to be successful when the labyrinthine lesion is stable but the patient is unable to compensate centrally.

Certain surgical procedures are applicable only for a particular diagnosis. Some of these operations are widely accepted as rational and effective, such as posterior semicircular canal occlusion for intractable BPPV. Other disease-specific operations, such as endolymphatic sac surgery for Ménière's disease, repair of perilymph fistula, and microvascular decompression of cranial nerve VIII, continue to generate controversy. Some surgeons have enthusiastically embraced and promoted such procedures, but others have minimized their application or abandoned them altogether. All of the operations in this group have as their unifying feature the desirable goal of correcting a pathologic process that is unique to the particular diagnosis while preserving or restoring inner ear function. Success in this setting hinges on making an exact diagnosis and selecting operations with proven efficacy.

Certain surgical procedures are designed to ablate unilateral vestibular function and may be applied successfully in the treatment of any peripheral vestibular disorder. Operations such as labyrinthectomy and vestibular nerve section fall into this category. In this setting, an exact etiologic diagnosis is less critical. Instead, the physician must be certain that the problem is attributable to ongoing fluctuant or rapidly progressive labyrinthine dysfunction and that the pathologic ear has been correctly identified. If the ongoing symptoms are caused by poor central vestibular compensation or late decompensation after a prior peripheral vestibular insult, ablative surgery is unlikely to be effective.

REPAIR OF PERILYMPHATIC FISTULA

Perilymphatic fistula is controversial because of a lack of reliable clinical diagnostic criteria, making patients vulnerable to overly zealous practitioners. However, this diagnosis must be considered in the patient with vertigo after head trauma, barotrauma, or prior stapedectomy surgery. It is particularly likely in cases of penetrating middle ear trauma with vertigo. Most physicians agree that perilymph fistulas usually heal spontaneously, and a short course of bed rest is appropriate in acute cases. In chronic cases suspected to have this condition, a trial of vestibular rehabilitation before middle ear exploration is appropriate if the diagnosis is uncertain, assuming that the patient's hearing is stable.

An exploratory tympanotomy for perilymph fistula is appropriate when a patient believed to have a fistula has not responded to more conservative management. Exploration should be undertaken using local anesthesia whenever possible. After a tympanomeatal flap is elevated, bone is removed from the posterior superior wall of the bony external auditory canal until the oval window is completely visible. It may be wise to remove any mucosal folds and the bony overhang of the round window niche to better visualize the round window membrane. It is rare to see a dramatic defect in the oval or round window in routine perilymph fistula explorations. The surgeon may suction fluid from the niche to see if it reaccumulates, although this phenomenon is common because of local anesthetic and tissue fluids. This finding alone does not verify the existence of a perilymph fistula. The surgeon should also inspect for abnormal fissures in the bony labyrinth, especially anterior to the oval window and inferior to the round window. Any suspicious area or obvious defect should be repaired by removing surrounding mucosa and patching with connective tissue that is then secured by packing. It is our practice to routinely patch the round window niche in explorations with negative results, but a more conservative approach is taken with the oval window region to avoid the risk of conductive hearing loss.

PROCEDURES FOR BENIGN PAROXYSMAL POSITIONAL VERTIGO

Gacek[17] popularized the singular neurectomy procedure for BPPV, which involves selective transection of the branch of the inferior vestibular nerve innervating the posterior semicircular canal. The nerve is interrupted within the singular canal, which travels from the posterior portion of the internal auditory canal to the posterior canal ampulla. This procedure is a highly rational choice for treatment of intractable BPPV, because it is safer and more specific than a complete section of the vestibular nerve. However, this procedure is quite demanding technically and should not be undertaken unless the surgeon has mastered the approach in the temporal bone dissection laboratory. A tympanomeatal flap is elevated using a transcanal approach, and the lip of the round window niche is removed to visualize the round window membrane itself. The singular canal is approached by drilling inferior to the round window. Ideally, the nerve is encountered and transected just before its point of entry into the ampulla. The ampulla and the vestibule are at risk during the procedure, and injury of either structure may result in severe vertigo and sensorineural hearing loss. This procedure, although safe and highly reliable in experienced hands, has largely been supplanted by the technically simpler posterior semicircular canal occlusion procedure.

Parnes[18] introduced the concept of surgical occlusion of the posterior semicircular canal for the relief of BPPV. Conceptually, the canal occlusion procedure is based on the assumption that otoconial debris, originally from the macula of the utricle, settles into the endolymphatic space of the posterior semicircular canal and produces the signs and symptoms of BPPV. The surgery is undertaken to obstruct the lumen of that portion of the bony labyrinth that contains the arch of the membranous posterior semicircular canal. After a complete mastoidectomy is performed, the dome of the posterior semicircular canal is identified between the horizontal semicircular canal and the posterior fossa dural plate. The lumen of the posterior canal is approached with a diamond drill until it is visible as a dark line through a thin layer of residual bone. The canal lumen is opened by removing the remaining bone with delicate instrumentation, taking care to avoid damaging the membranous canal or suctioning the perilymphatic fluid. The perilymph is then gently removed by placing a wick of absorbent material near the labyrinthotomy site. The membranous canal usually can be observed to collapse against the deep wall of the bony canal. The canal is then occluded by placing two small plugs of periosteum into the canal, one toward the ampulla and one toward the common crus. The labyrinthotomy is then repaired by filling the lumen with wet bone dust harvested during the mastoidectomy. This repair can be secured in position by placing bone wax or a larger piece of periosteum over the dome of the canal.

The patient may have mild to moderate unsteadiness after the procedure but is usually fit for discharge from the hospital within 24 to 48 hours. Although the risk of reactive labyrinthitis and sensorineural hearing loss from opening the bony labyrinth is recognized, it has rarely been a problem as clinical experience has been gained with the procedure. It appears that careful handling of the canal contents and preservation of the membranous labyrinth permits this intervention with an acceptably low incidence of sensorineural hearing loss.

ENDOLYMPHATIC SAC PROCEDURES

The complex of recurrent episodic vertigo, fluctuating sensorineural hearing loss, tinnitus, and aural fullness characterizes Ménière's disease. Histopathologically, Ménière's disease is associated with endolymphatic hydrops, producing distention of the membranous labyrinth. Although the specific physiologic defect causing the hydropic changes is unclear, some surgeons report a beneficial effect from endolymphatic sac surgery when patients are unresponsive to medical management.[19] Reported rates for control of vertigo are 50% to 70% with most procedures, with initial results deteriorating over time. Some suggest that the operation is ill conceived and the results are influenced by reporting bias or merely approximate the natural history of this spontaneously remitting condition. Complications of endolymphatic sac procedures include hearing loss, facial nerve paralysis, and cerebrospinal fluid leak, although they occur infrequently.

LABYRINTHECTOMY

Surgical labyrinthectomy may be considered when persistent or recurrent labyrinthine disability of any cause is associated with an ear that has severe to profound sensorineural hearing loss. The patient must concur with the assessment that the hearing is useless in the involved ear, because all residual hearing sensitivity is sacrificed by labyrinthectomy.

The transmastoid approach for labyrinthectomy allows complete visualization and removal of the entire semicircular canal system, utricle, and saccule, resulting in highly reliable relief of vertigo.[20] The transcanal oval window labyrinthectomy retains some popularity because it can be performed by approaching the inner ear through the external auditory canal, although complete ablation of vestibular neuroepithelium is less reliably accomplished.[21] These transtemporal procedures are technically demanding and require precise knowledge of the anatomy of the temporal bone generally and of the vestibular labyrinth particularly.

The disadvantage of labyrinthectomy is ipsilateral loss of hearing and a period of postoperative vertigo, followed eventually by vestibular compensation. Postoperative nystagmus is usually brisk and may persist for several days. Generally, the patient walks unassisted by the third or fourth postoperative day. Although much of vestibular compensation is complete by 2 months postoperatively, further gradual improvement over 12 to 18 months may be anticipated. In some patients, significant dysequilibrium persists. Complications of labyrinthectomy include incomplete destruction of the neuroepithelium resulting in persistent symptoms, cerebrospinal fluid leak, and facial nerve injury. In experienced hands, the overall occurrence of these complications is uncommon.

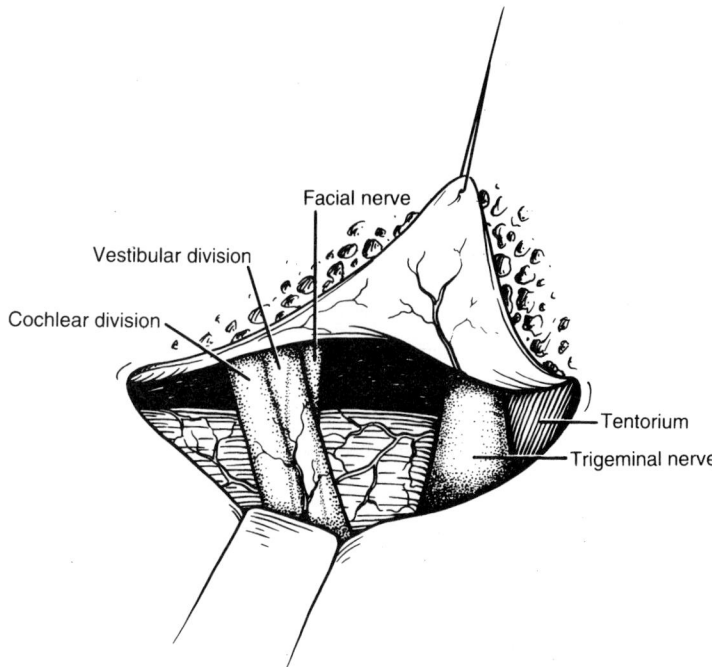

FIGURE 179–2. Surgeon's view of cranial nerve VIII in the left cerebellopontine angle during retrolabyrinthine surgery. After a complete mastoidectomy is performed, the posterior fossa dura and sigmoid sinus are widely decompressed. The dura is incised between the sigmoid sinus and the bony labyrinth, and the sinus is retracted along with the cerebellum. The vestibular fibers constitute the superior portion of the nerve. The facial nerve courses anteromedial to cranial nerve VIII.

VESTIBULAR NERVE SECTION

When useful hearing remains in the symptomatic ear, selective section of the vestibular nerve with structural preservation of the bony labyrinth and the auditory nerve fibers may be considered. In the 1930s, Dandy[22] and McKenzie[23] each reported early series of selective eighth cranial nerve sections performed through a lateral suboccipital craniotomy. Long-term follow-up of Dandy's suboccipital vestibular nerve sections demonstrated a 90% rate of complete relief of vertigo.[24] This approach continues to be widely used, but it is associated with a higher incidence of long-term headache problems postoperatively.

The middle cranial fossa approach to the vestibular nerve within the internal auditory canal was popularized in the 1970s by Fisch[25] and Glasscock.[26] This technically demanding procedure places the cochlear blood supply and the facial nerve at somewhat higher risk than with other approaches, but it permits a more definitive section of the vestibular fibers after they have divided from the main trunk of cranial nerve VIII. Relief of vertigo was accomplished in more than 90% of patients. Over the next decade, several surgeons reported successful series of retrolabyrinthine vestibular nerve sections, establishing this approach as a reliable method of selectively ablating unilateral vestibular function with a significantly lower chance of headache, hearing loss, and facial nerve injury.[27–29] The surgical view of cranial nerve VIII obtained by the retrolabyrinthine approach is shown in Figure 179–2.

The rate of control of vertigo by all routes to the vestibular nerve is 80% to 90%, making these procedures somewhat less reliable than a transmastoid labyrinthectomy. This situation results from the possibility of leaving functional vestibular neurons because of variability in the anatomic relationship between the auditory and vestibular portions of cranial nerve VIII in the posterior fossa. Postoperative sensorineural hearing loss and facial nerve paralysis are uncommon, especially with posterior fossa approaches. After vestibular nerve section, there is a period of vestibular compensation. We think that recovery from vestibular nerve section is more prolonged than that after labyrinthectomy, perhaps because of the intracranial nature of the operation. Most patients are able to return to their usual activities 2 to 4 months postoperatively.

Although the potential for catastrophic postoperative complications exists when using intracranial approaches, the overall complication rate is low. In most series, the incidence of sensorineural hearing loss is less than 10%. Cerebrospinal fluid leaks occur in 5% to 10% of cases. Stroke, subdural hematoma, facial nerve paralysis, meningitis, and wound infection have been rarely reported. It is the risk of these complications that has led to the increased popularity of intratympanic aminoglycoside administration.

NEUROVASCULAR DECOMPRESSION

Jannetta and colleagues[30] pioneered microvascular decompression of the cochlear-vestibular nerve complex for patients with disabling positional vertigo. This entity is distinct from Ménière's disease, vestibular neuritis, and BPPV and is described fully elsewhere in this volume.

REFERENCES

1. Baloh RW: Dizziness, Hearing Loss, and Tinnitus: The Essentials of Neurotology. Philadelphia, FA Davis, 1984.

2. Rubin AM, Gerard G, Bork C, et al: Central dizziness associated with cerebral blood flow disorders. Am J Otol 15:625–633, 1994.

3. Disher MJ, Telian SA, Kemink JL: Evaluation of acute vertigo: Unusual lesions imitating vestibular neuritis. Am J Otol 12:227–231, 1991.

4. Johnson GD: Medical management of migraine-related dizziness and vertigo. Laryngoscope 108(Pt 2):1–28, 1998.

5. Baloh RW: Neurotology of migraine. Headache 37:615–621, 1997.

6. Baloh RW: Paraneoplastic cerebellar disorders. Otolaryngol Head Neck Surg 112:125–127, 1995.

7. Paparella MM: The cause (multifactorial inheritance) and pathogenesis (endolymphatic malabsorption) of Ménière's disease and its symptoms (mechanical and chemical). Acta Otolaryngol (Stockh) 99:445–451, 1985.

8. Baloh RW, Honrubia V: Clinical Neurophysiology of the Vestibular System, 2nd ed. Philadelphia, FA Davis, 1990.

9. Shepard NT, Telian SA: Practical Management of the Balance Disorder Patient. San Diego, Singular Publishing, 1996.

10. Herdman S: Assessment and management of benign paroxysmal positional vertigo. In Herdman S (ed): Vestibular Rehabilitation. Philadelphia, FA Davis, 1994, pp 331–346.

11. Zee DS: Perspectives on the pharmacotherapy of vertigo. Arch Otolaryngol lll:609–612, 1985.

12. Schuknecht HF: Ablation therapy for the relief of Ménière's disease. Laryngoscope 66:859–870, 1956.

13. Balyan FR, Taibah A, DeDonato G, et al: Titration streptomycin therapy in Meniere's disease. Otolaryngol Head Neck Surg 118:261–266, 1998.

14. Hirsch BE, Kamerer DB: Role of chemical labyrinthectomy in the treatment of Meniere's disease. Am J Otol 13:18–22, 1992.

15. Blakely BW: Clinical forum: A review of intratympanic therapy. Am J Otol 18:520–526, discussion 527–531, 1997.

16. Smith-Wheelock M, Shepard NT, Telian SA: Physical therapy program for vestibular rehabilitation. Am J Otol 12:218–225, 1991.

17. Gacek RR: Technique and results of singular neurectomy for the management of benign paroxysmal positional vertigo. Acta Otolaryngol (Stockh) 115:154–157, 1995.

18. Parnes LS, McClure JA: Posterior semicircular canal occlusion in the normal hearing ear. Otolaryngol Head Neck Surg 104:52–57, 1991.

19. Shah DK, Kartush JM: Endolymphatic sac surgery in Meniere's disease. Otolaryngol Clin North Am 30:1061–1074, 1997.

20. Kemink JL, Telian SA, Graham MD, et al: Trans-mastoid labyrinthectomy: Reliable surgical management of vertigo. Otolaryngol Head Neck Surg 101:5–10, 1989.

21. Schucknecht HF: Transcanal labyrinthectomy. Oper Tech Otolaryngol Head Neck Surg 2:17–19, 1991.

22. Dandy WE: Treatment of Ménière's disease by section of only the vestibular portion of the acoustic nerve. Bull Johns Hopkins Hosp 53:52–55, 1933.

23. McKenzie KG: Intracranial division of the vestibular portion of the auditory nerve for Ménière's disease. Can Med Assoc J 34:369–381, 1936.

24. Green RE: Surgical treatment of vertigo with follow up on Walter Dandy's cases. In Proceedings of the Congress of Neurological Surgeons. Baltimore, Wilkins & Williams, 1958, pp 141–152.

25. Fisch U: Vestibular and cochlear neurectomy. Trans Am Acad Ophthalmol Otolaryngol 78:252–255, 1974.

26. Glasscock ME III, Miller GW: Middle fossa vestibular nerve section in the management of Ménière's disease. Laryngoscope 87:529–541, 1977.

27. Silverstein H, Norrell H: Retrolabyrinthine surgery: A direct approach to the cerebellopontine angle. Otolaryngol Head Neck Surg 88:462–469, 1980.

28. Kemink JL, Hoff JT: Retrolabyrinthine vestibular nerve section: Analysis of results. Laryngoscope 96:33–36, 1986.

29. House JW, Hitselberger WE, McElveen J, et al: Retrolabyrinthine section of the vestibular nerve. Otolaryngol Head Neck Surg 92:212–215, 1984.

30. Moeller MB, Moeller AR, Jannetta PJ, et al: Diagnosis and surgical treatment of disabling positional vertigo. J Neurosurg 64:21–28, 1986.

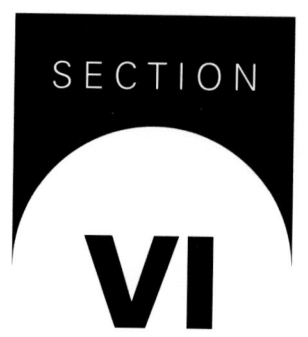

SECTION

VI

Pain

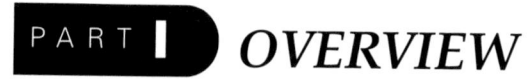

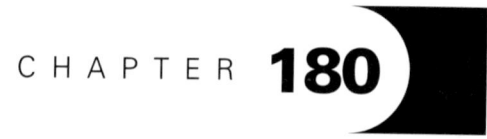

CHAPTER 180

Pain: General Historical Considerations

KIM BURCHIEL

The advent of the modern era in the neurosurgical management of pain can be traced to the start of the 19th century. In 1809 Walker[1] proposed that the anterior and posterior spinal roots serve distinct motor and sensory functions. Bell[2] subsequently expanded this idea, and Magendie[3] in 1822 provided evidence of the role of the posterior spinal roots in the transmission of pain. However, it was another 100 years until Spiller[4] and Schüller[5] described the pain conduction pathways in the anterolateral columns of the spinal cord. Although the debate concerning the anatomic and physiologic substrate serving pain continued, evidence for the specificity theory of pain gained momentum, and neurosurgeons exploited the existing knowledge of pain pathways to perform pain surgery, often with great success. Neurosurgeons were also quick to adapt new technology, most notably stereotaxy, radiofrequency generators, and the operating microscope, for pain procedures (Table 180–1).

Probably the first reported procedure for the relief of pain was in 1873, when Létiévant[6] published his description of peripheral and cranial nerve rhizotomies. Section of the posterior spinal roots for the relief of pain in humans was first proposed by Charles Dana in 1886 and performed by Bennet[7] in 1889 and also by Abbe[8, 9] in four patients. Otrid Foerster of Breslau, Poland, a neurologist by training, gained enough experience with the operation of posterior rhizotomy to perform it himself. Foerster later presented his landmark paper mapping the dermatomes in humans.[10]

TRIGEMINAL NEURALGIA

Early pain surgeons were also interested in cranial nerve pathologies, especially tic douloureux, a condition that had vexed patients and physicians alike for more than 2 centuries.[11] Bell had established the trigem-

inal nerve as the sensory nerve for the face in 1844.[12] Although Victor Horsley is credited with the first gasserian ganglionectomy and retrogasserian neurotomy in 1891,[13] in truth, the contributory efforts of several other neurosurgical pioneers helped transform the management of trigeminal neuralgia. Horsley used the extradural temporal approach described by Hartley[14] and Krause,[15] but because his patient died, retrogasserian neurotomy was abandoned until Tiffany[16] in 1896 and Spiller and Frazier[17] in 1901 revived it. Dandy[18] described the posterior fossa approach for retrogasserian neurotomy in 1925, although this was probably not his own original idea.[19] His experience led him to conclude that subtotal section spared significant sensation without a major increase in pain recurrence.[20] Although Dandy frequently observed the vascular loops compressing the trigeminal nerve and, like Gardner and Miklos some 30 years later,[21] suspected this to be the cause of the neuralgia, Dandy did not conceive of decompression as a solution. With the introduction of better medical therapy and percutaneous procedures using the Härtel approach to the foramen ovale,[22] open surgical procedures for trigeminal neuralgia fell into decline until Jannetta[23] in 1967 reported his experience with microvascular decompression, a procedure that has stood the test of time.

CORDOTOMY

Bell,[24] with the sole aid of the naked eye and the scalpel, had also traced the posterior spinal roots up the spinal cord into the brainstem and cerebrum. Accurately filling in the details would take the rest of the 19th century. Both Schiff and Brown-Séquard had performed numerous experiments trying to locate the sensory tracts in the spinal cord when, in 1871, Müller[25] cited a case of a stab wound involving one half of the

TABLE 180–1 ■ **Chronology of the Modern Neurosurgical Management of Pain**

YEAR	INVESTIGATOR	TECHNIQUE
1873	Létiévant	Neurotomies for facial and extremity neuralgias
1889	Abbe & Bennet	Spinal dorsal rhizotomy
1891	Horsley	Gasserian ganglionectomy for trigeminal neuralgia
1899	François-Franck	Conception of the potential of sympathectomy
1901	Spiller and Frazier	Open trigeminal rhizotomy (middle fossa)
1905	Spiller	Spinothalamic tract in the anterolateral cord
1912	Spiller & Martin	First cordotomy
1913	Leriche	Sympathectomy for painful extremities
1916	Jonnesco	Sympathectomy for angina pectoris
1923	Läwen	Diagnostic nerve blocks
1925	Dandy	Trigeminal rhizotomy (posterior fossa)
1927	Armour	Midline commissural myelotomy
1933	Foerster	Mapping of the spinal dermatomes in humans
1938	Sjöqvist	Trigeminal tractotomy
1941	Schwartz & White	Open medullary spinothalamic tractomy
1942	Walker	Open mesencephalic tractotomy
1953	Spiegel & Wycis	Stereotactic thalamotomy and mesencephalotomy
1960	Heath & Mickle	Deep brain (septal) stimulation for pain
1960	Mazars	Thalamic (VPL) stimulation for pain
1961	Sano	Posteromedial hypothalamotomy for pain
1962	Foltz & White	Bilateral cingulotomy for pain
1963	Mullan	First percutaneous cordotomy
1965	Melzack & Wall	Gate theory of pain
1965	Sweet	Peripheral nerve stimulation
1966	Kudo	Pulvinotomy
1967	Jannetta	Trigeminal microvascular decompression
1967	Shealy	Spinal cord stimulation
1968	Hitchcock	Extralemniscal myelotomy
1969	Kapur & Dalton	Hypophysectomy for cancer pain
1972	Sindou & Nashold	DREZ lesions
1973	Hitchcock	Stereotactic pontine spinothalamic tractotomy
1974	Sweet & Wepsic	Radiofrequency trigeminal rhizolysis
1979	Wang	Intrathecal morphine
1979	Behar	Epidural morphine
1981	Håkanson	Glycerol trigeminal chemoneurolysis
1983	Mullan & Lichtor	Trigeminal balloon microcompression
1991	Tsubokawa	Motor cortex stimulation

DREZ, Dorsal root entry zone; VPL, nucleus ventroposterolateralis.

spinal cord and the opposite dorsal column, producing bilateral anesthesia for touch but causing analgesia only on the side opposite the lesion. Gowers[26] later reported a case that he had seen in 1876 of a student who had shot himself through the mouth. The patient had intact tactile sensibility in his left limbs, but pain sensation was abolished. Postmortem examination revealed that the injury to the spinal cord was a spicule of bone that had effectively caused a unilateral cervical cord section, destroying the continuity of the anterior and lateral columns on the right side. Gowers concluded that this part of the cord carries the fibers for the transmission of contralateral pain impulses. Edinger[27] in 1889 demonstrated the existence of the spinothalamic tract in newborn cats and amphibians. It remained for Spiller,[4] however, to prove conclusively that the spinothalamic tract carries pain and temperature impulses. In 1905, he described a patient with pain and temperature loss in the lower part of the body who at autopsy was confirmed to have bilateral tuberculomas involving the lower thoracic anterolateral tracts. Schüller[5] in 1910 sectioned the anterolateral tract in monkeys. Martin performed the first "cordotomy" in a human being at the instigation of Spiller in 1911,

in another patient with a tuberculoma of the cord.[28] Their short- and long-term results were encouraging and established the technique for treating intractable pain. Stookey[29] was probably the first to perform a high cervical cordotomy in 1931 for pain in the chest and upper extremity. Mullan and colleagues[30] introduced a technique for percutaneous cordotomy at the C1-2 level using a radioactive needle tip in 1960. The lesioning utility of radiofrequency thermocoagulation was applied to the technique by Rosomoff and coworkers,[31] and cord penetration as determined by electrical impedance was described by Gildenberg and associates.[32] Kanpolat and colleagues[33] popularized the computed tomography–guided percutaneous procedure in use today.

STEREOTAXY

Pain affecting the face, head, and shoulder could not be managed effectively by cordotomy, so open brainstem spinothalamic tractotomies were attempted.[34–36] Unfortunately, the analgesic effects were short-lived, and morbidity and mortality rates were high. Spiegel and

Wycis,[37] the great pioneers of human stereotaxy, applied their technique to perform mesencephalotomy and thalamotomy with greater accuracy and success. Subsequently, Hitchcock[38, 39] introduced a stereotactic technique for pontine spinothalamic and trigeminal tractotomy.

Stereotaxy not only enabled more accurate localization of targets but also generated important insights into the pathophysiology of chronic denervation pain.[40] Lesions in the thalamic somatosensory ventrocaudal nuclei (receiving input from the neospinothalamic system) were not very successful at relieving chronic pain and were often associated with postoperative ataxia and dysesthesias.[41] Attention was focused on lesioning targets of the paleoreticulospinothalamic system, especially the nonspecific intralaminar nuclei[42, 43] and the pulvinar,[44] with greater success.

GATE THEORY OF PAIN

A major milestone in the neurosurgical management of pain came with the publication in 1965 of Melzack and Wall's gate theory.[45] Their proposal that afferent pain transmission might be modulated by a spinal gating mechanism introduced the possibility of pain management by *neuromodulation*. This motivated Sweet[46] in 1965 to perform peripheral nerve stimulation, the first augmentative procedure for pain relief. In 1967 Shealy and coworkers[47] performed the first trial of spinal dorsal column stimulation. Heath,[48] having observed pain relief in psychiatric patients with septal stimulation, repeated these findings in nonpsychiatric patients in 1960.[49] That same year, Mazars and associates[50] showed that thalamic nucleus ventroposterolateralis stimulation was also effective for chronic pain. As stimulation technology improved, other groups confirmed these results.[51, 52] Encouraged by the phenomenon of stimulation-produced analgesia in animals following electrical stimulation of the periaqueductal gray matter and the suggestion that this was mediated by endogenous opioids, Richardson and Akil[53, 54] implanted a stimulating electrode in the periventricular gray matter in humans and reported effective pain relief. Tsubokawa and colleagues[55] have since described the efficacy of motor cortex stimulation for deafferentation pain of thalamic origin.

Many ablative techniques have now been supplanted by augmentative techniques. One notable exception was the introduction by Sindou[56] in 1972 of dorsal root entry zone ablation for deafferentation pain associated with brachial plexus avulsion and traumatic paraplegia. This pain had remained intractable to all previously attempted ablative and augmentative techniques. Nashold and coworkers[57] further popularized this procedure using a radiofrequency thermocoagulation technique.

INTRASPINAL OPIOIDS

The discovery of morphine receptors in the central nervous system in 1973 and in the spinal cord in 1977 was soon followed by the display of their utility for analgesia in the spinal fluid and epidural space.[58, 59] Controlled opiate delivery from implanted pumps was introduced as an analgesic technique in the late 1970s for a variety of neuropathic pain syndromes and has become a mainstay neuromodulatory procedure. Pump technology has become more sophisticated, and drugs other than opioids have been delivered to the spinal fluid.

SUMMARY

Today's trend is to classify pain syndromes as nociceptive or neuropathic and to choose appropriate therapy tailored to the type of pain. In general, conservative, augmentative, or modulatory techniques are preferred to ablative ones. It is likely that the next great strides in the therapy of chronic pain will be the result of discoveries at the molecular level.

REFERENCES

1. Walker A: New anatomy and physiology of the brain in particular and of the nervous system in general. Arch Univ Sc 3:172, 1809.
2. Bell C: Idea of a New Anatomy of the Brain, Submitted for the Observation of His Friends. London, Strahan & Preston, 1811.
3. Magendie F: Experiénces sur les fonctíons des racines des nerfs rachidiens. J Physiol Exp et Path 2:336, 1822.
4. Spiller WG: The location within the spinal cord of the fibers for temperature and pain sensations. J Nerv Ment Dis 32:318–320, 1905.
5. Schüller A: Ueber operative Durchtrennung der Rückenmarkesstränge (Chordotomie). Wien Med Wochenschr 60:2292–2296, 1910.
6. Létiévant E: Traité des sections nerveuses. Paris, JB Balliere et Fils, 1873.
7. Bennet WH: A case in which acute spasmodic pain in the left lower extremity was completely relieved by subdural division of the posterior roots of certain spinal nerves. Med Chirurg Trans 72:329–348, 1889.
8. Abbe R: A contribution to the surgery of the spine. Med Rec 35:149–152, 1889.
9. Abbe R: Intradural section of the spinal nerves for neuralgia. Boston M & SJ 135:329–335, 1896.
10. Foerster O: The dermatomes in man. Brain 56:1–39, 1933.
11. Lewy FH: The first authentic case of major trigeminal neuralgia and some comments on the history of the disease. Ann Med Hist 10:247–250, 1938.
12. Bell C: The Nervous System, 3rd ed. London, Spottiswode, 1844, p 26.
13. Horsley V, Taylor J, Colman WS: Remarks on the various surgical procedures devised for the relief or cure of trigeminal neuralgia (tic douloureux). BMJ 2:1139–1143, 1191–1193, 1249–1252, 1891.
14. Hartley F: Intracranial neurectomy of the second and third divisions of the fifth nerve: A new method. NY Med J 55:317–319, 1892.
15. Krause F: Resection des Trigeminus innerhalb der Schädelhöhle. Arch Klin Chir 44:821–832, 1892.
16. Tiffany LM: Intracranial operations for the cure of facial neuralgia. Ann Surg 24:575–619, 736–748, 1896.
17. Spiller WG, Frazier CH: The division of the sensory root of the trigeminus for the relief of tic douloureux: An experimental, pathological and clinical study, with a preliminary report of one surgically successful case. Univ Pa Med Bull 14:341–352, 1901.
18. Dandy WE: Section of the sensory root of the trigeminal nerve at the pons. Bull Johns Hopkins Hosp 36:105–106, 1925.
19. Stookey B, Ransohoff J: Trigeminal Neuralgia: Its History and Treatment. Springfield, Ill, Charles C Thomas, 1959.

20. Dandy WE: An operation for the cure of tic douloureux: Partial section of the sensory root at the pons. Arch Surg 18:687–734, 1929.

21. Gardner WJ, Miklos MV: Response of trigeminal neuralgia to "decompression" of sensory root. JAMA 170:1773–1776, 1959.

22. Härtel F: Ueber die intracranielle injektionsbehandlung der trigeminusneuralgie. Med Klin 10:582–584, 1914.

23. Jannetta PJ: Arterial compression of the trigeminal nerve at the pons in patients with trigeminal neuralgia. J Neurosurg 26:159–162, 1967.

24. Bell C: The Nervous System, 3rd ed. London, Spottiswode, 1844, p 22.

25. Müller W: Beiträge zur patholocischen Anatomie und Physiologie des menschlichen Rückenmarks. Leipzig, Germany, L Voss, 1871.

26. Gowers WR: A case of unilateral gunshot injury to the spinal cord. Trans Clin Soc Lond 11:24–32, 1878.

27. Edinger L: Vorlesungen über den Bau der nervösen Centralorgane des Menschen und der Thiere für Aerzte und Studirende. Leipzig, Germany, FCW Vogel, 1900–1904.

28. Spiller WG, Martin E: The treatment of persistent pain of organic origin in the lower part of the body by division of the anterolateral column of the spinal cord. JAMA 58:1489–1490, 1912.

29. Stookey B: Chordotomy of the second cervical segment for relief from pain due to recurrent carcinoma of the breast. Arch Neurol Psychiatry 26:443, 1931.

30. Mullan S, Harper PV, Hekmatpanah J, et al: Percutaneous interruption of spinal pain tracts by means of a strontium-90 needle. J Neurosurg 20:931–939, 1963.

31. Rosomoff HL, Caroll F, Brown J, Sheptak P: Percutaneous radiofrequency cervical cordotomy: Technique. J Neurosurg 23:639–644, 1965.

32. Gildenberg PL, Zanes C, Flitter MA, et al: Impedance monitoring device for detection of penetration of the spinal cord in anterior percutaneous cervical cordotomy: Technical note. J Neurosurg 30:87–92, 1969.

33. Kanpolat Y, Deda H, Akyar S, Bilgic S: CT-guided percutaneous cordotomy. Acta Neurchir Suppl (Wien) 46:67–68, 1989.

34. Shwartz HG, O'Leary JL: Section of the spinothalamic tract in the medulla with observations on the pathway for pain. Surgery 9:183–193, 1941.

35. White JC: Spinothalamic tractotomy in the medulla oblongata. Arch Surg 43:113–127, 1941.

36. Walker AE: Relief of pain by mesencephalic tractotomy. Arch Neurol Psychiatry 43:284–298, 1942.

37. Spiegel EA, Wycis HT: Mesencephalotomy in the treatment of "intractable" facial pain. Arch Neurol Psychiatry 69:1–13, 1953.

38. Hitchcock E: Stereotactic pontine spinothalamic tractotomy. J Neurosurg 39:746–752, 1973.

39. Hitchcock ER: Stereotactic trigeminal tractotomy. Ann Clin Res 2:131–135, 1970.

40. Tasker RR, Kiss ZHT: The role of the thalamus in functional neurosurgery. Neurosurg Clin N Am 6:73–82, 1995.

41. Tasker RR, Organ LW, Hawrylshyn PA: The Thalamus and Midbrain of Man: A Physiological Atlas Using Electrical Stimulation. Springfield, IL, Charles C Thomas, 1982.

42. Spiegel EA, Wycis HT, Szekely EG, et al: Combined dorsomedial, intralaminar and basal thalamotomy for relief of so called intractable pain. J Int Coll Surg 42:160–168, 1964.

43. Sano K, Yoshioka M, Ogashiwa M, et al: Thalamolaminotomy: A new operation for relief of intractable pain. Conf Neurol 27:63–66, 1966.

44. Kudo T, Yoshii N, Shimizu S, et al: Effects of stereotactic thalamotomy on intractable pain and numbness. Keio J Med 15:191–194, 1966.

45. Melzack P, Wall PD: Pain mechanisms: A new theory. Science 150:971–978, 1965.

46. Sweet WH: Control of pain by direct electrical stimulation of peripheral nerves. Clin Neurosurg 23:103–111, 1976.

47. Shealy CN, Mortimer JT, Reswick JB: Electrical inhibition of pain by stimulation of the dorsal columns: A preliminary clinical report. Anesth Analg 46:489–491, 1967.

48. Heath RG: Studies in Schizophrenia. Cambridge, Mass, Harvard University Press, 1954.

49. Heath RG, Mickle WA: Evaluation of seven years experience with depth electrode studies in human patients. In Ramey ER, O'Doherty DS (eds): Electrical Studies in the Anesthetized Brain. New York, Harper & Row, 1960, pp 214–247.

50. Mazars G, Roge R, Mazars Y: Stimulation of the spinothalamic fasciculus and their bearing on the physiopathology of pain. Rev Neurol 103:136–138, 1960.

51. Hosobuchi Y, Adams JE, Rutkin B: Chronic thalamic stimulation for the control of facial anesthesia dolorosa. Arch Neurol 29:158–161, 1973.

52. Adams JE, Hosobuchi Y, Fields HL: Stimulation of internal capsule for relief of chronic pain. J Neurosurg 41:740–744, 1974.

53. Richardson DE, Akil H: Pain reduction by electrical stimulation in man. Part I. Acute administration in periaqueductal and periventricular sites. J Neurosurg 47:178–183, 1977.

54. Richardson DE, Akil H: Pain reduction by electrical stimulation in man. Part II. Chronic self-administration in the periventricular gray matter. J Neurosurg 47:184–194, 1977.

55. Tsubokawa T, Katayama Y, Yamamoto T, et al: Chronic motor cortex stimulation for the treatment of central pain. Acta Neurochir Suppl (Wien) 52:137–139, 1991.

56. Sindou M: Etude de la jonction radiculo-médullaire postérieure. La radicellotomie postérieure sélective dans la chirurgie de la doleur [thesis]. Villeurbanne, France, University of Lyon, 1972.

57. Nashold BS, Urban B, Zorub DS: Phantom pain relief by focal destruction of the substantia gelatinosa of Rolando. Adv Pain Res Ther 1:959, 1976.

58. Wang JK, Nauss LE, Thomas JE: Pain relief by intrathecally applied morphine in man. Anesthesiology 50:149–151, 1979.

59. Behar M, Magora F, Olshwang D, Davidson JT: Epidural morphine in treatment of pain. Lancet 1:257, 1979.

Physiologic Anatomy of Pain

THOMAS K. BAUMANN

Pain is an "unpleasant sensory and emotional experience associated with actual or potential tissue damage."[1] Pain is usually elicited by activation of nociceptive primary afferent neurons by noxious stimuli (i.e., nociceptive pain). However, pain may also result from nerve injury or damage of the central nervous system itself (i.e., neuropathic pain). This chapter describes the neuronal substrate—neurons and neuronal circuits—responsible for sensing peripheral tissue damage (i.e., nociception). Nociception is only one dimension of pain. The psychological dimension of pain is not explicitly addressed in this chapter, which starts by describing the properties of primary sensory neurons that transduce noxious stimuli and transmit the information to second-order neurons in the central nervous system.

NOCICEPTIVE PRIMARY AFFERENT NEURONS

Animals, including humans, have nociceptive primary afferent neurons that are specialized to transduce noxious stimuli. These neurons were first identified in the neurophysiologic experiments of the late 1960s.[2, 3] Nociceptive neurons behave very differently from neurons that transduce innocuous stimuli. Nociceptive neurons have the ability to code the intensity of noxious stimuli, whereas receptors for innocuous stimuli saturate, or seize, their response at noxious levels of stimulation. Most nociceptive primary afferent neurons have small-diameter, thinly myelinated axons or unmyelinated axons, which in the Erlanger-Gasser classification scheme for primary afferent neurons are referred to as Aδ and C fibers, respectively, and the corresponding muscle afferent fibers are called group III and group IV in the Lloyd-Hunt classification scheme (Table 180–1). Nociceptive primary afferent neurons with large-diameter myelinated axons (i.e., Aβ fibers) do exist[4] but are much less numerous. Table 180–1 gives a breakdown of the various nociceptive and non-nociceptive fiber groups in peripheral nerves and their conduction velocities.

Tissue-damaging stimuli can be thermal, chemical, or mechanical in nature. Collectively, nociceptive primary afferent neurons can sense all three submodalities of tissue-damaging stimulation, but nociceptive primary afferent neurons are by no means homogeneous. Some nociceptive fibers respond to only one submodality of nociceptive stimulation; others are *polymodal*, responding to more than one submodality. Even within a particular conduction-velocity group, there are several subtypes of nociceptive fibers that differ in their sensory and electrophysiologic properties. For instance, C fiber nociceptors differ in their ability to respond to thermal, mechanical, and chemical submodalities of nociceptive stimuli (Fig. 181–1). Some nociceptive fibers respond readily to mechanical stimuli, but others (i.e., mechanically insensitive afferents) do not. Differential sensitivity to submodalities of nociceptive stimulation is associated with differences in the electrophysiologic properties of the axons. When activated at a moderately high rate of electrical stimulation, the mechanically insensitive subtype is subject to a considerably higher degree of conduction-velocity slowing than the polymodal subtype.[5] This electrophysiologic difference indicates that the axons of different physiologic subtypes of nociceptive C fibers differ in their expression of voltage-gated ion channels.

NOCICEPTIVE TRANSDUCTION MECHANISMS

In recent years, the biophysical characteristics and molecular identity of some of the transducing elements for the different submodalities of noxious stimulation became known. All of the identified nociceptor transducer elements are membrane ion channels. Some of the specialized ion channels respond to only one sub-

T A B L E   1 8 1 – 1 ■ **Classification of Sensory Fibers in Peripheral Nerves**

FIBER GROUP	INNERVATION	MEAN DIAMETER (RANGE, μm)	MEAN CONDUCTION VELOCITY (RANGE, m/s)
Erlanger/Gasser Classification			
Cutaneous sensory			
Aβ	Low-threshold mechanoreceptors	8 (5–15)	50 (30–70)
Aδ	Low-threshold hair mechanoreceptors, mechano-heat nociceptors (Type I) AMH,* chemosensitive (Type II) AMH	<3 (1–4)	15 (12–30)
C	Mechano-, heat-, chemo-nociceptors	1 (0.5–1.5)	1 (0.5–2)
Sympathetic Efferent			
B	Preganglionic	3 (1–3)	7 (3–15)
C	Postganglionic	1 (0.5–1.5)	1 (0.5–2)
Lloyd/Hunt Classification			
Muscle sensory			
Ia	Primary muscle spindle	15 (12–20)	100 (70–120)
Ib	Tendon organ		
II	Secondary muscle spindle, Spray (Ruffini) endings, Lamellated (paciniform) endings	9 (4–12)	55 (25–70)
III	Mechanonociceptors	3 (1–4)	11 (10–25)
IV	Mechanoreceptors, chemonociceptors, and thermoreceptors	1 (0.5–1.5)	1 (0.5–2)

*AMH = A-fiber mechano-heat nociceptor.

modality of stimulation; others are polymodal in the sense that a given channel responds to thermal and chemical stimulation.

Noxious Heat

Moderately intense noxious heat stimuli are transduced by a cation-selective ion channel that is gated open by temperatures in excess of 42°C. The channel is called vanilloid receptor type 1 (VR-1) because it was derived by expression cloning and monitoring the response of the cells to capsaicin, a sensory irritant with a chemical structure related to vanillin.[6] A related molecule was cloned subsequently and named vanilloid receptor type 1–related channel (VRL-1). VRL-1 is not activated by capsaicin, but it responds to temperatures

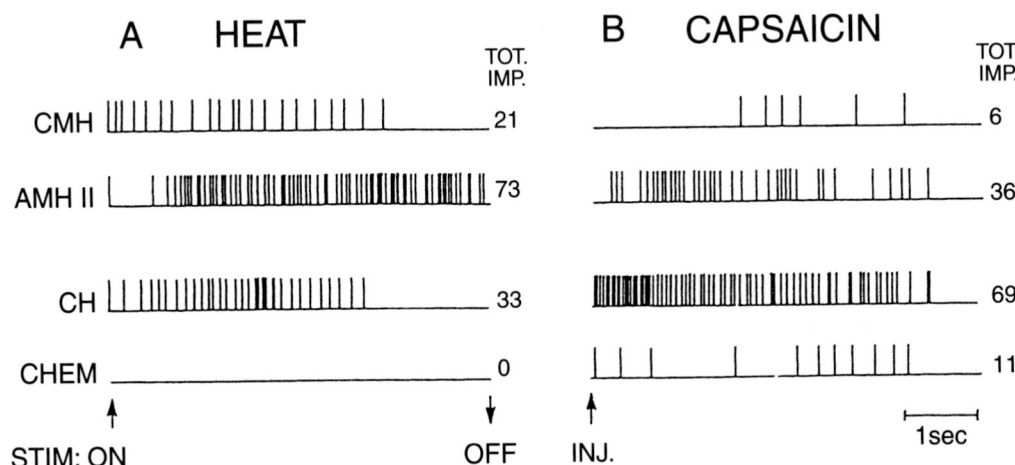

FIGURE 181–1. Comparison of responses of different physiologic types of nociceptors to heat and noxious chemical stimuli applied to the skin of an anesthetized monkey. *A*, Response to a 5-second heat stimulus of 51°C. *B*, Response during the first 5 seconds after intradermal injection of 100 μg of capsaicin. The number to the right of each trace is the total number of action potentials fired by the primary afferent neuron during the 5 seconds. The top three rows illustrate the responses of heat-sensitive nociceptive afferents. The bottom row shows the response of a chemonociceptive fiber (CHEM) that was insensitive to heat and mechanical stimuli but responded to capsaicin. Mechano-heat fibers responded more vigorously to heat than to capsaicin. The opposite was true for C fiber heat-nociceptor (CH) and CHEM fibers. AMH II, type II A fiber mechano-heat nociceptor; CMH, C fiber mechano-heat nociceptor. (From Baumann TK, Simone DA, Shain C, LaMotte RL: Neurogenic hyperalgesia: The search for the primary cutaneous afferent fibers that contribute to capsaicin-induced pain and hyperalgesia. J Neurophysiol 66:212–227, 1991.)

in excess of 51°C.[7] The heat-activation profiles of VR-1 and VRL-1 match nicely the response profile of certain C fiber and Aδ fiber heat nociceptors, respectively. All thermally sensitive ion channels that were cloned belonged to the transient receptor potential (TRP) family of ion channels.[8, 9]

Noxious Chemical Stimuli

Chemosensitivity of nociceptive primary afferent neurons is mediated by various ligand-gated ion channels (Fig. 181–2). Noxious chemicals that act directly on ligand-gated channels include metabolites of 12- and 15-lipoxygenase (VR-1 receptors), the endogenous cannabinoid anandamide (VR-1 receptors), adenosine triphosphate (P2X receptors), serotonin (5-HT₃ receptors), and protons (ASIC and VR-1 receptors).[10–19] Discharge of nociceptive primary afferent neurons is also controlled by modulation of voltage-gated ion channels through intracellular pathways that involve second messenger molecules such as inositol-1,4,5-triphos-phate (IP₃), diacylglycerol (DAG), or cyclic AMP.[15, 20] Inflammatory mediators with the ability for acting through G-protein–coupled second messenger pathways include prostaglandins, histamine, serotonin, and bradykinin.[15, 20] Chemosensitivity of primary afferent nociceptive neurons plays a central role in many forms of inflammatory pain.[21, 22]

Noxious Mechanical Stimuli

There are good reasons to believe that noxious mechanical stimuli are transduced by ion channels that are gated open by membrane stretch. Such channels were recorded with patch-clamp methods,[23, 24] but the molecular identity of the channels remains to be elucidated.

NOCICEPTOR ACTIVATION AND PAIN

Microneurographic recordings[25] with microelectrodes inserted in fascicles of peripheral nerves make possible

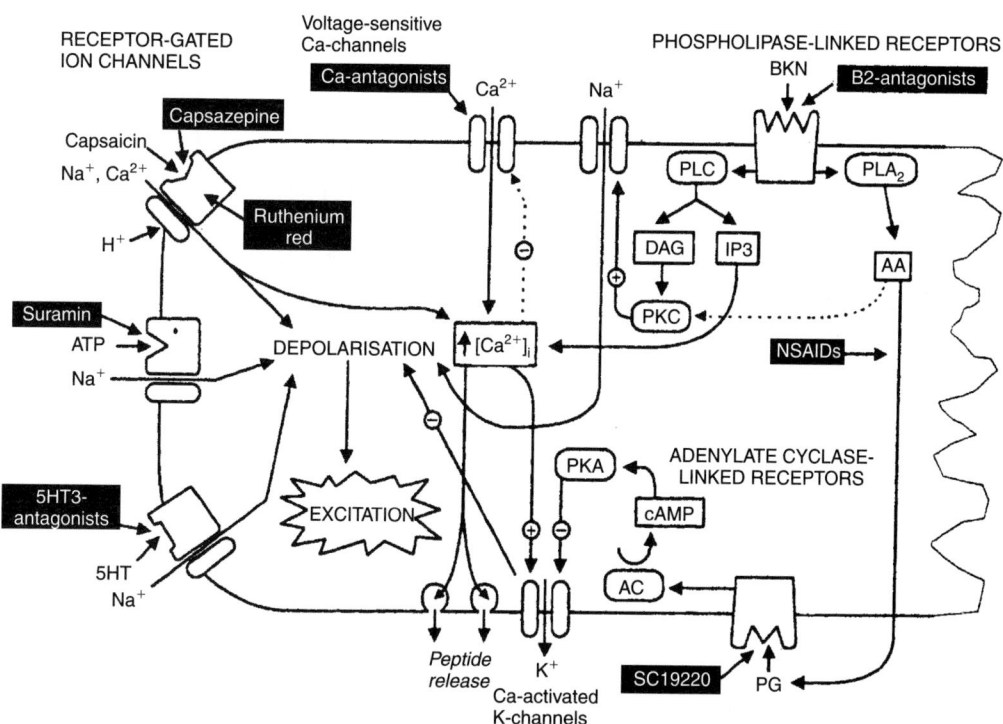

FIGURE 181–2. A simplified scheme shows some of the extracellular and intracellular processes involved in control of the excitability of nociceptive nerve terminals. *Left,* Cation channels gated extracellularly by pain-producing compounds such as capsaicin, protons, adenosine triphosphate (ATP), and serotonin (5-HT). *Right,* Receptors for inflammatory mediators such as bradykinin (BKN) and prostaglandin (PG). Activation of phospholipase-linked receptors (by BKN) and adenylate cyclase linked receptors (by PG) results in the production of intracellular messengers, such as diacylglycerol (DAG) or cyclic adenosine monophosphate (cAMP), which activate kinases that modulate the excitability of voltage- or calcium-gated ion channels. Generation of inositol-1,4,5-triphosphate (IP₃) increases the level of calcium coming from intracellular stores, which facilitates the release of neuropeptides by the nerve ending. SC19220 is a PG antagonist. The scheme is a composite of the excitatory pathways within the nociceptive terminal. Any given nociceptive terminal may express receptors for only a subset of the chemical mediators. AA, arachidonic acid; AC, adenyl cyclase; NSAIDs, nonsteroidal anti-inflammatory drugs; PKA, cAMP-dependent protein kinase; PKC, protein kinase C; PLA₂, phospholipase A₂; PLC, phospholipase C. (Adapted from Rang HP, Bevan S, Dray A: Chemical activation of nociceptive peripheral neurones. Br Med Bull 47:534–548, 1991.)

a direct correlation between action potential discharge in identified primary afferent neurons and concomitant reports of sensations in humans.[26–30] Microneurographic studies show that electrical activation of very few, perhaps even a single nociceptive primary afferent neuron, is sufficient to produce a pain sensation, but the initiation of the sensation requires temporal summation of several action potentials. Above this level, the intensity of the sensation is proportional to the stimulus frequency. The quality of pain evoked by electrical stimulation depends on the target tissue and the type of primary afferent that is stimulated. Activation of cutaneous Aδ nociceptor afferents typically evokes sharp, pricking pain, whereas stimulation of C fiber nociceptors causes dull or burning pain and, in some cases, itching.[31] Activation of nociceptive C fibers that innervate muscle gives rise to cramping pain.[32]

SENSITIZATION OF NOCICEPTORS: PRIMARY HYPERALGESIA

Chemical mediators that act through second messenger systems tend to lower the threshold of primary afferent nociceptive neurons for excitation. Mechanically insensitive afferents[33–35] can be quite insensitive in normal, healthy tissue, but they become markedly sensitized to mechanical stimuli by exposure to inflammatory mediators.[35] Chemical mediators that act through second messenger systems also increase nociceptor responses to suprathreshold stimuli. Such chemical mediators cause hyperalgesia at the site of tissue injury (i.e., primary hyperalgesia).[21] Endogenous compounds that sensitize nociceptive neurons are released locally from injured tissues or from inflammatory cells recruited to

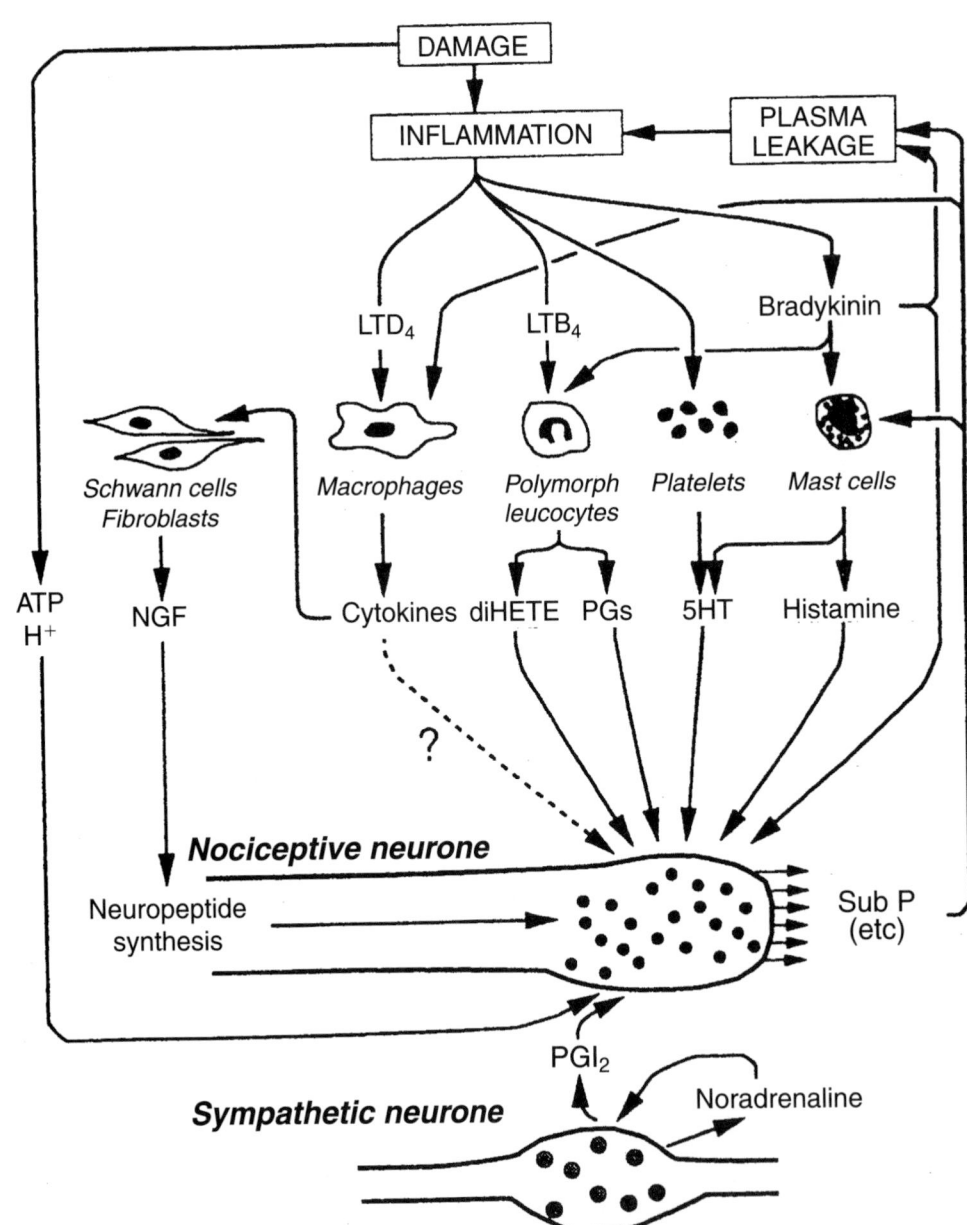

FIGURE 181–3. An overview of the factors and cells involved in activation and sensitization of nociceptive neurons after tissue damage and inflammation. Notice that substances released by inflammatory cells act on the nerve ending. Substances released by the nerve ending (e.g., substance P) may facilitate the inflammatory response. ATP, adenosine triphosphate; diHETE, 8(R),15(S)-dihydroxyeicosatetraenoic acid; H+, protons; LTB₄, leukotriene B₄; LTD₄, leukotriene D₄; NGF, nerve growth factor; PGs, prostaglandins E₁ or E₂, F₂; PGI₂, prostacyclin; 5-HT, 5-hydroxytryptamine. (Adapted from Rang HP, Bevan S, Dray A: Chemical activation of nociceptive peripheral neurones. Br Med Bull 47:534–548, 1991.)

the site of injury (Fig. 181–3). Among these compounds are eicosanoids (i.e., cyclooxygenase products prostaglandins E_1 and E_2 and the 15-lipoxygenase product 8(R),15(S)-dihydroxyeicosatetraenoic acid),[36, 37] kinins (i.e., bradykinin[38] and T-kinin[39]), 5-HT, low pH,[40, 41] and ATP.[42]

NEUROGENIC INFLAMMATION

Some small-diameter primary afferent neurons, when activated by stimuli in the noxious range, play a major efferent function in inflammatory processes through the release of proinflammatory (i.e., substance P) (see Fig. 181–3) and anti-inflammatory (i.e., somatostatin) neuropeptides.[43] There is some evidence that neurogenic release of substance P contributes to the severity of arthritis.[44] The contribution of meningeal neurogenic inflammation to migraine[45, 46] remains a controversial issue.

PROPERTIES OF NOCICEPTIVE INNERVATION

Nociceptors at the Body Surface

Because of easy accessibility to experimental manipulation, cutaneous[47] and corneal[48, 49] nociceptive neurons have been studied extensively. Collectively, these superficial nociceptors respond to noxious heat, noxious cold, noxious mechanical, and noxious chemical stimuli. Nociceptive neurons in general are fairly heterogeneous and may respond to one or more submodalities of noxious stimulation. Most ubiquitous are the so-called polymodal C fiber nociceptors. These fibers respond readily to mechanical and heat stimuli. Their average heat threshold of about 42°C is the same as that of specific heat nociceptors of C fibers. Mechano-heat nociceptors of Aδ fibers have higher thresholds: about 45°C for type II and in excess of 53°C for most type I A-mechano-heat nociceptors. Microneurographic recordings in humans, as well as correlative psychophysical studies in humans and neurophysiologic studies in anesthetized animals, have demonstrated that the intensity of burning pain evoked by heat is best matched by the frequency of action potential discharge in C-heat and C-mechano-heat nociceptor fibers.[50] The intense pain felt after an intracutaneous injection of the sensory irritant capsaicin is best matched by the level of discharge in heat nociceptors and chemospecific nociceptors (see Fig. 181–1).[51] Cutaneous nociceptive innervation is dense, and the pathways preserve a high degree of somatotopic organization, as shown by the small, projected receptive fields of the sensations that are evoked by electrical stimulation of primary afferent fibers through microneurographic electrodes, which agree rather well with the receptive fields determined by natural stimulation of the nerve endings.[31]

Deep Nociceptors of Muscle and Joints

Muscle pain occurs during sustained muscular contraction and ischemia, after trauma, or after eccentric exer-

cise.[52, 53] Slightly less than one half of the group III and IV fibers in muscle are thought to be nociceptors; the remainder are low-threshold afferents thought to signal deep pressure and thermosensitive afferents believed to be involved in thermoregulation. Mense[54] offers an extensive review of this topic. Pain is the major sensation ascribed to the joint.[55] Joints are frequently affected by inflammatory and degenerative disorders and by injury. Experimentally induced arthritis causes dramatic changes in the response properties of joint afferent fibers.[56] Sensitization has been directly documented in long-term electrophysiologic recordings from single, identified afferent fibers during the development of acute inflammation.[57] These experiments have shown that joints receive substantial innervation by the so-called silent, or mechanically insensitive, nociceptors, which begin to respond to moderate strength stimuli only after inflammation becomes established.

Visceral Nociceptors

Viscera are particularly sensitive to distention but may be quite insensitive to cutting or burning. The peripheral basis of visceral pain differs from other body regions.[58, 59] The distinction between responses to innocuous and noxious stimulation has been more difficult to draw for visceral neurons because there is a much

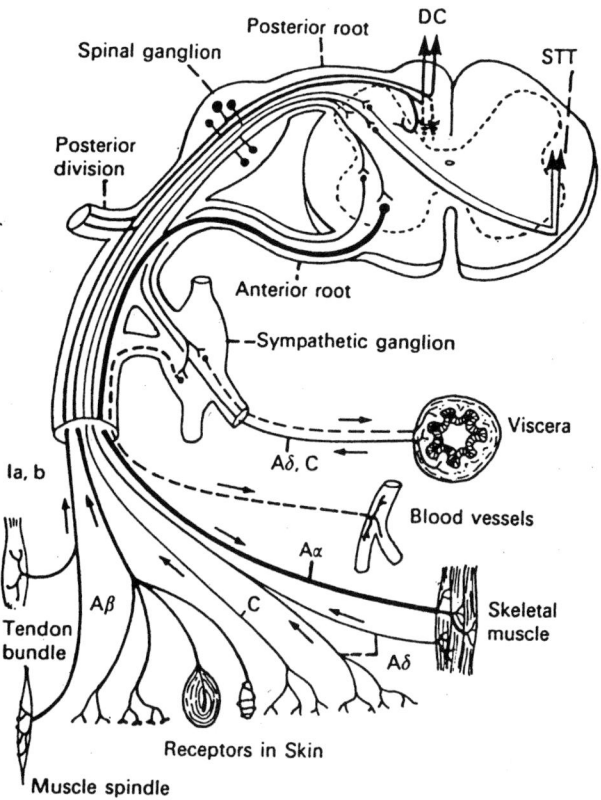

FIGURE 181–4. Spinal nerve and the different types of fibers it contains. DC, dorsal column; STT, spinothalamic tract. (From Bonica JJ: Anatomic and physiologic basis of nociception and pain. In Bonica JJ [ed]: The Management of Pain, vol 1. Philadelphia, Lea & Febiger, 1990, pp 28–94.)

wider overlap in their response properties and some neurons are spontaneously active even in the absence of obvious sensitization or intentional stimulation.[60] Compared with cutaneous tissues, pain from visceral tissues is more difficult to localize, most likely because of lower innervation density.

Centripetal Transfer of Nociceptive Information

All tissues of the body, with the exception of the neuraxis, are innervated by nociceptive primary afferent neurons. The cornea, teeth, internal surface of the tym-

panic membrane, dura, and venous and bony sinuses within the cranium are innervated mainly, if not exclusively, by nociceptive primary afferent neurons. Other tissues are innervated by nociceptive and non-nociceptive (i.e., low-threshold mechanoreceptor and thermoreceptor) neurons. Axons of nociceptive neurons project through peripheral nerves and dorsal roots accompanied by axons of non-nociceptive neurons (Fig. 181–4). Axons of visceral nociceptive neurons project through visceral nerves along with axons of sympathetic and parasympathetic neurons (see Fig. 181–4). The cell bodies of nociceptive primary afferent neurons are located in dorsal root ganglia or trigeminal ganglia,

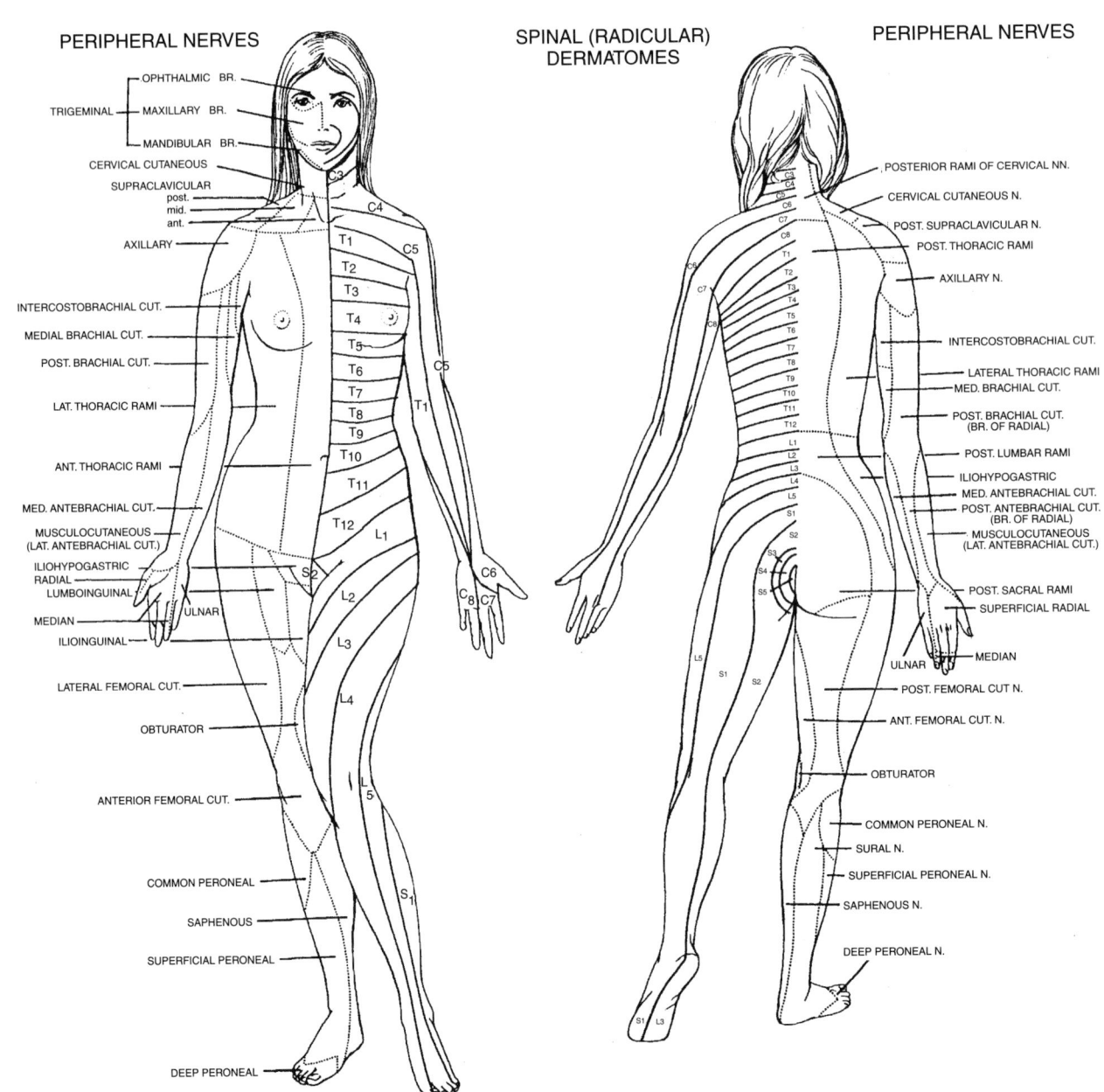

FIGURE 181–5. Comparison of peripheral nerve innervation territories and radicular dermatomes. C, cervical; L, lumbar; S, sacral; T, thoracic. (From Marcus EL: Clinical considerations of the spinal cord. In Curtis BA, Jacobson S, Markus EM [eds]: An Introduction to the Neurosciences. Philadelphia, WB Saunders, 1972, pp 150–206.)

mixed with the cell bodies of non-nociceptive neurons and arranged in a loosely somatotopic fashion. Innervation of the body surface follows the well-known pattern of radicular dermatomes (Fig. 181–5).

Spinal Nerve Roots

Figure 181–4 schematically depicts a spinal nerve root and its constituent axon types. As the spinal nerve root approaches the spinal cord, it splits into a group of smaller rootlets. Larger-diameter axons tend to aggregate in the medial and central rootlets, whereas small-diameter axons congregate in the lateral rootlets, although the separation is not absolute. Early workers reported that cutting the lateral rootlets abolishes some behaviors and reflexes that are normally triggered by nociceptive inputs.[61] However, subsequent studies showed that it is probably impossible to destroy nociceptive fibers selectively by cutting the lateral rootlets. Modern interpretation of the classic experiments is that the nociceptive deficits resulted from vascular damage associated with cutting dorsal roots.[62]

There are some exceptions to the general rule that sensory information enters the central nervous system through dorsal roots.[63] Some afferent axons enter through the ventral root.[63] About 30% of axons in the ventral root are unmyelinated, even in segments that contribute little to the autonomic outflow. These unmyelinated axons may mediate nociceptive information. Figure 181–6 shows the two possibilities for the ulti-

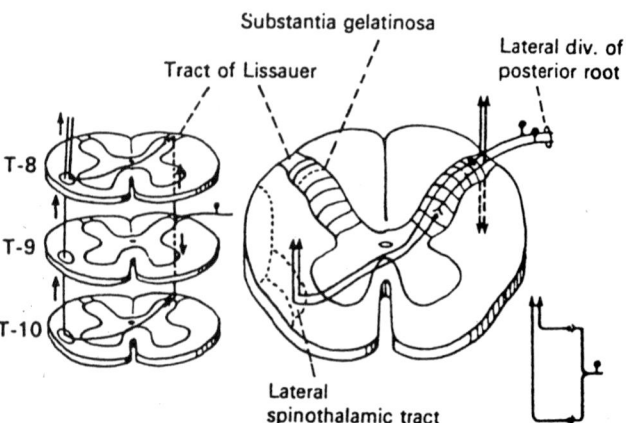

FIGURE 181–7. The tract of Lissauer, formed by axons of primary afferent neurons that enter by the dorsal (posterior) root, bifurcates and travels rostrally and caudally. Also indicated is the decussation and contralateral projection of dorsal horn neurons through the spinothalamic tract. (Adapted from Bonica JJ: Anatomic and physiological basis of nociception and pain. In Bonica JJ [ed]: The Management of Pain, vol 1. Philadelphia, Lea & Febiger, 1990, pp 28–94.)

mate course of these aberrant axons. Most fibers that enter ventral root turn back and then enter the spinal cord through the dorsal root as usual (see Fig. 181–6B). A few fibers also probably penetrate the cord from the ventral root and traverse the ventral horn to terminate in superficial layers of the dorsal horn (see Fig. 181–6A). These findings have been cited as one reason dorsal rhizotomy frequently fails to relieve pain[64] and why dorsal root ganglionectomy may be a better surgical strategy for the elimination of all nociceptive afferent fibers to a spinal segment.

Lissauer's Tract

As nociceptive axons in the dorsal roots enter the superficial root entry zone, they bifurcate into short ascending and descending branches, forming Lissauer's tract, which caps the dorsal horn (Fig. 181–7). The tract is formed predominantly by small, myelinated (Aδ) and unmyelinated (C) primary afferent fibers, although large, myelinated fibers are also intermixed. Many, if not most, of the fibers in Lissauer's tract mediate nociceptive information. From Lissauer's tract, the nociceptive primary afferent fibers enter the dorsal horn, where they synapse with local interneurons and projection neurons.

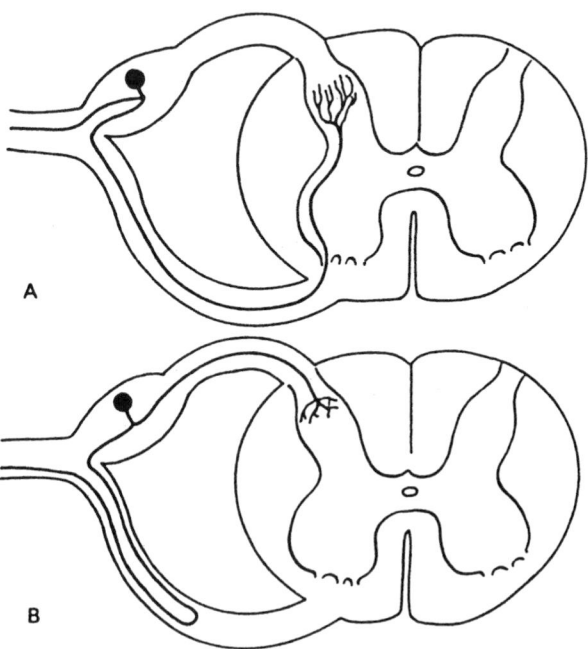

FIGURE 181–6. Aberrant course of some dorsal root ganglion neurons. *A,* Dorsal root ganglion (DRG) neuron has an axon projecting through the ventral root and ventral horn and then terminating in the dorsal horn of the spinal cord. *B,* The DRG neuron axon loops in the ventral root. (From Bonica JJ: Anatomic and physiological basis of nociception and pain. In Bonica JJ [ed]: The Management of Pain, vol 1. Philadelphia, Lea & Febiger, 1990, pp 28–94.)

Spinal Cord Gray Matter

On a cytoarchitectonic basis, the gray matter of the spinal cord can be divided into 10 rostrocaudally oriented laminae.[65] Reception, processing, and rostral transmission of nociceptive information occurs primarily in the two most superficial laminae (I and II) and three deeper laminae (V, VI, and X).[66] The nociceptive primary afferent neurons from all tissues terminate primarily in laminae I and V. The C fiber nociceptors from skin terminate in laminae I and II, and C fiber

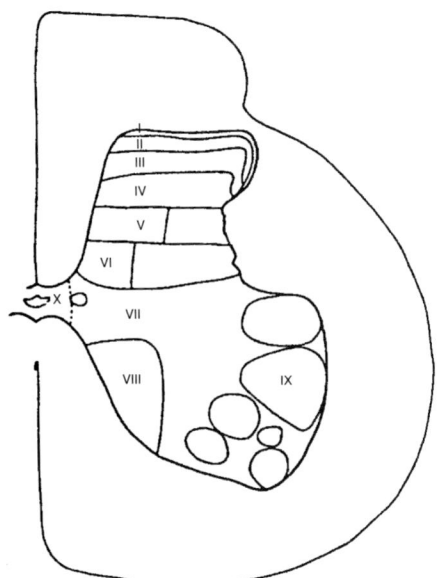

FIGURE 181–8. Laminae in the gray matter of the spinal cord. Cells in laminae I through VI make up the dorsal horn. Cells in laminae VII through IX constitute the ventral horn. Lamina X cells surround the central canal. The shape and relative size of the laminae in the cross section correspond to those in the L7 segment of cat spinal cord. (From Rexed BJ: A cytoarchitectonic atlas of the spinal cord of the cat. J Comp Neurol 96:415–466, 1954.)

nociceptors from deep tissues (i.e., muscles, joints, and viscera) terminate in lamina I and, to some extent, in laminae V and X.

The following paragraphs provide a brief description, in dorsoventral order, of each spinal cord lamina and its inputs and outputs, summarized from an article written by Willis and Coggeshall[64] and a book by

Brown.[67] Figure 181–8 shows the relative positions of the laminae of the gray matter. Figure 181–9 illustrates the shapes of the neurons in the various laminae, and Figure 181–10 depicts the typical shape and position of terminal arbors of different nociceptive and non-nociceptive primary afferent neurons.

Lamina I is the classic marginal zone. Lamina I is the only lamina that receives nociceptive inputs from all types of tissue (e.g., skin, muscle, joints, viscera). Spinal neurons in lamina I have a wide range of cell sizes: large, horizontal cells (i.e., marginal cells of Waldeyer) and much more numerous small neurons. The major dendrites of the Waldeyer cells are oriented horizontally, with dendritic fields forming flattened ovals with the long axis in the rostrocaudal direction. The dendrites of some cells may enter deeper laminae. Large numbers of fine fibers enter lamina I from the overlying tract of Lissauer and surrounding white matter (see Figs. 181–7 and 181–10, *left*). The fibers form the marginal plexus, a plexus of numerous horizontally arranged axons. Approximately one half of the synapses formed by this plexus is of primary afferent origin; the other half is propriospinal connections. There are two distinct types of nociceptive lamina I neurons. The nociceptive-specific neuron is fusiform and dominated by input from Aδ nociceptors. The other type of neuron has multipolar shape and is dominated by nociceptive input from C fibers. Lamina I is a main source of nociceptive output projections from the superficial dorsal horn.

Lamina II is sometimes called *substantia gelatinosa*. The gelatinous appearance of this layer is caused by the concentration of small neurons and their processes. The two predominant cell types are the stalked cells and the islet cells. The dendrites of stalked cells form a cone projecting from the cell body and passing ventrally into laminae II through IV. The major axon desti-

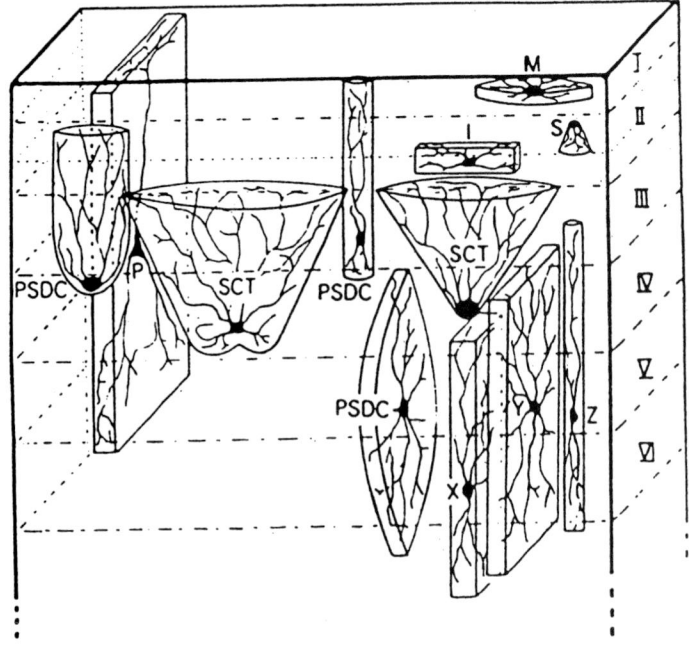

FIGURE 181–9. Schematic depiction of the dendritic tree shapes of the major cell types in the dorsal horn (parasagittal section). Laminae I through VI are shown. I, islet neuron, M, marginal neuron, P, pyramidal neuron, PSDC, post-synaptic dorsal column neuron, S, stalked neuron, SCT, spinocervical tract neuron; X, Y, and Z, interneurons. (From Brown AG: Organization in the Spinal Cord. Berlin, Springer Verlag, 1981.)

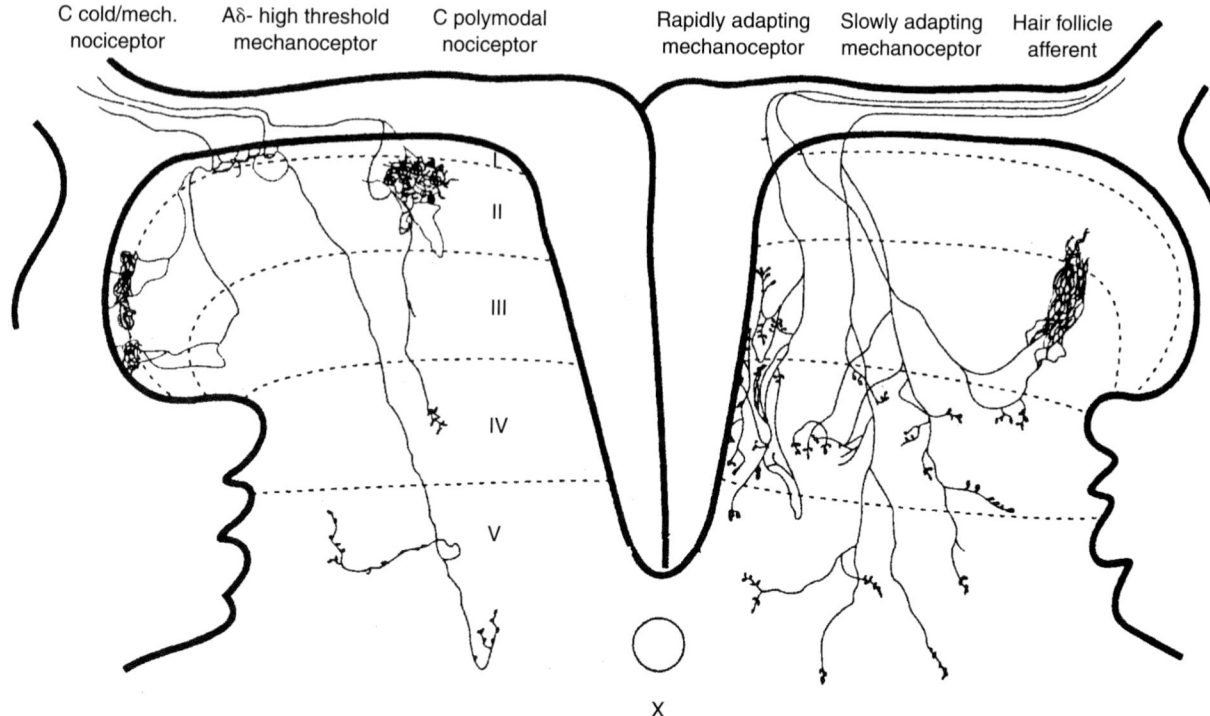

FIGURE 181–10. A schematic diagram of primary afferent terminals in a transverse cross section of lumbar spinal cord. *Left,* Terminal arbors of nociceptive fibers in the dorsal horn. *Right,* Typical terminal arbors of several subtypes of low-threshold mechanoreceptors. Notice the difference in the shape of terminal arbors and their location relative to laminae I through V. (Redrawn from Fitzgerald M: The course and termination of primary afferent fibres. In Wall PD, Melzack R [eds]: Textbook of Pain, 2nd ed. Edinburgh, Churchill Livingstone, 1989.)

nation of stalked cells is lamina I, and the synaptic targets are probably the nociceptive, long-projecting neurons of lamina I. The dendritic trees of islet cells are oriented in the rostrocaudal plane (i.e., flattened mediolaterally). The axons of islet cells end mainly in lamina II. The dendrites form dendrodendritic and dendroaxonic synapses. Lamina II neurons that receive C fiber nociceptive inputs are propriospinal interneurons. They have axons that extend, at most, three spinal segments.

Lamina III is distinguished from lamina II by having slightly larger and more widely spaced neurons. In contrast to lamina II, lamina III contains many myelinated axons and has major input from primary afferent fibers. Intracellular recordings from single, functionally identified axons employing intracellular markers have revealed inputs from low-threshold mechanoreceptor afferents (i.e., from hair follicles, Pacinian corpuscles, and rapidly adapting and slowly adapting mechanoreceptors) with distinct geometries of the terminal branches (see Fig. 181–10, *right*). Two types of projecting neurons have been identified in lamina III: postsynaptic dorsal column neurons and neurons projecting through the spinocervical tract.

Lamina IV differs from lamina III by the presence of some very large neurons (see Fig. 181–9), but small and medium-sized neurons are also present. The neuropil of lamina IV differs from lamina III by having axosomatic synapses. Projection neurons (i.e., postsynaptic

dorsal column neurons and spinocervical tract projecting neurons) have the same properties as those in lamina III. The dendrites of many neurons in lamina IV project into laminae I through III and can receive direct input from primary afferent neurons, which terminate in these upper laminae. Direct terminations of primary afferent neurons in lamina IV are from large-diameter, myelinated axons (see Fig. 181–10).

Lamina V neurons are even more varied in their cytoarchitecture than those in lamina IV. Compared with lamina IV, there are relatively more spinothalamic projection neurons and fewer spinocervical tract and postsynaptic dorsal column neurons. Analogous to lamina IV, lamina V receives direct terminations from low-threshold, large-diameter (Aβ) primary afferent neurons. Nociceptive input is from Aδ nociceptive primary afferent neurons (see Fig. 181–10, *left*) and from nociceptive C fibers. Lamina V neurons have relatively large receptive fields. Depending on the degree of convergence of non-nociceptive and nociceptive inputs, the postsynaptic neurons have the physiologic properties of low-threshold neurons, wide-dynamic-range neurons (i.e., those receiving inputs from low-threshold and nociceptive afferent fibers), or nociceptive-specific neurons (i.e., neurons that normally respond only to noxious stimuli). Low-threshold inputs to higher-order nociceptive neurons may become unmasked and highly effective, causing allodynia and hyperalgesia.

Lamina VI is present only in the cervical and lumbosacral enlargements of the spinal cord and has been studied less than the other laminae. Most neurons in this lamina are probably propriospinal, but some project to the thalamus or to the lateral cervical nucleus. Lamina VII occupies the intermediate zone of the gray matter and contains some well-defined nuclei, such as the dorsal nucleus of Clarke and the intermediolateral nucleus.

Laminae VIII and IX make up the ventral horn of the gray matter. Lamina VIII is restricted to the medial half of the ventral horn in the cervical and lumbar enlargements. Lamina IX harbors groups of motor nuclei that consist of α and γ motoneurons. Although these laminae serve major motor functions, they also harbor spinothalamic projection neurons.

Lamina X surrounds the central canal. Many of lamina X neurons receive convergent input from visceral afferents. Some spinothalamic projection neurons are also found in this lamina.

Trigeminal Nuclei

The axons of trigeminal primary afferent neurons project to the main nucleus and the spinal nucleus. The latter is made up of three subnuclei: oralis, interpolaris, and caudalis (Fig. 181–11). Although there are many similarities with the somatic system (e.g., lamination of trigeminal subnucleus caudalis resembles that of spinal dorsal horn), there are also some important differences in the organization of the trigeminal nuclei. One example is the multiple projection regions of trigeminal afferent neurons.[68] Direct nociceptive inputs are most firmly established for interpolaris and caudalis subnuclei of the trigeminal nuclear complex, but behav-

ioral studies indicate that more rostral nuclei (i.e., nucleus oralis and the main sensory nucleus of the trigeminal nerve) are also important for the processing of nociceptive information.[69] All four subdivisions of the trigeminal nucleus receive inputs from corneal and dental afferents, which are considered to be largely, perhaps exclusively, nociceptive. Neurons in the rostral and the caudal trigeminal nuclear complex respond to stimuli applied to cerebral vasculature. Nociceptive primary afferent neurons that innervate the cranial blood vessels may play a significant role in cluster and migraine headaches.[70-73] The trigeminal nuclear complex also receives input from cranial nerves VII, IX, and X.

Somatotopic Organization

The trigeminal nerve has three main divisions: ophthalmic, maxillary, and mandibular. In the spinal nucleus, the mandibular fiber projection is located most dorsally, the maxillary projection is in intermediate position, and the ophthalmic projection is located most ventrally (Fig. 181–12). In the subnucleus caudalis, fibers nearest to the lips and lower nose terminate highest in the subnucleus, and those located more peripherally terminate more caudad in the tract. This results in an "onion peel" distribution of sensation on the face, which may be revealed by lesions of the upper cervical spinal cord or after caudal trigeminal tractotomy.

SEGMENTAL FACILITATORY MECHANISMS

Allodynia and Secondary Hyperalgesia

Primary afferent neurons synthesize excitatory amino acids and a wide variety of neuropeptides, any of

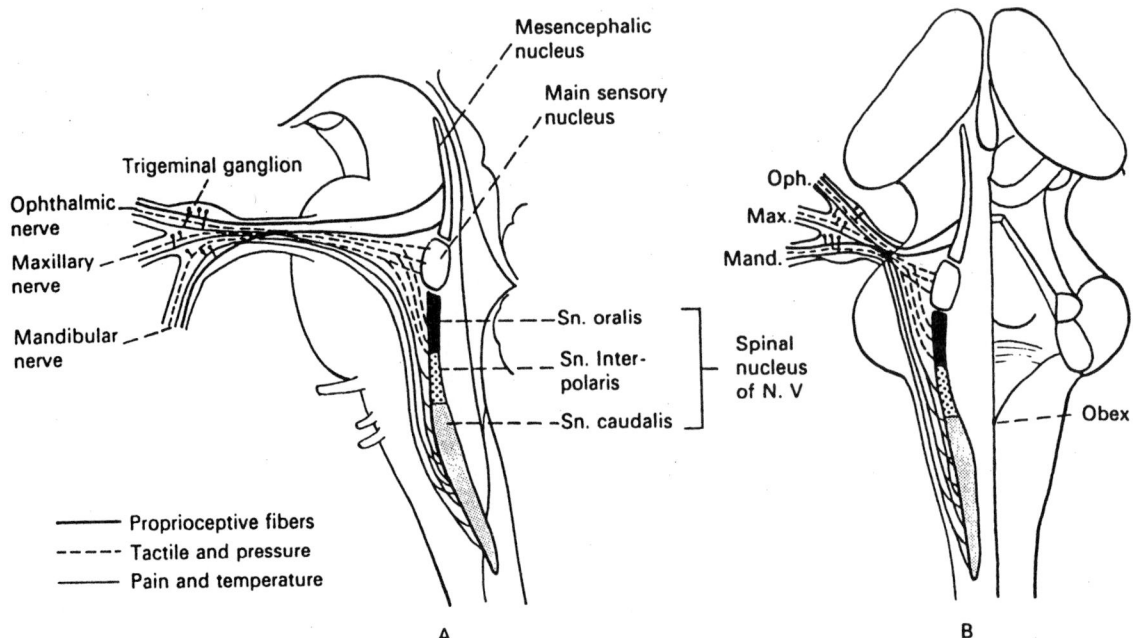

FIGURE 181–11. Schematic diagram of the trigeminal system. *A,* lateral view. *B,* Dorsal view. (From Bonica JJ: Anatomic and physiological basis of nociception and pain. In Bonica JJ [ed]: The Management of Pain, vol 1. Philadelphia, Lea & Febiger, 1990, pp 28–94.)

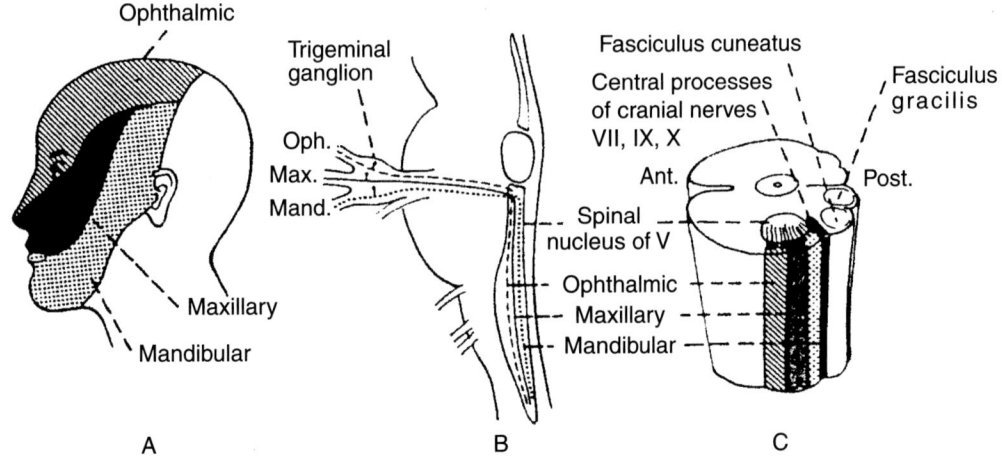

FIGURE 181–12. The cutaneous distribution of the three divisions of the trigeminal nerve in the spinal nucleus of the trigeminal nerve. *A,* Areas innervated by the ophthalmic, maxillary, and mandibular trigeminal divisions. *B* and *C,* Relative positions of the terminations in the spinal nucleus. (From Bonica JJ: Anatomic and physiological basis of nociception and pain. In Bonica JJ [ed]: The Management of Pain, vol 1. Philadelphia, Lea & Febiger, 1990, pp 28–94.)

which can act as a synaptic neurotransmitter or neuromodulator.[74] The excitatory acid glutamate is the substance most likely responsible for fast excitatory synaptic actions of primary nociceptive neurons. Substance P appears to mediate some of the slower synaptic actions. Other neuropeptides that are released from small-diameter primary afferent neurons (i.e., calcitonin gene–related peptide, vasoactive intestinal peptide, and somatostatin) may modulate synaptic transmission.[66] Intense activation of nociceptive inputs has profound effects on synaptic transmission in nociceptive pathways. Higher-order nociceptive neurons become sensitized and begin to respond vigorously to previously less effective or ineffective inputs from low-threshold sensory receptors.[75–81] Such activation of ascending nociceptive neurons is believed to be the cause of secondary hyperalgesia and allodynia, respectively.

Preemptive Anesthesia

The surgeon and the anesthesiologist need to take into consideration that, unless proper countermeasures are taken, surgical intervention is likely to trigger secondary hyperalgesia. General anesthesia does not prevent the activation of nociceptors, nor does it prevent the development of hyperalgesia. Discharge of nociceptive fibers and the development of hyperalgesia can be blocked effectively by infiltrating the surgical site with a local anesthetic (i.e., preemptive anesthesia). Controlled studies have shown that prevention of secondary hyperalgesia by preemptive anesthesia substantially lessens the requirement for analgesic medication after surgery and hastens patients' recovery.[82]

ASCENDING NOCICEPTIVE PATHWAYS

Preautonomic Projections

Lamina I spinal cord neurons project to the spinomedullary junction, the thoracolumbar sympathetic pregan-

glionic regions, and the sacral parasympathetic regions. In the lower brainstem, projections from spinal lamina I neurons terminate in preautonomic regions of the ventrolateral medulla and dorsolateral pons. Major projection from spinal lamina I neurons (through the spinomesencephalic tract) targets the parabrachial nucleus that is a major viscerosensory integration site connected to the periaqueductal gray, hypothalamus, and amygdala. These projections contribute to the integration of pain processing with homeostasis of bodily functions. This integrative concept of pain as an aspect of enteroreception has been emphasized in recent reports.[83] Lamina V neurons project to more medial, core regions of the lower brainstem, where they may affect behavioral state.[83]

Spinothalamic Tract

Figure 181–13 shows schematically the primary neural pathways for the transmission of nociceptive information from the various body structures to the brain. The main ascending pathway for pain sensation is the crossed lateral spinothalamic tract that carries information from lamina I neurons, courses in the middle of the lateral funiculus, and terminates in the posterolateral thalamus (VMpo) (Fig. 181–14).[84] This nucleus contains nociceptive-specific and thermoreceptive-specific neurons that have the ability to encode the location and intensity of stimulation. VMpo neurons project to the dorsal margin of the insular cortex. There is a collateral projection from the VMpo to area 3a in the central sulcus. Lamina I spinothalamic neurons also terminate in the ventral portion of the main somatosensory thalamic relay nucleus (i.e., ventral posterior inferior nucleus [VPI]). VPI neurons project to the secondary somatosensory cortex (SII). There is also a projection to the medial dorsal thalamic nucleus, which projects to the anterior cingulate cortex (Fig. 181–15).

Lamina V projection neurons carry nociceptive and

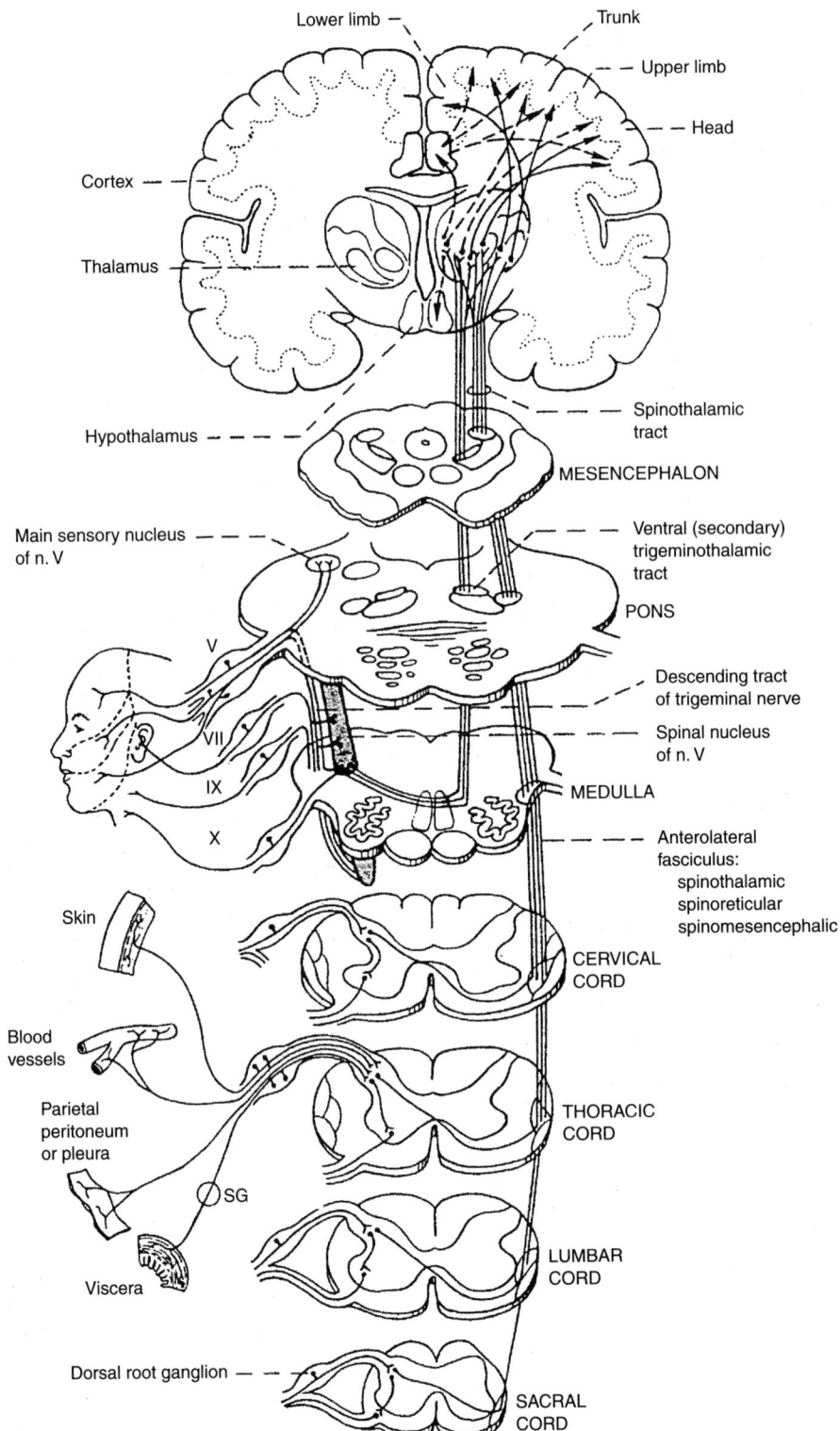

FIGURE 181–13. Principal pathways for the transmission of nociceptive information from various body structures to the brain. n. V, trigeminal nerve; SG, sympathetic ganglion. (From Bonica JJ: Anatomic and physiological basis of nociception and pain. In Bonica JJ [ed]: The Management of Pain, vol 1. Philadelphia, Lea & Febiger, 1990, pp 28–94.)

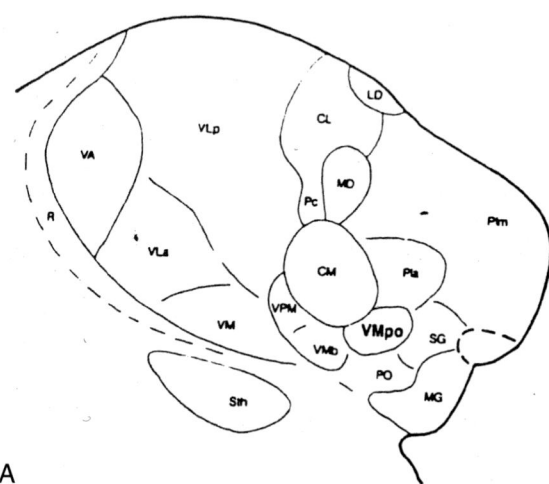

A

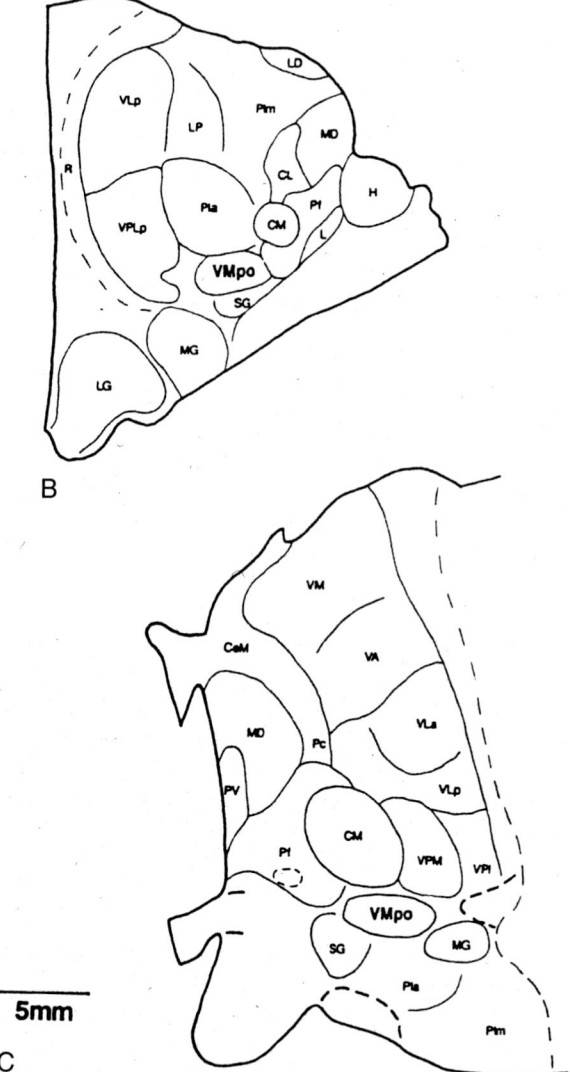

B

FIGURE 181–14. Drawings of the cytoarchitectonic location of the posterior part of the ventral medial nucleus of the human thalamus in three standard stereotactic planes. A, Sagittal plane, L + 14.0 mm. B, Frontal plane, A + 0.5 mm. C, Horizontal plane, H 0.0. CeM, central medial nerve; CL, central lateral nerve; H, habenula; L, limitans nerve; LD, lateral dorsal nerve; LG, lateral geniculate nerve; LP, lateral posterior nerve; MD, medial dorsal nerve; Pc, paracentral nerve; Plm, medial pulvinar nerve; PO, posterior complex; PV, paraventricular (thalamic) nerve; R, reticular nerve; SG, suprageniculate nerve; Sth, subthalamic nerve; VA, ventral posterior nerve; VLa, anterior part of the ventral lateral nerve; VLp, posterior part of the ventral lateral nerve; VM, ventral medial nerve; VMpo, posterior part of the ventral medial nerve; VPI, ventral posterior inferior nerve; VPLp, posterior part of the ventroposterior lateral nerve; VPM, ventroposterior medial nerve. (Adapted from Craig AD, Bushnell MC, Zhang ET, Blomqvist A: A thalamic nucleus specific for pain and temperature sensation. Nature 372:770–773, 1994.)

5mm

C

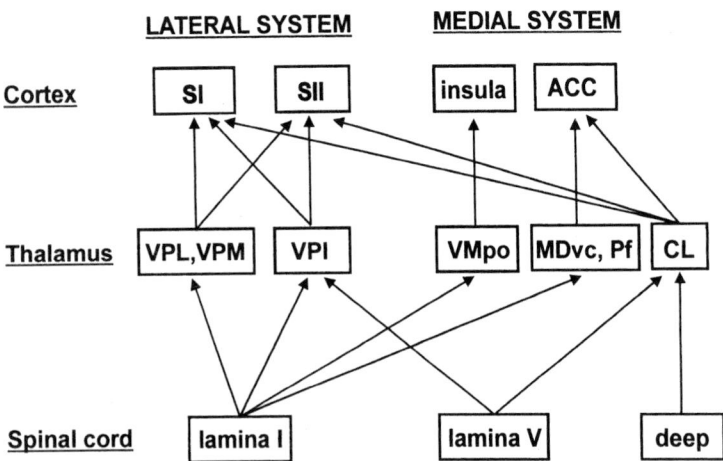

FIGURE 181–15. Cortical areas that receive information from the spinothalamic tract. The main spinothalamic and thalamocortical projections were summarized and simplified from several reports on the central nociceptive pathways in monkeys. Corticocortical connections are not shown. ACC, anterior cingulate cortex; CL, centrolateral nucleus; MDvc, ventrocaudal part of medial dorsal nucleus; Pf, parafascicular nucleus; SI, primary somatosensory cortex; SII, secondary somatosensory cortex; VMpo, posterior part of ventromedial nucleus; VPI, ventral posterior inferior nucleus; VPL, ventroposterior lateral nucleus; VPM, ventroposterior medial nucleus. (Adapted from Treede RD, Kenshalo DR, Gracely R, Jones AK: The cortical representation of pain. Pain 79:105–111, 1999.)

tactile information through the anterior spinothalamic tract to neurons in the main thalamic somatosensory relay nuclei (i.e., ventroposterior medial nucleus [VPM] and ventroposterior lateral nucleus [VPL]), which project to the primary somatosensory cortex (SI) in the postcentral gyrus (see Fig. 181–15).

Spinoreticular Tract

The reticular formation plays a role in nociceptive mechanisms by triggering arousal, contributing to the motivational and affective aspects of pain perception and to somatic and autonomic reflexes. The cells of origin of this tract are found in laminae VII and VIII, with some cells in other laminae, including I, V, and X.[85–87] In the lumbar area, the spinoreticular tract is predominantly contralateral, whereas, in the cervical area, cells from both sides of the cord make up the tract (Fig. 181–16).[85, 88] In the spinal cord, the spinoreticular tract accompanies the spinothalamic tract and the spinomesencephalic tract, but in the brainstem it is located medial to these tracts.

Spinomesencephalic Tract

The spinomesencephalic tract is similar to the spinoreticular tract in that most of its fibers terminate in the reticular formation. Like the spinoreticular tract, spinomesencephalic tract projections are probably involved autonomic reflexes and motivational or affective responses. The spinomesencephalic tract may also be involved in some discriminative functions, because it projects to the ventrobasal thalamus. The cells of origin are predominantly from lamina I, although lamina V and deeper laminae may also contribute.[89] Most of these cells project contralaterally in the anterolateral system and dorsolateral funiculus, although about 25% project ipsilaterally. At the level of the mesencephalon, the spinomesencephalic tract terminates in rostral subnuclei of the reticular formation, including the subnucleus lateralis of the periaqueductal gray and the intercollicularis, cuneiformis, superior colliculus, Darkschewitsch, and Edinger-Westphal nuclei (Fig.

181–17). More rostral projections include the ventrobasal and medial thalamus and the limbic system.

Other Ascending Systems

Several other ascending tracts are relevant to nociceptive sensation. A small number of neurons that make up the dorsal column postsynaptic system probably respond exclusively to noxious stimulation (Fig. 181–18). The cells of origin are in laminae III and IV. The dorsal column postsynaptic system projects to the dorsal column nuclei in a somatotopic fashion (i.e., lower extremity sensation to the nucleus gracilis and upper extremity to the cuneate nucleus). From there, the pathway principally courses to the ventroposterolateral nucleus of the thalamus. It has been suggested that this tract might play a discriminative or modulatory role in pain sensation.

The other pathway of interest is the propriospinal, multisynaptic ascending system. This polysynaptic network is thought to be located deep in the dorsal column and in lamina X, which receives prominent input from deep nociceptors and from midline structures. This pathway projects rostrally to the brainstem reticular formation and then to the medial and intralaminar thalamic nuclei. It has been speculated that disruption of this pathway might be responsible for the pain relief sometimes achieved by midline myelotomy performed well above the painful segment.

Pathways Ascending from the Trigeminal Nuclear Complex

Trigeminal brainstem nuclear complex neurons project to a large number of extratrigeminal structures, such as the thalamic nuclei, motor nuclei, superior colliculus, pretectal nucleus, parabrachial nucleus, inferior olive, nucleus of the solitary tract, reticular formation, periaqueductal gray, spinal cord, and cerebellum (Fig. 181–19).[69] Spinal trigeminal nuclei project to the thalamic VPM through a crossed pathway that merges with the spinothalamic tract.[69] Principalis neurons are major contributors of the thalamofugal projections. They syn-

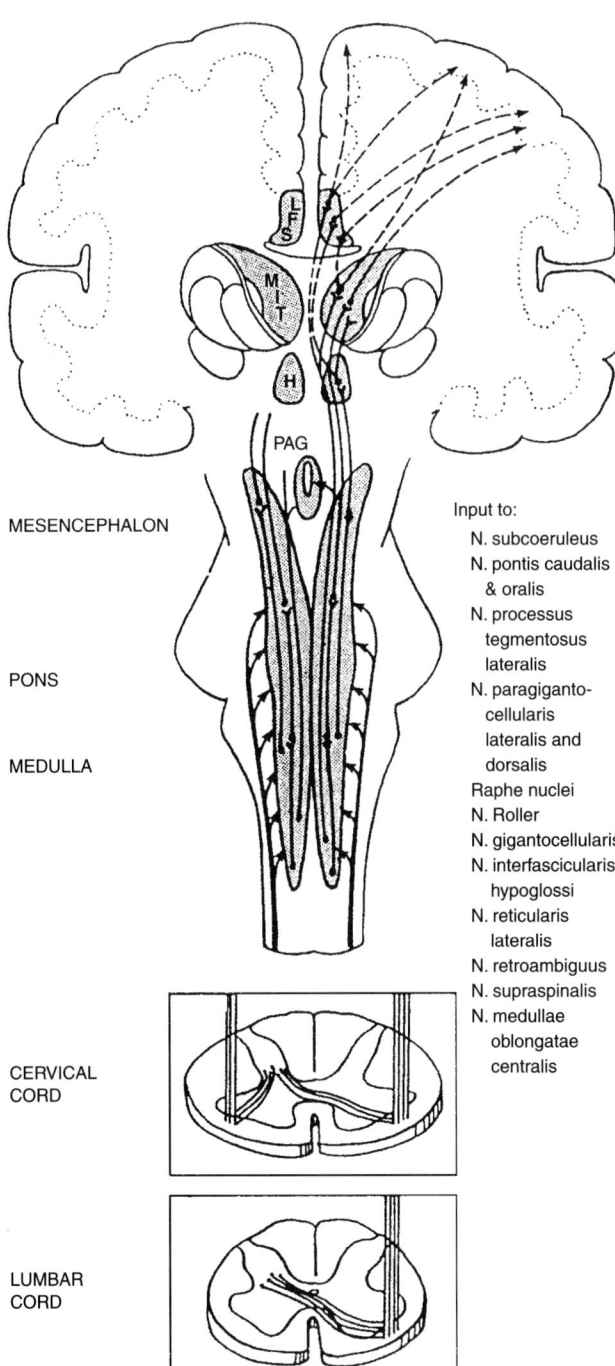

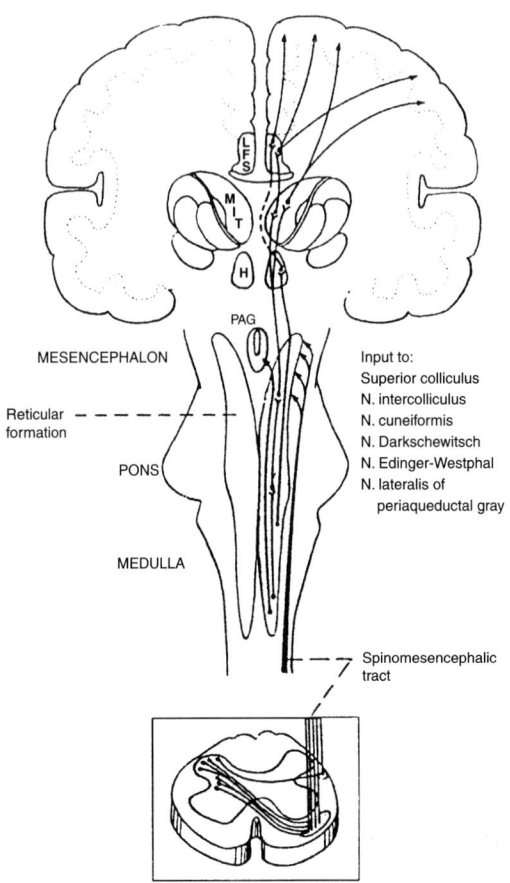

FIGURE 181–17. Diagram of the origin, course, and termination of the spinomesencephalic tract. H, hypothalamus; LFS, limbic forebrain structure; MIT, medial intrathalamic nuclei; PAG, periaqueductal gray matter. (From Bonica JJ: Anatomic and physiological basis of nociception and pain. In Bonica JJ [ed]: The Management of Pain, vol 1. Philadelphia, Lea & Febiger, 1990, pp 28–94.)

FIGURE 181–16. Diagram of the origin, course, and termination of the spinoreticular tract. H, hypothalamus; LFS, limbic forebrain structure; MIT, medial intrathalamic nuclei; PAG, periaqueductal gray matter. (From Bonica JJ: Anatomic and physiological basis of nociception and pain. In Bonica JJ [ed]: The Management of Pain, vol 1. Philadelphia, Lea & Febiger, 1990, pp 28–94.)

apse in the contralateral and ipsilateral medial subnucleus of the VPM. The contralateral projection originates in the ventral aspect of principalis, and it decussates caudal to the interpeduncular nucleus and ascends with the medial lemniscus. Projections from interpolaris, oralis, and caudalis neurons make a lesser contribution to the VPM projection. In addition to the VPM, the caudal subnuclei of the trigeminal brainstem nuclear complex project to the posterior thalamus and the internal medullary lamina. Particularly important for nociception may be a bilateral projection from the caudalis to the medial thalamus (a region called *nucleus submedius* in the cat).[90] A bilateral projection from trigeminal subnucleus caudalis to the parabrachial nuclei, which is part of a trigeminal-pontine-amygdaloid pathway, is likely to play an important role in affective and autonomic reactions to noxious stimuli.[69]

CORTICAL PROJECTIONS

Cortical structures that are activated by noxious stimuli most consistently include the SI, SII, anterior cingulate cortex, and insular cortex.[91–99]

Primary Sensory Cortex

The SI is located in the postcentral gyrus and extends from the interhemispheric fissure to the sylvian fissure.

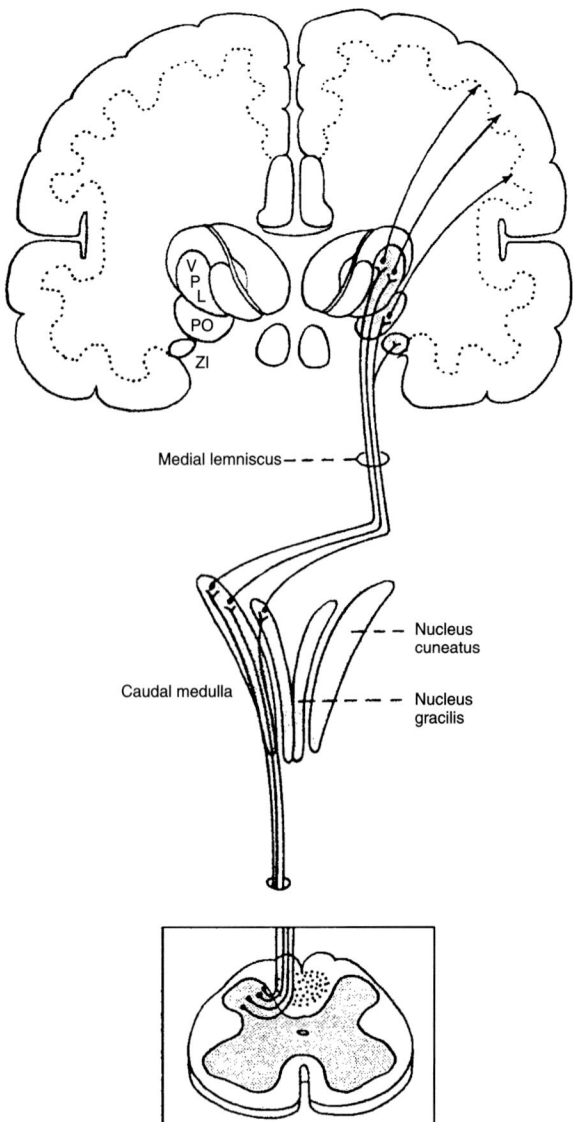

FIGURE 181–18. Diagram of the origin, course, and termination of the dorsal column postsynaptic system. *Stippled area* in the spinal cord cross section indicates the location of axons in the dorsal column. PO, posterior thalamic nuclear group; VPL, ventroposterior lateral nucleus; ZI, zona incerta. (From Bonica JJ: Anatomic and physiological basis of nociception and pain. In Bonica JJ [ed]: The Management of Pain, vol 1. Philadelphia, Lea & Febiger, 1990, pp 28–94.)

The SI receives direct nociceptive input from the ipsilateral nuclei in the ventrobasal thalamus (i.e., VPL and VPM), which are part of the lateral ascending system. Nociceptive information also reaches SI through the centrolateral nucleus (CL) of the thalamus (see Fig. 181–15). Single-cell neurophysiologic studies in the monkey show that SI nociceptive neurons are arranged in clusters confined to layers III through V in areas 3b and 1 (Fig. 181–20).[100] SI nociceptive neurons have the ability to encode graded stimulus intensities. The receptive fields are small, arranged in a somatotopic pattern along the postcentral gyrus.[101] Likewise, functional imaging studies in the human found that noci-

ceptive inputs to SI are arranged in a somatotopic fashion.[102] SI nociceptive neurons appear well suited to be the neural substrate for the discriminative aspects of nociception (i.e., estimation of stimulus intensity and fine localization of the area stimulated).[98]

Positron-emission tomography, function magnetic resonance imaging, and magnetoencephalographic or electroencephalographic studies have provided convergent evidence for participation of the SI in human pain processing.[103] However, clinical observations complicate the picture regarding involvement of the SI in pain processing. Electrical stimulation of the SI with macroelectrodes was found to rarely produce pain in patients undergoing surgery with local anesthesia.[104, 105] Attempts at resection of the somatosensory cortex to relieve pain have been disappointing. Although most patients who had the postcentral gyrus resected had initial pain relief, this effect persisted in only a minority of patients.[106] Somewhat paradoxically, lesions of the somatosensory cortex can produce a syndrome that strongly resembles so-called thalamic pain.[106] It has been reported that chronic macrostimulation of primary motor cortex can relieve deafferentiation pain related to subcortical or thalamic infarction, possibly mediated through cortical association connections to the somatosensory cortex or through corticofugal projections to the ventrobasal thalamus.[107]

Secondary Somatosensory Area

Another cortical area that is activated by noxious stimuli is SII. It is located in the cortex of the parietal lobe in the operculum just above the sylvian fissure (see Fig. 181–20). Like SI, the SII receives nociceptive inputs from thalamic nuclei that belong to the lateral (i.e., VPL and VPM) or the medial (i.e., CL) ascending systems (see Fig. 181–15).[98] The SII appears less well equipped than the SI to subserve the fine sensory-discriminative aspects of nociception. There are few nociceptive neurons in the center of the SII. Nociceptive neurons found in the border region between area 7b and the SII are not particularly proficient at coding stimulus intensity.[108] Because there is convergence with visual information about threatening stimuli approaching the nociceptive receptive field, it was suggested that SII neurons play a role in spatially directed attention toward noxious stimuli.[98]

Anterior Cingulate Cortex

The anterior cingulate cortex is part of the limbic system. It receives input from medial thalamic nuclei (i.e., ventrocaudal part of the medial dorsal nucleus and the parafascicular and centrolateral nuclei) (see Fig. 181–20). Nociceptive neurons in the anterior cingulate gyrus have properties that reflect the properties of nociceptive neurons that ascend to the medial thalamic nuclei. Anterior cingulate cortex neurons show some capacity for intensity coding, but they have large receptive fields that are not somatotopically organized and may encompass the entire body surface. The neurons therefore appear unsuitable for sensory-discrimi-

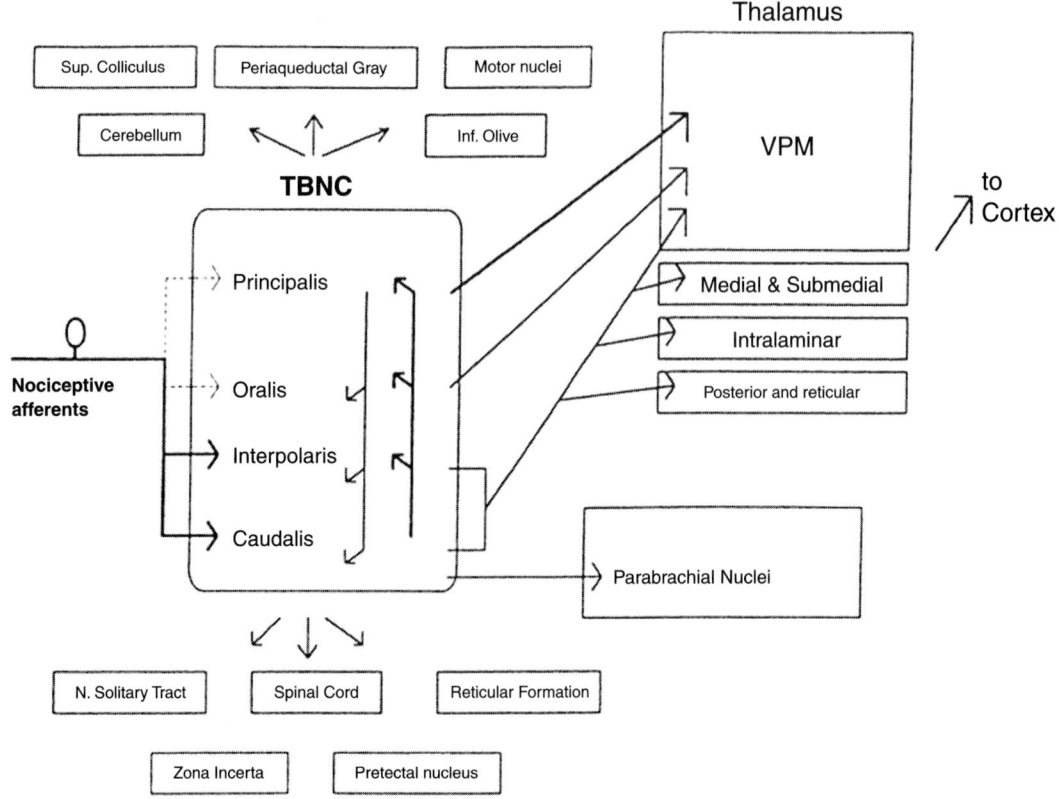

FIGURE 181–19. Diagram of the principal connections of the trigeminal brainstem nuclear complex. (Adapted from Renehan WE, Jacquin MF: Anatomy of central nervous system pathways related to head pain. In Olesen J, Tfelt-Hansen P, Welch MA [eds]. The Headaches. New York, Raven Press, 1993, pp 59–68.)

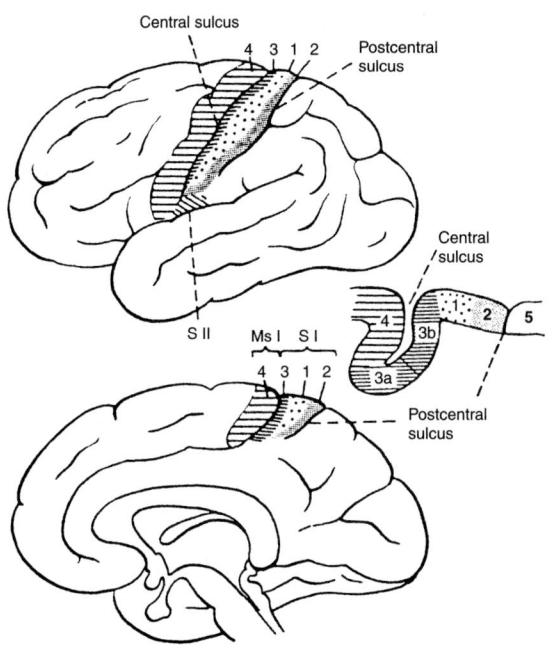

FIGURE 181–20. Location of somatosensory cortices. MsI, motor cortex; SI, primary somatosensory cortex; SII, secondary somatosensory cortex; 1 to 5, Brodman areas. *Inset,* Location of areas 1 and 3b. (From Bonica JJ: Anatomic and physiological basis of nociception and pain. In Bonica JJ [ed]: The Management of Pain, vol 1. Philadelphia, Lea & Febiger, 1990, pp 28–94.)

native processing of nociceptive information.[98] Anterior cingulate cortex neurons may encode the unpleasantness of pain.[103] Surgical lesions of the cingulate cortex reduce the emotional aspect of pain and the motivation to avoid painful stimuli. The lesions do not impair the ability to detect painful stimuli.[103]

Insular Cortex

The insular cortex is another cortical area with connections to the limbic system that receives nociceptive input through the medial spinothalamic system.[98] The insular cortex is considered to be a multisensory area that integrates nociceptive, tactile, and vestibular information, as well as taste and other visceral sensations.[109] The anterior part of insular cortex shows consistent pain-related activations.[103] There are direct connections to the middle and anterior insula from the thalamic relay nucleus VMpo (see Fig. 181–14), which contains a high density of neurons with specifically nociceptive and thermoreceptive properties.[110] It has been suggested that this area integrates information on the physiologic condition of the body, including the specific sensations of pain and temperature. The insulae integrate pain related input from the SII and the thalamus with contextual information from other sensory modalities before relaying this information to the limbic structures of the temporal lobe.[103]

CONCLUSIONS

An understanding of the physiologic basis of nociception is essential for the science of neurosurgery. Knowledge about the physiology and anatomy of nociception has increased dramatically in recent years. We now have a greater appreciation of the peripheral transduction and transmission of nociceptive information, as well as peripheral and spinal mechanisms of hyperalgesia. Functional imaging is beginning to provide important information about central structures that are activated by pain. The next decade will see major advances in our understanding of the central mechanisms of hyperalgesia and central pain. Increasing knowledge in this area will likely open new venues for the development of neurosurgical procedures for pain control.

REFERENCES

1. Merskey H, Bogduk N (eds): IASP Task Force on Taxonomy; Classification of Chronic Pain, vol I, 2nd ed. Seattle, IASP Press, 1994.
2. Burgess PR, Perl ER: Myelinated afferent fibres responding specifically to noxious stimulation of the skin. J Physiol 190:541–562, 1967.
3. Perl ER: Pain and nociception. In Handbook of Physiology. Bethesda, MD, American Physiological Society, 1984, pp 915–975.
4. Lawson SN: Phenotype and function of somatic primary afferent nociceptive neurones with C-, Adelta- or Aalpha/beta-fibres. Exp Physiol 87:239–244, 2002.
5. Weidner C, Schmidt R, Schmelz M, et al: Time course of postexcitatory effects separates afferent human C fibre classes. J Physiol 527(Pt 1):185–191, 2000.
6. Caterina MJ, Schumacher MA, Tominaga M, et al: The capsaicin receptor: A heat-activated ion channel in the pain pathway. Nature 389:816–824, 1997.
7. Caterina MJ, Rosen TA, Tominaga M, et al: A capsaicin-receptor homologue with a high threshold for noxious heat. Nature 398:436–441, 1999.
8. Clapham DE: Signal transduction. Hot and cold TRP ion channels. Science 295:2228–2229, 2002.
9. McKemy DD, Neuhausser WM, Julius D: Identification of a cold receptor reveals a general role for TRP channels in thermosensation. Nature 416:52–58, 2002.
10. Burnstock G: P2X receptors in sensory neurones. Br J Anaesth 84:476–488, 2000.
11. Gauldie SD, McQueen DS, Pertwee, R, Chessell IP: Anandamide activates peripheral nociceptors in normal and arthritic rat knee joints. Br J Pharmacol 132:617–621, 2001.
12. Hilliges M, Weidner C, Schmelz M, et al: ATP responses in human C nociceptors. Pain 98:59–68, 2002.
13. Hwang SW, Cho H, Kwak J, et al: Direct activation of capsaicin receptors by products of lipoxygenases: Endogenous capsaicin-like substances. Proc Natl Acad Sci U S A 97:6155–6160, 2000.
14. Olah Z, Karai L, Iadarola MJ: Anandamide activates vanilloid receptor 1 (VR1) at acidic pH in dorsal root ganglia neurons and cells ectopically expressing VR1. J Biol Chem 276:31163–31170, 2001.
15. Rang HP, Bevan, S, Dray A: Chemical activation of nociceptive peripheral neurones. Br Med Bull 47:534–548, 1991.
16. Roberts LA, Christie MJ, Connor M: Anandamide is a partial agonist at native vanilloid receptors in acutely isolated mouse trigeminal sensory neurons. Br J Pharmacol 137:421–428, 2002.
17. Robertson B, Bevan S: Properties of 5-hydroxytryptamine₃ receptor-gated currents in adult rat dorsal root ganglion neurones. Br J Pharmacol 102:272–276, 1991.
18. Sutherland SP, Cook SP, McCleskey EW: Chemical mediators of pain due to tissue damage and ischemia. Prog Brain Res 129:21–38, 2000.
19. Tominaga M, Caterina MJ, Malmberg AB, et al: The cloned capsaicin receptor integrates multiple pain-producing stimuli. Neuron 21:531–543, 1998.
20. Rang HP, Bevan, S, Dray A: Nociceptive peripheral neurons: Cellular properties. In Wall PD, Melzack R (eds): Textbook of Pain, 2nd ed. Edinburgh, Churchill Livingstone, 1994, pp 57–78.
21. Handwerker HO, Reeh PW: Pain and inflammation. In Bond MR, Charlton JE, Woolf CJ (eds): Proceedings of the VIth World Congress on Pain. Amsterdam, Elsevier, 1991, pp 59–70.
22. Levine J, Taiwo Y: Inflammatory pain. In Wall PD, Melzack R (eds): Textbook of Pain, 2nd ed. Edinburgh, Churchill Livingstone, 1994, pp 45–56.
23. Baumann TK, Burchiel KJ, Martenson ME: Mechanosensitive channels in adult human DRG neurons. Soc Neurosci Abstr 19:1072, 1993.
24. Cho H, Shin J, Shin CY, et al: Mechanosensitive ion channels in cultured sensory neurons of neonatal rats. J Neurosci 22:1238–1247, 2002.
25. Vallbo AB, Hagbarth K-E, Torebjörk HE, Wallin BG: Somatosensory, proprioceptive, and sympathetic activity in human peripheral nerves. Physiol Rev 59:919–957, 1979.
26. Handwerker HO, Forster, C, Kirchhoff C: Discharge patterns of human C-fibers induced by itching and burning stimuli. J Neurophysiol 66:307–315, 1991.
27. Handwerker HO, Kobal G: Psychophysiology of experimentally induced pain. Physiol Rev 73:639–671, 1993.
28. Ochoa J, Torebjörk HE: Sensations evoked by intraneural microstimulation of C nociceptor fibres in human skin nerves. J Physiol 415:583–599, 1989.
29. Torebjörk HE: Afferent C units responding to mechanical, thermal, and chemical stimuli in human non-glabrous skin. Acta Physiol Scand 92:374–390, 1974.
30. Torebjörk HE, Ochoa JL: Specific sensations evoked by activity in single identified sensory units in man. Acta Physiol Scand 110:445–447, 1980.
31. Ochoa J, Torebjörk E: Sensations evoked by intraneural microstimulation of C nociceptor fibres in human skin nerves. J Physiol 415:583–599, 1989.
32. Marchettini P, Simone DA, Caputi G, Ochoa JL: Pain from excitation of identified muscle nociceptors in humans. Brain Res 740:109–116, 1996.
33. Handwerker HO, Kilo S, Reeh PW: Unresponsive afferent nerve fibres in the sural nerve of the rat. J Physiol 435:229–242, 1991.
34. McMahon SB, Koltzenburg M: Novel classes of nociceptors: Beyond Sherrington. Trends Neurosci 13:199–201, 1990.
35. Meyer RA, Davis KD, Cohen RH, et al: Mechanically insensitive afferents (MIAs) in cutaneous nerves of monkey. Brain Res 561:252–261, 1991.
36. Cohen RH, Perl ER: Contributions of arachidonic acid derivatives and substance P to the sensitization of cutaneous nociceptors. J Neurophysiol 64:457–464, 1990.
37. Martin HA, Basbaum AI, Goetzl EJ, Levine JD: Leukotriene B₄ decreases the mechanical and thermal thresholds of C-fiber nociceptors in the hairy skin of the rat. J Neurophysiol 60:438–445, 1988.
38. Sugiura T, Tominaga M, Katsuya H, Mizumura K: Bradykinin lowers the threshold temperature for heat activation of vanilloid receptor 1. J Neurophysiol 88:544–548, 2002.
39. Cohen RH, Perl ER: Chemical factors in the sensitization of cutaneous nociceptors. In Hamann W, Iggo A (eds): Transduction and Cellular Mechanisms in Sensory Receptors, vol 74. Progress in Brain Research. New York, Elsevier, 1988.
40. Steen KH, Reeh PW: Sustained graded pain and hyperalgesia from experimental tissue acidosis in human subjects. Soc Neurosci Abstr 18:384, 1992.
41. Steen KH, Reeh PW, Anton F, Handwerker HO: Protons selectively induce lasting excitation and sensitization to mechanical stimulation of nociceptors in rat skin, in vitro. J Neurosci 12:86–95, 1992.
42. Tominaga M, Wada M, Masu M: Potentiation of capsaicin receptor activity by metabotropic ATP receptors as a possible mechanism for ATP-evoked pain and hyperalgesia. Proc Natl Acad Sci U S A 98:6951–6956, 2001.
43. Levine JD, Fields HL, Basbaum AI: Peptides and primary afferent nociceptor. J Neurosci 13:2273–2286, 1993.
44. Levine JD, Clark R, Devor M, et al: Intraneuronal substance P

contributes to the severity of experimental arthritis. Science 226: 547–549, 1984.

45. Markowitz S, Saito K, Moskowitz MA: Neurogenically mediated leakage of plasma protein occurs from blood vessels in dura mater but not brain. J Neurosci 7:4129–4136, 1987.

46. Moskowitz MA: The trigeminovascular system. In Olesen J, Tfelt-Hansen P, Welch MA (eds): The Headaches. New York, Raven Press, 1993, pp 97–104.

47. Meyer RA, Campbell JN, Raja SN: Peripheral neural mechanisms of nociception. In Wall PD, Melzack R (eds): Textbook of Pain, 2nd ed. Edinburgh, Churchill Livingstone, 1994, pp 13–44.

48. Belmonte C, Gallar J, Pozo MA, Rebollo I: Excitation by irritant chemical substances of sensory afferent units in the cat's cornea. J Physiol 437:709–725, 1991.

49. Belmonte C, Giraldez F: Responses of cat corneal sensory receptors to mechanical and thermal stimulation. J Physiol 321:355–368, 1981.

50. LaMotte RH, Campbell JN: Comparison of responses of warm and nociceptive C-fiber afferents in monkey with human judgments of thermal pain. J Neurophysiol 41:509–528, 1978.

51. Baumann TK, Simone DA, Shain C, LaMotte RH: Neurogenic hyperalgesia: The search for the primary cutaneous afferent fibers that contribute to capsaicin-induced pain and hyperalgesia. J Neurophysiol 66:212–227, 1991.

52. Mense S: Physiology of nociception in muscles. In Fricton JR, Awad E (eds): Advances in Pain Research and Therapy, vol 17. New York, Raven Press, 1990, pp 67–85.

53. Mense S: Considerations concerning the neurobiological basis of muscle pain. Can J Physiol Pharmacol 69:610–616, 1991.

54. Mense S: Nociception from skeletal muscle in relation to clinical muscle pain. Pain 54:241–289, 1993.

55. Schaible H-G, Grubb BD: Afferent and spinal mechanisms of joint pain. Pain 55:5–54, 1993.

56. Hanesch U, Heppelmann B, Messlinger K, Schmidt RF: Nociception in normal and arthritic joints. In Willis WD Jr (ed): Hyperalgesia and Allodynia. New York, Raven Press, 1992, pp 81–105.

57. Schaible H-G, Schmidt RF: Direct observation of the sensitization of articular afferents during an experimental arthritis. In Dubner R, Gebhart GF, Bond MR (eds): New York, Elsevier, 1988, pp 44–50.

58. Cervero F: Sensory innervation of the viscera: Peripheral basis of visceral pain. Physiol Rev 74:95–138, 1994.

59. Sengupta JN, Gebhart GF: Gastrointestinal afferent fibers and sensation. In Johnson LR (ed): Physiology of the Gastrointestinal Tract, 3rd ed. New York, Raven Press, 1994, pp 483–519.

60. McMahon SB: Mechanisms of cutaneous, deep and visceral pain. In Wall PD, Melzack R (eds): Textbook of Pain, 2nd ed. Edinburgh, Churchill Livingstone, 1994, pp 129–151.

61. Ranson SW, Billingsley PR: The conduction of painful afferent impulses in the spinal nerves. Am J Physiol 40:571–584, 1916.

62. Willis WD, Coggeshall RE: Sensory Mechanisms of the Spinal Cord, 2nd ed. New York, Plenum, 1991, p 575.

63. Coggeshall RE: Law of separation of function of the spinal roots [review]. Physiol Rev 60:716–755, 1980.

64. Coggeshall RE, Applebaum ML, Fazen M, et al: Unmyelinated axons in human ventral roots, a possible explanation for the failure of dorsal rhizotomy to relieve pain. Brain 98:157–166, 1975.

65. Rexed B: A cytoarchitectonic atlas of the spinal cord in the cat. J Comp Neurol 96:415–466, 1954.

66. Millan MJ: The induction of pain: An integrative review. Prog Neurobiol 57:1–164, 1999.

67. Brown AG: Organization in the Spinal Cord. Berlin, Springer, 1981, p 238.

68. Bereiter DA, Hirata H, Hu JW: Trigeminal subnucleus caudalis: Beyond homologies with the spinal dorsal horn. Pain 88:221–224, 2000.

69. Renehan WE, Jacquin MF: Anatomy of central nervous system pathways related to head pain. In Olesen J. Tfelt-Hansen P, Welch MA (eds): The Headaches. New York, Raven Press, 1993, pp 59–68.

70. Moskowitz MA: Cluster headache: Evidence for a pathophysiologic focus in the superior pericarotid cavernous sinus plexus. Headache 28:584–586, 1988.

71. Moskowitz MA: The visceral organ brain—implications for the pathophysiology of vascular head pain. Neurology 41:182–186, 1991.

72. Moskowitz MA, Buzzi MG: Neuroeffector functions of sensory fibres: Implications for headache mechanisms and drug actions. J Neurol 238:S18–S22, 1991.

73. Moskowitz MA, Saito K, Brezina L, Dickson J: Nerve fibers surrounding intracranial and extracranial vessels from human and other species contain dynorphin like immunoreactivity. Neurosci 23:731–737, 1987.

74. Carr PA, Nagy JI: Emerging relationships between cytochemical properties and sensory modality transmission in primary sensory neurons. Brain Res Bull 30:209–219, 1993.

75. Coderre TJ: Examination of the evidence that distinct excitatory amino acid receptors and intracellular messengers mediate thermal and mechanical hyperalgesia. Pain Forum 3:232–239, 1994.

76. Dougherty PM, Mittman S, Sorkin LS: Hyperalgesia and amino acids. Receptor selectivity based on stimulus intensity and a role for neuropeptides. Pain Forum 3:240–248, 1994.

77. Dougherty PM, Willis WD: Enhancement of spinothalamic neuron responses to chemical and mechanical stimuli following combined micro-iontophoretic application of N-methyl-D-aspartic acid and substance-P. Pain 47:85–93, 1991.

78. Henry JL, Radhakrishnan V: Hyperalgesia following noxious thermal, mechanical, or chemical stimulation involves overlapping spinal mechanisms and interactive participation of excitatory amino acids and neuropeptides. Pain Forum 3:249–256, 1994.

79. Meller ST: Thermal and mechanical hyperalgesia. Pain Forum 3:215–231, 1994.

80. Simone DA, Sorkin LS, Oh U, et al: Neurogenic hyperalgesia: Central neural correlates in responses of spinothalamic neurons. J Neurophysiol 66:228–246, 1991.

81. Yaksh TL, Malmberg AB: Central pharmacology of nociceptive transmission. In Wall PD (ed): Textbook of Pain, 2nd ed. Edinburgh, Churchill Livingstone, 1994, pp 165–200.

82. Kelly DJ, Ahmad M, Brull SJ: Preemptive analgesia II: Recent advances and current trends. Can J Anaesth 48:1091–1101, 2001.

83. Craig AD: Commentary on physiological anatomy of nociception by T. K. Baumann. In Burchiel KJ (ed): Surgical Management of Pain. New York, Thieme, 2002, p 992.

84. Blomquist A, Zhang E-T, Craig AD: Cytoarchitectonic and immunohistochemical characterization of a specific pain and temperature relay, the VMpo nucleus, in the human thalamus. Brain 123:601–619, 2000.

85. Haber LH, Moore BD, Willis WD: Electrophysiological response properties of spinoreticular neurons in the monkey. J Comp Neurol 207:75–84, 1982.

86. Netter FH: Nervous System: Anatomy and Physiology, vol 1. CIBA Collection of Medical Illustrations. West Caldwell, NJ, CIBA Foundation, 1983.

87. Willis WD: The Pain System: The Neural Basis of Nociceptive Transmission in the Mammalian Nervous System. Basel, Karger, 1985.

88. Kevetter GA, Haber L, Yezierski RP, et al: Cells of the origin of the spinoreticular tract in the monkey. J Comp Neurol 207:61–74, 1982.

89. Hylden JL, Hayashi H, Bennett GJ: Lamina I spinomesencephalic neurons in cat ascend via the dorsolateral funiculi. Somatosens Res 4:31–41, 1986.

90. Craig ADJ, Burton H: Spinal and medullary lamina I projection to nucleus submedius in medial thalamus: A possible pain center. J Neurophysiol 45:443–466, 1981.

91. Barreto JA, Gonzalez-Lima F: A landscape parametric profile approach for rat brain image analysis. Neuroimage 2:35–43, 1995.

92. Davis KD, Kwan CL, Crawley AP, Mikulis DJ: Functional MRI study of thalamic and cortical activations evoked by cutaneous heat, cold, and tactile stimuli. J Neurophysiol 80:1533–1546, 1998.

93. Derbyshire SWG, Jones AKP: Cerebral responses to a continual tonic pain stimulus measured using positron emission tomography. Pain 76:127–135, 1998.

94. Jones AKP, Brown WD, Friston KJ, et al: Cortical and subcortical localization of response to pain in man using positron emission tomography. Proc R Soc Lond B Biol Sci 244:39–44, 1991.

95. Porro CA, Cettolo V, Francescato MP, Baraldi P: Temporal and intensity coding of pain in human cortex. J Neurophysiol 80: 3312–3320, 1998.

96. Silverman DHS, Munakata JA, Ennes H, et al: Regional cerebral activity in normal and pathological perception of visceral pain. Gastroenterology 112:64–72, 1997.

97. Talbot JD, Marrett S, Evans AC, et al: Multiple representations of pain in human cerebral cortex. Science 251:1355–1358, 1991.

98. Treede R-D, Kenshalo DR, Gracely RH, Jones AKP: The cortical representation of pain. Pain 79:105–111, 1999.

99. Vogt BA, Derbyshire S, Jones AK: Pain processing in four regions of human cingulate cortex localized with co-registered PET and MR imaging. Eur J Neurosci 8:1461–1473, 1996.

100. Kenshalo DR, Isensee O: Responses of primate SI cortical neurons to noxious stimuli. J Neurophysiol 50:1479–1496, 1983.

101. Lamour Y, Willer JC, Guilbaud G: Rat somatosensory (SmI) cortex. I. Characteristics of neuronal responses to noxious stimulation and comparison with responses to non-noxious stimulation. Exp Brain Res 49:35–45, 1983.

102. Andersson JL, Lilja A, Hartvig P, et al: Somatotopic organization along the central sulcus, for pain localization in humans, as revealed by positron emission tomography. Exp Brain Res 117: 192–199, 1997.

103. Schnitzler A, Ploner M: Neurophysiology and functional neuro-anatomy of pain perception. J Clin Neurophysiol 17:592–603, 2000.

104. Penfield W, Boldrey E: Somatic motor and sensory representation in cerebral cortex of man as studied by electrical stimulation. Brain 60:389–443, 1937.

105. Penfield W, Jasper H: Epilepsy and the Functional Anatomy of the Human Brain. Boston, Little, Brown & Company, 1954.

106. Sweet WH: Cerebral localization of pain. In Thomson RA, Green JR (eds): New Perspectives in Cerebral Localization. New York, Raven Press, 1982, pp 205–242.

107. Tsubokawa T, Katayama Y, Yamamoto T, et al: Chronic motor cortex stimulation in patients with thalamic pain. J Neurosurg 78:393–401, 1993.

108. Dong WK, Salonen LD, Kawakami Y, et al: Nociceptive responses of trigeminal neurons in SII-7b cortex of awake monkeys. Brain Res 484:314–324, 1989.

109. Augustine JR: Circuitry and functional aspects of the insular lobe in primates including humans. Brain Res Brain Res Rev 22:229–244, 1996.

110. Craig AD, Bushnell MC, Zhang ET, Blomqvist A: A thalamic nucleus specific for pain and temperature sensation. Nature 372:770–773, 1994.

Approach to the Patient with Chronic Pain

JOEL L. SERES

There is a high rate of trial failure and apparent regression of initial benefit from pain-relieving operations and treatments.[1-4] All physicians and especially surgeons are motivated to reduce the suffering that they observe in their patients. Too often, however, treatments that seem at first to be effective fail to provide enough meaningful relief later.[5-9] The meaning of such regression of benefit is difficult for most to comprehend.

As physicians, we sometimes have difficulty integrating the real meaning of the pain behaviors we observe in patients. When we attend a patient with acute pain, the suffering and despair often melt before us when we provide curative care. We extinguish the abdominal pain of appendicitis and its attendant anguish with an operation that we consider relatively simple. We treat the apparent distress of the patient with an acute fracture of the humerus with dispatch. Many patients with acutely extruded lumbar disks, after the operation relives the pain, stop at their place of employment on the way home. However, when we try to treat the apparent fear, anxiety, and suffering observed in a patient with chronic pain, we often fail to achieve long-term benefit.[10, 11] Even when we control the physiologic mechanisms of nociception, we can still fail.[12] The operation works, pain relief is reported, but the patient somehow continues to suffer.

Chronic pain patients speak a language that stimulates the physician to action. When the patient indicates improvement, we feel validated in our efforts. When the patient continues to hurt or regresses after some improvement, we must strive again to respond to the patient's expressions. Sometimes, it is not only the patient's back that hurts but also the heart. Fixing the back does not necessarily help the back problem when the level of improvement does little to reduce the emotional suffering of the patient. A better back is not really of much help if the patient still cannot return to work or enjoy life with friends and family because of residual pain.[13]

We sometimes wonder what the patient really expects from us. There is a built-in expectation that patients are looking for relief of symptoms when they appear before us. That is a part of the story, but what many seem to need is a new way of relating to their world, which has become different because of the effects of injury or the ravages of age.[14-16] Suffering behaviors are the only way most patients know to express their myriad requests to health care providers or others. Some insights are gained when asking patients what they expect from a proposed procedure and what they plan to do with that outcome. Often, patients have expectations that are far more global than the procedure offers. The dichotomy between patient expectations and reality may be an important link in understanding why late failures occur. Patients offer additional insights when their level of enthusiasm for the effects of treatment is less than might be expected considering the improvement that has been provided.[17]

Physicians' expectations are even more variable than those of patients. Physicians often misjudge the extent of a patient's improvement and its meaning. Even more informative are patients who consider themselves to be treatment successes although the surgeons judged them as failures.[18] In approaching the chronic pain patient, surgeons must comprehend the expectations of the patient and of the significant others. Surgeons must also understand their own expectations and what they may mean to the patient.

The surgical concept that pain is a "thing" that we must attack and conquer may be the grist for repeated failures. This idea was expressed in a presentation reviewing the history of pain-relieving surgery: "At some point, the anatomy of pain and the secret to its defeat will be discovered."[19] The psychological issues, including the meaning that the pain has to the patient, are always going to transcend the anatomy of nocioception.[20, 21] The approach to the patient with chronic pain must always include an understanding of these principles.

In this chapter, I review the influence of outcomes on decision making for pain-relieving operations and explore the expectations of the patient, surgeon, and others who are affected by the patient's distress. The variety of medical, surgical, and social limitations of pain surgery is discussed, followed by presentation of a reasoned surgical approach to the patient with chronic pain.

SURGERY AS THE LAST RESORT

The operations done to treat chronic pain are often spoken of as "last resorts."[22] They are something to do when everything else has failed. However, our concepts of "last" seem to evolve. Not too long ago, a fusion for the patient with failed back surgery syndrome was considered a last resort. With the advent of newer technology, such procedures are considered *de rigeur* in the course of care for the patient. The use of a spinal stimulator constituted the last resort for a while, until development of the morphine pump, which acquired the designation. It is likely that, with the availability of an U.S. Food and Drug Administration (FDA)–approved brain electrode, we may see a resurgence of deep brain stimulation for pain relief, which will probably evolve to become the last resort treatment.

Why do last resorts fail so often? Why do failures ultimately occur so often after what initially appear to be successful outcomes? A pattern of remarkable improvement followed by progressive recurrence of pain and suffering seems to typify the patients failed by pain surgery.[23] Perhaps it is this type of past pattern that can teach us more about the likelihood of future success.

Denervation procedures for the facet joints and coagulation of the disk itself[24] cannot be any more effective than total denervation of one side of the motion segment by dorsal root ganglion resection. However, the lessons taught by the failure of that procedure[25] are not even mentioned in reports extolling the short-term benefit of what, for the time, seemed to be something to do for the patient.

Procedures are too often undertaken despite knowing that long-term benefit is unlikely. The expectations and the needs of the surgeon as decision maker seem sometimes to be more important than what is best for the patient. There are those for whom pain-relieving surgery is beneficial, but patients with long-term chronic pain are less common in the scheme of things. Regression of initial benefit is the norm, and late failure is a likely expectation, except in rare patients. Tragically, we have yet to define the patient who will succeed with neurosurgery. We study and report our successes; rarely do we study in detail our failures. However, the legacy of Cushing[26] and others of his generation was predicated on understanding the fail-

ures and complications far better than their successes. In the case of the patient with chronic pain, it often appears that we have lost our way.

Understanding the reasons for a negative outcome is important. In their classic tome, *Pain and the Neurosurgeon*, White and Sweet[27] make this clear. "We have made every effort to record the bad as well as the good results of our endeavors, keeping in mind the recent addition by Penfield, Lende, and Rasmussen (1961) to the Hippocratic oath: 'I will faithfully record and analyze my failures in the care of the sick, seeking the cause so that those who follow may be warned of danger.'"[27]

Our excitement for new and more technical approaches has jaded perceptions about our roles and the effects that our treatments produce. Sometimes, even when we clearly discern that a treatment has no prolonged efficacy in treating chronic pain, we extol its use as "satisfying."[28]

Chronic pain is defined as a biopsychosocial phenomenon. In functional terms, this means that, although the psychological and the social aspects are often the result of the biologic part,[29] eliminating the biologic part does not necessarily improve the other aspects. It is as though, after the psychosocial wheel is spinning, it does not need the biologic aspect to keep it moving. The surgical approach to the chronic pain patient therefore must include the essence of the patient's existence as she or he sees it, and improvement must be couched in terms that have meaning to the patient. This may not be something that a surgeon enamored by the latest operation wants to comprehend or to act on.[30]

OUTCOME EXPECTATIONS

Outcomes and our expectation of them temper our judgment as we approach the patient with chronic pain. However, factors that influence outcome are variable, and they change as time passes.[31] Sometimes, we emphasize positive conclusions that are not always borne out by the data. For example, in one study of 83 originally selected patients, only 4 indicated a satisfactory level of pain reduction about 12 months after treatment. With only about 49% of patients demonstrating a 1-cm analog scale reduction in pain, a reasonable conclusion might be that further research into patient selection and outcomes enhancement was needed. However, reading the study's conclusions might give an exaggerated view of the treatment's efficacy.[22]

Because we try to justify what we do, we sometimes may lose sight of the realities. Humility and objectivity are more appropriately based on the negative aspects of our results than on our efforts to justify a procedure. We often learn more by studying our failures than by concentrating on our successes.[27] When we document no meaningful outcome, we may have trouble saying that in our conclusions.[24, 32] The meaning of such conclusions becomes poignant when later we quote only the positive aspects of our interpretation to a patient suffering chronic pain who is desperate for assistance.

Offering a 50% reduction in pain to a patient may not be fair when the data suggest that this level of improvement offers little in terms of pain tolerance and return to work for most patients.[33] It also may not be the most common of results.

Even appropriately reported outcomes sometimes take on an importance that transcends the meaning of the outcome to the patient. A surgeon may be pleased by the patient who admits to 50% pain reduction as the outcome of an operation. However, the very fact that such an outcome level had been discussed beforehand might color the statements of the patient who in some way wants to thank the surgeon for trying to help.

Other questions need to be resolved. How does a patient interpret his or her pain? How is the pain measured and when? Patients do not remember pain well. Knowing that the preoperative pain level was designated as 9/10 might color the patient's answer postoperatively differently from knowing that the level was 6/10.

Outcome Expectations of the Physician

Besides the surgeon, the expectations of the referring physician deserve review. Patients are referred because they have reached the limits of the physician to provide help. The expectations are for the surgeon to "fix" the problem. Although this is possible in many situations, it often fails in chronic pain patients. However, there is rarely a preoperative fail-safe program in place to provide care afterward. Too often, we do procedures and then wait to see how the patient does before we respond, although with the number of failures that we see, it is always appropriate to consider what to do with any outcome, positive or negative, before the patient enters the surgical therapeutic arena. Are we ignoring our failures to the patient? More importantly, are we ignoring our failures to ourselves?

The surgical consultant must ask several questions. What will happen to this patient if my proposed treatment does not work? Who will take over the care of the patient at that point—the referring physician who did not know what else to do and had referred the patient? What will the consultant's role be then? If the surgeon judges the outcome successful, but the patient or the referring physician does not, how should the surgeon act? How should the surgeon educate referring physicians about the their role in patient selection and outcomes management?[34]

Outcome Expectations of the Patient and Family

Patients sadly often do not understand much of what we tell them. They conceptualize medical jargon in a variety of remarkable ways. It should be part of any preoperative interview to ask the patient to describe what is causing the suffering and pain, to describe what was done previously, and to explain why the treatments did not work. Done regularly, this approach elicits remarkable misconceptions. "My disks are gone,

and the bones are rubbing raw on each other." "They had to remove my vertebra—that's why I'm getting shorter." "My body is disintegrating from arthritis." "The doctor said I'll never work again." "I have fibromyalgia, and the doctor told me it's incurable." Patients often interpret what they have been told in terms that may justify their goals. If patients are interested in compensation or retirement rather than returning to work, they will understand the situation in a way that justifies being unable to work again. Motive plays an important role in outcome expectation and in planning treatment.[35–37]

Patients who present to the surgeon for relief may indicate that return to work is their goal. However, for a variety of reasons, such a goal may be too difficult for the patient to achieve. That does not mean that return to work is impossible; it does indicate that a reasonable outcome may not be enough for the patient. The negative aspects of the outcome then become more important to the patient in justifying an inability to return to work. Whatever success there might have been dissipates with the amplified importance of an unachievable goal. The success of the treatment therefore may have a variety of different meanings to the patient and to the physician. An appropriate approach to the patient with chronic pain is to define the goals before treatment starts.

The patient's family is under severe stress in contemplating another surgical odyssey. The surgeon may discuss with them that waiting for the surgical outcome may be harder for them than it is for the patient. This empathy often results in a remarkable sharing of concerns and fears, and such emotions can have a major impact on the meaning of outcomes for the patient.

It is important to review the responses of the family members to prior attempts at care. How did they feel when the patient had had a few months of progressive improvement? Was there a different response after regression of benefit? Is there any difference now? These are the important issues that speak to motivation and support. The usual psychological preoperative screening before pain surgery should include such matters.

When patients who have passed our selection criteria for treatment do not do well, it indicts the selection technique. Psychological screening does not adequately predict outcomes with pump and stimulator trials or insertions.[38–41] This means that we are not asking the proper questions. Would a more reasonable selection process mean fewer procedures? The outcomes data suggest that this should be the case.

Outcome Expectations of Third-Party Payer

Outcomes management and expectations have important roles in medical care costs.[42] The addition of another procedure that fails to reduce medical care contacts, costs, and consideration for further surgery is not viewed in a positive way by those who must pay for them.[43, 44] In many of our reviews, the issue of return to work is often missing or is treated shab-

TABLE 182–1 ■ **Major Compensation and Liability Systems in the United States**

Worker's Compensation. Each state, territory, and the District of Columbia has a no-fault system that covers injured workers. Scheduled disabilities vary considerably. Unscheduled disabilities take into consideration psychosocial and physical issues.

Federal Employees Compensation Act (FECA). This is similar to state systems, but it is only for employees of the federal government. The payments for disabilities are considerably larger than those provided by the state systems.

Federal Employers Liability Act (FELA). This a liability, not a compensation, system. It includes railroad workers. Unlike the state systems, each case is a potential federal court proceeding in front of a jury.

Supplemental Security Income (SSI). This federal system is designed to support people who, because of impairments, have not worked long enough to qualify for Social Security benefits. This system is administered by the Social Security Administration, but the funds come from the general U.S. treasury.

Social Security Disability Insurance (SSDI). This part of Social Security provides benefits for those who are unable to work anywhere in the U.S. economy because of physical, educational, or experiential impairments.

Social Security (SS). Social Security benefits may be obtained before 65 years of age based on a grid system of experience and impairments.

bily.[45, 46] This does not excite support from compensation systems, whose basic responsibility is to return the worker to employment.

Physicians often do not understand the differences that exist between the variety of compensation and liability systems under which their patients work. They are briefly reviewed in Table 182–1. How reports are expressed can mean different things in different systems of compensation. It is important to recognize these differences and how they may affect the patients and their compensation and disability ratings.

Third-party payers have increasingly adopted an adversarial position. Difficulties abound in obtaining authorization for treatment, getting timely payment for services, and squandering time tracing through a maze of communication systems. It may be best to consider the ways these companies work and the means we have to aid their efforts. After all, it is often the patient who is in the middle of disagreements between payers and physicians. It is possible to approach this problem without involving the patient by presenting some of the data that supports our treatments.[47, 48]

Outcome Expectations of Peers

The expectations of peers constitute an area that is not often explored. For a variety of reasons, some surgeons have a hard time saying that no further treatment is likely to be effective. They may feel pressured to do something for the patient in an effort to justify the referral. There is an expectation that a specialist knows best what should be done for the patient, and a referral may imply that something surgical will be done. If the surgeon offers nothing, she or he may be concerned about how the referring physician interprets this.

Many surgeons have skills and abilities that others in the specialty do not have. How easy is it for a surgeon to acknowledge this among peers in the community? How easy is it for the surgeon to refer patients who were referred to him or her to those others?

It is never wrong to offer no treatment unless it can be effective. Another failing experience can be even more harmful to the patient than doing nothing for the pain. It is never wrong to suggest referral to someone else who is more skilled, more experienced, or more interested in the patient's presenting predicament. Referral elsewhere should be considered part of treatment planning. No surgeon has the answer for every patient.

The difficulty in appearing less adequate before peers may keep surgeons performing treatments that sometimes do little for the patient.[49–51] As part of the approach to the chronic pain patient, the surgeon should consider what to say if the proposed treatment fails to provide benefit and reconsider whether the treatment is being prescribed because of feeling compelled to do something. If these pressures influence the decision, where do the patient's needs fit in?

REGRESSION OF BENEFIT

Outcomes expectations are often validated in the immediate post-treatment period. A variety of treatments can effectively improve the patient with chronic pain. Many patients do surprisingly well with alternative medical care. A characteristic of the patient with chronic pain is the regression of benefit that often follows initial benefit. The meaning of regression is often different for the patient, the surgeon, and the primary physician. It is important to understand the language of regression to avoid repetitions of past failures and to prevent imparting false hope.

Regression of Benefit with Laminectomy

The benefit of lumbar or cervical disk excision in the properly selected patient is well known.[52, 53] However, most of us do not truly understand the meaning of regression of benefits. Many patients do well after disk excision and seemingly never seek medical care for backache again. Others do well only for a time. Redevelopment of symptoms may have anatomic causes that require further treatment, including surgery.[54–56] Often, however, we find only scarring on imaging studies; vague, nonlocalized neurological symptoms and signs; and little to explain recurrence of the patient's problem.[57] It is important to approach carefully patients whose histories document regression, because there may be issues other than those of anatomic pathology that explain the truncation of benefit.[58]

Regression of Benefit with Behavioral Programs

Behavioral programs can give us remarkable insights into the causes and management of regression.[59] In managing chronic pain patients, the behavioral approach has documented that significant improvement in function, sense of well-being, cessation of narcotic analgesic use, and return to work could occur without making changes in the anatomic causes of the patient's distress.[60] Studies demonstrate that pain behaviors stop as long as the patient is appropriately supervised and motivated. Continued courses of wellness without recurrence of difficulties have been identified in a substantial group of patients treated with behavioral means alone. Similar to surgical patients, regression of benefit was also found in many. The emotional responses to improvement and to regression of benefit are also similar to those that are observed in failed surgical patients.

It is possible to conclude that it was not so much the anatomic (nociceptive) cause of pain that determined the patient's reaction. In the behavioral treatment situation and in the surgical situation, improvement occurs. The reasons for the improvement may be as much functional as anything else in both situations. Regression can be paired in both situations with motivational issues, incentives, and personal needs.[61] Chronic pain is the result of psychosocial issues that must first be controlled if long-term benefit is to be achieved,[62] and the method of treatment may matter little. Initial improvement followed by regression of benefit seems to occur no matter what we do to the chronic pain patient. We must therefore not extol our results until long after the initial blush of success. The approach to the chronic pain patient should be tempered by understanding this concept.

Regression of Benefit with Spinal Stimulation

Reports of the long-term effects of procedures for chronic pain relief are often tainted by surgeons' needs to maximize outcomes.[12] Although there has never been any real correlation between a 50% pain reduction and functional restoration, surgeons seem to accept the idea that good pain relief is about half.[33] Return to work is often judged to be an inappropriately harsh outcome measure, but that may be the goal of the patient contemplating neurological augmentative therapy. A reduction of pain enough to satisfy the surgeon's outcome criteria may not suffice for the patient.

Relief is obtained by many patients who undergo spinal stimulation, but it is unfair to suggest to each surgical candidate that most patients achieve enough relief to return to work. It is important to understand the patient's goals and their meanings, and this part of the preoperative psychological assessment is not given enough consideration in many situations.

Regression of Benefit with Morphine Pumps

Implanted drug delivery systems brought an initial wave of enthusiasm because they were technically simple to insert and theoretically should be able to handle any level of pain from any possible source in the spine and other areas. Enthusiastic reports documented ade-

quate pain relief in as many as 95% of patients.[63] However, only about 80% of patients reported improvements in daily activities. Although this is a small difference, it speaks to the disharmony between expressed pain relief and the impact of that relief. Even more dramatic evidence for this disparity was documented by the data showing that only 29 of the 427 patients returned to work.[63]

Issues other than pain cause patients not to work. With morphine pumps, as with other treatment approaches for the chronic pain, there is often initial success followed by accelerating doses and ultimate failure in many patients.[64] The lesson here is substantial. When all the morphine receptors of the spinal system are bathed in morphine, the continued suffering and complaints of some patients are not generated by nociceptive phenomena. This issue is further complicated by tolerance to analgesics. The intensive preoperative screening used further documents the nonbiologic aspects of chronic pain. Based on outcomes, it should be clear that we are not asking the right questions in selecting many patients for neuro-augmentative procedures.[39, 65]

Regression of Benefit with Any Form of Rehabilitation

Mental illness treatment; rehabilitation for substance abuse, alcoholism, or compulsive gambling; and therapies for a variety of other conditions have significant regression of benefit after rehabilitation. In each area studied, it appears that motivation, support, reinforcement, environmental factors, reward structure, and personal issues are implicated. This is also true for the patient with chronic pain. The appropriate approach to the chronic pain patient must be more than labeling the problem as biopsychosocial in its extent. We must understand and act on all aspects of the patient's predicament to maximize outcome. Labeling the patient, having them "cleared" by a psychologist as having no contraindications, and then dealing only with the biologic aspects with an operation that blocks the pain are not enough for a substantial population of sufferers. The failures in rehabilitation that are based on issues not directly related to the patient's impairment document the need for a more global approach to the patient.

Patients' fear and anxiety, as well as a variety of other possible psychological and thought processes, can influence pain perception.[66] Studies that document such relationships help to explain what surgeons observe clinically. The approach to the patient must include a mechanism to deal with these important findings.

UNDERSTANDING SURGICAL LIMITATIONS

Surgeons often view intervention as the ultimate fix. Although surgery often is remarkably effective, it does not follow that it is always worth a try to see if it works. In many patients who become chronic sufferers, such logic typified their first surgical adventure. Surgeons often see this when reviewing the records of many chronic patients, finding statements such as "the patient failed to respond to conservative management" when there are no other indications for the disk operation that was done.

We have become enamored with finding the "pain generator."[54] Reproducing the pain by diskography[67] or blocking the pain with a variety of injections continues to focus our attention on the biologic aspects of the patient. When we find such a spot, we tend to ignore the rest of the story. Initial success and short-term follow-up create a sense of security and belief that we can deal with the physical and ignore the psychosocial issues.[68, 69] However, even major denervation procedures that fail to document any long-term effects[25] do not dim our enthusiasm for finding the anatomic cause for the pain and eliminating it.

Limitations Intrinsic to the Disorder

A variety of factors related to the nature of the patient's condition influence the efficacy of treatments. There is abundant evidence that a multiplicity of factors cause chronic low back pain. It is unusual for degenerative changes to occur only at one level. Degenerative disk disease progresses to involve most of the vertebrae. Often, it is silent.[70] Sometimes, it may be associated with persistent symptoms that defy the efforts of the most aggressive surgeon.[13] Patients with solid fusions still hurt. Neurolysis works only some of the time and then usually not for long.[71] The multiple areas involved in the pain production make a focused surgical approach impossible in many patients.[72] Low back pain in the industrialized world is a major economic issue.[73]

People doing heavy physical labor generally do not reach their expected age of retirement.[74] Most societies accept medical disorders as an inevitable result of strenuous jobs. The worker is forced to ask for medical help to reverse the effects of their predicament. Physicians feel obliged to treat the condition. The facts given at the outset—that the worker will never return to her or his former occupation—are too often ignored. The medicalization of the need to step down from physically demanding work often worsens the situation.[75] Inappropriate therapeutic goals are often doomed before treatment starts. The limitations intrinsic to the medical disorder are ignored, as is the futility of some treatments. We then report our successes and explain away our failures by concluding that "better patient selection is needed."[76]

Limitations Imposed by the Patient

Much can be learned about patients and their motivation by asking them to comply with measurable therapeutic activities. Some patients, although expressing a desire for improvement, may have no plans after improvement occurs. It is reasonable to ask chronic pain patients to participate in exercises, discussions about future planning, and keeping a variety of diaries.

The office staff can implement and monitor most of these relatively simple activities, and participation can provide clues regarding the patient's motivation.[76, 77]

In some families, improvement may be interpreted negatively. Control issues can change when the patient improves and becomes less dependent. In some cases, independent functioning may be viewed as a threat to the integrity of the relationship. Sometimes, when there are adverse issues about the work environment, the patient may ask for help but tend to minimize any benefit, thereby avoiding the issues regarding return to work.[78–80]

Limitations Related to the Procedure

There is an inherent failure rate for every operation. As surgeons, we often tend to ignore this while looking for something to do for the patient. During a PAR, we do not often present the patient with factual statistics regarding the rate or meaning of success. Likewise, we do not present data regarding the meaning of failures. Patients tend to hear what they want to believe in, and sometimes, presenting all the objective data may confuse the patient enough so that he or she may not want the procedure done. We often do not follow our own reasonable indications for procedures[81] or consider carefully how comments are directed to the patient. Is the point to talk the patient who needs help into the procedure, or are the factual limits of the procedure being presented? Is 50% pain relief adequate for the patient? Is it adequate for this patient with this condition?

There has been a resurgence of interest in a variety of thermocoagulation procedures for treating spinal pain problems.[82, 83] Radiofrequency coagulation of nerves, facet capsules, disks, and nerve roots produces seemingly miraculous results in some patients. However, documentation of meaningful long-term benefit is lacking. If the procedure can answer the needs of the patient well enough and provide for long-term effect, it may be considered worthwhile, but too often, such procedures are offered as curative in themselves along with the idea that they can be repeated as needed. This situation is not much different from the repeated disk surgeries and fusions of past decades.[84]

Lumbar fusion can relieve pain in a group of patients, but there is no good evidence that the solidity of the fusion is directly related to outcome.[84] With the advent of newer technology promising a higher rate of solid fusions, we may be destined to repeat the mistakes of the past. Does a solid fusion make a difference to the chronic pain patient when returning to work is the patient's goal?

Corticosteroid injections, nerve root sleeve injections, and adhesiolysis all promise benefit but lack meaningful long-term outcome data and increased return to work potential for the patient.[33, 85–87] It is important to understand what patients are really asking for when they seek pain treatment. The approach must always be synchronous with the well-being that patients define for themselves.

WHEN IS SURGERY THE LAST RESORT?

Surgery is often performed when everything else has failed to offer enough benefit to the patient. Surgery for pain works best when it is specific to the source of the pain and the patient's reaction to it.[88, 89] The patient's reaction to any residual pain may in the long run be more important than what happens at the nociceptive level. I think that one of the functions of the surgeon is to define when the last resort is really the last one.[90]

Understanding Limitations

Limitations come from many sources, and all may impact our view of what constitutes the last resort. We often can deal more easily with the limitations of the operation than with those from a variety of other sources, including personal limits set by the patient to improve, limits set by the patient's environment to improve, limits set by the workplace for the patient to improve, and limits set by the patient's pathology to improve.

Too often, we grasp at the likelihood for a procedure to work without contemplating what else is going on. The patient's vocational and personal life might have passed the possibility for improvement with our surgical last resort to fix the pain problem. The predicament of the patient must be carefully considered before we use our last resort approach. If what we do does not solve the problems that transcend the patient's pain, the treatment is likely to fail. These limitations must be understood before the next approach. If the limits that truncated success in the past still exist, they will limit the efficacy of any proposed new approach or treatment.[91–93]

Learning to Accept Failure

One of the most difficult aspects of care for most surgeons is to accept failure. Acceptance means understanding failure and its meaning. In an effort to avoid responsibility for failures, we have evolved a set of acceptable outcomes that often have very little real meaning for the patient. The 50% pain reduction discussed previously is one example. Even when a procedure produces no improvement for any patient according the most minimal of our criteria, we invoke something as nebulous as "proper patient selection" rather than admit that the procedure does not work. Because of this denial, we see subsequent generations of neurosurgeons trying again with their nuances of patient selection. Personal experience of failure is often difficult to find in the literature, and this makes repeated attempts more acceptable. For example, the early enthusiasm for facet denervation was met with no long-term improvement, but there has been a renewal of interest in the procedure by younger surgeons. Cordotomy for low back pain is a classic example. The earlier failures of open cordotomy were

thought to be avoided with the advent of percutaneous procedures. We had to learn again that cordotomy performed in any manner is not likely to provide long-term benefit for chronic low back disorders.

There is nothing ignoble about failures. They probably teach us much more about who we really are and about the results of what we do than do our successes. However, the literature stresses the success rate. If this is so, how do we learn to make our failures an important part of our progressive education?

Although the suggestion I make is not easy to embrace, it is worthy of daily consideration in approaching a patient with chronic pain. One way to accept failure is to look for it in everything we do. Even in the face of apparent success, there is always an element that borders on failure. The aneurysm was successfully clipped, but there might be a slight change in the patient's cognitive powers if we look for it. The disk removal resulted in complete pain relief, but the patient might have some weakness of the back. The intradiskal procedure resulted in immediate pain relief, but the prognosis for recurrent pain is guarded. If we can contemplate the realities of issues of failure on a regular basis, we can desensitize to them. They become part of our lexicon. They become constant companions and not enemies, and they keep us humble about the appropriate application of our work.

Probably the best advice to a young surgeon is to never avoid the importance of failures, because a physician learns the most from them. Those who ignore their failures document the weaknesses of their personalities. Those who deny the existence of their failures cannot present an unbiased and honest list of options for the patient. The surgeon's best approach to patients with chronic pain may be to contemplate what to do if the treatment being offered does not relieve the suffering enough to make a difference. I believe that, if a surgeon cannot do this, he or she owes the patient the option of having others choose who that surgeon's patients will be.

Whose Responsibility is the Patient Now?

One way of looking at the meaning failure has for the surgeon is to observe how she or he deals with the failed patient. Patients who have failed to improve despite our best efforts are the most powerful responsibility we face. For some, the burden is so profound that the only tool available is for the surgeon to escape from the relationship by having the patient seen only by associates, by ignoring calls, or by spending as little time as possible with the patient. Sometimes, anger about failure becomes displaced toward the patient. People who have failed to benefit adequately quickly get the idea that the surgeon is no longer interested in their problem and stop going to the physician.

Surgeons sometimes offer additional treatments and interventions and then ask the patient make the choice. These offerings often have as little likelihood of benefit as those tried before. The patient may have reached the point at which only palliative care, narcotics, and behavioral pain control methods are appropriate, but for some of us, it is difficult to define such an end point in our efforts "to do something." It is not appropriate to do something else only because all previous efforts have failed. Interventions require consideration of appropriate patient selection and proof of efficacy before they are offered to the desperate, suffering pain patient.

Some of us can appropriately refer the patient to others who can help in what rehabilitation may be possible. Even then, the responsibility of the surgeon does not end. It is reasonable to follow such patients for several reasons. The information provided by others help to refine the decision-making skills of the surgeon. Other physicians may help the patient enough so that the patient can share some aspects of care with the surgeon, adding to her or his knowledge. Surgeons act honestly when they are willing to ask for the help of those more expert in certain aspects of the patient's care, and this adds to the humility that all must feel when patients have failed to thrive because of or in spite of what was done.[93, 94]

Implications for the Role of the Surgeon

The surgeon performing pain-relieving operations, as in most other situations, is the final arbiter of what is being offered to the patient. Surgeons commonly present a variety of treatment options and permit the patient to participate in making the decision. However, when asked to review a surgical decision, it has become clear that even well-educated patients are often naive about what is being suggested to them. When operations have failed to improve their conditions, patients have reported that they could not understand why the surgeon had undertaken the procedure even though the patients had indicated that they were improving spontaneously. Patients should be asked to repeat what was said at the last setting to ensure comprehension. It is important to educate the patient about treatment options, and the surgeon must be sure that the patient understands what is being done and for what reason.

In a long career in pain medicine, I have seen patients with a variety of misconceptions about their problems. One, who had a master's degree, was convinced that three of his lower vertebrae had been removed because of uncomplicated back pain. The operation had been a decompression of a purported stenotic lumbar canal although no symptoms or definite magnetic resonance imaging findings of spinal stenosis existed. A second patient, whose preoperative narcotics use was one or two hydrocodone pills weekly, had a morphine pump installed. Another patient had a spinal stimulator installed after the third operation, a fusion, had failed to relieve the pain. The patient had never been taught appropriate postural mechanics or exercises and marveled later at their effect.

Because the surgeon's pronouncements carry power, it is important to understand the patient completely. This includes the needs as seen by the patient that extend beyond pain relief. It includes what the patient plans to do with the relief offered. It most certainly includes what the surgeon plans to do with the successful or the failed patient. Holding out hope to a patient suffering great pain carries with it an awesome responsibility. In the surgical management of chronic pain, it is not appropriate to have an attitude of "let's wait and see how well you do after the operation." We know too much about outcomes, regression of benefit, and the meaning of success or failure to permit such a passive attitude.

It is important to understand what the past has taught. Although we continue to invent more technical procedures to treat pain, we must recognize the knowledge on which they are based. Despite a higher rate of back fusions, we still produce a coterie of pain-relief failures that belie the success rates found in the literature.[13] Despite significant pain relief from drug-delivery systems and stimulation, many patients continue to take oral narcotics, and few return to measurable work.[95] Although a new procedure suggests that new data should be collected, the already accumulated data must be considered as well. There is no objective literature that documents good long-term effects from facet denervation, epidural steroid injections, many intradiskal procedures, and sensory denervation at the dorsal root level. The implications of these facts must influence how we present possible treatments to the patient. Patients are often looking for the long-term "fix." It is important that we understand how they interpret what we say to them and consider how often we tell patients that more surgery is not the answer for their predicaments.

EXPECTATIONS AND NEEDS

Surgeons' Needs

Although the major thrust of this part of the discussion concerns the patient, it is necessary to first consider the needs of the surgeon. The social and economic pressures on the modern surgeon are greater and more malevolent than ever before. Consider the history of modern surgery and the deportment of the surgeon in each of its epochs. Modern surgical approaches are little more than 100 years old. Great pressures existed in the time of surgeons such as Cushing, Dandy, Sachs, or Peet, and their trainees faced many stresses. Surgeons of the next generation were the teachers of most of us now practicing. This generation of surgeons faces decreases in patient volume, income, and prestige that typify the managed-care environment. Surgical judgment and techniques of the past have changed to meet the needs of the modern surgical office.[96, 97]

For some surgeons, these pressures have created attitudes that would never have been accepted in the past. One surgical colleague suggested that, if the condition were not a surgical one, the patient would not have been referred. Others have stated that they offer all the treatments that can be done and tell the patient to decide. Most patients, however, are not educated well enough to participate intelligently.

Patients' Needs

People are complex, and they bring to the pain surgery theater an infinite array of presentations and needs.

Although there exists the commonality of pain relief, the true extent of their wants may be occult. It is not enough to assume we understand the desires of our patients just because they present suffering to our view. We must understand them as they see themselves. Their needs must become our goals of treatment. We cannot be as effective as we must unless we understand them.

We exist at an interesting time in the history of employment, when it has become acceptable for many that working until age 65 is not the norm. People do not last that long doing heavy physical work, truck driving, or millwork. They stop doing that type of work long before the end of their expected working years. Some go into lighter jobs, and others use their accrued knowledge to ease the physical aspects of their job. For many, however, disability remains the only acceptable and financially secure course.[98, 99] Because of factors dealing with social acceptability and expectations, the patient whose working years have ended commonly speaks in the language of recovery and restoration. This is the language that spurs the surgeon to action. For some time, someone else takes over the predicament for the patient, and expectations often abound that surpass any reasonable outcome; ultimate regression and failure are more likely than true recovery. Patients in chronic pain are so varied that treatment cannot become standard for all,[100, 101] and surgeons must consider this in the approach to the chronic pain patient.

Work History and Expectations

There are many incentives and pressures regarding work issues.[102] Work incentives are based on job satisfaction and on financial and societal issues.[103] The ubiquity of low back pain makes for an interesting study. The differences between those who suffer low back pain and those who make back injury claims are mostly psychological or psychosocial and not physical in nature.[104] Only certain types of physical work actually play a role in work disability resulting from low back pain. These workers are brick-layers and those who drive cable cars in San Francisco.[105, 106] There appears to be no bearing between these facts and the presence of disk degeneration due to work.[107–109] The person's relationship to the workplace and to the immediate supervisors better predicts claim making than the degree of physical impairment or pain.[73] The length of time out of work correlates with permanent disability, which also depends on the attitudes of those with whom the injured person works.[110]

Many workplaces require complete resolution of impairment before consideration of return to work. Despite the plethora of insightful employers who have developed alternative job options, there are many who remain firm in requiring a level of restoration not possible in most patients. Patients quickly realize that their working years are limited and that there are appropriate supports if they play the game of "disabled" well enough.[110] Some patients seem to work through courses of medical care toward total disability status

as other people work through courses of education toward college degrees. The goal is often visible at the outset, and it remains only for enough "courses" to be passed to achieve the goal.[110]

These observations may be viewed pejoratively, but that is not the purpose for their inclusion in a discussion of approaches to the chronic pain patient. In many ways, surgeons inadvertently encourage such a passage by suggesting that there is still something else to do. For some patients, the decision is confounded by the underlying thought that perhaps something does exist that could make the situation all better and by the implied pressure to undergo everything the doctor suggests. Some surgeons ignore this predicament of the patient; others seemingly exploit it.[13]

The Role of Psychology

Because of the extensive psychosocial aspects of the chronic pain syndrome, psychological clearance has become the norm before pain-relieving surgery. Studies have failed, however, to document that such screening is effective in improving outcomes.[111] A reasonable conclusion is that psychological evaluation is not effective in predicting outcomes and therefore may be abolished or curtailed. Although such a response may be based on a degree of logic, it begs the issue in this case.

Psychologists can be quite effective in predicting the outcomes of patients contemplating a variety of operations.[112] It is important, however, that the psychologist be given the tools for a proper determination. It is blatantly inappropriate to ask a psychologist to run a battery of tests and interviews to see whether there are psychological contraindications for an already promised procedure. Merely telling a patient in need that a treatment exists is enough to pressure the psychologist to look for only the grossest of psychological contraindications. This type of screening does not require the services of a psychologist. Most of us are adept enough in determining whether a patient is psychologically inept enough for us to not offer an operation.

The problem with the current method of psychological assessment is related to the question we ask of the psychologist and on which the psychologist's income is based. The operational question instead should be what the psychologist considers the patient's prognosis will be if the proposed procedure is done. This question loses its effectiveness if the procedure has already been discussed with the patient. In some circumstances, the patient may have already seen a video extolling the positive outcomes of the procedure without the appropriate balance of information on poor outcomes before the psychologist sees the patient.

For psychologists to become effective in decision making, they must be involved at the outset, before patients have developed biases. Surgeons should ask a psychologist only for her or his straightforward prognosis. Psychologists' decisions, just as ours, must be validated by the outcome. A poor outcome invalidates the preoperative decision; a good outcome validates it. From these examples, we learn how to become more reasonably selective and effective in approaching the chronic pain patient.

Identified psychological issues should not serve as excuses for our failures.[112-114] If we impugn psychological or psychosocial issues to explain our failures, we must accept that we had not understood their meaning beforehand. We might have missed their presence entirely before the operation in our enthusiasm to do something for the patient. Each time we identify psychosocial influences as important explanations for our failed attempts, we must acknowledge that they existed beforehand and should have provided more influence on our decisions. By ignoring these issues in our preoperative decisions, we sometimes permit ourselves an acceptable "out" when treatment fails to fulfill its promise.[115, 116] The psychological motivational and security needs of the patient are probably stronger predictors of long-term success than anything we do to modulate the effects of nociceptive input.

Satisfying Needs

Patients who complete behavioral pain management programs are often grateful to the point of tears when they finish. However, as with pain-relieving operations, there is a significant regression of benefit for many patients. An important part of maintaining appropriate perspective is teaching the staff of such programs how to respond to the patients' initial accolades. Initial praise has shallow meaning if regression occurs rapidly. Alternatively, the staff members can obtain their gratification in two different and special ways. The first is to tell patients who express their gratitude at the completion of care that a good result can only be acknowledged after a year has passed. Because of the frequency of regressed benefit, a short-term demonstration of efficacy means little. The second technique is for the staff to observe how each one of them works with these sometimes difficult patients. Regular, even scheduled peer encouragement and judgment of work quality can provide the validation needed by all professionals. In this way, the gratification that the staff achieves is based on the quality of work as judged by peers and by the patient doing well long enough after treatment to make a difference.

We must all find satisfaction in the work that we do, but that satisfaction must be borne on the real effects of what we do and our responsibility to the patient. Our neurosurgical tradition was based on this philosophy.[117] We must not lose sight of its importance as we become more technical in our endeavors. Each patient must be approached with a sense of responsibility, caring, and honest appraisal of what is accomplished.

A REASONED APPROACH TO PATIENTS WITH CHRONIC PAIN

Patients who present for pain-relieving operations represent the failure of prior treatments. In a very real sense, medicine has failed the patient. Any new attempts must carry a reasonable chance for success, or they do not belong in the patient's life. Dashing patients' hopes with another failure is not in their best interest and only amplifies their depressed state.[118] The approach to the chronic pain patient is different from approaching a patient who has an acute problem with a simple solution. The approach to the chronic sufferer goes beyond a short history, physical examination, and PAR.

Algorithms

Algorithms provide us with an approach to patients that can improve our comprehension of issues that influence outcome.[119] Algorithms can be simple or complex. The important point is that they must be used. They should be designed to provide stops along the way for consideration of alternative treatments. They must be regularly modified on the basis of results. Several already exist.[120, 121] However, it is best for surgeons to develop their own approaches. A good starting point is the algorithm presented in Figure 182–1. Surgeons can add their own approaches and experiences to this algorithm, which should be revised at least yearly.

A series of *red flags* should be set at each step.[122] It is not necessary to react to each of them, but it is important to acknowledge their presence and decide whether they are important to the decision. Examples of red flags may be found in Table 182–2. Surgeons should think about the problems they have had with former patients. Are there red flags from those cases that should be added to the list of things to look for? By creating a personal list, the surgeon progresses through a process that increases awareness of problems.

Many red flags are related to the personality of the patient and the style of relationship the patient develops with the treating team. Other red flags are related to the surgeon's personality and reactions to issues about patient compliance, improvement, or regression.

T A B L E   1 8 2 – 2 ■ **Possible Red Flags**

1. Patient's significant other calls the office for appointments or answers for the patient.
2. Patient has given no consideration to vocational issues.
3. History of remarkable improvement after prior treatments (e.g., operations, physical therapy, behavioral programs) followed by remarkable regression of benefit
4. General physical deconditioning
5. Depression that has pervaded patient's history of pain
6. Patient indicates that even a 50% reduction in pain would suffice.
7. Patient develops special relationships with the physician's staff.
8. Patient resists compliance-measuring activities, such as keeping records of activities, drug use, pain level, or vocational goals, and compliance with exercises or general physical conditioning.
9. Patient's repetition of the discussion at an earlier meeting is significantly distorted.
10. Patient does not comprehend what was done in prior operations when asked.

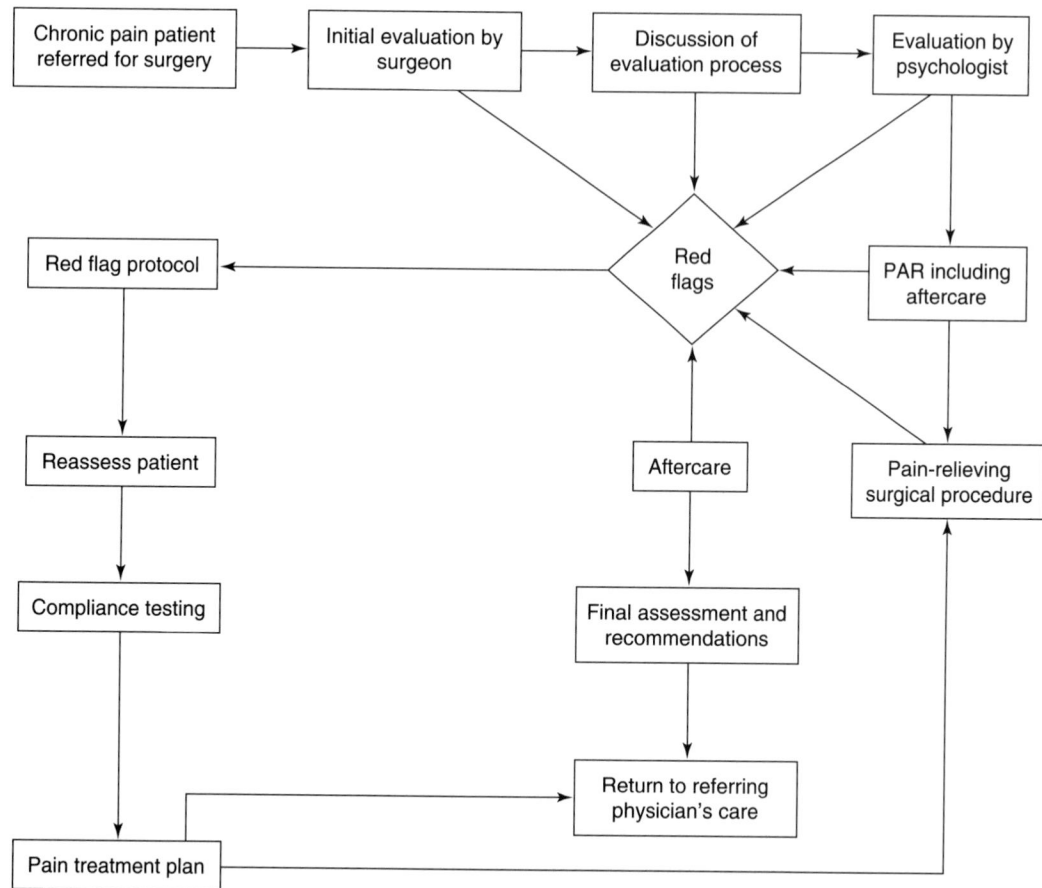

FIGURE 182–1. Algorithm for the patient with chronic pain who is referred for surgery. It stresses the importance of "red flags." These warnings may be as simple as a lack of comprehension by the patient or as complex as expectations that transcend the effects of any operation. Awareness of their presence at each and every stage of patient evaluation and treatment is important. Detection of each red flag requires a break in the protocol that leads to treatment and requires further evaluation, definition, and consultation before proceeding. Ignoring such red flags during preoperative planning is probably a major reason for poor results and for the regression of apparent initial benefit.

Some red flags are related to the way the surgeon runs the medical office and interacts with the personalities of the staff. For example, a red flag may be associated with the special relationships a staff member develops with some patients. Although some such liaisons may be productive, others are not. Identifying them as concerns helps the surgeon to recognize and analyze them, reducing their effects. The staff can help with the development of the surgeon's algorithm and list of red flags. The algorithm for treating chronic pain patients and the red flags should be reviewed at predetermined intervals for best effect.

The surgeon must decide what to do when she or he or a staff member identifies red flags. A protocol is necessary. It may be as simple as a discussion with the staff about identified issues. It may involve new, measurable compliance chores for the patient. It may suggest the need for a conference with all participants in the patient's care and a presentation of concerns to the patient.

Prognosis versus Goals

For many people suffering chronic pain, there is a dichotomy between the reality of the prognosis and their inferred or expressed goals.[2, 123] Surgeons often see people who express a desire to return to work. That goal may be reasonable after effective pain treatment, but patients commonly describe returning to heavy-duty work that they have not been able to do for many years. When challenged, patients may indicate that it is the only kind of work they know how to do. During the disabled phase, there typically has been no effort to explore reasonable alternatives, despite the efforts of vocational counseling. The patient's prognosis to return to work may be quite good for light-duty activities, but the goal to return to truck driving, logging, or millwork is not reasonable. This dichotomy in thinking influences the patient's interpretation of treatment results. It is remarkable that vocational issues are usually the last consideration in planning pain-relieving surgery for people injured in the workplace. Unless the treatment satisfies all the needs of the patient, it is more likely to fail.

Preoperative Planning of Postoperative Care and Direction

It is usually appropriate to see how a patient does after an operation before making postoperative care plans.

However, the method is different in treating the chronic pain patient because there is a high rate of regression of surgical pain-relieving benefit and an inordinate number of patients who do not prosper even after apparently effective surgery. Any approach to the care of these patients must therefore include preoperative planning and patient involvement. Many patients with chronic pain are relatively passive. Providing some form of homework and requiring compliance before proceeding can increase patient participation in efforts to maximize outcome.

Homework

A variety of measurable patient activities have been described, and their use preoperatively cannot be overstressed. It is a simple matter to consider what should be done by the patient who does not fare well after a pain-relieving operation. They should be asked to do some of those things before the operation. Several important measures should be considered:

1. *Diaries.* The patient should be asked to keep written records and to bring them to each office visit. Some items to consider are activity records, drug use and efficacy records, and diaries of job-seeking activities, activity plans, exercises, and progressive increase of activities such as walking, swimming, and getting out of the house. The use of diaries improves compliance.

2. *Demonstration of exercise principles.* It is easy to teach even the most pained patient some safe exercises that can be checked regularly by the surgeon or office staff.

3. *Plans for the future.* A 5-year plan, written with the help of a significant other or a mental health counselor, is a relatively simple exercise for the patient.

4. *Specific plans for return to work.* It is not appropriate to see how the patient does before resolving questions about return to work. Patients who have specific plans before treatment tend to do better than those with none. Patients who indicate their inability to consider any form of work must continue to hurt to maintain that frame of mind. It is an important part of rehabilitation to help the patient act more appropriately and to recognize reasonable limitations and residual abilities.[124] The best time to explore this area is before the operation.

5. *Psychological issues.* Pain-relieving operations do not treat depression, anger, frustration, or an inability to work.[125, 126] They do treat pain. Although pain is often the expressed reason for an inability to function before an operation, people consider many other aspects of their lives. Psychologists seem to do best when given true freedom to explore their own prognoses. Psychological testing by itself is not enough to appropriately select people for pain surgery. However, the prognosis expressed as an overall opinion by the psychologist can be more prophetic if included before the surgeon discusses the operation with the patient. Psychological issues have been shown repeatedly to be more important predictors of prognosis than the degree of pain relief. If negative attitudinal and motivational issues exist before the operation, it is likely that they will persist afterward. These forces drive the psychological components of chronic pain, and they can result in depression and in emotional and social impotence unless they can be changed.

PUTTING IT TOGETHER

The purpose of this discourse is to look at means of approaching the chronic pain patient in a way that helps to maximize outcome for the patient and satisfaction for the surgeon. A surgeon must consider the need to justify any new treatment approach for a patient who suffers from chronic pain. Justification must be based on a reasonable chance for success. The population of patients without malignancies has already experienced the failure of prior attempts at pain relief before considering pain-relieving surgery. As surgeons, we do not provide appropriate service when we merely continue the course of initial results, followed by repeated failure. The failures of previous efforts should help to educate us about the appropriate use of our current approaches. The demoralization precipitated by another failure is usually not in the patient's best interest, and the newest treatment may interfere with rehabilitative efforts that may be more appropriate for the patient in the long run.

Gaining Satisfaction for the Surgeon and Patient

Treatment must answer the needs of the patient. Satisfaction for the physician can come from several sources: satisfying the needs of the patient, satisfaction that the surgery was appropriate and went well, satisfaction that the patient does well, and accolades from peers, especially the referring physician. In treating the chronic pain patient, it is a good idea to delay feelings of satisfaction. Improvement for a short time may not matter much to the patient, and recurrence of symptoms may be seen as another failure by the patient or the patient's family. Surgeons can gain more satisfaction if they approach the patient somewhat in the same way the patient approaches them. A degree of healthy skepticism is appropriate on both sides. The surgeon is not sure about providing long-lasting relief, and the patient is not sure whether relief is another hollow promise. Satisfaction about treatment and reasonable efficacy can only become meaningful when viewed many months after the treatment. Any pain relief that does not last at least a year probably has very little meaning to the patient.

Dealing with Expectations

One of the best ways to handle everyone's expectations is to express them at the outset. For a patient with chronic pain, it is inappropriate to suggest that a procedure should be done in an effort to see what happens. There is too much literature and accumulated experience for such a naive approach. Pain relief for the patient with chronic pain requires a reasonable expectation of improvement at a meaningful level. Unless the procedure can satisfy this level of improvement, the surgeon should not proceed. Despite confidence about helping the patient, the surgeon should consider his or her role if the procedure fails and must be willing to be involved afterward, especially when the procedure fails. If surgeons cannot accept this responsibility, they must accept that they are defining their role as mechanics. Although most surgeons cringe at this suggestion, it is how many seem to behave. The physician and patient will be better off if the surgeon's role is chosen ahead of time.

Surgeons who feel they may be of some help but not enough to fully satisfy the patient should define who will later care for the patient. That person probably should be involved in the decision to operate. Pain-relieving surgery should have a good chance of relieving pain at a level that has meaning to the patient. A patient who experiences a 60% or 70% reduction in pain but continues to suffer has achieved little. For a third-party payer, continued oral narcotics and disability payments may indicate that the procedure has little consequence, although it was considered a success by the surgeon. The future of pain-relieving surgery is predicated on the honesty and responsibility of the physician who understands the meanings of outcomes. Patients should always be approached with outcomes, including failures, in mind.

Failure and Starting Over

Is it appropriate to try every treatment a surgeon knows if the first one fails? The answer will remain a source of controversy as long as there are surgeons who are convinced that their approach is the only valid one. The most functional answer is to ask a different question. Do the patients who have failed to improve after any procedure fail for the same reasons? Surgeons should never proceed with another operation unless the reasons for prior failures are understood. Are prior failures caused by the same issues of dashed expectations, even with the admission of prior improvement? Failure of pain relief may not have a medical cause. A psychologist who has been given reasonable latitude to assess the patient's predicament can explain these issues. After failure of one pain-relieving operation, it is important to reassess a patient, the person's needs and expectations, and the real meanings of outcomes.

Dealing with Frustration

The physician's frustrations are probably one of the most neglected aspects of patient care.[127] In the context of approaching the chronic pain patient, the frustrations of the physician and support staff often are important determinants of care, decision making, and ultimate patient satisfaction. The trick is to recognize that frustration in dealing with chronic pain patients is common and to recognize it early so that the frustration can be diffused.

Regular meetings for discussion about difficult patients provide a valuable tool for controlling frustration and dissatisfactions. The physician probably should not lead these meetings but should always be there. Absence of the physician can add to staff discontent. An early morning meeting or a working brown-bag lunch may be times when all can attend. The purpose of the meeting is to air frustrations about patients and working conditions and to develop actions to deal with them. By demanding that staff members direct the meeting and find a solution for each complaint, the meeting does not become a "bitch session." The responsibility for each member is to offer ways of dealing with frustrations.

The meeting should be planned at least monthly and can be part of a schedule of regular weekly staff team meetings. It is important to recognize particularly irritated staff members and to help them develop more effective coping styles.

Sharing frustrations with the patient can have a beneficial effect. When patients become aware of their negative impact on the physician or staff, they often change their behavior. In an especially difficult situation, the surgeon can consider a behavioral contract with the patient. It spells out clearly the behaviors that are the most obnoxious and extracts a promise of more reasonable efforts by the patient. Such an agreement should include specifics about diary keeping and other homework as discussed earlier in this chapter.

Surgeons should never let their frustrations with the patient, the lack of pain response, or pressure to "do something" deter them from sound medical judgment. An operation or treatment that is not likely to work is not acceptable to prevent or respond to frustration.

CONCLUSIONS

The approach to the chronic pain patient must carry a sense of empathy and support and must be based on reasonable decisions. These people have been through a lot. Patients with long-standing, nonmalignant pain have myriad, often occult expectations and needs that commonly transcend the relief of pain alone. In many circumstances, the patient may not be able to express them. It is important to understand the reality of these expectations before treatment is begun.

Psychologists can help to uncover the patient's needs as the patient perceives them and to help the person see the reality of the predicament. This comprehension requires a level of professional involvement by the psychologist that evaluates prognosis and psychological health.

Pain-relieving surgery succeeds in many cases, and this chapter has explored some of the reasons for failure in others. Understanding these issues and incorporating them into a comprehensive approach to pain management can better address the needs of the patient. A reasonable, studied approach to the suffering patient can provide increased rewards for the caring surgeon and for the patient. This approach to the chronic pain patient helps to explain the reason for prior treatment failures and helps to prevent their recurrence.

"Is medicine science or art? The obvious answer is that it is both, as it has always been—and that the real question is how to find the right balance between them."[128]

REFERENCES

1. Gatchel RJ, Gardea MA: Psychosocial issues: Their importance in predicting disability, response to treatment, and search for compensation. Neurol Clin 17:149–166, 1999.
2. Fishbain DA, Cutler RB, Rosomoff HL, et al: Prediction of "intent," "discrepancy with intent," and "discrepancy with non-intent" for the patient with chronic pain to return to work after treatment in a pain facility. Clin J Pain 15:141–150, 1999.
3. Brown J, Klapow J, Doleys D, et al: Disease-specific and generic health outcomes: A model for the evaluation of long-term intrathecal opioid therapy in noncancer low back pain patients. Clin J Pain 15:122–131, 1999.
4. Wright A, Mayer TG, Gatchel RJ: Outcomes of disabling cervical spine disorders in compensation injuries. A prospective comparison to tertiary rehabilitation response for chronic lumbar spinal disorders. Spine 24:178–183, 1999.
5. Randolph PD, Racz GB: Consider the uncertainty: Holistic and reductionist considerations in spinal cord stimulation trial and permanent implantation. Pain Forum 5:107–110, 1996.
6. Levy RM, Lamb S, Adams JE: Treatment of chronic pain by deep brain stimulation: Long term follow-up and review of the literature. Neurosurgery 21:885–893, 1987.
7. Burchiel KJ, Anderson VC, Brown FD, et al: Prospective, multicenter study of spinal cord stimulation for relief of chronic back and extremity pain. Spine 21:2786–2794, 1996.
8. Maron J, Loeser JD: Spinal opioid infusions in the treatment of chronic pain of nonmalignant origin. Clin J Pain 12:174–179, 1996.
9. Anderson VC, Burchiel KJ: A prospective study of long-term intrathecal morphine in the management of chronic nonmalignant pain. Neurosurgery 44:289–301, 1999.
10. Hildebrandt J, Pfingsten M, Saur P, Jansen J: Prediction of success from a multidisciplinary treatment program for chronic low back pain. Spine 22:990–1001, 1997.
11. Romano JM, Turner JA, Jensen MP, et al: Chronic pain patient–spouse behavioral interactions predict patient disability. Pain 63:353–360, 1995.
12. Turner JA, Loeser JD, Bell DG: Spinal cord stimulation for chronic low back pain: A systematic literature synthesis. Neurosurgery 37:1088–1096, 1995.
13. Robertson JT: The rape of the spine. Surg Neurol 39:5–12, 1993.
14. Jensen MP, Romano JM, Turner JA, et al: Patient beliefs predict patient functioning: Further support for a cognitive-behavioral model of chronic pain. Pain 81:95–104, 1999.
15. Fishbain DA, Rosomoff HL, Cutler RB: I. Do chronic pain patients' perceptions about their preinjury jobs determine their intent to return to the same type of job post–pain facility treatment? Clin J Pain 11:267–278, 1995.
16. Rosomoff HL, Fishbain DA, Cutler RB: II. Do chronic pain patients' perceptions about their preinjury jobs differ as a function of worker compensation and non–worker compensation status? Clin J Pain 11:279–286, 1995.
17. Crombez G, Vlaeyen JWS, Heuts PHTG, Lysens R: Pain-related fear is more disabling than pain itself: Evidence on the role of pain-related fear in chronic back pain disability. Pain 80:329–339, 1999.
18. Epstein NE, Hood DC, Bender JF: A comparison of surgeon's assessment to the patient's analysis (short form 36) after far lateral lumbar disc surgery. Spine 22:2422–2428, 1997.
19. Rawlings C, Rossitch E, Nashold BS: The history of neurosurgical procedures for the relief of pain. Surg Neurol 38:454–463, 1992.
20. McCracken LM, Spertus IL, Janeck AS, et al: Behavioral dimensions of adjustment in persons with chronic pain: Pain-related anxiety and acceptance. Pain 80:283–289, 1999.
21. Papageorgiou AC, Croft PR, Thomas E, et al: Influence of previous pain experience on the episode incidence of low back pain: Results from the South Manchester Back Pain Study. Pain 66:181–185, 1996.
22. Racz GB, Heavner JE, Raj P: Percutaneous epidural neuroplasty: Prospective one-year follow-up. Pain Digest 9:87–102, 1999.
23. Seres JL: The neurosurgical management of pain: A critical review. Clin J Pain 9:284–290, 1993.
24. Troussier B, Lebas JF, Chirossel JP, et al: Percutaneous intradiscal radio-frequency thermocoagulation: A cadaveric study. Spine 20:1713–1718, 1995.
25. North RB, Kidd DH, Campbell JN, Long DM: Dorsal root ganglionectomy for failed back surgery syndrome: A 5-year follow-up study. J Neurosurg 74:236–242, 1991.
26. Cushing H: Case 9. In Meningiomas. New York, Hafner Publishing, 1938, pp 217–219.
27. White JC, Sweet WH: Pain and the Neurosurgeon. Springfield, IL, Charles C Thomas, 1969, p 7.
28. McDonald GJ, Lord SM, Bogduk N: Long-term follow-up of patients treated with cervical radiofrequency neurotomy for chronic neck pain. Neurosurgery 45:61–68, 1999.
29. Long DM, BenDebba M, Torgerson WS, et al: Persistent back pain and sciatica in the United States: Patient characteristics. J Spinal Disord 9:40–58, 1996.
30. Postacchini F: Presidential address: The lumbar spine in the 2000s. Spine 24:991–995, 1999.
31. Woertgen C, Rothoerl RD, Holzschuh M, et al: Are prognostic factors still what they are expected to be after long-term follow-up? J Spinal Disord 11:395–399, 1998.
32. Devulder J, Deene P, De Laat M, et al: Nerve root sleeve injections in patients with failed back surgery syndrome: A comparison of three solutions. Clin J Pain 15:132–135, 1999.
33. Seres JL: The fallacy of using 50% pain relief as the standard for satisfactory pain treatment: Focus article. Pain Forum 8:183, 1999.
34. Deyo RA, Phillips WR: Low back pain: A primary care challenge. Spine 21:2826–2832, 1996.
35. Bhandari M, Louw D, Reddy K: Predictors of return to work after anterior cervical discectomy. J Spinal Disord 12:94–98, 1999.
36. Riley JL, Robinson ME, Geisser ME: Relationship between MMPI-2 cluster profiles and surgical outcome in low-back pain patients. J Spinal Disord 8:213–219, 1995.
37. Teasell RW, Harth M: Functional restoration: Returning patients with chronic low back pain to work—revolution or fad? Spine 21:844–847, 1996.
38. North RB, Kidd DH, Wimberly RL, et al: Prognostic value of psychological testing in patients undergoing spinal cord stimulation: A prospective study. Neurosurgery 39:301–311, 1996.
39. North RB: Psychological criteria are outcome measures as well as prognostic factors. Pain Forum 5:111–114, 1996.
40. Williams DA: Psychological screening and treatment for implantables: A continuum of care. Pain Forum 5:115–117, 1996.
41. Olson KA: Commentary. Pain Med J Club 3:31–33, 1997.
42. Bodenheimer T: Disease management—promises and pitfalls. N Engl J Med 340:1202–1205, 1999.
43. Franklin GM, Haug J, Heyer NJ, et al: Outcome of lumbar fusion in Washington State worker's compensation. Spine 19:1897–1904, 1994.
44. Hardy RW. Commentary. Neurosurg Q 6:73–75, 1996.
45. Hashemi L, Webster BS, Clancy EA, Volinn E: Length of disability and cost of workers' compensation low back pain claims. J Occup Environ Med 39:937–945, 1997.
46. Kupers RC, Van den Oever R, Houdenhove BV, et al: Spinal cord stimulation in Belgium: A nation-wide survey on the incidence, indications and therapeutic efficacy by the health insurer. Pain 56:211–216, 1994.
47. Malter AD, Larson EB, Urban N, Deyo RA: Cost-effectiveness of lumbar discectomy for the treatment of herniated intervertebral disc. Spine 21:1048–1054, 1996.
48. Wright A, Mayer TG, Gatchel RJ: Outcomes of disabling cervical spine disorders in compensation injuries. Spine 24:178–183, 1999.
49. Carette S, Leclaire R, Marcoux S, et al: Epidural corticosteroid injections for sciatica due to herniated nucleus pulposus. N Engl J Med 336:1634–1640, 1997.
50. Boduk N: Commentary. Pain Med J Club 4:29–31, 1998.
51. Fukusaki M, Kobayashi I, Hara T, et al: Symptoms of spinal stenosis do not improve after epidural steroid injection. Clin J Pain 14:148–151, 1998.

52. Weinstein JN (ed): Clinical Efficacy and Outcome in the Diagnosis of Low Back Pain. New York, Raven Press, 1992.

53. Bovin G, Schrader H, Sand T: Neck pain in the general population. Spine 19:1307–1309, 1994.

54. O'Neill C, Derby R, Kenderes : Precision injection techniques for diagnosis and treatment of lumbar disc disease. Semin Spine Surg 11:104–118, 1999.

55. Fritch EW, Heisel J, Rupp S: The failed back surgery syndrome: Reasons, intraoperative findings, and long-term results: A report of 182 operative treatments. Spine 21:626–633, 1996.

56. Snider RK, Krumwiede NK, Snider LJ, et al: Factors affecting lumbar spinal fusion. J Spinal Disord 12:107–114, 1999.

57. Lurie JD, Sox HC: Spine update: Principles of medical decision making. Spine 24:493–498, 1999.

58. Jamison RN, Matt DA, Parris WC: Treatment outcome in low back pain patients: Do compensation benefits make a difference? Orthop Rev 17:1210–1215, 1988.

59. Randolph PD, Caldera YM, Tacone AM, et al: The long-term combined effects of medical treatment and a mindfulness-based behavioral program for the multidisciplinary management of chronic pain in West Texas. Pain Dig 9:103–112, 1999.

60. Painter JR, Seres JL, Newman RI: Assessing benefits of the pain center: Why some patients regress. Pain 8:101–113, 1980.

61. Penny KI, Purves AM, Smith BH, et al: Relationship between the chronic pain grade and measures of physical, social and psychological well-being. Pain 79:275–279, 1999.

62. Asmundson GJ, Norton PJ, Norton GR: Beyond pain: The role of fear and avoidance in chronicity. Clin Psychol Rev 19:97–119, 1999.

63. Paice JA, Penn RD, Shott S: Intraspinal morphine for chronic pain: A retrospective multicenter study. J Pain Symptom Manage 11:231–241, 1996.

64. Gallagher RM: Treatment planning in pain medicine: Integrating medical, physical, and behavioral therapies. Med Clin North Am 83:823–849, 1999.

65. Anderson VC, Burchiel KJ: A prospective study of long-term intrathecal morphine in the management of chronic nonmalignant pain. Neurosurgery 44:289–301, 1999.

66. Ploghaus A, Tracey I, Gati JS, et al: Dissociating pain from its anticipation in the human brain. Science 284:1979–1981, 1999.

67. Heggeness MH, Watters WC, Gray PM: Discography of lumbar discs after surgical treatment for disc herniation. Spine 15:1606–1609, 1997.

68. Radanov BP, Begre S, Struzenegger M, et al: Course of psychological variables in whiplash injury—a 2-year follow-up with age, gender and education pair-matched patients. Pain 64:429–434, 1996.

69. Wallis BJ, Lord SM, Bogduk N: Resolution of psychological distress of whiplash patients following treatment by radiofrequency neurotomy: A randomised, double-blind, placebo-controlled trial. Pain 73:15–22, 1997.

70. Weishaupt D, Zanetti M, Hodler J, Boos N: MR imaging of the lumbar spine: Prevalence of intervertebral disk extrusion and sequestration, nerve root compression, end plate abnormalities, and osteoarthritis of the facet joints in asymptomatic volunteers. Radiology 209:661–666, 1998.

71. Heavner JE, Racz GB, Raj P: Percutaneous epidural neuroplasty: Prospective evaluation of 0.9% NaCl versus 10% NaCl with or without hyaluronidase. Reg Anesth Pain Med 24:202–207, 1999.

72. Nachemson A, Zdeblick TA, O'Brien JP: Lumbar disc disease with discogenic pain. What surgical treatment is most effective? Spine 21:1835–1838, 1996.

73. Fordyce WE: Pain in the workplace. Seattle, IASP Press, 1997.

74. Lavender SA, Oleske DM, Nicholson L, et al: Comparison of five methods to determine low back disorder risk in a manufacturing environment. Spine 24:1441–1448, 1999.

75. Hadler NM: Back pain in the workplace: What you lift or how you lift matters far less than whether you lift or when. Spine 22:935–940, 1997.

76. Turk DC, Rudy TE: Neglected topics in the treatment of chronic pain patients—relapse, noncompliance, and adherence enhancement. Pain 44:5–28, 1991.

77. Seres JL: Nonsurgical management of chronic pain. In Tindall GT, Cooper PR, Barrow (eds): The Practice of Neurosurgery. New York, Lippincott Williams & Wilkins, 1996, 2997–3008.

78. Papageorgiou AC, Macfarlane GJ, Thomas E, et al: Psychosocial factors in the workplace—do they predict new episodes of low back pain? Evidence from the South Manchester back pain study. Spine 22:113–1142, 1997.

79. Hazard RG, Haugh LD, Reid S, et al: Early prediction of chronic disability after occupational low back injury. Spine 21:945–951, 1996.

80. Hildebrandt J, Pfingsten M, Saur P, Jansen J: Prediction of success from a multidisciplinary treatment program for chronic low back pain. Spine 22:990–1001, 1997.

81. Porchet F, Vader JP, Larequi-Lauber T, et al: The assessment of appropriate indications for laminectomy. J Bone Joint Surg Br 81:234–239, 1999.

82. McDonald GJ, Lord SM, Bogduk N: Long-term follow-up of patients treated with cervical radiofrequency neurotomy for chronic neck pain. Neurosurgery 45:1494–1498, 1999.

83. Sluijter ME: Percutaneous intradiscal radio-frequency thermocoagulation. Spine 21:528–529, 1996.

84. Penta M, Fraser RD: Anterior lumbar interbody fusion: A minimum 10-year follow-up. Spine 22:2429–2434, 1997.

85. Carette S, Marcoux S, Truchon R, et al: A controlled trial of corticosteroid injections into facet joints for chronic low back pain. N Engl J Med 325:1002–1007, 1991.

86. Manchikanti L, Pakanati PR, Bakhit CE, Pampati V: Role of adhesiolysis and hypertonic saline neurolysis in management of low back pain: Evaluation of modification of the Racz protocol. Pain Dig 9:91–96, 1999.

87. Devulder J, Deene P, De Laat M, et al: Nerve root sleeve injections in patients with failed back surgery syndrome: A comparison of three solutions. Clin J of Pain 15:132–135, 1999.

88. Goodman RR: Surgical management of pain. Neurosurg Clin N Am 1:701–717, 1990.

89. Gybels JM: Indications for neurosurgical treatment of chronic pain. Acta Neurochir (Wein) 166:171–175, 1992.

90. Seres JL: The neurosurgeon's greatest responsibility in treating chronic pain: "Knowing when to quit." Pain Newslett 4:6, 1997.

91. Nachemson A: Chronic pain—the end of the welfare state? Qual Life Res 3(Suppl 1):S11–S17, 1994.

92. Krames ES, Olson K: Clinical realities and economic considerations: Patient selection in intrathecal therapy. J Pain Symptom Manage 14(Suppl):S3–13, 1997.

93. Noordenbos W, Wall PD: Implications of the failure of nerve resection and graft to cure chronic pain produced by nerve lesions. J Neurol Neurosurg Psychiatry 44:1068–1073, 1981.

94. Burns JW, Sherman ML, Devine J, et al: Association between workers' compensation and outcome following multidisciplinary treatment for chronic pain: Roles of mediators and moderators. Clin J Pain 11:94–102, 1995.

95. Price JA, Penn RD, Shott S: Intraspinal morphine for chronic pain: A retrospective multicenter study. J Pain Symptom Manage 11:231–241, 1996.

96. Loeser JD, Melzack R: Pain: An overview. Lancet 353:1607–1609, 1999.

97. McCarberg B, Wolf J: Chronic pain management in a health maintenance organization. Clin J Pain 15:50–57, 1999.

98. Butterfield PG, Spencer PS, Redmond S, et al: Low back pain: Predictors of absenteeism, residual symptoms, functional impairment, and medical costs in Oregon worker's compensation recipients. Am J Ind Med 34:559–567, 1998.

99. Gatchel RJ, Garea MA: Psychosocial issues: Their importance in predicting disability, response to treatment and search for compensation. Neurol Clin 17:149–166, 1999.

100. Schade V, Semmer N, Main CJ, et al: The impact of clinical, morphological, psychosocial and work-related factors on the outcome of lumbar discectomy. Pain 80:239–249, 1999.

101. Volinn E, Turczyn KM, Loeser JD: Theories of back pain and health care utilization. Neurosurg Clin N Am 2:739–748, 1991.

102. Hagen KB, Thune O: Work incapacity from low back pain in the general population. Spine 23:2091–2095, 1998.

103. Bendix AF, Bendix T, Haestrup C: Can it be predicted which patients with chronic low back pain should be offered tertiary rehabilitation in a functional restoration program? A search for demographic, socioeconomic, and physical factors. Spine 23:1775–1784, 1998.

104. Loeser JD, Henderlite SE, Conrad DA: Incentive effects of work-

er's compensation benefits: A literature synthesis. Med Care Res Rev 52:34–59, 1995.

105. Sturmer T, Luessenhoop S, Neth A, et al: Construction work and low back disorder. Preliminary findings of the Hamburg Construction Worker Study. Spine 222:2558–2563, 1997.

106. Krause N, Ragland DR, Fisher JM, Syme SL: Psychosocial job factors, physical workload, and incidence of work-related spinal injury: A 5-year prospective study of urban transit operators. Spine 23:2507–2516, 1998.

107. Luoma K, Riihimaki H, Raininko R, et al: Lumbar disc degeneration in relation to occupation. Scand J Work Environ Health 24:358–366, 1998.

110. Murphy PL, Volinn E: Is occupational low back pain on the rise? Spine 24:691–697, 1999.

108. Wood DJ: Design and evaluation of a back injury prevention program within a geriatric hospital. Spine 12:77–82,1987.

109. Donceel P, Du Bois M: Fitness for work after surgery for lumbar disc herniation: A retrospective study. Eur Spine J 7:29–35, 1998.

110. Voiss DV: Occupational injury. Fact, fantasy, or fraud? Neurol Clin 13:431–446, 1995.

111. North RB, Kidd DH, Wimberly RL, Edwin D: Prognostic value of psychological testing in patients undergoing spinal cord stimulation: A prospective study. Neurosurgery 39:301–310, 1996.

112. Burchiel KJ, Anderson VC, Wilson BJ, et al: Prognostic factors of spinal cord stimulation for chronic back and leg pain. Neurosurgery 36:1101–1110, 1995.

113. Snow-Turek AL, Norris MP, Tan G: Active and passive coping strategies in chronic pain patients. Pain 64:455–462, 1996.

114. Asghari MA, Nicholas MK: Personality and adjustment to chronic pain. Pain Rev 6:85–97, 1999.

115. Turk DC, Tudy TE: Neglected topics in the treatment of chronic pain patients—relapse, noncompliance, and adherence enhancement. Pain 44:5–28, 1991.

116. Turk DC, Tudy TE, Sorkin BA: Neglected topics in chronic pain

treatment outcome studies: Determination of success. Pain 53: 3–16, 1993.

117. Rawlings C, Rossitch E, Nashold BS: The history of neurosurgical procedures for relief of pain. Surg Neurol 38:454–463, 1992.

118. Dworkin SF, Von Korff M, LeResche L: Multiple pains and psychiatric disturbance: An epidemiologic investigation. Arch Gen Psychiatry 47:239–244, 1990.

119. Fishbain DA: Approaches to treatment decisions for psychiatric comorbidity in the management of the chronic pain patient. Med Clin North Am 83:737–760, 1999.

120. Zaza C, Stolee P, Prkachin K: The application of goal attainment scaling in chronic pain settings. J Pain Symptom Manage 17: 55–64, 1999.

121. Brady A, Cleeland C, Goldstein G, et al: Pain management guidelines: Implications for managed care—a roundtable discussion. Med Interface (Suppl):10–32, 1997.

122. Swensen R: Differential diagnosis: A reasonable clinical approach. Neurol Clin 17:43–63, 1999.

123. Brown J, Klapow J, Doleys D, et al: Disease-specific and generic health outcomes: A model for the evaluation of long-term intrathecal opioid therapy in noncancer low back pain patients. Clin J Pain 15:122–131, 1999.

124. Tait RC, Chibnall JT: Attitude profiles and clinical status in patients with chronic pain. Pain 78:49–57, 1998.

125. Fishbain DA, Cutler RB, Rosomoff HL, et al: Impact of chronic pain patients' job perception variables on actual return to work. Clin J Pain 13:197–206, 1997.

126. Burchiel KJ, Anderson VC, Brown FD, et al: Prospective, multicenter study of spinal cord stimulation for relief of chronic back and extremity pain. Spine 21:786–794, 1996.

127. Tait RC, Chibnall JT: Physician judgments of chronic pain patients. Soc Sci Med 45:1199–1205, 1997.

128. Boyle PJ, Callahan D: Physicians' use of outcomes data: Moral conflicts and potential resolutions. In Boyle PJ (ed): Getting Doctors to Listen: Ethics and Outcomes Data in Context. Washington, D.C., Georgetown University Press, 1998, p 18.

CHAPTER 183

Medical Management of Chronic Pain

JAIMIE M. HENDERSON ■ PAUL E. FEWINGS

Pain is the most common complaint for which patients seek medical attention. Chronic pain remains the most frequent cause of suffering and disability throughout the United States and the world. One of the great challenges for all physicians, particularly for neurosurgeons, is the rational treatment of the chronic pain patient. Although acute pain is relatively well understood and usually responds predictably to a variety of interventions, chronic pain is notoriously nonlinear in its response to medications and surgery. Although there are various causes for chronic pain, the original source of the pain may be less important than the factors that potentiate it. Because of this unpredictability, much of the literature on chronic pain treatment has been confusing, contradictory, and sometimes misleading.

The goal of this chapter is to examine the role of a number of established medications and several novel agents in the treatment of chronic pain and to consider their sites and mechanisms of action. In doing so, we hope to provide a framework for understanding the application of various neuromodulatory medications in the treatment of chronic pain.

SITES FOR MODULATION OF CHRONIC PAIN

Medications used for the treatment of pain fall into several categories, each with distinct sites and mechanisms of action. A brief review of the anatomy of the pain transmission pathways with emphasis on potential modulatory sites (Fig. 183–1) allows us to better understand the unique mechanisms of each pharmacologic agent.

Noxious cutaneous stimuli activate bare nerve endings in the dermis and in the dermal-epidermal boundary zone. These nociceptive impulses are conducted centrally by two major classes of nerve fibers: unmyelinated C fibers and small, myelinated A fibers. The primary receptors consist of bare nerve endings, which under normal circumstances are activated only by very strong heat or mechanical stimuli that are sufficient to cause tissue damage. Associated tissue damage produces a large variety of inflammatory substances and

begins a cascade of events that leads to increasing inflammation and pain. Modulation of this inflammatory cascade at the periphery provides one means for modulating pain.

Stimulation of peripheral nociceptors causes release of several neurotransmitters, including glutamate, substance P, and calcitonin gene–related peptide (CGRP), at their synapses within the central nervous system (CNS)[1] (Fig. 183–2). Tissue damage, which frequently accompanies intense noxious stimuli, can release a number of substances, including bradykinin, histamine, serotonin, prostaglandins, potassium, and protons, from the tissue and from platelets, macrophages, neutrophils, lymphocytes, and mast cells. Many of these substances are nociceptive by means of direct activation or sensitization of nociceptors. Substance P released from primary afferent neurons contributes to neurogenic inflammation by causing mast cell degranulation, which releases histamine, bradykinin, and serotonin (Fig. 183–3). These substances contribute to increasing vasodilatation with the extravasation of further inflammatory mediators and algogens into the tissue. The inflammatory mediators activate macrophages, monocytes, and lymphocytes, further amplifying the inflammatory response. The contribution of ongoing inflammation to the generation of certain chronic pain states is discussed further in later sections.

Myelinated Aδ and unmyelinated C fibers pass through the dorsal root to synapse on numerous interneurons and central transmission cells within the dorsal gray matter of the spinal cord. Although several theories have been advanced regarding the precise mechanisms of sensory processing that occur in the dorsal horn, most investigators agree that "wide dynamic range" cells in Rexed's lamina I and V serve as central transmission cells, with significant modulatory input supplied by interneurons in lamina II and III, also known as the *substantia gelatinosa*. This modulatory input of the substantia gelatinosa interneurons on central projection cells formed the basis of the influential *gate control theory* of Melzack and Wall[2] and remains a central element of modern theories of pain processing in the dorsal horn.[3, 4] It is clear from observation and experiment that complex processing of nociceptive stimuli occurs in the dorsal gray matter of the spinal

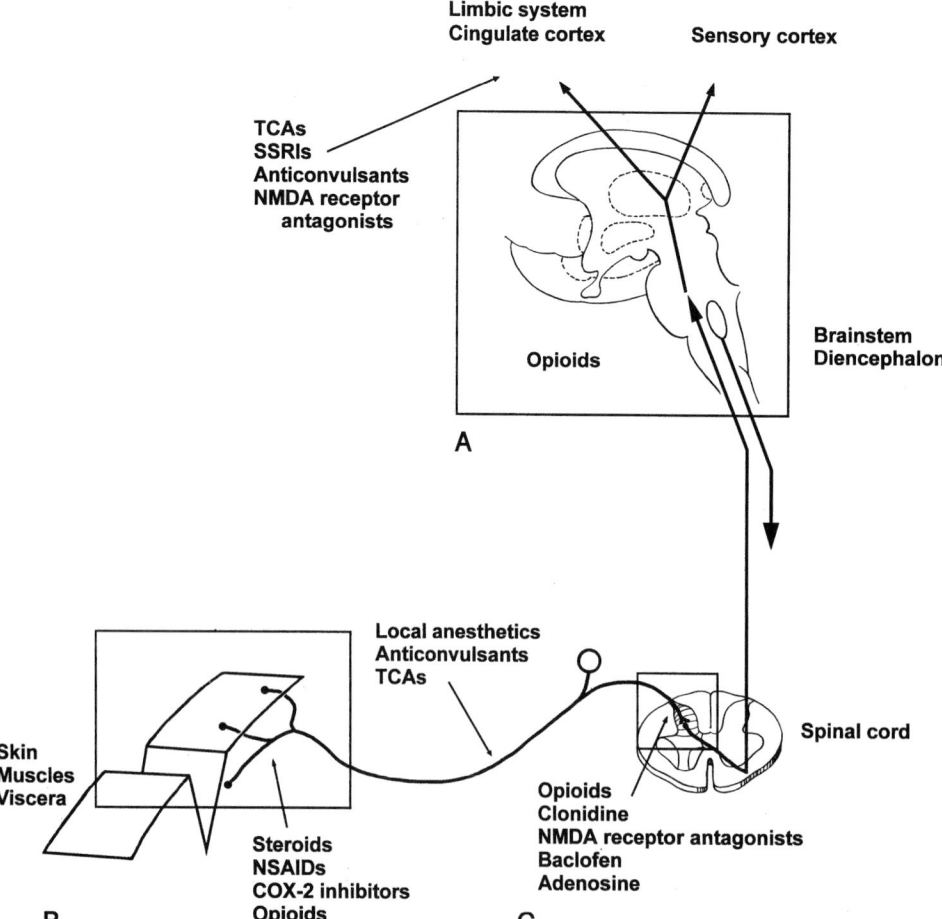

FIGURE 183–1. Pharmacologic targets for modulation of the pain transmission and perception pathways. A, Opioid-rich areas in the brainstem and diencephalon provide targets for opioid agonists. The limbic system, including cingulate cortex, amygdala, and connections through the thalamus, can be modulated by antidepressants and other agents. B, Tissue injury in skin, muscle, and viscera releases inflammatory substances that can be modulated by anti-inflammatory agents. C, Axonal conduction can be decreased by ion channel blockers, including local anesthetics, anticonvulsants, and tricyclic antidepressants. In the spinal cord, complex neurochemical circuitry can be modulated by a number of pharmacologic agents.

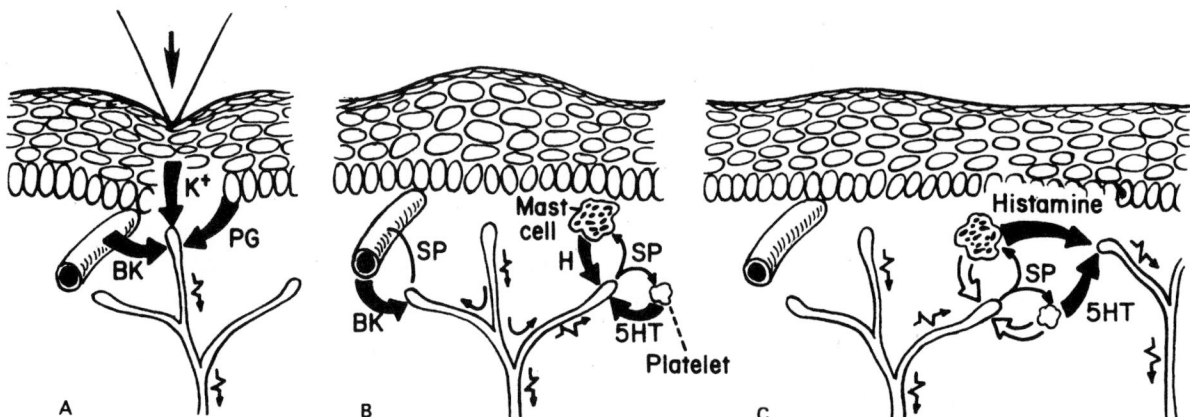

FIGURE 183–2. Events leading to activation, sensitization, and spread of sensitization of primary afferent nociceptor terminals. *A,* Direct activation by tissue damage, leading to release of potassium (K⁺) and the synthesis of prostaglandins (PGs) and bradykinin (BK). Prostaglandins increase the sensitivity of the terminal to bradykinin and other pain-producing substances. *B,* Secondary activation, showing that impulses generated in the stimulated terminal propagate to the spinal cord and into other terminal branches, where they induce the release of peptides including substance P (SP). Substance P causes vasodilation and neurogenic edema with further accumulation of bradykinin and causes release of histamine (H) from mast cells and serotonin (5-HT) from platelets. *C,* With continued liberation of substance P, the levels of histamine and serotonin continue to rise in the extracellular fluid and indirectly mildly sensitize nearby nociceptors. Sensitization leads to a gradual spread of hyperalgesia. (From Bonica JJ, Yaksh TL, Liebeskind JC, et al: Biochemistry and modulation of nociception and pain. In Bonica JJ (ed): The Management of Pain. Philadelphia, Lea & Febiger, 1990, p 98.)

Bulbospinal pathways

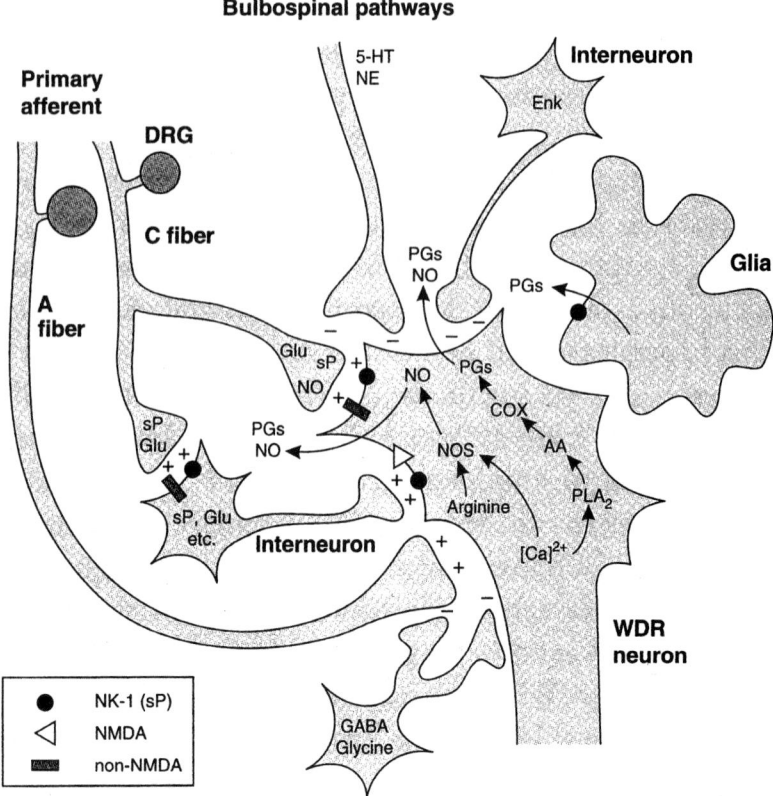

FIGURE 183–3. Neurochemical pathways in the dorsal horn of the spinal cord. Primary afferent fibers release substance P (sP), calcitonin gene–related peptide, and glutamate (Glu). These excitatory neurotransmitters stimulate second-order neurons, including interneurons and wide dynamic range (WDR) central transmission cells. Interneurons activated by nociceptive input excite central transmission cells through N-methyl-D-aspartate (NMDA) receptors and neurokinin (NK-1) receptors. This leads to increases in intracellular Ca^{2+}, which activates a number of second messenger systems. Prostaglandins (PGs) and nitric oxide (NO) are released into the extracellular space and facilitate nociceptive transmitter release. Modulatory control is exerted by a number of descending projection neurons and interneurons, modulated by serotonin (5-HT), norepinephrine (NE), and endogenous opioids such as enkephalin (Enk). (From Yaksh T: Central pharmacology of nociceptive transmission. In Wall PD, Melzack R (eds): Textbook of Pain. Edinburgh, Churchill Livingstone, 1999, p 265.)

cord. Modulation of this spinal circuitry provides a route for the pharmacologic treatment of pain. It has been demonstrated convincingly that opioid medications exert a strong influence on the dorsal horn circuitry, acting to impair central transmission of nociceptive impulses from the cells in lamina V, from which many of the spinothalamic tract fibers originate.[5]

Opioids act at a number of supraspinal sites, including the periaqueductal and periventricular gray matter, rostral ventral medulla, and nucleus raphe magnus.[6] These sites, as well as a number of other nuclei in the brainstem, form an important portion of the endogenous pain control system (Fig. 183–4). Descending projections from this system travel in the dorsolateral portion of the spinal cord, eventually exerting their influence on the dorsal horn through serotonergic, noradrenergic, and cholinergic synapses. Modulation, emulation, or enhancement of these endogenous mechanisms can provide fertile ground for the pharmacologic treatment of pain. Many of the beneficial effects of opioids seem to be based on activation of opioid receptors in these nuclei.

The limbic system, thalamus, hypothalamus, and neocortex contribute to the perception of pain, although the relative contributions of each system are still poorly understood. The limbic system is intimately connected with the endogenous pain control circuitry in the brainstem. Limbic activation can lead to widespread changes in cortical and subcortical activity, sensitizing or inhibiting areas that probably contribute to the perception of pain. Anxiety and depression frequently accompany chronic pain, and their treatment

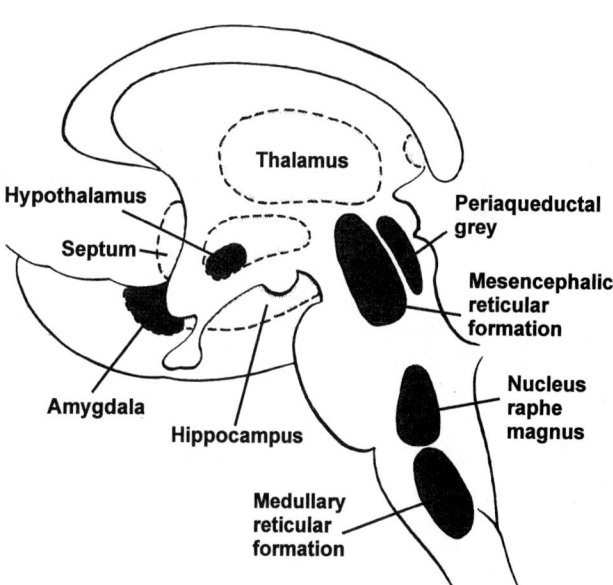

FIGURE 183–4. Supraspinal sites containing opioid receptors. The descending endogenous pain control system originates from neurons in the reticular formation, periaqueductal gray, and nucleus raphe magnus. Activation of opioid receptors in these regions can exert ascending and descending influences on the pain transmission and perception circuitry. (Adapted from Bonica JJ, Yaksh TL, Liebeskind JC, et al: Biochemistry and modulation of nociception and pain. In Bonica JJ (ed): The Management of Pain. Philadelphia, Lea & Febiger, 1990, p 98.)

is an important part of the overall treatment of chronic pain patients.

MECHANISMS IN THE TRANSITION FROM ACUTE TO CHRONIC PAIN

Acute pain is usually characterized by a relatively linear relationship between the degree of tissue damage and the intensity and duration of pain. This response drives the organism away from continued noxious stimuli, averting further tissue damage. In most cases, the pain resolves as tissue healing occurs. However, in some instances, there is maintenance of pain beyond the normal period of healing. This is called *chronic pain*, a poorly defined term that serves only to describe the ongoing nature of the pain but does not differentiate the cause or type of pain.

Various investigators have struggled to explain how a similar stimulus can cause chronic pain in one patient while another heals completely and reports no further pain. Several mechanisms seem to be involved in the development of chronic pain, with each affecting different portions of the pain transmission circuitry. Despite the fact that chronic pain is inherently complex and poorly localized within the neuraxis, the mechanisms can be logically divided into four categories:

1. Chronic activation of pain receptors, producing sensitization and persistent *nociceptive pain*
2. Damage to or derangement of small-diameter sensory fibers and their connections in the spinal cord, producing *neuropathic pain*
3. Damage to the CNS itself, causing *central pain*
4. Psychological and behavioral mechanisms that can augment or inhibit chronic pain or can produce *psychogenic pain*

Ongoing research has challenged many of our previous assumptions regarding mechanisms of pain perception, and there are a variety of competing theories regarding the genesis of chronic pain. The division between nociceptive and neuropathic pain has also been questioned as a means to classify painful syndromes. Despite these shortcomings, this fourfold scheme serves as a conceptual framework for the pharmacologic treatment of chronic pain and allows us to systematically examine potential sites of modulation of the pain pathways.

Peripheral or Nociceptive Mechanisms

Ongoing tissue damage and inflammation associated with various chronic inflammatory diseases can contribute to the development of a chronic pain state. Persistent noxious stimulation and sensitization of nociceptors may play a role in this type of chronic, nociceptive pain. Various products of tissue damage and inflammation stimulate afferent fibers to induce pain and hyperalgesia and to release neuropeptides. Nociceptive afferents are stimulated by a variety of inflammatory mediators, including bradykinin, serotonin, prostaglandins, and free protons. The sensory neuropeptides substance P, neurokinin-A and CGRP

play a critical role in the responses elicited by sensory nerves and are important in orchestrating a number of events that occur in inflammation.[7] The action of substance P on arterial endothelium causes vasodilation through the production of the freely diffusable second messenger nitric oxide. Substance P causes mast cell degranulation with further release of histamine, serotonin, and proteolytic enzymes; the latter catalyzes the production of further kinins and ultimately increases nociceptive input and perpetuates inflammation.[8] The effects of neurokinin release may be complemented or modified by the concomitant release of other sensory neuropeptides such as galanin, somatostatin, and neuropeptide Y, which may have inhibitory or regulatory actions on afferent excitability, ultimately reducing the release of substance P from sensory fibers during neurogenic inflammation.[9] With ongoing inflammation, nociceptors undergo changes in sensitivity that may be mediated by growth factors such as nerve growth factor (NGF).[10] Increased levels of NGF have been measured in severe inflammatory conditions, including pleurisy, rheumatoid arthritis, blister fluid, and skin after experimental inflammation.[11] NGF binds with tyrosine kinase receptors on small sensory neurons, entering the cell body and increasing production of mRNA coding for neurokinin precursor peptides.[12] Neuropeptide release then increases at the periphery and in the spinal cord,[13] and it induces nerve sprouting that amplifies these events.[14] As a result of these effects, NGF may promote a prolonged increase in afferent fiber sensitivity and synaptic activity leading to hyperalgesia. This viewpoint is strengthened by the observation that injection of NGF into tissues leads to increased sensitivity and responsiveness to noxious stimuli, responses that are attenuated by anti-NGF antibodies.[11]

Persistent stimulation and sensitization of nociceptive neurons appear to contribute to certain types of chronic pain. This suggests several strategies: control of inflammation, blocking of second messengers and growth factors, and direct blockade of hyperactive peripheral neurons. Removal of the source of inflammation, such as by joint replacement, can often markedly reduce inflammatory peripheral pain.

Peripheral-Central or Neuropathic Mechanisms

Whereas peripheral mechanisms are concerned mainly with the responses of intact nociceptive pathways to ongoing stimuli, peripheral-central mechanisms address states in which the primary nociceptive afferents have been damaged or are otherwise dysfunctional. This leads to a type of pain called *neuropathic pain*, which differs in its mechanism and clinical manifestations from other types. Peripheral neuropathic pain manifests as spontaneous pain (i.e., stimulus-independent pain) or painful hypersensitivity elicited by a stimulus after damage to or alterations in sensory neurons (i.e., stimulus-evoked pain). Normal functioning of a neuron depends on the integrity of the neuron itself, the supporting cells, and the surrounding chemical environment. Alteration of any of these components can bring about abnormal neuronal excitability, leading to neuropathic pain.

Abnormal impulse generation occurs in damaged nerves.[15] Ectopic discharges can be produced in nerve stump neuromas, demyelinated peripheral nerves, or injured dorsal root ganglia. Spontaneous volleys of high-frequency firing from ectopic "pacemaker sites" can produce long-lasting pain after even low-intensity mechanical stimuli. The increased input onto the dorsal horn can contribute to the phenomenon of *central sensitization*, potentiating the chronic pain state. The mechanisms of ectopic hyperexcitability most likely involve changes in the membrane properties of the damaged axons. Excess Na^+ channel accumulation has been demonstrated in neuroma end-bulbs, in demyelinated axons, and in aborted and regenerating axonal sprouts.[15] Numerous other metabolic changes also affect excitability, including K^+ and Ca^{2+} channel production, control of the functional properties of these ion channels, and the production of substances such as peptides that may have secondary excitatory activity. Medications that alter excitability of the axon by blocking ion channels may have a profound beneficial effect in reducing abnormal ectopic impulse generation in nociceptive fibers.

Central sensitization refers to the changes in neuronal firing in the dorsal horn that can develop in response to chronic stimulation of nociceptive fibers. These changes can include increases in neuronal responsiveness, a decrease in the firing threshold, or expansion of receptive fields.[16] Much attention has been focused on the role of *N*-methyl-D-aspartate (NMDA) glutamate receptors in the generation of this abnormal neuronal activity. Under normal circumstances, activation of the NMDA receptor is blocked by a magnesium ion. Continuous C-fiber input can cause progressive membrane depolarization, which then leads to loss of magnesium blockade of NMDA receptors. Synaptically released glutamate then binds to the activated receptors, causing an inward calcium flux, which leads to further activation of second messenger systems within the cell. One action of these second messengers is to phosphorylate the NMDA receptor, causing a decrease in the magnesium blockade at physiologic resting potentials and resulting in a net sensitization of the cell to glutamate activation. This propensity for central sensitization has led to the concept of *preemptive analgesia* to lessen the effect of massive C-fiber activation that occurs with surgery. NMDA receptor antagonists may allow modulation of this system in patients who have developed central sensitization.

Central Mechanisms

Injury to certain portions of the CNS can cause a severe type of chronic pain that has been referred to as *central pain*. The structures usually affected include the spinal cord, thalamus, and brainstem, although central pain has rarely been reported in the setting of cerebral cortical lesions. Patients typically describe burning and dysesthetic sensations, including tingling, numbness, or intense pressure. The mechanisms are unknown but may involve disinhibition of areas normally inhibited by the injured structures, or the sensations may represent changes in patterning or rearrangement of receptive fields in structures above the level of injury. Patients with central pain after spinal cord injuries exhibit increased spontaneous activity in the ventral posterior nuclei of the thalamus. Increased excitation involving NMDA receptors has been hypothesized to underlie this increased activity.[17] Neurons in the ventral posterior thalamus change their receptive fields within minutes of deafferentation.[18] Central nervous system plasticity almost certainly plays a role in the development of central pain states.

As we develop more sophisticated models to explain the integrative functions of the brain, it becomes increasingly clear that a delicate and complex homeostasis exists between the various brain systems. In an attempt to conceptualize these complex interactions, Melzack proposed the *neuromatrix theory of pain*,[19] which consists of three spheres: sensory-discriminative, affective-motivational, and evaluative-cognitive (Fig. 183–5). In this model, input from any of the three component networks can potentiate pain. Continued development of a systems approach to brain function may allow us to better conceptualize the phenomenon of central pain. Unfortunately, central pain remains poorly understood and difficult to treat pharmacologically.

Psychological and Environmental Mechanisms

Pain is by nature a subjective experience. The only method for measuring pain is by the report of the individual who is suffering it. Psychological and environmental mechanisms play a large role in defining the framework within which individual patients perceive their pain and in providing the verbal and nonverbal vocabulary with which they communicate their pain. Most patients who seek medical attention for chronic pain have significant psychological or social issues that must be addressed if treatment is to have any hope of succeeding.[20] Ignoring these factors dooms to failure the most well-intentioned and physiologically sound pharmacologic interventions.

The experience of chronic pain consists of numerous components that interact in complex and unpredictable ways. Nociceptive circuitry that may begin as a simple transmission pathway becomes quite complex as multiple levels of modulation are considered, with the brain representing the final gateway to the perception of pain. Psychological factors play a large role in the response of any individual to pain, including the possible development and maintenance of the chronic pain state.

In evaluating the patient with chronic pain, it is important to develop a sense of the personality traits that make up that patient's peculiar mechanisms for response to pain. Coping strategies play an important role in patients' adjustment to pain. Patients who have a more active coping style, choosing to control their own pain or participate in activities despite pain, tend

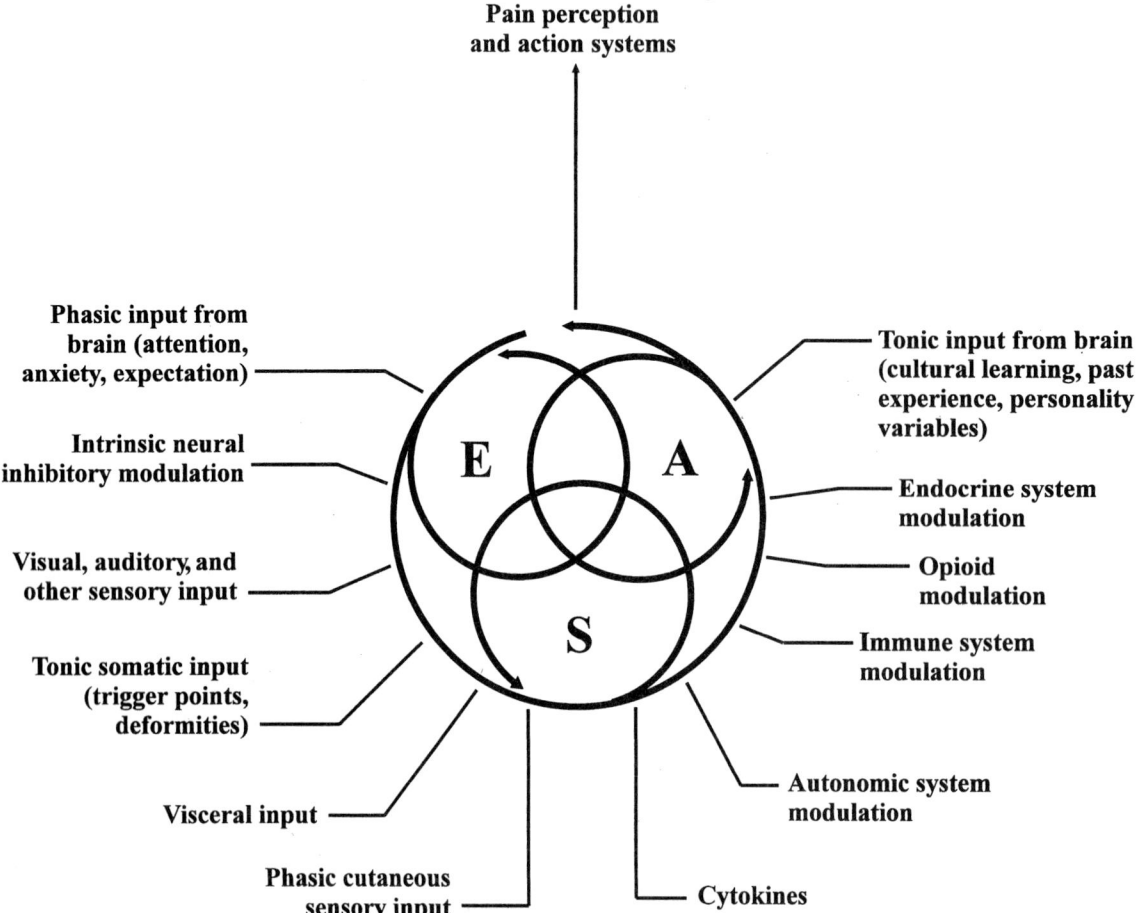

FIGURE 183–5. As described by Melzack, the body self-neuromatrix consists of a widely distributed neural network that includes somatosensory, limbic, and thalamocortical components. This is schematically depicted as a circle containing smaller parallel networks that contribute to the sensory-discriminative (S), affective-motivational (A), and evaluative-cognitive (E) dimensions of the pain experience. The synaptic architecture of the neuromatrix is determined by genetic and sensory influences. The neurosignature output of the neuromatrix—patterns of nerve impulses of various temporal and spatial dimensions—is produced by neural programs genetically built into the neuromatrix and determines the particular qualities of and other properties of the pain experience and behavior. Multiple inputs that act on the neuromatrix programs and contribute to the output neurosignature include (1) sensory inputs from somatic receptors; (2) visual and other sensory inputs that influence the cognitive interpretation of the situation; (3) phasic and tonic cognitive and emotional inputs from the other areas of the brain; (4) intrinsic neural inhibitory modulation inherent in all brain functions; and (5) the activity of the body's stress-regulation systems, including cytokines and the endocrine, autonomic, immune, and opioid systems. (From Melzack R: From the gate to the neuromatrix. Pain Aug(Suppl 6):S121-S126, 1999.)

to develop fewer maladaptive psychological sequelae than those whose passive coping style relinquishes control of their pain to others.[21] A tendency toward somatization is frequently observed in patients with chronic pain, although it is difficult to be certain whether this is cause or effect.[22] Anger and hostility may adversely affect adjustment among chronic pain patients,[23] and these patients have an increased tendency to suffer from depression and chronic pain.[22] Learning and conditioning can also play a role in the development and maintenance of chronic pain.

Because pain can only be evaluated by self-report and behavior, increasing pain behavior is often equated with increasing pain. If the pain behavior results in some reward for the patient, that behavior is reinforced and may persist despite resolution of the underlying painful stimulus.[24] By the same token, animal studies have demonstrated what appears to be increased sensitivity to painful stimuli through classic and operant conditioning.[25] There are also rare cases in which pain behavior is feigned for secondary gain or when the patient's true psychogenic pain is more readily explained by psychological rather than nociceptive terminology. However, the physician should be constantly vigilant to guard against the natural tendency to classify an exasperating patient as "psychogenic" without thoroughly evaluating all potential causes of pain.

If a thorough psychological and physical evaluation reveals a preponderance of psychological mechanisms over pathophysiologic mechanisms, behavioral and psychological interventions should take precedence over pharmacologic interventions. Patients should be encouraged to take an active role in their pain management and adopt an attitude of "learning to live with the pain." There is some evidence that this type of attitude allows the patient greater long-term adjustment and better quality of life.[20] However, a mix of pathophysiologic and psychological mechanisms are present in most cases. It is therefore important to be familiar with the psychological and behavioral aspects of pain treatment as well as the pharmacologic interventions.

PHARMACOLOGIC TARGETS

In considering the physiology of the pain perception pathways and the mechanisms of chronic pain, it is evident that there are several fruitful avenues of pharmacologic treatment available. Centrally and peripherally acting agents can be used, with the consequence that nociceptive systems can be modulated at various points.

The following principles of pharmacologic treatment of chronic pain have been suggested by Aronoff and Gallagher[26] and serve as a good starting point for the design of any medical treatment regimen for chronic pain:

1. Make safety a priority when treating nonmalignant chronic pain.

2. Make efficacy a priority when treating a terminally ill patient with pain.

3. Review potential interactions with medical conditions and with other medications.

4. Selectively choose drugs for pain disorder and comorbid psychiatric disorder according to efficacy and specific mechanism.

5. Balance the side-effect profile against efficacy.

6. Consider drugs' effects on the efficacy of other analgesics.

7. Consider behavioral effects when prescribing.

8. Select combinations of medications from different classes.

9. Establish a reliable method of monitoring pain and activity levels.

10. Avoid irrational polypharmacy.

As a prerequisite to any medication trial, a thorough evaluation of the patient must be performed, including a detailed history and physical examination, review of prior records and imaging studies, and formulation of a working differential diagnosis. Although a disease-specific diagnosis may not be reached, knowledge of the mechanisms of chronic pain and their clinical characteristics as discussed previously can help to guide the selection of initial modes of therapy.

Peripherally Acting Medications

ANTI-INFLAMMATORY AGENTS

Inflammatory mediators trigger arachidonic acid production in a variety of different cell populations, re-sulting in the formation of prostanoids (i.e., prostaglandins and thromboxanes) through the cyclooxygenase (COX) pathway and leukotrienes through the lipoxygenase pathway.

Inhibition of COX by nonsteroidal anti-inflammatory drugs (NSAIDs) results in the prevention of prostaglandin formation and therefore exerts analgesic and anti-inflammatory effects.[27] Two isoforms of COX have been identified: COX-1 and COX-2.[28] COX-1 influences a number of cellular housekeeping functions through its promotion of synthesis of prostaglandins and thromboxane A_2. Prostaglandins are involved in maintaining the integrity of the gastrointestinal mucosal lining, limiting gastric acid secretion, and regulating renal hemodynamics and water-electrolyte balance. Thromboxane A_2 stimulates platelet aggregation and mediates vasoconstriction, both of which are important in normal hemostasis. COX-2 metabolites are intimately involved in the induction of pain and inflammation. Conventional NSAIDs such as acetylsalicylic acid (aspirin) act as inhibitors of COX-1 and COX-2, although their anti-inflammatory and analgesic effects are expressed only through COX-2 inhibition. The COX-1 inhibition is responsible for the side effects commonly seen, including gastric mucosal lesions and ulceration, renal toxicity, blockade of platelet aggregation, and hepatic dysfunction.[29, 30]

Identification of COX-2 swiftly led to the development of COX-2–specific inhibitors,[31] of which celecoxib is perhaps the best known. Celecoxib has been shown to be effective in alleviating acute pain and chronic inflammatory pain,[32] with an adverse event profile similar to that of placebo.

Acetaminophen is included in the category of NSAIDs, and although it has good analgesic and antipyretic effects, it is only very weakly anti-inflammatory. There is, however, a well-known risk of hepatotoxicity with increasing cumulative dosage.[33-37] Acetaminophen acts on sites in the CNS that may mediate its efficacy as an analgesic agent.[38] Acetaminophen is equally effective and equipotent with aspirin in single-dose studies of pain due to carcinoma, postoperative pain, and headache, although it is far less effective in the treatment of inflammatory conditions such as rheumatoid arthritis.

Corticosteroids are very potent anti-inflammatories; however, when used in doses high enough to elicit their anti-inflammatory effects, they produce less desirable effects such as suppression of the hypothalamic-pituitary-adrenal axis, weight gain, skeletal muscle wasting, suppression of the immune response and diabetes mellitus. Their use is therefore limited in chronic pain conditions. Occasionally, rheumatoid patients are placed on steroids, although at the lowest possible dose and for the shortest time.

ANTICONVULSANTS AND OTHER ION CHANNEL BLOCKERS

Normal functioning of voltage-gated sodium channels in axons is vital for the conduction of neuronal signals.

Abnormal ion channel activity probably plays a prominent role in the genesis of chronic pain. Anticonvulsants probably exert their beneficial effect by blocking sodium channels and suppressing ectopic neuronal discharges. Phenytoin, carbamazepine, sodium valproate, and clonazepam suppress spontaneous neuronal firing.[39] Carbamazepine also exerts analgesic effects by the central potentiation of adrenoceptors and by increasing the noradrenergic output from the locus ceruleus, thereby enhancing descending inhibition.[40] Many studies[41–45] have demonstrated the efficacy of anticonvulsants in neuropathic, chronic dysesthetic, and cancer-related neuropathic pain; in post-herpetic and deafferentation neuralgia; and in pain from radiation fibrosis and surgical scarring.

Another anticonvulsant, gabapentin, initially developed as a γ-aminobutyric acid (GABA) analog, has proven efficacy in the treatment of neuropathic pain,[46] trigeminal neuralgia,[47] painful diabetic neuropathy,[48] and post-herpetic neuralgia.[49] It has a superior adverse event profile compared with other anticonvulsants, and its chief side effects are mild somnolence, dizziness, and fatigue.[50] Most actions of gabapentin are central, but it has been demonstrated to decrease sustained firing of sodium-dependent action potentials in vitro.[51]

Other drugs acting on sodium channels include local anesthetics for regional, local, and trigger-point blocks (see Chapter 184) and antiarrhythmics, specifically mexiletine, which has been successfully used to treat neuropathic pain[52] and painful diabetic neuropathy.[53]

TRICYCLIC ANTIDEPRESSANTS

In addition to their well-known central antidepressant activity, tricyclic antidepressants (TCAs) have a peripheral mechanism of action mediated by sodium channel blockade. A general feature of these drugs is the ability to selectively block ectopic discharges without affecting axonal conduction.[54] One explanation for this selectivity is that the activity-dependent action of many sodium channel blocking drugs[55] may result in inhibition of the tonic ongoing discharges at concentrations too low to interfere with action potential conduction under normal physiologic conditions.

Among the TCAs used in the treatment of chronic pain, amitriptyline is the most commonly prescribed and the most thoroughly studied. As well as the central effects and mood-altering effects on analgesia, amitriptyline has peripheral analgesic effects mediated in part by an interaction with endogenous adenosine.[56] Amitriptyline is also known to bind and block histamine H$_1$, α$_2$-adrenergic, and serotonin receptors in the periphery that may contribute to its antinociceptive effect.[57] Amitriptyline and other TCAs interact with opioid receptors,[58] and naloxone can block the antinociceptive action of systemically administered antidepressants.

OPIOIDS

As well as the established central analgesic effects of opioids, immune cells have been shown to produce endogenous opioids during inflammation,[59] and this is matched by increased expression of opioid receptors on primary afferent nociceptors where they exert analgesic activity.[60] Experimental models of inflammatory and neuropathic pain suggest that the antinociceptive effect of opioids in part results from their action on primary nerve terminals and sympathetic fibers. This is supported by the observation that the mechanical hyperalgesia induced by inflammatory mediators is attenuated by opioid agonists and that their effect is blocked by naloxone.

Centrally Acting Agents

OPIOIDS

The opioid analgesics are the oldest and still the most effective centrally acting medications prescribed for the treatment of pain. Opioids exert their profound analgesic effects by activation of opioid receptors located on primary nociceptive neurons, on transmission cells and interneurons in the spinal cord, and in supraspinal sites. The same opioid receptors are normally activated by the endogenous opioids, including the enkephalins, endorphins, and dynorphins. Opioid analgesics mimic the actions of these endogenous ligands by binding to opioid receptors (μ, δ, and κ), decreasing neurotransmission by several mechanisms. Binding of an opioid to its receptor causes a conformational change in the receptor, which causes activation of a G protein bound to the inner surface of the cell membrane. The G protein then dissociates into its two subunits (α and βγ), which subsequently interact with their targets. Opioid receptors act through several different G proteins, coupling directly and indirectly to ion channels and other effector systems. The μ and δ receptors are coupled to G protein–activated K$^+$ channels, with the consequence that activation of these receptors causes efflux of K$^+$ ions with resulting hyperpolarization of the cell and decrease in excitability of the membrane. Activation of μ and κ receptors inhibits Ca^{2+} influx by means of inhibitory G proteins, which couple directly to voltage-activated Ca^{2+} channels. Because intracellular Ca^{2+} is necessary for binding of synaptic vesicles to the cell membrane, a decrease in the intracellular calcium concentration causes decreased binding of synaptic vesicles and decreased neurotransmitter release, leading to a presynaptic inhibitory action. In addition to the direct actions on ion channels, opioid receptors and coupled G proteins also act on the membrane-bound enzyme adenylyl cyclase to increase intracellular concentrations of cyclic AMP (cAMP), which acts as a second messenger for a number of regulatory cell processes.

Sites of Action

Opioid receptors have been found at spinal and supraspinal sites, especially in the brainstem,[1] as part of the descending modulatory pathways and in the limbic system. The amygdala, nucleus accumbens, periaqueductal gray, mesencephalic reticular formation, substantia nigra, and the medial medulla contain opioid receptors that participate in complex modulatory pathways (see Fig. 183–4). The descending pain control circuitry that originates in these central structures is modulated by opioids, as are higher centers that participate in the perception of pain. The relationships between these various sites of opioid modulation are subjects of ongoing studies, which hope to exploit them with more specific ligands.

Treatment Dilemmas of Opioid Use for Chronic Pain

Opioid analgesics remain the most effective means of alleviating severe pain across a wide range of conditions that includes acute, persistent inflammatory, and neuropathic pain states.[61] Although numerous studies have demonstrated the benefits of opioid use in cancer pain, there is ongoing debate regarding the appropriate use of opioids in nonmalignant pain. Some investigators believe that the use of opioids in nonmalignant pain is never appropriate,[62] but others cautiously advocate their use in well-controlled circumstances. Personal experience and the results of several studies indicate that there is a subpopulation of patients with chronic nonmalignant pain who can benefit from long-term opioid use and who will not develop tolerance, addiction, or dose escalation. However, the use of opioids in this population requires a thorough understanding of several issues, including opioid responsiveness, side-effect profile, tolerance, dependence, and addiction.

Opioid Responsiveness

Opioid *responsiveness* can be defined as the balance between analgesia and dose-limiting side effects during dose titration.[63] Both of these end points can be difficult to identify and must be determined by the patient and pain practitioner. Whereas acute nociceptive pain and chronic pain related to tissue damage usually respond well to opioids,[64] chronic pain of musculoskeletal origin or idiopathic pain may not respond as well.[65] It was long thought that neuropathic pain was not opioid responsive,[65] but later studies have suggested otherwise.[66–69] Patient-related factors that influence responsiveness to opioids can include predisposition to side effects, ongoing psychological distress, or prior opioid exposure. Responsiveness may vary between different opioids for any individual patient.[66] If a decision is made to institute opioid therapy, titration with sequential agents may reveal one that exhibits a markedly better ratio of analgesic effect to side effects. Knowledge of an equianalgesic table is indispensable in this case. Overall, the use of opioids in chronic, nonmalignant pain can achieve analgesic benefit for at least some patients, although psychological and functional improvement may be much less likely.[70]

Side Effects

Although many patients experience transient side effects when first started on opioid therapy, the percentage of patients who experience persistent side effects is relatively low.[71] Tolerance usually develops

quickly to nausea, but a few patients have persistent nausea with all groups of opiates at effective doses. Tolerance to constipation develops slowly, if at all, but can be managed successfully with stimulant laxatives and stool softeners. Although all opioids act through a limited subset of receptors, each opioid medication has different affinities for each receptor and may exhibit different efficacy and side-effect profiles. At least one double-blind, crossover study has demonstrated differences in the side-effect profile between different opioids, although the mechanism for this remains unclear.[72] Sedation and cognitive impairment are often noticed by patients when receiving opiates for acute pain, and it is therefore not unreasonable to assume there may be long-term effects on psychomotor performance and cognition associated with chronic use. On the contrary, in most cases, significant cognitive and psychomotor changes do not usually persist after an individual has adapted to a particular dose of opioid,[70, 73, 74] and tolerance usually develops to the cognitive effects of opioid drugs. Regarding cognition and level of function, the practitioner must also recognize the deleterious effects of uncontrolled pain on concentration and performance. Insomnia, decreased sexual function, and persistent sweating have also been reported as side effects of chronic opioid use.[71]

Tolerance and Dose Escalation

When increasing doses of opioids become necessary to produce the same analgesic effect, the effect is referred to as *tolerance*. Tolerance to the analgesic effects of opioids has been readily demonstrated in animals[75]; however, painful stimuli given before opioid administration can prevent the development of tolerance. Most studies of chronic pain populations show that opioid dosage can remain stable for long periods with little or no dose escalation,[76–78] whereas there is some evidence from other series that tolerance does occur.[79] Studies of cancer patients have suggested that dose escalation is usually related to disease progression.[80] Rapid dose escalation suggests that the pain may be poorly opioid responsive, and tapering the medication dosage should be considered.

Physical Dependence

Physical dependence is defined as the development of withdrawal symptoms after abrupt discontinuation or substantial dose reduction of an opioid medication or after the administration of an antagonist. It is generally accepted that all patients who are treated with opioids for any significant length of time will exhibit some degree of physical dependence, although patients can sometimes be withdrawn from medication after lengthy treatment without undue side effects.[81] Common symptoms of opioid withdrawal include irritability, anxiety, sleeplessness, diarrhea, sweating, and piloerection. Patients may also complain of marked increase in pain, as well as generalized aching and deep pain throughout the body. An important theoretical concern is the development of a vicious cycle in which patients are maintained on opioid therapy only to avoid withdrawal symptoms rather than for relief of pain.[62] Patients may report that the medication does not help the pain so much as "take the edge off." For patients who were previously obtaining good pain relief, a small dose escalation may alleviate the problem. However, for patients who never achieved significant therapeutic efficacy, discontinuation of the medication should be considered.

Addiction

The fear of creating addicts underlies most of the reluctance to use opioids in patients with chronic pain; however, there are few hard data to substantiate this concern. *Addiction* can be defined as a maladaptive behavioral change whereby the patient loses control over the use of opioids, becomes preoccupied with their use despite adequate pain relief, and continues their use in the face of apparent adverse consequences.[82] Several studies have shown that the incidence of addiction in patients being treated for various types of pain is low, ranging from 0.1% to 0.04%. In one brief report, 4 of 11,582 patients without a history of substance abuse who were treated with opioids in hospital developed evidence of addiction.[83] A survey of burn units revealed no cases of addiction in more than 10,000 patients treated for burn pain,[84] and a survey of more than 2000 patients attending a headache clinic revealed only three cases of opioid abuse.[85] However, a number of studies have reported relatively high rates of aberrant drug use in multidisciplinary pain management programs.[71]

The contradictions in the literature prevent any de-finitive statement regarding addiction in patients being treated with long-term opioids. Constant vigilance and close follow-up are essential to identify patients who may have developed an addiction to their opioid medications. Several behaviors are more or less predictive of opioid addiction. The management of addiction is beyond the scope of this chapter, but it should include consultation with a specialist in the management of opioid addiction. The physician must be wary of patients who present to the clinic with a history of opioid use. Although many of these patients may have been treated properly for a legitimate pain complaint, others may be addicted to their medications, may be selling or diverting them, and may be obtaining medications from various physicians. In an attempt to decrease abuse or addiction and to detect such problems as soon as possible, patients should be counseled, and it is recommended that a contract be made between physician and patient (Fig. 183–6). Although such a written contract does not prevent abuse or addiction, it can help clarify the roles and responsibilities of the patient and the physician, and it may help to deter those who seek to exploit the system.

Practical Issues of Opioid Use for Chronic Pain Management

The use of long-term opioid therapy in nonmalignant chronic pain remains controversial. Although there are risks involved with the use of opioids, rational use in selected patients can greatly improve quality of life and produce gratifying outcomes. Portenoy[71] developed some useful guidelines for the use of opi-

---

**Consent for Opioid (Narcotic) Management
In Nonmalignant Pain**

Department of Surgery
Division of Neurosurgery
3635 Vista Ave. at Grand Blvd.
PO Box 15250
St. Louis, MO 63110-0250
Phone: 314-577-8795
Fax: 314-268-5061

_____
Patient Name

Jaimie M. Henderson, MD at the Saint Louis University Health Sciences Center (SLUHSC) has decided to use opioids (narcotics) to manage your chronic pain since other treatments have failed to bring relief. The goal of this treatment is to improve your functional ability as well as your social and work activities. This form of treatment has risks and potential side effects which are listed as follows:

1) Sedation
2) Constipation
3) Nausea and vomiting
4) Confusion or change in thinking abilities
5) Difficulty with balance which may make it unsafe to operate heavy equipment or motor vehicles
6) Sleepiness and drowsiness
7) Decreased respiration or breathing
8) Physical dependence, which means if you abruptly stop taking this medication you may withdraw. Signs of withdrawal include diarrhea, abdominal cramping, "goose flesh," and anxiety.
9) Psychological dependence or addiction
10) Tolerance, which means that you may need more drug to get the same effect
11) Risks regarding pregnancy; children born to mothers on opioids will likely be physically dependent to the drug at birth.

FIGURE 183–6. Pain contract and consent form as used at St. Louis University.

Jaimie M. Henderson, MD at SLUHSC is willing to treat you with opioids (narcotics) under the following guidelines and conditions:

1) Other reasonable non-opioid treatment measures have been ineffective or have produced intolerable side effects.
2) The patient does not have current problems with substance abuse or dependence.
3) The patient has never been involved in the sale, diversion, illegal possession or transport of controlled substances including narcotics, sleeping pills, nerve pills and/or pain killers.
4) The patient will obtain all narcotic prescriptions from the SLUHSC.
5) The patient will take the medications exactly as prescribed by the SLUHSC and under no circumstances allow any other individual to take these medications.
6) The patient will contact Dr. Henderson's office 5–7 days before refills are required.
7) The patient will provide Dr. Henderson's office with the name and phone number of their pharmacy. Dr. Henderson's office must be notified in advance with the reason of any proposed pharmacy change.
8) The patient allows any physician at the SLUHSC to communicate with the patient's referring physical and/or any pharmacists regarding the use of opioids. To this end, we will provide the referring and/or primary care physician with a copy of this contract.
9) The patient will follow the advice of Dr. Jaimie M. Henderson at the SLUHSC in regards to stopping controlled substances if it is felt that this will be necessary.
10) Patient consents to unannounced blood screen tests in order to properly assess the effect of narcotics and patient compliance.
11) If the patient is a female of child bearing years, the patient certifies that she is not pregnant and will use appropriate measures to prevent pregnancy during the course of this treatment.
12) The patient will keep all scheduled appointments at the SLUHSC and will bring medications with them for pill counts.
13) The patient understands that NO ALLOWANCE will be made for lost prescriptions of drugs.
14) Should the patient feel that they require more opioid (narcotic) than has been prescribed they must contact Dr. Jaimie M. Henderson PRIOR to increasing the dose. If this is not done, prescriptions will not be refilled early. *It is the patient's responsibility to call for refills. No telephone calls will be taken from family members.*
15) The patient understands that this treatment option will be discontinued if any of the following occur:
    a) if Dr. Jaimie M. Henderson feels that the opioids have not been effectively managing your pain.
    b) if the patient gives away, sells or misuses the drugs
    c) if the patient develops rapid tolerance or loss of effect from the opioid
    d) if the side effects become intolerable
    e) if the patient obtains opioids from any source other than SLUHSC.
16) If we choose to discontinue your opioid treatment, we will gradually lower the dose over several days to avoid withdrawal symptoms. If Dr. Jaimie M. Henderson feels you have a dependence problem, we may refer you elsewhere for management of that dependency.

I have read this document, understand it, and have had all questions answered satisfactorily. I consent to the use of opioids (narcotics) to help control my pain and understand that the treatment will be conducted in accordance with the conditions stated above.

_____   _____
Patient Signature   Date

_____   _____
Jaimie M. Henderson, MD   Date

FIGURE 183–6. *Continued.*

oids in nonmalignant pain. After the institution of opiate therapy, careful monitoring is required during the titration phase to assess the analgesic effect and side effects. Patients should be seen at regular intervals and compliance with functional goals ascertained, as well as remaining vigilant to the possibility of addiction or abuse.

Indications for the termination of opioid therapy include the opioid being ineffective in the treatment of the pain, intolerable side effects, or the development of aberrant use behavior. The dosage is tapered slowly to lessen the unpleasant side effects associated with physiologic dependency. Clonidine and benzodiazepines are often used to assist in the attenuation of these effects. In cases of chronic pain unrelated to progressive disease that is being successfully managed by multiple drugs or modalities, it is prudent to intermittently attempt opiate withdrawal.

Some patients, despite years of opioid treatment, can be withdrawn from medication with relatively few side effects. Patients may voluntarily request withdrawal from opioids after some time. This may not be caused by any lack of efficacy of the medication but instead may reflect the changing attitudes of the patient in finding alternative methods to control the pain.

TRICYCLIC ANTIDEPRESSANTS

The use of antidepressants is well established in the treatment of chronic pain states such as peripheral neuropathy, diabetic neuropathy, post-herpetic neuralgia, and chronic headache.[86] The effectiveness of the antidepressants may result from several potential mechanisms, including a direct analgesic effect, amelioration of comorbid psychiatric disorders, and reduction of pain-related symptoms such as poor appetite and disturbed sleep. There is relatively good evidence for a direct analgesic effect of TCAs, based on observations that analgesia can occur at doses lower than those generally used for antidepressant effect[87] and of their analgesic effectiveness even in the absence of depression.[88] TCAs may exert their antinociceptive activity through several mechanisms. They inhibit the central reuptake of norepinephrine and serotonin, enhancing the action of these neurotransmitters in descending inhibition.[89] Inflammatory models have implicated spinal antagonism of NMDA receptors in the action of amitriptyline.[90] The peripheral action of TCAs has already been reviewed. Amitriptyline also blocks activated sodium channels and therefore has the ability to inhibit pain-generating ectopic activity in the CNS,[91] an effect that may be important in the treatment of central pain.

An important observation, which is not explained by the proposed mechanisms of action of the TCAs, is that reuptake blockade occurs promptly, but pain relief often takes more than a week to manifest, and an antidepressant effect may take several weeks.[89] This is an important pharmacodynamic factor to consider when prescribing TCAs, and patients should be informed about the delay between initiation of therapy and beneficial effect.

The older TCAs have a significant side-effect profile because of their anticholinergic (muscarinic) action and antagonistic effects at histamine H_1 receptors and α_1 adrenoceptors.[91] The side effects commonly experienced are similar to other anticholinergic agents and include dry mouth, blurred vision, tachycardia, urinary retention, decreased gastric emptying, and ileus. Cardiovascular side effects include orthostatic hypotension and dysrhythmias, contraindicating the use of TCAs in patients with atrioventricular node conduction defects. CNS side effects are mainly those of sedation and reduced seizure threshold in patients with known epilepsy. TCAs interact with a number of other commonly prescribed medications, including sympathomimetics and anticholinergics. Concomitant use of TCAs and monoamine oxidase inhibitors can cause life-threatening side effects of hyperthermia, seizures, or coma.

SELECTIVE SEROTONIN REUPTAKE INHIBITORS

The selective serotonin reuptake inhibitors (SSRIs) are the most broadly prescribed drugs for the treatment of depression and are the drugs of choice for the treatment of mild to moderate depression. Compared with the TCAs, SSRIs have little effect on norepinephrine reuptake. SSRIs lack anticholinergic properties and therefore do not cause postural hypotension or delayed cardiac conduction, nor do they have any effect on seizure threshold. The common side effects of the SSRIs include insomnia, agitation, headache, nausea, diarrhea, and sexual dysfunction. Fluoxetine is a potent inhibitor of the cytochrome P450 enzyme system and therefore is prone to drug interactions with other drugs metabolized by cytochrome P450, including phenytoin, carbamazepine, and warfarin. The relatively benign side-effect and toxicity profile of SSRIs compared with the TCAs favors their use when there is no therapeutic advantage to using TCAs or when TCAs are relatively contraindicated because of the risks of cardiac conduction defects, seizures, and suicide.

Activation of descending antinociceptive serotonergic pathways by the SSRIs makes them an attractive choice in the treatment of chronic pain. Several placebo-controlled trials have shown the effectiveness of SSRIs in the treatment of neuropathic pain.[92] However, larger studies are required to accurately compare the efficacy of SSRI treatment with TCAs, which are the most effective antidepressant agents for the treatment of neuropathic pain.

Tramadol

Tramadol is an inhibitor of norepinephrine and serotonin reuptake (similar to some antidepressants) and a weak μ-opioid receptor agonist (approximately 1/6000 the potency of morphine). A double blind, placebo-controlled study demonstrated tramadol to provide better pain relief compared with placebo in the treatment of painful diabetic neuropathy.[93] Because of the weak opioid effect, mild withdrawal symptoms may occur on discontinuation. Seizures have been reported at high doses, especially in patients with a history of seizure activity.

GABAergic AGENTS

GABA is a major inhibitory amino acid neurotransmitter in the CNS. Its actions are mediated by two receptor types, $GABA_A$ and $GABA_B$, found throughout the CNS.[94] They are also found on primary afferents and dorsal horn neurons,[94, 95] with the latter contributing to inhibitory control at the spinal level.[96] $GABA_A$ agonists such as muscimol and $GABA_B$ agonists including baclofen have antinociceptive effects at the level of the spinal cord.[97, 98]

Baclofen

As well as antinociceptive actions mediated by virtue of its agonist action at $GABA_B$ receptors, baclofen can act as an agonist at opioid receptors. The antinociceptive effect of baclofen is reversed by pretreatment with naloxone, and systemically administered baclofen potentiates morphine-induced antinociception.[99] Baclofen has been used to some effect in the treatment of peripheral neuropathies and trigeminal neuralgia, phantom orofacial pain, migraine, and carcinoma pain as a second-line drug. One of the major uses of baclofen in the treatment of chronic pain states is in the treatment of coexisting spasticity or spasms.

Gabapentin

Gabapentin was developed to be structurally similar to GABA, but with increased lipophilicity to aid its entry into the CNS.[100] It was developed and subsequently approved for use as an anticonvulsant agent for add-on use with the well-established anticonvulsants. After clinical use, gabapentin was reported to have therapeutic activity against various chronic pain states.[101, 102] Studies have established the unequivocal efficacy of gabapentin in the treatment of chronic pain states, especially painful neuropathies. Two double-blind, placebo-controlled studies[46, 48] showed gabapentin to be significantly better than placebo in decreasing pain associated with diabetic peripheral neuropathy. Other studies have found gabapentin to be effective in the treatment of painful diabetic neuropathy,[103] trigeminal neuralgia,[47] reflex sympathetic dystrophy (i.e., complex regional pain syndrome),[104] and the pain and sleep disturbance associated with post-herpetic neuralgia.[49, 105]

Gabapentin does not interact with $GABA_A$ or $GABA_B$ receptors,[106] nor does it alter neuronal or glial uptake of GABA.[107] Gabapentin interacts with GABA-transaminase,[108] the enzyme catalyzing GABA degradation, and increases the activity of partially purified glutamic acid decarboxylase (GAD) in vitro,[109] producing both of these effects at high concentrations. The effect on GAD suggests that gabapentin may increase the synthesis of GABA from glutamate in brain tissues. In vivo, nuclear magnetic resonance spectroscopy in humans has indicated that brain levels of GABA are elevated after gabapentin treatment.[110, 111] Further animal in vivo experiments have indicated that the increase in GABA levels on treatment with gabapentin is caused by increased GABA synthesis by the promotion of activity of GAD.[112] Gabapentin seems to act as a weak blocker of ion channels.[51]

Most of the reporting of the side effects of gabapentin has come from studies investigating gabapentin as an add-on agent in the treatment of epilepsy.[50, 113, 114] In most cases, the side effects were mild and included mainly somnolence, dizziness, fatigue, headache, ataxia, and weight gain. The side effects tended to be dose dependent and transient. The side-effect profile of gabapentin is low compared with other antiepileptics. There is no documentation of long-term toxicity, active metabolites, hepatic enzyme induction, or major drug interactions associated with the use of gabapentin,[115] which led to its immediate and widespread use.[116]

Pregabalin

Further investigation of 3-alkylated GABA systems led to the identification of 3-isobutyl-GABA (pregabalin), which appears to have the same mechanism of action as gabapentin and similar pharmacologic profile, although with greater potency demonstrated in several preclinical models.[117] It has been identified as a novel anticonvulsant and a potential treatment for various pain states. Pregabalin is undergoing a number of clinical trials in this area.

OTHER AGENTS

Clonidine

Clonidine is a centrally acting partial α_2-adrenergic agonist that is typically used as an antihypertensive drug. It also has analgesic effects thought to be mediated by stimulation of inhibitory bulbospinal pathways[118] and by activation of postsynaptic α_2 receptors in the substantia gelatinosa of the spinal cord,[119] which results in membrane hyperpolarization and thereby reduces nociceptive ascending transmission. The α_2 receptors are located on the primary afferent terminals of neurons located in the superficial laminae of the spinal cord and within several brainstem nuclei implicated in analgesia,[120] supporting the possibility of analgesic action at peripheral, spinal, and brainstem sites.

Clonidine is more potent when administered intrathecally than when given systemically, indicating a spinal site of action and favoring neuraxial administration.[121, 122] Oral and transdermal preparations have been effective in the treatment painful diabetic neuropathy[123] and post-herpetic neuralgia.[124] Clonidine can be considered for these indications as a second-line drug to the anticonvulsants and antidepressants. Its use as an intrathecal agent is expanding, but a detailed discussion is beyond the scope of this chapter.

NMDA Receptor Antagonists

Glutamate is one of the major excitatory neurotransmitters, and glutamatergic NMDA and non-NMDA receptors are widely distributed throughout the central and peripheral nervous systems. NMDA receptors in the spinal cord dorsal horn may play a large role in the development and maintenance of neuropathic pain. Spinal administration of NMDA receptor antagonists has reduced or reversed the expansion of receptive fields and reduced the enhanced dorsal horn responses and the behavioral hyperalgesia observed after experimental inflammation.[125] Ketamine, a phencyclidine derivative that produces dissociative anesthesia, is a potent analgesic at subanesthetic concentrations, most likely as a result of its NMDA receptor antagonism, but it also interacts with opioid, monoaminergic, and muscarinic receptors.[126] Clinical studies have established the efficacy of NMDA receptor antagonists for hyperalgesic and allodynic pain states, but they also produce significant psychotomimetic effects,[127] cognitive impairment,[128] and neurotoxicity.[129] Accordingly, available NMDA receptor antagonists have not found widespread use for the management of chronic pain. However, this field represents an active area of research, and the modulation of NMDA receptors holds promise in the treatment of chronic pain because of their role in excitatory neurotransmission and neural plasticity.

Adenosine

Adenosine and ATP exert multiple influences on pain transmission at peripheral and spinal sites.[130] It has been postulated that the antinociception produced by supraspinal and spinal opioid administration is partly caused by the release of adenosine in the spinal cord.[131] In an animal model of neuropathic pain, spinal adenosine was found to potentiate the antinociceptive effects of spinal morphine in an additive manner.[132] Despite these theoretical advantages, systemic adenosine administration in humans appears to offer only transient pain relief.[133]

EMOTIONAL AND BEHAVIORAL ASPECTS OF PAIN AND THEIR MANAGEMENT

Treatment of the psychological sequelae of chronic pain cannot be overemphasized. All patients with chronic pain of significant duration experience some degree of adverse psychological effects. Truly effective management of chronic pain requires attention to analgesia and pain relief, as well as a decrease in the depression, anxiety, and social stressors that affect the patient's emotional well-being. Pain and depression are often self-perpetuating; inadequately treated pain can cause depression, and ongoing depression can worsen the perception of pain. Patients need pharmacologic and behavioral therapy to help with their depression and anxiety.

Antidepressants

If depression is identified, antidepressants should be commenced and titrated to the levels necessary for antidepressant effects over the course of 2 to 3 weeks. For neuropathic pain, TCAs are the drugs of choice, but in the absence of neuropathic pain, SSRIs are the drugs of choice because of their lower side-effect profile and fewer drug interactions. Specialist psychiatric consultation should be sought sooner rather than later in cases of identified depression, because there is considerable physical, psychological, and social morbidity associated with untreated depression.[134]

Anxiolytics

Anxiety is a psychological state associated with stress and is frequently comorbid with chronic pain, precipitating and perpetuating the pain. Anxiety can also induce deleterious autonomic effects such as increased arousal, tremor, increased muscle tension, and other psychophysiologic effects such as irritable bowel syndrome and stress headaches. Benzodiazepines are often used as anxiolytics. Their mechanism of action is suppression of serotonin release and stimulation of inhibitory GABA receptors. Benzodiazepines are effective in postoperative pain[135] and have been of some use in chronic pain states. Their long-term use for anxiolysis is not recommended because of tolerance, dependence, and cognitive effects. Antihistamines such as diphenhydramine are an alternative for the treatment of anxiety and sleep disturbance. Psychotherapy is also useful in anxiety states.

Behavioral and Physical Therapy

Several behavioral approaches, including relaxation techniques, biofeedback, hypnotic techniques, and cognitive behavioral treatments, can lead to long-term reductions in pain intensity and increases in physical functioning.[136] Physical therapy should be part of any chronic pain treatment regimen, with a focus on maintenance of conditioning, muscle tone, and proper posture. A structured program of therapy can also help motivate the patient, serving as a roadmap to improved functioning and eventual reintegration into the home and workplace. Heat, massage, ice, deep ultrasound therapy, and other treatments can help alleviate pain for short periods and may be useful during periods of increased pain.

CONCLUSIONS

The medical management of chronic pain is one of the most difficult challenges in medicine. It requires knowledge of myriad anatomic and chemical pathways; an ability to communicate effectively with patients who are angry, frustrated, and depressed; intimate familiarity with psychological aspects and personality traits; and strict attention to detail regarding treatment plans, follow-up evaluations, and medication administration. It has been suggested, and we would agree, that an attitude of compassionate skepticism be maintained when dealing with the patient with chronic pain. The physician must always be on guard against manipulation, secondary gain, narcotic abuse, and outright pathologic or criminal behavior that can sometimes be well hidden. However, this must be tempered with all the compassion that can be mustered, because as Milton wrote in *Paradise Lost*: "Pain is a perfect miserie, the worst of evils, and excessive, overturns all patience."

REFERENCES

1. Yaksh T: Central pharmacology of nociceptive transmission. In Wall PD, Melzack R (eds): Textbook of Pain. Edinburgh, Churchill Livingstone, 1999, pp 253–308.
2. Melzack R, Wall PD: Pain mechanisms: A new theory. Science 150:971–979, 1965.
3. LeBars D, Dickenson AH, Besson JM, et al: Aspects of sensory processing through convergent neurons. In Yaksh TL (ed): Spinal Afferent Processing. New York, Plenum Press, 1986, pp 467–504.
4. Kerr FWL: Pain: A central inhibitory balance theory. Mayo Clin Proc 50:685–690, 1975.
5. Henderson JM: Intrathecal opioids. I. Mechanisms of action. In Burchiel K (ed): Pain Surgery. New York, Thieme. (in press).
6. Bonica JJ, Yaksh TL, Liebeskind JC, et al: Biochemistry and modulation of nociception and pain. In Bonica JJ (ed): The Management of Pain. Philadelphia, Lea & Febiger, 1990, pp 95–121.
7. Dray A: Neurogenic mechanisms and neuropeptides in chronic

pain. In Carli G, Zimmerman M (eds): Progress in Brain Research, vol 110. New York, Elsevier, 1996, pp 85–94.

8. Bevan SJ: Nociceptive peripheral neurons: Cellular properties. In Wall PD, Melzack R (eds): Textbook of Pain. Edinburgh, Churchill Livingstone, 1999, pp 85–103.

9. Green PG, Basbaum AI, Levine JD: Sensory neuropeptide interactions in the production of plasma extravasation in the rat. Neuroscience 50:745–749, 1992.

10. Koltzenburg M: The changing sensitivity in the life of the nociceptor. Pain Aug(Suppl 6):S93–S102, 1999.

11. Woolf CJ, Safieh-Garabedian B, Ma QP, et al: Nerve growth factor contributes to the generation of inflammatory sensory hypersensitivity. Neuroscience 62:327–331, 1994.

12. Watson A, Ensor E, Symes A, et al: A minimal CGRP gene promoter is inducible by nerve growth factor in adult rat dorsal root ganglion neurons but not in PC12 phaeochromocytoma cells. Eur J Neurosci 7:394–400, 1995.

13. Valtschanoff JG, Weinberg RJ, Rustioni A: Central release of tracer after noxious stimulation of the skin suggests non-synaptic signaling by unmyelinated fibers. Neuroscience 64:851–854, 1995.

14. Diamond J, Holmes M, Coughlin M: Endogenous NGF and nerve impulses regulate the collateral sprouting of sensory axons in the skin of the adult rat. J Neurosci 12:1454–1466, 1992.

15. Devor M, Seltzer Z: Pathophysiology of damaged nerves in relation to chronic pain. In Wall PD, Melzack R (eds): Textbook of Pain. Edinburgh, Churchill Livingstone, 1999, pp 129–164.

16. Doubell TP, Mannion R, Woolf C: The dorsal horn: State-dependent sensory processing, plasticity and the generation of pain. In Wall PD, Melzack R (eds): Textbook of Pain. Edinburgh, Churchill Livingstone, 1999, pp 165–181.

17. Boivie J: Central Pain. In Wall PD, Melzack R (eds): Textbook of Pain. Edinburgh, Churchill Livingstone, 1999, pp 879–914.

18. Kiss ZHT, Davis KD, Tasker RR, et al: Human thalamic neurons develop novel receptive fields within minutes of deafferentation. Soc Neurosci Abstr 20:119, 1994.

19. Melzack R: From the gate to the neuromatrix. Pain Aug(Suppl 6):S121–S126, 1999.

20. Reitsma B, Meijler WJ: Pain and patienthood. Clin J Pain 13:9–21, 1997.

21. Snow-Turek AL, Norris MP, Tan G: Active and passive coping strategies in chronic pain patients. Pain 64:455–462, 1996.

22. Aigner M, Bach M: Clinical utility of DSM-IV pain disorder. Compr Psychiatry 40:353–357, 1997.

23. Burns JW, Johnson BJ, Mahoney N, et al: Anger management style, hostility, and spouse responses: Gender differences in predictors of adjustment among chronic pain patients. Pain 64:445–453, 1996.

24. Turk DC, Flor H: Pain greater than pain behaviors: The utility and limitations of the pain behavior construct. Pain 31:277–295, 1987.

25. Birbaumer N, Flor H: A leg to stand on: Learning creates pain. Behav Brain Sci 20:441–442, 1997.

26. Aronoff GM, Gallagher RM: Pharmacological management of chronic pain: A review. In Aronoff GM (ed): Evaluation and Treatment of Chronic Pain. Baltimore, Williams & Wilkins, 1998, pp 433–453.

27. Vane JR: Inhibition of prostaglandin synthesis as a mechanism of action of aspirin-like drugs. Nature 231:232–235, 1971.

28. Needleman P, Isakson PC: The discovery and function of COX-2. J Rheumatol 24(Suppl 49):6–8, 1997.

29. Allison MC, Howatson AG, Torrance CJ, et al: Gastrointestinal damage associated with the use of nonsteroidal antiinflammatory drugs. N Engl J Med 327:749–754, 1992.

30. Clive DM, Stoff JS: Renal syndromes associated with nonsteroidal antiinflammatory drugs. N Engl J Med 310:563–572, 1984.

31. Lefkowith JB: Cyclooxygenase-2 specificity and its clinical implications. Am J Med 106:435–505, 1999.

32. Simon LS, Lanza FL, Lipsky PE, et al: Preliminary study of the safety and efficacy of SC-58635, a novel cyclooxygenase 2 inhibitor: Efficacy and safety in two placebo-controlled trials in osteoarthritis and rheumatoid arthritis, and studies of gastrointestinal and platelet effects. Arthritis Rheum 41:1591–1602, 1998.

33. Prescott LF: Paracetamol (acetaminophen): A Critical Bibliographic Review. London, Taylor & Francis, 1996.

34. Whitcomb DC, Block GD: Association of acetaminophen hepatotoxicity with fasting and ethanol use. JAMA 272:1845–1850, 1994.

35. Maddrey WC: Hepatic effects of acetaminophen: Enhanced toxicity in alcoholics. J Clin Gastroenterol 9:180–185, 1987.

36. Zimmerman JH, Maddrey WC: Acetaminophen (Paracetamol) hepatotoxicity with regular intake of alcohol: Analysis of instances of therapeutic misadventure. Hepatology 22:767–773, 1995.

37. Slattery JT, Nelson SD, Thummel KE: The complex interaction between alcohol and acetaminophen. Clin Pharmacol Ther 60:241–246, 1996.

38. Urquhart E: Central analgesic activity of nonsteroidal antiinflammatory drugs in animal and human pain models. Semin Arthritis Rheum 23:198–205, 1993.

39. Maciewicz R, Bouckoms A, Martin JB: Drug therapy of neuropathic pain. Clin J Pain 1:39–49, 1985.

40. Goodman LS, Gilman A: The Pharmacological Basis of Therapeutics. New York, Pergamon Press, 1990.

41. Ellenberg M: Treatment of diabetic neuropathy with diphenylhydantoin. N Y State J Med 68:2653–2655, 1968.

42. Caccia MR: Clonazepam in facial neuralgia and cluster headache: Clinical and electrophysiological study. Eur Neurol 13:560–563, 1975.

43. Peiris JB, Perera GLS, Devendra SV, et al: Sodium valproate in trigeminal neuralgia. Med J Aust 2:278, 1980.

44. Dunsker SB, Mayfield FN: Carbamazepine in the treatment of flashing pain syndrome. J Neurosurg 45:49–51, 1976.

45. Bruera E, Navigante A, Barugel M, et al: Treatment of pain and other symptoms in cancer patients: Patterns in a North American and South American hospital. J Pain Symptom Manage 5:78–82, 1990.

46. Edwards KR, Bennington VT, Marykay S, et al: Gabapentin (Neurontin®) for pain associated with diabetic peripheral neuropathy: A double-blind, placebo-controlled study (945-210). Neurology 50(Suppl):A378–A379, 1998.

47. Valzania F, Strapela AP, Nassetti SA, et al: Gabapentin in idiopathic trigeminal neuralgia. Neurology 50(Suppl):A379, 1998.

48. Backonja M, Beydoun A, Edwards KR, et al: Gabapentin for the symptomatic treatment of painful neuropathy in patients with diabetes mellitus: A randomized controlled trial. JAMA 280:1831–1836, 1998.

49. Rowbotham M, Harden N, Stacey B, et al: Gabapentin for the treatment of postherpetic neuralgia: A randomized controlled trial. JAMA 280:1837–1842, 1998.

50. Anhut H, Ashman P, Feuerstein TJ, et al: Gabapentin (Neurontin) as add-on therapy in patients with partial seizures: A double-blind, placebo-controlled study. The International Gabapentin Study Group. Epilepsia 35:795–801, 1994.

51. Wamil AW, McLean MJ: Limitation by gabapentin of high frequency action potential by mouse central neurons in cell culture. Epilepsy Res 17:1–11, 1994.

52. Tanelian DL, Brose WG: Neuropathic pain can be relieved by drugs that are use-dependent sodium channel blockers: Lidocaine, carbamazepine and mexiletine. Anesthesiology 74:949–951, 1991.

53. Dejgard A, Petersen P, Kastrup J: Mexiletine for treatment of chronic painful diabetic neuropathy. Lancet 1:9–11, 1988.

54. Devor M, Wall PD, Catalan N: Systemic lidocaine silences ectopic neuroma and DRG discharge without blocking nerve conduction. Pain 48:261–268, 1992.

55. Raymond SA, Thalhammer JG, Popitz-Bergez F, et al: Changes in axonal impulse conduction correlate with sensory modality in primary apparent afferent fiber in the rat. Brain Res 526:318–321, 1990.

56. Sawynok J, Reid AR, Esser MJ: Peripheral antinociceptive action of amitriptyline in the rat formalin test: Involvement of adenosine. Pain 80:45–55, 1999.

57. Hall H, Ögren SO: Effects of antidepressant drugs on different receptors in the brain. Eur J Pharmacol 70:393–407, 1981.

58. Isenberg KE, Cicero TJ: Possible involvement of opiate receptors in the pharmacological profiles of antidepressant compounds. Eur J Pharmacol 103:57–63, 1984.

59. Schäfer M, Carter L, Stein C: Interleukin 1 beta and corticotropin-releasing factor inhibit pain by releasing opioids from immune cells in inflamed tissue. Proc Natl Acad Sci U S A 91:4219–4223, 1994.

60. Czlonkowski A, Stein C, Herz A: Peripheral mechanisms of opioid antinociception in inflammation: Involvement of cytokines. Eur J Pharmacol 242:229–235, 1993.

61. Yaksh TL: Pharmacology and mechanisms of opioid analgesic activity. Acta Anaesthesiol Scand 41:94–111, 1997.

62. Gildenberg PL: Medical management of chronic pain. In Youmans JR (ed): Neurological Surgery. Philadelphia, WB Saunders, 1996, pp 3327–3343.

63. Portenoy RK, Foley KM, Inturrisi CE: The nature of opioid responsiveness and its implications for neuropathic pain: New hypotheses derived from studies of opioid infusions. Pain 43:273–286, 1990.

64. Bonica JJ: Post-operative pain. In Bonica JJ (ed): The Management of Pain. Philadelphia, Lea & Febiger, 1990, pp 461–480.

65. Arner S, Meyerson BA: Lack of analgesic effect of opioids on neuropathic and idiopathic forms of pain. Pain 33:11–23, 1988.

66. Galer BS, Coyle N, Pasternak GW, et al: Individual variability in the response to different opioids: Report of five cases. Pain 49:87–91, 1992.

67. Portenoy RK, Foley KM: Chronic use of opioid analgesics in nonmalignant pain: Report of 38 cases. Pain 25:171–186, 1986.

68. Rowbotham MC, Reisner-Keller LA, Fields HL: Both intravenous lidocaine and morphine reduce pain of post-herpetic neuralgia. Neurology 41:1024–1028, 1991.

69. McQuay H: Opioids in pain management. Lancet 353:2229–2232, 1999.

70. Moulin DE, Iezzi A, Amireh R, et al: Randomized trial of oral morphine for chronic non-cancer pain. Lancet 347:143–27, 1996.

71. Portenoy RK: Opioid therapy for chronic nonmalignant pain: A review of the critical issues. J Pain Symptom Manage 11:203–217, 1996.

72. Kalso E, Vainio A: Morphine and oxycodone hydrochloride in the management of cancer pain. Clin Pharmacol Ther 47:639–46, 1990.

73. Foley K: Clinical tolerance to opioids. In Basbaum A, Besson J (eds): Towards a New Pharmacotherapy of Pain. New York, John Wiley & Sons, 1991, pp 181–203.

74. Zacny J: A review of the effects of opioids on psychomotor and cognitive functioning in humans. Exp Clin Psychopharmacol 3:432–466, 1995.

75. Louie AK, Way EL: Overview of opiate tolerance and physical dependence. In Almeida OF, Shippenberg TS (eds): Neurobiology of Opioids. New York, Springer-Verlag, 1991.

76. Portenoy RK, Foley KM: Chronic use of opioid analgesics in non-malignant pain: Report of 38 cases. Pain 25:171–186, 1986.

77. Hill HF, Chapman CR, Kornell JA, et al: Self-administration of morphine in bone marrow transplant patients reduces drug requirement. Pain 40:121–129, 1990.

78. Savage SR: Long-term opioid therapy: Assessment of consequences and risks. J Pain Symptom Manage 11:274–286, 1996.

79. Houde RW, Wallenstein SL, Beaver WT: Evaluation of analgesics in patients with cancer pain. In Lasagna L (ed): International Encyclopedia of Pharmacology and Therapeutics. Oxford, Pergamon Press, 1966, pp 59–98.

80. Twycross R: Clinical experience with diamorphine in advanced malignant disease. Int J Clin Pharmacol Ther Toxicol 9:184–198, 1974.

81. Melzack R: Humans versus pain: The dilemma of morphine. In Sicuteri F, Terenius L, Vecchiet L, et al (eds): Advances in Pain Research and Therapy, vol 20. New York, Raven Press, 1992, pp 149–159.

82. American Society of Addiction Medicine: Public policy statement on definitions related to the use of opioids in pain treatment. J Addict Dis 17:129–33, 1998.

83. Porter J, Jick H: Addiction: Rare in patients treated with narcotics. N Engl J Med 302:123, 1980.

84. Perry S, Heidrick G: Management of pain during debridement: A survey of U.S. burn units. Pain 13:267–280, 1982.

85. Medina JL, Diamond S: Drug dependency in patients with chronic headache. Headache 17:12–14, 1977.

86. Onghens P, Van Houdenhove B: Antidepressant-induced analgesia in chronic non-malignant pain: A meta-analysis of 39 placebo-controlled studies. Pain 49:205–219, 1991.

87. Bryson HM, Wilde MI: Amitriptyline: A review of its pharmacological properties and therapeutic use in chronic pain states. Drugs Aging 8:459–476, 1996.

88. Max MB, Culnane M, Schafer SC, et al: Amitriptyline relieves diabetic neuropathic pain in patients with normal and depressed mood. Neurology 37:589–596, 1987.

89. Max M: Antidepressants as Analgesics. Progress in Pain Research and Management, vol 1. Seattle, IASP Press, 1994.

90. Eisenach JC, Gebhart GB: Intrathecal amitriptyline acts as an N-methyl-D-aspartate receptor antagonist in the presence of inflammatory hyperalgesia in rats. Anesthesiology 83:1046–1054, 1995.

91. Dray A, Urban L, Dickenson A: Pharmacology of chronic pain. Trends Pharmacol Sci 15:190–197, 1994.

92. Sindrup SH, Jensen TS: Efficacy of pharmocological treatments of neuropathic pain: An update and effect related to mechanism of drug action. Pain 83:389–400, 1999.

93. Erdine S, Yucel A, Ozyalcin S: Efficacy of tramadol hydrochloride in chronic painful diabetic neuropathy: A double blind placebo controlled study. Paper presented at the 8th World Congress on Pain, August 1996, Vancouver, British Columbia, Canada.

94. Désarmenien M, Feltz P, Occhipinti G, et al: Coexistence of GABA_A and GABA_B receptors on A and C primary afferents. Br J Pharmacol 81:327–333, 1984.

95. Price GW, Wilkin GP, Turnbull MJ, et al: Are baclofen-sensitive GABA_B receptors present on primary afferent terminals of spinal cord? Nature 307:71–74, 1984.

96. Lin Q, Peng YB, Willis WD: Role of GABA receptor subtypes in inhibition of primate spinothalamic tract neurons: Difference between spinal and periaqueductal gray inhibition. J Neurophysiol 75:109–123, 1996.

97. Hammond DL, Washington JD: Antagonism of L-baclofen-induced antinociception by CGP 35348 in the spinal cord of the rat. Eur J Pharmacol 234:255–262, 1993.

98. Roberts LA, Beyer C, Komisaruk BR: Nociceptive responses to altered GABAergic activity at the spinal cord. Life Sci 39:1667–1674, 1986.

99. Aley KO, Kulkarni SK: GABAergic agents-induced antinociceptive effects in mice. Methods Find Exp Clin Pharmacol 11:597–601, 1989.

100. Bartoszyk GB, Meyerson N, Reimann W, et al: Gabapentin (pharmacology). Curr Probl Epilepsy 4:147–163, 1986.

101. Mellick GA, Mellicy LB, Mellick LB: Gabapentin in the management of reflex sympathetic dystrophy. J Pain Symptom Manage 10:265–266, 1995.

102. Rosner H, Rubin L, Westenbaum A: Gabapentin adjunctive therapy in neuropathic pain states. Clin J Pain 12:56–58, 1996.

103. Dallochio C, Buffa C, Ligure N, et al: Gabapentin vs amitriptyline in painful diabetic neuropathy of the elderly. American Academy of Neurology, annual meeting, April 1998. Neurology 50(Suppl):A-102, 1998.

104. Mellick GA, Mellick LB: Reflex sympathetic dystrophy treated with gabapentin. Arch Phys Med Rehabil 78:98–105, 1997.

105. Segal A, Rordof G: Gabapentin as a novel treatment for herpetic neuralgia. Neurology 46:1175–1176, 1996.

106. Taylor CP: Gabapentin: Mechanisms of action. In Levy RH, Mattson RH, Meldrum BS (eds): Antiepileptic Drugs. New York, Raven Press, 1995, pp 829–841.

107. Su TZ, Lunney E, Campbell G, et al: Transport of gabapentin, a gamma-amino acid drug, by system 1 alpha-amino acid transporters: A comparative study in astrocytes, synaptosomes, and CHO cells. J Neurochem 64:2125–2131, 1995.

108. Goldlust A, Su TZ, Welty DF, et al: Effects of anticonvulsant drug gabapentin on the enzymes in metabolic pathways of glutamate and GABA. Epilepsy Res 22:1–11, 1995.

109. Taylor CP, Vartanian MG, Andruskiewiecz R, et al: 3-Alkyl GABA and 3-alkylglutamic acid analogues: Two new classes of anticonvulsant agents. Epilepsy Res 11:103–110, 1992.

110. Petroff OAC, Rothman DL, Behar KL, et al: The effect of gabapentin on brain gamma-aminobutyric acid in patients with epilepsy. Ann Neurol 39:95–99, 1996.

111. Mattson RH, Rothman DL, Behar KL, et al: Gabapentin: A GABA active drug. Epilepsia 38:65–66, 1997.

112. Fichter N, Taylor CP, Feuerstein TJ: Nipecotate-induced GABA release from slices of the rate caudoputamen: Effects of gabapentin. Arch Pharmacol 354:R35, 1996.

113. Morris GL 3rd: Efficacy and tolerability of gabapentin in clinical practice. Clin Ther 17:891–900, 1995.

114. Chadwick D, Leiderman DB, Sauermann W, et al: Gabapentin in generalized seizures. Epilepsy Res 25:191–197, 1996.
115. Chadwick D: Gabapentin. Lancet 343:89–91, 1994.
116. Gallagher RM, Pasol E: Psychopharmacologic drugs in the chronic pain syndromes. Curr Rev Pain 1:138–152, 1997.
117. Bryants JS, Wustrow DJ: 3-Substituted GABA analogs with central nervous system activity: A review. Med Res Rev 19:149–177, 1999.
118. Viallancourt PD, Langevin HM: Painful peripheral neuropathies. Med Clin North Am 83:627–642, 1999.
119. Stoetling RK: Pharmacology and Physiology in Anesthetic Practice. Philadelphia, Lippincott-Raven, 1999, p 304.
120. Unnerstall JR, Kopajtic TA, Kuhar MJ: Distribution of alpha$_2$ agonist binding sites in the rat and human central nervous system: Analysis of some functional, anatomic correlates of the pharmacologic effects of clonidine and related adrenergic agents. Brain Res Rev 7:69–101, 1984.
121. Filos KS, Goudas LC, Patroni O, et al: Intrathecal clonidine as a sole analgesic for pain relief after cesarean section. Anesthesiology 77:267–274, 1992.
122. De Kock M, Crochet B, Morimont C, et al: Intravenous or epidural clonidine for intra- and postoperative analgesia. Anesthesiology 79:525–531, 1993.
123. Byas-Smith MG, Max MG, Muir J, et al: Transdermal clonidine compared to placebo in painful diabetic neuropathy using a two stage enriched enrollment design. Pain 60:267–274, 1995.
124. Max MB, Schafer, SC, Culnane M, et al: Association of pain relief with drug side effects in post-herpetic neuralgia: A single dose study with clonidine, codeine, ibuprofen and placebo. Clin Pharmacol Ther 43:363–371, 1988.
125. Urban MO, Gebhart GF: The glutamate synapse: A target in the pharmacologic management of hyperalgesic pain states. Prog Brain Res 116:382–395, 1998.
126. Hirota K, Lambert DG: Ketamine: Its mechanism(s) of action and unusual clinical uses. Br J Anesth 77:441–444, 1996.
127. Koek W, Woods JH, Winger GD: MK-801, a proposed noncompetitive antagonist of excitatory amino acid neurotransmission, produces phencyclidine like behavioral effects in pigeons, rats and rhesus monkeys. J Pharmacol Exp Ther 245:969–974, 1988.
128. Morris RGM, Anderson E, Lynch GS, et al: Selective impairment of learning and blockage of long term potentiation by N-methyl-D-aspartate receptor antagonist, AP5. Nature 319:774–776, 1986.
129. Olney JW, Labruyere J, Wang G, et al: NMDA antagonist neurotoxity: Mechanism and prevention. Science 254:1515–1518, 1991.
130. Sawynok J: Adenosine receptor activation and nociception. Eur J Pharmacol 317:1–11, 1998.
131. Sawynok J, Sweeney MI, White TD: Adenosine release may mediate spinal analgesia by morphine. Trends Pharmacol Soc 10:186–189, 1989.
132. Lavand'homme PM, Eisenach JC: Exogenous and endogenous adenosine enhance the spinal antiallodynic effects of morphine in a rat model of neuropathic pain. Pain 80:31–36, 1999.
133. Belfrage M, Sollevi A, Segerdahl M, et al: Systemic adenosine infusion alleviates spontaneous and stimulus evoked pain in patients with peripheral neuropathic pain. Anesth Analg 81:713–717, 1995.
134. Wells GB, Golding JM, Burnham MA: The functioning and well-being of depressed patients: Results from the Medical Outcomes Study. JAMA 262:914–919, 1989.
135. Singh PN, Sharma P, Gupta PK, et al: Clinical Evaluation of diazepam for relief of postoperative pain. Br J Anesth 53:831–836, 1981.
136. Integration of behavioral and relaxation approaches into the treatment of chronic pain and insomnia. NIH Technology Assessment Panel on Integration of Behavioral and Relaxation Approaches into the Treatment of Chronic Pain and Insomnia. JAMA 276:313–318, 1996.

CHAPTER 184

Management of Pain by Anesthetic Techniques

BRETT STACEY ■ ANTHONY COLANTONIO ■ JENNIFER VOOKLES ■ DAVID SIBELL ■ LYNDA KULAWIAK

Many health care providers associate the term *pain clinic* with a "place to get an injection" or "have a nerve blocked." Many pain clinics do provide pain relief primarily by means of injections of local anesthetics and steroids. However, others see anesthetic techniques as therapy with little proven efficacy. As the field of pain medicine has matured, the role for neural blockade techniques in the assessment and treatment of pain continues to be debated and refined.

This chapter reviews some of the more common techniques and related issues in the use of neural blockade, although it is not meant as a comprehensive review of all nerve block techniques.

CONSIDERATIONS FOR DIAGNOSTIC AND THERAPEUTIC INJECTIONS

Therapeutic Injection

Application of local anesthetics to nervous tissue decreases transmission of sensory and motor information by means of sodium channel blockade. In combination with knowledge of innervation patterns and nervous system anatomy, transient pain relief can be delivered by injection of local anesthetics. Temporary pain relief that lasts until the local anesthetic blockade is reversed provides the basis for diagnostic injections. Therapeutic injections are based on the well documented, frequently encountered, and not well understood phenomenon of prolonged pain relief after local anesthetic injection. Prolonged pain relief may result from altered central nervous system function, altered muscle tonicity at the affected area, morphology of peripheral nerve physiology, or some as yet undiscovered mechanism.

The rationale for including corticosteroids in therapeutic injections is based on the belief that perineural inflammation accompanies painful conditions. The numerous anti-inflammatory and membrane stabilizing properties of steroids may contribute to decreased sensitization, decreased edema, and pain relief when injected into the vicinity of painful nerves. Previous animal models have demonstrated that steroids can beneficially modify the effects of neurogenic inflammation by decreasing thermal hyperalgesia,[1] decreasing phospholipase A_2 activity,[2] inhibiting prostaglandin production,[3] and blocking normal C-fiber firing.[4]

Diagnostic Injection

When an injection or any interventional procedure is the basis for diagnosis or future treatment, careful attention to patient selection, technique, and process is critical. The patient must understand that the injection is intended as a diagnostic maneuver, not as therapy. Counseling the patient in this regard to facilitate cooperation and understanding is critical. Advance consideration of other factors that may confound interpretation of the injection should be a part of the diagnostic process. A general approach to diagnostic injections is summarized in Table 184–1.

Limitations of Neural Blockade and Therapeutic Injection

In many pain practices, the role of diagnostic and therapeutic injections is firmly entrenched; however, limited controlled studies, wide variations in technique, lack of standards, and inconsistent outcome assessment limit their acceptance in the era of evidence-based medicine. Many pain physician practices exist in which the treatment focus is injection therapy to the exclusion of other treatments, but very few pain practitioners would publicly advocate the use of neural blockade as unimodal treatment for chronic pain states. This type of practice has been condemned,[5] and some have even labeled the use of injection techniques as outdated or, at a minimum, less effective than other techniques.

Limitations Associated with Neural Blockade

Because pain is a subjective experience, patient cooperation and feedback is the basis for interpretation of diag-

TABLE 184-1 ■ **GUIDELINES FOR DIAGNOSTIC NEURAL BLOCKADE**

1. Document sensory and motor function before and after the injection.
2. Document a preprocedure pain score (baseline), taking into account provocation of pain with movement, positioning, touch, or other stimuli.
3. Track pain relief afterward with a pain diary extended over several hours, including pain at rest and with provocation.
4. Careful attention to technique and needle placement using
   a. Fluoroscopy for all injections with anatomic bony landmarks
   b. Nerve stimulation for localization of peripheral nerves
   c. Radiographic contrast to ensure a lack of vascular uptake and appropriate spread only to intended target
   d. Atraumatic technique (e.g., small needles, minimal repositioning)
   e. Minimal infiltration of subcutaneous tissues with local anesthetic
   f. Minimal volume of injectate (often less than 1 mL when the needle is placed accurately)
5. Consider two diagnostic injections, possibly with different local anesthetics.
6. Consider the possibility for a placebo response at any stage of the procedure. Some authorities advocate a separate placebo injection.
7. Consider alternative diagnoses or explanations for the pain and the patient's responses.

nostic block testing. There may be an incidence of placebo response as high as 35% with each injection[6, 7] that cannot be clinically differentiated from a true response. This response is not voluntary, may be delayed and profound, and does not tell the practitioner whether the patient has "real" pain. Physicians must be attentive to their word selection when discussing pending diagnostic procedures because the patient response may be influenced by physicians' suggestions, expectations, and interactions.[8, 9] The patient may have more than one type of pain or source of pain that may confound the patient's interpretation of the injection, leading to a partial response open to interpretation. Pain is a dynamic experience, and a patient's response on any given day to an injection may not predict a response on another day or in another situation.

Anatomic and physiologic variations may lead to incomplete block, block of unintended nerves, or lack of effectiveness.[10, 11] Vascular uptake resulting from unrecognized placement of the needle partially in an unappreciated vascular structure may limit the effect of the injection and confound interpretation of the results. Changes after surgery may obscure landmarks, limit flow of injectate, or result in moved or missing targets. The phenomenon of central sensitization may mean that even a few unblocked nerve fibers may leave significant pain and lead to the false conclusion that the injection was not in the correct nerve. Peripheral nerve blocks may relieve pain of a more central origin such as stroke or lumbar radiculopathy,[12–14] representing a state in which peripheral input sustains a central process.[15]

The effects of local anesthetic may not be as easily predicted as we believe. Local anesthetics that are systemically absorbed or administered relieve many types of chronic pain, especially neuropathic pain.[16–18] The

differential blockade concept, with low doses or concentrations of local anesthetic selectively blocking sympathetic fibers and higher doses or concentrations blocking somatic nerves, was widely held in the past. Later evidence suggests that this belief may be false, with unpredictability in the extent of block or types of fibers being blocked more common than previously believed.[19, 20] True differential block is more likely to be successful if anatomy assists in the process of selectivity rather than relying on varying nerve sensitivity to local anesthetic.

Limitations of Therapeutic Injections

The literature in support of therapeutic benefits to patients from neural blockade techniques is, unfortunately, quite limited. Documentation of case reports, retrospective reviews, and unblinded studies floods the literature. For almost every condition or technique, a "pro" and "con" position can be supported by the literature. Neural blockade techniques are often advocated by anesthesiologists and other "injectionologists" for use in conditions such as sciatica or herpes zoster that have a natural history favoring improvement. A variety of alternative treatments such as physical therapy, systemic analgesics, and psychological techniques are available for these conditions, but few studies compare nerve blocks with the other options.

It is a rare occurrence when we can attribute chronic pain conditions to a single cause. There may be numerous musculoskeletal factors initiating the pain, as well as psychosocial factors and functional issues that can influence the impact of the pain syndrome on the patient. If pain persists after an appropriate block, the procedure may be interpreted as having failed because of unappreciated or untreated components; successful blocks may reveal only one of several contributing factors.

Neural blockade technique standards do not exist. For example, a patient referred for nerve blocks for the diagnosis of complex regional pain syndrome (i.e., reflex sympathetic dystrophy) of an upper extremity could receive an impressive variety of nerve blocking techniques for this condition. Injection at the stellate ganglion with or without fluoroscopic guidance, a posterior paravertebral approach to the upper thoracic sympathetic chain, injection into the epidural space, performance of an intravenous regional anesthetic, and performance of a brachial plexus block are some of the options available for this condition. For each of these, local anesthetic, steroid, opioid, clonidine, guanethidine, reserpine, bretylium, or a variety of other medications could be employed.[21, 22] There is scant literature to support most of these techniques, and few have been compared with each other; all could be called nerve blocks. Which technique is applied to which patient becomes a matter of clinician preference, habit, convenience, and circumstance. Many clinicians do not perform all of these techniques, and there are few data comparing them.

Comprehensive treatment of chronic pain patients is strongly supported by scientifically sound literature.[23, 24]

Improvements in work status, mood, use of health care, and pain levels can be achieved. Unfortunately, such comprehensive outcome assessments of neural blockade treatment do not exist. The role of neural blockade techniques in facilitating other efforts at pain rehabilitation has not been studied. Most physicians who use these techniques believe they are not stand-alone treatments but that they should instead be part of a comprehensive treatment approach.

PREPARATIONS FOR PERFORMING THE TECHNIQUES OF NEURAL BLOCKADE

Training and Background

The association between anesthesiologists and neural blockade techniques has a long and rich history, but by no means can the anesthesiologist lay sole claim to this area. Multiple disciplines are represented by the membership of the International Spinal Injection Society (ISIS), with a focus on the development, implementation, and standardization of percutaneous techniques for diagnosing and treating spinal pain. ISIS has published standards about patient selection and technical considerations on their website (www.spinalinjection.com). Experienced and dedicated "injectionologists," "proceduralists," or "neural blockade specialists" represent many medical specialties. Because training in pain management and regional anesthetic techniques is a required component of the anesthesiology residency, most physicians with interest and practice in this area are anesthesiologists.

Many physicians are capable of placing needles and medications in the correct location. Some of these physicians have received specialized training in pain management and focus a significant portion of their practice on providing care to chronic pain patients. The procedure may be part of a comprehensive treatment plan developed by an anesthesiologist or other pain management specialist. Physicians with this background may take a more active role in the overall management of the patient or may perform the procedural aspect of care, leaving the remainder of care to the referring physician. Specialized training is not required for some neural blockade techniques, and these techniques may be performed as part of a practice primarily devoted to other types of care by anesthesiologists or radiologists. In this setting, the person performing the injection technique does not direct other aspects of patient care.

General Standards and Safety Guidelines

Similar to any invasive procedure, performance of anesthetic interventions in chronic pain management includes a risk of bleeding, infection, damage to structures, and allergic reaction. Each procedure also carries its own unique potential complications. For example, there are case reports of spinal anesthesia after facet joint injection.[25, 26] The benefits, alternatives, risks, and potential complications should be discussed with the patient, and informed consent must be obtained before procedures are started.

Because of the potentially devastating consequences of bleeding or infection proximal to the spinal cord, bleeding diatheses, systemic infection, and localized infection in the region of the procedure are considered absolute contraindications. A history of allergic reaction to iodinated radiographic contrast is only a relative contraindication, because this problem can usually be preempted by pretreatment with corticosteroids and histamine antagonists and with use of an alternative contrast material. Although patients occasionally report an allergy to a local anesthetic, true allergic reactions to local anesthetics are rare.[27] Many of these individuals report symptoms consistent with inadvertent intravenous injection of an epinephrine-containing anesthetic or signs of local anesthetic toxicity, which is not an allergic reaction. However, there are rare reports of allergic responses to amino-ester local anesthetics caused by cross-sensitivity between this group and methylparaben, a common preservative in other drugs, food, and cosmetics. If an actual allergic response is suspected after questioning the patient, selection of an alternate class of local anesthetics is advised.

Risks and Complications

Basic precautions should be taken to reduce risks. Intravenous access should be obtained if sedation is required or if there is a possibility of significant physiologic change. It is appropriate for patients to take nothing orally before and to avoid driving home after most procedures. Fluoroscopy can be used to ensure accurate positioning of needles, as is discussed later in this chapter. Standards for the performance of some procedures involving spinal injection are published by ISIS.[28] Similar guidelines are suggested for institutions using such procedures. They include physiologic monitoring of the patient and observation of aseptic technique with sterile skin preparation, drapes, and gloves. Sterile gowns are worn for intrathecal line placement; implantable pumps and spinal cord stimulators are placed in an operating room.

These safety principles regarding technique and other guidelines should be observed in using such interventions appropriately. The natural history of a patient's complaint must be considered before initiating an invasive diagnostic or therapeutic regimen. For example, acute-onset back pain without associated neurological findings typically resolves within 8 weeks, independent of any intervention.[29] Because the discussed procedures do entail risks and can be difficult to interpret, ISIS recommends that any invasive diagnostic or potentially therapeutic interventions be avoided for at least 4 weeks from the onset of symptoms and 3 weeks after initiation of more conservative, noninvasive measures.

FLUOROSCOPIC GUIDANCE

Fluoroscopy is an essential adjunct for performing neural blockade techniques. Fluoroscopy and radiopaque contrast material help to improve the safety and accuracy of needle placement before regional anesthetic or neurolytic interventions and to verify accurate neuraxial catheter or spinal cord stimulator electrode placement.

When high-velocity electrons are accelerated by a high voltage (i.e., kilovolt peak [kVp]) and allowed to crash into a material with a high atomic number, such as the tungsten target in an x-ray tube, x-rays are produced. Electrons in an x-ray tube are provided by passing a current, measured in milliamperes (mA), through an electrically heated filament. The electrons are then accelerated from the filament to the tungsten target by the application of a high voltage across the x-ray tube. Fluoroscopy is usually performed using 2 to 6 mA and 75 to 125 kVp of accelerating voltage.[30]

Most fluoroscopy units produce images with an image intensifier and have a "last image hold" function, which allows recalling the last image without having to again expose the patient to radiation. Many newer fluoroscopy units offer a "pulsed fluoro mode," which is often used to follow the spread of contrast material in real time. In pulsed mode, the x-ray beam is pulsed rapidly on and off, resulting in a lower radiation dose compared with continuous fluoroscopy.[30] Quick and easy correlation of surface anatomy with the radiographic image is allowed by use of a laser guidance system. This also decreases fluoroscopy time and radiation dose.

Electronic magnification, obtained by changing the field of view of the image intensifier, improves image sharpness. Magnification is especially helpful when anatomic landmarks are obscured by previous surgery, scarring, or surgical hardware.

During fluoroscopy, contrast material provides opacification of blood vessels and tissues. Contrast agents that are commonly used have a fully substituted tri-iodinated benzene ring structure and may have an ionic or nonionic formulation. Nonionic contrast agents such as iohexol, iotrolan, iomeprol, and iodixanol are water soluble and have a lower potential for central nervous system toxicity, renal impairment, or anaphylactoid reactions compared with ionic agents.[31–34] Using fluoroscopy in the anteroposterior, lateral, or oblique views, the pattern of spread visualized after injecting contrast agent can be used to delineate different tissue planes and proper needle placement before the introduction of local anesthetic, steroids, or neurolytic substances.

The celiac plexus neurolytic block demonstrates the advantages of fluoroscopy compared with the blind needle technique and highlights a major deficiency of this approach. This block is commonly performed with a two-needle technique at the L1 level. The aorta lies anterior and slightly to the left of the anterior margin of the L1 vertebral body. The inferior vena cava lies to the right of midline, and the kidneys are posterolateral to the great vessels. The pancreas is anterior to the celiac plexus. The celiac plexus is anterior to the diaphragmatic crura and extends anterior to and around the aorta. Accurate placement of the two needles is essential with such crucial organs and vessels sur-

rounding the celiac plexus. The needle to the left side is advanced until it lies just posterior to the aorta on the left, and the needle on the right side is advanced to the anterolateral aspect of the aorta on the right. If using fluoroscopy, a small volume of contrast material is injected through each needle and is observed with fluoroscopy as it spreads. On the fluoroscopic anteroposterior view, the contrast material is ideally confined to the midline and concentrated near the L1 vertebral body (Fig. 184–1). On the lateral view, a smooth posterior contour can be observed that corresponds to the psoas fascia (Fig. 184–2). Although these images increase confidence in the injection technique, many of the vital structures in the region are not radiopaque and cannot be directly observed. This limitation is the primary reason that some advocate computed tomography (CT) for guidance in performing injections in areas with nonbony landmarks.

The use of fluoroscopy and contrast material should not be limited to anatomically complicated procedures. Epidural steroid injections (ESIs) have traditionally been performed using a "blind" technique without fluoroscopic guidance. This blind technique introduces the potential for erroneous needle placement and subsequent injection of steroids into unintended areas such as the intrathecal space, leading to possible adhesive arachnoiditis. White and coworkers[35, 36] found that inaccurate needle placement occurred in 25% to 30% of blind injections, even in the hands of skilled and experienced proceduralists. Injecting variable amounts of radiologic contrast material under fluoroscopic observation before therapeutic injection improves safety and efficacy. In this way, the risk of unintended intrathecal injection and its consequences can be virtually eliminated. Moreover, the traditional practice with the blind ESI technique to proceed with a second and third ste-

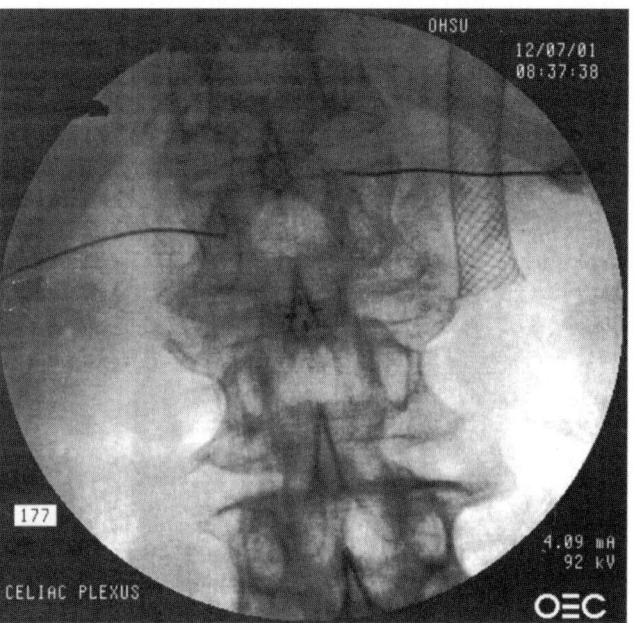

FIGURE 184–1. Anteroposterior view of a celiac plexus block. (Courtesy of Brett Stacey, Oregon Health & Science University School of Medicine, Portland, OR.)

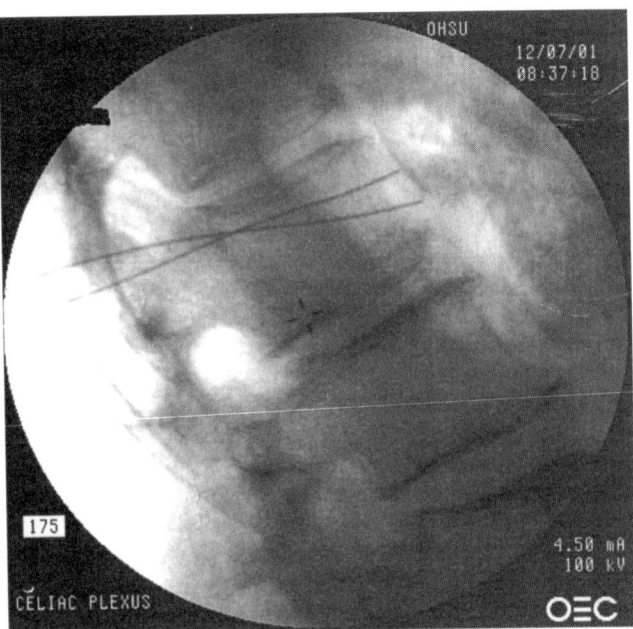

FIGURE 184–2. Lateral view of a celiac plexus block. (Courtesy of Brett Stacey, Oregon Health & Science University School of Medicine, Portland, OR.)

roid injection as a routine series to assess efficacy becomes unnecessary.[37] Documenting the distribution of injected materials may also explain a patient's response if a unilateral or limited epidural block is encountered.[38] Being able to visualize the target may allow placement of the needle with fewer corrections in trajectory, reducing the time and trauma involved. Even with negative needle aspiration results, a significant number of injections after blind needle placement have been shown to be intravascular.[39] Intravascular needle placement is quickly ascertained by rapid uptake and disappearance of contrast material injected under fluoroscopy before local anesthetic injection, diminishing the risk of toxicity.

EPIDURAL AND NERVE ROOT INJECTIONS

ESIs have been described as the "bread and butter" of injection treatment for back, neck, and extremity pain. They are frequently performed for a wide range of conditions involving spinal and radicular pain. Individual practitioners often perform the procedures consistently in their own way, but differences in technique between practitioners vary widely. The Agency for Health Care Policy and Research gave ESIs a classification of C, because there has been limited research-based evidence (at least one adequate scientific study in patients with low back pain).[40] Published studies and commentaries have emphasized the safety of ESIs but questioned the efficacy of the technique and highlighted the ubiquitous, nondiscriminant application of ESIs.[41] Different conclusions have resulted from attempts at distilling the literature by the use of meta-analyses.[42–44] Despite these controversies, ESIs probably

have an important role to play in selected patients, particularly those with radicular pain.[45] The success of this important therapeutic procedure depends on attention to patient selection, technique, and concomitant therapies.

Rationale for Epidural Steroid Injections

It is well known that a herniated disk pressing on a nerve root can produce radicular pain. However, significant abnormalities of the spine, spinal canal, and intervertebral disks are found in asymptomatic individuals.[46, 47] Compression of a nerve root by mechanical forces may not be sufficient in many cases to produce radicular pain, fueling the search for additional mechanisms.

Inflammation may play a role in symptomatic nerve root irritation that is associated with herniated intervertebral disks.[48] Proinflammatory substances are contained in extruded nucleus pulposus material and may produce an inflammatory response in the epidural space and in the underlying nerve roots.[49–51] It is likely that pain and other symptoms are produced by a combination of this inflammatory response, edema, and the mechanical pressure on nerve roots. Additional sources of spinal pain include degenerated, symptomatic areas of the spine that develop sensory nerve formation into the outer layer of abnormal intervertebral disks, vertebral end plates, and other structures.[52, 53]

Steroids can decrease neurogenic inflammation and produce membrane stabilization that results in pain relief. This steroid effect may evolve over a period of days. In symptomatic individuals, the epidural space can be very sensitive to any pressure or injection. Because of the delayed onset of this steroid effect, a rationale can be made for including a local anesthetic in the injection, decreasing the pain of the initial injection. The local anesthetic can provide pain relief that lasts beyond the duration of detectable sensory blockade and can produce a more sustained, but temporary, relief of pain.[54]

Indications, Contraindications, and Limitations

Radicular extremity pain that has not responded to more conservative treatments is the primary indication for ESI (Table 184–2). ESI is not indicated for the treatment of mechanical or muscular axial back pain. Outcome studies do not clearly support the use of ESIs in spinal stenosis patients,[55] but many clinicians feel they can be helpful in this population, particularly in patients with radicular symptoms. Benefit in patients with prior back surgery is less clear, but many feel a subset of these patients benefits from ESI as well.[45]

Prospective and retrospective studies have revealed several patient features associated with failure of ESIs to relieve pain or improve function.[56, 57] These factors also are summarized Table 184–2.

Injection Technique

The goal of the injection is to deliver steroid as a single agent or combined with local anesthetic to the

TABLE 184–2 ■ Selection for Epidural Steroid Injection

INDICATIONS	CONTRAINDICATIONS	FACTORS ASSOCIATED WITH FAILURE
Herniated nucleus pulposus with extremity pain in a radicular pattern	Anticoagulation	Smoking
Foraminal stenosis with radicular symptoms	Infection at the site	Unemployed
Spinal stenosis with extremity symptoms	Other pain that is more intense	Long duration
Imaging studies with concordant findings	Lack of consent	Unvarying pain despite activity or treatment
Pain present for weeks to months	Allergy to intended injectate	Psychological distress
	Relative contraindications include primarily back pain, failed prior epidural steroid injections, untreated anxiety or depression	Nonradicular pain

Adapted from Hopwood MB, Abram SE: Factors associated with failure of lumbar epidural steroids. Reg Anesth 18:238–243, 1993; Jamison RN, VandeBoncouer T, Ferrante FM: Low back pain patients unresponsive to an epidural steroid injection: Identifying predictive factors. Clin J Pain 7:311–317, 1991.

presumed source of pain and symptoms. Usually, the presumed source is the nerve root at the symptomatic level. Delivery techniques vary widely, and a variety of solutions and volumes are commonly used.[58] Two very common techniques in widespread use are interlaminar and transforaminal injections.

INTERLAMINAR INJECTION TECHNIQUE

For labor analgesia and perioperative anesthesia and analgesia, the epidural space is typically accessed using the loss of resistance technique with an interlaminar approach as the patient assumes a sitting or lateral decubitus position. The technique is simple, straightforward, familiar to most anesthesiologists, and does not require the use of specialized equipment such as fluoroscopy. For ESIs, this technique has the advantage of simplicity and familiarity, delivering most of the injectate directly into the epidural space. It also has the disadvantage of delivering the medication into the center of the posterior epidural space instead of focusing the medication directly at the level of presumed pathology. This approach to the epidural space is what most clinicians refer to as an ESI.

Classically, ESIs have been performed without the assistance of imaging techniques. When combined with the use of contrast injection and multiplanar fluoroscopy, the technique has diagnostic value (the patency of foraminal openings, scarring, and flow of injectate are all seen with fluoroscopy) and the ability to ensure that the injectate has been delivered to the epidural space. Without the use of fluoroscopic guidance, failure to achieve injection into the epidural space has been reported to be as high as 12% to 38%.[39, 59] A prospective study of patients with previous back operations demonstrated a failure rate of 53% in placing an epidural needle at the desired level based on surface anatomy alone and only a 26% success rate in delivering injectate to the level of pathology.[59] In a retrospective study, Johnson and colleagues[37] demonstrated that combining epidurography with ESI permitted safe and accurate therapeutic injections with an exceedingly low incidence of complications.

Commonly, a specialized epidural needle such as a 17- to 22-gauge Tuohy or a Crawford needle coupled with the loss of resistance technique is employed to locate the epidural space. Sometimes, an epidural catheter inserted through the needle is used to direct the medication delivery to the desired area.

TRANSFORAMINAL INJECTION TECHNIQUE

With the transforaminal technique, the epidural space is accessed at the level of the spinal nerve. In addition to *transforaminal epidural injection*, this approach is also known as *selective nerve root injection*, because the initial point of injection is at a specific nerve root. The injectate can be easily directed to the epidural space, particularly with medial placement, so the term *selective* may not always be accurate. Correct application of the technique requires the use of fluoroscopy because surface landmarks and tactile sensations are unreliable in ensuring appropriate final needle position.

With the patient in a prone position, the primary lumbar landmarks for performing this injection are the transverse process above the desired nerve root and the superior aspect of the nerve root foramen. The transverse process is best viewed on an anteroposterior projection, and the superior aspect of the nerve root foramen is best seen on a lateral projection. Sacral nerve root visualization may occasionally be difficult and may require a canted fluoroscopic projection. The target area is referred to as *the safe triangle* because it does not contain neural structures and therefore limits the opportunity for direct nerve damage from the needle[60] (see Fluoroscopic Guidance). Typically, a 3- to 6-inch, 20- to 25-gauge needle is used with or without an introducer needle. We use a curved needle technique, in which the distal aspect of the needle is curved away from the bevel opening. This technique provides improved steerability to the needle for localizing the precise end point and avoiding sensitive structures such as the nerve root. Needle position is confirmed using radiographic contrast injection; then, a combination of local anesthetic and steroid is injected. Often, a small volume injection with concentrated local anesthetic is used to place the medication at the area of pathology.

The transforaminal approach to the epidural space has become the standard approach for many injection therapists. The ability to deliver concentrated, small volumes precisely to the location of pain generation is the main reason for this popularity, but there are several additional advantages. A small-caliber needle (e.g., 25 gauge) can be used at a location remote from the intrathecal space and nerve root, minimizing the chance of damage to sensitive structures. Tissue trauma from this small needle is less than that produced by the larger, specialized epidural needles typically used for an interlaminar injection. The pressure of injection on the nerve root may reproduce the patient's radicular symptoms, confirming the likely source of the pain. Careful examination of contrast flow under pulsed or continuous fluoroscopy allows the clinician to visualize the patency of the neural foramen and confirm the spread medially to the epidural space. Prospective studies have shown transforaminal epidural injection to be effective in treating radicular pain from degenerative lumbar stenosis.

ADDITIONAL APPROACHES

Additional methods for medication delivery to the epidural space deserve comment. A technique for delivery of a variety of medications through a stiff, steerable catheter reportedly has an additional benefit.[61] This technique, known as *lysis of adhesions* or *neuroplasty* involves delivery of local anesthetic and steroid along with hyaluronidase or hypertonic saline, or both. In addition to anti-inflammatory benefits, this technique may relieve compression caused by scar or adhesions. Unfortunately, prospective studies comparing it with other treatments are not available to validate these claims.

The epidural space may also be accessed caudally through the sacral hiatus. A catheter (e.g., Racz) may then be used to advance the tip to within the epidural space to the lumbar level of pathology.

Epiduroscopy, with introduction of a fiber-optic scope through the sacral hiatus, allows direct visualization of the target and confirmation of drug delivery.[62] Direct visualization can confirm the presence of pathology and allow mechanical disruption of adhesions. This technique is not widely employed and requires the use of specialized equipment. No studies have compared this approach with more standard drug delivery methods.

OUTCOMES

Large, placebo-controlled randomized studies using perceived "best practice" standards do not exist for ESIs. Numerous editorials and meta-analyses have detailed the shortcomings of the literature and called for appropriate study.[45, 58, 63-67] An independently funded, multicenter, randomized, controlled trial was unable to enroll sufficient patients, primarily because referring physicians were unwilling to submit their patients to potentially inactive treatment.[68] Many of the prospective studies often quoted fail to use fluoroscopic guidance or even make an effort to localize medication injection to the level of presumed pathology. Few studies examine functional outcomes or control for other treatments, medications, or interventions. The patient populations studied most commonly have been mixed, with inconsistent diagnoses, symptom duration, and localization of symptoms.

Two outcome studies deserve comment. Carette and associates[69] published a randomized, double-blind trial of 158 subjects who received up to three injections of methylprednisolone acetate and saline versus a smaller volume of saline alone for patients with sciatica due to herniated nucleus pulposus. The steroid group had short-term improvements in leg pain, mobility, and sensory deficits with no long-term benefit or change in eventual surgical intervention rate. Drawbacks of the study include no fluoroscopic guidance, no effort to place the epidural needle at the corresponding level of disk herniation, unequal volumes of injectate in the groups, a patient population probably requiring surgery, less than ideal timing between injections, and no groups receiving local anesthetic. This study has been widely referenced by nonpain specialists as evidence that epidural steroids have little role in managing radicular pain, whereas pain physicians have noticed the ESI technique deficiencies.

A second study suffers from different limitations. Lutz and colleagues[70] performed a prospective, nonblinded, noncontrolled study of transforaminal epidural and local anesthetic injections in patients with lumbar herniated nucleus pulposus confirmed by history, physical examination, and magnetic resonance imaging. Sixty-nine patients received transforaminal injections at the level of their identified pathology in a manner similar to the previous description and were followed for an average of 80 weeks. Patients received an average of 1.8 injections, and 75% had more than 50% pain reduction. Formalized assessment of function was not performed. Limitations of this study primarily are related to the noncontrolled, nonrandom patient selection and the limited outcome assessment measures. The technique of injection, medication selection (i.e., radiographic contrast, 9 mg of betamethasone, and 15 mg of 2% lidocaine), and selection criteria fit with what many injection-oriented pain specialists feel are ideal for demonstrating a favorable outcome of ESIs.

Potential complications of ESIs include dural puncture headache, increased pain, vasovagal response, elevated blood glucose levels, systemic toxicity from the intravenous injection, unilateral administration of injectate, hematoma, bleeding, infection, and nerve damage.

MEDIAL BRANCH AND FACET PROCEDURES FOR DIAGNOSIS AND TREATMENT

During the past 25 years, the lumbar, cervical, and thoracic facet (or zygapophyseal) joints have been a topic of considerable interest as they pertain to axial spinal pain and its minimally invasive treatment. The technique of using selective denervation of the facet joints to reduce pain caused by facet joint arthropathy has gained much support because of an increasingly positive body of evidence in the medical literature.

History

For decades, the lumbar facet joint has been recognized as an important generator of axial spinal pain, although there is some controversy about this theory.[71, 72] Initially, surgical lumbar spine fusion with or without destruction of the facet joint (i.e., facetectomy) was the procedure of choice. In the past 3 decades, less destructive procedures have been researched, although the spinal fusion still has utility for some spinal disorders.[73]

INTRA-ARTICULAR FACET JOINT INJECTIONS

Injections into the lumbar facet joint were a popular, if somewhat understudied, modality of treating lumbar spinal pain in past decades. Advances in technology, specifically in the area of radiographic visualization, have made fluoroscopic identification of the facet joint and subsequent cannulation possible. Joint injections for diagnostic and therapeutic purposes were made convenient and cost-effective by this advance in technology. However, because of extravasation of injectate into the epidural space or surrounding musculature, the lack of specificity of this technique led to its discredit as a diagnostic tool.[74, 75] Further investigation into the utility of these injections as a therapy for acute back pain also diminished enthusiasm, because intra-articular injections of local anesthetic and corticosteroid were found to be similar to placebo injections several months after injections.[76]

LUMBAR MEDIAL BRANCH DENERVATION

Nikolai Bogduk and colleagues[77] clarified the neuroanatomy of the facet joint in the late 1970s. This improved understanding of anatomy, as well as improvements in the technology available for radiofrequency neurodestructive procedures, led to increased interest in the use of radiofrequency energy to lesion the nervous supply of the facet joints. Original research in this field was somewhat clouded by outdated techniques and materials. Several studies are in progress, and the initial work indicates that this technique of treating axial lumbar pain is more frequently successful and less frequently complicated than other means of treating pain mediated by lumbar facet arthropathy. Reassessment of this treatment found that it provides improvements in subjective pain rating and that activity tolerance is improved by lumbar medial branch denervation.[78]

CERVICAL AND THORACIC MEDIAL BRANCH DENERVATION

The same principles and techniques used in diagnosing and treating lumbar pain from facet arthropathy have been applied to the cervical spine. Because the procedure has a briefer history in this anatomic location, it appears that the literature involving these treatments is clearer than that of its predecessor. Early outcome studies involving intra-articular cervical facet injections of local anesthetic or corticosteroid have indicated disappointing results.[79] However, radiofrequency cervical medial branch denervation demonstrated prolonged benefits.[80, 81] McDonald and associates[82] reported significant pain relief after blocks with radiofrequency cervical medial branch denervation for 71% of treated patients. The patients with success had a median duration of relief of 422 days. Repeating the denervation procedure could successfully treat recurrent pain.[82]

There has been less interest in thoracic facet arthropathy for technical and anatomic reasons. This disease entity is less frequently encountered because there is a relative lack of motion in the thoracic spine. However, the referral patterns[83] and the anatomy[84-86] involving thoracic facet arthropathy have been elicited, and work involving thoracic medial branch denervation is ongoing.[87]

Neuroanatomy

There are facet joints in the human spine at each level between the C1-2 and L5-S1 joints. They are synovial joints, with the capsule and synovium extensively innervated with sensory fibers. Innervation includes mechanoreceptors,[88] fibers containing substance P,[89] and numerous other neurotransmitters linked to nociception.[90, 91] Their innervation is thought to be segmental and based primarily on the medial branch of the primary posterior ramus of each segmental spinal nerve[58] (Fig. 184–3). However, later research has shown that there is also nonsegmental and autonomic innervation of the facet joint.[92]

The medial branch innervates the multifidus muscle segmentally in addition to the facet joint capsule and its contents. This muscle, itself a significant pain generator, may account for some of the analgesia associated with lumbar medial branch blocks and denervations.[93, 94] Because of specific innervation, multifidus electromyelography may also be used as an outcome determinant in studies of lumbar medial branch denervation.[95]

Except for this muscle, there is no other significant structure for which the medial branch is the sole innervation. The anatomy of the cervical, thoracic, and lumbar medial branches is demonstrated in Figure 184–4.

Diagnosis

Diagnosis of pain due to facet arthropathy is based on an accurate history and physical examination. Unfortunately, neither is sufficiently specific to make decisions leading to definitive therapy.[72, 96] Several physical examination characteristics are used to select patients for diagnostic lumbar medial branch blocks; classic signs include localized low back pain exacerbated by extension and rotation[97] with referral in a stereotypical distribution (Fig. 184–5). Incorporating facet-loading maneuvers into the physical examination of the lumbar spine

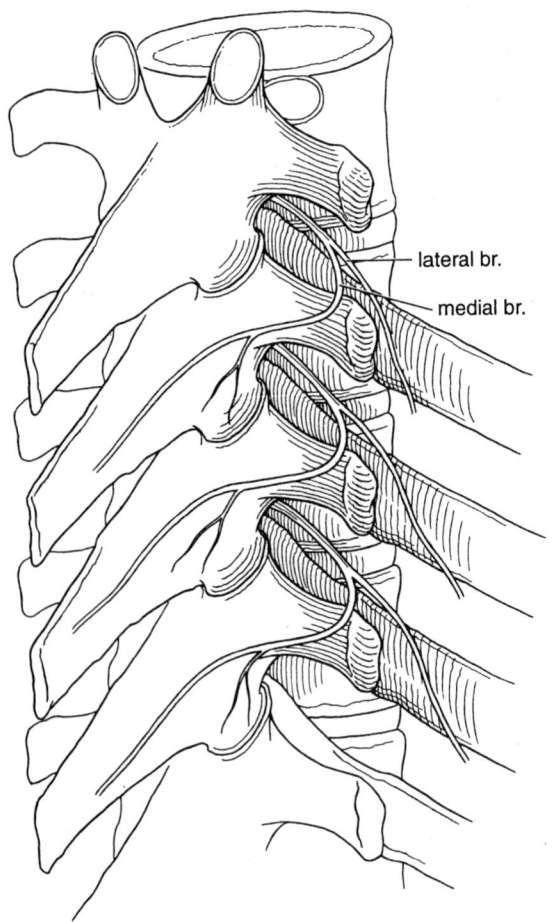

FIGURE 184–3. Thoracic space anatomy. (Courtesy of Brett Stacey, Oregon Health & Science University School of Medicine, Portland, OR.)

is recommended. Imaging evaluations, such as CT, are insufficiently sensitive and specific to be considered diagnostic.[98] A sequence of diagnostic injections of the medial branches is performed to help secure the diagnosis.

There was originally much speculation about the appropriate diagnostic regimen, but most clinicians use the so-called two-block paradigm. With this method, the patient is subjected to two sets of diagnostic, fluoroscopically guided medial branch injections.[99] These injections are usually single blinded (i.e., the clinician knows the contents of the injection; the patient does not) and contain a long-acting (e.g., 0.5% bupivacaine) or short-acting (2% lidocaine) local anesthetic. The patient is not sedated during the procedure. After the procedure, the patient is asked to complete a pain diary, recording numerical rating scale values representing the pain.

Pain relief in each of the two blocks that is concordant with the expected duration of the local anesthetic is required before the clinician makes a decision to perform a radiofrequency denervation. This technique has been validated,[99] and although definitive correlation with outcome studies is pending, pain reductions greater than 50% have been reported in up to 70% of patients using this diagnostic paradigm (Manning D: personal communication, 1997). Some controversy exists regarding the accuracy of this model,[100, 101] but no other single model has emerged as a validated model to replace it. Refinements in technique may lead to further improvements in the use of diagnostic injections in prognosis regarding the treatment of lumbar facet arthropathy.[102]

Radiofrequency Denervation Treatment
PROCEDURE

Neurolysis can be achieved using many techniques.[103] Various technical considerations have led to the use of

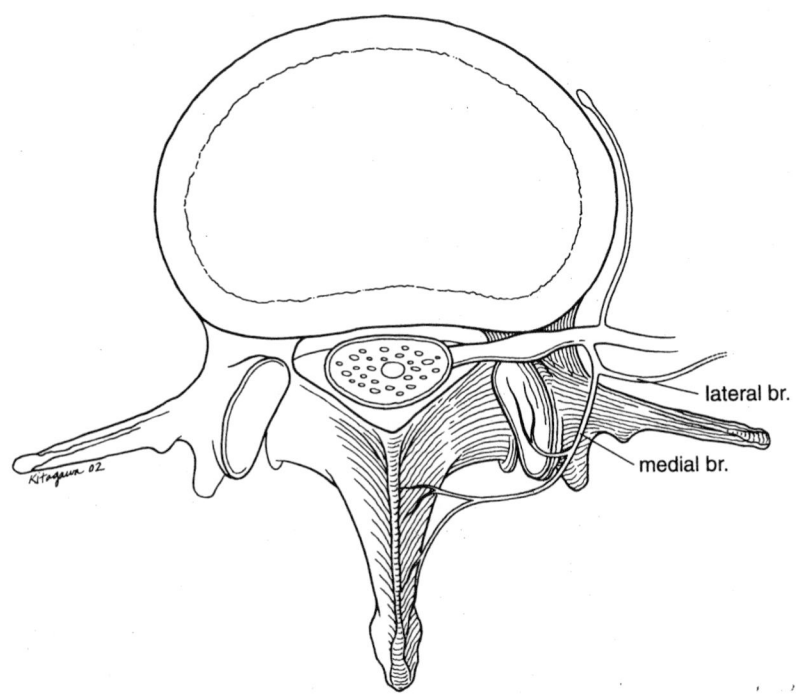

FIGURE 184–4. Lumbar vertebrae body anatomy with medial branch. (Courtesy of Brett Stacey, Oregon Health & Science University School of Medicine, Portland, OR.)

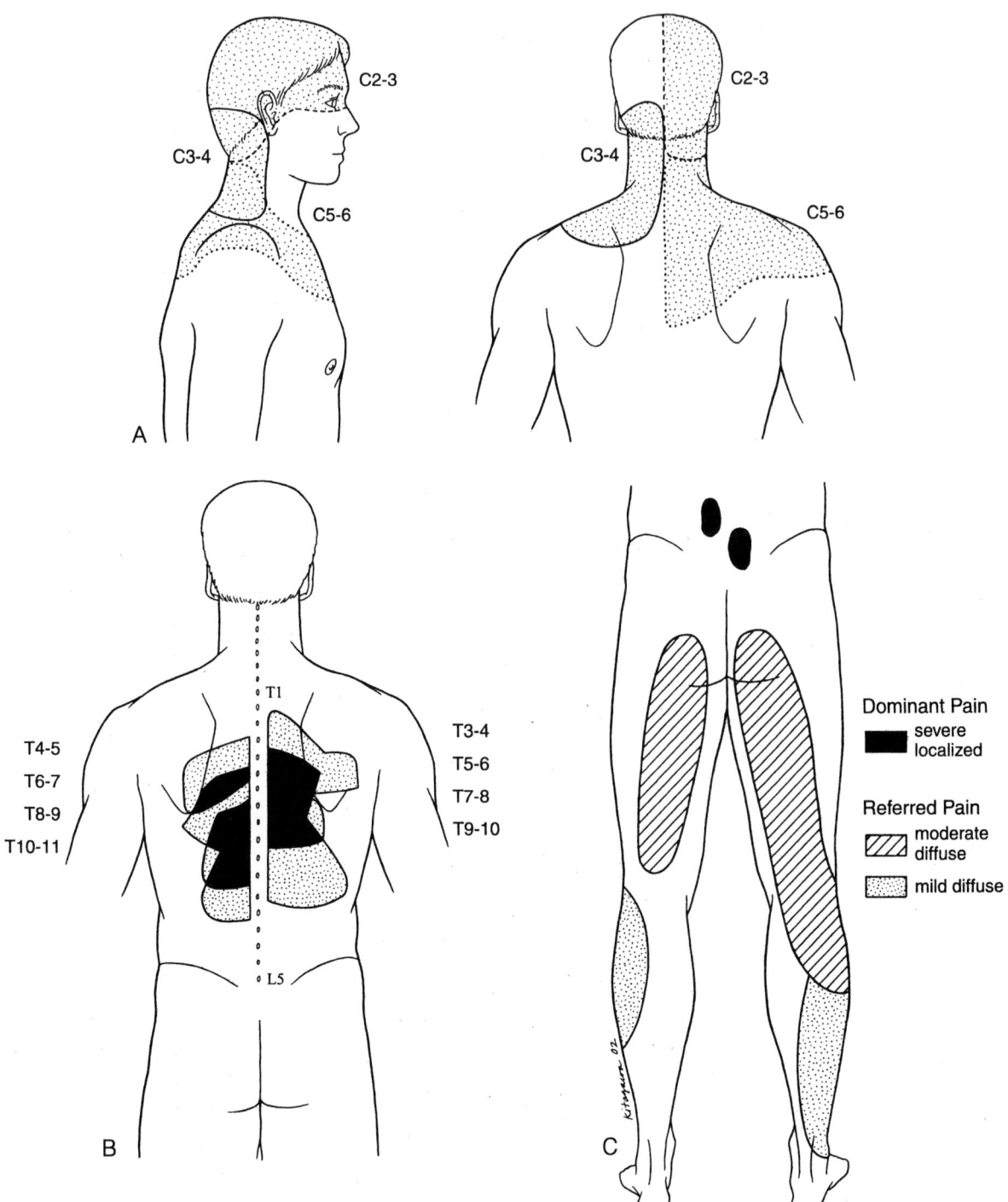

FIGURE 184–5. Referral patterns for cervical *(A)*, thoracic *(B)*, and lumbar facets *(C)*. (*A*, Adapted from Lord SM, Barnsley L, Wallis BJ, Bogduk N: Chronic cervical zygapophysial joint pain after whiplash. Spine 21:1737–1745, 1996; *B*, Adapted from Dreyfuss P, Tibiletti C, Dreyer SJ: Thoracic zygapophyseal joint pain patterns. Spine 19:807–811, 1994; *C*, Adapted from Fukui S, Ohseto K, Shiotani M, et al: Distribution of referred pain from the lumbar zygapophyseal joints and dorsal rami. Clin J Pain 13:303–307, 1997.)

radiofrequency energy as the method of choice for denervation of the medial branch (Table 184–3). Equipment improvements include small-diameter (22-gauge) and curved probes, which minimize tissue trauma and improve navigation. The lesion generator, which is also used for intracranial functional neurosurgery, allows multiple settings, depending on the procedure. Of greater importance is the ability to stimulate the adjacent structures with a harmless neurostimulating electrical field before denervation. Although not universally used, this is a potentially significant safety advantage of using this technique.

TABLE 184-3 ■ **Evaluation of Neurotomy Techniques**

TYPE OF NEUROTOMY	PRECISION OF LESION SIZE	COLLATERAL DAMAGE FROM DENERVATION	TRAUMA OF PROCEDURE	ABILITY TO ASSESS INTRAVASCULAR STATUS	ABILITY TO STIMULATE ADJACENT NERVES
Radiofrequency	5	5	5	5	5
Cryotherapy	5	3	2	0	5
Surgery	0–5	1–3	3	5	0–5
Injection of lytic chemicals	2	1–3	5	5	0

The rating scale is from 0 to 5: 0 (poor) 1   2   3   4   5 (good)

The radiofrequency-active cannula tip must be positioned within 2 mm of the nerve to denervate the medial branch. This precision requires an understanding of the anatomy of the adjacent bony structures plus the availability of high-quality fluoroscopy.

The medial branches of two segmental spinal nerves innervate each facet joint ipsilaterally (see Fig. 184–4). To affect anesthesia of the lumbar medial branch, the radiofrequency cannula has to be positioned precisely slightly inferior to the junction of the transverse process and the pedicle at each lumbar level. At the sacrum, it is the dorsal ramus of L5 that is denervated in the sacral alar notch.[102] Also commonly denervated is the S1 contribution to the L5-S1 joint, as is the nerve that exits the superior aspect of the ipsilateral S1 neural foramen.[104] Sensorimotor neurological lesions are extremely uncommon as a result of this procedure, because the medial branch is more than 2 mm from adjacent neurological structures at the point of lesioning.

At the cervical levels inferior to C3, the active tip must be positioned in the concave aspect of the lateral articular pillar of the transverse process at each segment. At C3, the anatomy is similar to the inferior segments, except that it has a superficial branch that runs immediately posterior to the C2-3 facet joint and becomes the third occipital nerve, which is partially responsible for the sensory innervation of the posterior skull and scalp. In denervating this nerve as it passes posterior to the C2 lateral articular pillar, the C2 component of the C2-3 joint and the third occipital nerve are lesioned.[80]

The third occipital nerve lesion can cause ataxia, because it is proprioceptive to the posterior scalp and skull. This complication is relatively common but rarely severe.[80] Up to 40% of patients having cervical denervation without neurostimulation before lesioning experience mild hypesthesia or dysesthesia in the distribution of portions of the deep or superficial cervical plexus[81] that are immediately adjacent to the lesioning target. In our experience, use of the stimulation mode before denervation can reduce this risk to approximately 20% without compromising the beneficial results.

The thoracic anatomy can be more involved, and facet-related pain is less common in this distribution. Successful medial branch denervations have, however, been performed in the thoracic spine after the discovery that, at several levels, the medial branch exists in a plane not adjacent to the transverse process. The course of the medial branches of the thoracic dorsal rami is lumbar in character at T11 and T12 only. The other thoracic levels assume a different anatomic distribution. A two-needle technique has been advocated for this region.[28] With the two-needle technique, one needle is inserted to contact the lateral third of the transverse process, and a second is positioned at the identical depth (as verified by lateral fluoroscopy) but cephalad, so as to be near the medial branch without puncturing the lung. Although based on the published literature mentioned previously, this technique has not yet been published in a peer-reviewed journal.

To facilitate performance of these neurolytic procedures, conscious sedation is often used. Cautious use of short-acting sedative agents should be considered to allow for rapid on and off titration. Intermittent feedback from the patient should be sought during innervation testing (motor and sensory) before neurolytic lesioning.

OUTCOMES

The prolonged effects of radiofrequency medial branch denervation have been demonstrated through numerous studies. The cervical region is the most thoroughly studied of these procedures. In this area, 75% of the treatment group had at least 50% analgesia for a median duration of 263 days.[81] With radiofrequency denervation, the neuronal contents are selectively coagulated, and neuronal function is interrupted. However, the neuronal substrate remains.[104] This allows regrowth of the nerve approximately 8 to 12 months after the procedure but prevents neuroma formation.

The pain relief from the procedure is sufficient to allow many of the patients to improve their activity tolerance and reduce other therapies for pain; however, various investigators have questioned the value of a "permanent" procedure that "wears off." There is no contraindication to repeating the denervation if the symptoms recur, nor is there any additional technical disadvantage presented by repeat denervation. Compared with surgical therapy, these considerations favor the minimally invasive route.

The literature on this subject has presented medial branch denervation as a single therapy. There may, however, be advantages to combining appropriate denervations with other multidisciplinary therapies, such as psychological and physical therapy. Although there are proven psychological benefits to successful denervation alone,[105] future research may show that the multidisciplinary approach to this clinical entity produces a more robust and long-lasting result.

SYMPATHETIC NERVE BLOCKS

Anatomy of the Sympathetic Nervous System

The sympathetic nervous system is one half of the autonomic nervous system. It is the *yin* to the parasympathetic nervous system's *yang*. Commonly described as the "fight or flight" part of the autonomic nervous system, it causes vasoconstriction, increased heart rate, decreased intestinal motility, and piloerection. Its function in maintaining vasoconstrictor tone was first described by Claude Bernard as early as 1852.

The sympathetic nervous system efferent fibers begin in the intermediolateral column of the spinal cord and exit along the ventral roots from T1 to L2. This distribution has some variability, and some people have contributions from lower cervical roots. These fibers then exit the ventral root as white rami communicantes and enter the sympathetic chains, which lie on the anterolateral aspect of the vertebral bodies. In the thoracic region, these chains are relatively close to the somatic nerves and are close to the neck of the ribs.

These preganglionic fibers, as the name implies, eventually synapse in one of the sympathetic ganglia. The ganglia may be part of the sympathetic chain, may be adjacent to it (e.g., celiac plexus), or may be relatively remote. Before they synapse, the preganglionic fibers travel a variable distance in the sympathetic chain, which makes it impossible to speak of sympathetic dermatomes. After synapsing, the postganglionic fibers then travel to their site of action.[106]

Pain and visceral sensation are carried by sympathetic afferent nerves. They are thin, unmyelinated nerves, commonly classified as C fibers. They transmit burning, aching pain. These fibers enter the spinal cord through the dorsal roots, and they have their cell bodies in the dorsal root ganglia. Afferent fibers travel along the somatic nerves (carrying somatic pain) or as hitchhikers with the sympathetic nerves (carrying visceral pain and sensation). Those providing visceral sensation and pain pass through the sympathetic ganglia but do not synapse there. Because these visceral sensory nerves travel beside the sympathetic efferent nerves, sympathetic nerve blocks inevitably anesthetize these nerves as well. This is part of the reason that sympathetic blocks are an important part of the pain management armamentarium.

Indications for Sympathetic Nerve Blocks

There are numerous reasons for choosing sympathetic nerve blockade, but almost all fall into one of two categories: pain control or vasodilation. Sympathetic blocks done for diagnosis are still common but have lately become somewhat controversial.[107]

For years, sympathetic blocks were used to diagnose reflex sympathetic dystrophy, now known as complex regional pain syndrome type I. Relief of pain was considered diagnostic of that disorder. As controversy about the diagnosis continues and we learn more about the heterogeneity of the pathophysiology, sympathetic blockade is no longer thought to be a powerful diagnostic tool.[108] However, even if the blocks are no longer the diagnostic tool they were once thought to be, they can still provide useful information.[109] Sympathetic blockade with local anesthetic can predict the effectiveness of a neurolytic sympathetic block, as in celiac plexus neurolysis for the pain of pancreatic carcinoma.

Sympathetic blockade, as the anatomy suggests, may be extremely helpful in treating a number of painful conditions. The simultaneous blockade of the C fibers can often yield tremendous pain relief even if the disorder is unrelated to the sympathetic nervous system. Sympathetic nerve blocks, if properly done, do not cause somatic numbness or motor blockade, unlike blockade of the somatic nerves. This can be an especially useful technique for patients who are unable to obtain acceptable pain relief from the more conventional methods or who are experiencing intolerable side effects. Some patients accept significant risk of morbidity or mortality from sympathetic blockade because it is such an effective treatment of their pain.

The literature is nearly void of well conducted, randomized, controlled studies of sympathetic blocks, but case reports and retrospective studies are numerous. This lack of definitive evidence has led some to question the role of these blocks in modern pain management.[107] Sympathetic block was long considered to be the gold standard in diagnosing complex regional pain syndrome type I.[110] Although it has fallen from that pedestal, sympathetic blockade still has a place in the therapy of complex regional pain syndrome and other painful conditions. Sometimes, the sympathetic fibers are not the target; instead, the small, unmyelinated pain nerves, when blocked, provide pain relief.

The vasodilation caused by a sympathetic block can also be helpful in treating certain disorders. Any condition that produces a significant amount of vasoconstriction can be relieved or moderated by sympathetic blockade. In these conditions, the sympathetic efferent fibers, rather than the C fibers, are the targets of the therapy. Ischemic pain, tissue breakdown, and slow healing can be reasons for performing sympathetic blocks. Diseases such as scleroderma that manifest with vasospasm and tissue ischemia may respond to sympathetic blockade. Extreme cases may warrant sympathetic neurolysis to give the patient pain relief and allow the tissues to heal.

Fixed vascular lesions, such as those caused by atherosclerosis, usually show little improvement with sympathetic block because the vessels are rigid and cannot dilate. The tissue ischemia may worsen with sympathetic blockade because of the steal phenomenon; dilation of relatively healthy vessels in the ischemic area can cause a drop in local blood pressure, reducing the flow of blood through the fixed stenosis. If a permanent sympathectomy is contemplated, the patient should first have a trial block with local anesthetic to ensure that the symptoms will not be worsened.

Peripheral vascular surgery is a special case in which temporary sympathetic blockade may make the difference between success and failure. In the anastomosis of small arteries, as is seen in repair of a traumatic amputation, the trauma of surgery (and the original injury, if traumatic) can lead to vasospasm and loss of circulation. The distal tissues are at risk for dying of ischemia when circulation is lost. A clot may form in the repaired vessel from the stagnation of blood and damaged or missing endothelium. In many cases, a sympathetic block can significantly reduce the degree of vasospasm and maintain blood flow through the repaired or damaged vessels. Another benefit of sympathectomy, which may be critical in patients who have peripheral vascular disease, is an increase in collateral circulation. However, the risk of steal phenomena and subsequent ischemia of marginal tissue must be considered.

Sympathetic Nerve Blocks

The sympathetic nervous system can be blocked at any point between the brainstem and the effector organs. Most effective are blocks that are done where the sympathetic nerves or ganglia are separated from the somatic nerves, so that there is little or no sensory or motor block. Other important considerations are proximity to delicate or sensitive structures and the ease of access.

Spinal (intrathecal) and epidural blocks are also sympathetic blocks, but they typically are not used as such. Rather, the sympathetic blockade that accompanies such blocks is a benefit or a liability, depending on the situation. These are examples of sympathetic blocks in which the sensory and motor nerves are equally affected. Peripheral nerve blocks, such as an ulnar nerve block, also produce a sympathetic blockade, because the sympathetic nerves hitchhike along the somatic nerves.

SPHENOPALATINE GANGLION BLOCK

The sphenopalatine or Meckel's ganglion usually is the most rostral of the sympathetic ganglia that are commonly blocked. The sphenopalatine block was rarely done until recently, but it is now thought to be effective in treating and preventing cluster headaches. The ganglion is a small triangular mass in the pterygopalatine fossa, medial and inferior to the maxillary nerve and lateral to the sphenopalatine foramen. The sphenopalatine ganglion is not made up of only sympathetic nerves; it receives two (or three) sensory fibers from the maxillary nerve and receives parasympathetic fibers from the nervus intermedius of the facial nerve through the greater superficial petrosal nerve. The sympathetic fibers arise from the carotid plexus and arrive through the deep petrosal nerve. Although this is a mixed ganglion, its sympathetic nerves supply the nose, orbit, and part of the face, making it a useful ganglion to block. The sensory components involve the mucosa of parts of the nose, palate, uvula, and tonsils. Numbness of these areas is often not readily noticed by the patient, because some of these regions have dual sensory innervation. In performing the block, the sphenopalatine ganglion can be approached extraorally, in the same way as the maxillary nerve, or it can be approached intranasally. It may also be blocked by insertion of a needle though the greater palatine foramen and by advancement of the needle along the pterygopalatine canal.

STELLATE GANGLION BLOCK

Moving down the body, the next major sympathetic block is the stellate ganglion block. The stellate ganglion supplies sympathetic fibers to the ipsilateral upper extremity and one half of the head. It is often used when vasodilation of the arm or face is desired or for treating certain painful conditions (e.g., complex regional pain syndrome type I) of the hand or arm. The greatest risks of doing the stellate ganglion block are related to puncturing or anesthetizing structures that pass near the cervical sympathetic trunk.

Horner's syndrome (i.e., ptosis, meiosis, and anhidrosis) is commonly seen after a stellate ganglion block and has often been taken as a sign of an effective block (it is not). There is usually no significant morbidity associated with this syndrome, although it may lead to increased intraocular pressure in patients with certain types of glaucoma. The most serious complications are injection of local anesthetic into the carotid or vertebral arteries; either mistake leads to an almost immediate seizure. The duration of the seizure and its severity depend on many factors, including the amount and type of local anesthetic injected. Another serious potential complication is high spinal anesthesia, which can occur if the local anesthetic is injected into a dural cuff. Potentially, a high-level epidural anesthesia could also occur if the local anesthetic went through the neural foramina.

The stellate ganglion block, as it is usually performed, is misnamed. With the usual techniques, the injection occurs at the middle cervical ganglion, and the drug spreads along fascial layers to the stellate ganglion and part of the superior cervical ganglion. A brief review of the anatomy of the sympathetic nervous system in the cervical region may elucidate this block. The neck has three sympathetic ganglia, called the middle and inferior cervical ganglia. The inferior cervical ganglion is usually fused to the first thoracic ganglion, and together, they are called the stellate ganglion. The stellate ganglion is 1 to 3 cm long and lies anterior to the transverse process of C7 and the first rib. Anterior to this ganglion is the vertebral artery, and anteromedial to it lies the carotid artery. Immediately inferior to the stellate ganglion is the dome of the pleura. The dural cuffs of the seventh and eighth cervical nerve roots are also in the immediate vicinity. The stellate ganglion is truly in a hazardous zone.

The middle cervical ganglion lies at the level of the vertebral body of C6 on the anteromedial border of the thyrocervical trunk of the inferior thyroid artery. Its size also varies, and in rare cases, it may be entirely absent. Its nerves are distributed between the superior and inferior ganglia. The superior cervical ganglion is huge, often up to 3 cm long and almost 1 cm thick. It may be shaped like an American football but can also be oval. It is the fusion of the superior three or four sympathetic ganglia. Its inferior border is usually at the level of C4 or C5.

The classic approach to the stellate ganglion block is to pierce the skin over the anterior tubercle of the C6 transverse process (i.e., Chassaignac's tubercle) and advance the needle to contact the anterior tubercle. After withdrawing the needle 2 or 3 mm to clear the periosteum, local anesthetic is injected. The needle tip is placed right at the middle cervical ganglion. Because the sympathetic chain lies in a fascial space between the longus coli muscle and the scalene muscle group, any liquid injected at the middle cervical ganglion level will likely travel along this narrow space and end up surrounding the stellate ganglion and at least the inferior portion of the superior cervical ganglion. The fact that this technique is routinely successful shows that this spread occurs.

THORACIC SYMPATHETIC BLOCK

The thoracic sympathetic chain, unlike the cervical sympathetic chain, is close to the spinal (segmental) nerves, and there is no muscle or fascial layer separating the two. This proximity limits the utility of the thoracic sympathetic block somewhat because of the higher probability of also having a somatic block. However, sensory and motor blockade in the thoracic dermatomes is extremely well tolerated by most patients, even when it is permanent.

Most often done for painful conditions of the chest wall, thoracic sympathetic blocks may also be effective for pain involving the heart and lungs. Intractable angina can often be effectively treated with this block, although the loss of the "cardiac accelerator" fibers can be a serious problem in this patient population. Pain due to primary or metastatic tumors of the lungs may also be relieved by a thoracic sympathetic block.

The thoracic sympathetic chain lies posterior to the vertebral bodies and anterior to the necks of the ribs. There is no muscle barrier equivalent to the longus coli in the cervical chain that separates the sympathetic chain from the spinal nerve roots. Immediately adjacent to the sympathetic chain is the parietal pleura, making pneumothorax a real danger when performing blocks. Because of the high risk of pneumothorax, most practitioners use epidural analgesia to deal with temporary painful disorders such as surgery or herpes zoster outbreaks. However, neurolytic sympathetic blocks are still performed for permanent conditions that can be treated by sympathectomy.

Thoracic sympathetic block is usually accomplished by inserting a long needle over the tip of the transverse process. The needle is then advanced to contact the tip of the transverse process and redirected to pass inferior to the rib while also directed slightly medially. The needle then is advanced to contact the vertebral body. Even when using local anesthetic, this procedure requires fluoroscopy to be successful and safe. Although there is a risk of damaging the spinal roots when performing a neurolytic sympathetic block, this technique still has less morbidity than the axillary surgical thoracic sympathectomy.

CELIAC PLEXUS BLOCK AND SPLANCHNIC NERVE BLOCK

The viscera of the upper abdomen obtain their innervation from sympathetic rami of T5 to T12. These fibers course along the lateral aspect of the thoracic vertebral bodies and the greater, lesser, and least splanchnic nerves. These nerves pass through the diaphragm at the thoracolumbar junction and enter the abdominal cavity, where they branch and rebranch to finally form the celiac plexus. The celiac plexus is a tangled net of nerve fibers that wraps around the aorta and inferior vena cava at the level of the celiac artery. This nerve net also wraps around the bases of the celiac artery and vein. From this plexus, sympathetic nerves travel to the organs of the upper abdomen, and C-fiber pain impulses return from those organs.

Because all sensation from the upper abdominal viscera passes through the celiac plexus, the celiac plexus block can be a powerful tool for controlling abdominal pain. Celiac plexus block, combined with local infiltration of the abdominal wall, has been used as a complete anesthetic for upper abdominal surgery. Because there are few or no somatic sensory or motor nerves that pass through the celiac plexus, neurolysis carries little liability. The celiac plexus may be the most common site of neurolytic nerve block. In patients with pain from pancreatic carcinoma, celiac plexus neurolysis is sometimes done on the first visit to a pain management center.

Although celiac plexus neurolysis is extremely common, there are also several indications for local anesthetic blocks. Almost every practitioner performs a local anesthetic block before neurolysis to ensure that the preprocedural assessment is correct. Patients with mysterious abdominal pain may also undergo celiac plexus blockade to differentiate visceral and somatic pain.

A disorder that is singularly resistant to celiac plexus block is chronic pancreatitis. This has been a puzzle to pain management specialists for many years. Because the pain of pancreatic carcinoma usually responds dramatically to celiac plexus blockade, it would seem logical that chronic pancreatitis should respond as well. Oddly enough, patients with chronic pancreatitis, no matter what the cause, usually get no relief or very brief or partial relief from celiac plexus block. There are many theories about why this occurs, but no studies have been done to validate any of them.

The usual approach for a celiac plexus block is posterior, although there are reports of an anterior approach. Long needles are inserted bilaterally at the L1 level, starting over the tips of the 12th ribs. To block the splanchnic nerves, the needles are directed toward the body of T12. To block the celiac plexus, the needles are directed toward the body of L1. There are numerous variations on this technique, but the aim of all of them is to direct the needles so that they graze the anterolateral aspect of the vertebral body. Although fluoroscopy can make the procedure much easier and quicker, it can be done blind, although few would do a neurolytic block without fluoroscopic guidance. The final position of the needle tips depends on the type of block; for splanchnic nerve blocks, the needle tips should be 0.5 cm posterior to the anterior margin of the vertebral body when viewed in the lateral projection.

Because the celiac plexus projects much further anterior than the splanchnic nerves, the needle tips should end up between 1 to 2 cm anterior to the anterior margin of the vertebral body. If the procedure is being done without fluoroscopic guidance, the left (patient's left) needle is advanced first while the operator feels and looks for the aortic pulsations transmitted through the needle. When the needle tip is in contact with the aortic wall, the needle can often be seen to twist slightly when not held. Pulsatile, bright red blood issuing from the needle hub is a sign that the needle is in too far.

LUMBAR SYMPATHETIC BLOCK

The lumbar sympathetic chains carry preganglionic fibers from the lower thoracic sympathetic chains. The lumbar sympathetic chains send rami communicantes to the first and second lumbar spinal nerve roots. The chains enter the abdomen posterior to the medial arcuate ligament and anterior to the psoas muscle. They then travel along the psoas fascia to reach the anterolateral aspect of the vertebral bodies, eventually running along the medial border of the psoas muscle. The left sympathetic chain lies posterior and lateral to the aorta, and the right sympathetic chain lies posterior to the vena cava. Both sympathetic chains are anterior to the segmental spinal vessels.

The rami communicantes of the lumbar ganglia are longer than those in the thoracic chain. They are contained in tunnels formed by the ligamentous attachments of the psoas muscle to the lateral aspects of each vertebral body. The resulting separation of the spinal roots and the sympathetic ganglia allows the sympathetic nerves to be blocked or destroyed by neurolysis with less risk to the somatic nerves. Some of the rami communicantes pass through the psoas muscle itself and synapse with accessory ganglia. These nerves are not affected by local anesthetic solution nor neurolysis and may account for the occasional incomplete sympathectomy.

There are many variations in the anatomy of the lumbar sympathetic chain. As many as three ganglia may send nerves to a single spinal root, or one ganglion may give off up to three nerves, each to a different spinal root. There are many small plexuses formed by the lumbar sympathetic chains, but the two major ones are the aortic plexus and hypogastric plexus.

There are two approaches to the lumbar sympathetic chains commonly in use: the paramedian approach and the lateral approach. In the paramedian approach, the needles enter the skin at approximately the level of the transverse process and 5 to 6 cm lateral to the midline. The lateral approach begins 9 to 10 cm lateral to the midline. These two different approaches have their own advantages and disadvantages, but they are essentially identical in their ease and risks.[111]

The paramedian approach is technically more difficult, because the needles must be "steered" to pass inferior to the transverse process and then directed to contact the anteromedial aspect of the vertebral body, where the sympathetic chain lies. Because of the angle of the needle, it is more difficult to position the tip of the needle to be in contact with the sympathetic chain.

The lateral approach can often be more painful to the patient, especially on the right side, where the needle may pass through the substance of the kidney. Although this sounds dangerous, it is important to remember that nephrologists routinely perform needle biopsies of the kidney using needles of 12 gauge and larger. Of course, the risk increases significantly if the patient is anticoagulated or suffering from a coagulopathy. However, because the angle of the needle is more perpendicular to the anterolateral aspect of the vertebral bodies (relative to the paramedian approach), it is much easier to hit the target with the lateral approach.

Another variation in the approach to the lumbar sympathetic chain is in the number of injections. Early descriptions of the procedure recommended three to four injections on each side, usually at the level of L1, L2, and L3 (and occasionally L4). These injections now are performed at a single level, L1 or L2. With the multiple-injection techniques, smaller injection volumes (2 to 3 mL) are used, and the single-injection technique uses volumes of 10 to 20 mL and relies on spread of the local anesthetic along fascial planes. Surprisingly, the incidence of spillover onto the spinal nerve roots is fairly low with the single-injection (per side) technique. When using a neurolytic agent such as phenol, however, the extra margin of safety of the multiple-injection technique is invaluable.

REFERENCES

1. Hayashi N, Weinstein JN, Meller ST, et al: The effect of epidural injection of betamethasone or bupivacaine in a rat model of lumbar radiculopathy. Spine 23:877–885, 1998.
2. Lee HM, Weinstein JN, Meller ST, et al: The role of steroids and their effects on phospholipase A2. Spine 23:1191–1196, 1998.
3. Kantrowitz F, Robinson DR, McGuire MB, Levine L: Corticosteroids inhibit prostaglandin production by rheumatoid synovia. Nature 258:737–739, 1975.
4. Johansson A, Hao J, Sjolund B: Local corticosteroid application blocks transmission in normal nociceptive C-fibers. Acta Anesthesiol Scand 34:335–338, 1990.
5. Merrill DG: Abuses and excesses in pain management. Am Soc Anesthesiol Newslett 61:22, 1997.
6. Mount BM: Psychological and social aspects of cancer pain. In Wall PD, Relzack R (eds): Textbook of Pain, 2nd ed. New York: Churchill Livingstone, 1989, p 619.
7. Turner JA, Deyo RA, Loaser JD, et al: The importance of placebo effects in pain treatment and research. JAMA 271:1609–1614, 1994.

8. Fine PG, Roberts WJ, Gillette RG, Child TR: Slowly developing placebo responses confound tests of intravenous phentolamine to determine mechanisms underlying idiopathic chronic low back pain. Pain 56:235–242, 1994.

9. Gracely RH, Dubner R, Deeter WR, Wolskee PJ: Clinicians' expectations influence placebo analgesia [letter]. Lancet 1:43, 1985.

10. Kirgis HD, Kuntz A: Inconsistent sympathetic denervation of the upper extremity. Arch Surg 44:95–102, 1942.

11. Cicala RS, Jones JW, Westbrook LL: Causalgic pain responding to epidural but not sympathetic nerve blockade. Anesth Analg 70:218–219, 1990.

12. Tajiri K, Takahashi K, Ikeda K, Tomita K: Common peroneal nerve block for sciatica. Clin Orthop Relat Res 347:203–207, 1998.

13. Crisologo PA, Neal B, Brown R, et al: Lidocaine-induced spinal block can relieve central poststroke pain: Role of the block in chronic pain diagnosis. Anesthesiology 74:184–185, 1991.

14. Xavier AV, McDanal J, Kissin I: Relief of sciatic radicular pain by sciatic nerve block. Anesth Analg 67:1177–1180, 1988.

15. Abram SE: Pain mechanisms in lumbar radiculopathy. Anesth Analg 67:1135–1137,1988.

16. Backonja MM: Local anesthetics as adjuvant analgesics. J Pain Symptom Manage 9:491–499, 1994.

17. Edwards WT, Habib F, Burney RG, Begin G: Intravenous lidocaine in the management of various chronic pain states: A review of 211 cases. Reg Anesth 10:1–6, 1985.

18. Wallace MS, Laitin S, Licht D, Yaksh TL: Concentration-effect relations for intravenous lidocaine infusions in human volunteers: Effects on acute sensory thresholds and capsaicin-evoked hyperpathia. Anesthesiology 86:1262–1272, 1997.

19. Murphy TM: Treatment of chronic pain. In Miller RD (ed): Anesthesia, 2nd ed. New York, Churchill Livingstone, 1986, p 2088.

20. Fink BR, Cairns AM: Lack of size-related differential sensitivity to equilibrium conduction block among mammalian myelinated axons exposed to lidocaine. Anesth Analg 66:948–953, 1987.

21. Dirkson R, Rutgers MJ, Coolen MW: Cervical epidural steroids in reflex sympathetic dystrophy. Anesthesiology 66:71–73, 1987.

22. Bloncherd J, Ramamurthy S, Walsh N, et al: Intravenous regional sympatholysis: A double-blind comparison of guanethidine, reserpine, and normal saline. J Pain Symptom Manage 5:357–361, 1990.

23. Flor H, Fydrich T, Turk DC: Efficacy of multidisciplinary pain treatment centers: A meta-analytic review. Pain 49:221–230, 1992.

24. Turk DC, Stacey BR: Multidisciplinary pain centers in the treatment of chronic back pain. In Frymoyer JW, Sucker TB, Hadler NM, et al (eds): Adult Spine: Principles and Practice, 3rd ed. New York, Lippincott Williams & Wilkins, 1997, pp 235–274.

25. Gallstone J, Pennant JH: Spinal anaesthesia following facet joint injection. Anaesthesia 42:754–756, 1987.

26. Marks R, Semple AJ: Spinal anaesthesia after facet joint injection. Anaesthesia 43:65–66, 1988.

27. Adriani J: Reactions to local anesthetics. JAMA 196:4305–4308, 1966.

28. International Spinal Injection Society (ISIS): Standards for the performance of procedures involving spinal injection. Available at: www.spinalinjection.com/ISIS/standard/stand1.htm

29. Bigos S, Bowyer O, Braen G, et al: Acute Low Back Problems in Adults. Clinical Practice Guideline, no. 14. AHCPR publication no. 95–0642. Rockville, MD, US Department of Health and Human Services, Public Health Service, Agency for Health Care Policy and Research, 1994.

30. Brown PH: Medical Fluoroscopy: Guide for Safe Usage. Portland, Oregon Health Sciences University, 1997.

31. Wagner A, Jensen C, Snebye A, Rasmussen TB: A prospective comparison of iotrolan and iohexol in lumbar myelography. Acta Radiol 35:182–185, 1994.

32. Skalpe IO, Bonneville JF, Grane P, et al: Myelography with a dimeric (iodixanol) and a monomeric (iohexol) contrast medium: A clinical multicentre comparative study. Eur Radiol 8:1054–1057, 1998.

33. Stacul F, Thomsen HS: Safety profile of new non-ionic contrast media: renal tolerance. Eur J Radiol 23(Suppl 1):S6–S9, 1996.

34. Hill JA, Winniford M, Cohen MB, et al: Multicenter trial of ionic versus nonionic contrast media for cardiac angiography: The Iohexol Cooperative Study. Am J Cardiol 72:770–775, 1993.

35. White AH, Derby R, Wynne G: Epidural injections for the diagnosis and treatment of low back pain. Spine 5:67–86, 1980.

36. White AH: Injection techniques for the diagnosis and treatment of low back pain. Orthop Clin North Am 14:553–567, 1983.

37. Johnson BA, Schellhas KP, Pollei SR: Epidurography and therapeutic epidural injections: Technical considerations and experience with 5334 cases. AJNR Am J Neuroradiol 20:697–705, 1999.

38. Fukushige T, Kano T, Sano T: Radiological investigation of unilateral epidural block after single injection. Anesthesiology 87:1574–1575, 1977.

39. Renfrew DL, Moore TE, Kathol MH, et al: Correct placement of epidural steroid injections: Fluoroscopic guidance and contrast administration. AJNR Am J Neuroradiol 12:1003–1007, 1991.

40. Agency for Health Care Policy and Research. Acute lower back problems in adults: Clinical Practice Guideline 14. Publication No. 95-0642, 1994.

41. Rydevik BL, Cohen DB, Kostuik JP: Controversy: Spine epidural steroids for patients with lumbar spinal stenosis. Spine 22:2313–2317, 1997.

42. Rapp SE, Haselkorn JK, Elamm JK, et al: Epidural steroid injection in the treatment of low back pain: A meta-analysis. Anesthesiology 81:923, 1994.

43. Koes BW, Scholten RJPM, Mens JMA, Bouter LM: Efficacy of epidural steroid injections for low-back pain and sciatica: A systemic review of randomized clinical trials. Pain 63:279–288, 1995.

44. Hopayian K, Mugford M: Conflicting conclusions from two systematic reviews of epidural steroid injections for sciatica: Which evidence should general practitioners heed? Br J Gen Pract 49:57–61, 1999.

45. Rowlingson JC: Epidural steroids: Do they have a place in pain management? Pain Forum 3:20–27, 1994.

46. Jensen MC, Brant-Zawadzki MN, Obuchowski N, et al: Magnetic resonance imaging of the lumbar spine in people without back pain. N Engl J Med 331:69–73, 1994.

47. Weishaupt D, Zanetti M, Hodler J, Boos N: MR imaging of the lumbar spine: Prevalence of intervertebral disk extrusion and sequestration, nerve root compression, end plate abnormalities, and osteoarthritis of the facet joints in asymptomatic volunteers. Radiology 209:661–666, 1998.

48. Goupille P, Jayson MI, Valat JP, Freemont AJ: The role of inflammation in disk herniation-associated radiculopathy. Semin Arthritis Rheum 28:60–71, 1998.

49. McCarron RF, Wimpee MW, Hudkins PG, Laros GS: The inflammatory effect of nucleus pulposus: A possible element in the pathogenesis of low-back pain. Spine 12:760–764, 1987.

50. Saal JS, Franson RC, Dobrow R, et al: High levels of inflammatory phospholipase A_2 activity in lumbar disc herniations. Spine 15:674–678, 1990.

51. Koch H, Reinecke JA, Meijer H, Wehling P: Spontaneous secretion of interleukin 1 receptor antagonist (IL-1ra) by cells isolated from herniated lumbar discal tissue after discectomy. Cytokine 10:703–705, 1998.

52. Coppes MH, Marani E, Thomeer RT, Groen GJ: Innervation of "painful" lumbar discs. Spine 22:2342–2349, 1997.

53. Brown MF, Hukkanen MV, McCarthy ID, et al: Sensory and sympathetic innervation of the vertebral endplate in patients with degenerative disc disease. J Bone Joint Surg Br 79:147–153, 1997.

54. Arner S, Lindblom U, Meyerson BA, Molander C: Prolonged relief of neuralgia after regional anesthetic blocks: A call for further experimental and systemic clinical studies. Pain 43:287–297, 1990.

55. Fukusaki M, Kobayashi I, Hara T, Sumikawa K: Symptoms of spinal stenosis do not improve after epidural steroid injection. Clin J Pain 14:148–151, 1998.

56. Hopwood MB, Abram SE: Factors associated with failure of lumbar epidural steroids. Reg Anesth 18:238–243, 1993.

57. Jamison RN, VandeBoncouer T, Ferrante FM: Low back pain patients unresponsive to an epidural steroid injection: Identifying predictive factors. Clin J Pain 7:311–317, 1991.

58. Bogduk N: Epidural steroids. Spine 20:845–848, 1995.

59. Fredman B, Nun MB, Zohar E, et al: Epidural steroids for treating "failed back surgery syndrome": Is fluoroscopy really necessary? Anesth Analg 88:367–372, 1999.

60. Derby R, Bogduk N, Kine G: Precision percutaneous blocking procedures for localizing spinal pain. Part 2. The lumbar neuraxial compartment. Pain Digest 3:175–188, 1993.

61. Heavner JE, Racz GB, Raj P: Percutaneous epidural neuroplasty: prospective evaluation of 0.9% NaCl versus 10% NaCl with or without hyaluronidase. Reg Anesth Pain Med 24:202–207, 1999.

62. Saberski LR, Kitahata LM: Review of the clinical basis and protocol for epidural endoscopy. Conn Med 60:71–73, 1996.

63. Hogan QH, Abram SE: Epidural steroids and the outcome movement. Pain Digest 1:269–270, 1992.

64. Abram SE: Risk versus benefit of epidural steroids: Let's remain objective. Pain Forum 3:20–27, 1994.

65. Hammonds WD: Epidural steroid injections: An unproven therapy for pain. Pain Forum 3:28–30, 1994.

66. Koes BW, Scholten RJPM, Mens JMA, Bouter LM: Efficacy of epidural steroid injections for low-back pain and sciatica: A systemic review of randomized clinical trials. Pain 63:279–288, 1995.

67. Watts RW, Silagy CA: A meta-analysis on the efficacy of epidural corticosteroids in the treatment of sciatica. Anaesth Intensive Care 23:564–569, 1995.

68. Hopwood MB, Manning DC: Lumbar epidural steroid injections: is a clinical trial necessary or appropriate? [editorial]. Reg Anesth 24:5–7, 1999.

69. Carette S, Leclaire R, Marcoux S, et al: Epidural corticosteroid injections for sciatica due to herniated nucleus pulposus. N Engl J Med 336:1634–1640, 1997.

70. Lutz GE, Vad VB, Wisneski RJ: Fluoroscopic transforaminal lumbar epidural steroids: An outcome study. Arch Phys Med Rehabil 79:1362–1366, 1998.

71. Murphy WA: The facet syndrome. Radiology 151:533, 1984.

72. Schwarzer AC, Aprill CN, Derby R, et al: Clinical features of patients with pain stemming from the lumbar zygapophysial joints: Is the lumbar facet syndrome a clinical entity? Spine 19:1132–1137, 1994.

73. Markwalder TM, Merat M: The lumbar and lumbosacral facet-syndrome: Diagnostic measures, surgical treatment and results in 119 patients. Acta Neurochir (Wien) 128:40–46, 1994.

74. Moran R, O'Connell D, Walsh M: The diagnostic value of facet joint injections. Spine 13:1408–1410, 1988.

75. Esses SI, Moro JK: The value of facet joint blocks in patient selection for lumbar fusion. Spine 18:185–190, 1993.

76. Carette S, Marcoux S, Truchon R, et al: Controlled trial of corticosteroid injections into facet joints for chronic low back pain. N Engl J Med 325:1002–1007, 1991.

77. Bogduk N, Long DL: The anatomy of the so-called "articular nerves" and their relationship to facet denervation in the treatment of low-back pain. J Neurosurg 51:172–177, 1979.

78. Van Kleef M, Barendse GA, Kessils A, et al: Randomized trial of radiofrequency lumbar facet denervation for chronic low back pain. Spine 24:1937–1942, 1999.

79. Barnsley L, Lord SM, Wallis BJ, Bogduk N: Lack of effect of intraarticular corticosteroids for chronic pain in the cervical zygapophyseal joints. N Engl J Med 330:1047–1050, 1994.

80. Lord SM, Barnsley L, Bogduk N: Percutaneous radiofrequency neurotomy in the treatment of cervical zygapophysial joint pain: A caution. Neurosurgery 36:732–739, 1995.

81. Lord SM, Barnsley L, Wallis BJ, et al: Percutaneous radio-frequency neurotomy for chronic cervical zygapophyseal-joint pain. N Engl J Med 335:1721–1726, 1996.

82. McDonald GJ, Lord SM, Bogduk N: Long-term follow-up of patients treated with cervical radiofrequency neurotomy for chronic neck pain. Neurosurgery 45:61–68, 1999.

83. Dreyfuss P, Tibiletti C, Dreyer SJ: Thoracic zygapophyseal joint pain patterns. Spine 19:807–811, 1994.

84. McLain RF, Pickar JG: Mechanoreceptor endings in human thoracic and lumbar facet joints. Spine 23:168–173, 1998.

85. Chua WH, Bogduk N: The surgical anatomy of thoracic facet denervation. Acta Neurochir (Wien) 136:140–144, 1995.

86. Stolker RJ, Vervest ACM, Groen GJ: Parameters in electrode positioning in thoracic percutaneous facet denervation: An anatomical study. Acta Neurochir (Wien) 128:32–39, 1994.

87. Stolker RJ, Vervest ACM, Groen GJ: Percutaneous facet denervation in chronic thoracic spinal pain. Acta Neurochir (Wien) 122:82–90, 1993.

88. McLain RF: Mechanoreceptor endings in human cervical facet joints. Spine 19:495–501, 1994.

89. Beaman DN, Graziano GP, Glover RA, et al: Substance P innervation of lumbar spine facet joints. Spine 18:1044–1049, 1993.

90. Ashton IK, Ashton BA, Gibson SJ, et al: Morphological basis for back pain: The demonstration of nerve fibers and neuropeptides in the lumbar facet joint capsule but not in ligamentum flavum. J Orthop Res 10:72–78, 1992.

91. Ahmed M, Bjurholm A, Kreicbergs A, et al: Sensory and autonomic innervation of the facet joint in the rat lumbar spine. Spine 18:2121–2126, 1993.

92. Suseki K, Takahashi Y, Takahashi K, et al: Innervation of the lumbar facet joints: Origins and functions. Spine 22:477–485, 1977.

93. Indahl A, Kaigle A, Reikeras O, et al: Electromyographic response of the porcine multifidus musculature after nerve stimulation. Spine 20:2652–2658, 1995.

94. Hides JA, Richardson CA, Jull GA: Multifidus muscle recovery is not automatic after resolution of acute, first-episode low back pain. Spine 21:2763–2769, 1996.

95. Dreyfuss P, Halbrook B, Pauza K, et al: An ISIS funded study evaluating lumbar radiofrequency neurotomy for chronic zygapophysial joint pain [abstract]. Presented at the 7th Annual Scientific Meeting of the International Spinal Injection Society, Las Vegas, NV, 1999.

96. Dreyer SJ, Dreyfuss PH: Low back pain and the zygapophysial (facet) joints [review]. Arch Phys Med Rehabil 77:290–300, 1996.

97. McCulloch JA: Percutaneous radiofrequency lumbar rhizolysis (rhizotomy). Appl Neurophysiol 39:87–96, 1976–1977.

98. Schwarzer AC, Wang S, O'Driscoll D, et al: The ability of computed tomography to identify a painful zygapophysial joint in patients with chronic low back pain. Spine 20:907–912, 1995.

99. Barnsley L, Lord S, Bogduk N: Comparative local anesthetic blocks in the diagnosis of cervical zygapophysial joint pain. Pain 55:99–106, 1993.

100. Schwarzer AC, Aprill CN, Derby R, et al: The false-positive rate of uncontrolled diagnostic blocks of the lumbar zygapophysial joints. Pain 58:195–200, 1994.

101. North RB, Kidd DH, Zahurak M, et al: Specificity of diagnostic nerve blocks: A prospective, randomized study of sciatica due to lumbosacral spine disease. Pain 65:77–85, 1996.

102. Dreyfuss P, Schwarzer AC, Lau P, et al: Specificity of lumbar medial branch and L5 dorsal ramus blocks. Spine 22:895–902, 1997.

103. Kline MT, Yin W: Radiofrequency techniques in clinical practice. In Waldman SD, Winnie AP (eds): Interventional Pain Management. Philadelphia, WB Saunders, 1996, p 167.

104. Kline MT: Radiofrequency techniques in clinical practice. In Waldman SD, Winnie AP (eds): Interventional Pain Management. Philadelphia, WB Saunders, 1996, pp 188, 191.

105. Wallis BJ, Lord SM, Bogduk N: Resolution of psychological distress of whiplash patients following treatment by radiofrequency neurotomy: A randomized, double-blind, placebo-controlled trial. Pain 73:15–22, 1997.

106. Rocco AG, Palombi D, Raeke D: Anatomy of the lumbar sympathetic chain. Reg Anesth 20:13–19, 1995.

107. Boas RA: Sympathetic nerve blocks: In search of a role. Reg Anesth Pain Med 23:292–305, 1998.

108. Harden RN, Bruehl S, Galer BS, et al: Complex regional pain syndrome: Are the IASP diagnostic criteria valid and sufficiently comprehensive? Pain 93:211–219, 1999.

109. Stanton-Hicks M, Kaigle A, Reikeras O, Holm S: Complex regional pain syndromes: Guidelines for therapy. Clin J Pain 14:155–166, 1998.

110. Dellemijn PL, Fields HL, Allen RR, et al: The interpretation of pain relief and sensory changes following sympathetic blockade. Brain 117(Pt 6):1475–1487, 1994.

111. Raj P, Nolte H, Stanton-Hicks M: Illustrated Manual of Regional Anesthesia. Berlin, Springer-Verlag, 1988, pp 85–92.

Diagnosis and Nonoperative Management

ANDREW S. YOUKILIS ■ OREN SAGHER

The diagnosis and medical management of trigeminal neuralgia can be one of the most frustrating and rewarding challenges in neurosurgical practice. Facial pain is an extremely vexing problem, with a wide variety of possible causes. It is therefore important for neurosurgeons to have a broad understanding of the underpinnings of the facial pain syndromes. Good outcome depends on proper diagnosis and patient selection for any treatment regimen being considered. Fortunately, with an improved understanding of entities such as trigeminal neuralgia, our ability to diagnose and treat facial pain syndromes has improved remarkably since the 1950s.

HISTORY OF FACIAL PAIN

In the 11th century, the Arab physician Jurjani described a facial pain syndrome that likely was trigeminal neuralgia. He wrote of "a type of pain which affects the teeth on one side and the whole of the jaw on the side which is painful."[1, 2] The first modern description of the syndrome was by physician John Locke in the 17th century. In letters to a friend, Locke provides a detailed account of the symptoms of the wife of the English ambassador to France. Faced with limited treatment options and the patient's excruciating pain, the physician opted for eight rounds of cleansing of the gastrointestinal tract, which reportedly resulted in remission of symptoms.[3]

In the era preceding the description of trigeminal neuralgia, there were incremental and ultimately converging studies of the anatomy of the cranial nerves as well as facial pain syndromes. In 1829, Bell was the first to elaborate on the gross anatomy of the fifth cranial nerve and perform experiments that defined it as a mixed motor and sensory nerve.[4] These experiments would establish the trigeminal nerve as the cranial nerve responsible for supplying facial sensation as well as innervation to the muscles of mastication. Before this, it was widely believed that the seventh cranial nerve was the source of facial pain syndromes. Bell's discovery shifted the focus of investigation into facial pain syndromes from the seventh to the fifth cranial nerve.

Perhaps the most important event in the modernization of facial pain treatment was the observation of Trousseau in 1853 that facial pain tended to be paroxysmal.[5] Trousseau hypothesized that the pathophysiology of trigeminal neuralgia was related to abnormal impulse conduction analogous to the epilepsies. The disorder was for a time even referred to as "neuralgia epileptiform."[5, 6] This serendipitous analogy eventually led Bergouignan in 1942 to use the newly introduced anticonvulsant diphenylhydantoin to treat trigeminal neuralgia.[7] In the 1950s, there were several promising case series using the hydantoin anticonvulsants.[2, 8–10] When carbamazepine, a new medication for epilepsy, was introduced in 1962, it was soon used in patients with trigeminal neuralgia.[11, 12] It was found to have greater efficacy and less toxicity than the hydantoins and remains the mainstay of therapy today. In recent years, many other agents have been tried and found to have efficacy in trigeminal neuralgia; the most effective of these are discussed in greater detail in this chapter.

CAUSE AND DIAGNOSIS OF TRIGEMINAL NEURALGIA

Many theories have been postulated to explain the cause of trigeminal neuralgia. One of the most common is based on the observation that demyelination of large-diameter A fibers is found at the trigeminal root entry zone in patents with trigeminal neuralgia. This theory holds that there is ephaptic transmission from these fibers to poorly myelinated A delta and unmyelinated C fibers, which results in paroxysmal facial pain. It has been widely speculated that this demyelination comes from compression of the trigeminal nerve by an artery or vein at the root entry zone. Interestingly, autopsy series have shown that vascular compression is absent in a significant percentage of patients with trigeminal neuralgia. Conversely, these studies also note that vascular compression of the trigeminal nerve is often present in patients who have never suffered from trigeminal neuralgia.

Regardless of the cause, patients with trigeminal neuralgia tend to present in a stereotypical fashion. The classic symptoms of trigeminal neuralgia include (1) paroxysmal, "electric" pain in the trigeminal distribution on one side of the face; (2) trigger areas that, when stimulated, bring on this classic type of pain; (3) periods of remission and exacerbation; (4) pain that is typically more severe in the morning and absent during sleep; and (5) periodic pain relief when treated with an adequate trial of carbamazepine.

Controversy exists over the epidemiology of trigeminal neuralgia. Multiple studies show a trend toward a female predominance, with a female-to-male ratio as high as 2:1. In addition, the overwhelming majority of patients with the disease present at age 50 or older. The paroxysmal attacks appear to have a slightly increased tendency to occur on the right side of the face, but this is controversial. Multiple case studies corroborate that the location of the pain is more frequent in the V2 and V3 distributions. Despite these trends, trigeminal neuralgia can appear in either sex, at any age, on either side of the face, and in any distribution of the trigeminal nerve. For these reasons, it is important to consider the diagnosis in any patient with paroxysmal facial pain. The neurological examination and imaging studies are generally without demonstrable abnormalities. It is important to remember, however, that patients with multiple sclerosis or tumors of the cerebellopontine angle can present with classic features of trigeminal neuralgia. For this reason, imaging studies, including magnetic resonance imaging of the brain and posterior fossa, should be standard before the various treatment modalities are considered.

DIFFERENTIAL DIAGNOSIS

When a patient presents with facial pain symptoms that do not follow the classic features of trigeminal neuralgia, the clinician must explore other possible causes. This is especially true for pain that is constant, pain that is not confined to the dermatomal distribution of the trigeminal nerve, and pain that does not respond initially to carbamazepine. Patients with glossopharyngeal neuralgia often present with deep-seated ear or throat pain. Postherpetic neuralgia is generally preceded by a vesicular rash and is most often confined to the ophthalmic branch of the trigeminal nerve. Other possibilities, such as temporal arteritis, cluster headache, temporomandibular joint dysfunction, and atypical odontalgia, can initially be mistaken for trigeminal

TABLE 185–1 ■ **Differential Diagnosis of Trigeminal Neuralgia**

CULPRIT	EXAMPLES
Nerve	Trigeminal neuralgia
	Postherpetic neuralgia
	Trigeminal neuropathic pain
	Glossopharyngeal neuralgia
	Sphenopalatine neuralgia
	Geniculate neuralgia (Ramsay Hunt syndrome)
	Multiple sclerosis
	Cerebellopontine angle tumor
Teeth and jaw	Dentinal, pulpal, or periodontal pain
	Temporomandibular disorders
Sinuses and aerodigestive tract	Sinusitis
	Head and neck cancer
	Tolosa-Hunt syndrome
Eyes	Optic neuritis
	Iritis
	Glaucoma
Vessels	Giant cell arteritis
	Migraine
	Cluster headache (?)
Psyche	Psychogenic facial pain
	Atypical facial pain (?)

neuralgia if the physician does not specifically rule out their identifying features.

The causes of facial pain are myriad but can be roughly classified into several categories (Table 185–1). Although many types of facial pain fall outside the expertise or practice of neurosurgery, it is important for neurosurgeons to consider the differential diagnosis before embarking on medical or surgical therapy.

The diversity of possible causes of facial pain represents the first (and sometimes most difficult) hurdle to treatment. When an anatomic cause can be found, such as cancer of the head or neck, efforts can focus on treatment of the lesion or on palliative treatment. However, when no such lesion is apparent, the neurosurgeon must rely on other, indirect diagnostic clues. Factors such as distribution of pain, pain triggers, and quality of pain provide important information about the origin of the pain as well as the most appropriate treatment. Table 185–2 summarizes some of the salient features of commonly encountered facial pain syndromes.

Diagnostic uncertainty may arise when a patient presents with what appears to be trigeminal neuralgia with atypical features. Certain authors differentiate between typical trigeminal neuralgia and atypical trigeminal neuralgia. Fromm and Sessle note that a certain percentage of patients initially presents with a prodromal continuous, dull, aching pain in the jaw or teeth that is not brought on by typical trigger zones.[6] These patients generally go on to develop more classic paroxysmal pain in the same division of the trigeminal nerve months or years later. It is important to note, however, that although patients with atypical trigeminal neuralgia may present with atypical features, their response to initial medical management does not differ from that of patients with the typical form.[6]

TABLE 185–2 ■ **Diagnostic Clues in Facial Pain**

DIAGNOSIS	PAIN CHARACTER	PAIN DISTRIBUTION	PAIN TRIGGERS	OTHER CLUES
Trigeminal neuralgia	Paroxysmal, lancinating	Trigeminal *only*, V2 most frequent	Touch, chewing, talking, etc.	
Glossopharyngeal neuralgia	Paroxysmal, lancinating	Ear, throat	Swallowing	
Trigeminal neuropathic pain	Constant, burning, dull throbbing	Trigeminal *only*	None	History of trigeminal nerve injury
Postherpetic neuralgia	Constant, crawling, may have paroxysmal component	Trigeminal *only*, V1 most frequent	Touch	History of herpes zoster ophthalmicus
Anesthesia dolorosa	Constant, burning, itching in an insensate region	Trigeminal *only*	None	History of trigeminal nerve lesion
Malignancy	Constant, but may have paroxysmal component	In area of neoplasm or referable to nerve compression	Possible if trigeminal nerve involved	Head or neck neoplasm
Atypical facial pain	Constant	Nonanatomic, often bilateral	None	Prominent psychiatric component

GENERAL PRINCIPLES OF MEDICAL TREATMENT

The initial treatment of most facial pain syndromes is medical, but treatment must be diagnosis driven. Therefore, pain due to a head or neck neoplasm may be best treated by treatment of the lesion. Similarly, psychogenic pain is best addressed by treatment of the underlying psychiatric condition.

Medical treatment of facial pain is guided by the characteristics of the pain as much as it is by the underlying diagnosis. The primary differentiation that needs to take place is between nociceptive pain and neuropathic pain. Nociceptive pain is caused by normal and appropriate neuronal activity in the setting of local tissue damage. The primary example of nociceptive facial pain is that caused by head and neck cancer. Nociceptive pain is typically constant and aching, although it may sometimes have a paroxysmal component as well. Nociceptive pain is usually best treated by the use of opioid medications, although one should consider treatment of the offending neoplasm as the first option.

Neuropathic pain is thought to result from abnormal and inappropriate neuronal activity and may occur in the absence of any anatomic lesion. Neuropathic pain frequently follows injury to the nervous system and is thought to involve aberrant regeneration or conduction. Neuropathic pain may be either paroxysmal or constant, and it is frequently described as electrical, burning, itching, or crawling. Neuropathic pain is thought to be relatively opioid insensitive; its treatment usually focuses on reducing abnormal neuronal activity through the use of anticonvulsants or psychotropic medications.

In addition to the important distinction between nociceptive and neuropathic pain, the differentiation between paroxysmal and constant pain plays a key role in medical treatment. Paroxysmal pain, commonly seen in neuralgias, is thought to represent abnormal sensitization of the nerve, which leads to attacks of lancinating pain in the distribution of the affected nerve. Constant neuropathic pain, in contrast, is thought to occur in the setting of damage to the nerve or central nervous system. In the latter case, the pain is thought to result from an abnormal balance of inputs in neuromodulatory circuits. It is frequently described as pain that is burning, itching, or crawling in nature. Paroxysmal neuropathic pain is usually treated with anticonvulsants, whereas constant pain is best treated with psychotropic medications, such as tricyclic antidepressants. The distinction between the two types of neuropathic pain is useful when deciding on treatment options for facial pain. However, it is likely that this type of distinction represents a vast oversimplification of the differential causes of neuropathic pain.

The character of pain as well as its presumed cause guide the medical treatment of facial pain. Figure 185–1 summarizes the general principles that apply when choosing a medical therapy. In the next section, we discuss the specific classes of medications used to treat the various facial pain syndromes.

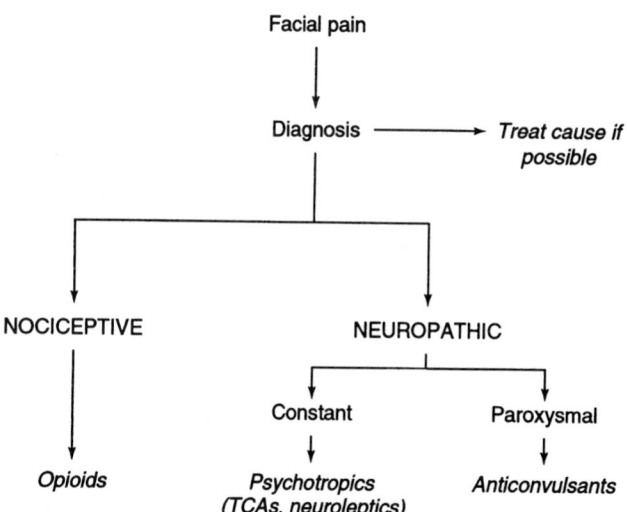

FIGURE 185–1. General guidelines in the medical management of facial pain.

MEDICATIONS USED

Classes of Medication

ANTICONVULSANTS

Following Trousseau's observation that trigeminal neuralgia resembles the epilepsies in its paroxysmal presentation, a number of anticonvulsants have been used in its treatment. Potassium bromide was first used successfully in the treatment of trigeminal neuralgia.[13] In 1942 Bergouignan described the use of phenytoin for the treatment of trigeminal neuralgia.[7] However, it was the development of a new Ciba-Geigy anticonvulsant in 1961 that revolutionized the treatment of facial pain.[12] Later known as carbamazepine, this medication still constitutes the linchpin of medical therapy in many facial pain syndromes. Other anticonvulsants have been developed and tested in the treatment of facial pain. Among these, only baclofen has remained a first-line therapy in trigeminal neuralgia. Table 185–3 outlines the typical anticonvulsant medications used in the treatment of facial pain.

The mode of action of anticonvulsants in the treatment of facial pain is not entirely clear. However, animal studies indicated that both carbamazepine and baclofen act to enhance inhibitory neuronal activity in the trigeminal nucleus oralis.[14] Because this sensory nucleus appears to play an important role in trigeminal neuralgia, it is likely that the action of anticonvulsants at the level of the brainstem sensory nuclei is at least partially responsible for their beneficial effects.

In addition to their important therapeutic role in trigeminal neuralgia, anticonvulsants are used to treat other paroxysmal facial pain syndromes. Paroxysmal components in trigeminal neuropathic pain, malignant facial pain, and postherpetic neuralgia are typically treated with anticonvulsants.

ANTIDEPRESSANTS

The antidepressants have found a prominent role in the treatment of neuropathic pain from a variety of causes. Although the precise mechanism by which they relieve pain is unclear, it is though to involve alterations in monoamine levels in the central nervous system.[15] In particular, elevations in brain and cerebrospinal fluid levels of serotonin, norepinephrine, and dopamine are thought to be important. Because the monoamines are believed to play a prominent role in chronic neuropathic pain, it is no surprise that these medications should prove useful.

In addition to their independent analgesic effects, the antidepressant effect of these drug is probably beneficial. Because chronic pain is often compounded by a depressive component, these medications may work, in part, by improving mood. Finally, they may improve pain partially through their sedative activity by improving sleep.

The beneficial alteration of monoamine neurotransmitters is sometimes accompanied by anticholinergic and psychomimetic effects. It is an unfortunate reality that efficacy and side effects go hand in hand with the use of antidepressants; the most consistently effective antidepressants are among the most poorly tolerated. Nevertheless, the antidepressants are extremely useful in the treatment of constant neuropathic pain. Table 185–4 outlines some of the antidepressants commonly used in facial pain.[16]

NEUROLEPTICS

Neuroleptics are a class of psychotropic medications traditionally used for their antipsychotic effects. Like

TABLE 185-3 ■ **Anticonvulsants Used for Facial Pain**

DRUG	DOSING	COMMON ADVERSE REACTION	SEVERE ADVERSE REACTION	CONTRAINDICATION
Carbamazepine (Tegretol)	Starting dose: 100–300 mg/day Therapeutic range: 800–1200 mg/day	Dizziness, somnolence, nausea, vomiting, diplopia, rash	Hematopoietic (aplastic anemia), dermatologic (Stevens-Johnson syndrome), congestive heart failure	Previous myelosuppression, adverse reaction to tricyclic medications
Phenytoin (Dilantin)	Starting dose: 200 mg/day Therapeutic range: 5–7 mg/kg/day	Nystagmus, ataxia, dizziness, lethargy, incoordination, dysarthria, rash, gingival hyperplasia	Hepatitis, Stevens-Johnson syndrome	Hydantoin hypersensitivity
Baclofen (Lioresal)	Starting dose: 30 mg/day Therapeutic range: 50–80 mg/day	Lethargy, ataxia, gastrointestinal distress, nausea	Withdrawal, seizures, hallucinations	
Clonazepam (Klonopin)	1.5–6 mg/day (divide dose to minimize sedation)	Central nervous system depression	Lethargy, rash, fatigue, thrombocytopenia	Benzodiazepine sensitivity, liver disease, narrow-angle glaucoma
Oxcarbazepine (Trileptal)	Starting dose: 300 mg/day Therapeutic range: 800–1200 mg/day	Dizziness, somnolence, nausea, vomiting	Unknown	Unknown
Sodium valproate (Depakote)	Starting dose: 600 mg/day Therapeutic range: 600–1200 mg/day	Tremor, nausea, vomiting, weight gain, alopecia, irritability	Hepatotoxicity	Liver disease

TABLE 185–4 ▪ **Antidepressants Used for Facial Pain**

CLASS	EXAMPLES	TYPICAL DOSE (MG/DAY)	SEROTONIN EFFECT	NOREPINEPHRINE EFFECT	ANTICHOLINERGIC EFFECT	SEDATION
Tricyclic	Amitriptyline	10–150	High	Mild	High	Moderate
	Desipramine	75–100	Mild	High	Minimal	None
	Doxepin	30–200	Mild	Minimal	Moderate	High
	Imipramine	20–150	Moderate	High	Mild	Minimal
	Nortriptyline	50–150	Mild	Moderate	Mild	Minimal
Monoamine oxidase inhibitor	Phenelzine	45–75	Minimal	Minimal	Minimal	None

the antidepressants, neuroleptics modify neurotransmitter levels in the central nervous system. Their mode of action is similarly nebulous and is thought to be related to a combination of direct neurotransmitter effects, antipsychotic activity, and sedative effects.[17, 18] Unlike the antidepressants, however, they work predominantly to alter dopaminergic transmission. They have little effect on the other monoamines.

Neuroleptics have found a role in the treatment of facial pain in several special circumstances. The phenothiazine fluphenazine has been reported to be effective in treating the "crawling" pain of postherpetic neuralgia.[19, 20] Neuroleptics may also be used as adjuncts to narcotic analgesia in malignant facial pain. In addition, neuroleptics may be helpful in the treatment of the psychotic features that accompany severe or psychogenic facial pain.

OPIOIDS

Nociceptive facial pain, such as that seen with malignancy, is usually treated with opioid medications. When treatment of the offending lesion with surgery, radiotherapy, or chemotherapy is not possible, opioids should be used routinely and liberally. In these cases, the guidelines developed by the World Health Organization and the Agency for Health Care Policy and Research are relevant and useful.[21, 22] When adequate systemic opioids result in unacceptable sedation, the drugs may be delivered intrathecally or intraventricularly.[23, 24]

The use of chronic opioids to treat facial pain not related to malignancies is fraught with difficulties. First, many nonmalignant facial pain syndromes are neuropathic or neuralgic and therefore respond poorly to opioid analgesics. Second, treating facial pain that has a prominent psychiatric component (e.g., atypical facial pain) with opioids is usually counterproductive. Finally, the issue of opioid tolerance plagues the long-term administration of these medications.

Mechanism of Action

Experimental studies evaluating the mechanism of action of drugs that are effective in treating trigeminal neuralgia have helped elucidate a theory for the pathophysiology of the disorder. However, the definitive cause of trigeminal neuralgia remains to be determined. Theories of the pathogenesis of trigeminal neu-

ralgia are addressed more comprehensively elsewhere; drug actions are briefly reviewed here.

Most experimental studies have focused on neurons in the nucleus oralis of the trigeminal nuclear complex.[6] This region receives heavy input from the perioral region, a frequent trigger zone for the paroxysms of pain in trigeminal neuralgia. Carbamazepine and phenytoin have been shown to facilitate inhibition of input to the nucleus oralis after electrical stimulation of the maxillary nerve in experimental animals. Testing of baclofen in the animal model has also shown this effect.[14] This led to the clinical testing and successful use of baclofen in the treatment of trigeminal neuralgia. Taken together, these lines of evidence support the hypothesis that there is a deficiency in segmental inhibition at the trigeminal nucleus, contributing to the pathogenesis of trigeminal neuralgia. There is also evidence that peripheral nerve irritation or injury contributes to or results in loss of the central inhibitory mechanisms.[25, 26]

Specific Medications Used

CARBAMAZEPINE

Carbamazepine is a tricyclic drug that is structurally related to the antidepressant imipramine. It was first synthesized in 1961[27] and was subsequently found to be effective in seizure disorders, affective disorders, and trigeminal neuralgia. After oral ingestion, the drug is absorbed from the gastrointestinal tract, with peak blood levels generally achieved 2 to 8 hours after the dose. The drug is distributed to all tissues and is approximately 70% to 80% protein bound in blood. Initially, there is a linear relationship between dose and plasma concentration. During chronic therapy, carbamazepine typically causes autoinduction of hepatic metabolism. Therefore, although the initial elimination half-life is 20 to 40 hours, later in treatment it can become as short as 11 hours. This effect on metabolism is thought to be responsible for significant fluctuations in serum concentrations of the drug during maintenance therapy. Side effects and drug efficacy are known to correlate with serum concentrations of the drug. In the past, a divided dosing strategy was used to limit peak serum concentrations of the drug. More recently, a new formulation of controlled-release carbamazepine has been marketed, which allows less frequent dosing and achieves more stable blood levels of the drug. A study using the controlled-release formulation showed a significant reduction in serum concentration fluctuations.[28]

The first reports of the use of carbamazepine for the treatment of trigeminal neuralgia were published in 1962.[11, 12] Following this, there were many open trials initially in Europe and later in the United States. The early trials were frequently uncontrolled and difficult to interpret. Further, follow-up periods were short, and patients with atypical facial pain were often included in the treatment groups. Better controlled studies later confirmed the efficacy of carbamazepine in the treatment of trigeminal neuralgia.[29–33]

The initial response of trigeminal neuralgia to carbamazepine is virtually universal. Lack of response should lead the clinician to reassess the diagnosis. Despite the initially good response, a small percentage of patients are unable to tolerate the side effects of the medication. In addition, long-term studies have demonstrated a gradual decline in efficacy over time. The initial response rate is usually in the 80% range,[33] but by 10 years from the start of therapy, only about 50% of patients respond to carbamazepine therapy.[34]

Currently, carbamazepine is the initial drug of choice for the management of trigeminal neuralgia. The initial dose in an average-sized adult is 200 mg/day, increasing by 200 to 300 mg/day until pain relief is achieved. Early dose-related side effects may be minimized by a gradual escalation to the therapeutic dose range. A typical dose that results in pain control is between 800 and 1200 mg/day. The dose may need to be increased after several weeks of therapy because of hepatic enzyme induction. At this point, it may also prove beneficial to take a greater proportion of a divided dose in the evening to ensure adequate serum concentration of drug for pain control the following morning.

Before initiating therapy with carbamazepine, a baseline complete blood count and liver and renal function tests should be obtained. These studies should be repeated every 2 weeks for the first 2 months of therapy and then four times a year thereafter. The drug should be discontinued if the peripheral white cell count drops below 3000 cells/μL (see later).

Between 20% and 40% of patients treated with carbamazepine experience some form of drug-related side effect. Early dose-related side effects commonly include somnolence, dizziness, nausea, and nystagmus. These occur more commonly in the elderly and when the dose escalates rapidly. Dermatologic reactions occur in approximately 5% to 10% of patients and include rash, erythema multiforme, and, rarely, Stevens-Johnson syndrome. The most common idiosyncratic side effects are hematologic, and they occur in 2% to 6% of patients. The most serious of these is aplastic anemia, which, though rarely encountered, necessitates the regular monitoring of a hematologic profile, as described previously. Other infrequent side effects include hepatotoxicity, hyponatremia, and congestive heart failure.

Because carbamazepine induces hepatic drug metabolism, it has interactions with and effects on many commonly used drugs. Serum concentrations of clonazepam, valproate, primidone, and other antiepileptic drugs are often decreased owing to enzyme induction. Carbamazepine has no significant interaction with baclofen. Phenytoin and carbamazepine compete for a common catabolic pathway. Therefore, phenytoin levels typically rise in combination therapy with carbamazepine, although the autoinduction of hepatic catabolic pathways makes the effect somewhat unpredictable, requiring careful monitoring of blood levels. Lamotrigine and valproate have been shown to inhibit metabolism of the bioactive carbamazepine epoxide, thus potentiating toxicity without necessarily changing the serum concentration of drug. A comprehensive review of interactions is beyond the scope of this chapter, and the reader is encouraged to refer to one of the numerous sources available.[6, 13, 35]

PHENYTOIN

Phenytoin (diphenylhydantoin) was first synthesized in 1908 and tested for use as a hypnotic. It is a white crystalline powder, insoluble in water. After oral absorption, peak serum concentration is generally reached in 4 to 8 hours. The time taken to reach peak serum concentration is independent of dose. Phenytoin is absorbed in the small intestine and bound 90% to serum proteins, primarily albumin. The drug is metabolized in the liver. When the catabolic pathway becomes saturated, phenytoin levels rise with zero-order kinetics. Therefore, small increments in dose can result in large changes in serum concentration.

The efficacy of phenytoin in trigeminal neuralgia was initially reported in 1942.[7] Patients who respond to therapy generally experience pain relief within 2 days of beginning therapy. The dose to achieve pain control is usually 5 to 7 mg/kg per day. There have been no controlled trials to date comparing phenytoin with carbamazepine for trigeminal neuralgia.[36, 37] Reports of phenytoin's efficacy describe a response rate of anywhere from 25% to 60% of patients.[38] These are certainly less than the response rates reported in the literature for carbamazepine. Thus, phenytoin is not typically the initial drug of choice for the treatment of trigeminal neuralgia.

The most frequently encountered dose-dependent side effects of phenytoin are ataxia, drowsiness, nystagmus, and diplopia. Other common side effects include gingival hyperplasia, acne, and hirsutism. Morbilliform rash occurs commonly. Manifestations of systemic hypersensitivity include Stevens-Johnson syndrome, hepatitis, a lupus-like syndrome, and folate-responsive megaloblastic anemia.

Drug interactions with phenytoin are frequent. The drug is loosely bound to hepatic cytochrome P450 and thus is susceptible to competitive displacement. Because phenytoin is a potent hepatic enzyme inducer, the metabolism of numerous drugs is altered. Serum levels of phenytoin should be carefully monitored when medications with known interactions are added or withdrawn.[13]

BACLOFEN

Baclofen became available in 1972. Structurally, it is an analog of the inhibitory neurotransmitter γ-aminobutyric acid. After oral ingestion, baclofen is rapidly absorbed via the gastrointestinal tract, and peak serum concentration is achieved in 2 to 3 hours. It has a variable half-life, generally ranging from 3 to 4 hours. The drug is excreted unchanged by the kidneys.[6]

In laboratory studies, baclofen has similar features to carbamazepine and phenytoin. In a cat model, baclofen was found to promote segmental inhibition at the nucleus oralis of the trigeminal brainstem complex.[39] After this encouraging experimental data, baclofen was used in a series of clinical trials and was found to have efficacy in trigeminal neuralgia. To date, there have been several trials, including a blinded crossover trial with carbamazepine, that have shown the efficacy of baclofen.[39–42] In long-term follow-up, 30% of patients develop resistance to therapy with baclofen.[39] There appears to be a synergism between baclofen and either carbamazepine or phenytoin; therefore, in specific cases, combination therapy is a reasonable option.[43] Because baclofen is formulated as a racemic mixture, the issue of which isomer is most effective has been examined. In these experimental series, the L-baclofen isomer was found to be significantly more effective and better tolerated than the racemic form.[44, 45]

The initial dose of baclofen is 10 mg three times per day. The dose should be incrementally increased until pain relief is achieved or toxicity is encountered. The typical daily maintenance dose required in trigeminal neuralgia is 50 to 60 mg/day.

Common side effects of baclofen include somnolence, dizziness, and gastrointestinal distress. These are usually dose dependent. Baclofen does not have the potentially life-threatening adverse effects of carbamazepine or phenytoin, and it is typically well tolerated. Because of the low toxicity profile, some clinicians use it as first-line therapy in trigeminal neuralgia despite its lower efficacy. Withdrawal of the medication should be gradual to prevent seizures or hallucinations. Baclofen does not have known interactions with other medications.[6]

CLONAZEPAM

Clonazepam is a benzodiazepine derivative that was introduced for use in epilepsy and myoclonus in 1973.[46] It has been used in trigeminal neuralgia since 1975.[47] Several clinical trials have shown its efficacy in trigeminal neuralgia, usually in the 60% to 70% range.[47–49] A typical maintenance dose of clonazepam for trigeminal neuralgia is 6 to 8 mg/day. The major dose-related side effect of the drug is sedation, which at the typical maintenance dose is prevalent. This has limited the usefulness of the medication.

SODIUM VALPROATE

Sodium valproate, although first synthesized in the 19th century, was not used in the treatment of epilepsy until 1964.[50] In 1980 it showed efficacy in a trial in the treatment of trigeminal neuralgia, but it is not as effective as the other anticonvulsants.[51] It is only occasionally used in the management of the disorder. Side effects include tremor, weight gain, alopecia, and dependent edema. A more threatening side effect is thrombocytopenia, which is typically reversible by altering the dosage. The initial dose is generally 600 mg/day, with maintenance therapy in the 800 to 1200 mg/day range.[13]

OXCARBAZEPINE

Oxcarbazepine is a derivative of carbamazepine and has been marketed outside the United States since 1991. The drug is metabolized rapidly to a pharmacologically active compound whose half-life is 14 to 26 hours. Clinical studies, primarily in epilepsy, have shown less significant toxicity when compared with carbamazepine.[52–54] The degradation pathway for oxcarbazepine differs from that for carbamazepine and does not induce hepatic enzyme systems.

Most studies evaluating the efficacy of oxcarbazepine have been directed at patients with epilepsy. There was a small trial of oxcarbazepine in patients with trigeminal neuralgia refractory to carbamazepine therapy, and all patients had a good response.[55] A second crossover trial from carbamazepine to oxcarbazepine also showed promising results.[56]

Dosing with oxcarbazepine is similar to that for carbamazepine. Higher doses of oxcarbazepine are often tolerated owing to an improved side effect profile.

OPHTHALMIC ANESTHETICS

There have been several reports of patients achieving symptomatic relief of trigeminal neuralgia with instillation of proparacaine ophthalmic drops.[57, 58] The only controlled trial published to date showed no efficacy with the treatment regimen tested.[59]

LOCAL ANESTHETICS

Local anesthetics, such as lidocaine, have a minor role in the treatment of facial pain. They have been reported to be useful in temporarily halting paroxysms of trigeminal neuralgia.[57] Mexiletine, an oral anesthetic related to lidocaine, may be tried in cases of lidocaine-sensitive pain. Tocainide, another oral anesthetic, has been reported to be effective in the treatment of trigeminal neuralgia, but it was associated with serious hematologic complications.[60]

CAPSAICIN

The neurotoxin capsaicin is used primarily in the treatment of painful neuropathies (e.g., diabetic neuropathy). Its mechanism of action is presumed to be related to a depletion of substance P in the dorsal horn. Capsaicin is used in the treatment of postherpetic neuralgia, but there have been few reports of its use in the treatment of other types of facial pain.[61–63]

SALICYLATES

Salicylates may have a role in the treatment of facial pain with an inflammatory component. Disorders of the temporomandibular joint, for example, may be treated with salicylates. Topical salicylates may also be used in neuropathic pain syndromes such as postherpetic neuralgia.

APPROACH TO TREATMENT

It is important to stress that even classic trigeminal neuralgia can be elicited by a posterior fossa mass or a multiple sclerosis plaque. For that reason, diagnostic imaging should be part of nearly every workup for facial pain syndromes.

For patients who have been carefully evaluated and diagnosed with trigeminal neuralgia, the appropriate initial therapy is carbamazepine. It would be reasonable to consider baclofen initially, especially in elderly or frail patients, with the understanding that efficacy, along with toxicity, is less. Either drug should be titrated until pain relief is achieved or side effects ensue. If pain remains refractory, combination therapy with baclofen and carbamazepine or phenytoin should be tried, given the synergism of these medications. If combination therapy proves ineffective, consideration should be given to either a second-line medication or surgical therapy. Once pain relief is achieved for a period of several months, attempts can be made to wean the patient from medical therapy. If pain recurs, therapy must be reinstituted. Medication trials are also appropriate for patients who develop recurrent pain after surgical procedures. As previously mentioned, the diagnosis of trigeminal neuralgia should also be reconsidered in patients who do not show the typical initial response to medical therapy.

Although the results of medical and surgical treatment of trigeminal neuralgia have improved exponentially since the 1950s, our ability to diagnose atypical facial pain syndromes is still poor. It is important for neurosurgeons to recognize that patients who present with atypical symptoms generally respond poorly to the routine medical and surgical management aimed at patients with more classic signs of trigeminal neuralgia. These patients may respond more favorably to antidepressants, and psychiatric consultation should be offered early to them.

CONCLUSION

Trigeminal neuralgia is a disease with relapses and remissions whose symptoms are not relieved by traditional medical approaches to pain management. Although there is no cure for the disorder, effective medical and surgical interventions are available. Thus, it is a disease that requires rational medical decision making and a close alliance between those practitioners specializing in medical and surgical therapies.

Neurosurgeons are frequently called on to diagnose and treat facial pain. Although surgical options for specific facial pain syndromes are quite attractive, it is crucial that neurosurgeons be familiar with the myriad facial pain syndromes that do not respond to surgery. Moreover, it is important to arrive at a rational treatment regimen that addresses not only the cause of pain but its character as well. A better appreciation of the neuroanatomic and chemical changes that occur in chronic pain has allowed us to rationalize our medical treatment of different pain syndromes. As our understanding of the neuroanatomy and pathophysiology of facial pain improves, so will our ability to offer more effective treatment, both medical and surgical.

REFERENCES

1. Ameli N: Avicenna and trigeminal neuralgia. J Neurol Sci 2: 105–107, 1965.
2. Wilkins R: Historical perspectives. In Rovit RL, Murali R, Jannetta PJ (eds): Trigeminal Neuralgia. Baltimore, Williams & Wilkins, 1990.
3. Stookey BR: Trigeminal Neuralgia. Springfield, Ill, Charles C Thomas, 1959.
4. Bell C: On the nerves of the face, being a second paper on that subject. Phil Trans R Soc (Lond) 1:317–330, 1829.
5. Trousseau A: De la neuralgie epileptiforme. Arch Gen Med 1: 33–44, 1853.
6. Fromm GH, Sessle BJ: Trigeminal Neuralgia: Current Concepts Regarding Pathogenesis and Treatment. Boston, Butterworth-Heinemann, 1991.
7. Bergouignan M: Cures hereuses de neuralgie faciales essentielles par le diphenylhydantoinate de soude. Rev Laryngol Otol Rhinol 63:34–41, 1942.
8. Lemoyne J: Le Traitment de la neuralgie faciele essentielle par le dimethyldithiohydantoine. Concours Med 73:461–462, 1951.
9. White JC, Sweet WH: Pain and the Neurosurgeon: A Forty Year Experience. Springfield, Ill, Charles C Thomas, 1969.
10. Jensen H: Die Behandlung der trigeminus-neuralgie mit Diphenylhydantoin. Arztl Wochensch 9:105–108, 1954.
11. Blom S: Trigeminal neuralgia: Its treatment with a new anticonvulsant drug (G-32883). Lancet 1:839–840, 1962.
12. Blom S: Tic douloureux treated with a new anticonvulsant. Arch Neurol 9:285–290, 1962.
13. Zakrzewska JM: Trigeminal neuralgia. In Warlow CP, van Gijn J (eds): Major Problems in Neurology, vol 28. London, WB Saunders, 1995.
14. Terrence CF, Sax M, Fromm GH, et al: Effect of baclofen enantiomorphs on the spinal trigeminal nucleus and steric similarities of carbamazepine. Pharmacology 27:85–94, 1983.
15. Richelson E, Nelson A: Antagonism by antidepressants of neurotransmitter receptors of normal human brain in vitro. J Pharmacol Exp Ther 230:94–102, 1984.
16. Monks R: Psychotropic drugs. In Bonica J, et al (eds): The Management of Pain. Philadelphia, Lea & Febiger, 1990, pp 1676–1689.
17. Bodnar RJ, Nicotera N: Neuroleptic and analgesic interactions upon pain and activity measures. Pharmacol Biochem Behav 16: 411–416, 1982.
18. Merskey H: Pharmacological approaches other than opioids in chronic non-cancer pain management. Acta Anaesthesiol Scand 41(1 Pt 2):187–190, 1997.
19. Hurtig HI: Fluphenazine and postherpetic neuralgia. JAMA 263: 2750, 1990.
20. Milligan NS, Nash TP: Treatment of post-herpetic neuralgia: A review of 77 consecutive cases. Pain 23:381–386, 1985.
21. Cancer Pain Relief and Palliative Care. Geneva, World Health Organization, 1990.
22. Jacox AK, Carr DB, Payne R: Management of Cancer Pain: Clinical Practice Guideline No. 9. Rockville, Md, Agency for Health Care Policy and Research, 1990.
23. Donnadieu S, Nguyen S, Bertrand J, et al: Evaluation and treat-

ment of chronic pain after cervicofacial cancer surgery. Ann Otolaryngol Chir Cervicofac 109:211–214, 1992.

24. Karavelis A, Foroglan G, Selviaridis P, et al: Intraventricular administration of morphine for control of intractable cancer pain in 90 patients. Neurosurgery 39:57–61, 1996.

25. Burchiel K: Ectopic impulse generation in focally demyelinated trigeminal nerve. Exp Neurol 69:423–429, 1980.

26. Burchiel K: Abnormal impulse generation in focally demyelinated trigeminal roots. J Neurosurg 53:674–683, 1980.

27. Shindler W: 5H-Dibenz [b,f] azepines. Chem Abstr 55:1671, 1961.

28. Mckee PB, Blacklaw J, Gillham RA: Monotherapy with conventional and controlled release carbamazepine. Br J Clin Pharmacol 32:99–104, 1991.

29. Campbell F, Killian JM, Fromm GH: Clinical trial of carbamazepine in trigeminal neuralgia. J Neurol Neurosurg Psychiatry 29:265–267, 1966.

30. Killian JM: Carbamazepine in the treatment of trigeminal neuralgia: Use and side effects. Arch Neurol 19:129–136, 1968.

31. Rockliff BD, Davis EH: Controlled sequential trials of carbamazepine in trigeminal neuralgia. Arch Neurol 15:129–136, 1966.

32. Sturman ROB, O'Brien FH: Non-surgical treatment of douloureux with carbamazepine. Headache 9:88–91, 1969.

33. Rasmussen P, Riishede J: Facial pain treated with carbamazepine. Acta Neurol Scand 46:385–408, 1970.

34. Taylor JC, Braver S, Espir ML: Long-term treatment of trigeminal neuralgia with carbamazepine. Postgrad Med J 57:16–18, 1981.

35. Masdeu J: Medical treatment and clinical pharmacology. In Rovit RL, Murali R, Jannetta PJ (eds): Trigeminal Neuralgia. Baltimore, Williams & Wilkins, 1990.

36. Swedlow M, Cundill JG: Anticonvulsant drugs used in the treatment of lacerating pain. Anesthesia 36:1129–1132, 1981.

37. Chinitz A, Seelinger DF, Greenhouse AH: Anticonvulsant therapy in trigeminal neuralgia. Am J Med Sci 252:62–67, 1966.

38. Braham JS: Phenytoin in the treatment of trigeminal and other neuralgias. Lancet 2:892–893, 1960.

39. Fromm GH, Terrence CF, Chatta AS, Glass JD: Baclofen in trigeminal neuralgia. Arch Neurol 37:768–771, 1980.

40. Fromm GH, Terrence CF, Chatta AS: Baclofen in the treatment of trigeminal neuralgia: Double blind study and long-term follow-up. Ann Neurol 15:240–244, 1984.

41. Parmar BS, Shah KH, Gandhi IC: Baclofen in trigeminal neuralgia—a clinical trial. Ind J Dent Res 1:109–113, 1989.

42. Steards L, Leo A, Marano E: Efficacy of baclofen in trigeminal neuralgia and some other painful conditions. Eur Neurol 23:51–55, 1984.

43. Baker KA, Taylor JW, Lilly GE: Treatment of trigeminal neuralgia: Use of baclofen in combination with carbamazepine. Clin Pharmacol 4:93–96, 1985.

44. Fromm GH, Terrence CF: Comparison of L-baclofen and racemic baclofen in trigeminal neuralgia. Neurology 37:1725–1728, 1987.

45. Sawynok J, Dickson C: D-Baclofen is an antagonist at baclofen receptors mediating antinociception in the spinal cord. Pharmacology 31:248–259, 1985.

46. Browne R, Perry JK: Benzodiazepines in the treatment of epilepsy. Epilepsia 15:277–310, 1973.

47. Caccia M: Clonazepam in facial neuralgia and cluster headache: Clinical and electrophysiological study. Eur Neurol 13:560–563, 1975.

48. Court JE, Kase CS: Treatment of tic douloureux with a new anticonvulsant. J Neurol Neurosurg Psychiatry 39:297–299, 1976.

49. Smirne S, Scarlato G: Clonazepam in cranial neuralgias. Med J Aust 1:93–94, 1933.

50. Carraz GF, Chateau G: First clinical trials of the antiepileptic activity of N-dipropylacetic acid. Ann Med Psychol 122:577–584, 1964.

51. Peiris JB, Perera GL, Devendra SV, et al: Sodium valproate in trigeminal neuralgia. Med J Aust 2:278, 1980.

52. Houtkooper MA, Lammertsma A, Meyer JW, et al: Oxcarbazepine: A possible alternative to carbamazepine. Epilepsia 28:693–698, 1987.

53. Reinikainen KJ, Keranen T, Halonen T, et al: Comparison of oxcarbazepine and carbamazepine: A double-blind study. Epilepsy Res 1:284–289, 1987.

54. Dam M, Ekberg R, Loyning Y, et al: A double-blind study comparing oxcarbazepine and carbamazepine in patients with newly diagnosed, previously untreated epilepsy. Epilepsy Res 3:70–76, 1989.

55. Zakrzewska JM, Patsalos PN: Oxcarbazepine: A new drug in the management of trigeminal neuralgia. J Neurol Neurosurg Psychiatry 52:472–476, 1989.

56. Remmilard G: Oxcarbazepine and intractable trigeminal neuralgia. Epilepsia 35:528–529, 1994.

57. Spaziante R, Cappabianca P, Saini M, et al: Topical ophthalmic treatment for trigeminal neuralgia. Neurosurg 82:993–997, 1995.

58. Vassilouthis J: Relief of trigeminal neuralgia by proparacaine. J Neurol Neurosurg Psychiatry 57:121, 1994.

59. Kondziolka D, Lemley T, Kestle JR, et al: The effect of single-application topical ophthalmic anesthesia in patients with trigeminal neuralgia: A randomized double-blind placebo controlled trial. J Neurosurg 80:993–997, 1994.

60. Lindstrom P, Lindblom U: The analgesic effect of tocainide in trigeminal neuralgia. Pain 28:45–50, 1987.

61. Hersh EV, Pertes RA, Ochs HA: Topical capsaicin—pharmacology and potential role in the treatment of temporomandibular pain. J Clin Dentistry 5:54–59, 1994.

62. Epstein JB, Marcoe JH: Topical application of capsaicin for treatment of oral neuropathic pain and trigeminal neuralgia. Oral Surg Oral Med Oral Pathol 77:135–140, 1994.

63. Lincoff NS, Rath PP, Hirano M: The treatment of periocular and facial pain with topical capsaicin. J Neuroophthalmol 18:17–20, 1998.

CHAPTER 186

Percutaneous Techniques

JEFFREY A. BROWN

This chapter is intended to serve as a guide to students, residents, and practitioners with an interest in trigeminal neuralgia. It is organized progressively from the clinical diagnosis through the selection of a treatment option. It discusses the potential problems and solutions for each technique described. Although it is not possible to fully explore every nuance of the subject in a single chapter, this discussion provides a solid, informative basis for exploring the percutaneous treatment of tic douloureux.

DIAGNOSIS

The diagnosis of classic trigeminal neuralgia is usually made by listening carefully to the patient's history. It is primarily a disease of older adults. Typically, a 65-year-old woman describes intermittent, unilateral electric shock–like pains in the jaw and cheek triggered by lightly touching the face or by a cool breeze, chewing, or speaking. When the description is longer or more complex, the diagnosis becomes less clear. Some patients may describe an underlying burning component to the pain or a dull aching pain that persists beyond the electric shock–like pain. This burning component is called neuropathic pain. When both shocking and burning pain are present, it generally means that the disease has progressed from the simple form of tic douloureux to the stage of trigeminal neuropathy, the treatment of which is usually more complex. Often, the lancinating component (tic pain) and the neuropathic (burning) pain must be addressed separately. The practitioner should keep in mind that the percutaneous treatment of tic douloureux usually addresses only the lancinating component. It is possible that the trigeminal neuropathy will resolve secondarily, but this issue has not been thoroughly studied. Be aware that if it is severe enough, the neuropathic pain may be aggravated by percutaneous injury.

Thus, it is important to keep in mind that the condition of trigeminal neuralgia is not static. The pain intensity progresses from infrequent shocks separated by long pain-free intervals to agonizing, often lengthy or continuous periods of shock (tic) accompanied by aching or burning pain (neuropathy). In a long-suffering patient, there is often a significant psychological component to the discomfort, making treatment complicated. Patience and support are key elements to a successful outcome.

Medical treatment with an anticonvulsant can delay disease progression, but once trigeminal neuralgia exists, drugs will not cure it. Once medical treatment is necessary (usually beginning with carbamazepine at gradually increasing doses from 100 to 600 mg daily), it cannot be stopped, although the initial intermittent nature of the pain would lead one to think so.

Modern medicine first clearly described trigeminal neuralgia when philosopher John Locke corresponded with colleagues in London regarding the terrible facial pains of the wife of the ambassador to France: "When the fit came, there was, to use my Lady's own expression of it, as it were a flash of fire all of a sudden shot into all those parts . . . which made her shreeke out. . . . These violent fits terminated on a suddaine, and then my Lady seemed to be perfectly well, excepting only a dull pain which ordinarily remained in her teeth on that side." The letter, written on December 4, 1677, no longer exists, but the response from Dr. Mapletoft can still be found in the Oxford Library. One hundred years later, Nicolas Andre, a French physician, argued that the term *cynical spasm*, which had been applied to the disorder, fit less well than the words *tic douloureux*. This term remains popular, though there is much to be said for the emotional impact of a term that implies that the sufferer's facial expression is that of a dog about to bite.

ANATOMY

The trigeminal nerve is the largest of the cranial nerves. Similar to a spinal nerve, it has a ganglion developed from its posterior root. Its function is also comparable because it is a compound nerve. The trigeminal nerve mediates sensation to the mucosa of the mouth, the anterior two thirds of the tongue, the anterior and middle cranial fossa dura, the tooth pulp, and the surrounding gingiva and periodontal membrane. The first and second divisions are entirely sensory, and the third division is partially motor. The motor innervation is to the muscles of mastication (masseter and ptery-goid muscles), the anterior belly of the digastric muscle, and the mylohyoid, tensor tympani, and palati muscles. The nerve originates at the upper ventral pons. Its true origin is from the gasserian ganglion, corresponding to the ganglion in a spinal nerve. Each peripheral fiber has an associated autonomic component. The ciliary ganglion is associated with the ophthalmic division, the sphenopalatine ganglion with the maxillary division, and the otic ganglion with the mandibular division. Sympathetic fibers have cell bodies in the superior cervical ganglion, whose axons are along the external carotid artery. These autonomic fibers do not associate with the nerve root, only with the peripheral branches of each division.[1]

The portio major of the trigeminal root is somatotopically organized. The ophthalmic division fibers are dorsal, the mandibular division fibers are ventral, and the maxillary fibers are intermediate. There is considerable variation in the somatotopic organization of the root. As the fibers move from ganglion to brainstem, the root rotates randomly.[2, 3] To some extent, this explains the unpredictable degree of sensory loss after partial trigeminal rhizotomy. Half of the 125,000 fibers in the sensory root are myelinated. Spinal dorsal roots, however, are 80% unmyelinated.[4] This may account for the fine discriminative ability of the facial structures.

The hypothesis that classic trigeminal neuralgia is caused by vascular compression and secondary demyelination has been confirmed by biopsies of the trigeminal nerves of patients who had caudal rhizotomy performed for trigeminal neuralgia. There is a zone of chronic demyelination in the proximal and centrally myelinated part of the root near the entry zone. The zone contains closely packed axons with no intervening glial cytoplasm. Sometimes a single thin myelin sheath encircles several adjacent axons that are still in close opposition.[5] Autopsy studies of normal cadavers do not show the presence of neurovascular contact as often as it is noted at surgery for trigeminal neuralgia.[6]

TREATMENT OPTIONS

Thermal rhizotomy, glycerol rhizolysis, balloon compression, and gamma knife radiosurgery are the percutaneous treatments most commonly performed for trigeminal neuralgia that no longer responds to anticonvulsant therapy. Percutaneous neurectomy approaches are still used when appropriate. These procedures, their historical origins, the results, and the potential problems associated with them are discussed.

Thermal Rhizotomy

In 1965 Sweet introduced the first modern percutaneous technique for the treatment of trigeminal neuralgia.[7] He used controlled thermocoagulation of trigeminal rootlets to differentially injure pain fibers. Two approaches using thermal rhizotomy are currently used. The first, developed by Sweet, uses a thin, straight or curved electrode that heats fibers over timed intervals, often while the patient is awake and the blink reflex is repeatedly assessed. The second technique, developed by Tew[8], uses an electrode to measure the temperature at which the retrogasserian fibers are being heated while the patient is anesthetized with a short-acting anesthetic.

Later studies showed that compound action potentials of nociceptive fibers were selectively blocked at lower temperatures than were those of myelinated fibers, which mediate tactile sensation.[9, 10] Although these electrophysiologic studies suggest that, in the early stages of heating, this differential injury occurs, histologic evaluation of injured trigeminal ganglia and roots in animal studies has shown only nonspecific fiber injury.[11] Thermal rhizotomy, like other percutaneous treatments, may be effective because it reduces the overall sensory input to the demyelinated peripheral site of ephaptic transmission.

TECHNIQUE

Patients are premedicated with 0.4 mg atropine intramuscularly. The procedure is performed in the radiology suite with the patient lying supine in the neutral position. In the technique described by Tew,[8] a portable imaging unit is positioned for a lateral view of the skull. The patient is anesthetized with 30 to 50 mg of intravenous methohexital. Propofol can also be used, and anesthesiologists tend to be more familiar with it, but with methohexital, patients awaken more rapidly. As a ground, a spinal needle is placed in the soft tissue of the deltoid. A 21-gauge spinal needle is placed through the cheek while the physician stands on the patient's right side. Standard landmarks are used: 2.5 cm lateral to the angle of the lip, 3 cm anterior to the external auditory meatus, just below the medial aspect of the pupil. When the foramen ovale is engaged, the patient usually winces, and the surgeon can feel the cannula entering the foramen. When this approach is chosen, a series of lateral fluoroscopic images should be obtained when the needle is close to the foramen. Nugent[12] advocates using a modified anteroposterior image at this point. Here the petrous bone is aligned in the radiographic center of the orbit. The needle is directed to the midpoint of the dip in the petrous bone that corresponds to the entrance of Meckel's cave. Third-division fibers are positioned more laterally. First-division fibers are more medial and superior. The entrance point may be varied in order to approach the desired retrogasserian fibers. Tew[8] has documented lateral radiographic landmarks for localizing each division. The 5-mm conductive electrode tip is directed to a point 5 to 10 mm caudal to a line drawn through the floor of the sella turcica, intersecting with the clival line (Fig. 186–1).[8] If a curved electrode is used, the curve is directed superomedially for first-division and inferiorly for third-division selection. In this technique, a single approach can be used to treat all three divisions.

When the patient has awakened, the retrogasserian fibers are stimulated with 0.1 to 0.4 V at 50 to 75 cycles/second and a 1-msec pulse duration to identify

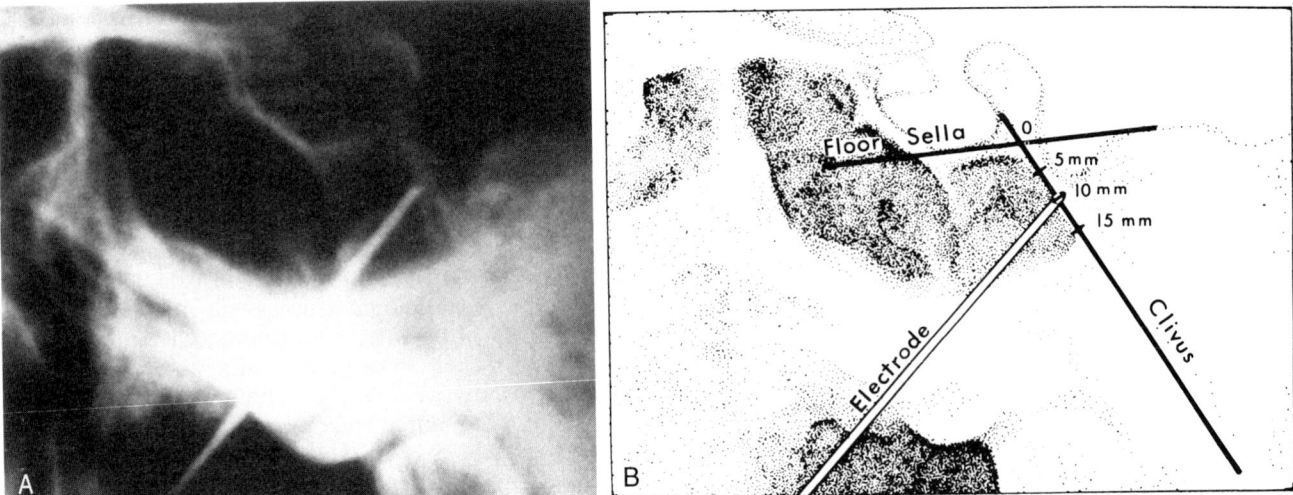

FIGURE 186–1. *A,* Position of the electrode for thermal coagulation. *B,* The point 5 to 10 mm below the intersection of a line drawn from the floor of the sella turcica to the clival line, or the intersection of the petrous ridge with the clivus. (From Tew JM: Treatment of trigeminal neuralgia by percutaneous rhizotomy. In Youmans JR [ed]: Neurological Surgery, 2nd ed. Philadelphia, WB Saunders, 1982, p 3568.)

the site where the lesion is to be located. The electrode position is then adjusted according to where in the face the patient feels the stimulation. Anesthesia is induced again, and a series of lesions is made. If the thermocouple probe is used, the initial lesions are made over a 1-minute interval at 60°C. The patient is then awakened and sensation is evaluated. Next, lesions are made over 60 to 90 seconds, increasing the temperature by 5°C with each lesion. When there is partial numbness, it may be possible to create additional lesions while the patient is awake and while continuously testing for the extent of sensory loss. This is especially important when treating a patient with a first-division trigger. Tew emphasizes that the goal is dense hypalgesia, not analgesia. At this stage, the patient can still determine that a safety pin feels sharp, but the degree of sharpness is considerably reduced.

Nugent's approach uses a smaller straight or curved cordotomy electrode. The bared tip of this electrode is 0.4 mm in diameter and 3 mm long. In this approach, the hub of the spinal needle is used as a ground. Temperature monitoring is not used. Nugent emphasizes that the lesion is usually complete in the first 15 to 20 seconds. Early lesions are made at 10 V and 60 mA for 15 to 20 seconds. He lengthens the duration to 40 seconds with later lesions, finally increasing the current by several units until a range of 18 to 20 V and 90 to 100 mA is reached. During the later phases of lesion generation, Nugent recommends repeatedly drawing a piece of sponge or tissue across the eyelashes of the closed eye to check the blink reflex. First, the consensual reflex is diminished, and then the direct reflex is lost, if first-division fibers are injured.[12]

DISCUSSION

The benefits of thermal rhizotomy depend on how much numbness is created. Large series, such as those

discussed here, show that the greater the numbness, the longer the patient is free of recurrence but the higher the risk of discomfort from the nerve injury itself. A balance between extremes is necessary. This trade-off has to be emphasized in discussions with patients.

Taha and colleagues[13] summarized Tew's series of 154 consecutive patients with trigeminal neuralgia treated by thermal rhizotomy and prospectively followed for 15 years. Ninety-nine percent of the patients obtained initial pain relief after one procedure. Overall, dysesthesia occurred in 23% of the patients; it occurred in only 7% with mild initial hypalgesia, in 15% with dense hypalgesia, and in 36% with analgesia. Dysesthesia was mild and did not require treatment in "most patients." The corneal reflex was absent or depressed in 19%, and keratitis developed in three patients. Motor weakness was present in 15% of the treated patients, but this resolved within 1 year in 86% of those patients. Of the 21% who had pain recurrence, 15% required additional surgical treatment. Kaplan-Meier analysis showed that the 14-year recurrence rate was 25% in the total group: 60% in patients with mild hypalgesia, 25% in those with dense hypalgesia, and 20% in those with analgesia. It was interesting to note that the timing of pain recurrence varied according to the degree of sensory loss. All pain recurrences in patients with mild hypalgesia occurred within 4 years after surgery; among the patients with dense hypalgesia, 10% more had pain recurrence within the first 10 years compared with patients with analgesia. The median pain-free survival was 32 months for patients with mild hypalgesia and more than 15 years for patients with either analgesia or dense hypalgesia. Of the 100 patients followed for 15 years after one or two procedures, 95% rated the procedure excellent or good. Dense hypalgesia in the painful trigger zone, rather than analgesia, is recommended as the target lesion.

Taha and Tew[14] also retrospectively reviewed Tew's series of 500 patients. They compared results to 6305 patients reported in the literature who underwent thermal rhizotomy, 1217 patients who underwent glycerol rhizotomy, 1417 patients who underwent microvascular decompression (MVD), and 759 patients who underwent balloon compression. MVD had the lowest rate of technical success. Thermal rhizotomy and MVD had the lowest rates of numbness and dysesthesias. Glycerol rhizotomy led to the highest reported recurrence rate, and balloon compression had the highest rate of motor weakness. Percutaneous procedures had similar dysesthesia rates. MVD had the highest rate of associated cranial nerve injury.

Nugent's[12] summary experience in treating 1070 patients with a 9-year mean follow-up showed an overall 27% recurrence rate and 12% fair to poor results. Six percent of patients had annoying dysesthesias, although they may still have rated their procedures as providing good to excellent results. Neurolytic keratitis occurred in 0.4% of patients, and two patients experienced loss of vision. There were two postoperative deaths in his series, each a consequence of an older treatment population with medical infirmities.

PROBLEMS AND SOLUTIONS

The difficulty of communicating with older patients who are awakening from fast-acting barbiturates may hinder the decision to continue radiofrequency heating. The patient may be confused, uncooperative, or agitated, making the task more difficult. Success depends on the neurosurgeon's or anesthetist's expertise in the pharmacology of sedation and in communication. Airway protection may also be an issue during the deeper moments of sedation.

Localization of the foramen ovale should be the easiest part of this procedure. With experience, it can be entered in seconds. If it cannot be entered using a lateral image for assistance, a modified submental view directly demonstrates the foramen. In this view, the foramen is seen superior to the petrous ridge, lateral to the maxillary sinus, and medial to the mandible (Fig. 186–2). If the foramen still cannot be entered, the endovascular suite can be used to obtain better imaging quality.

It is important to remember that carotid puncture can occur. If this happens, the procedure should be discontinued, the needle withdrawn, and pressure placed on the cheek. No morbidity occurs because of this event.

There may be a range of autonomic effects from injury to the trigeminal system. Hypertensive intracerebral hemorrhages have occurred.[15] In a series of 126 patients who had thermal rhizotomy, Kuchta and coworkers[16] observed significant bradycardia (<50 beats/minute) in 20% of patients ($P < 0.0002$) during or immediately after penetration of the foramen ovale. A significant rise in blood pressure (180 mm Hg systolic) was observed in 36% of patients. One should be prepared to deal with an elevation in blood pressure, usually by adjusting the depth of anesthetic.

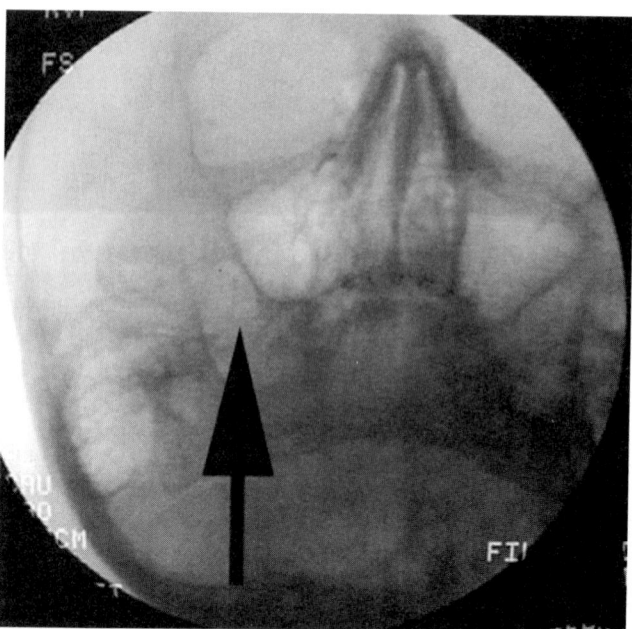

FIGURE 186–2. Modified submental view demonstrating the foramen ovale *(arrow)* above the petrous ridge, medial to the maxillary sinus and lateral to the mandible.

Another problem is that subtemporal placement of the electrode is possible if it is positioned lateral to Meckel's cave. This is avoidable by using an anteroposterior image to localize electrode placement.

Glycerol Rhizotomy

Hakanson[17] introduced percutaneous glycerol rhizotomy in 1981. The discovery of glycerol's effectiveness was serendipitous. Glycerol was thought to be a harmless carrier for the tantalum powder used to outline the trigeminal cistern in preparation for gamma knife treatment. It had been used as a medium for mixing phenol, a neurolytic agent commonly used for injuring the trigeminal nerve.

TECHNIQUE

The principle of treatment by glycerol rhizotomy is that a measured volume of water-soluble radiopaque dye is injected with a 22-gauge spinal needle into the trigeminal cistern to accurately measure its capacity. A variable volume of anhydrous glycerol is then injected, depending on the division selected for injury and the volume of Meckel's cave. For multidivision pain, up to 0.3 mL is used. Lesser amounts can be injected for selectivity by layering glycerol over higher-density dye to avoid injury to the third or second divisions. It is unclear why larger volumes of fluid spill preferentially into the posterior fossa and not along the subarachnoid space surrounding the entering nerve roots; however, to adequately fill the cistern, the patient is positioned sitting upright, head slightly flexed forward. The position is maintained for 1 hour. Afterward, the glycerol is evacuated, and fluoroscopic confirmation of this is obtained. Hakanson recommends using a mixture of 2 mL of glycerol and 0.5 mg of tantalum, which is then used to mark the cistern permanently. This makes it easier to identify the cistern should a repeat procedure be needed.

DISCUSSION

In the most recently published large series, 191 patients were treated over 7 years using Hakanson's method of glycerol rhizotomy, with minor modifications.[18] The technical failure rate was 15%. In 6%, the surgeon could not pass a needle through the foramen ovale, and in 9%, cerebrospinal fluid was not obtained.

In 65% of successful cases, pain relief was immediate; in 28%, relief occurred within 6 days. There was an overall failure rate of 7%. Postoperative sensory evaluation showed no sensory loss in 17%, hypalgesia in 4%, and mild hypesthesia in 46%. Analgesia was confined to the affected divisions in 24% and exceeded it in 23%. There was moderate hypesthesia in 33%; this was restricted to the target divisions in 19% and exceeded them in 14%. No anesthesia dolorosa occurred. Herpes simplex eruptions occurred in 33%, but these regressed spontaneously and completely. Minor dysesthesia, seldom reported as painful, was seen in 17%; impairment of corneal reflex occurred in 10%; masseter weakness in 6%; and aseptic meningitis in 1%.

Follow-up ranged from 1 to 7 years. In 8%, a partial relapse occurred, well controlled by drug therapy and not requiring further surgical treatment; in 15%, a new percutaneous procedure was required. The mean time until recurrence was 31 months. The overall recurrence rate at the end of the follow-up period was 23%.

A broad range of recurrence rates has been published for the procedure. Eliminating the extremes, the range is 23% to 45% recurrence at less than 2 years' follow-up and 25% to 72% after 2 years.[19] More significant than static recurrence would be a Kaplan-Meier survival curve for pain-free days after rhizotomy. Clearly, in all percutaneous procedures, there is a gradually increasing recurrence rate. The incidence of slight hypesthesia is also variable, ranging from 4% to 72%. Less numbness is associated with greater early recurrence. In North and associates' series,[20] a recurrence rate of 55% after 2 years was associated with only 4% slight hypesthesia. Kaplan-Meier survival analysis showed a median time to recurrence of 2 years for medical intervention and 3 years for surgical therapy. Young,[21] however, had a 34% recurrence rate after 2 years but a much higher rate of dysesthesia (12%) and hypesthesia (72%).

It is logical to conclude that recurrence is associated with remyelination of the injured zones. Glycerol injures myelin. Lunsford and coworkers[22] demonstrated this in studies of cat trigeminal ganglia 4 to 6 weeks after injection. Eide and Stubhaug[23] found that there are impaired thin fiber (C and A delta)– and thick fiber (A beta)–mediated sensations and abnormal temporal pain summation in the trigger zones of patients with trigeminal neuralgia. When pain is relieved by glycerol injection, the temporal summation normalizes.

PROBLEMS AND SOLUTIONS

How much glycerol should be instilled? More than 0.3 mL is discouraged because of the risk of sensory deficit.[19] How long should it remain in contact with the nerve? Usually a duration of 1 hour is recommended. Hakanson[17] is concerned that short-duration contact with the nerve can cause extensive and less well-controlled injury, whereas Linderoth and Hakanson[19] believe that contact with the first division of the nerve for longer than 12 minutes can cause corneal anesthesia. Other issues regarding glycerol include incomplete pain relief and cisternal adhesions preventing adequate cisternography or third-division selectivity. If adhesions prevent complete contrast drainage from the cistern, the glycerol will not contact the more inferior third-division fibers, and they will be selectively protected, not injured. Like other techniques, the success of the glycerol technique depends on inherent subtleties in needle position.

Balloon Compression

Percutaneous balloon compression is a technique derived from mechanical injury to the trigeminal ganglion originally performed during temporal craniotomies in the 1950s by Shelden and Pudenz. Their original intent was to decompress the ganglion or peripheral divisions; however, they learned that results were better when there was facial numbness after surgery. Results were marred by their inability to control the degree of compression. Mullan, who in earlier work developed an open percutaneous technique for cervical cordotomy, introduced percutaneous compression in 1983.[24]

TECHNIQUE

Selection criteria for balloon compression are similar to those for other percutaneous procedures. Balloon compression is usually performed with the patient under general anesthesia, although intravenous anesthesia combined with local anesthesia at the ganglion level has been used. Patients should be able to tolerate a brief period of general anesthesia. Contralateral jaw weakness is not a contraindication, despite the possibility of temporary masseter and pterygoid muscle weakness.

The procedure is easiest if performed in the endovascular suite, where excellent multiplane imaging is available. Atropine is not used preoperatively. The presence of a trigeminal depressor response confirms trigeminal injury. After induction, placement of a transcutaneous pacemaker blocks the brief but significant bradycardia that may occur in two thirds of patients. A transesophageal pacemaker is also acceptable, but it must be turned on and off by the anesthesiologist rather than automatically, based on preset parameters. Anesthesia is induced with isoflurane and nitrous oxide. Anesthetic depth may need to be increased during compression to avoid a reflex hypertensive response.

The patient is positioned supine, and a roll is placed

beneath the shoulder. The first image obtained is a modified submental view. A nick, parallel to a skin crease, is made in the cheek with a scalpel blade; a 14-gauge cannula with a sharp obturator (Brown Access Needle; Cook, Inc, Bloomington, IN) then punctures through the external soft tissues. A blunt obturator replaces the sharp one as the foramen ovale is approached so the cannula cannot lacerate the external carotid artery. When the foramen ovale is engaged, there is a brief bradycardia, and the masseter and pterygoid muscles contract. The obturator is removed, and a straight guiding stylet is inserted. A modified anteroposterior image is then obtained. The thin guiding stylet is directed to the midpoint of the entrance to Meckel's cave for second-division or multidivision pain, to the lateral portion for third-division selection, or to the medial portion for first-division selection. If needed, a curved guiding stylet is used to direct the stylet medially. The stylet is removed, and the balloon catheter is directed to the same location as demonstrated on the anteroposterior image intensifier (Fig. 186–3). Finally, a lateral view is reviewed. This image is accurately obtained by aligning the external auditory canals on the image intensifier. For third-division pain, the balloon catheter is aligned parallel to the petrous ridge. For second-division pain, it is angled cephalad at the same angle advocated for thermal rhizotomy electrode positioning. For first-division pain, the angle is slightly greater, in addition to the more medial direction on anteroposterior viewing.

The balloon is inflated to a pressure of 1.3 to 1.5 atmospheres using an insufflation syringe (Merit Medical, Salt Lake City, UT) with an attached transducer calibrated up to 2 atmospheres as read on a separate digital monitor. When the balloon is correctly positioned, bradycardia may occur briefly, triggering the pacemaker. On the lateral image intensifier, the balloon appears to be pear shaped once it is inflated, because

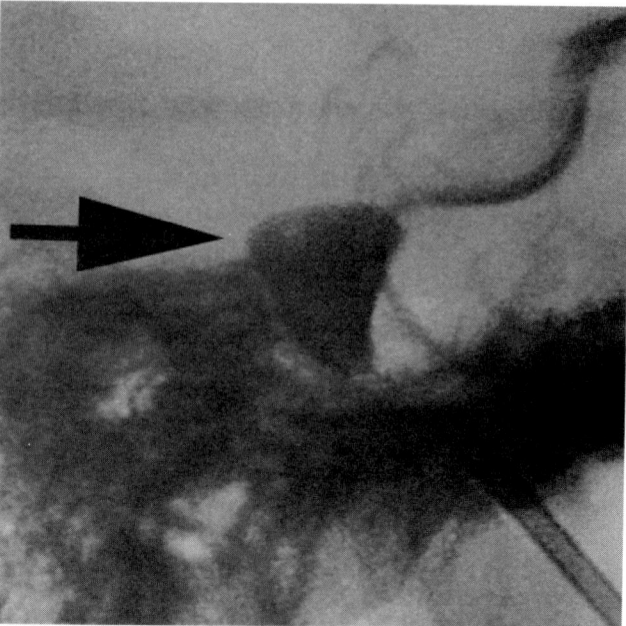

FIGURE 186–4. Lateral view of the inflated balloon forming an ideal pear shape. The *arrow* points to the constriction in the tip of the balloon that corresponds to the portion lying within the elliptical porus trigeminus.

the tip is contained in the porus trigeminus, a 3 mm × 11 mm opening bordered by the firm edge of the dura and the petrous ridge (Fig. 186–4). The retrogasserian nerve fibers are compressed for 1 minute in the medial porus against the dural edge and petrous bone. The pressure and duration of compression may be varied, but compression should not be maintained for more than 1.5 minutes, or the risk of dysesthesias will increase. The procedure can be performed with a tuberculin syringe and a volume-controlled injection of 0.75 to 1 mL, but the additional control provided by the pressure measurement prevents overinflation, severe dysesthesias, or diplopia from cavernous sinus and fourth nerve compression. After compression, the balloon catheter and cannula are removed, and the cheek is compressed for several minutes. Blood-tinged cerebrospinal fluid may be obtained if the catheter is removed separately from the cannula, but its presence has no significant effect on the likelihood of success.

Patients may be discharged after an overnight stay. The procedure can also be performed on an outpatient basis, depending on the physician's experience and the patient's other health factors. It is important that patients be informed of the risk of herpetic eruptions, be instructed in proper eye care, and be given a tapering schedule for the anticonvulsants used to treat their neuropathic pain.

DISCUSSION

Balloon compression is distinct from thermal rhizotomy and glycerol injection because it is performed on anesthetized patients. It is a simple technique that can be performed efficiently in a short period, and the results are comparable.

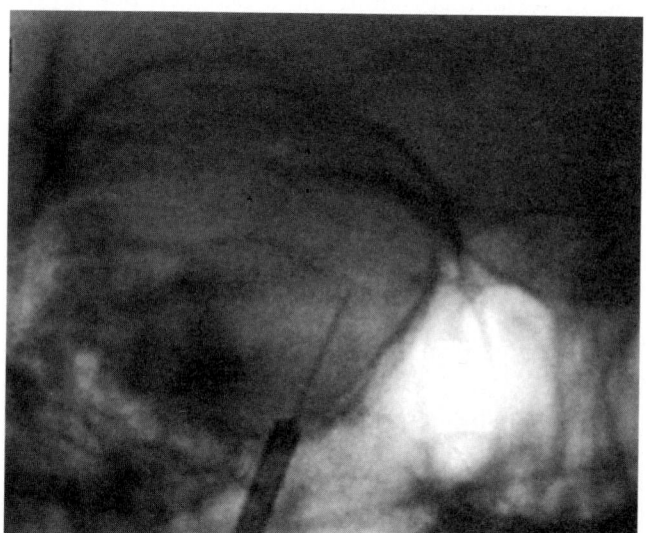

FIGURE 186–3. Anteroposterior view demonstrating the balloon catheter positioned in the center of the entrance to Meckel's cave at the petrous ridge.

Compression selectively injures large myelinated fibers, removing the "trigger" to the presumed ephaptic transmission of pain.[25] Because unmyelinated fibers, which control the corneal reflex, are preserved, compression may be advantageous in the treatment of first-division pain, because the corneal reflex is mediated by the small unmyelinated fibers.

The trigeminal depressor response that occurs during compression consists of sympathetic inhibition and parasympathetic stimulation. This leads to bradycardia and brief hypotension. It is likely caused by injury to large myelinated trigeminal fibers.[26] Glutamate receptor antagonists block the response, which is likely mediated through the brainstem trigeminal nucleus interpolaris.[27]

Between 1983 and 1997, I treated 183 patients by percutaneous compression. First-division pain was present in 37% of the patients studied. Previous destructive procedures had been performed on 30% of patients. Multiple sclerosis was associated with trigeminal neuralgia in 7% of the patient population. The mean follow-up was 4 years, and the range was 2 months to 13 years. Ninety-three percent of the patients had initial pain relief, and 61% had subjective numbness; 80% of patients described this numbness as mild, 14% described it as moderate; and 6% described it as severe. Nineteen percent had masseter or pterygoid weakness documented after compression. In one patient, the corneal reflex was absent. Anesthesia dolorosa did not occur, nor was there neurokeratitis.

The overall recurrence rate was 25%. The recurrence rate for the last 42 patients, treated in the last 2 years of the series, was 12%, with an initial success rate of 95%. Among those 42 patients, 50% had postoperative numbness, 26% had temporary masseter weakness, and in 74%, the balloon formed a pear shape. Among patients with recurrent pain who underwent repeat balloon compression, 68% had pain relief from the repeat procedure. Sixty-nine percent of patients with first-division pain alone or in combination with other sensory divisions had pain relief without a recurrence requiring medication or surgery; 62% of 115 patients without first-division pain had successful pain relief without medication or surgery.

PROBLEMS AND SOLUTIONS

If the balloon fails to form a pear shape or it is not possible to achieve adequate inflation pressure, it is likely that the balloon is not properly positioned in the entrance to Meckel's cave. The anteroposterior image should be reviewed to determine whether the tip of the balloon catheter is positioned at the edge of the petrous ridge, within the margins of the dip in the petrous bone that represents the porus trigeminus. If the balloon is inflated only over the ganglion, it will merely elevate the dura off the ganglion at a pressure inadequate to cause a lasting benefit. If the balloon is inflated lateral to the ganglion, beneath the temporal lobe, there will be no benefit. The surgeon should know that introduction of the balloon catheter is not likely to rupture or tear the dura.[28]

How is it possible to injure divisions selectively when the patient is asleep? Balloon compression is selective according to the site of the balloon tip. Fibers that are closer to it are compressed more. By manipulating the catheter tip to the lateral, mid-, or medial porus, fiber divisions can be selected. The duration and pressure of compression need not vary; this simplifies the issues of judgment but sometimes prolongs the operation because of the need to adjust the angle of catheter entry and the site of the catheter tip. Facial soft tissue anatomy is variable, making the entry site selection—between 2 and 3 cm lateral to the edge of the lip and at, above, or below the horizontal from the lip's edge—variable and subject to surgical judgment.

Because the balloon selectively preserves the small myelinated and unmyelinated fibers that mediate the corneal reflex, the balloon may make treatment of first-division pain safer, especially for neurosurgeons without lengthy experience in thermal rhizotomy.

There may be epidural venous oozing if the cannula is positioned just outside the foramen ovale. This bleeding can be stopped by holding the cannula against the foramen while inserting or removing the stylets or catheter, or by advancing the cannula several millimeters until it is within the foramen.

The trigeminal depressor response may be blocked by infusing 1 mL of 1% lidocaine to the retrogasserian fibers; however, the presence of the response provides a useful cue to monitor successful compression and is easily controlled by the external pacemaker.[29] Should the initial compression fail to alleviate the pain, it is possible to repeat the compression within a few days. If pain relief is not achieved, it is unlikely that the procedure will succeed.

The population with trigeminal neuralgia generally consists of aged patients with a variety of medical concerns. They may require anticoagulation for atrial fibrillation, coronary artery disease, or stroke prevention. The risk of discontinuing warfarin anticoagulation must be carefully assessed in such cases. There is a low risk of hemorrhage from these percutaneous procedures. The length of time that reversal of anticoagulation is allowed and the risks of reversal are variable and are best reviewed in conjunction with a cardiologist and hematologist. Patients with a high risk of stroke may not tolerate a long reversal; heparin infusion must be initiated soon after the procedure has been completed, usually the next day.

Trigeminal neuralgia is rarely caused by compressive masses. When there is an associated mass lesion, the decision to treat the tic pain is distinct from the decision to excise the mass, as decompression and percutaneous injury are both effective.

Gamma Knife

Radiosurgery for trigeminal neuralgia has been performed since the 1950s, when Leksell introduced the technique of radiosurgery. At first, the target was the trigeminal ganglion, but because results were inconsistent, the target became the nerve root entry zone of the trigeminal root near the pons.[30] It is important to understand that pain relief from radiosurgery is not immediate. Patients with intractable pain that prevents them from eating are not candidates for this treatment. However, because of its relatively noninvasive nature, patients with cardiovascular disease who take anticoagulants do not need to discontinue them in preparation for this treatment.

TECHNIQUE

A magnetic resonance imaging–compatible stereotactic frame is applied to the skull, and 1-mm axial images of the trigeminal root are obtained, centered at the level of the midpons. Arterial compression may be identified, but this is not a contraindication to proceeding with treatment. The vessel may be included in the 4-mm 50% isocenter to which a maximal dose of 70 to 90 Gy is delivered. The target is located 2 to 4 mm anterior to the junction of the nerve and the pons. This plan delivers less than 20% of the dose to the brainstem. Patients are discharged within 24 hours and are told that pain relief may take up to 10 weeks. Tapering of anticonvulsant medication begins after there has been consistent pain relief for several days.

DISCUSSION

As the following data indicate, the results from gamma knife treatment are preliminary and mixed, but they suggest that the success rate may be less than that for thermal rhizotomy or balloon compression. However, as with any new treatment, patients who have failed standard therapies may represent a larger component of the treated population. It is clear that the degree of postoperative numbness with gamma knife therapy is less than with other percutaneous procedures.

In a series of 106 patients treated using this technique, 60% were initially pain free and required no further medication.[31] An additional 17% required some medication and achieved 50% to 90% pain reduction. At a median follow-up of 18 months by an independent examiner, 77% had excellent or good results. A lower percentage of patients (10%) developed numbness. Postoperative imaging at 6 to 9 months demonstrated enhancement of the nerve at the targeted site. It has been shown that the trigeminal nerve is more tolerant of radiation than the optic nerve is. Doses of 5 to 30 Gy do not cause neuropathy to any of the nerves in the cavernous sinus.[32]

Young and colleagues[33] treated 110 patients with a mean follow-up of 20 months. They noted that pain relief was less in patients who did not have typical trigeminal neuralgia or who had undergone previous procedures. Patients with classic pain had only a 3% recurrence rate during this period and 95% initial relief. The incidence of sensory loss was 3%. A Mayo Clinic series of 20 patients with trigeminal neuralgia and follow-up for more than 2 months noted that 70% were free of pain after radiosurgery.[34]

PROBLEMS AND SOLUTIONS

Imaging of the trigeminal nerve may be difficult, especially in patients who have undergone microvascular decompression. The felt placed around the trigeminal nerve may mimic a mass lesion and make it difficult to identify the nerve. In patients who have had rhizotomies, the nerve can be atrophic and difficult to identify.

It is not yet known whether a repeat dose of radiation is possible and safe when there is a recurrence. A more anterior target on the nerve could be selected in such cases, and perhaps delivering a lower dose, such as 50 Gy.

Peripheral Neurectomy

Peripheral neurectomies are performed infrequently because of the high recurrence rate. However, some patients, such as those who are aged and medically debilitated, may not be candidates for a procedure directed at the trigeminal root. The supraorbital and infraorbital nerves can be easily exposed surgically, often with the patient receiving local anesthetic and intravenous sedation. The nerve is grabbed with a small hemostat, twisted, and sectioned at its base. A neurolytic agent such as phenol can be peripherally injected at the exiting neural foramen. Pain recurrence is high with peripheral procedures, and dysesthesias are more common after several repeated procedures.

In a series of older patients (mean age, 74 years), 18 patients were treated with 10% phenol injection. Although initial pain relief was 87%, at 2 years only 30% had lasting relief.[35] Oturai and colleagues[36] reported a 78% to 84% recurrence from alcohol block or peripheral neurectomy after a mean follow-up of 8 years. Nevertheless, peripheral neurectomy may be effective in elderly patients with pain in the first or second divisions, especially when the patient's life span is limited and early recurrence is less of a concern.[37]

MICROVASCULAR DECOMPRESSION AND NUMBNESS

Historically, there has been debate whether operative trauma to the trigeminal nerve is the reason for pain relief after MVD. Barker and coworkers'[38] series of 1205 patients who underwent MVD over 20 years was analyzed for a relationship between postoperative numbness and relief of pain. Seventeen percent of patients had postoperative numbness, which correlated with the absence of arterial compression and findings of venous compression. In fact, outcome was worse in such patients ($P = 0.3$). The numbness was associated with burning and aching facial pain. Bergenheim and colleagues[39] prospectively studied 37 patients for sensory changes before and after MVD. Forty-three percent of patients had elevated sensory thresholds when measured by electrical stimulation, and 32% had clinical evidence of sensory deficits. However, all 51% of patients without sensory deficits had excellent results after MVD. The benefit of MVD is clearly not because of injury to the trigeminal nerve.

CONCLUSION

The procedures discussed in this chapter represent the percutaneous techniques for trigeminal neuralgia treatment that are most commonly recommended by neurosurgeons when medical therapy has failed. It is important that neurosurgeons who treat this disease be knowledgeable regarding the full range of surgical options available for their patients.

The most important question for a surgeon reading this chapter is, Why use percutaneous therapy for trigeminal neuralgia? At this point, the answer should be clear. The treatment is advantageous because it has a low incidence of significant morbidity, can be performed inexpensively, and has comparable results to MVD. Simply, it is a solid and valid treatment technique.

REFERENCES

1. Gray H: Anatomy, Descriptive and Surgical. New York, Bounty Books, 1977, pp 725–738.
2. Gudmundsson K, Rhoton AL, Rushton JG: Detailed anatomy of the intracranial portion of the trigeminal nerve. J Neurosurg 35:592–600, 1971.
3. Pelletier VA, Poulos DA, Lende RA: Functional localization in the trigeminal root. J Neurosurg 40:504–513, 1974.
4. Young RF: Unmyelinated fibers in the trigeminal motor root: Possible relationship to the results of trigeminal rhizotomy. J Neurosurg 49:538–543, 1978.
5. Love S, Hilton DA, Coakham HB: Central demyelination of the Vth nerve root in trigeminal neuralgia associated with vascular compression. Brain Pathol 8:1–11, discussion 11–12, 1998.
6. Hamlyn PJ: Neurovascular relationships in the posterior cranial fossa, with special reference to trigeminal neuralgia. 2. Neurovascular compression of the trigeminal nerve in cadaveric controls and patients with trigeminal neuralgia: Quantification and influence of method. Clin Anat 10:380–388, 1997.
7. Sweet WH, Wepsic JG: Controlled thermocoagulation of trigeminal ganglion and rootlets for differential destruction of pain fibers. J Neurosurg 39:143–156, 1974.
8. Tew JM: Treatment of trigeminal neuralgia by percutaneous rhizotomy. In Youmans JR (ed): Neurological Surgery, 2nd ed. Philadelphia, WB Saunders, 1982, p 3568.
9. Letcher FS, Goldring S: The effect of radiofrequency current and heat on peripheral nerve action potential in the cat. J Neurosurg 29:42–47, 1968.
10. Frigyesi TL, Siegfried J, Broggi G: The selective vulnerability of evoked potentials in the trigeminal sensory root to graded thermocoagulation. Exp Neurol 49:11–21, 1975.
11. Smith HP, McWhorter JM, Challa VR: Radiofrequency neurolysis in a clinical model: Neuropathological correlation. J Neurosurg 55:246–253, 1981.
12. Nugent GR: Radiofrequency treatment of trigeminal neuralgia using a cordotomy-type electrode: A method. Neurosurg Clin N Am 8:41–52, 1997.
13. Taha JM, Tew JM Jr, Buncher CR: A prospective 15-year follow up of 154 consecutive patients with trigeminal neuralgia treated by percutaneous stereotactic radiofrequency thermal rhizotomy. J Neurosurg 83:989–993, 1995.
14. Taha JM, Tew JM Jr: Comparison of surgical treatments for trigeminal neuralgia: Reevaluation of radiofrequency rhizotomy. Neurosurgery 38:865–871, 1996.
15. Sweet WH, Poletti CE, Robert JT: Dangerous rises in blood pressure upon heating of trigeminal rootlets: Increased bleeding times in patients with trigeminal neuralgia. Neurosurgery 17:843–844, 1985.
16. Kuchta J, Koulousakis A, Decker A, Klug N: Pressor and depressor responses in thermocoagulation of the trigeminal ganglion. Br J Neurosurg 12:409–413, 1998.
17. Hakanson S: Trigeminal neuralgia treated by the injection of glycerol into the trigeminal cistern. Neurosurgery 9:638–646, 1981.
18. Cappabianca P, Spaziante R, Graziussi G, et al: Percutaneous retrogasserian glycerol rhizolysis for treatment of trigeminal neuralgia: Technique and results in 191 patients. J Neurosurg Sci 39:37–45, 1995.
19. Linderoth B, Hakanson S: Retrogasserian glycerol rhizolysis in trigeminal neuralgia. In Schmidek HH, Sweet WS (eds): Operative Neurosurgical Techniques. Philadelphia, WB Saunders, 1995, pp 1523–1536.
20. North RB, Kidd DH, Piantadosi S, Carson BS: Percutaneous retrogasserian glycerol rhizotomy: Predictors of success and failure in treatment of trigeminal neuralgia. J Neurosurg 72:851–856, 1990.
21. Young RF: Glycerol rhizolysis for treatment of trigeminal neuralgia. J Neurosurg 69:39–45, 1988.
22. Lunsford LD, Bennett MG, Martinez AJ: Experimental trigeminal glycerol injection: Electrophysiologic and morphologic effects. Arch Neurol 42:146–149, 1985.
23. Eide PK, Stubhaug A: Relief of trigeminal neuralgia after percutaneous retrogasserian glycerol rhizolysis is dependent on normalization of abnormal temporal summation of pain, without general impairment of sensory perception. Neurosurgery 43:462–472, discussion 472–474, 1998.
24. Mullan S, Lichtor T: Percutaneous microcompression of the trigeminal ganglion for trigeminal neuralgia. J Neurosurg 59:1007–1012, 1983.
25. Brown JA, Hoeflinger B, Long PB, et al: Axon and ganglion cell injury in rabbits after percutaneous trigeminal balloon compression. Neurosurgery 38:993–1003, 1996.
26. Brown JA, Preul MC: Trigeminal depressor response during percutaneous microcompression of the trigeminal ganglion for trigeminal neuralgia. Neurosurgery 23:745–748, 1988.
27. McCulloch PF, Paterson IA, West NH: An intact glutamatergic trigeminal pathway is essential for the cardiac response to simulated diving. Am J Physiol 269(3 Pt 2):R669–R677, 1995.
28. Urculo E, Martinez L, Arrazola M, Ramirez R: Macroscopic effects of percutaneous trigeminal ganglion compression (Mullan's technique): An anatomic study. Neurosurgery 36:776–779, 1995.
29. Dominguez J, Lobato RD, Rivas JJ, et al: Changes in systemic blood pressure and cardiac rhythm induced by therapeutic compression of the trigeminal ganglion. Neurosurgery 34:422–427, 1994.
30. Kondziolka D, Lunsford LD, Habeck M, Flickinger JC: Gamma knife radiosurgery for trigeminal neuralgia. Neurosurg Clin N Am 8:79–85, 1997.
31. Kondziolka D, Perez B, Flickinger JC, et al: Gamma knife radiosurgery for trigeminal neuralgia: Results and expectations. Arch Neurol 55:1524–1529, 1998.
32. Leber KA, Bergloff J, Pendl G: Dose-response tolerance of the visual pathways and cranial nerves of the cavernous sinus to stereotactic radiosurgery. J Neurosurg 88:43–50, 1998.
33. Young RF, Vermulen S, Posewitz A: Gamma knife radiosurgery for the treatment of trigeminal neuralgia. Stereotact Funct Neurosurg 70(Suppl 1):192–199, 1998.
34. Pollock BE, Gorman DA, Schomberg PJ, Kline RW: The Mayo Clinic gamma knife experience: Indications and initial results. Mayo Clin Proc 74:5–13, 1999.
35. Wilkinson HA: Trigeminal nerve peripheral branch phenol/glycerol injections for tic douloureux. J Neurosurg 90:828–832, 1999.
36. Oturai AB, Jensen K, Eriksen J, Madsen F: Neurosurgery for trigeminal neuralgia: Comparison of alcohol block, neurectomy, and radiofrequency coagulation. Clin J Pain 12:311–315, 1996.
37. Murali R, Rovit RL: Are peripheral neurectomies of value in the treatment of trigeminal neuralgia? An analysis of new cases and cases involving previous radiofrequency gasserian thermocoagulation. J Neurosurg 85:435–437, 1996.
38. Barker FG 2nd, Jannetta PJ, Bissonette DJ, Jho HD: Trigeminal numbness and tic relief after microvascular decompression for typical trigeminal neuralgia. Neurosurgery 40:39–45, 1997.
39. Bergenheim AT, Shamsgovara P, Ridderheim PA: Microvascular decompression for trigeminal neuralgia: No relation between sensory disturbance and outcome. Stereotact Funct Neurosurg 68(1–4 Pt 1):200–206, 1997.

CHAPTER 187

Trigeminal Neuralgia: Microvascular Decompression of the Trigeminal Nerve for Tic Douloureux

PETER J. JANNETTA ■ ELAD I. LEVY

HISTORY

Only recently has microvascular decompression become a recognized treatment for tic douloureux, or trigeminal neuralgia. Like other cranial rhizopathies, trigeminal neuralgia has long defied categorization, clarification of pathophysiology, and effective treatment, despite efforts by clinicians in several disciplines. Although the clinical presentation of disorders such as trigeminal neuralgia, hemifacial spasm, glossopharyngeal neuralgia, tinnitus, spasmodic torticollis, and disabling positional vertigo are quite different, these problems all share a common underlying pathology: vascular compression of the respective cranial nerve exit zone near the brainstem.

Descriptions of trigeminal neuralgia first emerged by the end of the first millennium. According to a recent historical article by Rose, Aretaeus of Cappadocia was thought to have been referring to trigeminal neuralgia when he described a headache in which "spasm and distortion of the countenance take place."[1, 2] Several centuries later, facial syndromes were described by Avicenna (died AD 1037). In 1677, John Locke described the Countess of Northumberland, wife of the English ambassador to France, who had "a fit of such violent and exquisite torment that it forced her to . . . cries and shrieks . . . which extended itself all over the right side of her face and mouth." Some credit Nicolas André for coining the term *tic douloureux.*[3] In his 1756 text, *Observations pratiques sur les maladies de l'urethre et sur pluysiers faits convulsifs*, he discussed the surgical treatment of five patients with tic douloureux, though it is believed that only two of the five had true trigeminal neuralgia.[3] He described "a cruel and obscure illness, which causes . . . in the face some violent motions, some hideous grimaces which are an insurmountable obstacle to the reception of food, which put off sleep." In 1773, John Fothergill presented his series of 14 patients with trigeminal neuralgia to the Medical Society of London.[2] His descriptions of typical triggers and lancinating pain are still considered accurate and representative of trigeminal neuralgia.[4]

Despite these early historical accounts, more than 2 centuries would pass before a definitive surgical intervention would prove efficacious. In 1934, Dandy suggested that anomalies in the posterior fossa might be responsible for trigeminal neuralgia, but it was not until the early 1960s that patients with known trigeminal neuralgia were noted to have compression of the trigeminal nerve by a small artery near the brainstem. Based on early reports by Taarnhøg, Gardner performed posterior fossa explorations in search of pathology compressing the trigeminal nerve and facial nerve in patients with trigeminal neuralgia and hemifacial spasm, respectively. In his early reports he described mobilizing a vessel away from the nerve and placing Gelfoam between the vessel and the nerve.[5] Following several more operations to relieve vascular compression of the trigeminal nerve, it became apparent that pulsatile, mechanical forces from a blood vessel were the pathophysiologic mechanism responsible for the cranial hyperactive syndromes such as trigeminal neuralgia. The trigeminal nerve, like all the cranial nerves, is subject to the forces of vascular compression, such as arteriosclerosis, dolichoectasia, and parenchymal atrophy.

In this chapter, we describe the patient selection criteria, perioperative management, operative technique, postoperative results, and complications following microvascular decompression for trigeminal neuralgia.

PATIENT SELECTION

Patients with trigeminal neuralgia are selected for microvascular decompression based on their symptoms, history, ability to undergo general anesthesia, and failure of medical management. Exceptions include patients with a known diagnosis of multiple sclerosis, because they are thought to be poor candidates for microvascular decompression. For patients unable to tolerate general anesthesia, treatment with percutaneous radiofrequency rhizotomies, percutaneous glycerol rhizotomies, trigeminal balloon microcompression, stereotactic radiosurgery, or peripheral balloon microcompression is recommended.[6, 7] A brief discussion of these other surgical techniques is imperative to clarify why microvascular decompression is the surgical procedure of choice for most patients.

Radiofrequency gasserian ganglion lesions, created by a percutaneous needle-stick into the trigeminal ganglion, have an initial success rate of 90% or greater; over the long term, 20% to 80% of patients are pain free.[8–10] Approximately 10% of patients suffer from facial dysesthesias following radiofrequency rhizotomies. In a recent series of 1600 patients who underwent a total of 2138 procedures, immediate pain relief was achieved in 97%, but only 58% had sufficient pain relief at 5-year follow-up after a single procedure. At 20-year follow-up, only 41% of patients who had undergone a single procedure had pain relief. Complications included, but were not limited to, diminished corneal reflex in 91 patients (6%), masseter weakness and paralysis in 66 (4%), dysesthesia in 16 (1%), and anesthesia dolorosa in 12 (<1%).[11]

Glycerol rhizotomies cause facial dysesthesias less frequently than radiofrequency rhizotomies do. Although glycerol rhizotomies have initial success rates between 80% and 90%, median time to recurrence is 16 to 36 months.[12–15] Peripheral neurectomies, though less invasive, typically have a short duration of tic relief and may be indicated for those with a short life expectancy. Balloon microcompression of the trigeminal ganglion has initial success rates ranging from 78% to 100%, with a mean time to recurrence of 3.5 years.[16, 17] Minor dysesthesias occur in approximately 20% of patients, and mild temporary masseter weakness is seen in the majority of those treated with balloon microcompression.[16, 17]

Stereotactic radiosurgery for trigeminal neuralgia is the least invasive of the aforementioned procedures. This modality of treatment targets the nerve root entry zone with 60 to 90 Gy of single-dose radiation.[18–21] Benefits are seen within 1 to 8 weeks of initial treatment, and more than 60% of patients are pain free. A recent study of 220 patients with trigeminal neuralgia treated with radiosurgery demonstrated complete pain relief in 65% of patients at 6 months, 70% at 1 year, and 75% at 33 months, with a 13.4% recurrence rate over a median follow-up of 15 months.[22]

The choice between microvascular decompression and other procedures should be based on the patient's preference and his or her ability to tolerate a small craniotomy under general anesthesia. Advantages of microvascular decompression include consistently higher long-term success rates with a substantially lower incidence of facial dysesthesias. Another advantage of microvascular decompression over other ablative techniques is the ability to restore normal or near-normal function to the nerve itself. In one study of 10 patients, direct root and scalp electrode recordings showed significant improvement in seven patients following microvascular decompression. Although all patients were pain free following surgery, seven showed improved neurophysiologic parameters immediately after decompression of the offending vessel, suggesting the condition of "rapid reversible physiologic block" or a class 1 nerve injury. Such injuries are potentially reversible with treatment of the causative agent—in this case, a vessel compressing the nerve root.[23] Others have demonstrated normalization of elevated sensory perception thresholds for touch, pinprick, warmth, and coolness sensations following microvascular decompression. These findings provide evidence that this surgery preserves nerve integrity rather than causing superficial trauma to the nerve at the entry zone.[24]

The advantages of a high success rate, a lower recurrence of pain, and the normalization of nerve function are significant, given that the average life expectancy of the patients treated by the primary author (PJJ) was 34 years from the initial onset of symptoms.[25]

PATIENT HISTORY AND PHYSICAL EXAMINATION

A careful history and physical examination are imperative for selecting the patients who will benefit most from microvascular decompression. The classic symptom of typical trigeminal neuralgia is unilateral, lancinating pain in one or more distributions of the trigeminal nerve. Wind, talking, eating, and shaving often precipitate symptoms due to trigeminal distribution trigger points. Typically, patients describe an abrupt and memorable onset of symptoms, with a variable duration of intermittent remission. A history of trigger points and a sudden onset of symptoms was described in 87% of the primary author's patients (based on a review of 1820 electronic medical records of patients treated with microvascular decompression for trigeminal neuralgia). There is often a positional component to the pain, such that some patients find temporary relief by lying supine or with the affected side up. Burning, aching pain without specific trigger points characterizes atypical trigeminal neuralgia, which differs from the typical form in the expected area of vascular compression on the trigeminal nerve. Although surgery is less successful in patients with atypical trigeminal neuralgia than in those with typical symptoms, there are currently no alternative treatments with equal or better outcomes.

The physical findings in patients with trigeminal neuralgia may range from subtle to striking. These patients frequently have decreased sensation in the ipsilateral trigeminal distribution. In the primary author's series, 30% of patients had hypalgesia, hypesthesia, or both elicited on physical examination.[26] A careful neurological examination in these patients involves light touch and sharp sensory testing in the pure distribution of the trigeminal nerve, including the corneal reflex. Sensory abnormalities are best elicited by beginning from the area of sensory dysfunction and progressing carefully to the area of intact function. One area of common sensory dysfunction is around the ipsilateral nasolabial fold. Repetitive pinprick testing involves starting in this region and radiating out in other directions like the spokes of a wheel. This usually elicits hypalgesia, hypesthesia, or both. Additionally, a careful clinician may note a decreased corneal reflex in patients with trigeminal neuralgia of the first division. Occasionally, patients may be noted to have asymmetrical jaw motion. It is unknown whether this is due to voluntary guarding against an attack of pain or to mild denervation of the motor-proprioceptive fascicles of the trigeminal nerve. These changes usually revert to normal after successful microvascular decompression.[26, 27]

It is important that preoperative surgical planning accurately determine the distribution of the trigeminal pain. For example, in lower trigeminal neuralgia (third division or second and third divisions), the superior cerebellar artery is commonly found compressing the entry zone of the nerve from the anterocephalad direction. Upper trigeminal neuralgia (first division or first and second divisions) is commonly caused by nerve compression from the caudolateral direction. Isolated second-division symptoms are typically associated with medial or lateral venous compression of the nerve. In a review of electronic medical records from patients with first-time microvascular decompression for typical trigeminal neuralgia treated before January 1999, combination second- and third-division trigeminal neuralgia was the most common distribution of symptoms, found in 34.7% of 1810 patients (unpublished data; Table 187–1). This percentage is similar to that previously reported by Barker and coworkers in a series of similar patients.[28] Although preoperative symptoms point to the area of likely compression, the surgeon must take care to inspect the nerve in all directions.

Before considering surgical options, it is important to demonstrate that patients have not found satisfactory relief with medical therapy. Some patients have initial success with medical management using agents such as carbamazepine, phenytoin, baclofen, valproic acid, clonazepam, and gabapentin, but long-term success is uncommon. Historically, carbamazepine has been most effective, but only 56% of patients maintain satisfactory pain relief after 10 years.[29] Allergic reactions, side effects, and the development of symptoms

refractory to medication necessitate early surgical intervention.

PREOPERATIVE EVALUATION WITH NEUROPHYSIOLOGY

Preoperative testing for every patient involves otologic examination, audiometry (pure tone and speech), acoustic middle ear reflexes, and brainstem auditory evoked potentials. All patients have preoperative magnetic resonance imaging and computed tomographic scans to rule out tumors, cysts, and vascular or bony anomalies.

The audiometric tests are performed preoperatively to obtain a baseline for determining quantitative changes in hearing function. Additionally, preoperative brainstem auditory evoked potentials provide baseline information for the neurophysiology team members, so that they can warn the surgeon of any deviations observed during intraoperative monitoring. Deviations, such as delays or shifts in interpeak latencies of more than 1.5 to 2 msec, can signify potential stretch-induced injury to the eighth nerve.[30–36]

Audiometric tests are typically repeated on postoperative day 6 to detect any hearing changes. Fluid effusions in the mastoid air cells cause some patients to experience transient conductive hearing loss. This typically resolves spontaneously within 2 to 5 weeks, at which point the test can be repeated (up to 3 months postoperatively).

SURGICAL TECHNIQUE

As in any operation, patient positioning is imperative for surgical success. The patient is placed on the operating table such that his or her head is at the foot of the bed. This provides the surgeon with maximal working room during the microscopic portion of the case. A three-point head fixation device is applied, and the patient is placed in the lateral decubitus position. An axillary roll is used, and padding is placed on other pressure points. The head is rotated slightly away from the affected side and then flexed, always maintaining two fingerbreadths between the patient's chin and sternum. The vertex of the head is positioned parallel to the floor, placing the seventh-eighth nerve complex at a more inferior position relative to the trigeminal nerve.[37] The patient is then secured to the bed, and the head fixation device is fastened into position. The patient's shoulder is taped caudally for maximal working room[37] (Fig. 187–1).

Following satisfactory positioning, a 3- by 3-cm area behind the ear is shaved, and bony landmarks are identified. These include the mastoid eminence, digastric groove, and inion. The iniomeatal line identifies the transverse sinus, and the digastric groove identifies the sigmoid sinus. The intersection of these two lines correlates well with the transverse-sigmoid junction. Once these landmarks are visualized, the field is prepared in the usual sterile fashion. The incision, approxi-

T A B L E   1 8 7 – 1 ■ Distribution of Symptoms in 1810 Previously Unoperated Patients with Typical Trigeminal Neuralgia

DISTRIBUTION	NO. OF PATIENTS	PERCENTAGE
V1 only	47	2.6
V2 only	291	16
V3 only	271	15
V1+2	327	18
V1+3	0	0
V2+3	628	34.7
V1+2+3	246	13.7

From Burchiel KJ (ed): Surgical Management of Pain. New York, Thieme, 2002.

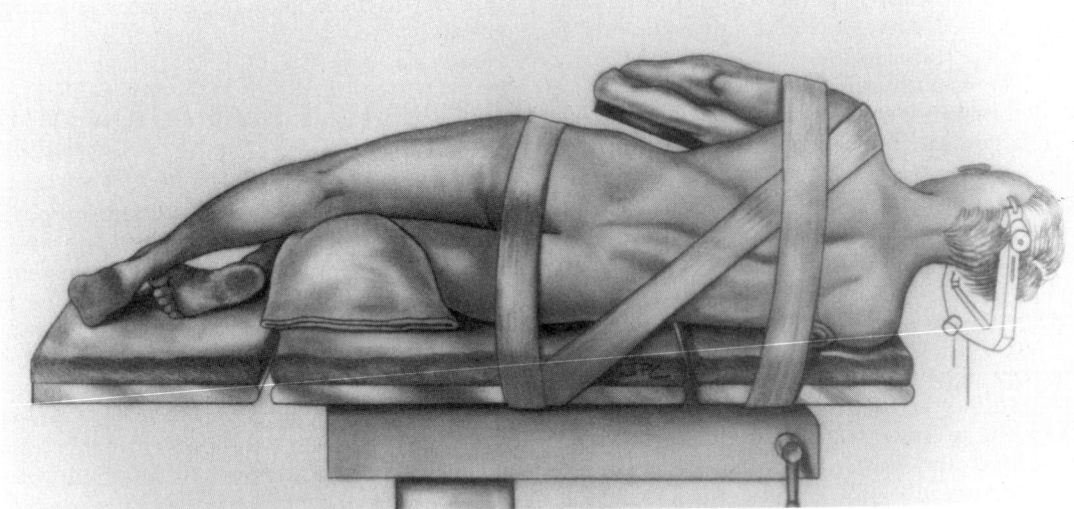

FIGURE 187–1. The patient is placed on the operating table such that his or her head is at the foot of the bed. A three-point head fixation device is then applied, and the patient is placed in the lateral decubitus position. An axillary roll and padding for other pressure points are placed. The head is rotated slightly away from the affected side and then flexed, always maintaining two fingerbreadths between the patient's chin and sternum. The vertex of the head is positioned parallel to the floor. The patient is then secured to the bed, and the head fixation device is fastened into position. (From Burchiel KJ [ed]: Surgical Management of Pain. New York, Thieme, 2002.)

mately 3 to 5 cm long, is placed 0.5 cm posterior to the hairline, extending one quarter above the iniomeatal line and three quarters below. Electrocautery is used to dissect and clear soft tissue until the mastoid eminence is adequately visualized. Often the occipital artery and mastoid emissary vein are encountered and can be used as landmarks. The occipital artery is typically cauterized and sacrificed.

Before beginning the craniectomy, the digastric groove should be visualized and the soft tissues adequately dissected. Using a high-speed drill or perforator, a bur hole is placed over the mastoid emissary vein (which does not lie directly over the sigmoid sinus), which is a good landmark for the junction between the sigmoid and transverse sinuses. The craniectomy is expanded until the junction of the transverse and sigmoid sinuses is definitively appreciated, with the apex of the triangular craniectomy pointed at this junction (Fig. 187–2). All air cells are then waxed diligently, and meticulous hemostasis is obtained to prevent blood from running over the cerebellum, brainstem, and cranial nerves. A minimal or partial mastoidectomy has been advocated by some surgeons in select cases to provide greater lateral exposure and potentially minimize cerebellar retraction (which in turn minimizes the risk of hearing loss due to excessive tension on the eighth nerve). This may be especially useful when attempting microvascular decompression of multiple nerves or the lower cranial nerves.[38]

A curvilinear or T-shaped durotomy is performed, exposing a direct corridor along the petrotentorial bone down to the brainstem[37] (Fig. 187–3). The dura is pulled taught and sutured back, and cerebrospinal fluid is aspirated (Fig. 187–4). While gently retracting the cerebellum with a cottonoid on a sterile piece of latex

(rubber dam), the surgeon must allow adequate cerebrospinal fluid to drain so that the cerebellum falls away, minimizing the need for much cerebellar retraction. The operating microscope with a 250-mm focal length objective is now used to "turn the corner," or

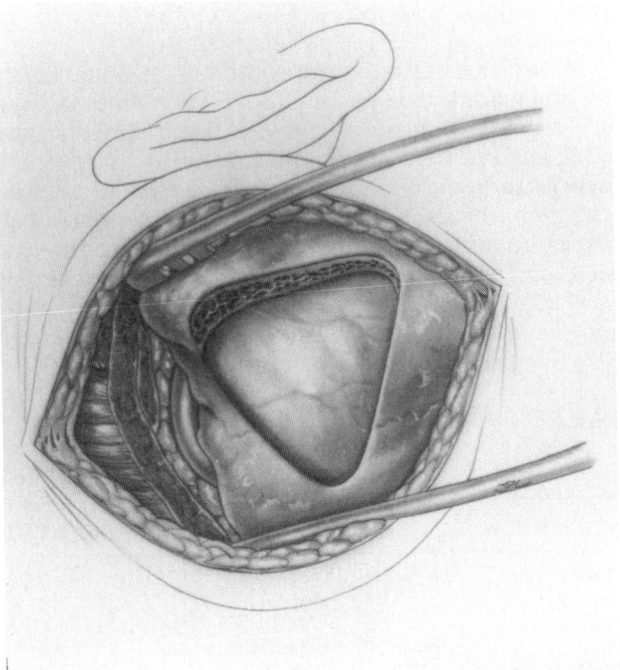

FIGURE 187–2. A craniectomy is expanded until the junction of the transverse and sigmoid sinuses is definitively appreciated, with the apex of the triangular craniectomy aimed at this junction. (From Burchiel KJ [ed]: Surgical Management of Pain. New York, Thieme, 2002.)

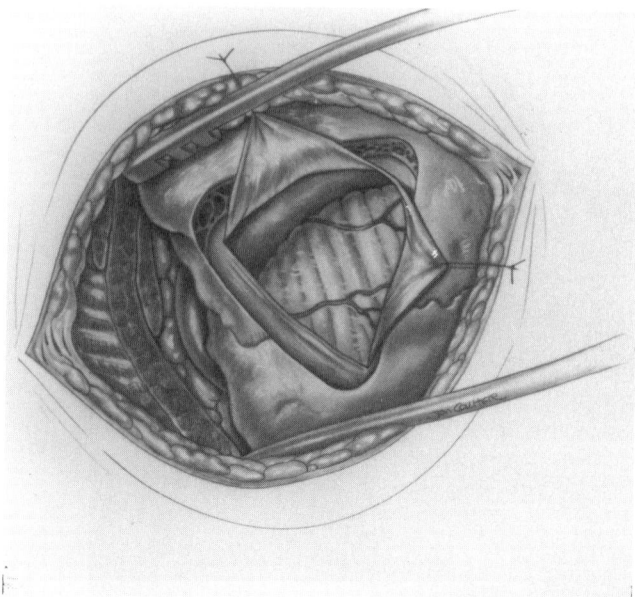

FIGURE 187–3. A curvilinear or T-shaped durotomy is performed, exposing a direct corridor along the petrotentorial bone down to the brainstem. (From Burchiel KJ [ed]: Surgical Management of Pain. New York, Thieme, 2002.)

expose the cerebellopontine angle. Penetration of the trigeminal cistern and sharp dissection of arachnoid adhesions with an arachnoid knife greatly reduce the need for significant cerebellar retraction medially. The cottonoid and a precisely flexible, curved, self-retaining brain retractor are placed on the superolateral portion of the cerebellum for trigeminal exposures. The cerebel-

lum is then retracted up and medially, attempting to elevate it slightly toward the surgeon. Often, the first vessel encountered is the petrosal vein complex, which is coagulated and cut.[37] If the petrosal vein is not intrusive or can easily be mobilized away from the field of view, efforts should be made to preserve it to avoid the risk (albeit very low) of venous infarction.

Before performing microvascular decompression of the trigeminal nerve, the surgeon must be cognizant of the fact that the dorsal root exit zone of the trigeminal nerve extends to a more distal portion of the nerve. The nerve must be meticulously inspected from the brainstem throughout its course to Meckel's cave, and all offending vessels must be decompressed. It is important to keep in mind that no vessel is too small to cause trigeminal neuralgia. Often a dental mirror is useful to assist the surgeon in inspecting the ventral and distal portions of the dorsal root entry zone. Recent studies described the use of endoscopic techniques for visualizing around tortuous vessels. These investigators believe that retraction may be minimized in some situations by endoscope-assisted techniques. However, with increased experience and familiarity with the anatomy of the posterior fossa, the need for endoscopy may be limited to a few select cases.[39, 40]

Performing the actual decompression requires that all arachnoid over the nerve be dissected away, freeing the nerve from any tethering points (Fig. 187–5). Shredded Teflon felt is placed between the vessel and the nerve in a proximal-to-distal fashion. The vessel is

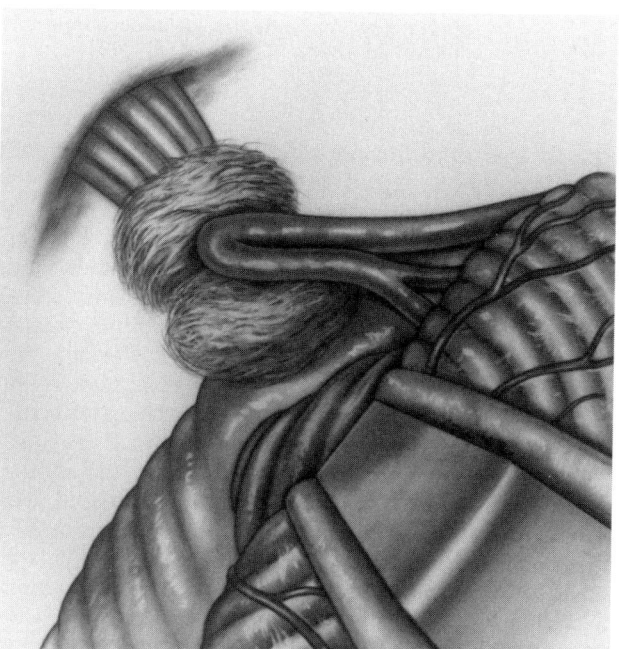

FIGURE 187–5. Performing the actual decompression requires that all arachnoid over the nerve be dissected away, freeing the nerve from any tethering points. Shredded Teflon felt is placed between the vessel and the nerve in a proximal-to-distal fashion. The vessel is then flipped onto the dorsal aspect of the nerve, with shredded Teflon placed between the vessel and the nerve. (From Burchiel KJ [ed]: Surgical Management of Pain. New York, Thieme, 2002.)

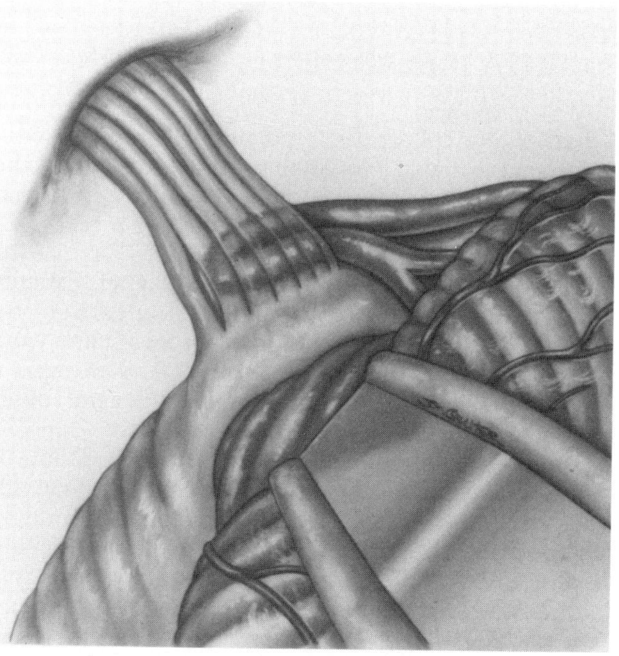

FIGURE 187–4. The dura is pulled taut and sutured back, and cerebrospinal fluid is aspirated. (From Burchiel KJ [ed]: Surgical Management of Pain. New York, Thieme, 2002.)

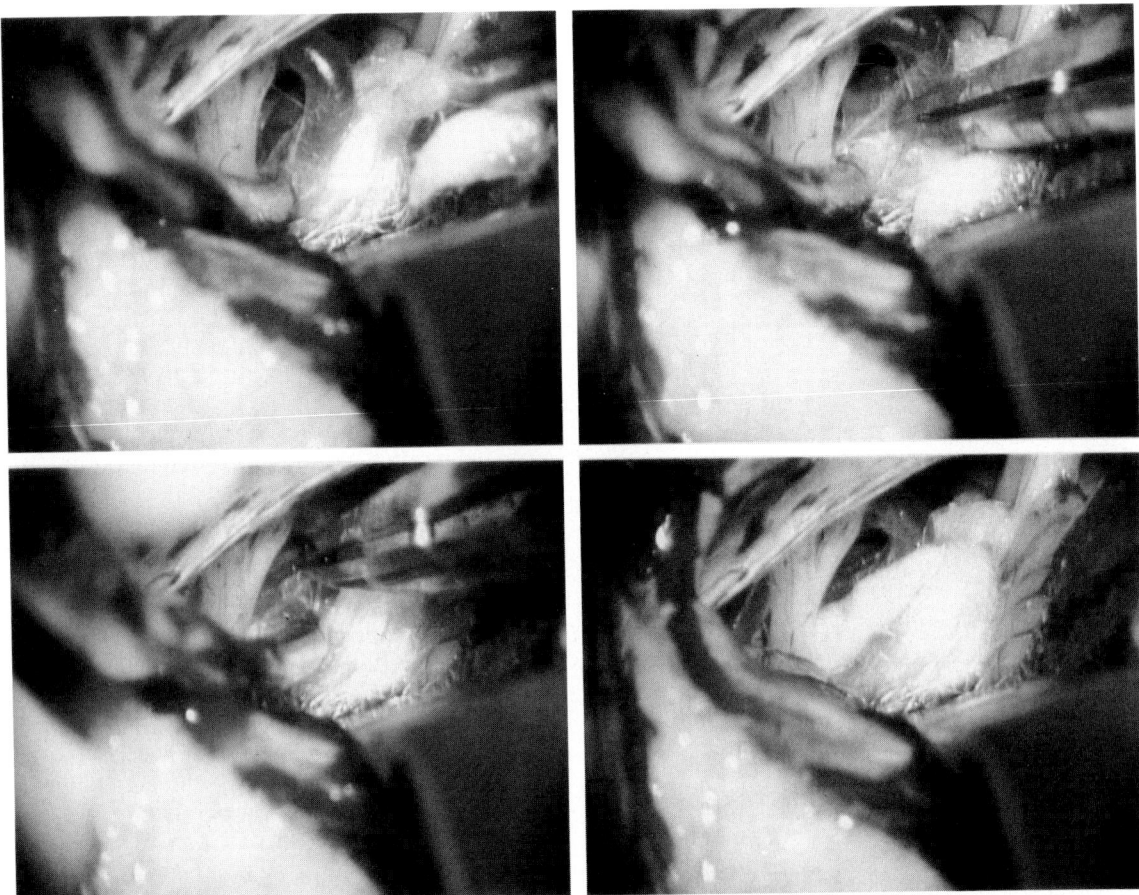

FIGURE 187–6. Intraoperative photograph of the superior cerebellar artery being lifted away with a suction device (*a*) and Teflon felt being placed in a proximal-to-distal fashion (*b, c*), lifting the vessel off the root entry zone (see color section in this volume). (From Burchiel KJ [ed]: Surgical Management of Pain. New York, Thieme, 2002.)

then flipped onto the dorsal aspect of the nerve, with shredded Teflon placed between the vessel and the nerve (Fig. 187–6; see color section in this volume). The surgeon must take great care not to push smaller vessels into the nerve with the Teflon pledgets. Often veins and venules can be coagulated, but arteries must never be sacrificed. The most frequent vessel found causing compression of the trigeminal nerve is the superior cerebellar artery. Multiple pieces of shredded Teflon felt are used to decompress looping arteries affecting more than one side of the trigeminal nerve.[37]

Before closure, the surgeon must be satisfied that the trigeminal nerve is completely decompressed. Valsalva's maneuver is performed to ensure hemostasis. The durotomy is closed carefully in a watertight fashion to prevent cerebrospinal fluid leakage. If a watertight closure cannot be obtained, cadaveric, synthetic, or muscle (if the leak is small) graft material is used to patch the leak. In repeat procedures, some advocate the use of a fibrin sealant to repair small holes in friable dura. The bone edges are waxed for a second time, and a cranioplasty is performed using wire mesh or methyl methacrylate placed over a piece of Gelfoam. Fascia, subcutaneous tissue, and skin are closed in standard fashion.

PATIENT OUTCOME FOLLOWING MICROVASCULAR DECOMPRESSION

In Barker and colleagues' report of 1204 patients who underwent initial microvascular decompression at the University of Pittsburgh, 80% were pain free at 1 year, and an additional 8% had greater than 75% relief, for a total success rate of 88%.[28] At 10 years, 70% remained pain free, and 4% had greater than 75% relief. Patients with persistent or recurrent pain (11%) underwent repeat microvascular decompression. Of these, 96% were either pain free or had greater than 75% pain relief a year after surgery (89% at 10 years). Several other groups have demonstrated similar results.

A more recent review by the primary author of 1820 electronic medical records of patients treated with microvascular decompression for trigeminal neuralgia demonstrated similar findings immediately following surgery (this group excluded patients with multiple decompressions). Of these patients, 83% had immediate complete relief, and another 15% had partial relief. Only 2% had no relief (these percentages are based on available data from 1811 patients). Patient satisfaction following microvascular decompression is quite high.

In the authors' series of patients with excellent outcomes, 99.7% considered their results successful, and 93% of patients with partial relief considered their outcomes successful.

A recent report by Tronnier and coworkers examined the results of 378 patients who underwent microvascular decompression for trigeminal neuralgia over a 20-year period.[41] These results were compared with those of a similar cohort of 316 patients who underwent radiofrequency lesions for the same indication over the same time interval. Complications following microvascular decompression included complete hearing loss in 2.6%, vertigo persisting longer than 14 days in 2.2%, and mortality, facial paresis, tinnitus, and cerebrospinal fluid leak in approximately 1% each. However, the results clearly demonstrated that microvascular decompression provided superior rates of long-term pain relief compared with radiofrequency rhizotomy. Patients treated with radiofrequency rhizotomy had a 75% chance of pain recurrence 4.5 years after the procedure. In the group of patients who underwent microvascular decompression, 76% were pain free after 2 years, and 63% were pain free after 20 years.

The recurrence rate of trigeminal neuralgia following microvascular decompression has been reported in many different series. Some of the larger series are listed in Table 187–2. In the authors' series, the annual recurrence rate fell below 2% by 5 years postoperatively and below 1% by 10 years postoperatively.[28] Using multivariate Cox analysis, four factors correlated with long-term recurrence of trigeminal neuralgia: female sex, preoperative symptoms lasting longer than 8 years, venous compression, and failure of immediate postoperative relief.[28] Several other reports noted similar findings.[42–48] When pain recurs following successful

microvascular decompression, repeat exploration is suggested if the pain recurs in the perioperative period. However, if there is mild to moderate recurrence of pain following a pain-free interval of months to years, a second trial of medical therapy may be warranted. Should this fail, microvascular decompression should be considered. Although reoperation can be more challenging owing to obscuration of the trigeminal nerve by scar tissue and Teflon, it is safe and yields satisfactory results. In a report of 80 patients who were successfully treated with microvascular decompression, 5 patients experienced severe recurrent disease that was intractable to medication. These five patients underwent repeat microvascular decompression; three were found to have vascular compression of the nerve, and the other two were believed to have symptoms related to felt placement. Four of these patients had excellent pain relief, and the fifth had only partial relief following the second surgery.[49] Cho and associates reported a large series of 376 patients, 31 of whom underwent repeat microvascular decompression for pain recurrence.[50] Half of these patients had a negative re-exploration, which correlated with early recurrence of pain at less than 1 year. Among the others, seven (22%) had arterial loop compression, four (13%) had venous compression, and four (13%) had Teflon compression or adhesion. It is interesting to note that these series differ substantially from the findings of Bederson and Wilson,[42] who found only one patient with an abnormal neurovascular relationship.

A caveat to performing less invasive ablative procedures is the increased risk of failure, despite eventual surgical decompression. In one review of 135 patients, 36 had unsatisfactory results following microvascular decompression, and 16 elected to have repeat microvas-

T A B L E 1 8 7 – 2 ■ Long-Term Rate of Recurrence or Unsatisfactory Relief Following Microvascular Decompression

AUTHOR	YEAR	NO. OF PATIENTS	UNSATISFACTORY RELIEF OR RECURRENCE (%)	MEAN FOLLOW-UP (mo)
Apfelbaum[48]	1988	300	31	63
Barker et al[28]	1996	1204	30	74
Bederson & Wilson[42]*	1989	252	17	61
Dahle et al[63]	1989	57	44	37
Klun[64]	1992	178	12	62
Kolluri & Heros[43]	1984	72	22	59
Kondo group A[65]	1997	127	20	151
Kondo group B[65]	1997	154	17	84
Lee et al[66]	1997	146	12	86
Piatt & Wilkins[67]	1984	103	23	48
Sun et al[47]	1994	61	18	80
Van Loveren et al[68]	1982	50	16	36
Zorman & Wilson[69]	1984	92	12	26
Tronnier et al[41]	2001	225	25	131
Barba & Alksne[44]	1984	37	41	43
Liao et al[49]	1997	80	6	9–58 (range)†
Cho et al[50]	1994	376	14	76
Rath et al[51]	1996	135	27	30
Broggi et al[53]	2000	148	15	38
Total		**3797**	**mean = 21**	**mean = 67.5**

* Includes some patients with partial sensory rhizotomy with or without microvascular decompression.
† Range not used to calculate mean follow-up duration.
From Burchiel KJ (ed): Surgical Management of Pain. New York, Thieme, 2002.

cular decompression. Of these 16, 9 were found to have either new or missed vessels impinging on the trigeminal nerve. Twelve of the 16 patients had good long-term pain relief. The other four patients who remained symptomatic had all had prior neuroablative procedures. A previous ablative procedure and prolonged symptoms before seeking treatment were found to be statistically significant predictors of poor outcome.[51]

Recurrent trigeminal neuralgia following microvascular decompression may share a common pathophysiology. Lee and colleagues reported that of 393 patients identified as having venous compression of the trigeminal nerve, 121 (31%) developed recurrent pain[52] (Fig. 187–7; see color section in this volume). Approximately 75% of the patients who developed recurrent pain did so in the first 24 months. Of the 32 patients who underwent repeat microvascular decompression, 28 (88%) were found to have venous compression of the nerve. Based on these findings and the knowledge that veins can regrow, venous compression should be treated with Teflon decompression rather than bipolar electrocautery techniques. Following a second surgery, 81% had pain improvement, perhaps suggesting that re-exploration and repeat decompression are warranted in the setting of early pain recurrence.

Patient outcomes following microvascular decompression may be worse in those with a prolonged history of trigeminal pain before surgical intervention or a prior ablative procedure.[45] In a review of 148 patients who underwent microvascular decompression between 1991 and 1996, Broggi and coworkers found that patients with a preoperative duration of symptoms of 7 years or longer had a statistically significant shorter duration of postoperative pain relief.[53] We too found that a prior ablative procedure, in addition to a prolonged history of trigeminal neuralgia, correlates with a lower probability for long-term success following microvascular decompression. Broggi's group also found that 5 of 10 patients with trigeminal neuralgia

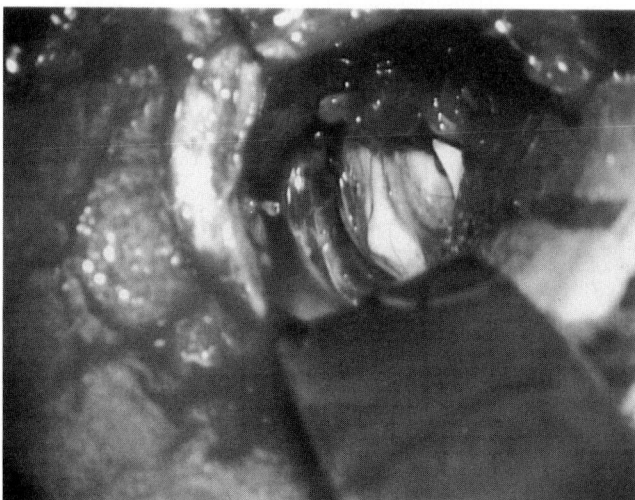

FIGURE 187–7. Intraoperative photograph demonstrating venous compression of the trigeminal nerve resulting in trigeminal neuralgia (see color section in this volume). (From Burchiel KJ [ed]: Surgical Management of Pain. New York, Thieme, 2002.)

and multiple sclerosis improved following microvascular decompression. In another series of 15 patients with multiple sclerosis and trigeminal neuralgia, only 7 patients had excellent pain relief following microvascular decompression.[54]

There is much controversy regarding the efficacy of microvascular decompression in the setting of trigeminal neuralgia associated with multiple sclerosis. The pathology in the setting of multiple sclerosis may be one of demyelination rather than isolated compression. A recent electron microscopy study demonstrated that trigeminal nerve specimens from patients with trigeminal neuralgia and concomitant multiple sclerosis have areas of demyelination in the entry zone, with associated gliosis and variable inflammation. These areas of demyelination are conductive to both spontaneous impulse activity and ephaptic spread of excitation.[55] Other therapies such as radiosurgery or other percutaneous procedures may be indicated.[56]

In addition to patients with multiple sclerosis, patients with atypical trigeminal neuralgia tend to have lower rates of long-term pain relief following microvascular decompression. In a review of 672 microvascular decompressions (107 of which involved multiple surgeries), excellent postoperative pain relief was achieved in 47% of patients, and an additional 40% had partial pain relief. At the time of long-term follow-up (>5 years), 51% continued to have excellent or partial relief. This is significantly less than a similar cohort of patients with typical trigeminal neuralgia, in which 80% still had good pain relief at long-term follow-up. In the group of patients with atypical trigeminal neuralgia, preoperative hypesthesia was a negative predictor for long-term pain relief. Although the outcomes of microvascular decompression for atypical trigeminal neuralgia are less than satisfactory, no alternative interventions have demonstrated superior long-term results.[57]

In a study by Resnick and associates, microvascular decompression for pediatric-onset trigeminal neuralgia had a lower success rate than that for adults.[58] At the time of discharge, 73% of patients had complete pain relief, with an additional 18% having greater than 75% diminution of pain. At last follow-up, at a mean of 105 months, 57% of patients had either complete relief or greater than 75% pain relief. The lower therapeutic response is most likely due to a difference in the pathophysiology of the disease in the pediatric population. Venous compression was found in 86% of cases and was the sole offending vessel in 18%. This is significantly greater than in the adult population. Venous compression often results in recurrence of pain due to revascularization. In 393 cases of trigeminal neuralgia caused by veins, 31% developed recurrence (most within 1 year of operation) after initial improvement of pain.[58]

As mentioned earlier, vessel elongation and ectasia, along with atherosclerotic disease, may contribute to the pathogenesis of vascular compression of cranial nerves. Therefore, the elderly tend to present with this disease. Some clinicians fear that general anesthesia, combined with a posterior fossa craniotomy, may be poorly tolerated in the elderly. Age older than 65 years is not an absolute contraindication to microvascular decompression, but patients should be considered for alternative treatments based on the presence of significant comorbidities such as severe congestive heart failure, pulmonary dysfunction, and myasthenia gravis. In a report of 42 patients older than 65 years, no significant morbidity or significant prolongation of hospital stay (mean duration, 9 days) was ascribed to the advanced age of the patient population. Others have described similar results.[59, 60] It is often easier to perform the surgery in an older patient, because the cerebellum tends to be more relaxed, requiring less retraction for proper visualization of the trigeminal nerve. Additionally, the risk of cerebellar swelling and herniation is less than in younger patients.

Overall, the small craniectomy required for microvascular decompression is well tolerated by the majority of patients. In a review of 320 patients who returned a questionnaire (65% response rate), 50% of patients had returned to their preoperative level of activity by 1 month. By 3 months, 90% were at their baseline level of activity. A total of 98% claimed eventual return to their preoperative activity level.[61]

INTRAOPERATIVE FINDINGS: THE OFFENDING VESSELS

The most frequent operative finding was trigeminal nerve compression by the superior cerebellar artery in 75.5% of patients without a prior history of microvascular decompression. Venous compression was observed in 68.2% of patients but was the sole offending vessel in only 12.5% (see Fig. 187–7 and color section in this volume).[28] Compression by the vertebral or basilar artery was noted in 1.6% and 0.7%, respectively, and was more prevalent in the elderly, in males, and in patients with hypertension (Table 187–3).[28] In patients with recurrent trigeminal neuralgia found to have venous compression at the time of initial surgery, intraoperative findings at the second surgery confirmed the presence of venous pathology in 88% of patients. The most common location of venous compression was anterior to the trigeminal nerve at the dorsal root entry zone.[52]

PERIOPERATIVE COMPLICATIONS

The complication rate for microvascular decompression of the trigeminal nerve is low for surgeons who are experienced with the procedure and with posterior fossa anatomy. In a review of 1336 microvascular decompressions performed by the principal author, operative mortality occurred twice (0.15%). One death was due to a postoperative hemispheric stroke, and the other was due to infarction resulting from superior cerebellar artery occlusion by the implant. Both deaths occurred before the use of intraoperative monitoring of brainstem evoked potentials. In a review by McLaughlin and coworkers, hearing loss was noted in 31 of 3196 patients (0.97%) following microvascular decompression for trigeminal neuralgia.[37] Before 1990, the incidence of hearing loss was 1.33%, but it has decreased substantially to 0.59% with the use of brainstem auditory evoked response monitoring by neurophysiologists.[37] Facial paresis occurred in nine patients but was permanent and severe in only one. Postoperative facial dysesthesia was reported in less than 5% of patients after single microvascular decompression in the absence of ablative procedures.[28] Cerebrospinal fluid leaks were noted in 20 patients (1.5%). Other postoperative complications are listed in Table 187–4. It should be stressed that low complication rates result from intraoperative monitoring by an experienced neurophysiologist who communicates effectively with the neurosurgeon.

POSTOPERATIVE CARE

The postoperative care of these patients involves routine overnight observation in the neurosurgical stepdown (intermediate care) or continuous care unit. Vigilant monitoring is essential, because some clinicians reported postoperative mortality before the routine use of modern continuous monitoring instruments in inten-

T A B L E 1 8 7 – 3 ■ Vessels Found Compressing the Trigeminal Nerve in 1336 Consecutive Microvascular Decompressions

VESSEL	FIRST OPERATION (*N* = 1204)	PERCENTAGE	REOPERATION (*N* = 132)	PERCENTAGE
SCA	909	75.5	27	20.5
AICA	116	9.6	4	3
PICA	8	0.7	0	0
Vertebral	19	1.6	0	0
Basilar	9	0.7	0	0
Labyrinthine	3	0.2	1	1
Unnamed artery	186	15.4	47	35.6
Vein	822	68.2	95	72
Vein only	151	12.5	49	37.1
Artery and vein	671	55.7	46	34.8
Unnamed small artery and vein	223	18.5	102	77.3

AICA, anterior inferior cerebellar artery; PICA, posterior inferior cerebellar artery; SCA, superior cerebellar artery.
Adapted from Barker FG, Jannetta PJ, Bissonette DJ, et al: The long-term outcome of microvascular decompression for trigeminal neuralgia. N Engl J Med 334:1077–1083, 1996; see comments.

TABLE 187-4 ■ **Complications Following 1336 Consecutive Microvascular Decompressions for Trigeminal Neuralgia**

COMPLICATION	NO. OF PATIENTS	PERCENTAGE
Brainstem infarct	1	0.07
Operative death	2	0.15
Permanent facial paresis	2	0.15
Transient facial paresis	10	0.75
Severe ipsilateral hearing loss	15	1.12
Mild ipsilateral hearing loss	1	0.07
Severe facial numbness	22	1.65
Permanent extraocular palsies	2	0.15
Hydrocephalus	2	0.15
Cerebrospinal fluid leak	20	1.50
Pseudomeningocele	4	0.30
Bacterial meningitis	5	0.37
Cerebellar hematoma	2	0.15
Supratentorial hematoma	2	0.15
Cerebellar edema	4	0.30
Other		<1

Adapted from Barker FG, Jannetta PJ, Bissonette DJ, et al: The long-term outcome of microvascular decompression for trigeminal neuralgia. N Engl J Med 334:1077–1083, 1996; see comments.

sive care or step-down units.[62] Blood pressure is monitored continuously with an arterial line, and pressures greater than 160 mm Hg are treated with intravenous antihypertensive medications. Antiemetics are also given routinely. The next morning, most patients are transferred from the intermediate care unit to the ward, where they are encouraged to ambulate and begin oral intake. Typically, patients are discharged home 72 hours from the time of surgery. Some patients may complain of bifrontal headaches that are not alleviated by narcotic pain medication. This complaint necessitates an urgent computed tomographic scan of the brain to rule out a posterior fossa hemorrhage. If the scan is negative for a hemorrhage, a lumbar puncture is performed and cerebrospinal fluid is drained, often relieving the postoperative headache pain.

SUMMARY

Atherosclerosis, elongation of vessels, and cerebellar atrophy place an aging population at risk for developing trigeminal neuralgia. An understanding of the cerebellopontine angle anatomy with respect to the cranial nerves enables trained neurosurgeons to offer patients a nondestructive cure for their disease, with good long-term success and a low risk of morbidity. Favorable outcomes are dependent primarily on patient selection, preoperative and intraoperative monitoring, and surgical experience. A careful history and physical examination are imperative for proper patient selection and preoperative planning. In experienced hands, many patients find long-term relief of their pain. We believe that microvascular decompression for trigeminal neuralgia is the treatment of choice for patients with a normal life expectancy who are able to endure approximately 2 hours of general anesthesia.

REFERENCES

1. Stookey B, Ransohoff J: Trigeminal Neuralgia: Its History and Treatment. Springfield, IL, Charles C Thomas, 1959.
2. Rose FC: Trigeminal neuralgia. Arch Neurol 56:1163–1164, 1999.
3. Brown JA, Coursaget C, Preul MC, et al: Mercury water and cauterzing stones: Nicolas André and tic douloureux. J Neurosurg 90:977–981, 1999.
4. Fothergill J: Of a Painful Affection of the Face: Medical Observation and Inquiries by a Society of Physicians in London. London, 1776, pp 129–142.
5. Gardner WJ: Trigeminal neuralgia. Clin Neurosurg 15:1–56, 1968.
6. Sweet WH, Poletti CE: Problems with retrogasserian glycerol in the treatment of trigeminal neuralgia. Appl Neurophysiol 48:252–257, 1985.
7. Mullan S, Lichtor T: Percutaneous microcompression of the trigeminal ganglion for trigeminal neuralgia. J Neurosurg 59:1007–1012, 1983.
8. Broggi G, Franzini A, Lasio G, et al: Long-term results of percutaneous retrogasserian thermorhizotomy for "essential" trigeminal neuralgia: Considerations in 1000 consecutive patients. Neurosurgery 26:783–786, 1990.
9. Taha JM, Tew JMJ, Buncher CR: A prospective 15-year follow up of 154 consecutive patients with trigeminal neuralgia treated by percutaneous stereotactic radiofrequency thermal rhizotomy. J Neurosurg 83:989–993, 1995.
10. Taha JM, Tew JMJ: Treatment of trigeminal neuralgia by percutaneous radiofrequency rhizotomy. Neurosurg Clin N Am 8:31–39, 1997.
11. Kanpolat Y, Savas A, Bekar A, Berk C: Percutaneous controlled radiofrequency trigeminal rhizotomy for the treatment of idiopathic trigeminal neuralgia: 25-year experience with 1600 patients. Neurosurgery 48:524–532, discussion 532–534, 2001.
12. Lunsford LD, Bennett MH: Percutaneous retrogasserian glycerol rhizotomy for tic douloureux. Part 1. Technique and results in 112 patients. Neurosurgery 14:424–430, 1984.
13. Lunsford LD, Apfelbaum RI: Choice of surgical therapeutic modalities for treatment of trigeminal neuralgia: Microvascular decompression, percutaneous retrogasserian thermal, or glycerol rhizotomy. Clin Neurosurg 32:319–333, 1985.
14. Burchiel KJ: Percutaneous retrogasserian glycerol rhizolysis in the management of trigeminal neuralgia. J Neurosurg 69:361–366, 1988.
15. Slettebo H, Hirschberg H, Lindegaard KF: Long-term results after percutaneous retrogasserian glycerol rhizotomy in patients with trigeminal neuralgia. Acta Neurochir (Wien) 122:231–235, 1993.
16. Lichtor T, Mullan JF: A 10-year follow-up review of percutaneous microcompression of the trigeminal ganglion. J Neurosurg 72:49–54, 1990.
17. Brown JA, Gouda JJ: Percutaneous balloon compression of the trigeminal nerve. Neurosurg Clin N Am 8:53–62, 1997.
18. Kondziolka D, Lunsford LD, Flickinger JC, et al: Stereotactic radiosurgery for trigeminal neuralgia: A multiinstitutional study using the gamma unit. J Neurosurg 84:940–945, 1996.
19. Kondziolka D, Flickinger JC, Lunsford LD, et al: Trigeminal neuralgia radiosurgery: The University of Pittsburgh experience. Stereotact Funct Neurosurg 66(Suppl 1):343–348, 1996.
20. Kondziolka D, Perez B, Flickinger JC, et al: Gamma knife radiosurgery for trigeminal neuralgia: Results and expectations. Arch Neurol 55:1524–1529, 1998.
21. Kondziolka D, Lunsford LD, Flickinger JC: Gamma knife radiosurgery as the first surgery for trigeminal neuralgia. Stereotact Funct Neurosurg 70(Suppl 1):187–191, 1998.
22. Maesawa S, Salame C, Flickinger JC, et al: Clinical outcomes after stereotactic radiosurgery for idiopathic trigeminal neuralgia. J Neurosurg 94:14–20, 2000.
23. Leandri M, Eldridge P, Miles J: Recovery of nerve conduction following microvascular decompression for trigeminal neuralgia. Neurology 51:1641–1646, 1998.
24. Miles JB, Eldridge PR, Haggett CE, Bowsher D: Sensory effects of microvascular decompression in trigeminal neuralgia. J Neurosurg 86:193–196, 1997.
25. National Center for Health Statistics: Fast Stats. Available at http://www.cdc.gov/nchs/fastats/lifexpec.htm.
26. Jannetta PJ: Treatment of trigeminal neuralgia by suboccipital

and transtentorial cranial operations. Clin Neurosurg 24:538–549, 1977.

27. Saunders RL, Krout R, Sachs E Jr: Masticator electromyography in trigeminal neuralgia. Neurology 21:1221–1225, 1971.

28. Barker FG, Jannetta PJ, Bissonette DJ, et al: The long-term outcome of microvascular decompression for trigeminal neuralgia. N Engl J Med 334:1077–1083, 1996; see comments.

29. Taylor JC, Brauer S, Espir ML: Long-term treatment of trigeminal neuralgia with carbamazepine. Postgrad Med J 57:16–18, 1981.

30. Moller AR, Jannetta PJ: Auditory evoked potentials recorded intracranially from the brain stem in man. Exp Neurol 78:144–157, 1982.

31. Moller AR, Jannetta P, Moller MB: Intracranially recorded auditory nerve response in man: New interpretations of BSER. Arch Otolaryngol 108:77–82, 1982.

32. Moller AR, Jannetta PJ: Compound action potentials recorded intracranially from the auditory nerve in man. Exp Neurol 74:862–874, 1981.

33. Moller AR, Jannetta PJ: Interpretation of brainstem auditory evoked potentials: Results from intracranial recordings in humans. Scand Audiol 12:125–133, 1983.

34. Moller AR, Jannetta PJ: Monitoring auditory functions during cranial nerve microvascular decompression operations by direct recording from the eighth nerve. J Neurosurg 59:493–499, 1983.

35. Moller AR, Jannetta PJ: Auditory evoked potentials recorded from the cochlear nucleus and its vicinity in man. J Neurosurg 59:1013–1018, 1983.

36. Moller AR, Jannetta PJ, Sekhar LN: Contributions from the auditory nerve to the brain-stem auditory evoked potentials (BAEPs): Results of intracranial recording in man. Electroencephalogr Clin Neurophysiol 71:198–211, 1988.

37. McLaughlin MR, Jannetta PJ, Clyde BL, et al: Microvascular decompression of cranial nerves: Lessons learned after 4400 operations. J Neurosurg 90:1–8, 1999.

38. Rizvi SS, Goyal RN, Calder HB: Hearing preservation in microvascular decompression for trigeminal neuralgia. Laryngoscope 109:591–594, 1999.

39. Abdeen K, Kato Y, Kiya N, et al: Neuroendoscopy in microvascular decompression for trigeminal neuralgia and hemifacial spasm: Technical note. Neurol Res 22:522–526, 2000.

40. Jarrahy R, Berci G, Shahinian HK: Endoscope-assisted microvascular decompression of the trigeminal nerve. Otolaryngol Head Neck Surg 123:218–223, 2000.

41. Tronnier VM, Rasche D, Hamer J, et al: Treatment of idiopathic trigeminal neuralgia: Comparison of long-term outcome after radiofrequency rhizotomy and microvascular decompression. Neurosurgery 48:1261–1267, discussion 1267–1268, 2001.

42. Bederson JB, Wilson CB: Evaluation of microvascular decompression and partial sensory rhizotomy in 252 cases of trigeminal neuralgia. J Neurosurg 71:359–367, 1989.

43. Kolluri S, Heros RC: Microvascular decompression for trigeminal neuralgia: A five-year follow-up study. Surg Neurol 22:235–240, 1984.

44. Barba D, Alksne JF: Success of microvascular decompression with and without prior surgical therapy for trigeminal neuralgia. J Neurosurg 60:104–107, 1984.

45. Puca A, Meglio M, Cioni B, et al: Microvascular decompression for trigeminal neuralgia: Prognostic factors. Acta Neurochir Suppl (Wien) 58:165–167, 1993.

46. Kleineberg B, Becker H, Gaab MR, et al: Essential hypertension associated with neurovascular compression. Neurosurgery 30:834–841, 1992.

47. Sun T, Saito S, Nakai O, et al: Long-term results of microvascular decompression for trigeminal neuralgia with reference to probability of recurrence. Acta Neurochir (Wien) 126:144–148, 1994.

48. Apfelbaum RI: Surgical management of the disorders of the lower cranial nerves. In Schmidek HH, Sweet WH (eds): Operative Neurosurgical Techniques, 2nd ed. New York, Grune & Stratton, 1988, pp 1097–1109.

49. Liao JJ, Cheng WC, Chang CN, et al: Reoperation for recurrent trigeminal neuralgia after microvascular decompression. Surg Neurol 47:562–568, discussion 568–570, 1997.

50. Cho DY, Chang CGS, Wang YC, et al: Repeat operations in failed microvascular decompression for trigeminal neuralgia. Neurosurgery 35:665–670, 1994.

51. Rath SA, Klein HJ, Richter HP: Findings and long-term results of subsequent operations after failed microvascular decompression for trigeminal neuralgia. Neurosurgery 39:933–938, discussion 938–940, 1996.

52. Lee SH, Levy EI, Scarrow AM, et al: Recurrent trigeminal neuralgia attributable to veins after microvascular decompression. Neurosurgery 46:356–361, discussion 361–362, 2000.

53. Broggi G, Ferroli P, Franzini A, et al: Microvascular decompression for trigeminal neuralgia: Comments on a series of 250 cases, including 10 patients with multiple sclerosis. J Neurol Neurosurg Psychiatry 68:59–64, 2000.

54. Broggi G, Ferroli P, Franzini A, et al: Role of microvascular decompression in trigeminal neuralgia and multiple sclerosis. Lancet 354:1878–1879, 1999.

55. Love S, Gradidge T, Coakham HB: Trigeminal neuralgia due to multiple sclerosis: Ultrastructural findings in trigeminal rhizotomy specimens. Neuropathol Appl Neurobiol 27:238–244, 2001.

56. Bonicalzi V, Canavero S: Role of microvascular decompression in trigeminal neuralgia [letter; comment]. Lancet 355:928–929, 2000.

57. Tyler-Kabara EC, Kassam AB, Horowitz MH, et al: Predictors of outcome in surgically managed patients with typical and atypical trigeminal neuralgia: Comparison of results following microvascular decompression. J Neurosurg 96:527–531, 2002.

58. Resnick DK, Levy EI, Jannetta PJ: Microvascular decompression for pediatric onset trigeminal neuralgia. Neurosurgery 43:804–807, 1998.

59. Ogungbo BI, Kelly P, Kane PJ, Nath FP: Microvascular decompression for trigeminal neuralgia: Report of outcome in patients over 65 years of age. Br J Neurosurg 14:23–27, 2000.

60. Jodicke A, Winking M, Deinsberger W, Boker DK: Microvascular decompression as treatment of trigeminal neuralgia in the elderly patient. Minim Invasive Neurosurg 42:92–96, 1999.

61. Lovely TJ, Lowry DW, Jannetta PJ: Functional outcome and the effect of cranioplasty after retromastoid craniectomy for microvascular decompression. Surg Neurol 51:191–197, 1999.

62. Romansky K, Stoianchev N, Dinev E, Iliev I: Results of treatment of trigeminal neuralgia by microvascular decompression of the Vth nerve at its root entry zone. Arch Physiol Biochem 106:392–396, 1998.

63. Dahle L, von Essen C, Kourtopoulos H, et al: Microvascular decompression for trigeminal neuralgia. Acta Neurochir (Wien) 99:109–112, 1989.

64. Klun B: Microvascular decompression and partial sensory rhizotomy in the treatment of trigeminal neuralgia: Personal experience with 220 patients. Neurosurgery 30:49–52, 1992.

65. Kondo A: Follow-up results of microvascular decompression in trigeminal neuralgia and hemifacial spasm. Neurosurgery 40:46–51, 1997.

66. Lee KH, Chang JW, Park YG, et al: Microvascular decompression and percutaneous rhizotomy in trigeminal neuralgia. Stereotact Funct Neurosurg 68:196–199, 1997.

67. Piatt JHJ, Wilkins RH: Treatment of tic douloureux and hemifacial spasm by posterior fossa exploration: Therapeutic implications of various neurovascular relationships. Neurosurgery 14:462–471, 1984.

68. van Loveren H, Tew JMJ, Keller JT, et al: A 10-year experience in the treatment of trigeminal neuralgia: Comparison of percutaneous stereotaxic rhizotomy and posterior fossa exploration. J Neurosurg 57:757–764, 1982.

69. Zorman G, Wilson CB: Outcome following microsurgical vascular decompression or partial sensory rhizotomy in 125 cases of trigeminal neuralgia. Neurology 34:1362–1365, 1984.

Alternative Surgical Treatments for Trigeminal Neuralgia

WAYEL KAAKAJI ■ KIM BURCHIEL

The preceding chapters dealt with the standard surgical therapies for trigeminal neuralgia. In the overwhelming majority of patients with this disorder, these therapies—singly or in combination—are sufficient to bring about effective and long-lasting pain relief. This chapter discusses other surgical modalities that have been used in the past and continue to be used today. These modalities are not considered first-line or even second-line treatments. They are alternative therapies, with varying degrees of efficacy, that may be used after careful consideration of the standard treatments or in patients who have failed the other, more traditional, treatments.

It is worth noting at the outset that a clinician caring for a patient with trigeminal neuralgia should reconsider the diagnosis if the patient is refractory to the standard treatments. There are a variety of conditions that present with facial pain (Table 188–1). A careful history taking, more than any other method of clinical evaluation, can distinguish these entities and help the clinician attain a proper diagnosis.

In this chapter we discuss the roles of open partial rhizotomy, peripheral neurectomy, and stereotactic radiosurgery in treating trigeminal neuralgia.

PARTIAL SENSORY RHIZOTOMY

This procedure involves sectioning fibers of the trigeminal root. Typically, 30% to 50% of the lower fascicles of the portio major are sectioned via a retromastoid craniectomy. This procedure is most commonly indicated when no convincing vascular compression is noted on exploration of the posterior fossa; however, it may also be performed in conjunction with microvascular decompression.[1-5] This method has also been used to treat patients with a recurrence of pain following microvascular decompression.[1] The origins of the procedure date back to the trigeminal nerve root section popularized by Frazier.[6] Whereas Frazier used a middle fossa extradural approach, today this procedure is performed through a retromastoid intradural approach. Dandy described this suboccipital approach in 1929.[2]

The approach is similar to the one typically used for microvascular decompression. Once the trigeminal nerve is identified and significant vascular compression has been ruled out, the lower and lateral fascicles of the portio major are sectioned. This should be done 2 to 5 mm from the surface of the brainstem. The surgeon must avoid cutting the medial portion of the nerve containing the motor fibers. Despite aggressive nerve sectioning in this fashion, postoperative facial anesthesia is rare; however, facial paresthesias and dysesthesias are common. The sensory deficit produced by this lesion is typically mild. Impairment of the corneal reflex is not uncommon, but loss of the reflex and subsequent keratitis are unusual.[4]

Bederson and Wilson[1] reported results of partial sensory rhizotomy in 86 patients. Fifty-six patients were found to have some vascular elements in proximity to the nerve, but no deformation of the nerve was noted. These patients underwent microvascular decompression in addition to partial sensory rhizotomy. The remaining 30 patients had no vascular compression. At an average 5-year follow-up, the outcome in this group of patients was not statistically different from the outcome of patients treated with microvascular decompression by the same surgeon. Seventy-five percent had excellent relief, 8% had good relief, and 12% were pain free for at least 1 month before they had recurrence of pain; 5% had no benefit from the surgical procedure. Corneal hypesthesia occurred in four patients, and anesthesia dolorosa occurred in two patients. The incidence of seventh or eighth nerve injury was lower than that seen with microvascular decompression. Delayed hydrocephalus occurred in two patients. No operative mortality was noted.

Klun[7] reported the results of open partial rhizotomy in 42 patients. He compared the outcome to the results obtained with microvascular decompression in 178 patients. The immediate pain relief after rhizotomy was 86%, dropping to 50% at 5-year follow-up; these numbers were 96% and 93%, respectively, in the microvascular decompression group. He attributed the high recurrence rate to overcautious division of the nerve. No corneal anesthesia and no anesthesia dolorosa were encountered. Only one patient had motor weakness.

TABLE 188–1 ■ Differential Diagnosis of Facial Pain

Trigeminal Neuralgia (Tic Douloureux)
Idiopathic trigeminal neuralgia
Secondary trigeminal neuralgia

Atypical Trigeminal Neuralgia

Trigeminal Neuropathic Pain
Post-traumatic trigeminal pain
Postherpetic neuralgia

Other Cranial Neuralgias
Glossopharyngeal neuralgia
Geniculate neuralgia
Sphenopalatine (Sluder's) neuralgia
Auriculotemporal neuralgia
Nasociliary neuralgia

Constant Facial Pain
Cancer-related pain
Paratrigeminal (Raeder's) syndrome
Painful ophthalmoplegia (Tolosa-Hunt) syndrome
Petrous apex (Gradenigo's) syndrome
Anesthesia dolorosa

Central Deafferentation Syndromes
Lateral medullary plate (Wallenberg's) syndrome
Thalamic pain syndrome

Atypical Facial Pain
Orofacial pain
Temporomandibular joint syndrome
Headache and migraine syndrome

Young and Wilkins[8] reported a series of 83 patients with an average follow-up of 72 months. Only 48% had an excellent outcome, and 22% had initial relief but experienced partial return of the pain; 30% had persistent pain or complete pain recurrence. In this group, the majority of patients had less than 50% of the root fibers sectioned. This might explain the comparatively low rate of excellent outcomes reported in this series. Other authors have reported outcomes equivalent to those achieved with microvascular decompression.[9–11] In these reports, the majority of patients received aggressive resection (50% to 90%) of the trigeminal sensory rootlets.

These published series demonstrate that partial sensory rhizotomy is a safe and effective procedure for the treatment of trigeminal neuralgia. The degree of efficacy is proportional to the extent of rhizotomy, with aggressive sectioning leading to excellent outcomes. This procedure is an important adjunct in the treatment of patients with recurrent pain and in patients who have little or no compression upon posterior fossa exploration.

PERIPHERAL NEUROTOMY AND NEURECTOMY

These procedures involve the ablation of peripheral branches of the trigeminal nerve. Before the wide adoption of microvascular decompression and the discovery of the benefit of percutaneous gasserian gangliolysis, neurectomy was the main surgical treatment of trigeminal neuralgia.[12] The goal of the nerve ablation is to denervate the trigger zone region, as opposed to denervating the area of pain distribution. The ablation can be carried out chemically or surgically. Most frequently, the supraorbital-supratrochlear, infraorbital, and inferior alveolar nerves are targeted.

These procedures are not commonly used in the treatment of trigeminal neuralgia today.[13] Because of the safety and efficacy of other methods, such as percutaneous radiofrequency gangliolysis and glycerol injections, these peripheral ablative procedures have been superseded. However, there are patients who may be better served by these techniques. Elderly patients, cognitively impaired patients who cannot cooperate with the physician to undergo radiofrequency lesioning, or patients who prefer a quick temporizing measure might be good candidates for these procedures. Patients must be made aware through preoperative education that these procedures will result in complete or near-complete anesthesia in the distribution of the ablated nerves. The high incidence of pain recurrence after these procedures must also be stressed to patients. Because of these drawbacks, these procedures are rarely indicated as first-line treatment of trigeminal neuralgia.

Alcohol Injections

Absolute alcohol is highly neurotoxic, and when injected, it causes partial destruction of the nerve. The main advantage of this method of ablation is that the treatment can be performed at the patient's bedside, in an outpatient setting, or in a fluoroscopy suite. This procedure plays a very limited role in the modern management of trigeminal neuralgia, but it is a quick and highly effective palliative procedure for elderly patients. Alcohol injection may also be used to predict the results of more permanent ablative procedures such as neurectomy or rhizotomy.[14]

General anesthesia is not necessary for this procedure. Using surface bony anatomic landmarks or fluoroscopic guidance, the branches of the trigeminal nerve can be localized within their bony foramina.[15] Figure 188–1 shows the needle orientations needed for placement of the injected material within the appropriate bony canals. Once the needle is in proper position—confirmed by paresthesias in the nerve distribution—the nerve is injected with 0.5 to 1.5 mL of absolute alcohol. A small injection of air following the alcohol injection reduces the chances of developing a sinus tract.

Before alcohol injection, some authors recommend using a test injection of a local anesthetic agent.[16] This is done to ensure that pain relief is indeed obtained from denervating the particular region of the face targeted by the injection. Additionally, this maneuver acquaints the patient with the facial anesthesia that can be anticipated following the procedure. The local block should be administered separately from the alcohol

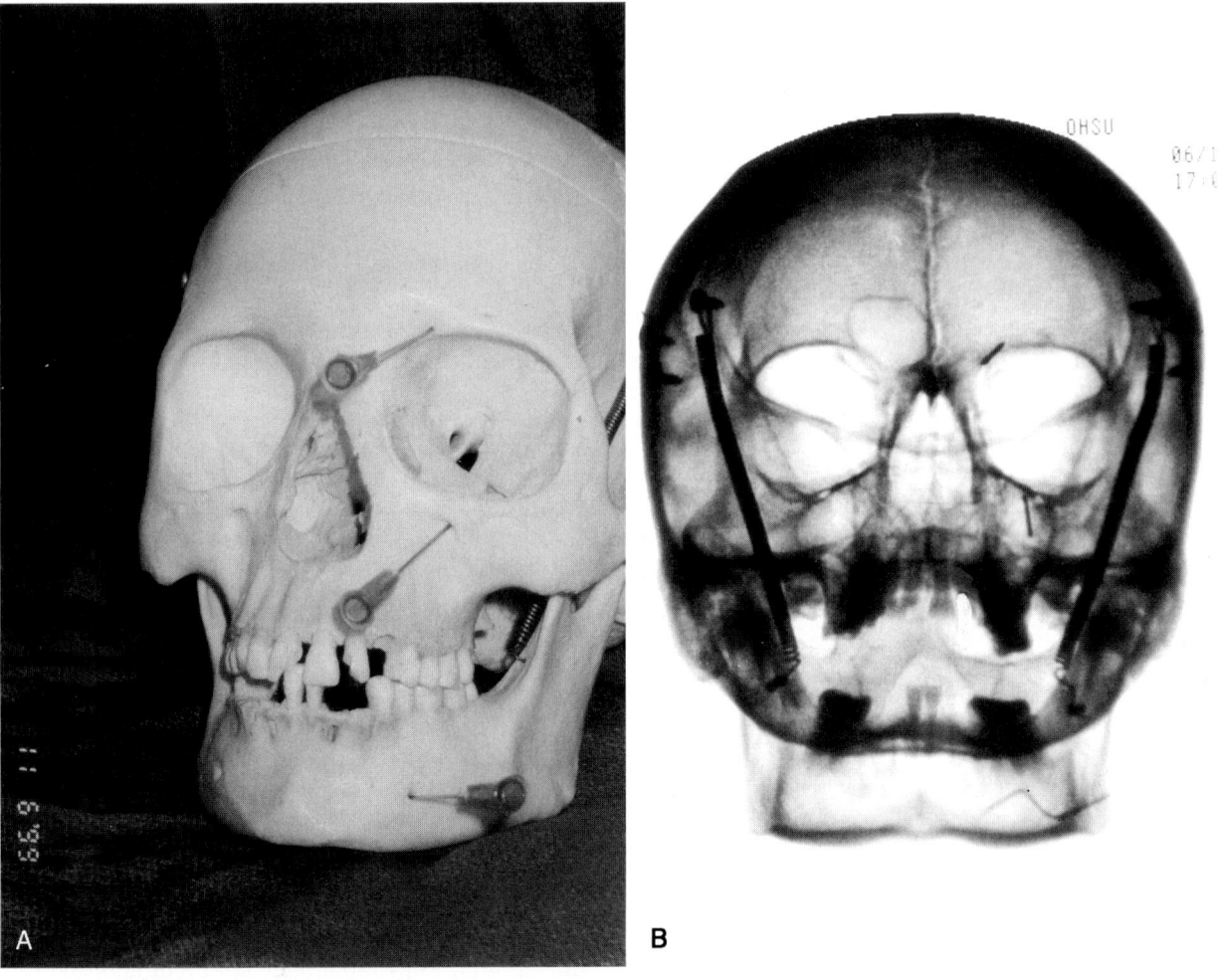

FIGURE 188–1. *A,* Cadaveric skull photograph with needles inserted into the bony foramina housing the trigeminal nerve branches. Note the orientation of the needles in the bony canals. *B,* Radiograph of the same cadaveric skull with needles used to mark the location of the bony foramina.

block so as not to dilute the concentration of alcohol and its chemical effect.[14]

Although the injection itself is painful, pain relief and anesthesia follow shortly, but complete pain relief may be delayed for 24 to 72 hours. The average duration of pain relief following alcohol injection ranges from 8.5 to 16 months.[17] This is a shorter duration than that obtained with surgical ablation, which is explained by the fact that alcohol neurotomy does not result in as complete a lesion as surgical neurectomy does, possibly sparing some nerve fibers.

The complications of this procedure are typically mild. Facial paresthesias and dysesthesias are not uncommon. Tissue necrosis might result from the intraarterial injection of alcohol, but this can be avoided by following proper injection technique.[14]

Surgical Neurectomy

For trigeminal pain triggered in the V1 distribution, supraorbital and supratrochlear neurectomy results in pain relief. With the patient in the supine position, the incision can be made through the eyebrow or through the supratarsal fold of the upper eyelid.[18] The supraorbital nerve is easily identified as it exits the supraorbital foramen. A nerve hook is used to elevate all the nerve fascicles from the periosteum. The nerve is subsequently cut, and the proximal end is used to avulse the nerve using a hemostat. Care should be taken to coagulate the supraorbital vessels. The supratrochlear nerve is found medial to the supraorbital foramen and is similarly ablated. This procedure does not result in any corneal anesthesia.

For V2-triggered pain, infraorbital neurectomy is chosen. Although pain in the distribution of the cheek and upper lips is well controlled with this procedure, pain in the roof of the mouth is not as responsive. The incision is made either in the lower eyelid or intraorally through the mucosa overlying the labiogingival fold.[13] The infraorbital foramen is easily identified near the medial half of the lower orbital ridge. The nerve is sectioned and avulsed as described previously. In patients who describe pain in their teeth, the nerve is dissected into the canal and followed onto the orbital floor. In this manner, the superior alveolar nerves are included in the ablation. Bone wax may be impacted into the foramen to delay nerve regeneration.

For V3-triggered pain involving the lower jaw, inferior alveolar neurectomy can be performed. The incision is made behind the angle of the mandible. The masseter muscle fibers are retracted and dissected in a subperiosteal fashion. A bur hole is made through the outer table of bone, exposing the inferior alveolar nerve in its canal. The nerve is sectioned and avulsed. This procedure is not effective in relieving pain originating from the tongue. Alternatively, the nerve can be exposed using an intraoral approach. The incision is made in the oral mucosa on the medial aspect of the mandible. The nerve is avulsed at its point of entry into the bony canal.[19]

Figure 188–2 demonstrates the typical incisions we use for peripheral neurectomy of trigeminal nerve branches.

Although pain relief is typically immediate following neurectomy procedures, recurrence rates are high. Pain relief was reported to last 26 to 38 months, depending on the nerve avulsed. Within 5 years of the procedure, 27% of patients require reoperation for recurrent pain.[14, 20, 21] Complications of this procedure are rare; anesthesia dolorosa and corneal anesthesia have not been reported with this procedure.

STEREOTACTIC RADIOSURGERY

This therapy has been offered as first-line therapy or for treatment of recurrent pain.[22] It is particularly attractive for patients who cannot tolerate surgery. In the last 5 years, there has been a resurgence of interest in using the gamma knife for the treatment of trigeminal neuralgia. The advent of improved imaging techniques that allow clear visualization of the trigeminal nerve and the ability to deliver precisely focused, highly conformal radiation doses have led to this resurgence. The procedure involves delivering a stereotactic radiosurgical dose to the trigeminal nerve as it courses from the brainstem to its entry into Meckel's cave. A single isocenter is typically used. The maximal doses delivered range from 70 to 90 Gy. Patients are discharged on the same day in most instances. In patients who respond to the therapy, there is a delay in pain relief typically ranging from 1 day to 6.7 months, with a median delay of 1 month.[23]

The mechanism of action is not completely understood. Some authors have postulated that the radiation energy interrupts the ephaptic electrical transmission that is thought to underlie the pathophysiology of trigeminal neuralgia pain. Interestingly, only a small minority of patients experience changes in facial sensation after gamma knife treatment for trigeminal neuralgia. This lack of clinical sensory deficit, in the setting of demonstrable pain relief, suggests little or no physiologic alteration in the sensory function of the nerve as a result of radiation. This observation is in sharp contrast to the lessons learned from percutaneous radiofrequency and glycerol lesioning procedures. The extent and duration of pain relief following these procedures seem to depend to a large degree on the amount of induced facial hypesthesia. Further studies may elicit more tangible explanations for the mechanism of action of radiosurgical treatment. Several centers found that post–gamma radiation magnetic resonance imaging scans revealed contrast enhancement of the trigeminal nerve in some patients.[23, 24] The significance of this finding is not clear.

Leksell initially developed the gamma knife for the specific purpose of using it in functional neurosurgical procedures. The first use of the gamma knife was in patients with trigeminal neuralgia.[25] In 1991 Lindquist and coworkers[26] reported the use of the gamma knife to treat trigeminal neuralgia in 46 patients who had stereotactic radiosurgery to the gasserian ganglion. They reported a success rate of 60%. Rand and colleagues[27] reported similar results in 1993. They treated 12 patients using the retrogasserian segment of the nerve, its root entry zone, and the surface of the brainstem as targets. These encouraging results prompted a multicenter study in which the proximal trigeminal

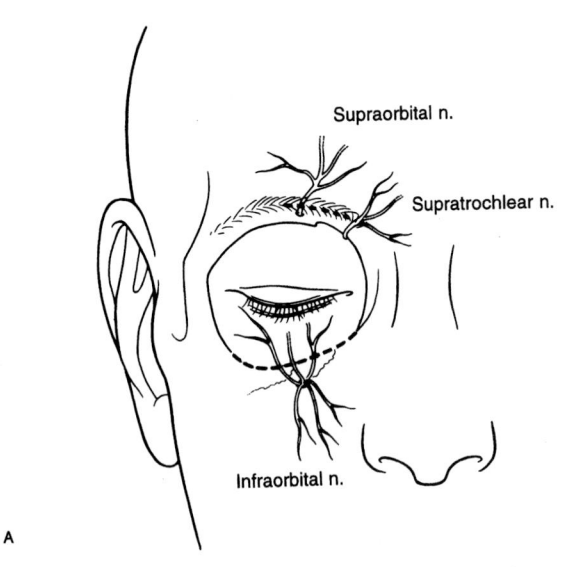

A

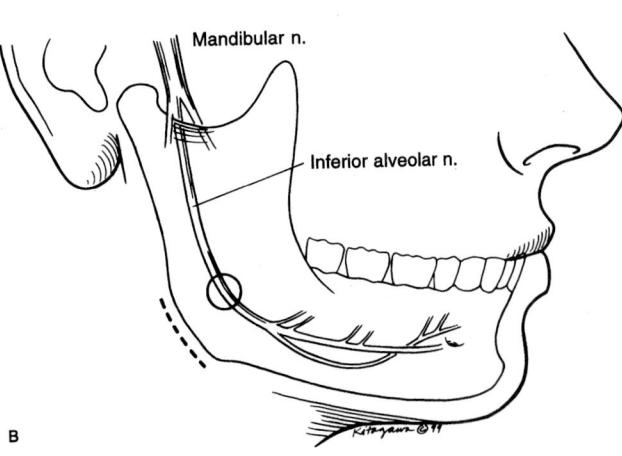

B

FIGURE 188–2. Artist's depiction of incisions used for peripheral neurectomy. Dashed lines represent incision location.

nerve (the nerve root entry zone) was targeted.[23] Most centers used a single 4-mm isocenter, magnetic resonance imaging guidance, and doses between 60 and 90 Gy. The nerve was targeted at a point 2 to 4 mm away from its point of entry into the pons. The isocenter was positioned so that the brainstem received less than 20% of the prescribed dose.

The initial results of the study were reported in 1996. Fifty patients were enrolled in five centers, and all patients had at least 3 years follow-up. Excellent results were obtained in 58% (pain free), and 36% had good control (at least 50% improvement with medication). Six percent failed to get any benefit, and an additional 6% had pain recurrence in less than 1 year. Six percent developed delayed loss of facial sensation. The study indicated that a dose of 70 Gy or more was needed for effective treatment.

Since this initial study, many centers have published their own experiences. Young and associates[28] published their series of 110 patients, with a mean follow-up of 19.8 months. Overall, 76.4% had an excellent response, 11.8% had a good response, and another 11.8% failed treatment. They noted an initial response of 95.5% in patients who had had no prior surgery. Recurrence was reported in 3.3%. Among patients who had had prior surgical intervention, the initial response rate was 88%, with the success rate dropping off to 69% at long-term follow-up. The only complication encountered was loss of facial sensation, which occurred in 2.7% of patients. They noted a mean latency of response of 14 days. Kondziolka and coworkers[29] published results for 66 patients who received a radiosurgical dose of 70 to 90 Gy. They had an initial success rate of 92%, and the success rate after a mean follow-up of 18 months was 82%.

Although the initial results of gamma knife treatment for trigeminal neuralgia are promising, recurrence rates seem to be high. Young and associates[28] calculated a recurrence rate of 34% using Kaplan-Meier analysis of their results. They noted that recurrence was higher in patients with atypical trigeminal neuralgia and in patients who had had multiple procedures before gamma knife therapy. Kondziolka and coworkers[29] showed a similar trend in their report. Studying the rate of recurrence at extended follow-up—the longest available being 3 years—will be critical in determining the place of stereotactic radiosurgery among the more established treatment methods. At this point, this procedure is reserved for patients who cannot tolerate conventional surgical treatment and for those who are willing to accept a delay in pain relief.

CONCLUSION

Microvascular decompression remains the gold standard in the treatment of trigeminal neuralgia, and the percutaneous techniques have proved to be an important adjunct in the treatment of this condition. When these therapies fail, partial sensory rhizotomy, peripheral neurectomy, and stereotactic radiosurgery may be beneficial. A number of techniques, such as tractotomy, nucleotomy, thalamotomy, and chronic electrical stimulation of the trigeminal ganglion and nerve, the thalamus, and the motor cortex, have been proposed for the treatment of facial pain. These procedures should not be used in the treatment of trigeminal neuralgia. They are reserved for the treatment of other conditions such as neuropathic facial pain, including postherpetic neuralgia and traumatic lesions, anesthesia dolorosa, and other deafferentation syndromes.

REFERENCES

1. Bederson JB, Wilson CB: Evaluation of microvascular decompression and partial sensory rhizotomy in 252 cases of trigeminal neuralgia. J Neurosurg 71:359–367, 1989.
2. Dandy WE: An operation for the cure of tic douloureux: Partial section of the sensory root at the pons. Arch Surg 18:687–734, 1929.
3. Matsushima T, Fukui M, Suzuki S, Rhoton AL Jr: The microsurgical anatomy of the infratentorial lateral supracerebellar approach to the trigeminal nerve for tic douloureux. Neurosurgery 24:890–895, 1989.
4. Burchiel KJ: Surgical management of trigeminal neuralgia: Major operative procedures. In Fromm G (ed): Medical and Surgical Management of Trigeminal Neuralgia. Mt Kisco, NY, Futura, 1987, pp 101–119.
5. Piatt JH, Wilkins RH: Treatment of tic douloureux and hemifacial spasm by posterior fossa exploration: Therapeutic implication of various neurovascular relationships. Neurosurgery 14:462, 1984.
6. Frazier CH: Subtotal resection of sensory root for relief of major trigeminal neuralgia. Arch Neurol Psychiatry 13:378–384, 1925.
7. Klun B: Microvascular decompression and partial sensory rhizotomy in the treatment of trigeminal neuralgia: Personal experience with 220 patients. Neurosurgery 30:49–52, 1992.
8. Young JN, Wilkins RH: Partial sensory trigeminal rhizotomy at the pons for trigeminal neuralgia. J Neurosurg 79:680–687, 1993.
9. Adams CBT, Kaye AH, Teddy PJ: The treatment of trigeminal neuralgia by posterior fossa microsurgery. J Neurol Neurosurg Psychiatry 45:1020–1026, 1982.
10. Hussein M, Wilson LA, Illingworth R: Patterns of sensory loss following fractional posterior fossa Vth nerve section for trigeminal neuralgia. J Neurol Neurosurg Psychiatry 45:786–790, 1982.
11. Pelletier VA, Poulos DA, Lende RA: Functional localization in the trigeminal root. J Neurosurg 40:504–513, 1974.
12. Grantham EG, Segerberg LH: An evaluation of palliative surgical procedures in trigeminal neuralgia. J Neurosurg 9:390–392, 1952.
13. Murali R, Rovit R: Are peripheral neurectomies of value in the treatment of trigeminal neuralgia? An analysis of new cases and cases involving previous radiofrequency gasserian thermocoagulation. J Neurosurg 85:435–437, 1996.
14. Burchiel KJ: Surgical treatment of trigeminal neuralgia: Minor operative procedures. In Fromm G (ed): Medical and Surgical Management of Trigeminal Neuralgia. Mt Kisco, NY, Futura, 1987, pp 101–119.
15. Jenkner FL: Peripheral Nerve Block. New York, Springer-Verlag, 1977, p 90.
16. Murali R: Peripheral nerve injections and avulsions in the treatment of trigeminal neuralgia. In Rovit RL, Murali R, Jannetta PJ (eds): Trigeminal Neuralgia. Baltimore, Williams & Wilkins, 1990, pp 95–108.
17. Stookey B, Ransohoff J: Trigeminal Neuralgia: Its History and Treatment. Springfield, Ill, Charles C Thomas, 1959.
18. Persing JA, Jane JA: Surgical treatment of V1 trigeminal neuralgia: Technical refinement. Neurosurgery 17:660–662, 1985.
19. White JC, Sweet WH: Pain and the Neurosurgeon: A Forty-Year Experience. Springfield, Ill, Charles C Thomas, 1969.
20. Quinn JH: Repetitive peripheral neurectomies for neuralgia of second and third division of trigeminal neuralgia (tic douloureux). Clin Neurosurg 24:550, 1977.
21. Freemont AJ, Millac P: The place of peripheral neurectomy in the management of trigeminal neuralgia. Postgrad Med J 57:75, 1981.
22. Kondziolka D, Lunsford LD, Flickinger JC: Gamma knife radio-

surgery as the first surgery for trigeminal neuralgia. Stereotact Funct Neurosurg 70(Suppl 1):187–191, 1998.

23. Kondziolka D, Lunsford LD, Flickinger JC, et al: Stereotactic radiosurgery for trigeminal neuralgia: A multi-institutional study using the gamma unit. J Neurosurg 84:940–945, 1996.

24. Urgosik D, Vymazal J, Vladyka V, Liscak R: Gamma knife treatment of trigeminal neuralgia: Clinical and electrophysiological study. Stereotact Funct Neurosurg 70(Suppl 1):200–209, 1998.

25. Leksell L: Stereotaxic radiosurgery in trigeminal neuralgia. Acta Chir Scand 37:311–314, 1971.

26. Lindquist C, Kihlstrom L, Hellstrand E: Functional neuro-surgery—a future for the gamma knife? Stereotact Funct Neurosurg 57:72–81, 1991.

27. Rand RW, Jacques DB, Melbye RW, et al: Leksell gamma knife treatment of tic douloureux. Stereotact Funct Neurosurg 61(Suppl):93–102, 1993.

28. Young RF, Vermeulen S, Posewitz A: Gamma knife radiosurgery for the treatment of trigeminal neuralgia. Stereotact Funct Neurosurg 70(Suppl 1):192–199, 1998.

29. Kondziolka D, Lunsford LD, Habeck M, Flickinger JC: Gamma knife radiosurgery for trigeminal neuralgia. Neurosurg Clin N Am 8:79–85, 1997.

Neurosurgical Management of Intractable Pain

KENNETH A. FOLLETT

Neurosurgeons have a long history of accomplishments in the field of pain management, and neurosurgery, as a specialty, holds an important position within this discipline. The development of ablative pain therapies, which were the mainstay of surgical treatment for intractable pain for many years, was facilitated by neurosurgeons' understanding of the physiology and anatomy of nociception and their ability to access surgically the peripheral and central nervous systems. Over the past 2 to 3 decades, the treatment of intractable pain has undergone evolutionary change as neuroaugmentative therapies (e.g., spinal cord and peripheral nerve stimulation, intrathecal analgesic administration, deep brain stimulation) have largely replaced the historically important, and still clinically important, neuroablative therapies. Neurosurgeons have had a significant role in guiding this evolution.

Neurosurgeons continue to occupy a critical niche within pain management, even though individuals in other specialties are entering the field of interventional pain management in growing numbers. In contrast to the other specialists involved in the management of intractable pain, neurosurgeons have the training, expertise, and opportunity to provide the full range of neuroaugmentative and neuroablative therapies to patients with intractable pain. Neurosurgeons should take advantage of this special position but must recognize that the successful treatment of intractable pain requires more than good surgical skills alone. Successful outcomes also require the ability to select patients properly for surgical treatment and an understanding of patient management. Many surgeons do not have a strong interest in managing complex pain problems long term. Even so, neurosurgeons can participate actively in the treatment of pain disorders by establishing good collaborative relationships with the physicians who coordinate the long-term care of these patients. This multidisciplinary interaction helps surgeons better understand the treatments they provide and promotes good long-term outcomes.

PRELUDE TO SURGICAL TREATMENT

The most fundamental requirement for successful pain management, whether the treatment is surgical or nonsurgical, is to understand the nature of the pain. Different types of pain respond differently to treatment; the cause and characteristics of a patient's pain must be understood in order to develop a rational treatment plan. In general, pain can be classified as acute or chronic, and nociceptive or neuropathic. Classification of a pain complaint into these simple categories facilitates formulation of a proper treatment scheme.

Acute pain signals acute tissue injury. It is generated by activation of nociceptors in tissue that has sustained an injury or insult. Acute pain resolves as the injured tissues heal. Chronic pain is that which outlasts the typical period required for healing of an acute injury. Some definitions of chronic pain are based on the duration of pain (e.g., pain that lasts longer than 3 or 6 months). This is not always an accurate distinction, because different types of acute injuries require different healing times, and the transition of acute pain to chronic pain can vary according to the nature of the injury.[1]

The distinction between acute and chronic pain is important. Acute pain reflects acute tissue injury, and treatment should be aimed at promoting tissue healing. Treatment might include rest or immobilization, analgesics, and passive physical therapy modalities.[2] In contrast, chronic pain does not always serve a useful physiologic purpose (unless tissue injury is ongoing). In some instances, chronic pain no longer reflects disease but may itself be considered a disease.[3] Physical deconditioning is a common accompaniment of many chronic pain disorders (e.g., failed back surgery syndrome). Many individuals with chronic pain require physical reactivation and rehabilitation, rather than the rest and relaxation used for the treatment of acute pain. In this regard, chronic pain often dictates a treatment program opposite to the treatment of acute pain. This basic distinction between acute and chronic pain is critical, because when physicians treat chronic pain as acute pain, this only promotes further disuse and deconditioning.[2] Differentiation of acute and chronic pain is also important because psychological and social factors that complicate a pain complaint may be more common in the setting of chronic pain. In some instances, psychosocial factors may be the primary cause of persistent pain.

Pain can also be classified as nociceptive or neuropathic. This is an important distinction, because the two types of pain usually respond differently to specific treatments. Nociceptive pain is generated by activation of nociceptors subsequent to injury or disease (e.g., a broken arm, cancer pain with local tissue invasion). Stimulation of nociceptors, in turn, activates central nervous system nociceptive pathways. Nociceptive pain represents normal activity of peripheral and central nociceptive systems. Patients use characteristic descriptors for nociceptive pain, such as throbbing, aching, or dull.[4] In contrast, neuropathic pain is the result of a pathologic process (injury or disease) affecting the peripheral or central nervous system. Neuronal injury leads to abnormal neuronal excitability, spontaneous discharges, and ephaptic transmission, which may lead to the generation of pain. In contrast to nociceptive pain, which reflects normal activity within the nervous system, neuropathic pain reflects abnormal neuronal activity. Neuropathic pain may be continuous or paroxysmal (lancinating). Patients use characteristic descriptors for neuropathic pain, such as burning, shooting, tingling, or shocklike.[4] Although nociceptive pain usually responds to opioid analgesic treatment (e.g., the pain of a broken arm can be treated with morphine), neuropathic pain tends to be relatively resistant to opioid treatment (at least at typical doses) and frequently requires treatment with adjuvant nonopioid medications.

Pain is sometimes classified according to its association with cancer (i.e., cancer-related or malignant pain) or the lack of such an association (benign pain or nonmalignant pain). This classification can be useful, because cancer pain may respond differently from noncancer pain to specific interventions. In practical terms, the differences in response to treatment are most likely related to the general predominance of nociceptive pain in the setting of cancer (although neuropathic pain can occur, such as with tumor invasion of the nervous system) and the relative predominance of neuropathic pain in the absence of cancer (e.g., poststroke pain, phantom limb pain, leg pain associated with failed back surgery syndrome, complex regional pain syndromes). The shorter life expectancies of individuals with cancer also become a consideration, because

we do not typically require that surgical procedures performed for cancer pain yield many years of relief.

Surgical treatment of intractable pain is not usually the first treatment option. In most cases, treatment of intractable pain should follow a rational process, with the simplest, safest methods being used first, and interventional treatments being reserved for later in the course.[4] A simple way of picturing this approach is to imagine a pain treatment ladder, similar to that proposed by the World Health Organization.[5] On the lowest rungs are the simplest, safest measures. Each higher rung reflects a more invasive treatment that, like climbing to higher rungs on a ladder, entails greater risk should complications arise. Medical therapy should generally precede surgical interventions, beginning typically with nonopiate analgesic agents (e.g., nonsteroidal anti-inflammatory medications) in conjunction with adjuvant therapies when appropriate. If adequate pain control is not obtained with nonopiate medications, mild opiate analgesics might be required, followed by strong opiate analgesics if necessary. In most cases, pain relief is most readily achieved using scheduled rather than "as needed" dosing of analgesic medications.[6, 7] Neuropathic pain frequently requires treatment with nonopioid medications, although opioid analgesics can be helpful for some individuals. For continuous neuropathic pain (e.g., constant burning, dysesthetic pain), useful adjuvant medications include antidepressants (e.g., tricyclic antidepressants such as amitriptyline), clonidine, local anesthetics (e.g., mexiletine), and capsaicin cream.[7] Paroxysmal, lancinating, or evoked neuropathic pain may improve with anticonvulsant medications (e.g., carbamazepine, phenytoin, gabapentin) or baclofen.[7]

Nonpharmacologic adjuvant therapy can be useful in the treatment of either nociceptive or neuropathic pain. Nonpharmacologic adjuvants include psychological support, relaxation therapies, coping strategies, passive physical therapy modalities (e.g., massage, heat or cold), transcutaneous electrical nerve stimulation, and orthoses.[6, 7]

Simple interventional therapies (e.g., nerve blocks, peripheral nerve ablations) may be useful supplements to medication. In most instances, more aggressive surgical interventions are best reserved for patients who fail treatment with medications. Failure includes either inadequate pain relief with medication therapy or the occurrence of intolerable medication side effects. Augmentative therapies (e.g., spinal cord stimulation, neuraxial analgesic infusion) are typically the next step, followed by ablative therapies if augmentative approaches are not successful or are inappropriate. An element of flexibility should be maintained in the approach to patients with pain, and treatment should be tailored to meet the needs of each individual. For example, dorsal root entry zone (DREZ) lesioning can relieve pain associated with spinal nerve root avulsion and, for some patients, is preferable to more conservative neuroaugmentative techniques. A patient with intractable pain related to late-stage cancer might be treated most appropriately with cordotomy rather than implantation of an intrathecal drug infusion system.

PATIENT SELECTION FOR SURGICAL PAIN THERAPIES

In general, surgical treatment of intractable pain is appropriate for individuals in whom more conservative therapies have not provided adequate pain relief or in whom other treatments are associated with unacceptable side effects (e.g., medication side effects). Further direct treatment of the underlying cause of pain should not be possible or practical, or it may be inappropriate.[4] For example, an individual with radicular leg pain from lumbar spinal stenosis can be treated with decompressive lumbar laminectomy; however, if the individual has severe coronary artery disease, spinal cord stimulation might be a safer and more appropriate treatment.[8] There should be no medical contraindications to surgery.

The pain should have a definable organic cause. This is especially important in the setting of chronic pain of nonmalignant origin, because it reduces the likelihood that significant psychological dysfunction exists. Psychological dysfunction is common in patients with chronic pain disorders and may preclude good outcomes of surgical treatment. Formal psychological evaluation may be appropriate for many (or most) individuals being considered for surgical treatment of intractable pain. Overt dysfunction such as active psychosis, suicidal or homicidal behavior, major uncontrolled depression or anxiety, serious alcohol or drug abuse, and serious cognitive deficits contraindicates surgical intervention. Other psychological factors may be viewed as "risk factors." Potential psychological risk factors include somatization disorders, personality disorders (e.g., borderline or antisocial personality), history of serious abuse, major issues of secondary gain, nonorganic signs on physical examination, unusual pain ratings (e.g., 12 on a 10-point scale), inadequate social support, unrealistic outcome expectations, and, in the case of implantable augmentative devices, an inability to understand the device or its use. Patients with psychological risk factors are not necessarily precluded from surgical treatment, but the treatment program should address the psychological issues to facilitate a good outcome.[9]

NEUROSURGICAL THERAPIES FOR INTRACTABLE PAIN

Procedures used by neurosurgeons include anatomic, neuroaugmentative (or neuromodulative), and neuroablative therapies (Table 189–1).[10] Augmentative therapies have largely replaced ablative techniques as the procedures of choice for pain management and are generally preferred as initial surgical treatments because of their relative safety and reversibility; however, ablative therapies still have a role in the treatment of certain pain syndromes. The specific treatment offered, whether ablative or augmentative, should be chosen according to the needs of each individual patient and the skills of the treating physician. Patient-related factors that must be taken into consideration when selecting a therapy include the cause of the pain, its distribution and characteristics (nociceptive or neuropathic), patient life expectancy, and psychological, social, and economic issues relevant to the pain complaint. The relative advantages and disadvantages of augmentative and ablative therapies should be weighed in view of these factors, and a choice between these two general approaches should be made. A specific intervention can then be selected. Specific interventions vary in their appropriateness as treatment for pain in specific body regions (Tables 189–2 to 189–5). Successful outcomes are facilitated by selecting the right treatment for the right patient at the right time (D. Doleys, personal communication, 1999).

Augmentative therapies fall into two categories: stimulation (spinal cord, peripheral nerve, motor cortex, and deep brain stimulation) and neuraxial (intrathecal and intraventricular) drug infusion. Ablative therapies have been developed that target almost every level of the peripheral and central nervous systems. Ablative therapies can be directed at preventing the transmission of nociceptive information into the central nervous system at the level of peripheral nerves (neu-

T A B L E 1 8 9 – 1 ■ Neurosurgical Pain Therapies

ANATOMIC	ABLATIVE	AUGMENTATIVE
Correction of structural deformity	Neurectomy	**Stimulation**
	Sympathectomy	Peripheral nerve
	Ganglionectomy	Spinal cord
	Rhizotomy	Thalamus (Vc, PVG-PAG)
	Spinal DREZ lesion	Motor cortex
	Cordotomy	
	Myelotomy	**Neuraxial Drug Infusion**
	Nucleus caudalis DREZ lesion	Intrathecal or epidural
	Trigeminal tractotomy	Intraventricular
	Mesencephalotomy	
	Thalamotomy	
	Cingulotomy	
	Hypophysectomy	

DREZ, Dorsal root entry zone; PVG-PAG, periventricular-periaqueductal gray matter; Vc, ventrocaudalis.
Modified from North R, personal communication, 1999.

T A B L E 1 8 9 – 2 ■ Procedures for Treatment of Head and Neck Pain

Augmentative
Peripheral nerve stimulation
Intraventricular analgesic administration
Deep brain or motor cortex stimulation

Ablative
Sympathectomy
Cranial or cervical rhizotomy or ganglionectomy
Caudalis DREZ
Trigeminal tractotomy
Mesencephalotomy
Thalamotomy
Cingulotomy

DREZ, Dorsal root entry zone.

TABLE 189-3 ■ **Procedures for Treatment of Upper Trunk, Shoulder, and Arm Pain**

Augmentative
Peripheral nerve stimulation
Spinal cord stimulation
Intraspinal or intraventricular analgesic administration
Deep brain or motor cortex stimulation

Ablative
Sympathectomy
Neurectomy
Ganglionectomy or rhizotomy
Spinal DREZ lesion
Mesencephalotomy
Thalamotomy
Cingulotomy
Hypophysectomy

DREZ, Dorsal root entry zone.

rectomy), roots (ganglionectomy, rhizotomy), and spinal cord dorsal horn (DREZ lesioning, including nucleus caudalis DREZ lesioning). Ascending nociceptive pathways can be disrupted at the level of the spinal cord or brainstem (cordotomy, myelotomy, tractotomy) or within the brain (thalamotomy, cingulotomy). These therapies are reviewed briefly to provide a broad perspective of the applications of neurosurgical pain therapies. Detailed discussions of indications, techniques, and outcomes of many of these techniques are available in other chapters.

Augmentative Therapies

Augmentative therapies offer the advantages of relative safety, reversibility, and "adjustability." For example, intraspinal analgesic infusion can be adjusted to meet the changing needs of a patient who has progressively worsening or spreading cancer pain. Some major disadvantages of augmentative therapies are their cost (initial device costs and upkeep), the need for maintenance (e.g., refilling of infusion pumps, replacement of stimulation system battery packs), and the potential for

TABLE 189-4 ■ **Procedures for Treatment of Lower Trunk and Leg Pain**

Augmentative
Peripheral nerve stimulation
Spinal cord stimulation
Intraspinal or intraventricular analgesic administration
Deep brain or motor cortex stimulation

Ablative
Sympathectomy
Neurectomy
Ganglionectomy or rhizotomy
Spinal DREZ lesion
Cordotomy
Myelotomy
Thalamotomy
Cingulotomy
Hypophysectomy

DREZ, Dorsal root entry zone.

TABLE 189-5 ■ **Procedures for Treatment of Diffuse Pain**

Augmentative
Intraspinal or intraventricular analgesic administration
Ablative
Thalamotomy
Cingulotomy
Hypophysectomy

device-related complications. General indications for augmentative therapies are those for neurosurgical pain treatment in general. In addition, especially for the treatment of cancer pain, estimated patient life expectancy should be sufficient to warrant implantation of a neuroaugmentative device (e.g., >3 months for a cancer patient being considered for implantation of a drug delivery system).

Stimulation therapies currently approved for use in the United States include spinal cord stimulation (SCS) and peripheral nerve stimulation (PNS). The prototypical indication for SCS is treatment of neuropathic pain in an extremity. Pain should be relatively focal (e.g., localized to one or two extremities or focal on the trunk) and static in nature. Common applications include treatment of persistent radicular pain associated with failed back surgery syndrome[11-14] or neuropathic pain related to a complex regional pain syndrome (reflex sympathetic dystrophy).[15-17] In the failed back surgery syndrome population, the success rate (typically defined as >50% reduction in pain) is approximately 60% at 5 years.[8, 12, 13, 15] Patients with complex regional pain syndromes have similar outcomes, although success rates as high as 70% to 100% have been reported.[15-17] Neuropathic pain affecting the trunk (e.g., postherpetic neuralgia or some types of post-thoracotomy pain) may improve with SCS. SCS can also be effective for the treatment of extremity pain related to peripheral neuropathy,[18] root injury, phantom limb pain[15] (but postamputation stump pain does not improve consistently with SCS), and ischemic extremity pain due to peripheral vascular disease.[19, 20] SCS is gaining acceptance as a treatment for refractory angina pectoris[21, 22] but has not been approved by the U.S. Food and Drug Administration for this indication.

The indications for PNS are similar to those for SCS, except that the distribution of pain should be limited to the territory of a single peripheral nerve.[23] Overlap exists between applications of SCS and PNS. Extremity pain that might be appropriate for PNS treatment can sometimes be treated equally well with SCS, and many surgeons find it easier to implant an SCS lead (which can be done percutaneously) than to implant a PNS lead (which usually requires an open procedure). Some situations clearly require PNS rather than SCS; for example, treatment of occipital neuralgia or cranial postherpetic neuralgia, for which PNS can be accomplished with percutaneously inserted leads.[24]

Intracranial stimulation therapies include deep brain stimulation (DBS) of somatosensory thalamus and periventricular-periaqueductal gray matter (PVG-PAG)[25–28] and motor cortex stimulation.[29–32] These therapies are used primarily to treat pain of nonmalignant origin, such as pain associated with failed back surgery syndrome, neuropathic pain following central or peripheral nervous system injury, or trigeminal pain. Neither DBS nor motor cortex stimulation is currently approved by the U.S. Food and Drug Administration for the treatment of pain, although DBS has been used clinically for more than 2 decades.

Targets for focal electrical stimulation of the brain include the ventrocaudal nucleus (nucleus ventroposterolateralis and ventroposteromedialis) and PVG-PAG. Stimulation sites for DBS are generally chosen on the basis of pain characteristics. Nociceptive pain and paroxysmal, lancinating, or evoked neuropathic pain (e.g., allodynia, hyperpathia) tend to respond best to PVG-PAG stimulation, which may activate endogenous opioid systems. Continuous neuropathic pain responds most consistently to paresthesia-producing stimulation of the sensory thalamus (nucleus ventrocaudalis).[28] Because many pain syndromes (e.g., cancer pain, failed back surgery syndrome) have mixed components of nociceptive and neuropathic pain, some physicians prefer to place electrodes in both regions, subject the patient to a trial of stimulation using externalized leads, and internalize the electrode that provides the best pain relief. Patients may be given a morphine-naloxone test to clarify the extent of nociceptive and neuropathic pain components and thus facilitate selection of the best stimulation target.[26]

Success rates of DBS for the treatment of intractable pain are difficult to determine from the literature, because patient selection, techniques, and outcome assessments vary substantially among studies. Overall, approximately 25% to 35% of individuals undergoing a trial of DBS have good long-term pain relief,[10, 25–28] although success rates as high as 80% have been reported.[25–28] In general, approximately 60% to 80% of patients undergoing a screening trial of DBS have pain relief sufficient to warrant implantation of a permanent stimulation system. Of those who receive a permanent stimulation system, approximately 25% to 80% (generally 50% to 60%)[25] have acceptable long-term pain relief.[10, 25–28] Patients with pain related to cancer,[28] failed back surgery syndrome, peripheral neuropathy, or trigeminal neuropathy (not anesthesia dolorosa)[25, 26, 28] tend to respond to DBS more favorably than do patients with central pain syndromes (e.g., thalamic pain, spinal cord injury pain, anesthesia dolorosa, postherpetic neuralgia, phantom limb pain).[25, 26, 28] The incidence of serious complications of DBS is generally low, but the combined incidences of morbidity, mortality, and technical complications can approach 25% to 30%.[10, 25]

Motor cortex stimulation has recently received attention as an alternative to thalamic and PVG-PAG stimulation.[29–32] Approximately 50% of patients undergoing motor cortex stimulation have good long-term pain relief. It is used primarily for the treatment of neuropathic pain syndromes and may be particularly effective for certain varieties of intractable facial pain (e.g.,

trigeminal neuropathic pain).[32] As with DBS, motor cortex stimulation appears to be most effective when used in the absence of anesthesia in the distribution of pain being treated. The overall clinical efficacy is similar to that of DBS, but complications may be less serious because the electrode is placed epidurally rather than within the brain parenchyma. Motor cortex stimulation is a promising therapy, but its long-term efficacy has not been determined. It is under active investigation at several centers.

Neuraxial drug infusion has become a popular interventional treatment for intractable pain.[33–38] In keeping with the idea that nociceptive pain tends to be responsive to opioid therapy, the primary indication for neuraxial analgesic administration is for the treatment of pain syndromes with a significant nociceptive pain component (e.g., cancer-related pain). However, neuropathic pain may improve with intrathecal analgesic administration.[35, 38] Accordingly, the most common indication for intrathecal analgesic administration is for pain related to failed back surgery syndrome, which typically includes both nociceptive (low back) and neuropathic (extremity) pain components. The use of intrathecal analgesics for the treatment of cancer-related pain is well accepted. In contrast, the use of this therapy for chronic nonmalignant pain is more controversial.[39] In part, this reflects concern that neuropathic pain (common in chronic nonmalignant pain syndromes) does not respond adequately to opioids. In addition, the efficacy and cost-effectiveness of the therapy have not been determined in controlled trials.

The key advantage of neuraxial analgesic administration is its versatility. It has a wide range of indications, including nociceptive and mixed nociceptive-neuropathic pain syndromes. It can be used to treat focal or diffuse pain (e.g., pain related to diffuse metastatic bone lesions) and to treat axial or extremity pain. It is commonly used to treat pain below the cervical level, but it can be effective for head and neck pain, especially if the analgesic agents are delivered intraventricularly.[40, 41] Neuraxial analgesics can be used in the setting of changing pain (e.g., in a patient with progressive cancer whose sites and intensity of pain are expected to change over time). Significant disadvantages include the cost (for the device and medications) and the need for maintenance (e.g., refilling and, in the case of programmable pumps, replacement of the battery). In general, approximately 60% to 80% of patients achieve good long-term pain relief. Despite controversy about the use of neuraxial analgesics for noncancer pain, outcomes (degree of pain relief, patient satisfaction, dose requirements) are similar for patients with cancer-related and noncancer pain.[34, 35] Serious complications of the therapy are uncommon.

Ablative Therapies

Augmentative therapies are becoming increasingly common techniques for pain management, but ablative therapies still have an important role in the treatment of intractable pain. Ablative therapies are often viewed as the top rung on the pain treatment ladder (i.e., the last resort), but in some instances, they are the procedures of choice. For example, phantom limb pain in the setting of root avulsion or "end-zone" pain arising from spinal cord injury can be treated effectively by DREZ lesioning. Cordotomy might be more appropriate than intrathecal analgesic administration via an implanted infusion system for the treatment of cancer-related pain in a patient with a short life expectancy. Therapy must be tailored to meet the needs of each individual patient.

Ablative therapies include peripheral techniques that interrupt or alter nociceptive input into the spinal cord (e.g., neurectomy, ganglionectomy, rhizotomy), spinal interventions that alter afferent input or rostral transmission of nociceptive information (e.g., DREZ lesioning, cordotomy, myelotomy), and supraspinal intracranial procedures that may interrupt the transmission of nociceptive information (e.g., mesencephalotomy, thalamotomy) or influence the perception of painful stimuli (e.g., cingulotomy). As with augmentative techniques, a successful outcome requires that the appropriate patient and appropriate intervention be selected. Ablative therapies tend to be most appropriate for the treatment of nociceptive pain rather than neuropathic pain. Neuropathic pain can be treated with ablative therapies, but improvement is limited primarily to intermittent, paroxysmal, or evoked (allodynia, hyperpathia) neuropathic pain; continuous neuropathic pain remains relatively unchanged in long-term follow-up.[42]

Sympathectomy can alleviate visceral pain associated with certain cancers.[43, 44] It can also be an effective treatment for noncancer pain, such as pain associated with vasospastic disorders or sympathetically maintained pain (when sympathetic blocks reliably relieve the pain). However, sympathectomy has generally fallen into disfavor as a treatment for intractable pain of nonmalignant origin because of inconsistent results.[43–46] Some data indicate that SCS provides a better long-term outcome with lower morbidity, and SCS may replace sympathectomy in the treatment of sympathetically maintained pain of noncancer origin.[47]

Neurectomy may be a useful treatment for individuals who develop pain following peripheral nerve injury, including that associated with limb amputation. If an identifiable neuroma is the cause of pain, its resection can provide significant relief.[48] Neurectomy is not useful for the treatment of nonspecific stump pain after amputation, and it is generally not useful for the treatment of other nonmalignant peripheral pain syndromes. The utility of neurectomy is limited because pain arising from a pure sensory nerve is not common, and mixed sensory-motor nerves cannot be sectioned without risk of functional impairment. Some specific exceptions to this general observation exist. For example, sectioning of the lateral femoral cutaneous nerve may provide good long-lasting relief of meralgia paresthetica,[49] and sectioning of the ilioinguinal or genitofemoral nerve (or both) may provide good relief in some inguinal pain syndromes (e.g., postherniorrhaphy pain) in properly selected individuals.[50]

Dorsal rhizotomy and ganglionectomy serve similar purposes in denervating somatic or visceral tissues, but ganglionectomy may produce more complete denervation. Some afferent fibers enter the spinal cord through the ventral root[51] and are not affected by dorsal rhizotomy. In contrast, ganglionectomy effectively eliminates input from dorsal and ventral root afferent fibers by removing their cell bodies, which are located within the dorsal root ganglion. Rhizotomy and ganglionectomy can be used to treat pain in the trunk or abdomen. Neither procedure is useful for the treatment of pain in the extremities unless function of the extremity is already lost, because denervation removes proprioceptive as well as nociceptive input and produces a functionless limb. Limited denervation does not provide adequate pain relief, probably because of overlap of segmental innervation of dermatomes. These procedures are most appropriate for the treatment of cancer-related pain; noncancer pain does not improve consistently.[52, 53] In the setting of cancer, these procedures can be useful for thoracic or abdominal wall pain; for perineal pain in patients with impaired bladder, bowel, and sex function; or for the treatment of pain in a functionless extremity.[54] Multiple sacral rhizotomies can be performed (e.g., to treat pelvic pain from cancer) by passing a ligature around the thecal sac below S1.[55] Rhizotomy may be useful for the treatment of craniofacial pain[56] of nontrigeminal origin as well as for classic trigeminal neuralgia.

DREZ lesioning of the spinal cord (for trunk or extremity pain)[57–59] or nucleus caudalis (for facial pain)[58, 60, 61] can provide significant pain relief in properly selected individuals; 70% to 80% of patients report improvement in pain. These techniques are best reserved for localized pain. Certain types of cancer pain can be treated effectively with DREZ lesioning (e.g., neuropathic arm pain associated with Pancoast's tumor), but the most successful applications are related to the treatment of neuropathic pain arising from root avulsion (cervical or lumbosacral) and "end-zone" or "boundary" pain following spinal cord injury. These pain syndromes sometimes respond adequately to SCS or intrathecal drug infusion, but DREZ lesioning can provide a similar result without the need for long-term maintenance of an augmentative device. DREZ lesioning has been used for the treatment of other neuropathic pain syndromes (e.g., postherpetic neuralgia), but good pain relief is not achieved consistently. Nucleus caudalis lesioning is most useful for deafferentation pain affecting the face (including postherpetic neuralgia) and is less helpful for facial pain of peripheral origin (e.g., traumatic trigeminal neuropathy). As with other ablative procedures, DREZ lesioning is most effective for relieving paroxysmal rather than continuous pain.[59]

Cordotomy is a valuable procedure for pain management, especially when pain is related to malignancy. Intrathecal analgesic administration has largely replaced cordotomy for the treatment of cancer pain, but cordotomy offers several advantages. As a one-time procedure, it requires no long-term follow-up or maintenance. This is important for individuals who would have difficulty returning to a medical facility for refilling of an infusion system or for whom the costs of ongoing medical care have become burdensome. Individuals with short life expectancies (for whom it is difficult to justify the costs of an implanted drug infusion system) may be candidates for cordotomy if their pain is located in an appropriate distribution.

Cordotomy is used most commonly for the treatment of cancer-related pain below the mid to low cervical dermatomes. It is used less frequently for the management of noncancer pain because of concern about the potential loss of pain relief over time, the occurrence of postcordotomy dysesthesias, and the risk of complications.[62] Cordotomy can be performed as an open[62] or closed (percutaneous)[63, 64] procedure. Percutaneous techniques are less invasive, but open techniques remain viable options because some surgeons lack the expertise and equipment required for percutaneous procedures.

In general, the level of analgesia produced by cordotomy falls over time, such that within 3 weeks after the procedure, the level has fallen three to six spinal levels, and by 6 months, the level may have fallen six to eight segments. Consequently, the procedure is best for pain below the midcervical levels.[62, 63] Lancinating, paroxysmal neuropathic pain and evoked (allodynic or hyperpathic) pain that sometimes occurs after spinal cord injury or as part of peripheral neuropathic pain syndromes can improve following cordotomy, but continuous neuropathic pain does not improve.[63] Laterally located pain responds better than does midline or axial (e.g., visceral) pain, which may require bilateral procedures. The utility of bilateral cordotomy is compromised by the attendant risk of weakness; bladder, bowel, and sexual dysfunction; and respiratory depression (if the procedure is performed bilaterally at cervical levels).[62, 63] The risk of respiratory depression subsequent to a unilateral cervical procedure mandates that pulmonary function be acceptable on the contralateral side. For example, a patient who has undergone previous pneumonectomy for lung cancer should not be subject to cordotomy that would compromise pulmonary function on the side of the remaining lung.[63]

Bilateral cordotomies may be necessary in some patients. Bilateral high (C1-2) percutaneous cordotomies are generally not recommended, owing to the relatively high risk of sleep apnea and other complications. An alternative approach is to perform a unilateral high cervical procedure followed by a contralateral low cervical procedure or open thoracic cordotomy.[62] Open cordotomy may be advantageous if a bilateral procedure is required, because both sides can be treated safely at one time by separating the operated levels by several spinal segments. In contrast, percutaneous (cervical) procedures are typically staged at least 1 week apart.[62]

Cordotomy provides good pain relief in approximately 60% to 80% of patients,[63, 65] but loss of pain relief tends to occur over time. Approximately one third of patients have recurrent pain in 3 months, half at 1 year, and two thirds at longer follow-up intervals.[54, 65, 66]

The gradual recurrence of pain over months to years and the potential development of postcordotomy dysesthetic pain limit the use of this technique in patients with pain syndromes of nonmalignant origin, who typically have long life expectancies.[62]

Myelotomy has also fallen into disuse since the advent of intrathecal drug infusion therapy, but it can provide significant pain relief in properly selected individuals, including some who fail treatment with intrathecal analgesics.[67] Commissural myelotomy was developed to provide the benefits of bilateral cordotomy without the inherent risks of lesioning both anterior quadrants of the spinal cord.[67–69] This is accomplished by sectioning spinothalamic tract fibers as they decussate in the anterior commissure. Subsequently, it was observed that a limited midline myelotomy[70] or high cervical myelotomy[65, 71] could be equally effective. Recent identification of a dorsal column visceral pain pathway has led to the development of punctate midline myelotomy.[69]

These procedures are indicated primarily for the treatment of cancer-related pain, generally in the abdomen, pelvis, perineum, and legs. The advantage over cordotomy is that bilateral and midline pain can be treated with a single operative procedure, with lower morbidity and mortality. The procedures are most effective for nociceptive rather than neuropathic pain. Myelotomy techniques are straightforward, and the anatomy is familiar to most neurosurgeons. Early complete pain relief is achieved in most patients (>90%), but pain tends to recur over time; approximately 50% to 60% of patients have good long-term pain relief.[65] Although the risk of bladder, bowel, and sexual dysfunction is less than that associated with bilateral cordotomy, it is sufficiently high that use of this procedure is usually restricted to patients with cancer-related pain who have preexisting dysfunction.[54]

Ablative neurosurgical procedures directed at the brainstem are not in widespread use, in part because relatively few patients require such interventions and because relatively few neurosurgeons have the expertise to perform them. As with other ablative procedures, however, they can provide significant benefit in carefully selected patients. Mesencephalotomy is indicated for the treatment of intractable pain involving the head, neck, shoulder, and arm.[42, 72] It can be viewed as a supraspinal version of cordotomy.[42] Most commonly, the procedure is used for the treatment of pain related to cancer, for which long-term pain relief is achieved in 85% of patients.[65] It does not provide consistent long-term relief of central neuropathic pain.[72] Side effects and complications can be frequent, especially oculomotor dysfunction.[42, 65, 72] The utility of mesencephalotomy has diminished since the advent of neuraxial analgesic administration; intraventricular morphine infusion can provide good pain relief, with a lower incidence of complications. Mesencephalotomy may be preferable for some individuals, however; for example, those with short life expectancies or for whom the costs of neuraxial analgesic administration or the long-term follow-up required has become burdensome.

Thalamotomy has been used for the treatment of cancer-related and noncancer-related pain.[73] The procedure can be accomplished via stereotactic radiofrequency[42, 65, 74–76] or radiosurgical[77] techniques. In the setting of cancer, thalamotomy is most appropriate for individuals who have widespread pain (e.g., from diffuse metastatic disease) or who have midline, bilateral, or head or neck pain for which other procedures are unlikely to provide relief.[73] Thalamotomy can be useful for individuals who are not candidates for cordotomy; for example, those with pain above the C5 dermatome or with pulmonary dysfunction.[76] The success rate of thalamotomy in relieving pain is slightly lower than that achieved with mesencephalotomy, but the incidence of complications is lower with thalamotomy.[76] The lateral thalamus (nucleus ventrocaudalis) is not considered an acceptable target for ablation because of the risk of dysesthesias and sensory loss,[42] but the subjacent parvicellular ventrocaudal nucleus, which may be a relay site for spinothalamic afferents, has been used as a target. Results of thalamotomy directed to this structure may be similar to those achieved with cordotomy.[74] Medial thalamotomy appears to be most effective for treating nociceptive pain (e.g., cancer pain), with acceptable long-term pain relief obtained in approximately 30% to 50% of patients.[42, 73, 75] Overall, neuropathic pain syndromes respond less consistently to thalamotomy, with only about one third of patients improving long term.[42, 75] Patients with paroxysmal, lancinating neuropathic pain or neuropathic pain with elements of allodynia and hyperpathia may improve significantly following thalamotomy, whereas those with continuous neuropathic pain tend not to benefit.[42]

Cingulotomy is used less commonly for the treatment of intractable pain than for the management of psychiatric disorders. It is applied most often to the treatment of cancer pain but has been used for noncancer pain as well.[65, 78, 79] Approximately 50% to 75% of patients benefit from the procedure, at least short term. In the cancer population, pain relief is generally maintained for at least 3 months. The utility of cingulotomy for chronic noncancer pain is less apparent, with some studies indicating relatively good long-lasting pain relief[65, 79] and others indicating only 20% long-term success.[73] Cingulotomy may be a reasonable option for individuals, especially those with cancer-related pain, in whom other treatments have not worked. Because cingulotomy is used to treat psychiatric disease and carries the stigma of "psychosurgery," formal review by institutional ethics committees may be warranted if this procedure is being considered as a treatment for intractable pain.

Hypophysectomy (surgical, chemical, or radiosurgical) can provide good relief of cancer-related pain. It is most effective for hormonally responsive cancers (e.g., prostate, breast) but may relieve pain associated with other tumors as well. This treatment is most appropriate for individuals with widespread disease and diffuse pain. Pain is alleviated in 45% to 95% of patients. Pain relief occurs independent of tumor regression; the specific mechanism of pain relief is unknown.[65, 74, 80, 81]

SUMMARY

Successful treatment of intractable pain requires that the right therapy be offered to the right patient at the right time. Candidates for neurosurgical treatment must be selected carefully, with full recognition of chronic pain as a biopsychosocial disorder. Undue emphasis on "pain generators" without consideration of the psychosocial factors that contribute to pain complaints can lead to treatment failure. The surgical intervention should be matched carefully to the needs of the patient. Outcomes of augmentative therapies in properly selected patients are good, and the risk of serious or permanent complications is low, making neuromodulation therapies the first choice for many patients. Augmentative techniques, especially the stimulation therapies of SCS and DBS, are superior to ablative techniques for the treatment of neuropathic pain with a continuous, dysesthetic component. Ablative therapies may be more appropriate for some individuals; for example, those with cancer-related pain who do not have long life expectancies. Patients with a predominant nociceptive component of pain, and those with neuropathic pain with paroxysmal or evoked components, can also benefit from ablative techniques.

Neurosurgeons are unique within the discipline of pain medicine by virtue of their knowledge, skills, and access to the nervous system. These attributes enable neurosurgeons to provide pain treatments chosen from the entire spectrum of pain therapies, including augmentative and ablative techniques. As more attention is focused on augmentative therapies for the treatment of intractable pain, ablative therapies that might be appropriate for some individuals may be overlooked, especially by nonsurgical specialists who are unfamiliar with the role of ablative neurosurgical therapies in the management of intractable pain. Neurosurgeons must remain knowledgeable about pain therapies and stay actively involved in the field of pain medicine to ensure the continued availability of the entire spectrum of pain therapies. By accepting this responsibility, neurosurgeons will continue to fulfill their important role in the management of intractable pain.

REFERENCES

1. Bonica JJ: Definitions and taxonomy of pain. In Bonica JJ (ed): The Management of Pain, 2nd ed. Philadelphia, Lea & Febiger, 1990, pp 18–27.
2. Loeser JD, Bigos SJ, Fordyce WE, et al: Low back pain. In Bonica JJ (ed): The Management of Pain, 2nd ed. Philadelphia, Lea & Febiger, 1990, pp 1448–1483.
3. Bonica JJ: General considerations of chronic pain. In Bonica JJ (ed): The Management of Pain, 2nd ed. Philadelphia, Lea & Febiger, 1990, pp 180–196.
4. Krames ES: Intraspinal opioid therapy for chronic nonmalignant pain: Current practice and clinical guidelines. J Pain Symptom Manage 11:333–352, 1996.
5. World Health Organization Expert Committee: Cancer pain relief and palliative care. World Health Organ Tech Rep Ser 804:1–73, 1990.
6. American Pain Society: Principles of Analgesic Use in the Treatment of Acute Pain and Cancer Pain, 3rd ed. Glenview, Ill, American Pain Society, 1992.

7. Cherny NI, Portenoy RK: The management of cancer pain. CA Cancer J Clin 44:262–303, 1994.

8. North RB, Kidd DH, Lee MS, et al: A prospective, randomized study of spinal cord stimulation versus reoperation for failed back surgery syndrome: Initial results. Stereotact Funct Neurosurg 62:267–272, 1994.

9. Doleys DM, Olson K: Psychological Assessment and Intervention in Implantable Pain Therapies. Minneapolis, Minn, Medtronic, 1997.

10. North RB, Levy RM: Consensus conference on the neurosurgical management of pain [review]. Neurosurgery 34:756–761, 1994.

11. Deer TR: The role of neuromodulation by spinal cord stimulation in chronic pain syndromes: Current concepts. Tech Regional Anesth Pain Manage 2:161–167, 1998.

12. North RB, Kidd DH, Zahurak M, et al: Spinal cord stimulation for chronic, intractable pain: Experience over two decades. Neurosurgery 32:384–395, 1993.

13. Turner J, Loeser J, Bell K: Spinal cord stimulation for chronic low back pain: A systematic literature synthesis. Neurosurgery 37:1088–1096, 1995.

14. Burchiel KJ, Anderson VC, Brown FD, et al: Prospective, multicenter study of spinal cord stimulation for relief of chronic back and extremity pain. Spine 21:2786–2794, 1996.

15. Spiegelmann W: Spinal cord stimulation: A contemporary series. Neurosurgery 28:65–70, 1991.

16. Barolat G, Schwartzman R, Woo R: Epidural spinal cord stimulation in the management of reflex sympathetic dystrophy. Stereotact Funct Neurosurg 53:29–37, 1989.

17. Kumar K, Nath R, Toth C: Spinal cord stimulation is effective in the management of reflex sympathetic dystrophy. Neurosurgery 40:503–508, 1997.

18. Kumar K, Nath R: Spinal cord stimulation for chronic pain in peripheral neuropathy. Surg Neurol 46:363–364, 1996.

19. Kumar K, Toth C, Nath R, et al: Improvement of limb circulation in peripheral vascular disease using epidural spinal cord stimulation: A prospective study. J Neurosurg 86:662–669, 1997.

20. Huber S, Vaglienti R, Midcap M: Enhanced limb salvage for peripheral vascular disease with the use of spinal cord stimulation. W V Med J 92:89–91, 1996.

21. Sanderson JE, Ibrahim B, Waterhouse D, et al: Spinal electrical stimulation for intractable angina—long-term clinical outcome and safety. Eur Heart J 15:810–814, 1994.

22. De Jongste MJL, Hautvast RWM, Hillege HL, et al: Efficacy of spinal cord stimulation as adjuvant therapy for intractable angina pectoris: A prospective, randomized clinical study. J Am Coll Cardiol 23:1592–1597, 1994.

23. Hassenbusch SJ, Stanton-Hicks M, Schoppa D, et al: Long-term results of peripheral nerve stimulation for reflex sympathetic dystrophy. J Neurosurg 84:415–423, 1996.

24. Weiner RL, Reed KL: Peripheral neurostimulation for control of intractable occipital neuralgia. Neuromodulation 2:217–221, 1999.

25. Levy RM, Lamb S, Adams JE: Treatment of chronic pain by deep brain stimulation: Long term follow-up and review of the literature. Neurosurgery 21:885–893, 1987.

26. Kumar K, Toth C, Nath RK: Deep brain stimulation for intractable pain: A 15-year experience. Neurosurgery 40:736–747, 1997.

27. Richardson DE: Deep brain stimulation for the relief of chronic pain. Neurosurg Clin N Am 6:135–144, 1995.

28. Tasker RR, Filho OV: Deep brain stimulation for the control of intractable pain. In Youmans JR (ed): Neurological Surgery, 4th ed. Philadelphia, WB Saunders, 1996, pp 3512–3527.

29. Nguyen J-P, Lefaucheur J-P, Decq P, et al: Chronic motor cortex stimulation in the treatment of central and neuropathic pain: Correlations between clinical, electrophysiological and anatomical data. Pain 82:245–251, 1999.

30. Ebel H, Rust D, Tronnier V, et al: Chronic precentral stimulation in trigeminal neuropathic pain. Acta Neurochir (Wien) 138:1300–1306, 1996.

31. Tsubokawa T, Katayama Y, Yamamoto T, et al: Chronic motor cortex stimulation in patients with thalamic pain. J Neurosurg 78:393–401, 1993.

32. Meyerson BA, Linderoth B, Lind G, et al: Motor cortex stimulation as a treatment of trigeminal neuropathic pain. Acta Neurochir Suppl (Wien) 58:150–153, 1993.

33. Follett KA, Hitchon PW, Piper J, et al: Response of intractable pain to continuous intrathecal morphine: A retrospective study. Pain 49:21–25, 1992.

34. Paice JA, Penn RD, Shott S: Intraspinal morphine for chronic pain: A retrospective, multicenter study. J Pain Symptom Manage 11:71–80, 1996.

35. Winkelmüller M, Winkelmüller W: Long-term effects of continuous intrathecal opioid treatment in chronic pain of nonmalignant etiology. J Neurosurg 85:458–467, 1996.

36. Schuchard M, Krames ES, Lanning R: Intraspinal analgesia for nonmalignant pain: A retrospective analysis for efficacy, safety, and feasibility in 50 patients. Neuromodulation 1:46–56, 1998.

37. Hassenbusch SJ, Pillay PK, Magdinec M, et al: Constant infusion of morphine for intractable cancer pain using an implanted pump. J Neurosurg 73:405–409, 1990.

38. Hassenbusch SJ, Stanton-Hicks M, Covington EC, et al: Long-term intraspinal infusions of opioids in the treatment of neuropathic pain. J Pain Symptom Manage 10:527–543, 1995.

39. Maron J, Loeser JD: Spinal opioid infusions in the treatment of chronic pain of nonmalignant origin [review]. Clin J Pain 12:174–179, 1996.

40. Dennis GC, DeWitty RL: Long-term intraventricular infusion of morphine for intractable pain in cancer of the head and neck. Neurosurgery 26:404–408, 1990.

41. Karavelis A, Foroglou G, Selviaridis P, et al: Intraventricular administration of morphine for control of intractable cancer pain in 90 patients. Neurosurgery 39:57–62, 1996.

42. Tasker RR: Stereotactic surgery. In Wall PD, Melzack R (eds): Textbook of Pain, 3rd ed. Edinburgh, Churchill Livingstone, 1994, pp 1137–1158.

43. Hardy RW Jr, Bay JW: Surgery of the sympathetic nervous system. In Schmidek HH, Sweet WH (eds): Operative Neurosurgical Techniques: Indications, Methods, and Results, 3rd ed. Philadelphia, WB Saunders, 1995, pp 1637–1646.

44. Wilkinson HA: Sympathectomy for pain. In Youmans JR (ed): Neurological Surgery, 4th ed. Philadelphia, WB Saunders, 1996, pp 3489–3499.

45. Johnson JP, Obasi C, Hahn MS, et al: Endoscopic thoracic sympathectomy. J Neurosurg 91:90–97, 1999.

46. Schwartzman RJ, Liu JE, Smullens SN, et al: Long-term outcome following sympathectomy for complex regional pain syndrome type I (RSD). J Neurol Sci 150:149–152, 1997.

47. Kumar K, Nath RK, Toth C: Spinal cord stimulation is effective in the management of reflex sympathetic dystrophy. Neurosurgery 40:503–509, 1997.

48. Burchiel KJ, Johans TJ, Ochoa J: The surgical treatment of painful traumatic neuromas. J Neurosurg 78:714–719, 1993.

49. Van Eerten PV, Polder TW, Broere CAJ: Operative treatment of meralgia paresthetica: Transection versus neurolysis. Neurosurgery 37:63–65, 1995.

50. Starling JR, Harms BA: Diagnosis and treatment of genitofemoral and ilioinguinal neuralgia. World J Surg 13:586–591, 1989.

51. Hosobuchi Y: The majority of unmyelinated afferent axons in human ventral roots probably conduct pain. Pain 8:167–180, 1980.

52. Onofrio BM, Campa HK: Evaluation of rhizotomy: Review of 12 years' experience. J Neurosurg 36:751–755, 1972.

53. North RB, Kidd DH, Campbell JN, et al: Dorsal root ganglionectomy for failed back surgery syndrome: A 5-year follow-up study. J Neurosurg 74:236–242, 1991.

54. Taha JM, Favre J, Burchiel KM: Management of malignant chronic pain. In Grossman RG, Loftus CM (eds): Principles of Neurosurgery, 2nd ed. Philadelphia, Lippincott-Raven, 1999, pp 435–442.

55. Saris SC, Silver JM, Vieira JFS, et al: Sacrococcygeal rhizotomy for perineal pain. Neurosurgery 19:789–793, 1986.

56. Tew JM Jr, Taha JM: Percutaneous rhizotomy in the treatment of intractable facial pain (trigeminal, glossopharyngeal, and vagal nerves). In Schmidek HH, Sweet WH (eds): Operative Neurosurgical Techniques: Indications, Methods, and Results, 3rd ed. Philadelphia, WB Saunders, 1995, pp 1469–1484.

57. Rath SA, Seitz K, Soliman N, et al: DREZ coagulations for deafferentation pain related to spinal and peripheral nerve lesions: Indication and results of 79 consecutive procedures. Stereotact Funct Neurosurg 68:161–167, 1997.

58. Nashold JRB, Nashold BS Jr: Microsurgical DREZotomy in treatment of deafferentation pain. In Schmidek HH, Sweet WH (eds):

Operative Neurosurgical Techniques: Indications, Methods, and Results, 3rd ed. Philadelphia, WB Saunders, 1995, pp 1623–1636.

59. Sindou MP: Microsurgical DREZotomy. In Schmidek HH, Sweet WH (eds): Operative Neurosurgical Techniques: Indications, Methods, and Results, 3rd ed. Philadelphia, WB Saunders, 1995, pp 1613–1621.

60. Bullard DE, Nashold BS Jr: The caudalis DREZ for facial pain. Stereotact Funct Neurosurg 68:168–174, 1997.

61. Gorecki JP, Nashold BS: The Duke experience with the nucleus caudalis DREZ operation. Acta Neurochir Suppl (Wien) 64:128–131, 1995.

62. Poletti CE: Open cordotomy and medullary tractotomy. In Schmidek HH, Sweet WH (eds): Operative Neurosurgical Techniques: Indications, Methods, and Results, 3rd ed. Philadelphia, WB Saunders, 1995, pp 1557–1571.

63. Tasker RR: Percutaneous cordotomy. In Schmidek HH, Sweet WH (eds): Operative Neurosurgical Techniques: Indications, Methods, and Results, 3rd ed. Philadelphia, WB Saunders, 1995, pp 1595–1611.

64. Kanpolat Y, Akyar S, Caglar S, et al: CT-guided percutaneous selective cordotomy. Acta Neurochir (Wien) 123:92–96, 1993.

65. Gybels JM, Sweet WH: Neurosurgical Treatment of Persistent Pain: Physiological and Pathological Mechanisms of Human Pain. Basel, Karger, 1989.

66. Rosomoff HL, Papo I, Loeser JD, et al: Neurosurgical operations on the spinal cord. In Bonica JJ (ed): The Management of Pain, 2nd ed. Philadelphia, Lea & Febiger, 1990, pp 2067–2081.

67. Watling CJ, Payne R, Allen RR, et al: Commissural myelotomy for intractable cancer pain: Report of two cases. Clin J Pain 12:151–156, 1996.

68. King RB: Anterior commissurotomy for intractable pain. J Neurosurg 47:7–11, 1977.

69. Nauta HJW, Hewitt E, Westlund KN, et al: Surgical interruption of a midline dorsal column visceral pain pathway: Case report and review of the literature. J Neurosurg 86:538–542, 1997.

70. Hirshberg RM, Al-Chaer ED, Lawand NB, et al: Is there a pathway in the posterior funiculus that signals visceral pain? Pain 67:291–305, 1996.

71. Hitchcock ER: Stereotactic cervical myelotomy. J Neurol Neurosurg Psychiatry 33:224–230, 1970.

72. Bullard DE, Nashold BS Jr: Mesencephalotomy and other brain stem procedures for pain. In Youmans JR (ed): Neurological Surgery, 4th ed. Philadelphia, WB Saunders, 1996, pp 3477–3488.

73. Jannetta PJ, Gildenberg PL, Loeser JD, et al: Operations on the brain and brain stem for chronic pain. In Bonica JJ (ed): The Management of Pain, 2nd ed. Philadelphia, Lea & Febiger, 1990, pp 2082–2103.

74. Tasker RR: Intracranial ablative procedures for pain. In Tindall TG, Cooper PR, Barrow DL (eds): The Practice of Neurosurgery. Baltimore, Williams & Wilkins, 1996, pp 3115–3128.

75. Tasker RR: Thalamic stereotaxic procedures. In Schaltenbrand G, Walker AE (eds): Stereotaxy of the Human Brain: Anatomical, Physiological and Clinical Applications. Stuttgart, Germany, Georg Thieme Verlag, 1982, pp 484–497.

76. Tasker RR: Thalamotomy. Neurosurg Clin N Am 1:841–864, 1990.

77. Young RF, Vermeulen SS, Grimm P, et al: Gamma knife thalamotomy for the treatment of persistent pain. Stereotact Funct Neurosurg 64(Suppl 1):172–181, 1995.

78. Hassenbusch SJ, Pillay PK, Barnett GH: Radiofrequency cingulotomy for intractable cancer pain using stereotaxis guided by magnetic resonance imaging. Neurosurgery 27:220–223, 1990.

79. Bouckoms AJ: Limbic surgery for pain. In Wall PD, Melzack R (eds): Textbook of Pain, 3rd ed. Edinburgh, Churchill Livingstone, 1994, pp 1171–1187.

80. Levin AB, Katz J, Benson RC, et al: Treatment of pain of diffuse metastatic cancer by stereotactic chemical hypophysectomy: Long term results and observations on mechanism of action. Neurosurgery 6:258–262, 1980.

81. Ramirez LF, Levin AB: Pain relief after hypophysectomy. Neurosurgery 14:499–504, 1984.

CHAPTER 190

Dorsal Rhizotomy and Dorsal Root Ganglionectomy

JAMAL M. TAHA ■ KHALED M. ABDEL AZIZ ■ NORBERTO ANDALUZ

HISTORY

The treatment of chronic pain by dorsal root rhizotomy is based on the work of Bell,[1] who demonstrated that dorsal spinal roots mediate sensory functions and motor spinal roots mediate motor functions. The first clinical application of this theory was reported in 1896 by Abbe,[2] who independently sectioned the intradural dorsal rootlets for the treatment of pain disorders. Early enthusiasm for the procedure was replaced by skepticism after reports of long-term failure in several patients and after the advent of spinothalamic cordotomy and sympathectomy.[3] However, several investigators maintained that rhizotomy produced better results than did cordotomy.[4] Subsequent surgical modifications and proper patient selection encouraged others to use dorsal rhizotomy increasingly for the treatment of pain disorders. In 1966 Scoville[5] reported on the technique of extradural spinal dorsal root section. In 1970 Smith[6] combined dorsal rhizotomy with section of the sympathetic rami communicans to eliminate the sensory input through the sympathetic chain. In 1974 Uematsu[7] described the technique of percutaneous radiofrequency spinal rhizotomy.

The discovery that motor roots contain unmyelinated sensory fibers[8] provided an explanation for the long-term failure of dorsal rhizotomy and set the theoretical basis for offering ganglionectomy as a means of eliminating all sensory input.[9] Alternatively, some investigators combined dorsal rhizotomy with section of the motor rootlets.[10] Currently, dorsal rhizotomy and ganglionectomy are both accepted procedures for the treatment of selected pain disorders.[11]

ANATOMY OF SPINAL ROOTS AND NERVES

Generally 3 to 5 anterior spinal rootlets emerge from the anterolateral sulcus, and 3 to 10 posterior spinal rootlets penetrate the posterolateral sulcus. Along the length of the spinal cord, the anterior spinal rootlets lie ventral and the posterior rootlets lie dorsal to the dentate ligament. Within the outer arachnoid layer, tiny anastomotic branches pass from one rootlet to another, increasing the extent of innervation of the root from which they arise. As the anterior and posterior rootlets approach the intervertebral foramen in the spinal canal, they group together within a common dural sleeve but remain separated by a thin fibrous septum. This separation continues throughout the intervertebral foramen, with the sensory root and ganglion lying dorsal to the fibrous septum and the motor root lying ventral to it, within a common dural sheath. The subarachnoid space accompanies the dural sheath several millimeters before it is sealed off by arachnoid trabeculae at varying distances proximal to the ganglion. Outside the intervertebral foramen, the anterior and posterior roots join just distal to the spinal ganglion to form the spinal nerve. At that level, the dural sheath is replaced by epineurium.

The spinal nerve quickly gives rise to several branches (Fig. 190–1). The white ramus communicans containing preganglionic sympathetic fibers from the anterior root joins the corresponding sympathetic ganglion; the gray ramus communicans containing postganglionic sympathetic fibers from the sympathetic ganglion rejoins the spinal nerve. Both white and gray rami communicans contain afferent fibers, including some for pain. Just distal to the intervertebral foramen, a small branch leaves the spinal nerve to anastomose with another small branch originating from the adjacent white ramus communicans to form the sinu-vertebral nerve, also known as the ramus meningeus of Luschka. The sinu-vertebral nerve, which also contains nociceptive fibers, returns through the intervertebral foramen anterior to the spinal nerve and terminates in the spinal canal, innervating spinal meninges, blood vessels, intervertebral ligaments, and vertebral joint surfaces. Outside the intervertebral foramen, the spinal nerve bifurcates into ventral and dorsal branches. The dorsal branch provides sensory innervation to the adjacent facet joints, ligaments, periosteum, and fascia.

Each spinal root is accompanied by an anterior and posterior radicular artery. Six to 8 arteries supplying the anterior spinal arterial trunk and 10 to 23 arteries

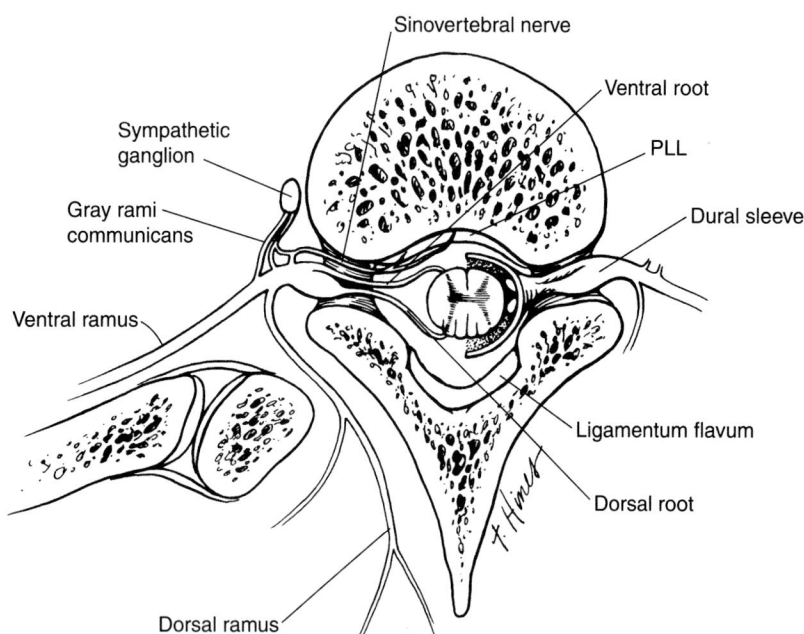

FIGURE 190–1. Anatomic illustration of thoracic roots, ganglion, and spinal nerve. PLL, posterior longitudinal ligament. (Courtesy Mayfield Clinic, Cincinnati, OH.)

supplying the posterolateral spinal arterial trunk are of functional significance in adults.

In humans, 13% to 51% of the total fiber spectrum of the ventral roots from C1 to S4 is unmyelinated.[8] There is evidence that at least some of these fibers are nociceptive. Not all afferent fibers in the ventral roots enter the spinal cord through the ventral roots. Some fibers that originate in dorsal root ganglion cells loop into the ventral roots and reenter the dorsal roots for access to the spinal cord.[12] Occasionally, ganglion cells are not exclusive to the ganglion but taper into the proximal and distal roots.[13] Aberrant dorsal root ganglion cells within the ventral roots have also been described.[14]

INDICATIONS

In 1994 the Joint Section on Pain of the American Association of Neurological Surgeons and the Congress of Neurological Surgeons outlined valid indications for the application of dorsal rhizotomy and ganglionectomy.[11] Based on the authors' experience, the recommendations of the Joint Section on Pain, and a review of the literature, the following recommendations are endorsed.

Indications for Rhizotomy or Ganglionectomy in the Treatment of Cancer Pain

1. Multilevel cervical dorsal rhizotomy to denervate a functionally useless limb in patients with brachial plexus involvement.

2. Extradural sacral rhizotomy for cancer pain of the pelvis, rectum, vulva, or cervix in patients with nonfunctional anal and vesicular sphincters and in whom a diversionary procedure has been performed.

3. Thoracic rhizotomy or ganglionectomy for localized thoracic pain secondary to invasion of the chest wall by pleural-based or other chest wall malignancy, or for pain related to tumor compression or invasion of thoracic nerves.

Indications for Dorsal Rhizotomy or Ganglionectomy in the Treatment of Noncancer Pain

1. Pain related to greater or lesser occipital neuralgia is best treated by a C2 or C3 ganglionectomy, respectively, although upper intradural cervical rhizotomy has been used successfully.

2. For allodynia and evoked pain of neuropathic pain syndromes, such as postherpetic neuralgia, pain following thoracotomy and laparotomy, and pain from thoracic roots caught in fractures, there is some evidence that ganglionectomy provides better results than does dorsal rhizotomy.

3. Cervical intradural rhizotomy is used to treat pain in a functionally useless extremity.

4. Percutaneous radiofrequency lumbar median branch rhizotomy is used for the treatment of facet arthropathy pain.

The role of dorsal rhizotomy and ganglionectomy in the treatment of other pain conditions remains unclear. Some series propose a beneficial role for percutaneous radiofrequency ganglionectomy in the treatment of monoradicular pain in an upper extremity[7, 15] and for dorsal root ganglionectomy in the treatment of monoradicular pain in a lower extremity.[16] These recommendations should be validated by other investigators.

DIAGNOSTIC EVALUATION

For rhizotomy or ganglionectomy to be successful, the surgeon must determine the proper level and number of roots or ganglia to be sectioned. This determination may be relatively simple in cases of tumor involvement of a single spinal nerve. The determination may be more complex in cases of widespread tumor invasion or in cases of pain involving multiple sensory dermatomes. Additional compounding factors include overlap of root innervation,[17] intradural root-to-root anastomosis,[18] individual anatomic and functional variation, poor correlation between cutaneous and deep structure sensory innervation, and rich anastomoses between the sympathetic system and the ventral root sensory fibers.[3]

Local anesthetic blockade of the affected nerve roots or spinal ganglia should temporarily render the patient pain free. A spinal subarachnoid anesthetic block or caudal epidural block may be performed as a screening test before sacral rhizotomy. Diagnostic blocks of the cervical region should be performed in a unit with resuscitation equipment in the rare event of subarachnoid injection of the local anesthetic. Placebo control is important, and repetition of the block is advisable. If a satisfactory block at the appropriate level fails to relieve pain, the patient will not benefit from surgery.[19] Pain relief following block, however, does not guarantee a successful surgical outcome.[20]

SURGICAL TECHNIQUE

Ganglionectomy is, by definition, an extradural operation. Dorsal rhizotomy can be performed intra- or extradurally. In addition, both rhizotomy and ganglionectomy can be performed by a percutaneous technique using radiofrequency current. Chemical rhizotomy is an alternative to open rhizotomy, but it is less selective.[21]

Dorsal Root Ganglionectomy

Thoracic Ganglionectomy. The technique for T6 ganglionectomy in the thoracic region is described. After administration of general anesthesia, the patient is placed prone, and the T6 transverse process is localized by intraoperative posterior-anterior fluoroscopy or radiography. A midline incision is made, and unilateral subperiosteal dissection is carried out laterally to expose the T6 and T7 laminae, the lateral edge of the T6-7 facet joint, and the T6 and T7 transverse processes (Fig. 190–2A). Under microscopic vision, the primary dorsal ramus of the T6 spinal nerve, which originates just distal to the ganglion, is identified in the intrans-

verse space lateral to the outer edge of the T6-7 facet joint. The primary dorsal ramus is found either attached to the retracted muscles or divided with its stump lying dorsal to the intertransverse ligament. A high-speed drill is used to remove the inferior edge of the proximal part of the T6 transverse process and the lateral half of the superior facet of T7, creating a lateral facetectomy and foraminotomy. Attention is directed to the primary dorsal ramus, which is followed through the intertransverse ligament to the T6 ganglion lying within the dural sheath. Dissection is carried out proximally, around the T6 pedicle, to identify the T6 nerve roots as they exit through the dura of the spinal cord. The dorsal and motor roots are usually enclosed within the same dural sheath but may occasionally be contained in separate dural sheaths. Care should be taken to avoid injuring the feeding segmental arteries that pass through the foramen. The dural sheath enclosing the ganglion is sharply incised longitudinally at its dorsal aspect, starting at the origin of the primary dorsal ramus, and dissection is carried proximally until the ganglion is encompassed proximally. The gross contour of the ganglion can be identified by its bulging appearance and by its yellowish color, which separates it from the whitish nerve roots. A hemoclip is placed on the proximal sensory root to prevent possible cerebrospinal fluid leakage as the sensory root is divided proximal to the ganglion, just distal to the clip. The ganglion is grasped, elevated, and bluntly dissected off the fibrous septum, which separates it from the dorsal root (see Fig. 190–2B). Distally, the ganglion is amputated after coagulation and section of its distal connection to the spinal nerve.

Cervical Ganglionectomy. In the lower cervical region, a similar technique for ganglionectomy is performed; however, ganglionectomy in the cervical region is hampered by extensive venous plexus in the lateral part of the intervertebral foramen. Because the ganglion lies in the lateral part of the intervertebral foramen, a relatively large portion of the facet joint must be removed to gain access, thus risking postoperative spinal instability. This difficulty does not apply to the C3 ganglion. For C2 ganglionectomy, the C2 ganglion can be readily visualized between the laminae of C1 and C2 (Fig. 190–3). The inferior edge of the C1 lamina is drilled laterally to expose the proximal part of the C2 ganglion as it winds around the C1 pedicle. The ganglion is surrounded by a copious venous plexus, which requires thorough coagulation using a bipolar cautery. The motor and sensory roots at C2 are usually enclosed within separate dural sheaths as they exit the dura of the spinal cord. This anatomic arrangement allows early transection of the proximal sensory roots distal to a hemoclip. Dissection is then carried out distally, elevating the ganglion from the underlying motor root and transecting it from the distal nerve. The motor C2 root, which occasionally supplies nerves to the muscles of swallowing function, should be preserved.

Lumbar Ganglionectomy. In the lumbar region, the L5 ganglion usually lies within the intervertebral fora-

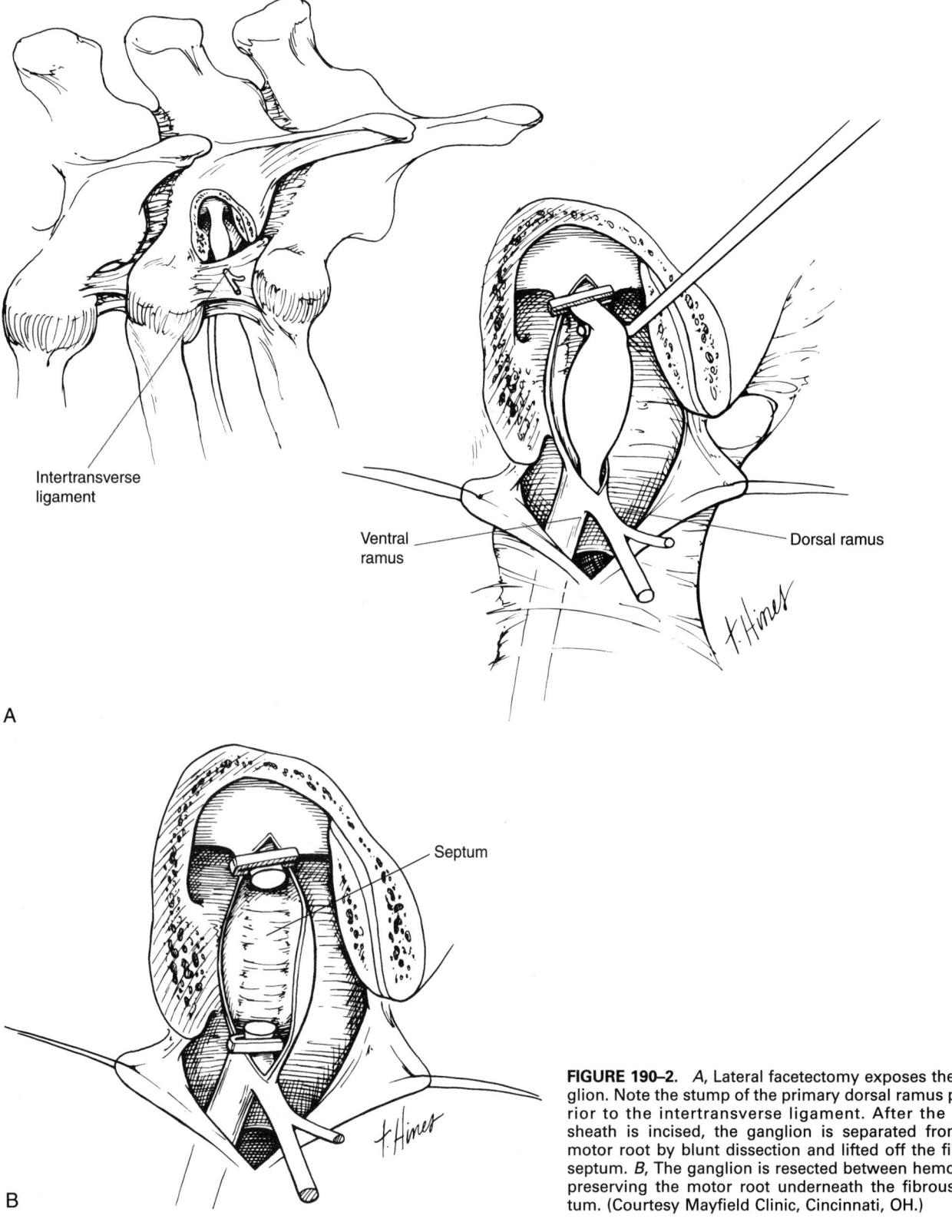

Intertransverse ligament

Ventral ramus

Dorsal ramus

Septum

A

B

FIGURE 190–2. *A,* Lateral facetectomy exposes the ganglion. Note the stump of the primary dorsal ramus posterior to the intertransverse ligament. After the dural sheath is incised, the ganglion is separated from the motor root by blunt dissection and lifted off the fibrous septum. *B,* The ganglion is resected between hemoclips, preserving the motor root underneath the fibrous septum. (Courtesy Mayfield Clinic, Cincinnati, OH.)

men, and the S1 ganglion usually lies within the spinal canal.[16, 22] The technique for L5 ganglionectomy requires resection of the lateral margin of the zygapophyseal joint and several millimeters of the inferolateral margin of the overhanging pars interarticularis. For an

S1 ganglionectomy, a standard L5-S1 hemilaminectomy and foraminotomy are performed. The dural sheath is incised longitudinally, and the ganglion is freed distally by transection of its attachment to the spinal nerve. The ganglion is elevated and dissected proximally off

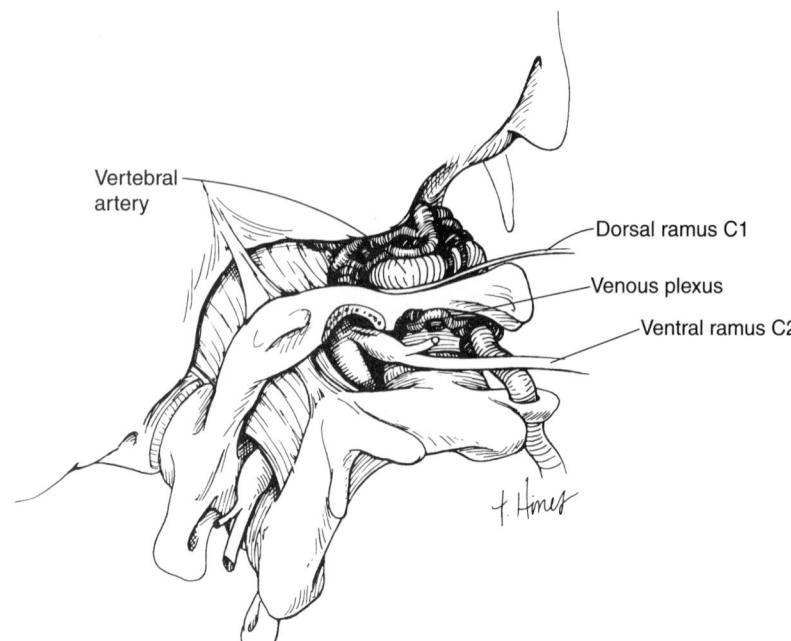

FIGURE 190–3. The C2 ganglion is exposed between the lamina of C1 and C2 and is surrounded by extensive venous plexus. Frequently, the motor and sensory roots can be separated proximally without incising open the dural sheath. (Courtesy Mayfield Clinic, Cincinnati, OH.)

the fibrous septum, which separates it from the ventral motor root, and is excised distal to a hemoclip applied to the proximal dorsal root.

Intradural Rhizotomy

The technique for intradural rhizotomy is accomplished through a standard multilevel laminectomy. In general, at least a three-level rhizotomy is required to accommodate overlap innervation.[23] After the dura is opened, the appropriate sensory roots are identified at their respective intervertebral foramina and followed rostrally. They are then transected between hemoclips or after coagulation. In the thoracic region, care must be taken to preserve the segmental blood supply, which can enter along the posterior roots.[24] At the cervical to midthoracic levels, the relatively horizontal egress of the roots allows a relatively limited surgical exposure. In the midthoracic to lumbar levels, the roots can lie several segments above their respective foramina, requiring a larger exposure. Although intraoperative physiologic monitoring, such as dermatomal somatosensory evoked potentials, may aid in identifying the appropriate roots to be sectioned, the most definitive method is to trace the nerve roots rostrally from their respective intervertebral foramina.

Extradural Rhizotomy

In the cervical, thoracic, and lumbar regions, the technique for extradural rhizotomy is similar to that for extradural ganglionectomy, except that the ganglion is not resected. After lateral facetectomy and foraminotomy are performed, dissection is carried out toward the dura to identify the proximal spinal roots. Occasionally, the proximal dorsal sensory roots and the ventral motor roots are enclosed within separate dural

sheaths. In such cases, the operation simply entails transection of the sensory root between two hemoclips. When the proximal and distal sensory roots are enclosed within the same dural sheath, the dural sheath should be incised longitudinally to identify the junction between the white dorsal root and the yellowish dorsal root ganglion. The dorsal root is dissected a few millimeters proximal and transected between two hemoclips. Care should be taken to preserve the underlying motor root, which is separated from the proximal root by a thin fibrous septum. Intraoperative nerve stimulation may be helpful in identifying the proximal motor root.

In the sacral region, extradural rhizotomy is performed as originally described by Crue and Todd.[25] Through a midline incision at the lumbosacral junction, a bilateral upper sacral laminectomy is performed, exposing the S1 and S2 nerve roots. The thecal sac is then double-ligated, using a nonabsorbable suture material such as silk. One tie is passed around the thecal sac just caudal to the S1 nerve root axilla, and a second tie is passed around the thecal sac just rostral to the S2 nerve root axilla. The thecal sac is sharply transected with its contents between the two ties, preserving the S1 nerve roots (Fig. 190–4).

Percutaneous Radiofrequency Rhizotomy and Ganglionectomy

The theory behind radiofrequency lesions of the dorsal roots and dorsal root ganglia is based on the work of Letcher and Goldring,[26] who demonstrated a relatively selective destruction of unmyelinated and small myelinated fibers by graded thermal lesions. The procedure is performed percutaneously, using local anesthesia and intravenous sedation. Through a posterior paraspinal approach in the thoracic and lumbar regions

S1 nerve root

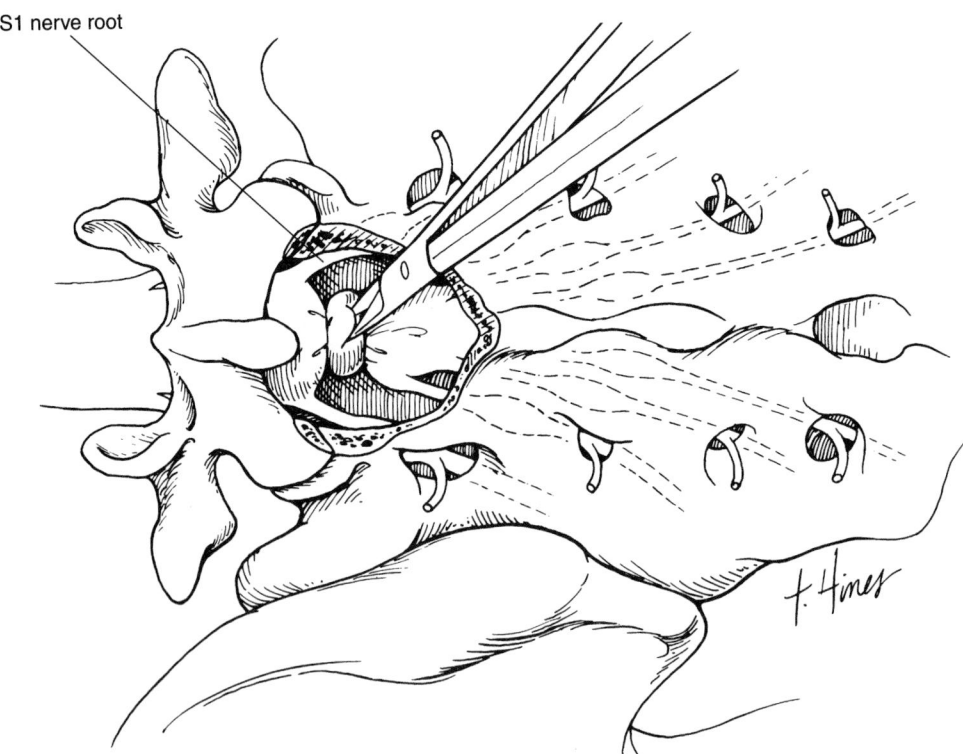

FIGURE 190–4. The thecal sac is transected between two ligatures applied caudal to the S1 axilla and rostral to the S2 axilla. (Courtesy Mayfield Clinic, Cincinnati, OH.)

and an anterior approach in the cervical region, a 2-mm uninsulated-tip electrode is placed percutaneously within the neural foramen, guided by fluoroscopy. Proper location of the electrode is confirmed by eliciting paresthesia in the region of the patient's pain at less than 1 V with 50-Hz stimulation. Stimulation with 2 Hz should not produce motor contraction at thresholds less than 1.5 times the threshold for sensory stimulation.[15] A test lesion is made at 42°C for 15 seconds. A more permanent lesion is created using a temperature of 65°C to 90°C for 60 to 90 seconds. Intravenous sedation is administered during lesion creation to minimize the patient's discomfort.

Percutaneous Lumbar Radiofrequency Median Branch Rhizotomy

Lumbar facet rhizotomy refers to the ablation of the medial branch of the posterior primary ramus, which innervates the synovial facet joint. The procedure is extended to one level above and one level below the targeted facet joint to denervate contributing sensory branches.

The patient is placed in the prone position on two chest rolls with all pressure points padded. Intravenous short-acting sedatives are administered periodically to keep the patient comfortable during needle placement but sufficiently awake to allow proper neurological examination during the procedure. A grounding pad is attached to the patient's skin. Bony landmarks are visualized to locate the median branches. The L2 through L4 median branches wind around the junction of the transverse process and the superior articular

process of the lower vertebral level. For example, the L4 median branch winds around the junction of the L5 transverse process and the superior articular process. The L5 median branch winds around the junction of the sacral ala and the S1 superior articular process. The S1 median branch travels along the superior-lateral border of the S1 foramen. The entry point for targeting the L2 through L4 median branches overlies the lateral third of the transverse process of the lower level. The entry point for targeting the L5 median branch is similar to that of the L4 median branch. The entry point for targeting the S1 median branch overlies the L5 target point.

After a skin weal is raised that overlies the entry point, a stab incision is made, through which a 14-gauge needle is introduced down to the transverse process. A 10-mm tip electrode (Radionics, Burlington, MA) is introduced through the needle and slid medially over the superior edge of the transverse process until it engages the groove between the transverse process and the superior articular process. For the S1 median branch, the electrode is directed toward the S1 foramen and redirected toward its superior-lateral border.

Once the electrode lies in its proper anatomic position, electrostimulation is performed at a pulse of 1-msec duration and a frequency of 2 and 50 Hz. With proper targeting, the patient should experience reproduction of back pain at less than 1 V at 50-Hz stimulation, motor contractions of back muscles at 1 to 2 V at 2-Hz stimulation, and no motor contractions in the extremities at less than 5 V at 2-Hz stimulation.

Each radiofrequency lesion is created at 80°C for 80

seconds. The limb is examined for motor strength during and after each lesion. The lesion should be stopped immediately if the patient reports any sensory changes in the limb.

After all lesions are created, the needle entry points are covered with sterile gauze. Patients are observed for 2 hours before discharge, and they are prescribed muscle relaxants and warned of the potential for increased back pain and back muscle spasms for several days postoperatively. Most patients can return to work 3 to 4 days after the procedure. Relief of back pain is noticed 1 to 4 weeks after surgery.

The use of facet rhizotomy has become popular, but the results are varied and sometimes confusing, with success rates ranging from 20% to 90%.[27] Recently, Tzaan and Tasker reported their experience with 118 consecutive percutaneous radiofrequency facet rhizotomies performed on 90 patients. For patients undergoing their first or only procedure, there was 41% overall improvement of symptoms (>50% relief). There was no statistically significant difference in success rates for procedures performed on the cervical, thoracic, or lumbosacral facets; with unilateral versus bilateral denervations; when two or three, versus more than three, facets were denervated; or for operations in patients who had undergone previous spinal surgery compared with those who had not. Results were unaffected by whether hyperextension of the spine aggravated the patient's preoperative pain. When the procedures were repeated in the same patients, outcomes tended to be consistent, arguing against repetition of failed facet denervations. The morbidity was low, with the chief problem being sensory loss and transient neuropathic pain in the distribution of cutaneous branches of posterior rami in the cervical and thoracic areas. The authors concluded that percutaneous radiofrequency facet denervation is still worth considering in patients with disabling spinal pain that fails to respond to conservative treatment.[27] In our experience with facet rhizotomy in 20 patients, there was an overall 70% improvement. Careful patient selection and evaluation of symptom relief after diagnostic facet blocks are key factors in the success of percutaneous facet rhizotomy.

MODIFICATIONS OF DORSAL RHIZOTOMY AND GANGLIONECTOMY

Since it was first described, dorsal rhizotomy has undergone a number of modifications in attempts to improve its results, based on several factors. First, extensive overlap exists between adjacent spinal segments. In the monkey, at least three adjacent roots supply each dermatome.[28] Experimental studies demonstrate an increase in dorsal horn cell receptive fields following sensory denervation, possibly due to loss of presynaptic inhibition in which the C-fiber afferents play a special role.[29] Sensory loss after dorsal rhizotomy can be reversed pharmacologically by strychnine, an agent that increases synaptic effectiveness, and by levodopa.[30] These findings suggest that extensive rhizotomy is necessary for effective denervation of a single

dermatome. At least one or two roots or ganglia above and below the desired level must be sectioned for effective sensory denervation.

Second, after dorsal rhizotomy, the excitability of dorsal horn cells increases as a result of decreased afferent-mediated inhibition. Hypersensitivity to substance P develops, the number of opiate receptors decreases, and abnormal spiking appears in dorsal root horn cells.[31] These changes have been linked to the development of gliosis in the dorsal horn following rhizotomy.[20] To reduce gliosis, Kato and colleagues[32] developed a novel approach—suicidal chemical rhizotomy. In this approach, doxorubicin is transported by the dorsal root in a retrograde manner to produce cell death, without producing gliosis.

Third, nociceptive afferents may ascend the sympathetic chain, bypassing the dorsal root and spinal cord segment.[6, 33] This hypothesis forms the basis for sectioning the white ramus communicans during extradural rhizotomy.[6]

The discovery of unmyelinated fibers in the ventral roots, some of which are nociceptive,[8] provided an explanation for some failures of dorsal rhizotomy and an impetus to investigate the hypothesis that spinal ganglionectomy might improve the results of posterior rhizotomy. Indeed, Hosobuchi[34] in 1980 removed the thoracic dorsal root ganglia of three patients who had not obtained relief after posterior rhizotomy for pain from thoracotomy or trauma to the chest wall. Two of the three patients were pain free 5 years later. Subsequently, Hosobuchi[34] successfully treated 13 of 18 patients by ganglionectomy. Osgood and coworkers[9] in 1976 described 18 patients who were successfully treated by posterior rhizotomy combined with ganglionectomy and followed for 2 to 20 months. However, Hosobuchi[34] concluded in 1982 that the addition of ganglionectomy to posterior rhizotomy did not improve long-term pain control.

In general, the results of ganglionectomy in the treatment of chronic pain have been variable, with some series demonstrating a benefit,[5, 35, 36] and others not.[23, 37, 38] The success of ganglionectomy in the treatment of pain depends partly on patient selection, pain cause and location, and duration of follow-up. Better results were reported in patients with cancer pain who had a relatively short life expectancy and in patients who underwent thoracic ganglionectomy in which multiple levels (no more than five) could be sacrificed with relative impunity and in which intersegmental connections between intradural roots were lacking.[6, 9, 34, 39]

COMPLICATIONS

The most serious complication of sensory denervation at any neural level is the development of deafferentation pain or anesthesia dolorosa. This complication is reportedly uncommon following dorsal rhizotomy, with an estimated risk of 4% to 5%[40]; however, a more recent report estimates that the risk is as high as 53%.[41] Deafferentation pain after ganglionectomy is usually transient, and currently, there is no uniformly beneficial treatment. In a rat model, dysesthetic pain following cervical ganglionectomy was reduced by a dorsal root entry zone lesion.[42]

In several pain syndromes, dorsal rhizotomy or ganglionectomy must include multiple levels for pain relief. Section of the dorsal roots of the upper cervical, thoracic, and upper lumbar roots results in little functional deficit, partly because there is extensive sensory overlap from adjacent dorsal roots. Lower cervical rhizotomy can lead to functional paralysis because of the absence of sensory input to the upper extremity. To avoid complete sensory loss to the arm, C6 or C7 or both C5 and C8 must be left intact.[17] In the thoracic region, motor roots can often be sacrificed without major morbidity, but extensive motor denervation of the intercostal muscles may lead to atrophy, with undesirable cosmetic results, or it may further decrease pulmonary function in patients with compromised ventilatory capacity. Extensive denervation of thoracic roots (T6-10) that supply abdominal muscles can result in disfiguring bulging of the abdominal contents.[39] Section of the sacral posterior roots interferes with sphincter and sexual function.

An uncommon but serious complication of dorsal rhizotomy or ganglionectomy is compromise of blood supply to the spinal cord.[20] This can occur after sacrifice of several radicular feeding arteries or a single large artery, resulting in spinal cord ischemia or infarction. This complication has also been reported following percutaneous radiofrequency ganglionectomy.[43]

Other complications of dorsal rhizotomy or ganglionectomy can usually be prevented by proper patient selection and surgical technique. Cervical ganglionectomy requires extensive removal of the facet joint, resulting in possible instability. Leakage of cerebrospinal fluid can be prevented by proper closure of the dura after intradural rhizotomy and by proper application of a hemoclip after extradural rhizotomy or ganglionectomy.

RESULTS

Pain Related to Malignancy

There are no prospective studies that analyze the results of dorsal rhizotomy and ganglionectomy in the treatment of cancer pain; however, considerable evidence supports the use of these procedures. The evidence consists primarily of well-designed studies that include comparative and descriptive case studies.[44] Retrospective reviews of large series demonstrate varied success rates: 25% to 72% for dorsal rhizotomy,[17, 23, 37, 45, 46] and 56% to 79% for ganglionectomy[6, 9, 10, 19, 47] (Table 190–1).

A relatively high success rate (50% to 90%) has been reported for dorsal rhizotomy in the treatment of pain related to pelvic neoplasms.[21, 25, 39, 48] Because interruption of S2 and S3 sensory input results in a neurogenic bladder and bowel, as well as an insensate anal sphincter, sacral rhizotomy is restricted to patients with a urinary diversion procedure or an indwelling catheter, a colostomy, and an inactive sex life.

Dorsal rhizotomy can relieve limb pain caused by tumor spread to the brachial plexus,[49] but extensive sensory denervation leads to a functionally useless limb. This may not be a concern in patients who have already developed profound motor and sensory deficits from tumor invasion.

Ganglionectomy or rhizotomy can be useful in the treatment of localized thoracic pain associated with tumor invasion of the chest wall or thoracic nerves. Because a three- to five-level ganglionectomy or rhizotomy is usually required, to allow for the overlap in segmental thoracic innervation, this treatment is considered for pain restricted to one or two dermatomes. In one series, pain was improved in 90% of patients who underwent open extradural ganglionectomy combined with ventral rhizotomy.[10] Our results using ganglionectomy to treat cancer pain are excellent, with a 100% rate of long-standing pain relief in a series of three patients. These patients had significant improvements in their quality of life and a decreased need for narcotics for pain management.

Pain Unrelated to Malignancy

Dorsal rhizotomy or ganglionectomy has a limited role in the treatment of noncancer pain; however, these procedures can be highly effective in selected conditions[4, 5, 16, 17, 23, 34, 35, 37, 50–52] (Table 190–2). Occipital neuralgia has been successfully treated by upper cervical intradural rhizotomy[25] or C2 ganglionectomy.[53, 54] Taha

TABLE 190–1 ■ Results of Dorsal Rhizotomy and Ganglionectomy in the Treatment of Cancer Pain in Selected Series

AUTHOR	YEAR	NO. OF PATIENTS	SURGERY	SUCCESS (%)
White & Sweet[17]	1969	33	Rhizotomy	58
Smith[6]	1970	2	Ganglionectomy	100
Loeser[23]	1972	7	Rhizotomy	43
Onofrio & Campa[37]	1972	18	Rhizotomy	28
Paillas & Pellet[51]	1972	6	Rhizotomy	0
Barrash & Leavens[45]	1973	71	Rhizotomy	70
Sindou & Larpas[46]	1976	585	Rhizotomy	47
Nash[47]	1986	3	Ganglionectomy	67
Arbit et al[10]	1989	14	Ganglionectomy	64
Young[19]	1996	33	Ganglionectomy	79
Taha (unpublished)	2000	3	Ganglionectomy	100

T A B L E 1 9 0 - 2 ■ **Results of Rhizotomy and Ganglionectomy in the Treatment of Noncancer Pain in Selected Series**

AUTHOR	YEAR	NO. OF PATIENTS	SURGERY	SUCCESS (%)
Scoville[5]	1966	12	Rhizotomy	50
Echols[35]	1969	62	Rhizotomy	60
White & Sweet[17]	1969	19	Rhizotomy	63
Loeser[23]	1972	29	Rhizotomy	25
Onofrio & Campa[37]	1972	211	Rhizotomy	37
Paillas & Pellet[51]	1972	42	Rhizotomy	76
White & Kjellberg[4]	1973	62	Rhizotomy	65
Hosobuchi[34]	1980	3	Ganglionectomy	75
North et al[50]	1991	13	Ganglionectomy	7
Taub et al[16]	1995	61	Ganglionectomy	59
Wetzel et al[52]	1997	37	Ganglionectomy	19
Taha (unpublished)	2000	7	Ganglionectomy	71

achieved success with C2 or C3 ganglionectomy in the treatment of selected patients with craniocervical headache (unpublished data); patients whose pain responded well included those with dull or shooting pains over the suboccipital (C2) or postauricular (C3) areas associated with decreased sensation to pinprick and who experienced total pain relief after unilateral C2 or C3 blockade, respectively. In 1998 Lozano and colleagues[55] described their results with microsurgical C2 ganglionectomy in 39 patients with medically refractory chronic occipital pain. Those who described their pain as shocklike, electric, shooting, jabbing, or sharp generally experienced a favorable outcome after a C2 ganglionectomy. Patients who described their pain as dull, pounding, aching, throbbing, or pressure-like did not achieve favorable results; nor did those with migraine, tension, and vascular headaches involving the occipital area. The procedure failed to relieve occipital neuralgia pain in 17 patients who had undergone a previous occipital neurectomy or C2 rhizolysis.[55] Our experience with C2 ganglionectomy has been satisfactory in carefully selected patients, with a 90% relief of symptoms after follow-up periods as long as 5 years. Blume recently achieved a 79% relief of symptoms in 100 patients by using radiofrequency rhizotomy of C2.[56] Results of the most recent clinical series on occipital neuralgia are presented in Table 190–3.[55–59]

The role of dorsal rhizotomy or ganglionectomy in the treatment of intercostal neuralgia, postherpetic neuralgia pain, and pain following thoracotomy or laparotomy is less clear. Although some series have had success using these procedures in such conditions,[53, 60, 61] others have reported disappointing results.[3, 24] The discrepancy may be related partly to the fact that dorsal rhizotomy or ganglionectomy can alleviate allodynia (an exquisite, evoked sensitivity to touch) and evoked pain but not the deep-seated, spontaneous pain of neuropathic pain syndromes. However, rhizotomy of roots caught in thoracic fractures has been beneficial in more than 60% of cases.[3] Four patients in our series of seven experienced excellent results after ganglionectomy; one patient reported moderate improvement, and two had no change in symptoms after surgery.

Dorsal rhizotomy or ganglionectomy has a limited role in the treatment of neck and arm pain. Although Wetzel[62] concluded that rhizotomy and ganglionectomy had no role in the treatment of chronic benign cervical pain, Harris[3] reported that some of his best results (50% chance of pain relief) with posterior rhizotomy were in patients with cervical and arm pain of post-traumatic origin. In a double-blind study, van Kleef and coworkers[15] documented the value of percutaneous radiofrequency ganglionectomy at a single level in relieving neck and arm pain 8 weeks after surgery. This procedure is based on the fact that somatic and visceral afferent fibers from all potentially nociceptive cervical structures have cell bodies in the dorsal root ganglion. Van Kleef and coworkers recom-

T A B L E 1 9 0 - 3 ■ **Clinical Series on the Treatment of Occipital Neuralgia with Rhizotomy and Ganglionectomy**

AUTHOR	YEAR	NO. OF PATIENTS	SURGERY	SUCCESS (%)
Stechison & Mullin[57]	1994	4	C2 ganglionectomy	100
Dubuisson[58]	1995	11	C1–3 rhizotomy	71
Lozano et al[55]	1998	39	C2 ganglionectomy	82*
Jansen[59]	2000	38	C2 ganglionectomy	84
Blume[56]	2000	100	C2 percutaneous radiofrequency rhizotomy	79
Taha (unpublished)	2000	10	C2 ganglionectomy	90

* Results in selected patients (see text).

mend this procedure for patients who experience at least 1 year of cervicobrachial pain (i.e., continuous dull, aching pain in the middle or lower cervical region that radiates either to one shoulder, beyond the gleno-humeral joint or the lateral margin of the acromion and deltoid muscle, or to the arm). They also recommend the procedure for those who have unilateral localized tenderness to direct palpation in the middle and lower regions of the cervical spine or pain on direct palpation of the trapezius muscle, patients without a definite surgically remediable abnormality, and those with a successful diagnostic block. In another study by van Kleef and associates,[63] however, 75% of the patients improved initially after percutaneous radiofrequency ganglionectomy, but 44% experienced recurrence of pain.

The role of ganglionectomy in the treatment of failed back syndrome is unclear; however, recent well-designed studies have documented its low success rate in the long-term control of chronic radiculopathy. In 1991 North and colleagues[50] reported the results of 13 patients who underwent dorsal root ganglionectomy for failed back syndrome and were followed by an unbiased third party for an average of 5.5 years. Only one patient (7%) had greater than 50% pain relief at long-term follow-up. Another well-designed study by Wetzel and coworkers,[52] involving 37 patients followed for at least 2 years, demonstrated a success rate of only 19%. Despite other studies[29] that demonstrate low success rates of ganglionectomy in treating failed back syndrome, Taub and associates[16, 64] repeatedly endorsed ganglionectomy for the treatment of chronic radiculopathy of the lower extremity associated with failed back syndrome. They emphasize the technique of preoperative selective root blockade as a relatively successful screening test for proper patient selection. A 19-gauge needle, inserted just lateral to the intervertebral foramen, should not produce paresthesia. Selective sensory block without blocking intraradicular sympathetic or motor fibers is created by injecting 7.5 mL of 0.5% lidocaine. The patient should report complete pain relief within 10 to 15 minutes, with a duration of 1.5 to 2 hours. Using this screening test, they reported a 59% success rate in 61 patients. Postoperative dysesthesia, which occurred in up to 59% of patients, was rarely permanent and usually resolved in 2 to 6 weeks. These results, including pain relief and postoperative complications, improved further when patients with exclusive monoradiculopathy were selected.

Dorsal rhizotomy and ganglionectomy seem to have no beneficial role in the treatment of perineal pain of benign origin, coccygodynia,[65] visceral pain syndromes,[3] and postparaplegic pain.[24] Paraplegic patients may experience significant relief of muscular spasm with bilateral L4-S1 dorsal rhizotomy. The procedure has benefited cerebral palsy patients, with reports of decreased motor spasms and improved strength.[66–69] Recently, brachial plexus dorsal rhizotomy has been documented to be an effective treatment for upper limb spasticity, resulting in functional improvement with no loss of sensation in the hand.[70]

CONCLUSION

Dorsal rhizotomy and ganglionectomy have a definite role in the treatment of some pain syndromes related to malignancy. In properly selected patients, these procedures can help patients with noncancer pain as well.

To produce a zone of hypesthesia, typically three or more contiguous roots must be surgically sacrificed. We recommend ganglionectomy for C2 or C3 denervation, intradural rhizotomy for lower cervical denervation, extradural ganglionectomy for thoracic and lumbar denervation, and extradural ligation rhizotomy for sacral denervation.

REFERENCES

1. Bell C: Idea of a New Anatomy of the Brain. London, Strahan & Preston, 1811, pp 17–19.
2. Abbe R: Intradural section of the spinal nerves for neuralgia. Boston Med Surg J 135:329–335, 1896.
3. Harris AB: Dorsal rhizotomy for pain relief. In Tindall G (ed): The Practice of Neurosurgery. Philadelphia, Lippincott Williams & Wilkins, 1995, pp 4029–4032.
4. White JC, Kjellberg RN: Posterior spinal rhizotomy: A substitute for cordotomy in the relief of localized pain in patients with normal life expectancy. Neurochirurgia (Stuttg) 16:141–170, 1973.
5. Scoville WB: Extradural spinal sensory rhizotomy. J Neurosurg 25:94–95, 1966.
6. Smith FP: Trans-spinal ganglionectomy for relief of intercostal pain. J Neurosurg 32:574–577, 1970.
7. Uematsu S: Percutaneous electrothermocoagulation of spinal nerve trunk, ganglion, and rootlets. In Schmidek HH, Sweet WS (eds): Operative Neurosurgical Techniques: Indications, Methods, and Results, 2nd ed. New York, Grune & Stratton, 1988, pp 1207–1221.
8. Coggesshall RE, Ito H: Sensory fibers in ventral roots L7 and S1 in the cat. J Physiol (Lond) 267:215–235, 1977.
9. Osgood CP, Dujovny MD, Faille R, Abassy M: Microsurgical ganglionectomy for chronic pain syndromes. J Neurosurg 45:113–115, 1976.
10. Arbit E, Galicich JH, Burt M, Mallya K: Modified open thoracic rhizotomy for treatment of intractable chest wall pain of malignant etiology. Ann Thorac Surg 48:820–823, 1989.
11. North R, Levy R: Consensus conference on the neurosurgical management of pain. Neurosurgery 34:756–761, 1994.
12. Risling M, Hildebrand C: Occurrence of unmyelinated axon profiles at distal, middle, and proximal levels in the ventral root L7 of cats and kittens. J Neurol Sci 56:219–225, 1982.
13. Coggeshall RE: Afferent fibers in the ventral root. Neurosurgery 4:443–448, 1979.
14. Yamamoto T, Takahashi K, Satomi H: Origins of primary afferent fibers in the spinal ventral roots in the cat as demonstrated by horseradish peroxidase method. Brain Res 126:1350–1357, 1977.
15. van Kleef M, Liem L, Lousberg R, et al: Radiofrequency lesion adjacent to the dorsal root ganglion for cervicobrachial pain: A prospective double blind randomized study. Neurosurgery 38:1127–1132, 1996.
16. Taub A, Robinson F, Taub E: Dorsal root ganglionectomy for intractable monoradicular sciatica. In Schmidek HH, Sweet WH (eds): Operative Neurosurgical Techniques: Indications, Methods, and Results, vol 2, 3rd ed. Philadelphia, WB Saunders, 1995, pp 1585–1593.
17. White JC, Sweet WH: Pain and the Neurosurgeon: A Forty-Year Experience. Springfield, Ill, Charles C Thomas, 1969, pp 633–660.
18. Schwartz HG: Anastomoses between cervical nerve roots. J Neurosurg 13:190–194, 1956.
19. Young RF: Dorsal rhizotomy and dorsal root ganglionectomy. In Youmans JR (ed): Neurological Surgery, vol 5, 4th ed. Philadelphia, WB Saunders, 1996, pp 3442–3451.
20. Gybels JM, Sweet WH: Neurosurgical Treatment of Persistent Pain. Basel, Karger, 1989, pp 109–124.
21. Rodriguez-Bigas M, Petrelli MJ, Herrera L, West C: Intrathecal

phenol rhizotomy for management of pain in recurrent unresectable carcinoma of the rectum. Surg Gynecol Obstet 173:41–44, 1991.

22. Hasue M, Kunogi J, Konno S, Kikuchi S: Classification by position of dorsal root ganglia in the lumbosacral region. Spine 14: 1261–1264, 1989.

23. Loeser JD: Dorsal rhizotomy for the relief of chronic pain. J Neurosurg 36:745–750, 1972.

24. Loeser JD, Sweet WH, Tew JM, et al: Neurosurgical operations involving peripheral nerves. In Bonica JJ (ed): The Management of Pain. Philadelphia, Lea & Febiger, 1990, pp 2044–2066.

25. Crue BL, Todd EM: A simplified technique of sacral rhizotomy for pelvic pain. J Neurosurg 21:835–837, 1964.

26. Letcher FS, Goldring S: The effect of radiofrequency current and heat on peripheral nerve action potential in the cat. J Neurosurg 29:42–47, 1968.

27. Tzaan WC, Tasker RR: Percutaneous radiofrequency facet rhizotomy: Experience with 118 procedures and reappraisal of its value. Can J Neurol Sci 27:125–130, 2000.

28. Denny-Brown D, Kirk EJ: Hyperesthesia from spinal and root lesions. Trans Am Neurol Assoc 93:116–120, 1968.

29. Koerber HR, Brown PB: Quantitative analysis of dorsal horn cell receptive fields following limited deafferentation. J Neurophysiol 74:2065–2076, 1995.

30. Hodge CJ, King RB: Medical modification of sensation. J Neurosurg 44:21–28, 1976.

31. Stevens CW, Seybold VS: Changes of opioid binding density in the rat spinal cord following unilateral dorsal rhizotomy. Brain Res 687:53–62, 1995.

32. Kato S, Otsuki T, Yamamoto T, et al: Retrograde Adriamycin sensory ganglionectomy: Novel approach for the treatment of intractable pain. Stereotact Funct Neurosurg 54–55:86–89, 1990.

33. Chung K, Lee BH, Yoon YW, Chung JM: Sympathetic sprouting in the dorsal root ganglia of the injured peripheral nerve in a rat neuropathic pain model. J Comp Neurol 376:241–252, 1996.

34. Hosobuchi Y: The majority of unmyelinated afferent axons in human ventral root probably conduct pain. Pain 8:167–180, 1980.

35. Echols DH: Sensory rhizotomy following operation for ruptured intravertebral disc: A review of 62 cases. J Neurosurg 31:335–338, 1969.

36. Hoppenstein R: A new approach to the failed back syndrome. Spine 5:371–379, 1980.

37. Onofrio BM, Campa HK: Evaluation of rhizotomy: Review of 12 years' experience. J Neurosurg 36:751–755, 1972.

38. Strait TA, Hunter SE: Intraspinal extradural sensory rhizotomy in patients with failure of lumbar disc surgery. J Neurosurg 54: 193–196, 1981.

39. Young RF: Dorsal rhizotomy and dorsal root ganglionectomy. In Youmans JR (ed): Neurological Surgery, vol 6, 3rd ed. Philadelphia, WB Saunders, 1990, pp 4026–4035.

40. Sweet WH: Deafferentation pain after posterior rhizotomy, trauma to a limb, and herpes zoster. Neurosurgery 15:928–932, 1984.

41. Pagni CA, Lanotte M, Canavero S: How frequent is anesthesia dolorosa following spinal posterior rhizotomy? A retrospective analysis of fifteen patients. Pain 54:323–327, 1993.

42. Rossitch E, Abdulhak M, Ovelmen-Levitt J, et al: The expression of deafferentation dysesthesias reduced by dorsal root entry zone lesions in the rat. J Neurosurg 78:598–602, 1993.

43. Koening HM, Koster HG, Niemeijer RP: Ischemic spinal cord lesion following percutaneous radiofrequency spinal rhizotomy. Pain 45:161–166, 1991.

44. Jacox A, Carr DB, Payne R: Management of Cancer Pain. Clinical Practice Guideline No. 9. Bethesda, Md, US Department of Health and Human Services, 1994.

45. Barrash JM, Leavens ME: Dorsal rhizotomy for the relief of intractable pain of malignant tumor origin. J Neurosurg 38:755–757, 1973.

46. Sindou M, Larpas C: Neurosurgical treatment for pain in the Pancoast-Tobias syndrome: Selective posterior rhizotomy and open anterolateral C2 cordotomy. In Bonica JJ (ed): Advances in Pain Research and Therapy, vol 4. New York, Raven Press, 1982, pp 199–206.

47. Nash TP: Percutaneous radiofrequency lesioning of dorsal root ganglia for intractable pain. Pain 24:67–73, 1986.

48. Swerdlow M: Neurolytic blocks of the neuraxis. In Patt RB (ed): Cancer Pain. Philadelphia, JB Lippincott, 1993, pp 427–442.

49. Kori SH: Diagnosis and management of brachial plexus lesions in cancer patients. Oncology (Huntingt) 9:756–760, 1995.

50. North RB, Kidd DH, Campbell JN, Long DM: Dorsal root ganglionectomy for failed back surgery syndrome: A 5-year follow-up study. J Neurosurg 74:236–242, 1991.

51. Paillas JW, Pellet W: Dorsal nerve root section in the treatment of refractory peripheral pain. In Janzen E (ed): Pain. Stuttgart, Thieme, 1972, pp 209–213.

52. Wetzel FT, Phillips FM, Aprill CN, et al: Extradural sensory rhizotomy in the management of chronic lumbar radiculopathy: A minimum 2-year follow up study. Spine 22:2283–2291, 1997.

53. Arguelles J, Burchiel K: Ablative neurosurgical procedures for the treatment of pain: Peripheral. In Tindall G (ed): The Practice of Neurosurgery. Baltimore, Williams & Wilkins, 1996, pp 3153–3175.

54. Stechison MT, Mullin RB: Surgical treatment of greater occipital neuralgia: An appraisal of strategies. Acta Neurochir (Wien) 131: 236–240, 1994.

55. Lozano AM, Vanderlinden G, Bachoo R, Rothbart P: Microsurgical C-2 ganglionectomy for chronic intractable occipital pain. J Neurosurg 89:359–365, 1998.

56. Blume HG: Cervicogenic headaches: Radiofrequency neurotomy and the cervical disc and fusion. Clin Exp Rheumatol 18(Suppl 19):S53–S58, 2000.

57. Stechison MT, Mullin BB: Surgical treatment of greater occipital neuralgia: An appraisal of strategies. Acta Neurochir (Wien) 131: 236–240, 1994.

58. Dubuisson D: Treatment of occipital neuralgia by partial posterior rhizotomy at C1-C3. J Neurosurg 82:581–586, 1995.

59. Jansen J: Surgical treatment of non-responsive cervicogenic headache. Clin Exp Rheumatol 18(Suppl 19):S67–S70, 2000.

60. Garcia Cosamalon PJ, Mostaza A, Fernandez J, et al: Dorsal percutaneous radiofrequency rhizotomy guided with CT scan in intercostal neuralgias: Technical note. Acta Neurochir (Wien) 109: 140–141, 1991.

61. Stolker RJ, Vernest AC, Groen GJ: The treatment of chronic thoracic segmental pain by radiofrequency percutaneous partial rhizotomy. J Neurosurg 80:986–992, 1994.

62. Wetzel FT: Chronic benign cervical pain syndromes: Surgical considerations. Spine 17(Suppl 10):S367–S374, 1992.

63. van Kleef M, Spaans F, Dingemans W, et al: Effects and side effects of a percutaneous thermal lesion of the dorsal root ganglion in patients with cervical pain syndrome. Pain 52:49–53, 1993.

64. Taub A: Relief of chronic intractable sciatica by dorsal root ganglionectomy. Trans Am Neurol Assoc 105:340–343, 1980.

65. Saris SC, Silver JM, Viera JFS, Nashold BS: Sacrococcygeal rhizotomy for perineal pain. Neurosurgery 19:789–793, 1986.

66. Steinbok P, Reiner AM, Beauchamp R, et al: A randomized clinical trial to compare selective posterior rhizotomy plus physiotherapy with physiotherapy alone in children with spastic diplegic cerebral palsy. Dev Med Child Neurol 39:178–184, 1997.

67. Loewen P, Steinbok P, Holsti L, MacKay M: Upper extremity performance and self-care skill changes in children with spastic cerebral palsy following selective posterior rhizotomy. Pediatr Neurosurg 29:191–198, 1998.

68. Fukuhara T, Najm IM, Levin KH, et al: Nerve rootlets to be sectioned for spasticity resolution in selective dorsal rhizotomy. Surg Neurol 54:126–133, 2000.

69. Engsberg JR, Ross SA, Park TS: Changes in ankle spasticity and strength following selective dorsal rhizotomy and physical therapy for spastic cerebral palsy. J Neurosurg 9:727–732, 1999.

70. Bertelli JA, Ghizoni MF, Michels A: Brachial plexus dorsal rhizotomy in the treatment of upper-limb spasticity. J Neurosurg 93: 26–32, 2000.

Dorsal Root Entry Zone and Brainstem Ablative Procedures

JOHN P. GORECKI

Ablative surgical procedures performed in the dorsal root entry zone (DREZ) have the primary objective of permanently destroying second-order neurons involved in the nociceptive afferent pathway. The nucleus caudalis, found in the brainstem, is similar to the DREZ. Ablative procedures performed in the spinothalamic tract destroy the axons of second-order neurons rather than cell bodies and interneurons. The spinothalamic tract for the contralateral body is uniquely located in contact with the spinothalamic tract for the contralateral face in the midbrain, providing an opportunity to treat pain that overlaps the head and neck. Because both midbrain tractotomy and nucleus caudalis DREZ (NCD) ablation treat pain in the face by destroying second-order neurons, it is appropriate to compare and contrast these procedures in one chapter. DREZ ablation and microsurgical DREZotomy are considered together. NCD, trigeminal nucleotomy, and descending trigeminal tractotomy are all used to treat facial pain of benign origin. This chapter reviews the indications, techniques, and outcomes for all these ablative procedures that focus on second-order neurons.

Midbrain tractotomy is the procedure of choice for unilateral cancer pain that extends above the fifth cervical dermatome level. The DREZ operations are unique exceptions to the generalization that ablative procedures are limited to the management of cancer pain. DREZ ablation or microsurgical DREZotomy are effective procedures for the central pain associated with plexus avulsion and the nociceptive pain associated with spinal cord injury (SCI). In addition, NCD, trigeminal nucleotomy, and descending tractotomy are effective for facial pain associated with anesthesia dolorosa, atypical facial pain, postherpetic pain, trauma-induced pain, and some deafferentation pains.

The mechanism of action for these destructive procedures is based on straightforward assumptions. The pain perceived in response to nociceptive stimuli should be eliminated if the normal nociceptive pathway is ablated. Cancer pain should be effectively and permanently removed if ablation occurs at the level of the second-order neurons within the central nervous system. Ablation within the peripheral nervous system

is often ineffective owing to nerve regeneration. The perception of pain, in addition to being a response to nociceptive input, is influenced by spontaneous neuronal activity within the central nervous system. In many central pain syndromes, abnormally increased electrophysiologic activity is identified within the dorsal horn.[1, 2] This abnormal activity is causally related to pain. Destruction of the DREZ eliminates dorsal horn electrical activity, helping to manage such central pain syndromes.

Cranial nerves V, VII, IX, and X carry somatic sensory input from the face. The fibers that carry somatic sensory input centrally are located in the descending trigeminal tract, which terminates in the nucleus caudalis. The nucleus caudalis is one of three subdivisions within the nucleus of the spinal tract. The nucleus caudalis contains second-order neurons for nociception from the head and face. The descending trigeminal tract and nucleus caudalis are targets for a number of ablative surgical procedures. The axons from the nucleus caudalis normally cross, travel in the quintothalamic tract, and terminate in synapses on third-order neurons in the thalamus or periaqueductal gray matter.

Ablative procedures that target the descending trigeminal tract and nucleus caudalis are presently performed either as open microsurgical operations or as operations using stereotactic methods. The ablative lesions consist of a series of lesions that coalesce over a length of the medulla and upper spinal cord, a single cylindrical or spherical lesion, or a single transverse incision. NCD ablation, trigeminal nucleotomy, and descending trigeminal tractotomy refer to these ablative operations.

DREZ ABLATION AND MICROSURGICAL DREZOTOMY

Anatomy and Physiology

Rolando is credited with describing the H-shaped central gray structure in the spinal cord.[3] He also identified the substantia gelatinosa, which corresponds to the second layer of the laminae later described by Rexed.[4] The first synaptic relay within the sensory system occurs in the dorsal horn. Larger afferent fibers project to laminae III and IV. Fine fibers project to laminae I, II, and V. The afferent nociceptive signal is modified within the dorsal horn by interneuronal and descending connections.

Indications

DREZ ablation has been used to treat painful conditions with many different causes. Conclusions regarding the indications for DREZ coagulation are drawn from more than 800 patients who have undergone DREZ ablation at Duke since 1976. These conclusions are supported by independent reports from other centers. DREZ ablation is effective for the relief of spontaneous pain due to brachial or lumbosacral plexus avulsion and for nociceptive-induced pain due to SCI located in an "end zone" pattern. DREZ ablation has a limited role for postherpetic pain. The indications for and limitations of DREZ coagulation in these conditions are well defined, but only by retrospective data.

The rate of satisfactory outcome following DREZ coagulation for pain due to brachial plexus avulsion is between 66% and 87%.[5-12] A retrospective review of 91 patients undergoing DREZ coagulation at Duke for brachial plexus avulsion confirms that 90% of patients were pain free at the time of hospital discharge.[13] Long-term outcome results were available for 55 patients. Complete pain relief was obtained in 18 patients (33%), good relief in 22 (40%), fair relief in 8 (14%), and poor pain relief in 7 (13%). The incidence of routine opiate intake diminished from 85% preoperatively to 38% following DREZ ablation. Five patients reported pain recurrence 6 to 9 years after DREZ coagulation; however, pain usually recurs within the first 6 months after surgery. A retrospective review of 39 patients who underwent surgery for pain due to conus medullaris and cauda equina trauma found that 54% of patients were pain free and off medication following DREZ ablation.[14]

DREZ ablation is effective for nociceptive-type end-zone pain but not for the more diffuse, spontaneous, central pain associated with SCI.[11, 15-17] A retrospective review of patients with SCI was carried out in which 105 patients underwent 127 DREZ operations; follow-up data were available for 45 subjects.[18] Reduced pain was evident at the time of discharge; 62% of the patients were pain free, and 21% had reduced pain. Sindou and Daher reported good relief of end-zone pain in 71% of patients.[15] Friedman and Nashold reported good relief of end-zone pain in 74% of patients, but only 20% of patients with diffuse pain had good relief.[16] Likewise, cordotomy provided effective control of end-zone pain in 62% of 34 patients.[19] Another way of describing end-zone pain, rather than by its anatomic location, is to refer to its induced and intermittent character. In contrast, the diffuse pain that is less responsive to ablation is constant, spontaneous, and often dysesthetic.

The outcome results of DREZ ablation in patients with postherpetic neuralgia is less clear. The complication rate is higher following DREZ surgery for postherpetic pain because shingles occurs more commonly in the elderly and often involves thoracic dermatomes. The thoracic cord is smaller in cross-sectional area than either the cervical or the lumbar expansions of the cord. Consequently, the incidence of inadvertent injury to the dorsal column or the corticospinal tract is higher. The DREZ operation has been performed at Duke 96 times on 86 patients with postherpetic neuralgia. Discharge pain evaluations revealed complete relief in 53% and partial relief in 33%. Pain relief at 6- to 12-week follow-up was complete in 47% and partial in 28%. In another study, pain relief at follow-up was complete in 18% and incomplete in less than 50%.[20] Earlier literature revealed much more favorable results with the DREZ operation for postherpetic neuralgia. Friedman and Bullitt reported good pain relief in 8 of 12 patients with postherpetic neuralgia.[21] In a follow-up study of 32 patients, 29 reported immediate relief, and 8 had excellent pain relief lasting 18 months; there was incomplete pain relief in 10.[22] The pain relief obtained following DREZ ablation for postherpetic neuralgia is not consistently maintained.

Fewer cases are available to evaluate the role of DREZ ablation for postamputation pain, but the conclusions are clearer than for postherpetic neuralgia. Results indicate good relief in six of nine patients with phantom pain and in five of six with amputation associated with root avulsion, but results were poor for patients with stump pain alone or stump pain associated with phantom pain.[23] DREZ coagulation is a reasonable intervention for phantom pain as well as root avulsion pain. Whenever DREZ ablation is offered to treat stump pain, however, the patient should be warned of a possible poor outcome, and the surgery should be performed as part of an outcome study.

DREZ coagulation is not indicated for other conditions. The results following DREZ ablation for 7 patients with brachial plexus radiation, 12 with brachial plexus stretch, 6 with cancer, 13 with post-thoracotomy pain, and 10 with reflex sympathetic dystrophy (now classified as complex regional pain syndrome) were unrewarding. All 113 patients with peripheral nerve injury who underwent DREZ coagulation were still experiencing pain at the time of follow-up.[24]

Preoperative Management

The incidence of pain immediately following plexus avulsion is initially 90% but may drop to 30% by 3 years.[25, 26] Therefore, DREZ ablation should be delayed 12 months. Motor vehicle accidents, especially those involving motorcycles, are the most common cause of brachial plexus avulsion. Most victims describe burning spontaneous pain that begins within 3 days in 50% of patients and is almost always present by 4 months. Magnetic resonance imaging and computed tomography–myelography are the primary diagnostic tools. Diagnostic studies may or may not show pseudomeningoceles.[27] Patients commonly undergo procedures aimed at improving motor function and improving the rate of reinnervation, such as neurolysis, nerve grafting, or tendon transfer.

Before considering DREZ ablation for patients with SCI, stability of the spine and adequate decompression must be demonstrated. Syringomyelia complicates some SCIs. Whenever a cyst is identified in a patient with SCI, Nashold recommends simultaneous treatment of the syringomyelia and DREZ ablation. An alternative approach is to treat the cyst first and perform a second operation for DREZ coagulation only when necessary. In this way, DREZ coagulation can be avoided in some patients, but at the risk of having to perform the DREZ operation in a scarred field. Presently, useful data comparing the two approaches are not available.

Before considering DREZ ablation for avulsion or SCI pain, patients should undertake a trial of analgesics, tricyclic antidepressants, and antiepileptics. The regimen currently used in our clinic for neuropathic pain includes the following: tricyclic antidepressants, carbamazepine, gabapentin, phenytoin, intravenous and topical lidocaine, topical aspirin, clonidine via any route, topical dimethyl sulfoxide, capsaicin, nonsteroidal anti-inflammatory drugs, mexiletine, steroids, and narcotics.[28] Almost all the patients referred for intervention have tried narcotic agents, usually to the point of side effects. The average time between injury and DREZ coagulation performed at Duke was 3.8 years, with a range of 3 months to 41 years.

Surgical Technique

DREZ is performed as a microsurgical procedure with the patient under general anesthesia. Perioperative intravenous steroids are used; the dose corresponds to the standard dose used for acute SCI (30 mg/kg bolus of methylprednisolone over 15 minutes, followed by a maintenance dose of 5.4 mg/kg per hour infusion for 23 hours). The patient is positioned prone, with the head held in Mayfield pins for the cervical laminectomy. A laminectomy is performed to expose the area in the spinal cord that corresponds to the dermatomal pattern of pain. For pain due to brachial plexus avulsion, DREZ lesions are normally performed at cord levels corresponding to C5-T1. The laminectomy extends from the top of C3 to a slight undercutting of T1, because the spinal cord segment levels are displaced relative to the vertebral body levels. When roots have been avulsed, the specific location of the pathology within the spinal cord is obvious to direct visual examination through the operating microscope. A change in color and size identifies stretched or partially avulsed roots or rootlets. Pseudomeningoceles are often but not always present. With or without the aid of electrophysiologic recordings, anatomic landmarks identify the location of the DREZ. The DREZ corresponds to the lateral edge of the dorsal column, or the dorsolateral sulcus. The sensory rootlets enter the spinal cord at the DREZ. Identifying the dorsolateral sulcus can be difficult when the roots are absent. The upper and lower location of the sulcus can be identified by the entry point of normal rootlets rostral and caudal to the pathology. The position of the rootlets exiting from the contralateral normal side can help the surgeon determine the location of the dorsolateral sulcus.

A series of cylindrical lesions is made using radiofrequency current passed through the DREZ electrode. The electrode has a diameter of 0.25 mm and an exposed tip that is 2 mm long. There is thick plastic insulation around the electrode that reaches down to the exposed tip. This plastic covering abuts the surface of the spinal cord when the electrode has penetrated to the correct depth. The temperature at the tip of the electrode and the time that the temperature is maintained control the size of the lesion. The standard lesion is made at a target temperature of 75°C for 15 seconds. Timing begins after the target temperature is achieved. The lesions are made as close together as possible. The cylindrical areas of coagulation are located in a plane perpendicular to the long axis of the cord. These coagulation sites coalesce to form a single flattened, sausage-shaped lesion along the length of the dorsal horn within the cord. The individual lesions are 1 mm apart. Therefore, approximately 50 lesions should be made over a length of cord measuring 50 mm.

Electrophysiologic monitoring during DREZ coagulation can assist in segmental localization and reduce the incidence of complications. A stimulus is applied to a peripheral nerve, and the electrical signal is recorded from an electrode placed directly over the cord. Recording must be done on the normal contralateral side of the cord when roots are avulsed. The peak electrical signal deflection is recorded from the DREZ of the dermatome level corresponding to the nerve being stimulated. An intraoperative x-ray taken with a radiopaque marker at the foramen is often sufficient for anatomic localization. Alternatively, the ventral motor root is stimulated with hook electrodes, and an electromyogram (EMG) is recorded to confirm the segmental level. EMG recording following motor root stimulation is the more accurate method of localization. Before a lesion is made, the EMG is recorded while electrical current is passed through the lesioning electrode. The electrode is assumed to be too close to the corticospinal tract if an EMG response is obtained in the leg at a threshold of less than 1 volt; in that case, the DREZ electrode is repositioned before making a lesion.

The dura is closed in a watertight fashion once the lesions are completed. The wound is closed using the routine techniques of intradural spinal surgery.

Microsurgical DREZotomy

Sindou first reported microsurgical DREZotomy in 1972.[29, 30] This operation is also an open microsurgical procedure. The goal of this technique is the specific destruction of the small, unmyelinated fibers that make up the substantia gelatinosa.

An opening is made in the dorsal portion of the spinal cord, starting at the lateral edge of the sensory nerve root. The lesion is carried down to the dorsal horn gray matter, which can be recognized visually. A blade is used to make a sharp incision that is extended using microcoagulation. The lesion is directed 45 degrees ventromedially and is 2 to 3 mm deep.

Microsurgical DREZotomy accomplishes the following: (1) interrupts small nociceptive fibers laterally and large myotatic fibers centrally, while sparing large medial lemniscal fibers; (2) destroys the excitatory medial part of Lissauer's tract; and (3) destroys cells of the dorsal-most layer of the dorsal horn (i.e., Rexed's laminae I to III).

Microsurgical DREZotomy is indicated for the following conditions: (1) localized pain associated with cancer; (2) neuropathic pain from brachial plexus avulsion, cauda equina and spinal cord lesions (segmental), peripheral nerve injury, herpes (allodynia and paroxysmal), and amputation; (3) spasticity; and (4) neurogenic hyperactive bladder. Good relief was reported in 87% of 46 cancer patients and in 87% of 139 patients with neurogenic pain. Microsurgical DREZotomy is most effective for radiculometameric pain due to SCI. Just as with DREZ ablation, pain relief is optimal when microsurgical DREZotomy is used to treat avulsion, paroxysmal pain, and allodynia. Results are inconsistent when treating stump pain.[12]

Dreval, who used an ultrasonic aspirator to produce a DREZ sulcomyelotomy,[5] modified Sindou's technique. A trough is made in the DREZ in the dorsolateral sulcus at the appropriate rostral to caudal level, based on the level of the pain. In a 1993 report, pain relief was described in 96% of patients treated for plexus avulsion pain with this modified procedure.[5]

Postoperative Principles

After surgery, patients are routinely observed for 8 to 12 hours in the neurosurgical intensive care unit, where blood pressure is monitored and manipulated aggressively to optimize cord perfusion. Patients are maintained on bed rest for an arbitrary period to reduce the risk of cerebrospinal fluid leak. If a new neurological deficit is noted, urgent radiologic imaging of the operated level of the spine using either computed tomography or magnetic resonance imaging is undertaken. Perioperative hematoma, infection, and instability are uncommon. The hospital stay is rarely more than 4 days in total.

Pitfalls and Complications

DREZ ablation and microsurgical DREZotomy are both open and invasive procedures. Risks of DREZ ablation include the general complications associated with intradural spinal surgery. After more than 800 DREZ operations at Duke, there have been two postoperative deaths. Complete sensory denervation in a segmental pattern that corresponds to the lesioned levels is a side effect rather than a complication specific to DREZ ablation. Patients who undergo DREZ ablation for SCI pain routinely describe a sensory level that is two to four levels more cephalad than that reported preoperatively. SCI is a potential complication following DREZ ablation; the most common deficit involves injury to the ipsilateral dorsal column. The ipsilateral corticospinal tract is also at risk for injury, which results in ipsilateral leg weakness. Some of the neurological findings in the lower extremities of patients who underwent DREZ coagulation can be explained by injury to the spinocerebellar tract. The incidence of leg weakness is reported to be 5%. Leg weakness is more common following surgery involving the thoracic cord.

NUCLEUS CAUDALIS DREZ ABLATION, DESCENDING TRIGEMINAL TRACTOTOMY, AND TRIGEMINAL NUCLEOTOMY

Anatomy and Physiology

The trigeminal nerve is the main sensory nerve for the face and head. Cranial nerves VII, IX, and X, in addition to the upper cervical sensory branches, also transmit sensation for the head and face. The nuclei of the trigeminal nerve include the motor nucleus of V, the chief sensory nucleus, the mesencephalic nucleus, and the nucleus of the spinal tract. The nucleus of the spinal tract is located in the medulla and is divided into three parts, based on the work of Olszewski[31]: pars caudalis, pars interpolaris (or oralis), and pars rostralis. The histology is indistinguishable between the nucleus of the trigeminal tract and the gray matter of the dorsal horn of the upper cervical cord. The nucleus of the spinal tract receives input from the descending trigeminal tract. Fibers transmitting pain and nociceptive signals originating from cranial nerves V, VII, IX, and X are included in the descending trigeminal tract. Some of the fibers in the spinal tract mingle within Lissauer's zone in the uppermost three segments of the cervical cord. Nociceptive fibers terminate in the nucleus caudalis within the medulla. The nucleus caudalis is a rostral extension of the dorsal horn of the spinal cord.

Cell bodies of trigeminal primary sensory neurons are located within the gasserian ganglion and the mesencephalic nucleus. The gasserian ganglion corresponds anatomically to segmental dorsal root ganglia. The mesencephalic nucleus contains unipolar primary sensory neurons involved in proprioception. The mesencephalic nucleus, which is made up of primary sensory neuronal cell bodies, is located beneath the lateral edge of the fourth ventricle. The location of these cell bodies within the central nervous system instead of within ganglia is anatomically unique.

The neurons in the sensory trigeminal nuclei represent second-order neurons. Efferent fibers from these neurons terminate in the nucleus ambiguus, hypoglossal nucleus, reticular formation, cerebellum, and both the ventral and dorsal trigeminothalamic tracts to the thalamus.

Somatotopic organization is described within the descending trigeminal tract and the nucleus caudalis. Two different patterns describe this segmental organization of sensory representation. The first is a pattern of concentric rings that have been compared to "onion rings." Sensation from the middle portion of the face immediately surrounding the mouth is represented at more rostral levels within the medulla. The difficulty in achieving dense analgesia close to the midline of the face with nucleotomy or tractotomy supports this theoretical pattern. When nucleotomy is performed at more caudal levels within the medulla, preservation of pain appreciation occurs in the midline of the face. The second pattern is based on the segmental trigeminal divisions. Fibers that originate in the first trigeminal division reach a more caudal level within the nucleus caudalis and descending tract than do fibers that originate in the third division. Direct sensory evoked potential recording performed during surgery confirms this anatomy. Observations following nucleotomy or tractotomy also confirm that dense analgesia is much easier to achieve in the first trigeminal division than in the third division. The third division of the trigeminal nerve is not represented as far caudally in the medulla. Based on trigeminal divisions, segmentation is also present from medial to lateral within the medulla. Immediately adjacent to the dorsal column and most medially in the descending tract are fibers from cranial nerves VII, IX, and X. Fibers from the third trigeminal division are located immediately lateral to fibers from nerves VII, IX, and X next to the dorsal column. Fibers from the first trigeminal division are located most laterally within the descending tract, farthest from the dorsal columns and closer to the motor roots of the vagus and spinal accessory nerves. The lesion must be made close to the dorsal column and relatively rostral in the medulla to achieve dense analgesia that includes the third trigeminal division. The risk of undesired injury to the dorsal column and the corresponding risk of proprioceptive deficit are increased when the lesion is in the location described.

Indications

NCD ablation is indicated for the treatment of medically intractable pain in the face. The operation is performed with the patient under general anesthesia and involves exposure of the upper spinal cord and lower brainstem. Offering such an invasive procedure to patients debilitated by malignancy is unnecessary, because many stereotactic and percutaneous techniques are appropriate for cancer pain. Bilateral pain can and has been treated by NCD ablation. Patients with "end-stage" trigeminal neuralgia are offered NCD ablation; these patients have failed all medical intervention and at least one of the more common surgical procedures for trigeminal neuralgia, such as microvascular decompression, radiofrequency retrogasserian rhizolysis, glycerol, balloon compression, avulsion, alcohol ablation, and open nerve section. NCD ablation is especially effective for first-division pain that is difficult to treat with the operations listed. The development of corneal anesthesia following surgery is unlikely when a patient has a preserved corneal reflex before NCD ablation.

NCD ablation is used to treat postherpetic neuralgia, atypical facial pain, anesthesia dolorosa, and various deafferentation pain syndromes in the face due to prior surgery or trauma. Nociceptive-type pain is most sensitive to NCD ablation. Pain from tumors compressing the fifth nerve is an indication for NCD ablation, although few cases have been performed. Several authors specifically state that there is no benefit derived from trigeminal tractotomy for postherpetic neuralgia,[32, 33] but early reports about NCD ablation indicate a high incidence of pain relief for postherpetic neuralgia.[34, 35] Longer follow-up with unbiased evaluation has not consistently supported this finding (see Table 191–2). Cluster headache and migraine are also treated with NCD ablation. Table 191–1 summarizes the results for NCD ablation.

Since 1982, 113 operations have been performed at Duke. The lesion-making technique has been consistent since January 1990. Fifty-eight NCD operations performed since 1990 were reviewed. Follow-up evaluation consisted of an interview by a disinterested third party. Complete information was available for 51 patients; 7 patients were lost to follow-up. The mean age in the group of 42 female and 16 male patients was 55.9 years. Mean follow-up was 23.7 months, with a range of 11 to 84 months. The cause of the pain was classified as follows: postherpetic neuralgia in 12, atypical facial pain in 10, stroke in 5, trauma in 10, trigeminal neuralgia in 18, cluster headache in 1, multiple sclerosis with tic douloureux in 1, and schwannoma in 1. The outcome was classified as excellent in 9, good in 2, fair in 14, and poor in 26. The outcome results are shown in Tables 191–2 and 191–3. When patients were asked to subjectively evaluate quality of life, 16 described it as improved, 6 as somewhat improved, 16 as unchanged, and 13 as worse. The mean preoperative verbal score for pain was 9 (range, 6 to 10). Such a high mean score suggests incapacitating pain. The mean postoperative score was 5.2. Before surgery, 100% of the patients were using narcotic medications on a regular basis. Following NCD ablation, only 19 (37%) were still using narcotics.

Caudalis DREZ ablation consistently results in analgesia in the absence of anesthesia. Following the procedure, the incidence of anesthesia dolorosa or painful dysesthesia is very low, and the corneal reflex is preserved. For these two reasons, lesions at the level of the nucleus caudalis are preferable to sectioning of the nerve or root. NCD ablation is most effective at producing analgesia in V1, while at the same time avoiding corneal ulceration. NCD ablation should be considered for the treatment of V1 pain. This surgical procedure is most effective for pain that is intermittent and induced, or nociceptive, in character. If dental pain is present, it may be necessary to include lesions of the pontine trigeminal nucleus or to use midbrain tractotomy to achieve dense dental analgesia. Owing to inconsistent long-term outcome data, it is difficult to define the usefulness of NCD ablation for postherpetic neuralgia.

Preoperative Management

NCD ablation is considered only when pharmacologic management fails and the patient's quality of life is negatively impacted by the pain's severity. Patients

TABLE 191-1 ■ **Summary of Reports on Nucleus Caudalis DREZ Ablation**

AUTHOR	PROCEDURE	NUMBER	OUTCOME	COMPLICATION	COMMENT
Siqueira[75]	Caudalis DREZ	2			First published report
Nashold[76]	Caudalis DREZ				Abstract
Nashold[34]	Caudalis DREZ	13	3 mo: 13 good–excellent 6 mo: 5 good, 1 fair, 7 poor		5/6 with postherpetic pain good at 6 mo
Bernard[77]	Caudalis DREZ	18 (5 postherpetic)	11 excellent 6 good 1 fair 1 poor	Incoordination in 17/21 procedures	Better outcome with less preoperative sensory loss
Nashold[78]	Caudalis DREZ				V1 ventrolateral, V3 dorsomedial
Bernard[35]	Caudalis DREZ	27	Immediate relief in 85%, delayed in 52%	20 with dysmetria	67% relief for herpetic pain; no benefit for 5 repeat procedures
Ishijima[79]	Caudalis DREZ	4	2 with herpetic pain completely relieved	3/4	
Rossitch[80]	Caudalis DREZ	5	5 immediate relief		Cancer
Rawlings[81]	Caudalis DREZ			3%–5%	Dense packing, two rows, proximal electrode insulation
Young[50]	Caudalis DREZ				Proximal insulation technique
Rossitch[82]	Caudalis DREZ	5 cancer			
Sampson[83]	Caudalis DREZ	2			Vascular lesions
Nashold[84]	Caudalis DREZ	Postherpetic, anesthesia dolorosa, tic, oropharyngeal, visceral pain		3%–5%	Nashold/El-Naggar electrode
Chen[85]	Caudalis DREZ	2	100%	None	4- and 5-yr follow-up
Nashold[51]	Caudalis DREZ	21	48% excellent 5% good 5% fair 43% poor	33% ataxia	New electrode
El-Naggar[86]	Caudalis DREZ	10	5 excellent	0%	New electrode
Friedman[87]	Caudalis DREZ			33% ataxia	Best results for postherpetic pain
Grigoryan[88]	Caudalis DREZ	14	11 pain free	1 paresis, 3 ataxia, 1 Brown-Sequard, 1 hypesthesia	Ultrasound
Bullard[89]	Caudalis DREZ	27	7/18 excellent, 5/18 good	50% ataxia, 2 meningitis	
Bullard[90]	Redo caudalis DREZ	20		60% ataxia	Redo
Gorecki[91]	Caudalis DREZ	35	12 excellent 14 good 3 fair 6 poor		Greatest benefit in atypical facial pain
Gorecki[92]	Caudalis DREZ	46	3/39 completely pain free		
Sjoqvist[36]	Intramedullary tractotomy	9	7/9 successful	Vocal cord paralysis, ataxia	
Grant[37]	Intramedullary tractotomy	20		Eliminated risk to restiform	Moved lesion caudal
Hamby[93]	Intramedullary tractotomy	48 (35 tic, 13 neoplasm)	10/28 pain free	5.7% mortality (tic) 46% mortality (neoplasm)	Corneal reflex preserved
Falconer[43]	Intramedullary tractotomy	20			Bilateral possible
Guidetti[94]	Intramedullary tractotomy	124	Pain recurred in 46 (37.1%)	Cerebellar problems in 19% of those operated caudally	Dysesthesia occurred in only 8

(continued)

TABLE 191-1 ■ Continued

AUTHOR	PROCEDURE	NUMBER	OUTCOME	COMPLICATION	COMMENT
McKenzie[95]	Intramedullary tractotomy	42	25% residual spots of pain	No corneal anesthesia	Developed medullary spinothalamic tractotomy
Moffie[96]	Intramedullary tractotomy	8	4 pain free, 4 slight pain		13–15 yr follow-up
Hosobuchi[38]	Intramedullary tractotomy	6	All	No lemniscal	SEP
Young[39]	Intramedullary tractotomy				Dental pain may be in pons
Hitchcock[97]	Trigeminal nucleotomy	7			
Hitchcock[98]	Trigeminal nucleotomy	3	All good for herpes	Spinothalamic tract, dorsal column	Short follow-up
Crue[47]	Trigeminal nucleotomy				
Fox[48]	Trigeminal nucleotomy				Free hand
Schvarcz[99]	Trigeminal nucleotomy	104	Herpetic 87.5%, anesthesia dolorosa 57%, dysesthesia 72%, cancer 83.3%		Procedure of choice for postherpetic pain
Hitchcock[100]	Trigeminal nucleotomy	13	4/4		Pontine trigeminal nuclei
Kanpolat[45]	Trigeminal nucleotomy	30	24 satisfactory	4 ataxia	Done in CT suite

CT, computed tomography; DREZ, dorsal root entry zone; SEP, somatosensory evoked potential.

being considered for NCD ablation undergo psychological evaluation to verify that no underlying psychiatric illness requiring therapy coexists. This validates the patient's understanding of informed consent.

Surgical Technique

NUCLEUS CAUDALIS DREZ ABLATION

Surgery is performed with the patient under general anesthesia and positioned prone; the head is supported by pin fixation. Muscle relaxation is not continued to permit EMG recording. An eccentric craniectomy is performed on the side ipsilateral to the pain to expose the cerebellar tonsils. The arch of C1 is removed on the same side, but the bone of C2 is left intact. Following an eccentric curvilinear or Y-shaped incision, the dura is held open more widely on the symptomatic side. The obex; rootlets of C1, C2, and cranial nerve XI; vertebral artery; and dorsolateral sulcus are the landmarks included in the exposure. A series of radiofrequency lesions is made extending cephalad from the uppermost sensory rootlet of C2, along the dorsolateral sulcus. The lesions are made by applying the electrode at a temperature of 80°C for 15 to 20 seconds. The lesioning electrode diameter is 0.25 mm. The electrodes incorporate insulation on the most proximal segment that penetrates the central nervous system. The purpose of the insulation is to prevent coagulation of the central nervous system close to the surface. Especially at the more cephalad locations, the spinocerebellar tract overlies the descending trigeminal tract. Two different sized electrodes are used, with the longer one being used to make lesions more cephalad, beyond the rootlet

of C1. The nucleus caudalis has a larger cross-sectional diameter at more cephalad levels, and the pyramidal tract does not lie in immediate contact with the deep surface of the nucleus caudalis at more cephalad levels, so the longer electrode can be used safely. Using the shorter electrode at more caudal levels reduces the chance of injury to the pyramidal tract. To make the procedure more ergonomic for the surgeon, the electrodes contain a curve close to the active tip.

We have introduced more aggressive electrophysiologic monitoring during the operative technique. The anatomy is mapped by recording trigeminal somatosensory evoked potentials (TSEPs) directly from the electrode tip that penetrates the cord and medulla. Simultaneously TSEPs are recorded from the scalp. The evoked potentials arise from electrical triggers passed through bipolar needle electrodes placed adjacent to the mental nerve, infraorbital nerve, and supraorbital nerve. The threshold stimulus required to produce a minimal response and the amplitude of the TSEP along the dorsolateral sulcus are recorded. It is therefore possible to localize the portion of the nucleus caudalis or descending tract that corresponds to various divisions of the trigeminal nerve. The lesion is tailored based on symptoms. The number of lesions made in each patient is reduced; consequently, the incidence of complications is reduced, because each time a lesion is created, there is a finite risk of complications.

The lateral margin of the cuneate nucleus can be mapped by recording somatosensory evoked potentials (SEPs) induced by a stimulus applied to the ipsilateral median nerve. As the recording electrode is progressively moved to a more lateral position, a point is

T A B L E 1 9 1 – 2 ■ **Outcome Following Nucleus Caudalis DREZ Ablation Based on Retrospective Evaluation of 58 Patients Treated at Duke: Classified by Cause of Pain**

CAUSE OF PAIN	NUMBER	OUTCOME*	CHANGE IN VDS	WILLING TO REPEAT[†]
Anesthesia Dolorosa				
Tic[‡]	18	Excellent 1 Good 0 Fair 3 Poor 12 Lost 2	Decrease 0.3	No 10 Yes 5 Unsure 1 Lost 2
Stroke	5	Excellent 0 Good 0 Fair 2 Poor 2 Lost 1	Decrease 0.5	No 3 Yes 1 Lost 1
Schwannoma	1	Excellent 0 Good 0 Fair 0 Poor 1 Lost 0	Decrease 0	No 1 Yes 0 Unsure 0
Multiple sclerosis	1	Excellent 0 Good 0 Fair 0 Poor 0 Lost 1	Lost	No 0 Yes 0 Lost 1
Trauma§—deafferentation	4	Excellent 0 Good 0 Fair 1 Poor 3 Lost	Decrease 0	No 3 Yes 0 Unsure 1
Nociceptive Trauma§	6	Excellent 4 Good 2 Fair 0 Poor 0 Lost 0	Decrease 5.0	No 0 Yes 5 Unsure 1
Cluster headache	1	Excellent Good Fair Poor Lost 1	Lost	Lost 1
Postherpetic neuralgia	12	Excellent 3 Good 0 Fair 3 Poor 4 Lost 2	Decrease 3.5	No 4 Yes 6 Lost 2
Other Atypical facial pain	10	Excellent 1 Good 0 Fair 5 Poor 4 Lost	Decrease 2.5	No 3 Yes 4 Unsure 3 Lost 0

*Excellent, pain free on no medication; good, pain free on some medication; fair, reduced pain and reduced narcotic intake; poor, pain no better or worse.
†Patient's response to the question: Given the outcome you actually experienced, would you have agreed to undergo the procedure?
‡Trigeminal neuralgia that failed to respond to prior surgical treatment.
§Injury from accident or surgery.
DREZ, dorsal root entry zone; VDS, verbal score for pain.

reached beyond which evoked potentials are no longer recorded unless the intensity of the stimulus is increased substantially. The amplitude of the recorded SEP drops sharply at this point. This line corresponds to the location from which low-threshold TSEPs are recorded.

Passing a stimulating current directly through the electrode while it is penetrating the central nervous system identifies the proximity of the pyramidal tract. When the electrode is close to the pyramidal tract, stimulation results in an EMG response that can be recorded from a leg or arm muscle with a threshold of less than 1 volt. Lesions should not be performed at these locations. We are actively evaluating techniques to record from or demonstrate the location of the spinocerebellar tract.

DESCENDING TRIGEMINAL TRACTOTOMY

Descending trigeminal tractotomy was first performed by Sjoqvist and reported in 1938.[36] His goal was to produce analgesia in the entire ipsilateral face without anesthesia and the accompanying complications of cor-

T A B L E 1 9 1 – 3 ■ **Outcome Following Nucleus Caudalis DREZ Ablation Based on Retrospective Evaluation of 58 Patients Treated at Duke: Classified by Character of Pain**

CHARACTER PAIN	NUMBER	OUTCOME*	WILLING TO REPEAT?[†]
Anesthesia Dolorosa‡			
Trigeminal neuralgia Stroke Trauma Multiple sclerosis Tumor	29	Excellent 1 Good 0 Fair 6 Poor 18 Lost 4	No 17 Yes 6 Unsure 2 Lost 4
Nociceptive§			
Trauma Postherpetic Cluster headache	19	Excellent 7 Good 2 Fair 3 Poor 4 Lost 3	No 4 Yes 11 Unsure 1 Lost 3
Other			
Atypical facial pain	10	Excellent 1 Good 0 Fair 5 Poor 4 Lost 0	No 3 Yes 4 Unsure 3 Lost 0
Total	58	Excellent 9 Good 2 Fair 14 Poor 26 Lost 7	No 24 Yes 23 Unsure 4 Lost 7

*Excellent, pain free on no medication; good, pain free on some medication; fair, reduced pain and reduced narcotic intake; poor, pain no better or worse.
†Patient's response to the question, Given the outcome you actually experienced, would you have agreed to undergo the procedure?
‡Constant, spontaneous pain associated with sensory loss.
§Intermittent, induced pain, usually sharp.

neal anesthesia. He was seeking an alternative to the trigeminal transection as described by Frazier. Descending tractotomy takes advantage of the fact that fibers that terminate in the nucleus caudalis are segregated and carry only the sensation of pain and temperature. The operation results in entire unilateral face analgesia without anesthesia. Descending trigeminal tractotomy has never enjoyed widespread application.

The operation may be carried out with the patient under either general or local anesthesia and in either the prone or sitting position. The advantage of local anesthesia is that the patient can be examined immediately to determine the extent of analgesia; when analgesia is inadequate, the location or depth of the lesion can be modified. Cutting the descending tract is very painful, however.

The exposure involves a small posterior fossa craniectomy and removal of the arch of C1. With a small blade, a transverse incision extending a length of 3 to 4 mm is made to a depth of 3 to 4 mm. The lesion is made between the dorsolateral sulcus (lateral edge of the cuneate nucleus) and the exit point of the rootlets of cranial nerve XI. The exact location of the lesion in a cephalad to caudal direction varies among surgeons. Sjoqvist indicated that the lesion should be made immediately caudal to the lowest rootlets of the vagus. This location corresponds to the junction of the middle and lower third of the olive, where the descending trigeminal tract is no longer covered by the restiform body. Grant and Weinberger later fortuitously discovered that analgesia is still produced throughout the face by a lesion located caudal to the obex.[37] Before cutting the descending tract, TSEPs have been recorded directly from an electrode penetrating the brainstem. The ophthalmic division is represented all the way down to C2; the maxillary division is represented no lower than 12 mm below the obex; and the mandibular division can be recorded only down to 2 to 3 mm below the obex.[38] Evidence from both animal and human studies suggests that pain sensation from the teeth may not exclusively involve the descending tract and nucleus caudalis.[39–41] This information would support creating lesions within the trigeminal nucleus in the pons for pain that includes the gums and teeth (see the next section).

McKenzie's experience with descending trigeminal tractotomy led to two interesting developments.[42] First, the observation of spinothalamic tract deficit in 10 patients led to medullary tractotomy for pain in the body. Second, a high recurrence rate for pain was correctly predicted in patients with residual spots of pinprick appreciation, in contrast to those with complete analgesia.

Bilateral tractotomy is possible and is, in fact, tolerated better than bilateral trigeminal root sections, which would result in unacceptable anesthesia of the entire face.[43]

TRIGEMINAL NUCLEOTOMY

Coagulation of the nucleus caudalis without injury to the adjacent tract is the primary goal of trigeminal

nucleotomy. This operation is performed stereotactically. Kanpolat has re-evaluated the role of trigeminal nucleotomy,[44, 45] which never achieved wide acceptance.

Hitchcock developed a special frame and stereotactic map for use in the posterior fossa and used ventriculography for localization. The target is selected relative to the fourth ventricle and confirmed by electrical stimulation. Stimulation within the nucleus produces ipsilateral painful paresthesia affecting the entire face. Stimulation parameters are unipolar square waves of 0.1-msec duration. Impedance is monitored. The electrode is passed through a bur hole and through the cerebellum, or through the ligament between the occiput and C1 or C2. The selected target is 3 mm anterior to the posterior margin of the spinal cord and 6 mm from the midline at the level of C1.[46] Fractionated lesions are sequentially enlarged with radiofrequency current. The electrode is made of tungsten, with a 0.5-mm diameter sharpened to 50 μm and a 2-mm exposed tip. The average lesion is 3 mm by 3 mm.

Crue and coworkers independently described a similar procedure,[47] and Fox reported a free-hand technique.[48] Today, localization is achieved with both computed tomography and magnetic resonance imaging (MRI). Kanpolat adapted computed tomographic localization and performs surgery in the computed tomography suite.[44] Frameless stereotactic methodology has not yet been adapted to this technique, but at Duke, we are exploring the utility of frameless stereotactic methodology during open nucleus caudalis DREZ ablation. Separately, we are exploring the value of temporary electrodes placed at the time of open surgery to be used for postoperative recording and lesioning in patients who are awake. Endoscopic techniques are being evaluated to allow the creation of lesions in the nucleus caudalis while the patient is awake.

When pain involves the teeth, Hitchcock suggested adding stereotactic lesions of the trigeminal nucleus within the pons. Hitchcock and Teixeira in 1987 deliberately made lesions in the descending tract and pontine trigeminal nucleus in four patients with facial pain.[49]

Postoperative Principles

Patients are monitored for at least 12 hours in the neurosurgical intensive care unit. Level of consciousness and blood pressure are monitored closely. Once the patient is alert, the resulting level of facial analgesia can be readily documented. Based on the residual level of pain, the systemic narcotic intake is modified for a rapid taper. Stereotactic procedures performed without general anesthesia allow for an immediate narcotic taper. Open posterior fossa exposure results in modest postsurgical pain in its own right.

Pitfalls and Complications

Pain relief is not universally achieved by any of these operations. Although the diligence of complication reporting should be viewed with a healthy skepticism, very few complications have been described for stereotactic nucleotomy. This reflects one clear advantage of producing lesions in patients who are awake and cooperative.

Sjoqvist reported that the most common complication was ataxia and blamed the clinical picture on injury to the spinocerebellar tract and restiform body. Ataxia is also the most common complication following NCD ablation. Usually the ipsilateral arm is affected, but sometimes the leg is also affected, resulting in gait impairment. The patient may report an inability to use the affected arm. This complaint is often out of proportion to the physical findings, especially if the patient has completed a course of physiotherapy. Patients may report significant disability even though the residual symptoms are only subjective. Deficits that may be identified include the following: ataxia, past pointing, loss of two-point discrimination, and weakness. Modest weakness is often present as the patient is emerging from anesthesia that resolves completely. We place all patients on high doses of systemic steroids. This complication results from injury to the spinocerebellar tract. Less commonly injured adjacent tracts include the cuneate tract and nucleus, as well as the pyramidal tract.

In an effort to reduce the risk of ataxia, the NCD ablation procedure has been modified three times. The addition of proximal insulation to the electrode was the first modification. The second modification was the introduction of electrodes with two different lengths for lesions in different parts of the nucleus. The so-called Nashold/El-Naggar electrode also includes a bend in the electrode to make the placement of lesions more accurate. Third, precise and rigid electrophysiologic monitoring has now been added. In the earliest reports of NCD ablation, the incidence of ataxia was 90%.[50] With use of the Nashold/El-Naggar electrode, the incidence of ataxia was reported to be 33%.[51]

NCD ablation was performed in 113 patients at Duke. In these patients, there were no episodes of serious wound complication, cerebrospinal fluid leak, infection, or death. Of the 58 patients treated with the Nashold/El-Naggar electrode system, 29 (50%) reported no untoward effect at all. Reported complications included ataxia in 21 (36%), hemiparesis in 1, aseptic meningitis in 1, retinal artery thrombosis in 1, hearing loss in 2, neck pain in 1, "turtle neck" tightness in 3, vertigo in 1, suicide in 1, and a suicide attempt in 1. The suicide and attempted suicide occurred in patients who did not experience any relief. The suicide attests to the severity of the underlying pain. Patients who experienced complications but also enjoyed pain relief were willing to repeat the operation, expecting the same outcome. This patient population suffered greatly before surgery.

MIDBRAIN TRACTOTOMY

Anatomy and Physiology

Nerve fibers with pain and temperature information from the contralateral body are located immediately lateral to the quintothalamic tract within the midbrain. This unique anatomic feature of the spinothalamic tract within the midbrain allows a single lesion to relieve pain from the face and body. Fibers within the spinothalamic and quintothalamic tracts are axons of second-order neurons that terminate in the ventral posterior lateral nucleus and ventral posterior medial nucleus of the thalamus. At the level of the midbrain, fibers transmitting pain data within the paleospinothalamic tract terminate with synapses in the periaqueductal gray matter. The face is represented most medially, and the leg is represented most laterally, within the spinothalamic tract. The dorsal column terminates within the medial lemniscus, which is made up of axons of neurons located in the nucleus gracilis and cuneatus. The lemniscus is located medial and ventral yet also adjacent to the spinothalamic tract.

The midbrain is located between the thalamus and the pons and is divided into three distinct parts. The cerebral peduncles are located ventrally and contain the pyramidal tract. The tegmentum surrounds the aqueduct of Sylvius, and the tectum is the dorsal part of the midbrain, which also contains the quadrigeminal plate. The brachium of the inferior colliculus runs to the medial geniculate body, which is functionally a relay station in the acoustic pathway. The brachium of the superior colliculus, which is involved in the visual reflex, ends in the lateral geniculate body. The midbrain contains the nuclei involved in the control of eye movements: Edinger-Westphal nucleus, trochlear nucleus, and abducens nucleus. The nucleus of the fourth nerve is located within the tegmentum at the level of the inferior colliculus. The medial longitudinal fasciculus is ventral to the fourth nerve nucleus within the midbrain. The red nucleus, the substantia nigra, and the nucleus of cranial nerve III are found at the level of the superior colliculus. The posterior commissure is the readily identified landmark located at the superior end of the midbrain that marks the junction between the third ventricle and the aqueduct. The red nucleus and the aqueduct can be easily identified on MRI.

Indications

Midbrain tractotomy is the surgical procedure of choice for unilateral intractable pain secondary to malignancy that extends above the C5 dermatome. Achieving and sustaining analgesia above C5 are difficult with percutaneous cordotomy. Midbrain tractotomy is especially effective for pain located on the side of the neck, shoulder, and upper extremity on the same side. Pain due to head and neck cancer is particularly responsive to midbrain tractotomy. It is unwise to persist with the aggressive use of systemic narcotic agents to the point of side effects when midbrain tractotomy is so effective. Midbrain tractotomy is more beneficial than a morphine pump for such high unilateral pain. Blond and colleagues recommended midbrain tractotomy over intraspinal narcotic analgesia.[52] Midbrain tractotomy can be performed bilaterally.

Voris and Whistler reviewed 90 patients treated for pain with stereotactic procedures, including 32 with malignancy.[53] Midbrain tractotomy was performed in 27 patients. All but one experienced immediate relief, and 85% maintained relief from pain due to cancer until death. The same authors reported 40 midbrain tractotomies done in 38 patients with cancer and found that 35 patients were pain free until death.[54] Tasker reviewed 33 patients with cancer who underwent 39 procedures and found that 74% were pain free until death.[55] Beauvillain and coworkers reported excellent pain relief in 10 of 11 patients treated with midbrain tractotomy.[56] Frank and colleagues treated 109 patients with cancer, and 83.5% were pain free until death, which occurred up to 7 months later.[57–59]

Preoperative Management

The underlying cause of the pain must be clearly defined. In the setting of cancer, radiologic imaging, particularly MRI, can almost always define any pathology in question. The World Health Organization ladder of pain management is normally followed.[60–62] Until unpleasant side effects outweigh the benefits, systemic oral narcotics are effective. For unilateral pain, midbrain tractotomy should be considered earlier rather than later. It is often possible to eliminate all narcotic agents following successful tractotomy.

Surgical Technique

Stereotactic midbrain tractotomy is performed with the patient under monitored anesthesia. MRI is currently the localization modality of choice, with the target selection being confirmed on axial images plus at least one additional plane of view, preferably coronal. The target is located at the axial level between the superior and inferior colliculi, which often corresponds to a point about 5 mm below the posterior commissure. The target is located lateral to the aqueduct in line with this structure in an anteroposterior direction. This location is often described as 5 mm posterior to the posterior commissure based on ventriculographic localization. The target is located 5 to 10 mm lateral to the midline. Within the spinothalamic tract, fibers that represent the face are located most medial, and fibers that represent the foot are located most lateral. The lesion of midbrain tractotomy is targeted to include the periaqueductal gray matter immediately medial to the spinothalamic tract. The periaqueductal gray matter, which is located within 5 mm of the midline, is recognized on MRI.

With the patient awake, the lesion is created by means of a radiofrequency current using a thalamotomy electrode with a 2-mm-diameter tip exposed over a length of 3 mm. Lesions are progressively enlarged by applying the electrode at 80°C for 60 seconds. A twist drill is used to penetrate the skull. The target localization is confirmed by electrophysiologic stimulation carried out at 2 and 100 Hz. Stimulation at 2 to 5 Hz allows for easier confirmation of induced hallucinations. At this rate of stimulation, the patient easily recognizes a change in the frequency of an auditory hallucination or clicking. With a frequency of 100 Hz,

TABLE 191–4 ■ Electrophysiologic Response to Electrical Stimulation at Various Anatomic Locations in the Brain

LOCATION OF ELECTRODE	RESPONSE TO STIMULATION AT 100 HZ
Spinothalamic tract	Very low threshold, contralateral sensation in face, arm, and leg—usually unpleasant and well localized, may have temperature component
Superior colliculus, MLF	Diplopia, blurred vision, visible involuntary version
Inferior colliculus	Auditory hallucination, ranging from distinct clicking to buzz
Periaqueductal gray matter	Fear, anxiety, indescribable sensation, alerting response, involuntary mastication
Medial lemniscus	Contralateral, poorly localized paresthesia in arm, trunk, and leg

other phenomena activated by stimulation are most easily recognized. Table 191–4 documents the observed responses following stimulation at different anatomic locations within the midbrain. Ocular phenomena consist of forced version away from the electrode, blurred vision due to divergence, or frank diplopia. The presence of ocular phenomena indicates that the electrode is ventral or rostral to the ideal target site. Lesions are not made when ocular findings are induced with stimulation at a threshold below 1 volt. Auditory hallucinations indicate that the electrode is caudal to, or caudal and lateral to, the ideal target location. At the ideal target, a discrete, sharp temperature or painlike sensation occurs in the contralateral face and body with a threshold below 0.2 volt.

Postoperative Principles

Postoperative monitoring focuses on level of consciousness, neurological function, and blood pressure. In some cases, the blood pressure should be monitored with an indwelling arterial line. Blood pressure is aggressively maintained within the normal range based on the individual patient's preoperative hemodynamic status. Poorly controlled blood pressure correlates with a higher incidence of hemorrhage. Patients are evaluated for diplopia and provided with an eye patch if necessary. Initial ambulating is initiated with physiotherapy. The hospital stay can be as short as 24 hours.

Following successful pain elimination, systemic narcotics may be rapidly tapered. The maintenance dose of systemic narcotics is reduced by 50% every day until narcotics are discontinued. Intermittent dosing of narcotics may be continued as needed.

Pitfalls and Complications

Risks include the general complications associated with stereotactic surgery and the specific complications related to midbrain tractotomy. Hemorrhage, diplopia, hearing loss, post-tractotomy dysesthesia, and decreased level of consciousness are the specific risks associated with midbrain tractotomy. Post-tractotomy dysesthesia deserves the most discussion. After only six cases and a 50% incidence of dysesthesia, Drake and McKenzie abandoned open midbrain tractotomy.[63] Zapletal described a similar incidence of dysesthesia of 47.3%.[64] After open tractotomy, Walker reported the incidence of post-tractotomy dysesthesia to be 10%.[65] Although the evidence is anecdotal, it appears that dysesthesia is described more often after open procedures than after stereotactic ones. Perhaps open lesions produce more complete spinothalamic tract denervation, or maybe they also impact the lemniscal system. It also appears that dysesthesia is less common after medullary tractotomy (8.5%)[66] and even less common after cordotomy (4.3%).[67] Six of 54 mesencephalotomies resulted in dysesthesia in the experience of Voris and Whistler.[53, 54] In eight patients, Columbo was able to correlate loss of sensory evoked potentials with the occurrence of dysesthesia.[68] When the lemniscal system is included in the lesion, evoked potentials are lost, suggesting that loss of lemniscal function has a role in the development of dysesthesia. Similar to symptoms of spontaneous dysesthesia, some patients and authors describe odd sensations associated with lost dorsal column function. Future reports about midbrain tractotomy and cordotomy may be clarified by the consistent recording of sensory evoked potentials.[69] Frank and colleagues found that only 3 of 109 patients who underwent midbrain tractotomy and cordotomy had anesthesia dolorosa.[57]

Diplopia is another complication specific to midbrain tractotomy. Diplopia occurs when the lesion includes the superior colliculus, medial longitudinal fasciculus, or nuclei for cranial nerves III and IV. Amano and colleagues reduced the incidence of extraocular movement abnormalities by moving the lesion to a more dorsal position.[70] Schieff and Nashold reported that the incidence of ocular movement abnormalities was 83.3% and the incidence of binocular vision abnormalities was 50% when lesions were made at the level of the superior colliculus; the incidence of these complications fell to 20% and 0%, respectively, for lesions at the inferior colliculus.[71] Frank and colleagues found that in 109 patients, transient oculomotor disorders occurred in 20%, and permanent disorders occurred in 2.75%; Parinaud's syndrome occurred in 4.6%.[57] A contralateral field cut, due to retraction on the temporal lobe, occurs with open tractotomy, which may be accompanied by hemiparesis.[65] The risk of ocular complications is avoided by Hitchcock's pontine lesions.[72, 73]

Because the inferior colliculus is involved in the auditory pathway, hearing loss is a potential complication. This was more prominent with open operations and earlier procedures. Hearing loss was avoided by moving the lesion more cephalad toward the superior colliculus.[74]

Owing to involvement of the reticular activating system, somnolence is described in some reports. In the last 10 cases performed at Duke, this occurred once in a severely debilitated, emaciated patient with postherpetic neuralgia.

Bilateral midbrain tractotomy can be safely carried out. Frank and coworkers included five such patients in their report,[57] and Whistler and Voris described two patients who underwent bilateral midbrain tractotomy.[54]

Hemorrhage, stroke, infection, and cerebrospinal fluid leak are other potential complications, but these have not been experienced at Duke University Medical Center.

CONCLUSIONS

DREZ coagulation is a definitive surgical intervention for intractable pain secondary to brachial or lumbosacral plexus avulsion. For patients with SCI and intractable pain, DREZ ablation provides definitive management of the nociceptive pain that is usually located in a dermatomal pattern close to the level of injury. The role of DREZ ablation in the management of phantom pain warrants further investigation. DREZ ablation and microsurgical DREZotomy are largely similar.

Stereotactic midbrain tractotomy is the procedure of choice for nociceptive pain due to cancer above the C5 dermatome. This surgery should be offered sooner rather than later, owing to the high success rate.

NCD ablation, descending trigeminal tractotomy, and trigeminal nucleotomy should be considered together. These procedures are particularly effective for pain located in the V1 distribution. If corneal anesthesia is not present before surgery, the corneal reflex should be preserved after these procedures. The risk of denervation dysesthesia is less after these procedures than after operations that result in peripheral deafferentation. Nucleus caudalis lesioning is more effective for nociceptive-type pain than for central pain. The development of ipsilateral ataxia is the major risk associated with these procedures, but this risk has been substantially reduced with the use of TSEPs to direct placement of the lesions. Not a single case of ataxia has been experienced since the introduction of routine TSEP monitoring. It may be possible to eliminate the risk to adjacent white matter tracts by lesioning the nucleus caudalis with neurotoxins that directly attack the perikaryon and spare passing axons.

ACKNOWLEDGMENT

Support for this work was obtained from the Durham Veterans Administration Medical Center.

REFERENCES

1. Lombard MC, Larabi Y: Electrophysiological study of cervical dorsal horn cells in partially deafferentiated rats. Adv Pain Res Ther 5:147–154, 1983.
2. Ovelmen-Levett J, Johnson B, Bedenbaugh P: Dorsal root rhizotomy and avulsion in the cat: A comparison of the long term effects on the dorsal horn neuronal activity. Neurosurgery 15: 921–927, 1984.
3. Rolando L: Ricerche Anatomiche sulla Structura del Midollo Spinale. Dizionario Periodico di Medicina. Torino, Italy, Staperia Reale, 1824.
4. Rexed B: The cytoarchitectonic organization of the spinal cord in the cat. J Comp Neurol 96:414–495, 1952.

5. Dreval ON: Ultrasonic DREZ—operations for treatment of pain due to brachial plexus avulsion. Acta Neurochir (Wien) 122: 76–81, 1993.

6. Friedman AH, Nashold BS, Bronec PR: Dorsal root entry zone lesions for the treatment of brachial plexus avulsion injuries: A follow-up study. Neurosurgery 22:369–373, 1988.

7. Thomas DGT, Kitchen ND: Long term follow-up of dorsal root entry zone lesions in brachial plexus avulsion. J Neurol Neurosurg Psychiatry 57:737–738, 1994.

8. Chen H: Dorsal root entry zone lesions in the treatment of pain following brachial plexus avulsion and herpes zoster. J Formos Med Assoc 91:508–512, 1992.

9. Samii M, Moringland JR: Thermocoagulation of the dorsal root entry zone for the treatment of intractable pain. Neurosurgery 15:953–955, 1984.

10. Krause BL, Balakrishnan V: Dorsal root entry zone radiofrequency lesions for pain relief in brachial plexus avulsion. N Z Med J 99:851–853, 1986.

11. Powers SK, Barbaro NM, Levy RM: Pain control with laser produced dorsal root entry zone lesions. Appl Neurophysiol 51: 243–254, 1988.

12. Sindou M: Microsurgical DREZotomy (MDT) for pain, spasticity, and hyperactive bladder: A 20-year experience. Acta Neurochir (Wien) 137:1–5, 1995.

13. Ostdahl OH: DREZ surgery for brachial plexus avulsion. In Nashold BS Jr, Pearlstein RD (eds): The DREZ Operation. Park Ridge, Ill, AANS, 1996, pp 105–124.

14. Sampson JH, Cashman RE, Nashold BS Jr, Friedman AH: Dorsal root entry zone lesions for intractable pain after trauma to the conus medullaris and cauda equina. J Neurosurg 82:28–34, 1995.

15. Sindou M, Daher A: Spinal cord ablation procedures for pain. In Dubner R, Gebhart GF, Bond MR (eds): Proceedings of the Fifth World Congress on Pain. Elsevier Science, 1988, pp 477–495.

16. Friedman AH, Nashold BS Jr: DREZ lesions for relief of pain related to spinal cord injury. J Neurosurg 65:465–469, 1986.

17. Friedman AH, Nashold BS Jr: Pain of spinal cord origin. In Youmans JR (ed): Neurological Surgery, 3rd ed. Philadelphia, WB Saunders, 1990, pp 3950–3959.

18. Bullitt E, Friedman AH: DREZ lesions in the treatment of pain following spinal cord injury. In Nashold BS Jr, Pearlstein RD (eds): The DREZ Operation. Park Ridge, Ill, AANS, 1996, pp 125–135.

19. Porter RW, Hohmann GW, Bors E: Cordotomy for pain following cauda equina injury. Arch Surg 92:765–770, 1996.

20. Friedman AH: Post herpetic neuralgia. In Nashold BS Jr, Pearlstein RD (eds): The DREZ Operation. Park Ridge, Ill, AANS, 1996, pp 189–198.

21. Friedman AH, Bullitt E: Dorsal root entry zone lesions in the treatment of pain following brachial plexus avulsion, spinal cord injury, and herpes zoster. Appl Neurophysiol 51:164–169, 1988.

22. Friedman AH, Nashold BS Jr, Ovelmen-Levitt J: Dorsal root entry zone lesions in the treatment of post herpetic neuralgia. J Neurosurg 60:1258–1262, 1984.

23. Saris SC, Iacono RP, Nashold BS Jr: Dorsal root entry zone lesions for post amputation pain. J Neurosurg 62:72–76, 1985.

24. Iacono RP, Pearlstein RD, Fierro R, Gonzales A: Pain syndromes treated by the DREZ operation. In Nashold BS Jr, Pearlstein RD (eds): The DREZ Operation. Park Ridge, Ill, AANS, 1996, pp 199–209.

25. Wynn-Parry CB: Pain in avulsion lesions of the brachial plexus. Pain 9:41–53, 1980.

26. Wynn-Parry CB: Pain in avulsion of the brachial plexus. Neurosurgery 15:960–965, 1984.

27. Carvlho GA, Nikkhah G, Matties C, et al: Diagnosis of root avulsion in traumatic brachial plexus injury: Value of computerized tomography myelography and magnetic resonance imaging. J Neurosurg 86:69–76, 1997.

28. Gorecki JP, Rubin LL, Villavicencio AT: Complex regional pain syndrome (CRPS): A systematic approach to treatment. In Meadows P (ed): Proceedings from INS/IFESS. La Canada Flintridge, Calif, 1999 (CD-ROM).

29. Sindou M: Etude de la jonction radiculo-meullaire. La radicellotomie posterieure selective dans le chirurgie de la douleur [thesis]. Lyon, France, 1972.

30. Sindou M, Fisher G, Goutelle A: La radicellotomie posterieure selective. Premiers resultats dans la chirurgie de la douleur. Neurochirurgie 20:397–408, 1974.

31. Olszewski J: On the anatomical and functional organization of the spinal trigeminal nucleus. J Comp Neurol 92:401–413, 1950.

32. Dogliotti M: First surgical sections, in man, of the lemniscus lateralis (pain-temperature path) at the brain stem, for the treatment of diffuse rebellious pain. Anesth Analg 17:143–145, 1938.

33. Kanpolat Y, Deda H, Akyar S, et al: CT guided trigeminal tractotomy. Acta Neurochir (Wien) 100:112–114, 1989.

34. Nashold BS Jr, Lopez H, Chodakiewitz, Bronec P: Trigeminal DREZ for craniofacial pain. In Samii M (ed): Surgery in and around the Brainstem. Heidelberg, Germany, Springer-Verlag, 1986, pp 54–59.

35. Bernard EJ, Nashold BS Jr, Caputi F: Clinical review of nucleus caudalis dorsal root entry zone for deafferentation pain. Appl Neurophysiol 51:175–187, 1988.

36. Sjoqvist O: Studies on pain conduction in the trigeminal nerves: A contribution to the surgical treatment of facial pain. Acta Psychiatr Neurol Suppl 17:1–139, 1938.

37. Grant FC, Weinberger LM: Experiences with intramedullary tractotomy, surgery of the brainstem and its operative complications. Surg Gynecol Obstet 72:742–754, 1941.

38. Hosobuchi H, Rutkin B: Descending trigeminal tractotomy. Arch Neurol 25:115–125, 1971.

39. Young RF: Effect of trigeminal tractotomy on dental sensation in humans. J Neurosurg 56:812–818, 1982.

40. Young RF, Perryman KM: Pathways for orofacial pain sensation in the trigeminal brain-stem nuclear complex of the macaque monkey. J Neurosurg 61:563–568, 1984.

41. Young RF, Oleson TD, Perryman KM: Effect of trigeminal tractotomy on behavioral response to dental pulp stimulation in the monkey. J Neurosurg 55:420–430, 1981.

42. McKenzie KG: Trigeminal tractotomy. Clin Neurosurg 2:50–70, 1955.

43. Falconer MA: Intramedullary trigeminal tractotomy and its place in the treatment of facial pain. J Neurol Neurosurg Psychiatry 12:297–311, 1949.

44. Kanpolat Y, Deda H, Akyar S, et al: CT guided trigeminal tractotomy. Acta Neurochir (Wien) 100:112–114, 1989.

45. Kanpolat Y: CT guided percutaneous procedures. In Sindou M, Gildenburg P, Franklin PO (eds): World Society for Stereotactic and Functional Neurosurgery: Summaries of Lectures. Basel, Karger, 1997, p 8.

46. Hitchcock E, Teixeira MJ: Pontine stereotactic surgery and facial nociception. Neurol Res 9:13–117, 1987.

47. Crue BL, Todd EM, Carregal EJ: Percutaneous radiofrequency stereotactic trigeminal tractotomy. In Crue BL (ed): Pain and Suffering. Springfield, Ill, Charles C Thomas, 1970, pp 69–79.

48. Fox JL: Percutaneous trigeminal tractotomy for facial pain. Acta Neurochir (Wien) 29:83–88, 1973.

49. Hitchcock E, Teixeira MJ: Pontine stereotactic surgery and facial nociception. Neurol Res 9:113–117, 1987.

50. Young JN, Nashold BS Jr, Cosman ER: A new insulated caudalis nucleus DREZ electrode: Technical note. J Neurosurg 70:283–284, 1989.

51. Nashold BS Jr, El-Naggar AO, Ovelmen-Levitt J, Abdul-Hak M: A new design of radiofrequency lesion electrodes for use in the caudalis nucleus DREZ operation. J Neurosurg 80:1116–1120, 1994.

52. Blond S, Assaker R, Meynadier J, Merienne L: La tractotomie pedonculaire sterotaxique:sa place dans le traitement des alties cervico-faciales neoplastiques. Agressologie 29:77–80, 1988.

53. Voris HC, Whistler WW: Results of stereotactic surgery for intractable pain. Confin Neurol 37:86–96, 1975.

54. Whistler WW, Voris HC: Mesencephalotomy for intractable pain due to malignant disease. Appl Neurophysiol 41:52–56, 1978.

55. Tasker RR. Neurological concepts of pain management in head and neck cancer. Can J Otolaryngology 1975;4:480–484.

56. Beauvillain de Montreuil C, Lajat Y, Resche F: Use of stereotactic neurosurgery in the treatment of pain in the cervicofacial cancers. Ann Otolaryngol Chir Cervicofac 100:181–186, 1983.

57. Frank F, Fabrizi AP, Gaist G: Stereotactic mesencephalotomy versus multiple thalamotomies in the treatment of chronic cancer pain syndromes. Appl Neurophysiol 50:314–318, 1987.

58. Frank F, Frank G, Gaist G: Rostral stereotactic mesencephalotomy in treatment of cancer pain: A survey of 40 treated patients. Acta Neurochir Suppl (Wien) 33:437–443, 1984.

59. Frank F, Tognetti F, Gaist G: Stereotactic mesencephalotomy in treatment of malignant facial brachial pain syndromes: A survey of 14 treated patients. J Neurosurg 56:807–811, 1982.

60. Sternsward J, Colleua SM, Ventafridda V: The World Health Organization Cancer Pain and Palliative Care Program: Past, present, and future. J Pain Symptom Manage 12:65–72, 1996.

61. World Health Organization: Cancer Pain and Palliative Care. Technical report series 804. Geneva, WHO, 1990.

62. Ventafridda V, Saita L, Ripamonti C, DeConno F: WHO guidelines for the use of analgesia in cancer pain. Int J Tissue React 7:93–96, 1985.

63. Drake CG, McKenzie KG: Mesencephalic tractotomy for pain: Experience with six cases. J Neurosurg 10:457–462, 1953.

64. Zapletal B: Open mesencephalotomy and thalamotomy for intractable pain. Acta Neurochir Suppl (Wien) 18:1–119, 1969.

65. Walker AE: Relief of pain by mesencephalic tractotomy. Arch Neurol Psychiatry 48:865–883, 1942.

66. Crawford AS: Medullary tractotomy for relief of intractable pain in upper levels. Arch Surg 55:53–529, 1947.

67. White JC, Sweet WH: Pain, Its Mechanisms and Neurosurgical Control. Springfield Ill, Charles C Thomas, 1955.

68. Columbo F: Somatosensory-evoked potentials after mesencephalic tractotomy for pain syndromes: Neuroradiologic and clinical correlations. Surg Neurol 21:453–458, 1984.

69. Lieberson WT, Voris HC, Uematsu S: Recording of somatosensory evoked potentials during mesencephalotomy for intractable pain. Conf Neurol 32:185–194, 1994.

70. Amano K, Kawamura H, Tanikawa T: Long term follow up study of rostral mesencephalac reticulotomy for pain relief: Report of 34 cases. Appl Neurophysiol 49:105–111, 1986.

71. Schieff C, Nashold BS Jr: Stereotactic mesencephalic tractotomy for the relief of thalamic pain. Neurol Res 9:101–104, 1987.

72. Hitchcock ER, Sotelo MG, Kim MC: Analgesic levels and technical methods in stereotactic pontine spinothalamic tractotomy. Acta Neurochir (Wien) 39:746–752, 1973.

73. Hitchcock ER: Stereotactic pontine spinothalamic tractotomy. J Neurosurg 39:746–752, 1973.

74. Wycis HT, Spiegel EA: Long-range results in the treatment of intractable pain by stereotactic midbrain surgery. J Neurosurg 101–107, 1962.

75. Siqueira JM: A method for bulbospinal trigeminal nucleotomy in the treatment of facial deafferentation pain. Appl Neurophysiol 48:277–288, 1995.

76. Nashold BS Jr, Caputi F, Bernard E: Trigeminal DREZ: Caudalis nuclear lesions for relief of facial pain. Neurosurgery 20:348, 1987.

77. Bernard EJ, Nashold BS Jr, Caputi F, Moossy JJ: Nucleus caudalis DREZ lesions for facial pain. Br J Neurosurg 1:81–92, 1987.

78. Nashold BS Jr: Neurosurgical technique of the dorsal root zone operation. Appl Neurophysiol 51:136–145, 1988.

79. Ishijima B, Shimoji K, Shimizu H, et al: Lesions of spinal and trigeminal dorsal root entry zone for deafferentation pain. Appl Neurophysiol 51:175–187, 1988.

80. Rossitch E Jr, Zeidman SM, Nashold BS Jr: Nucleus caudalis DREZ for facial pain due to cancer. Br J Neurosurg 3:45–49, 1989.

81. Rawlings CE III, El-Naggar AO, Nashold BS Jr: The DREZ procedure: An update on technique. Br J Neurosurg 3:633–642, 1989.

82. Rossitch E Jr, Young NJ, Nashold BS Jr: Nucleus caudalis and dorsal root entry zone lesions for pain relief: An update. In Wilkins RH, Rengachary SS (eds): Neurosurgery Update II. Vascular Spinal, Pediatric and Functional Neurosurgery. New York, McGraw-Hill, 1990, pp 360–365.

83. Sampson JH, Nashold BS Jr: Facial pain due to vascular lesions of the brain stem relieved by dorsal root entry zone lesions in the nucleus caudalis. Neurosurgery 77:473–475, 1992.

84. Nashold BS Jr, El-Naggar A: Dorsal root entry zone (DREZ) lesioning. In Rengachary SS (ed): Neurosurgical Operative Atlas. Lebanon, NH, AANS Publications, 1992, pp 9–24.

85. Chen HJ: Facial pain relieved by dorsal root entry zone lesions in the trigeminal nucleus caudalis: Report of two cases. J Formos Med Assoc 92:583–585, 1993.

86. El-Naggar AO, Nashold BS Jr: Nuleus cadalis DREZ lesions for relief of intractable facial pain. In Wilkins RR, Rengachary SS (eds): Neurosurgery, 2nd ed. New York, McGraw-Hill, 1995, pp 4047–4054.

87. Freidman AH, Nashold JRB, Nashold BS Jr: DREZ lesions for treatment of pain. In North RB, Levy RM (eds): Neurosurgical Management of Pain. Heidelberg, Germany, Springer-Verlag, 1997, pp 176–190.

88. Grigoryan YUA, Slavin KV, Ogleznev KYA: Ultrasonic lesion of the trigeminal nucleus caudalis for deafferentation facial pain. Acta Neurochir (Wien) 131:229–235, 1994.

89. Bullard D: Experience with the caudalis DREZ in the treatment of facial pain. In Sindou MP, Gildenberg PL, Franklin PO (eds): Twelfth Meeting of the World Society for Stereotactic and Functional Neurosurgery. Basel, 1997.

90. Bullard DE, Nashold BS: DREZ for recurrent head and neck pain. Paper presented at Joint Section on Pain, 47th Annual Congress of Neurological Surgeons, Sept 27–Oct 2, New Orleans.

91. Gorecki JP, Nashold BS Jr: The Duke experience with the nucleus caudalis DREZ operation. Acta Neurochir Suppl (Wien) 64:128–131, 1995.

92. Gorecki JP, Nashold BS Jr, Rubin LL, Ovelmen-Levitt J: The Duke experience with nucleus caudalis coagulation. Stereotact Funct Neurosurg 65:111–116, 1995.

93. Hamby WB, Shinners BM, Marsh IA: Trigeminal tractotomy: Observations on forty-eight cases. Arch Surg 57:171–177, 1949.

94. Guidetti B: Tractotomy for the relief of trigeminal neuralgia. J Neurosurg 7:499–508, 1950.

95. McKenzie KG: Trigeminal tractotomy. Clin Neurosurg 2:50–70, 1955.

96. Moffie D: Late results of bulbar trigeminal tractotomy: Some remarks on recovery of sensibility. J Neurol Neurosurg Psychiatry 34:270–274, 1971.

97. Hitchcock E: Stereotactic trigeminal tractotomy. Ann Clin Res 2:131–135, 1970.

98. Hitchcock ER, Schvarcz JR: Stereotaxic trigeminal tractotomy for post-herpetic facial pain. J Neurosurg 37:412–417, 1972.

99. Schvarcz JR: Spinal cord stereotactic techniques re: trigeminal nucleotomy and extralemniscal myelotomy. Appl Neurophysiol 41:99, 1978.

100. Hitchcock E, Teixeira MJ: Pontine stereotactic surgery and facial nociception. Neurol Res 9:113–117, 1987.

CHAPTER 192

Cordotomy for Pain

YÜCEL KANPOLAT

HISTORY

The first discoveries about the anatomy and function of the spinal cord by means of clinical and experimental studies were made by Galen in the second century AD.[1] Additional clinical suggestions about the function of the spinal cord came from empirical observations. In 1871, Muller reported a case in which isolated analgesia was observed after lesioning of the spinal cord. A few years later, Gowers reported a case of localized injury to the anterolateral column at the level of the third cervical segment, resulting in complete analgesia with preservation of tactile sensation of the opposite half of the body. Gowers concluded that the afferent pathway for pain was located in the anterolateral column.[2] The spinothalamic tract was first identified by Edinger in 1889 while conducting experiments on amphibians and newborn cats. In 1905, Spiller reported that pain and temperature sensations ascend in the anterolateral spinal cord, based on autopsy findings in patients with tuberculoma at the thoracic level of the spinal cord.[3] In 1910, Schüller sectioned the anterolateral tract in monkeys and named the procedure "chordotomie."[4] The first cordotomy in humans was carried out by Martin at Spiller's instigation, with many technical difficulties.[5] In 1920, Frazier published a series of six cordotomy patients, five of whom experienced postoperative pain relief.[6] After this publication, cordotomy was accepted as an important type of pain surgery. Since it was first described, open cordotomy has usually been performed using the posterior approach. The anterior approach was described by Collis and Cloward but has not been widely used because of technical difficulties.[7, 8]

Cordotomy is typically performed in cancer patients, who do not tolerate open surgery well owing to their poor health. Thus, clinicians have sought noninvasive treatments to accommodate these patients. Percutaneous cordotomy is a relatively new treatment modality performed using a needle electrode system and, conventionally, radiographic guidance. This procedure was first described and performed by Mullan in 1963 using a radioactive-tipped strontium needle.[9] Because of the unwanted effects of the radioactive source, Mullan began making unipolar, anodal, electrolytic lesions

in 1965.[10] In the same year, Rosomoff and colleagues described the technique of percutaneous cordotomy using a radiofrequency (RF) electrode system,[11] which allows one to make small, discrete lesions in the pain-conducting system of the spinal cord. With the help of impedance measurements and stimulation, evaluation of the target's neurophysiologic function became possible. The percutaneous method was performed in the lower cervical region via an anterior approach by Lin and associates in 1966.[12]

Radiography, the conventional visualization system in stereotactic pain procedures, cannot demonstrate patients' spinal cord morphology. In 1988, Kanpolat and coworkers published the first experience with computed tomography (CT) visualization in a stereotactic pain procedure, later using CT guidance as a visualization method in percutaneous cordotomy.[13, 14] CT visualization offers the advantage of topographic orientation. Using this contribution, Kanpolat and coworkers described selective unilateral and bilateral cordotomy in the following years.[15, 16] Morphologic orientation and neurophysiologic evaluation of the target allowed the use of this truly stereotactic method with RF energy. This defines the recent concept of cordotomy.

ANATOMY OF THE TARGET AND ITS ENVIRONS

Morphometric studies of the spinal cord at the level of the surgical approach provide the most critical information pertaining to anatomic orientation for cordotomy. At the C1-2 level, the diameters of the spinal cord have been reported by Mullan as being 10 mm anteroposteriorly and 13 mm transversely.[17] Kanpolat and colleagues measured the spinal cord diameters of 63 patients who underwent CT-guided percutaneous cordotomy at the C1-2 level and found them to be 7 to 11.4 mm (mean, 8.66 ± 0.72 mm) anteroposteriorly and 9 to 14 mm (mean, 10.9 ± 1.56 mm) transversely.[18] Kameyama and associates found the spinal cord diameters at the C2 level to be 6.4 ± 0.4 mm anteroposteriorly and 10.5 ± 0.8 mm transversely; at the C5 level, 6 ± 0.4 mm anteroposteriorly and 12.2 ± 0.8 mm transversely; and at the T1 level, 5.5 ± 0.5 mm anteroposteriorly and 10.6 ± 0.7 mm transversely.[19] By contrast, Poletti found the transverse diameter of the spinal cord of a cancer patient at the T2 level to be 5.2 mm.[20]

The target in cordotomy is the lateral spinothalamic tract, which is located in the anterolateral part of the spinal cord.[21-24] This ascending tract carries information chiefly about pain and temperature and relays some tactile information. The distribution of the pain-conducting fibers within the anterolateral spinal tract is such that the small, ventrally located fibers conduct mainly pain sensation. The organization of fibers from the outside inward is superficial pain, temperature, and deep pain.[25] Because most of the fibers in the anterolateral system decussate over two to five segments before entering the anterolateral columns, spinothalamic cordotomy aims to interrupt the spinothalamic tract ascending contralaterally to the painful side. Although the majority of pain-transmitting fibers decussate normally, the decussated axon rate and position may vary considerably among individuals; thus, unilateral cordotomy can, on rare occasions, produce ipsilateral analgesia owing to nondecussated neurons in some individuals.[23]

The anterolateral sensory system has a somatotropic relationship, with fibers from higher levels laminating medially and ventrally, and fibers from lower levels laminating laterally and dorsally within the lateral spinothalamic tract.[21, 22, 25] In 1926, Peet stated that deeper cordotomy incisions, particularly in the anterior portion of the anterolateral tract, caused analgesia in the upper parts of the body.[24] In 1939, Hyndman and Van Epps suggested the possibility of producing high-level analgesia with preservation of pain and temperature sensibility in the lower half of the body.[21] Segmentation of the fibers provides the opportunity for selective cordotomy, given that anteromedial lesions denervate the contralateral arm and upper chest region, while posterolateral lesions denervate the sacral and lumbar areas (Fig. 192–1).

Between the anterior extent of the pyramidal tracts and the posterior aspect of the lateral spinothalamic tracts is a narrow "safety zone" of white matter. The pyramidal tract is usually located posterior to the dentate ligament. It must be remembered, however, that in rare instances the dentate ligament is located posterior to its normal place.[23] Moreover, there is much variation in the size and location of the ventral corticospinal tract; sometimes it does not decussate at all. Because motor decussation may extend from the obex to the C1 level, contralateral leg weakness may also occur if the lesion is too high.[25] The ventral spinocerebellar tract is located in the lateral part of the lateral spinothalamic tract. Lesions of this tract cause ipsilateral ataxia of the arm. Autonomic fibers related to bowel and bladder function are found in the lateral part of the lateral horn of gray matter. Immediately posterior to the autonomic fibers are vasomotor fibers; bilateral lesioning of these fibers causes hypotension.[25]

The most important region related to upper cervical cordotomy practice is the medial aspect of the lateral spinothalamic tract, where the descending respiratory pathway is located. Nathan emphasized the importance of this region as follows: "The descending respiratory pathway may be considered to be the most important tract of the spinal cord; yet its position in

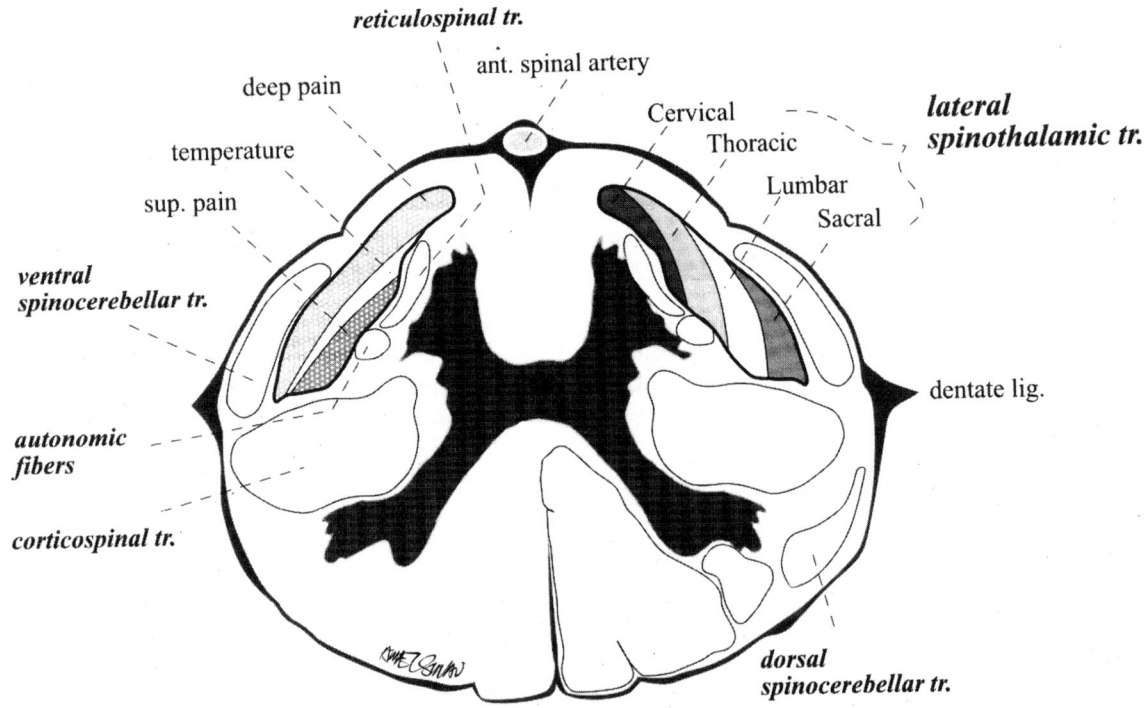

FIGURE 192–1. Schematic representation of the target (lateral spinothalamic tract) and its environs at the C1-2 level.

man is unknown. It is important to work out the location of these descending fibers not only to complete anatomic knowledge but also to provide those practicing surgery on the cervical cord with essential information. The absence of this knowledge contributed to the death of some of our patients after cordotomy and this has also been a cause of death in patients from other series of cordotomies."[26] Belmusto and colleagues concluded that fibers associated with respiration in humans occupied an area from C1 to C3, 3 to 5.5 mm from the lateral margin of the cord.[27] Hitchcock and Leece suggested that the anterior portion of the respiratory tract is largely related to diaphragmatic function, whereas the posterior portion of this tract supplies the remainder of the respiratory musculature—namely, the intercostal muscles as well as the abdominal and lumbar musculature used in respiration.[28]

PATIENT SELECTION

Cordotomy is the preferred method if the surgeon is certain that the patient's intractable pain is transmitted in the lateral spinothalamic tract. The best candidates for cordotomy are patients with unilateral somatic cancer pain and compression of the plexus, roots, or nerves.[29] Tasker mention defined two types of pain as indications for cordotomy: intermittent, neuralgia-like, shooting pain into the legs associated with a spinal cord injury, which is typically at the thoracolumbar level, and evoked pain—allodynia or hyperpathia—associated with neuropathic pain syndromes that arise from peripheral neurological lesions.[29, 30]

The indications for open and percutaneous cordotomy involve the same types of patients. Although percutaneous cordotomy is generally preferable, open cordotomy is recommended if the necessary equipment is not available or if the surgeon's experience is inadequate to perform percutaneous cordotomy. If the patient has anomalies or other diseases of the upper cervical region, open cordotomy is also recommended.[29, 30] Anterior open cordotomy for bilateral upper body pain is better tolerated than is the posterior approach. It must be emphasized that performance of this procedure should be reserved for experienced surgeons.[31]

Contrary to popular opinion, unilateral upper body pain (secondary to lung carcinoma, mesothelioma, or Pancoast's tumor) and bilateral somatic intractable pain in the lower body and extremities can be controlled by CT-guided unilateral or bilateral selective cordotomy.[15, 16] Standard practice is to use neurodestructive procedures only after narcotic analgesics prove to be inadequate.[32, 33] Gybels proposed administering cerebrospinal fluid opioid infusions and performing percutaneous neurolytic procedures instead of percutaneous cordotomy if the patient has only a 2- to 5-month life expectancy.[34] Today, with the help of imaging techniques and the recent contribution of electrode technology, cordotomy can be performed safely and effectively. Thus, CT-guided percutaneous cordotomy should be considered the treatment of choice even be-

fore morphine therapy.[15, 16] I believe that the new version of percutaneous cordotomy is simple and safe and is the preferred procedure, especially for intractable pain states due to malignancy. It stops patients' dependence on pumps, stimulation systems, drugs, and doctors and provides a last chance for patients to take a breath in the final stage of life.

Cordotomy is contraindicated in patients with severe pulmonary dysfunction, those who are unable to stay in a supine position for 30 to 40 minutes, and patients whose partial oxygen saturation is less than 80%. For patients with bilateral intractable pain of the chest and arms, bilateral high cervical cordotomy is not recommended. For this group, the anterior approach must be used—open or percutaneously, unilaterally or bilaterally.[15, 16, 29, 35, 36]

PERCUTANEOUS CORDOTOMY TECHNIQUE

Instrumentation and Calibration of Electrode Systems

Percutaneous cordotomy is routinely performed using an RF system consisting of a generator, specially designed needles, and electrodes. The generator system must comprise an impedance measurement system, stimulation capabilities, and temperature monitoring of the electrode system. Several systems are available on the market, manufactured by Diros Technology (Toronto, Canada), Electa (Stockholm, Sweden), Howmedica-Leibinger (Freiburg, Germany), and Radionics (Burlington, MA). The diameter and length of the uninsulated tip of the electrode are critical, because the lesion size is directly related to these parameters; thus, all parameters must be calibrated by making lesions in egg white before applying the electrode intraoperatively. I recommend using an electrode kit (KCTE Kanpolat CT Electrode Kit; Radionics, Inc, Burlington, MA) with 20-gauge, thin-walled needles and plastic hubs designed to avoid imaging artifact problems. Demarcations on the cannula indicate the depth of insertion (Fig. 192–2). The kit also includes two open-tip thermocouple electrodes with 2-mm tips and diameters of 0.3 and 0.4 mm (one straight-tip electrode and one curved-tip). The smaller-caliber electrode (0.3 mm) is usually used for bilateral cordotomy, and the 0.4-mm-diameter electrode is preferred for unilateral cordotomy.[37]

Preoperative Preparation

Before the procedure, cranial CT or magnetic resonance imaging must be performed to rule out brain metastasis, because cerebrospinal fluid loss during the procedure could theoretically result in brain herniation. The patient should have been fasting for 5 hours preoperatively. Before the procedure, the required dose of analgesic should be given parenterally. At this stage, patients should be reinformed of the details of the procedure. Clear communication and development of

Kanpolat CT Cannula & Electrodes

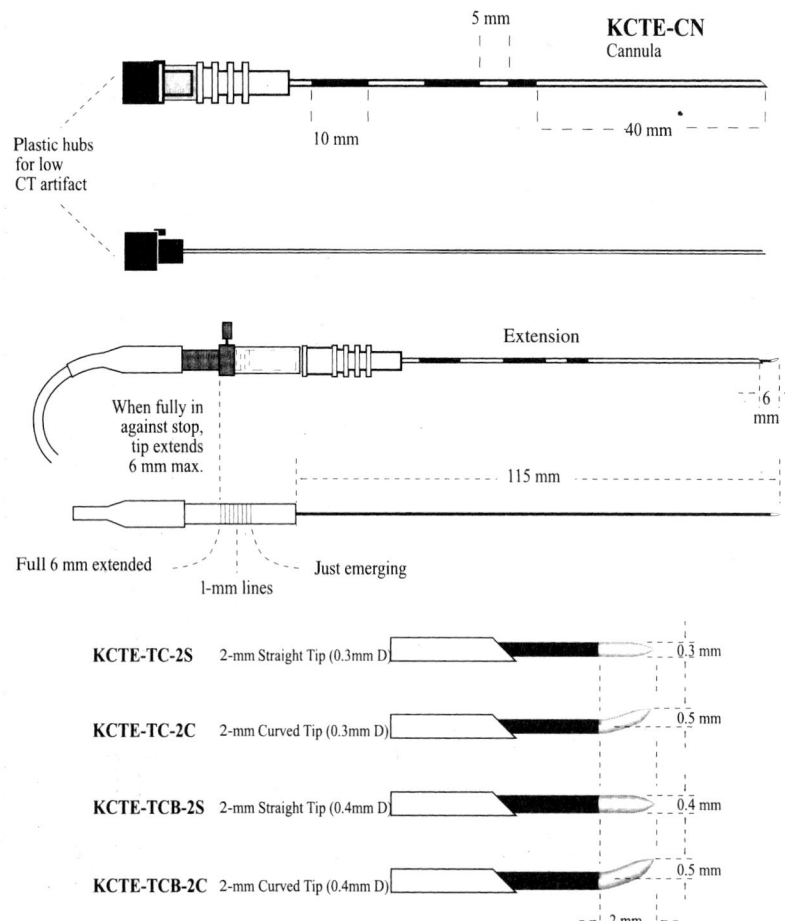

FIGURE 192–2. Drawing of the Kanpolat cannula and electrodes. KCTE, Kanpolat CT electrode.

a good rapport with the patient are crucial, because the success of the procedure is dependent on intraoperative feedback from the patient. In CT-guided percutaneous cordotomy, contrast material should be administered into the subarachnoid space of the spinal cord via lumbar puncture (7 to 8 mL of 240 mg/mL iohexol) 20 to 30 minutes before the operation. If the general condition of the patient does not permit lumbar puncture, contrast material (5 mL iohexol) is injected at the C1-2 level.

Positioning and Anesthesia

The patient is placed in the supine position. The upper cervical spine must be kept in a horizontal position, particularly for x-ray–guided cordotomy. In conventional lateral and anterior cordotomy, the head is flexed and fixed. In CT-guided cordotomy, the procedure is performed in the CT unit. The patient is placed in the CT machine in the supine position. The head is placed on the head holder, flexed, and fixed with a fixation band. In clinical practice, local anesthesia is adequate, but neuroleptic anesthesia may be used if necessary. Some surgeons use general anesthesia on rare occa-

sions,[38] but because of the need to communicate with the patient during the procedure, it is not recommended.

Anatomic Localization

The electrode system is placed on the anterolateral aspect of the anterolateral spinal cord with the assistance of an imaging method (Fig. 192–3). CT shows the morphology of the spinal cord segment directly, whereas in the conventional method, visualization of the spinal cord is obtained indirectly by radiograph without demonstration of the relationship between the spinal cord and the needle electrode.

In conventional C1-2 lateral cordotomy, the needle is inserted perpendicularly, 1 cm below and behind the mastoid process after deep local anesthetic infiltration. I recommend confirmation of the infiltration site by repeated aspiration to avoid subarachnoid or vertebral artery puncture. The local anesthetic needle is used as a guide needle before the initial puncture if a radiograph or CT image is taken. As a safety precaution, I use a special cannula (Kanpolat cannula; Radionics, Burlington, MA) with demarcations demonstrating the amount penetrated.

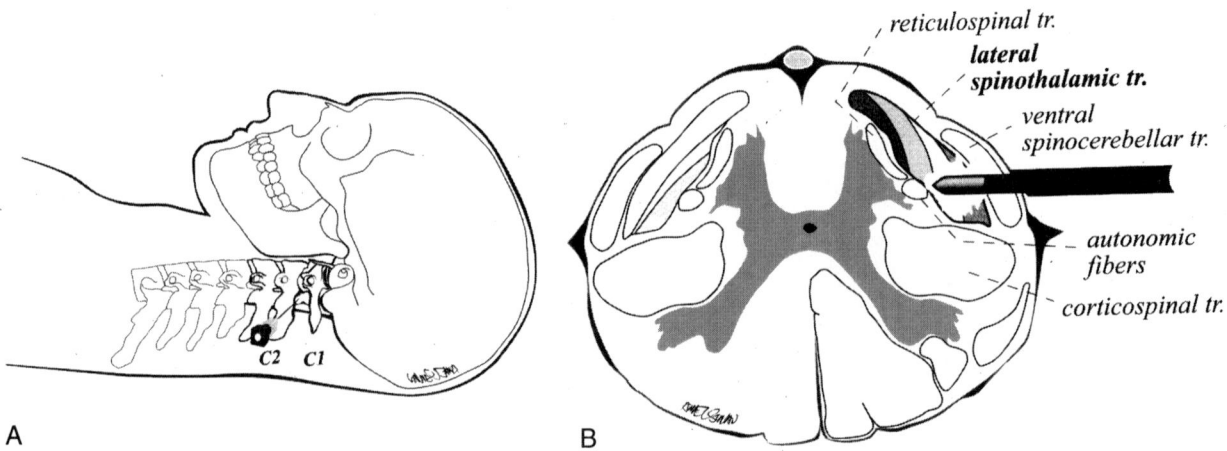

FIGURE 192–3. Schematic representation of lateral percutaneous cordotomy at the C1-2 level. *A*, Position of the needle at the C1-2 level. *B*, Ideal position of the needle electrode system in the target.

In CT-guided cordotomy, the skin-dura distance must now be measured. At this stage, the skin-dura distance and direction of the needle are well demonstrated by the CT image. Lahuerta and colleagues measured this distance as 57 ± 3 mm in males and 52 ± 2 mm in females.[39] This distance was measured as 46 to 66 mm (mean, 52.1 ± 4.3 mm) in males and 43 to 56 mm (mean, 48.4 ± 3.1 mm) in females in my series. The next step is to place the needle 1 to 2 mm anterior to the dentate ligament. Because lateral puncturing of the dura usually causes pain, a small amount of local anesthetic infiltration is recommended. The needle position is seen at every step of manipulation on lateral scanogram and axial computed tomographic scan, using a 1-mm slice thickness at the needle level (Fig. 192–4A). Multiple maneuvers under CT guidance may be needed to fix the needle in this position (see Fig. 192–4B). The active electrode is then inserted into the cannula using one insertion (see Fig. 192–4C). The location of the electrode in the spinal cord and displacement or rotation of the spinal cord can be visualized. Finally, the electrode is placed in the proper position. I do not recommend multiple puncturing with the active electrode at this stage, as it increases the risk of spinal cord injury and other complications (Fig. 192–5).

If conventional cordotomy is performed using x-ray guidance, use of an image intensifier is recommended. Some authors use Polaroid film for quick development. Visualization of the dentate ligament in the lateral radiograph is mandatory (Fig. 192–6A). Because water-soluble dyes do not demonstrate the dentate ligament,[29, 30] oil-based contrast material must be used; however, the risk of arachnoiditis with such dyes remains a problem. Theoretically, the anterior part of the spinal cord could be visualized by air myelogram, and the posterior part by oil-based contrast material. Tasker stated, "With image intensification it should now be possible to identify the dorsal margin of the subarachnoid space, the anterior cord margin, the dentate ligament, and sometimes, the ventral and dorsal root lines. Confusion can arise with images of contralateral structures, but the most common error is to mistake anterior or posterior root lines for the dentate ligament. In some patients the cord is unusually positioned either anteriorly or posteriorly, adding to the confusion, and this situation may be elucidated only with physiological corroboration."[29] Anteroposterior imaging is usually used to demonstrate the position of the needle in the lateral margin of the odontoid process (see Fig. 192–6B). Tasker stated, "The tip of a properly positioned cordotomy electrode should not pass the contralateral margin of the dens."[29]

In the anterior approach, the skin, subcutaneous tissues, and paravertebral fascia are infiltrated with local anesthetic. An 18-gauge, thin-walled spinal needle is inserted opposite the cordotomy site, medial to the carotid sheath and lateral to the trachea and esophagus at the C4-5, C5-6, or C6-7 level (Fig. 192–7). With the help of radiographic imaging, the needle passes through the disk space and is placed in the anterolateral part of the spinal cord. After reaching the subarachnoid space, only the anterior part of the spinal cord can be indirectly visualized on air myelogram. The location of the target has been reported as 4 to 6 mm from the midline for cervicothoracic pain and 8 to 9 mm from the midline for lumbosacral pain.[40, 41] In my opinion, however, these figures are not realistic because they indicate that the transverse diameter of the spinal cord at this level is greater than 18 mm, which has never been documented.

Physiologic Localization

To confirm whether the electrode is in the cerebrospinal fluid or the spinal cord, the surgeon obtains impedance values and determines the neurophysiologic response of the compartment where the electrode is located. Impedance measurements are an important indication of passage into a new medium along the path of the electrode. Impedance values are approximately 400 ohms in the cerebrospinal fluid; an increase of approximately 200 ohms is observed when there is contact between the electrode tip and the pia. The value is

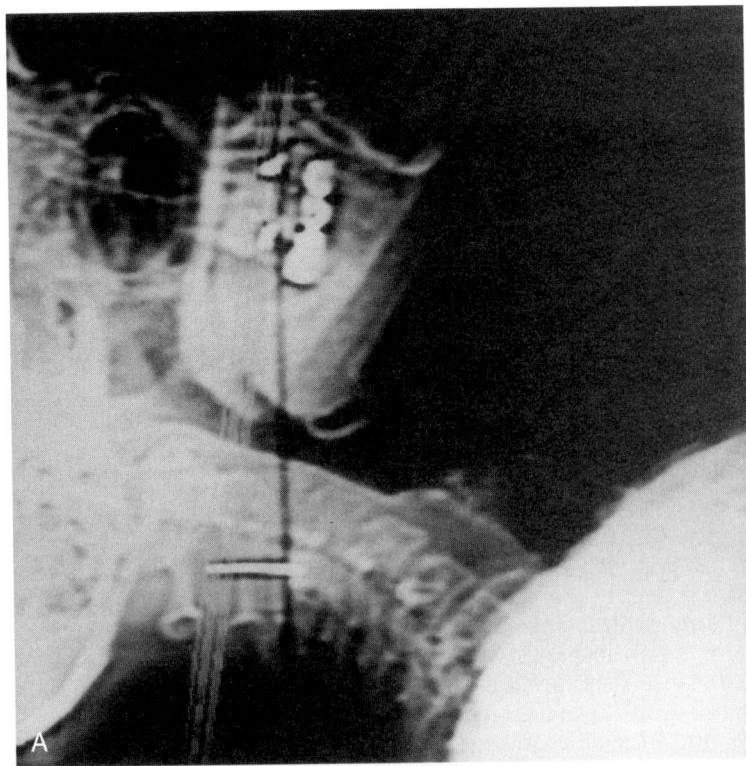

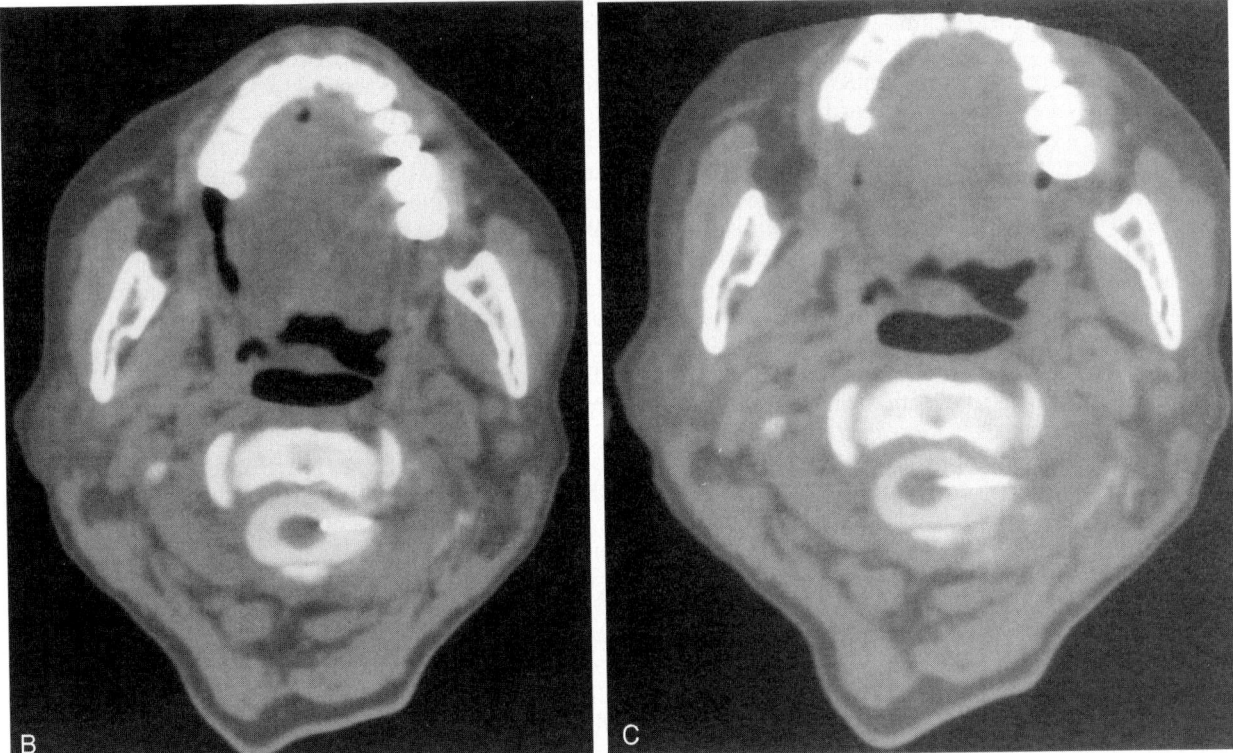

FIGURE 192–4. Stages of computed tomography–guided percutaneous left C1-2 cordotomy. *A,* Position of the needle at the C1-2 level on lateral scanogram. *B,* Final position of the needle on axial computed tomographic scan. *C,* Final position of the electrode in the target on axial computed tomographic scan.

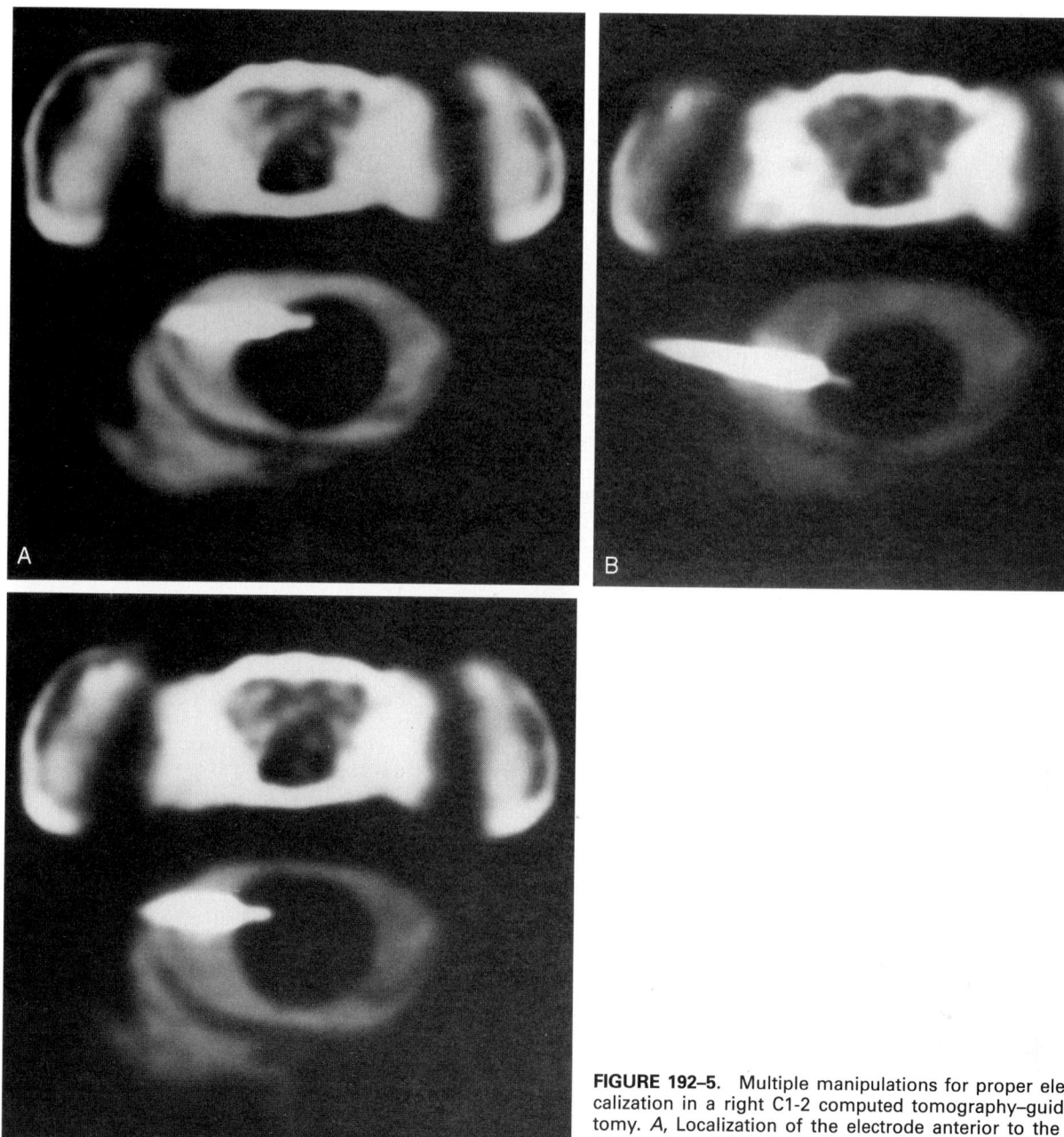

FIGURE 192–5. Multiple manipulations for proper electrode localization in a right C1-2 computed tomography–guided cordotomy. *A,* Localization of the electrode anterior to the target. *B,* Localization of the electrode posterior to the target. *C,* Electrode is in the target.

almost always greater than 1000 ohms after insertion into the spinal cord.

Real neurophysiologic confirmation of the target is obtained by stimulation, necessitating that the patient be alert and cooperative. As a rule of functional neurosurgery, stimulation must be initiated at minimal voltage values: 2- to 5-Hz stimulation with 0.4 to 1.5 V causes ipsilateral trapezius muscle contraction, indicating that the electrode is within or near the anterior gray matter of the lateral spinothalamic tract. Ipsilateral motor responses in the arm or leg indicate that the electrode is in the corticospinal tract. Stimulation of 100 Hz with 0.2 to 1.5 V causes pain, paresthesia, or warmth in the spinothalamic tract. Use of a curved

electrode allows the surgeon to rotate the needle 0.5 mm anteriorly or posteriorly in order to place the electrode in a specific part of the tract in the lateral-to-medial plane. In CT-guided cordotomy, the position of the electrode must be confirmed by new CT images. If stimulation is confirmed by the CT image, the effectiveness, safety, and selectivity of percutaneous cordotomy are ensured.

Lesion Making

The final step of the procedure is to make controlled RF lesions. By confirming the neurophysiologic function of the patient during CT-guided cordotomy using new

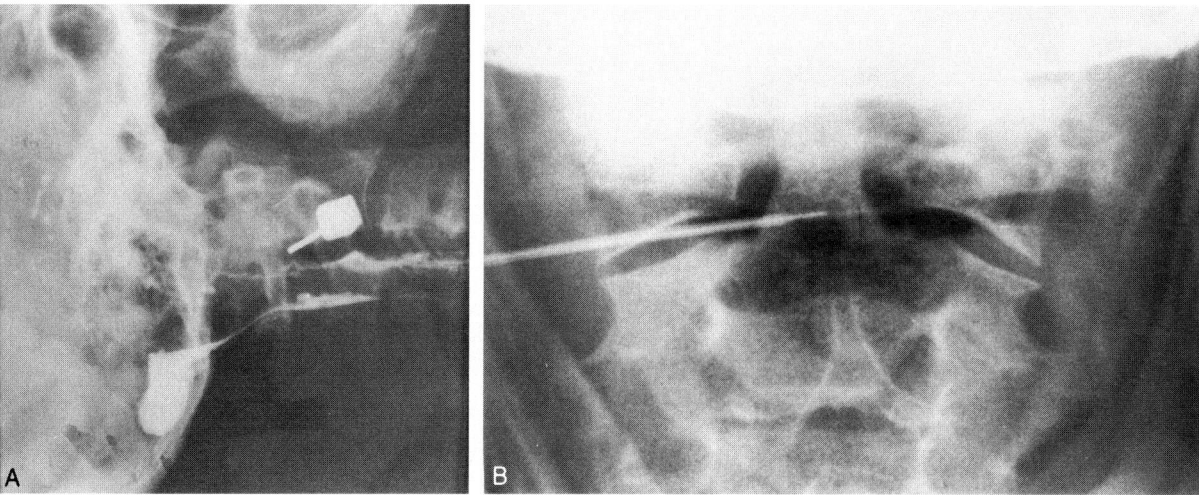

FIGURE 192–6. Position of the needle and electrode in conventional x-ray–guided percutaneous cordotomy. *A,* Needle located anterior to the dentate ligament at the C1-2 level. *B,* Final localization of the electrode with anteroposterior projection.

electrode systems, the surgeon can decide whether to stop or continue the lesioning and whether to change the direction of lesioning. I believe that temperature monitoring of the electrode is now mandatory. Lesions cannot be standardized according to certain RF power and milliampere values. These values change according to the impedance of the tissue and the caliber and length of the electrode. Moreover, the surgeon must test each electrode system by making lesions in egg white before applying it to patients. A test lesion should be made at 55°C to 60°C for 60 seconds before

making the final lesions. I then recommend making two to three lesions at 70°C to 80°C for 60 seconds. The patient's neurological function, particularly analgesia level and motor function, should be checked after making each lesion.

Bilateral Cordotomy

Bilateral percutaneous cordotomy is usually performed with a 1-week interval. I recommend using bilateral selective cordotomy for intractable pain in the lower

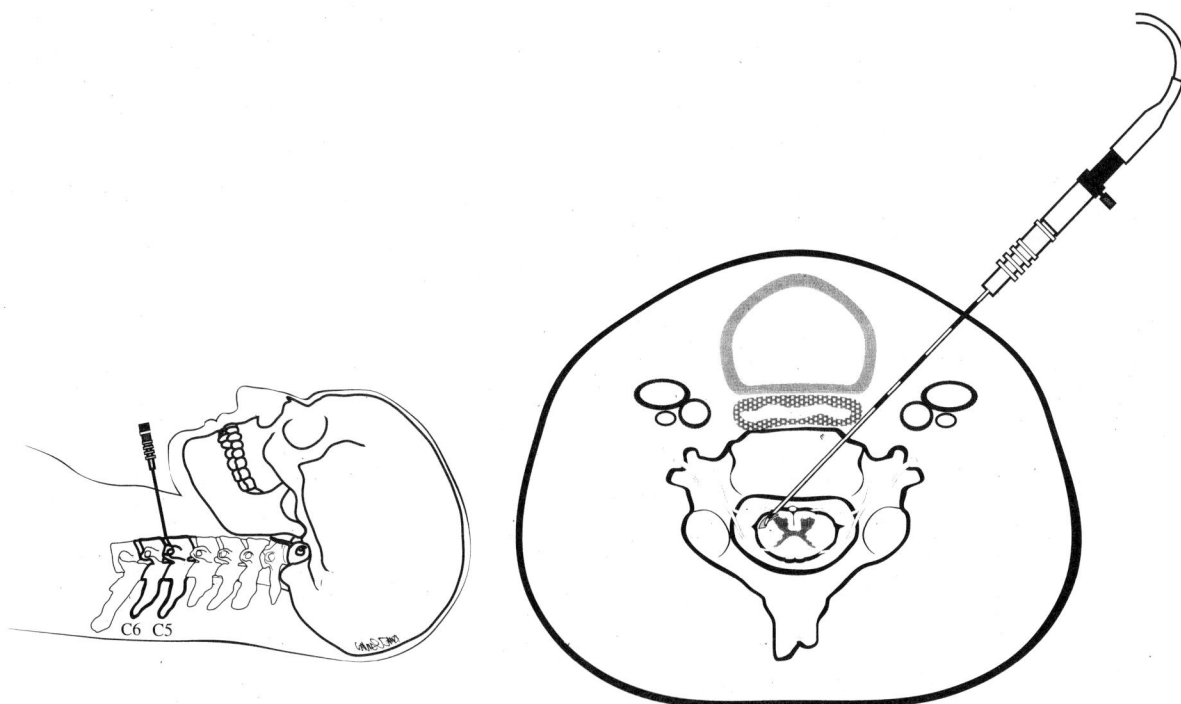

FIGURE 192–7. Schematic representation of anterior percutaneous cordotomy at the C5-6 level.

T10 dermatome. If the pain is located in the upper segment, C1-2 percutaneous lateral cordotomy is performed on one side, and percutaneous anterior cordotomy is performed on the other side,[36, 40, 41] although bilateral procedures may present technical difficulties.

I prefer to use a small-caliber electrode for CT-guided bilateral cordotomy only in patients with somatic lower body pain. The pain-dominant side is selected for the first denervation. After the test lesion is made, one or two lesions are made at a temperature of 70°C to 80°C.

Postoperative Period

The patient is kept in the supine position with the head elevated for 1 hour. After an observation period of 6 hours, unilateral cordotomy patients can go home if their condition permits. Bilateral cordotomy patients must be observed in the intensive care unit. Blood pressure must be monitored carefully because of the risk of hypotension, especially on the day of the procedure. Other important problems are related to lesions of the reticulospinal tract, which controls the rhythm and depth of ventilation. Blood gases must be evaluated, and sleep patterns monitored. If respiratory complications occur, injection of corticosteroids is advised. Patients with respiratory complications are kept in the hospital for 2 to 3 weeks. After successful cordotomy and pain control, one must not stop morphine therapy suddenly. Most patients reduce their dosages progressively and discontinue morphine use over time.

OPEN CORDOTOMY TECHNIQUE

Posterior Open Cordotomy

Posterior open cordotomy is usually performed at the T1-2 level in patients with pain below the T5 level. If unilateral upper body pain is located in the upper chest or arm region, unilateral open cordotomy is performed at the C2-3 level. It is essential that diameter measurements at the cordotomy level be evaluated preoperatively. Most patients are in moderate or poor condition and need blood, electrolyte, and protein replacement. Full-leg elastic stockings must be used during surgery to avoid induced orthostatic hypotension. Poletti proposed the use of wake-up anesthesia to allow identification of the spinothalamic tract by stimulation, to monitor bilateral motor function as the lesion is being made, and to test the extent of the induced sensory deficit before it is too late to enlarge the lesion.[20] He proposed placing the patient in the swimmer position with the thorax rotated 45 degrees up from horizontal. I recommend the prone position for unilateral or bilateral posterior cordotomy.

In percutaneous open cordotomy, a skin incision is made such that the T2 lamina and spinous process are located in the middle of the incision. The T1 and T3 lamina are also exposed. Total T2 laminectomy is performed, extending 2 to 3 mm into T1 and T3. At this stage, an operating microscope is necessary for better orientation. The dura is opened longitudinally and carefully tacked. I prefer bilateral exploration of the spinal cord with adequate exposure of the spinal cord segment to facilitate turning of the cord. Some authors prefer a dural opening with a curved incision via hemilaminectomy. Care must be taken not to open the arachnoid at the same time as the dura to avoid epidural bleeding. The arachnoid is opened later, and the posterior and anterior roots are dissected free to prevent stretching during spinal cord rotation. The width of the spinal cord is reconfirmed under the microscope. The dentate ligament is cut bilaterally. A cotton pledget is inserted contralateral to the cordotomy incision, and slight pressure is exerted on the contralateral part of the spinal cord (Fig. 192–8). The spinal cord is rotated

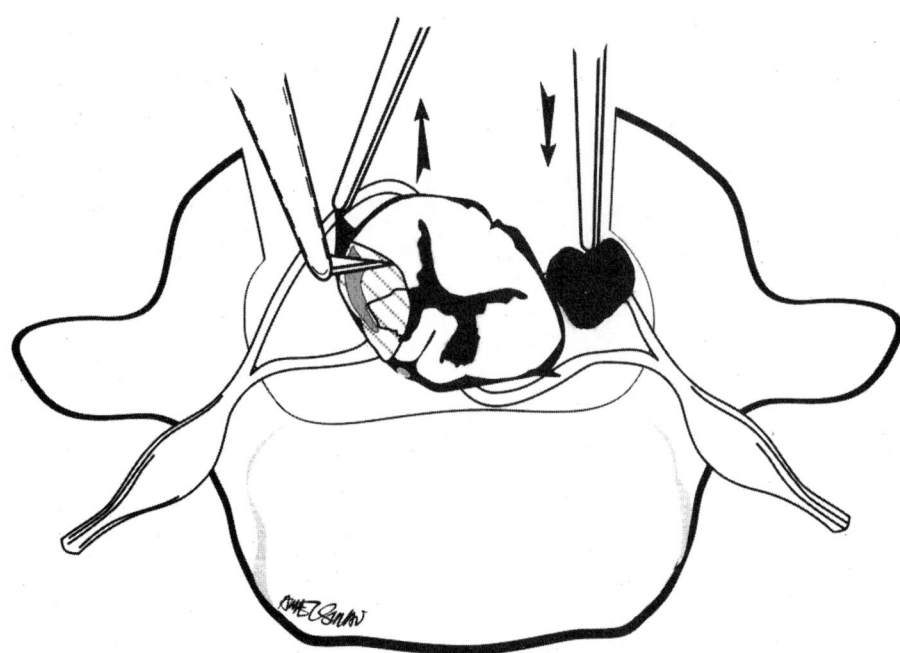

FIGURE 192–8. Schematic representation of posterior open cordotomy at the T1-2 level.

toward the cordotomy side by elevating the dentate ligament ipsilaterally, and a section is then made between the dentate ligament and the anterior root. The tract should be cut with one incision in an avascular area.[20] Some authors prefer to make a sharp incision with a knife, even in the anteromedial part of the incision. I recommend using a microspatula to sever the anteromedial pain fibers. The incision depth ranges from 3 to 5 mm, depending on the diameter measurement of the spinal cord, the severity of intractable pain, and the level of the spinal cord incision.[20, 42] In bilateral cordotomy, the second cordotomy site should be one segment up or down from the first cordotomy level. I do not recommend bilateral high cervical posterior open cordotomy. If necessary, anterior open cordotomy can be performed at the C4-5 and C5-6 levels.

Anterior Open Cordotomy

The anterior intervertebral approach is usually performed at the C5-6 or C6-7 level. If a higher level of analgesia is necessary, C4-5 is preferred. The disk space is removed at the level of the approach (i.e., C4-5, C5-6, or C6-7). An 18-mm trephine is used, and a hole is enlarged with a high-speed drill in the shape of a square. The posterior longitudinal ligament is removed. Epidural bleeding is sometimes a problem, but it can be controlled with gentle microcoagulation and microcompression with Gelfoam; aggressive compression usually increases the epidural bleeding. The dura is opened in the shape of an *X* and tacked with sutures only after epidural hemostasis has been established.

The arachnoid is incised and opened over the total operative region. A small arachnoid opening may cause a cerebrospinal fluid fistula with the valve mechanism. The anterior spinal artery is seen in the midline (Fig. 192–9). If the spinal cord is retracted gently, the dentate ligament is easily identified. If bilateral cordotomy is performed in the same session, it is better to make a second incision one segment inferior to the initial section. The depth of the incision is usually 3 to 5 mm but is determined by the incision level, the diameter measurement of the spinal cord, and the location of the pain. The dura is very difficult to close at this stage. Hardy and coworkers prefer to close the dura with silver clips.[31] I have performed five anterior open cordotomy procedures, leaving the dura open in three cases with no problem. Care is taken to ensure hemostasis, but no drain is used if the dura is left open.

RESULTS AND COMPLICATIONS

It is difficult to give results for open versus percutaneous cordotomy performed using an anterior, posterior, or lateral approach. Results depend on the volume of the destroyed part of the spinal cord at the approach level, and complications are related to spreading of the lesion in the area surrounding the target. In open cordotomy, the surgeon's ability to see the spinal cord segment directly is considered an advantage; however, mislocalization of the lesion and excessive or insufficient lesion size cannot be corrected intraoperatively. With percutaneous techniques, in contrast, controlled

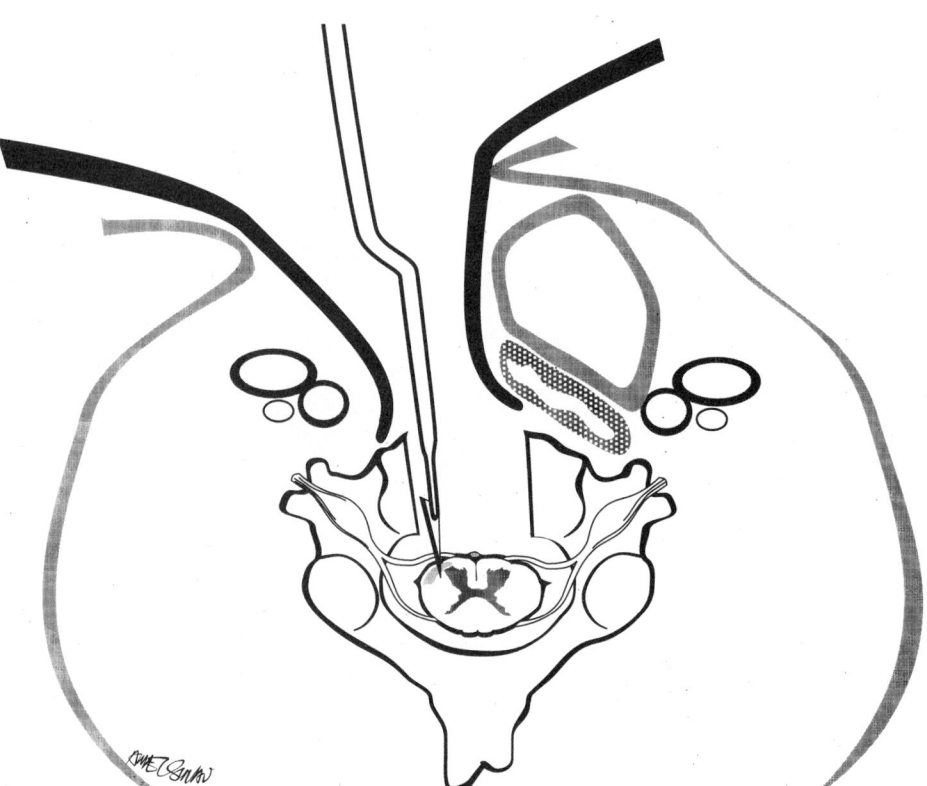

FIGURE 192–9. Schematic representation of anterior open cordotomy at the C4-5 level.

lesions are made with the help of morphologic and functional monitoring of the target.

Sindou and Daher reviewed 37 series in the literature comprising 5770 cordotomy cases.[43] Among patients with cancer (2022 cases), early pain relief was achieved after open anterolateral cordotomy in 30% to 97% of patients (mean, 70.9%) and after percutaneous anterolateral cordotomy in 76% to 100% of patients (mean, 88.3%). Long-term pain relief was experienced by 75% of patients at 6 months and by 40% after 1 year. Among noncancer patients, they reported 21.4% to 75% pain relief (mean, 47%). The best results were obtained in lower spinal cord pain or cauda equina injuries and in painful amputation stumps or phantom limbs. Long-term results have not been described by many authors, but cordotomy results after 3 months to 10 years, as reported by Rosomoff and colleagues, were as follows: the success rate was 84% at 3 months (495 patients), 61% between 3 months and 1 year (185 patients), 43% for years 1 to 5 (127 patients), and 37% for years 5 to 10 (32 patients).[44]

The outcome and complication rate associated with cordotomy are related to proper placement of the lesion and lesion diameter. Lahuerta and associates reported that the best results were obtained by creating lesions that extended 5 mm into the cord and destroyed about 20% of the hemicord.[39] This is a critical aspect of the success of cordotomy. If the location of the destruction is established using a direct imaging technique such as CT, confirmed by stimulation, and destroyed with controlled lesions, the best results can be obtained with no or minimal complications.

The mortality rate of cordotomy is related to the level of the procedure and whether it is unilateral or bilateral. This rate has been reported as 5.1% for open and 3% for percutaneous procedures in collected series.[43] Mortality is particularly increased in bilateral cervical cordotomy cases above the C4 level. Death occurs most commonly with destruction of a large portion of the anterolateral column of the reticulospinal tract, especially in bilateral lesions at the C1-2 level.[27, 41, 44, 45] This group of patients usually dies because of sleep-induced apnea. Lahuerta and colleagues reported 12 deaths after high cervical cordotomy[46]; 9 died after unilateral cordotomy and 3 after bilateral procedures. The researchers concluded that the cause of death was destruction of not only the descending respiratory pathway but also the ascending "pain pathways," which does not adequately explain the cause of respiratory complications. They advised lesions at a depth of 5 mm from the surface, but my clinical and experimental studies indicate that this depth is too medial to the target. On autopsy, the lesion area was found to be greater than 20% of the hemicord among the 9 patients who died after unilateral cordotomy.[39, 46]

Motor weakness is another important complication, and it usually occurs when lesions are made in the posterior part of the target area. The complication rate is higher in the open cordotomy group, especially in bilateral cordotomy patients. The overall motor complication rate in collected percutaneous series is 3.5%.[43] Two percent of patients in Lipton's series of 710 patients and 3%

in Rosomoff's series did not recover their motor function.[44, 47] Ataxia usually occurs secondary to destruction of the spinocerebellar tract. In percutaneous cordotomy, ataxia usually disappears within 2 weeks. Permanent ataxia was reported at a rate of 3% by Rosomoff and 0.5% by Lipton.[44, 47] Postcordotomy dysesthesia occurs due to sectioning of the lateral spinothalamic tract, especially in patients with intractable pain from benign disorders, due to their extended life spans. The incidence is given as 1% in large series.[44, 47] Horner's syndrome is frequently observed in cervical cordotomies, but it usually disappears in the long term.[43] Orthostatic hypotension as well as urinary and sexual disturbances are usually seen in bilateral lesions.

I believe that these series and figures do not provide sufficient documentation of the real status of cordotomy, because most cordotomies have been performed using the technical status of medicine 30 to 40 years ago. I thus present my series of 163 CT-guided percutaneous lateral cordotomies performed since 1987 in 144 patients at the C1-2 level. Of these, 138 patients had intractable pain caused by malignancy. Contrary to conventional criteria, most patients had intractable pain in the chest or arm region and were considered poor candidates for conventional percutaneous cordotomy. The majority of patients (75 cases, 54.3%) had malignancy of the chest and breast, including pulmonary carcinoma (40 cases, 29%), mesothelioma (16 cases, 11.6%), Pancoast's tumor (13 cases, 9.4%), and breast carcinoma (6 cases, 4.3%). The other malignancies consisted of gastrointestinal malignancies (12 cases, 8.7%), metastatic lesions (15 cases, 10.9%), prostatic carcinoma (3 cases, 2.2%), fibrosarcoma (3 cases, 2.2%), malignant melanoma (3 cases, 2.2%), and others (27 cases, 19.5%). In the group with cancer pain, pain control was obtained in 131 patients (94.9% initial success rate). Pain relief was obtained selectively in 82.7% and nonselectively in 17.3% of cases. Bilateral selective cordotomy was performed on 10 patients with intractable pain in the lower trunk and lower extremities, with achievement of pain control in 9 of them (90% initial success rate). However, most of the patients with malignancy could not be followed until the end of their lives, and no clear data could be obtained regarding the pain recurrence rate after cordotomy.

CT-guided percutaneous cordotomy was performed in six patients who had some form of intractable pain originating from benign pathologic states. Pain control was obtained in two patients with painful rhizopathy after disk surgery and gunshot and spinal cord injuries. Partial pain control was obtained in one patient with right perineural cysts at T9 and T10 and in another patient with Pott's disease who had postoperative painful neuropathy of the right cervicothoracic region. The procedure was ineffective for one patient with C5 root avulsion.

Overall, no mortality or important complications were encountered. Short-term complications included transient paresis in five cases (3.5%) and transient ataxia in four cases (2.8%). Postcordotomy hypotension was observed in three patients (bilateral cordotomy performed in two), but they stabilized with medical treatment on the first postoperative day. In two patients who underwent bilateral cordotomy, urinary retention was observed within 2 days. The only true postcordotomy complication was dysesthesia, which was observed in four patients (2.8%).

CONCLUSION

Cordotomy is not a new procedure, and in principle, it has not changed since its first application by Martin in 1911.[5] The goal of cordotomy is to interrupt pain transmission in the lateral spinothalamic tract. Conventionally, it has been performed with open techniques, and some surgeons continue to use these methods. In experienced hands, the open technique can be safe and effective, but it has two main disadvantages: first, open approaches, whether anterior or posterior, are not well tolerated by cancer patients in poor health; and second, this functional procedure is performed under general anesthesia. Although current technology enables us to monitor some spinal cord functions, an unconscious patient cannot cooperate with the surgeon during the operation.

Since Mullan's discovery of the percutaneous method, it has been routinely used with an RF system. The percutaneous application is performed under local anesthesia, which allows cooperation with the patient during the procedure and facilitates neurophysiologic monitoring and controlled lesioning of the target. In conventional percutaneous cordotomy, the most critical problem is that the visualization system—radiographic imaging—demonstrates the spinal cord indirectly. Even with the use of contrast material, only the dentate ligament plus the anterior and posterior borders of the spinal cord are visualized, not the spinal cord segment at the approach level. With radiographic imaging, individual spinal cord diameters—which are necessary for calibration of the depth of insertion of the active electrode—are not measured. The needle direction cannot be superimposed on the target, which facilitates insertion of the active electrode using morphologic orientation. Finally, the target-electrode relation is not directly demonstrated.

The new version of cordotomy—CT-guided, percutaneous cordotomy—is a stereotactic, real-time, functional procedure. Three-dimensional, stereotactic localization is obtained by the CT image. The patient's spinal cord diameters are measured, and those measurements are used to adjust the depth of insertion of the active electrode.[18] Direct visualization averts the need for multiple maneuvers when placing the electrode with the help of impedance measurements. Demonstration of mislocalization or improper insertion of the electrode, as well as torsion of the spinal cord, is possible.[14–16] Functional evaluation of the target with stimulation allows selective cordotomy to be performed unilaterally or bilaterally using controlled lesions made in close cooperation with the patient.

We are living in a new age—the technology and information age. The average life span has increased as a result of the successes of science and technology,

and the outcome is that we are living among a more elderly population with an increased incidence of cancer and degenerative diseases. Intractable pain remains a great problem in this group, despite recent advancements in technology and dramatic discoveries in pharmacology. The National Cancer Society estimates that approximately 8 million Americans alive today have a history of cancer; an estimated 564,800 Americans died of cancer in 1998, 28.6% of whom had lung cancer.[48] Twenty-five percent of cancer patients die without relief of severe pain,[33] despite the fact that many types of intractable cancer pain—especially that associated with mesothelioma and some unilateral bronchogenic carcinomas (conditions traditionally considered risky for conventional cordotomy)—can be denervated easily and effectively with CT-guided cordotomy. Pain palliation is necessary for terminal cases as well as for other patients with intractable pain, some of whom can return to their active lives once the pain is relieved.

Cordotomy is indisputably an effective procedure in neurosurgery practice and is still used by a number of surgeons, but there is some resistance to the new version of cordotomy. A tremendous number of patients worldwide could benefit from this procedure. Thanks to recent advancements in electrode and visualization technology, this technique can be performed easily and effectively. The best results are obtained in properly selected patients using the proper technique.

ACKNOWLEDGMENTS

Special thanks to Helen Stevens, RNC, for her editing skills; to Ahmet Sinav, MD, for his creative drawings; and to Ali Savas, MD, PhD, for his assistance in preparing this chapter. I would also like to acknowledge Professor Nurhan Avman, Professor Ziya Guner, and Professor William H. Sweet, who have been mentors throughout my career and have inspired me in the pursuit of excellence.

REFERENCES

1. Clarke E, O'Malley CD: Function of the spinal cord. In Clarke E, O'Malley CD (eds): The Human Brain and the Spinal Cord. San Francisco, Norman Publishing, 1996, pp 291–322.
2. Sjöqvist O: Discussion on the conduction of pain from the face. In Sjöqvist O (ed): Studies on Pain Conduction in the Trigeminal Nerve. Helsingfors, Finland, Mercators Tryckeri, 1938, pp 85–93.
3. Spiller WG: The location within the spinal cord of the fibers for temperature and pain sensations. J Nerv Ment Dis 32:318–320, 1905.
4. Schüller A: Über operative Durchtrennung der Rückenmarksstrange (Chordotomie). Wien Med Wochenschr 60:2292–2295, 1910.
5. Spiller WG, Martin E: The treatment of persistent pain of organic origin in the lower part of the body by division of the anterolateral column of the spinal cord. JAMA 58:1489–1490, 1912.
6. Frazier CH: Section of the anterolateral columns of the spinal cord for the relief of pain. Arch Neurol Psychiatry 4:137, 1920.
7. Collis JS: Anterolateral cordotomy by an anterior approach: Report of a case. J Neurosurg 20:445–446, 1963.
8. Cloward RB: Cervical cordotomy by the anterior approach: Technique and advantages. J Neurosurg 21:19–25, 1964.
9. Mullan S, Harper PV, Hekmatpanah J, et al: Percutaneous interruption of spinal-pain tracts by means of a strontium needle. J Neurosurg 20:931–939, 1963.

10. Mullan S, Hekmatpanah J, Dobben G, et al: Percutaneous, intramedullary cordotomy utilizing the unipolar anodal electrolytic lesion. J Neurosurg 22:548–555, 1965.
11. Rosomoff HL, Carroll F, Brown J, et al: Percutaneous radiofrequency cervical cordotomy: Technique. J Neurosurg 23:639–644, 1965.
12. Lin PM, Gildenberg PL, Polacoff PO: An anterior approach to percutaneous lower cervical cordotomy. J Neurosurg 25:553–560, 1966.
13. Kanpolat Y, Atalag M, Deda H, et al: CT-guided extralemniscal myelotomy. Acta Neurochir (Wien) 91:151–152, 1988.
14. Kanpolat Y, Deda H, Akyar S, et al: CT-guided percutaneous cordotomy. Acta Neurochir Suppl (Wien) 46:67–68, 1989.
15. Kanpolat Y, Akyar S, Çaglar S, et al: CT-guided percutaneous selective cordotomy. Acta Neurochir (Wien) 123:92–97, 1993.
16. Kanpolat Y, Savas A, Çaglar S, et al: Computerized tomography–guided percutaneous bilateral selective cordotomy. Neurosurg Focus 2:Article 5, 1997.
17. Mullan S: Percutaneous cordotomy. J Neurosurg 35:360–366, 1971.
18. Kanpolat Y, Akyar S, Çaglar S: Diametral measurements of the upper spinal cord for stereotactic pain procedures. Surg Neurol 43:478–483, 1995.
19. Kameyama T, Hashizume Y, Sobue G: Morphologic features of the normal human cadaveric spinal cord. Spine 21:1285–1290, 1996.
20. Poletti CE: Open cordotomy and medullary tractotomy. In Schmidek HH, Sweet WH (eds): Operative Neurosurgical Techniques. Philadelphia, WB Saunders, 1995, pp 1557–1571.
21. Hyndman OR, Van Epps C: Possibility of differential section of the spinothalamic tract: A clinical and histological study. Arch Surg 38:1036–1053, 1939.
22. Walker EA: The spinothalamic tract in man. Arch Neurol Psychiatry 43:284–298, 1940.
23. White JC, Sweet WH: Pain and the Neurosurgeon: A Forty Year Experience. Springfield, Ill, Charles C Thomas, 1969.
24. Peet MM: The control of intractable pain in the lumbar region, pelvis and lower extremities. Arch Surg 13:153–204, 1926.
25. Taren JA, Davis R, Crosby EC: Target physiologic corroboration in stereotaxic cervical cordotomy. J Neurosurg 30:569–584, 1969.
26. Nathan PW: The descending respiratory pathway in man. J Neurol Neurosurg Psychiatry 26:487–499, 1963.
27. Belmusto L, Brown E, Owens G: Clinical observations on respiratory and vasomotor disturbance as related to cervical cordotomies. J Neurosurg 25:225–232, 1963.
28. Hitchcock E, Leece B: Somatotopic representation of the respiratory pathways in the cervical cord of man. J Neurosurg 27:320–329, 1967.
29. Tasker RR: Cordotomy for pain. In Youmans JR (ed): Neurological Surgery, 4th ed. Philadelphia, WB Saunders, 1996, pp 3463–3476.
30. Tasker RR, North R: Cordotomy and myelotomy. In Tasker RR, North R (eds): Neurological Management of Pain. New York, Springer, 1997, pp 191–220.
31. Hardy J, LeClercq TA, Mercky F: Microsurgical cordotomy by the anterior approach. J Neurosurg 41:640–643, 1974.
32. World Health Organization: Cancer pain relief and palliative care. Geneva, World Health Organization, 1990.
33. Foley KM: The treatment of cancer pain. N Engl J Med 313:84–95, 1985.
34. Gybels JM: Indications for the use of neurosurgical techniques in pain control. In Bond MR, Charlton JE, Wolf J (eds): Proceedings of the Sixth World Congress on Pain. Amsterdam, Elsevier, 1995, pp 475–482.
35. Amano K, Kawamura H, Tanikawa T, et al: Bilateral versus unilateral percutaneous high cervical cordotomy as a surgical method of pain relief. Acta Neurochir Suppl (Wien) 52:143–145, 1991.
36. Fenstermaker RA, Sternau LL, Takaoka Y: CT-assisted percutaneous anterior cordotomy. Surg Neurol 43:147–150, 1995.
37. Kanpolat Y, Cosman E: Special radiofrequency electrode system for computed tomography–guided pain-relieving procedures. Neurosurgery 38:600–603, 1996.
38. Izumi J, Hirose Y, Yazaki T: Percutaneous trigeminal rhizotomy and percutaneous cordotomy under general anesthesia. Stereotact Funct Neurosurg 59:62–68, 1992.
39. Lahuerta J, Bowsher D, Lipton S, et al: Percutaneous cervical cordotomy: A review of 181 operations on 146 patients with a study on the location of "pain fibres" in the C-2 spinal cord segment of 29 cases. J Neurosurg 80:975–985, 1994.
40. Lin MP: Percutaneous lower cervical cordotomy. In Gildenberg PL, Tasker RR (eds): Textbook of Stereotactic and Functional Neurosurgery. New York, McGraw-Hill, 1998, pp 1403–1409.
41. Gildenberg PL: Percutaneous cervical cordotomy. Clin Neurosurg 21:246–256, 1974.
42. Ehni BL, Ehni G: Open surgical cordotomy. In Wilkins HR, Rengachary SS (eds): Neurosurgery. New York, McGraw-Hill, 1985, pp 2439–2445.
43. Sindou M, Daher A: Spinal cord ablation procedures for pain. In Dubner R, Gebhart GF, Bond MR (eds): Proceedings of the Vth World Congress on Pain. Amsterdam, Elsevier, 1988, pp 477–495.
44. Rosomoff HL, Papo I, Loeser JD: Neurosurgical operations on the spinal cord. In Bonicca JJ (ed): The Management of Pain. Philadelphia, Lea & Febiger, 1990, pp 2067–2081.
45. Rosomoff H: Bilateral percutaneous cervical radiofrequency cordotomy. J Neurosurg 31:41–46, 1969.
46. Lahuerta J, Buxton P, Lipton S, et al: The location and function of respiratory fibers in the second cervical spinal cord segment: Respiratory dysfunction syndrome after cervical cordotomy. J Neurol Neurosurg Psychiatry 55:1142–1145, 1992.
47. Lipton S: Percutaneous cordotomy. In Wall PD, Melzac R (eds): Textbook of Pain. Edinburgh, Churchill Livingstone, 1989, pp 832–839.
48. American Cancer Society: Cancer Facts & Figures. Atlanta, GA, American Cancer Society, 1998.

CHAPTER 193

Brainstem Procedures for Management of Pain

PHILIP L. GILDENBERG

Alleviation of pain has long been a goal of neurosurgery. The earliest attempts involved cutting peripheral or cranial nerves to trade numbness for pain. Later procedures involved cutting the lateral spinothalamic tract to interrupt pain perception but leave touch and proprioception sensations in tact. It was only when pain pathways within the brainstem were targeted that the importance of interruption of the extralemniscal pathways was established. A review of brainstem procedures for the management of pain provides a perspective on how pain treatment concepts have changed through the years.

It is difficult to glean meaningful conclusions from reports of the treatment of pain using various procedures. Especially in the older literature, the clinical type of pain is rarely defined adequately, confounding psychological and addiction factors are rarely taken into account, the location and duration of pain are often not stated, the influence of prior treatments (especially denervation procedures) is ignored, many do not relate the type of neuropathic pain to peripheral versus central denervation versus neuropathy, and there is no standard measure of either pain or pain relief. Many papers do not even make a distinction between cancer pain and chronic pain of noncancer origin. Despite this imperfect information, there has been considerable progress in pain management in the past 5 decades.

MESENCEPHALOTOMY

The use of mesencephalotomy for pain management began before the introduction of stereotactic surgery, but it was only with that technique that it became feasible. The gradual evolution and modification of mesencephalotomy were instrumental in solidifying concepts of the anatomy of the diffusely projecting pain system within the brain, and it remains a useful technique for pain management for limited indications.

Anatomy of the Mesencephalon

The mesencephalon constitutes only a 1.5-cm length of the brainstem, but it contains more important relays and neural structures than any comparably sized area of the nervous system. It correlates and coordinates input from the somatosensory, touch, proprioceptive, and pain systems; coordinates auditory, visual, and oculomotor functions; supports basic reflexes related to sympathetic responses, food, and sexual drives; and is important in consciousness and alertness.

The aqueduct runs through the mesencephalon, surrounded by a central gray that consists of small nuclei with short axons constituting a multisynaptic reticular system.

The mesencephalon is divided anterodorsally into three regions (Fig. 193–1A). The area dorsal to the aqueduct is the quadrigeminal plate. The bilateral superior colliculi occupy the superior half and are involved with coordination of the head and eyes in response to visual, auditory, and somatic stimuli. Injury to this structure can produce loss of upward gaze, Parinaud's syndrome, or disruption of reflexes that turn vision toward a stimulus. Although Parinaud's syndrome may occur after mesencephalotomy, it is usually not of great clinical significance, and most patients are unaware of it until it is discovered on testing.

The inferior quadrigeminal plate consists of the inferior colliculi, which receive auditory fibers from the lateral lemniscus and are involved with acoustic reflexes. Lesions can inconsistently cause impairment of auditory perception. Because the brachium lies just lateral and dorsal to the spinothalamic tract, lesions made for pain management may interrupt input to the inferior colliculus.

The most ventral part of the mesencephalon is formed by the two large crura cerebri or peduncles, which consist of fibers running from the cerebrum to lower structures, with minimal direct communication with the relay structures within the mesencephalon. The medial three fifths contain somatotopically arranged corticospinal and corticobulbar fibers. The most medial and lateral fifths contain corticopontine axons. Although these structures have been approached for nonstereotactic surgery for movement disorders, they are a distance from the usual sites of stereotactic targets and are not usually involved with mesencephalotomy.

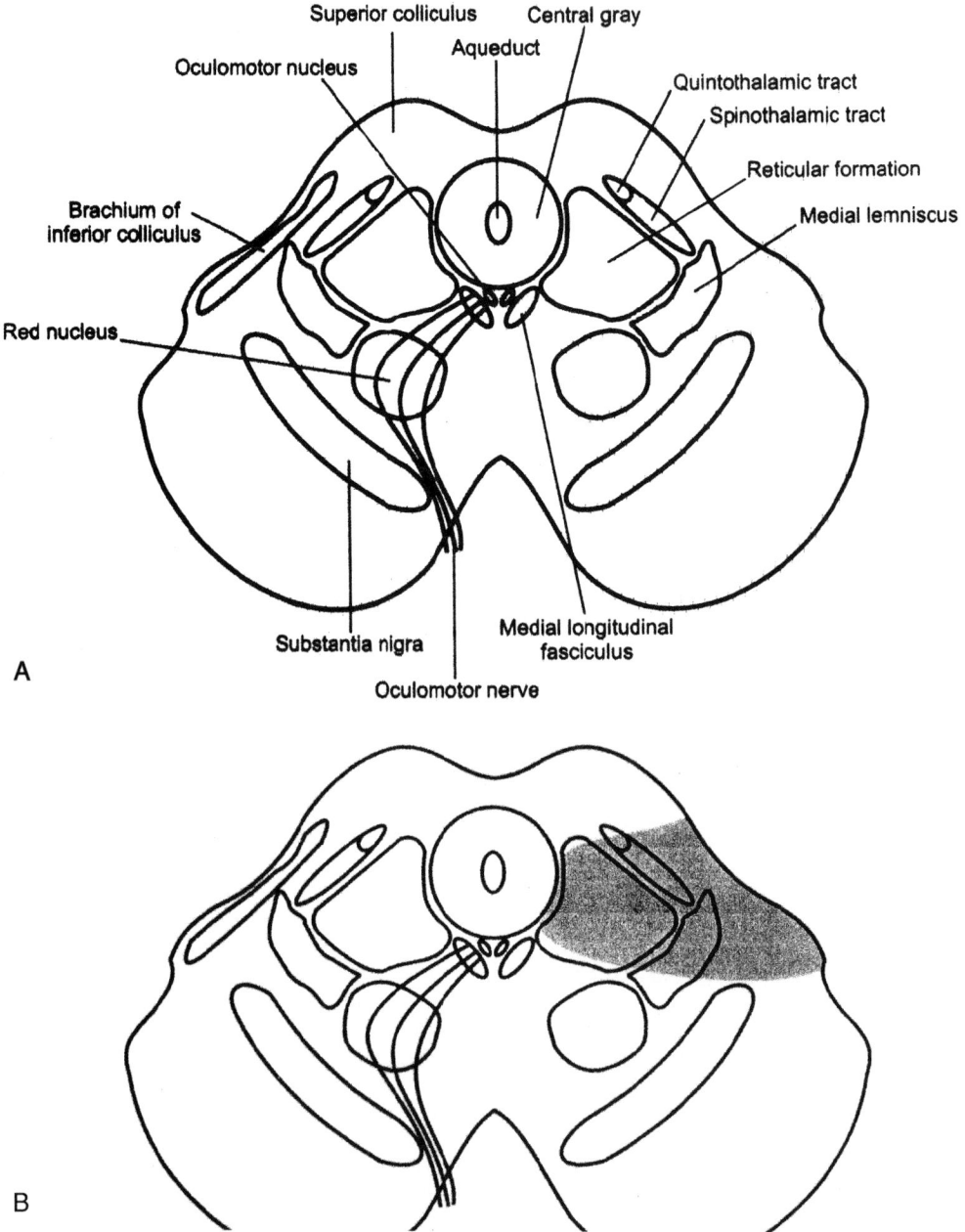

FIGURE 193–1. Anatomy of the mesencephalon. *A,* Structures of clinical significance are labeled. Section at the level of the superior colliculus dorsally and the inferior colliculus ventrally. *B,* Illustration of a typical section for Walker open surgical mesencephalotomy.[13] (From Burchiel K: Pain Surgery. New York, Thieme, 2000.)

The tegmentum lies just dorsal to the peduncles and ventral to the tectum and is a compact area containing nuclear structures, relay centers, and fibers passing through. The rostral tegmentum lies ventral to the superior colliculi.

The oculomotor nuclei lie in the rostral tegmentum just anterior to the central gray on both sides adjacent to the midline. The emerging fibers splay out through the red nuclei, which are at the level of the inferior colliculus, and come together again just as they leave the mesencephalon between the peduncles to form the oculomotor nerves. The trochlear and abducens nuclei are also at the level of the inferior colliculi and are connected with the oculomotor nuclei through the medial longitudinal fasciculus to coordinate eye movements.

The medial lemniscus carries somatosensory information from the dorsal columns. It lies just anterolateral to the spinothalamic tract and dorsolateral to the red nucleus. It lies close enough to the spinothalamic tract that it can be damaged when the latter is sectioned for pain management. Indeed, with prestereotactic mesencephalotomy that involved an incision in the dorsolateral mesencephalon to interrupt the spinothalamic tract, the medial lemniscus was invariably damaged, which may have contributed to the high incidence of dysesthesia from that procedure, whereas stereotactic procedures are targeted to avoid the medial lemniscus.

The spinothalamic tract lies just medial to the medial lemniscus near the dorsolateral surface of the mesencephalon. It is arranged somatotopically, with the higher levels more medial. Just medial to the spinothalamic tract lies the quintothalamic tract, which continues the somatotopy with the sensation from the head and face lying more medial still. Nashold and coworkers[1] mapped these areas by stimulating over several days with electrodes that had been inserted before mesencephalotomy. There is some irregularity in the organization of the medial structures, however, in that some facial areas have bilateral representation; some somatic sensory information conveyed by the seventh, ninth, and tenth cranial nerves is also represented; and there is some sensation from internal body cavities.

There are only 1500 fibers in the spinothalamic tract at the level of the mesencephalon, compared with 15,000 fibers in the upper cervical spinal cord.[2] Those few remaining fibers continue to the ventral posterolateral nucleus of the thalamus, which is also the terminus of the medial lemniscus.

As the spinothalamic tract ascends through the brainstem, individual fibers leave the direct pathway to synapse with the spinoreticular system or mesencephalic reticular formation. That multisynaptic pathway projects to two areas bilaterally. One contribution is the intralaminar and centromedian areas of the thalamus,[3] which are also targets for stereotactic ablation for the treatment of pain.[4, 5] The spinoreticular system also projects to the hypothalamus,[6] and that area has also been the target for severe, intractable chronic pain with a significant emotional component.[7] It has been postulated that the somatosensory thalamic projections are concerned with the discriminative aspects of pain, whereas the hypothalamic and limbic route subserves motivational aspects of pain, that is, the suffering that accompanies persistent pain.[5, 8]

Verification of these concepts of the various contributions of the direct and indirect pain pathways resulted to a large extent from stimulation studies done in patients to map the ideal target for mesencephalotomy.

Development

The spinothalamic tract was identified as early as 1878 as the pathway for pain perception after postmortem study of a patient who had lost unilateral pain sensation with preservation of touch after a gunshot wound.[9] This was followed by an observation by Spiller[10] in 1905 of a patient with a spinal tuberculoma who had similar loss of only pain and temperature sensation, which was the basis for Spiller and Martin[11] to perform the first anterolateral cordotomy for the treatment of pain in 1912. However, pain in the upper extremity required section of the spinothalamic tract at levels higher than could be produced at that time with spinal

cordotomy. Pain in the head and face required section of the quintothalamic tract, the cranial nerve equivalent of the spinothalamic tract. Although Dogliotti[12] sectioned the spinothalamic tract in the pons in 1938, results were inconsistent, and neurological complications were common.

The spinothalamic tract was reasonably accessible as it lay superficially in the dorsolateral mesencephalon, with the quintothalamic tract just medial to it. This led Walker,[13] in 1942, to perform open mesencephalotomy via a subtemporal craniotomy. A pie-shaped incision was made through the pia to interrupt the spinothalamic pathway, which resulted in good hemianalgesia and usually pain relief. It also often interrupted the medial lemniscus, so it left a feeling of numbness on the entire contralateral side and often significant dysesthesia. The illustration in that article demonstrated that the lesion also involved the brachium of the inferior colliculus, the lateral edge of the periaqueductal gray, and the intervening reticular formation (Fig. 193–1*B*). Similar complications were noted by Drake and McKenzie.[14] White and Sweet[15] stated that the procedure was not acceptable because of the occurrence of severe dysesthesia, a high postoperative mortality rate, and the tendency of the analgesia to diminish with time.

It was only a few years after the introduction of Walker's procedure that stereotactic surgery was introduced by Spiegel and colleagues.[16] As early as 1947, they performed a stereotactic mesencephalic spinoquintothalamic tractotomy for facial dysesthetic pain of iatrogenic origin, and stereotactic techniques have become the standard for mesencephalotomy since then.[17] They reported that pain relief in that patient lasted for 18 years. The medial lemniscus was avoided, and dysesthesia was not produced. The lesion was designed to interrupt both the spinothalamic and quintothalamic tracts, but it also probably encroached on the reticular formation dorsal to the red nucleus as it entered the central gray. They also made a lesion in the dorsomedial nucleus of the thalamus, which helped verify the concept of the suffering component of pain being projected via the spinoreticular system to limbic structures.[18] In those days of prefrontal lobotomy, they combined lesions for a variety of indications with dorsomedial lesions to blunt the affective component of the neurological dysfunction by interruption of the projections to the prefrontal area.[19]

Further evidence indicated that damage to the medial lemniscus was responsible for the severe dysesthesia. Frank and coworkers[20] correlated injury to that structure with dysesthesia after Walker's mesencephalotomy. Colombo[21] recorded sensory evoked potentials before, during, and after mesencephalotomy in eight patients to map the extent of the lesion and also concluded that dysesthesia correlated with abolition of the medial lemniscus response.

Other neurosurgeons targeted mainly the spinothalamic and spinoreticular pathways. Leksell[22] initially advocated including the medial lemniscus along with the spinothalamic tract for cancer pain. Mark and associates[23] advocated combining a thalamic with a mesencephalic lesion. Roeder and Orthner[24] noted marked reduction in the affective response to pain when the spinoreticulothalamic area was included in the lesion.

In 1954 Spiegel and colleagues[25, 26] demonstrated both in the laboratory and in patients with thalamic syndrome that pain was transmitted via the spinoreticular pathways. Thereafter, they advocated that the mesencephalotomy lesion extend medially to include spinoreticular areas, but they expressed caution about the extent of such lesions, especially in patients with a strong emotional component to their pain syndromes.[26, 27] They did, however, advise dorsomedial nucleus lesions in those patients and later obtained good relief of chronic pain by making lesions in the centromedianus and intralaminar thalamus without involving the somatosensory or spinothalamic areas.[28] Whisler and Voris,[29] however, involved the spinoreticular area freely and even made bilateral lesions, with excellent results and no adverse effects.

The study that best defined the physiologic anatomy and the best mesencephalotomy targets was done by Nashold and colleagues[1] in 1969 (Fig. 193–2). They inserted electrodes into the mesencephalon and stimulated over a period of several weeks to define the optimal location for the mesencephalotomy lesion. In doing so, they made critical observations about the organization of the mesencephalon in humans. They verified that the somatotopic organization of the spinothalamic and quintothalamic tracts extended from lateral to medial, and they were the first to demonstrate that the thorax and abdomen are represented medially, near the central gray. High-frequency stimulation in the central gray produced unpleasant sensations involving midline structures, as well as a strong negative or fearful emotional reaction, sometimes with hyperventi-

lation, a feeling of panic, involuntary verbalization or flushing, and slowed pulse and respiration, which have since been related to projections to the hypothalamus.[25, 30] Such stimulation at the level of the superior colliculus produced sensations in the face, arm, chest, and trunk, but stimulation at the level of the inferior colliculus produced sensations in just the arm and face, with little emotional response to stimulation. Complex ocular movements defined oculomotor or superior collicular areas in which lesions should be avoided. Low-frequency stimulation of the medial lemniscus produced a contralateral tremor. Stimulation of the spinothalamic tract produced burning pain, numbness, or a cold sensation localized contralaterally. By such stimulation, they localized that tract between 5 and 10 mm lateral to the midline.

On the basis of these stimulation studies, Nashold and Wilson[31] defined their target. They moved it medial to the original site directly overlying the spinothalamic tract, so they would encroach on the medial reticular area and lateral edge of the central gray. The result was improved relief of intractable pain with less sensory loss and no dysesthesia.[32] In addition, they noted that the pain relief was often bilateral, confirming the concept of projection from the midbrain reticular formation to the intralaminar thalamus bilaterally. Shieff and Nashold[33] later wrote that chronic pain is invariably associated with emotional distress, which is not purely a secondary psychological phenomenon but results from intrinsic neural changes. Interruption of the extralemniscal pathways alleviated the emotional aspect of pain and consequently the pain perception itself.

Tasker[34] also performed extensive mapping of stimu-

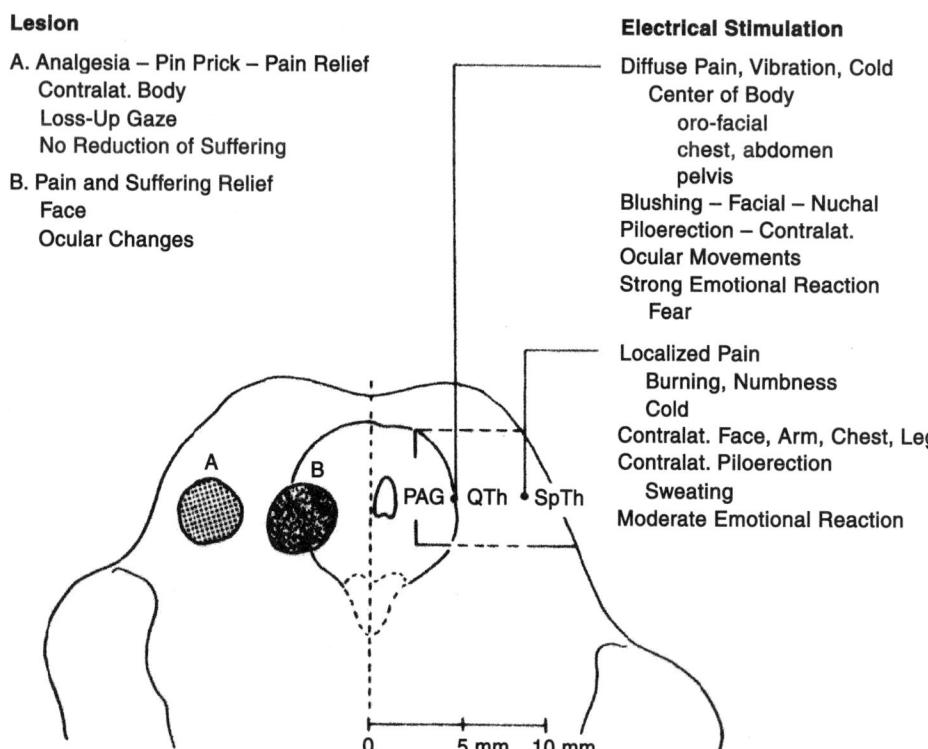

Lesion

A. Analgesia – Pin Prick – Pain Relief
   Contralat. Body
   Loss-Up Gaze
   No Reduction of Suffering

B. Pain and Suffering Relief
   Face
   Ocular Changes

Electrical Stimulation

Diffuse Pain, Vibration, Cold
   Center of Body
      oro-facial
      chest, abdomen
      pelvis
Blushing – Facial – Nuchal
Piloerection – Contralat.
Ocular Movements
Strong Emotional Reaction
   Fear

Localized Pain
   Burning, Numbness
   Cold
Contralat. Face, Arm, Chest, Leg
Contralat. Piloerection
   Sweating
Moderate Emotional Reaction

FIGURE 193–2. Effects produced by stimulation and stereotactic lesions at two sites in the mesencephalon. (From Nashold BS Jr: Brainstem stereotaxic procedures. In Schaltenbrand G, Walker AE [eds]: Stereotaxy of the Human Brain. New York, Stuttgart, Thieme, 1982, pp 475–483.)

lation of the mesencephalon in awake patients during stereotactic surgery. He identified the medial lemniscus as lying 10 to 12 mm lateral and the spinothalamic tract 7 to 9 mm lateral. Stimulation of the reticulothalamic tract 5 to 7 mm from the midline produced no effect unless the current were sufficient to affect the periaqueductal gray, which produced bizarre emotional responses.

The most distressing complication is disturbance of ocular motility. This was particularly common, occurring in 50% of cases, at Spiegel and Wycis's[18] original lesion site at the level of the superior colliculus or at the intercommissural plane. Shieff and Nashold[33, 35] and Amano[36] recommended moving the target caudally to the level of the inferior colliculus, 5 mm below the intercommissural plane, which significantly alleviated this complication.

Spiegel and Wycis's[18] original technique involved insertion of the electrode parasagittally from the parieto-occipital region, in anticipation that the electrode would intersect the spinothalamic system at an angle that would increase the chance of complete interruption. However, the electrode traversed the posterior limb of the internal capsule, which was blamed for the weakness of the contralateral leg seen in several patients. Also, the pia was pierced at the mesencephalon, so potential distortion of the target occurred. Nashold and colleagues,[37] however, advocated inserting the electrode from the coronal area, so it was introduced along the long axis of the brainstem, angulating medially by 2 to 4 degrees. This has become the most commonly used approach.

Indications

Types of mesencephalotomy were done in the prestereotactic era for the treatment of movement disorders, but this discussion involves only pain management, so they are not considered here.

The primary indication for mesencephalotomy is management of cancer pain of the head, face, neck, or upper extremity. If there is a great emotional component, as there often is in patients with extensive facial or pharyngeal cancer, an additional lesion in the dorsomedial, intralaminar, or basal thalamus may add considerably to success (Fig. 193–3).[28] Although cingulotomy has also been cited as being a helpful lesion site,[38] a lesion in the thalamus is just as effective, a smaller lesion can be used, and the target is near the primary target. I have found that the neuropathic pain of Pancoast's syndrome responds well to an intralaminar thalamotomy without the addition of a mesencephalotomy lesion.

Nashold and colleagues[37] reported considerable benefit from mesencephalotomy for central pain due to central nervous system pathologic involvement of the ascending pain pathways within the medulla, midbrain, or thalamus, the so-called lateral medullary plate syndrome and the thalamic syndrome. Mesencephalotomy is effective in many cases, whether the primary pathology lies above or below the mesencephalon, as though the addition of spinothalamic and spinoreticulothalamic input drives the pain sensation.

Postherpetic facial or upper extremity pain may benefit from mesencephalotomy if the symptoms are so

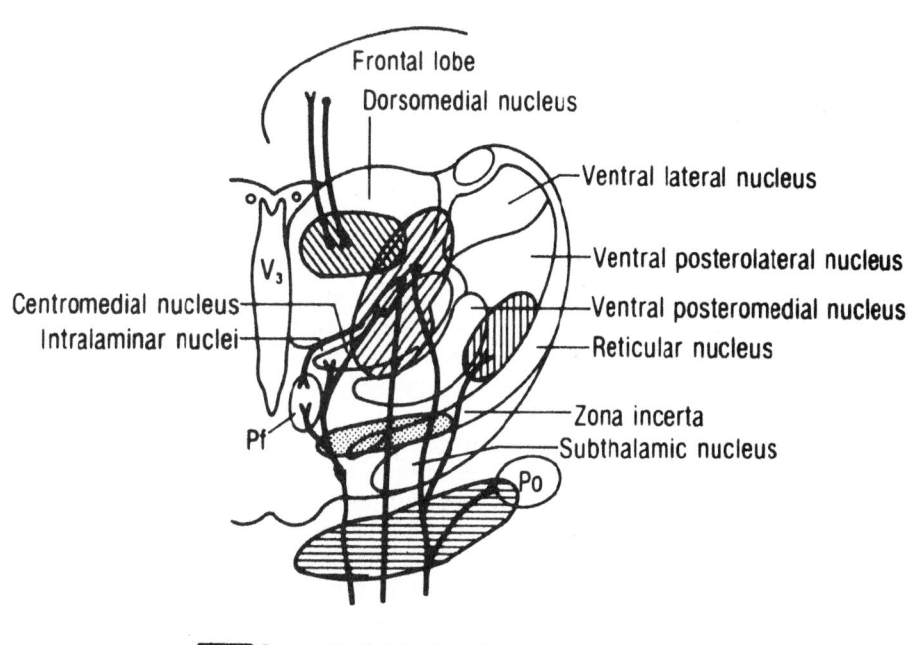

FIGURE 193–3. Targets for intralaminar and basal thalamotomy and mesencephalotomy. (Adapted from Spiegel EA, Wycis HT, Szekely EG, Gildenberg PL: Medial and basal thalamotomy in so-called intractable pain. In Knighton RS, Dumke PR [eds]: Pain. Boston, Little, Brown, 1966, pp 503–517.)

disabling that the risk is justified. Facial dysesthesia following denervation after unsuccessful surgery for trigeminal neuralgia may benefit from mesencephalotomy. So-called atypical facial neuralgia is not likely to benefit from any surgical procedure, because this ill-defined syndrome is often a distortion of somatosensory sensation rather than a sensation carried along the classic pain pathways.

Nashold[5] reported that patients who had been taking large doses of narcotics for their pain syndromes may be withdrawn abruptly after mesencephalotomy with minimal withdrawal effects. I have noted the same phenomenon after basal or intralaminar thalamotomy,[39] which involves interruption of the same spinoreticulothalamic pathway at a slightly higher level. It can also be observed in narcotic-addicted rats after a lesion in the centromedianus causes a decrease in drug-seeking behavior.[40] The results are not consistent enough, comprehensive enough, or dramatic enough to advocate the use of such lesions to treat narcotic addiction, however.

Technique

Mesencephalotomy is performed with the same care as any other functional stereotactic procedure. Perhaps the most important aspect of surgery is the selection of appropriate patients, which must be done with care. Psychological and addiction factors must be considered, and a comprehensive psychological evaluation of the patient is advisable.[41]

Because mesencephalotomy as currently practiced is an extralemniscal procedure, both the pain and suffering components of somatic pain may benefit. This is particularly helpful in patients undergoing the stress of head and facial carcinoma or in patients with central neuropathic pain. Surgery alone is rarely sufficient to deal with the emotional components of persistent pain, but successful surgery may open the door to a successful supportive psychological program. If psychological factors are the overwhelming component, the patient may benefit more from an intralaminar or basal thalamotomy[28] or a cingulotomy[42] than from a mesencephalotomy.

Patients with chronic pain not related to cancer must be selected with particular care. Before any procedure, a multidisciplinary noninvasive program that involves both the psychiatric and rehabilitation needs of the patient should be attempted.[41, 43]

The procedure must be explained to the patient in detail, and the patient's participation in intraoperative monitoring must be practiced before entering the operating room. During surgery, the patient is awake, usually in the semireclining position. There are currently a variety of imaging procedures that can be used to define the stereotactic target. Some authors use intraoperative ventriculography, but more and more are using computed tomography, magnetic resonance imaging (MRI), or a combination. I prefer to use axial MRI to measure the targets. First the anterior and posterior commissures are identified on a T2-weighted sagittal scan. The targeting measurements are made

on an axial scan, using the image recovery sequence technique developed at Emory Medical Center.[44] The midpoints of both commissures are identified by correlating the three-dimensional MRI console coordinates with the sagittal scan to establish the intercommissural line. Measurements are made on the MRI console to establish the target coordinates, and identical measurements are drawn on graph paper to verify the targeting. Correction for minor rotation error is made on the axial scan, and correction for minor tilt error is made on the coronal scan, both of which are verified by manually graphing the corrections. Lately, I have also used the StealthStation Framelink for additional verification of the target point and have found it very helpful.

The anatomic target is 5 mm behind the posterior commissure, 5 to 10 mm lateral to and 5 mm below the intercommissural plane, which is an amalgam of the target points of several authors.[5, 18, 24, 35, 37]

Stimulation is done at various frequencies between 2 and 300 Hz to identify the location of the tip of the 1.2-mm-diameter electrode.[5] The surgeon looks for those responses described earlier that indicate stimulation of the surrounding structures, particularly extraocular movements (too high, in the emerging oculomotor fibers), fear or emotional outburst (central gray, too medial if at low current), or projection of spinothalamic sensation to the contralateral body (the lesion is just medial to this site). Stimulation of the target area produces some emotional response, and sensation in general is projected to the central core of the body. Amano and associates[45] reported observations with microelectrode recording, with neurons in the target reticular area responding only to peripheral pinprick stimulation with a latency of 250 to 1000 msec.

The lesion is made at 70°C for 30 seconds.[46] There is usually no discernible analgesia except with critical testing, but even in the stressful operating room environment, many patients report pain relief. Even if the pain is bilateral, it is best to make only a lesion contralateral to the more severe pain. Many patients do not need a second lesion. Those who do can have the procedure done more safely after waiting at least 3 weeks.

Results

Several compilations of numerous articles about mesencephalotomy have been published by Nashold,[5] Tasker,[47] and Gybels and Sweet.[48] Because all three reviewed essentially the same prior series,[21, 27, 29, 32, 37, 49–55] only a summary is presented here. The individual reports are tabulated most clearly in the Gybels and Sweet book.[48]

To tabulate results, it is important to divide patients into those with cancer pain and those without. Most of the patients with noncancer pain in the various mesencephalotomy series had neuropathic or denervation pain, but usually the specific cause was not given. It is therefore difficult to draw conclusions about noncancer, non-neuropathic pain except to say that long-term relief cannot be expected, so a procedure fraught with significant risk should not be considered.

Considerable success was reported in a total of 270 patients treated for cancer pain. Cumulative reports indicated that 86% of patients had significant pain relief, usually for life. However, mortality rates varied between 1.8% and 8%. Oculomotor dysfunction was seen in 13% to 20% of patients, even after the lesion was placed at the safer, lower mesencephalic location. Dysesthesia occurred in 15% to 21%. One study reported 15.8% "lemniscal damage," with 42.1% dysesthesia.[56]

Most authors did not recommend mesencephalotomy for chronic noncancer pain, except for neuropathic pain. Nashold and colleagues[37] reported 15 patients with central neuropathic pain. Although 11 had short-term pain relief, the pain relief lasted longer than 10 years in 8 (53%), which was consistent with the 50% long-term success rate in 24 patients in a more recent report.[35] In contrast, Voris and Whisler[50] reported long-term relief in only 5 of 23 patients (18%).[56] With an average 42-month follow-up, Amano and coworkers[51] reported successful alleviation of chronic pain in 28 of 34 patients (82%). Tables illustrating results from series involving mesencephalotomy and other brainstem procedures have been published.[48, 57]

Present Status

Mesencephalotomy continues to be a valuable procedure in carefully selected patients, particularly for cancer pain in the upper extremity or head that is too high to be treated with a spinal morphine pump or percutaneous cervical cordotomy. Many neurosurgeons, including myself, preferentially use a target in the thalamus, where a basal or intralaminar thalamotomy may be as beneficial as mesencephalotomy without the risk of extraocular palsy. If there is a very strong somatic component to the pain, particularly involving the head or face, mesencephalotomy may be the procedure of choice.

Mesencephalotomy has been documented to be of particular value in central denervation pain. Lesions at other sites have not achieved the same success as mesencephalotomy. Especially in pain following a stroke, the thalamus may be damaged, leaving the mesencephalon as the best remaining target.

The use of mesencephalotomy in chronic noncancer pain has not been as well defined. This is a particularly difficult group of patients to evaluate, as well as to treat, and generally a less destructive approach is preferred. Psychological factors must be considered, because they might contraindicate surgery in general or suggest that another target may be of benefit with less risk.

THALAMOTOMY

Thalamotomy was not done until stereotactic techniques made it possible. Its role in pain management was realized early, and one of the first patients treated by Spiegel and Wycis[58] had denervation facial pain treated by mesencephalotomy plus a dorsal medial thalamotomy. As early as 1952 they advocated extending the mesencephalotomy lesion medially to include spinoreticulothalamic fibers,[18] and soon thereafter they advocated interrupting this same pathway higher as it entered the intralaminar thalamic nuclei, in the hope of avoiding the risks of a mesencephalic lesion.[4] There have been many attempts since then to find an ideal thalamic target for the management of pain, but at present, there is no completely satisfactory procedure.

Anatomy of the Sensory Thalamus

Our understanding of the pain pathways above the level of the mesencephalon is far from complete or even comprehensive. The present discussion is confined to only those issues that concern thalamotomy for pain management.

The medial lemniscus carries touch and proprioception information to the ventrolateral nuclear group of the thalamus, where it ends in a somatotopically organized fashion in Hassler's VCpc nucleus, with cranial sensation represented medially and caudal sensation more laterally. Tasker and associates[59] confirmed this somatotopy with exhaustive stimulation mapping in awake patients and also demonstrated a second somatotopic organization oriented vertically, the nature of which has not been elaborated.

Most of the axons of the lateral spinothalamic tract synapse with spinoreticulothalamic extralemniscal fibers before they reach the thalamus, so there appear to be very few direct connections within the thalamus. However, it is clear that the incoming information interacts with the lemniscal information at the thalamic level. It is not known how the reticulothalamic input is represented or how it relates to the lemniscal input in the ventrolateral area, although Hassler and Riechert[60] identified the nucleus ventrocaudalis parvicellularis, a thalamic relay area for the neospinothalamic tract in humans, as receiving significant reticulothalamic input. There are reticulothalamic connections with the intralaminar nuclei, as well as with the periaqueductal and periventricular gray, the parafascicularis, and the centromedianus, which lie medial to the ventrolateral nucleus. These same areas receive input from the nonsomatotopically organized paleospinothalamic tract, which ascends through the spinal cord within the central gray. Those areas then project to the hypothalamus and limbic system, which constitutes an anatomic basis for the "suffering" that accompanies pain.

The dorsomedial nucleus reacts reciprocally with the frontal and prefrontal areas. Indeed, the original impetus for the development of human stereotactic surgery was Spiegel's abhorrence of prefrontal lobotomy as it was practiced in the early 1940s.[61] Lesions in this structure are thought to produce an effect similar to that of prefrontal lobotomy, but without the tremendous risk to mentation.

Development

From the first stereotactic operation, Spiegel and Wycis[30] made lesions in the dorsomedial nucleus to dampen the exaggeration of symptoms of motor disorders and pain that occurs with emotional distress. This target was more useful for cancer pain, when the patient's life expectancy was limited and there was a great deal of emotional turmoil associated with the disease itself. However, cingulotomy has generally replaced the dorsomedial nucleus as the preferred target.[42, 62]

Naturally occurring lesions of the ventral posterior nuclei, the most likely terminus of spinothalamic fibers, may produce the pain of a thalamic syndrome, which made neurosurgeons reluctant to lesion that area to attempt pain treatment.[63] Paradoxically, relief of pain could sometimes be attained by enlarging the preexisting lesion.[60] Lesioning the ventrolateral (VL) thalamus was quickly recognized to be ineffective in relieving chronic or cancer pain, and it might leave the patient with disagreeable contralateral sensory loss.[61]

In general, there are five groups of procedures involving lesions in or around the thalamus for the management of pain[64, 65]: (1) thalamotomy of the ventral posterior nuclei, interrupting the lemniscal projections, which has limited value, and only for denervation pain; (2) medial thalamotomy, or thalamolaminotomy, interrupting the extralemniscal projections within the intralaminar nuclei and the centromedianus nucleus; (3) basal thalamotomy, interrupting the extralemniscal fibers before they enter the intralaminar nuclei and the centromedianus nucleus; (4) dorsomedial thalamotomy, interrupting the projection to and from the frontal lobe; and (5) lesions in the pulvinar nuclei.

As early as 1949 Hécaen and colleagues[66] suggested adding a centromedianus lesion to one in the ventral posterolateral (VPL) or ventral posteromedial (VPM) nuclei for the treatment of pain. Although the somatosensory ventrolateral thalamus alone proved to be a poor target for pain management, adding a lesion in the medial intralaminar thalamus, involving the intralaminar and centromedianus areas, provided better pain relief.[67] This is a similar observation to that made in mesencephalotomy, where the results were much better if the extralemniscal area were included in the target area, rather than lesioning the spinothalamic tract alone.[32] In fact, better results were observed even if the somatosensory thalamus were spared.[50, 68–70]

This led Spiegel and coworkers[4] to advocate intralaminar and basal thalamotomy alone for pain relief, with sparing of the lemniscal and extralemniscal areas. Intralaminar thalamotomy, involving both centromedianus and parafascicular nuclei (later termed *thalamolaminotomy* by Sano and associates[71]), proved to be disappointing for the treatment of neuropathic or chronic noncancer pain in several series.[50, 72] Results in cancer pain are somewhat better, but not as good as those with mesencephalotomy. Although there is no discernible loss of sensation after combined basal and intralaminar thalamotomy, some patients have confusion that is usually transient. In addition, I have observed a number of patients who had relief of their cancer pain and were able to discontinue narcotics abruptly with no withdrawal effects.

Dorsomedial thalamotomy was used in the early stereotactic days for pain relief,[4] but the limbic target that later gained more popularity was the cingulate gyrus.[42, 62] Lesions in such limbic structures, without including other extralemniscal fibers, have limited use in cancer pain, except when depression or addiction is the overwhelming symptom.

There is some evidence in the cat that cells in the medial pulvinar respond to painful stimulation.[73] This was based on Richardson's[74] observation of good pain relief after making lesions in the medial pulvinar in five of six patients with cancer pain. Although this prompted other neurosurgeons to use this procedure for both cancer and chronic pain,[75–77] it has never gained much popularity.

Indications

There are fewer indications for thalamotomy for the treatment of pain than for procedures involving more caudal structures, such as mesencephalotomy or cordotomy.[41, 78] Even many of those procedures have been supplanted by nondestructive procedures, such as spinal cord stimulation for chronic noncancer pain and implantation of intraspinal morphine pumps for cancer pain.[41, 79]

It has generally been conceded that thalamotomy (and most other destructive procedures) produces inadequate long-term relief of chronic noncancer pain, so there is little use for thalamotomy except in cancer pain.[78, 80, 81] My subjective experience is that thalamotomy can be useful in patients with cancer pain in whom other alternatives have been exhausted, but there is no controlled series to support this observation. There are patients for whom no other treatment seems appropriate and who may benefit from combined intralaminar and basal thalamotomy, such as those with Pancoast's tumor or severe involvement with head or neck cancer. If there is extreme emotional distress, extending the lesion to include the dorsomedial nucleus may provide additional benefit. The advantages are that the risk of neurological sequelae is less than with mesencephalotomy, and a unilateral procedure may be beneficial for bilateral or widespread pain.

Technique

Thalamotomy for pain relief is performed the same as for movement disorders, except that different targets are used. There is no particular response to stimulation of the intralaminar structures or dorsomedial nucleus, so stimulation is used primarily to indicate if the electrode is out of the target. A 1.8- to 2-mm electrode with a 3-mm bared tip is used. The coordinates are related to the posterior commissure. For basal thalamotomy, they are anterior 1, lateral 12, and extending vertically from 0 to 11 mm with a series of multiple lesions. For medial thalamotomy, they are anterior 4, lateral 11, and vertical from +2 to +13, plus anterior 9, lateral 9, and vertical +2 to +13. Dorsomedial thalamotomy lies at anterior 4, lateral 4, and vertical +2 to +10. These are large lesions distributed in several flat planes. Because the lesions are placed purely by anatomic and not physiologic targeting, the use of stereotactic radiosurgery for medial thalamotomy has recently been advocated, although not without some risk.[82]

STEREOTACTIC TRIGEMINAL TRACTOTOMY

A chance observation a century ago of a patient with complete unilateral trigeminal analgesia with preservation of touch sensation, probably caused by a small infarct near the inferior olive, led to the concept that pain input from the trigeminal nerve descends through the medulla before it synapses with the next-order sensory neurons.[83] Its position just below the surface invited surgical interruption of these pain fibers, equivalent to the spinothalamic axons conducting pain sensation from the body.[84]

Development

Nonstereotactic trigeminal tractotomy was introduced by Sjöqvist[84] in 1938. The procedure did not gain popularity because of the difficulty of identifying the tract to obtain adequate analgesia without injuring the overlying and adjacent medullar tracts, which often led to significant neurological problems, such as ataxia or recurrent laryngeal nerve paralysis. The excellent results reported by Kunc[85] have not been reported by others. White and Sweet[15] improved the procedure by extending the incision ventral to the descending trigeminal tract, which also produced some analgesia in the opposite leg, but with better results. Nevertheless, the procedure never became popular because of the inconsistent results and great risk.[86]

This led to the observation that the lesion might be made more consistently if it were done stereotactically. Unfortunately, most stereotactic frames do not allow the very low approach through the foramen magnum that this procedure requires, but the Hitchcock apparatus is particularly well designed for this.[86] He and Schvarcz,[87, 88] who had trained with Hitchcock, became the two proponents of this stereotactic procedure, although it never became widely used.

There has recently been renewed interest in this procedure. Kanpolat and colleagues[89] developed a series of procedures involving computed tomography guidance of needle-electrodes into the cervical spinal column for percutaneous cervical cordotomy or into the medulla to direct lesions to the descending trigeminal tract. Although this technique has not yet become widespread, it may lead to renewed interest in trigeminal tractotomy.

Indications and Results

Those who use this procedure have published small series. Hitchcock[86] reported pain relief in four of five patients with pain caused by head or neck malignancy, in one of two with neuralgia-like facial pain, and in two of three patients with postherpetic trigeminal neuralgia. Schvarcz[87] reported on 100 patients and achieved 87.5% successful pain relief in patients with postherpetic neuralgia, 57% in those with anesthesia dolorosa, 72% in patients with dysesthesia, and 83.8% in those with cancer pain. Kanpolat and colleagues[89] reported good to excellent results in six patients with vagoglossopharyngeal neuralgia and in three patients with trigeminal neuralgia, with two patients experiencing transient ataxia.

In general, this procedure may be of help for patients with carcinoma of the head and neck, but its use for other types of pain has not been established.

Technique

The procedure of stereotactic trigeminal tractotomy requires a stereotactic frame that allows an insertion through the foramen magnum angulated 30 degrees craniad. The target is 6 mm from the midline, where the trigeminal fibers lie 4 mm beneath the pial surface. A fine, sharpened electrode is used to penetrate the pia sharply and introduce the bared tip beyond the overlying fibers. Verification of electrode position is obtained with 50-Hz stimulation, which produces sensation projected to the face at low voltage, with no interference with fine motor function.

CONCLUSION

Stereotactic techniques for pain management have had only modest use. In general, mesencephalotomy may be helpful in denervation pain, but the efficacy of these procedures for other chronic noncancer pain has not been established. Ablation procedures at the brainstem can be of use for cancer pain, especially that involving the upper extremity, head, face, or neck, where other techniques cannot reach. Such pain is often associated with severe emotional turmoil, which can also be addressed, and life expectancy is usually limited.

REFERENCES

1. Nashold BS Jr, Wilson WP, Slaughter DG: Sensations evoked by stimulation in the midbrain of man. J Neurosurg 30:14–24, 1969.
2. Glees P, Bailey EA: Schichtung und Fasergrösse des Tractus spinothalamicus des Menschen. Mschr Psychiat Neurol 122:129–141, 1951.
3. Hécaen H, Talairach J, David M, Dell MD: Coagulations limitées du thalamus dans les algies du syndrome thalamique. Rev Neurol (Paris) 81:917–931, 1949.
4. Spiegel EA, Wycis HT, Szekely EG, et al: Combined dorsomedial, intralaminar and basal thalamotomy for relief of so-called intractable pain. J Int Coll Surg 42:160–168, 1964.
5. Nashold BS Jr: Brainstem stereotaxic procedures. In Schaltenbrand G, Walker AE (eds): Stereotaxy of the Human Brain. New York, Stuttgart, Thieme, 1982, pp 475–483.
6. Sano K, Sekino H, Hashimoto I, et al: Postero-medial hypothalamotomy in the treatment of intractable pain. Conf Neurol 37:285–290, 1975.
7. Sano K: Sedative neurosurgery with special reference to postero-medial hypothalamotomy. Neurol Med Chir(Tokyo) 4:112–114, 1962.

8. Gildenberg PL, DeVaul RA: Management of chronic pain refractory to specific therapy. In Youmans JR (ed): Neurological Surgery. Philadelphia, WB Saunders, 1982, pp 3749–3768.
9. Gowers WR: A case of unilateral gunshot injury to the spinal cord. Trans Med Soc Lond 11:24–32, 1878.
10. Spiller WG: The location within the spinal cord of the fibers for temperature and pain sensations. J Nerv Ment Dis 32:318–320, 1905.
11. Spiller WG, Martin E: The treatment of persistent pain of organic origin in the lower part of the body by division of the anterolateral column of the spinal cord. JAMA 58:1489–1490, 1912.
12. Dogliotti M: First surgical sections, in man, of the lemniscal lateralis (pain-temperature path) at the brain stem, for the treatment of diffuse rebellious pain. Anesth Analg 17:143–145, 1938.
13. Walker AE: Relief of pain by mesencephalic tractotomy. Arch Neurol Psychiatry 48:865–883, 1942.
14. Drake CG, McKenzie KG: Mesencephalic tractotomy for pain: Experience with six cases. J Neurosurg 10:457–462, 1953.
15. White JC, Sweet WH: Pain, Its Mechanism and Neurosurgical Control. Springfield, Ill, Charles C Thomas, 1955.
16. Spiegel EA, Wycis HT, Marks M, Lee AStJ: Stereotaxic apparatus for operations on the human brain. Science 106:349–350, 1947.
17. Spiegel EA, Wycis HT: Present status of stereoencephalotomies for pain relief. Conf Neurol 27:7–17, 1966.
18. Spiegel EA, Wycis HT: Mesencephalotomy in the treatment of "intractable" facial pain. Arch Neurol 69:1–13, 1953.
19. Spiegel EA, Wycis HT, Baird HW: Effect of thalamic and pallidal lesions upon involuntary movements in choreoathetosis. Trans Am Neurol Assoc 75:234, 1950.
20. Frank F, Tognetti F, Gaist G, et al: Stereotaxic rostral mesencephalotomy in treatment of malignant faciothoracobrachial pain syndromes: A survey of 14 treated patients. J Neurosurg 56:807–811, 1982.
21. Colombo F: Somatosensory-evoked potentials after mesencephalic tractotomy for pain syndromes: Neuroradiologic and clinical correlations. Surg Neurol 21:453–458, 1984.
22. Leksell L: Gezielte Hirnoperationen. In Hassler R, Riechert T (eds): Handbuch der Neurochirurgie. Berlin, Springer, 1957, pp 178–192.
23. Mark VH, Ervin FR, Hackett TP: Clinical aspects of stereotactic thalamotomy in the human. Arch Neurol 3:17–32, 1960.
24. Roeder F, Orthner H: Über zentrale Schmerzoperationen, insbesondere mediale Mesencephalotomie bei thalamischer Hyperpathie und bei Anaesthesia dolorosa. Conf Neurol 21:51–67, 1961.
25. Spiegel EA, Kletzkin M, Szekely EG, Wycis HT: Pain reactions upon stimulation of the tectum mesencephali. J Neuropathol Exp Neurol 13:212–220, 1954.
26. Spiegel EA, Kletzkin M, Szekely EG, Wycis HT: Role of hypothalamic mechanisms in thalamic pain. Neurology 4:739–745, 1954.
27. Wycis HT, Spiegel EA: Long-range results in the treatment of intractable pain by stereotaxic midbrain surgery. J Neurosurg 19:101–107, 1962.
28. Spiegel EA, Wycis HT, Szekely EG, Gildenberg PL: Medial and basal thalamotomy in so-called intractable pain. In Knighton RS, Dumke PR (eds): Pain. Boston, Little, Brown, 1966, pp 503–517.
29. Whisler WW, Voris HC: Mesencephalotomy for intractable pain due to malignant disease. Appl Neurophysiol 41:52–56, 1978.
30. Spiegel EA, Wycis HT: The central mechanism of emotions. Am J Psychiatry 109:426–431, 1951.
31. Nashold BS Jr, Wilson WP: Central pain: Observations in man with chronic implanted electrodes in the midbrain tegmentum. Conf Neurol 27:30–44, 1966.
32. Nashold BS Jr: Extensive cephalic and oral pain relieved by midbrain tractotomy. Conf Neurol 34:382–388, 1972.
33. Shieff C, Nashold BS Jr: Stereotactic mesencephalotomy. Neurosurg Clin N Am 1:825–839, 1990.
34. Tasker RR: Identification of pain processing systems by electrical stimulation of the brain. Human Neurobiol 1:261–272, 1982.
35. Shieff C, Nashold BS Jr: Stereotactic mesencephalic tractotomy for the relief of thalamic pain. Br J Neurosurg 1:305–310, 1987.
36. Amano K: Destructive central lesions for persistent pain: Outcome. In Gildenberg PL, Tasker RR (eds): Textbook of Stereotactic and Functional Neurosurgery. New York, McGraw-Hill, 1998, pp 1425–1429.
37. Nashold BS, Wilson WP, Slaughter DG: Stereotaxic midbrain

lesions for central dysesthesia and phantom pain: Preliminary report. J Neurosurg 30:116–126, 1969.
38. Turnbull IM: Cingulotomy. In Voris HC, Whisler WW (eds): Treatment of Pain. Springfield, Ill, Charles C Thomas, 1975, pp 143–150.
39. Gildenberg PL, Frost EAM: The effect of neurological disease on narcotic actions. In Adler MW, Manara L, Samanin R (eds): Factors Affecting the Action of Narcotics. New York, Raven Press, 1978, pp 703–716.
40. Gildenberg PL, Murthy KS: Modification of thalamic evoked activity by dorsal column stimulation. Acta Neurochir (Wien) 272:159–161, 1977.
41. Gildenberg PL: General principles and selection of techniques in the management of pain of benign origin. In Gildenberg PL, Tasker RR (eds): Textbook of Stereotactic and Functional Neurosurgery. New York, McGraw-Hill, 1998, pp 1321–1336.
42. Hurt RW, Ballentine HT Jr: Stereotactic anterior cingulate lesions for persistent pain: A report of 68 cases. Clin Neurosurg 21:334–351, 1974.
43. Gildenberg PL, DeVaul RA: The Chronic Pain Patient: Diagnosis and Management. Basel, Karger, 1985.
44. Starr PA, Vitek JL, Delong M, Bakay RA: Magnetic resonance imaging–based stereotactic localization of the globus pallidus and subthalamic nucleus. Neurosurgery 44:303–313, 1999.
45. Amano K, Tanikawa T, Kawamura H, et al: Single neuron analysis of the human midbrain tegmentum. Appl Neurophysiol 41:66–78, 1978.
46. Gorecki JP: Stereotactic midbrain tractotomy. In Gildenberg PL, Tasker RR (eds): Textbook of Stereotactic and Functional Neurosurgery. New York, McGraw-Hill, 1998, pp 1651–1660.
47. Tasker RR: Stereotactic surgery. In Wall PD, Melzack R (eds): Textbook of Pain. Edinburgh, Churchill Livingstone, 1994, pp 1137–1157.
48. Gybels JM, Sweet WH: Neurosurgical Treatment of Persistent Pain, vol 11. Basel, Karger, 1989.
49. Schvarcz JR: Periaqueductal mesencephalotomy for facial central pain. In Sweet WH (ed): Neurosurgical Treatment in Psychiatry, Pain, and Epilepsy. Baltimore, University Park Press, 1977, pp 661–667.
50. Voris HC, Whisler WW: Results of stereotaxic surgery for intractable pain. Conf Neurol 37:86–96, 1975.
51. Amano K, Kawamura H, Tanikawa T: Long-term follow-up study of rostral mesencephalic reticulotomy for pain relief: Report of 34 cases. Appl Neurophysiol 49:105–111, 1986.
52. Shieff C, Nashold BS Jr: Mesencephalotomy for thalamic pain. Neurol Res 9:101–104, 1987.
53. Helfand MH, Leksell L, Strang RR: Experiences with intractable pain treated by stereotaxic mesencephalotomy. Acta Chir Scand 129:573–580, 1965.
54. Mazars G: Etat actuel de la chirurgie de la douleur. Neurochir 22:Suppl 1:1976.
55. Frank F, Sturiale C, Gaist G, et al: Stereotactic mesencephalic tractotomy in the treatment of Pancoast syndrome. Appl Neurophysiol 48:274–276, 1985.
56. Laitinen LV: Mesencephalotomy and thalamotomy for chronic pain. In Lunsford LD (ed): Modern Stereotactic Neurosurgery. Boston, Martinus Nijhoff, 1988, pp 269–277.
57. Jannetta PJ, Gildenberg PL, Loeser JD, et al: Operations on the brain and brain stem for chronic pain. In Bonica JJ (ed): The Management of Pain. Philadelphia, Lea & Febiger, 1990, pp 2082–2103.
58. Spiegel EA, Wycis HT: Stereoencephalotomy: Part II. Philadelphia, Grune & Stratton, 1962.
59. Tasker RR, Organ LW, Hawrylyshyn PA: The Thalamus and Midbrain of Man: A Physiologic Atlas Using Electrical Stimulation. Springfield, Ill, Charles C Thomas, 1982.
60. Hassler R, Riechert T: Klinische und Anatomische Befunde beid Stereotaktischen Schmerzoperationen im Thalamus. Arch Psychiat Z Gesamte Neurol 200:93–122, 1959.
61. Spiegel EA: Guided Brain Operations. Basel, Karger, 1982.
62. Hassenbusch SJ: Cingulotomy for cancer pain. In Gildenberg PL, Tasker RR (eds): Stereotactic and Functional Neurosurgery. New York, McGraw-Hill, 1998, pp 1447–1451.
63. Riechert T: Die chirurgische Behandlung der zentralen Schmerzzustande. Acta Neurochir (Wien) 8:136–152, 1960.

64. Gildenberg PL: Functional neurosurgery. In Schmidek HH, Sweet WH (eds): Operative Neurosurgical Techniques, vol 2. New York, Grune & Stratton, 1982, pp 993–1043.

65. Gorecki JP: Destructive central lesions for persistent pain. Part I, an overview. In Gildenberg PL, Tasker RR (eds): Stereotactic and Functional Neurosurgery. New York, McGraw-Hill, 1998, pp 1417–1429.

66. Hécaen H, Talairach T, David M, Dell MB: Mémoires originaux. Coagulations limitées du thalamus dans les algies du syndrome thalamique. Rev Neurol 81:917–931, 1949.

67. Mark VH, Ervin FR, Yakovlev PI: Stereotactic thalamotomy. Part III. Arch Neurol 8:528–538, 1963.

68. Fairman D: Evaluation of results in stereotactic thalamotomy for the treatment of intractable pain. Conf Neurol 27:67–70, 1966.

69. Urabe M, Tsubokawa T, Kikuchi M, et al: Relation of the lesion site in the human thalamus to the thalamic syndrome and the effect of thalamotomy. No To Shinkei 17:933–944, 1965.

70. Hitchcock E: The surgical relief of pain. Practitioner 198:777–786, 1967.

71. Sano K, Yoshioka M, Ogashiwa M, et al: Thalamolaminotomy: A new operation for relief of intractable pain. Conf Neurol 27:63–66, 1966.

72. White JC, Sweet WH: Pain and the Neurosurgeon: A Forty Year Experience, Springfield, Ill, Charles C Thomas, 1969.

73. Richardson DE, Zorub DS: Sensory function in the pulvinar. Conf Neurol 32:165–172, 1970.

74. Richardson DE: Thalamotomy for intractable pain. Conf Neurol 29:139–143, 1967.

75. Laitinen LV: Pulvinotomy for cancer pain. In Gildenberg PL, Tasker RR (eds): Stereotactic and Functional Neurosurgery. New York, McGraw-Hill, 1998, pp 1445–1446.

76. Laitinen LV: Anterior pulvinotomy in the treatment of intractable pain. In Sweet WH (ed): Neurosurgical Treatment in Psychiatry, Pain, and Epilepsy. Baltimore, University Park Press, 1977, pp 669–672.

77. Whittle IR, Jenkinson JL: CT-guided stereotactic antero-medial pulvinotomy and centromedian-parafascicular thalamotomy for intractable malignant pain. Br J Neurosurg 9:195–200, 1995.

78. Hitchcock E: A comparison of analgesic ablative and stimulation techniques. Zentralbl Neurochir 42:189–202, 1981.

79. Hassenbusch SJ, Pillay PK, Magdinec M, et al: Constant infusion of morphine for intractable cancer pain using an implanted pump. J Neurosurg 73:405–409, 1990.

80. Tasker RR: Thalamotomy. Neurosurg Clin N Am 1:841–864, 1990.

81. Gildenberg PL, DeVaul RA: Treatment of chronic pain refractory to specific therapy. In Youmans JR (ed): Neurological Surgery. Philadelphia, WB Saunders, 1990, pp 4144–4166.

82. Young RF: Functional neurosurgery with the Leksell gamma knife. Stereotact Funct Neurosurg 66:19–23, 1996.

83. Hun H: Analgesia, thermic anaesthesia, and ataxia resulting from softening in medulla oblongata etc. N Y Med J 65:513, 581, 613, 1897.

84. Sjöqvist O: Studies on pain conduction in the trigeminal nerve. Acta Psychiat Neurol Suppl 17:1–139, 1938.

85. Kunc Z: Treatment of essential neuralgia of the 9th nerve by selective tractotomy. J Neurosurg 23:494–500, 1965.

86. Hitchcock E: Stereotactic cervical myelotomy. J Neurol Neurosurg Psychiatry 33:224–230, 1970.

87. Schvarcz JR: Stereotactic trigeminal tractotomy. Conf Neurol 37:73–77, 1975.

88. Hitchock ER, Schvarcz JR: Stereotaxic trigeminal tractotomy for post-herpetic facial pain. J Neurosurg 37:412–417, 1972.

89. Kanpolat Y, Savas A, Batay F, Sinav A: Computed tomography–guided trigeminal tractotomy-nucleotomy in the management of vagoglossopharyngeal and geniculate neuralgias. Neurosurgery 43:484–489, 1998.

CHAPTER 194

Caudalis Nucleus Dorsal Root Entry Zone Procedure for the Treatment of Intractable Facial Pain

DENNIS E. BULLARD ■ BLAINE S. NASHOLD

Pain involving the face is a complex problem clinically and surgically. This is especially true when prior ablative procedures have been performed. After a central surgical procedure for facial pain has been performed, the chance of success for peripheral procedures or medical management is generally limited. Other approaches to primary facial pain are outlined in earlier chapters.

In the 1960s, Kerr[1, 2] proposed the theory that a selective caudalis nucleus and tract lesion from the obex to the C2 dorsal root level might relieve facial pain in humans by destruction of the secondary neurons. The spinal cord dorsal root entry zone (DREZ) procedure evolved at Duke University Medical Center in the early 1970s and was based on the premise that intractable deafferentation pain could be attributed to spontaneous neuronal discharge.[3–7] In the 1980s, this assumption was expanded to include facial pain modulated by the nucleus caudalis. The caudalis DREZ procedure has been remarkably effective in treating many patients with facial, head, or neck pain.[7, 8]

ANATOMY

The spinal trigeminal nucleus appears to be a rostral extension of the dorsal horn.[9, 10] Significant evidence suggests an overlap between the cervical and trigeminal afferent projections.[11, 12] The spinal nucleus has been anatomically divided into three major portions based on the cytoarchitecture: the nucleus oralis, the nucleus interpolaris, and the nucleus caudalis.[13] However, there appear to be multiple bidirectional pathways among the three portions of the spinal nucleus, although it appears that the nucleus caudalis is the major area for the integration and processing of nociceptive components from the face.[14] The structure and electrophysiologic pattern of response of the spinal nucleus is analogous to the substantia gelatinosa, with both synapses of A-delta and C fibers providing the substrate for presynaptic inhibition and interconnection with first-

order neurons of the upper level of the cervical cord.[14,15] In cases of facial pain, there are also contributions from cranial nerves VII, IX, and X,[1, 16, 17] which have input to the adjacent reticular formation, medial and lateral cuneate nuclei, contralateral nucleus caudalis, and eventually, the cerebral cortex.[18]

Pain involving the central area of the face and the intraoral structures provides a more complex and difficult anatomic problem. Kunc[19] observed that providing analgesia to the midline of the face required interruption of the spinal tract at a level 12 to 15 mm above the second dorsal root. Pain and temperature pathways of the trigeminal nerve are present in the upper cervical cord, but there is significant animal and human evidence to suggest that the more rostral aspects of the spinal and brainstem nuclear complex are also involved.[9] Several aspects of this arrangement are unclear, however, and many investigators have found that the induction of analgesia in the mandibular division and in the areas innervated by cranial nerves VII, IX, and X are especially difficult to treat by tractotomy.[20–23]

SURGICAL PROCEDURES

In 1936, Serra and Neri[24] reported the first attempt at interruption of the trigeminal system in the brainstem using a diathermy electrode. Sjoqvist[20] reported the results of an open trigeminal tractotomy in 1937. Using a suboccipital craniotomy, Sjoqvist exposed the brainstem, and a section was made 3.5 to 4 mm deep and 8 to 10 mm above the obex in the region of the restiform body. The olive and the last vagal rootlet were used as anatomic references. The operation generally resulted in ipsilateral thermoanalgesia of the face, with preservation of light touch and other sensory modalities. The complications reported were ipsilateral ataxia, lateropulsion, contralateral analgesia, paralysis of the vocal cords, and damage of the recurrent laryngeal nerve with gait dysfunction and impairment of position sense in the limbs.[25]

Subsequently, Grant and Weinberger[25] made a lesion below this target site at 4 to 5 mm below the obex and confirmed analgesia over all three facial divisions with fewer complications.[26, 27] Olivecrona[22] also altered the operation to make the incision at the level of the obex to spare the restiform body and the fibers of the dorsal spinocerebellar tract, believing that lesions made at or below the obex would spare this pathway. Complication rates were less at this level, but the facial analgesia reported was often incomplete, sparing the third division of the trigeminal nerve and the distributions of cranial nerves VII, IX, and X in the descending nociceptive spinal tract.[23] In comparing these procedures, it was noticed that anesthesia of the mandibular division was possible only with lesions above those for the ophthalmic division and that lesions at the level of the obex often failed to include the third division.[20, 22, 28–30]

It is difficult to compare the results from these studies because of individual variations and the variable anatomic landmarks. Most surgeons used the obex as the primary landmark, although McKenzie[27] and others thought that this structure was not consistent with the brainstem pathways. The success rate of trigeminal tractotomy varied among surgeons, ranging from 17% to 61% for some patient series[22, 31–33] to a rate of 90% to 100% for others[3, 21, 34–36] with trigeminal neuralgia. A relatively high recurrence rate of 29% to 37% was reported.[22, 27, 34, 36, 37]

Many complications of open tractotomies were seen. Ataxia was the most common complication associated with open trigeminal tractotomy.[3, 21, 34, 37] It was thought to be associated with sectioning of the spinocerebellar tract. In the initial operations done above the obex, ataxia occurred in approximately 60% of patients, but after alteration in the technique, the rate was reported to have dropped to less than 5%.[32, 35, 36, 38] Neuropathic keratitis developed in a few patients.[21, 37] Paresthesias in the analgesic facial area was reported but was generally less severe than the preoperative pain.[25] Other infrequently reported symptoms included personality changes, Horner's syndrome, headaches, and other distal dysfunction.[22, 25, 37] The overall mortality rate was 0% to 16.6%.[22, 29, 35–37, 39] With benign problems, the rate generally was less than 5%,[21, 29, 36, 37] whereas with cancer-related problems, the rate was as high as 30%.[22, 38] Trigeminal tractotomy was technically complex, and after initial evaluation by the neurosurgical community, the procedure was discarded because of the complications, inconsistent sensory response,[21, 23] high recurrence rate,[40] and potential morbidity and mortality.

Subsequently, stereotactic procedures were developed to provide radiofrequency (RF) lesions without the morbidity of the open procedure.[31] However, none of these techniques gained wide acceptance.

Kerr (personal communication), in collaboration with Nashold, developed the theory that a selective caudalis lesion might potentially relieve facial pain in humans by destruction of the secondary neurons in the caudalis nucleus and portions of the tract from the obex to the C2 dorsal root level. Initially, the caudalis DREZ operation was made with a straight electrode in a single row of RF lesions.[39, 41] Later, this approach was modified to use a double row of lesions in an attempt to provide more complete coverage of the caudalis nucleus. In 1989, the standard DREZ electrode was modified by Young[42] to reduce involvement of the overlying spinocerebellar complex. This second-generation electrode increased the length to 3 mm, with insulation of the proximal 1 mm to reduce the RF lesion effect on the spinocerebellar tract. This change reduced the rate of postoperative ataxia from 90% to 50%. Subsequently, El-Naggar[7] designed a third generation of caudalis electrodes. These right-angled electrodes with 2- or 3-mm lesion tips further reduced the incidence of ataxia by sparing the dorsospinocerebellar tract. They are now the standard electrodes used.

PATIENT SELECTION

Primary diagnoses reported for the caudalis nucleus DREZ procedure include refractory trigeminal neuralgia, atypical headaches or facial pain, post-traumatic closed head injuries, postsurgical anesthesia dolorosa, multiple sclerosis, brainstem infarction, postherpetic neuralgia, and cancer-related pain. The procedure has proved to be effective for many but not all patients with these types of facial pain.[7, 8] The fair to excellent response rates from prior studies using essentially the same overlapping patient population have ranged from 46% to 60%, depending on the method of treatment.[7, 43] The evolution of this operation through several modifications and the complex nature of the procedure itself have largely been responsible for this variation and have made it somewhat difficult to evaluate the true benefits and risks of the procedure. Pain in cranial nerve V_1 and V_2 branches and areas of hyperpathia usually has resolved after surgery, but oral and mucosal pain have been the most difficult to treat.[44]

TREATMENT

Surgical Technique

The current surgical protocol has been modified from that previously reported.[45] Patients are placed in the prone position or semi-lateral position on a Wilson frame after application of a Mayfield head holder (Fig. 194–1). Inferiorly, a hemilaminectomy is performed on C1 and, if needed, on a portion of C2; superiorly a small, unilateral, suboccipital craniectomy is extended to the midline. The upper cervical roots and the obex are consistently well visualized (Fig. 194–2). The extent of DREZ lesioning depends on the distribution of pain and the results of intraoperative surface evoked potential results.

Impedance values are recorded before each DREZ lesion is made. The DREZ lesions are made at 75°C for 15 to 20 seconds. The lesions are made 1 mm apart and perpendicular to the surface of the spinal cord and medulla (Fig. 194–3). Below C2, the straight, 2.0-mm

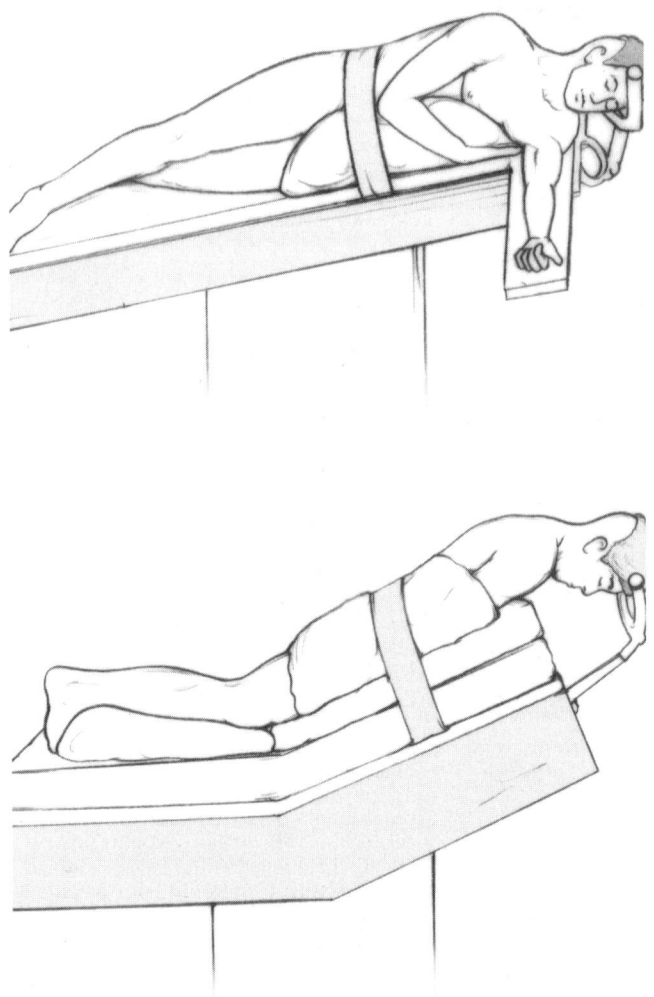

FIGURE 194–1. General positioning for the caudalis dorsal root entry zone procedure. The modified park bench or the prone position may be used. For both, the neck must be optimally flexed to allow exposure of the C2 through suboccipital areas on the involved side.

exposed-tip DREZ electrode is used. At C2, the small, 1.2-mm, right-angled nucleus caudalis electrode is used until reaching a level 10 mm above the superior aspect of the C2 sensory fibers. This is approximately the level of the C1 sensory rootlets. The longer, 2-mm, right-angled electrode is employed for all more cephalad lesions. Lesions in the lower one half of the nucleus are made along the line of the root entry zone, and lesions in the upper half of the nucleus are made in a curvilinear fashion, just posterior to the point of emergence of the rootlets of the spinal accessory nerve (see Fig. 194–3). These variations are done in an attempt to best approximate the shape of the caudalis nucleus while sparing the surrounding structures. After completion of the lesioning, the evoked potentials are again recorded. In general, the pre-DREZ evoked potential is replaced by a flat-line or dominant p-wave pattern before termination of the procedure (Fig. 194–4).

Lesions are extended only to the obex in patients with V_1 and V_2 pain. Lesions are generally extended 1 to 15 mm above the obex in patients with mucosal, oral, or V_3 pain (see Fig. 194–3).

Recording Technique

Somatosensory evoked potentials are routinely recorded during caudalis nucleus procedures.[44, 45] The three divisions of cranial nerve V are localized before surgery with transcutaneous nerve stimulation with a bipolar probe with 2-mm interelectrode distance. The supraorbital nerve is localized and used for V_1, the infraorbital nerve for V_2, and the mental nerve for V_3. These peripheral stimulation sites are stimulated intraoperatively before lesions with paired platinum subdermal needle electrodes with an interelectrode distance of 10 mm. Stimulation currents are adjusted according to the requirements of particular patient and vary by level of pathology by 10 to 40 mA. A 50-μsec pulse duration is used to avoid baseline shift due to stimulus artifact of the recorded responses at 2.11 cycles per second. The peripherally generated responses are recorded directly for the cervicomedullar junction from 5 to 10 mm above the obex to the C2 dorsal root level. The recording electrode is a Silastic-coated platinum array with 5-mm interelectrode distance. Recordings are displayed and averaged using a Cadwell Excel protocol (Cadwell Laboratories, Kenewrite, WA) with 20-msec sweep and 20-μV gain. The evoked potential consisted of a tract volley, followed by aggregate neuronal firing for the caudalis nucleus, displayed for the surgeon and printed for comparison with postlesion responses with respect to changes in wave morphology for prospective evaluation of the complete ablation of neuronal responses from the affected divisions.

Impedance recording is done from the lesioning electrode before all lesions. A Radionics RFG-3B RF Lesion Generator (Radionics, Inc., Burlington, MA) was used for impedance recording and lesion generation. The technique and rationale have previously been reported by Bullard 1998.[46]

Complications

The major consideration for any surgical procedure is risk. Most prior open brainstem procedures for pain failed to gain widespread acceptance because of the considerable potential risks.[19, 20, 28] The same concerns have been expressed about the caudalis DREZ procedure, although a high mortality or morbidity rate has not been reported.[7, 8, 43] The more serious complications reported, including paralysis, cranial nerve dysfunction and keratitis, have not exceeded 10% in any large series, and the most frequently reported disability associated has been an ataxia-dysmetria syndrome.

Ataxia-dysmetria is a complex problem with components of incoordination, sensory loss, reduced joint position sense, and weakness of the ipsilateral upper extremity and is related to the multiple structures adjacent to the DREZ; the spinocerebellar tract, cuneate tract, and nucleus; and the pyramidal tract. In early

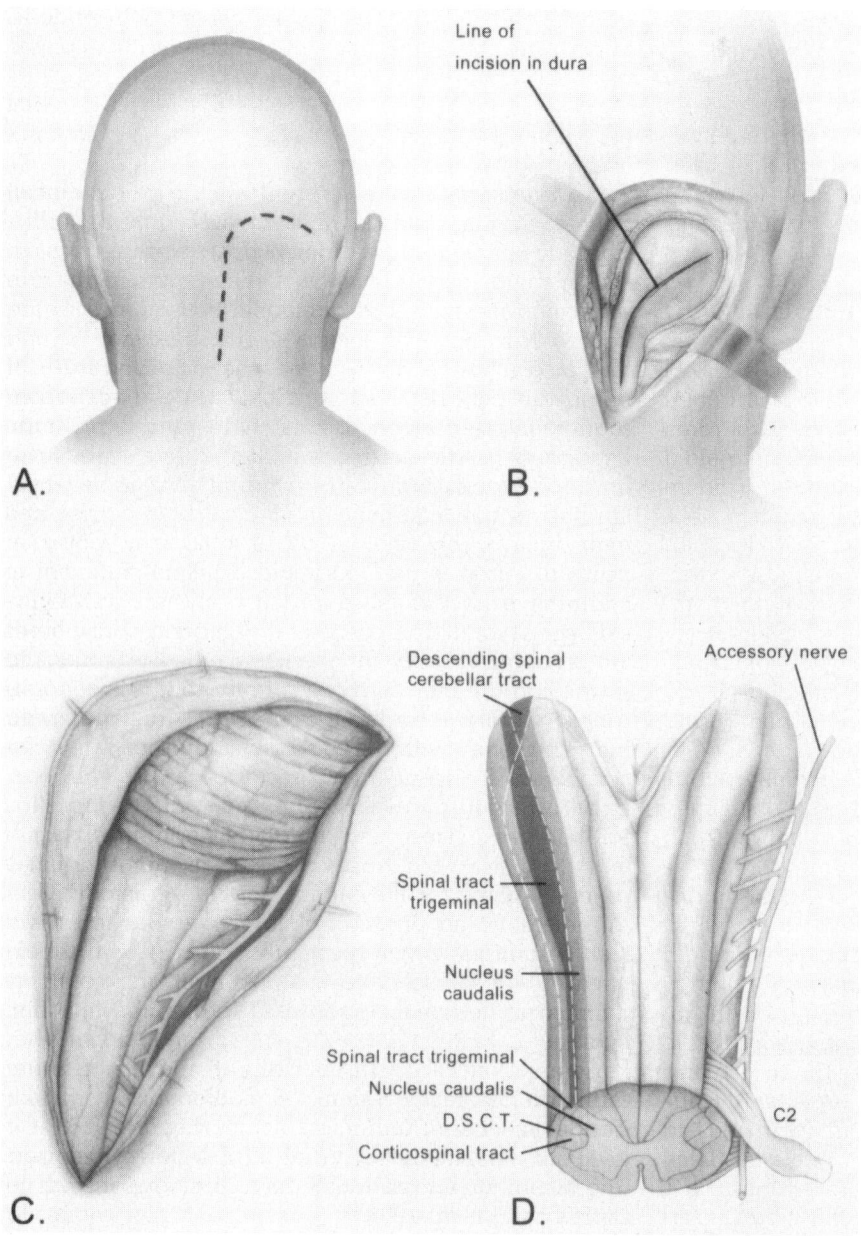

A.

B.

Line of
incision in dura

C.

D.

Descending spinal
cerebellar tract

Accessory nerve

Spinal tract
trigeminal

Nucleus
caudalis

Spinal tract trigeminal
Nucleus caudalis
D.S.C.T.
Corticospinal tract

C2

FIGURE 194–2. Surgical exposure for the caudalis dorsal root entry zone procedure. *A,* A standard curvilinear incision can be made, starting at the midline of C2-3 and extending up to the midline at the level of the inion. The incision is incurved to the involved side. A cuff of muscle can be left, if desired. The anatomic dissection should allow the muscles to be dissected down to the spinous processes of C1 and C2 and laterally to the aspect of the mastoid groove. The venous structures and vertebral artery must be carefully avoided. *B,* The dural opening is curved, extending from the midposition of the bony opening of C2 up through the lateral aspect over the cerebellum. The major posterior fossa sinuses, including the transverse and sigmoid sinuses, should be avoided. Smaller venous channels can be temporarily clipped and the dura retracted with sutures. The arachnoid is preserved until all bleeding is controlled. *C,* The arachnoid is opened, exposing the C2 roots inferiorly extending up through the spinal accessory nerve, the vertebral artery, and the lateral aspects of the brainstem superiorly. Medially, the obex must be seen. *D,* A diagram of the superficial anatomic landmarks is superimposed on the underlying descending spinal cerebellar (DSCT), spinal trigeminal, and corticospinal tracts and the nucleus caudalis.

studies using variable techniques, ataxia was reported in up to 90% of patients in the initial postoperative period.[39] In the most recent retrospective reviews of studies using right-angled electrodes and a single row of lesions, the incidence of this as a subjective complaint had dropped to 35% postoperatively and 23% at 1 year.[7, 8] In most later reports, most patients were functional on discharge examination and did not complain of ataxia as a major disability.[8] Increased surgical experience, the use of the right-angled electrodes, and the routine use of intraoperative high-dose steroids may all have played a role in reducing the incidence and severity of the ataxia-dysmetria syndrome in the postoperative period. The current percentage, however, may reflect a relatively absolute rate based on the proximity of the spinocerebellar and other tracts to the DREZ.

Outcome

The pattern of pain relief has been variable among reported DREZ cases. With multiple techniques included, the overall rate of long-term good to excellent results has ranged from 36% to 60%.[7, 8] In the longest followed series, 16 (43%) of the 37 patients had recurrence of their pain.[7] The time of recurrence ranged from 1 week to 4 years, with a median of 3 months. Two thirds of patients reported that the pain recurrence had been gradual. In this same study, 21 (60%) of 35 patients interviewed in a retrospective telephone survey reported fair to excellent pain relief at 1 year, although 56% reported that a portion of their original pain had returned. Most failures had recurrence in the full preoperative anatomic distribution. This is similar to the pattern of distribution and time of recurrence.

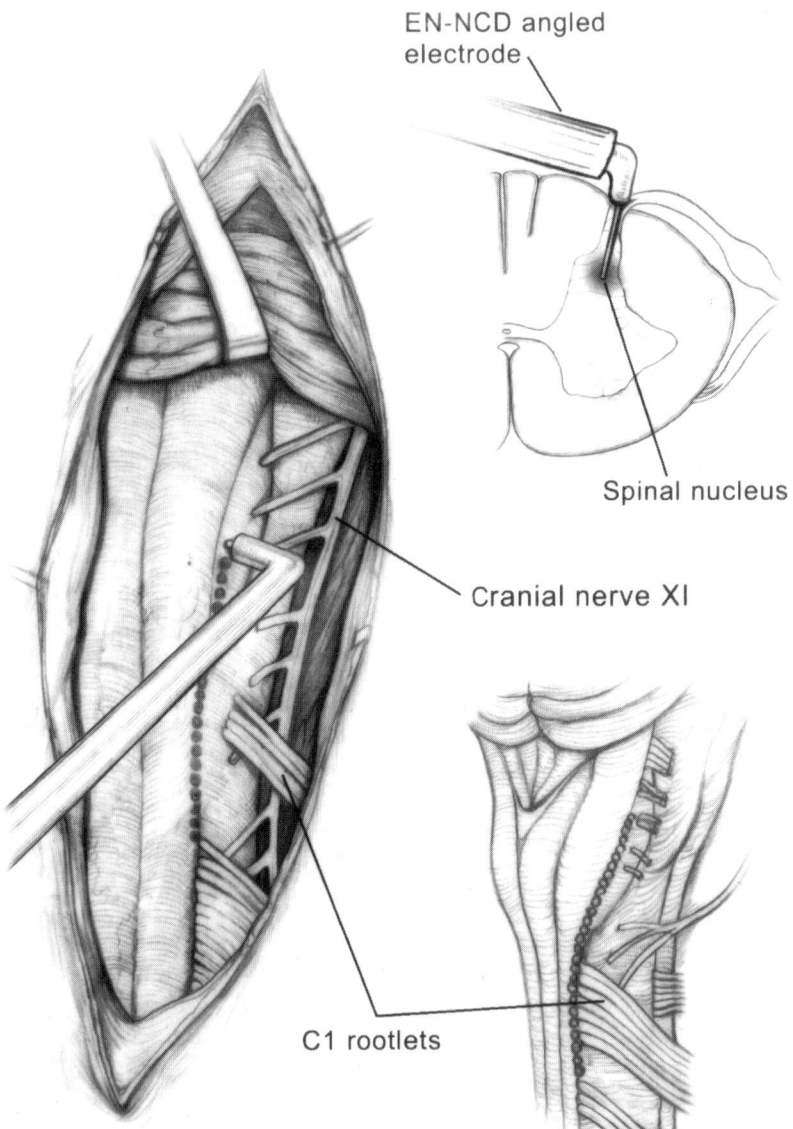

EN-NCD angled electrode

Spinal nucleus

Cranial nerve XI

C1 rootlets

FIGURE 194–3. Positioning of the right-angled EN-NCD electrode in relation to the dorsal columns and the underlying cranial nerves. The general position of the lesion is shown in cross section.

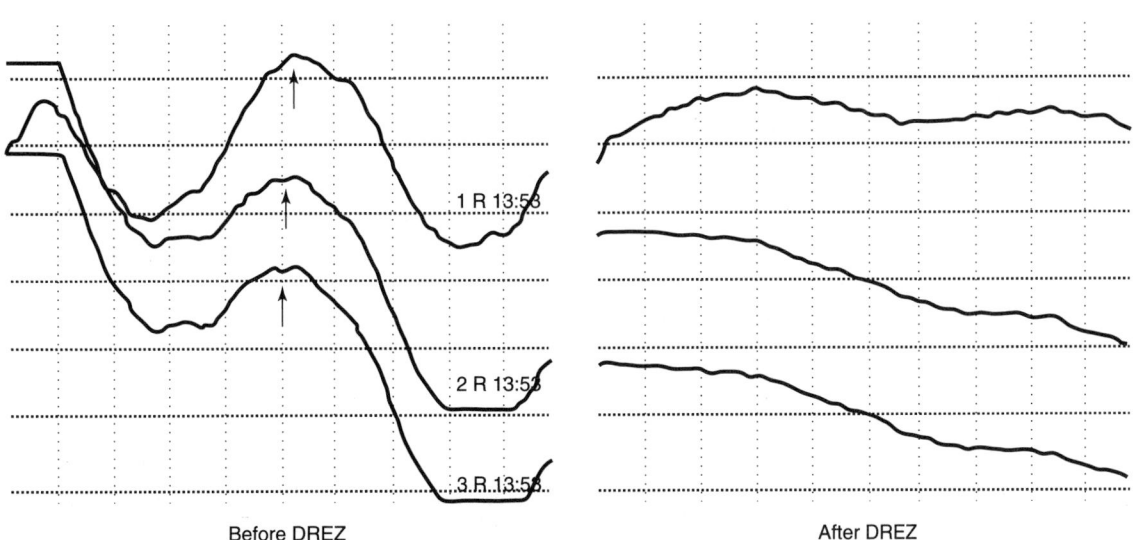

Before DREZ

After DREZ

1 R 13:53

2 R 13:53

3 R 13:53

FIGURE 194–4. A somatosensory evoked potential (SSEP) shows a pattern of waveforms before a dorsal root entry zone (DREZ) procedure and after DREZ ablation.

Thomas and Kitchen[47] had reported with cervical DREZ for brachial plexus avulsion. This suggests that the pain pathways in some patients are temporarily blocked and that the pain later recurs because of the recovery of the partially ablated tissue and the reemergence of a hyperactive focus.

Recurrence in these patients is a complex phenomenon. Virtually all patients have been on high doses of narcotic analgesics and multiple other non-narcotic medications. A reasonable evaluation of the benefits of the surgery would appear to be long-term assessment of the patient's functional level and lifestyle, including reduction in the amount and strength of their maintenance medications. In one report, the retrospective subjective assessment of improved quality of life was only 38%, but the objective parameters, including activity level and narcotic use, suggested a more substantial improvement, with a drop in patient narcotic use from 100% preoperatively to only 38% postoperatively.[43] In our experience, two thirds of patients have significant pain relief 1 year after surgery, their narcotic use has generally dropped substantially, and the level of functioning improved in most.[8]

CONCLUSIONS

The results from caudalis nucleus DREZ are variable, ranging from good to excellent in most cases. Attempts to improve results are aimed toward evaluating the parameters for extent of lesion making. The lesions are now made from the C2 root to the level of the obex, based on the pattern of preoperative pain distribution. The success rate for such tailored lesions appears initially to be higher. A set temperature, 75°C, and a set time, 15 to 20 seconds, control the size of the lesions. This approach has remained fixed. Attempts to increase the size of the lesions by changing these parameters have been met with an increased incidence of neurological dysfunction.[26] We have begun to evaluate somatosensory evoked potential (SSEP) ablation as a predictor of short- and long-term response and an intraoperative predictor of anatomic location. In our series of 43 patients, ablation of the SSEP signal intraoperatively had a high correlation with short-term pain relief and appropriate lesion localization, but it has not allowed prediction of long-term pain relief.

The degree of success achieved in some patients is very encouraging, considering the poor response rates reported by virtually all other methods of treatment for refractory facial pain. Results support the role of the caudalis DREZ procedure as an option in the treatment of refractory facial pain. There are many questions about patient selection and size of lesions that are still unanswered. The surgical learning curve, however, is high, and prior training and the ability to do detailed intraoperative monitoring are crucial for success.

ACKNOWLEDGMENTS

We wish to thank Mr. Thomas S. Binford, PAC; Mrs. Elizabeth Murphy; Mrs. Joanne Wall; and Mrs. Judy Harrell for assistance and advice in the preparation of this manuscript.

REFERENCES

1. Kerr FWL: Structural relation of the trigeminal spinal tract to upper cervical roots and the solitary nucleus in the cat. Exp Neurol 4:134–148, 1961.
2. Kerr FWL: Spinal Vth nucleolysis: Intractable craniofacial pain. Surg Forum 17:419–421, 1966.
3. Anderson L, Black RG, Abraham J, Ward AA Jr: Neuronal hyperactivity in experimental trigeminal deafferentation. J Neurosurg 35:444–452, 1971.
4. Crue BL, Todd EM, Carregal EJA, Kilham O: Percutaneous trigeminal tractotomy: Case report utilizing stereotactic radiofrequency lesions. Bull Los Angeles Neurol Soc 32:86–92, 1967.
5. King RB: Electrophysiology of trigeminal neurons under normal and epileptogenic conditions. In Hassler R, Walker AE (eds): Trigeminal Neuralgia. Stuttgart, Thieme, 1970, pp 78–85.
6. Loeser JD, Ward AA Jr, White LE Jr: Chronic deafferentation of human spinal cord neurons. J Neurosurg 29:48–50, 1968.
7. Nashold BS Jr, El-Naggar AO, Gorecki JP: The microsurgical trigeminal caudalis nucleus DREZ procedure. In Nashold BS Jr, Pearlstein RD (eds): The DREZ Operation. Park Ridge, American Association of Neurological Surgeons, 1996, pp 159–189.
8. Bullard DE, Nashold BS Jr: The caudalis DREZ for facial pain. Stereotact Funct Neurosurg 68(Pt 1):168–174, 1997.
9. Dallel R, Raboisson P, Auroy P, Woda A: The rostral part of the trigeminal sensory complex is involved in orofacial nociception. Brain Res 448:7–19, 1988.
10. Crosby EC, Yoss RE: The phylogenetic continuity of neural mechanisms as illustrated by the spinal tract of V and its nucleus. Res Publ Assoc Res Nerv Ment Dis 33:174–208, 1954.
11. Thelander HE: The course and distribution of the radix mesencephalica trigemini in the cat. J. Comp Neurol 37:207–220, 1924.
12. Taren JA, Kahn EA: Anatomic pathways related to pain in face and neck. J Neurosurg 19:116–121, 1962.
13. Olszewski J: On the anatomical and functional organization of the spinal trigeminal nucleus. J Comp Neurol 92:401–413, 1950.
14. Azerad J, Woda A, Albe-Fessard D: Physiological properties of neurons in different parts of the cat trigeminal sensory complex. Brain Res 246:7–21, 1982.
15. Darian-Smith I, Yokota T: Cortically evoked depolarization of trigeminal cutaneous afferent fibers in the cat. J Neurophysiol 29:170–178, 1966.
16. Brodal A: Central course of afferent fibers for pain in facial, glossopharyngeal and vagus nerves. Arch Neurol Psychiatry 57:292–306, 1947.
17. Kerr FWL: Facial, vagal and glossopharyngeal nerves in the cat: Afferent connections. Arch Neurol 6:264–281, 1962.
18. Brodal A, Szabo T, Torvik A: Corticofugal fibers to sensory trigeminal nuclei and nucleus of solitary tract: An experimental study in the cat. J Comp Neurol 106:527–555, 1956.
19. Kunc Z: Significance of fresh anatomic data on spinal trigeminal tract for possibility of selective tractotomies. In Knighton RS, Dumke PR (eds): Pain. Henry Ford Hospital International Symposium. Boston: Little, Brown, 1966, pp 351–363.
20. Sjoqvist O: Studies on pain conduction in the trigeminal nerve: A contribution to the surgical treatment of facial pain. Acta Psychiatr Neurol Scand Suppl 17:1–139, 1938.
21. Falconer MA: Intramedullary trigeminal tractotomy and its place in the treatment of facial pain. J Neurol Neurosurg Psychiatry 12:297–311, 1949.
22. Hamby WB, Shinners BM, Marsh IA: Trigeminal tractotomy. Arch Surg 57:171–177, 1948.
23. Grant FC: Complications accompanying surgical relief of pain in trigeminal neuralgia. Am J Surg 75:42–47, 1948.
24. Serra A, Neri V: Die elekrto-chirurgische Unterbrechung der Zentralbahnen das V. Paares am lateralen ventralen Rand des Pons Varoli als erster Behandlungsversuch von hartnackigen Neuralgien des Trigeminus durch Tumoren der Schadelbasis. Zentralbl Chir 63:2248–2251, 1936.
25. Grant FC, Weinberger LM: Experiences with intramedullary tractotomy. IV. Surgery of the brain stem and its operative complications. Arch Surg 42:747–754, 1941.

26. Spiegelmann R, Friedman WA, Ballinger WE, Tedeschi H: Anatomic examination of a case of open trigeminal nucleotomy (nucleus caudalis dorsal root entry zone lesions) for facial pain. Stereotact Funct Neurosurg 56:166–178, 1991.

27. McKenzie KJ: Trigeminal tractotomy. Clin Neurosurg 2:50–70, 1955.

28. White JC, Sweet WH: Pain and the Neurosurgeon: A Forty-Year Experience. Springfield, IL, Charles C Thomas, 1969.

29. Raney R, Raney AA, Hunter C: Treatment of major trigeminal neuralgia through section of the trigeminospinal tract in the medulla. Am J Surg 80:11–17, 1950.

30. Grant FC: Surgical methods for relief of pain. Bull N Y Acad Med 19:373–385, 1943.

31. Schvarcz JR: Spinal cord stereotaxic techniques for trigeminal nucleotomy and extralemniscal myelotomy. Appl Neurophysiol 41:99–112, 1978.

32. Plangger CA, Fischer J, Grunert V, Moshsenipour I: Tractotomy and partial vertical nucleotomy for treatment of special forms of trigeminal neuralgia and cancer pain of face and neck. Acta Neurochir Suppl (Wien) 39:147–150, 1987.

33. Bernard EJ, Nashold BS Jr, Caputti F: Clinical review of nucleus caudalis dorsal root entry zone lesions for facial pain. Appl Neurophysiol 51:218–224, 1988.

34. Olivecrona H: Tractotomy for relief of trigeminal neuralgia. Arch Surg 47:544–654, 1942.

35. Kunc Z: Vertical trigeminal partial nucleotomy. Adv Pain Res Ther 3:325–329, 1979.

36. Penzholz H, Menzel J, Hagenlocher HU: Results of surgical treatment of idiopathic trigeminal neuralgia using different operative techniques (a cooperative study). Adv Neurosurg 3:320–327, 1975.

37. Guidetti B: Tractotomy for relief of trigeminal neuralgia: Observations in 124 cases. J Neurosurg 7:499–508, 1950.

38. Kunc Z: Treatment of essential neuralgia of the 9th nerve by selective tractotomy. J Neurosurg 23:494–500, 1965.

39. Bernard EJ Jr, Nashold BS Jr, Caputti F, Mossy JJ: Nucleus caudalis DREZ lesions for facial pain. Br J Neurosurg 1:81–92, 1987.

40. Moffie D: Late results of bulbar trigeminal tractotomy: Some remarks on recovery of sensibility. J Neurol Neurosurg Psychiatry 34:270–274, 1971

41. Nashold BS Jr, Lopes H, Chadokiewitz J, et al: Trigeminal DREZ for craniofacial pain. In Samii M (ed): Surgery in and around the Brainstem. Heidelberg, Springer, 1986, pp 53–58.

42. Young JN, Nashold BS Jr, Cosman ER: A new insulated caudalis nucleus DREZ electrode: Technical note. J Neurosurg 70:283–289, 1989.

43. Gorecki JP, Nashold BS Jr, Rubin LL, Ovelmen-Levitt J: The Duke experience with nucleus caudalis DREZ coagulation. Stereotact Funct Neurosurg 65:111–116, 1996.

44. Sharpe R, Pearlstein RD: Recordings of somatosensory evoked cord dorsum potentials and electromyograms during the DREZ operation. In Nashold BS Jr, Pearlstein RD (eds): The DREZ Operation. Park Ridge, IL, American Association of Neurological Surgeons, 1996, pp 27–39.

45. Bullard DE, Nashold BS Jr: The DREZ Operation. Atlas Neurosurg Tech (submitted).

46. Bullard DE, Nashold BS Jr: Impedance recording in functional neurosurgery. Stereotact Funct Neurosurg 98:949–953, 1998.

47. Thomas DGT, Kitchen ND: Long-term follow-up of dorsal root entry zone lesions in brachial plexus avulsion. J Neurol Neurosurg Psychiatry 57:737–738, 1994.

Sympathectomy for Pain

ANTONIO A. F. DE SALLES ■ JOHN PATRICK JOHNSON

The popularity of surgical sympathectomy for the treatment of pain has decreased over the years. This reduction reflects the improvement of medical management and the development of less invasive and nondestructive surgical techniques: radiofrequency percutaneous sympathectomy and dorsal column stimulation.[1-3] The invasive nature of thoracic or lumbar sympathectomy, requiring thoracotomy, posterior costotransversectomy, large retroperitoneal dissection, or laparotomy, has made this approach less desirable for treating mild cases of sympathetic-mediated pain (SMP). Severe cases of causalgia that failed to respond to all less invasive treatments are the ones that still undergo the large, invasive approaches to the sympathetic chain. There is great interest in the endoscopic approach to the sympathetic nervous system.[4-6] In 1994, a symposium dedicated to thoracic endoscopic sympathectomy summarized the main clinical issues and technical advances of this technique.[7] The thoracic and lumbar sympathetic ganglia can be readily visualized and severed or electrocoagulated through minimal incisions with the use of several endoscopic ports. This chapter discusses the historical landmarks, rationale, results, and latest techniques for surgery of the sympathetic system to curtail SMP.

HISTORY

Claude Bernard and Brown Sequard described the physiology of the sympathetic nervous system in 1852. Bernard showed that the removal of the stellate ganglia in rabbits led to an increased temperature in that side of the animal's face, contrary to his own theory that the temperature should decrease. Gaskell and Langley mapped the sympathetic ganglia distribution, although in a rudimentary fashion, in 1859. The true segmental distribution of the sympathetic nervous system became available only much later.[4] When surgeons became aware of the anatomic distribution and physiologic consequences of this curious system, their creative minds found numerous reasons to surgically intervene in the sympathetic nervous system.[8] In 1889, Alexander performed the first cervical sympathectomy for the treatment of epilepsy.[9] The result was marginal, as were the results of several other surgical interventions in the sympathetic system. Jaboulay and Jonnesco tried stellectomy for treatment of exophthalmic goiter in 1896.[10] Other applications with marginal results were described in the late 1800s and early 1900s, including glaucoma in 1889, trigeminal neuralgia in 1902, optical nerve atrophy in 1905, and angioma of the external carotid artery in 1917.[9]

Leriche, the famous French vascular surgeon, dedicated his research to the enervation of large arteries such as the femoral and axillary arteries. He was interested in surgical procedures to improve peripheral vascular insufficiency. He was a student of Jaboulay, who in the late 1800s described the stripping of large arteries from their nerve supply to improve distal circulation. Leriche found that sympathectomy was a more effective procedure than artery denervation.[11] Vascular surgeons treating peripheral vascular insufficiency largely used this procedure. Two Australian scientists, Royle and Hunter, believed that sympathectomy improved spasticity. They thought that sympathetic fibers maintained skeletal muscle tonus.[8] Their work became widely know, but their results could not be reproduced.[12] The interest on the physiology of the sympathetic nervous system was greatly enhanced by the theory of Royle and Hunter. The clinical observations of Royle and Hunter were important to support the vascular effects of sympathectomy.

Similar to the operation of Royle and Hunter, another application of sympathectomy that fell into disuse was for the treatment of arterial hypertension by resection of the splanchnic plexus.[13, 14] Sympathectomy was settled as a treatment of peripheral vascular disease. In 1925, Adson and Brown described the posterior approach for removal of the second thoracic sympathetic ganglion. Davis and Kanavel reported the anterior approach to the upper thoracic sympathetic chain in the same year.[8] Atkins developed the transaxillary approach in 1954.[15] After 1920, sympathectomy also gained acceptance for treatment of hyperhidrosis through the work of Kotzareff.[9] Cloward[16] described the dorsal midline approach to both sides of the sympathetic chain in 1969, and the approach gained popularity among neurosurgeons. After Wilkinson[17] described the fluoroscopic approach to the thoracic sympathetic chain, Adler and coworkers[18] described the computed tomography (CT)–guided approach. Chuang and colleagues[18] described a stereotactic approach to the upper thoracic ganglia for treating hyperhidrosis.

In 1928, Spurling[19] resected the stellate and first thoracic ganglion for the treatment of causalgia of the upper extremity resulting from a partial lesion of the axillary artery by a gunshot wound. He hypothesized that vascular insufficiency of the arm led to the pain and that posterior sympathectomy as described by Adson and Brown improved the circulation and pain.[19] Since then, the treatment of causalgia and sympathetic dystrophy with sympathectomy has been encouraging. Rates of 59% to 74% for excellent results and of 9% to 17% for fair control of pain have appeared in the literature.[20–22] The term *causalgia* was derived from two Greek words, *kausos,* meaning heat, and *algos,* meaning pain.[23] The term describing burning pain was coined from the work of Weir Mitchell[24] because of his detailed description of the syndrome after major nerve injuries identified during the United States Civil War, although Pare probably described the first case of causalgia in the 16th century.

NOMENCLATURE

Several terms have been used to describe pain related to the sympathetic nervous system, such as reflex sympathetic dystrophy, causalgia, and SMP. An organized nomenclature for the pain phenomenon is necessary to allow comparison of treatment results and to define appropriate treatment for the various forms of pain related to the sympathetic nervous system. The term *sympathetic-mediated pain,* introduced by Roberts in 1986, is a general term indicating that surgery on the sympathetic nervous system may lead to important control of the patient's chronic pain.[25] The term *reflex sympathetic dystrophy,* describing a chronic pain syndrome of a limb out of proportion in severity to the original injury and implying sympathetic hyperactivity, became widely popular and often has been used in an inconsistent and misleading fashion.[26] The same fate has ensued for facial pain syndromes that are difficult to treat and that do not fall in the recognized diagnoses of facial pain such as trigeminal neuralgia, cluster headaches, and anesthesia dolorosa. Certain types of facial pain also may be included in the category of reflex sympathetic dystrophy,[27] but facial pain syndromes are not included in the classification of complex regional pain syndrome.

A consensus workshop in 1993 suggested the term *complex regional pain syndrome* (CRPS).[26] It describes a variety of painful situations that follow injury, appear regionally, have a distal predominance of abnormal findings, exceed in magnitude and duration the expected clinical course of the inciting event, often result in significant impairment of motor function, and show variable progression over time. CRPS is further divided into CRPS type I, which traditionally was referred to as reflex sympathetic dystrophy, and CRPS type II,

previously known as causalgia. The only difference between them is that type II has a known nerve injury.

Clinically, it is useful to define whether the CRPS is dependent or independent of the sympathetic activity. The terms SMP and sympathetic-independent pain (SIP) complement the term CRPS. Sympathectomy can help only patients with SMP and is contraindicated for patients with sympathetic-independent pain. The challenge for the clinician is to determine whether a particular patient with CRPS has SMP and, if so, properly select patients for clinical or surgical treatment. For the purpose of this chapter oriented to the surgical approach, SMP is widely used, leaving the terminology of CRPS for situations in which it becomes necessary.

PATHOPHYSIOLOGY OF SYMPATHETIC-MEDIATED PAIN

The pathophysiology of SMP is poorly understood. Some theories suggest ephaptic transmission between somatic afferents and sympathetic efferents at the level of the spinal cord, leading to the release of chemical mediators known to cause pain in inflammatory reactions, such as substance P, prostaglandin, and bradykinin. These substances produce the classic symptoms of vascular instability and temperature changes.[28–31] Supporting this theory, the results of dorsal column stimulation in suppressing SMP appear to occur because of stimulation-induced suppression of efferent sympathetic hyperactivity.[2, 32, 33] Conversely, an experiment of electrical stimulation of distal sympathetic stumps after sympathectomy for SMP reproduced presympathectomy pain.[34] This classic, well-controlled experiment in humans with stimulation of the sympathetic chain between the second and third thoracic sympathetic ganglia reproduced symptoms of SMP such as burning, tingling, and pricking sensations in the fingers, hand, or arm. Before the sensation of discomfort, subjects could observe a pilomotor response over the entire arm and shoulder. After stimulation, a chronic aching sensation lasted for 24 hours. Patients undergoing sympathectomy for causalgia appear to have more of a painful response to stimulation than patients undergoing sympathectomy for other causes.[34]

Leriche[35] developed the vicious cycle hypothesis to explain causalgic pain, and Livingstone expanded it.[36] Self-sustained, abnormal firing of loops in the dorsal horn provoked by an irritative focus in small nerve endings or major nerve trunks activates central projection fibers, leading to pain. Others also embraced this theory, and the popular reflex sympathetic dystrophy denomination came to be. Resolution of pain with sympathetic blocks gives support to this theory. Bonica[37] gave further support to this approach with his detailed accounts of the syndrome variables and with special emphasis on objective assessment of the efficacy of block techniques. Taken together, the studies of dorsal column stimulation and stimulation of stumps of sympathectomized patients, as well as the results of sympathectomy and sympathetic blocks, support the hypothesis of ephaptic hyperactivity at the level of dorsal horn between sensory afferent and sympathetic efferent elements.

DIAGNOSTIC ASSESSMENTS AND PATIENT EVALUATION

Clinical Diagnosis

SMP must be differentiated from chronic pain syndromes with similar features but different maintaining factors, such as secondary gain, psychological problems, viral infections, neuropathic processes, and peripheral nerve injury. True SMP implies that, despite multiple triggering events in the pain syndrome, an abnormal response of the sympathetic system mediating the pain can be documented. Although the clinical features of advanced cases of causalgia are easily identifiable, mild cases are difficult to diagnose. Classically, SMP is associated with burning pain hypersensitivity in the distribution of the injured somatic nerve, signs of autonomic imbalance, and ultimately secondary trophic changes. Many patients do not have an identifiable trauma triggering sympathetic dystrophy. In a large series, 10% of the patients were diagnosed as having sympathetic dystrophy without a previous history of trauma.[38] This pattern has also been largely identified in smaller series.[20] Sudeck's atrophy and Sudeck's syndrome focus on the associated osteoporosis observed in late cases, an inconsistent finding that may result from a neurovascular reflex or disuse. Numerous manifestations of the disorder by different causes and in different regions of the body have been reported.[3, 27, 39–42]

The onset and progression of the SMP syndromes have been divided in three stages. Stage I (i.e., early or acute) is characterized by constant, intense, and burning pain that is disproportionate to the injury and that is accompanied by vasomotor instability, edema, and swelling. Stage II (i.e., intermediate or dystrophy) is characterized by severe pain with skin sensitivity, shiny and discolored skin, and dystrophic nails. Stage III (i.e., late or atrophic) shows signs of wasting, atrophy of skin and subcutaneous tissues, stiffness of joints, and osteoporosis.[38, 43]

Wilkinson[44] mentioned several sympathetic pain syndromes. He grouped them as syndromes with principally SMP but little dystrophy or vasculopathy, including minor causalgia, shoulder-hand syndrome, and

TABLE 195–1 ■ **Summary of 112 Sympathectomy Procedures in Which Unilateral and Bilateral Approaches Were Used in 65 Patients**

APPROACH	NO. OF PATIENTS	NO. OF PROCEDURES
Unilateral	20	22
Bilateral (staged)	11	22
Bilateral (same day)	34	68

diabetic burning foot syndrome; syndromes with significant dystrophy and variable SMP, including major causalgia, reflex sympathetic dystrophy, and Sudeck's atrophy; and syndromes with significant vasculopathy and variable SMP, including vasospasm of postacute vascular occlusion, peripheral occlusive vasculopathy, vasospastic vasculopathy such as Raynaud's syndrome, and Prinzmetal's angina.[17, 44]

The clinical diagnosis of SMP must be always confirmed by an objective test, usually relief of pain with sympathetic blockade.

Laboratory Tests

Although SMP is a clinical diagnosis confirmed with nerve block, certain laboratory studies may be confirmatory. Thermography may reveal a temperature difference between extremities or regions in the same extremity. Regular radiographs of the extremity in question may show patchy demineralization of epiphyses and the short bones of the hands and feet.[45, 46] Soft tissue swelling may be detected. In advanced phases of the disease, fine-detail x-ray films show subperiosteal bone resorption, striation, and tunneling in the cortices, as well as large excavations and tunneling of the endosteal surface.[47, 48] These changes are not specific for SMP; they may occur in hyperparathyroidism, thyrotoxicosis, and other conditions associated with rapid bone turnover.[49, 50]

A bone scintilogram usually reveals increased periarticular uptake in the involved limb, and higher sensitivity may be achieved with triple-phase bone scan.[51–53] Kozin and colleagues[54] compared the sensitivity and specificity of radiographs and scintilography in cases of reflex sympathetic dystrophy. The specificity of radiographs was 71% and that of scintilography was 86%. The sensitivity of radiographs was 69% and that of scintilography was 60%.[54] Magnetic resonance imaging (MRI) has been described as a more sensitive study than radiographic examination and radionuclide assessment for detection of changes in the bones of patients with SMP. It also has the advantage of detecting soft tissue changes such as edema and muscle atrophy. MRI allows a differential diagnosis between SMP and other bone lesions.[55] Doppler flow studies and plethysmography may also be used as adjunctive studies, but they are not always reliable.[56]

Although the blood flow through the affected extremity tends to be lower than the normal extremity in stress conditions, in a warm and resting environment, the temperature of the affected extremity tends to approach that of the normal extremity.[56] Jeng and associates[57] observed an increase in cerebral blood flow after T2 sympathectomy, and they suggested the possibility of using such a surgical approach to improve cerebral blood flow in patients with cerebral vascular insufficiency.

Patient Selection

Not all patients with SMP require sympathectomy. Early and frequent use of sympathetic blockade may carry the patient through a milder and self-limited episode of causalgic pain.[58] Other clinical measures of controlling pain must be exhausted before considering sympathectomy. Withholding surgery too long, however, my decrease chances of complete pain relief afforded by a sympathectomy. The patients must have a reliable and objective response to regional sympathetic block encompassing the affected extremity. Good pain relief with sympathetic nerve block confirms that the complex regional pain is mediated by the sympathetic nervous system. Blockade of α_1-adrenergic receptors by intravenously administered phentolamine correlates with subjective pain relief.[59] Use of saline as a placebo control minimizes the chance of a false response, and objective findings such as temperature change should be documented.[60] Bier block with guanethidine can be employed to provide regional sympathetic blockade.[61] Guanethidine displaces norepinephrine in presynaptic vesicles and prevents its reuptake. Reserpine also depletes norepinephrine stores by interfering with its storage, and it can be administered intra-arterially to achieve regional block.[49, 50]

Paravertebral sympathetic block is the most widely used diagnostic and therapeutic modality for SMP.[62, 63] For upper extremity pain, the target is the stellate ganglion, which is readily accessible percutaneously. Although the sympathetic innervation to the arm is mainly from T2, anesthetic agents readily diffuse through paravertebral space to block the sympathetic outflow to the arm.[64] The lower extremity sympathetic outflow can be blocked at L2 and L3 levels, sources for most of the sympathetic innervation for the legs. Results of the blockade must be carefully evaluated clinically by observing for Horner's syndrome when the upper extremity is blocked and for changes in skin temperature and color when the upper or lower extremity is blocked. Objective changes in temperature and blood flow to the skin can be detected by careful measurements.[56] Patients must remain naive of the result expected, and placebo must be used when there is suspicion of secondary gain. The visual digital scale must be used as a hard record of the effects of the sympathetic blockade. Patients with unequivocal pain relief with sympathetic blockade are sympathectomy candidates.

SURGICAL TREATMENT

There are several approaches for upper thoracic and lower cervical sympathectomy and fewer options for splanchnic and lumbar sympathectomy. The transaxillary and posterior paravertebral approaches are advocated by a few authorities for exposure of the upper thoracic and lower cervical ganglia. The most acceptable open procedure is the modification of MacKay's paravertebral approach described in 1955.[65] Cloward[66] described a similar approach in 1957. This approach has the advantage of bilateral exposure through a single incision. It provides a more direct exposure of the sympathetic ganglia and their rami communicantes.[16] The retroperitoneal flank approach is predominantly used for the lumbar chain, and the splanchnic chain

is reached by means of a lower thoracic paramedian incision. This surgery involves rib removal and retraction of the pleura.[12] These procedures are frequently too invasive for the patient's symptoms, which is why minimally invasive approaches to the sympathetic ganglia are becoming prevalent. This section discusses endoscopic approaches to the lower cervical, upper thoracic, and lumbar sympathetic ganglia. The splanchnic procedure is usually indicated for very debilitated patients with cancer pain who are being treated mostly medically or with phenol injection of the splanchnic chain.[12]

Thoracoscopic Sympathectomy

Jacobaeus[67] first performed thoracic endoscopic procedures in 1910 for the diagnosis of pulmonary tuberculosis and neoplastic diseases. Thoracoscopic sympathectomy procedures were originally described by Hughes[11] in 1942 and Kux[61] in 1951, using a ureteroscope for the treatment of hyperhidrosis. Jacobaeus[67] reported a series of more than 1400 endoscopic procedures. There was little interest in this technique until recently.[6, 68–74] Minimally invasive treatment of sympathetic-mediated syndromes affecting the extremities with endoscopic techniques has expanded because of the refinement of techniques and clarification of the indications and applications.[69, 71–73, 75–77] The most common indications for thoracic sympathectomy include hyperhidrosis, SMP syndromes, Raynaud's syndrome, postamputation syndrome (i.e., phantom pain), and refractory cardiac tachyarrhythmias. Percutaneous sympathectomy procedures have limited efficacy, and the long-term successes are not optimal.[17, 68] Thoracoscopic resection of the sympathetic ganglia appears to have a lower incidence of morbidity than open thoracotomy or a posterior paraspinal approach. This result may reflect the magnified endoscopic view of the sympathetic chain and adjacent anatomy, leading to a more precise resection.[6, 28, 74, 78] Subsequently, patient demand and improved satisfaction due to shortened hospital stay with reduced costs and morbidity made minimally invasive thoracoscopic sympathectomy an attractive choice for treatment of SMP syndromes of the upper extremities.

INDICATIONS

The thoracoscopic paraspinal approach is useful for sympathectomy and for biopsies and thoracic spinal work. Besides the indications of sympathectomy for SMP, the most common indications for sympathectomy using the endoscopic approach are discussed.

Sympathetic–Mediated Pain Syndrome

Constant burning pain and atrophic skin changes in the extremity are typical signs and symptoms of SMP syndromes. Medical therapy with narcotics, neuroleptics, or anticonvulsants usually has only limited use and temporary benefit. Similarly, stellate blocks provide temporary relief, allowing the patient to pursue rehabilitation in an attempt to resolve the problem. A

T1-4 sympathectomy provides good initial relief, but there is a variable rate of recurrence that is difficult to predict.[20, 49, 62]

Vasculitis and Raynaud's Syndrome

Ischemic vascular disorders have episodes of severe, painful skin blanching, primarily in the hands and fingertips, that are exacerbated by cold temperatures or emotional response. Extreme cases may cause ischemic and gangrenous ulceration of the digits. The initial treatment is avoidance of cold and use of α-adrenergic medications that are effective for less severe cases. Refractory cases may achieve good initial relief from sympathectomy, but the long-term results may be somewhat less optimal.[6, 78, 79]

Cardiac Arrhythmia

Malignant tachyarrhythmias may result from stress and "sympathetic imbalance" due to disproportionate left-right sympathetic outflow.[72, 80] A right stellate ganglion block coupled with left stellate ganglion stimulation lengthens the QT interval on the electrocardiogram, and conversely, a left stellate ganglion block with right stellate ganglion stimulation shortens the QT interval. Accordingly, a left T1-4 sympathectomy produces a "β-adrenergic effect" that shortens the QT interval and may reduce the incidence of medically refractory tachyarrhythmias associated with dangerous, prolonged QT interval syndromes. Despite this cardiac function, the hemodynamics and catecholamine concentrations may not be altered significantly after sympathectomy.[57, 80, 81]

Hyperhidrosis

Palmar and axillary hyperhidrosis is the primary indication for thoracoscopic sympathectomy. Hyperhidrosis is characterized by excessive sweating, primarily in the hands, that is exacerbated by minor stresses such as handshaking. The cause is unknown. Hyperhidrosis has an incidence of approximately 1% in Western populations, but the incidence may be higher in Asian populations.[68] The sympathetic nervous system innervates eccrine sweat glands through cholinergic nerve fibers arising from the intermediolateral column of the thoracic and upper lumbar spinal cord. Increased sympathetic tone results in vasoconstriction, and skin cooling exacerbates the excessive sweating.[16, 78, 80] Stellate ganglion blocks result in temporary drying and decreased sweating in the ipsilateral hand and armpit. The warming effect is caused by increased blood flow through cutaneous arteriovenous fistulas and cholinergic blockage. Resection of the T2-3 sympathetic ganglia that provide sympathetic innervation to the upper extremity through the lower trunk of the brachial plexus provides lasting relief from hyperhidrosis.[16] Details of this syndrome and surgical approaches are discussed elsewhere in this volume.

SURGICAL AND ANESTHETIC CONSIDERATIONS

Endoscopic thoracic sympathectomy procedures require an anesthesiologist and operating room staff familiar with thoracic endoscopy. Double-lumen endotracheal tube placement for contralateral lung ventilation and ipsilateral lung deflation is essential. The patient

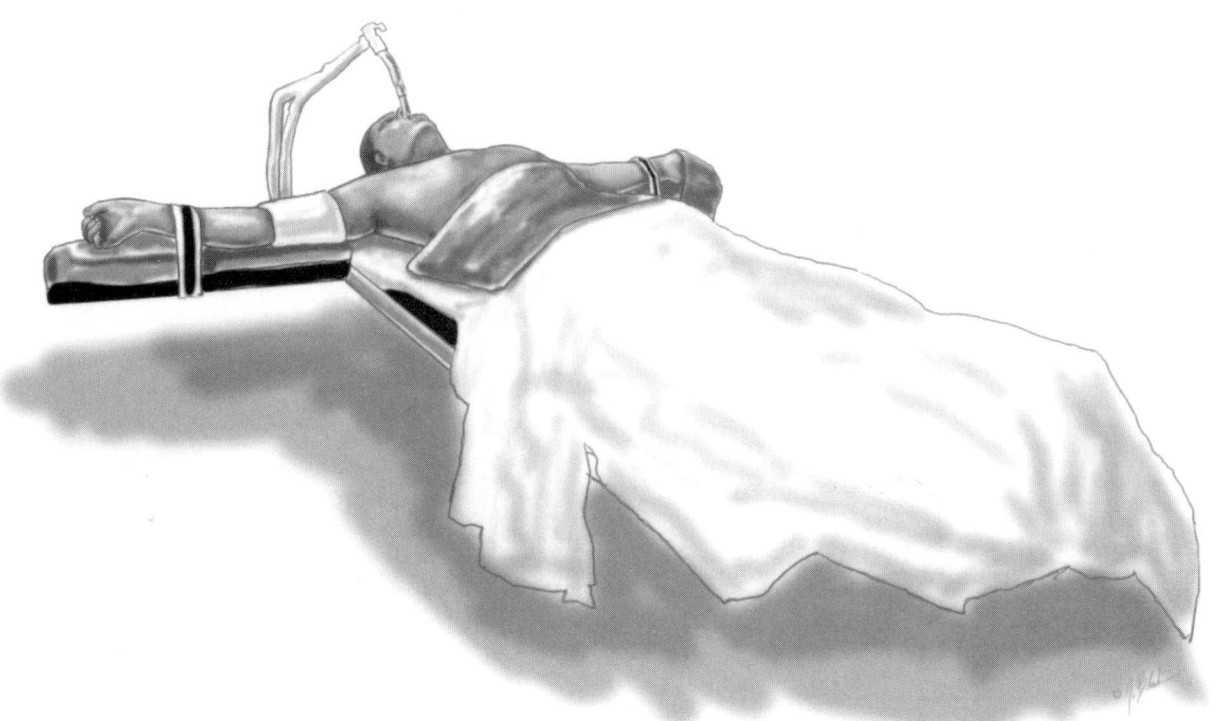

FIGURE 195–1. Supine positioning of the patient undergoing sequential bilateral thoracoscopic sympathectomies. Right and left selective bronchi intubation is performed during the operation on each side.

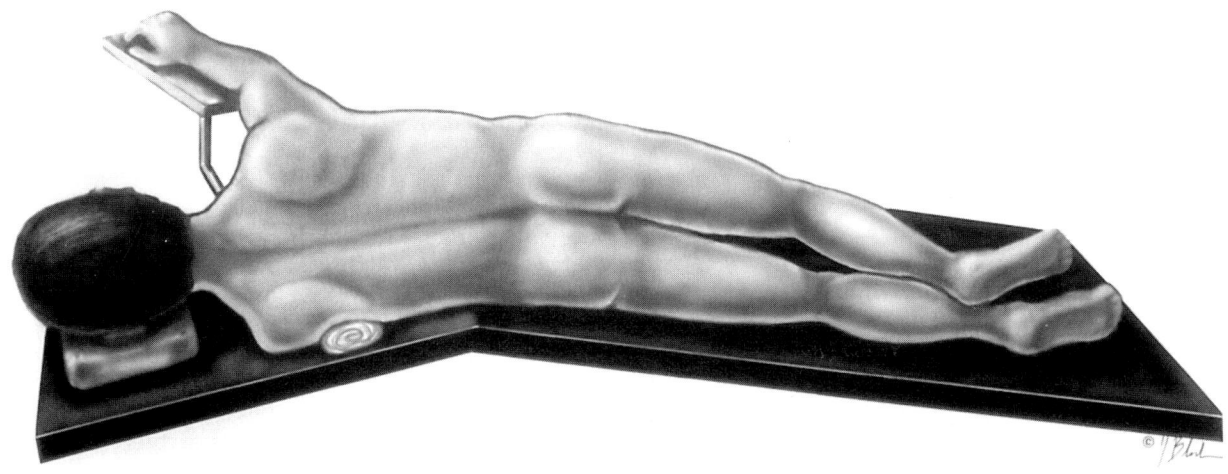

FIGURE 195–2. Lateral positioning of the patient undergoing right thoracoscopic sympathectomy is the same as for a thoracotomy. Notice the exposure of the axillary region, including the upper intercostal spaces, which are important for the endoscope and instrumentation portals.

is positioned supine for bilateral thoracoscopic procedures (Fig. 195–1), and the lateral decubitus position (Fig. 195–2) can be used for unilateral procedures. The operating table positioning is important to allow the lung to fall away from the upper thorax and open the intercostal spaces for access into the thorax.

Instruments

Thoracoscopic sympathectomy equipment and instruments are similar to those used in general and obstetric-gynecologic procedures. A standard endoscopic video-monitoring system with a 5- to 10-mm-

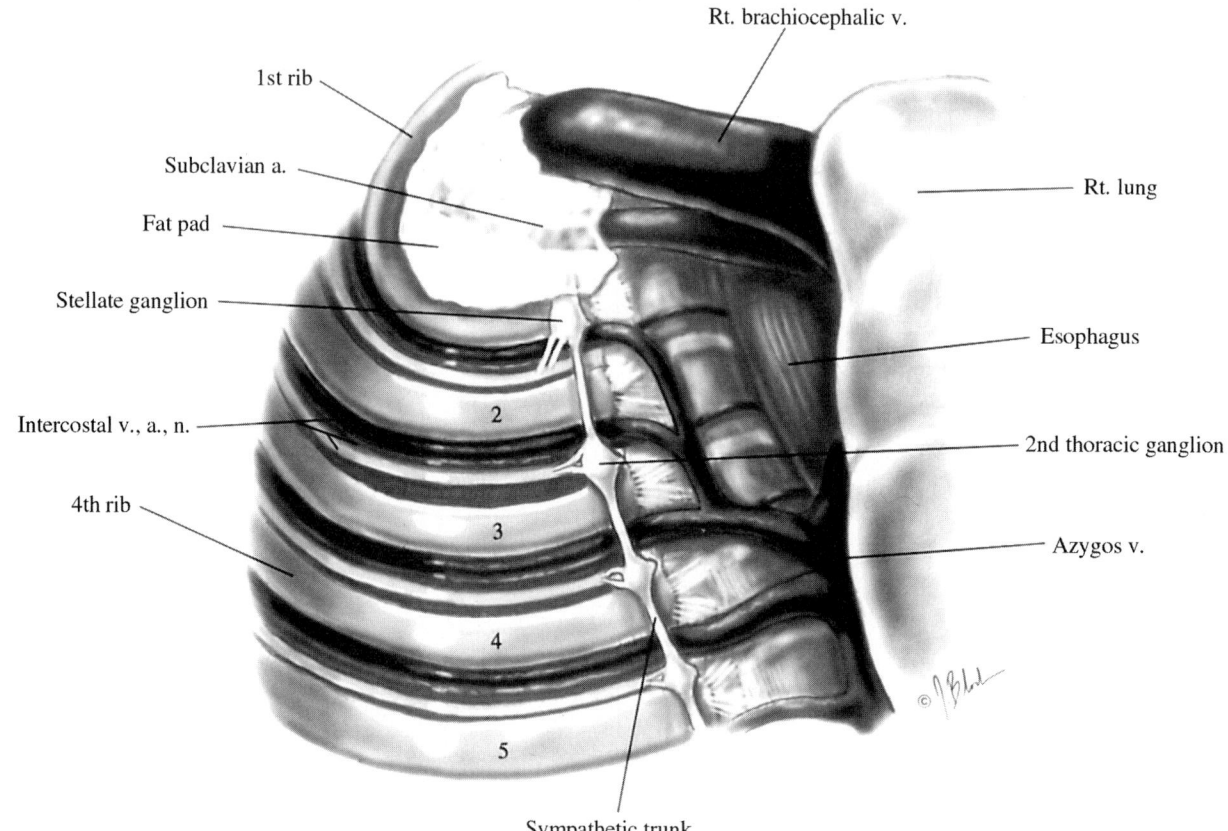

FIGURE 195–3. View of the intrathoracic anatomy of the right upper thorax shows the location of the sympathetic ganglia and chain. Notice the subclavian artery and the first rib, landmarks for determination of the stellate ganglion.

diameter, rigid laparoscope is needed. Basic endoscopic surgical instruments include 5-mm-diameter mini-Metzenbaum scissors with monopolar electrocautery, a 10-mm-diameter curved hemostat, and a 5-mm-diameter suction-irrigator. Endoscopic vascular clips and a retractable fan-type retractor should be available if needed.

Ports and Port Placement

Two or three ports are used to perform the sympathectomy procedure. One port is for the endoscope, and one or two ports are for the instruments. Port insertion is similar to chest tube placement, with a 2-cm skin incision and blunt dissection with a curved hemostat over the rib into the thorax, avoiding the intercostal neurovascular bundle. The 15-mm-diameter ports (Ethicon Flexi-path, Cincinnati, OH) are soft, flexible endoscopic cannulas inserted through the chest wall with an introducer. The anesthesiologist deflates the lung, and the first port is placed. The endoscope is placed through the port in the fifth intercostal space in the posterior axillary line. An instrument port is placed in the same fifth intercostal space. If another working port is needed, it is placed in the fourth intercostal space in the anterior axillary line.

Steps of the Procedure

The endoscope provides a panoramic view of the upper thoracic cavity, and the working ports can be rearranged according to the surgeon's preference (Fig. 195–3). A 0-degree endoscope usually provides good visualization for most sympathectomy procedures, but the 30-degree endoscope lens occasionally is needed. Endoscopic exploration of the thoracic cavity is performed after the ports are placed, and any adhesions to the parietal pleura are coagulated and divided, allowing the lung to be retracted. Additional lung retraction can be accomplished by rotating or elevating the operating table so that the lung falls away from the vertebral column.

Important intrathoracic anatomic landmarks for a sympathectomy are the first and second ribs. The sympathetic chain is a whitish, glistening, raised, longitudinal structure that courses over each rib head (see Fig. 195–3). The pleura overlying the sympathetic chain should not be pressed excessively with endoscopic instruments, because repetitive touch leads to pleural hyperemia that obscures visualization of the chain. The cephalad aspect of the sympathetic chain and limit of the surgical resection is the stellate ganglion. The stellate ganglion is immediately below the subclavian artery. Other major vascular structures, such as the azygous vein, subclavian veins, and the highest (supreme) intercostal artery and veins, should be avoided during dissection of the sympathetic chain.

The sympathectomy begins with a pleural incision over the sympathetic chain at T3 using curved scissors and continuing cephalad above T2 but remaining short of the inferior aspect of the stellate ganglion (Fig. 195–4). The sympathetic chain is mobilized from T3 with scissors by dividing the rami communicantes at the T2-3 levels (Fig. 195–5). It is important to maintain the

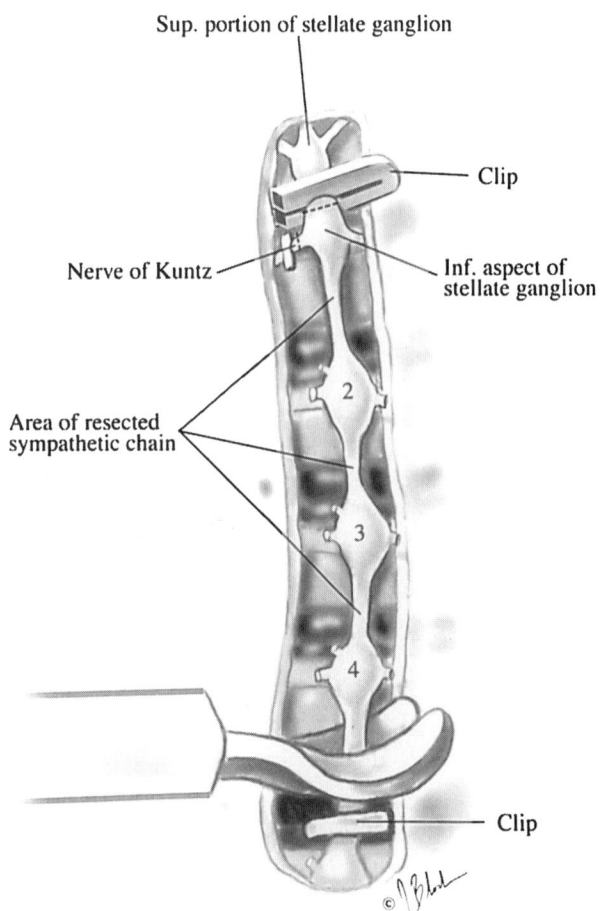

FIGURE 195–4. Division of the rami communicants at each level (left) and division of the sympathetic chain at the inferior aspect of the stellate ganglion and T4 *(right)*. Notice sectioning of the nerve of Kuntz, which is important to achieve sympathetic denervation of the upper extremity, and preservation of the upper part of the stellate ganglion, which is important to avoid Horner's syndrome.

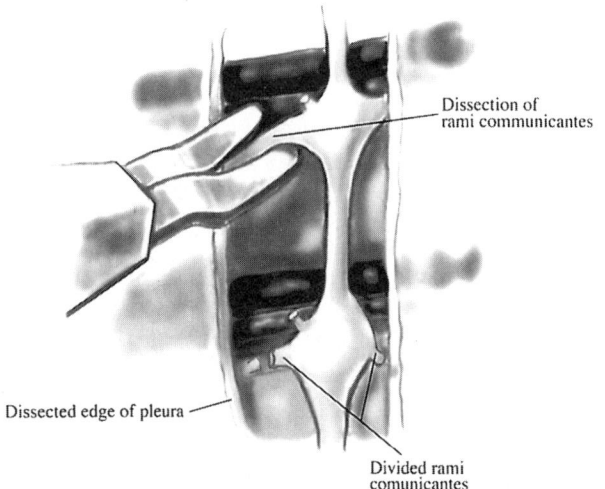

FIGURE 195–5. Detailed dissection of the rami communicants for complete release of the sympathetic chain to be removed. Notice the proximity to the intercostal vessels, which should be avoided during this dissection. The intercostal nerve must be preserved to avoid postoperative chest wall deafferentation pain.

TABLE 195–2 ■ Diagnosis of Patients Undergoing Thoracoscopic Sympathectomy

DISORDER	NO. OF PATIENTS
Hyperhidrosis	48
RSD/CRPS	12
Raynaud's syndrome	5

CRPS, complex regional pain syndrome; RSD, reflex sympathetic dystrophy.

TABLE 195–4 ■ Patient Satisfaction and Willingness to Undergo a Repeat Procedure

DISORDER	PATIENT SATISFACTION RATE (%)	WILLINGNESS TO REPEAT (%)
Hyperhidrosis	96	98
RSD/vasculitis	66	65

RSD, reflex sympathetic dystrophy.

dissection plane immediately beneath the sympathetic chain to avoid the underlying intercostal vessels. If bleeding is encountered, clip ligation or cautery of the vessel achieves the necessary meticulous hemostasis. Most intercostal vessels are small, but occasionally, they are enlarged or course over the sympathetic chain and require division.

A large ramus arising laterally from the T2 ganglion is the nerve of Kuntz, which is slightly larger than other rami (see Fig. 195–4). It provides important sympathetic innervation to the lower trunk of the brachial plexus.[82] The nerve of Kuntz and the stellate ganglion are usually found beneath the fat pad that envelops the subclavian artery (see Fig. 195–3). The stellate ganglion should remain undisturbed to avoid injury and possible Horner's syndrome. The dissected T2-3 sympathetic chain is then divided proximally and distally and sent for histologic evaluation. The dissection bed is irrigated, and hemostasis is ensured. A 16-French (16F) chest tube is inserted and positioned endoscopically through one of the ports. The instrument ports are then removed, and the lung is re-inflated with positive pressure by the anesthesiologist. The port incisions are closed in two layers using absorbable sutures and Steri-Strips. The operative procedure requires approximately 1 hour, depending on the anatomic complexity of the individual patient and the experience of the surgeon.

Postoperative Care

The chest tube is placed on 15 cm H_2O of suction until the patient reaches the recovery room, where the patient is placed on a water-seal drainage system with suction. A chest radiograph is obtained to ensure proper lung expansion, and one chest tube is removed, followed by a repeat chest radiograph. The procedure is repeated for the second chest tube. Pneumothorax is uncommon and requires chest tube replacement until the leak resolves. Oral analgesics are adequate for pain control, and the hospital stay is typically 1 or 2 days.

Patients with chronic pain syndromes may require a slow taper of preoperative medications, which is managed on an outpatient basis.

OPERATIVE EXPERIENCE

Patient Population

The experience of the first 100 procedures performed at the University of California–Los Angeles (UCLA) is presented. These data represent the use of modern technology and the learning curve resulting when using the thoracic endoscopic approach. Sixty-five patients underwent 112 thoracoscopic sympathectomy procedures at UCLA Medial Center for sympathetic-mediated disorders between 1993 and 1999. The procedures were performed for unilateral or bilateral symptoms. Twenty patients underwent unilateral procedures, and 11 patients with bilateral symptoms underwent staged procedures several weeks apart in the early part (1993–1995) of this series. In recent years, 34 patients with bilateral symptoms had staged procedures on the same day (see Table 195–1).

Outcome Analysis

The follow-up period was 6 months to 6 years, with assessment performed by a clinical examination or telephone interview, or both. An independent observer collected clinical outcome questionnaires, and a retrospective analysis was performed. Patients with hyperhidrosis were evaluated for the presence or absence of sweaty palms, surgery-related complications, and delayed-onset complications of compensatory hyperhidrosis or gustatory sweating. Patients with pain disorders were evaluated with the Oswestry Pain Scale to quantify the severity of their preoperative and postoperative symptoms. The incidence and severity of recurrent pain symptoms were evaluated, and all patients were questioned about their "overall satisfaction" and "willingness to undergo a repeat procedure."

TABLE 195–3 ■ Outcomes for 48 Patients with Hyperhidrosis

DISORDER	RELIEF OF SYMPTOM	PARTIAL RELIEF OF SYMPTOM	RECURRENT SYMPTOMS	LOST TO FOLLOW-UP
Hyperhidrosis	47	1	0*	0

* Although no patients experienced recurrent palmar hyperhidrosis, 11 had mild compensatory sweating in the trunk, and 2 patients suffered gustatory sweating.

TABLE 195–5 ■ Outcomes for 17 Patients with Pain and Vasculitis Disorders

	NUMBER OF PATIENTS		
DISORDER	Relief of Symptoms	Recurrence of Symptoms	Lost to Follow-up
RSD/CRPS	7	4	1
Raynaud's syndrome/ vasculitis (5 patients)	4	1	0

CRPS, complex regional pain syndrome; RSD, reflex sympathetic dystrophy.

Results

Patients with hyperhidrosis were the largest group treated by thoracoscopic sympathectomy (Table 195–2). They had very high success rates (Tables 195–3 and 195–4), but they also had the highest complication rates. Complications were usually related to compensatory hyperhidrosis manifested as sweating in the trunk or torso. However, most patients were sufficiently satisfied with the result, as indicated by their willingness to repeat the procedure. Patients treated for pain syndromes or vascular disorders had a positive initial response to treatment (see Table 195–2), however, outcomes were diminished for some patients after more than 6 months by variable recurrence of symptoms (Tables 195–5 and 195–6; see also Table 195–4). The overall satisfaction and willingness to repeat the operative treatment was similarly decreased (see Table 195–4). No patients had worsened pain symptoms after sympathectomy. The hospital length of stay for thoracoscopic sympathectomy patients was usually 1 or 2 days (Table 195–7). The patients considered historical cohorts at our institution who were treated with posterior paraspinal sympathectomies had a hospital length of stay that typically ranged from 3 to 6 days. The overall complication rates for thoracoscopic procedures were also comparable with those of previous treatment modalities (Table 195–8).

Complications

Complications from endoscopic sympathectomy procedures are usually minor and self-limited. Horner's syndrome from injury to the stellate ganglion in thoracoscopic procedures occurred more often early in the series, probably reflecting the learning curve for

TABLE 195–7 ■ Length of Stay after Thoracoscopic Sympathectomy

DURATION	UNILAT SYMPATHECTOMY (DAYS)	BILAT SYMPATHECTOMY (DAYS)
Median	1	2
Mean	1.5	1.8
Range	0–4	1–3

TABLE 195–8 ■ Postoperative Complications after Sympathectomy

COMPLICATION	NO. OF PATIENTS
Horner's syndrome	
Transient	7
Permanent	1
Compensatory hyperhidrosis*	11
Gustatory sweating	2
Pneumothorax (requiring chest tube)	1
Pleural effusion (not requiring thoracocentesis or chest tube)	4
Wound infection	1
Intercostal neuralgia	
Transient	3
Permanent	1
Death†	1

* Only patients with hyperhidrosis experienced compensatory sweating symptoms.
† An elderly patient with intractable Raynaud's died. The patient suffered a myocardial infarction 1 month after an uncomplicated, unilateral sympathectomy.

endoscopic surgical techniques. Horner's syndrome is usually transient and rarely permanent. Endoscopic visualization should minimize the incidence of Horner's syndrome, because only the rami caudal to the stellate that provide sympathetic innervation to the upper extremity are divided, with preservation of the rostrally ascending fibers that innervate the ocular and pupillary muscles.[49, 83] Intercostal neuralgia can result from intercostal nerve injury during port placement or from pressure during the procedure. This problem has been reduced with the use of soft, flexible ports and a 5-mm endoscope. Hashmonai and colleagues[76] cited the lower incidence of intercostal neuralgia as the major difference between open supraclavicular and endoscopic sympathectomy procedures; however, this re-

TABLE 195–6 ■ Outcomes for Pain and Vasculitis Disorders as Measured by the Oswestry Pain Scale*

DISORDER	PREOPERATIVE STATUS	1 MONTH POSTOPERATIVE STATUS (%)	> 6 MONTHS POSTOPERATIVE STATUS (%)
RSD/CRPS	42	92	65
Raynaud's syndrome/vasculitis	51	96	88

* Oswestry Pain Scale score is derived from a 10-item questionnaire administered to each patient preoperatively and 6 months postoperatively, with a scale of 1 to 100. Patient data are presented as a percentage of the mean.
CRPS, complex regional pain syndrome; RSD, reflex sympathetic dystrophy.

port did not reflect the use of flexible ports and smaller instruments.

Small pleural effusions do not require drainage but should be followed with repeated chest radiographs.[6, 77, 83] Pneumothorax indicates a parenchymal or port-site leak. Most cases can be observed, although a large pneumothorax may require chest tube placement. The one death that occurred in the series was several weeks after surgery for severe Raynaud's with significant pre-existing cardiovascular risk factors, and the patient was doing well after surgery.

Endoscopic Lumbar Sympathectomy

Open lumbar sympathectomy procedures have been used effectively to treat lower extremity vasculitis and pain syndromes but are being supplanted by minimally invasive laparoscopic retroperitoneal techniques.[84, 85] The most frequent indications for splanchnic sympathectomy procedures include lower extremity reflex sympathetic dystrophy (or CRPS) and Raynaud's syndrome. Pelvic and visceral pain syndromes have also been treated with splanchnic sympathectomy, although less frequently. Similar to thoracoscopic sympathectomy, minimally invasive endoscopic techniques can reduce the surgical morbidity, hospital stay, and return to activity due to small surgical incisions and reduced tissue injury.[86–88] A limited number of published reports with small series suggest results similar to those for open procedures, but reduced morbidity and hospitalization are the major differences.[1, 89–91]

PATIENT SELECTION

Patients with autonomic lower extremity pain syndromes require similar medical evaluation and man-

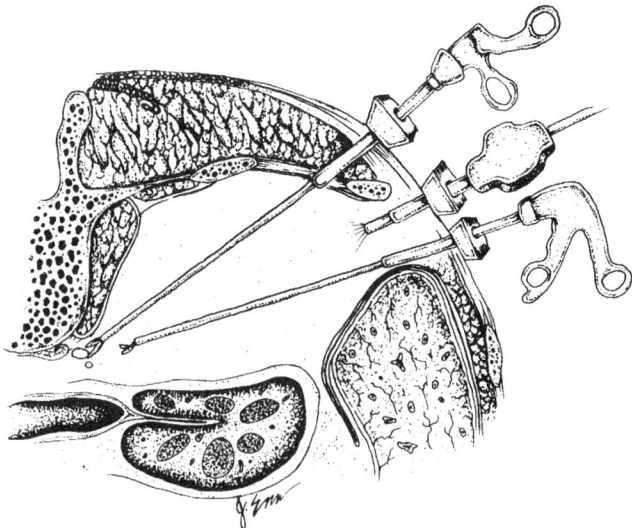

FIGURE 195–7. Lumbar retroperitoneal endoscopic exposure of the lumbar sympathetic chain for a sympathectomy. Notice the direct reach of the sympathetic ganglia with this approach.

agement before consideration of a lumbar sympathectomy procedure. For most patients with lower extremity pain syndromes, pelvic and lumbar imaging studies are necessary to exclude other treatable disorders. Peripheral vascular abnormalities should be evaluated with noninvasive methods or angiography to exclude treatable vascular lesions. Provocative testing with anesthetic lumbar sympathetic blocks can provide confirmation of diagnosis and useful predictive outcome assessment.

SURGICAL TECHNIQUE

The patient is placed in the prone position under general anesthesia, and ports are placed in the midaxillary line at the level of the intended sympathectomy. Blunt digital dissection is applied into the retroperitoneum to create an endoscopic working space with a balloon tissue expander or direct carbon dioxide insufflation (Fig. 195–6). Laparoscopic gas-tight ports are placed for the endoscope and working ports. Exposure and resection of the lumbar sympathetic chain proceed in a manner similar to that for open procedures (Fig. 195–7).

CONCLUSION

Minimally invasive endoscopic sympathectomy techniques have surgical goals that are similar to those for open procedures with equivalent outcomes; however, the associated morbidity is substantially reduced because of reduced tissue injury. We recommend that surgeons receive formal training for these procedures, including didactic and laboratory training, followed by work with an experienced surgeon who performs these operations on a regular basis. These endoscopic procedures have learning curves that necessitate precise knowledge of the anatomy and an understanding of endoscopic surgical techniques.

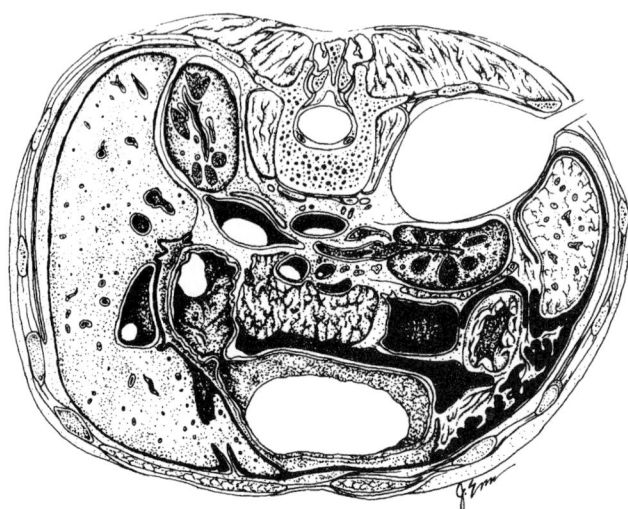

FIGURE 195–6. Cross-sectional anatomy through the midlumbar level demonstrates where the retroperitoneal dissection occurs. Notice the expansion of the retroperitoneal space, with anterior dislocation of the kidney and lateral dislocation of the spleen. There is a direct approach to the anterolateral aspect of the vertebrae where the sympathetic chain is visualized. The patient is in the prone position.

ACKNOWLEDGMENTS

We wish to thank Joe Bloch and Josh Emerson for their illustrations.

REFERENCES

1. Hourlay P, Vangertruyden G, Verduyckt F, et al: Endoscopic extraperitoneal lumbar sympathectomy. Surg Endosc 9:530–533, 1995.
2. Kumar K, Toth C, Nath RK, et al: Improvement of limb circulation in peripheral vascular disease using epidural spinal cord stimulation: a prospective study. J Neurosurg 86:662–669, 1997.
3. Richards RL: Causalgia: A centennial review. Arch Neurol 16:339–350, 1967.
4. Drott C: The history of cervicothoracic sympathectomy. Eur J Surg Suppl 572:5–7, 1994.
5. Johnson JP, Ahn SS, Choi WC, et al: Thoracoscopic sympathectomy: Techniques and outcome. Neurosurg Focus 4:1–8, 1998.
6. Ahn SS, Machleder HI, Concepcion B, et al: Thoracoscopic cervicodorsal sympathectomy: Preliminary results. J Vasc Surg 20:511–519, 1994.
7. Drott C, Claes G, Olsson-Rex L, et al: Successful treatment of facial blushing by endoscopic transthoracic sympathiotomy. Br J Dermatol 138:639–643, 1998.
8. Greenwood B: The origins of sympathectomy. Med Hist 11:165–169, 1967.
9. Kotzareff A: Resection partielle de trone sympathetique cervical droit pour hyperhidrose unilaterale. Rev Med Suisse Romande 40:111–113, 1920.
10. Jonnescu T: Rescetia totala di bilaterala a simpaticului cervical in cazuri de epilepsie si gusa exoftalmica. Romania Med 4:479–481, 1896.
11. Hughes J: Endothoracic sympathectomy. Proc R Soc Med 35:585–586, 1942.
12. Hardy RW, Bay JW: Surgery of the sympathetic nervous system. In Schimidek HH, Sweet WH (eds): Operative Neurosurgical Techniques: Indications, Methods and Results, 3rd ed. Boston, WB Saunders, 1995, pp 1637–1646.
13. Peet MM: Splanchnic resection for hypertension. Univ Hosp Bull Ann Arbor Mich 1:17, 1935.
14. Smithwick RH: A technique for splanchnic resection for hypertension. Surgery 7:1, 1940.
15. Atkins HBJ: Sympathectomy by the axillary approach. Lancet 1:538–539, 1954.
16. Cloward RB: Hyperhidrosis. J Neurosurg 30:545–551, 1969.
17. Wilkinson HA: Percutaneous radiofrequency upper thoracic sympathectomy: A new technique. Neurosurgery 15:811–814, 1984.
18. Adler OB, Engel A, Rosenberger A, Dondelinger R: Palmar hyperhidrosis CT guided chemical percutaneous thoracic sympathectomy. Fortschr Rontgenstr 153:400–403, 1990.
19. Spurling RG: Causalgia of the upper extremity: Treatment by dorsal sympathetic ganglionectomy. Arch Neurol Psychiatry 23:794, 1930.
20. Mockus B, Rutherford RB, Rosales C, Pearce WH: Sympathectomy for causalgia. Arch Surg 122:668–672, 1987.
21. Monart FD, Sadler TR, Schmitt EA, Reiner GW: Upper dorsal sympathectomy. Am J Surg 150:762–766, 1985.
22. Olcott C, Eltherington LG, Wilcosky BR, et al: Reflex sympathetic dystrophy: The surgeon's role in management J Vasc Surg 14:488–495, 1991.
23. Mitchell SW, Morehouse GR, Kern WW: Gunshot Wounds and Other Injuries of Nerves. New York, JB Lippincott, 1869, p 164.
24. Mitchell SW: On the disease of nerves, resulting from injuries. In Flint A (ed): Contributions Relating to the Causation and Prevention of Disease and of Camp Diseases. New York, US Sanitary Commission Memoirs, 1867, p 412.
25. Roberts WJ: A hypothesis of the physiological basis of causalgia and related pains. Pain 24:297–311, 1986.
26. Stanton-Hicks M, Janing W, Hassenbusch S, et al: Reflex sympathetic dystrophy: Changing concepts and taxonomy. Pain 63:127–133, 1995.
27. Jaeger B, Singer E, Kroening R: Reflex sympathetic dystrophy of the face: Report of two cases and review of the literature. Arch Neurol 43:693–695, 1986.
28. Janig W: The sympathetic nervous system in pain: Physiology and pathophysiology. In Stanton-Hicks M (ed): Pain and the Sympathetic Nervous System. Boston, Kluwer Academic, 1990, pp 17–89.
29. Mackinnon SE, Dellon AL: Painful sequelae of peripheral nerve injury. In Mackinnon SE, Dellon AL (eds): Surgery of the Peripheral Nerve. New York, Thieme Medical Publishers, 1998, pp 492–504.
30. Szolcsanyi J: A pharmacological approach to elucidation of the role of different nerve fibers and receptor endings in mediation of pain. J Physiol 73:251–259, 1977.
31. Yaksh TL, Hammond DL, Peripheral and central substrates involved in the rostrad transmission of nociceptive information. Pain 13:1–85, 1982.
32. Kumar K, Spinal cord stimulation is effective in the management of reflex sympathetic dystrophy. Neurosurgery 40:503–509, 1997.
33. Linderoth B, Meyerson BA: Dorsal column stimulation: Modulation of somatosensory and autonomic function. In McMahon SB, Wall PD (eds): The Neurobiology of Pain: Seminars in the Neurosciences, vol 7. London, Academic Press, 1995, pp 263–277.
34. Walker AE, Nulson F: Electrical stimulation of the upper thoracic portion of the sympathetic chain in man. Arch Neurol Psychiatry 59:559–560, 1948.
35. Leriche R: De la causalgie envisagee comme une nevrite du sympathique et son treitement par la denudation et lexcision des plewus nerveux peri-arteriels. Presse Med 24:178–180, 1916.
36. Livingstone WK: Pain mechanisms: A Physiological Interpretation of Causalgia and its Related States. London, Macmillan, 1943.
37. Bonica JJ: Causalgia and other reflex sympathetic dystrophies. In JJ Bonica (ed): The Management of Pain. Philadelphia, Lea & Febiger, 1990, pp 230–243.
38. Veldman PH, Reynen HM, Arntz IE, Goris RJ: Signs and symptoms of reflex sympathetic dystrophy: Prospective study of 829 patients. Lancet 342:1012–1016, 1993.
39. Escobar PL: Reflex sympathetic dystrophy. Orthop Rev 15:646–651, 1986.
40. Poplawski ZJ, Wiley AM, Murray JF: Post-traumatic dystrophy of the extremities. J Bone Joint Surg Am 65:642–646, 1983.
41. Saddison DK, Vanek VW: Reflex sympathetic dystrophy after modified radical mastectomy: A case report. Surgery 114:116–120, 1993.
42. Veldman PH, Jacobs PB: Reflex sympathetic dystrophy of the head: case report and discussion of diagnostic criteria. J Trauma 36:119–121, 1994.
43. Bickerstaff DR, O'Doherty DP, Kanis JA: Radiographic changes in algodystrophy of the hand. J Hand Surg Br 16:47–52, 1991.
44. Wilkinson HA: Surgery for hyperhydrosis and sympathetically mediated pain syndromes. In WH Sweet, Schmideck HH (eds): Operative Neurosurgical Techniques, Indications, Methods and Results, 3rd ed. Boston, WB Saunders, 1995, pp 1573–1583.
45. Helms CA, O'Brien ET, Katzberg RW: Segmental reflex sympathetic dystrophy syndrome. Radiology 135:67–68, 1980.
46. Herrmann LG, Reineke HG, Caldwell JA: Post-traumatic painful osteoporosis: A clinical and roentgenological entity. AJR Am J Roentgenol 47:353–361, 1942.
47. Kozin F, Genant HK, Bekerman C, et al: The reflex sympathetic dystrophy syndrome. II. Roentgenographic and scintilographic evidence of bilateral and of periarticular involvement. Am J Med 60:332–338, 1976.
48. Genant HK, Kozin F, Bekerman C, et al: The reflex sympathetic dystrophy syndrome. Radiology 117:21–32, 1976.
49. Herz DA, Looman JE, Ford RD, et al: Second thoracic sympathetic ganglionectomy in sympathetic maintained pain. J Pain Symptom Manage 8:483–491, 1993.
50. Schwartzman RJ, McLellan TL: Reflex sympathetic dystrophy: A review. Arch Neurol 44:555–561, 1987.
51. Campbell JN Raja SN, Selig DK, et al: Diagnosis and management of sympathetically maintained pain. In Fields HL, Liebeskind JK (eds): Progress in Pain Research and Management. Seattle, IASP Press, 1994, pp 85–100.
52. Mackinnon SE, Holder LE: The use of three-phase radionuclide bone scanning in the diagnosis of reflex sympathetic dystrophy. J Hand Surg Am 9:556–563, 1984.

53. Simon H, Carlson DH: The use of bone scanning in the diagnosis of reflex sympathetic dystrophy. Clin Nucl Med 5:116–121, 1980.

54. Kozin F, Ryan LM, Carrera GF, et al: The reflex sympathetic dystrophy syndrome. III. Scintilographic studies, further evidence of therapeutic efficacy of systemic corticosteroids, and proposed diagnostic criteria. Am J Med 70:23–30, 1981.

55. Sintzoff S, Sintzoff S Jr, Stallenberg B, Matos C: Imaging in reflex sympathetic dystrophy. Hand Clin 13:431–442, 1997.

56. Baron R, Maier C: Reflex sympathetic dystrophy: Skin blood flow, sympathetic vasoconstrictor reflexes and pain before and after surgical sympathectomy. Pain 67:317–326, 1996.

57. Jeng JS, Yip PK, Huang SJ, et al: Changes in hemodynamics of the carotid and middle cerebral arteries before and after endoscopic sympathectomy in patients with palmar hyperhidrosis: Preliminary results. J Neurosurg 90:463–467, 1999.

58. Thompson JE: The diagnosis and management of post-traumatic pain syndromes (causalgia). Aust N Z J Surg 49:299–304, 1979.

59. Raja SN, Treede RD, Davis KD, et al: Systemic alpha-adrenergic blockade with phentolamine: A diagnostic test for sympathetically maintained pain. Anesthesiology 74:691–698, 1991.

60. Valley MA, Rogers JN, Gale DW: Relief of recurrent upper extremity sympathetically-maintained pain with contralateral sympathetic blocks: Evidence for crossover sympathetic innervation? J Pain Symptom Manage 10:396–400, 1995.

61. Hannington-Kiff JG: Relief of causalgia in limbs by regional intravenous guanethidine. Br Med J 2:367–368, 1979.

62. Abu Rahma AF, Robinson PA, Powell M, et al: Sympathectomy for reflex sympathetic dystrophy: Factors affecting outcome. Ann Vasc Surg 8:372–379, 1994.

63. Noppen M, Sevens C, Gerlo E, et al: Plasma catecholamine concentrations in essential hyperhidrosis and effects of thoracoscopic D2-D3 sympathicolysis. Eur J Clin Invest 27:202–205, 1997.

64. Wallace MS, Milholland AV: Contralateral spread of local anesthetic with stellate ganglia block. Reg Anesth 18:55–59, 1993.

65. MacKay HJ: Improved approach for posterior upper thoracic sympathectomy. J Am Med Ass 159:1261–1263, 1955.

66. Cloward RB: Treatment of hyperhidrosis. Hawaii Med J 16:381–387, 1957.

67. Jacobaeus HC: Uber die Moglichkeith die zystoskopie bei untersuchung seroser Hohlungen anzuwenden. MMW Munch Med Wochenschr 40:2090–2092, 1910.

68. Chuang KS, Liou NH, Liu JC: New stereotactic technique for percutaneous thermocoagulation of upper thoracic ganglionectomy in cases of palmar hyperhidrosis. Neurosurgery 22:600–604, 1988.

69. Dumont P, Hamm A, Skrobala D, et al: Bilateral thoracoscopy for sympathectomy in the treatment of hyperhidrosis. Eur J Surg 11:774–775, 1997.

70. Johnson JP, Obasi CN, Hahn MS, et al: Endoscopic thoracic sympathectomy. J Neurosurg Suppl 91:90–97,1999.

71. Nicholson ML, Hopkinson BR, Dennis MJS: Endoscopic transthoracic sympathectomy: Successful in hyperhidrosis but can the indications be extended? Ann R Coll Surg Engl 76:311–314, 1994.

72. Noppen M, Dendale P, Hagers Y, et al: Changes in cardiocirculatory autonomic function after thoracoscopic upper dorsal sympathicolysis for essential hyperhidrosis. J Autonom Nerv Syst 60:115–120, 1996.

73. Reardon PR, Preciado A, Scarborough T, et al: Outpatient endoscopic thoracic sympathectomy using 2-mm instruments. Surg Endosc 13:1139–1142, 1999.

74. Samuelsson H, Claes G, Drott C: Endoscopic electrocautery of the upper thoracic sympathetic chain: A safe and simple technique for treatment of sympathetically maintained pain. Eur J Surg Suppl 572:55–57, 1994.

75. Goetz RH, Marr JAS: The importance of the second thoracic ganglion for the sympathetic supply of the upper extremities, with a description of two new approaches for its removal in cases of vascular disease: Preliminary report. Clin Proc 3:102–114, 1944.

76. Hashmonai M, Kopelman D, Schein M: Thoracoscopic versus open supraclavicular upper dorsal sympathectomy: A prospective randomized trial. Eur J Surg Suppl 572:13–16, 1994.

77. Johnson JP, Ahn SS, Moosy JJ, et al: Surgery of the sympathectomy nervous system. In Benzel EC (ed): Spine Surgery: Techniques, Complication Avoidance and Management, vol 2. New York, Churchill Livingstone, 1999.

78. Edwards JM, Porter JM: Associated diseases with Raynaud's syndrome. Vasc Med Rev 1:51–58, 1990.

79. Landry GJ, Edwards JM, Porter JM: Current management of Raynaud's syndrome. Adv Surg 30:333–347, 1997.

80. Kao MC, Tsai JC, Lai DM, et al: Autonomic activities in hyperhidrosis patients before, during, and after endoscopic laser sympathectomy. Neurosurg 34:262–268, 1994.

81. Noppen M, Herrogodts P, Dendale P, et al: Cardiopulmonary exercise testing following bilateral thoracoscopic sympathicolysis in patients with essential hyperhidrosis. Thorax 50:1097–1100, 1995.

82. Kuntz A: Distribution of the sympathetic rami to the brachial plexus. Arch Surg 15:871–877, 1928.

83. Lai YT, Yang LH, Chio CC, et al: Complications in patients with palmar hyperhidrosis treated with transthoracic endoscopic sympathectomy. Neurosurg 41:110–113, 1997.

84. Elliott TB, Royle JP: Laparoscopic extraperitoneal lumbar sympathectomy: Technique and early results. Aust N Z J Surg 66:400–402, 1996.

85. Wattanasirichaigoon S, Ngaorungsri U, Wanishayathanakorn A, et al: Laparoscopic transperitoneal lumbar sympathectomy: A new approach. J Med Assoc Thai 80:275–281, 1997.

86. Beglaibter N, Berlatzky Y, Zamir O, et al: Retroperitoneoscopic lumbar sympathectomy. J Vasc Surg 35:815–817, 2002.

87. Tseng MY, Tseng JH: Endoscopic extraperitoneal lumbar sympathectomy for plantar hyperhidrosis: Case report. J Clin Neurosci 8:555–556, 2001.

88. Watarida S, Shiraishi S, Fujimura M, et al: Laparoscopic lumbar sympathectomy for lower-limb disease. Surg Endosc 16:500–503, 2002.

89. Bannenberg JJ, Hourlay P, Meijer DW, et al: Retroperitoneal endoscopic lumbar sympathectomy: Laboratory and clinical experience. Endosc Surg Allied Technol 3:16–20, 1995.

90. Katkhouda N, Wattanasirichaigoon S, Tang E, et al: Laparoscopic lumbar sympathectomy. Surg Endosc 11:257–260, 1997.

91. Lacroix H, Vander Velpen G, Penninckx F, et al: Technique and early results of videoscopic lumbar sympathectomy. Acta Chir Belg 96:11–14, 1996.

BIBLIOGRAPHY

Adson AW: Changes in technique of cervico-thoracic ganglionectomy and trunk resection. Am J Surg 3:287–288, 1934.

Drott C, Gothberg G, Claes G: Endoscopic procedures of the upper-thoracic sympathetic chain. Arch Surg 128:237–241, 1993.

Ghostine SY, Comair YG, Turner DM, et al: Phenoxybenzamine in treatment of causalgia: Report of 40 cases. J Neurosurg 60:1263–1268, 1984.

Kozin F, Soin JS, Ryan LM, et al: Bone scintilography in reflex sympathetic dystrophy syndrome. Radiology 138:437–443, 1981.

Kux E: The endoscopic approach to the vegetative nervous system and its therapeutic possibilities. Dis Chest 20:139–147, 1951.

Kux E: Thorakoskopiche eingriffe am Nervensystem. Stuttgart, Thieme, 1954.

Kux M: Thoracic endoscopic sympathectomy in palmar and axillary hyperhidrosis. Arch Surg 113:264–266, 1978.

Lee DY, Yoon YH, Shin HK, et al: Needle thoracic sympathectomy for essential hyperhidrosis: Intermediate-term follow-up. Ann Thorac Surg 69:251–253, 2000.

Leriche R: La chirurgie del la Douleur. Paris, Masson, 1940.

Levine DZ: Burning pain in an extremity. Postgrad Med 90:175–178, 1991.

Lin TS, Fang HY: Transthoracic endoscopic sympathectomy in the treatment of palmar hyperhidrosis—with emphasis on perioperative management (1,360 case analyses). Surg Neurol 52:453–457, 1999.

Linderoth B, Fedorcsak I, Meyerson BA: Peripheral vasodilation after spinal column stimulation: Animal studies of putative effector mechanisms. Neurosurgery 28:187–195, 1991.

Linderoth B, Gunasekera L, Meyerson BA: Effects of sympathectomy on skin and muscle microcirculation during dorsal column stimulation: Animal studies. Neurosurgery 29:874–879, 1991.

Munn JS, Baker WH: Recurrent sympathetic dystrophy: Successful treatment by contralateral sympathectomy. Surgery 102:102–105, 1987.

Nathan PW, Smith MC: The location of descending fibers to sympathetic preganglionic vasomotor and sudomotor neurons in man. J Neurol Neurosurg Psychiatry 50:1253–1262, 1987.

Noppen M, Herrogodts P, D'Haese J, et al: A simplified T2-3 thoracoscopic sympathicolysis technique for the treatment of essential hyperhidrosis: Short-term results in 100 patients. J Laparoendosc Surg 6:151–159, 1996.

Roos DB: Transaxillary extrapleural thoracic sympathectomy. In Bergan JJ, Yao JST (eds): Operative Techniques in Vascular Surgery. New York, Grune & Stratton, 1980, p 115.

Schwartzman RJ, Liu JE, Smullens SN, et al: Long-term outcome following sympathectomy for complex regional pain syndrome type 1 (RSD). J Neurol Sci 150:149–152, 1997.

Telford ED: The technique of sympathectomy. Br J Surg 23:448–450, 1935.

Wang JK, Johnson DA, Ilstrup DM: Sympathetic blocks for reflex sympathetic dystrophy. Pain 23:13–17, 1985

Wattanasirichaigoon S, Katkhouda N, Ngaorungsri U: Totally extraperitoneal laparoscopic lumbar sympathectomy: An initial case report. J Med Assoc Thai 79:49–54, 1996.

White JC, Smithwick RH, Allen AW, et al: A new muscle splitting incision for resection of the upper thoracic sympathetic ganglia. Surg Gynecol Obstet 56:651–657, 1933.

CHAPTER 196

Spinal Cord and Peripheral Nerve Stimulation for Chronic, Intractable Pain

RICHARD B. NORTH

The 1965 publication of the "gate theory" of pain transmission in the dorsal horn of the spinal cord provided a rationale for using electrical stimulation in the treatment of pain.[1] Technology that had been developed for cardiac pacing—in particular, compact, implantable, solid-state electronic devices—was readily adapted for electrical stimulation of the nervous system. The initial favorable experience prompted widespread use of this technique before patient selection criteria for these procedures and the multidisciplinary management of chronic pain were completely understood. Accordingly, results in many cases were disappointing. In recent years, however, patient selection criteria and management techniques have been refined, and implanted stimulation devices have become more reliable, leading to significantly better long-term results.[2, 3]

MECHANISMS OF PAIN RELIEF BY ELECTRICAL STIMULATION

The gate theory proposed that the activity of cells in the dorsal horn of the spinal cord, which signaled the central transmission of pain, is governed by the balance of small- and large-fiber afferent activity in the peripheral nervous system. The "gate" opens in response to an excess of small-fiber activity and closes in response to predominantly large-fiber activity. It happens that large fibers have a lower threshold for depolarization by an electrical field applied to a mixed peripheral nerve, so they can be recruited selectively. The motor threshold in a mixed peripheral nerve, however, may be very close to the sensory threshold, making amplitude adjustment critical. Further, most pain problems encountered clinically involve the distribution of more than one peripheral nerve. Electrical stimulation applied to the spinal cord can overcome both these problems. Large-diameter primary afferents are conveniently segregated in the dorsal columns. These can be activated antidromically and, through collaterals to the

dorsal horn, can influence segmental activity in the distribution of multiple peripheral nerves.

The gate theory has always been controversial,[4] and there are certain pathologic, painful conditions that it does not explain. For example, hyperalgesia can be signaled by large fibers.[5] In this circumstance, it may be that relief of pain by electrical stimulation of peripheral nerve or spinal cord is due to a frequency-related conduction block, acting at primary afferent branch points where dorsal column fibers and dorsal horn collaterals diverge. Our clinical experience is consistent with such a mechanism, in that patients show a significant preference for a minimal stimulation pulse repetition rate of 25 pulses per second.[3] Of course, alternative mechanisms involving interneurons in the dorsal horn, or involving descending fibers or sympathetic mechanisms, may be frequency dependent.[6–9]

In experimental studies of the therapeutic effects (and side effects) of spinal cord stimulation (SCS) in humans and in animal models, it is important to scale the stimulation amplitude to clinically relevant levels, between the amplitude producing first perception and that producing discomfort or motor threshold.[10] Animal models of SCS have, until recently, been limited in clinical relevance owing to the lack of a chronic or neuropathic pain model. Meyerson and coauthors described a sciatic nerve ligation model in the rat, using stimulation parameters that were adjusted to a clinically relevant range; this showed that stimulation relieved the manifestations of chronic pain or hyperalgesia.[11] There is evidence in animal models, also using parameters scaled to the clinical range, that some of the effects of SCS pertinent to the management of ischemic pain caused by peripheral vascular disease, as well as neuropathic pain, are mediated by the sympathetic nervous system and by GABAergic interneurons.[9, 12]

The relief of ongoing, chronic pain by SCS or any other treatment may be accompanied by undesirable effects on normal sensation. Careful psychophysical studies have shown only modest effects, however. As might be expected with a vibratory stimulus, vibratory sensation is impaired,[13] but acute pain sensation is not affected to a degree that would lead to insensible injury, such as Charcot's joints.[14, 15]

The electrical fields produced within the spinal cord by SCS have been modeled by computerized finite element techniques.[16, 17] These models predict distributions of voltages and currents within the spinal cord that are in general agreement with actual measurements in primate and cadaver spinal cord.[18] An electrode's longitudinal position is most important to achieving the desired effect at a particular segmental level; bipolar stimulation is most selective for longitudinally oriented midline fibers. A contact separation of 1.4 times the thickness of meninges and cerebrospinal fluid, or 6 to 8 mm, is optimal.[17] Entering dorsal root fibers are relatively superficial within the first few segments of the fasciculus gracilis,[19] and as they ascend, they decrease in mean diameter.[20] These and other anatomic factors determine the appropriate position and spacing of spinal cord electrodes; positioning electrodes more cephalad, which might be expected to achieve more widespread effects, instead elicits unwanted local segmental effects, which become excessive at the amplitudes necessary to achieve widespread paresthesias.[21, 22] Adding lateral anodes may mitigate this, and with a suitably designed pulse generator, right-left steering becomes possible.[23]

Analysis of cerebrospinal fluid in patients undergoing SCS has shown some changes in neurotransmitter and neurotransmitter metabolite concentrations.[24] Administration of the narcotic antagonist naloxone had no effect on the relief of pain by SCS or by any other form of transcutaneous or peripheral nerve stimulation.[25]

IMPLANTABLE DEVICES

Spinal Cord Stimulation Electrodes

Figure 196–1 shows representative spinal cord stimulating electrodes, including arrays that can be inserted percutaneously through a Tuohy needle, and arrays requiring laminectomy. When SCS was introduced in 1967, and for several years thereafter, the available electrodes required a laminectomy for introduction into the epidural, endodural, or subarachnoid space.[26–29] Laminectomy placement limited longitudinal access to the spinal canal, particularly under local anesthesia. This compromised the technical objective of eliciting paresthesias overlapping a patient's usual distribution of pain, a necessary condition for pain relief. Even with technically adequate placement of the electrode, pain relief did not necessarily occur, and the need for a less invasive test configuration became apparent.

These problems were addressed by the development of percutaneous techniques for electrode introduction in the 1970s.[30–32] High thoracic levels had been used in early implants,[27, 28] but this tended to cause excessive and unpleasant local segmental effects before recruitment of more caudal segments. Overlap of the patient's

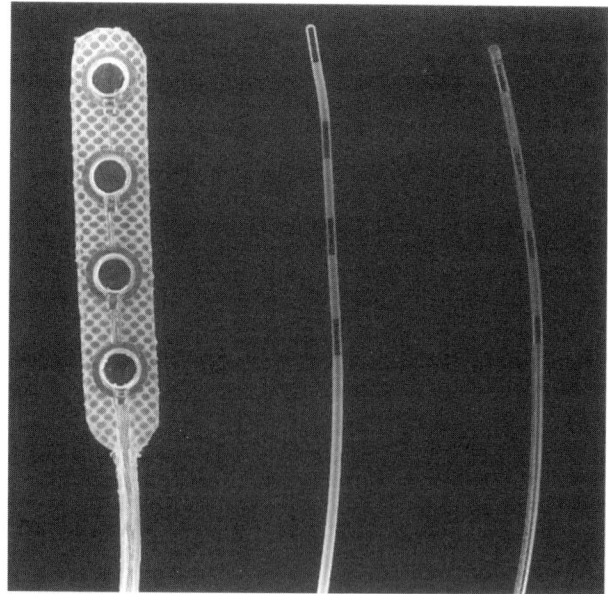

FIGURE 196–1. Spinal cord stimulation electrode arrays in contemporary use have multiple contacts. Some may be placed percutaneously through a Tuohy needle; others require laminectomy.

distribution of pain by stimulation paresthesias must, of course, be achieved below the discomfort threshold to be clinically useful. Percutaneous electrode placement allows free longitudinal access to the spinal canal and determination of the optimal level for electrode placement. In the common clinical application of failed back surgery syndrome, with low back and lower extremity pain, low thoracic electrode placement has proved to be most effective for isolating the painful segments.[33]

Percutaneously placed electrodes, initially used to establish clinical benefit before implanting a permanent system, were adapted quickly to chronic use.[15, 34] The earliest such electrodes were single contacts; insertion of multiple electrodes to achieve bipolar stimulation was often complicated by movement of one electrode with respect to another, necessitating operative revision.[15] Arrays of electrodes on a single carrier, which could be inserted as an assembly through a Tuohy needle, were developed in the early 1980s. This development was accompanied by improvements in methods of anchoring the electrodes and by the development of programmable implanted pulse generators, permitting the selection of active anodes and cathodes noninvasively. This allows postoperative adjustment of the stimulating anode and cathode positions with the patient in the supine or erect position, in which the device will be used, not the artifactual prone position in which it is routinely implanted. These technical improvements have resulted in a statistically significant improvement in clinical results[2, 3]; contemporary multicontact, programmable devices require surgical revision less frequently, and long-term efficacy has improved.

The performance of different electrode designs was

compared in a series of studies in which patients underwent trials with temporary single, percutaneous, quadripolar electrodes, followed by permanent implantation with new electrodes (either the same or a different design), using each patient as his or her own control. These studies used blinded, quantitative computerized methods, with adjustment of stimulation parameters to specific psychophysical thresholds.[35]

Insulated electrodes (requiring a small laminectomy) were compared with percutaneous electrodes—both designs featuring four contacts with nearly identical contact areas and spacing.[36] The insulated array performed significantly better than the percutaneous electrode in the same patients by most technical measures; it required half the power. Clinical outcome was significantly better short term (1 to 2 years) but not long term (3 years).

"Dual electrode" percutaneous arrays, created by inserting two electrodes in parallel, have been reported to have advantages in the treatment of axial low back pain.[10, 37–39] A prospective study comparing dual electrodes with two different spacings with single, midline electrodes showed no technical advantages (and some significant disadvantages), although clinical outcome was worthwhile.[40] A recent multicenter trial suggests that intractable low back pain can be treated effectively with a 16-contact insulated array, with two columns of contacts in parallel.[41]

Analysis of hardware and clinical failures over the last 20 years is presented in Figures 196–2 and 196–3. Contemporary "multichannel" systems (technically, single-channel generators gated to multiple outputs) are significantly more reliable than single-channel systems, in technical as well as clinical terms. Surgical revision of electrode position is required significantly less often, and clinical failure is significantly less frequent.[3]

Peripheral Nerve Stimulation Electrodes

Unlike SCS, peripheral nerve stimulation was tested percutaneously in the earliest reported cases.[42] Chronically implanted electrodes generally employed a cuff design, which encircled the involved nerve (Fig. 196–4). However, even with allowance for postoperative edema on the order of 150% of the original nerve diameter, there was still the potential for constrictive injury, so more recent implants use a flat array of electrodes, which can be separated from the nerve by a fascial graft.[43–47] Specialized electrode geometries and

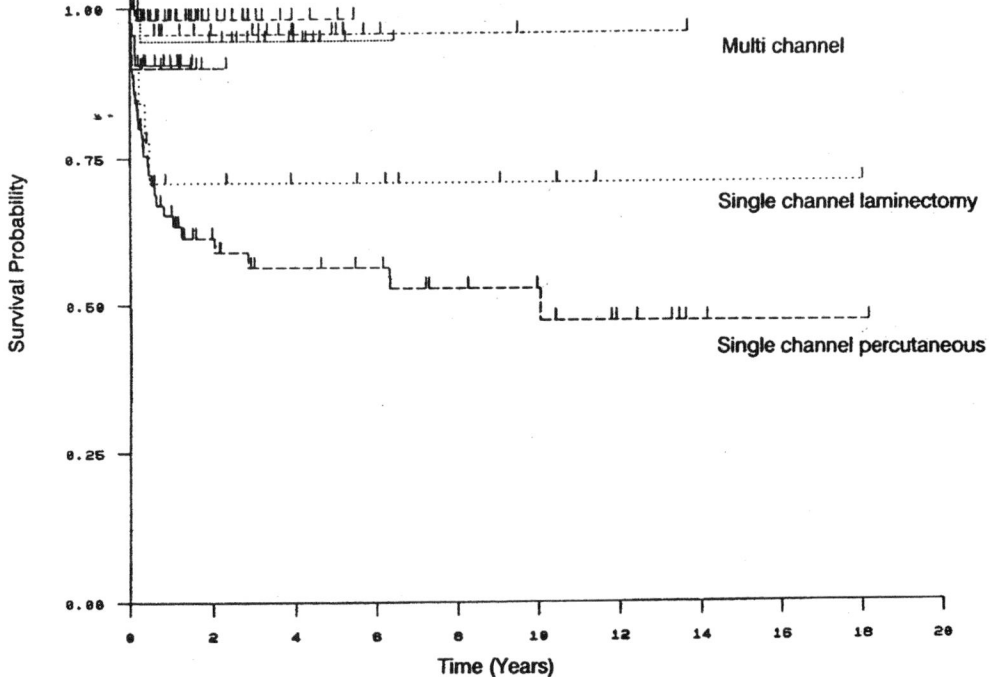

FIGURE 196–2. Survival analysis, using Kaplan-Meier techniques, for different electrode configurations used over the past 2 decades for spinal cord stimulation. A technical failure requiring return to the operating room for surgical revision of electrode position is the statistical end point for this analysis. Electrode migration, unless radiographically obvious, can be difficult to distinguish from malposition such that stimulation paresthesias do not satisfactorily overlap the patient's distribution of pain; for purposes of this analysis, the two are equivalent. The uppermost curves represent contemporary multicontact percutaneous and laminectomy electrodes, which have been significantly more reliable than any bipolar single-channel configuration. The lowest curve, which shows eventual technical failure in a majority of patients, represents dual, independently inserted percutaneous electrodes, which were vulnerable to migration as well as malposition. The middle curve represents bipolar electrodes implanted by laminectomy. Neither of these single-channel systems allowed noninvasive adjustment of anode and cathode positions.

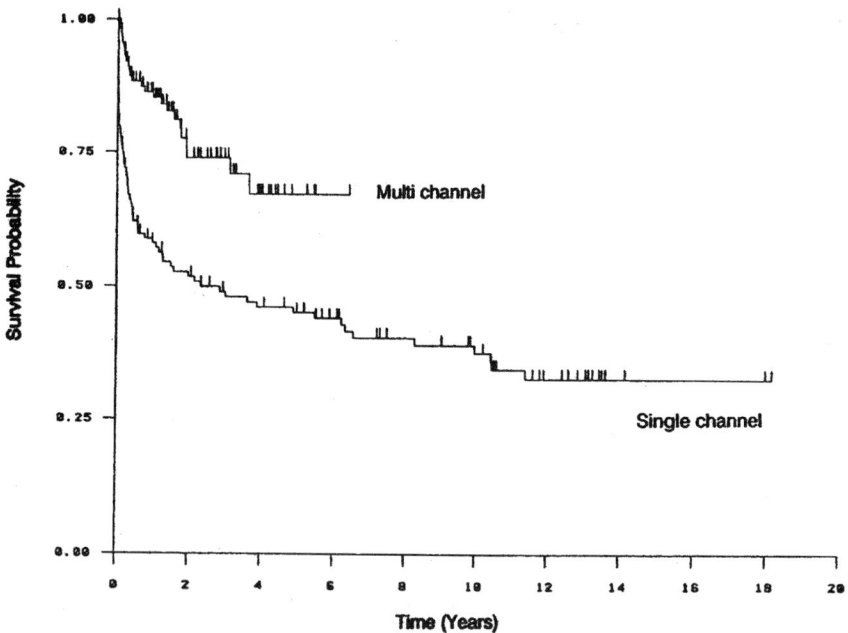

Survival Probability (y-axis)

Time (Years) (x-axis)

Multi channel

Single channel

FIGURE 196–3. The clinical reliability of single-channel and multichannel systems is represented as a Kaplan-Meier survival curve. The end point for this statistical analysis is a clinical failure, defined as the patient no longer using device, for any reason. This includes electromechanical failure of the device, without replacement, and failure of the device to relieve pain (which may occur independently of technical failure). Programmable, multichannel systems were significantly more reliable ($P < 0.001$). (From North RB, Kidd DH, Zahurak M, et al: Spinal cord stimulation for chronic, intractable pain: Two decades' experience. Neurosurgery 32:384–395, 1993.)

stimulus waveforms have been developed for functional peripheral nerve stimulation to achieve effects such as unidirectional propagation of action potentials,[48] but these have not been used in the management of pain. Electrodes placed over a mixed peripheral nerve may recruit motor fibers at an amplitude very close to the amplitude necessary to produce paresthesias and resulting pain relief. Fortunately, the mobility of a peripheral nerve with respect to the electrodes is less than the mobility of the normal spinal cord, so

positional effects are less pronounced with peripheral nerve implants.

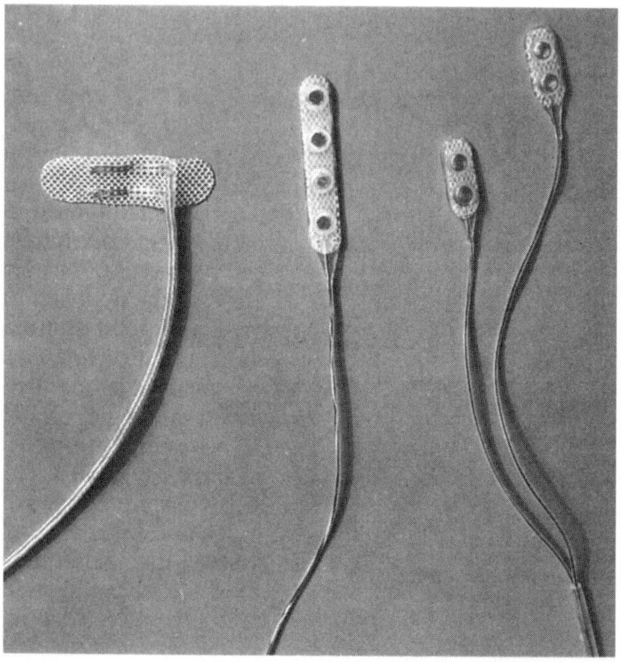

Implanted Pulse Generators

During the first decade of experience with implanted spinal cord and peripheral nerve stimulators, radiofrequency-coupled passive implants were used exclusively. These devices functioned as simple AM radio demodulators, delivering the envelope of radiofrequency bursts as stimulation energy. Their advantage is that they use no implanted batteries or other limited-life components, so pulse generator replacement, with its attendant expense and potential morbidity, is not required routinely. The patient may be inconvenienced, however, by the need to wear an external device, and variable coupling between the external antenna and the implant may lead to fluctuations in the stimulation amplitude.

Since the 1980s, implanted pulse generators have been available. More significant than implantation of the pulse generator—which arguably is implanted even with radiofrequency-coupled systems—is implantation of the battery; thus, they might more appropriately be called internally powered generators. These devices have obvious advantages in terms of convenience, cosmesis, and perhaps patient compliance. They are, however, limited in longevity; this may require compromises in the adjustment of stimulation parameters and in the pattern of usage by the patient to maximize battery life. The patient still requires an external device (e.g., a magnet) to control the unit, so the system is not totally implanted. Magnet control suffices for on-off operation and may control amplitude within limits; a more elaborate external programming device is necessary to adjust other parameters. In individual patients, the power requirements and patient performance during the temporary, percutaneous test phase indicate the

FIGURE 196–4. Peripheral nerve stimulating electrode arrays include cuffs that encircle the nerve, as well as flat arrays, derived from spinal cord stimulating electrodes.

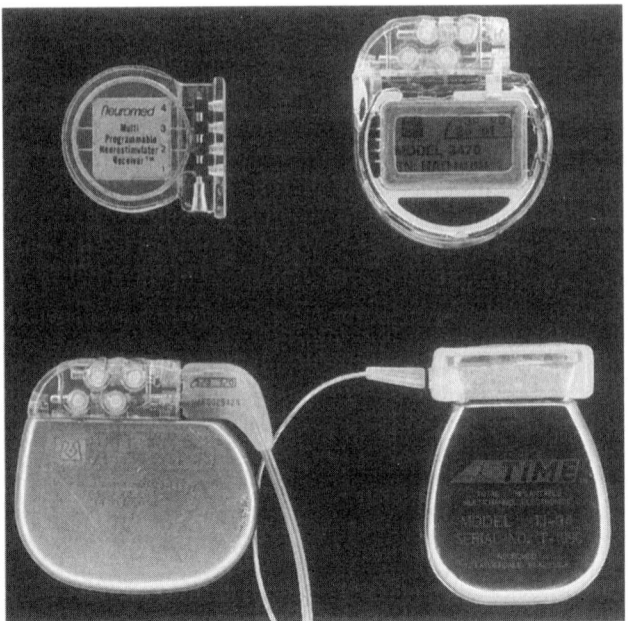

FIGURE 196–5. Implanted pulse generators used for spinal cord and peripheral nerve stimulation allow noninvasive assignment of anode and cathode positions from an array of multiple electrodes. Some require or accept power from an externally worn device, and others are powered by implanted primary cells (visible in this figure); one can use power from either source.

feasibility of an implanted device. Figure 196–5 shows representative implanted pulse generators, including "totally implanted" as well as radiofrequency-coupled externally powered devices.

SCREENING PROTOCOLS

As a "neuroaugmentative" technique, SCS has inherent advantages over other pain-relieving techniques, including anatomic procedures that attempt to address the structural problem causing pain, and ablative procedures that attempt to block pain transmission by destroying portions of the nervous system. Neuroaugmentative techniques not only are reversible but also are amenable to preoperative testing in a manner that reproduces the proposed long-term treatment exactly. (By comparison, preoperative bracing to determine a patient's candidacy for fusion, or a preoperative temporary nerve block to predict the results of an ablative procedure, provides, at best, indirect evidence of potential long-term benefit from the procedure.) A temporary epidural electrode may be placed percutaneously for a therapeutic trial of SCS. This allows longitudinal mapping of the epidural space for potential electrode positions to optimize the technical effect. The patient can then be followed during a therapeutic trial to establish whether permanent implantation is warranted.

In the United States, third-party payers routinely require demonstration of pain relief with a temporarily implanted electrode before permanent implantation. Technically, this requirement may be met by stimulation during implantation, proceeding directly to inter-

nalization.[49] A more prolonged trial with a temporary, percutaneous electrode has a number of advantages, however. First, a temporary electrode that exits percutaneously can be placed in a fluoroscopy room, as opposed to an operating room, minimizing expense and allowing assessment of a greater number of anode and cathode positions and pulse parameters. Second, the clinical effects of stimulation can be assessed by the patient outside the operating room under everyday conditions of activity and posture. Third, experience by the patient and the physician with the temporary system expedites implantation of the permanent device (assuming the temporary electrode is removed rather than internalized for chronic use).

A temporary electrode may emerge through the needle track at the site of insertion, secured by a single skin suture; alternatively, an incision can be made around the needle, and the lead anchored as for a permanent implant and tunneled subcutaneously. A percutaneous extension cable, intended for later removal, allows conversion of this electrode for use with a permanent system. This saves the expense of an additional electrode, but it incurs several disadvantages. First, the patient and physician are committed to two trips to the operating room—the first for electrode placement and anchoring, and the second for either removal or internalization. By comparison, a simple percutaneous lead requires one trip to the operating room, and only for those patients undergoing permanent implants. Second, the necessity of returning to the operating room may influence the patient (if not the physician) to implant a pulse generator, even in dubious circumstances. A temporary electrode destined for removal at the bedside involves no such commitment on the part of the patient and physician and therefore does not partially defeat the purpose of the trial. Third, a temporary electrode that is anchored subcutaneously, so that it can be implanted permanently, does not allow bedside adjustment to assess alternative electrode positions as the patient gains more experience with stimulation. I routinely insert a temporary array percutaneously, to the most cephalad position that gives promising results, in naive patients. Incremental withdrawal of the electrode array at the bedside allows repeated testing at more caudal positions. This time-consuming process is removed from the operating room and the fluoroscopy room; plain radiographs are taken as required to document electrode position. Fourth, the results of the therapeutic trial may be confused by incisional pain associated with placement of a lead anchor and subcutaneous tunneling. Fifth, percutaneous lead extensions increase the risk of infection around the permanent system.[21, 50]

The criteria for proceeding from a temporary to a permanent implant vary considerably, as reported in the clinical literature on SCS. Some authors implant in a single stage, with only intraoperative testing,[49] and others require a percutaneous test phase as long as 2 months.[51] Some require as little as 30% reported relief,[52] and others require as much as 70% to 75% reported relief.[53–55] Long-term "success," if defined simply as a minimal reported percentage of pain relief (commonly

50%), will obviously be increased by requiring a high reported percentage during the test phase. An extended trial can be expected to have the same effect. This may unduly and arbitrarily emphasize only one of a number of potentially important outcome measures. I offer a permanent implant to patients who, after a 2.5- to 3-day trial with a temporary electrode, report at least 50% relief of pain while demonstrating improved or stable analgesic requirements and activity levels. Other outcome measures, such as return to work or productive activity or use of other health care resources, are difficult to assess or predict on the basis of a therapeutic trial, however prolonged. A prolonged trial may incur additional morbidity—not only infection but also epidural scarring, which may compromise implantation of a permanent device.

GENERAL INDICATIONS FOR SPINAL CORD STIMULATION

Interventional or invasive techniques of pain management, particularly for chronic, nonmalignant pain, are appropriate under the conditions outlined here.

A specific diagnosis should be established as an objective basis for the complaint of pain. In the common example of failed back surgery syndrome, there should be abnormalities on diagnostic imaging studies or objective physical findings consistent with the patient's pattern of pain, and objective findings on examination should predominate over nonphysiologic or functional signs.[56] Postsurgical epidural fibrosis is seen commonly in asymptomatic patients, and neurological abnormalities such as diminished deep tendon reflexes also occur after successful surgery; it should therefore be borne in mind that these findings are nonspecific. When the patient's original records and imaging studies are available, the indications for the original operation in a patient with failed back surgery syndrome are often unclear.[57]

SCS should be undertaken as a late or last resort, after acceptable alternative treatments have been exhausted. In failed back surgery syndrome, for example, surgical options should have been exhausted (although one may consider that reoperation offers lower yield and greater potential risks in some cases).[58]

Multidisciplinary evaluation of the patient is important, particularly with regard to psychological issues. Major psychiatric comorbidities, significant drug habituation, and issues of secondary gain should be addressed.[10] Standardized psychological testing reportedly has some value in identifying poor candidates for SCS.[59]

Relief of pain should be demonstrated by temporary electrode placement before a permanent pulse generator is implanted. The technical feasibility of achieving overlap of pain by paresthesias, and resulting relief, may require special electrode geometries; this can be determined during this phase.

SPECIFIC INDICATIONS FOR SPINAL CORD AND PERIPHERAL NERVE STIMULATION

In the United States, the most common indication for SCS has been failed back surgery syndrome. These patients commonly have associated axial low back pain, which poses a technical problem: achieving overlap of the low back by stimulation paresthesias is difficult. Complex electrode arrays and detailed psychophysical testing methods may be helpful.[10, 60] In fact, axial low back pain may be nociceptive or mechanical and thus may not respond as well as neuropathic or deafferentation pain.[61] Axial pain is more difficult to cover than radicular pain,[3, 10, 33, 38, 58] but new technical methods (electrodes, adjustments) are helpful.[10, 37–39, 58, 62] I generally select patients in whom axial low back pain is not the chief complaint. In those so selected and treated, there have been only minor associations between outcome and the reported percentage of low back pain; in one series selected specifically for axial low back pain, the results were similar.[3, 40, 58] Patients with unilateral lower extremity pain are reportedly more easily treated than those with bilateral pain[29, 54, 63, 64]; this has not been my experience, however.[3]

A meta-analysis by Turner and colleagues included 57 articles related to the treatment of failed back surgery syndrome by SCS from 1966 to 1994.[65] Papers were included if they met the following criteria: original data on return to work, pain, medication use, reoperations, functional disability, and stimulator use after permanent implantation of spinal cord stimulators in patients with chronic low back or leg pain despite previous back surgery, and follow-up greater than 30 days for all patients. Of the 39 studies identified, at follow-up (mean, 16 months; range, 1 to 45 months), an average of 59% of patients had more than 50% pain relief (range, 15% to 100% of patients). Complications occurred in 42% of patients, with 30% experiencing one or more stimulator-related complication. All studies were case controlled. Most studies did not separate reported outcomes from reported dimensions of pain and function, and many included little detail concerning the length of follow-up. Additionally, many reported patient outcomes that were averaged across time from implantation. Based on these data, the authors concluded that there was insufficient evidence from the literature to draw conclusions about the efficacy of SCS relative to no treatment or other treatments or about the effects of SCS on patient work status, functional disability, and medication use.

In a randomized, controlled trial comparing SCS with repeated lumbar spine surgery, North and coworkers selected candidates for repeated decompression, with or without fusion.[62] Patients were excluded from randomization if they presented with severe canal stenosis; extremely large disk fragments; a major neurological deficit, such as footdrop; or radiographic evidence of gross instability. Additionally, patients were excluded for untreated dependency on narcotic analgesics or benzodiazepines, major psychiatric comorbidity, the presence of any significant or disabling chronic pain problem, or a chief complaint of low back pain exceeding lower extremity pain. In a preliminary report, 27 patients were included at 6-month follow-up, at which point they became eligible for crossover. Of the 15 who underwent reoperation, 10 (67%) crossed over to SCS. Of the 12 who underwent SCS, 2 (17%) opted for crossover to reoperation ($P = 0.018$). Additionally, of the 19 patients who reached the 6-month follow-up after reoperation, outside of the study, 8 (42%) opted for SCS. Long-term (3-year) follow-up of 90% of patients (unpublished as of this writing) has shown that SCS continues to be more effective than reoperation, with significantly better outcomes by standard measures and significantly lower rates of crossover to the alternative procedure. Additionally, patients randomized to reoperation used significantly more opiate analgesics than did those randomized to SCS ($P < 0.025$). Other measures of activities of daily living and work status did not differ significantly.

In 1996, Burchiel and colleagues published the results of a multicenter prospective study of SCS.[66] After psychological screening, 219 patients were entered in the study. Following a percutaneous trial, 182 patients were implanted with permanent systems. Patient evaluation of pain and functional levels was performed before implantation and at 3, 6, and 12 months after implantation. Complications, medication usage, and work status also were monitored. One-year follow-up was available on 70 patients. All pain and quality-of-life measures showed statistically significant improvement during the treatment year. Complications requiring surgical intervention were experienced by 17% (12 of 70). Medication usage and work status were not changed significantly.

A recent multicenter trial suggests that intractable low back pain can be treated effectively with a dual-lead 16-contact laminotomy system.[41] Sixty patients were included in the intent-to-treat group. All patients in the group had undergone previous unsuccessful spinal surgery, although this was not a prerequisite for enrollment. Reversible compressive pathology or instability was ruled out. Patients with confounding medical conditions, arachnoiditis, or severe psychological dysfunction were excluded. Patients were screened with an extended percutaneous trial for at least 3 days. A greater than 50% reduction in pain was required for permanent implantation. Standard outcome measures, including the visual analog scale, the Oswesty Disability Questionnaire, and the sickness impact profile, were used. At 1 year, 44 patients were available for follow-up. All patients reported a decrease in the visual analog scale. At 6 months, 91.6% of patients reported fair to excellent relief in the legs, and 80.7% of patients reported fair to excellent relief in the low back. At 1 year, these numbers dropped to 88.2% and 68.8%, respectively. Improvement in functional quality of life was found at 6-month and 1-year follow-ups using the Oswesty Disability Questionnaire and sickness impact profile. The majority of patients reported that the procedure was worthwhile (would you have it again?)—92% at 6 months, and 88% at 1 year. The

laminotomy electrodes offer certain theoretical advantages: more focused ventral stimulation, and a fixed relationship between multiarray systems. The authors speculated that these features were important in the treatment of low back pain with SCS.

In Europe, ischemic pain associated with peripheral vascular disease in the lower extremities has been the most common application of SCS in recent years.[67, 68] This application is unique among painful conditions treated with SCS, in that there are measurable changes in response to treatment, as opposed to subjective reports of pain relief alone. Improvement in red blood cell flow velocity, capillary density, and perfusion pressure has been reported; rates of limb salvage, by comparison with best medical therapy, approach statistical significance in the small series reported.[68–70]

Since the first reports by Murphy and Giles 15 years ago,[71, 72] SCS has become an attractive treatment for intractable angina pectoris. This is a logical extension of the use of SCS for pain relief in peripheral vascular disease. In randomized, controlled clinical trials, it has been shown to be superior to nonoperative therapy, as reflected in symptom relief as well as anti-ischemic effects.[73, 74] Experimental models support the clinical findings that it exerts not only analgesic but also anti-ischemic effects.[73, 75] Potential unwanted effects of SCS on biologically useful, nociceptive pain are minimal.[14] SCS does not mask the pain of myocardial infarction.[76, 77] By comparison with coronary artery bypass grafting, it offers equivalent pain relief, with lower mortality and cerebrovascular morbidity at lower risk, albeit with less apparent anti-ischemic effects.[78]

Segmental pain confined to the level of a spinal cord injury is amenable to treatment with SCS. In our institutional experience over 20 years, more than 90% of these patients had successful percutaneous trials and proceeded to implantation of a permanent device.[3] The same patients may be candidates for dorsal root entry zone lesions, an ablative procedure. The latter is an irreversible procedure, which may preclude subsequent SCS and may sacrifice useful residual sensation; for these reasons, SCS should be considered first. Patients with postcordotomy dysesthesias and those with pain due to other spinal cord lesions (such as multiple sclerosis) commonly respond to SCS; the yield is lower, but this may be addressed by percutaneous trial.

Peripheral nerve injury or neuralgia, causalgia, and so-called reflex sympathetic dystrophy commonly respond to SCS or to peripheral nerve stimulation.[79, 80] In our experience over 20 years, patients with these pain syndromes proceeded from temporary, trial electrodes to permanent implants significantly less often than did those with other conditions.[3] Most of these patients did proceed to permanent implantation, however, so this observation, though statistically significant, is of limited clinical significance.

One of the few randomized prospective studies of SCS involves reflex sympathetic dystrophy (complex regional pain syndrome), as reported by Kemler and coworkers.[81] Thirty-six patients were assigned to receive a standardized physical therapy program plus

SCS, and 18 were assigned to receive therapy alone. In all cases, the sympathetic dysfunction involved the upper extremities, and all patients underwent a percutaneous trial lasting at least 7 days. Outcomes were assessed using standard visual analog scale, global perceived effect, functional status, and health-related quality-of-life instruments. In 24 of the 36 patients randomized to SCS plus physical therapy, the trial was successful, and permanent implantation was performed. At 6-month follow-up, patients in the SCS group had a significantly greater reduction in the visual analog scale, and a significantly higher percentage was graded much improved for global perceived effect. There were no clinically significant improvements in functional status. Based on these data, the authors concluded that, in the short term, SCS can reduce pain and improve the quality of life for patients with autonomic dysfunction involving the upper extremities.

Patients with the same conditions are also candidates for peripheral nerve stimulation when the pain is in the distribution of or is attributable to injury of a single nerve. A number of investigators have reported satisfactory results with chronic peripheral nerve stimulation in 45% to 79% of patients at up to 10 years' follow-up.[42-46, 82] The best results are achieved in patients who are temporarily relieved by blocks proximal to the injury and whose electrodes are likewise implanted proximally.[83] The treatment of radiating pain with electrodes implanted distal to the site of nerve injury (e.g., sciatica in failed back surgery syndrome) has not been successful.[43, 84]

Postamputation pain syndromes, including phantom limb and stump pain, respond in most cases to SCS.[85] Stump neuroma pain often coexists with, and may be difficult to distinguish from, other postamputation pain syndromes. When postamputation pain occurs in the distribution of a single peripheral nerve, peripheral nerve stimulation may be applicable.

Other applications of SCS for pain include the management of angina pectoris[86] and the management of intractable pain associated with lower extremity spas-ticity.[87] Beyond the scope of this chapter are other applications such as evoked potential monitoring, cerebral blood flow, autonomic hyperreflexia, and management of motor disorders.

OUTCOME STUDY INTERPRETATION

The clinical results of SCS, as reported in a number of series over the last 30 years, were summarized earlier. Reported rates of "success" range from 12%[30] to 88%,[88] at various follow-up times ranging from 6 months to 8 years. The most common criterion for "success" is a minimum of 50% reported pain relief, as rated by the patient.

The source of follow-up data in published reports should be considered; when obtained by a disinterested third-party interview, it may yield very different results from hospital charts and physician office records.[2, 3, 30] Third-party interviews are reported increasingly in the literature on SCS.[2, 3, 26, 50, 63, 89-93]

Apart from ratings of pain and its relief, other outcome measures are considered criteria for success in the management of pain. These include patient satisfaction with treatment (would you do it again for same result?), which would seem a sine qua non for "success"; activities of daily living; work status; medication requirements; and changes in neurological function. Figure 196–6 presents these outcome measures for a series of patients accumulated over 2 decades.[3]

Results are often reported in terms of the number of devices permanently implanted, as opposed to the number of patients undergoing trial electrode placement. When the rate of implantation of a permanent device is as low as 40%,[94] adjustment for this factor is important; when the implantation rate exceeds 75%, it is less so.[3] Other neurosurgical procedures for the relief of pain are reported routinely for the population undergoing the definitive procedure, as opposed to those undergoing screening tests such as temporary nerve blocks or myelography. The morbidity of these diagnostic tests may be comparable to that of temporary

Spinal Cord Stimulation: Two Decades' Experience

Permanent implants only: n=171

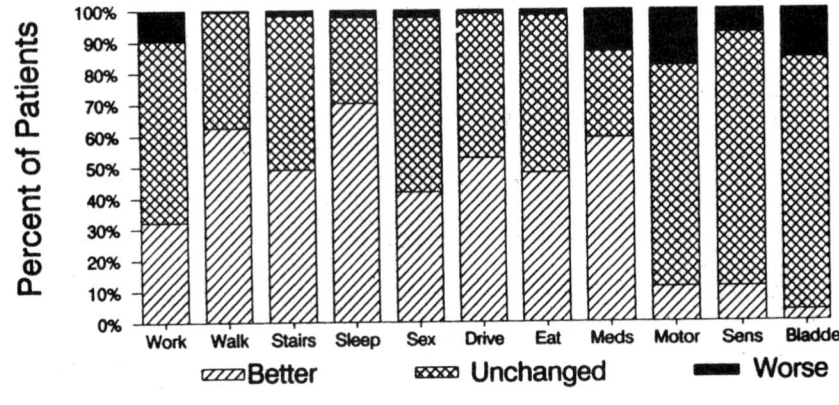

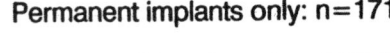

FIGURE 196–6. In our experience over 2 decades, improvement in many activities of daily living has been reported by a majority of patients. Most report a decrease in daily medication usage. Neurological symptoms progress infrequently and independently of treatment. (From North RB, Kidd DH, Zahurak M, et al: Spinal cord stimulation for chronic, intractable pain: Two decades' experience. Neurosurgery 32:384–395, 1993.)

percutaneous electrode placement. Like other neuroaugmentative procedures, such as lumbar subarachnoid drug infusion, SCS has the advantage (or disadvantage, if accounting methods include all patients) of being a simple screening test with low morbidity that emulates the permanent procedure exactly.

Is SCS cost-effective? A collaborating center of the World Health Organization reported, "SCS appears to be cost-effective versus alternative therapies costing $20,000 per year or more, with 78% or less efficacy."[95] An economic model developed by our group in cooperation with Charles River Associates, a Boston-based economic consulting firm, reached similar conclusions after considering (1) the initial screening and implantation costs; (2) the cost of periodic battery replacements in "totally implanted" systems; (3) the frequency of complications and hardware failure, and the costs of dealing with the consequences; and (4) the cost of periodic physician visits to adjust stimulation parameters, the regular annual cost of medications, and so forth.[52]

CONTRAINDICATIONS AND COMPLICATIONS

Tables 196–1 and 196–2 present contraindications to SCS and potential complications and adverse effects, respectively.

COMPUTERIZED METHODS OF STIMULATOR ADJUSTMENT

Arrays of multiple electrodes, supported by programmable implanted pulse generators, have significantly improved the technical as well as clinical results of SCS. However, the number of possible cathode and anode assignments for an array grows rapidly as the number of contacts increases. Each useful combination of electrodes requires study in a detailed, quantitative fashion over a range of amplitudes, from first perception to discomfort; the amplitude at which paresthesias overlap the distribution of pain may be measured

TABLE 196–1 ■ Contraindications to Spinal Cord Stimulation

Medical
  Coagulopathy
  Sepsis

Psychological or Behavioral
  Untreated, major comorbidity (e.g., depression)
  Serious drug-related behavioral issues
  Inability to cooperate, control device
  Secondary gain

Technical
  Demand cardiac pacemaker (requires electrocardiogram monitoring or changing pacemaker mode to fixed rate)
  Magnetic resonance imaging needs

TABLE 196–2 ■ Potential Complications and Adverse Effects of Spinal Cord Stimulation

General Spinal Surgical and Interventional
  Spinal cord or nerve injury
  Cerebrospinal fluid leak
  Infection
  Bleeding

Specific to Spinal Cord Stimulation
  Hardware failure (e.g., generator failure, electrode fatigue fracture)
  Electrode migration or malposition

Extraneous Influences
  Electromagnetic fields (e.g., diathermy, security systems)

along this scale. This facilitates comparison between different configurations of electrodes and different pulse parameters.

Quantitative study of these effects for contemporary multicontact devices generates a large volume of data, necessitating computerized methods.[33, 60, 96, 97] Computer data entry may be performed by a health care professional working with the patient.[33, 60] Alternatively, the patient can interact directly with a computer to perform these adjustments.[96-98] We have developed a sys-

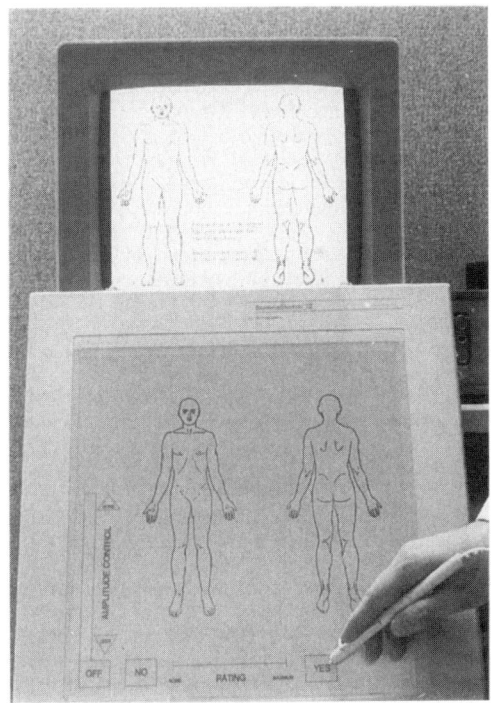

FIGURE 196–7. A graphics tablet and a personal computer are used by patients to control standard radiofrequency-coupled spinal cord stimulation implants. This system's controls were developed for easier operation than the standard unit. "Pain drawings," corresponding drawings of the location of stimulation paresthesias, and associated 100-mm visual analog ratings are entered directly by the patient. Quantitative measures of stimulator performance are derived, to select settings for everyday clinical use.[96-98]

tem for this purpose, whereby the patient uses a graphic input device to control stimulus amplitude, enter analog ratings, and enter "pain drawings." This is illustrated in Figure 196–7. Computerized methods of stimulator control facilitate optimization of SCS settings for individual patients, as well as systematic study across patients to establish general principles.

CONCLUSION

Since the 1980s, the development of programmable, implanted stimulation devices, which allow noninvasive selection of anodes and cathodes from electrodes with multiple contacts, has significantly enhanced both technical and clinical results of the treatment of pain. With the development of percutaneous placement of electrode arrays, SCS has evolved into a relatively easily implemented, reversible neuroaugmentative technique with low morbidity. Implantation of contemporary devices achieves successful long-term treatment of chronic, intractable pain in a majority of patients.

REFERENCES

1. Melzack R, Wall PD: Pain mechanisms: A new theory. Science 150:971–978, 1965.
2. North RB, Ewend MG, Lawton MT, Piantadosi S: Spinal cord stimulation for chronic, intractable pain: Superiority of "multichannel" devices. Pain 44:119–130, 1991.
3. North RB, Kidd DH, Zahurak M, et al: Spinal cord stimulation for chronic, intractable pain: Two decades' experience. Neurosurgery 32:384–395, 1993.
4. Nathan PW: The gate-control theory of pain: A critical review. Brain 99:123–158, 1976.
5. Campbell JN, Raja SN, Meyer RA, Mackinnon SE: Myelinated afferents signal the hyperalgesia associated with nerve injury. Pain 32:89–94, 1988.
6. Duggan AW, Foong FW: Bicuculline and spinal inhibition produced by dorsal column stimulation in the cat. Pain 22:249–259, 1985.
7. Handwerker HO, Iggo A, Zimmerman M: Segmental and supraspinal actions on dorsal horn neurons responding to noxious and non-noxious skin stimuli. Pain 1:147–165, 1975.
8. Lindblom U, Tapper R, Wiesenfeld Z: The effect of dorsal column stimulation on the nociceptive response of dorsal horn cells and its relevance for pain suppression. Pain 4:133–144, 1977.
9. Linderoth B, Gunasekera L, Meyerson BA: Effects of sympathectomy on skin and muscle microcirculation during dorsal column stimulation: Animal studies. Neurosurgery 29:874–879, 1991.
10. Law JD, Kirkpatrick AF: Pain management update: Spinal cord stimulation. Am J Pain Management 2:34–42, 1991.
11. Meyerson BA, Herregodts P, Linderoth B: Enhanced flexor reflex in the mononeuropathic rat is attenuated by spinal cord stimulation. Acta Neurochir (Wien) 117:88, 1992.
12. Linderoth B, Meyerson BA: Spinal cord stimulation. I. Mechanisms of action. In Burchiel K (ed): Surgical Management of Pain. New York, Thieme, 2002, pp 505–526.
13. Lindblom U, Meyerson BA: Influence on touch, vibration and cutaneous pain of dorsal column stimulation in man. Pain 1:257–270, 1975.
14. Marchand S, Bushnell MC, Molina-Negro P, et al: The effects of dorsal column stimulation on measures of clinical and experimental pain in man. Pain 45:249–257, 1991.
15. North RB, Fischell TA, Long DM: Chronic stimulation via percutaneously inserted epidural electrodes. Neurosurgery 1:215–218, 1977.
16. Coburn B, Sin W: A theoretical study of epidural electrical stimulation of the spinal cord. Part I. Finite element analysis of stimulus fields. IEEE Trans Biomed Eng 32:971–977, 1985.
17. Holsheimer J, Struijk JJ: How do geometric factors influence epidural spinal cord stimulation? A quantitative analysis by computer modeling. Stereotact Funct Neurosurg 56:234–249, 1991.
18. Sances A, Swiontek TJ, Larson SJ, et al: Innovations in neurologic implant systems. Med Instrum 9:213–216, 1975.
19. Dyck PJ, Lais A, Karnes J, et al: Peripheral axotomy induces neurofilament decrease, atrophy, demyelination and degeneration of root and fasciculus gracilis fibers. Brain Res 340:19–36, 1985.
20. Ohnishi A, O'Brien PC, Okazaki H, Dyck PJ: Morphometry of myelinated fibers of fasciculus gracilis of man. J Neurol Sci 27:163–172, 1976.
21. Law J: Spinal stimulation: Statistical superiority of monophasic stimulation of narrowly separated, longitudinal bipoles having rostral cathodes. Appl Neurophysiol 46:129–137, 1983.
22. Holsheimer J: Effectiveness of spinal cord stimulation in the management of chronic pain: Analysis of technical drawbacks and solutions. Neurosurgery 40:990–999, 1997.
23. Holsheimer J, Nuttin B, King GW, et al: Clinical evaluation of paresthesia steering with a new system for spinal cord stimulation. Neurosurgery 42:541–547, 1998.
24. Linderoth B: Dorsal Column Stimulation and Pain: Experimental Studies of Putative Neurochemical and Neurophysiological Mechanisms. Stockholm, Kongl Carolinska Medico Chirurgiska Institutet, 1992.
25. Freeman TB, Campbell JN, Long DM: Naloxone does not affect pain relief induced by electrical stimulation in man. Pain 17:189–195, 1983.
26. Burton C: Dorsal column stimulation: Optimization of application. Surg Neurol 4:171–176, 1975.
27. Nashold BS Jr, Friedman H: Dorsal column stimulation for control of pain: Preliminary report on 30 patients. J Neurosurg 36:590–597, 1972.
28. Shealy CN, Mortimer JT, Reswick JB: Electrical inhibition of pain by stimulation of the dorsal columns: Preliminary clinical report. Anesth Analg 46:489–491, 1967.
29. Sweet W, Wepsic J: Stimulation of the posterior columns of the spinal cord for pain control. Clin Neurosurg 21:278–310, 1974.
30. Erickson DL: Percutaneous trial of stimulation for patient selection for implantable stimulating devices. J Neurosurg 43:440–444, 1975.
31. Hoppenstein R: Percutaneous implantation of chronic spinal cord electrodes for control of intractable pain: Preliminary report. Surg Neurol 4:195–198, 1975.
32. Hosobuchi Y, Adams JE, Weinstein PR: Preliminary percutaneous dorsal column stimulation prior to permanent implantation. J Neurosurg 37:242–245, 1972.
33. Barolat G, Massaro F, He J, et al: Mapping of sensory responses to epidural stimulation of the intraspinal neural structures in man. J Neurosurg 78:233–239, 1993.
34. Zumpano BJ, Saunders RL: Percutaneous epidural dorsal column stimulation. J Neurosurg 45:459–460, 1976.
35. North RB: Quantitative studies of spinal cord stimulation electrode designs. In International Neuromodulation Society Abstracts. Lucerne, Switzerland, 1998, p 212.
36. North RB, Olin JC, Kidd DH, Sieracki JN: Spinal cord stimulation electrode design: A prospective, randomized controlled trial comparing percutaneous and laminectomy electrodes. Part I. Technical Outcomes. Neurosurgery 51:381–390, 2002.
37. Alo KM, Yland MJ, Kramer DL, et al: Computer assisted and patient interactive programming of dual electrode spinal cord stimulation in the treatment of chronic pain. Neuromodulation 1:30–45, 1998.
38. Law JD: Spinal stimulation in the "failed back surgery syndrome": Comparison of technical criteria for palliating pain in the leg vs. in the low back. Acta Neurochir (Wien) 117:95, 1992.
39. Rossi U: Technical advances in neuromodulation: State of the art hardware technology in neurostimulation. In Abstracts of the 3rd International Congress, International Neuromodulation Society, 1996, p 11.
40. North RB: Spinal cord stimulation for axial low back pain: Single versus dual percutaneous electrodes. In International Neuromodulation Society Abstracts. Lucerne, Switzerland, 1998, p 212.
41. Barolat G, Oakley JC, Law JD, et al: Epidural spinal cord stimulation with multiple electrode paddle leads is effective in treating intractable low back pain. Neuromodulation 4:59–66, 2001.

42. Wall PD, Sweet WH: Temporary abolition of pain in man. Science 155:108–109, 1967.

43. Campbell JN, Long DM: Peripheral nerve stimulation in the treatment of intractable pain. J Neurosurg 45:692–699, 1976.

44. Law JD, Swett J, Kirsch WM: Retrospective analysis of 22 patients with chronic pain treated by peripheral nerve stimulation. J Neurosurg 45:692–699, 1980.

45. Long DM, Erickson D, Campbell J, North R: Electrical stimulation of the spinal cord and peripheral nerves for pain control. Appl Neurophysiol 44:207–217, 1981.

46. Picaza JA, Cannon BW, Hunter SE, et al: Pain suppression by peripheral nerve stimulation. Surg Neurol 4:105–114, 1975.

47. Racz GB, Lewis R, Heavner JE, Scott J: Peripheral nerve stimulator implant for treatment of causalgia. In Stanton-Hicks M (ed): Pain and the Sympathetic Nervous System. Dordrecht, The Netherlands, Kluwer Academic, 1990, pp 225–239.

48. Van den Honert C, Mortimer J: Generation of unidirectionally propagated action potentials in a peripheral nerve by brief stimuli. Science 206:1311–1312, 1979.

49. Feler C, Kaufman S: Spinal cord stimulation: One stage? Acta Neurochir (Wien) 117:91, 1992.

50. Koeze TH, Williams AC, Reiman S: Spinal cord stimulation and the relief of chronic pain. J Neurol Neurosurg Psychiatry 50:1424–1429, 1987.

51. Meglio M, Cioni B, Rossi GF: Spinal cord stimulation in management of chronic pain: A 9-year experience. J Neurosurg 70:519–524, 1989.

52. Bel S, Bauer BL: Dorsal column stimulation (DCS): Cost to benefit analysis. Acta Neurochir Suppl (Wien) 52:121–123, 1991.

53. Leibrock L, Meilman P, Cuka D, Green C: Spinal cord stimulation in the treatment of chronic low back and lower extremity pain syndromes. Nebr Med J 69:180–183, 1984.

54. Meilman PW, Leibrock LG, Leong FTL: Outcome of implanted spinal cord stimulation in the treatment of chronic pain: Arachnoiditis versus single nerve root injury and mononeuropathy. Clin J Pain 5:189–193, 1989.

55. De la Porte C, Van de Kelft E: Spinal cord stimulation in failed back surgery syndrome. Pain 52:55–61, 1993.

56. Waddell G, McCulloch JA, Kummel EG, Venner RM: Non-organic physical signs in low back pain. Spine 5:117–125, 1980.

57. Long DM, Filtzer DL, BenDebba M, Hendler NH: Clinical features of the failed-back syndrome. J Neurosurg 69:61–71, 1988.

58. North RB, Ewend MG, Lawton MT, et al: Failed back surgery syndrome: Five-year follow-up after spinal cord stimulator implantation. A prospective, randomized study design. Neurosurgery 28:692–699, 1991.

59. Daniel M, Long C, Hutcherson M, Hunter S: Psychological factors and outcome of electrode implantation for chronic pain. Neurosurgery 17:773–777, 1985.

60. Law JD: Targeting a spinal stimulator to treat the "failed back surgery syndrome." Appl Neurophysiol 50:437–438, 1987.

61. Sanchez-Ledesma MJ, Garcia-March G, Diaz-Cascajo P, et al: Spinal cord stimulation in deafferentation pain. Stereotact Funct Neurosurg 53:40–55, 1989.

62. North RB, Kidd DH, Lee MS, Piantadosi S: Spinal cord stimulation versus reoperation for the failed back surgery syndrome: A prospective, randomized study design. Stereotact Funct Neurosurg 62:267–272, 1994.

63. Kumar K, Nath R, Wyant GM: Treatment of chronic pain by epidural spinal cord stimulation: A 10-year experience. J Neurosurg 75:402–407, 1991.

64. Ray CD, Burton CV, Lifson A: Neurostimulation as used in a large clinical practice. Appl Neurophysiol 45:160–206, 1982.

65. Turner JA, Loeser JD, Bell KG: Spinal cord stimulation for chronic low back pain: A systematic literature synthesis. Neurosurgery 37:1088–1096, 1995.

66. Burchiel KJ, Anderson VC, Brown FD, et al: Prospective, multicenter study of spinal cord stimulation for relief of chronic back and extremity pain. Spine 21:2786–2794, 1996.

67. Broseta J, Barbera J, DeVera J, et al: Spinal cord stimulation in peripheral arterial disease. J Neurosurg 64:71–80, 1986.

68. Jacobs MJ, Jorning PJ, Beckers RC, et al: Foot salvage and improvement of microvascular blood flow as a result of epidural spinal cord electrical stimulation. J Vasc Surg 12:354–360, 1990.

69. Augustinsson LE, Carlsson CA, Holm J, Jivegard L: Epidural electrical stimulation in severe limb ischemia: Evidence of pain relief, increased blood flow and a possible limb-saving effect. Ann Surg 202:104–111, 1985.

70. Jacobs MJ, Jorning PJ, Joshi SR, et al: Epidural spinal cord electrical stimulation improves microvascular blood flow in severe limb ischemia. Ann Surg 207:179–183, 1988.

71. Murphy DF, Giles KE: Intractable angina pectoris: Management with dorsal column stimulation (case report). Med J Aust 146:260, 1987.

72. Murphy DF, Giles KE: Dorsal column stimulation for pain relief from intractable angina pectoris. Pain 28:365–368, 1987.

73. de Jongste MJL, Hautvast RV, Hillege HL, Lie KI: Efficacy of spinal cord stimulation as adjuvant therapy for intractable angina pectoris: A prospective, randomized clinical study. J Am Coll Cardiol 23:1592–1597, 1994.

74. Hautvast RW, de Jongste MJL, Staal MJ, et al: Spinal cord stimulation in chronic intractable angina pectoris: A randomized, controlled efficacy study. Am Heart J 136:1114–1120, 1998.

75. Foreman RD: Neurophysiological mechanisms of pain relief by spinal cord stimulation in angina pectoris. In Horsch S, Claeys L (eds): Spinal Cord Stimulation: An Innovative Method in the Treatment of PVD and Angina. Darmstadt, Germany, Steinkopff Verlag, 1995, pp 155–164.

76. Andersen C, Hole P, Oxhj H: Does pain relief with spinal cord stimulation for angina pectoris conceal myocardial infarction? Br Heart J 71:419–421, 1994.

77. Eliasson T, Augustinsson LE, Mannheimer C: Spinal cord stimulation in severe angina pectoris—presentation of current studies, indications and clinical experience. Pain 65:169–179, 1996.

78. Mannheimer C, Eliasson T, Augustinsson L, et al: Electrical stimulation versus coronary artery bypass surgery in severe angina pectoris: The ESBY study. Circulation 97:1157–1163, 1998.

79. Barolat G, Schwartzman RJ, Woo R: Epidural spinal cord stimulation in the management of reflex sympathetic dystrophy. Stereotact Funct Neurosurg 53:29–39, 1989.

80. Kumar K, Toth C, Nath RK, Laing P: Epidural spinal cord stimulation for treatment of chronic pain—some predictors of success: A 15-year experience. Surg Neurol 50:110–121, 1998.

81. Kemler MA, Barendse GAM, van Kleef M, et al: Spinal cord stimulation in patients with chronic reflex sympathetic dystrophy. N Engl J Med 343:618–624, 2000.

82. Picaza JA, Hunter SE, Cannon BW: Pain suppression by peripheral nerve stimulation. Appl Neurophysiol 40:223–234, 1978.

83. Nashold BS: Dorsal column stimulation for control of pain: A three year follow up. Surg Neurol 4:146–147, 1975.

84. Meyer GA, Fields HL: Causalgia treated by selective large fiber stimulation of peripheral nerve. Brain 95:163–168, 1972.

85. Krainick JU, Thoden U, Riechert T: Pain reduction in amputees by long-term spinal cord stimulation: Long-term follow-up study over 5 years. J Neurosurg 52:346–350, 1980.

86. Augustinsson LE: Spinal cord electrical stimulation in severe angina pectoris: Surgical technique, intraoperative physiology, complications and side effects. Pace 12:693–694, 1989.

87. Barolat G, Myklebust JB, Wenninger W: Effects of spinal cord stimulation on spasticity and spasms secondary to myelopathy. Appl Neurophysiol 51:29–44, 1988.

88. Klin M-T, Winkelmller W: Chronic pain after multiple lumbar discectomies—significance of intermittent spinal cord stimulation. Pain 5:S241, 1990.

89. Erickson DL, Long DM: Ten-year follow-up of dorsal column stimulation. In Bonica JJ (ed): Advances in Pain Research and Therapy. New York, Raven Press, 1983, pp 583–589.

90. Long DM, Erickson DE: Stimulation of the posterior columns of the spinal cord for relief of intractable pain. Surg Neurol 4:134–141, 1975.

91. Nielson KD, Adams JE, Hosobuchi Y: Experience with dorsal column stimulation for relief of chronic intractable pain. Surg Neurol 4:148–152, 1975.

92. Shatin D, Mullett K, Hults G: Totally implantable spinal cord stimulation for chronic pain: Design and efficacy. Pace 9:577–583, 1986.

93. Spiegelmann R, Friedman WA: Spinal cord stimulation: A contemporary series. Neurosurgery 28:65–71, 1991.

94. De la Porte C, Siegfried J: Lumbosacral spinal fibrosis (spinal arachnoiditis): Its diagnosis and treatment by spinal cord stimulation. Spine 8:593–603, 1983.
95. ECRI: Spinal cord (dorsal column) stimulation for chronic intractable pain. Health Technology Assessment Information Service. Plymouth Meeting, Pa, ECRI, 1993.
96. North RB, Fowler KR, Nigrin DA, Szymanski RE: Patient-interactive, computer-controlled neurological stimulation system: Clinical efficacy in spinal cord stimulation. J Neurosurg 76:689–695, 1992.
97. North RB, Fowler KR, Nigrin DA, et al: Automated "pain drawing" analysis by computer-controlled, patient-interactive neurological stimulation system. Pain 50:51–58, 1992.
98. North RB, Sieracki JM, Fowler KR, et al: Patient-interactive, microprocessor-controlled neurological stimulation system. Neuromodulation 1:185–193, 1998.

CHAPTER 197

Deep Brain Stimulation for Chronic Pain

MICHAEL G. KAPLITT ■ ALI R. REZAI ■ ANDRES M. LOZANO ■ RONALD TASKER

Chronic electrical stimulation of subcortical brain targets is becoming increasingly popular in stereotactic and functional neurosurgery. In contrast to traditional lesioning procedures, deep brain stimulation (DBS) is adjustable and reversible. This maximizes clinical efficacy while minimizing the complications traditionally associated with lesioning, such as deafferentiation syndromes and poor long-term results. The most common application of DBS is in movement disorder surgery. Thalamic DBS has long been a successful treatment for essential tremor, and the improved safety and striking benefits of DBS have expanded the possibilities of intervention in novel targets, including the subthalamic nucleus and the globus pallidus.[1-7] The technical and scientific advances that led to a renaissance in movement disorder surgery now permit reexamination of the use of DBS in the treatment of pain.

HISTORY

Based on the observation of positive reinforcement and "pleasure centers" identified by brain stimulation in rodents,[8] neurosurgeons ventured into the field of electrical stimulation of the brain for the relief of pain. Early efforts using temporarily implanted electrodes were eventually replaced by chronic brain stimulation through permanently implanted electrodes coupled to battery-powered pulse generators.

DBS for chronic pain began almost 50 years ago. Health[9] and Pool[10] first reported implantation of temporary electrodes in the septum pellucidum in a region anterior and inferior to the foramen of Monro. They used DBS to treat patients with schizophrenia and pain from metastatic carcinoma. Subsequently, Pool[11] in 1956 and Heath and Mickle[12] in 1960 reported pain relief with septal stimulation in chronic pain patients without psychiatric disorders. Stimulation of the caudate nucleus was performed by Ervin and colleagues[13] to produce analgesia in a patient with intractable facial pain from carcinoma of the pharynx and skull base. Pain relief occurred for up to 8 hours after discontinua-

tion of stimulation. Gol[14] combined these approaches, stimulating the caudate nucleus and the septal region in six patients with intractable pain. No clear benefit from this approach was observed, because clinically significant pain relief was obtained in only one patient.

In 1965, Melzack and Wall[15] developed the gate theory of pain. It was based on observations that stimulation of large, myelinated fibers of peripheral nerves that result in paresthesias block the activity in small, nociceptive projections. Wall and Sweet confirmed this observation in humans, which led to development of central nervous system (CNS) stimulation to treat pain. CNS stimulation began in the spinal cord at the dorsal columns, followed by stimulation of more rostral brain structures to activate the lemniscal pathways, including thalamic sensory relay nuclei (i.e., entralis caudalis [VC] or ventralis posterior [VP]), and the sensory portion of the internal capsule (IC).[16] The goal of this approach was to induce paresthesias in the area of pain, thereby producing chronic pain relief.

Even before development of this theory, surgeons began to explore the concept of thalamic stimulation to relieve chronic pain. In 1960, Mazars and coworkers[17] treated chronic intractable deafferentation pain using paresthesia-producing stimulation of the ventroposterolateral (VPL) nucleus. Hosobuchi and associates[18] also described chronic ventroposteromedial (VPM) stimulation as an effective treatment for patients with refractory facial pain. Both groups[18, 19] subsequently reported long-term success with chronic VP stimulators implanted in patients with deafferentation pain. Similarly, the IC was explored as a target for paresthesia-producing stimulation. Adams and colleagues[16, 20] observed pain relief with chronic stimulation near the IC or within the posterior limb. Cooper and coworkers[21] also reported pain relief in a spinal cord injury patient with lower extremity pain after IC stimulation.

During the same period, a different approach to brain stimulation for pain relief was being explored. Reynolds[22] demonstrated that stimulation of the lateral margin of the periaqueductal gray (PAG) in rats induced analgesia, enabling abdominal operation to be

TABLE 197–1 ■ **International Association for the Study of Pain: Recommended Definitions of Common Pain Syndromes**

TERM	DEFINITION
Central pain	Pain from a primary dysfunction of the central nervous system
Anesthesia dolorosa	Pain in a region which is anesthetic
Neurogenic pain	Pain from a primary dysfunction or disruption of fibers in the peripheral or central nervous system
Hyperalgesia	Increased response to an ordinarily painful stimulus
Allodynia	Pain from a stimulus that is not usually painful
Hyperpathia	Abnormally painful reaction and increased threshold to a stimulus, particularly a repetitive stimulus

performed on awake animals without the use of anesthetics. In 1977, Richardson and Akil[23, 24] adapted this method for use in humans. Pain relief was achieved using frequencies of 10 to 75 Hz and pulse widths of 200 to 250 milliseconds. Hosobuchi and colleagues[25] reported similar findings after periventricular gray (PVG) stimulation. These effects were reversible with the opiate antagonist naloxone, suggesting that the mechanism of pain relief was opioid mediated. Boivie and Meyerson[26] and Young and Rinaldi[27] also showed that stimulation involved the dorsal medial nucleus and the parafascicular nucleus.

GENERAL CONSIDERATIONS

Pain Characteristics

Several terms used to describe pain have resulted in conflicts or confusion within the literature. As a result, a task force of the International Association for the Study of Pain suggested specific definitions for a variety of terms.[28] They are described in Table 197–1. The term *thalamic pain* has often been used to describe a variety of syndromes now called *central pain. Thalamic pain* should more appropriately be reserved for patients with a central pain syndrome and a demonstrated thalamic lesion.

Various types of chronic pain can be divided into two groups based on the mechanism of pain generation (Table 197–2). Nociceptive or somatic pain is caused by direct activation of the nociceptors (i.e., mechanical, chemical, and thermal) found in various tissues. The afferent somatosensory pathways are intact in nociceptive pain. Examples include cancer pain from bone or tissue invasion and noncancer pain from degenerative bone and joint disease or osteoarthritis.

Neuropathic pain occurs in the absence of activation of peripheral nociceptors. It is has also been called nonnociceptive or deafferentation pain. This type of pain results from an injury or dysfunction of the CNS or peripheral nervous system. This damage can occur anywhere along the neuraxis. Examples include thalamic pain, stroke, traumatic or iatrogenic brain or spinal cord injuries, phantom limb or stump pain, postherpetic neuralgia, and various peripheral neuropathies.

Patient Selection

The initial choice for treating the chronic pain patient is a conservative approach involving medications (e.g., narcotic and non-narcotic analgesics, antidepressants, anticonvulsants), physical therapy, biofeedback, transcutaneous electrical nerve stimulation, and less conventional or alternative therapies. After conservative approaches have been exhausted, more invasive procedures can be considered. This may involve blocks, neurolysis, or other ablative procedures. Neuroaugmentative techniques such as spinal cord stimulation or intrathecal pumps may also be beneficial. With failure of these measures and persistent, incapacitating pain, the patient becomes a candidate for DBS.

Before DBS, patients must satisfy general selection criteria (Table 197–3). Treatment by a multidisciplinary pain management team, including medical pain specialists and neuropsychologists, can often be helpful for identifying optimal surgical candidates and maximizing the chance of postoperative success. A mini-

TABLE 197–2 ■ **Characteristics of Chronic Pain**

CHARACTERISTIC	NOCICEPTIVE PAIN	NEUROPATHIC PAIN
Mechanism	Activation of nociceptors Intact somatosensory afferents	Activation of non-nociceptors Lesion, injury or dysfunction of central and peripheral nervous systems
Symptoms	Aching, dull, throbbing pain	Steady, burning or dysesthetic pain Sharp, shooting (neuralgic) pain Stimulation induced (evoked) pain
Examples	Failed back, cancer	Allodynia, hyperpathia, central pain postherpetic neuralgia, stroke pain, anesthesia dolorosa, brachial plexus injury, spinal cord injury
Best medical therapy	Narcotics, NSAIDs	Antidepressants
Best surgical therapy	Medical (PVG or PAG)	Paresthesia-producing (VC, ML, IC)

IC, internal capsule; NSAIDs, nonsteroidal anti-inflammatory drugs; ML, medial lemniseus; PAG, periaqueductal gray; PVG, periventricular gray; VC, ventralis candalis.

TABLE 197-3 ■ Chronic Pain Patient Selection Criteria for Deep Brain Stimulation Therapy

Severe, incapacitating pain as primary complaint (6 or more on analog scale)

All other therapy (e.g., medical, external stimulation, psychotherapy) exhausted or ruled out

No major psychological component

Realistic patient expectations (e.g., no cure, expect 50% chance of pain reduction, possible recurrence)

Patient proximity to center familiar with deep brain stimulation programming

Patient can tolerate long, awake procedure

No medical contraindications; cardiac pacemaker is a relative contraindication

---

mum of 6 months should have passed after pain onset before considering DBS. We generally reserve DBS for patients who have pain that they regard as severe and incapacitating and that scores 6 or higher (of a maximum of 10) in intensity on a visual analog pain scale. The patients must have persistent, severe, incapacitating pain despite exhausting all previous, less invasive treatment modalities. The pain should be the predominant problem causing disability and suffering for which the patient seeks relief. Patients with long-standing pain complaints without a clearly defined cause are not candidates.

Psychiatric evaluation by an experienced team can help exclude patients with significant psychological or psychosocial overlay and the possibility of secondary gain. In general, patients with psychosis or strong psychopathology should be encouraged to undergo further psychological treatment. However, most patients with refractory, chronic pain have mild psychological disturbances such as depression and anxiety, and this should not exclude patients as candidates for DBS. Specific psychological tests, such as the Minnesota Multiphasic Personality Inventory (MMPI),[29] can be helpful in the selection process, although this is certainly not necessary in all cases. Among potential complicating psychological factors, high hypochondriasis and hysteria indexes have been associated with a poorer outcomes after surgery.[30]

Choice of Target

Various chronic neuropathic and nociceptive conditions have been treated with DBS (Tables 197-4 and

Table 197-5; see Table 197-2). The choice of stimulation site is determined by the pathophysiology of the patient's pain. In general, patients with refractory neuropathic pain should undergo paresthesia-producing stimulation, and those with nociceptive pain should undergo PVG or PAG stimulation. Because most pain syndromes have mixed components of nociceptive and neuropathic pain, both paresthesia-evoking and PVG or PAG stimulation trials may be indicated. In the context of neuropathic pain, the steady component responds best to paresthesia-producing stimulation, and the evoked (i.e., allodynia and hyperpathia) and neuralgic elements of neuropathic pain may also be helped by PVG or PAG stimulation. Overall, DBS is an option for carefully selected patients with chronic, refractory, incapacitating nociceptive and neuropathic pain. Evaluation of the patients by a multidisciplinary pain center and strict adherence to the selection criteria can optimize responses. This is important because a significant percentage of failures can be attributed to improper patient selection.

MECHANISMS OF PAIN MODULATION

Paresthesia-Producing Stimulation

The exact mechanism by which paresthesia-evoking thalamic stimulation results in pain relief is unknown, but it is most likely a nonopioid mechanism. One concept is that deafferentation causes an abnormal firing pattern in thalamic neurons and that thalamic stimulation inhibits this abnormal neural activity. Gerhardt and coworkers[31] showed that stimulation of the VPL, the primary somatosensory relay nucleus, in monkeys caused inhibition of spinothalamic neurons' evoked responses to noxious cutaneous stimulation. Thalamic stimulation caused a greater reduction of the response to C-fiber volleys than A-fiber volleys.

In studies of chronic pain patients, an abnormal pattern of neuronal firing was shown in the sensory thalamus in those with central deafferentation pain.[32] This led to the suggestion that an abnormal bursting of thalamic neurons might mediate the pain sensation of deafferentiation syndromes. Lenz and associates[33] showed that areas in the somatosensory thalamus that had lost their normal innervation had abnormal spontaneous bursting activity, with electrical stimulation inducing burning dysesthesias. Similarly, Rinaldi and

---

TABLE 197-4 ■ Published Results of Periaqueductal Gray and Periventricular Gray Stimulation–Induced Pain Relief by Diagnosis*

Study	Richardson and Akil[51]	Meyerson et al[59]	Levy et al[60]	Hosobuchi[52]	Plotkin[62]	Kumar et al[61]
No. of patients	14	13	57	65†	38	43
Failed back*	60%		32%	80%	80%	74%
Cancer	75%	23%	33%	71%	100%	
Osteoarthritis				0%	0%	
Overall	64%	23%	32%	77%	89%	74%

* Data represent the percentage of all patients treated for each diagnosis who had long-term benefit (usually more than 6 months) of generally greater than 50% improvement on analog pain scale.

† Nineteen patients had periaqueductal gray and thalamic electrodes.

TABLE 197–5 ■ **Published Results of Paresthesia-Producing Pain Relief from Deep Brain Stimulation by Diagnosis**

Study	Turnbull et al[57]	Levy et al[60]	Hosobuchi[52]	Siegfried[65]	Plotkin[62]	Kumar et al[61]
No. of patients	18	84	95†	119	12	16
Thalamic syndromes*		24%	47%		0%	20%
Brachial plexus avulsion	100%		33%	53%	0%	
Stroke	100%			63%		
Postherpetic neuralgia			40%	72%		0%
Postcordotomy dysesthesia		50%	89%	100%		
Spinal cord injuries		0%	25%	60%	0%	0%
Peripheral neuropathies	88%	50%	90%	71%		100%
Anesthesia dolorosa		18%	33%	67%	60%	
Phantom limb pain		20%	50%	77%	50%	100%
Overall‡	72%	32%	58%	68%	33%	38%

* Data represent the percentage of all patients treated for each diagnosis who had long-term benefit (usually more than 6 months) of generally greater than 50% improvement on analog pain scale.
† Nineteen patients had periaqueductal gray and thalamic electrodes.
‡ Percentages reflect all patients who underwent surgery. May include some patients who were not tested or not internalized and are therefore not reflected within any of the diagnostic categories for long-term follow-up.

colleagues[34, 35] demonstrated an increased number of bursting neurons in the medial and lateral thalamic nuclei in deafferented rats compared with controls and an increase in the number of nociceptive responsive neurons in the medial thalamus. However, bursting cells have been identified within the sensory thalamus of nonpain patients.[36] Because the incidence of these cells in nonpain patients is comparable to that in pain patients, the predictive value of identifying bursting cells in pain patients is unclear.

Functional imaging has been applied to examine pain patients undergoing DBS.[37] Functional magnetic resonance imaging (fMRI) analysis of three pain patients with VC stimulators (one of whom also had a PVG stimulator) demonstrated activation of the primary sensory cortex when VC stimulation was performed at a level above threshold for producing paresthesias. At subthreshold intensities, primary sensory cortex activation was not observed. In contrast, PVG stimulation in the one patient did not induce paresthesias but did induce a warm sensation, which was coincident with activation of the medial thalamus and cingulate gyrus but not the primary sensory cortex. Study with positron emission tomography (PET) of five pain patients during VC or medial lemniscus (ML) DBS revealed activation of the contralateral anterior portion of the anterior cingulate cortex (ACC) throughout a 40-minute period of DBS, whereas the ipsilateral posterior ACC was activated after a period of delay after the onset of stimulation.[38] The anterior ACC has been associated with cognitive or awareness aspects of pain, and the posterior ACC has been related to direct pain responses or processing. This suggests that both functions are influenced by paresthesia-inducing stimulation, although not necessarily in the same temporal pattern.

Periventricular or Periaqueductal Stimulation

The mechanism of pain modulation with PVG or PAG stimulation is most likely through an opioid-dependent pathway. Elevations of endogenous opioids such as β-endorphin and met-enkephalin have been demonstrated in cerebrospinal fluid samples from the third ventricle after PVG or PAG stimulation but not with VC stimulation.[39, 40] Several intralaminar thalamic nuclei, including the CM with the parafascicular nucleus and centralis lateralis nucleus, may also contribute to pain modulation.[41, 42]

The neural substrates of the endogenous analgesia pathway include the PVG, PAG, nucleus raphe magnus (NRM), the locus ceruleus, and the magnocellular part of the nucleus reticularis gigantocellularis.[43] These pathways involve descending projections from the midbrain to the dorsal horn and to various thalamic intralaminar and medial nuclei. Further evidence for ascending and descending endogenous opioid pathways has been provided by Peschanski and Besson,[44] who demonstrated projections form the NRM to the intralaminar nuclei and the nucleus submedius. Stimulation of the dorsal NRM has been shown to inhibit the responses to noxious stimuli of parafascicular neurons.[45]

The ACC has been associated with nociceptive and neuropathic pain. The anterior ACC may be more closely associated with nociceptive pain. Although PET has demonstrated ACC activation after stimulation of areas associated with neuropathic pain, fMRI failed to duplicate this but instead demonstrated ACC activation after PVG stimulation.[37, 38] Microelectrode recording has also identified cells within the ACC that represent the first human cortical neurons identified that are directly responsive to pain.[46] These cells were nociceptive specific, with some neurons responsive to restrictive receptive fields and some with more complex responses that may be related to higher integrative or cognitive functions.

TECHNIQUE

Patients are usually admitted on the day of the procedure, and no special preoperative preparation or testing is generally necessary. Unlike movement disorder cases, pain patients may continue all preoperative pain medication on the day of surgery. Sedation should be avoided, however, to permit maximal cooperation of the patient during surgery. We have found that sedation or general anesthesia can alter the firing of thalamic neurons, thereby compromising the integrity of microelectrode recordings.

Head Frame Application and Stereotactic Imaging

The head frame is usually placed under local anesthesia immediately before obtaining a localizing scan on the morning of surgery. We use the Leksell G head frame (Elekta Instruments, Atlanta, GA), which has a long history of use in stereotactic procedures and which some studies have shown to be more accurate than other systems, although any commercially available system is usually adequate.

Accurate placement of the frame is necessary to maximize the likelihood of success for any stereotactic procedure. Most practitioners prefer that the frame be angled parallel to the intercommissural line. This often places the anterior commissure (AC) and posterior commissure (PC) within a single axial section, although they may often be separated by one or two sections without compromising the outcome. Another factor that can influence accuracy is the coronal tilt or axial rotation of the frame with respect to the brain, also referred to, respectively, as the roll or yaw. Often, this problem can be minimized with careful visual inspection, but many surgeons prefer to use ear bars during frame placement to prevent roll and yaw. Because the patient is usually awake for several hours and may be asked to interact with the surgeon, frame placement should consider the patient's comfort and ability to speak and breathe easily.

After frame fixation with local anesthesia, the localizer is secured to a base that secures the head position during computed tomography (CT) or MRI. Rotation of the patient's head within the scanner (MRI or CT) can represent a possible source of error, which can be minimized by confirming proper alignment with the laser positioners available on all modern scanners. At the Toronto Hospital, we use a Signa 1.5-tesla magnet (General Electric, Milwaukee, WI) for initial acquisition, and the anterior-posterior boundaries of AC and PC are demarcated on a midline sagittal slice. A volumetric scan is then performed along the AC-PC line, and an axial slice is generally used to identify the positions of AC and PC. If direct visual targeting is used, coronal or sagittal sections may also be obtained, but AC and PC information is sufficient for indirect coordinate or map-based targeting methods.

Target Localization

Targets may be chosen from among the thalamic sensory nuclei (i.e., VC, ML, IC, PVG, or PAG), based on criteria described elsewhere in this chapter. As with other stereotactic neurosurgical procedures, imaging can be used to identify targets by direct or indirect methods. Direct targeting uses visual identification of a structure on an image to obtain target coordinates. Indirect targeting is based on the identification of the AC, PC, and resulting intercommissural line, as well as calculation of the middle commissural point. This information can then be input into a computer, and a standardized brain atlas (e.g., the Schaltenbrand and Wahren atlas) is adjusted to the intercommissural distance of the patient. Sagittal sections can be printed, and targets can be identified on this map along with the coordinates specific for the patient. The laterality of the sagittal maps vary based on the location of pain, particularly for VC and ML targets, with facial pain 12 to 14 mm from the midline, upper extremity pain 14 to 15 mm, and 15 to 17 mm lateral for lower extremity pain. Alternatively, standard distances from the midcommissural point or PC have been reported for each structure, and these can be used without a map for targeting. All of these techniques can be performed manually, with trajectories and individual tracks mapped on a millimeter grid after the angles of the stereotactic arc are obtained. Several commercial systems permit automatic target localization by all three methods, along with computerized trajectory or track generation and recording of all data on a single workstation.

Surgical Procedure

After frame placement and imaging are complete, the patient is taken to the operating room. Given the length of the procedure, care should be taken to place the operating table in a comfortable "dental chair" position, and the head position should not be excessively flexed or extended in a way that could compromise breathing or communication over time. After prophylactic antibiotics are given and sterile scalp preparation is performed, the linear incision site is infiltrated with local anesthetic. The incision is positioned two-thirds anterior and one-third posterior to the coronal suture; we place the incision approximately 1.5 to 2 cm lateral to the midline, at roughly the same distance from the midline as the target so that a relatively straight trajectory is taken. A 14-mm bur hole is then placed immediately anterior to the coronal suture. Care should be taken to create an even and complete bur hole, because modern DBS electrodes are secured in a plastic ring and cap that are machined to seat snuggly within the 14-mm bur hole. After coagulation and penetration of the dura and cortical surface, the hole in the meninges is filled with fibrin glue to prevent cerebrospinal fluid leakage and brain shift during the extended procedure. The stereotactic arc is then applied, and coordinates in x, y, and z directions are set for the image-defined target. Before initiation of physiologic localization, a guide tube with a blunt-tipped stylet is passed to within 10 to 15 mm above the image-defined target. Through this guide tube, microelectrodes or stimulating macroelectrodes are passed for physiologic target localization.

Physiologic Target Localization

In our experience, physiologic localization is mandatory for definitive target determination in DBS for pain. No study has directly examined the value of any given method of target localization in optimizing outcome. Each imaging modality is subject to variable degrees of error, and deep brain targets are often difficult to identify even with the most optimal modern imaging technique. It is also unclear the degree to which even the most perfect imaging correlates with the physiology of a given pain syndrome. Because we often find the initial target to be suboptimal for maximizing pain relief, use of some form of physiologic confirmation appears warranted in most cases. Physiologic corroboration can be achieved with microelectrode recording and microstimulation or macrostimulation, or both. Macroelectrode stimulation is rapid and requires minimal equipment, but the inability to record single neurons limits spatial resolution, and discrimination between axons and neurons is not possible.

Microelectrodes provide exquisite physiologic identification of receptive fields and neuronal firing patterns by direct measures of individual single unit neuronal activity. This is particularly useful for thalamic targets, which can have specific firing patterns. Microelectrode recording can also differentiate somatodendritic from axonal activity, which can assist mapping by determining boundaries between gray and white matter structures, and it can confirm localization within white matter for targets such as the IC. An initial target is chosen based on imaging with the stereotactic frame in place and usually from a point on an atlas adjusted to the intercommissural distance of the patient. After the anteroposterior angle for the frame is chosen, we use this information to draw a line to the target on an appropriate parasagittal atlas section. We use this graphic representation of the microelectrode tract to record the activity of single units at each point along the tract and to note appropriate receptive and projected fields for specific cells. This allows rapid analysis of the total data generated along an individual tract to determine whether another tract is necessary or whether DBS insertion may proceed, and it also provides an excellent archival data record. The characteristic physiologic mapping findings of microelectrode recording and microstimulation or macrostimulation for specific target are discussed in the following sections.

Paresthesia-Evoking Targets

The paresthesia-producing targets are the thalamic sensory relay nucleus (VC), the ML, and the IC. The target in the VC is typically 12 to 14 mm from the midline for the stimulation of the face, 14 to 15 mm for the upper limb, and 15 to 17 mm for the lower limb (Figs. 197–1 and 197–2). The ML can be targeted inferior to the intercommissural line 12 to 14 mm from the midline. Electrodes are generally placed contralateral to the area of pain. For focal neuropathic pain, the somatotopic representation of the patient's pain area in the VC is targeted. For more diffuse or hemibody pain,

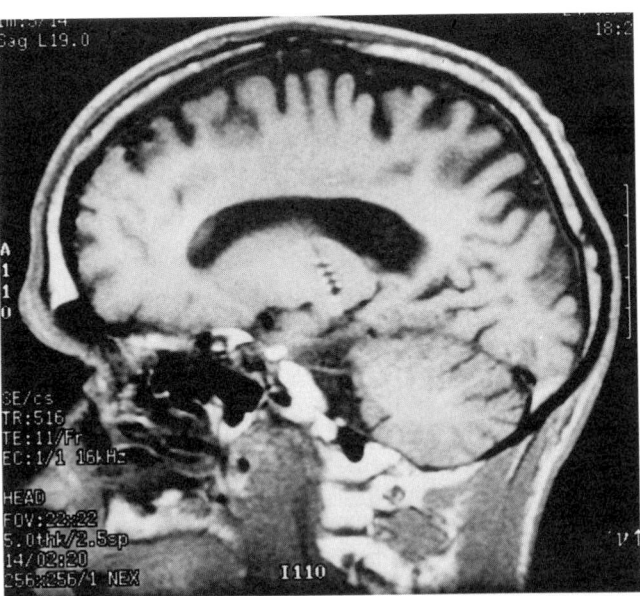

FIGURE 197–1. Sagittal view of a lateral thalamic electrode for deep brain stimulation. This is a T1-weighted image 14 mm lateral to midline, with the tip of the electrode posterior to the cerebellar and pallidal thalamic nuclei and adjacent to the rostral medial lemniscus.

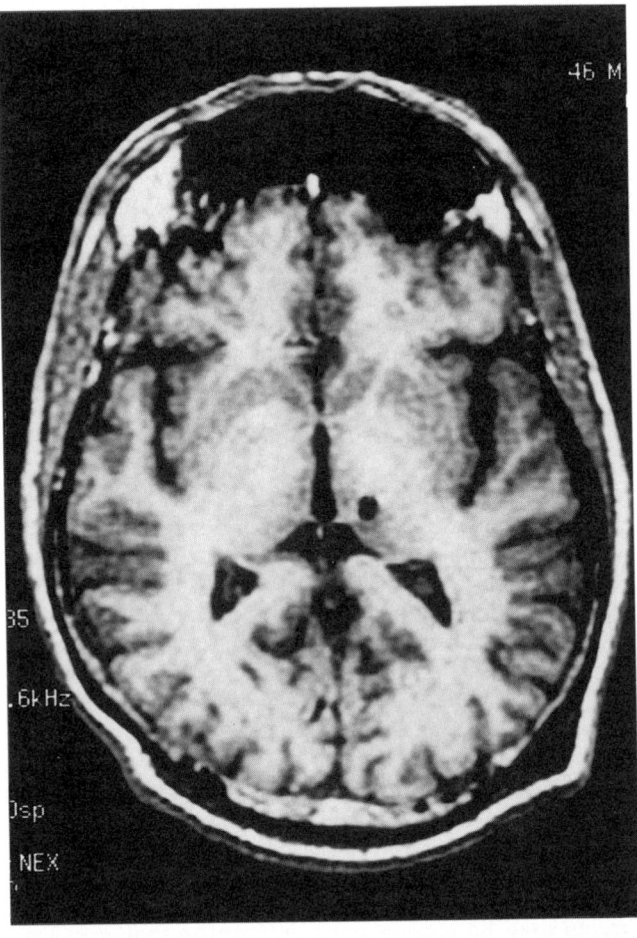

FIGURE 197–2. Axial view of a lateral thalamic electrode for deep brain stimulation. Notice the location of the posterior commisure just slightly posterior to the electrode tip but at the same ventral level.

the ML or IC is chosen to obtain more widespread paresthesia coverage. With pain resulting from destructive thalamic lesions, microelectrode mapping of the thalamus have a poor yield,[47] and the thalamic afferent or efferent projections (e.g., IC, ML) can be targeted for stimulation.[18]

Microelectrode recording in the VC reveals a somatotopic representation of body parts expressed with discrete tactile receptive fields. With microstimulation, patients experience somatotopically organized paresthesias, defining a projected field for these thalamic neurons. As an alternative to microstimulation, macrostimulation can be performed every 1 to 2 mm from about 10 mm above to 10 mm below the expected target.

Physiologic mapping in patients with stroke or major deafferentation may vary from the normal observations as a result of neuronal loss, structural anatomic changes, or plasticity. Causes include absence of neurons and their corresponding receptive or projected fields, mismatch between the fields, somatotopic reorganization, widened or shrunken receptive fields, neuronal bursting activity, and projected fields that evoke burning or pain rather than paresthesias. This can be particularly true of stroke pain, spinal cord lesion or injury pain, and phantom limb pain after amputation, with the receptive field for the residual stump within the thalamus massively expanding to include the area that represented the amputated limb.[48] In these situations, microstimulation can reproduce the phantom sensation or pain. When physiologic mapping does not provide a clear receptive field definition, particularly for stroke or thalamic lesions, stimulation can be performed at a distal site such as the motor cortex.[49, 50] PVG or PAG stimulation can be an alternative, particularly in patients with the evoked features of neuropathic pain.

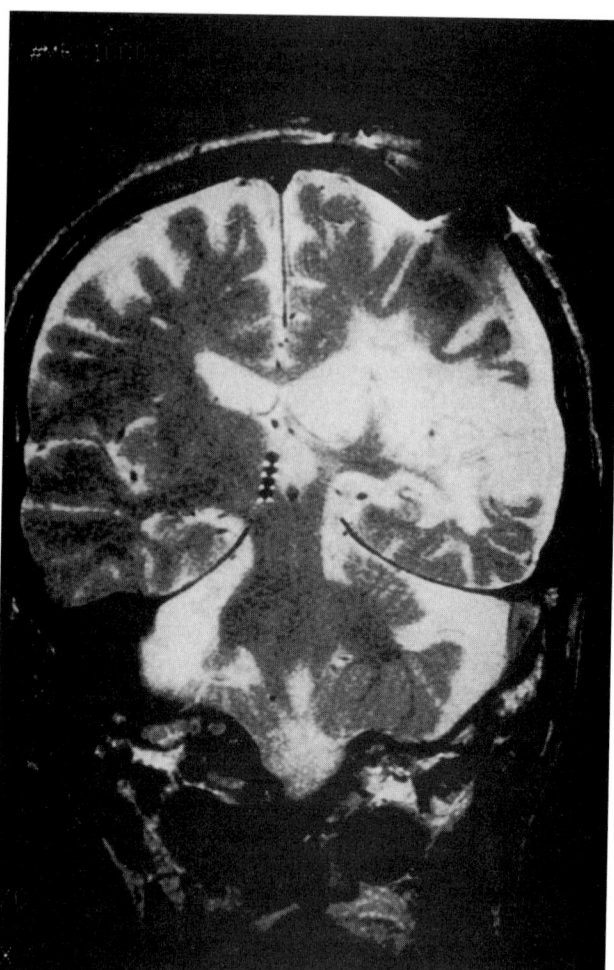

FIGURE 197–3. Coronal view of a medial thalamic electrode for deep brain stimulation. This is a T2-weighted image of a periventricular gray electrode placed just lateral to the medial wall of the third ventricle.

Periaqueductal Gray and Periventricular Gray Targets

The anatomic target for the PVG is typically 2 to 5 mm anterior to the PC, 2 mm lateral to the medial wall of the third ventricle, and at the level of the PC[23, 24, 51] (Fig. 197–3). The microelectrode recordings from the PVG region in humans are not well characterized. PVG stimulation can result in pleasant sensations or warmth and well-being with stimulation frequencies of 25 to 50 Hz. At higher intensities, PVG stimulation may evoke feelings of diffuse burning or anxiety. The typical stereotactic coordinates for the PAG are 2 to 3 mm lateral to the midline, just lateral to the aqueduct (1 to 2 mm), at the level or 1 to 2 mm behind the PC, and 2 to 3 mm below the AC-PC line.[52, 53] With ventral PAG stimulation, sensations similar to those of PVG stimulation are experienced, but dorsal PAG stimulation typically evokes unpleasant sensations of fear, doom, anxiety, and agitation. Current spread from increased stimulation settings can cause vertical gaze or other gaze abnormalities. In general, we prefer the placement of the electrode in the PVG because of the increased adverse effects associated with PAG stimulation.

PVG or PAG stimulation typically causes elevations in the heart rate and blood pressure.[54] Because these cardiovascular changes are not always seen and are seen with higher stimulation thresholds, they should not be routinely relied on.

Electrode Implantation for Deep Brain Stimulation

After physiologic mapping is complete, the final target of the permanent DBS electrode is determined. The information from the map is used to identify an optimal target that maximizes paresthesias or nonpainful sensations while minimizing side effects. This is confirmed with test stimulation after insertion and securing of the DBS electrode. Because true pain relief often is difficult to elicit within the operating room, physiologic mapping permits localization of the DBS electrode within an region of maximal receptive and projected fields for the body area with pain.

The DBS electrode in use is a quadripolar electrode (Medtronic, Minneapolis, MN). Each 1.5-mm-long contact is made of cylindrical platinum or iridium, with a distance between contacts of 1.5 or 0.5 mm, depending on the model and preference (see Fig. 197–1). The diameter of the electrode is 1.27 mm, and the entire electrode length is 28 or 40 cm, depending on the model. A specially provided plastic ring designed to fit in a 14-mm bur hole is secured into the bur hole, and the DBS electrode is fixed in place by pushing the extracranial portion into a slot within the ring, which prevents lead migration. The bur hole is then covered, and the electrode is further secured by insertion of a plastic cover into the ring. The position and trajectory of the DBS electrode is confirmed by intraoperative stereotactic radiography or fluoroscopy. All electrode manipulations are then performed under flouroscopy, including securing the electrode to the bur hole ring, to prevent migration from the final target before permanent fixation. Intraoperative test stimulation begins before permanent fixation of the electrode and uses a hand-held pulse generator (Screener). Various pole combinations and stimulation frequencies, pulse widths, and intensities are used to determine the thresholds for therapeutic and adverse effects. After securing the electrode to the bur hole ring, the proximal portion of the DBS lead is attached to a transcutaneous pacing wire for a trial period.

Stimulation Trial Period

In movement disorder surgery, test stimulation is often performed postoperatively for study purposes, but it may not always be therapeutically necessary. However, a trial period of 3 to 7 days is absolutely necessary to determine the value of DBS to the individual pain patient. During this time, various stimulation parameters are used while a detailed pain diary is compiled using visual analogy and verbal pain scores. Typical stimulation parameters include unipolar or bipolar stimulation, frequencies of 25 to 75 Hz, pulse widths of 60 to 500 microseconds, and variable voltage intensities. A successful trial consists of more than 33% reduction in the patient's pain with stimulation. If successful, the patient undergoes implantation of a pulse generator or radiofrequency-coupled receiver. If unsuccessful, DBS at that location is unlikely to benefit the patient, and the DBS electrode and the transcutaneous wires are removed. Occasionally, a persistent insertional or lesioning effect from placing the DBS electrode is observed, with significant, sustained, postoperative pain relief without stimulation. In these situations, we often leave the DBS electrode in place, cut the transcutaneous wires at the skin, and close the wound at the bedside. After several weeks, the preoperative pain usually returns, and we use a second period of test stimulation or connect the DBS electrode to a permanently implanted pulse generator.

Pulse Generator or Radiofrequency Receiver Implantation

Implantation is usually carried out under general anesthesia, because it involves a painful tunneling procedure from the frontal incision to the infraclavicular region. The patient is positioned in a fashion similar to that for a ventriperitoneal shunt. An implantable pulse generator (IPG) device (Itrel III) or radiofrequency receiver (Xtrel, Medtronic) is placed in the subcutaneous tissue in the infraclavicular space. The IPG device is powered by a lithium battery and is fully programmable by telemetry, but only clinicians can adjust IPG settings; the patient control is limited to turning the device on or off with a supplied magnet. The radiofrequency device, however, can be activated by an external transmitter using an antenna placed on the skin overlying the receiver. This permits greater patient control over stimulation parameters, which can be adjusted as necessary to a given level of pain. Such control requires adequate levels of patient cognition and motivation, and patients with severe physical limitations such as quadriplegia may be poor candidates for radiofrequency receivers. Batteries can last 3 to 5 years or longer, depending on the intensity of stimulation and method of use.

OUTCOMES

Results for Various Applications

DBS has been used in clinical practice for pain patients for decades before the technique was applied to movement disorders or other functional disorders. This has resulted in the publication of several case series, some spanning 10 to 15 years, that examined the outcome of DBS for pain relief.[51, 52, 55–65] Even the best case series have not systematically examined a single method of treatment with a particular piece of equipment using standardized outcome measures. This is partially the nature of pain therapy, but it also reflects the long periods necessary to acquire data on a large series, which necessarily results in technical variabilities due to improved equipment. Changing practice patterns, such as the development of intrathecal opiate pumps, have also resulted in varying enthusiasm for particular DBS targets or applications. Many series have grouped patients differently, with some grouped by diagnosis and others grouped by surgical target. Although surgical targets and techniques have been modified only modestly over the past 25 years, the lack of a large recent series creates some difficulties in assessing the relevance of any outcome analysis to modern practice. Nonetheless, a sufficient number of large or defined case series have been published to provide some guidance regarding patient selection and potential outcomes based on target site and diagnosis.

The best results from DBS in published reports have been for patients with nociceptive pain (see Table 197–4). Within this group, cancer pain and pain from failed back syndrome appear to respond best to DBS. Failed back syndrome usually has been diagnosed in patients who have had multiple lumbosacral operations for herniated disks, spinal stenosis, or sponydlolisthesis. Patients have often undergone two or three operations, with variable success, but they develop severe, refractory back and leg pain over time that cannot be resolved with further local surgery. Medial DBS (PAG or PVG) has been the target of choice for most of these cases. In some instances of failed back syndrome, paresthesia-producing stimulation has been performed along with PAG or PVG stimulation because many cases of failed back syndrome have nociceptive and neuropathic (evoked) components, particularly if there is severe back pain and shooting leg pain. Cancer pain has been reported to respond to PAG or PVG DBS with more than 50% long-term pain reduction in 25% to 100% of patients, whereas 30% to 80% of failed back syndrome patients appear to respond. The variability in both situations may in part reflect patient selection and reporting methods. One study of cancer pain with poorer response rates involved patients with only trunk pain, and it is possible that appendicular or pelvic pain may respond better to medial DBS. There is also a trend toward better results for both disorders in larger and later series (see Table 197–4), suggesting that technical improvements and more experience may improve outcomes. The long-term data for cancer pain and potential surgical impact in this patient population are limited by the fact that most cancer pain patients have disseminated disease, and as a result, they have often unacceptably poor life expectancies.

Subsets of neuropathic pain appear to respond well to DBS, whereas certain disorders appear unlikely to respond to stimulation. In most instances, paresthesia-producing stimulation was used (see Table 197–5). Brachial plexus injuries, peripheral neuropathies, and phantom limb pain show significant long-term improvement in 50% to 100% of patients, although lesser responses have been reported. Patients with stroke pain, pain from spinal cord injuries, and postherpetic neuralgia are among the poorest responders. As with nociceptive pain, there is a trend toward better results in later and larger series. Even in the most difficult situations, such as stroke pain, there are some reports of significant responses to paresthesia-inducing DBS, suggesting that exploration in severe, completely refractory cases may be warranted as long as the patient recognizes the likelihood that stimulation may not provide relief. Every series that compared short-term (perioperative testing) and long-term results found a substantial decrease in the percentage of patients responding to DBS over time, regardless of site of insertion or mechanism of pain relief. Unfortunately, this is typical of most other therapies used to treat chronic pain.

Toronto Hospital Experience

To gain further insight into the long-term efficacy of DBS for pain in an almost exclusively neuropathic population of pain patients, we evaluated the long-term follow-up data of 80 patients who underwent attempted DBS at the Toronto hospital from 1979 to 1997. The patient characteristics and the diagnoses are shown in Table 197–6. All patients had the steady (e.g., burning, aching, dysesthetic) component of neuropathic pain, 58% had evoked pain (e.g., allodynia, hyperpathia), and 47% had intermittent or neuralgic pain.

T A B L E   1 9 7 – 6 ■ Diagnosis in 80 Patients Treated with Deep Brain Stimulation for Pain at the Toronto Hospital Between 1979 and 1997

DIAGNOSIS	NO. OF PATIENTS
Central lesions	40
Brain	22
Ischemic stroke	21
Hemorrhage	1
Spinal cord	18
Trauma	14
Arteriovenous malformation	1
Multiple sclerosis	1
Postcordotomy dysesthesia	1
Myelopathy	1
Peripheral lesions	38
Peripheral nerve—anesthesia dolorosa	20
Peripheral nerve—trauma	4
Multiple iatrogenic	3
Postherpetic neuralgia	3
Brachial plexus lesions or avulsion	2
Phantom pain	2
Stump pain	2
Phantom and stump pain	1
Traumatic cauda equina	1
Nociceptive pain	2

All patients had microelectrode-guided stereotactic electrode placement, with microstimulation in 90% and macrostimulation in 10% of the patients. Twenty-five patients had single electrodes placed in the VC, 43 had simultaneous electrodes placed in the VC and PVG, 5 in the VC and ML, 6 in the ML, and 1 in the VC and IC. Figures 197–2 and 197–3 show the typical locations of VC and PVG electrodes. After the initial electrode implantation, all patients underwent a stimulation trial for 3 to 14 days. Results were graded as excellent (>67% reduction in pain), good (33% to 67% reduction in pain), fair (≤33% reduction in pain), or failures (no pain relief), based on analog pain scale reports from patients, reports of others concerning evidence of pain, and influence of pain on daily activities. We usually considered patients for surgical intervention if they reported a pain level of greater than 6 on a scale of 1 to 10. Although the goal of surgery was more than 50% pain relief, a patient with a preoperative pain level of 8, for example, reduced to 5 with stimulation would be considered successful, despite a reduction of only 37%.

Of the initial 80 patients undergoing DBS implantation, 71 proceeded to the test stimulation stage. Nine patients did not proceed to the test stimulation because the procedure was stopped (e.g., concern over hemorrhage, acute medical problem) or because the patient could not tolerate and complete the entire surgical procedure. Of the 71 patients who completed the surgical procedure, 48 had a successful test stimulation (>33% pain relief) and subsequently received a permanent subcutaneous implant of a radiofrequency-coupled device or an IPG in a second procedure. The other 23 patients failed to obtain significant pain relief during the trial period, and their electrodes were removed. Results of the last follow-up assessment are shown in

T A B L E 1 9 7 – 7 ■ **Long-Term Outcome of Pain Reduction from Deep Brain Stimulation Performed at the Toronto Hospital from 1979 to 1997**

	DEGREE OF PAIN RELIEF*			
PATIENTS	**67% to 100%**	**33% to 67%**	**≤33%**	**Failure**
All patients (N=80)	14 (18%)	9 (11%)	5 (6%)	52 (65%)
Internalized patients (N=48 [60%])	14 (29%)	9 (19%)	5 (10%)	20 (42%)

* Long-term is pain relief based on analog patient pain scales taken at last follow-up (range, 9–131 months; mean, 61 months).

Table 197–7. Fifty-eight percent of those who underwent permanent implantation had satisfactory pain relief at the last follow-up examination, although this represented only 35% of those who were initially explored.

In summary, approximately 60% of patients pass the trial stimulation (i.e., derive at least 33% pain relief with stimulation), and approximately 60% of this group derive long-term benefit. The results also indicated that paresthesia-producing stimulation was more effective for the steady component and that medial stimulation (i.e., PVG) was more efficacious for the evoked element of neuropathic pain. Successful pain control appeared to be more likely in patients with lesser degrees of preoperative sensory loss. The patient's age, sex, or duration of pain did not significantly influence outcome.

COMPLICATIONS

The major complications of DBS for pain are similar to those associated with DBS for movement disorders. They include insertional or neurological, technical or hardware, and stimulation-related complications.[51, 52,] [55–64, 66] The most serious complications are in the insertional or neurological category, including hemorrhage, stroke, permanent neurological deficit, seizures, and pneumocephalus. Most large series report a hemorrhage rate of 1% to 4%, although larger rates have been reported (Table 197–8). Death from hemorrhage has occurred in 1% to 2% of patients, although several large series reported no deaths. Significant, permanent neurological deficits have similarly occurred in 1% to 2% of patients, but several studies have not reported long-term deficits. There appears to be a trend toward reduced hemorrhage rates in more recently treated patients, and this may reflect improvements in DBS electrode design and increased use of advanced imaging modalities for preoperative planning. The use of microelectrode or microstimulation versus macrostimulation has not been correlated with incidence of significant hemorrhage. The other major neurological complication related to insertion is diplopia or occulomotor problems. This is most often seen with stimulators placed in the PAG or PVG and can be sufficiently problematic that repositioning or removal of electrodes may be necessary even with good pain relief.

The major hardware-related complications are infection and technical failures. Overall, infection rates

T A B L E 1 9 7 – 8 ■ **Published Reports of Complications from Deep Brain Stimulation for Pain in Several Large Series**

COMPLICATION	HOSOBUCHI[52] 1970–1984 (N=122)	LEVY ET AL[60] 1972–1987 (N=141)	YOUNG ET AL[56] 1978–1983 (N=48)	TASKER AND VILELA FILHO[66] 1978–1991 (N=62)	KUMAR ET AL[61] 1982–1997 (N=68)
Hemorrhage	4.1%*	3.5%	2.1%	13.2%†	1.5%
Death	1.6%	0.8%	0%	0%	0%
Permanent deficit	0%	1.6%		1.6%	1.5%
Infection	4.9%	12.1%	6.3%	12.9%	5.9%
Removal	0.8%	7.8%	2.1%	9.7%	1.5%
Death	0%	0%	0%	1.6%	0%
Hardware failure (lead migration, fracture, device failure)		24.0%	12.5%	43.5%	7.4%
Skin erosion	1.6%	7.1%			8.1%
Foreign body reaction		3.5%			
Seizure				3.0%	2.9%
Diplopia	4.2%	14.2%	1.4%		2.9%
Headache		51.5%			22.1%
Local pain		5.0%	8.3%	3.2%	
Transient confusion		7.8%		1.6%	

* Complications are reported as percentages of the patient population.
† Represents asymptomatic, radiographically demonstrated hemorrhages in addition to symptomatic hemorrhages.

range from 5% to 13%, and this has been consistently observed in all series, regardless of hardware used (see Table 197–8). Prophylactic antibiotic use before surgery and in the immediate perioperative period was not standard practice in the early years of DBS for pain, and its introduction has likely contributed to decreased rates of infection. There has been no correlation between externalization of hardware for perioperative testing and increased incidence of infection.[60] A sufficiently serious infection leading to death has only rarely been reported. Even superficial infections usually require hardware removal, although in some instances when the DBS was providing substantial pain relief, infections have been successfully treated with antibiotics alone. In patients with bilateral DBS but unilateral infections, the contralateral hardware is usually spared and rarely requires revision if it is functioning satisfactorily. Hardware failure represents the most common complication, with rates of 5% to 25% reported (see Table 197–8). This category of complications includes lead migration, lead or hardware fracture, and device failure. Usually, these problems require revision or replacement of part or all of the hardware. Most seizures reported in the neurological category have been attributed to lead migration. Both of these complications have been significantly reduced with the advent of modern DBS electrodes and fixation techniques, as described previously.

Stimulation-related complications are usually transient and resolve with adjustment of stimulation parameters or repositioning of electrodes. Diplopia can result from the position of the electrode in the PVG or PAG without stimulation, but this problem can also occur or worsen with stimulation. Uncomfortable paresthesias, local pain, headaches, and motor dysfunction have occurred after stimulation. Reduction in stimulation intensity can resolve many of these effects, and the use of multiple contact electrodes permits adjustment of the region of stimulation to maximize benefits and minimize side effects without the need for reoperation. Occasionally, repositioning of the electrode may be necessary. With PAG DBS, feelings of anxiety, fear, or discomfort may accompany the onset of stimulation. This is one reason that most practitioners favor PVG stimulation, because these side effects are rarely seen if electrode placement in maintained above the intercommissural line. Failure to resolve severe stimulation-induced side effects, particularly if pain relief is inadequate, is one reason for complete hardware removal after test stimulation.

CONCLUSIONS

DBS continues to be a viable surgical option for many pain patients. As with any surgical procedure, the risk-benefit ratio favors use of DBS only in patients who are refractory to nonsurgical alternatives. The long history of using DBS in pain patients provides some guidance about risks and about which disorders might best respond to DBS. Experience suggests that PVG stimulation is better tolerated and has fewer side effects than PAG stimulation. Although some series have demonstrated impressive results using PVG or PAG stimulation to treat nociceptive pain, the popularity of intrathecal opiate pumps probably will continue to limit the use of DBS in these cases. Some subsets of neuropathic pain, particularly brachial plexus avulsion and peripheral neuropathy, respond to paresthesia-inducing stimulation (sometimes in combination with medial stimulation). Bipolar stimulation from electrodes with multiple lead contacts permits greater flexibility during postoperative testing, and this may limit the need for surgical revision.

Advances in pain research and in functional neurosurgery techniques should continue to improve the risk-benefit ratio of DBS for pain. The advent of burhole rings for fixation of DBS electrodes has largely eliminated lead migration and seizures due to this complication, and the use of prophylactic antibiotics has reduced hardware-related infections. Development of smaller components should improve patient tolerance to hardware and possibly minimize skin erosions. Increasing use of computerized workstations, which permit preoperative integration of multiple imaging modalities and trajectory planning, may reduce the length of procedures and possibly reduce risks such as hemorrhage. For testing and outcome analyses, there is a major need for improved pain monitoring techniques and rating systems with greater uniformity and more generalized acceptance. This is true for all pain research but would certainly aid in improving outcome measures of DBS for particular disorders. More widespread application of functional imaging to pain patients, including fMRI, PET, and magnetoencephalography, should enhance our insight into the anatomic substrates of DBS therapy for pain and may provide previously unidentified CNS targets for stimulation to relieve chronic pain.

REFERENCES

1. Tasker RR: Deep brain stimulation is preferable to thalamotomy for tremor suppression. Surg Neurol 49:145–153, discussion 153–154, 1998.
2. Limousin P, Krack P, Pollak P, et al: Electrical stimulation of the subthalamic nucleus in advanced Parkinson's disease. N Engl J Med 339:1105–1111, 1998.
3. Kumar R, Lozano AM, Kim YJ, et al: Double-blind evaluation of subthalamic nucleus deep brain stimulation in advanced Parkinson's disease. Neurology 51:850–855, 1998.
4. Krack P, Pollak P, Limousin P, et al: Subthalamic nucleus or internal pallidal stimulation in young onset Parkinson's disease. Brain 121:451–457, 1998.
5. Krack P, Limousin P, Benabid AL, et al: Chronic stimulation of subthalamic nucleus improves levodopa-induced dyskinesias in Parkinson's disease [letter]. Lancet 350:1676, 1997.
6. Benabid AL, Pollak P, Seigneuret E, et al: Chronic VIM thalamic stimulation in Parkinson's disease, essential tremor and extrapyramidal dyskinesias. Acta Neurochir Suppl 58:39–44, 1993.
7. Benabid AL, Pollak P, Hoffmann D, et al: Stimulators of the central nervous system. Rev Prat 43:1129–1139, 1993.
8. Olds J, Milner B: Positive reinforcement produced by electrical stimulation of the septal area and other regions of the rat brain. J Comp Physiol Psychol 47:419, 1954.

9. Heath R: Studies in Schizophrenia: A Multidisciplinary Approach to Mind-Brain Relationships. Cambridge, MA, Harvard University Press, 1954.

10. Pool JL: Psychosurgery in older people. J Am Geriatr Soc 2: 456–465, 1954.

11. Pool J, Clark W, Hudson P, et al: Hypothalamic-Hypophyseal Interrelationships. Springfield, IL, Charles C Thomas, 1956.

12. Heath R, Mickle W: Evaluation of 7 years' experience with depth electrode studies in human patients. In Ramey E, O'Doherty D (eds): Electrical Studies in Unanesthetized Brain. New York, Harper & Brothers, 1960, pp 214–217.

13. Ervin F, Brown C, VH M: Striatal Influence on facial pain. Confin Neurol 27:75–86, 1966.

14. Gol A: Relief of pain by electrical stimulation of the septal area. J Neurol Sci 5:115–120, 1967.

15. Melzack R, Wall R: Pain mechanisms: A new theory. Science 150: 971–979, 1965.

16. Adams JE, Hosobuchi Y Fields HL: Stimulation of internal capsule for relief of chronic pain. J Neurosurg 41:740–744, 1974.

17. Mazars G, Roge R, Mazars Y: Stimulation of the spinothalamic fasciculus and their bearing on the pathophysiology of pain. Rev Neurol 103:136–138, 1960.

18. Hosobuchi Y, Adams J, Rutkin B: Chronic thalamic stimulation for the control of facial anesthesia dolorosa. Arch Neurol 29: 158–161, 1973.

19. Mazars GL, Merienne L Ciolocca C: Treatment of certain types of pain by implantable thalamic stimulators. Neurochirurgie 29: 117–124, 1974.

20. Fields HL, Adams JE: Pain after cortical injury relieved by electrical stimulation of the internal capsule. Brain 97:169–178, 1974.

21. Cooper IS, Upton AR, Amin I: Reversibility of chronic neurologic deficits: Some effects of electrical stimulation of the thalamus and internal capsule in man. Appl Neurophysiol 43:244–258, 1980.

22. Reynolds D: Surgery in the rat during electrical analgesia induced by focal brain stimulation. Science 164:444–445, 1969.

23. Richardson DE, Akil H: Pain reduction by electrical brain stimulation in man. Part 1. Acute administration in periaqueductal and periventricular sites. J Neurosurg 47:178–183, 1977.

24. Richardson DE, Akil H: Pain reduction by electrical brain stimulation in man. Part 2. Chronic self-administration in the periventricular gray matter. J Neurosurg 47:184–194, 1977.

25. Hosobuchi Y, Adams JE, Linchitz R: Pain relief by electrical stimulation of the central gray matter in humans and its reversal by naloxone. Science 197:183–186, 1977.

26. Biovie J, Meyerson B: Correlative anatomical and clinical study of pain suppression by deep brain stimulation. Pain 13:113–126, 1982.

27. Young R, Rinaldi P: Brain stimulation in pain. In Levy RM, North R (eds): The Neurosurgery of Chronic Pain. New York, Springer-Verlag.

28. Taxonomy ITFO: Classification of Chronic Pain: Description of Chronic Pain Syndromes and Definitions of Pain Terms. Seattle, IASP Press, 1994.

29. Long C: The relationship between surgical outcome and MMPR profiles in chronic pain patients. J Clin Psychol 37:744–749, 1981.

30. Wiltse L, Rocchio P: Preoperative psychological tests as predictors of success of chemonucleolysis in the treatment of the low-back syndrome. J Bone Joint Surg Am 57:478–483, 1975.

31. Gerhart K, Yezierski R, Fang Z, et al: Inhibition of primate spinothalamic tract neurons by stimulation in ipsilateral or contralateral ventral posterior lateral (VPL) thalamic nucleus: Possible mechanisms. J Neurophysiol 59:406–423, 1983.

32. Hirayama T, Dostrovsky J, Gorecki J, et al: Recordings of abnormal activity in patients with deafferentation and central pain: Proceedings of the microelectrode meeting. Stereotact Funct Neurosurg 52:120–126, 1989.

33. Lenz F, Tasker R, Dostrovsky J, et al: Abnormal single-unit activity recorded in the somatosensory thalamus of a quadriplegic patient with central pain. Pain 31:225–236, 1987.

34. Rinaldi P, Young R, Albe-Fessard D, et al: Spontaneous neuronal hyperactivity in the medial and intralaminar thalamic nuclei of patients with deafferentation pain. J Neurosurg 74:415–421, 1991.

35. Lis-Planells M, Tronnier V, Rinaldi P, et al: Neural activity of medial and lateral thalamus in a deafferentation model. Soc Neurosci Abstr 18:288, 1992.

36. Radhakrishnan V, Tsoukatos J, Davis KD, et al: A comparison of the burst activity of lateral thalamic neurons in chronic pain and non-pain patients. Pain 80:567–575, 1999.

37. Rezai AR, Lozano AM, Crawley AP, et al: Thalamic stimulation and functional magnetic resonance imaging: Localization of cortical and subcortical activation with implanted electrodes. Technical note. J Neurosurg 90:583–590, 1999.

38. Davis KD, Taub E, Duffner F, et al: Activation of the anterior cingulate cortex by thalamic stimulation in patients with chronic pain: A positron emission tomography study. J Neurosurg 92: 64–69, 2000.

39. Hosobuchi Y, Adams J, Bloom F, et al: Stimulation of human periaqueducta gray for pain relief increases immunoreactive beta endorphin in ventricular fluid. Science 203:279–281, 1979.

40. Young R, Bach F, Van Norman A, et al: Release of beta-endorphin and methionine-enkephalin into the cerebrespinal fluid during deep brain stimulation for chronic pain. J Neurosurg 79:816–825, 1993.

41. Bushnell M, Duncan G: Sensory and affective aspects of pain perception: Is medial thalamus restricted to emotions issues? Exp Brain Res 78:415–418, 1989.

42. Guilbaud G, Peschanski M, Besson J: Experimental data related to pain at the supraspinal level. In Wall P, Malzack R (eds): Textbook of Pain. London, Churchill Livingstone, 1989, pp 149–153.

43. Basbaum AI, Fields HL: Endogenous pain control mechanisms: Review and hypothesis. Ann Neurol 4:451–462, 1978.

44. Peschanski M, Besson JM: Diencephalic connections of the raphe nuclei of the rat brainstem: An anatomical study with reference to the somatosensory system. J Comp Neurol 224:509–534, 1984.

45. Andersen E, Dafny N: An ascending serotonergic pain modulation pathway from the dorsal raphe nucleus to the parafascicularis nucleus of the thalamus. Brain Res 269:57–67, 1983.

46. Hutchison WD, Davis KD, Lozano AM, et al: Pain-related neurons in the human cingulate cortex. Nat Neurosci 2:403–405, 1999.

47. Parrent AG, Lozano AM, Dostrovsky JO, et al: Central pain in the absence of functional sensory thalamus. Stereotact Funct Neurosurg 59:9–14, 1992.

48. Davis KD, Kiss ZH, Luo L, et al: Phantom sensations generated by thalamic microstimulation. Nature 391:385–387, 1998.

49. Tsubokawa T, Katayama Y, Yamamoto T, et al: Chronic motor cortex stimulation for the treatment of central pain. Acta Neurochir Suppl 52:137–139, 1991.

50. Tsubokawa T, Katayama Y, Yamamoto T, et al: Chronic motor cortex stimulation in patients with thalamic pain. J Neurosurg 78:393–401, 1993.

51. Richardson DE, Akil H: Long term results of periventricular gray self-stimulation. Neurosurgery 1:199–202, 1977.

52. Hosobuchi Y: Subcortical electrical stimulation for control of intractable pain in humans. J neurosurgery. 64:543–553, 1986.

53. Hosobuchi Y, Adams JE, Linchitz R: Pain relief by electrical stimulation of the central gray matter in humans and its reversal by naloxone. Science 197:183–186, 1977.

54. Young R: Effects of PAG stimulation upon cardiovascular function in humans: Relation to analgesic effects. NATO Advanced Research Workshop in the Midbrain Periaqueductal Gray Matter. Casteraverduzan, France, 1990.

55. Meyerson BA: Biochemistry of pain relief with intracerebral stimulation. Few facts and many hypotheses. Acta Neurochir Suppl 30:229–237, 1980.

56. Young RF, Kroening R, Fulton W, et al: Electrical stimulation of the brain in treatment of chronic pain. J Neurosurg 62:389–396, 1985.

57. Turnball IM, Shulman R, Woodhusst WB: Thalamic stimulation for neuropathic pain. J Neurosurg 52:486–493, 1980.

58. Meyerson BA: Recent advances in neurosurgical treatment of chronic pain. Acta Neurol Scand Suppl 78:15–23, 1980.

59. Meyerson BA, Boethius J, Carlsson AM: Alleviation of malignant pain by electrical stimulation in the periventricular region: Pain relief as related to stimulation sites. Adv Pain Res Ther 3:525–533, 1979.

60. Levy RM, Lamb S, Adams JE: Treatment of chronic pain by deep brain stimulation: Long term follow-up and review of the literature. Neurosurgery 21:885–893, 1987.

61. Kumar K, Toth C, Nath RK: Deep brain stimulation for intractable pain: A 15-year experience. Neurosurgery 40:736–746, 1997.
62. Plotkin R: Results in 60 cases of deep brain stimulation for chronic intractable pain. Appl Neurophysiol 45:173–178, 1982.
63. Dieckmann G, Witzmann A: Initial and long-term results of deep brain stimulation for chronic intractable pain. Appl Neurophysiol 45:167–172, 1982.
64. Tasker RR, Vilela Filho O: Deep brain stimulation for neuropathic pain. Stereotact Funct Neurosurg 65:122–124, 1995.
65. Siegfried J: Therapeutical neurostimulation—indications reconsidered. Acta Neurochir Suppl (Wien) 52:112–117, 1991.
66. Tasker RR, Vilela Filho O: Deep brain stimulation for the control of intractable pain. In Youmans JR (ed): Neurological Surgery. Philadelphia, WB Saunders, 1996, pp 3512–3527.

CHAPTER 198

Intrathecal Drug Infusion for Pain

RICHARD D. PENN

More than 35,000 drug pumps have been implanted to treat patients with severe pain since their introduction in the early 1980s. Initially, intrathecal morphine was used only in cancer patients, but currently a majority of patients have other causes of pain, such as failed back surgery syndrome. The reasons for this rapid application of new technology are the advantages of intrathecal medications and the unmet needs of patients with severe, chronic, incapacitating pain. Experience indicates that intrathecal morphine provides adequate pain relief in well over 60% of patients and possibly as high as 75% (Table 198–1). If new medications are developed to deal with opiate-nonresponsive pain or central pain syndromes, the use of pumps will be greatly expanded. This chapter covers the issues of patient selection and screening, implantation, and medications for intrathecal use. The pharmacokinetics of drug delivery are very similar to those of intrathecal baclofen, which is covered in Chapter 177.

PATIENT SELECTION

Cancer Pain

Use of implanted drug pumps for cancer pain is a well-proven therapy. More than a decade of clinical experience has provided abundant evidence that it is safe and effective. Table 198–1 lists a series of studies, all of which conclude that a majority of patients can get adequate pain relief after other treatments have failed.[1–13] The percentage of pain relief varies, and the patient groups are different at each center, but in general, two thirds to three fourths of patients have good to excellent pain control.

The criteria for using intrathecal morphine are straightforward. The patient must have failed to respond to an adequate trial of oral narcotics or have unacceptable side effects such as mental confusion or somnolence. In the past, many physicians were reluctant to give adequate doses of narcotics for fear of addiction. Fortunately, this attitude has gradually changed, and more patients are being given appropriate oral medications. Also, more long-acting opiate preparations are available. If these drugs are used properly, 90% of patients will get good pain relief. This

means that only the most difficult patients on high opiate doses who are not responding or who have side effects are likely to be referred for evaluation of drug pump therapy.

Once a patient has failed oral narcotics, the second consideration is how long the patient is expected to live. On a cost basis, at least 3 to 6 months' longevity is needed to justify the expense of device implantation.[14] If the time is shorter, a percutaneous catheter and external pump should be employed.[15] Destructive neurosurgical procedures are rarely used. However, in selected cases, percutaneous cordotomy for unilateral pain is very effective and should be considered (see Chapter 192). Clearly, open rhizotomies or myelotomies are rarely justified because of the magnitude of the surgery in a terminally ill patient.

The key to success is selecting patients who are clearly responsive to intrathecal morphine. For that reason, a trial is necessary. This can be done with a bolus injection of intrathecal or epidural morphine or with placement of an intraspinal catheter for continuous infusion using a temporary external pump. If the epidural route is used for a trial, the correct intrathecal dose is 10% of the lowest effective epidural dose. The

TABLE 198–1 ■ **Intrathecal Drug Therapy for Pain: Selected Studies**

AUTHOR	TYPE OF PAIN	NUMBER OF PATIENTS
Brazenor, 1987[1]	Cancer	25
Follet et al, 1992[2]	Cancer	37
Hassenbusch et al, 1990[3]	Cancer	41
Onofrio et al, 1981[4]	Cancer	53
Penn & Paice, 1987[5]	Cancer	35
	Nonmalignant	8
Shetter, 1986[6]	Cancer	24
Krames & Lanning, 1993[7]	Nonmalignant	16
Tutak & Doleys, 1996[8]	Nonmalignant	26
Winkelmüller & Winkelmüller, 1996[9]	Nonmalignant	120
Van Buyten, 1998[10]	Nonmalignant	32
Erdine & Yücel, 1996[11]	Cancer	54
Paice et al, 1996[12]	Cancer	140
	Nonmalignant	289
Schuchard et al, 1998[13]	Nonmalignant	50

trial period is important for both physician and patient. The physician can get to know the responses of the patient over a number of days, and the patient can find out the degree of pain relief to be expected and how that relief affects activities of daily living. A common problem is that many patients have been given escalating amounts of oral or intravenous morphine and tolerance has developed. However, a trial of intrathecal morphine is sometimes effective even in this setting. Systemic opiate therapy should not be suddenly stopped after an intrathecal trial is begun because of possible withdrawal symptoms or severe pain that occurs before the right intraspinal dose is found. By letting the patient manage his or her own supplementary opiate therapy, the physician can judge from the amounts taken how effective the intraspinal drug is.

Because most patients considered for intraspinal morphine are already taking systemic opiates, the likelihood of respiratory depression or nausea and vomiting is low. However, an apnea monitor is recommended throughout the trial, particularly at night, when respiratory drive may decrease. If an overdose of intrathecal morphine is given, it can be managed by using an opiate antagonist, but it must be carefully titrated so as not to produce a full withdrawal syndrome or recurrent pain. Intraspinal morphine can produce constipation and, particularly in the first few days, urinary retention. Itching can also occur; it may clear in 12 to 24 hours, but occasionally itching persists, and treatment has to be discontinued. Myoclonus is a rare problem, often appearing after some months of treatment. Changing to another opiate, such as hydromorphone, may be helpful in some cases.

A major concern with the use of intrathecal morphine has been the development of tolerance. Animal experiments show that repeated daily boluses of intrathecal morphine lead to rapid loss of analgesia, as judged by tail-flick tests of pain.[16] If these tests were predictive of the human situation, intrathecal morphine would be of little value after 2 or 3 days. Fortunately, that is not the case, and the reason may be the comparatively higher doses used in the animal experiments. However, if a patient reports the gradual loss of pain relief over weeks or months, the question of tolerance arises. It is often difficult to tell whether this decrease in effectiveness is caused by true biologic tolerance or by progression of the cancer. Clinical experience has demonstrated a need for increasing dosages over months or years (Fig. 198–1), but this overall effect hides the fact that many patients can be maintained on a steady dose for a long time.[12] An alternative explanation for the need for increasing doses in some patients is that the pain is neuropathic. Typically, opiates initially reduce neuropathic pain, but the pain reappears over weeks; then, even very high doses of opiates are relatively ineffective.

Severe Chronic Pain

The most controversial area of drug pump use is the treatment of severe chronic pain. For these patients, the risks of opiate side effects, pump and catheter

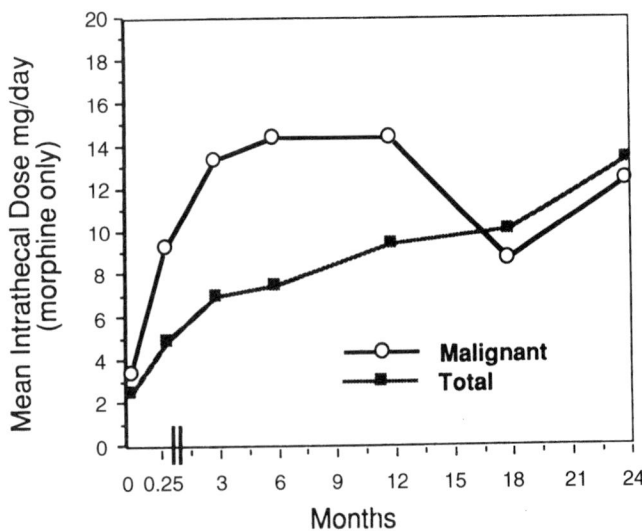

FIGURE 198–1. Mean intrathecal morphine dose progression from the initial dose to 24 months (mean intrathecal morphine doses for all patients and those diagnosed with malignancy included). (From Paice J, Penn R, Shott S: Intrathecal morphine for chronic pain: A retrospective, multicenter study. J Pain Symptom Manage 11:71–80, 1996.)

malfunctions, and drug tolerance become more important because of the long treatment period. Effective pain relief for these patients is difficult to achieve, however, and if intraspinal opiates work, the expense of the operation, equipment, and maintenance is certainly justified. In a survey of 35 physicians and more than 429 patients, two thirds of patients implanted with pumps had noncancer pain, and of these, more than 60% had failed back surgery syndrome as a cause for the pain.[12] These current practice patterns suggest that pain from failed back surgery will be the diagnosis for the vast majority of patients treated. If the results of treatment are compared between the cancer and noncancer patients, the overall rating of pain relief is similar in both groups (Fig. 198–2). In general, patients with pain characterized as somatic did better than those with neurogenic pain; however, even 50% of the patients with neurogenic pain had what they and their physicians judged to be good pain relief. A more recent single-center prospective study suggests similar results.[9] Both the neurogenic and nociceptive groups had significant pain relief (Fig. 198–3). Besides improvement in visual analog ratings of pain, about half the patients had increased their activities and were less depressed. Ninety-six percent were satisfied with their therapy. These results appear to compare favorably with dorsal column stimulation, but undoubtedly the patients with drug pump implants were different in many ways from those treated with stimulation.

If dose escalation is taken as a sign of tolerance—a reasonable assumption in noncancer patients—tolerance is definitely seen, but it often has a slow course over many years. The averages hide the individual patients who can be maintained without increased dosages, such as one patient with postherpetic pain

Cancer

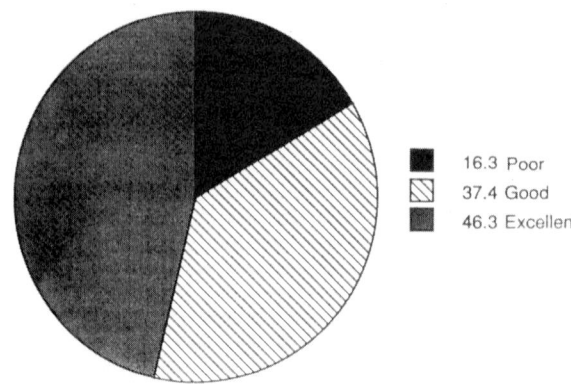

■ 16.3 Poor
▨ 37.4 Good
▨ 46.3 Excellent

Non-Cancer

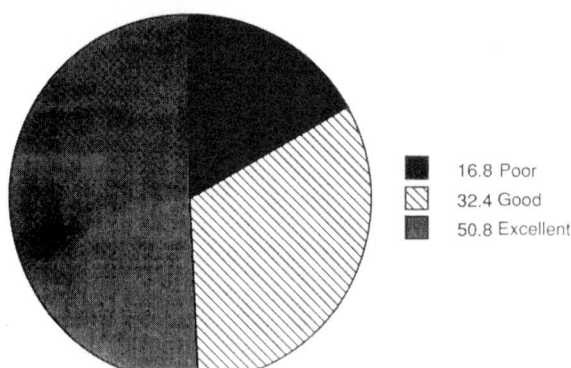

■ 16.8 Poor
▨ 32.4 Good
▨ 50.8 Excellent

FIGURE 198–2. Pain relief reported in a survey of 425 patients with implanted pumps. Note the same degree of response in cancer and noncancer patients. (From Paice J, Penn R, Shott S: Intrathecal morphine for chronic pain: A retrospective, multicenter study. J Pain Symptom Manage 11:71–80, 1996.)

who was treated for more than 8 years on the same dose.[17]

In contrast, some patients who respond to screening require rapidly increasing doses and clearly are poor long-term opiate responders. The impression has been that these patients have neurogenic pain, but this is being questioned.[9] More prospective, controlled trials are needed in well-defined neurogenic pain syndromes to resolve this issue.

Because the question of which type of pain is most likely to be helped by intrathecal morphine has not been answered, guidelines for implantation have to be empirical. As with any pain procedure, a candidate has to be evaluated preoperatively for psychological problems. Patients with severe personality disorders or psychosis should not undergo implantation. Depression almost always accompanies chronic pain, so depression alone is not a reason to withhold therapy. However, antidepressants should be tried before pump therapy is initiated.

A trial of intrathecal narcotics is mandatory. The trial period allows an assessment in the hospital of not only the response to intrathecal medication but also the changes in the patient's behavior, activity level, and oral narcotic consumption. Although a positive response is encouraging to both the patient and the physician, experience has shown that eventually about a third of selected patients do not get good long-term pain relief from intrathecal morphine.[12] No study has been done to see whether patients who fail to respond to an acute trial of intrathecal morphine would respond to chronic infusion (the false-negative group). If a trial is equivocal, an intrathecal catheter can be implanted and attached to an external pump. Then placebo and medication periods can be compared. Also, the dose can be gradually changed with a continuous infusion to optimize the effect (as would be achieved with an implanted pump). When nonopiates become available, longer trial periods to test several drugs and combinations will be necessary.

FIGURE 198–3. Mean pain scores according to the visual analog scale (VAS) before and during treatment. The best initial pain reduction (77%) was observed in the "nociceptive" group, which subsequently diminished to 48% at the last follow-up examination. The best long-term reduction (68%) occurred in the "deafferentation" pain group. (From Winkelmüller M, Winkelmüller W: Long-term effects of continuous intrathecal opioid in chronic pain of nonmalignant etiology. J Neurosurg 85: 458–467, 1996.)

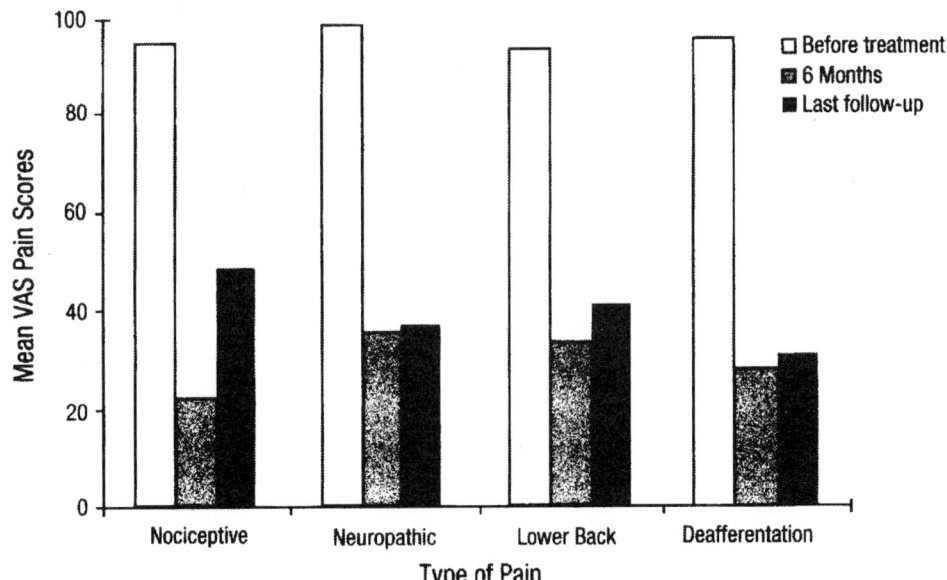

EQUIPMENT AND TECHNIQUES

Pumps and Catheters

For spinal analgesia, morphine has to reach opiate receptors in the superficial layers of the dorsal horn.[18] This is accomplished by delivering morphine into the cerebrospinal fluid for distribution.[19] After it reaches the spinal cord, it diffuses slowly into the tissue. To achieve a steady diffusion gradient, the level of morphine in the fluid must be maintained by a constant infusion. A number of devices have been employed to provide a steady perfusion of drug. They include simple catheters connected to external pumps; complex, totally implanted programmable devices; and capsules that produce analgesic substances. Each type of system has advantages and drawbacks, and choosing the best one for an individual patient depends on many factors, including the expected length of treatment, support at home, activities of daily living, available nursing care, and cost.

Several catheter systems for intrathecal or epidural infusion are available.[20, 21] For long-term treatment, the system is placed subcutaneously and then tunneled underneath the skin for at least 5 cm. A wide variety of external perfusion pumps can be connected to the catheter. Some are small enough to be easily carried by the patient. Any system that is used should contain an in-line bacteriostatic filter to protect the patient from contamination of the injected fluid. Careful maintenance of the catheter and use of prophylactic antibiotics at the time of placement lower the chance of infection. For many cancer patients who need only a few months of therapy, this is an excellent approach. In some settings, with visiting nurses and good support at home, catheters have been maintained for a year or more with only a low rate of infection or dislodgment.[15, 21]

With external pumps, epidural catheters are employed for a number of reasons; the most compelling is that direct intrathecal injections could result in meningitis. Another advantage of the epidural route is that high-dose local anesthetics and clonidine can be combined with morphine if morphine tolerance develops. The basic problem with the epidural route is that only a small percentage of morphine diffuses from the epidural space into the cerebrospinal fluid; more than 90% goes into the systemic circulation through absorption by epidural vessels.[19] This means that the patient is receiving both systemic and intraspinal analgesics at the same time.

Cost seems to favor the use of an external pump connected to a percutaneous catheter over an implanted pump. However, the epidural route requires about 10 times the intrathecal morphine dose, and home health care to maintain treatment is expensive. Cost calculations indicate that after 3 to 6 months, an implanted pump can be the less expensive treatment.[14]

If the expected duration of treatment is longer than 3 to 6 months, most physicians choose to use a totally implanted system. Implanted reservoirs are mentioned here only to eliminate them from consideration. Such systems do not have bacteriostatic filters, and the frequent percutaneous needle sticks required to give medication result in a high rate of serious infection. Further, intermittent injection has a much greater risk because of the sudden high levels of morphine that are created in the cerebrospinal fluid. In addition, drug distribution from such a bolus injection does not reach a steady state, so the patient does not have steady analgesia.[19] Redistribution of a bolus of morphine to the brainstem can result in vomiting and respiratory depression, which are rarely seen with a steady infusion.[22]

The first totally implanted pump available for infusion was made by Infusaid and, in slightly modified form, is still in use.[4] Its design incorporates a renewable energy source (Fig. 198–4). Filling of the 50-mL pump reservoir compresses Freon gas surrounding a metal bellows. The compressed gas then produces a pressure on the bellows, and fluid in the reservoir is forced through an outflow path of metal tubing. The small gauge of the tubing and its length create enough resistance to slow the flow to 1 to 3 mL/day. The exact rate varies from pump to pump, but any particular pump provides a constant flow. If the pump is overfilled or if the amount of fluid in the reservoir is less than 5 mL, the rate will be higher or lower, respectively. Increases in temperature increase the flow rate because the Freon gas pressure increases. Likewise, an increase in altitude may increase the rate. For most patients, these changes in rate of delivery do not produce any perceivable consequences, because small changes in morphine levels do not drastically change analgesia. The Infusaid pump has been used for more than 20 years and is a reliable system. The pump may slow its rate of delivery gradually over many years, but this can be easily compensated for by adjusting the concentration of morphine used. The most dangerous problems occur subsequent to drug leakage out of the reservoir. The Silastic refill system can be damaged by multiple sticks with a coring needle. A Tuohy needle, provided by the company, avoids the problem but makes refills more difficult. In summary, the constant-flow Infusaid device is a simple, reliable, sturdy, and effective pump for intrathecal morphine delivery.

A more complex device, based on cardiac pacemaker technology, has also proved safe and effective. The major advantage of this system is that it can be programmed by a radiofrequency link to provide different infusion rates. Rather than changing the concentration of medication in the pump reservoir to provide a different dosage, the physician can simply program the Medtronic pump to do so; this allows rapid and accurate dose titration. A rotary, peristaltic pump is controlled by electronic circuits, and both are powered by a lithium battery (Fig. 198–5). The device is very accurate, to within ± 5% or better. It may be the most accurate device ever designed to give medication to patients. This type of precision is not needed for morphine but can be of considerable value in delivering other drugs that must be more carefully titrated. Having a battery means that the pump has to be replaced in 5 to 7 years. Replacement of the pump is easy and can be done under local anesthesia on an outpatient basis. The pump failure rate is 0.5% per year or less, and when it

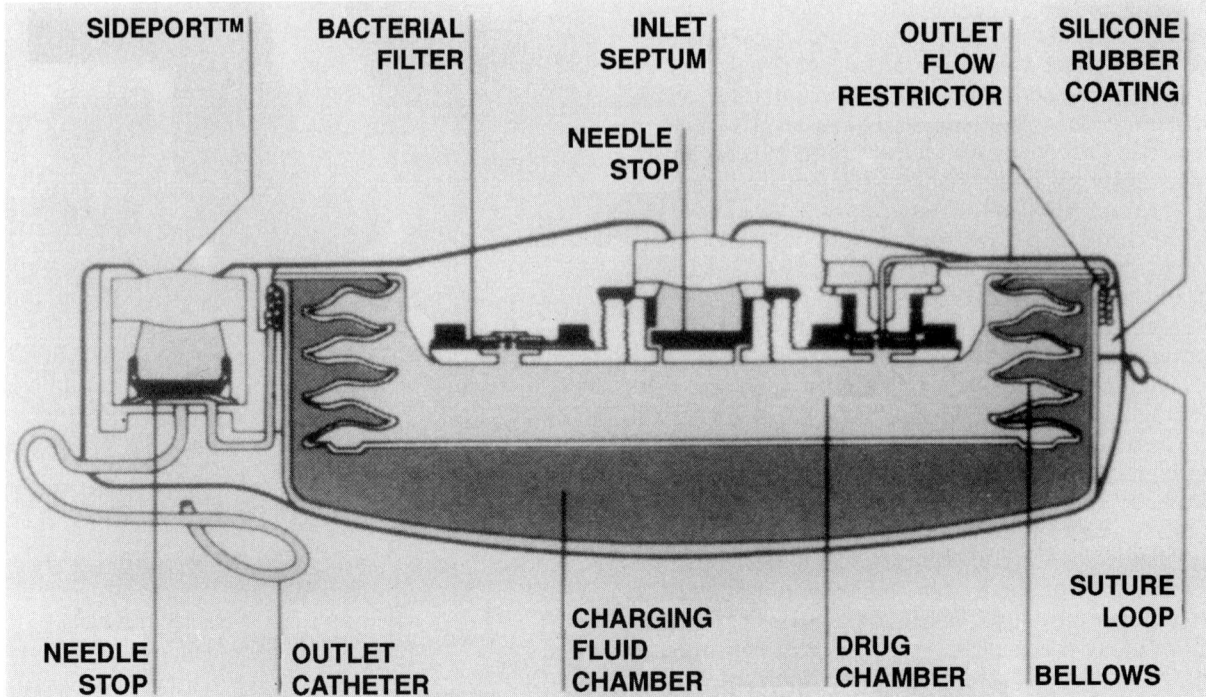

FIGURE 198–4. Infusaid constant-flow implanted pump. Note the charging fluid chamber, which holds Freon gas to provide pressure against the drug chamber. (Courtesy of Infusaid, Pfizer Hospital Products Group, Norwood, MA.)

fails, it almost always stops delivering medication. Pump overdoses due to mechanical failure are very rare.

Both constant-flow and programmable pumps have optional side access ports to inject directly into the catheter for bolus administration or patency testing. These ports are potentially dangerous, and the risk is higher in an obese patient whose pump is deep in subcutaneous tissue and difficult to feel. Two patients have died from morphine overdoses after the side port was injected with a refill intended for the reservoir. A mechanical device has been added over the side port to avoid this problem.

Another implanted pump is in clinical design trials in the United States. The pump is patient activated and has a one-way valve, a reservoir for morphine, and a catheter. This arrangement provides a single bolus injection of a small amount of drug and has a lockout

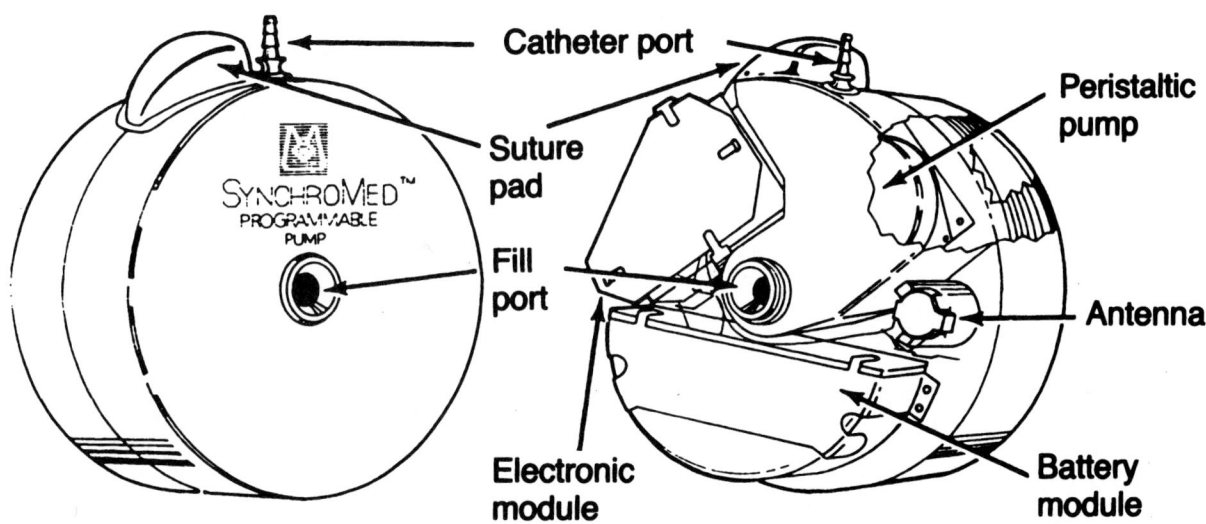

FIGURE 198–5. Medtronic programmable pump showing the electronic module battery and peristaltic pump. The computer (not shown) signals the unit via a radiofrequency link to control the drug dosage. (Courtesy of Medtronic Neurological, Minneapolis, MN.)

period. This system is less expensive and could be an important alternative to the more complex pumps now available. The fact that it is patient activated may be an advantage in some clinical situations. In other situations, it may be a problem because a steady level of morphine in the cerebrospinal fluid cannot be obtained, and the onset of anesthesia is delayed. Typically, it takes 90 minutes for an intrathecal bolus to maximally reduce pain, so a patient who is having pain during that delay period may activate the pump too many times and produce an overdose.

The catheters that go from the pump to the sub-arachnoid space are made of Silastic. They have to be soft enough to avoid injury when introduced and flexible enough so as not to damage the roots or the spinal cord when in place. The resulting low mechanical strength means that they can break or be torn. Catheters are also subjected to considerable stress when anchored because of relative movements of the subcutaneous tissue, fascia, and muscles. They are the most vulnerable part of the system and the most likely to fail with long-term use. The more active the patient, the more likely it is that the catheters will fail. In most series, the majority of drug delivery failures are caused by catheter kinks, dislodgment, tears, and breaks.[5] In a few cases, the catheter has been enclosed in a fibrous layer that slowly stops fluid flow or diverts fluid distribution. Newer thick-walled catheters have fewer problems but require a larger-bore needle for introduction. Other materials might provide better performance, but they remain to be tested.

Pump Implantation

Implantation of a drug pump and catheter system for delivery of morphine is an easy procedure. It usually can be done with local anesthetics and sedation. As with other surgical implants, prophylactic antibiotics are frequently given, although no study has been done to prove that they reduce infection rates with implanted pumps. The specifics of preparing the pump for implantation depend on which type of pump is used. After the pump is loaded with medication, the tubing inside the pump must be filled by running it until the medication reaches the outport. Likewise, the dead space inside the catheter going to the intrathecal space must be calculated so that the amount of time for the medicine to reach the end of the catheter is known. These dead spaces are important factors in determining the time it will take a new concentration of morphine to reach the spinal subarachnoid space after the concentration of morphine in the reservoir is changed. Often, a delay of a day or more occurs with slow infusion rates.[23]

The patient is placed in the lateral position so that the abdomen and lumbar region can be prepared in continuity and so that a fluoroscopy unit can be brought in to view the lumbar spine in an anteroposterior direction (Fig. 198–6). Some surgeons use lateral fluoroscopy, which also works well. The lumbar sub-arachnoid catheter is introduced percutaneously through a Tuohy needle under fluoroscopic control

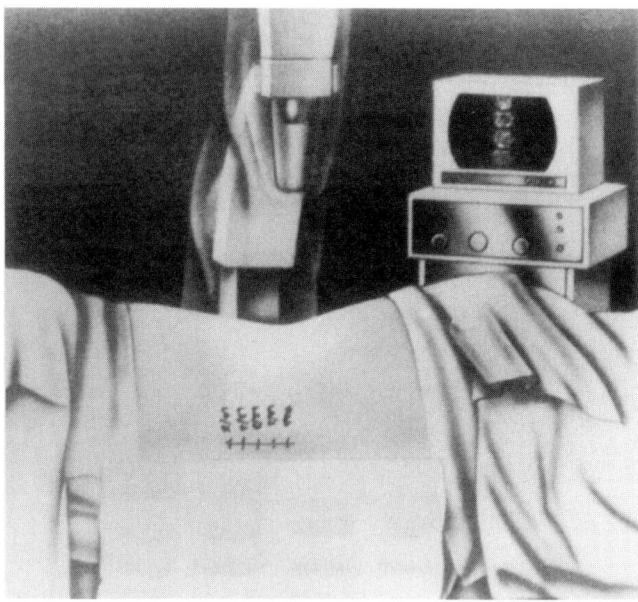

FIGURE 198–6. Position for pump implantation and fluoroscopy. (Courtesy of Medtronic, Minneapolis, MN.)

(Fig. 198–7). A laminectomy is not necessary. An oblique cephalad angle, beginning 2 to 4 cm away from the midline, is used. The oblique angle allows the catheter to be easily advanced after it is within the subarachnoid space; the off-midline approach means that the thin-walled catheter will not be compressed by the spinous processes or ligaments. If backflow of cerebrospinal fluid is poor, or if there is any question

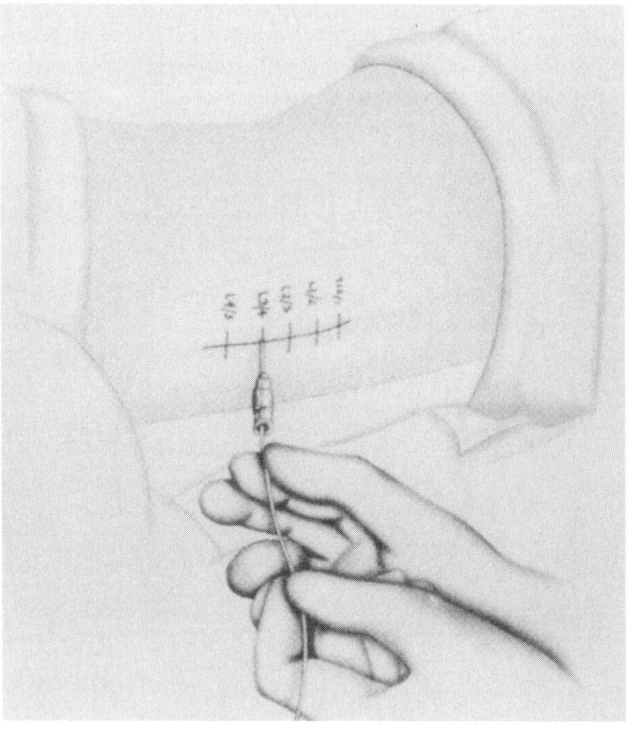

FIGURE 198–7. Placement of the intrathecal catheter. (Courtesy of Medtronic, Minneapolis, MN.)

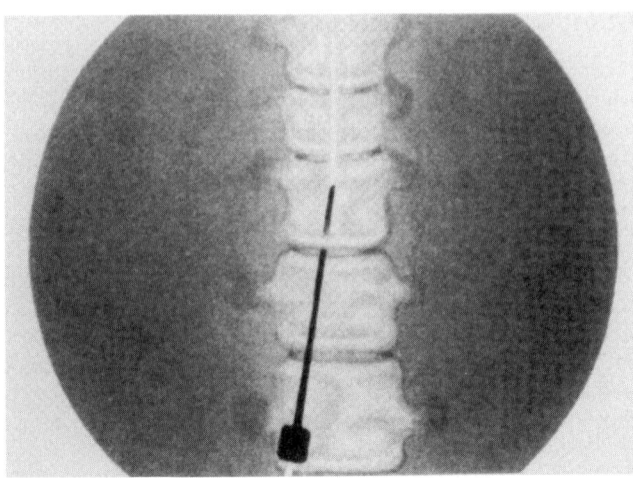

FIGURE 198–8. Fluoroscopic picture of catheter placement. (Courtesy of Medtronic, Minneapolis, MN.)

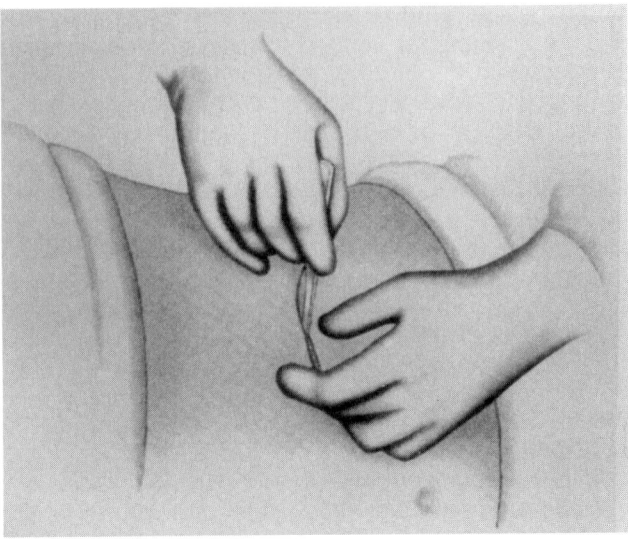

FIGURE 198–10. Subcostal incision for the pump pocket. (Courtesy of Medtronic, Minneapolis, MN.)

about correct placement, contrast material is injected to visualize the position (Fig. 198–8). The catheter is usually introduced at a low lumbar level, and the tip is placed at Ll or L2. This leaves enough catheter in the subarachnoid space so that it will not pull out with movement and still allows for the mixing of morphine in a large cerebrospinal fluid space below the conus. There is no need to place the catheter at the dermatomal level of the pain; flow of the fluid will provide adequate distribution to that level of the spinal cord. Even arm pain can be managed by a lumbar placement. After the catheter is in position, a lumbar incision is made, and the catheter is held by Silastic holders to the lumbar fascia. Care must be taken to ensure that the

catheter does not kink when set in place. An absorbable suture is put around the catheter as it exits from the fascia to avoid a cerebrospinal fluid leak around the outside of the catheter (Fig. 198–9). After the suture is placed, flow of cerebrospinal fluid is rechecked.

The subcutaneous pocket for the pump is placed below the costal margin (Fig. 198–10). Too lateral a placement in a thin person forces the pump against the superior iliac crest, causing pain when the patient is sitting. A medial and superior position is usually preferable. The pocket should be at most 1 cm below the skin, so that the pump reservoir port can be felt (Fig. 198–11). The less pressure the pump exerts against the incision site, the less likely it is that wound dehiscence will occur. A large pocket is therefore better, and an incision away from the edge of the pump is helpful. In

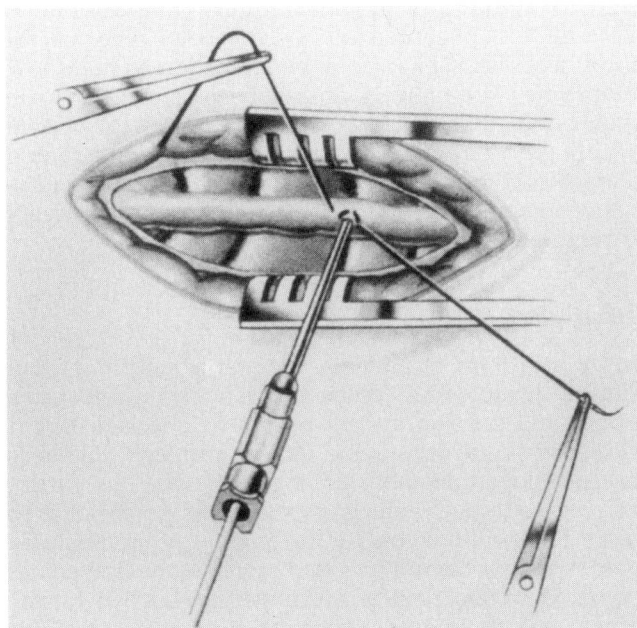

FIGURE 198–9. Placement of purse-string suture (absorbable) around the catheter at the lumbar sacral fascia to avoid leakage of cerebrospinal fluid. (Courtesy of Medtronic, Minneapolis, MN.)

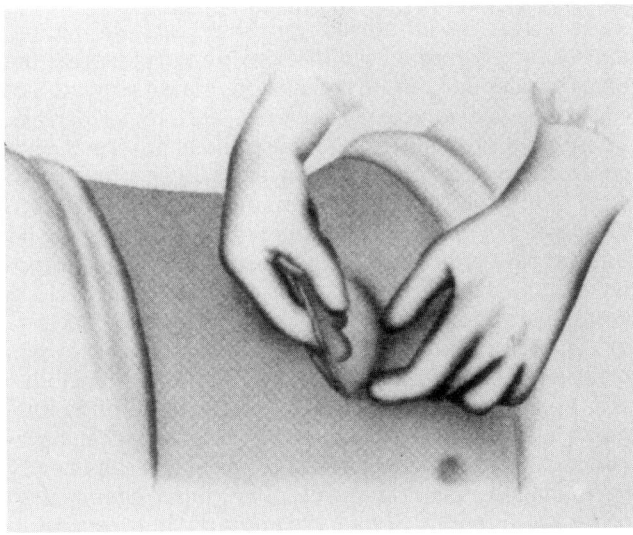

FIGURE 198–11. Development of a pump pocket approximately 1 cm in depth. (Courtesy of Medtronic, Minneapolis, MN.)

a thin person, gradual skin erosion over the edge of the metal pump or outport can be a problem. The pump is held in place by permanent sutures to fascia. A Dacron pouch may be used for the programmable pump, which is held in place by sutures, or loops on the pump can be used for anchoring. Passing the catheter from the abdominal pocket to the lumbar incision is done with a shunt tube passer. If the route for passage was infiltrated with local anesthetic at the beginning of the case, pain from placement of the passer can be minimized. Good solid connections of the catheter are needed, and kinks must be avoided, as in shunt surgery. Because the only bacteriostatic filter is within the pump, injections directly through the tubing into the subarachnoid should be avoided. Preloading the catheter with medication is not necessary.

Because the operation is performed under local anesthesia and sedation, the patient can return to the hospital room directly. The procedure can also be done on an outpatient basis, as long as medication is started at a low level. A headache from leakage of cerebrospinal fluid is not uncommon and can be managed by an increase in the patient's fluid intake, the use of analgesics, and avoidance of the upright position. A blood patch can be done if headache persists. If leaking fluid fills the abdominal pocket, it may slowly resolve. If it does not, a suture around the catheter track at the lumbar region is necessary.

Most of the mechanical problems with the catheter can be diagnosed by plain film radiography or a flow study using contrast material or indium 111 in the pump.[24] Repair of the catheter is done under local anesthesia, and the pump can be replaced on an outpatient basis if necessary. After initial adjustments to find the best dosage for a patient, subsequent dosage adjustments and refills are done on an outpatient basis.

COMPLICATIONS

Side Effects of Intrathecal Morphine

Acute effects of intrathecal morphine include itching, nausea and vomiting, sedation, respiratory depression, urinary retention, and hypotension. Massive overdoses can cause apnea, coma, seizures, and hyperthermia. These side effects are much less likely to occur with chronic, slow lumbar infusion via a drug pump than with bolus injections. However, the long-term infusion of spinal opiates is associated with a number of significant late side effects. Decreased libido and impotence in men and disturbance in the menstrual cycle in women are frequent.[25] These neuroendocrine effects of intraspinal morphine must be recognized, and for men, testosterone replacement may be necessary. Myoclonus can occur and is difficult to treat. High intraspinal doses may produce constipation and bladder incontinence or urinary retention. These problems can usually be managed symptomatically. Peripheral edema may occur in up to 10% of patients and may not respond to diuretics; in severe cases, this may necessitate stopping the morphine infusion.

Complications of Surgery

Numerous problems can arise from pump and catheter placement. A cerebrospinal fluid leak can cause severe spinal headache, requiring bed rest, fluids, and sometimes an epidural blood patch. If a leak extends along the catheter track, fluid accumulation in the pump pocket can occur. If it persists for months, surgery may be necessary to close off the track around the catheter at the lumbar site. Seromas often occur simply as a reaction to the pump itself, but they usually resolve on their own. An infection rate similar to that for other implanted devices is expected, about 3%. Pump pocket or catheter track infection requires removal of the system. Meningitis is rare and can be treated with intrathecal antibiotics using the pump.

Catheter placement rarely causes a problem. Too high a placement can cause injury to the spinal cord due to the large Tuohy needle used to introduce the catheter. The soft Silastic catheter tip does not usually cause root irritation with insertion. Inappropriate placement of the catheter into the subdural or epidural space is possible. A flow of cerebrospinal fluid does not always indicate that subarachnoid placement has been accomplished, because the Tuohy needle can tear the dura and arachnoid, causing cerebrospinal fluid to flow into the subdural or epidural space. Checking the catheter position with fluoroscopy at the time of surgery will detect a bad placement.

Long-term complications of the pump are rare. Catheters, in contrast, may dislodge, kink, break, or be occluded by fibrous scarring.[5] Any unexpected reduction in pain control, if it persists, may indicate a drug delivery problem. A rare, serious catheter complication is the formation of a granuloma at the catheter tip. This has been reported in a number of patients and is associated with increased pain and then symptoms and signs of spinal cord or cauda equina compression.[26–29] Because this phenomenon has not been reported for intrathecal baclofen, it may be a reaction to high-dose morphine. Alternatively, an indolent infection or toxin may be at fault. A change in pain control associated with a new neurological complaint or finding should alert the clinician to this possibility. Magnetic resonance imaging will reveal the granuloma, and surgery is required to remove it.

Tolerance

In up to a third of patients, long-term morphine infusion is unsuccessful. When the pain relief is lost, the pump and catheter system should be checked. If it is clear that the drug is being infused properly, tolerance has developed. A more potent opiate such as hydromorphone (approximately five times as potent) can be tried. This will help only if the amount of opiate delivered is the problem. If marked morphine tolerance has occurred or the pain is no longer responsive to any opiate, switching drugs will fail. A test for true biologic tolerance is a drug holiday over several weeks, which restores sensitivity to morphine. Unfortunately, reintroduction of morphine rapidly induces tolerance again.

The only solution to tolerance or lack of sensitivity to opiates is to use alternative intrathecal medications. A number of non–μ-receptor classes of compounds are available.[30] Local anesthetics are frequently tried with morphine, similar to their use in operative and postoperative pain control. Bupivacaine has been used most frequently because of its potency and availability in a preservative-free form. Another class of drugs is the α$_2$ agonists. These act on descending pathways in the spinal cord and are known to modify nociception. Clonidine is used for chronic epidural infusion for chronic pain. This preservative-free preparation has been used in combination with morphine for intrathecal infusion. Unfortunately, the available preparations of both bupivacaine and clonidine are at too low a concentration for practical application in a drug pump, which at most will deliver 1 mL/day. Therefore, appropriate concentrations have to be made to order for pump use. Because these are "off-label" uses, many physicians are reluctant to do so. Until long-term stability, toxicity, and efficacy studies are done, the use of these medications will be empirical. They should be offered to patients who fail to respond to morphine in whom such off-label use is justified by the clinical situation. Clearly, the patient needs to be informed.

Other classes of drugs are being investigated for intrathecal use. Somatostatin has been effective in reducing postoperative pain.[31] A stable, long-acting analog, octreotide, can be used in the pump and has shown clinical efficacy in cancer patients tolerant to morphine and in two patients with allodynic pain.[32, 33] The cost of this medicine is its major limiting factor. Calcitonin and N-methyl-D-aspartate antagonists have been tried in animal pain models and limited human trials. SNX-111, an N-channel calcium blocker, has had clinical trials and continues to be investigated for safety and efficacy. It is a potent medication and can lead to adverse central nervous system side effects as it ascends to the brainstem and cortical areas. Considering the widely differing classes of medications and the active clinical investigations taking place, new nonopiates should soon be available for intrathecal use. Once a choice is possible, clinicians will be able to empirically test patients with different intrathecal agents to optimize outcome.

ALTERNATIVE APPROACHES

The studies summarized in Table 198–1 support the use of lumbar intrathecal morphine for cancer and chronic nonmalignant pain. However, drug pump techniques are not the only approach. Transplanted tissue has been placed intrathecally to provide pain-relieving substances in the cerebrospinal fluid. Trials in animals have demonstrated that adrenal medullary tissue placed in the lumbar space significantly decreases pain.[34] This effect is only partially antagonized by naloxone, so more than one substance is responsible. All the chemicals released from the medullary tissue are not known, but enkephalins and adrenergics undoubtedly account for some of the response. According to

one report, patients who received an autotransplant of medullary tissue for Parkinson's disease had much less pain than expected.[35] A few cancer patients have had cadaver adrenal medullary tissue injected into the lumbar space to control their pain.[36] A variation of this approach is to use a selective membrane to encapsulate and protect implanted calf adrenal tissue from immunologic destruction. Testing in animals and in humans has demonstrated the feasibility of such an implanted system and suggests that it may be effective, although much more development is needed.

The use of controlled delivery of medication directly into the brain, rather than into the cerebrospinal fluid, is also a possibility. Implanted pumps have been used to deliver morphine into the third ventricle for control of pain from head and neck tumors.[37] The effect is probably mediated by the periaqueductal gray matter, where the morphine receptors are located. Direct placement of a catheter into this region, similar to deep brain stimulation, may be a useful strategy. Other areas in the thalamus or limbic system may also be good targets for intervention. Functional imaging of pain pathways in individual patients may indicate which regions are overactive in chronic pain and where suppression of activity by infusion would relieve pain.

Regardless of future developments, the delivery of chronic intrathecal morphine has an important place in pain control at present, and many patients can be expected to benefit from this technologic advance.

REFERENCES

1. Brazenor G: Long-term intrathecal administration of morphine: A comparison of bolus injection via reservoir with continuous infusion by implanted pump. Neurosurgery 21:484–491, 1987.
2. Follet K, Hitchon P, Piper J, et al: Response of intractable pain to continuous intrathecal morphine: A retrospective study. Pain 49: 21–25, 1992.
3. Hassenbusch S, Pillay P, Magdinec M, et al: Constant infusion of morphine for intractable cancer pain using an implanted pump. J Neurosurg 73:405–409, 1990.
4. Onofrio B, Yaksh T, Arnold P: Continuous low-dose intrathecal morphine administration in the treatment of chronic pain of malignant origin. Mayo Clin Proc 56:526–530, 1981.
5. Penn R, Paice J: Chronic intrathecal morphine for intractable pain. J Neurosurg 67:182–186, 1987.
6. Shetter A: Administration of intraspinal morphine sulfate for the treatment of intractable cancer pain. Neurosurgery 18:740–747, 1986.
7. Krames E, Lanning R: Intrathecal infusional analgesia for nonmalignant pain: Analgesic efficacy of intrathecal opioid with or without bupivacaine. J Pain Symptom Manage 8:539–548, 1993.
8. Tutak U, Doleys D: Intrathecal infusion systems for treatment of chronic low back and leg pain of noncancer origin. South Med J 89:295–300, 1996.
9. Winkelmüller M, Winkelmüller W: Long-term effects of continuous intrathecal opioid treatment in chronic pain of nonmalignant etiology. J Neurosurg 85:458–467, 1996.
10. Van Buyten J: Outcomes of intrathecal morphine. Paper presented at advanced interventional pain therapies meeting, European Continuing Medical Training (ECMT) Symposium, Tenerife, Spain, May 1998.
11. Erdine S, Yücel A: Intrathecal morphine delivered by implanted manual pump for cancer pain. Pain Digest 6:161–165, 1996.
12. Paice J, Penn R, Shott S: Intrathecal morphine for chronic pain: A retrospective, multicenter study. J Pain Symptom Manage 11: 71–80, 1996.
13. Schuchard M, Krames E, Lanning R: Intraspinal analgesia for

nonmalignant pain: A retrospective analysis for efficacy, safety, and feasibility in 50 patients. Neuromodulation 1:45–56, 1998.

14. Mueller-Schwefe G, Hassenbusch S, Reig E: Cost effectiveness of intrathecal therapy for pain. Neuromodulation 2:77–84, 1999.

15. Gestin Y, Vainio A, Pègurier A: Long-term intrathecal infusion of morphine in the home care of patients with advanced cancer. Acta Anaesthesiol Scand 41:12–17, 1997.

16. Yaksh T, Noueihed R: The physiology and pharmacology of spinal opiates. Annu Rev Pharmacol Toxicol 25:433–462, 1985.

17. Penn R, Paice J: Chronic intrathecal morphine for intractable pain. J Neurosurg 67:182–186, 1987.

18. Yaksh T: Opioid receptor systems and the endorphins: A review of their spinal organization. J Neurosurg 67:157–176, 1987.

19. Nordberg G, Hedner T, Mellstrand T, et al: Pharmacokinetic aspects of intrathecal morphine analgesia. Anesthesiology 60: 448–454, 1984.

20. Staren E, Cullen M: Epidural catheter analgesia for the management of postoperative pain. Surg Gynecol Obstet 162:389–404, 1986.

21. Zenz M, Schappler-Scheele B, Neuhaus R, et al: Long-term peridural morphine analgesia in cancer pain. Lancet 1:91, 1981.

22. Penn R: Use and abuse of drug pumps in cancer pain. Clin Neurosurg 35:409–421, 1989.

23. Gianino J, York M, Paice J: Intrathecal Drug Therapy for Spasticity and Pain: Practical Patient Management. New York, Springer-Verlag, 1996.

24. Rosenson A, Ali A, Fordham E, et al: Indium-111 DPTA flow study to evaluate surgically implanted drug pump delivery system. Clin Nucl Med 15:154–156, 1990.

25. Paice J, Penn R, Ryan W: Altered sexual function and decreased testosterone in patients receiving intraspinal opioids. J Pain Symptom Manage 9:126–131, 1994.

26. Blount J, Remley K, Yue S, et al: Intrathecal granuloma complicat-

27. Cabbell K, Taren J, Sagher O: Spinal cord compression by catheter granulomas in high-dose intrathecal morphine therapy: Case report. Neurosurgery 42:1176–1181, 1998.

28. Bejjani G, Karim N, Tzortzidis F: Intrathecal granuloma after implantation of a morphine pump: Case report and review of literature. Surg Neurol 48:288–291, 1997.

29. Schuchard M, Lanning R, North R, et al: Neurologic sequelae of intraspinal drug delivery systems: Results of a survey of American implanters of implantable delivery systems. Neuromodulation 1:137–148, 1998.

30. Hassenbusch S, Garber J, Buchser E, et al: Alternative intrathecal agents for the treatment of pain. Neuromodulation 2:85–91, 1999.

31. Chrubasik J, Meynadier J, Blond S, et al: Somatostatin, a potent analgesic. Lancet 2:1208–1209, 1984.

32. Penn R, Paice J, Kroin J: Octreotide: A potent new non-opiate analgesic for intrathecal infusion. Pain 49:13–19, 1992.

33. Paice J, Penn R, Kroin J: Intrathecal octreotide for relief of intractable nonmalignant pain: 5-year experience with two cases. Neurosurgery 38:203–207, 1996.

34. Sagen J, Wang H: Prolonged anesthesia by enkephalinase inhibition in rats with spinal cord adrenal medullary transplants. Eur J Pharmacol 179:427–433, 1990.

35. Penn R, Goetz C, Tanner C, et al: The adrenal medullary transplant operation for Parkinson's disease: Clinical observations in five patients. Neurosurgery 22:999–1104, 1988.

36. Winnie A, Pappas G, Gupta T, et al: Subarachnoid adrenal medullary transplants for terminal cancer pain. Anesthesiology 79: 644–653, 1993.

37. Lenzi A, Galli G, Gandolfini M, et al: Intraventricular morphine in paraneoplastic painful syndrome of the cervicofacial region: Experience in 38 cases. Neurosurgery 17:6, 1985.

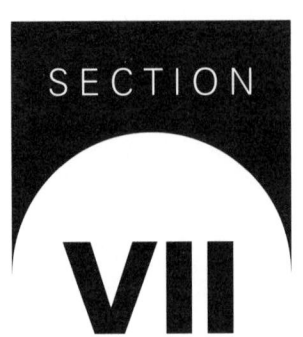

SECTION

VII

Pediatric

CHAPTER **199**

Neurological Surgery in Childhood: General and Historical Considerations

JAMES TAIT GOODRICH

Pediatric neurosurgery as a field has developed only recently, but significant antecedents can be traced to antiquity. This chapter reviews some of the historical developments on which the creation of this subspecialty rests, taking note of the individuals who brought them about. I examine three problems that are the province of pediatric neurosurgery: hydrocephalus, spinal dysraphism, and craniosynostosis.

HYDROCEPHALUS

Hardly any other pathologic condition has been accorded more determined attention on the part of the medical profession with the aim of finding a cure for it than has hydrocephalus. And in hardly a single other condition have cures been so illusive or so often wrecked on purely mechanical obstacles. Yet the outlook is certainly not hopeless. Especially during the past twenty years, during which surgery of the nervous system has improved so remarkably, frequent reports of cures by surgical means have appeared.[1]

Descriptions of hydrocephalus and its associated pathologic changes are among the oldest in medicine. Ancient illustrations of the condition still exist. The early Olmec peoples of Meso-America, for example, described young children with large heads, prominent foreheads, and findings consistent with untreated hydrocephalus[2] (Figs. 199–1 and 199–2), and achondroplastic dwarfs are illustrated in early texts (Fig. 199–3).

In Western medical writings, hydrocephalus first appeared in the works of Hippocrates (ca. 460–368 BC), who described clinical examples. He believed that the accumulation of cerebrospinal fluid (CSF) was caused by the excess *pituita* of chronic epilepsy. Hippocrates described symptoms associated with hydrocephalus: headache, vomiting, visual loss, diplopia, and squinting. He appropriately noted that outcome and prognosis in hydrocephalus were extremely poor.[3] He suggested little in the way of treatment other than laxatives and dietary supplements. Although he was not a surgeon, it has been suggested that he advocated trephination over the anterior fontanelle to relieve pressure. However, my examination of the Hippocratic corpus failed to disclose any recommendations of surgical treatment in his discussion of internal hydrocephalus; at best, Hippocrates[4] might have advocated this form of trephination in a case of external hydrocephalus (i.e., fluid outside the brain).

Galen of Pergamon (130–200 AD), the great Alexandrian anatomist and surgeon, gave several early descriptions of hydrocephalus.[5] He categorized the disorder into four types according to the site of fluid accumulation: between brain and meninges, between meninges and bone, between bone and pericranium, and between pericranium and skin. The condition in which fluid accumulated below the meninges was not curable, whereas fluid above the pericranium could be drained.

Galen was a superb anatomist and appreciated that CSF was in free communication within the ventricular system (i.e., flowed freely throughout the ventricles). He was the first to describe the structure whose discovery was later erroneously attributed to Franciscus de le Boë, or Sylvius (1614–1672), a professor of medicine at Leyden.[6] Galen also provided a complete anatomic description of the foramen of Monro, the communication between the two lateral ventricles; Alexander Monro Secundus (1733–1817), whose credit for the discovery is conveyed by the eponym, did not publish his anatomic findings (which were accurate) until 1783.[7] Galen also provided the first anatomic description of the choroid plexus as well as its name.

Galen incorporated into his humoral theory of hydrocephalus the idea that the "animal spirit" is an

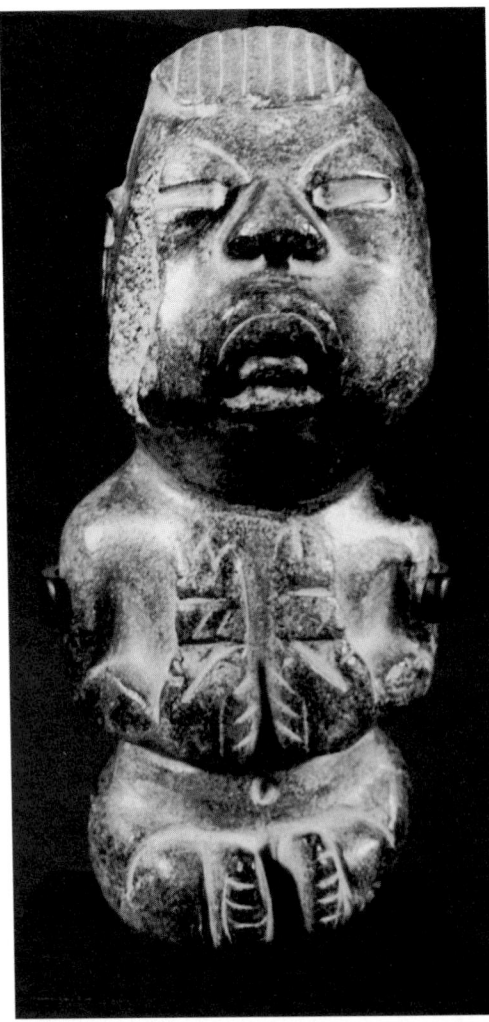

FIGURE 199–1. The serpentine stone statue of a Meso-American achondroplastic dwarf is from the Olmec period (1500–500 BC). The figure shows the typical characteristics of foreshortened arms and legs. These children were held in high regard by the Olmec society. A number of original carvings still exist in collections around the world. (Courtesy of James Tait Goodrich, Montefiore Medical Center, Bronx, NY.)

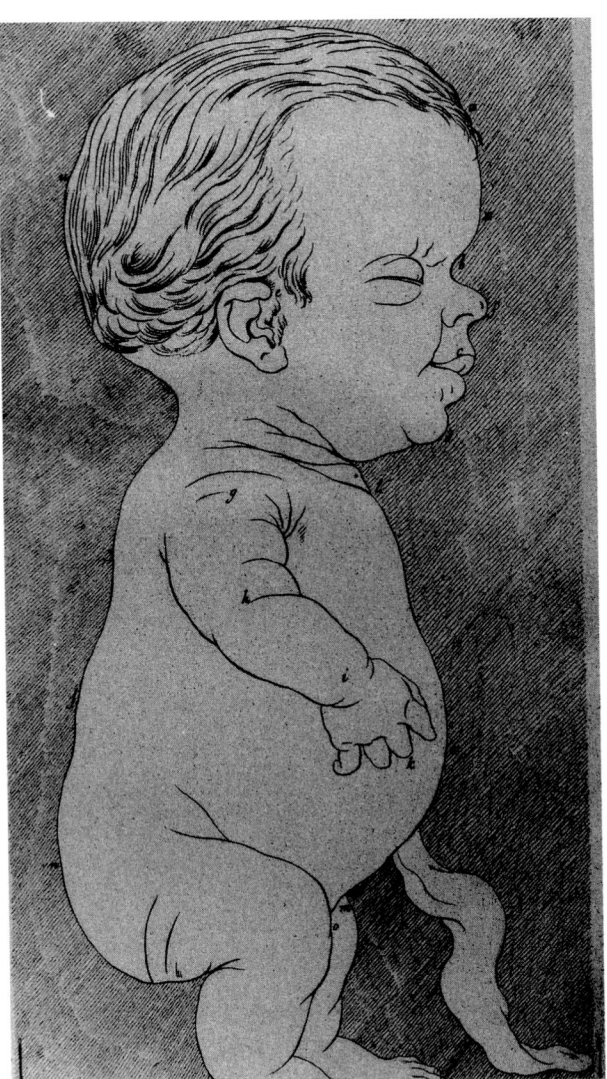

FIGURE 199–3. This illustrated example of an achondroplastic dwarf with hydrocephalus first appeared in a work by S. T. Soemmerring in 1791. (From Soemmerring ST: Abbildungen und Beschreibungen einiger Misgeturten die sich ehemals auf dem anatomischen Theater zu Cassellell befanden. Maninz, Universitäts Buchhanlung, 1791, plate XI.)

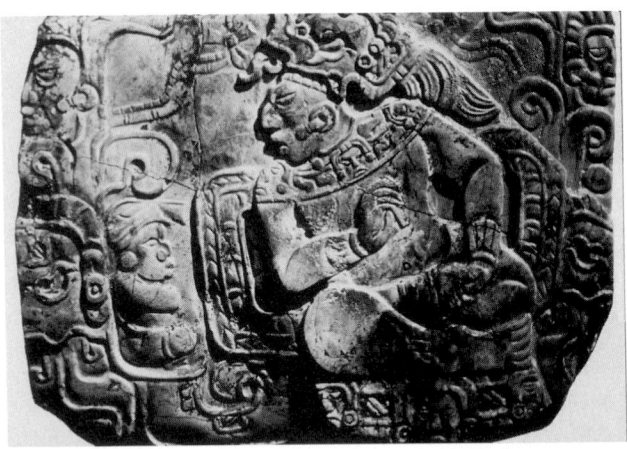

FIGURE 199–2. The carved jadeite stone is from the Mayan classic period (300–800 AD). The dwarf figure on the left side shows evidence of hydrocephalus, and a Mayan noble is looking on.

entity residing within the ventricles. This spirit, he maintained, is purified by its passage through pores in the brain. The waste products then pass through the pituitary gland and are discharged by the nose as *pituita*. In Galen's view, hydrocephalus is caused by a defect in the formation of the animal spirit that results in a backup of fluid. This concept remained in force until well into the 16th century, when it was challenged for the first time by Vesalius in his classic work of 1543.[8] After Galen's animal spirit had been called into question, a number of later investigators characterized the contents of the ventricles as air, vacuum, vapor, or water. These views dominated medical thinking until well into the 18th century.

Oribasius (325–403), a fourth century Byzantine surgeon, classified hydrocephalus into three types. Fluid collections between brain and meninges were not operable, whereas those between bone and pericranium and between pericranium and scalp could be drained.[9] Classifications and views on the surgical treatment of hydrocephalus such as those cited remained intact until just recently. Taking into account an inadequate understanding of the cause plus infection and meningitis from contaminated surgical instruments, it is easy to understand why the outcomes of hydrocephalus surgery were almost invariably lethal until the beginning of the 20th century.

In the Arab tradition, Albucasis (Al-Zahrawi, 936–1013) was a great compiler, scholar, and surgeon, whose writings (about 30 volumes) were focused mainly on surgery, dietetics, and materia medica.[10] His *Compendium* contains an interesting discussion of hydrocephalus:

On the cure of hydrocephalus: This disease occurs most commonly in infants upon delivery when the midwife grasps the child's head roughly. It also sometimes happens from some hidden and unknown cause. I have never seen this disease except in very small children; and death very quickly overtook all those that I have seen; therefore I have preferred not to undertake operation in these cases. I have seen a child whose head was filled with fluid and daily growing in size, until the child could not sit upright on account of the size of his head, and the humidity increased till he died.[11]

In cases of external hydrocephalus, in which the fluid is between the scalp and the skull or the dura and the skull, Albucasis argued for making a T-type incision to drain off the "humidity," and in such cases, he had good results. He cautioned against incising over an artery lest hemorrhage result; the patient can die from that, he pointed out, at the same time that the physician is trying to remove the humidity. An additional treatment in the child with hydrocephalus is to "bind" the head with a wrap and then put the child on a "dry diet" with little fluid—a rather thoughtful and progressive treatment plan for its time.[10]

Albucasis was one of the earliest to popularize the frequent use of emetics as prophylaxis against disease, a concept that has survived in the prescription of "purging" that continued in medical and surgical practice until late into the 19th century. Albucasis's *Compendium* was used extensively in the schools of Salerno and Montpellier and had an important influence in the medieval period. Illustrations of surgical instruments were a unique feature. Many of the instruments were designed by Albucasis; the text describes them, along with technical aspects of their use. One of the instruments was a specially designed scalpel for puncturing the ventricle in children with hydrocephalus.[12]

Albucasis provided an elegant discussion of the infant "ping-pong" fracture of the skull:

This is a fracture due to a fall or a blow from a stone and the like, making a dent in the surface of the bone and a hollow at the site as occurs in a bronze bowl when a blow falls on it and a portion of it is pushed in. This mostly occurs in heads whose bones are soft, as those of children.[13]

One of the most interesting historical examples of hydrocephalus appears in the great anatomic work of

Andreas Vesalius (1519–1564), *De Humani Corporis Fabrica*, published in Basel in 1543.[8] In Book I, in a discussion of "Heads of other shape," he gave the following clinical description:

. . . at Genoa a small boy is carried from door to door by a beggar woman, and was put on display by actors in noble Brabant in Belgium, whose head, without any exaggeration, is larger than two normal human heads and swells out on either side.[14]

In the second edition of *De Humani Corporis Fabrica*, Vesalius described another case of hydrocephalus in a young girl whom he noted to have a head "larger than any man's."[15] In this case, he made the important observation that the fluid had collected within the ventricles and not between the dura and the skull. He reported removing 9 pounds of water from the ventricles at autopsy.[16] These two interesting clinical observations were made by a very skillful early anatomist who offered no insight into the cause or the treatment of the condition that resulted in such remarkably large heads. In 1632, the first illustration of a child with hydrocephalus appeared in an early book on surgical pathology by Marco Aurelia Severino[17] (1580–1656) (Fig. 199–4).

In the 17th and 18th centuries, the first steps were taken, although the path was circuitous, toward what eventually emerged as an understanding of hydrocephalus. Views about CSF production and hydrocephalus contained as many errors as correct observations. Thomas Willis[18] (1621–1675), the prominent London physician and anatomist, believed that the choroid plexus acted only as a "blood filterer," which he stated in his monograph *Pathologiae Cerebri* (1670). Contrary to this view were the writings of Contanzo Variolio[19] (Varolius, 1543–1575), Professor of Anatomy at the University of Bologna and physician to the Pope. Variolio believed that the choroid plexus merely absorbed ventricular fluid. Adding confusion to the picture was Jean Riolan (1580–1657), a Paris anatomist who noted the exceptional vascularity of the choroid plexus and called its constituent vessels the *rete mirablile*, thereby reintroducing an erroneous anatomic concept first postulated by Galen in the second century.[20, 21] However, the brilliant Dutch anatomist Frederik Ruysch[22] (1638–1731) offered a more accurate view, suggesting that choroid plexus was a gland that formed CSF. Albrecht von Haller[23] (1708–1777), one of the intellectual giants of the 18th century, incorporated the recently discovered concept of the circulation of the blood into his theory. He thought that the contents of the ventricles were formed by the vapor produced by the exhalation of the arteries and its subsequent inhalation by the veins.

A bizarre sidelight in the evolution of ideas of CSF circulation was introduced by Antoni Pacchioni[24] (1665–1726), who in 1701 described what are now called the pacchionian granules. Pacchioni suggested that the dura mater was in reality a layer of muscle designed to move fluid around the brain. Pacchioni had no concept of the physiologic role of the granules he described; this had to await the work of Key and Retzius (Fig. 199–5).

One of the best early pathologic descriptions of hy-

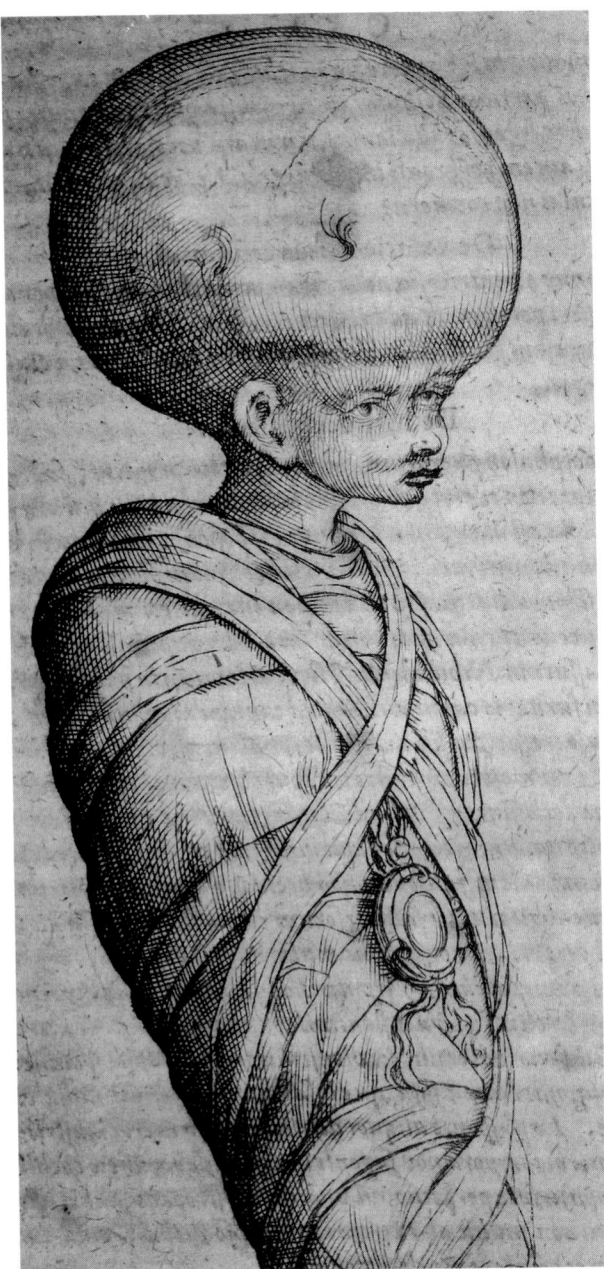

FIGURE 199–4. One of the earliest known illustrations of hydrocephalus appeared in Severino's classic monograph of 1632. (From Severino MA: De Recondita Abscessum Natura, libri VII. Napoli, Beltranum, 1632.)

observations on the various clinical stages, but it offers little in innovative treatment. He categorized hydrocephalus in three stages: stage 1, quickened pulse; stage 2, slow irregular pulse; and stage 3, rapid pulse. In stage 3, the pupils become dilated and are no longer responsive even "in the greatest light."[28] The treatments offered by Whytt were standard for the day: emetics, purging, blisters, and the like. No surgical treatment was discussed, but this was appropriate for the time. Whytt made a pessimistic observation about the late stages of hydrocephalus:

> [When] so much water is accumulated as, by its pressure on the sides of the ventricles, to disturb the action of the brain, we have little to hope from medicine"

—an observation that remained essentially correct for the next 150 years.[27] Other work on understanding the anatomic distribution of CSF was carried out by Domenico Cotugno[29] (1736–1822). His study[29] of experimental animals, published in 1764, showed that CSF

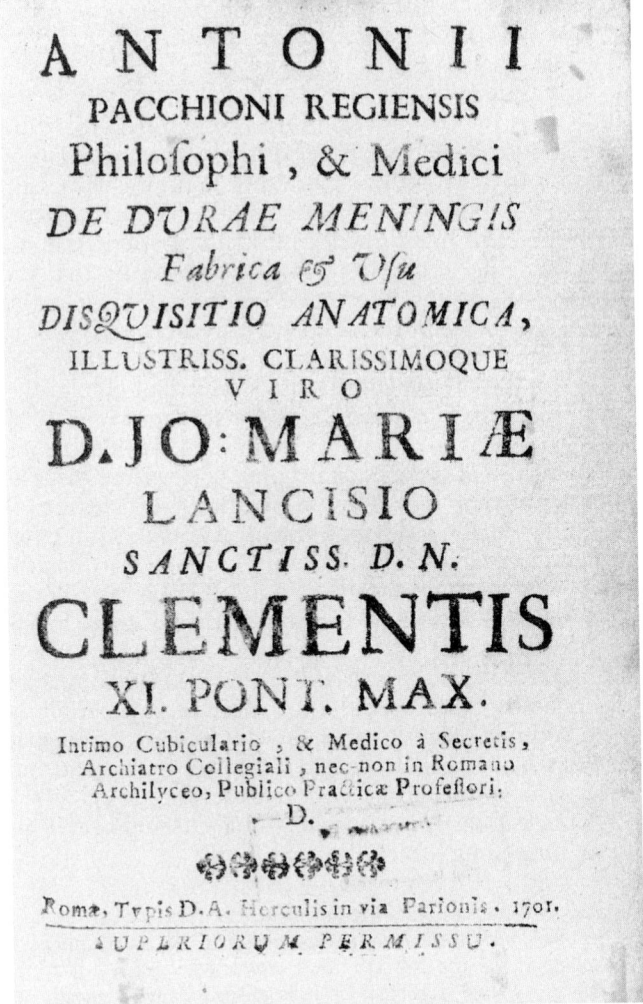

FIGURE 199–5. Title page from Pacchioni's classic work in which he described pacchionian granules. (From Pacchioni A: De Durae Meningis Fabrica & Usu Disquisitio Anatomicae. Rome, DA Herculis, 1701.)

drocephalus was that of G. B. Morgagni[25] (1682–1770) in his classic work of 1761, in which he described a case "Of the hydrocephalus and watery tumour of the spine." This clinical description appears to be the first in which hydrocephalus and spina bifida were associated. Because this was a report of postmortem examinations, no clinical observation or treatment recommendations were offered.[26]

An important early monograph, *Observations on the Dropsy in the Brain*, by the English physician Robert Whytt[27] (1714–1766) appeared in 1768, 2 years after his death. Within this work is an extensive discussion of hydrocephalus with a number of remarkable clinical

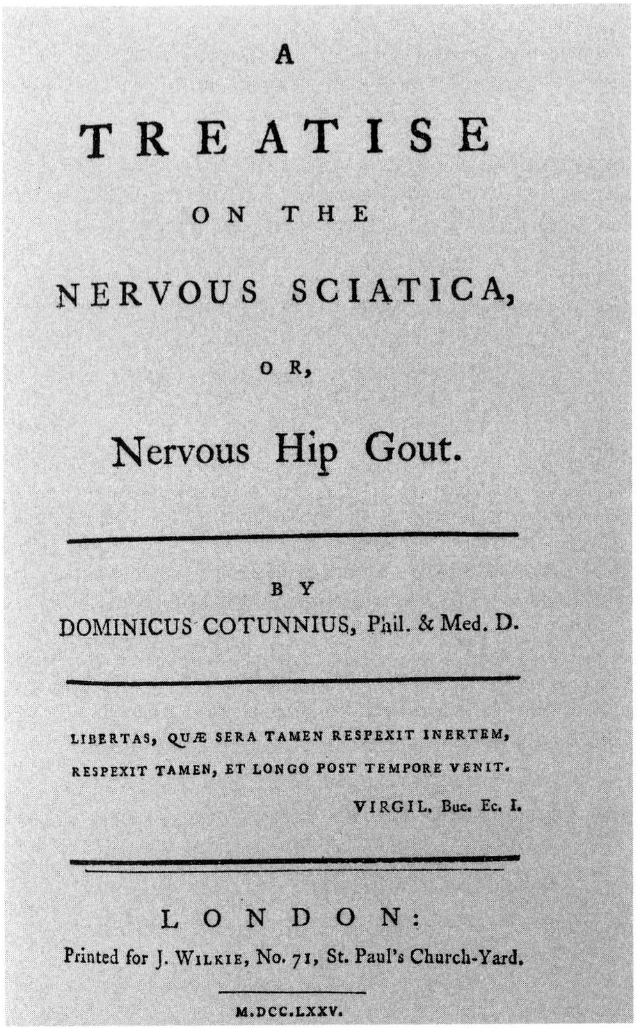

A

TREATISE

ON THE

NERVOUS SCIATICA,

O R,

Nervous Hip Gout.

BY

DOMINICUS COTUNNIUS, Phil. & Med. D.

LIBERTAS, QUÆ SERA TAMEN RESPEXIT INERTEM,

RESPEXIT TAMEN, ET LONGO POST TEMPORE VENIT.

VIRGIL. Buc. Ec. I.

LONDON:

Printed for J. WILKIE, No. 71, St. Paul's Church-Yard.

M.DCC.LXXV.

FIGURE 199–6. Title page from Cotugno's classic work that described spinal fluid. (From Cotugno D: De Ischiade Nervosa Commentarius. Napoli, Fratres Simmonos, 1764.)

was a liquid, not a gas or vapor as first proposed. His description from the 1775 English translation follows:

This water, which fills the tube of the Dura Mater even to the Os sacrum, does not entirely enclose the spinal marrow, but even abounds in the cavity of the skull, and fills all the spaces which are between the brain and the ambitus of the Dura Mater. Some of these spaces are always to be met with about the basis of the brain; and it is not uncommon to find a considerable space between the ambitus itself of the brain, and the surrounding Dura Mater. This is principally to be found in consumptive persons, and old men.[30]

Cotugno was also the first to outline the subarachnoid space accurately (Fig. 199–6). However, Albrecht Haller's vapor theory was firmly in vogue, and years passed before Cotugno's work was accepted. Galen's view of the animal spirit had been eliminated by this time, but his view that the pituitary body was the exit portal of the ventricular contents was still strongly maintained by a number of 18th century physicians. Alexander Monro Secundus argued that hydrocephalus

occurred when sclerosis of the pituitary body prevented egress of CSF, resulting in a backup of fluid, or hydrocephalus.[31] Other contemporary views on hydrocephalus were no further advanced, as is evidenced in one of the most prominent works by John Cheyne (1777–1836), a well-known Scottish physician. In a monograph devoted solely to hydrocephalus, Cheyne attempted to provide a better clinical understanding of this disease and its manifestations.[32] His work, like that of his predecessors, offered little in the way of effective medical or surgical treatment. The standard regimen of bleeding, purging, vomiting, leeches, and the like was used, mainly with the idea of removing "excess water." Cheyne did, however, offer an excellent clinical description of the stages (i.e., degrees of severity of the condition in a child) (Figs. 199–7 and 199–8):

In the first stage, every stimulus produces a sensation more than proportioned to its common effects. There is great aversion to light and to sounds; there is watching, sickness, pain, a quick pulse. In the second stage, the child is not easily roused, his pupil dilated, his pulse slow, he is lethargic, with

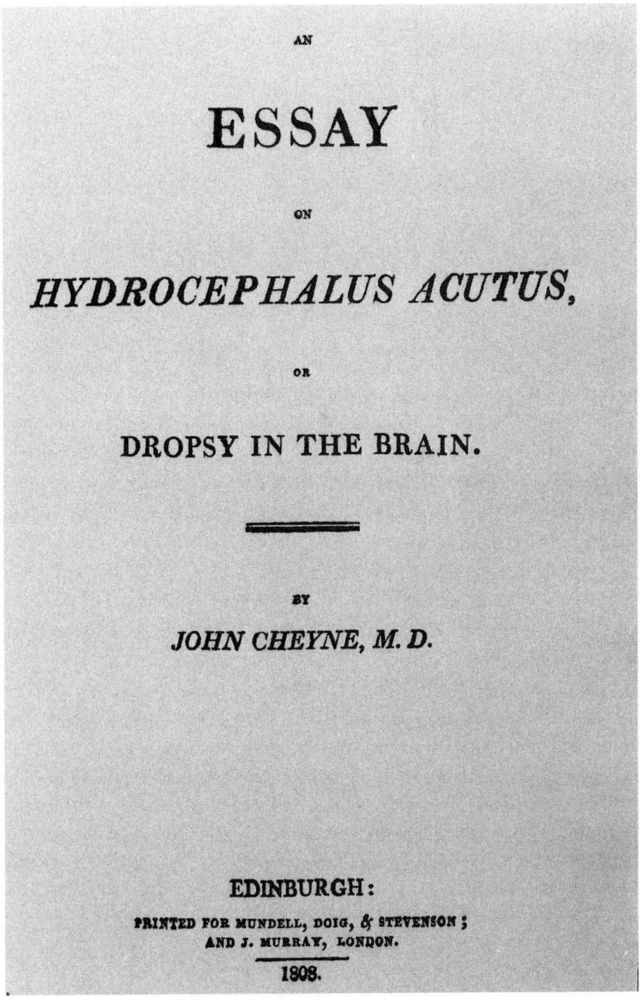

AN

ESSAY

ON

HYDROCEPHALUS ACUTUS,

OR

DROPSY IN THE BRAIN.

BY

JOHN CHEYNE, M. D.

EDINBURGH:

PRINTED FOR MUNDELL, DOIG, & STEVENSON;

AND J. MURRAY, LONDON.

1808.

FIGURE 199–7. Title page from Cheyne's 1808 monograph on hydrocephalus. (From Cheyne J: An Essay on Hydrocephalus Acutus, or Dropsy in the Brain. Edinburgh, Mundell, Doig, & Stevenson, 1808.)

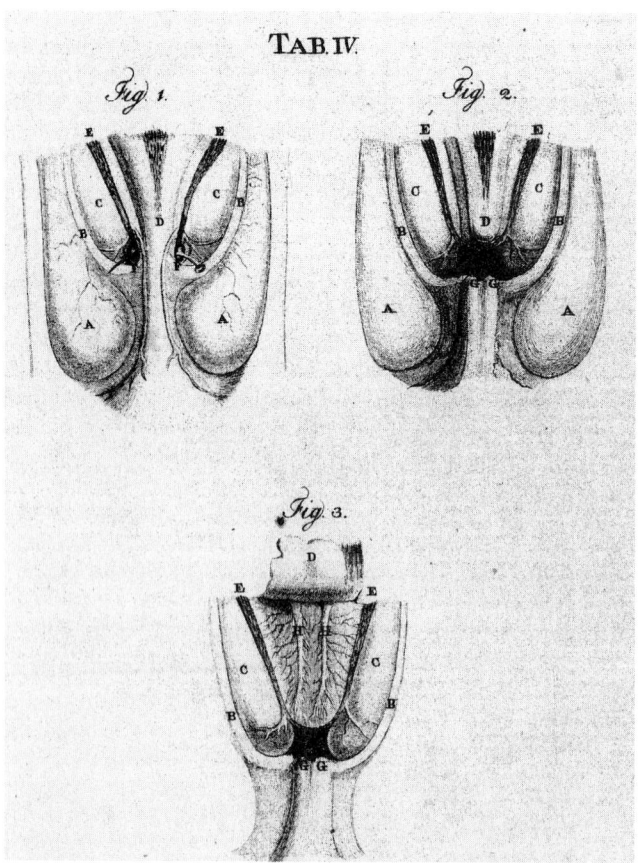

FIGURE 199–8. The original illustration of the foramen of Monro. (From Monro A: Observations of the Structure and Function of the Nervous System. Edinburgh, Creech-Johnson, 1783.)

often an obstinately costive belly. In the third stage, which perhaps may be considered as a continuation of the second, there is squinting, rolling of the head, raving, stupor, convulsions, with a rapid thready pulse.[32]

During this period, debates on the anatomic features of CSF pathways were being conducted by a number of anatomists and physicians. Alexander Monro Secundus accurately described the foramen of Monro.[7] This great anatomist denied the existence of the foramen of Magendie, whereas Haller and Cotugno affirmed it. Monro based his claim on his postmortem examination of a hydrocephalic child in whom he found no communication between the fourth ventricle and the spinal subarachnoid space because this space was occluded by the choroid plexus. Ironically, this lack of communication is what most likely caused the hydrocephalus.[31]

François Magendie[33] (1783–1855) clarified this anatomic point (i.e., foramen of Magendie) in his classic study of 1842. Although Magendie described the foramen that bears his name, Herbert von Luschka (1820–1875), Professor of Anatomy at Tübingen, clearly documented its existence in a series of animals studies in 1854 and named it after Magendie.[34] These anatomic findings were supported by the work of John Hilton (1804–1878), who provided the first anatomic drawings of these pathways and showed that internal hydrocephalus could occur because of obstruction along

these CSF pathways.[35] Axel Key (1832–1901) and Gustav Retzius (1842–1919) were the first to demonstrate conclusively, in their classic studies published in 1875,[36] that CSF flows through the foramen of Magendie (Fig. 199–9).

Magendie made other important contributions to understanding hydrocephalus. In studies making use of an animal model of the condition,[33] he demonstrated that the ventricles and subarachnoid space in living subjects were filled with a watery fluid that communicated freely between the ventricles and the spinal subarachnoid space through the foramen of Magendie—a view first postulated by Cotugno in 1764 but not accepted! Magendie described cases of hydrocephalus resulting from obstruction at the aqueduct of Sylvius and the foramen of Magendie. In an autopsy, he demonstrated that a puerperal thrombosis had led to a thrombosis of the vein of Galen and dural sinuses, resulting in hydrocephalus. The hydrocephalus was postulated to have occurred because of reduced absorption of CSF resulting from venous obstruction.

An interesting error—that CSF is produced by the pia—was perpetuated in Magendie's view, a view that continued to be asserted by others, including Lewan-

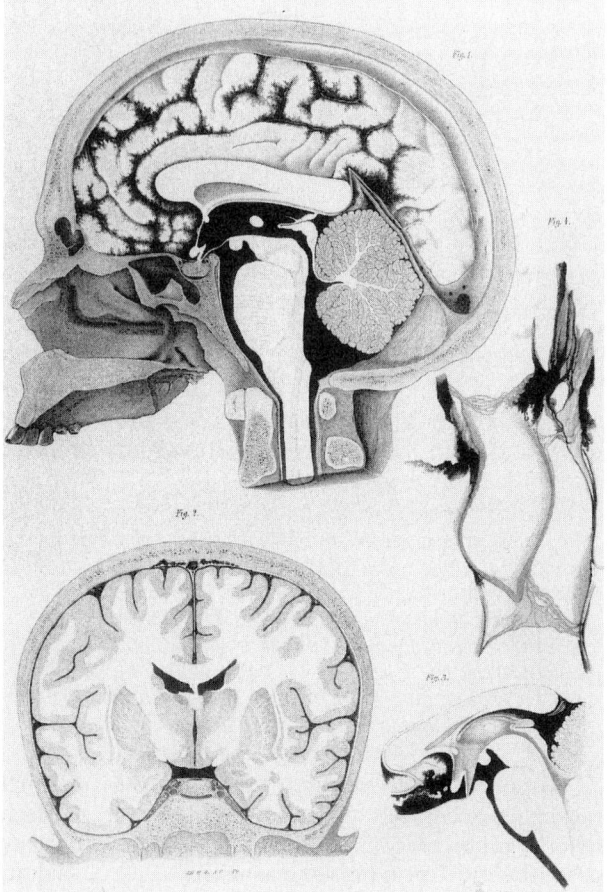

FIGURE 199–9. Cerebrospinal fluid circulation was illustrated by Key and Retzius in 1875. In the original illustration, blue is used to show the dye resorption seen by these investigators. (From Key A, Retzius G: Studien in der Anatomie des Nervensystems und des Dindesgewebes. Stockholm, Norstedt & Söner, 1875.)

dowsky,[37] Spina,[38] and Schmorl,[39] until well into the 20th century. Max Lewandowsky[37] (1876–1918) of Berlin declared that CSF was primarily a brain secretion, only a small portion of which was produced by the pia. Spina[38] argued that CSF was a transudation product of brain capillaries and the pia. Georg Schmorl[39] stated that CSF was formed by the ventricles and the pia. He believed there was no anatomic communication between the ventricles and the spinal subarachnoid space. It was not until the publication by Walter Dandy (1886–1946) and Kenneth D. Blackfan (1883–1941) of their classic study[40] of 1914 using a series of artificial blockages in dogs and phenolsulfonphthalein dye that the true pathways of communication were conclusively established. Equally important, Dandy and Blackfan[41] demonstrated how blockage of the pathways at one or another site caused the various forms of hydrocephalus, resolving the centuries-old dispute.

The importance of Dandy and Blackfan's work was not restricted to the anatomic features relevant to hydrocephalus. A number of anatomic errors regarding CSF foramina had been published in the 19th century. The foramen of Bichat had been described in 1819 as a communication between the space around the vein of Galen and the third ventricle.[1] Bichat later described a foramen (i.e., lateral foramen of Bichat) at the tip of each lateral ventricle. Even the prominent pathologist Rudolf Virchow (1821–1902) had questioned the open flow of CSF between the cerebral subarachnoid space and the spinal subarachnoid space and expressed strong doubts about the existence of the foramen of Luschka and foramen of Magendie as part of these communication pathways:

> There is no direct communication between the subarachnoid spaces, either between each other or with the cavities of the brain, and the fluid contained in them cannot simply rise or fall. (Die subarachnoidealen Raüme stehen in keiner offenen Verbindung, weder unter sich, noch mit de Hirnhöhlen, und die in ihnen enthaltene Flüssigkeit könne daher nicht einfach in ihnen auf oder absteigen.)[42]

The correction of these errors required the efforts of several major figures in the neurosciences. The foramina of Bichat were proved to be artifacts in a series of studies that included the work of Magendie and Luschka and the dye studies of Key and Retzius. Key and Retzius[36] demonstrated the pathways of CSF flow through the foramen of Magendie in their classic studies published in 1875. They attributed CSF absorption to the pacchionian granulations. After injecting colored dye under pressure into the subarachnoid space, they observed the dye entering into the pacchionian bodies along the sagittal sinus. The definitive proof of the nonexistence of the foramina of Bichat was accomplished by Dandy and Blackfan[40] using phenolsulfonphthalein flow studies in 1914.

We cannot leave the topic of the origin and nature of hydrocephalus without revisiting the question of the source of CSF. The concept that the choroid plexus produces CSF was recognized as early as 1854, when Ernest Faivre[43, 44] (1827–1879) published his findings on

CSF production. This source of CSF production was not readily accepted by all. As late as 1912, William Mestrezat[45] (1883–1928) proposed the view that the choroid plexus was not a glandular structure and did not secrete CSF. The secretory activity of the choroid plexus was finally established by the anatomic studies of Dixon and Halliburton,[46] Weed,[47–50] and Cushing.[51, 52] The insights of Dandy and Blackfan[40] into the production of CSF by glandular secretion and filtration revolutionized the concept of hydrocephalus and its treatment:

> The pia is almost exclusively a tissue of blood-vessels, and resembling very closely the pulmonary parenchyma, offers the most favorable conditions for a secretion, prompt and considerable. Everything, therefore, leads us to suppose the pia to be the secretory organ of the cerebrospinal fluid.

This concept was refined in the classic studies summarized in Cushing's Cameron Lectures given in 1925 on the "Third Circulation."[52] In this work and earlier papers, Cushing clarified the active secretion of CSF by the choroid plexus and other details of this so-called third circulation.

Medical Treatment of Hydrocephalus

Medical treatments over the years for hydrocephalus have included blood letting and the application of external vesicants, leeches, aperients, and caustics. Laxatives and medicines for the treatment of dropsy also have been used. Some rather remarkable treatments, such as the use of sneezing agents (e.g., asafoetida), were advocated by William Buchan[53] (1729–1805), a widely read 18th century English physician. By hearty sneezing, the *pituita* or accumulation of fluid in the brain would be removed through the nose—an outrageous treatment but certainly less lethal than the clinical application of the trephine to the anterior fontanelle.

One of the most popular books on pediatrics in the 18th century, *A Treatise on the Treatment of Diseases of Children*, was written Michael Underwood[54] (1732–1820). He reduced the classification of hydrocephalus to two categories: *internal*, which occurred within the ventricles, and *external*, which occurred outside the brain. The first form was invariably lethal, whereas the latter had a better outcome in some cases. Underwood applied vesicants along the sagittal sinus (and on the body) in the hope of "drying out" the fluid. Underwood also used a combination of mercurial derivatives and diuretics to treat hydrocephalus; the concept of using diuretics was remarkably advanced although rarely curative.

Surgical Treatment of Hydrocephalus

Except for cases that cure themselves, i.e., those that undergo spontaneous arrest, the outlook is almost hopeless. The majority die within the first four years of life, the first year claiming most of them. . . . At the present time, even the best-intentioned surgery can hardly serve other than to delay to some few cases the possibility of a spontaneous recovery by subjecting them to an operation and a surgical death.[55]

As expected, the surgical treatment of hydrocephalus has continued to evolve over the centuries. Innovative surgeons have introduced trocars of various types into the ventricles through the anterior fontanelle to drain CSF. An Italian surgeon, Dominico Galvani[56] (d. 1649), developed an ingenious drainage system in the 17th century. Included in this system was a device to hold the drainage tube in place, various receptacles for collecting CSF, a trocar used to place the drain, and a cap to prevent air entering and getting into the ventricles.[56] Another trocar-type system was described by Claude Nicholas Le Cat[57] (1700–1768) in the *Philosophical Transactions of the Royal Society (London)* in 1753, which had an illustration of a child with hydrocephalus. Le Cat noted that his outcomes were dismal and that the mortality rate eventually reached 100%. Alexander Monro Secundus[31] also advocated drainage through a trocar but only in cases of "external hydrocephalus"; otherwise, he declared, the outcome was invariably lethal. All subsequent experience proved him correct; the only outcome of such treatment has been death due to sepsis and meningitis. Antoine Chipault[58] (1866–1920) also employed a trocar. In his technique (1894), the trocar was placed into the ventricle through the nose. He did not discuss the outcomes, but it is reasonable to assume that the results were not good. Langenbeck and Hahn[59] (1859) introduced an innovative technique in which the trocar was passed through the orbital roof into the ventricle; however, the mortality rate remained 100% (Fig. 199–10).

In the next 75 years, many new approaches were recorded. In 1891, Heinrich Quincke[60, 61] (1842–1922) introduced the lumbar puncture, offering one of the earliest modern methods for reducing CSF fluid accumulation, but the results were temporary at best. Quincke[60, 61] showed that CSF was constantly produced so that removed fluid was replaced in a matter of hours.

In the ensuing developments, two principal threads are important: the neurosurgical procedure to be performed on the brain and what was to be done with the excess CSF. The concept of moving CSF fluid from one anatomic space to another was introduced by A. H. Ferguson[62] (1853–1912) in 1898, when he described a technique for connecting the lumbar thecal sac to the peritoneal cavity by a wire passed through a vertebral body. This concept was enhanced in 1908 by Heile,[63] who anastomosed the lumbar thecal sac to the greater

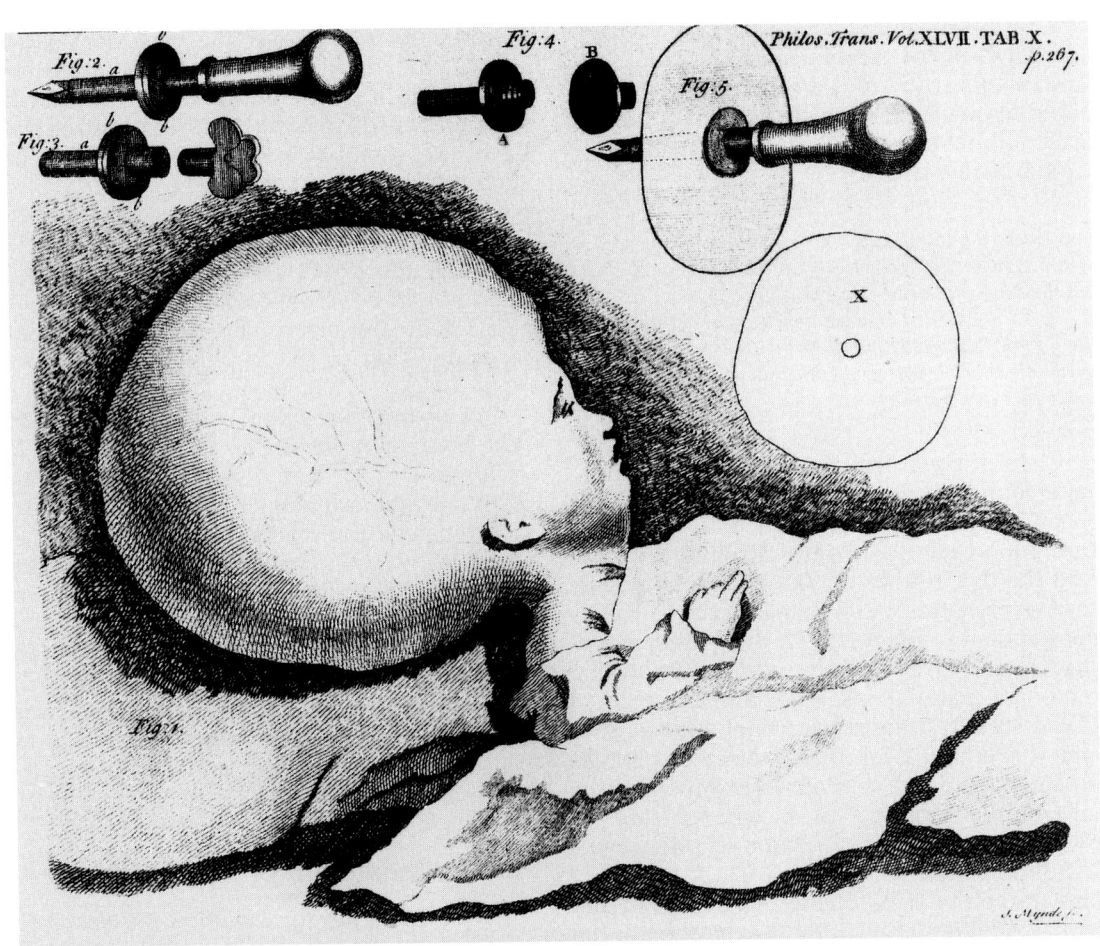

FIGURE 199–10. In 1753, Le Cat described a new trocar system for the treatment of hydrocephalus. (From Le Cat CN: A new trocart [sic] for the puncture in the hydrocephalus, and for other evacuations, which are necessary to be made at different times. Philos Trans R Soc Lond 47:267–272, 1753.)

omentum with a vein graft. Draining CSF from the ventricle to the subaponeurotic space of the scalp was proposed by Kanusch[64] in 1908. Early in the 20th century, several investigators[65, 66] suggested draining CSF from the ventricles into neck veins. A lumbar ureteral shunt was described in 1925 by Heile[67] and later revised by Donald Matson[68] in 1949. Matson further modified this approach by placing polyethylene tubes in the lumbar subarachnoid space and "tunneling" them into the peritoneal cavity, a technique still used in treating pseudotumor cerebri. Virtually every space imagined has been used for diversion of CSF from the ventricles to the chest, ureter, fallopian tubes, mastoid cells, jejunum, various veins, and gallbladder.

An internal technique for diverting CSF was introduced by Arne Torkildsen[69] in 1939. The ventriculocisternostomy initially proved to be extremely effective for bypassing stenosis of the aqueduct. Nevertheless, this procedure fell out of favor later as diversion shunts came into greater use.

As early as 1895, Gardner[70] had suggested that hydrocephalus could be treated by creating a communication between the lateral ventricle and the lymphatic or venous system. Although the idea was good, continuous clotting of the communicating tube made it impractical until Nulsen and Spitz[71] treated a 14-month-old child with a ball valve–regulated subcutaneous system. This system was refined in 1951, when Holter, an engineer, and Spitz, a neurosurgeon, introduced a unilateral valve (i.e., Spitz-Holter valve) that regulated CSF flow in a diversion system—the ventriculocaval shunt. This approach eliminated the problem of clotting within the diversionary tube.[71]

The early results with shunts of these types were encouraging because of the lower mortality rates. Spitz,[72] working at the Children's Hospital of Philadelphia, summarized his results for more than 400 patients using the Holter system. This group had only 15 deaths, and the shunt revision rate was reduced from 37% to 22%, a remarkable improvement over the early techniques.

These concepts were refined in 1957 by Robert Pudenz,[73] who introduced a single, one-way valve system for diversion of CSF from the ventricle to the atrium. This system was predicated on a simple but critical concept: one-way flow of CSF into the atrium during diastole (i.e., without reverse flow of blood into the catheter during systole). However, it rapidly became apparent that ventriculoatrial shunts had high complication rates because of catheter emboli, leading to cor pulmonale and renal emboli. As a result, most shunts are now placed in the peritoneal cavity.[74]

According to Loyal Davis,[75] the first plexectomy was performed by Lespinasse in Chicago in 1910, when he introduced a small cystoscope into the ventricle and fulgurated the structure bilaterally. One infant treated in this way died postoperatively, and another lived for 5 years. Regrettably, these cases were reported only in the form of a presentation at a local medical society meeting.

The studies of Dandy[76–79] and others led to an understanding of the various CSF blocks and flow patterns and to more rational surgical treatments. Dandy, Putnam, Scarff, and others[76–87] initially advocated the removal of the choroid plexus by endoscopic resection. Dandy refined this technique by converting it into an open procedure, exposing the ventricle, removing the CSF, and then fulgurating the choroid plexus. Recourse to an open technique was necessitated by the heavy debris left behind by the endoscopic approach, which sometimes led to blockage of the foramen of Monro or the aqueduct of Sylvius.

In addition to obliteration of the choroid plexus, Dandy[76–79] developed other surgical treatments for hydrocephalus, including cannulation of the aqueduct of Sylvius and the third ventriculostomy. Both treatments were developed in the hope of correcting newly understood abnormalities in the pathways of CSF movement. By the end of the 1940s, the plexectomy had become the primary treatment of choice for hydrocephalus.[88]

The third ventriculostomy, popularized by Dandy in 1922, had one serious disadvantage—sacrifice of an optic nerve when a transtemporal approach was followed.[78] It was not until 1945 that Dandy[89] reported his results for 92 cases: a 12% mortality rate and 50% success rate in arresting hydrocephalus, with follow-up ranging from 6 months to 23 years. Scarff and Stookey[87] modified the third ventriculostomy by using a transfrontal approach and puncturing the floor of the third ventricle through the lamina terminalis. They reported six cases, with one operative death, one failure to arrest the hydrocephalus, and four good results. By 1951, Scarff[85] was able to report follow-up results for 34 cases, with an operative mortality rate of 12% and successful arrest of hydrocephalus in 54%. Putnam,[82] another pioneer of choroid plexectomy, also reported good results: 49 operations in 26 patients, with 10 operative deaths, a strikingly high number, but surviving patients appeared to do well and had normal mentation. At a meeting of the Société de Neurologie de Paris in 1936, De Martel and others reported a single case of a subfrontal third ventriculostomy with relief of obstructive hydrocephalus.[86]

In 1954, Ransohoff and colleagues[90] described the ventriculopleural shunt and its use in six patients, with no morbidity and success in diverting CSF to the pleural space. He and his colleagues followed up this study in 1960 with a report[91] of 83 patients, with a 4% operative mortality rate and 65% success rate in controlling hydrocephalus.

By the 1940s, the subspecialty of pediatric neurosurgery was rapidly developing techniques for treatment of complex CSF production pathways. The introduction of internally placed, regulated one-way valve systems allowed successful treatment of a benign disease that previously had very high morbidity and mortality rates. The concept of pediatric subspecialization was extended to the areas of spina bifida and craniosynostosis, two disorders that were truly within the domain of the subspecialist in pediatrics and neurosurgery.

SPINAL DYSRAPHISM

Alius morbus oritur ex defluxione capitis per venas in spinalem medullam. Inde autem in sacrum os impetum facit, quo medulla ipsa fluxionem perducit.[92]

Spinal dysraphism is illustrated in a number of small terra-cotta sculptures from the Meso-American period. Descriptions of the malformation are found in the early writings of Hippocrates, Galen, and others, although these writers lacked any formal comprehension of the disorder. The earliest definitive description was probably that of Peter van Forest[93] (1522–1597), a Dutch clinician who gave an account of a child with a neck malformation that appears to be a form of spina bifida. An early illustrated example of spinal dysraphism appeared in 1641 in the writings of Nicholas Tulp[94] (1593–1674), to whom we owe the term *spina bifida*. In this work, Tulp described six cases, one of which was that of a child with a large lumbar myelomeningocele arising from a narrow pedicle (Fig. 199–11). He dissected the sac and ligated the pedicle, but the patient soon died of infection. Tulp's text illustration shows the sac and dissected nerves at autopsy. The descriptive term *spina bifida* is used in the plate's legend.[95]

Frederik Ruysch[22, 96] (1638–1731) published 10 cases of spina bifida in 1691:

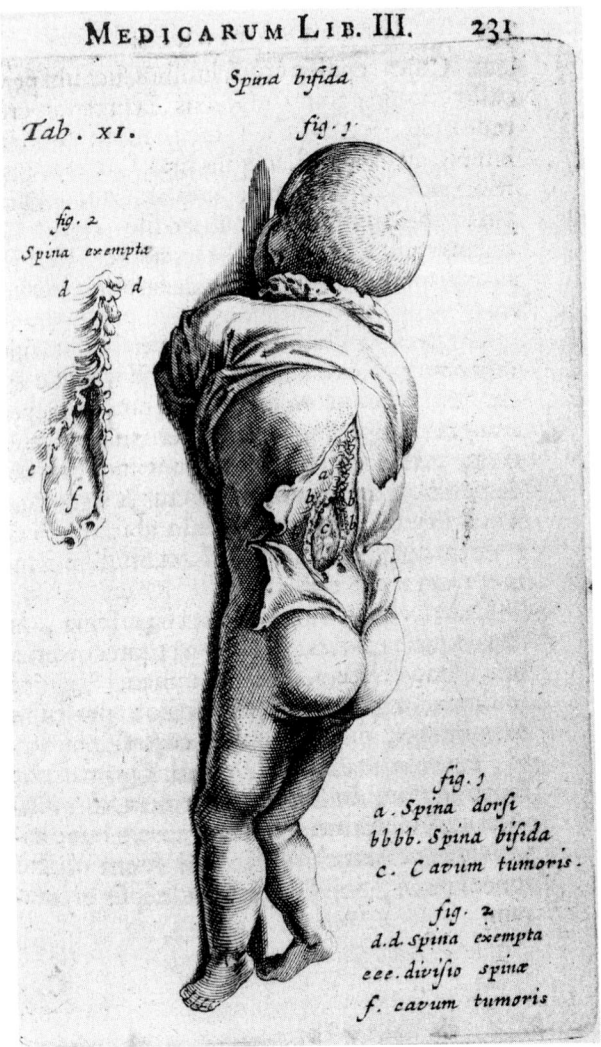

FIGURE 199–11. This illustration is considered to be one of the earliest examples of spina bifida. (From Tulpius N: Observations Medicae, libri III. Amsterdam, Elzeririum, 1641, p 231.)

A tumor frequently arises in the loins of a foetus, while it is yet an inhabitant of the uterus. . . . if we rightly examine this tumor, it will appear as plain as the Noon Sun to be a dropsy, in part of the spinal medulla and is almost the same disorder, allowing for the difference of situation with that which in the head of the foetus is commonly called an hydrocephalus. Whereas, it is surprising that I should often find the spinal medulla well conditioned below the tumor; whence some children retain the motion of their lower limbs, whereas I have found others with their lower limbs paralytic for want of the spinal medulla. With respect to the cure of this disorder, little or nothing can be done toward it.[96]

Some of the finest and earliest illustrated examples of spina bifida were prepared by Jean Cruveilhier (1791–1874) and published in his series of fascicles published over 15 years.[97] He believed that this abnormality resulted from a defect of development, a remarkably early insight (Fig. 199–12).

The first and still classic classification of spina bifida, based on a characterization of the contents of the thecal sac, was developed by Friedrich Daniel von Recklinghausen[98] (1833–1910) in 1886. A few years earlier (1875), Rudolf Virchow[99] (1821–1902) had coined the term *spina bifida occulta*, a term that is now part of our standard nomenclature. In Recklinghausen's illustrated example (Fig. 199–13), the accuracy of his description can still be appreciated. von Recklinghausen also described a case of spina bifida occulta with an associated congenital clubfoot with hypertrichosis.

Baxter,[100] unaware of the findings of Morgagni of 1761, described the association of hydrocephalus with meningocele in 1882. Another anomaly associated with spina bifida was described in 1881 by Lebedeff[101] in a case of spina bifida associated with anencephaly.

Spina bifida was further elucidated in the classic anatomic studies by Kermauner,[102] Keiller,[103] and Bohnstedt.[104] The term *myelodysplasia* was coined by Fuchs[105] in 1910 to denote spina bifida, enuresis, and associated deformities of the feet. This clinical syndrome was further refined in the classic paper by de Vries[106] in 1928. Lichtenstein[107] used the term *spinal dysraphism* to describe a pleomorphic group of disorders of cutaneous, mesodermal, or neural origin. Lichtenstein[108] also discussed the neuroanatomic effects of spina bifida on distant parts of the central nervous system.

The treatment of spina bifida has varied over the years and in most cases involved nothing more than ligation or amputation of the sac. The outcome was usually fatal because of leakage and infection or the resultant hydrocephalus. A typical 18th century case of surgical treatment of spina bifida was described by Benjamin Bell[109] (1749–1806). He placed a tight snare ligature around the base of the sac. Bell appreciated that hydrocephalus was commonly associated with this disorder. The outcome was fatal in all the cases Bell described, leading him to comment:

This is perhaps the most fatal disease to which infancy is liable; for as yet no remedy has been discovered for it. . . . Experience shows, however, that every attempt of this kind should be avoided; for hitherto the practice has uniformly proved unsuccessful. The patient has either died suddenly, or in the course of a few hours after the operation.[109]

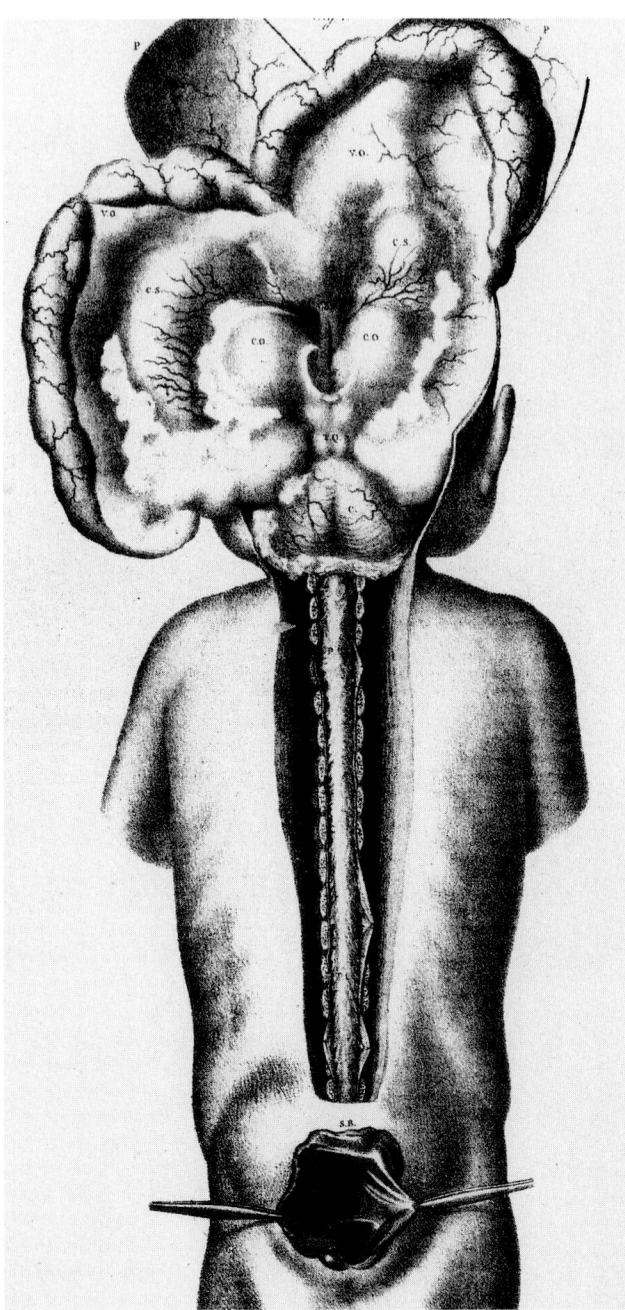

FIGURE 199–12. Some of the finest illustrations of spina bifida were published by Cruveilhier in a series of fascicles in the early 19th century. (From Cruveilhier J: Anatomie pathologique du corps humain. Paris, JB Baillière, 1829.)

A 19th century clinical view of spina bifida was provided by Samuel Cooper[110] (1780–1848), a prominent English surgeon who summed up the clinical problems with this disorder and the lack of successful treatment:

> The generality of children, affected with spina bifida, are deficient in strength, and subject to frequent diarrhoea [sic]. Incontinence of urine and the feces, emaciation, weakness, and even complete paralysis, are sometimes the concomitants of this serious complaint. However, some of the patients are,

in every respect, except the tumor, perfectly healthy, and well formed.[110]

Discussing surgery, Cooper remarked,

> Experience has fully proved that puncturing the tumor with a lancet and thus discharging the fluid, either at once or gradually, cannot be done without putting the patient in the greatest danger, the consequences being for the most part fatal in a very short space of time.[110]

Other techniques for treating spina bifida included injecting the sac with sclerosing solutions, typically iodine or potassium iodide. The reported mortality was less in such cases, but the neurological deficits were increased.[111]

Palasciano[112] proposed a new method to treat spina bifida cystica and encephalocele in the 1850s. He emptied the dysraphic sac of CSF and concentrically compressed it to bring together the cranial or vertebral margins of the defect and then injected iodine into the sac to induce sclerosis. This technique was refined by Francesco Rizzoli[113] (1809–1880) in 1869. In his cases, sclerosing iodine was abandoned as too damaging to the nervous elements. To treat myelomeningoceles, he designed and applied a "Rizzoli enterotome" to the dysraphic sac and slowly closed it, allowing the sac to slough off. Rotated flaps of musculofascial tissues were first used in 1892, when Bayer[114] reported on surgical repair of an open myelomeningocele using flap techniques. This new concept of replacing the neural elements within the canal and covering them with surrounding tissues was a remarkable advance (Figs. 199–14 and 199–15).

In the modern period, ideas about the timing of surgery for spina bifida changed several times. In 1943, Ingraham and Hamlin[115] stated that surgery should be delayed until 18 months of age to allow adequate assessment of the patient's neurological outcome. If the neurological impairment was not too severe and the IQ was normal, surgical closure was recommended. In the 1960s, earlier surgery was advocated by Lorber, Matson, Sharrard, and others within the first week of life to avoid complications. Such timing has become routine in most countries.[116] As a result of the complexity of these newborn disorders and their long-term follow-up, these lesions have come into the domain of the pediatric neurosurgeon. There are still rare exceptions; in some parts of the world, these surgical cases are still handled by pediatric surgeons.

CRANIOSYNOSTOSIS AND RELATED CRANIOFACIAL ANOMALIES

Craniosynostosis is one of the oldest known clinical anomalies. Remarkably, its intentional induction has been recorded in many cultures around the world, placing it in a category shared with few other diseases and disorders.[117, 118] The concept of cranial deformation as a means of bestowing indicia of tribal identity and of beautification is truly ancient. Terra-cotta and stone

Untersuchungen

über die

Spina bifida.

Von

Prof. F. v. Recklinghausen

in Strassburg.

Mit 2 Tafeln und 1 Zinkographie.

Berlin.

Druck und Verlag von Georg Reimer.

1886.

A

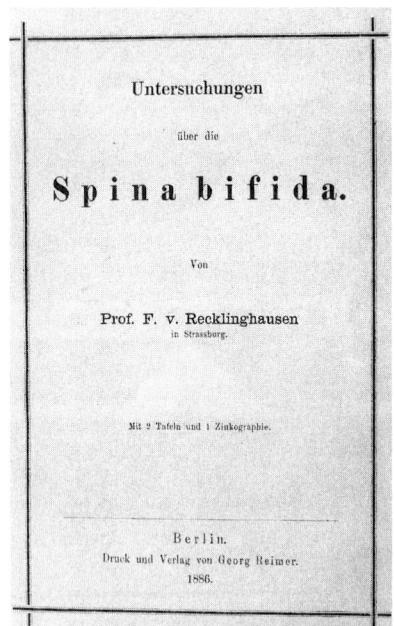

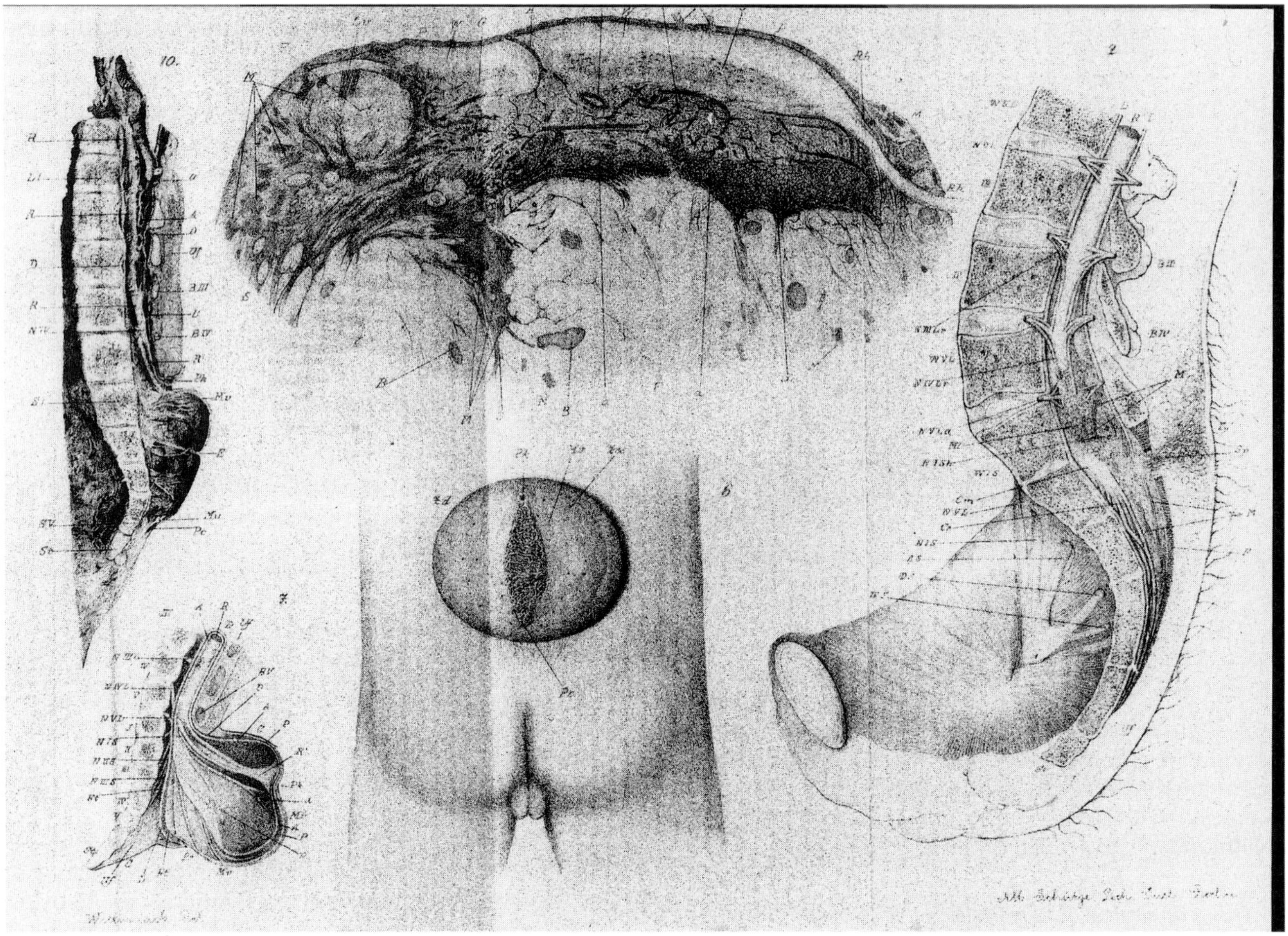

B

FIGURE 199–13. *A* and *B,* One of the earliest anatomically accurate illustrations of spina bifida was from a monograph by von Recklinghausen. (From von Recklinghausen F: Untersuchungen über die Spina Bifida. Berlin, Druck & Verlag von Georg Reimer, 1886.)

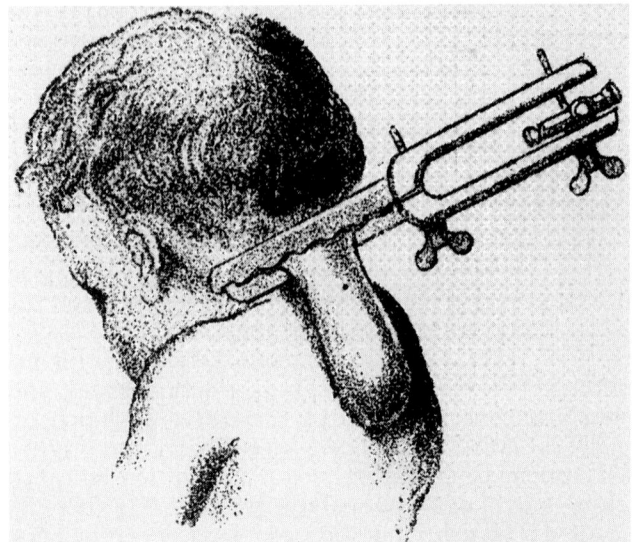

FIGURE 199–14. Innovative treatment of myelomeningocele was introduced by Rizzoli, an Italian surgeon. The Rizzoli enterotome is illustrated. (From Rizzoli F: Memoires de Chirurgie et d'Obstétrique. Paris, Delahaye, 1872.)

figures of cranial disfigurement and artificially induced craniosynostosis date from several thousand years ago and have been found in many parts of the world. The practice of severe head binding and its consequence of impaired mental development are thought to have been partially responsible for the disappearance of the Mayan civilization.[119]

Craniosynostosis was described in Hippocratic writings, which mentioned that it had been detected by observers from different cultures (Fig. 199–16). In his surgical writings, Hippocrates described several aspects of craniofacial malformation. His elegant clinical description of cranial sutures is included in his *Collected Works* (also known as his *Genuine Works*, so labeled by Francis Adams, his English translator).[3]

Men's heads are by no means all like to one another, nor are the sutures of the head of all men constructed in the same form. Thus, whoever has a prominence in the anterior part of the head, in him the sutures of the head take the form of the Greek letter tau T: for the head has the shorter line running transverse before the prominence, while the other line runs through the middle of the head, all the way to the neck. . . . But whoever has a prominence of the head both before and behind, in him the sutures resemble the Greek letter eta H [in the Greek text, the letter H is rotated 90 degrees and laid sideways]; for the long lines of the letter run transverse before each prominence while the short one runs through the middle and terminates in the long lines. But whoever has no prominence on either part he has the sutures of the head resembling the Greek letter χ; for the one line comes transverse to the temple while the other passes along the middle of the head.[3]

Some cranial malformations were intentional. In the *De Aere, Locis, et Aquis (Airs, Waters, and Places)*, Hippocrates described the techniques used by a local community to shape the heads of children of high social status.[120] The desired shape was acquired by applying

On voit que, théoriquement, la conduite à suivre serait facile à préciser.

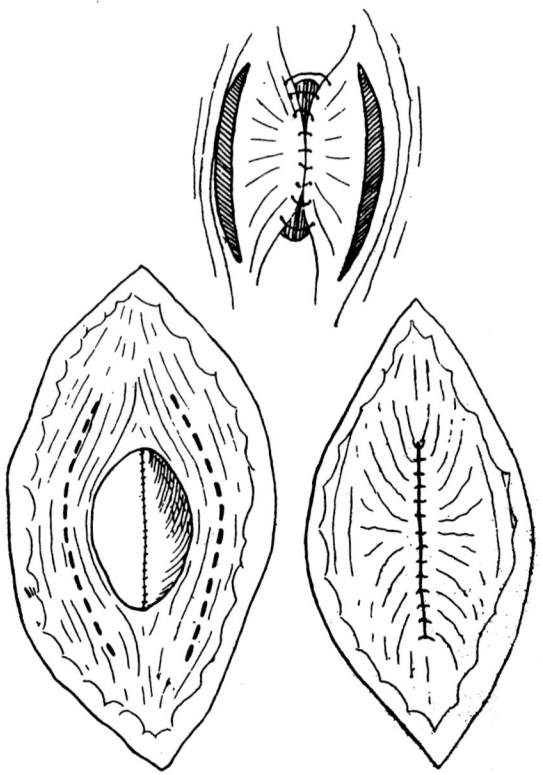

Fig. 7, 8 et 9. — Consolidation de la paroi rachidienne postérieure à l'aide de lambeaux musculo-aponévrotiques (d'après Bayer).

Dans les cas de la première catégorie : **éléments nerveux**

FIGURE 199–15. One the first techniques for closing a myelomeningocele defect with a series of anatomic layers was introduced by Bayer in 1892. (From Bayer C: Zur Technik der Operation der Spina Bifida und Encephalocele. Prag Med Wochenschr 17:317, 332, 345, 1892.)

a mold to the head of the child shortly after birth. Hippocrates described this as follows:

I will pass over the smaller differences among the natives, but will now treat of such as are great either from nature or custom; and first, concerning the macrocephali. . . . At first, usage was the principal cause of the length of their head, but now nature cooperates with usage. They think those the most noble who have the longest heads. It is thus with regard to the usage: immediately after the child is born, and while its head is still tender, they fashion it with their hands, and constrain it to assume a lengthened shape by applying bandages and other suitable contrivances whereby the spherical form of the head is destroyed and it is made to increase in length.[3]

The binding of heads to bring about an artificial form of craniosynostosis is an ancient one, whereas the surgical correction of craniosynostosis is of relatively recent origin. Several illustrated examples of craniosynostosis come from the 16th and 17th centuries. The

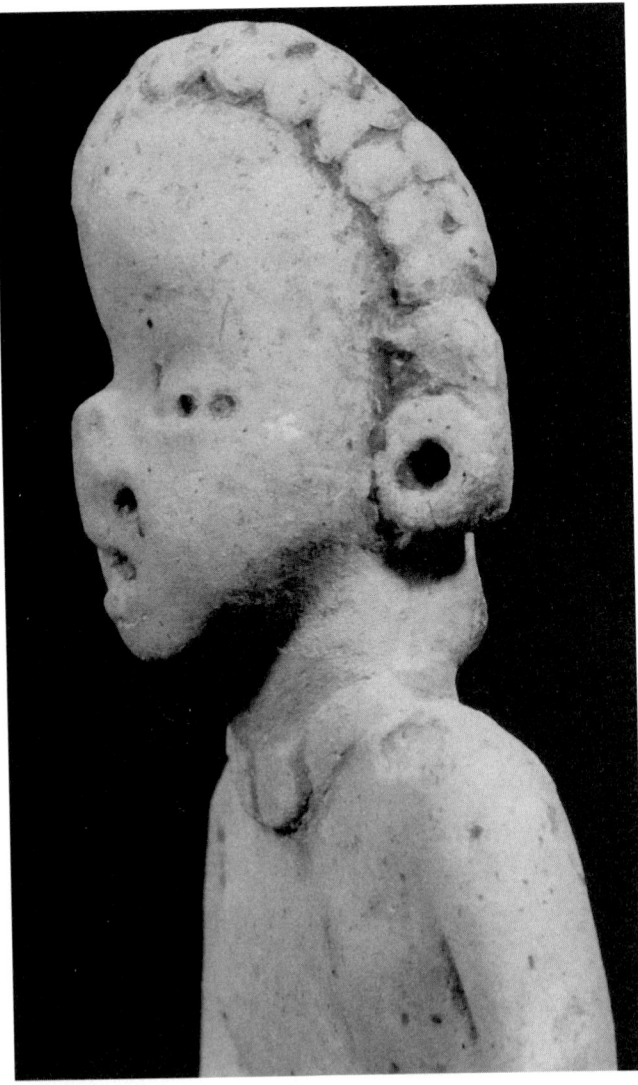

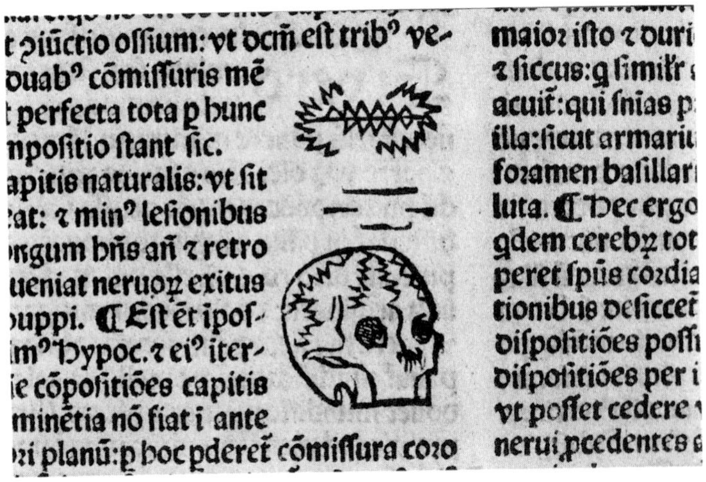

FIGURE 199–16. The terra-cotta figure from the Olmec period (1500–500 BC) in Meso-America is one of the earliest examples of a child with the clinical stigmata of Crouzon's syndrome, and it displays the typical findings of brachycephaly and midface retrusion. The child also appears to have ocular hypertelorism. (Courtesy of James Tait Goodrich, Montefiore Medical Center, Bronx, NY.)

most primitive of these cases was described by the medieval physician and founder of French surgery, Lanfrancho of Milan (Lanfranc, fl. 1290–1296). In his *Cyrurgia Parna*, first published in 1490, Lanfranco[121] described the cranial suture; later, it was illustrated in a 16th century edition.[122] The text reveals little understanding of the suture's purpose, nor is the illustration sophisticated (Fig. 199–17).

The appreciation of an abnormal cranial suture and its consequences for the skull by an observer trained in anatomy and illustration dates back to at least the 16th century. In his magnum opus, Andreas Vesalius depicted several skulls with craniosynostosis; his examples included scaphocephaly, plagiocephaly, and even one consistent with a Crouzon-type brachycephalic skull.[8] To him we owe several early and original descriptions of craniosynostosis, a condition he called "sutures in skulls of unnatural shape"[14] (Fig. 199–18). Chapter 5 of his publication provided an explanation in the legends for five figures:

> *Figure 1 of Chapter 5 portrays the shape of the normal head or skull; it is like an elongated sphere slightly depressed on either side and swelling out at the front and back. Figure 2 demonstrates the first unnatural shape, in which the anterior eminence is missing. Figure 3 shows the second unnatural shape of skull, in which the anterior (posterior) eminence is lost. Figure 4 depicts the third unnatural shape of skull, in which both swellings, anterior and posterior, are missing. In figure 5 we have illustrated the fourth unnatural shape of head, in which the two eminences are at the sides, not the front or back.*[14]

Vesalius provided one of the earliest printed descriptions of a craniofacial anomaly, in this case oxycephaly. In discussing various skull shapes, he commented,

> *Then there is a third one, yet more unlike the natural shape, in which both eminences of the head, both the prior at the forehead and the posterior at the occiput, are abolished and the head is exactly round like a perfect sphere. Thersites is related by Homer to have possessed this shape, for some assert that he describes the head of this shape as* phoxos; *though the majority are pleased to describe all persons with heads of peaked shape by this name or* oxykephalos.[14]

t ꝯiūctio ossium: vt dcm̄ est trib⁹ ve-
duab⁹ cōmissuris mē
t perfecta tota p hunc
npositio stant sic.
apitis naturalis: vt sit
:at: ⁊ min⁹ lesionibus
ngum hn̄s an̄ ⁊ retro
ueniat neruoꝝ exitus
uppi. ¶ Est ēt ipos-
im⁹ hypoc. ⁊ ei⁹ iter-
ie cōpositiōes capitis
minētia nō fiat i ante
ri planū: p hoc pderet cōmissura coro

maioꝛ isto ⁊ duri
⁊ siccus: q simil'r
acuit: qui snias p
illa: sicut armariu
foꝛamen basillari
luta. ¶ Hec ergo
qdem cerebꝝ tot
peret spūs coꝛdia
tionibus deficcet
dispositiōes possi
dispositiōes per i
vt posset cedere
nerui pcedentes

FIGURE 199–17. One of the earliest illustrated examples of a cranial suture. (From de Cavliaco CG: Et Cyrvrgia Brvni, Teodorici, Rolandi, Lanfranci, Rogerii, Bertapalie. Venice, Bernarinus Venetus de Vigalibus, 1519.)

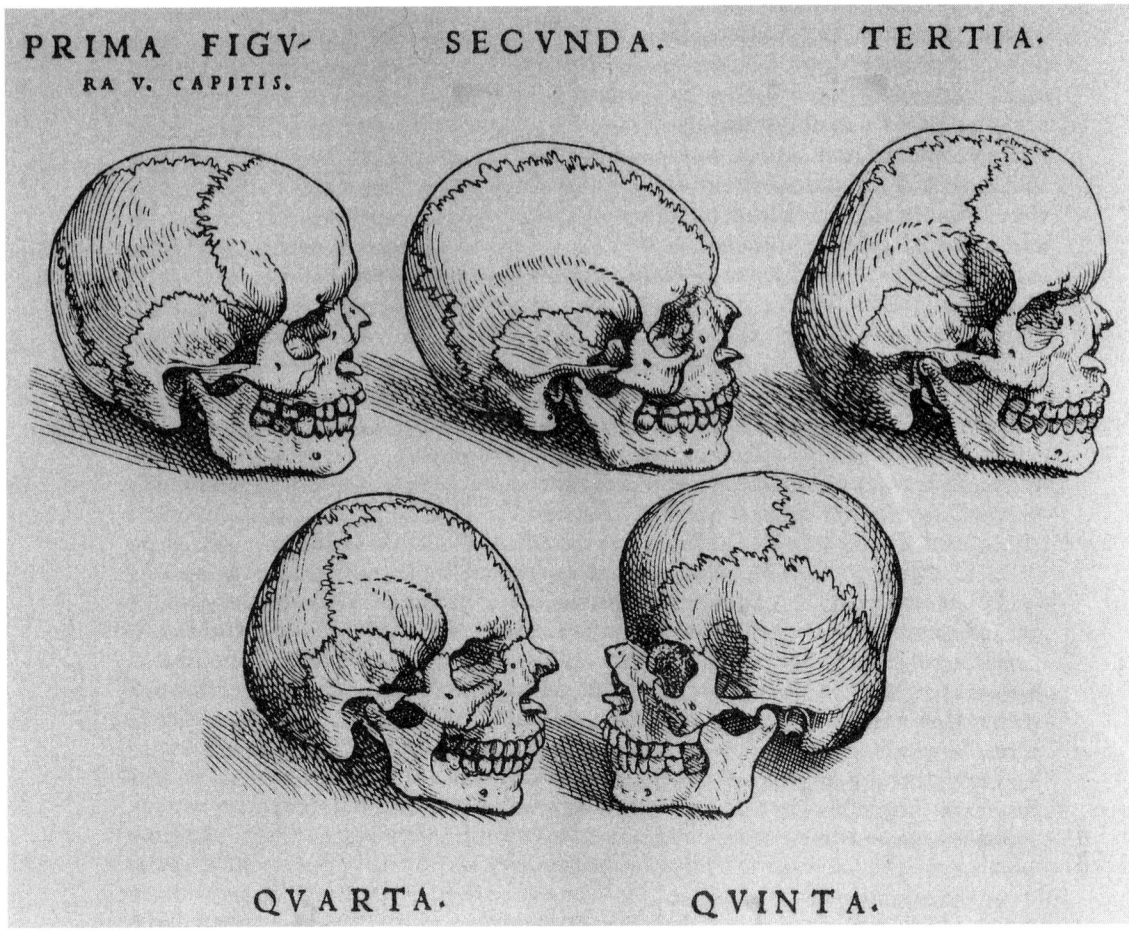

PRIMA FIGV-
RA V. CAPITIS.   SECVNDA.   TERTIA.

QVARTA.   QVINTA.

FIGURE 199–18. A series of skulls with several cranial suture anomalies appeared in Vesalius' monograph of 1543. (From Vesalius A: De Humani Corporis Fabrica. Basel, Oporinus, 1543.)

Applying a modern concept, Vesalius argued that the skull's truly important function was to protect the brain (and keep the plastic surgeons away!). In *Domicile Provided by Nature for the Brain*, Vesalius described the anatomic functions of the skull:

Controller and governor of two concupiscible souls, the brain is the seat of reason and sits enthroned like a queen at the summit of the body. That it be guarded by some sort of protective bulwark is therefore in the highest degree expedient; so the provident Creator of everything did not entrust its protection solely to skin and areas of flesh (as in the abdomen) or to bones spaced well apart from each other (as in the chest) but enveloped it completely in bone like a helmet.[14]

In the 16th century, Giovanni A. D. Croce[123] (1514–1590), an Italian surgeon, also published descriptions of a series of abnormal skulls with evidence of craniosynostoses (Fig. 199–19). The literature is replete with examples of craniosynostosis up to the present day. The early anatomists had no concept of the function of the suture nor any appreciation of craniosynostosis, buy they bequeathed to us many beautifully illustrated examples that are of historical interest. In 1800, Samuel T. Soemmerring[124] (1755–1830) first investigated the

cranial suture. He postulated that the suture's function was to allow for brain growth and that, if the suture closed prematurely, abnormal head growth would result; he described a case of lambdoidal synostosis. In subsequent work, the great German pathologist Rudolf Virchow[125] (1821–1902) postulated what is now called Virchow's law: The outward growth of the skull is restricted in a direction perpendicular to the prematurely fused suture, and compensatory growth occurs in the patent sutures. Virchow[126] provided one of the earliest descriptions of craniosynostosis in 1851. In 1866, von Graefe[127] reported a case of craniosynostosis with optic nerve involvement and subsequent blindness.

Surgical treatment of craniosynostosis was introduced in the 19th century by several pioneers: Lannelongue in France (1890), Padula and Dumont (1890), and L. C. Lane (1892).[128–131] Other reports appeared in the 1890s on surgical craniectomies were by John Wyeth, Karl Beck, and W. W. Keen.[132–134] The classic American case remains that reported by the San Francisco head and neck surgeon, L. C. Lane (1830–1902), who described the case of a child with microcephaly whose mother had written from the country: "My child's brain is locked up, and can you not unlock it?" Lane[135] operated on the child in May 1888, performing a series

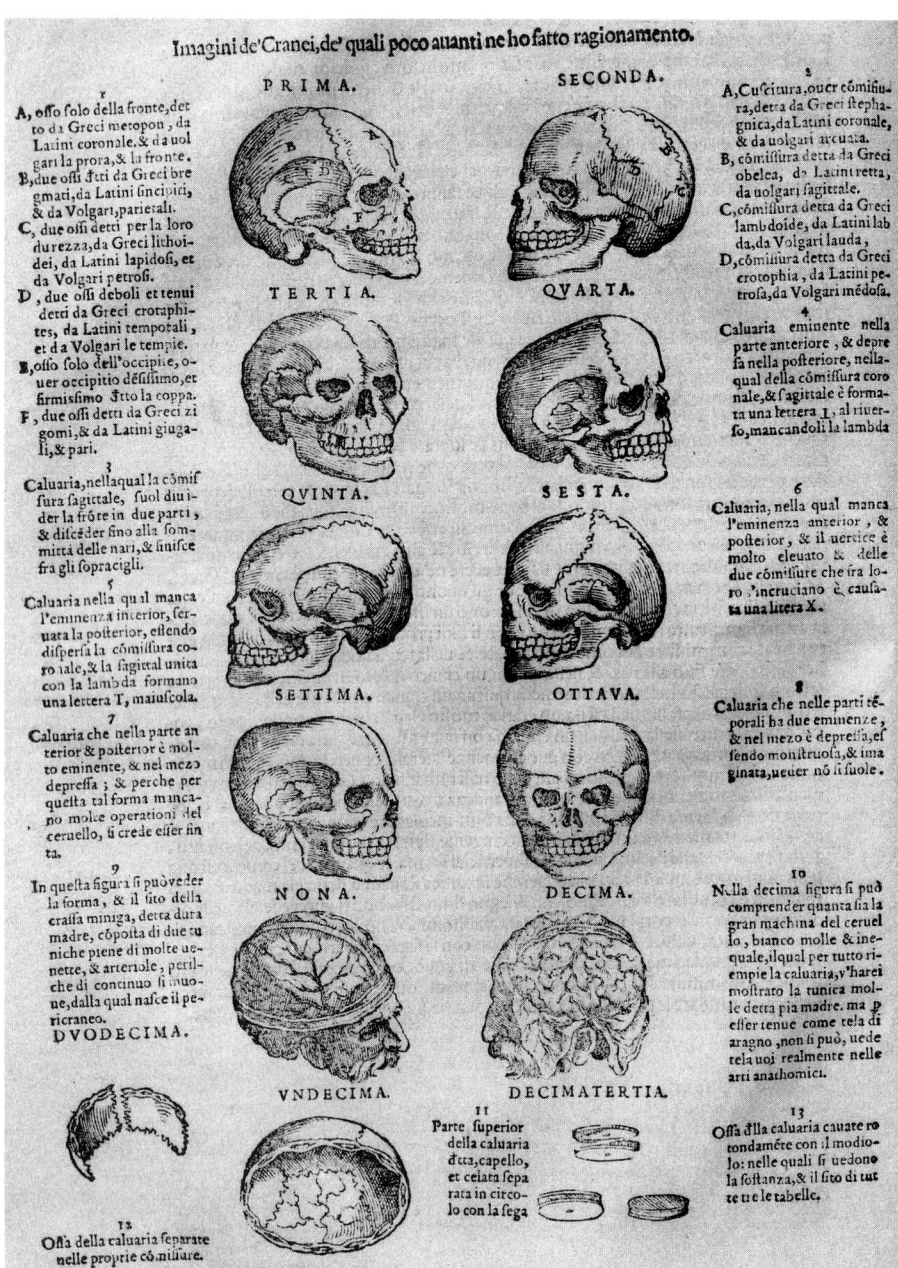

FIGURE 199–19. Croce's monograph on surgery in 1583 contained several examples of skulls with craniosynostosis. (From Croce GAD: Cirugia Universale e Perfetta. Venice, Giordana Ziletti, 1583.)

of strip craniectomies to "release" the brain, but the child died within 48 hours of anesthetic complications, an unfortunate but very common problem (Figs. 199–20 to 199–23).

By 1894, 33 linear craniectomies had been reported,[136] most of them performed on microcephalic children; the mortality rate was high, with 14 deaths. Abraham Jacobi[136] (1830–1919), a prominent New York pediatrician, published a paper called *"Non Nocere"* (Do No Harm) strongly denouncing this operation and its unacceptably high mortality rate.

> *The last subject I dare to discuss before you is that of linear craniotomy, craniotomie à lambeaux, and circular craniotomy. The two former have been introduced by Lannelongue, who, in 1891, published twenty-five cases of 'Enfants arri-*

> *érés et jeunes sujets présentant, avec ou sans crises épileptiformes, des troubles moteurs ou psychiques.' The results he claimed, not only as far as recovery from the operation was concerned, but also as to the improvements in mind which was said to have taken place in a remarkably short time, were so striking and novel that physicians began to hope, surgeons to glory—and the idiotic children? Let us see. When the brains of operative surgeons were taken with the furor operandi on the brains of luckless children, the war-cry was: microcephalus and idiocy. By many the two were identified. Nothing henceforth was required but to open the heads in order to admit light.[136]*

Later in the same address, he said:

> *I hold in my hand, Mr. President, the reports of cases operated upon for so-called idiocy, or for so-called microceph-*

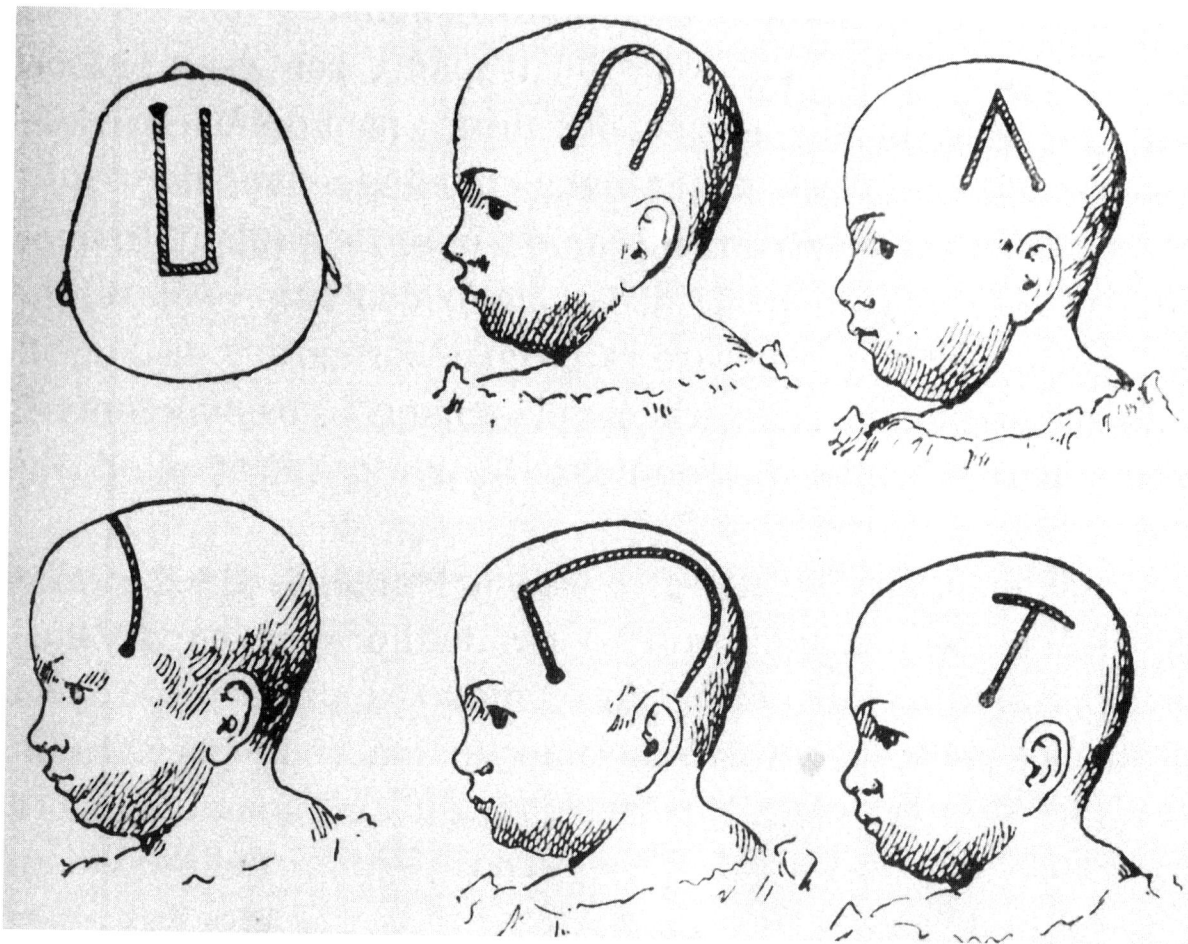

FIGURE 199–20. One of the earliest advocates for craniosynostosis surgery was Lannelongue, a French surgeon who performed various synostectomies to treat the condition. (From Lannelongue L: De la craniectomie dans la microcéphalie. C R Acad Sci 110:1382–1386, 1890.)

alus, by such American surgeons as I could reach personally, so as to have their tales verified from their own lips. The cases I command are 3 of Dr. Charles McBurney, of New York, 2 of Dr. Willy Meyer, of New York, 8 of Dr. John A. Wyeth, of New York, 14 of Dr. W. W. Keen, of Philadelphia, 3 of Dr. Burney Sachs, operated upon by Dr. Arpad Gerster, of New York, and 2 of Dr. I. Vander Veer, of Albany, N.Y. On these 33 cases 41 operations were performed. Of 33 there were 14 deaths and 19 recoveries. The deaths did not occur in the very young ones alone, but also in those four, five, and six years of age. Most of them occurred soon after the operation, six within a day. . . . The final report as to their mental and general condition was as follows: No history obtained, 1; uncertain, 1; no improvement, 7; slight improvement, 7; "some," 1; much improved, 2.[137]

These results led Jacobi to end the *Non Nocere* address with a scathing attack on craniofacial surgeons of this period:

Such rash feats of indiscriminate surgery, if continued, moreover in the presence of fourteen deaths in thirty-three cases, are stains on your hands and sins on your souls. No ocean of soap and water will clean those hands, no power of corrosive sublimate will disinfect the souls. Goethe once said the most interesting book that could written would be a

treatise on the errors of mankind. Let us see to it that our mistakes may not swell that book.[138]

Another therapeutic approach to craniosynostosis was the morcellation technique of Joseph King of New York and William MacEwen (1848–1927) of Scotland (Fig. 199–24).[139–142] For patients with oxycephaly (i.e., King's misnomer, because the patients were a mixed group of craniosynostoses-scaphocephaly and craniofacial problems such as Crouzon's syndrome), King[139] advocated the morcellation technique (first proposed by MacEwen[142]) in a preliminary report issued in 1937. In a summary[140] of his work published in 1942, he reviewed his results in two cases (and those of Barnes Woodhall in two others) and reported favorable aesthetic outcomes and, even more important, correction of developmental problems (i.e., blindness and retardation). Dandy[143] reviewed King's morcellation technique and found fault with his concept of not opening the dura. Maintaining that the dura was not elastic, Dandy[143] offered a technique in which two large bone flaps were elevated (without recourse to the morcellation advocated by King) on each side of the calvarium in two stages. The dura was opened below the flaps so that the brain could expand.

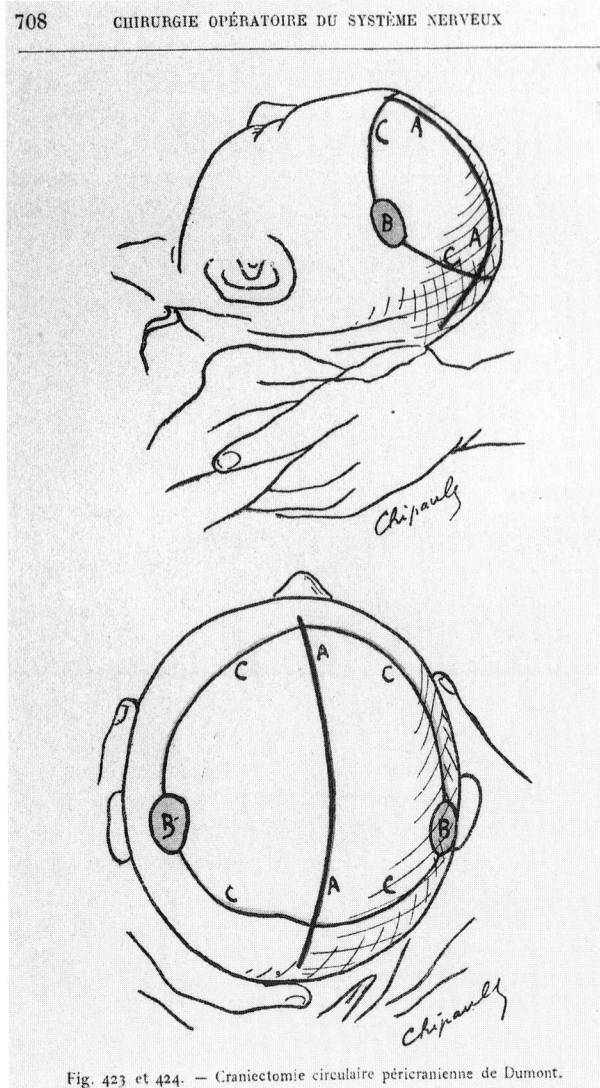

708 CHIRURGIE OPÉRATOIRE DU SYSTÈME NERVEUX

Fig. 423 et 424. — Craniectomie circulaire péricranienne de Dumont.

FIGURE 199–21. A contemporary of Lannelongue was a surgeon by the name of Dumont, who introduced the circular craniectomy for the treatment of craniosynostosis. (From Padula F: Chirurgia Cranica. Le Operazioni che si Praticano Sulle Ossa del Cranio Methodi e Processi Operatorii Relativi. Roma, Alighiere, 1895, pp 296–297.)

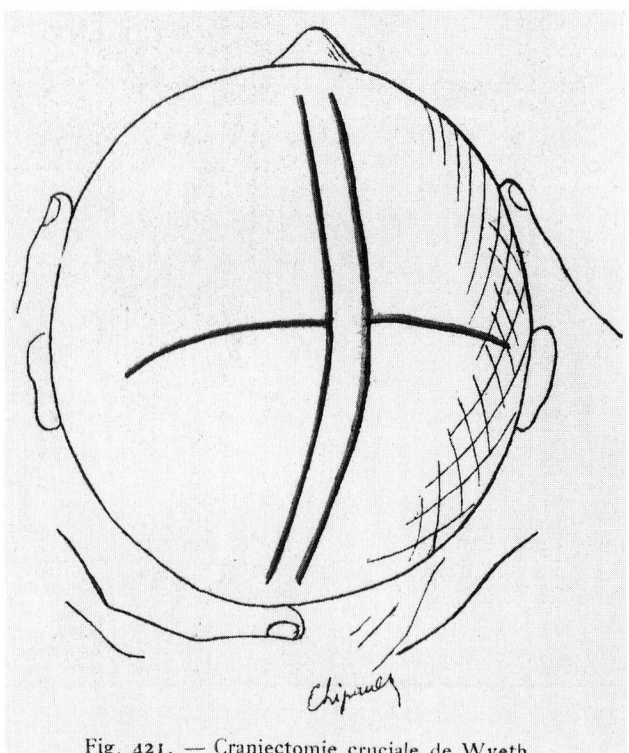

Fig. 421. — Craniectomie cruciale de Wyeth.

FIGURE 199–22. One of the first American surgeons to perform a craniectomy for craniosynostosis was James Wyeth, whose technique is illustrated here. (From Padula F: Chirurgia Cranica. Le Operazioni che si Praticano Sulle Ossa del Cranio Methodi e Processi Operatorii Relativi. Roma, Alighiere, 1895.)

In 1927, Faber and Towne[144] reintroduced the linear craniectomy in treating oxycephaly to prevent blindness. Differentiation of craniosynostosis from microcephaly remained a major problem over the next 25 years. It was not until Sear's[145] classic paper in 1937 that craniosynostosis was finally classified on the basis of radiographic findings. Faber and Towne[146] reemphasized the concept of early surgery in craniosynostosis in 1943, as did Lester Mount[147] in 1947. Strip craniectomies were popularized again in the 1940s by the Boston group of Ingraham, Alexander, and Matson.[148–151]

In another classic paper in 1952, McLaurin and Matson[152] made the best case for early surgical treatment in craniosynostosis. They argued that such surgery was prophylactic rather than curative. Early treatment also appeared to provide a better aesthetic result. These surgeons had long advocated strip craniectomies with placement of polyethylene film over the cut bone edges. They reported the results for 120 patients, one third (36 cases) of whom were operated on before 6 months of age. Further modifications included taking more bone, changing the direction of the osteotomies, and adding interpositional polyurethane sheets; these techniques were as ingenious as their designers.[151]

Hoffman and Mohr[153] recognized the inadequacy of craniotomy for the correction of craniosynostoses in 1976. They introduced the concept of mobilization of a supraorbital bar with an osteotomy of the orbital process. The space obtained by advancement was fixed and stabilized with a bone graft. Marchac and Renier[154, 155] supplemented craniofacial techniques with the "bandeau and floating forehead" concept, applying the principle that a bilateral potentially compressive problem should be treated in a bilateral decompressive fashion.

Octave Crouzon[156, 157] (1874–1938) presented his classic findings regarding what is now called Crouzon's syndrome in 1912 to the Medical Society of the Hospitals of Paris, with a follow-up paper in 1915. He presented the cases of a mother of 29 years old and her 3-year-old son who had "strange" malformations of the face and head (Fig. 199–25). He called this syndrome a "hereditary craniofacial dysostosis." He characterized it as a cranial malformation in which the skull is in the shape of a boat (i.e., scaphocephaly) or a wedge (i.e.,

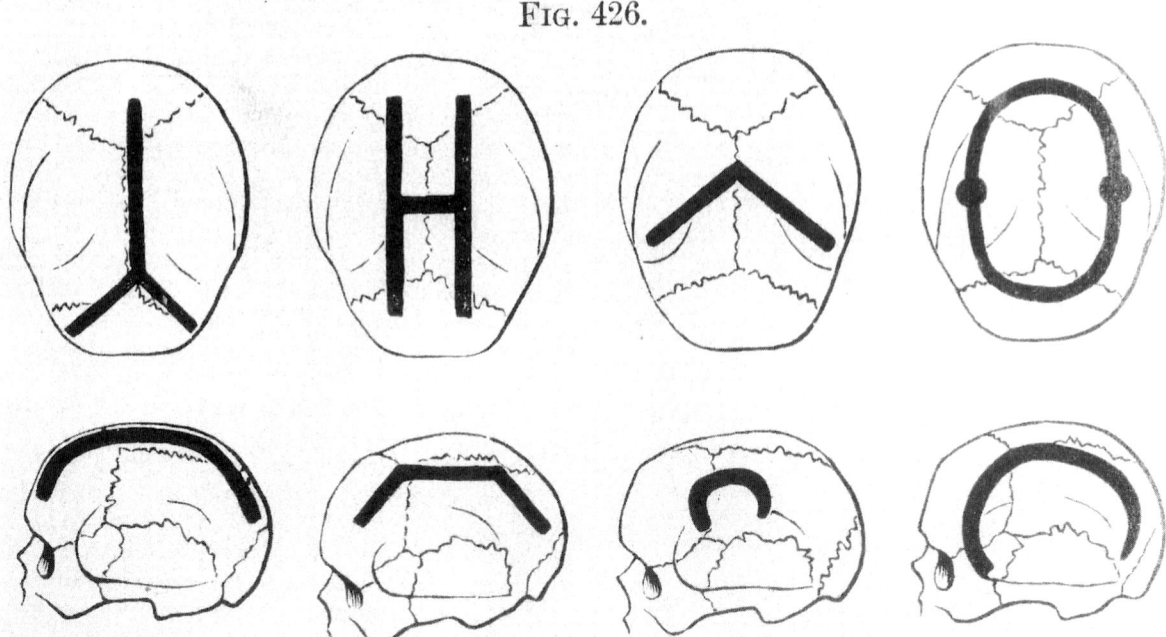

Fig. 426.

Lines of removal of bone as practised by the author, by Lannelongue, and by others.

FIGURE 199–23. Craniosynostosis surgery was illustrated in a 19th century American surgical text and reflects a contemporary view of treatment of this surgical disorder. (From Park RS: A Treatise on Surgery by American Authors, vol 2. Philadelphia, Lea Bros, 1896, p 68.)

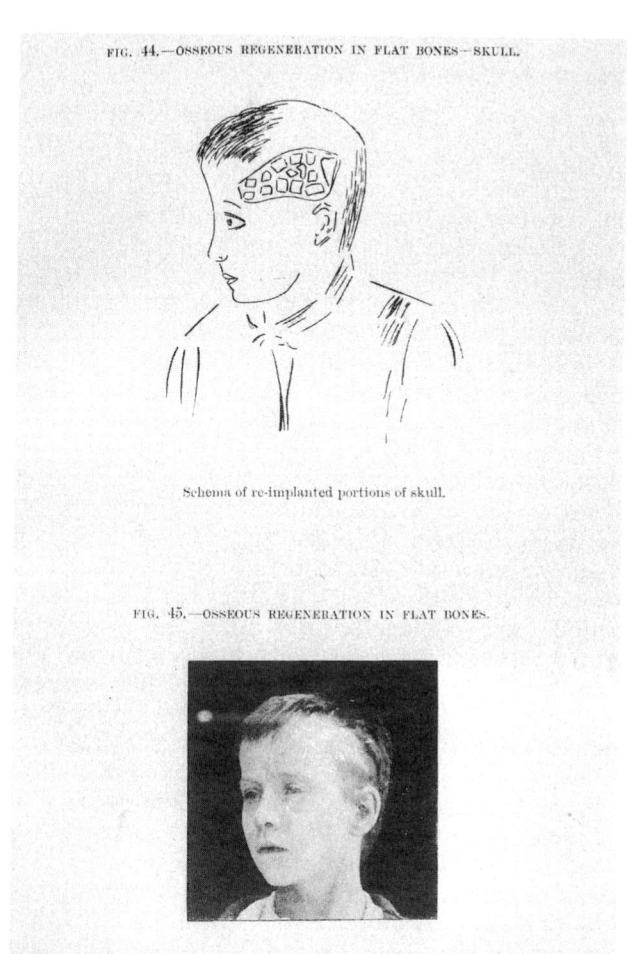

FIG. 44.—OSSEOUS REGENERATION IN FLAT BONES—SKULL.

Schema of re-implanted portions of skull.

FIG. 45.—OSSEOUS REGENERATION IN FLAT BONES.

Mosaic work of bones of skull by re-implantation. Boy aged 9 years—result when completed.

FIGURE 199–24. William MacEwen, an innovative Scottish surgeon, introduced the morcellation technique for treating children with craniosynostosis. (From MacEwen W: The Growth of Bone: Observations on Osteogenesis. Glasgow, MacLehose, 1912, pp 142–145.)

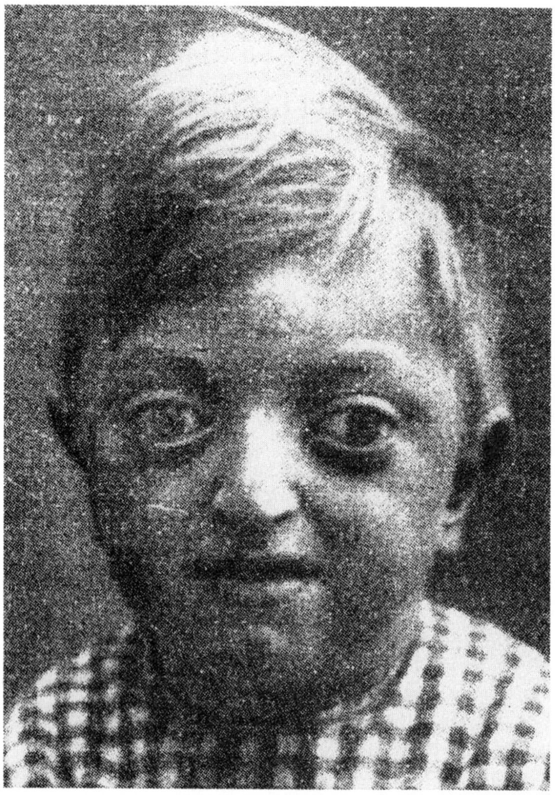

FIGURE 199–25. In a 1912 monograph, Octave Crouzon illustrated one of his patients who had Crouzon's syndrome. (From Crouzon O: Dysostose cranio-faciale héréditaire. Bull Mem Soc Med Hop Paris 33:545–555, 1912.)

trigonocephaly). Included also was a malformation of the face with an arched nose resembling a parrot's beak and marked forward protrusion of the mandible relative to the maxilla. Patients have bilateral exophthalmos with an external strabismus. This syndrome exhibited a familial inheritance pattern.

In 1894, S. W. Wheaton[158] described two infants with the congenital abnormalities of craniosynostosis associated with fusion of the fingers and toes. In a French publication of 1906, the definition of the syndrome was refined by Eugène Apert[159] (1868–1940), by whose name it is now identified. Apert's syndrome is one of the more common craniofacial disorders seen by pediatric neurosurgeons. Among the other craniofacial syndromes, Saethre-Chotzen syndrome was first described in two separate publications by Saethre[160] in 1931 and by Chotzen[161] in 1932. It is a relatively common form of craniosynostosis but is often confused with other syndromes (e.g., Crouzon's syndrome, Pfeiffer's syndrome). Clinical features include craniosynostosis (e.g., brachycephaly, acrocephaly, coronal suture synostosis, plagiocephaly), low-set frontal hairline, facial asymmetry, hypertelorbitism, eye abnormalities, brachydactyly, and partial cutaneous syndactyly, especially of the second and third fingers, along with various skeletal anomalies. In 1976, Jackson and colleagues[162] described the syndrome now known as Jackson-Weiss syndrome (i.e., craniosynostosis, mid-

face hypoplasia, and abnormalities of the feet) in a large kindred of 138 affected individuals.

Carpenter's syndrome was first described by Carpenter[163, 164] in 1901 and later refined in a 1909 paper. It is characterized by craniosynostosis (i.e., primarily the sagittal and lambdoidal sutures close first and the coronal sutures last), preaxial polysyndactyly of the feet, short fingers with clinodactyly, and variable soft tissue syndactyly.

Antley-Bixler syndrome is a craniofacial syndrome involving craniosynostosis (i.e., brachycephaly), dysplastic ears, arachnodactyly, radiohumeral synostosis, femoral bowing, and joint contractures; skeletal fractures also occur.[165] Patients typically develop a trapezoidal head shape (when viewed from the vertex) with fusion of the coronal and lambdoidal sutures.

Pfeiffer's syndrome was first described by Pfeiffer[166] in 1964. It involves craniosynostosis, broad thumbs, broad great toes, and partial soft tissue syndactyly of the hands and joints, the features of which are variable in severity. The head shape is typically turribrachycephalic, although the syndrome of cloverleaf head occurs sporadically.

After an understanding of craniosynostosis developed, it did not take long for surgeons to develop treatment techniques.[117] Unfortunately, in the early period, the selection of patients was poor (i.e., mostly microcephalic children) and the surgical outcomes even poorer, leading to Jacobi's lament. However, after the disease was better appreciated and the techniques improved, surgeons had far better results with significantly lower morbidity. Pediatric neurosurgeons are continuing, in collaboration with plastic surgical colleagues, to modify and improve on these complex surgical corrections. An understanding of the genetic bases of these disorders promises even more improvements in treatment results.

CONCLUSIONS

Pediatric neurosurgery began with little understanding of the surgical problems or the concepts of treatment. Our profession, as late as 100 years ago, lacked any formal understanding of hydrocephalus, spina bifida, or craniosynostosis. After the concepts became better understood, surgeons began to introduce techniques necessary to correct these ominous congenital lesions and to treat these complex problems in the "little people," our children.

REFERENCES

1. Davidoff LM: Treatment of hydrocephalus. Arch Surg 18:1737–1762, 1929.
2. von Winning H: Portrayal of pathological symptoms in pre-Columbian Mexico. Springfield, IL, Pearson Museum, Southern Illinois University School of Medicine, 1987.
3. Hippocrates: The Genuine Works of Hippocrates, vol 1. Adams F, trans. New York, William Wood, 1925, pp 353–391.
4. Hippocrates: The Genuine Works of Hippocrates, vol 2. Adams F, trans. New York, William Wood, 1925, pp 1–19.
5. Galen of Pergamon: Omnia quae Extant Opera in Latinum Sermonem Conversa, 5th ed. Venice, Juntas, 1576–1577.

6. de le Boë F (Sylvius): Disputationes Medicarum pars Prima, Primatias Corporis Humani Functiones Naturales en Anatomicis, Practicis et Chymicis Experimentils Deductas Complectens. Amstelodami, van den Berg, 1663.

7. Monro A: Observations of the Structure and Function of the Nervous System. Edinburgh, Creech-Johnson, 1783.

8. Vesalius A: De Humani Corporis Fabrica. Basel, Oporinus, 1543.

9. Oribasius: Opera quae Extant Omnia, Tribus Tomis Digesta. Basel, Michaëlem Isingrinium, 1557.

10. Albucasis (Abu al-Quasim): Liber Theoricae Necnon Practicae Alsaharavii. Augsburg, Impensis Sigismundi Grimm & Marci Vuirsung, 1519.

11. Albucasis (Abu al-Quasim): On Surgery and Instruments. Spink MS, Lewis GL, trans. Berkeley, CA, University of California Press, 1973, pp 170–72.

12. Albucasis (Abu al-Quasim): On Surgery and Instruments. Spink MS, Lewis GL, trans. Berkeley, CA, University of California Press, 1973, p 173.

13. Albucasis (Abu al-Quasim): On Surgery and Instruments. Spink MS, Lewis GL, trans. Berkeley, CA, University of California Press, 1973, pp 698–99.

14. Vesalius A: On the Fabric of the Human Body. Book 1. The Bones and Cartilages. (De Humani Corporis Fabica.) Richardson FW, Carman JB, trans. San Francisco, Norman, 1998, pp 45, 48, 60.

15. Vesalius A: De Humani Corporis Fabrica. Basel, Oporinus, 1555.

16. Ashwal S (ed): The Founders of Child Neurology. San Francisco, Norman, 1990, p 109.

17. Severino MA: De Recondita Abscessum Natura, libri VII. Napoli, Beltranum, 1632.

18. Willis R: Pathologiae Cerebri et Nervosi Generis Specimen. Amsterdam, Danielem Elzevirium, 1670.

19. Varolio C: De Neruis Opticis, Nonullisque Aliis Praeter Communem Opinionem in Humano Capite Obseruatis. Frankfurt, Ioannem Wechelum & Petrum Fischerum, 1591.

20. Riolan J: Opuscula Anatomica Nova. Instauratio Magna Physicae et Medicinae. London: Typis Milonis Flesher, 1649.

21. Riolan J: A Sure Guide, or the Best and Nearest Way to Physick and Chyrurgery, Being an Anatomical Description of the Whole Body of Man, and Its Parts [in Latin], 3rd ed. Culpeper N, trans. London, John Streater, 1671.

22. Ruysch F: Observationum anatomico-chirurgicarum centuria. Amsterdam, Henricum & Viduam Theodori Boom, 1691, p 86.

23. Haller A: Elementa Physiologiae Corporis Humani. Bern, Sumptibus Societatis Typographicae, 1757–1766.

24. Pacchioni A: De Durae Meningis Fabrica & Usu Disquisitio Anatomicae. Rome, DA Herculis, 1701.

25. Morgagni GB: De Sedibus et Causis Morborum per Anatomen Indagatis. Venice, 1761.

26. Morgagni GB: The Seats and Causes of Diseases Investigated by Anatomy [in Latin], vol 1. Alexander B, trans. London, A. Miller, 1769, pp 244–274.

27. Whytt R: Observations on the Dropsy in the Brain. Edinburgh, Balfour, 1768.

28. Ashwal S (ed): The Founders of Child Neurology. San Francisco, Norman, 1990, pp 87–88.

29. Cotugno D: De Ischiade Nervosa Commentarius. Napoli, Fratres Simmonos, 1764.

30. Cotugno D: A Treatise on the Nervous Sciatica, or Nervous Hip Gout. London, J. Wilkie, 1775, pp 16–17.

31. Monro A: Observations on the Communication of the Ventricles of the Brain with Each Other; and on the Internal Hydrocephalus. Edinburgh, Adam Neil, 1797.

32. Cheyne J: An Essay on Hydrocephalus Acutus, or Dropsy in the Brain. Edinburgh, Mundell, Doig, & Stevenson, 1808, p 25.

33. Magendie F: Recherches Physiologiques et Cliniques sur le Liquide Céphalo-Rachidien ou Cérébrospinal. Paris, Mequignon-Marvis, 1842.

34. Luschka H: Zur Lehre von der Secretionzelle. Arch Physiol Heilk 13:1, 1854.

35. Hilton J: On the Influence of Mechanical and Physiological Rest in the Treatment of Accidents and Surgical Diseases, and the Diagnostic Value of Pain. London, G Bell, 1863.

36. Key A, Retzius G: Studien in der Anatomie des Nervensystems und des Dindesgewebes. Stockholm, 1875.

37. Lewandowsky M: Zur Lehre von der Cerebrospinalflüssigkeit. Z Klin Med 40:480–490, 1900.

38. Spina A: Untersuchungen über die Resorption des Liquors bei normalen und erhalten intercraniellen Druck. Neurol Centralbl 20:224–234, 1901.

39. Schmorl D: Liquor Cerebrospinalis und Ventrikelflüssigkeit. Verh Dtsch Pathol Ges Erlangen, 1910.

40. Dandy WE, Blackfan KD: Internal hydrocephalus: An experimental, clinical and pathological study. Am J Dis Child 8:406–482, 1914.

41. Dandy WE: Experimental hydrocephalus. Ann Surg 70:129–142, 1919.

42. Virchow R: Einfall von angeborenem Hydrocephalus internus. Leipzig, Fest Schr Albert v Kölliker, 1887, p 37.

43. Faivre, E. Recherches sur la structure du conarium et des plexus choroides chez l'homme et chez les animaux. C R Acad Sci 34:424–434, 1854.

44. Faivre E: Etude sur le conarium et les plexus choroides de l'homme et des animaux. Ann Sci Nat Paris 7:52–62, 1857.

45. Mestrezat W: Le liquide céphalo-rachidien normal et pathologique. J Physiol Pathol Gen 14:504–514, 1912.

46. Dixon WE, Halliburton WD: The cerebrospinal fluid. 1. Secretion of the fluid. J Physiol 47:215–225, 1913.

47. Weed LH: The cerebrospinal fluid. Physiol Rev 2:171–182, 1922.

48. Weed LH: Studies on cerebrospinal fluid. J Med Res 31:21–118, 1914.

49. Weed LH: The development of the cerebrospinal spaces in pig and in man. Carnegie Inst Contrib Embryol 5:1–10, 1917.

50. Weed LH: Certain anatomical and physiological aspects of the meninges and cerebrospinal fluid. Brain 58:383–397, 1935.

51. Cushing H: Studies on the cerebrospinal fluid and its pathways. J Med Res 31:1–19, 1914.

52. Cushing H: Studies in Intracranial Physiology and Surgery. The Third Circulation, the Hypophysis, the Gliomas: The Cameron Prize Lecture. Oxford, Oxford University Press, 1925.

53. Buchan W: Domestic medicine, or A Treatise on the Prevention and Cure of Diseases by Regimen and Simple Medicines, 8th ed. London, W Strahan, 1784.

54. Underwood M: A Treatise on the Treatment of Diseases of Children. London, J Mathews, 1784.

55. Bucy PC: Hydrocephalus. In Brenneman (ed): Practice of Pediatrics, vol 4. Hagerstwon, MD, WF Prior, 1932, pp 23–27.

56. Galvani D: Della Fontanele Trattato: Diuiso in duo Libri. Padua, G Crivellari, 1620.

57. Le Cat CN: A new trocart [sic] for the puncture in the hydrocephalus, and for other evacuations, which are necessary to be made at different times. Philos Trans R Soc Lond 47:267–272, 1753.

58. Chipault A: Chirurgie Opératoire du Système Nerveux. Paris, Rueff, 1894–95, pp 717–718.

59. Graniere U: Il trattamento dell'idrocefalo infantile net secolo XIX. Rass Int Clin Ter 49:327–37, 1969.

60. Quincke H: Die lumbalpunktion des hydrocephalus. Berl Klin Wochenschr 28:929–933, 965–968, 1891.

61. Quincke H: About hydrocephaLus. Verh Kongr Inn Med 10:321–339, 1901.

62. Ferguson AH: Intraperitoneal diversion of the cerebrospinal fluid in cases of hydrocephalus. N Y Med J 67:902, 1898.

63. Heile B: Zur Behandlung des Hydrocephalus. Dtsch Med Wochenschr 34:1468–1470, 1908.

64. Kanusch W: Die Behandlung des hydrocephalus der kleinen Kinder. Arch Klin Chir 87:709, 1908.

65. Payr E: Ueber Ventrikeldrainage bei Hydrocephalus. Verh Dtsch Ges Chir 40:515, 1911.

66. McClure RD: Hydrocephalus treated by drainage into a vein of the neck. Bull Johns Hopkins Hosp 20:110, 1909.

67. Heile B: Uber neue operative Wege zur Druckentlastung bei angbornem Hydrocephalus (ureter-Dura-Anatomose). Zentralbl Chir 52:2229–2236, 1925.

68. Matson D: A new operation for the treatment of communicating hydrocephalus: Report of a case secondary to generalized meningitis. J Neurosurg 6:238–247, 1949.

69. Torkildsen A: A new palliative operation in cases of inoperable occlusion of the Sylvian aqueduct. Acta Chir Scand 82:117–24, 1939.

70. Gardner (1895), cited in Pudenz RH, Russell FE, Hurd AH, Shelden CH: Ventriculo-auriculostomy: A technique for shunting cerebrospinal fluid into the right auricle: Preliminary report. J Neurosurg 14:171–179, 1957.

71. Nulsen F, Spitz EB: Treatment of hydrocephalus by direct shunt from ventricule to jugular vein. Surg Forum 2:399–409, 1951.

72. Spitz EB: Neurosurgery in the prevention of exogenous mental retardation. Pediatr Clin North Am 6:1215–1235, 1959.

73. Pudenz RH, Russell FE, Hurd AH, Shelden CH:. Ventriculo-auriculostomy: A technique for shunting cerebrospinal fluid into the right auricle: Preliminary report. J Neruosurg 14:171–179, 1957.

74. Noonan JA, Ehmke DA: Complications of ventriculovenous shunts for control of hydrocephalus: Report of three cases with thromboemboli to the lungs. N Engl J Med 269:70–74, 1963.

75. Davis L: Neurological Surgery. Philadelphia, Lea & Febiger, 1936, p 405.

76. Dandy WE: Extirpation of the choroid plexus of the lateral ventricles in communicating hydrocephalus. Ann Surg 68:569–579, 1918.

77. Dandy WE: The diagnosis and treatment of hydrocephalus resulting from strictures of the aqueduct of Sylvius. Surg Gynecol Obstet 31:340–358, 1920.

78. Dandy WE: Operative procedure for hydrocephalus. Bull Johns Hopkins Hosp 33:188–190, 1922.

79. Dandy WE: The operative treatment of communicating hydrocephalus. Ann Surg 108:194–202, 1938.

80. Putnam TJ: Treatment of hydrocephalus by endoscopic coagulation of the choroid plexus: Description of a new instrument and preliminary report of results. N Engl J Med 210:1373–1376, 1934.

81. Putnam TJ: Results of the treatment of hydrocephalus by endoscopic coagulation of the choroid plexus. Arch Pediatr 52:676–685, 1935.

82. Putnam TJ: Mentality of infants relieved of hydrocephalus by coagulation of choroid plexus. Am J Dis Child 55:990–999, 1938.

83. Putnam TJ: The surgical treatment of infantile hydrocephalus. Surg Gynecol Obstet 76:171–182, 1943.

84. Scarff JE: Endoscopic treatment of hydrocephalus: Description of a ventriculoscope and preliminary report of cases. Arch Neurol Psychiatry 35:853–861, 1936.

85. Scarff JE: Treatment of obstructive hydrocephalus by puncture of the lamina terminalis and floor of the third ventricle. J Neurosurg 8:204–213, 1951.

86. Scarff JE: Treatment of hydrocephalus: An historical and critical review of methods and results. J Neurol Neurosurg Psychiatry 26:1–26, 1963.

87. Stookey B, Scarff JF: Occlusion of the aqueduct of Sylvius of neoplastic and non-neoplastic processes with a rational surgical treatment for relief of the resultant obstructive hydrocephalus. Bull Neurol Inst N Y 5:348–377, 1936.

88. Davidoff LM: Hydrocephalus and hydrocephalus with meningocele: Their treatment with choroid plexectomy. Surg Clin North Am 416–431, 1948.

89. Dandy WE: Diagnosis and treatment of stricutres of the aqueduct of Sylvius (causing hydrocephaus). Arch Surg 51:1–14, 1945.

90. Ransohoff J: J Neurosurg 11:295, 1950.

91. Ransohoff J, Shulman K, Fishman RA: . J Pediatr 56:399, 1960.

92. Hippocrates: Medicorum Graecorum Opera quae Exstant. Kühn DCG (ed). Leipzig, C Cnoblochius, 1925, p 500.

93. van Forestus P: Observationum et Curationum Chirurgicarum Libri Quinque Lugduni Batavorum. Leiden, ex Officina Plantiniana Raphelengii, 1610.

94. Tulpius N: Observationes Medicae, libri III. Amsterdam, Elzeririum, 1641, p 231.

95. Furukawa T: First description of spina bifida by Nicolaas Tulp. Neurology 37:1816–1828, 1987.

96. Walker AE (ed): A History of Neurological Surgery. Baltimore, Williams & Wilkins, 1951, pp 352–353.

97. Cruveilhier J: Anatomie pathologique du corps humain. Paris, JB Baillière, 1829.

98. von Recklinghausen F: Untersuchungen über die Spina Bifida. Berlin, Druck & Verlag von Georg Reimer, 1886.

99. Virchow R: Ein fall von Hypertrichosis Circumscripta Mediana, Kombiniert mit Spina Bifida Occulta. Z Ethnol 7:280, 1875.

100. Baxter: Chronic hydrocephalus with meningocele. Med Times Gaz 1:239–249, 1882.

101. Lebedeff A: Über die entstehung der anecephalie and spina bifida be Vögeln und menschen. Virchows Arch 86:263–273, 1881.

102. Kermauner F: . In Schwalbes (ed): Die Morphologie der Missbildungen des Menschen und der Tiere, III. Jena, Gustav Fischer, 1909, p 86.

103. Keiller VH: A contribution to the anatomy of spina bifida. Brain 45:31–41, 1922.

104. Bohnstedt G: Beitrag zur Kasuistik der Spinal Bifida Occulta. Arch Pathol Anat 140:47–57, 1895.

105. Fuchs A: Über Beziehungen der Enuresis nocturna zu Rudimentärformen der Spina Bifida Occulta (Myelodysplasie). Wien Med Wochenschr 60:1569–1573, 1910.

106. de Vries E: Spina bifida occulta and myelodysplasia with unilateral clubfoot beginning in adult life. Am J Med Sci 175:365–371, 1928.

107. Lichtenstein BW: Spinal dysraphism: Spina bifida and myelodysplasia. Arch Neurol Psychiatry 44:792–809, 1940.

108. Lichtenstein BW: Distant neuroanatomic complications of spina bifida (spinal dysraphism): Hydrocephalus, Arnold-Chiari deformity, stenosis of aqueduct of Sylvius, etc; pathogenesis and pathology. Arch Neurol Psychiatry 47:195–214, 1942.

109. Bell B: A System of Surgery. Edinburgh, C Elliott, 1787, pp 245–249.

110. Cooper S: The Practice of Surgery, vol 2. Philadelphia, John Grigg, 1830, pp 346–347.

111. Morton J: Case of spina bifida cured by injection. Br Med J 1:632–633, 1872.

112. Palasciano F: Memorie ed osservazioni del Prof. Ferdinando Palasciano. Napoli, Trani, 1897.

113. Rizzoli F: Memoires de Chirurgie et d'Obstétrique. Paris, Delahaye, 1872.

114. Bayer C: Zur Technik der Operation der Spina Bifida und Encephalocele. Prag Med Wochenschr 17:317, 332, 345, 1892.

115. Ingraham FD, Hamlin H: Spina bifida and cranium bifidum: Surgical treatment. N Engl J Med 228:631–641, 1943.

116. Sharrard WJ, Zachary RB, Lorber J: The long-term evaluation of a trial of immediate and elayed closure of spina bifida cystica. Clin Orthop Res 50:197–207, 1967.

117. Matson DD: Craniosynostosis. In Matson DD, Ingraham FD (eds): Neurosurgery of Infancy and Childhood. Springfield, IL, Charles C Thomas, 1969, pp 138–143.

118. Dingwall EJ: Artificial Cranial Deformation. A Contribution to the Study of Ethnic Mutilations. London, John Bale & Sons, 1931.

119. Feindel W: Cranial clues to the mysterious decline of the Maya civilization: The hippocampal hypothesis. Neuroimage 3:1–5, 1986.

120. Hippocrates: Magni Hippocratis Medicorvm Omnivm Facile Principis, Opera Omnia Quae Extant in VIII Sectionis. Anvtio Foesio Mediomatrico (ed). Frankfurt, And. Wecheli, 1596, pp 265, 918.

121. Lanfranchi of Milan (Lanfrac): La Chirurgie d'Alanfranc. Traduit du Latin par Guillaume Yvone. Lyon, Jean de la Fontaine, 1490.

122. de Cavliaco CG: Et Cyrvrgia Brvni, Teodorici, Rolandi, Lanfranci, Rogerii, Bertapalie. Venice, Bernarinus Venetus de Vigalibus, 1519, p 175.

123. Croce GAD: Cirugia Universale e Perfetta. Venice, Giordana Ziletti, 1583.

124. Soemmerring ST: Vom Baue des Menschlichen Körpers. Frankfurt am Main, 1800.

125. Virchow R: Ueber den cretinisms namentlich in Franken und über pathologischen Schädelformen. Verh Phys Med Ges 2:230–271, 1851.

126. Virchow R: Handbuch der speziellen Pathologie und Therapie. Erlangen 1:112–122, 1851.

127. von Graefe A: Ueber Neuroretinitis und Gewisse. Fälle fulminirender Erblindung. Arch Ophthalmol 12:114–149, 1866.

128. Lannelongue L: De la craniectomie dans la microcéphalie. C R Acad Sci 110:1382–1386, 1890.

129. Padula F: Chirurgia Cranica. Le Operazioni che si Praticano Sulle Ossa del Cranio Methodi e Processi Operatorii Relativi. Roma, Alighiere, 1895.

130. Padula F: Chirurgia Cranica. Le Operazioni che si Praticano Sulle Ossa del Cranio Methodi e Processi Operatorii Relativi. Roma, Alighiere, 1895, pp 296–297.
131. Lane LC: Pioneer craniectomy for relief of the mental imbecility due to premature sutural closure and microcephalus. JAMA 18: 49–50, 1892.
132. Wyeth J: Craniosynostosis. N Y Med Rec Feb 21, 1891.
133. Beck K: Craniotomy in microcephalus. JAMA 22, 1894.
134. Keen WW: Linear craniotomy (miscalled craniectomy) for microcephalus. Am J Med Sci 101:549–555, 1891.
135. Lane LC: The Surgery of the Head and Neck, 2nd ed. Philadelphia, Blakiston, 1899, pp 279, 281.
136. Jacobi A: Medical Addresses, vol VI. New York, Critic & Guide, 1909, p 26.
137. Jacobi A: Medical Addresses, vol VI. New York, Critic & Guide, 1909, p 33.
138. Jacobi A: Medical Addresses, vol VI. New York, Critic & Guide, 1909, p 43.
139. King JEJ: Oxycephaly: A new operation and its results (a preliminary report). Arch Neurol Psychiatry 40:1205–1219, 1937.
140. King JEJ: Oxycephaly. Ann Surg 115:488–506, 1942.
141. Woodhall B: Oxycephaly: Results of treatment by the King "morcellation" method. J Pediatr 20:585–595, 1942.
142. MacEwen W: The Growth of Bone: Observations on Osteogenesis. Glasgow, MacLehose, 1912, pp 142–145.
143. Dandy WE: An operation for scaphocephaly. Arch Surg 47: 247–249, 1943.
144. Faber HK, Towne EB: Early craniectomy as a preventive measure in oxycephaly and allied conditions with special reference to the prevention of blindness. Am J Med Sci 173:701–711 1927.
145. Sear HR: Some notes on craniosynostosis. Br J Radiol 10:445–487, 1937.
146. Faber HK, Towne EB: Early operation in premature cranial synostosis for prevention of blindness and other sequelae. J Pediatr 22:286–296, 1943.
147. Mount LA: Premature closure of sutures of cranial vault: Plea for early recognition and early operation. N Y State J Med 47: 270–276, 1947.
148. Ingraham FD, Alexander E Jr, Matson DD: Polyethylene, a new synthetic plastic for use in surgery: Experimental application in neurosurgery. JAMA 113:82–92, 1947.
149. Ingraham FD, Matson DD, Alexander E Jr: Experimental observations in the treatment of craniostenosis. Surgery 23:252–268, 1948.

150. Ingraham FD, Alexander E Jr, Matson DD: Clinical studies in craniosynostosis: Analysis of fifty cases and description of a method surgical treatment. Surgery 24:518–541, 1948.
151. Shillito J Jr, Matson DD: Craniosynostosis: A review of 519 surgical patients. Pediatrics 41:829–853, 1968.
152. McLaurin RL, Matson DD: Importance of early surgical treatment of craniostenosis: Review of thirty-six cases treated ruing the first six months of life. Pediatrics 10:637–652, 1952.
153. Hoffman HJ, Mohr G: Lateral canthal advancement of the supraorbital margin: A new corrective technique in the treatment of coronal synostosis. J Neurosurg 45:376–381, 1976.
154. Marchac D: Radial forehead remodeling for craniostenosis. Plast Reconstr Surg 61:823, 1978.
155. Marchac D, Renier D: Craniofacial Surgery for Craniosynostosis. Boston, Little, Brown, 1982.
156. Crouzon O: Dysostose cranio-faciale héréditaire. Bull Mem Soc Med Hop Paris 33:545–555, 1912.
157. Crouzon O: Une nouvelle famille atteinte de dysostose cranio-faciale héréditaire. Arch Med Enf 18:540–550, 1915.
158. Wheaton SW: Two specimens of congenital cranial deformity in infants associated with fusion of fingers and toes. Trans Pathol Soc Lond 45:238–241, 1894.
159. Apert E: De l'acrocéphalosyndactylie. Bull Soc Med Paris 23: 1310–1330, 1906.
160. Saethre H: Ein beitrag zum Turmschädelproblem (Pathogenese, Erblichkeit und Symptomologie). Dtsch Z Nervenheilkd 117: 533–555, 1931.
161. Chotzen F: Eine eigenartige familiare Entwicklungsstörung: Akrocephalosyndaktylie, Dysostosis, Craniofacialis und Hypertelorismus. J Monatschr Kinderheilkd 55:97–122, 1932.
162. Jackson CE, Weiss L, Reynolds WA, et al: Craniosynostosis, mid-facial hypoplasia, and foot abnormalities: An autosomal dominant phenotype in a large Amish kindred. J Pediatr 88: 963–968, 1976.
163. Carpenter G: Two sisters showing malformations of the skull and other congenital abnormalities. Rep Soc Study Dis Child (Lond) 1:110–118, 1901.
164. Carpenter G: Case of acrocephaly with other congenital malformations. Proc R Soc Med 2(Pt 1):45–53, 199–201, 1909.
165. Antley R, Bixler D: Trapezoidocephaly, midfacial hypoplasia and cartilage abnormalities with multiple synostoses and skeletal fractures. Birth Defects 11:387–401, 1983.
166. Pfeiffer RA: Dominant erbliche Akrocephalosyndaktylie. Z Kinderheilkd 90:301–320, 1964.

CHAPTER 200

Neurological Examination in Infancy and Childhood

WILLIAM J. LOGAN

The neurological evaluation of infants and children is different from that of older children and adults, principally because of the phenomenon of development. The process of development alters the neurological behaviors and functions expected at different ages, and development changes the findings of physical examination. The natural history and manifestation of abnormal function and disease are very often different at different stages of development. Development is an important variable in the evaluation of infants and young children.

Another important difference in the pediatric age group is that the medical history is usually provided by parents or other caregivers. These individuals can also assist with the physical examination. Older children and adolescents, even if accompanied by parents, should be asked to describe the chief complaint and symptoms, which may be different from that given by the parents. They should also be given the opportunity and courtesy of meeting with the physician in private to discuss more personal concerns.

The goal of the neurological assessment is to detect abnormalities, to localize them, and to monitor their changes. After a complete and successful neurological evaluation, it is possible to establish a diagnosis and recommend treatment, if indicated, or determine what further diagnostic testing is indicated.

The primary emphasis in this chapter is on the neurological examination but some suggestions regarding the neurological history are discussed. The examination described is more detailed than would be routinely performed, but in an individual patient such detail may be required in the area of suspected or actual abnormality. A different approach to the examination of specific age groups is recommended, and this is described at the end of the chapter.

HISTORY

The history is considered to be the most essential part of the evaluation. Usually, the attentive clinician formulates an appropriate differential diagnosis, if not the actual diagnosis, after completing the history. It seems reasonable to allot ample time to this part of the evaluation if the diagnosis has not already been established. Most clinicians also take advantage of the interview time to observe the patient's interaction with the parent or caregiver, the environment, and the examiner and to scrutinize the patient's spontaneous activity and function. The interview can provide an opportunity for the patient to become more comfortable with the examiner and to begin to interact socially. This time provides much of the information necessary to judge whether the patient's mental, visual, and motor functions are grossly normal.

Current Status

It is important to have a complete description of the chief complaint. This should include the onset (i.e., acute or insidious) and the duration of the problem, as well as determining whether the course has been acute, chronic, or intermittent and whether it is static or progressive. Based on the complaints and relevant solicited information, the physician can usually determine which system is likely to be involved. It may be possible to implicate the cognitive and behavioral system, the cranial nerve and special sensory system, the pain and sensory system, the neuromuscular system, or the motor control system or to determine whether there are multiple areas affected or there is more general or diffuse involvement. Identifying the pattern of involvement can help to narrow the diagnostic possibilities.

It is useful to summarize for the parents their concerns and complaints and reiterate what is perceived to be the most important of the problems. This reassures the parents that the clinician has heard and understood their history, and it allows the clinician to determine whether there are other areas of concern not previously mentioned.

Birth History

For the neonate or the older infant and child whose symptoms date to early infancy, a detailed birth history is essential. Many of the neurological disorders present at birth began with damage or a developmental abnormality occurring during gestation. A complete pregnancy history should include gestation time, maternal illness, exposure to legal and illicit drugs (including alcohol), and any history of spontaneous abortions. The history taker notes the occurrence during the pregnancy of infections, vaginal bleeding, symptoms of toxemia, and polyhydramnios or oligohydramnios. The history should determine whether there was prenatal care, whether the infant was monitored, whether fetal ultrasonography and other diagnostic tests were performed, and whether there was evidence of fetal distress. An increasing number of congenital malformations involving the nervous system are being identified with prenatal ultrasound imaging.

It is important to know the type and duration of delivery, whether it was difficult, whether the presentation was unusual, whether there was evidence of abruptio placentae or malpositioned placenta, and whether there was premature rupture of membranes. It should be determined whether there was a prolapsed cord at birth, and the condition of the newborn should be documented (e.g., Apgar scores, cyanosis, breathing, requirement for resuscitation). Did the infant feed well after birth, develop an infection, or become jaundiced? The examiner should record the infant's birth weight, head circumference, and any obvious birth defects. Respiratory distress, apneic episodes, seizures, bleeding, and duration of stay in the nursery may all be helpful clues to an abnormal neurological state of the newborn.

Developmental History

The developmental milestones are an extremely important measure of the preschool child's neurological

TABLE 200–1 ■ Language Development

AGE*	BEHAVIOR
4 mo	Cooing (vowel-like sounds)
6 mo	Babbling (one-syllable sounds)
8 mo	Responds to name
12 mo	Speaks at least one word
	Responds to simple commands such as "no"
18 mo	Speaks more than three words
	Knows two or three body parts
2 yr	Has two- to three-word sentences
	Follows two- or three-word commands
	Points to pictures as requested
3 yr	Speaks three- or four-word sentences
	Uses pronouns and plurals
	Knows age, sex, and full name
	Asks questions
4 yr	Has four- to five-word sentences
	Can tell story
	Knows one color
	Uses past tense
	Responds to two-part commands
5 yr	Responds to three-part commands
	Has more than five-word sentences
	Uses future tense
	Knows four colors
	Counts 10 or more objects
	Recalls parts of story

* Ages at which most children achieve the language milestones listed.

TABLE 200–2 ■ Adaptive Development

AGE*	BEHAVIOR
6 wk	Smiles responsively
3 mo	Follows visually 180 degrees
5 mo	Reaches for object
6 mo	Holds one block or toy in each hand
9 mo	Has stranger awareness or anxiety
12 mo	Waves bye-bye
	Plays peek-a-boo
	Finds object hidden in presence
15 mo	Places one block on top of another
	Throws items
18 mo	Mimics examiner
	Finger-feeds self
	Helps undress self
2 yr	Copies vertical line
	Builds tower of three blocks
	Uses utensil for eating
	Turns single book pages
2.5 yr	Copies horizontal line
	Completely feeds self
3 yr	Mostly dresses self
	Copies circle
	Builds tower with four blocks
	Produces horizontal line of blocks
3.5 yr	Plays interactively with other children
4 yr	Copies cross
	Draws person with two to four parts
	Uses scissors
	Knows concepts of length, height, and weight
5 yr	Copies triangle and square
	Draws a person with body
6 yr	Copies diamond

* Ages at which most children can demonstrate the listed behaviors.

development. For the older child, school performance also becomes an important indicator of development. It is convenient to consider the developmental milestones in four categories: motor behavior, adaptive behavior, language behavior, and personal-social behavior. Normal motor development is reassuring regarding any underlying motor abnormality. Normal language development (Table 200–1) and adaptive behavior (Table 200–2) are strong predictors of normal cognitive outcome. Normal personal-social behavior is less significant in terms of prediction than is the presence of abnormal development in this area. With the possible exception of motor development, most of these factors can be heavily influenced by the patient's cultural, social, and educational environment. Because school is such an intense and demanding experience, existing cognitive deficits are magnified, and minor unrecognized problems (e.g., learning disability) are initially manifested at this time. Good school achievement and function is a reassuring sign of normal cognitive development, and deterioration in school performance can be a very sensitive and early sign of a newly acquired or progressive neurological abnormality.

Family History

The family history is important for identifying several neurological disorders. The ages and health of siblings and parents are noted, and the cause of death of any immediate relative should be ascertained. The parents should be questioned about consanguinity and the presence of any neurological or familial disease. The social status of the family and child should be ascertained, including the living conditions, the integrity of the family, who the usual caregivers are, and the presence of drug usage by the patient or other family members.

In the review of past health, the history of injuries, hospitalizations, operations, illnesses, medications, immunizations, and allergies may be important for understanding the patient's current problems. A review of systems should include general and systemic organ dysfunction, as well as neurological dysfunction. Some relevant neurological symptoms are seizures, headaches, weakness, development delay, regression, visual disturbance, hearing loss, enuresis, and incontinence.

PHYSICAL EXAMINATION

Because the nervous system interacts with so many other organ systems in the body, it is important to know whether other areas are dysfunctional. The physical examination is usually performed at the same time as the neurological examination, and the examination is adjusted to the age of the child. It is often most effective if the patient is initially examined in the parent's lap. At some time during the examination, male patients should be disrobed to their shorts, and female patients should be disrobed to their shorts and tops to detect skin marks or other abnormalities that would be concealed by the clothing. Older female patients must always be examined in the presence of a parent or female aide.

The minimal equipment for a routine examination for all patients includes a tape measure, a stethoscope, a light, an ophthalmoscope, an otoscope, a tuning fork, a reflex hammer, wooden tongue depressors, cotton or tissue wipes, a bright and squeaky toy, paper and pencil or crayon, and items such as coins, paper clips, round balls, safety pins, and keys.

In addition to the routine examination, the following physical characteristics are of particular interest in the neurological assessment:

Measurements: height, weight, length, and vital signs
Skin: birthmarks, rashes, sinus tracts, and unusual tufts of hair
Head and face: cranial sutures, fontanelles, shape, deformity, dysmorphic features, and bruits (requires auscultation)
Neck and spine: scoliosis, kyphosis, palpable, or visible spine defect and meningeal signs (e.g., Kernig sign, Brudzinski sign)
Cardiovascular system: cardiomegaly, heart murmurs, and peripheral pulses
Abdomen: hepatomegaly, splenomegaly, and distended bladder
Musculoskeletal system: atrophy, hemihypertrophy, contractures, muscle tenderness, pes cavus, clubfoot, and other deformities

Mental Status Examination

Mental status can be evaluated in children of all ages. The usual adult approach may be taken with children older than 6 years of age with consideration of the different capacities of patients in the younger age groups. Assessment of the mental state must consider language and culture differences. Primary sensory deficits (e.g., deafness, blindness) or motor deficits (e.g., cerebral palsy) must be recognized, and their effects on the assessment of mental function should be considered. To accurately assess the mental state, the patient should be alert and awake. *State* is one of the components of consciousness. The second component, *awareness*, reflects cognitive functioning. It ranges from full orientation and cognitive function to confusion and to total lack of awareness. *Delirium* describes an acute, active confusional state with disordered thinking, cognition, and perception, often with agitation. Decreased levels of alertness or arousal are associated with depressed awareness, but abnormal awareness may be seen in an awake individual.

The approach to mental status evaluation should be adjusted to the age of the patient. Up to approximately 6 months of age, mental status is assessed through review of the history and, to a lesser extent, by observation of the early developmental milestones (see Tables 200–1 and 200–2). The clinician notes the patient's attentiveness and awareness of the environment as well as his or her responsiveness to social stimulation (e.g., smile). The early foundations of speech, with cooing of vowel sounds, begin at this age and evolve into babbling at the next stage.

After 6 months, mental status is evaluated by determining the levels of development of language and adaptive behavior (see Tables 200–1 and 200–2). These levels are determined by review of the developmental history provided by the parents and by observation of the patient in spontaneous activity and in response to the parents or examiner.

Normal language development follows an age-determined sequence, and the developmental level that the patient has achieved can be assessed by comparison to this scale (see Table 200–1). It is practical to ask the parents about the milestones that most children of the same chronologic age have reached to determine whether there is any developmental lag for the patient. If the patient has not demonstrated language function at the expected age level, the level of function that best describes their language development is determined. A 3-year-old child who is just beginning to put words together in phrases or sentences is considered to be functioning at an approximately 2-year-old level regarding language. Attempts should be made to confirm the parent's description by observing and speaking with the patient during the entire examination.

Another measure of cognitive development is adaptive behavior, which refers to the faculties that reflect a child's ability to initiate new experiences and to learn from them. This includes understanding, concept formation, and imagery. As with language, there is a series of developmental sequences, and patients can be assessed to determine what level in this sequence they best fit and how this level compares with normal expectations (see Table 200–2). This measure has a fairly good correlation with overall intelligence. The patient's level is estimated by review of the history provided by the parent and by the observation of spontaneous or elicited behaviors and functions at the time of examination. The examination can be facilitated by some accessories, including several 1-inch building blocks of different colors; toys of interest to a child, including ones with which he or she can interact (e.g., doll, truck); a book with pictures and simple text; and a container into which the child can put a pellet or other object.

After the age of 6 years, the more standard mental status examination can be performed. Cognition can be considered to consist of functions that are lateralized and those that have more general or bilateral distribution. Language is lateralized to the dominant hemisphere, which is usually the left hemisphere. Visuospatial analysis is thought to have greater representation in the nondominant hemisphere.

It is important initially to determine the general level of orientation of the older child. This is an indication of the level of cognitive ability and of awareness. Patients should be asked questions that measure their orientation to time, including the day, date, month, season, and year. Do they know where they are located in terms of the building, room, city, region, and country? They should be asked whether they recognize the other people in attendance, including the examiner, and this questioning should include individuals whom they would be expected to recognize. Right-left orientation should be included. Handedness of the patient may be determined at this stage and should be recorded. Most children demonstrate a hand preference by 4 years of age. If a child younger than 1 year of age shows strong hand preference, it usually indicates motor abnormality involving the other hand.

Memory consists of short-term memory and long-term memory. The former includes working memory, the function of which is to hold information while it is being processed. This type of memory can be tested by digit span, immediately repeating three items, or spelling a word backward. At 4 to 5 years, the child should be able to remember four digits, and at 10 years, the child should remember six digits. The normal adult can remember seven or eight digits.

Long-term memory can be considered to be explicit or implicit. Explicit refers to memory of specific events or episodes (i.e., episodic memory) or facts, concepts, words, and meanings (i.e., semantic memory). This type of memory has bilateral representation involving diencephalic, hippocampal, and limbic structures. Semantic memory also involves the temporal neocortex, particularly in the dominant hemisphere. Explicit memory refers to knowing *that*, whereas implicit or procedural memory refers to knowing *how*. Implicit memory refers to the kinds of memory traces that are required when learning skills of procedures such as riding a bicycle or playing a musical instrument. This type of memory seems to involve mainly the basal ganglia, certain parts of the cerebral cortex, and probably the cerebellum.

The clinician tests memory at the bedside by asking the patient to recall three or more items, a name and an address, a short story, or a complex figure that was presented more than 5 minutes previously. Particularly in cases of head injury, it may be useful to assess retrograde memory. This is generally not possible in younger children.

Language includes speech, reading, and writing. Loss of language results in aphasia or dysphasia, which can be described as global, expressive, or receptive. Wernicke's area in the posterior superior temporal lobe is important for language comprehension and reception. Broca's area in the inferior frontal lobe is involved in speech production and fluency. The connection between these areas, the arcuate fasciculus, couples comprehension and reception to expression. Damage here produces a disorder (i.e., conduction aphasia) in which repetition is disturbed and speech, although fluent, has paraphasic errors such as substitution of letters, syllables, and words. Articulation, fluency, prosody (i.e., intonation and stress), vocabulary, and word substitution errors should be assessed during spontaneous speech. Further testing should include naming of objects, pictures, or colors. Comprehension should be tested first with the use of three-part commands such as "close your eyes, turn your head to the left, and touch your left hand to your right ear" or simpler commands if this is not possible. The clinician can test for repetition by using single words and then progressing to a longer test phrase such as the popular "no ifs, ands, or buts."

Reading aloud is a good screening test because it requires several neurological abilities in addition to reading. Writing also tests several neurological functions, particularly if it is a spontaneous composition by the patient about a person, place, or event. If this spontaneous composition is not possible, writing in response to dictation can give some indication of the patient's ability in this area. Spelling is also a useful bedside test of language function and level of cognitive ability.

Calculation is considered to be another dominant-hemisphere function, residing in the angular gyrus region. A simple screening test is to ask the patient to subtract numbers such as 21 minus 17 or 31 minus 9. More difficult calculations may require paper and pencil.

The most easily demonstrated abnormality of the nondominant (usually right) hemisphere is the phenomenon of neglect. This abnormality is detected by having the patient draw from memory a picture of a clock face or of a daisy flower. In cases of obvious neglect, there is much poorer construction of the picture on the left side. However, a visual field deficit cannot be considered evidence of neglect. Visuospatial function may also have nondominant hemisphere localization. In any event, it is a useful mental function to be examined. Copying complex designs and drawing a person are useful bedside tests for which developmental age standards are available (e.g., Greek cross, 8 years; cylinder, 9 years; three-dimensional cube, 12 years).

Cranial Nerve Examination

CRANIAL NERVE I: OLFACTORY NERVE

Although children and infants, including neonates, can detect olfactory stimuli, an olfactory test is often not included in the routine cranial nerve examination. For more formal testing, a supply of materials that have distinct but not strongly aromatic odors, such as coffee, orange, vanilla, and mint, may be used to test each nostril separately. With one nostril occluded, the patient is asked to sniff to detect an odor. During one of the sniffs, the test substance is brought close to the nostril. The ability to first detect and then identify the test substance and the number of sniffs needed to do that reflect different levels of sensitivity. Testing of neonates and infants requires more specialized testing procedures.

CRANIAL NERVE II: OPTIC NERVE

In premature and full-term neonates, infants, or the less cooperative patient, the blink response and the pupillary responses to light should be detectable. There should be a direct and a consensual pupillary response. The clinician should evaluate the presence of a relative afferent pupillary defect (i.e., Marcus Gunn pupillary sign) by swinging a light from one pupil to the other and back. The pupil with the relative afferent pupillary defect dilates when the light is immediately directed to it from the other pupil. Even the neonate should show visual fixation and visual following if vision is intact and if the patient is alert and not crying. Lack of fixation and following is nonlocalizing and can be caused by a lack of attention, cognitive impairment, decreased level of consciousness, or visual pathway dysfunction anywhere from the eye to the occipital cortex. The size of the pupil and the possibility of pupillary anisocoria should be noted.

Visual acuity can be formally tested in cooperative children older than 4 years of age with the use of a visual chart for near and far vision. A note should be made about whether the patient wears glasses and whether they were used for the testing. If the patient does not know the alphabet, the clinician can use a chart with toy diagrams that the child can name or the letter E chart and have the child indicate the direction in which the arms of each E are pointing. Each eye should be tested separately. A simple bedside test of acuity is to use a very small piece of tissue into a ball approximately 1 mm in diameter. The patient is asked to pick up the small object. If the patient can do this with the object at least 18 inches away, the near vision in at least one eye is at the level of 20/40 to 20/60. If the patient cannot see that object, larger items can be used. At birth, vision is about 20/150, and it matures to 20/20 after 12 months of age. Infants can follow a face or bright object, such as a multicolored ball or toy. The clinician can test for color vision informally by asking the child to pick up a specific color from a collection of different-colored items (e.g., crayons) or more formally by using an Ishihara color chart.

The visual fields are tested by confrontation of each eye separately. The cooperative patient is instructed to look at the examiner's eyes or nose and to report when a moving object comes into view. Moving fingers are brought in from each visual quadrant randomly until each quadrant and each eye are tested. A more sensitive method for picking up relative field defects is double, simultaneous visual stimulation. The clinician simultaneously presents two targets to different quadrants, and the patient is asked to point to the hand or hands with moving fingers. Older patients can be asked to count the number of fingers that are presented simultaneously in the different quadrants. For less cooperative patients, the clinician may grossly assess visual fields by using visual threat, in which the hand is rapidly moved toward the eye from different directions, and noting a blink response. To test infants, the clinician brings an interesting object from behind the infant's head into a visual quadrant and ascertains the patient's response as the target comes into view. The lack of visual response in the presence of a normal pupillary response to light suggests a cortical deficit or cortical blindness.

Funduscopic examination may be facilitated by instillation of a drop of 2.5% phenylephrine hydrochloride and 0.5% or 1.0% tropicamide or similar ophthalmic preparation on the cornea to dilate the pupils. For routine testing, the disk and adjacent retina often can be seen without pupillary dilation, particularly if the examination is done in a somewhat darkened room. Newborns are often more easily examined than are somewhat older infants, who are more likely to resist examination. An assistant or a parent standing behind the examiner should try to attract the attention of the patient away from looking at the ophthalmoscope so that the examiner can get a good view of the optic disk. If the patient does look at the ophthalmoscope, it may be an opportunity to view the macula. The vessels and the peripheral retina should be examined for lesions such as chorioretinitis and retinitis pigmentosa. The margins, color, and shape of the optic disk should be assessed. In early papilledema, there is blurring of the margins, venous distention, and hyperemia of the optic nerve head. In more advanced papilledema, there is elevation of the disk, obliteration of the optic cup, hemorrhage, and exudates. Optic nerve pallor indicates optic atrophy, which may be difficult to recognize in the normally pale optic disk of the young infant.

The clinician begins the examination of the fundus with a high plus lens at a distance from the eye looking for a red reflex and for abnormalities such as cataract. The examiner moves closer to the eye, decreasing the plus power toward the minus side until the fundus structures come into view. In the newborn and the younger infant, a high minus reading such as 8 or 15 often gives the best visualization.

CRANIAL NERVES III, IV, AND VI: OCULOMOTOR, TROCHLEAR, AND ABDUCENS NERVES

Cranial nerves III, IV, and VI subserve eye movement, and the cranial nerve III also mediates pupillary constriction and lid elevation. The clinician should observe spontaneous movements of the eyes, looking for conjugate movements, abnormal movements, or limitations in movement. In newborns and in unresponsive patients, the oculocephalic reflex (i.e., doll's eye maneuver) produces lateral eye movements that should be conjugate and full. In this test, if the head is rapidly rotated to one side, the eyes temporarily deviate to the opposite side. Infants can follow a bright object or toy. Older children can cooperate with formal testing of eye movement. Such testing should be done with both eyes moving in the vertical and the horizontal meridians and in intermediate directions in each quadrant. If there is a question of abnormality, each eye must be tested separately. The child should be asked if there is any evidence of diplopia and, if so, in which direction of gaze the diplopia is most severe. The child should also be questioned about the position of the two objects relative to each other.

Infants may have strabismus with esotropia, exotropia, hypotropia, or hypertropia. This deviation may be obvious or may be detected by the reflection of the light on the pupil. If the eyes are aligned, the light reflection should be in the same part of the pupil of both eyes. The clinician may detect subtle weakness or evidence of a tendency for strabismus by performing the cover-uncover test. In this test, the vision of one eye is blocked from the target by the examiner's hand, and the hand is then moved to the other eye, thereby blocking it from the target. The examiner watches the movement of the eye that is uncovered as the hand moves to cover the second eye. An inward movement, for example, indicates exophoria or weakness of the medial rectus muscle in that eye. In cases of diplopia, it is useful first to determine in which direction the double vision is greatest, because this indicates that one of the muscles most responsible for movement in that direction is involved. The most distal image belongs to the eye that has the abnormal function. The clinician can determine which eye is abnormal by covering one of the eyes with a red filter and determining whether the most lateral spot of light from a penlight is perceived by the child as red or white.

Cranial nerve III innervates the medial rectus, the superior and inferior rectus, the inferior oblique, and the levator muscles of the upper eyelid and supplies the parasympathetic constrictor fibers to the pupil. The superior rectus muscle elevates the eye, the inferior rectus muscle depresses the eye, and the medial rectus muscle adducts the eye. The inferior oblique elevates the eye and rotates it outward. Weakness of the levator palpebrae results in ptosis, or drooping of the eyelid. Involvement of the parasympathetic fibers results in pupil dilation. Lack of pupillary constriction to light reflects blindness, efferent third cranial nerve abnormality, or pupillary sphincter dysfunction. A small pupil may be associated with Horner's syndrome (i.e., miosis, ptosis, enophthalmos, and ipsilateral facial anhidrosis) because of disruption of sympathetic innervation. A large pupil may reflect pupillary constrictor dysfunction caused by lesions of the Edinger-Westphal nucleus or cranial nerve III. Pupillary constriction or dilatation can also result from a pharmacologic effect.

Cranial nerve IV innervates the superior oblique muscle, which primarily rotates the eye inward (i.e., intorsion) and depresses the eye. Weakness of this muscle may result in a head tilt to the opposite side to compensate for the lack of intorsion. Cranial nerve VI innervates the lateral rectus muscle, which abducts the eye. Internal ophthalmoplegia is paralysis of the pupillary sphincter and ciliary muscle (i.e., accommodation) only. Paralysis of the extraocular muscles only is called external ophthalmoplegia, and paralysis of both is referred to as complete ophthalmoplegia.

In addition to abnormalities of the nerves or muscles they innervate, there can be internuclear abnormalities. The medial longitudinal fasciculus yokes the movement of the two eyes in a conjugate fashion. Unilateral medial longitudinal fasciculus lesions produce an internuclear ophthalmoplegia consisting of ipsilateral medial rectus involvement and contralateral lateral rectus involvement when the patient looks to the contralateral side. This condition manifests as a lack of adduction of the ipsilateral eye and nystagmus in the abducting eye.

Supranuclear abnormalities produce gaze disturbances in which the conjugate movement of both eyes during gaze vertically up or down or horizontally left or right is impaired. Vertical upward gaze is controlled at the pretectal dorsal midbrain level. Parinaud's syndrome consists of impaired conjugate upward gaze with pupillary and convergence abnormalities. Lateral gaze is controlled by the pontine gaze center, which is responsible for gaze ipsilaterally. Higher cortical gaze centers control gaze contralaterally. Convergence is also mediated by internuclear mechanisms and is generally associated automatically with accommodation. Eye movements can be described as *pursuit* when they smoothly and steadily follow an object or *saccadic* when they jump quickly from one target to another. The latter is more of a ballistic type of movement. Pursuit movements may not be smooth, but instead show a jerky irregularity as the movement is fragmented into individual and multiple saccadic jumps (i.e., saccadic pursuit).

Nystagmus is a repetitive to-and-fro movement of the eyes. In jerk nystagmus, movements in one phase are saccadic, and movements in the opposite direction are slow and smooth. In pendular nystagmus, both phases are the smooth. In jerk nystagmus, the direction is named according to the direction of the saccadic phase. Vestibular nystagmus is a jerk nystagmus. Disorders affecting the visual pathways, however, can produce pendular nystagmus. The roving eye movements of a blind infant are somewhat different but may be accompanied by pendular nystagmus. In congenital nystagmus, both jerk and pendular nystagmus occur. Nystagmus can be further described by the eye position in which it is apparent. Gaze-evoked nystagmus may be present only when the patient is looking in one direction. Unilateral gaze-evoked jerk nystagmus implies unilateral labyrinthine or vestibular abnormality. Vertical jerk nystagmus indicates central, usually brainstem, dysfunction. Opsoclonus, a rapid, nystagmus-like oscillation of the eyes that occurs episodically, is caused by rapid volleys of saccadic conjugate-appearing movements in any direction, giving the appearance of dancing eyes. This pattern is seen in children in conjunction with the opsoclonus-myoclonus-ataxia syndrome, which is sometimes associated with neuroblastoma.

CRANIAL NERVE V: TRIGEMINAL NERVE

Cranial nerve V has sensory and motor components. Sensory testing in the neonate and infant relies on the infant's reflex or other response to stimulation. The corneal reflex can be elicited by touching the cornea with a wisp of cotton or a puff of air. There is a bilateral blink response. In the older infant, tickling the ear, nose, and face with a piece of cotton or paper tissue usually causes the infant to bring the hand to the site of stimulation. Sometimes, a sneeze is elicited when the nose is stimulated. For the older child, the clinician can make this sensory test more precise by having the child localize it with eyes closed by touching the site of stimulation. This test requires detection of the stimulation and point localization. The clinician can test for pain with a clean, sharp disposable object (e.g., wooden applicator stick) by stimulating areas in each region of the trigeminal distribution—the ophthalmic, maxillary, and mandibular divisions. Stimulating the forehead or just above the hairline (i.e., ophthalmic division), the cheek (i.e., maxillary division), and the chin (i.e., mandibular division) elicits withdrawal and crying in newborns and young infants. This stimulation can be localized, and the intensity reported by the cooperative older patient, who should be able to detect any differences between the left and right side of the face and between the face and other parts on the body. Sensation within the mouth has a cranial nerve distribution corresponding to that of the overlying external surface.

A sucking or biting response in neonates or young infants and their forceful opening of the mouth against resistance enable the motor function of cranial nerve V to be tested. Opening of the mouth, which is caused by the action of the external pterygoid muscles, is more easily overcome in testing strength than is jaw closure, which is mediated by the masseter muscles. During the latter motion, however, masseter contraction and bulk can also be palpated.

CRANIAL NERVE VII: FACIAL NERVE

In newborns and young infants, the acts of smiling and crying provide a gross estimate of the function of cranial nerve VII, which innervates the facial musculature. Forceful eye closure with crying or on request allows the strength of eye closure to be tested and compared on each side. In the patient at rest, weakness of the orbicularis oculi may manifest as a widened palpebral fissure on the affected side. Lower facial weakness manifests as a loss or decrease of the nasolabial fold on the affected side. The older child can make rapid lip movements, whistle, and smile on request. Lower motoneuron weakness of cranial nerve VII involves all muscles to a similar degree. Weakness due to an upper motoneuron lesion involving cranial nerve VII generally spares the muscles in the upper part of the face, and wrinkling of the brow is unaffected. Some infants, particularly those with congenital cardiac disease, have a developmental absence or hypoplasia of the depressor anguli oris on one side. This deficiency gives rise to an asymmetrical mouth during crying and apparent weakness of depression of the angle of the mouth. In patients with facial weakness, there can also be some alteration in articulation of speech.

Sensory and autonomic fibers originate with the facial nerve but branch off early. The lacrimal gland innervation passes through the nervus intermedius root of the facial nerve and branches off at the geniculate ganglion. Abnormalities of these parasympathetic fibers can produce a decrease in tearing. Fibers for taste sensation of the anterior two thirds of the tongue leave the facial nerve through the chorda tympani and join the lingual nerve. Although taste is not tested routinely in infants, the clinician can test for it in older, cooperative children by using solutions of sweet, salty, sour, and bitter substances. One of these solutions is dabbed on the protruded tongue, and the patient should report the taste before the tongue is brought back into the mouth, where other receptors with cranial nerve IX innervation may detect it.

CRANIAL NERVE VIII: AUDITORY NERVE

Cranial nerve VIII has two components. The cochlear nerve deals with auditory function, and the vestibular nerve mediates labyrinthine function. Newborns respond to a loud whistle by alerting, opening the eyes, crying, or otherwise changing their behavior. After several months of life, normal infants orient themselves to the sound and, after 6 months, can localize the sound. A squeaky toy, whistle, spoken word, or tuning fork can be used to demonstrate this reaction. In the older child, the detection of whisper or the sound of rubbing fingers can be used to estimate hearing acuity. A tuning fork of 256 Hz or higher is useful for hearing tests and for comparing hearing on the two sides. This instrument is also used for the Weber test, in which the stem of the tuning fork is placed at the vertex of the head, and the patient is asked to localize the sound to one ear or the other or to the midline. Lateralization of the sound to the side of decreased hearing indicates that it is a conductive hearing loss, whereas lateralization to the side with normal hearing indicates that the contralateral hearing loss is of the sensorineural type. The Rinne test examines the relative efficiency of air conduction compared with that of bone conduction. The tuning fork stem is held against the mastoid bone for testing bone conduction, and the vibrating end is held near the external ear for the air conduction test. Normally, air conduction is more sensitive than bone conduction. A reverse of that relationship indicates conduction abnormalities in the middle ear. For more detailed testing of hearing, particularly in the newborn, the auditory brainstem-evoked response is useful. Audiometry using behavioral responses in the younger infant and cooperative responses in the older child provides more detailed information on hearing acuity at different frequencies.

Vestibular function is not tested routinely but should be evaluated if abnormalities in vestibular function are suspected or patients have vertigo or nystagmus. The clinician examines for positional nystagmus and vertigo by quickly moving the patient's body and head into a recumbent position with the head turned with one ear down and then repeating the maneuver with the other ear down to see if any of these positions exacerbates the symptoms and the nystagmus. Caloric stimulation of the external auditory canal is not generally done at the bedside in the awake patient but can be performed as a more detailed vestibular test in special laboratories. Ice water caloric testing of the unconscious patient with intact tympanic membranes is useful to assess the brainstem pathways from the labyrinth to the cranial nerves that control eye movement. Cold stimulation causes a deviation of the eyes to the stimulated side when the patient is in a recumbent position with the head tilted 30 degrees above horizontal. Newborns and young infants can be held by and facing the examiner, and when the examiner rotates with the infant, he or she may show eye deviation toward the direction of rotation. This response is mediated by the vestibular system. Oculocephalic reflexes also require vestibular activation.

CRANIAL NERVES IX AND X: GLOSSOPHARYNGEAL AND VAGUS NERVES

Cranial nerves IX and X are usually tested together. Cranial nerve IX appears to provide much of the pharyngeal somatosensory and taste sensation innervation, and cranial nerve X integrates and controls the pharyngeal constrictor action, palate elevation, and vocal cord action, but there is much overlap in innervation for these nerves. In patients of all ages, these nerves are examined by the eliciting the gag response by stimulation of the pharyngeal wall. The gag response demonstrates constriction of the pharyngeal musculature and elevation of the palate by the levator palatini muscle. Older children can also detect and report the sensation produced by stimulating the pharyngeal wall. The clinician can also assess pharyngeal constrictor function by observing swallow. This is particularly useful in newborns and infants. During speech, the vocal cord phonatory function is assessed for vowel sounds, and nasal pharyngeal closure is examined when vocal sounds are made that maximally elevate the palate, such as the word *key*. Hypernasality of speech indicates an incomplete separation of the nasal and pharyngeal cavities during palate elevation.

CRANIAL NERVE XI: SPINAL ACCESSORY NERVE

Cranial nerve XI innervates the sternocleidomastoid and trapezius muscles. The clinician evaluates the sternocleidomastoid by having the patient rotate the head to the opposite side against resistance; at the same time, the contracting muscle can be palpated. Trapezius strength is evaluated by having the patient shrug the shoulders up against resistance. These muscles are also involved in head flexion and extension. In the newborn, sternocleidomastoid strength can be indirectly evaluated by observing head flexion on the traction response (i.e., lifting the head and trunk from supine by pulling the arms) and by observing the resting head posture and spontaneous head rotation. In older infants and children, resistance to head rotation gives some indication of sternocleidomastoid strength.

CRANIAL NERVE XII: HYPOGLOSSAL NERVE

Cranial nerve XII provides motor control to the tongue. In patients of all ages, the clinician ascertains the position of the tongue at rest and on protrusion. A protruded tongue deviates to the weaker side. Tongue movements are tested by observing the patient produce lingual speech sounds such as "takataka" and "lalala." The patient is asked to move the tongue from side to side very quickly and to push the tongue into the inside of the cheek against resistance applied by the examiner's finger on the outside of the cheek. The tongue should be examined when it is totally at rest for evidence of fibrillations or fasciculations. As the newborn sucks on the examiner's finger, lingual tone, movement, and strength can be gauged.

Speech Assessment

After the child has developed the ability to talk, spontaneous speech should be observed. A more cooperative child can repeat phrases and sentences for speech assessment. Infants initially coo, then babble, and then say single words, some of which may be intelligible. Speech is assessed for its clarity, accuracy, and rhythm. Immature speech has characteristic substitutions of certain sounds such as "w" for "r" in "wabbit." If there are other abnormalities of articulation and no structural explanation (e.g., cleft palate), an attempt should be made to localize the neurological deficit. Abnormalities of the cranial nerves VII (i.e., labials), X (i.e., phonation and nasopharyngeal closure), and XII (i.e., lingual function) can produce characteristic speech abnormalities. Dysarthria, or slurring of speech, generally is caused by cerebellar or extrapyramidal disorders. Cerebellar speech is typically a telegraphic or scanning type of speech, whereas extrapyramidal disorders produce a monotonous slow speech with poor breath control. Speech abnormalities must be distinguished from language abnormalities.

Motor Examination

In the child of any age, motor evaluation should begin with observation of the patient's posture and spontaneous movements. Lack or asymmetry of movement can be a manifestation of abnormality. Assessment of function of the newborn infant or young child occurs within the context of the expected age-appropriate motor abilities. By the age of 6 years, the motor performance of normal children should include most of the repertoire of a mature nervous system, although not necessarily the skill and facility.

POSTURE

The clinician should inspect posture with infants in a supine and sitting position and with older children in the standing position. The normal posture of the preterm infant is one of extension, whereas that of a full-term infant is one of flexion of the extremities. In younger children who are beginning to sit, there is some slumping forward, which improves with maturation. In older children, there is the tendency for a lordotic posture during standing, which also improves with maturity. There should be no asymmetry, and the sitting and standing posture should be erect. When older children are asked to hold the arms horizontally outstretched in front of the body with the hands supinated, they should hold the arms steadily and symmetrically. Pronation and downward drifting of one of the limbs indicate motor impairment on that side (i.e., pronator drift).

Several other postural abnormalities may be apparent. In the newborn, the frog-leg posture in which the legs are externally rotated and abducted at the hips with flexion at the knees is frequently seen in cases of profound weakness, such as with anterior horn cell disease. Slumping of the child in a sitting position can indicate motor dysfunction at several areas of the nervous system. Head posturing can be associated with a variety of local or neuropathologic processes, or both. Excessive lumbar lordosis may indicate weakness of the muscles of the girdle or spine. Many postures are sufficiently characteristic to be recognized. The decerebrate posture with opisthotonus, extensor posturing of the limbs, and decorticate posture in which there is flexion of the upper limbs is fairly well known. The typical hemiplegic posture with flexion at the elbow and wrist and internal rotation of the arm along with extension of the leg on the hemiplegic side is also readily recognized. Mild forms of this type of posture or a tendency to assume this posture during activities such as walking can be a sign of mild hemiparesis. In younger infants, the scissoring posture of the legs is caused by increased adductor tone and crossing of the legs, and it is frequently seen in children with spastic diplegia. Dystonia can result in unusual postures at the neck, spine, and limbs, but these characteristically are quite variable. The posture of internal rotation of the arm and cupping of the hand (i.e., waiter's-tip position) is characteristic of lesions of the upper brachial plexus (i.e., Erb's palsy).

MUSCLE TONE

Muscle tone is the palpable resistance to movement that is experienced by the examiner when the limbs or spine of the patient are passively manipulated by the examiner. Tone may be normal, increased (i.e., hypertonia), or decreased (i.e., hypotonia). Flaccidity is the complete absence of tone, and it is always accompanied by weakness or total paralysis. To assess tone, the patient should be at rest, offering no voluntary resistance or help while the examiner actively moves the joints through their range of motion. Tone reflects the resting neural activation of the agonist-antagonist muscle groups. In addition to range of motion, muscle tone can be tested by observing the inertial lag of the limb when it is suddenly displaced by the examiner. This test is conveniently performed in a supine patient by lifting the knee up quickly and observing the position and movement of the heel, which should normally stay on the surface. In hypertonia, there is failure of the leg extensors to relax quickly, and the heel lifts off the surface. The clinician can also assess tone in most limbs by observing the motion of the unsupported part of the limb when it is shaken in a flapping motion. Flappability is increased in hypotonia and decreased in hypertonia.

During early development, the tone of the normal infant changes considerably. The resting tone and resting posture are interrelated. The posture of the newborn preterm (28 to 30 weeks' gestation) is one of extension, and as the gestational age of the newborn increases to full term (40 weeks' gestation), there is a progressively increasing flexion posture. The limb tone is decreased in the preterm, progressing to increased flexion tone in the full-term newborn. Tone in the newborn is also assessed by range of movement tests such as the scarf maneuver, in which the extent to which the arm can be gently pulled across the chest to the opposite side is determined. The degree of extension of the leg (i.e., popliteal angle), dorsiflexion of the foot, and other maneuvers are also used to assess tone (and gestational age) in newborn infants. Muscle tone in the newborn can be judged by assessing the degree and speed of limb recoil from an extended position after it is released. Shaking of the arm or leg by the clinician while he or she observes the amplitude of movement of the more distal hand or foot (i.e., flappability) is particularly useful in assessing the newborn and young infant. The flexed tone and posture of the newborn gradually decreases until normal mature tone is seen by about the age of 6 months. In addition to appendicular tone, the clinician can assess axial tone in the infant by supporting the trunk in ventral suspension and observing the position of the infant draped over the suspending hand. The examiner observes the head and trunk posture and movement when the infant is held in an upright sitting position. These maneuvers and the traction response assess active tone (i.e., power) and passive tone. The clinician elicits the traction response by grasping the hands and pulling the supine infant to a sitting position while observing normal head support (or head lag) and normal reflex contraction of the biceps. In the very hypotonic (or weak) infant, care must be taken to avoid injury by excessive movement of limbs or head during these tests. Infants may have a discrepancy between axial and appendicular tone. Tone also can be markedly influenced by drugs, stress, excitement, or systemic illness.

Hypertonia is abnormally increased tone that usually is a sign of a central nervous system defect. In children, this condition is frequently spastic hypertonia, which is characterized by a velocity-dependent increase in tonic stretch reflexes (i.e., muscle tone). If the limb is passively moved slowly, the resistance is less, but if it is moved more rapidly, there is correspondingly increased resistance (i.e., tone) until a sudden lessening occurs (i.e., clasp-knife response). Spasticity is caused by an upper motoneuron abnormality, but it does not equate precisely with cortical spinal tract disturbance, as is often assumed.

Rigidity is muscle hypertonia and stiffness appreciated as a persistent resistance to passive movement throughout the range of movement. Plastic rigidity is increased resistance in agonist and antagonist muscles that is not velocity dependent. Its presence often is an indication of extrapyramidal or basal ganglia dysfunction. Nuchal rigidity, with stiffness of the neck and resistance to neck flexion, frequently is a reflex rigidity caused by meningeal irritation. Extension of this rigidity into the musculature of the spine produces opisthotonus, which is primarily a form of extensor rigidity. Decerebrate rigidity results from the release of brainstem centers from higher control. This type of rigidity is a sustained muscle contraction of antigravity muscles, with the spine and all four limbs being rigidly extended.

Rarely, hypertonia is caused by peripheral mechanisms that result in continuous muscle fiber activity (i.e., neuromyotonia) or impaired and delayed muscle relaxation after contraction (i.e., myotonia). Myotonia can be demonstrated by the inability of the patient to release a handshake quickly or may be elicited by the percussion of muscles, producing an exaggerated contraction. This percussion myotonia can be elicited from several muscles, including the tongue, but perhaps the most dramatic is percussion of the belly of the opponens pollicis muscle in the thenar eminence, which causes sustained contraction of this muscle for several seconds.

Hypotonia should be characterized by degree (i.e., mild, moderate, or severe) and distribution (i.e., focal, axial, appendicular, or generalized). The distribution has little localizing value unless it is focal. Hypotonia can be associated with dysfunction of virtually any part of the central and peripheral nervous system or musculoskeletal system. Still, an attempt should be made to determine whether the hypotonia is central (i.e., related to central nervous system pathology) or peripheral (i.e., related to peripheral nervous system pathology), or both. Associated neurological manifestations, such as altered reflexes, are helpful in making this distinction.

MUSCLE BULK AND POWER

Muscle bulk should be evaluated using inspection and palpation. The degree and distribution of atrophy, absence, hypertrophy, or pseudohypertrophy of muscle should be evaluated. The presence of atrophy suggests decreased innervation, particularly if it is focal atrophy. Absence of muscle is generally a developmental abnormality. Hypertrophy may indicate overuse, over-

growth, or underlying muscle pathology. Pseudohypertrophy describes the selectively enlarged but weak muscles seen in disorders such as Duchenne's muscular dystrophy. It is difficult to judge muscle bulk in newborns and young infants because of the large amount of adipose tissue on the limbs at this age. The tongue, however, is a muscle in which bulk is more easily assessed. Atrophy or hypertrophy may be prominent in this muscle when it is not apparent in others.

Power or strength can be determined in the older child using the formal Medical Research Council (MRC) of the United Kingdom scale, in which power is graded from 0 to 5. The grades are defined in Table 200–3.

Individual muscles or muscle groups should be formally tested when indicated. For routine neurological examination in infants and children, a greater emphasis is placed on functional strength and on how patients use this strength in the various muscular activities of their bodies. The activities of standing up from a supine position, walking, hopping, pulling away, "making a muscle," and squeezing an object can be easily understood by the patient, and their observation by the clinician can provide a fairly good indication of the patient's strength. In infants and young children, strength is often estimated by the power of withdrawal from a noxious stimulus or away from the examiner. Assessment of active tone, such as by observing head support in ventral suspension when the patient is held in a sitting position and during the traction response, indicates power as much as tone. The older infant can be observed holding the head up in the prone position (2 months old), then crawling, and later walking (12 to 15 months old). As children become older, they can be expected to cooperate more with formal testing. By age 4 to 6 years, the normal child can cooperate well enough for a good assessment of power. In older children, detailed muscle strength testing can be performed using the MRC scale for individual muscles when indicated.

In younger children and as a screening neurological evaluation in older children, tests of function can provide a gross estimate of strength in several muscle groups at once. During the first year, the clinician can observe the functions of reaching (4 to 5 months old), sitting when placed (5 to 7 months old), crawling (9 to 12 months old), and pulling to stand. Asymmetry of muscle function is also noted. After the age of 1 year,

TABLE 200–3 ■ **Medical Research Council Scale for Determining Strength**

SCORE	POWER OR STRENGTH
0	No contraction
1	Flicker or trace of contraction
2	Active movement with gravity eliminated
3	Active movement against gravity
4	Active movement against gravity and resistance*
5	Normal power

* It is customary to use 4–, 4, and 4+ to indicate movement against slight, moderate, and strong resistance, respectively.

walking, running, and then climbing can be observed. At about 3 years of age, the young child may begin to ride a tricycle. At 4 years, hopping with both feet and, at 5 years, hopping on one foot may be possible. Strong preference for using one hand in infants younger than 1 year of age suggests weakness or other impairment of the opposite side. Useful information about motor function can also be obtained from observing how the uncooperative child actively resists the examination or holds on to items that are being retrieved.

COORDINATION

Coordination is the smooth integration of all elements involved in the accurate and efficient performance of movement. Incoordination is seen in pyramidal and extrapyramidal disorders of motor control, in sensory abnormalities, and in cerebellar disturbances. Ataxia is incoordination not caused by weakness, altered tone, or involuntary movements. The most important form of ataxia, cerebellar ataxia, is caused by a disturbance of the cerebellum and its afferent or efferent pathways. Sensory ataxia results from altered sensory feedback regarding motion and position of the limbs.

Coordination is tested by examination of the speed, regularity, and accuracy of movement. It is difficult to evaluate in the infant until sufficient voluntary control has developed, such as the ability to reach for objects (4 to 5 months old). Coordination is formally tested in the limbs and trunk and during walking.

The finger-to-nose test of the upper extremity and the heel-to-shin test of the lower extremity are used to evaluate the ability to stop on target rather than bypass the target or miss it altogether. Loss of this ability, dysmetria, is a form of ataxia. The patient is instructed to rapidly touch the tip of the finger to two targets alternately: the examiner's finger, which should be moved to different positions during the test, and the tip of the patient's nose. Other targets may be used. This test may also bring out another sign of cerebellar dysfunction, intention tremor, in which, as the patient's finger approaches the target, it oscillates with increasing amplitude. The heel-to-shin maneuver is most easily performed when the patient is in a supine position. The patient is instructed to raise one leg and bring the heel of the foot of that leg down accurately onto the knee of the resting leg and, after touching it, move the heel smoothly down the shin to the foot and back again. This maneuver is done several times, and the smoothness and accuracy of the movement from the knee down to the foot are observed. In cases of cerebellar disease, this movement is slow and irregular, and the heel may fall off the shin. Having the patient perform these tests with the eyes closed also allows the clinician to evaluate sensory ataxia. In the young child, reaching for an object or touching a light or other interesting target can substitute for the finger-to-nose test. The clinician can also ask the child to touch various parts of their body, such as the nose.

Dysdiadochokinesis is impairment of rapid and alternating movements due to a cerebellar abnormality. The clinician can identify this abnormality by observing the speed, accuracy, rhythm, and regularity of any repetitive movement. The usual tests for dysdiadochokinesis are rapid finger-to-thumb tapping, patting movements of the hand, toe tapping, and the more complex movement of patting something with the palm of the hand and then the dorsum of the hand in an alternating pronation-supination movement.

The aforementioned tests measure coordination in the extremities. Unsteadiness of the patient while standing or sitting is referred to as truncal ataxia, which is frequently seen with caudal vermis abnormalities. The clinician observes the patient while he or she is sitting and standing, with and without the arms extended in front, and notes the patient's inability to hold a steady position. The patient may have a wide-based stance. For older children, a more sensitive test is standing on one leg.

ABNORMAL MOVEMENTS

A variety of abnormal movements occur in children and, less frequently, in infants. The movements are usually involuntary and are abnormal in their pattern or time of occurrence compared with normal, voluntary movement. The dyskinesias include tremor, tics, myoclonus, and the involuntary movements of chorea, hemiballismus, dystonia, and athetosis. Ataxia, epileptic movements, fasciculations, hemifacial spasm, and sleep-associated movements, although involuntary, are by convention considered under other categories of neurological abnormality. Repetitive movements such as mannerisms, self-stimulation, and stereotypies are not considered to be motor abnormalities. The clinician assesses for dyskinesias by observing the patient at rest and during voluntary action. Because these movements are usually obvious on visual inspection, video technology allows the clinician to document the degree and pattern of abnormality and the caregiver to record movements that occur intermittently or infrequently. Dyskinesias usually only occur when the patient is awake and frequently can be voluntarily modulated but not totally controlled.

The characteristic feature of tremor is rhythmic oscillation of a body part. In children, this oscillation usually occurs in the upper extremity or, less commonly, the head. The clinician determines whether the tremor occurs mainly at rest, with sustained posture (e.g., with arms extended) or with action, and whether the frequency is greater or less than 6 Hz. The patient should be asked to copy a spiral or other figure and to write a sentence to demonstrate the effects of the tremor on these fine motor activities. Myoclonus is a sudden, brief, involuntary contraction of a muscle or group of muscles. Myoclonus produces a movement that is not synergistic or stereotyped. Tics are sudden, repetitive, synergistic, stereotyped movements that may be simple, complex, or phonatory. Choreic movements are brief, arrhythmic, asymmetrical, and synergistic; they appear to be fragments of normal movements. Hemiballismus is a severe form of chorea with large-amplitude movements involving an entire limb. Dystonic movements are characterized by sustained muscle co-contraction of agonist and antagonist muscles. The abnormal muscle activity in dystonia produces twisting movements or abnormal postures. The movements and postures of dystonia typically fluctuate during the examination. Athetotic movements are more rapid and the postures are more transient than dystonia. Speech is affected more often in athetosis than in the other dyskinesias. The clinician should observe for abnormal movement in the child in different positions at rest and while performing voluntary movements, such as walking, extending the arms in front, and reaching for objects.

GAIT

Before the infant begins to walk, there is a period (11 to 13 months old) when "cruising," or walking with support, occurs. Asymmetries can be seen at this stage. Initially, there is hesitancy and unsteadiness, which progresses to a wide-based "toddlers gait" as part of normal maturation. Specialized variations of the gait, such as running and climbing stairs, provide additional dimensions to the gait assessment. In the older child, associated movements such as arm swing should be assessed, particularly for the presence of asymmetry. The base, size, and speed of the steps and the posture should he observed during gait observation. The ability to independently ambulate and the use of walking aids are recorded. The sounds of the footfall, particularly with the shoes on, can provide additional information, but gait should generally be observed with the patient barefoot as well. Excessive wearing of one shoe sole or part of the sole on one or both feet can indicate abnormal gait.

Several gaits are characteristic of neurological impairment. The hemiplegic gait has some degree of footdrop and circumduction, or lateral swinging movement, of the foot. The spastic paraparetic or tetraparetic gait is a bilateral shuffling gait with a tendency for the legs to pull together in adduction (i.e., scissoring). There can be a tendency to walk on the toes, or the patient may walk in a crouched position. Gait ataxia frequently is related to rostral cerebellar vermis dysfunction. The patient has difficulty in maintaining a narrow-based gait and spontaneously may have a wide-based gait. Most normal children older than 5 years can perform tandem gait with one foot directly in front of the other in the midline and with toe touching heel. Children are able to walk on a narrow path before they are able to walk tandem. Narrow-path walking should be tested if the patient is too young to perform the tandem test. The ataxic gait is wide based and unsteady, with staggering, lurching, or swaying. Tandem walk is particularly difficult. A unilateral ataxic gait produces much less disturbance, but there may be a tendency to deviate to the ataxic side. The waddling gait of girdle weakness is caused by weakness of the gluteus medius bilaterally, creating pelvic instability that leads to an exaggerated vertical movement of the pelvis with gait, producing the waddling appearance. Footdrop results in scraping of the toe on the floor or a steppage gait in which there is compensatory, excessive lifting of the lower extremity with the foot being swung forward and slapped down to prevent the toe from dragging. This type of abnormality may be unilateral or bilateral. The antalgic gait results from the patient's attempts to avoid pain by performing maneuvers to limit the time that weight is put on the affected side during walking.

Reflex Testing

Reflex testing is important in the pediatric examination because it does not require conscious or voluntary responses or even cooperation. Many primitive reflexes are described in the section on neonatal examination. Others are stretch reflexes, superficial reflexes, and pathologic reflexes.

The muscle stretch reflexes or deep tendon reflexes are evoked by stimulation of sensory organs in the muscle by stretch. There is a reflex contraction of the muscle being stretched. These reflexes are easily elicited in newborns and young infants with the tomahawk-style percussion hammer or a miniaturized version of the Queen's Square or other reflex hammers.

The jaw, or masseter, stretch reflex (i.e., testing the trigeminal nerve) is readily seen in the newborn infant but may be difficult to elicit in the older child. The clinician elicits this reflex by placing an index finger horizontally over the chin of the patient's slightly open and relaxed jaw and then tapping the index finger. This causes a stretch of the masseter muscle, and the reaction is a contraction of that muscle. Newborns may demonstrate clonus with this maneuver, which may be normal or an indication of a corticobulbar abnormality.

Maneuvers to elicit the biceps reflex (C5-6, musculocutaneous nerve), the brachioradialis reflex (C5-6, radial nerve), and the triceps reflex (C7-8, radial nerve) are performed on the upper extremity. The method is the same for infants and older children. The examiner percusses his or her thumb or finger placed over the biceps tendon at the antecubital fossa for the biceps reflex. Percussion of the brachioradialis tendon near the styloid process or of the triceps tendon just proximal to the olecranon may be done directly with the hammer or indirectly through the overlying digits of the examiner. Percussion of the examiner's fingers overlying the slightly flexed distal fingers can elicit the finger flexor reflex (C6-T1, median and ulnar nerves). Maneuvers to elicit the patellar reflex (L2-4, femoral nerve), the ankle reflex (L5-S2, tibial nerve), and the adductor reflex (L2-4, obturator nerve) are performed in the lower extremity. The patellar reflex is elicited by percussing the subpatellar tendon with the knee slightly flexed, thereby producing a quadriceps muscle stretch and then contraction. The ankle reflex is elicited by tapping the Achilles tendon, producing a contraction of the gastrocnemius, soleus, and plantaris muscles, and the adductor reflex is elicited by tapping the adductor tendon near the medial epicondyle of the distal femur, producing adductor muscle contraction.

Reflexes are graded from 0 to 4+; an absent reflex is 0, a normal reflex is 2+, and a hyperactive reflex is 3 or 4+. If there is reduplication of the reflex or if clonus is elicited by the testing, the reflex usually is graded 4+. It may be possible for the examiner to elicit otherwise undetectable reflexes by using the Jendrassik maneuver, in which the patient clasps the fingers of both hands together and attempts to pull the hands apart at the same time the reflex is tested. A similar reinforcement may be possible if the patient makes a very tight fist of both hands or clenches the jaw at the same moment the reflex is tested. In addition to grading the reflex, the clinician should observe the spread of reflex to adjacent joints as a sign of increased reflex activity. The crossed adductor response is elicited on patellar testing. When this reflex is present, the contralateral adductor also contracts, which is evidence of increased reflex activity.

The superficial (cutaneous) reflexes are present in young children. The abdominal reflexes are elicited by stroking the upper and then lower quadrants of the abdomen. The reflex consists of a contraction of the abdominal musculature beneath the stimulus, usually resulting in a movement of the umbilicus toward that quadrant. A slightly blunted stick, such as a split tongue depressor, can be used as an effective stimulus. If the object is too blunt, a reflex will not be elicited, but the stimulus should not be painful. The superficial abdominal reflexes are mediated by the nerve segments that innervate the abdominal wall, approximately T7 to T10 in the upper quadrants and T11 to L2 in the lower quadrants. These reflexes disappear after certain upper motoneuron lesions have occurred.

The cremasteric reflex is elicited by stimulating the skin of the upper inner thigh and observing the contraction of the cremasteric muscle resulting in ipsilateral elevation of the testicle. This reflex is innervated by L1-2 nerves. The bulbocavernous reflex is sometimes useful. Stimulation of the dorsum of the glans penis causes a palpable contraction of the bulbocavernous muscle and the external anal sphincter. The bulbocavernous reflex is mediated by the S3-4 nerve segments. Anal tone can conveniently be assessed at the same time. The cutaneous anal reflex is a contraction of the external anal sphincter in response to stroking or pricking the skin or mucous membrane in the perianal region. This reflex can be seen as a contraction of the anus (i.e., anal wink) in response to the stimulus. This reflex is mediated by the S2-4 nerve segments.

Pathologic cutaneous reflexes include the classic Babinski sign and other reflexes that elicit an extensor response of the great toe. These responses have various eponymous names. The stimulation for the Babinski response is a somewhat noxious stroking of the plantar surface of the foot from the heel forward. The normal response is a plantarflexion of the toes, particularly the great toe, but this does not always occur. The abnormal response is a dorsiflexion or extensor response of the great toe and fanning of the other toes. This reflex is mediated through the tibial nerve and involves nerve segments L4 through S2. To avoid a grasp response with flexion of the toes in the neonate, it is often better to stimulate from the toes downward to the heel. Extensor responses of the toe are frequently seen in normal newborns and infants during the first year of life, but the quality of these responses seems different from the usual Babinski sign. Nevertheless, an important aspect is asymmetry of response between the two sides. Another response that is sometimes seen in comatose or paraplegic individuals is the triple flexion response, in which stimulation of the sole of the foot gives rise to dorsiflexion of the toe, flexion of the knee, and flexion of the hip. This is a spine-mediated response, and its presence does not indicate voluntary withdrawal.

Withdrawal is often seen when the Babinski sign is elicited in children. Sometimes, the response can be minimized by simultaneous elicitation of the Oppenheim sign, which produces a Babinski-like response but is elicited by heavy pressure with the thumb and index finger on the anterior surface of the tibia, stroking from the knee to the ankle. Another maneuver that may minimize withdrawal is flexion of the hip and knee and dorsiflexion of the foot in infants or children before eliciting the Babinski sign. Some clinicians are concerned that this may inhibit a valid Babinski response when one is present. The Gonda sign is elicitation of the Babinski sign by flicking the distal tip of the second or fourth toe. This approach can be useful when there is a cast on the foot.

Clonus is a reflex response that indicates hyperreactivity of the cortical spinal tract. This reflex can sometimes be seen in normal newborns or young infants, but it usually is not sustained. Ankle clonus is elicited by rapid and sustained dorsiflexion of the foot by the examiner when the leg is slightly flexed at the knee. Rhythmic, alternating contraction and relaxation of the gastrocnemius muscle produces rhythmic ankle plantarflexion movements against the examiner's hand. This reflex is usually elicited most easily by a rapid stretch, but it may require several repetitions to elicit the clonus. The clonus may be unsustained, in which case it attenuates, or sustained, in which case it is maintained for many seconds or indefinitely. Clonus may occur spontaneously when the patient places the foot in certain positions. Clonus can also be elicited from other sites, and the mechanism is similar.

Developmental Reflexes

Near-term premature infants, full-term neonates, and young infants have many reflexes that disappear with time or are replaced by voluntary movements and cannot be elicited in the older infant. The Moro response, seen in preterm and full-term neonates, disappears by the fifth or sixth month of life. The infant's head and body are held, and the head is allowed to drop quickly a very short distance before being gently supported again. In response to this and other maneuvers that suddenly displace the head and trunk relationship, there is a sudden extension and abduction of the upper limbs with opening of the hands. These responses are immediately followed by flexion and adduction of the limbs toward the midline. The Moro response reflects the general level of excitability of the infant's nervous system; an infant with a depressed nervous system, for example, has a decreased or absent response. Asymmetry of the response can be significant and usually indicates a peripheral problem (e.g., Erb's palsy, fracture of the clavicle). In the less responsive newborn, some indication of the level of nervous system depression can be determined by the nasal closure response. Lightly pinching the nostrils together briefly elicits an extensor posturing of the arms in the normal newborn. This response may persist even when the Moro response can no longer be elicited in the neonate with a severely depressed nervous system.

Premature and mature newborns and young infants demonstrate an involuntary grasp response. This reflex persists until the time that they begin to make voluntary reaching movements (3 to 5 months old), and it then gradually diminishes and is replaced with a voluntary grasp. The clinician elicits the grasp response by putting his or her finger into the palms of the infant's hands or the soles of the infant's feet, producing involuntary closure of the infant's digits around the finger. The toe grasp may persist until later in the first year.

The sucking reflex is a robust primitive response that reflects the level of excitability of the infant's nervous system and oral function. This reflex can often best be estimated by the use of a gloved finger. The vigor and degree of suction and the absence of an abnormal biting movement should be evaluated as the infant suckles the finger. The effectiveness of an infant's sucking can also be observed during bottle-feeding, which also offers the opportunity for evaluation of swallow. The clinician tests for the rooting response by stimulating the lateral margins of the infant's lips and noticing an orientation and turning of the face and mouth to the stimulus in an attempt to suckle it. This reflex, which requires intact face sensation, disappears as the nervous system becomes depressed.

The traction response is elicited by taking the supine infant by the hands and pulling him or her up to a sitting position. The response is flexion of the arms and stabilization of the head. Head lag and lack of arm flexion are abnormal responses. The placing response is elicited by holding the infant vertically and bringing the dorsum of the foot and leg up to the edge of a tabletop or a bed rail. The limb is flexed, then pulled forward, and extended almost as if the infant is stepping over the obstacle. This reflex diminishes during the second half of the first year. The supporting reaction is variably present in the first 6 months. The infant is held erect and lowered so that feet touch a surface. When the supporting reaction is present, the infant extends the leg and supports his or her weight somewhat. The stepping response is elicited by holding the infant erect and then leaning the infant forward with the feet lightly touching the surface. The response is a stepping forward movement of the legs, which may continue for several steps. This reflex is often present during the first 6 weeks of age, but it can be seen later in some infants.

When the infant is held in a horizontal, prone position (i.e., ventral suspension), the truncal incurvature response (i.e., Galant's reflex) can be elicited by superficial stimulation of the back along the paraspinal musculature of the infant from birth to 2 months of age. This stimulation causes twisting and curving of the body toward the stimulus. This reaction should be compared on both sides. The Landau response is also elicited with the infant in ventral suspension. A normal infant has some extension of the head and legs in this prone position. Flexion of the head results in flexion of the hips. This response appears around 3 months of age and persists throughout infancy.

The tonic neck response may normally be present in the first 4 or 5 months of life and is most easily elicited between 2 and 4 months. Turning the head to one side produces a tendency for flexion of the limbs of the contralateral side and extension of the ipsilateral limbs. Rotating the head back to the other side causes a reversal of this posture to its mirror image. The normal response is never obligate, persists past 6 months, or is significantly different from one side to the other. There is persistent or obligate posturing of the flexed arm on the side of an existing hemiparesis. With maturation, the tonic neck response is replaced by the neck-righting reflex in which the infant's body and limbs automatically follow when the head is turned to the side as the patient attempts to roll over. This normal response becomes obvious around the ages of 4 to 8 months when rolling over develops.

The clinician elicits the parachute response by holding the infant in ventral suspension and moving the body downward rapidly. The reflex is an extension of the arms forward as if to break a fall. This response appears at the age of 8 to 10 months in all normal infants. The clinician should assess its presence and any asymmetry, which may indicate the presence of a hemiparesis or other motor abnormality.

Sensation

The sensory system includes the primary modalities of pain and temperature; touch, proprioception, and vibration of the somatosensory system; and the higher cortical processes of perception and discrimination of more complex sensory stimuli. This system also includes special senses such as smell, vision, taste, and hearing, which are evaluated during the cranial nerve examination. The normal child of 5 or 6 years should be able to cooperate for a fairly complete sensory examination. Because a refined examination depends on the subjective and qualitative judgment of the patient, examination of the younger child must be cruder and more creative.

In the somatosensory examination of the newborn, virtually all that can be assessed is response to pain or to tickle, which are probably mediated by similar pathways. When the clinician tests for pain sensation in a patient of any age, a clean, sharp stick that is disposed of after the examination is preferable to a pin, which can transmit disease, or to a sterile needle, which often draws blood. This stick is used to test cutaneous pain sensation. Deep pressure over bones or tendons can cause diffuse, aching (deep) pain, which is less well localized but can be used to test the level of responsiveness of the individual. For a child of any age, the clinician tries to determine the location of the sensory abnormality and whether it has the pattern of dermatome (segmental) or nerve distribution. In the older infant, tickle is preferable to painful stimulation during the initial stages of the examination. The examiner observes whether the infant notices a touch or tickle that is performed surreptitiously. The infant may look at the stimulus or brush it away. Some older infants may respond to a vibratory stimulus. The clinician places the stem of the tuning fork on the extremity when the fork is not vibrating and allows the infant to adapt to this sensation. The examiner then observes the response of the infant to the initiation of vibration while the fork is still in place on the limb.

For older children, the examination can be more formal. Response to pain is usually tested with a sharp, disposable stick, but response to tickle can be used in the overreactive and oversensitive child. In an otherwise normal child with no sensory complaints, a screening test with detection and comparison of responses to a sharp stick distally in the feet and in the hands and comparison between distal and proximal responses may be all that is required. Any indication of spinal cord abnormality requires a detailed search for a sensory level. The sharp stick is touched and quickly withdrawn, with the clinician taking care to apply the same pressure with each stimulus. The cooperative patient is asked to report whether the stimulation is sharp or dull and whether the quality or sharpness is different from that of the comparison stimulus. It is preferable to move from an area of loss or lesser sensation to the normal area to detect a change, the location of which is then marked on the skin. In the extremities, the sensory loss may be peripheral, occurring in a stocking-glove distribution, or may follow the distribution of a root or nerve. There is much overlap between adjacent dermatomes, which may make minor sensory losses difficult to identify.

In less responsive individuals, deep pressure over a bone, tendon, or nailbed can produce a noxious and painful stimulus that may be more arousing to the obtunded patient. This test is generally not useful in a conscious, cooperative child.

Temperature is mediated by the same pathways as pain and, when necessary, can be tested more formally with cold and hot tubes of water applied to the skin briefly to determine if the patient can detect cold or hot. Many examiners use, as a simple screening test for temperature, a cold metal object applied to the skin to see whether it is recognized as cold. The metal tuning fork is often used for this purpose. Pain and temperature are carried by afferent fibers with cell bodies in the dorsal root ganglion that enter the dorsal spinal cord and, after ascending several segments, cross over near the central canal to spinothalamic tracts in the lateral part of the cord and ascend to the thalamus.

Touch or tactile sensibility is tested with a wisp of cotton or a paper tissue. This stimulus must be a touch and not a moving or wiping stimulus, because such stimuli activate other neural pathways. It is useful to ask the patient, whose eyes are closed, to touch where the examiner has touched. This approach ensures that the stimulus was detected and provides a higher cortical assessment of point localization. Children are encouraged to view this type of examination as a game, and this is reinforced with praise when they succeed. Alternatively, the patient can be asked to say "now" whenever the stimulus is felt. Patients can consciously or subconsciously alter the results of the sensory examination. In that event, repeat testing usually shows discrepancies in the location of sensory loss. Other strategies, such as having the patient say "yes" when he or she feels it and "no" when nothing is felt, are sometimes revealing. The sensations are compared between peripheral and proximal sites, between left and right sides, between levels of the trunk, and between the different sides of an extremity. The cooperative patient can give a subjective assessment of qualitative differences between two stimuli that are both detected when the examiner is testing in an area of deficit. Fibers carrying tactile or touch sensibility enter the zone of Lissauer and synapse with neurons in the dorsal horn. Tactile sensibility uses two pathways. One of these pathways crosses over near the central canal to the opposite side and ascends in the ventral spinothalamic tract to reach the ventral posterolateral nucleus of the thalamus. The other pathway follows the dorsal column ipsilaterally, crosses over to the opposite side in the medulla, and terminates in the ventral posterolateral nucleus of the thalamus.

The sense of vibration is tested with a 128-Hz tuning fork, and most children can detect and recognize the stimulus. Older children are able to report thresholds. The stimulus is usually placed on the distal finger or toe, but vibration can be tested over any bony prominence, including the iliac crest, spinous processes, sternum, and skull. In cooperative patients, the test is usually done only distally, unless there are sensory complaints or findings. To detect a sensory loss, the threshold of the vibration stimulus is compared from distal to proximal, from left to right, and with the same site on the examiner. So that the younger child can understand what is expected, the tuning fork is first placed on the digit without vibration. Often, the cooperative, younger child says "yes" to any stimulation, including the pressure of the tuning fork, and must be coached in proper discrimination. Vibration is mediated through large and medium-sized myelinated nerve fibers and is believed to ascend the spinal cord in the dorsal columns ipsilaterally, but other pathways may also be used. Because the sound and the vibration produced by the tuning fork are compelling stimuli for some children, it can be used as a novelty that can attract their attention and induce them to reach, touch, or want to play with it.

Proprioception, or position sense, is not easily examined in infants and young children and is not usually tested. Older, cooperative children can be fully evaluated. Testing is done initially in the distal digits, usually the great toe and the thumb or index finger. The digit is held on either side of the joint to be tested, usually the distal joint. The proximal part is held fixed while the distal part is moved in extension or flexion during the testing. The digits are held on the side so as not to provide pressure clues on the direction of movement. The clinician demonstrates the motion to the patient, indicating which direction is up or down (or forward or backward), so that both examiner and examinee agree on this point. Alternatively, the patient can indicate the direction of movement by pointing. Small-amplitude, single movements are made in one direction, with the patient's eyes closed, to determine whether he or she can detect movement and, if so, the direction of the movement. The amplitude of excursion required for detection can be used to quantitate the response. A series of movements in random directions are done until the examiner is convinced that the patient is accurately identifying the direction. Proprioception on left and right sides should be compared, and testing of the toes should be compared with that of the fingers. If a deficit is found, the clinician should test the same limb at a joint more proximal, similarly holding the limb proximal and distal to the new joint being tested.

Proprioception also is indirectly tested during other parts of the neurological examination. On finger-to-nose testing done with the patient's eyes closed, proprioceptive mechanisms are indirectly being evaluated. Testing for the Romberg sign also assesses proprioception. Even younger children can cooperate with this test; the child stands with feet as close together as possible and still maintains a steady stance and then closes the eyes. If there is increased swaying or falling when the eyes close, the Romberg sign is positive, indicating a sensory abnormality, often in peripheral nerve or dorsal columns, that affects proprioception.

Testing of higher cortical sensory perception and discrimination (i.e., gnosis) can be done as part of the mental status examination or the sensory examination. Most of these tests are possible only in older children or very cooperative younger children. The tests measure contralateral parietal lobe function. Point localization is a form of perception that can be tested as part of the routine examination even in younger children, because it is easy for them to understand the concept. As part of sensory testing, the examiner can ask the patient to "touch where I touched." This documents that the touch has been felt and measures the accuracy of the patient's point localization. Younger infants are not precise, but they can localize touch to the approximate vicinity of the stimulus. Older children and adults should demonstrate very precise localization.

Graphesthesia is easily tested at the bedside. Letters or numbers can be used. It is often helpful to initially trace the number or letter in the palm of the child's hand with a pointed object while he or she is watching to ensure that the instructions are understood. If that seems acceptable, a different symbol is drawn with the patient's eyes closed to see if he or she can identify it. Younger children may not be able to recognize all numbers, but there should not be asymmetry in the responses for the two hands. Stereognosis testing uses common objects such as coins, keys, safety pins, paper clips, or small balls. These objects are placed in the patient's hand, but she or he should not look at them and should be prevented from manipulating the objects

with the fingers. If these objects cannot be identified, finger manipulation of the item can be allowed, but the results are not considered normal except in younger children. The responses of the two sides of the body must be compared. Testing for two-point discrimination is best done with the use of a special caliper manufactured for that purpose, but a paper clip can be readjusted to provide two tips whose separation can be varied. Distal fingers and lips are very sensitive in discriminating small separations. In older children, a 3- to 4-mm separation should be readily detected. Comparison of the responses of the two sides is most useful.

EXAMINATION OF SPECIFIC AGE GROUPS

Neonates and Young Infants

Examination of premature and full-term neonates or young infants is limited to observation, palpation, and reflex testing, but it can generally be done without great resistance from the infants if they are not hungry or have other discomforts. The examination can be approached systematically, as in the older child and adult, or it can be coupled with the general physical examination for convenience. In the following description, the sequence listed is one possible approach to the examination.

Any deformity of the face, head, spine, or feet should be noted. The shape of the head and the anterior fontanelle dimension (from one frontal bone margin to the opposite parietal bone margin) should be recorded. The clinician should look for separated sutures, a posterior fontanelle, an overriding suture or fusion, and any palpable swelling, such as a soft tissue caput or periosteal cephalhematoma. The blink reflex, pupillary reaction, and visual following and eye movements (i.e., spontaneous and with oculocephalic reflex) are tested, and a funduscopic examination is performed. The examiner assesses the corneal response to stimulation with a cotton wisp or puff of air, the sucking response, the jaw jerk, and the rooting response. Evaluation of facial contraction, including eyelid closure, may be postponed until the infant begins to cry. Testing for the gag response should also be deferred until the end of the examination. Sucking can be examined using a soother or finger stimulus. Sucking and swallowing may be evaluated during the infant's feeding. The response to a loud whistle or a bell should be noted. The grasp responses are tested, and the resting tone and posture are noted. The clinician should test for biceps, triceps, and brachioradialis stretch reflexes in the upper extremities and for the patellar and ankle jerk reflexes and the Babinski response in the lower extremities. The stepping, placing, and supporting reactions, as well as the truncal incurvature and Landau responses, are tested next. Testing for the infant's head support, Moro response, response to nasal closure, and traction response can be done together. The clinician can test for the tonic neck and neck-righting responses in the older infant and the parachute response in the still older infant.

Testing of the sensory response to painful stimulation is best done at the end of the examination. A sharp stick should provoke arousal, a grimace, or crying, depending on how noxious the stimulus is. Comparison of the responses from both sides of the head, body, and extremities should be made, and a sensory level should be sought, particularly if there is an obvious spinal malformation. The superficial anal reflex is then elicited, and if a neurological deficit is suspected, the anal tone can be evaluated with a gloved finger.

Infants 4 to 6 months of age can hold on to objects that are handed to them and may even begin to transfer them from one hand to the other. There should be no preference for the use of one hand over the other at this age; a preference probably indicates hemiparesis or some other abnormality. The clinician observes the older infant's ability to lift the head when she or he is in the prone position (2 months old), ability to roll over (4 to 6 months old), sitting when placed (6 to 8 months old), or moving into a sitting position independently (8 to 10 months old).

Older Infants and Young Children

For older infants and young children, the nervous system is not systematically examined, and the examination results are recorded in the standard outline. This approach is most appropriate for infants who have developed stranger anxiety (6 to 9 months old). In older children, a more systematic approach can be taken, as in adults.

OBSERVATION DURING HISTORY TAKING

The clinician can estimate the patient's mental status by reviewing the history; by observing the patient's interactions with parents, toys, the environment, and the examiner; and by noticing the patient's actions during feeding and playing. The examiner ascertains whether the patient is alert and aware, visually attentive, and socially interactive and comfortable or fearful. The examiner observes the patient's response to the caregiver's verbal stimuli, comments, and requests and notices the patient's level of speech. The clinician assesses how the patient performs complicated actions that require a certain level of cognitive development and sensorimotor ability. To perform many simple activities, the patient uses several neurological functions, and these activities therefore constitute a gross screening test for dysfunctions in those systems. For example, picking up a very small object requires a certain level of vision, a degree of fine motor control, and steadiness.

HANDS-OFF EXAMINATION

Without touching the patient, the clinician can assess the child's visual fields, vision, eye movements, and sometimes, the pupils. Facial movements during spontaneous smiling or crying can be evaluated, and hearing can be checked. Head support and trunk support

can be observed. The use of the limbs spontaneously in walking, crawling, and the manipulation of objects such as toys gives some indication of coordination and motor control. It is often useful to hand the patient a toy or other interesting object, if this has not been done previously. If the patient refuses the object from the examiner, he or she may accept it from the parent. Playing with an item distracts the infant's attention so that he or she may overcome fear of the examiner. As the patient reaches for the toy, the clinician further observes his or her motor control. Small blocks may be offered to the child, and designs for arranging them can be suggested to see whether the child can mimic them. A penlight can be used to play the "put out the light" game. The examiner demonstrates how the light can be extinguished by touching it, and then the infant is invited to try the same thing. This game provides a very good approximation of elements of the finger-to-nose test. During these observations, handedness should be identified. The child's response to requests and the child's own speech are noted during this part of the examination. At the end of this stage of the examination, the infant may have walked or crawled, but if not, the parent or caregiver can put the infant on the floor or table to encourage this movement. Observation of how the infant rises from the floor to a standing position and then walks can be informative.

HANDS-ON EXAMINATION

The hands-on examination can be done along with the rest of the general pediatric physical examination. There are two sections: the nonthreatening examination and the possibly threatening examination.

Nonthreatening Examination

The clinician can check the infant's response to sensory stimulation by tickling or touching various parts of the body to see if the infant notices it. The face, particularly around the ears and nose, and the extremities are good areas to test with a wisp of cotton or tissue. Vibration from a tuning fork is often of interest to the infant, and the examiner can often tell from the patient's response that the vibration is detected.

Reflex testing is usually nonthreatening, and reflexes can be examined along with muscle tone at this time. Strength can be tested as the infant pulls a toy away from the examiner, as the infant stands up, or as the infant withdraws from a tickle or perhaps noxious stimulus. The clinician should examine for cutaneous lesions, scoliosis, and organomegaly at this time.

Possibly Threatening Examination

When the nonthreatening examination has been completed, it is appropriate to examine the areas that were resisted by the infant. These and anything uncomfortable or noxious to the child should be postponed until this time, much as the examination of the ears may be postponed until the end of the general pediatric examination. Some infants allow a funduscopic examination fairly early and permit pupillary responses to be tested without complaint. Having an assistant or family member hold interesting objects behind the examiner often successfully directs the vision of the infant away from the ophthalmoscope.

The clinician can test the gag response and observe palate and tongue movement and position in addition to pharyngeal contraction. The infant often facilitates parts of the examination by crying, at which time symmetrical facial contraction with good eye closure can be observed. The tongue and palatal position and movement also can be assessed during crying or vocalization. If gait has not been tested previously, the examiner should take the infant away from the parent and then observe how the patient crawls or stands up from the floor and walks or runs to the parent.

If measurements such as head circumference have not previously been done, they should be obtained before the end of the examination. It may be best to postpone the measurement of head circumference until the end of the examination, because many infants do not like the sensation of the tape on their heads.

BIBLIOGRAPHY

Baird HW, Gordon EC: Neurological Evaluation of Infants and Children. Clinics in Developmental Medicine, nos. 84 and 85. , Spastic International Medical Publications, 1983, pp 1–249.

Brett EM (ed): Paediatric Neurology, 2nd ed. New York, Churchill Livingstone, 1991.

Dubowitz LMS, Dibpwotz V, Mercuri E: The Neurological Assessment of the Preterm and Full-term Newborn Infant, 2nd ed. Clinics in Developmental Medicine, no.148. London, MacKeith Press, 1999, pp 1–155.

Haerer AF (ed): Dejong's the Neurologic Examination, 5th ed. Philadelphia, JB Lippincott, 1992.

Levine MD, Carey WB, Crocker AC (eds): Developmental-Behavioral Pediatrics, 3rd ed. Philadelphia, WB Saunders, 1999.

Pollack M: Textbook of Developmental Pediatrics. New York, Churchill Livingstone, 1993.

Swaiman KF, Ashwal S: Pediatric Neurology: Principles and Practice, 3rd ed. St. Louis, Mosby, 1999.

CHAPTER 201

Neuroanesthesia in Children

SULPICIO G. SORIANO ■ ELIZABETH A. ELDREDGE ■ MARK A. ROCKOFF

The perioperative management of infants and children undergoing neurosurgical procedures presents challenges to neurosurgeons and anesthesiologists alike. The aim of this chapter is to highlight clinically relevant differences between children and adults that relate to the perioperative management of patients undergoing neurosurgical procedures.

PREOPERATIVE EVALUATION AND PREPARATION

Pediatric patients present for surgery with special issues that may affect their perioperative management. Because many children are either preverbal or do not fully understand their medical condition, parents or primary caretakers should be interviewed carefully to obtain information regarding coexisting medical prob-

lems. A thorough review of the patient's history can reveal conditions that may increase the risk of adverse reactions to anesthesia and perioperative morbidity and identify patients who need more extensive evaluation or whose medical condition needs to be optimized before surgery. Certain medical problems may require that the anesthetic be modified (Table 201–1). There are also special perioperative concerns regarding children with neurological abnormalities (Table 201–2). Preoperative fasting is necessary to minimize aspiration of gastric contents during the operative procedure, and guidelines are listed in Table 201–3.[1]

The management of pediatric patients is unique in that the anesthesiologist and neurosurgeon have to manage the infant or child, who may not have the cognitive ability to rationalize the gravity of the situation, and interact with the parents as well. Patients and family members are usually frightened by the strange

TABLE 201–1 ■ Common Perioperative Concerns in Infants and Children

CONDITION	ANESTHETIC IMPLICATIONS
Congenital heart disease	Hypoxia and cardiovascular collapse
Prematurity	Postoperative apnea
Gastrointestinal reflux	Aspiration pneumonia
Upper respiratory tract infection	Laryngospasm and postoperative hypoxia or pneumonia
Craniofacial abnormality	Difficulty with airway management

TABLE 201–2 ■ Common Perioperative Concerns in Infants and Children with Neurologic Problems

CONDITION	ANESTHETIC IMPLICATIONS
Denervation injuries	Hyperkalemia after succinylcholine
	Resistance to nondepolarizing muscle relaxants
Chronic anticonvulsant therapy for epilepsy	Hepatic and hematologic abnormalities
	Increased metabolism of anesthetic agents
Arteriovenous malformation	Potential congestive heart failure
Neuromuscular disease	Malignant hyperthermia
	Respiratory failure
	Sudden cardiac death
Chiari's malformation	Apnea
	Aspiration pneumonitis
Hypothalamic/pituitary lesions	Diabetes insipidus
	Hypothyroidism
	Adrenal insufficiency

TABLE 201-3 ■ **Guidelines for Fasting before Surgery or Anesthesia**

No food after midnight the night before surgery
Formula may be given 6 hr before surgery
Breast milk may be offered up to 4 hr before surgery
Clear liquids may be offered up to 2 hr before surgery

surroundings of the hospital and operating room, exposure to unfamiliar hospital workers, the possibility of painful stimuli, and the thought of separation from each other and treasured comfort objects. Therefore, the approach to the pediatric patient should take into account the patient's developmental age. Table 201–4 lists the cognitive stages of pediatric patients and age-appropriate concerns.

Preoperative sedatives given before the induction of anesthesia can ease the transition from the preoperative holding area to the operating room. Midazolam given orally is particularly effective in relieving anxiety and producing amnesia. If an indwelling intravenous (IV) catheter is in place, midazolam can be slowly administered to achieve sedation. Alternatively, sedatives (such as barbiturates) can be given rectally to induce sleep in preschool children who are uncooperative; this avoids the use of intramuscular injections. However, methohexital administered rectally has been shown to induce seizures in patients with epilepsy.[2] Preoperative sedation should be withheld or administered only with close observation in patients with deteriorating findings on neurological examination or lethargy, because it can induce vomiting or apnea and interfere with serial neurological examinations.

INTRAOPERATIVE MANAGEMENT

Induction of Anesthesia

The infant's or child's neurological status and coexisting abnormalities dictate the most appropriate technique and drugs for induction of anesthesia. Generally, alert patients should be able to tolerate any type of induction technique. If there is no IV access, general anesthesia can be established by inhalation of sevoflurane and nitrous oxide with oxygen. This can be facilitated by having one parent present in the operating room during induction to help calm small children. Once the patient is unresponsive, the parent is escorted out of the operating room, and IV access is rapidly established. A nondepolarizing muscle relaxant

such as pancuronium is then injected to facilitate intubation of the trachea. Despite the widespread use of this induction technique in pediatric anesthesia, complications such as laryngospasm or vomiting may occur and lead to airway obstruction, hypoxia, or hypotension. The use of sevoflurane has been shown to decrease the incidence of these complications.[3, 4] Alternatively, if the patient has IV access, anesthesia can be rapidly induced with sedative-hypnotic drugs such as thiopental (5 to 8 mg/kg) or propofol (3 to 5 mg/kg).

Intracranial hypertension, hypoxia, hemodynamic instability, vomiting, and seizures can rapidly develop and have deleterious consequences if an inappropriate anesthetic technique is used. For example, patients with severe intracranial hypertension often present with nausea or vomiting and decreased airway reflexes. These patients are at risk for aspiration pneumonitis and should have a rapid-sequence induction of anesthesia performed with thiopental or propofol, immediately followed by a rapid-acting muscle relaxant such as succinylcholine or rocuronium. To minimize the risk of pulmonary aspiration of gastric contents, cricoid pressure is used to compress the esophagus. Induction of anesthesia can also depress myocardial function in patients who are hemodynamically unstable. Therefore, the dose of induction agents should be decreased to minimize cardiovascular depression. Etomidate and ketamine are frequently used to induce anesthesia in hemodynamically compromised patients. However, central nervous system excitation and increased intracranial pressure have been associated with these drugs, respectively, and they may not be appropriate for many neurosurgical patients.

Airway Management

Anatomic differences between the pediatric and the adult airway are primarily due to the size and orientation of the components of the upper airway, larynx, and trachea. Neonates and infants have the greatest differences from adults in this respect. However, the configuration of the larynx begins to become similar to that of the adult after the second year of life. Table 201–5 highlights the major differences between pediatric and adult airway anatomy.

These developmental differences in the cricothyroid and tracheobronchial tree have a significant impact on the management of the pediatric airway. The cricoid and thyroid cartilages almost overlap in the neonate and infant, resulting in a relatively small cricothyroid membrane. The infant's larynx is also funnel-shaped and narrowest at the level of the cricoid, making this

TABLE 201-4 ■ **Preoperative Concerns in Pediatric Patients**

AGE GROUP	CONCERNS
Infants (0–9 mo)	None; separate easily from parents
Preschoolers (9 mo–5 yr)	Stranger anxiety, difficulty with parental separation
Grade schoolers (6–12 yr)	Fear of needles and pain
Adolescents (>12 yr)	Anxious about surgery and self-image

TABLE 201–5 ■ **Differences between Pediatric and Adult Airway Anatomy**

	INFANT	ADULT
Tongue	Relatively large	Normal
Epiglottis	Floppy, angled posteriorly	Firm, less posterior angle
Vocal cord angle	Inclined	Flat
Glottis	C3–C4 level	C5 level
Cricothyroid membrane	Small	Normal
Trachea	Mobile, posterior displacement into thorax	Stationary, vertical descent into thorax

the smallest cross-sectional area in the infant airway. This feature places the infant at risk for life-threatening subglottic obstruction secondary to mucosal swelling after prolonged intubation with tight-fitting endotracheal tubes. An endotracheal tube can migrate into a mainstem bronchus if the infant's head is flexed for a suboccipital approach to the posterior fossa or the cervical spine. Therefore, the anesthesiologist should auscultate both lung fields to rule out inadvertent intubation of a mainstem bronchus after positioning the patient.

Given the pediatric patient's developmental anatomy and the inaccessibility of the head and airway during most neurosurgical procedures, tracheal intubation requires careful planning. Tracheal intubation by the oral route is acceptable for most neurosurgical cases, especially for surgical approaches to the supratentorial area and when transsphenoidal exposure is planned. Two potential problems with the orotracheal route are kinking of the endotracheal tube at the base of the tongue when the head is flexed and direct pressure injury to the tongue caused by the tube, especially when the patient is in a prone position. Nasotracheal tubes can prevent these problems and therefore are better suited for situations in which the patient will be prone and the head inaccessible to the anesthesiologist, such as suboccipital and cervical surgical approaches and when postoperative mechanical ventilation or endotracheal intubation is anticipated.

Maintenance of Anesthesia

The choice of anesthetic agents for maintenance of anesthesia has been shown not to affect the outcome of neurosurgical procedures.[5] Table 201–6 lists commonly used anesthetic drugs. The most frequently used technique for neurosurgery consists of the opioid fentanyl administered at a rate of 1 to 2 μg/kg/hr intravenously, along with inhaled nitrous oxide (70%) and low-dose isoflurane (0.2% to 0.5%). Deep neuromuscular blockade is maintained during most neurosurgical procedures to avoid patient movement. Patients receiving chronic anticonvulsant therapy require larger doses of muscle relaxants and narcotics because of induced enzymatic metabolism of these agents (Fig. 201–1).[6] Muscle relaxation should be withheld or not maintained when assessment of motor function during seizure and spinal cord surgery is planned.

Hemodynamic stability during intracranial surgery requires careful maintenance of the patient's fluids and electrolytes. Small patients have a greater percentage (up to 25%) of their cardiac output directed toward the head. Fluid restriction and diuretic therapy may lead to hemodynamic instability and even cardiovascular collapse if sudden blood loss occurs during surgery. Therefore, normovolemia should be maintained throughout the procedure. Normal saline is commonly used as the maintenance fluid during neurosurgery because it is mildly hyperosmolar (308 mOsm/kg) and it theoretically attenuates brain edema. However, rapid infusion of normal saline (30 mL/kg per hour) is associated with hyperchloremic acidosis.[7] Table 201–7 provides guidelines for IV fluid administration in pediatric patients. Hyperventilation and careful patient positioning to maximize venous drainage of the brain can

TABLE 201–6 ■ **Pharmacologic Agents Used in Anesthesia**

Inhaled Anesthetics
Halogenated agents
Isoflurane
Sevoflurane
Desflurane
Halothane
Nitrous oxide

Intravenous Anesthetics
Opioids (Narcotics)
Fentanyl
Sufentanil
Remifentanil
Morphine
Barbiturates
Thiopental
Methohexital
Benzodiazepines
Midazolam
Diazepam
Lorazepam
Other Sedative-Hypnotics
Ketamine
Propofol
Etomidate

Muscle Relaxants
Nondepolarizing
Pancuronium
Vecuronium
Rocuronium
Cisatracurium
Mivacurium
Depolarizing
Succinylcholine

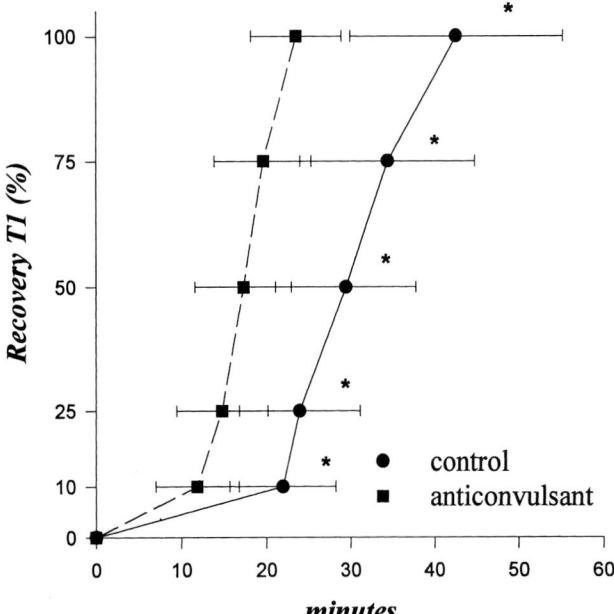

FIGURE 201–1. Patients on chronic anticonvulsant therapy have increased requirements for nondepolarizing muscle relaxants. The recovery time for return of muscle function was significantly faster in the anticonvulsant group than in the control group. *P <0.05, mean ± SD. (From Soriano SG, Kaus SJ, Sullivan LJ, Martyn JAJ: Onset and duration of action of rocuronium in children receiving chronic anticonvulsant therapy. Paediatr Anaesth 10:133–136, 2000.)

minimize brain swelling. Should these maneuvers fail, mannitol can be given at a dose of 0.25 to 1 g/kg intravenously. This transiently alters cerebral hemodynamics and raises serum osmolality by 10 to 20 mOsm/kg.[8] However, repeated dosing can lead to extreme hyperosmolality, renal failure, and further brain edema.[9] Furosemide is a useful adjunct to mannitol for decreasing acute cerebral edema and has been shown in vitro to prevent rebound swelling due to mannitol.[9] All diuretics interfere with the ability to use urine output as a guide to intravascular volume status.

Local Anesthesia

Neurosurgeons usually infiltrate subcutaneous epinephrine before the surgical incision to minimize cutaneous bleeding. If 0.25% bupivacaine is administered with epinephrine, prolonged analgesia can also be achieved. However, all local anesthetics have the potential for cardiac and neurological toxicity. Limiting

TABLE 201–7 ■ **Guidelines for Maintenance of Intravenous Fluids in Infants and Children**

WEIGHT (kg)	MAINTENANCE FLUIDS PER HOUR
<10	4 mL/kg
10–20	40 mL + 2 mL/kg for every kg between 10 and 20 kg
>20	60 mL + 1 mL/kg for every kg > 20

the total dose to 0.5 mL/kg delivers a maximum of 1.25 mg/kg of bupivacaine and 2.5 μg/kg of epinephrine; both are generally safe dosages in all patients. Dilution of the bupivacaine with saline increases the spread of the local anesthetic without increasing toxicity.

Vascular Access

Owing to limited access to the child during neurosurgical procedures, optimal IV access is mandatory before the start of surgery. Typically, two large-bore venous cannulas are sufficient for most craniotomies. Should initial attempts fail, access to central veins may be necessary. The femoral vein is best suited for this purpose because it is easy to cannulate in all patients, avoids the risk of pneumothorax associated with subclavian catheters, and does not interfere with cerebral venous return.

Monitoring

Standard monitoring equipment used for all anesthesia includes a stethoscope (precordial or esophageal), electrocardiograph, pulse oximeter, blood pressure gauge, end-tidal carbon dioxide analyzer, and thermometer. Given the potential for sudden hemodynamic instability due to venous air embolus (VAE), hemorrhage, herniation syndromes, or manipulation of cranial nerves, placement of an intra-arterial cannula for continuous blood pressure monitoring is appropriate for most neurosurgical procedures. An arterial catheter also provides access for sampling serial blood gases, electrolytes, and hematocrit. Normal age-dependent vital signs are listed in Table 201–8. Central venous pressures may not accurately reflect vascular volume, especially in a child in the prone position. Therefore, the risks of a central venous catheter may outweigh the benefits.

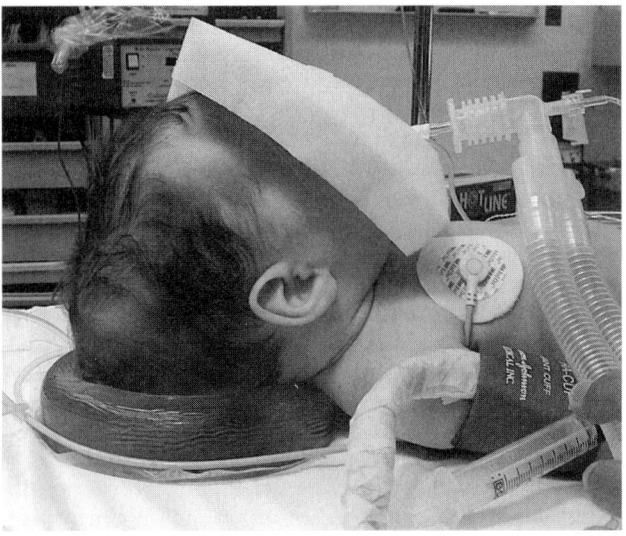

FIGURE 201–2. Supine infant. Note that the infant's head lies at a higher plane than the rest of his body. This increases the likelihood of venous air embolism during craniotomies.

TABLE 201–8 ■ **Approximate Vital Signs in Healthy Pediatric Patients**

AGE	WEIGHT (kg)	BLOOD PRESSURE (mm Hg)	HEART RATE
Premature	<2.5	60/30	140–180
Term neonate	>2.5	70/40	140–170
1 yr	10	90/55	110–130
6 yr	20	100/60	90–100

Venous air embolism is a common occurrence during craniotomies in infants.[10] This is because the head of a small child is large in relation to the rest of the body and rests above the heart, even in the supine position (Fig. 201–2). Standard neurosurgical technique may elevate the head of the table to improve venous drainage and is conducive to air entrainment into the venous system through open venous channels in bone and sinuses.[11] Patients with cardiac defects, such as patent foramen ovale or patent ductus arteriosus, are at risk for arterial air emboli through these defects and should be monitored carefully. Precordial Doppler ultrasonography can detect minute VAE and should be used routinely in conjunction with an end-tidal carbon dioxide analyzer and arterial catheter in all craniotomies. The Doppler probe is best positioned on the anterior chest, usually just to the right of the sternum at the fourth intercostal space. An alternative site on the posterior thorax can be used in infants weighting approximately 6 kg or less.[12]

Recent advances in neurophysiologic monitoring have enhanced the ability to safely perform more definitive neurosurgical resections in functional areas of the brain and spinal cord. However, the depressant effects of many anesthetic agents limit the utility of these monitors. A major part of preoperative planning should include a thorough discussion of the modality and type of neurophysiologic monitoring to be used during any surgical procedure. In general, electrocorticography and electroencephalography require low levels of volatile anesthetics and barbiturates. Somatosensory evoked potentials used during spinal and brainstem surgery can be depressed by volatile agents and, to a lesser extent, nitrous oxide. An opioid-based anesthetic is the most appropriate agent for this type of monitoring. Spinal cord and peripheral nerve surgery many require electromyography and detection of muscle movement as an end point. Therefore, muscle relaxation should be avoided or not maintained during the monitoring period. Table 201–9 lists common anesthetic agents and their effects on various neurophysiologic monitors.

Thermal Homeostasis

Infants and children are susceptible to hypothermia during any surgical procedure. Active heating of the patient by increasing the ambient temperature and using radiant light warmers during induction of anesthesia, catheter insertion, and preparation and positioning of the patient are prophylactic measures against hypothermia. Mattress warmers, forced hot air blankets, and humidification of inspired gases can also prevent temperature loss and postoperative shivering.

Positioning

Patient positioning for surgery requires careful preoperative planning to allow adequate access to the patient

TABLE 201–9 ■ **Neurophysiologic Effects of Common Anesthetic Agents**

	MEAN ARTERIAL PRESSURE	CEREBRAL BLOOD FLOW	CEREBRAL PERFUSION PRESSURE	INTRACRANIAL PRESSURE	CEREBRAL METABOLIC RATE OF OXYGEN	SOMATOSENSORY EVOKED POTENTIAL	
						Amplitude	Latency
Inhaled Agents							
Halothane	↓↓	↑↑↑	↑↑	↑↑	↓↓	↓	↑
Enflurane	↓↓	↑↑	↑↑	↑↑	↓↓	↓	↑
Isoflurane	↓↓	↑	↑↑	↑	↓↓↓	↓	↑
Sevoflurane	↓↓	↑	↑	↑	↓↓↓	↓	↑
Desflurane	↓↓	↑	↑	↑	↓	↓	↑
Nitrous oxide	ø–↓	↑–↑↑	↓	↑–↑↑	↓↑	↓	↑/ø
Intravenous Agents							
Thiopental	↓↓	↓↓↓	↑↑↑	↓↓↓	↓↓↓	↓	↑
Propofol	↓↓↓	↓↓↓	↑↑	↓↓	↓↓↓	↑	↑
Etomidate	–↓	↓↓↓	↑↑	↓↓↓	↓↓↓	↑	ø
Ketamine	↑↑	↑↑↑	↓	↑↑↑	↑	↑	ø
Benzodiazepine	–↓	↓↓↓	↑	ø–↓	↓↓	↓	↑/ø
Narcotics	–↓	↓	↑↓	ø–↓	↓	↓	↑

ø, No change; ↑, increase; ↓, decrease.

TABLE 201–10 ■ **Physiologic Effects of Patient Positioning**

POSITION	PHYSIOLOGIC EFFECT
Head elevated	Enhanced cerebral venous drainage
	Decreased cerebral blood flow
	Increased venous pooling in lower extremities
	Postural hypotension
Head down	Increased cerebral venous and intracranial pressure
	Decreased functional residual capacity (lung function)
	Decreased lung compliance
Prone	Venous congestion of face, tongue, and neck
	Decreased lung compliance
	Increased abdominal pressure can lead to venocaval compression
Lateral decubitus	Decreased compliance of down-side lung

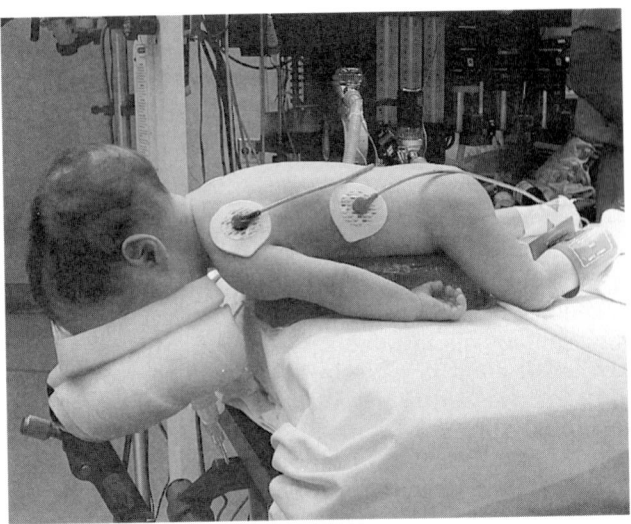

FIGURE 201–3. Prone infant. Lateral rolls are used to elevate the infant and minimize thoracic and abdominal pressure.

for both the neurosurgeon and the anesthesiologist. Table 201–10 describes various surgical positions and their physiologic sequelae. These issues should be considered because the duration of most neurosurgical procedures can lead to significant physiologic impairment or injury if positioning problems occur. Before placement of the sterile drapes, all pressure points should be padded and peripheral pulses checked to prevent compression or pressure injury. It is also important to avoid stretching peripheral nerves and to prevent skin and soft tissue injury due to improper contact with surgical accessories such as instrument stands and grounding wires. Given the limited access to the patient's airway once surgery begins, the endotracheal tube must be secured carefully to the patient's head.

The prone position is commonly used for posterior fossa and spinal cord surgery. In addition to the physiologic sequelae of this position, a whole spectrum of compression and stretch injuries has been reported. Padding under the chest and pelvis can support the torso. It is important to ensure free abdominal wall motion, because increased intra-abdominal pressure can impair ventilation, cause venocaval compression, and increase epidural venous pressure and bleeding. Figure 201–3 demonstrates proper positioning for these patients. Soft rolls are used to elevate and support the lateral chest wall and hips in order to minimize any increase in abdominal and thoracic pressure. In addition, this allows a Doppler probe to be placed on the chest without pressure. The head must be carefully flexed to avoid kinking of the endotracheal tube, inadvertently advancing the tube into an endobronchial position, or compressing the chin on the chest. Too much flexion for an extended time can cause lower brainstem and upper spinal cord ischemia, as well as head and tongue swelling from blockage of venous or lymphatic drainage. This can lead to postextubation airway obstruction or croup.

HEAD POSITIONING

Positioning of the patient's head can be a contentious issue between the anesthesiologist and the neurosur-

geon. Many neurosurgical procedures are performed with the head slightly elevated to facilitate venous and cerebrospinal fluid drainage from the surgical site. However, superior sagittal sinus pressure decreases with greater head elevation, and this increases the likelihood of VAE.[11] Extreme head flexion can cause brainstem compression in patients with pathologic conditions of the posterior fossa, such as mass lesions or Arnold-Chiari malformations. It can also cause endotracheal tube problems, including obstruction from kinking or displacement to the carina or the right mainstem bronchus. Extreme rotation of the head can impede venous return through the jugular veins and lead to impaired cerebral perfusion, increased intracranial pressure, and cerebral venous bleeding.

Emergence from Anesthesia

Prompt emergence from general anesthesia is important so that neurological function can be assessed after neurosurgical procedures. Therefore, one of the goals of neurosurgical anesthesia is to time the duration of anesthesia to allow smooth awakening with spontaneous respiration and hemodynamic stability. A drawback of rapid emergence from anesthesia is coughing on the endotracheal tube, leading to arterial and intracranial hypertension. This can be prevented if small doses of fentanyl are given before emergence. Premature extubation of the trachea can lead to laryngospasm or apnea, which can progress to hypoxia and cardiac arrest if not treated promptly. Hypertension during emergence from anesthesia can be controlled with vasodilator drugs; these include labetalol, an α- and β₂-antagonist, or a direct vasodilator such as sodium nitroprusside. Neuromuscular blockade should be fully antagonized, and all the anesthetic agents should be discontinued. Once the patient exhibits spontaneous ventilation, and appropriate responses to verbal commands are demonstrated, the trachea can be extubated. Failure to achieve these two criteria should

TABLE 201–11 ■ **Conditions Leading to Delayed Emergence from Anesthesia**

Residual Anesthetic Drugs
Volatile anesthetics
Intravenous anesthesia
Residual neuromuscular blockade

Metabolic Abnormalities
Hypothermia
Electrolyte imbalances
Hypoglycemia
Hypothyroidism

Neurologic Abnormalities
Hypoxia
Cerebral ischemia (stroke or venous air embolism)
Intracranial hemorrhage
Extensive surgical resection

prompt a search for additional problems (Table 201–11), and extubation of the trachea should be delayed. If anesthetic causes for delayed awakening are not apparent, neurological conditions should be strongly considered and evaluated with a computed tomographic scan of the head. Transportation to the computed tomography suite requires maintenance of general anesthesia and continuous hemodynamic monitoring. In certain circumstances, consideration should be given to keeping the patient's trachea intubated. These include procedures in which several blood volumes have been lost and replaced with crystalloid and blood, especially with the patient in the prone position for a prolonged period. This frequently results in airway and facial edema and may lead to postextubation airway obstruction. In addition, operations that result in disruption of cranial nerve nuclei or brainstem function can lead to impairment of airway reflexes and respiratory drive. However, residual anesthetic and neuromuscular blockade should always be ruled out before making the diagnosis of neurological injury. Antagonism of residual narcotic by naloxone can lead to uncontrolled hypertension and coughing on the endotracheal tube and should be avoided.

POSTOPERATIVE MANAGEMENT

Close observation in an intensive care unit with serial neurological examinations and invasive hemodynamic monitoring is helpful for the prevention and early detection of postoperative problems. Respiratory dysfunction is the leading complication after posterior fossa craniotomies.[13] Airway obstruction after a craniotomy can be due to airway edema or cranial nerve dysfunction after surgical manipulation of the cranial nerves or nuclei. Airway edema is usually self-limited and may require endotracheal intubation as a stent. Occasionally, ischemia or edema of the respiratory centers in the brainstem interferes with respiratory control and leads to postoperative apnea. Residual narcotics can also produce apnea, but this is transient and can be pharmacologically antagonized with naloxone. Acute

changes in the neurological examination may be due to mass effect secondary to intracranial bleeding, hydrocephalus, or cerebral infarction. An emergent computed tomographic scan of the head may be helpful to confirm the diagnosis and guide management of the inciting event. Derangements in sodium concentration in the postoperative period are typically due to over- or underproduction of antidiuretic hormone and result in the syndrome of inappropriate antidiuretic hormone secretion or diabetes insipidus, respectively. Diabetes insipidus commonly occurs after operations in the region of the hypothalamus and pituitary gland and can be managed acutely with an IV vasopressin infusion. Postoperative seizures may be a clinical manifestation of an intracranial hemorrhage or acute hyponatremia and should be treated rapidly with anticonvulsants and correction of the initiating process. Analgesia with morphine is often required in the postoperative period to minimize stress and discomfort. However, postcraniotomy patients are frequently lethargic, and excessive administration of narcotics and sedatives may interfere with serial neurological examinations. Postoperative nausea and vomiting can cause sudden increases in intracranial pressure and should be treated with a nonsedating antiemetic such as ondansetron. However, prophylactic administration of ondansetron during surgery is not effective in decreasing the incidence of vomiting following craniotomies in children.[14]

SPECIAL ISSUES

Neonatal Emergencies

Most neonatal surgery is performed on an emergent basis.[15] There is more than a 10-fold increase in perioperative morbidity and mortality in neonates when compared with other pediatric age groups.[16] The major concern in managing neonates is uncovering congenital anomalies, primarily of the cardiovascular and respiratory systems. Depending on the lesion, congenital heart disease may not be apparent immediately after birth, but it is frequently associated with intraoperative hypoxia and hemodynamic instability. Echocardiography can be helpful in the assessment of the heart, and a pediatric cardiologist should evaluate patients with suspected problems in order to help optimize cardiac function before surgery. Perinatal cardiovascular physiology is an evolving process; the fetal circulation is primarily a parallel circuit that converts to a serial one after birth. Hypoxia, hypercarbia, hypothermia, acidosis, and stress can precipitate regression to a fetal circulation in neonates during the intraoperative period. Congestive heart failure can occur in neonates with large cerebral arteriovenous malformations, and this condition requires aggressive hemodynamic support. Management of the neonatal respiratory system may be difficult because of the diminutive size of the airway, craniofacial anomalies, laryngotracheal lesions, and acute (hyaline membrane disease, retained amniotic fluid) or chronic (bronchopulmonary dysplasia) disease. Because these conditions are in a state of flux,

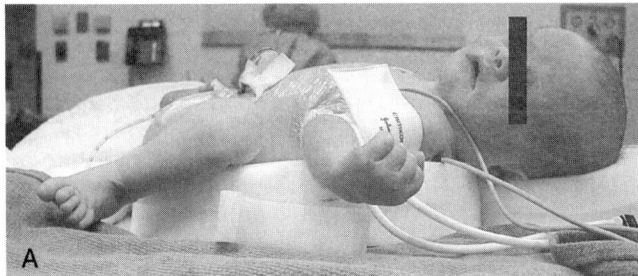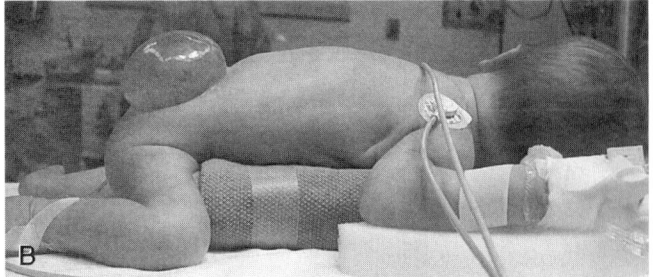

FIGURE 201–4. Positioning of a neonate with a myelomeningocele. *A,* Before induction of general anesthesia, the neonate is elevated on soft padding with a center cutout to relieve pressure on the myelomeningocele. *B,* Positioning of the neonate for closure of the myelomeningocele. (Courtesy of Robert T. Wilder, MD, PhD.)

they should be addressed preoperatively to minimize perioperative morbidity.

The neonatal central nervous system is capable of sensing pain and mounting a stress response after a surgical stimulus.[17] Therefore, it is imperative that neonates receive adequate anesthesia for surgical procedures. Yet immature neonatal organ systems are highly sensitive to anesthetic agents. Neonatal myocardial function is particularly sensitive to both inhaled and IV anesthetics, and these agents must be used judiciously to block surgical stress without causing myocardial depression. Use of an opioid-based anesthetic is generally the most stable hemodynamic technique for neonates. However, the hepatic and renal systems are not fully developed, and neonates anesthetized with a narcotic technique often have delayed emergence and may require postoperative mechanical ventilation.

Closure of a myelomeningocele or encephalocele presents special problems. Positioning the patient for tracheal intubation may rupture the membranes covering the spinal cord or brain. Therefore, careful padding of the lesion (Fig. 201–4) and, in some cases, intubation of the neonate's trachea in the left lateral decubitus position may be necessary.

Craniosynostosis

Repair of craniosynostosis is likely to have the best result if performed early in life. However, these procedures are associated with loss of a significant percentage of an infant's blood volume, with great losses occurring when more sutures are involved. VAE frequently occurs and should be minimized by mainte-

nance of intravascular blood volume and early detection with continuous precordial Doppler ultrasonography. When hemodynamic instability does occur, the operating table can be placed in the Trendelenburg position. This maneuver augments the patient's blood pressure and prevents further entrainment of intravascular air. Special risks exist in neonates and young infants with potential right-to-left cardiac shunts that cause arterial emboli.

Tumors

Because the majority of intracranial tumors in children occur in the posterior fossa, cerebrospinal fluid flow is often obstructed, and intracranial hypertension and hydrocephalus are often present. Most neurosurgeons approach this region with children in the prone position. The patient's head is often secured with a Mayfield head frame. Pins used in small children can cause skull fractures, dural tears, and intracranial hematomas. During elevation of the bone flap, the transverse and straight sinuses can be inadvertently lacerated, and massive blood loss or VAE can occur. Therefore, both the anesthesiologist and the neurosurgeon should be alerted to sudden changes in monitors for VAE and arterial blood pressure. Surgical resection of tumors in the posterior fossa can lead to brainstem or cranial nerve damage. Table 201–12 lists some of the signs of encroachment on these structures. Damage to the cranial nerves innervating the vocal cords and soft tissues of the upper airway can lead to airway obstruction after extubation of the patient's trachea. Furthermore, edema or damage to the respiratory centers can cause apnea in the postoperative period. Seizures frequently

TABLE 201-12 ■ **Effect of Surgical Brainstem Manipulation**

BRAINSTEM AREA	SIGNS	CHANGES IN MONITOR
CN V	Hypertension, bradycardia	Arterial pressure, ECG
CN VII	Facial muscle movement	EMG
CN X	Hypotension, bradycardia	Arterial pressure, ECG
Pons, medulla	Arrhythmias, hypotension, Hypertension, tachy- or bradycardia, Irregular breathing pattern	ECG, arterial pressure, end-tidal carbon dioxide

CN, cranial nerve; ECG, electrocardiogram; EMG, electromyogram.

occur in patients with supratentorial lesions. Phenytoin can be administered in the perioperative period until oral intake is resumed.

Tumors in the hypothalamic-pituitary region present special problems. Craniopharyngiomas are the most common lesions in this area and are often accompanied by derangements in the neuroendocrine axis. These patients should therefore receive a thorough endocrine evaluation. Steroids should be administered if there is impairment in the hypothalamic-pituitary-adrenal axis. Thyroid function should also be evaluated. Preoperative diabetes insipidus may lead to severe hypovolemia and electrolyte imbalances and should be corrected before surgery. The routine use of mannitol is not advised, because it may mask the diagnosis of diabetes insipidus intraoperatively. Diabetes insipidus can be managed intraoperatively with an IV infusion of aqueous vasopressin and strict control of IV fluids. Diabetes insipidus rarely occurs in the intraoperative period but frequently presents in the postoperative period; this occurs because the posterior pituitary gland's store of antidiuretic hormone lasts several hours.

Epilepsy

Surgical treatment has become a viable option for many patients with medically intractable epilepsy. Two major considerations should be kept in mind. First, chronic administration of the anticonvulsant drugs phenytoin and carbamazepine induces rapid metabolism and clearance of several classes of anesthetic agents, including neuromuscular blockers and opioids.[6, 18] Therefore, the anesthetic requirements for patients taking these drugs are increased; close monitoring of the anesthetic's effect is required, along with frequent redosing. Second, various neurophysiologic monitors can be used to guide the actual resection of the epileptogenic focus, and general anesthetics can compromise the sensitivity of these devices.[19] Table 201–9 lists the anesthetic effects of anesthetic agents on the electroencephalogram and electrocorticogram.

Because some epileptogenic foci are in close proximity to cortical areas controlling speech, memory, and motor or sensory function, monitoring of the patient's electrophysiologic responses is frequently used to minimize iatrogenic injury to these areas.[20, 21] Cortical stimulation of the motor strip in a child under general anesthesia requires either electromyography or direct visualization of muscle movement. Neuromuscular blockade should not be used in this situation. Neural function is best assessed in an awake and cooperative patient. We reported a series of children undergoing awake craniotomy for resections in eloquent areas of the brain with local anesthesia and propofol and fentanyl for sedation and analgesia, respectively.[22] Positioning of the patient was critical for the success of this technique. The patient should be in a semilateral position to allow both patient comfort and surgical and airway access to the patient. We found that propofol, when discontinued 20 minutes before monitoring, did not interfere with the electrocorticogram and that cooperative children older than 10 years of age were able

to withstand the procedure without incident. However, it is imperative that candidates for an awake craniotomy be mature and psychologically prepared to participate in this procedure. Therefore, patients who are developmentally delayed or have a history of severe anxiety or psychiatric disorders are not appropriate candidates. Very young patients cannot be expected to cooperate for these procedures and usually require general anesthesia with extensive neurophysiologic monitoring to minimize inadvertent resection of the motor strip and eloquent cortex.

Vascular Anomalies

Vascular anomalies are rare in infants and children. Most of these conditions are congenital anomalies and present early in life. Large arteriovenous malformations in neonates may be associated with high-output congestive heart failure and require hemodynamic support. Initial treatment of large arteriovenous malformations often consists of intravascular embolization in the radiology suite.[23] Operative management is commonly associated with massive blood loss, and these patients require several IV access sites and invasive hemodynamic monitoring. Ligation of an arteriovenous malformation can lead to sudden hypertension with hyperemic cerebral edema.[24] Vasodilators such as labetalol or nitroprusside can be used to control a hypertensive crisis.

Moyamoya syndrome is a rare, chronic vaso-occlusive disorder of the internal carotid arteries that presents as transient ischemic attacks or recurrent strokes in childhood. The cause is unknown, but the syndrome can be associated with previous intracranial radiation, neurofibromatosis, Down syndrome, and a variety of hematologic disorders. The anesthetic management of these patients is directed at optimizing cerebral perfusion.[25] This includes ensuring generous preoperative hydration and maintaining the blood pressure within the patient's preoperative range. Maintenance of normocapnia is essential in patients with Moyamoya syndrome because both hyper- and hypocapnia can lead to steal phenomenon from the ischemic region and further aggravate cerebral ischemia.[26] A nitrous oxide– and narcotic-based anesthetic provides a stable level of anesthesia for these patients and is compatible with intraoperative electroencephalographic monitoring. Once the patient emerges from anesthesia, the same maneuvers that optimize cerebral perfusion should be extended into the postoperative period. These patients should receive IV fluids to maintain adequate cerebral perfusion and adequate narcotics to avoid hyperventilation induced by pain and crying.

Trauma

Pediatric head trauma requires a multiorgan approach to minimizing morbidity and mortality.[27] A small child's head is often the point of impact in injuries, but other organs can also be damaged. Basic life support algorithms should be applied immediately to ensure a patent airway, spontaneous respiration, and adequate circulation. Immobilization of the cervical spine is essential to avoid secondary injury caused by manipulation of the patient's airway until radiologic clearance is confirmed. Blunt abdominal trauma and long bone fractures frequently occur with head injury and can be major sources of blood loss. To ensure tissue perfusion during the operative period, the patient's blood volume should be restored with crystalloid solutions or blood products, or both. Ongoing blood loss can lead to coagulopathies and should be treated with specific blood components.

Occasionally, a repeat craniotomy must be performed in a child shortly after the primary procedure. This can be emergent for evacuation of intracranial hemorrhages. Indications for elective repeat craniotomies include removal of electrocorticographic leads and depth electrodes used for chronic invasive electroencephalographic monitoring and subsequent resection of the seizure focus. It is important to avoid nitrous oxide until the dura is opened, because intracranial air can persist up to 3 weeks after a craniotomy.[28]

Spine Surgery

Spinal dysraphism is the primary indication for laminectomies in pediatric patients. Many of these patients have had meningomyelocele closure followed by several corrective surgical procedures. These patients have been exposed to latex products and may develop hypersensitivity to latex. Latex allergy can manifest as a severe anaphylactic reaction heralded by hypotension and wheezing and should be rapidly treated by removal of the source of latex and administration of fluid and vasopressors.[29] Patients at risk for latex allergy should have a latex-free environment.

Tethered cord releases require electromyographic monitoring to help identify functional nerve roots. An electromyogram of the anal sphincter and muscles of the lower extremities is performed intraoperatively to minimize inadvertent injury to nerves innervating these muscle groups. Muscle relaxants should be discontinued or antagonized to allow accurate monitoring.

Neuroradiology

Advances in imaging technology have provided less invasive procedures to diagnose and treat lesions in the central nervous system. The major issues in providing anesthesia in radiology suites are (1) availability of anesthetic equipment outside the operating room and compatibility in a magnetic environment, (2) training of ancillary staff in the radiology suite to appreciate anesthetic issues and concerns, and (3) transport of the patient to and from the radiology suite. These issues require thorough planning among the radiologist, neurosurgeon, and anesthesiologist and an established set of guidelines to provide a safe environment for the patient. Most neuroradiologic studies such as computed tomography and magnetic resonance imaging can be accomplished with light sedation. Recommendations have been published by consensus groups of

anesthesiologists and pediatricians and can serve as guidelines for managing these patients.[30, 31] General anesthesia is typically used for uncooperative patients, patients with coexisting medical problems, and patients undergoing potentially painful procedures such as embolization of lesions. Some patients with neurovascular problems are at risk for hemorrhage and hemodynamic instability and require invasive monitoring. Children requiring stereotactic-guided radiosurgery or craniotomies need general anesthesia in order to tolerate the procedure. Special head frames devised to allow airway manipulations should be used in these patients.[32]

CONCLUSION

The perioperative management of pediatric neurosurgical patients presents many challenges to neurosurgeons and anesthesiologists. Many conditions are unique to pediatrics. Thorough preoperative evaluation and open communication among members of the health care team are important. A basic understanding of age-dependent variables and the interaction of anesthetic and surgical procedures is essential for minimizing perioperative morbidity and mortality.

REFERENCES

1. Ferrari LR, Rooney FM, Rockoff MA: Preoperative fasting practices in pediatrics. Anesthesiology 90:978–980, 1999.
2. Rockoff MA, Goudsouzian NG: Seizures induced by methohexital. Anesthesiology 54:333–335, 1981.
3. Sarner JB, Levine M, Davis PJ, et al: Clinical characteristics of sevoflurane in children: A comparison with halothane. Anesthesiology 82:38–46, 1995.
4. Holzman RS, van der Velde ME, Kaus SJ, et al: Sevoflurane depresses myocardial contractility less than halothane during induction of anesthesia in children. Anesthesiology 85:1260–1267, 1996.
5. Todd MM, Warner DS, Sokoll MD, et al: A prospective, comparative trial of three anesthetics for elective supratentorial craniotomy. Anesthesiology 78:1005–1020, 1993.
6. Soriano SG, Kaus SJ, Sullivan LJ, Martyn JAJ: Onset and duration of action of rocuronium in children receiving chronic anticonvulsant therapy. Paediatr Anaesth 10:133–136, 2000.
7. Scheingraber S, Rehm M, Sehmisch C, Finsterer U: Rapid saline infusion produces hyperchloremic acidosis in patients undergoing gynecologic surgery. Anesthesiology 90:1265–1270, 1999.
8. Soriano SG, McManus ML, Sullivan LJ, et al: Cerebral blood flow velocity after mannitol infusion in children. Can J Anaesth 43:461–466, 1996.
9. McManus ML, Soriano SG: Rebound swelling of astroglial cells exposed to hypertonic mannitol. Anesthesiology 88:1586–1591, 1998.
10. Harris MM, Yemen TA, Davidson A, et al: Venous embolism during craniectomy in supine infants. Anesthesiology 67:816–819, 1987.
11. Grady MS, Bedford RF, Park TS: Changes in superior sagittal sinus pressure in children with head elevation, jugular venous compression, and PEEP. J Neurosurg 65:199–202, 1986.
12. Soriano SG, McManus ML, Sullivan LJ, et al: Doppler sensor placement during neurosurgical procedures for children in the prone position. J Neurosurg Anesthesiol 6:153–155, 1994.
13. Meridy HW, Creighton RE, Humphreys RB: Complications during neurosurgical procedures in the prone position. Can J Anaesth 21:445–452, 1974.
14. Furst SR, Sullivan LJ, Soriano SG, et al: Effects of ondansetron

on emesis in the first 24 hours after craniotomy in children. Anesth Analg 83:325–328, 1996.

15. Koka BV, Soriano SG: Anesthesia for neonatal surgical emergencies. Semin Anesth 9:309–316, 1992.

16. Cohen MM, Cameron CB, Duncan PG: Pediatric anesthesia morbidity and mortality in the perioperative period. Anesth Analg 70:160–167, 1990.

17. Anand KJ, Hickey PR: Pain and its effects in the human neonate and fetus. N Engl J Med 317:1321–1329, 1987.

18. Tempelhoff R, Modica PA, Spitznagel EL: Anticonvulsants therapy increases fentanyl requirements during anaesthesia for craniotomy. Can J Anaesth 37:327–332, 1990.

19. Eldredge EA, Soriano SG, Rockoff MA: Neuroanesthesia. In Adelson PD, Black PM (eds): Surgical Treatment of Epilepsy in Children. Philadelphia, WB Saunders, 1995, pp 505–520.

20. Black PM, Ronner SF: Cortical mapping for defining the limits of tumor resection. Neurosurgery 20:914–919, 1987.

21. Penfield W: Combined regional and general anesthesia for craniotomy and cortical exploration. Part I. Neurosurgical considerations. Anesth Analg 33:145–155, 1954.

22. Soriano SG, Eldredge EA, Wang FK, et al: The effect of propofol on intraoperative electrocorticography and cortical stimulation during awake craniotomies in children. Paediatr Anaesth 10:29–34, 2000.

23. Burrows PE, Robertson RL: Neonatal central nervous system vascular disorders. Neurosurg Clin North Am 9:155–180, 1998.

24. Morgan MK, Sekhon LH, Finfer S, Grinnell V: Delayed neurological deterioration following resection of arteriovenous malformations of the brain. J Neurosurg 90:695–701, 1999.

25. Soriano SG, Sethna NF, Scott RM: Anesthetic management of children with Moyamoya syndrome. Anesth Analg 77:1066–1070, 1993.

26. Kuwabara Y, Ichiya Y, Sasaki M, et al: Response to hypercapnia in Moyamoya disease: Cerebrovascular response to hypercapnia in pediatric and adult patients with Moyamoya disease. Stroke 28:701–707, 1997.

27. Lam WH, MacKersie A: Paediatric head injury: Incidence, aetiology and management. Paediatr Anaesth 9:377–385, 1999.

28. Reasoner DK, Todd MM, Scamman FL, Warner DS: The incidence of pneumocephalus after supratentorial craniotomy: Observations on the disappearance of intracranial air. Anesthesiology 80:1008–1012, 1994.

29. Holzman RS: Clinical management of latex-allergic children. Anesth Analg 85:529–533, 1997.

30. American Academy of Pediatrics Committee on Drugs: Guidelines for monitoring and management of pediatric patients during and after sedation for diagnostic and therapeutic procedures. Pediatrics 89:1110–1115, 1992.

31. Practice guidelines for sedation and analgesia by non-anesthesiologists: A report by the American Society of Anesthesiologists Task Force on Sedation and Analgesia by Non-Anesthesiologists. Anesthesiology 84:459–471, 1996.

32. Stokes MA, Soriano SG, Tarbell NJ, et al: Anesthesia for stereotactic radiosurgery in children. J Neurosurg Anesthesiol 7:100–108, 1995.

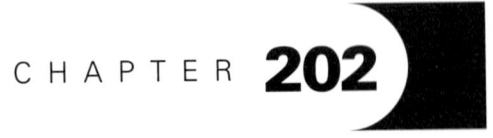

CHAPTER **202**

Encephaloceles

JAMES T. RUTKA ■ CARLOS CARLOTTI ■ MARK IANTOSCA

A cephalocele is defined as a protrusion of cranial contents beyond the normal confines of the skull.[1-3] In this definition, the term *cephalocele* includes meningocele (herniation of meninges and cerebrospinal fluid [CSF]), encephalomeningocele (herniation of brain tissue and meninges), and hydroencephalomeningocele (herniation of a portion of the ventricle, brain tissue, and meninges) (Fig. 202–1). Today, the terms *cephalocele* and *encephalocele* are used almost interchangeably to include all these lesions. In this chapter, we use the term *encephalocele* throughout, as this is the term used most frequently in the neurosurgical literature.

CLASSIFICATION

Most classifications of encephaloceles are based on the location of the defects in the cranium.[4] Six main groups have been proposed: occipital, occipitocervical, parietal, sincipital, basal, and temporal. Further subclassifications of parietal, sincipital, and basal encephaloceles have also been suggested (Table 202–1). Based on high-resolution computed tomographic and magnetic resonance imaging (MRI) scanning, most encephaloceles can be accurately classified according to this scheme, and also with respect to whether the encephalocele contains CSF, meninges, or brain substance.

EPIDEMIOLOGY AND INCIDENCE

Encephaloceles account for approximately 10% to 20% of all craniospinal dysraphisms.[5, 6] The prevalence ranges from 0.8 to 4 per 10,000 live births,[1, 7–9] although the true incidence is considerably greater because about 70% of encephaloceles result in loss of pregnancy.[10, 11] Racial and geographic factors influence both frequency and site. In Southeast Asia, lesions visible in the nasofrontal region (also known as sincipital defects) are nine times more common than posteriorly placed lesions.[7, 12] As another example, sincipital lesions make up only 2.2% of encephaloceles in the Australian white population but 50% of those occurring in Aboriginals.[1] In contrast, encephaloceles are much less frequent in North America and Europe, but 66% to 95% occur in the occipital region.[1, 5, 6, 13] Basal defects are rare in all racial groups, accounting for only 2% to 10% of encephaloceles.[5, 14]

Almost all encephaloceles are sporadic, although a small percentage occur as part of recognized conditions such as frontonasal dysplasia or aberrant tissue band syndrome.[15] Although occipital encephaloceles may occur in association with a spinal meningocele,[9] intracranial dermoid cyst,[16] Chiari type II malformation,[17] or diastematomyelia,[1] frontal and basal lesions are not associated with other neural tube defects, nor are they more prevalent with advancing maternal age.[2] There is no significant increase in the incidence of central nervous system anomalies in the siblings or offspring of patients with sincipital encephaloceles,[1] even in monozygotic twins.[12] Most of the time these lesions are sporadic, but they can occur in families[18] or be related to syndromes such as the Knobloch[19] and Walker-Warburg syndromes.[20]

Although sincipital and basal defects are present at birth, they may not manifest until well into adult life. The encephalocele may contain only meninges and CSF or dysplastic cerebral tissue that retains a basic but deranged cytoarchitecture. Other cephalic anomalies associated with sincipital or basal encephaloceles include cleft lip, cleft palate, malformation of the nasal tip, microphthalmia, corneal opacity, coloboma, craniosynostosis, and corpus callosum agenesis or lipoma.[1, 21–23]

EMBRYOPATHOGENESIS

The pathogenesis of encephaloceles is still not completely understood. The first theory postulated by von

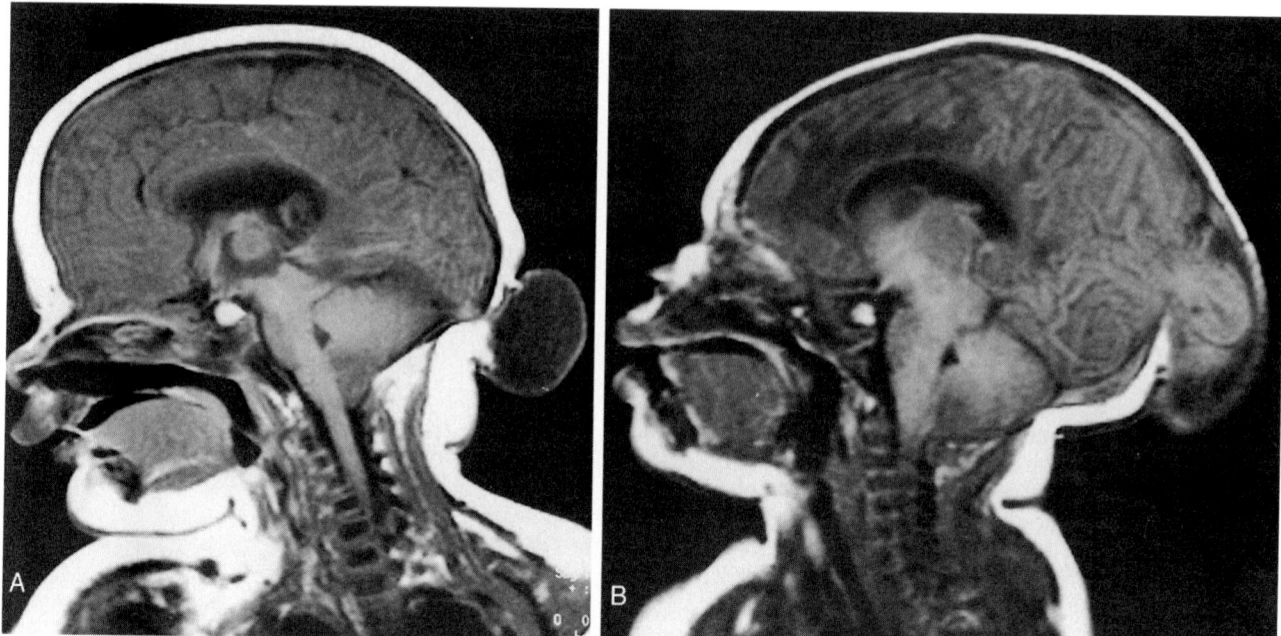

FIGURE 202–1. *A,* Sagittal magnetic resonance imaging (MRI) scan of a newborn with a predominantly cerebrospinal fluid (CSF)–filled encephalocele sac. Note the descent of the cerebellar tonsils through the foramen magnum and the bright pituitary gland. *B,* Sagittal MRI scan of a newborn with a predominantly brain-filled encephalocele sac. Knowledge of the contents of the sac helps the neurosurgeon plan the repair.

Recklinghausen, based on his clinical observations, suggested that there was a defect in primary cranial neurulation.[24] If this were the case, however, important neural structural anomalies and skin defects would be expected within all encephaloceles,[25] and the location of all the defects would be rostral.[24]

Studies of animal models and human embryos support a theory based on a disturbance in the separation of neural and surface ectoderm after neurulation.[26–28] The mesoderm usually forms in a progressive, sequential, and segmental cephalocaudal direction, beginning in the cephalic region and ending in the coccygeal area. Studies of the skeletal, neural, and oropharyngeal morphology in human encephalocele material suggest that a para-axial mesodermal insufficiency affecting the formation of the occipital bone, neurocranium, and dura mater may be the primary anomaly in some types of encephaloceles. The neural tissue defects associated with encephaloceles may thus be secondary to this anomaly rather than primary.[25]

As for encephaloceles of the anterior cranial fossa, the developmental arrest hypothesis suggests a similarity to myeloschisis in that the neural tube fails to close at the anterior neuropore. This generally occurs around day 24 of gestation in the region of the foramen cecum. The theory was built around the case of a sincipital encephalocele associated with agenesis of the corpus callosum, a structure that also originates from this site. However, this is unlikely to be the cause of frontal or basal encephaloceles for two reasons. First, these anomalies are not associated with other neural tube defects.[2] Second, immunohistochemical morphologic analysis of surgical and neonatal autopsy material, using neuron-specific enolase, demonstrated that there is no dysraphism of the underlying brain. Although exencephalic neonates with exposed neural placodes have brain remnants that fail to stain with neuron-specific enolase, the herniated brain in sincipital encephalocele retains a distorted cytoarchitecture that is neuron-specific enolase–positive.[29] This indicates that anencephaly, rather than encephalocele, is the cranial equivalent of myeloschisis.

TABLE 202–1 ■ **Classification of Encephaloceles**

Posterior Encephaloceles
Occipital
  Supratorcular
  Infratorcular
Occipitocervical
Parietal
  Interfrontal
  Interparietal
  Anterior fontanelle
  Posterior fontanelle

Anterior Cranial Fossa Encephaloceles
Sincipital
  Frontoethmoidal
  Nasofrontal
  Nasoethmoidal
  Naso-orbital
  Interfrontal
  Craniofacial cleft
Basal
  Sphenopharyngeal
  Spheno-orbital
  Sphenomaxillary
  Sphenoethmoidal
  Transethmoidal

An alternative hypothesis is that secondary hernia-tion of the brain and meninges occurs through either developmental failure of ossification of the anterior skull base[7, 30, 31] or persistence of the craniopharyngeal canal.[21] Contributing factors might include overdisten-tion of the primitive neural tube[32–34] or increased intra-cranial pressure during delivery.[31] Unfortunately, this notion is inconsistent with embryologic and anatomic studies, which indicate that the meningeal and neural protrusions are present from the outset and that failure of skeletal development occurs around them.[35, 36]

The most widely accepted theory is that of Geoffrey St. Hillaire (1827), proposing that neuroschisis occurs after neural tube closure. As the fissure heals, adhe-sions develop between neuroectoderm and cutaneous ectoderm, thereby preventing interposition of the mesoderm destined to form the cranium.[34] New in-sights into the pathogenesis of encephaloceles have come from molecular studies. The formation of the neural tube is a process controlled by genes and their respective proteins, which can be transcription factors, membrane receptors, or ligands. Several genes have been identified thus far, such as *sonic hedgehog*, that are expressed in the notochord and induce the formation and cytoarchitecture of the ventral spinal cord. It is now known that bone morphogenic protein is one fac-tor that induces the formation of the dorsal spinal cord. These newly described phenomena will undoubtedly enhance our understanding of the pathogenesis of en-cephaloceles.[27, 37]

POSTERIOR ENCEPHALOCELES

Occipital, Occipitocervical, and Parietal Encephaloceles

Occipital, occipitocervical, and parietal encephaloceles are frequently classified as posterior encephaloceles and are considered together here because they share several characteristics.[38] In general, posterior encepha-loceles are more common than anterior cranial fossa encephaloceles, except in some Asian populations.[1, 38–41] Parietal encephaloceles are classified as those that oc-cur between the bregma and lambda, inclusive of these two sites. Occipital encephaloceles are found between the lambda and foramen magnum and are subdivided into infratorcular and supratorcular types.[38, 42] Occipi-tocervical encephaloceles occur when the bone defect includes the cervical vertebrae.[1] The herniation of the hindbrain into a low occipital or high cervical encepha-locele in combination with pathologic and imaging features of Chiari II malformations is called the Chiari type III malformation,[43] or iniencephaly.[44] In general, for posterior encephaloceles, the occipital location is more common than the parietal location.

Prenatal Diagnosis

Prenatal diagnosis of encephaloceles is now possible through amniocentesis[45] and, more commonly, ultraso-nography (Fig. 202–2).[1, 46] Amniocentesis enables the

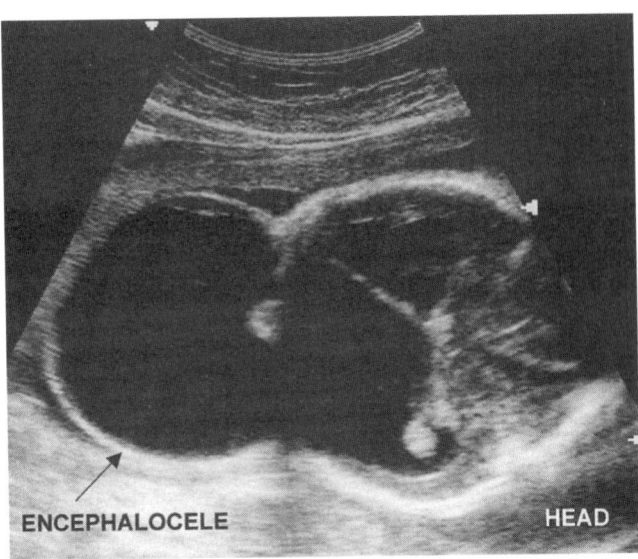

FIGURE 202–2. Fetal ultrasonography reveals a large cystic en-cephalocele in a second-trimester fetus. Limited normal cerebral tissue is identified in this severe case.

determination of alpha fetoprotein and acetylcholines-terase. Although these methods are more sensitive in the detection of open neural tube defects such as anen-cephaly and spina bifida aperta, a high percentage of encephaloceles can also be detected.[45] Ultrasonography has become a routine practice during pregnancy to rule out major congenital malformations of the nervous system. Advances in ultrasonography such as three-dimensional image reconstruction have improved its diagnostic accuracy.[46] Fetal MRI studies are now possi-ble, and the images are improving in terms of clarity and details provided (Fig. 202–3).

Imaging Studies

Imaging studies are important in the diagnosis and management of an infant or child with an encephalo-cele. High-resolution CT and MRI can now be per-formed, with MRI arguably being the gold standard for identifying the contents of the sac and their rela-tionship to neighboring neural and vascular structures (see Fig. 202–1).[13, 47] Magnetic resonance angiography and magnetic resonance venography (MRV) sequences are frequently helpful in delineating the whereabouts of the draining venous sinuses, information that is important to know before embarking on neurosurgical repair.[48–50] Other features that can be gleaned from im-aging studies include certain intracranial and extracra-nial malformations that may be associated with differ-ent clinical syndromes (Fig. 202–4).[15] The presence of hydrocephalus is a poor prognostic factor.[42] CT and MRI have also shown partial agenesis of the corpus callosum, cysts, agenesis of the cerebellar vermis, agy-ria, gray matter heterotopia, and other venous drainage anomalies (Fig. 202–5).[51–53]

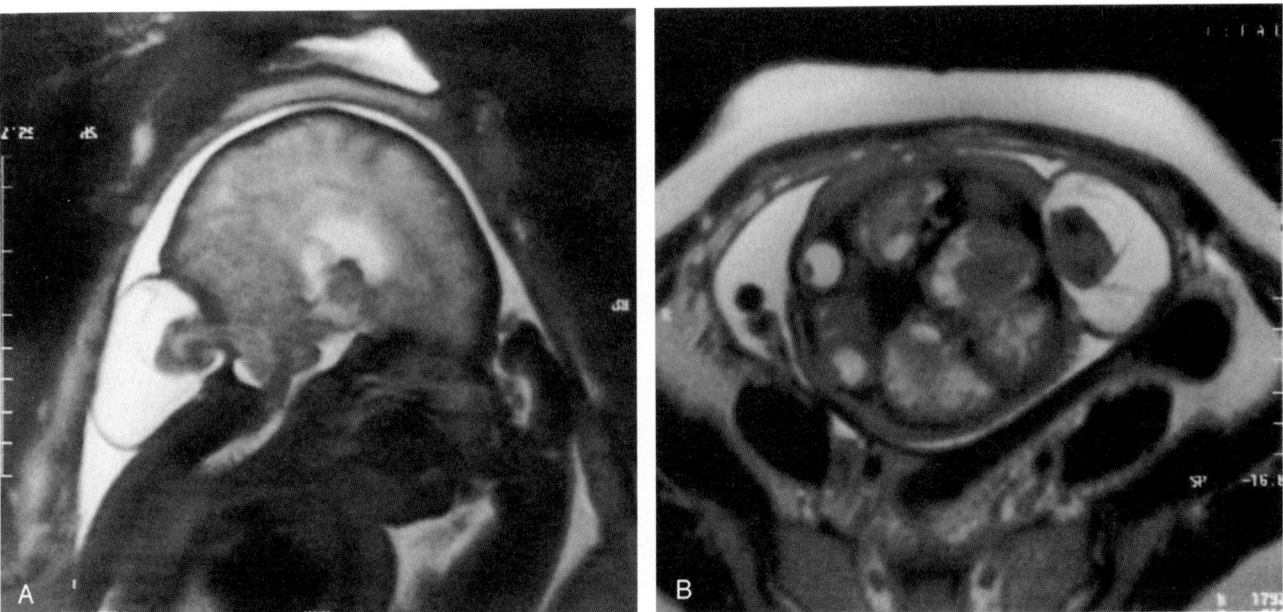

FIGURE 202–3. *A,* Fetal sagittal MRI scan showing a posterior occipital encephalocele in a third-trimester fetus. A large sac containing CSF is observed. In addition, herniation of neural tissue is seen in the sac. *B,* Fetal axial MRI scan of the same patient showing the CSF-containing sac and a round nodule of neural tissue within.

Associated Findings with Posterior Encephaloceles

Occipital encephaloceles located below the torcula present a remarkable array of morphologic features.

The most common findings are distortion of the brainstem, usually with an S-shaped kink; abnormalities in the cerebellum, which can be absent, rudimentary, lacking the vermis, or even "inverted," with the cerebellar hemispheres rotated ventrally around the pons and the brainstem displaced posteriorly; small poste-

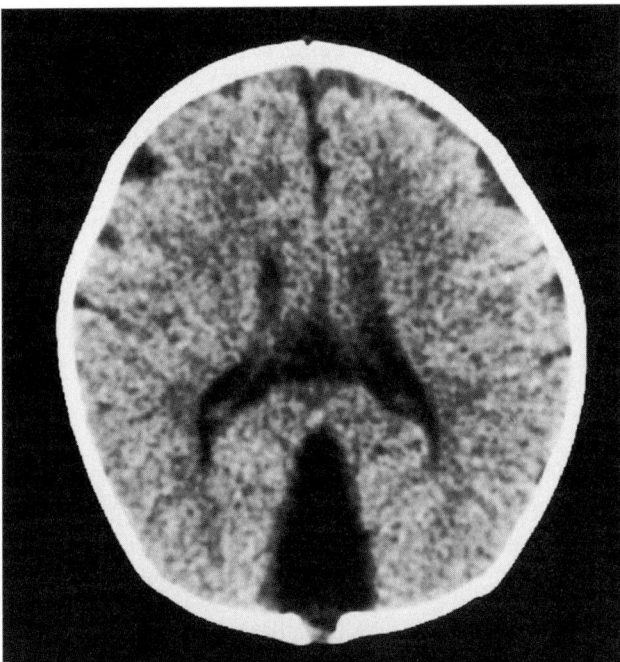

FIGURE 202–4. Axial computed tomographic scan showing a bony defect at the site of previous small, atretic encephalocele. This lesion was associated with a Dandy-Walker malformation, one of several known malformations found with encephaloceles in this region.

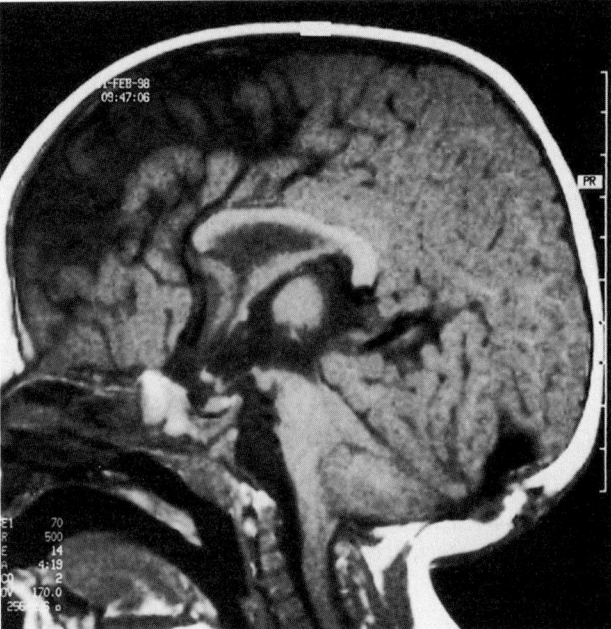

FIGURE 202–5. Sagittal MRI scan of a patient with a repaired occipital encephalocele. Note the low-lying torcular, small posterior fossa and associated polymicrogyria of the occipital lobes. Occipital encephaloceles are frequently accompanied by these and other cerebral malformations.

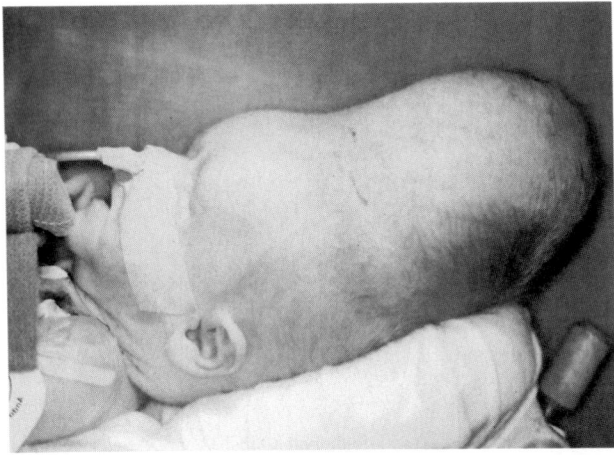

FIGURE 202–6. A large encephalocele is seen at the vertex of the infant's head. The lesion is totally covered by skin, and it stretches along the midline from the lambda to the bregma.

rior fossa (see Fig. 202–5); posterior fossa cysts similar to a Dandy-Walker malformation (see Fig. 202–4); elevation of the tentorium and dural venous sinuses; and caudal displacement of the occipital and temporal lobes.[13, 54] Encephaloceles in this region that contain only CSF and meninges, so-called meningoceles, actually represent an evagination of the ventricular system of the brain into the sac (ventriculocele) and are often associated with important malformations of the cerebellum.[13]

Parietal encephaloceles often have a worse prognosis than their occipital counterparts. This is because the brain malformations associated with parietal encephaloceles often include dorsal cysts that communicate directly with the ventricular system and holoprosencephaly, a major midline cerebral hemispheric fusion anomaly (Fig. 202–6). In these cases, the venous drainage system is characterized by a split sagittal sinus and anomalies in the galenic veins[14, 47] (Fig. 202–7).

In contrast to patients with anterior cranial fossa encephaloceles, who present with facial and ocular manifestations, patients with posterior encephaloceles present with extracranial malformations. These malformations may be associated with other syndromes but can also occur in sporadic cases. The most frequent malformations include cardiac anomalies, cystic kidneys, limb reduction defect, and polydactyly.[55]

Associated Syndromes

Although rare, syndromes associated with posterior encephaloceles must be recognized because they permit one to forecast a prognosis and provide genetic counseling.

MECKEL-GRUBER SYNDROME

In a series of 446 encephaloceles, 26 (5.8%) presented as part of a syndrome, and the most common syndrome was Meckel-Gruber syndrome.[55] Meckel's syndrome or the Meckel-Gruber syndrome is characterized by central nervous system malformations such as occipital exencephalocele; prosencephalic dysgenesis; rhombic roof and cerebellar vermis dysgenesis; enlarged kidneys, with multicystic dysplasia and fibrotic changes in the liver in the portal area with ductal proliferation; and postaxial polydactyly. Other malformations described include microphthalmia, cleft lip and palate, bowing of long bones, situs inversus, heart defects, and genital anomalies. Intra- and interfamilial variability have long been recognized. Today, most pregnancies are terminated, or the fetus is so severely affected that it is stillborn or dies shortly after birth.[15, 56, 57]

The transmission of Meckel-Gruber syndrome is autosomal recessive, with a 25% recurrence rate in subsequent pregnancies. The prevalence of the syndrome ranges from 1 in 9000 births in Finland to 1 in 20,000 births in the United Kingdom.[58] The syndrome is genetically heterogeneous, as two genes have been identified within patient populations. The first is on chromosome 17q21-q24,[59] and the second is on chromosome 11q13.[58]

KNOBLOCH'S SYNDROME

Knobloch's syndrome is a rare syndrome comprising severe myopia, vitreoretinal degeneration with retinal detachment in childhood, and an occipital encephalocele that is usually small and contains small amounts of dysplastic glial and neuronal tissue.[19, 60] Other congenital midline scalp defects such as hemangioma, tuft of hair, and dark hair can be found in lieu of the encephalocele.[61] Patients with Knobloch's syndrome have ocular anomalies, but their intelligence is normal, and imaging studies show falx and tentorium defects but an almost normal brain. The transmission is autosomal recessive, and the gene involved is localized to chromosome 21q22.3.[62]

WALKER-WARBURG SYNDROME

Walker-Warburg syndrome, or cerebro-ocular muscular syndrome, is characterized by central nervous system malformations including hydrocephalus and lissencephaly type II, cerebellar malformations, ocular malformations, and congenital muscular dystrophy. Encephaloceles can also be present. The mechanism of inheritance is autosomal recessive.[15, 20, 63]

Neurosurgical Repair

Most encephaloceles can be effectively repaired following the general principles outlined later. However, if the amount of dysplastic brain within the sac exceeds that within the cranium, the neurologic outcome will be poor. In this situation, the option of not closing the encephalocele can be considered. However, this course of nonoperative management should be undertaken only after extensive discussions with the family and the medical personnel directly caring for the infant.

In general, the goals of surgery are to remove the sac, preserve functional neural tissue, and obtain clo-

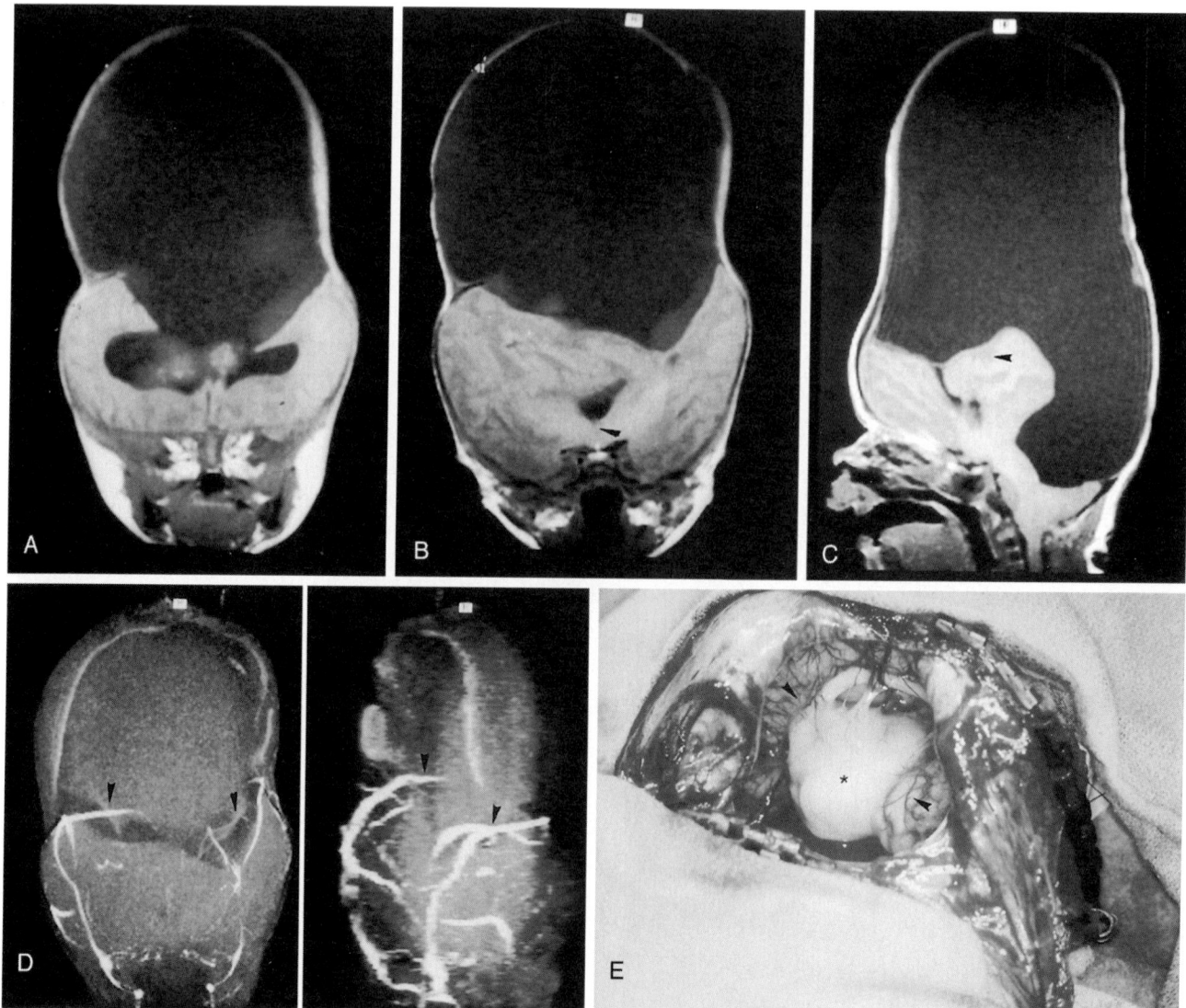

FIGURE 202–7. MRI investigation in a neonate (same case as Fig. 202–6). *A,* Coronal T1-weighted MRI scan demonstrates a huge dorsal cyst and anterior horns without septum pellucidum. *B,* Fused thalami are seen *(arrowhead). C,* The sagittal midline T1 image shows extensive gray matter crossing in the dysgenetic midline *(arrowhead).* Note also a malformation of the mesencephalic tegmentum and the lack of the aqueduct. *D,* Magnetic resonance venographic coronal and oblique reconstructions show wide splitting of the superior sagittal sinus *(arrowheads),* as well as a lack of a deep venous system. *E,* Intraoperative view of the inside of the cranium demonstrates the laterally displaced hemispheres *(arrowheads)* and the abnormally formed midline cerebral structures, which correspond partly to the topical hemisphere and thalami fusion *(asterisk).*

sure of the wound with the nondysplastic skin. Neurosurgical planning is facilitated by careful review of the preoperative imaging studies, especially the MRI. The presence of CSF inside the encephalocele is a favorable factor, because its presence means that less of the sac will be taken up by herniated, dysplastic cerebral tissue.

Neurosurgical repair of these often large lesions is possible only with skillfully administered neuroanesthesia. Essential monitoring information must be obtained throughout the case, including temperature, blood pressure, pulse, electrocardiogram, oxygen saturation, and end-tidal carbon dioxide levels. The infant's temperature must be maintained near 37°C. Through-

out the procedure, strict hemostasis must be maintained, as inadequate estimation of blood loss can lead to hypotension.

Posterior encephaloceles are usually repaired with the patient in the prone or sometimes the lateral decubitus position (Fig. 202–8). The neonate is placed facedown within an infant horseshoe headrest. The face is padded. For large lesions with excess amounts of redundant skin, we use "sky hooks" to hold the sac upright while dissection of the encephalocele is undertaken (Fig. 202–9).

Neurosurgical repair begins with the skin incision, which may be either horizontal or vertical, depending on the configuration of the sac and its dimensions. It

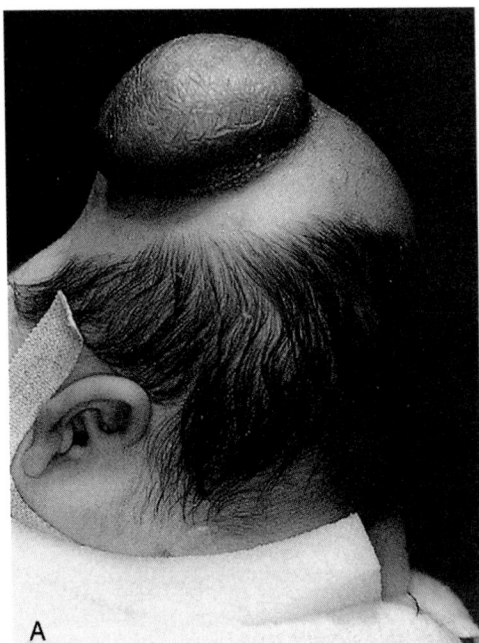
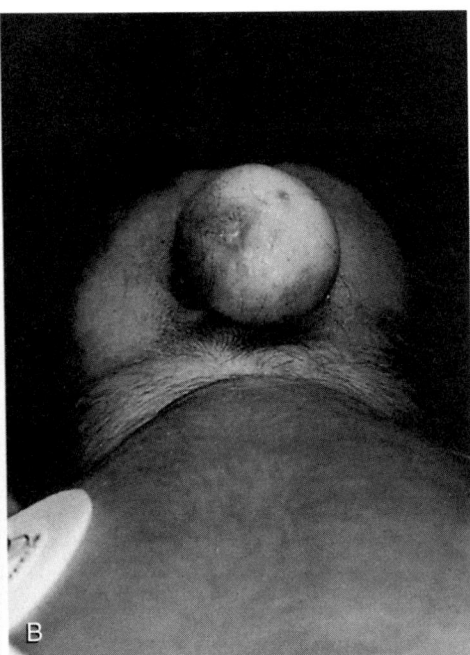

FIGURE 202–8. In preparation for surgery, the neonate is placed face-down on a padded headrest. *A,* View of occipital encephalocele from the side. *B,* View of occipital encephalocele from below.

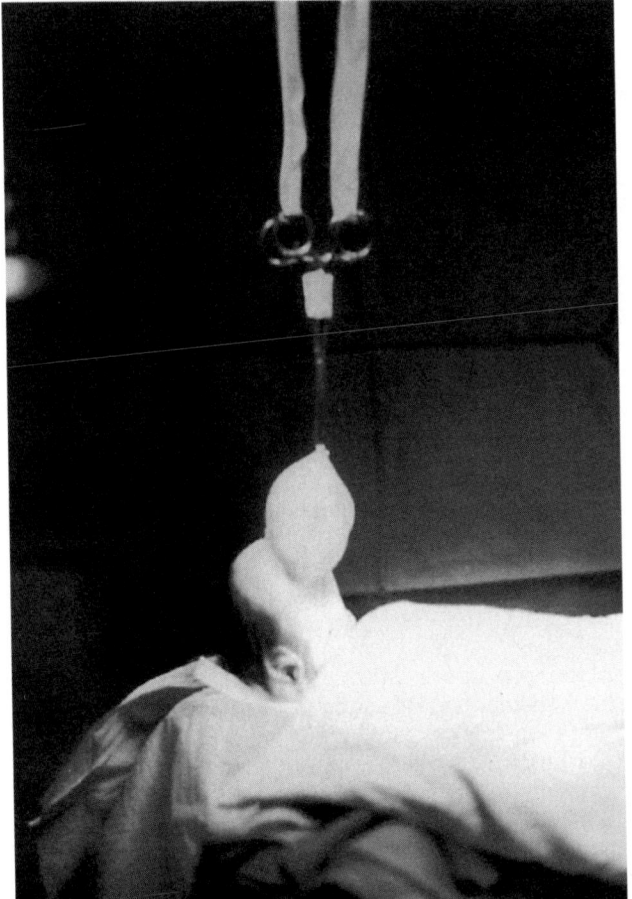

FIGURE 202–9. For large encephaloceles with redundant skin, we prefer to suspend the sac using tissue clamps that connect the sac to an overhead pole. Once the skin of the sac has been circumferentially dissected and the tissues freed, the tissue clamps holding the redundant skin are elevated away from the operative field by the anesthesiologist.

is important to mark the extent of scalp resection at the beginning of the case, erring on the side of leaving too much skin rather than too little (additional skin can always be removed). The skin should be circumferentially incised above the base of the encephalocele. The plane between the soft tissues of the scalp and the dura mater is then identified by blunt dissection. Dissection is again carried out circumferentially in this plane. The sac is opened and drained of CSF. The contents of the sac can then be inspected. If neural tissue is present and appears dysplastic, preventing adequate closure, this tissue can be resected flush with the bony opening. However, the decision to resect this tissue should be made only after weighing the intraoperative findings with the information on the MRI scan. Redundant dura can then be excised, and the remaining dura can be closed with a running stitch, trying to achieve a watertight closure at this level. It is essential to maintain hemostasis when cutting the dura and to know where the large venous sinuses are located before dural excision. The subcutaneous layers and skin are closed with interrupted sutures. The bony defects found with most posterior encephaloceles are not large. After routine closure of these lesions, new bone formation is frequently induced by the dura mater, and the bony defects usually get smaller over time.

In rare situations, the repair of encephaloceles with large amounts of brain herniation associated with microcephaly is difficult, and different techniques have been described to avoid the resection of neural elements in these cases. Gallo[64] described the use of a fine tantalum mesh to create a rigid extracranial compartment to protect the herniated brain. Whenever possible, we prefer to close large bony defects in a delayed fashion using autogenous split-thickness cranial bone grafts (Fig. 202–10).[65]

In the postoperative period, patients with repaired

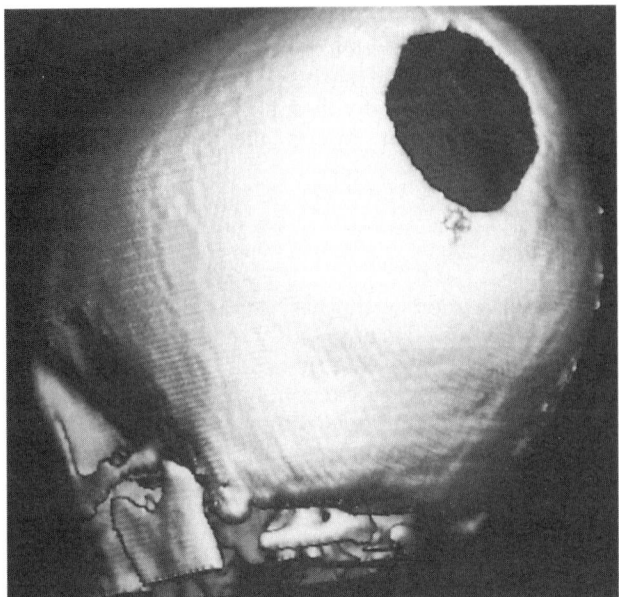

FIGURE 202–10. Posterior view of a three-dimensional reconstruction of a computed tomographic scan showing a large bony defect associated with a repaired occipital encephalocele. At a later age, defects this size can be repaired using autogenous split-thickness cranioplasties.

posterior encephaloceles need to be watched for the onset of symptomatic hydrocephalus and central nervous system infection. The treatment for progressive hydrocephalus is insertion of a ventriculoperitoneal shunt. The best way to minimize the morbidity of CSF shunting in the neonatal period is to delay shunt insertion until it is absolutely necessary. CSF leakage through a properly repaired encephalocele usually suggests the diagnosis of hydrocephalus, but a brief period of external ventricular drainage and antibiotic therapy may be warranted in this situation to avoid shunt infections.

Outcome after Repair of Posterior Encephaloceles

Several factors predict a worse outcome in patients with posterior encephaloceles, including the presence and amount of neural tissue in the sac, posterior location, microcephaly, and hydrocephalus requiring ventriculoperitoneal shunting. Other factors that bode poorly for the patient include the presence of major brain malformations. In a study of 16 cases, 8 patients had normal neurologic examinations and 8 were hydrocephalic and hypotonic (5 with Walker-Warburg syndrome). The follow-up showed eight with normal development, two mildly retarded, two severely handicapped, and four deaths. In this series, the patients with occipital encephaloceles had a worse prognosis than the patients with parietal ones.[52] In another series with five cases of encephaloceles located in the parietal region, the imaging studies showed porencephalic cysts and corpus callosum agenesis, and the follow-up found retardation in all patients.[14] In a study of eight children with parietal lesions, six were normal, one had mild motor delay, and one died at age 3.[66]

Atretic Encephalocele

An atretic encephalocele, also called *occult* or *rudimentary encephalocele*, or *mesencephalic meningocele manqué*,[67] is characterized by a small, noncystic, skin-covered, flat or nodular subscalp lesion in the midline occipital or parietal region. It is composed of meninges, blood vessels, and sometimes foci of neural or glial elements. The skin characteristics over the lesion are variable and can present with regions of alopecia, excessive hair growth, and angiomatous or discolored skin.[14, 52, 66, 67]

The differential diagnosis of these lesions includes dermoid cyst and sinus pericranium. A clinical finding favoring sinus pericranium is deflation of the lesion when the patient is in the upright position. The bone defect is oval or elongated and narrow from the inside outward in atretic encephalocele and is round and narrow from the outside inward in dermoid cyst. The atretic encephalocele enhances with contrast, but the dermoid cyst does not. CT and MRI show venous anomalies of the straight sinus and tentorium, with a stalk of tissue leading directly to the suprapineal recess in most instances. These lesions can often be explored and repaired using a horseshoe-shaped incision and careful dissection within the tissue planes (Fig. 202–11). Periosteum can usually be mobilized around the small amount of protruding tissue in the repair.[52]

ANTERIOR CRANIAL FOSSA ENCEPHALOCELES

Although encephaloceles of the anterior cranial fossa are present at birth, they may not manifest until well into adult life. The encephalocele may contain only meninges and CSF, or it may contain dysplastic cerebral tissue that retains a basic but deranged cytoarchitecture. Other cephalic anomalies associated with anterior cranial fossa encephaloceles include cleft lip, cleft palate, malformation of the nasal tip, microphthalmia, corneal opacity, coloboma, craniosynostosis, and corpus callosum agenesis or lipoma.[1, 21–23]

Several classifications have been proposed for encephaloceles of the anterior cranial fossa.[4, 68] Most systems divide these encephaloceles into sincipital and basal encephaloceles[4, 68–73] (see Table 202–1). Sincipital encephaloceles demonstrate an internal defect through the foramen cecum placed anteriorly with respect to the cribriform plate, whereas basal encephaloceles protrude through the cribriform plate or body of the sphenoid (Fig. 202–12). Both sincipital and basal encephaloceles are further subdivided into different subgroups, depending on the location of the bony defect and anatomic course of the encephalocele sac (see Table 202–1).

Although the emergence of the sac in the nasal cavity or orbit may be similar whether the internal defect is sincipital or basal, the clinical distinction between them is important. Because of the proximity of a sphenoidal defect to the suprasellar cistern, basal

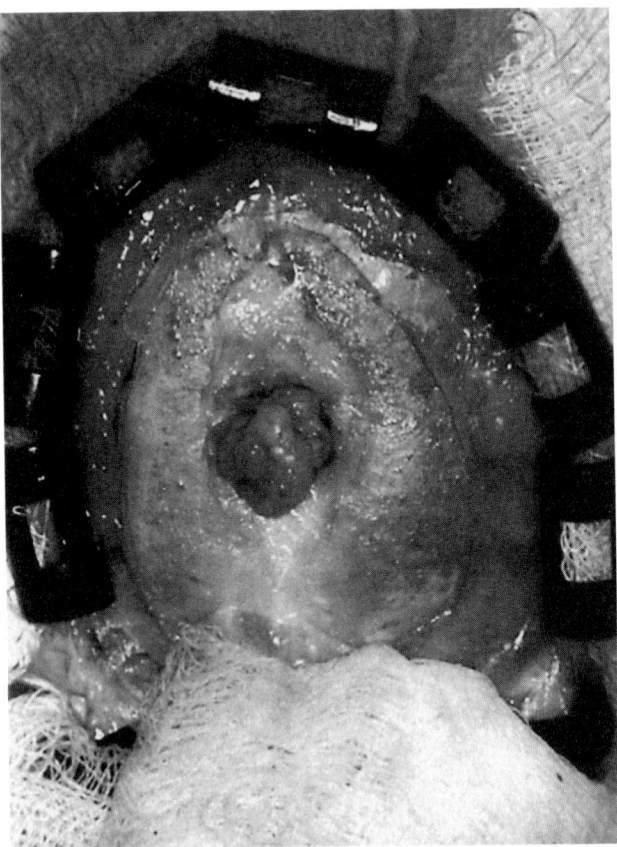

FIGURE 202–11. Operative view of an atretic encephalocele. In repairing this atretic encephalocele, a horseshoe incision was used. The periosteum was incised circumferentially and used to close the defect protruding through the small bony defect.

encephaloceles are much more likely to contain vital structures than are sincipital lesions.

Despite numerous publications on the results of treatment of this condition, controversy remains whether the defect should be repaired intradurally[7, 9] or extradurally.[74–77] Other debates center around whether minor degrees of hypertelorism will correct themselves once the encephalocele has been removed[8] and whether orbital translocation involving maxillotomy and nasoethmoidal resection impairs anterior facial growth in young children.[78]

Diagnosis

With the exception of the nasoethmoidal subtype, sincipital encephaloceles are readily diagnosed because of the evident facial swelling (Fig. 202–13). The mass may enlarge with crying or, exceptionally, cross-fluctuation with the anterior fontanelle may be apparent.[76] Dermoid cyst, sinus pericranium, nasal glioma, teratoma, ethmoid meningioma, and angioma should be considered in the differential diagnosis of such lesions.[79, 80] There are a number of reports in the literature of nasal masses that have been snared as polyps, resulting in immediate or delayed CSF rhinorrhea, meningitis, or a histologic diagnosis of encephalocele (Fig. 202–14).[21, 68] It should be remembered that nasal polyps are uncommon lesions in children. In a review of 10,000 such lesions, only 6 occurred in the pediatric age group.[80] Clinical features that may help differentiate an encephalocele from a polyp include pulsation and a positive Furstenberg sign (swelling of the mass on jugular vein compression).[81] Furthermore, because polyps emanate from the turbinates, their origin lies laterally in the nasal cavity. Encephaloceles, by contrast, usually emerge through a midline defect and are likely to be attached to the nasal septum.[82] Radiographic demonstration of downward bowing of the cribriform plate or the planum sphenoidale is further evidence that the lesion may be an encephalocele.[21] Encephalocele was considered in the differential diagnosis of the two cases in our series that were thought preoperatively to be polyps but was dismissed on the basis of 5-mm computed tomographic images, which failed to detect the

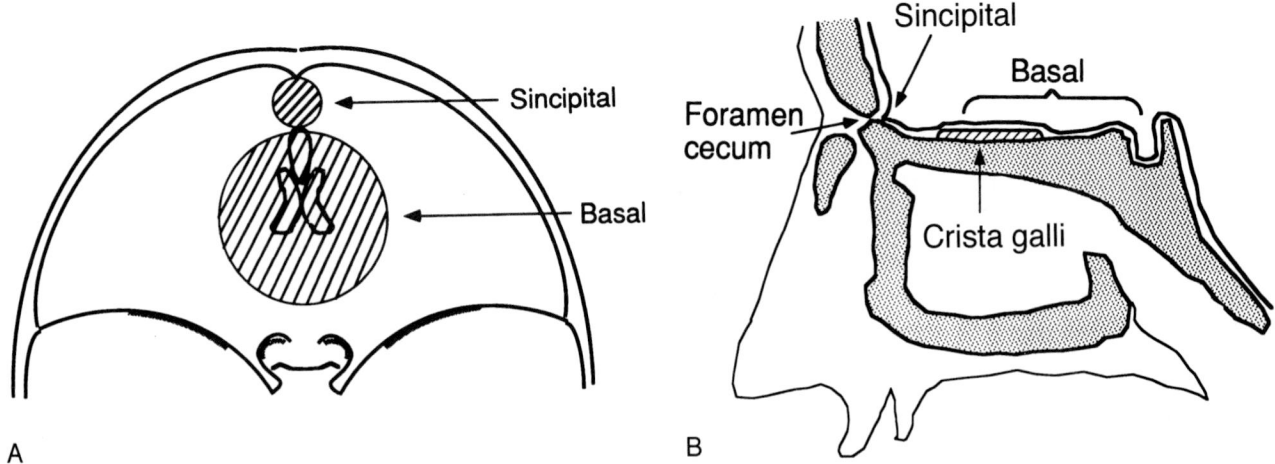

FIGURE 202–12. Anatomic differentiation of sincipital and basal encephaloceles as shown on anterior cranial base *(A)* and sagittal *(B)* diagrams. A sincipital encephalocele is closely associated with a defect in the foramen cecum anterior to the crista galli. A basal encephalocele may protrude through a defect in the sphenoid bone and sinus.

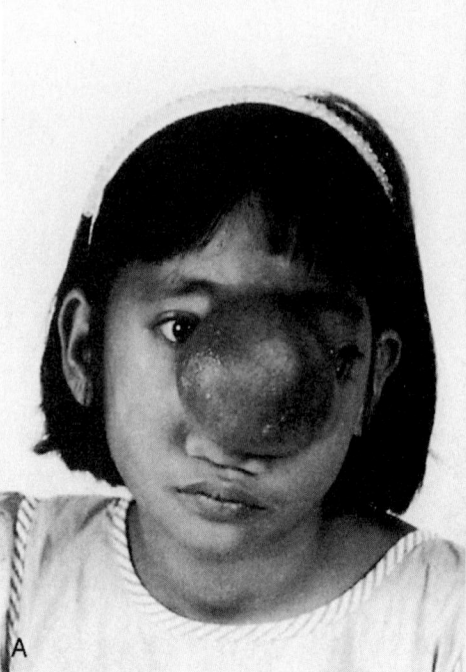 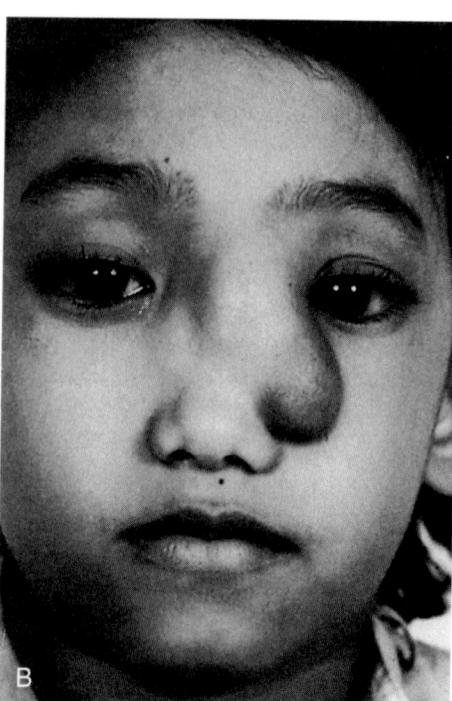

FIGURE 202–13. *A,* Twelve-year-old girl with a large nasofrontal encephalocele associated with hypertelorism. *B,* Eleven-year-old girl with a nasoethmoidal encephalocele with predominance of tissue protruding to the left of midline. Hypertelorism is mild.

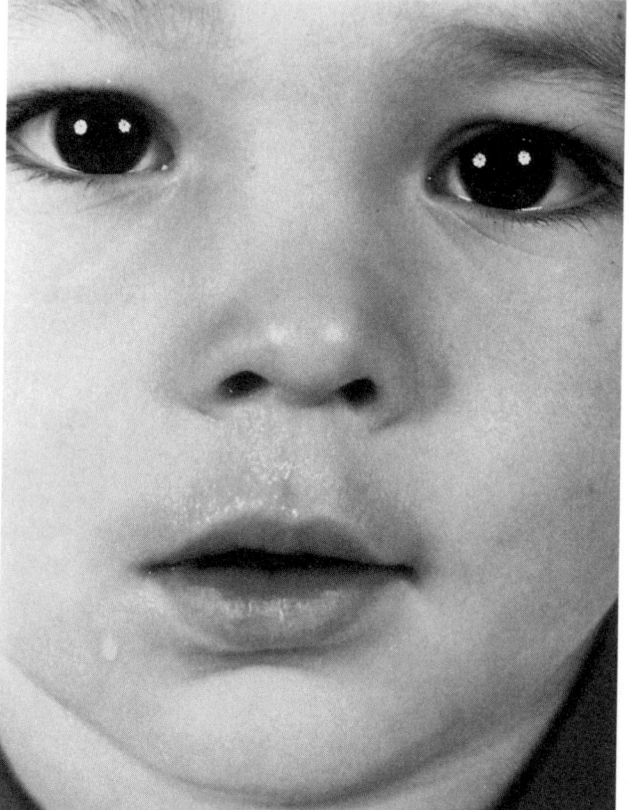

FIGURE 202–14. A 4-year-old boy presenting with persistent CSF rhinorrhea. Despite an active CSF leak for several months, the child never developed signs or symptoms of meningitis. His nasoethmoidal encephalocele was repaired through a bifrontal craniotomy and combined extradural and intradural repair of the dural defect.

cranial defect.[45] Both patients developed CSF rhinorrhea 5 to 6 months after polypectomy.

We now image all anterior cranial fossa encephaloceles by both CT and MRI—CT to delineate the bony anatomy and measure the intraocular diameter, and MRI to demonstrate the sac contents and to assess the brain for the presence of other anomalies (Figs. 202–15 and 202–16). CT alone may be inadequate, because small openings can be missed through the partial volume effect, and the demonstration of a small opening does not prove that a communication exists between the nasal mass and the intracranial compartment. MRI is more sensitive than CT at determining continuity between the nasal and cranial cavities when there is a lesion with a very narrow neck, as well as differentiating herniated brain from an inflammatory nasal mass.[81]

Nasal obstruction, mouth breathing, snoring, and nasal discharge are characteristic features of a basal encephalocele projecting into the nasopharynx.[21] These are common symptoms in infants and may initially be overlooked.[17] Two of our patients suffered CSF rhinorrhea for 6 to 8 weeks before the correct diagnosis was established (see Fig. 202–14). Rarely, basal encephaloceles are diagnosed only after repeated bouts of meningitis.[36]

Timing of Repair

The timing of surgery may be dictated by the nature of the encephalocele. Absence of skin cover or the presence of hemorrhage, CSF leakage, or impending ulceration all necessitate expeditious repair. Airway obstruction or visual impairment are further indications for early intervention.[83] However, in the absence of these, and when a complex craniofacial abnormality

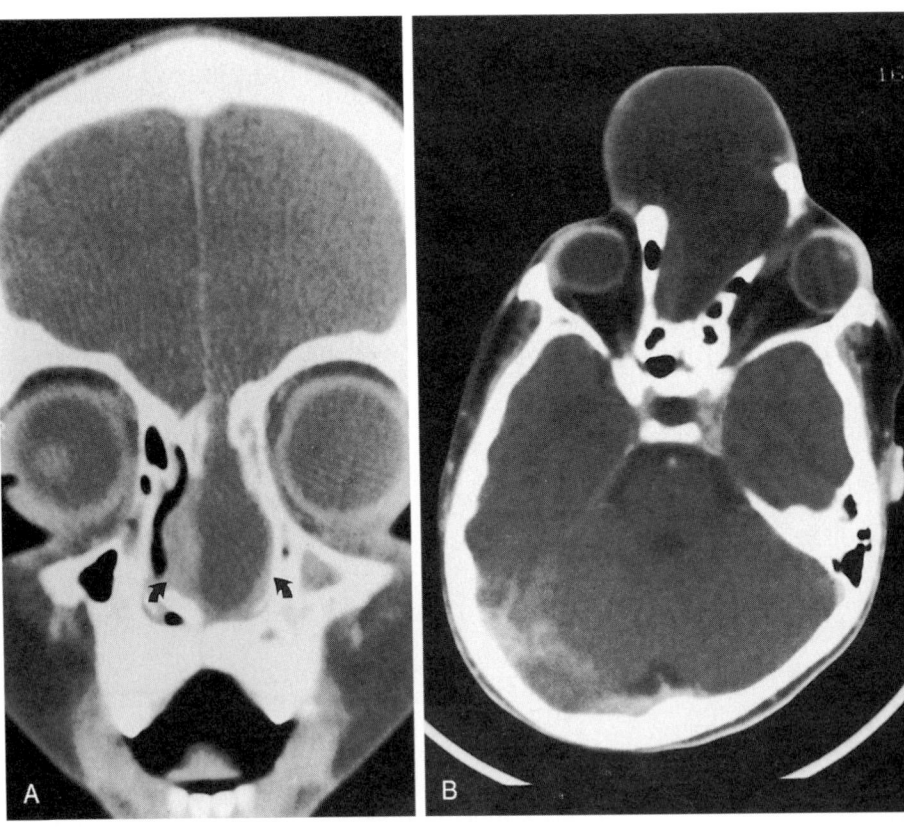

FIGURE 202–15. Computed tomographic appearance of sincipital encephaloceles. *A,* Coronal computed tomographic scan of a 2-year-old girl presenting with nasal obstruction. A nasoethmoidal sincipital encephalocele is apparent *(arrows).* The unilateral bony defect in the anterior fossa floor adjacent to the crista galli is appreciated on these scans with bone windows. *B,* Axial computed tomographic scan showing tertiary hypertelorism in a patient with a large nasofrontal encephalocele (same patient as in Figure 202–13*A*).

is present, treatment may be delayed until the patient's age and general condition are considered optimal.

When the developing eyes separate as diverticula from the diencephalon, they lie initially in the lateral position. The eyes rotate forward as the face matures, and the angle reduces from 180 degrees to about 71

degrees by birth and 68 degrees by maturity. Hypertelorism is a frequent accompaniment of frontobasal encephalocele because the presence of such a lesion obstructs this migration. In addition, the nasal cartilages may be displaced caudally, elongating the face and producing so-called long nose hypertelorism.[84, 85] Be-

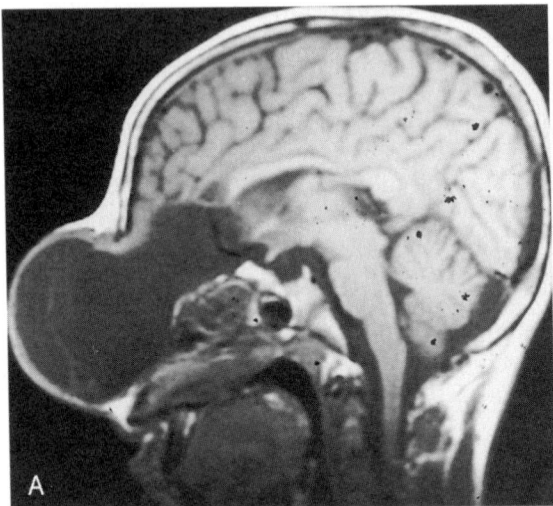
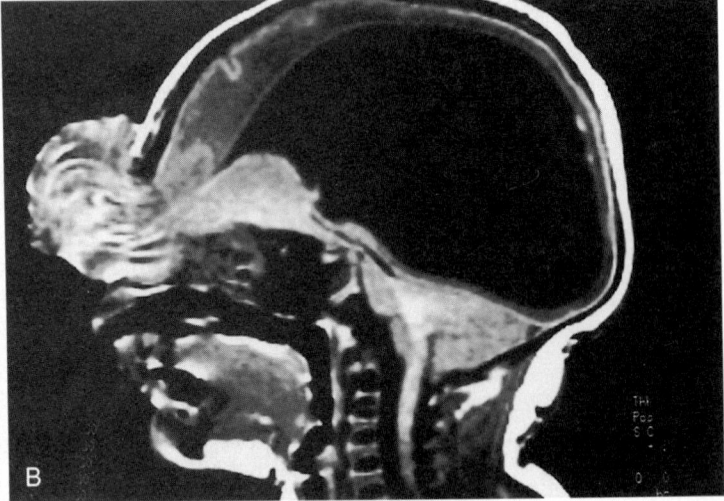

FIGURE 202–16. *A,* Sagittal MRI of an 8-year-old girl with a large nasofrontal sincipital encephalocele. The large sac of the encephalocele is filled with CSF and a small amount of brain tissue. The path of the anterior cerebral arteries coursing toward the corpus callosum can be appreciated. *B,* Sagittal MRI scan of male infant born with an extensive nasofrontal sincipital encephalocele. There is prominent cerebral herniation into the sac of the encephalocele. The brain is dysgenetic, and there is marked ventriculomegaly. This patient required a ventriculoperitoneal shunt. The neurologic outcome was poor.

cause the skeletal deformity is secondary to the encephalocele rather than an intrinsic problem with the tissues, and because the early months of life are a period of rapid growth for the brain and facial skeleton, some authors argue that removal of the encephalocele allows for resumption of normal morphology provided that the degree of deformity is slight.[12] Based on their experience treating 130 cases of sincipital encephalocele, Charoonsmith and Suwanwela[12] suggested that only the encephalocele and associated soft tissue mass need be removed initially, in the hope that the facial deformity would regress. In particular, they advised that surgery to the developing nasal capsule and facial bones be kept to a minimum in infancy. Concomitant treatment of hypertelorism was advised only in patients older than 3 years of age, because facial deformity tended to persist after that age.

In contrast, others believe that the best aesthetic results are produced by one-stage reconstruction within the first 3 months of life[1, 30, 86] using the technique of total orbital translocation pioneered by Tessier.[87] Their rationale is that early complete correction allows the rapidly expanding brain and eyes to model the reconstructed facial skeleton; left untreated, the soft tissue mass and facial deformities would progress rather than diminish with age. A further theoretical argument for early correction is the restoration of binocular vision,[87] although some authors claim that this does not occur.[78, 88]

There are three major arguments against one-stage reconstruction. The first is the duration of the procedure and the degree of blood loss in a very young child. Second, early total correction of hypertelorism was found in one study to interfere with anterior facial growth, and this was attributed to maxillotomy and nasoethmoidal resection.[78] For this reason, Mulliken and coworkers[78] advocate that orbital reconstruction be postponed until adolescence. However, maxillary hypoplasia did not occur in two other series,[89] and it has been found to develop in untreated sincipital and basal encephaloceles as well.[12, 90] A third concern regarding early craniofacial surgery is whether corrections will tend to regress with growth and the medial canthi will drift laterally. McCarthy and colleagues[89] studied 20 patients who underwent orbital translocation when they were younger than 5 years and found evidence of relapse in 3 (15%). When deterioration in the intercanthal distance occurs, it does so within the first 6 months of surgery and remains stable thereafter.[91]

An alternative to total orbital translocation is to transpose only the medial walls.[75, 86, 92, 93] This may provide adequate correction because some patients have only displacement of the medial orbital walls or medial canthal ligaments, that is, they have telecanthus rather than true hypertelorism.[85–87] Tessier[87] believed that this procedure was likely to fail because only part of the orbit is moved, and it therefore has little opportunity to displace the globes. However, several other groups reported good results with this technique.[1, 75, 85]

The question, then, is whether to undertake an early one-stage correction or to repair only the encephalocele in infancy and defer correction of the facial abnormalities until after the age of 5. Certainly, the evidence suggests that hypertelorism in the absence of an encephalocele is best treated in later childhood or adulthood. However, the desire both to avoid a second cranial procedure and to improve the facial appearance as much as possible, preferably before school age, favors early combined repair. Our experience is that primary and secondary hypertelorism often regresses if the encephalocele is repaired within 2 to 3 years of birth, and early orbital translocation is therefore generally inappropriate. Cases of tertiary hypertelorism and midline facial cleft require reduction of the intraocular diameter, the timing of which is dictated largely by whether the encephalocele requires urgent repair. Modern craniofacial techniques and anesthesia make one-stage correction both possible and safe, and we prefer this to separate treatment of the encephalocele and hypertelorism. However, the total blood volume of infants is small, and careful attention is needed to ensure adequate volume replacement.

Neurosurgical Repair

We agree with Matson[6] that extracranial operations are unsatisfactory for the treatment of sincipital encephaloceles. Surgery is performed through a contaminated field, the dural margins are harder to define, and it is more difficult to obtain a watertight closure. Furthermore, about 25% of dural defects are multiple,[68] and the cribriform plate may lie 1 to 2 cm below the more lateral elements of the anterior cranial fossa floor.[92] In addition, the dura may on occasion be deficient over an area much wider than that of the bony defect.[85] Nasoethmoidal and naso-orbital encephaloceles have sacs with long necks, adding to the difficulty of obtaining adequate closure at the internal orifice when approached from below.[4] The risk of recurrence is therefore greater than with an intradural approach.[7, 9] When using a combination of intradural and extradural delineation of the defect, and either primary dural closure reinforced with an intradural patch or combined intra- and extradural grafts when primary closure was not possible, none of our sincipital encephaloceles leaked CSF (Fig. 202–17).[45] In contrast, 7 of 86 lesions repaired extradurally developed rhinorrhea, and 2 patients died from meningitis.[94] The CSF leakage rate reported by others advocating extradural repair is also around 10%.[75] The only case of rhinorrhea we encountered in our series was in a child with a midline facial cleft, a basal encephalocele, and a large third ventriculocele within the sphenoid and nasopharynx.[45] Adherence of the optic chiasm and hypothalamus to the walls of the sac precluded an intradural patch. The extradural repair leaked 14 days after surgery but settled within 2 days of lumbar drain insertion.

In a review of the literature on basal encephaloceles, Yokota and colleagues[17] noted that the operative mortality in infancy was almost 50%, but that death was exceptional if repair was undertaken after the age of 3 years. The major causes of death in infancy were from

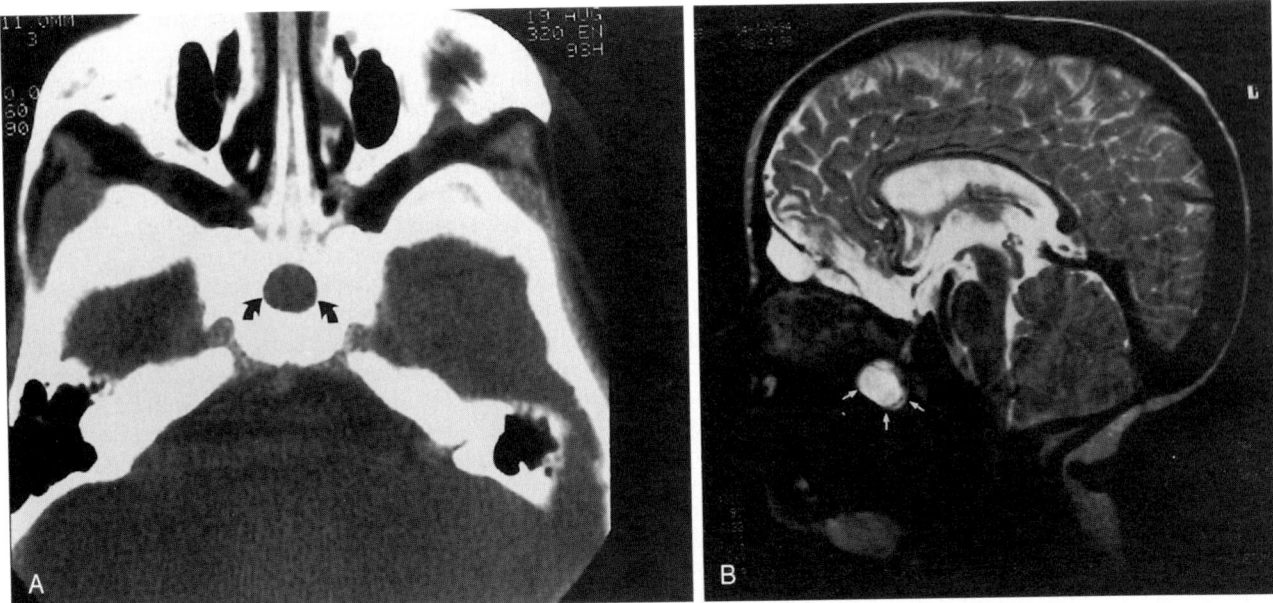

FIGURE 202–17. Infant with a basal sphenopharyngeal encephalocele. *A,* Axial computed tomographic scan demonstrating the midline defect in the sphenoid bone *(arrows).* *B,* Sagittal MRI scan showing CSF signal intensity on T2-weighted images of the nasopharyngeal contents of the sac *(arrows).*

general debility, hypothalamic dysfunction, and meningitis. These authors advocated delayed repair of basal encephaloceles unless there were life-threatening complications such as respiratory obstruction or meningitis. Lewin[74] also reported a 50% mortality from intracranial repair of such encephaloceles and suggested that extracranial repair may be advantageous if there is already a large cleft palate. He argued that this approach lessens the risk to the diencephalic structures, optic apparatus, and circle of Willis, all of which may be adherent to the sac. In addition, the risk of cerebral edema from excessive retraction is avoided.[74] Although cleft palate was present in two of our patients, we prefer intracranial exploration and encountered difficulty in repairing only one of five cases. Adequate preoperative imaging by MRI and CT is essential to identify the sac contents, as is angiography to establish the relationship between the major branches of the circle of Willis and the internal orifice.

Neurosurgical repair usually begins with the anesthetized patient in the supine position. A bicoronal incision is used to expose the anterior calvaria and frontal regions. A bifrontal craniotomy is then tailor-made to suit the exposure required for repair of the lesion (Fig. 202–18). When attempting to reduce the hernia or to excise the sac contents from above, every effort should be made to ensure that the nasal cavity is not entered, because of the risk of postoperative infection.[7] In four of our patients, the nasal component was removed by snaring, but only after completion of the dural repair and closure of the craniotomy.[45] Interestingly, Mattox and Kennedy[77] reported two cases in which they excised encephaloceles and repaired the dural defect by nasal endoscopy alone.

Unlike with occipital lesions, pre- and postoperative

hydrocephalus is uncommon, probably because the anterior subarachnoid space is a less important conduit for CSF transport. Preoperative hydrocephalus is likely only when the defect is extremely large and the inferior aspect of the frontal lobes is displaced anteriorly. This draws the diencephalon forward and may cause kinking of the cerebral aqueduct. Only two of our patients required shunting (9%), both 2 to 3 months after surgery.[95] The incidence of hydrocephalus in other series is 8.5% to 17%.[12]

The olfactory apparatus may form part of the hernia

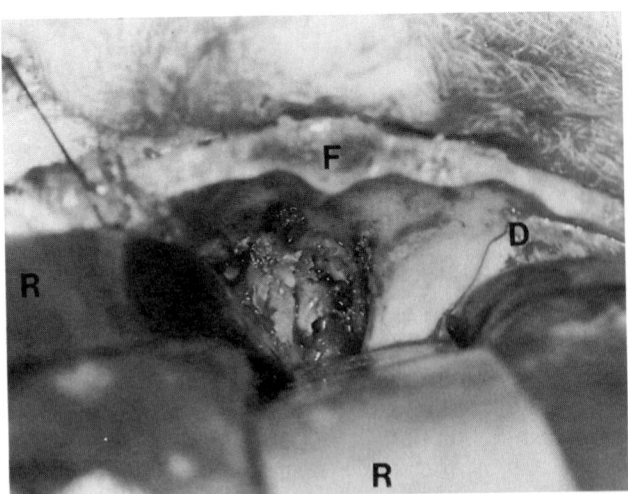

FIGURE 202–18. Intraoperative photograph, viewed from the top of the head, with the frontal lobes retracted posteriorly, showing a bony defect in a 2-year-old boy presenting with nasal obstruction from an encephalocele. The large defect required a bilateral exploration and closure with a combined extradural and intradural patch graft. D, dura; F, frontal bone; R, retractor.

sac in sincipital lesions. Although it has been claimed that complete and permanent anosmia is an almost inevitable consequence of sincipital encephalocele,[94] 2 of the 10 patients in whom assessment was possible retained olfaction after surgery,[95] as have some patients in other series.[30] An attempt should therefore be made to preserve the olfactory apparatus unless it is grossly dysplastic or if sparing it would compromise adequate dural closure. Small bone defects in the floor of the anterior cranial fossa may be left, but larger ones should be grafted because this helps support the dural repair and thereby lessens the risk of CSF leak. Although the graft sometimes incorporates into the surrounding skull base,[40, 65, 94] in some of our patients, the bone resorbed progressively.[95] However, despite its absence, there were no cases of recurrent encephalocele. Lewin[74] also noted sequential enlargement of skull defects after grafting, but the bone is replaced by fibrous tissue, which prevents recurrent prolapse.

Prognosis

The prognosis for both survival and intellectual development is better for anteriorly placed than for posteriorly placed encephaloceles. In the literature, overall mortality is 7% to 20% for sincipital defects,[3, 5, 7, 9, 26, 35] almost 50% for basal encephaloceles repaired in infancy,[17] and 25% to 60% for parietal and occipital lesions.[1, 9, 96] Many of these reports are now outdated, and mortality is currently low in patients considered appropriate candidates for surgery. There were no deaths in our series.[95] However, disability in survivors remains high. Although 59% of our patients are developing normally, 18% have mild disability, and 23% are severely impaired. Developmental outcome reported in two other studies is broadly similar. An assessment of 12 patients with sincipital encephaloceles found that 3.3% had severe disabilities and 17% mild developmental delays.[97] Simpson and colleagues[1] reported that 5% of patients with sincipital encephaloceles were severely delayed mentally, with a further 28% significantly affected and 67% either normal or slightly impaired. With the exception of massive lesions associated with microcephaly, the outcome of anterior encephaloceles is not related to the size of the defect, the presence or absence of brain tissue within it, or the age of the patient at the time of diagnosis.[78, 97]

Other than developmental delay, the major morbidity of anterior encephaloceles relates to cosmetic deformity, visual abnormalities, and anosmia.[97] Although correction of the facial malformation improves the cosmetic appearance, many children still suffer psychosocial problems in adolescence.[98] Although some children "blossom" after treatment to correct their facial anomalies, others show no appreciable social or psychological change, probably because few malformations can be corrected to the extent that a normal appearance is attained.[99]

Conclusion

The comparative rarity of anterior encephaloceles in the Western Hemisphere and the complex management issues they present suggest that they should be managed in a few specialized centers offering a multidisciplinary approach to treatment. The extent of surgery and its optimal timing depends on both the nature of the lesion and the presence of associated anomalies. With adequate facilities, the operative morbidity and mortality are low, but a significant percentage of children will be impaired by associated malformations. Long-term follow-up is required to ensure that a satisfactory cosmetic result is achieved.

REFERENCES

1. Simpson DA, David DJ, White J: Cephaloceles: Treatment, outcome, and antenatal diagnosis. Neurosurgery 15:14–21, 1984.
2. Naidich TP, Altman NR, Braffman BH, et al: Cephaloceles and related malformations. AJNR Am J Neuroradiol 13:655–690, 1992.
3. Emery JL, Kalhan SC: The pathology of exencephalus. Dev Med Child Neurol 12(suppl 22):51–64, 1970.
4. Suwanwela C, Suwanwela N: A morphological classification of sincipital encephalomeningoceles. J Neurosurg 36:201–211, 1972.
5. Ingraham FD, Swan H: Spina bifida and cranium bifida. I. A survey of five hundred and forty-six cases. N Engl J Med 228:559–563, 1943.
6. Matson DD: Neurosurgery of Infancy and Childhood. Springfield, Ill, Thomas, 1969.
7. Suwanwela C, Hongsaprabhas C: Fronto-ethmoidal encephalomeningocele. J Neurosurg 25:172–182, 1966.
8. Karch SB, Urich HL: Occipital encephalocele: A morphological study. J Neurol Sci 15:89–112, 1972.
9. Mealey JJ, Dzenitis AJ, Hockley AA: The prognosis of encephaloceles. J Neurosurg 32:209–218, 1970.
10. Field B: The child with an encephalocele. Med J Aust 1:700–703, 1974.
11. Sever LE, Sanders M, Monsen R: An epidemiologic study of neural tube defects in Los Angeles County. I. Prevalence of birth based on multiple sources of case ascertainment. Teratology 25:315–321, 1982.
12. Charoonsmith T, Suwanwela C: Frontoethmoidal encephalomeningocele with special reference to plastic reconstruction. Clin Plast Surg 1:27–47, 1974.
13. Chapman PH, Swearingen B, Caviness VS: Subtorcular occipital encephaloceles: Anatomical considerations relevant to operative management. J Neurosurg 71:375–381, 1989.
14. Yokota A, Kajiwara H, Kohchi M, et al: Parietal cephalocele: Clinical importance of its atretic form and associated malformations. J Neurosurg 69:545–551, 1988.
15. Cohen MM Jr, Lemire RJ: Syndromes with cephaloceles. Teratology 25:161–172, 1982.
16. Sedano HO, Cohen MM, Jirasek J, Gorlin RJ: Frontonasal dysplasia. J Pediatr 76:906–913, 1970.
17. Yokota A, Matsukado Y, Fuwa I, et al: Anterior basal encephalocele of the neonatal and infantile period. Neurosurgery 19:468–477, 1986.
18. Martinez-Lage JF, Martinez Robledo A, Poza M, Sola J: Familial occurrence of atretic cephaloceles. Pediatr Neurosurg 25:260–264, 1996.
19. Wilson C, Aftimos S, Pereira A, McKay R: Report of two sibs with Knobloch syndrome (encephalocoele and vitreoretinal degeneration) and other anomalies. Am J Med Genet 78:286–290, 1998.
20. Martinez-Lage JF, Garcia Santos JM, Poza M, et al: Neurosurgical management of Walker-Warburg syndrome. Childs Nerv Syst 11:145–153, 1995.
21. Pollock JA, Newton TH, Hoyt WF: Transsphenoidal and transethmoidal encephaloceles: A review of clinical and roentgen features in 8 cases. Radiology 9:442–453, 1968.
22. Goldhammer Y, Smith JL: Optic nerve anomalies in basal encephalocele. Arch Ophthalmol 93:115–118, 1968.
23. Zee CS, McComb JG, Segall HD, et al: Lipomas of the corpus callosum associated with frontal dysraphism. J Comput Assist Tomogr 5:201–205, 1981.
24. Van Allen MI, Kalousek DK, Chernoff GF, et al: Evidence for

multi-site closure of the neural tube in humans. Am J Med Genet 47:723–743, 1993.

25. Marin-Padilla M: Cephalic axial skeletal-neural dysraphic disorders: Embryology and pathology. Can J Neurol Sci 18:153–169, 1991.
26. Kjaer I, Hansen BF, Keeling JW: Axial skeleton and pituitary gland in human fetuses with spina bifida and cranial encephalocele. Pediatr Pathol Lab Med 16:909–926, 1996.
27. McLone DG: The biological resolution of malformations of the central nervous system. Neurosurgery 43:1375–1380, 1998; discussion 1380–1381.
28. Gluckman TJ, George TM, McLone DG: Postneurulation rapid brain growth represents a critical time for encephalocele formation: A chick model. Pediatr Neurosurg 25:130–136, 1996.
29. Oi S, Matsumoto S: Morphological evaluation for neuronal maturation in anencephaly and encephalocele in human neonates: A proposal of reclassification of cephalic dysraphism. Childs Nerv Syst 6:350–353, 1990.
30. David DJ, Sheffield L, Simpson D, White J: Fronto-ethmoidal meningoencephaloceles: Morphology and treatment. Br J Plast Surg 37:271–284, 1984.
31. Leblanc R, Tampieri D, Robataille Y, et al: Developmental anterobasal temporal encephalocele and temporal lobe epilepsy. J Neurosurg 74:933–939, 1991.
32. Gardner WJ: Diastematomyelia and Klippel-Feil syndrome: Relationship to hydrocephalus, syringomyelia, meningocele, meningomyelocele, and iniencephalus. Cleve Clin Q 31:19–34, 1964.
33. Gardner WJ: Hydrodynamic mechanism of syringomyelia: Its relationship to myelocele. J Neurol Neurosurg Psychiatry 28:247–259, 1965.
34. Padget DH: Neuroschisis and human embryonic maldevelopment: New evidence on anencephaly, spina bifida, and diverse mammalian defects. J Neuropathol Exp Neurol 29:192–216, 1970.
35. Whatmore WJ: Sincipital encephalomeningoceles. Br J Surg 60:261–270, 1973.
36. Nager GT: Cephaloceles. Laryngoscope 97:77–84, 1987.
37. Kerszberg M, Changeux JP: A simple molecular model of neurulation. Bioessays 20:758–770, 1998.
38. David DJ, Proudman TW: Cephaloceles: Classification, pathology, and management. World J Surg 13:349–357, 1989.
39. Alembik Y, Dott B, Roth MP, Stoll C: Prevalence of neural tube defects in northeastern France, 1979–1992: Impact of prenatal diagnosis. Ann Genet 38:49–53, 1995.
40. Alembik Y, Dott B, Roth MP, Stoll C: Prevalence of neural tube defects in northeastern France, 1979–1994: Impact of prenatal diagnosis. Ann Genet 40:69–71, 1997.
41. David DJ: Cephaloceles: Classification, pathology, and management—a review. J Craniofac Surg 4:192–202, 1993.
42. Date I, Yagyu Y, Asari S, Ohmoto T: Long-term outcome in surgically treated encephalocele. Surg Neurol 40:125–130, 1993.
43. Castillo M, Quencer RM, Dominguez R: Chiari III malformation: Imaging features. AJNR Am J Neuroradiol 13:107–113, 1992.
44. Erdincler P, Kaynar MY, Canbaz B, et al: Iniencephaly: Neuroradiological and surgical features. Case report and review of the literature. J Neurosurg 89:317–320, 1998.
45. Crandall BF, Chua C: Detecting neural tube defects by amniocentesis between 11 and 15 weeks' gestation. Prenat Diagn 15:339–343, 1995.
46. Bell WO, Nelson LH, Block SM, Rhoney JC: Prenatal diagnosis and pediatric neurosurgery. Pediatr Neurosurg 24:134–137, 1996.
47. Hoving E, Blaser S, Kelly E, Rutka JT: Anatomical and embryological considerations in the repair of a large vertex cephalocele: Case report. J Neurosurg 90:537–541, 1999.
48. Bartels RH, Thijssen HO, Rotteveel JJ, Bakker Niezen SH: Abnormal venous system in occipital meningoencephalocele: MR angiography. Pediatr Neurosurg 23:270–272, 1995.
49. Martinez-Lage JF, Poza M, Sola J, et al: The child with a cephalocele: Etiology, neuroimaging, and outcome. Childs Nerv Syst 12:540–550, 1996.
50. Maas K, Barkovich AJ, Dong L, et al: Selected indications for and applications of magnetic resonance angiography in children. Pediatr Neurosurg 20:113–125, 1994.
51. Saatci I, Yelgec S, Aydin K, Akalan N: An atretic parietal cephalocele associated with multiple intracranial and eye anomalies. Neuroradiology 40:812–815, 1998.

52. Martinez-Lage JF, Sola J, Casas C, et al: Atretic cephalocele: The tip of the iceberg. J Neurosurg 77:230–235, 1992.
53. Martinez-Lage JF, Piqueras C, Poza M: Atretic cephalocele in the adult. Acta Neurochir 139:585–586, 1997.
54. Demaerel P, Kendall BE, Wilms G, et al: Uncommon posterior cranial fossa anomalies: MRI with clinical correlation. Neuroradiology 37:72–76, 1995.
55. Kallen B, Robert E, Harris J: Associated malformations in infants and fetuses with upper or lower neural tube defects. Teratology 57:56–63, 1998.
56. Sepulveda W, Sebire NJ, Souka A, et al: Diagnosis of the Meckel-Gruber syndrome at eleven to fourteen weeks' gestation. Am J Obstet Gynecol 176:316–319, 1997.
57. Gazioglu N, Vural M, Seckin MS, et al: Meckel-Gruber syndrome. Childs Nerv Syst 14:142–145, 1998.
58. Roume J, Genin E, Cormier-Daire V, et al: A gene for Meckel syndrome maps to chromosome 11q13. Am J Hum Genet 63:1095–1101, 1998.
59. Paavola P, Salonen R, Weissenbach J, Peltonen L: The locus for Meckel syndrome with multiple congenital anomalies maps to chromosome 17q21-q24. Nat Genet 11:213–215, 1995.
60. Seaver LH, Joffe L, Spark RP, et al: Congenital scalp defects and vitreoretinal degeneration: Redefining the Knobloch syndrome. Am J Med Genet 46:203–208, 1993.
61. Passos-Bueno MR, Marie SK, Monteiro M, et al: Knobloch syndrome in a large Brazilian consanguineous family: Confirmation of autosomal recessive inheritance. Am J Med Genet 52:170–173, 1994.
62. Sertie AL, Quimby M, Moreira ES, et al: A gene which causes severe ocular alterations and occipital encephalocele (Knobloch syndrome) is mapped to 21q22.3. Hum Mol Genet 5:843–847, 1996.
63. Miny P, Holzgreve W, Horst J: Genetic factors in lissencephaly syndromes: A review. Childs Nerv Syst 9:413–417, 1993.
64. Gallo AE Jr: Repair of giant occipital encephaloceles with microcephaly secondary to massive brain herniation. Childs Nerv Syst 8:229–230, 1992.
65. Posnick JC, Goldstein JA, Armstrong D, Rutka JT: Reconstruction of skull defects in children and adolescents by the use of fixed cranial bone grafts: Long-term results. Neurosurgery 32:785–791, 1993; discussion 791.
66. Patterson RJ, Egelhoff JC, Crone KR, Ball WS Jr: Atretic parietal cephaloceles revisited: An enlarging clinical and imaging spectrum? AJNR Am J Neuroradiol 19:791–795, 1998.
67. McLone DG, De Leon G: Atretic encephalocele. Pediatr Neurosurg 28:326, 1998.
68. French BN: Midline fusion defects and defects of formation. In Youmans JR (ed): Neurological Surgery, 3rd ed. Philadelphia, WB Saunders, 1990, pp 1081–1135.
69. Yeoh GPS, Bale PM, de Silva M: The so-called nasal glioma or sequestered encephalocele and its variants. Pediatr Pathol 9:531–549, 1989.
70. Tessier P: Anatomical classification of facial, cranio-facial, and latero-facial clefts. J Maxillofac Surg 4:69–92, 1976.
71. Hoffman HJ: Craniofacial anomalies. In Wilkins RH, Rengachary SS (eds): Neurosurgery, vol 3. New York, McGraw-Hill, 1985, pp 2192–2203.
72. Grubben C, Fryns JP, De Zegher F: Anterior basal encephalocele in the median cleft face syndrome. Genet Couns 1:103–109, 1990.
73. McLaurin RL: Cranium bifidum and cranial cephaloceles. In Vinken PJ, Bruyn GW (eds): Handbook of Clinical Neurology, vol 30. Amsterdam, Elsevier, 1977, pp 209–218.
74. Lewin MJ: Sphenoethmoidal cephalocele with cleft lip: Transpalatal versus transcranial repair. Report of two cases. J Neurosurg 58:924–931, 1983.
75. Lello GE, Sparrow OC, Gopal R: The surgical correction of fronto-ethmoidal meningoencephaloceles. J Craniomaxillofac Surg 17:293–298, 1989.
76. Shah AK, Desai AA, Sharma SN: Frontoethmoidal meningoencephalocystocele. Ann Plast Surg 22:523–527, 1989.
77. Mattox DE, Kennedy DW: Endoscopic management of cerebrospinal fluid leaks and cephaloceles. Laryngoscope 100:857–862, 1990.
78. Mulliken JB, Kaban LB, Evans CA: Facial skeletal changes following hypertelorbitism correction. Plast Reconstr Surg 77:7–16, 1986.

79. Griffith BH: Frontonasal tumors: Their diagnosis and management. Plast Reconstr Surg 57:692–699, 1976.

80. Robinson RG: Anterior encephalocele. Br J Surg 45:36–40, 1958.

81. Zinreich SJ, Borders JC, Eisele DW: The utility of magnetic resonance imaging in the diagnosis of intranasal meningoencephaloceles. Head Neck Surg 118:1253–1256, 1992.

82. Raffel C, McComb JG: Encephalocele. In Apuzzo ML (ed): Brain Surgery, vol 2. New York, Churchill Livingstone, 1993, pp 1433–1447.

83. Hockley AD, Goldin JH, Wake MJC: Management of anterior encephalocele. Childs Nerv Syst 6:444–446, 1990.

84. Ortiz-Monasterio F, Fuente-del-Campo A: Nasal correction in hypertelorbitism: The short and the long nose. Scand J Plast Reconstr Surg 15:277–286, 1981.

85. Jackson IT, Tanner NSB, Hide TA: Frontonasal encephalocele—long nose hypertelorism. Ann Plast Surg 11:490–500, 1983.

86. Sargent LA, Seyfer AE, Gunby EN: Nasal encephaloceles: Definitive one stage reconstruction. J Neurosurg 68:571–575, 1988.

87. Tessier P: Experience in the treatment of orbital hypertelorism. Plast Reconstr Surg 53:1–18, 1974.

88. Hoffman WY, McCarthy JG, Cutting CB: Computerized tomographic analysis of orbital hypertelorism repair: Spatial relationship of the globe and the bony orbit. Ann Plast Surg 25:124–131, 1990.

89. McCarthy JG, La Trenta GS, Breitbart AS: Hypertelorism correction in the young child. Plast Reconstr Surg 86:214–225, 1990.

90. Ortiz-Monasterio F, Medina O, Musolas A: Geometrical planning for the correction of orbital hypertelorism. Plast Reconst Surg 86:650–657, 1990.

91. Yaremchuk MJ, Whitaker LA, Grossman R: An objective assessment of treatment of orbital hypertelorism. Ann Plast Surg 30:27–34, 1993.

92. Converse JM, Ransohoff J, Mathews ES: Ocular hypertelorism and pseudohypertelorism: Advances in surgical treatment. Plast Reconstr Surg 45:1–13, 1970.

93. Dhawan IJ, Tandon PN: Excision repair and corrective surgery for fronto-ethmoidal meningocele. Childs Brain 9:126–136, 1982.

94. Rahman N-Y: Nasal encephalocele: Treatment by transcranial operation. J Neurol Sci 42:73–85, 1979.

95. Macfarlane R, Rutka JT, Armstrong D, et al: Encephaloceles of the anterior cranial fossa: Management and outcome. Pediatr Neurosurg 23:148–158, 1995.

96. Lorber J: The prognosis of occipital encephalocele. Dev Med Child Neurol 13:75–86, 1967.

97. Brown MS, Sheridan-Pereira M: Outlook for the child with a cephalocele. Pediatrics 90:914–919, 1992.

98. Pertschuk MJ, Whitaker LA: Psychosocial outcome of craniofacial surgery in children. In Marchac D (ed): Craniofacial Surgery. Berlin, Springer, 1987, pp 486–487.

99. Mahapatra AK, Tandon PN, Dhawan IK: Anterior encephaloceles: A report of 30 cases. Childs Nerv Syst 10:501–504, 1994.

Myelomeningocele and Myelocystocele

ALAN R. COHEN ■ SHENANDOAH ROBINSON

Myelomeningocele is just one manifestation of a malformation that affects the entire central nervous system (CNS) in 2500 to 6000 newborns per year in the United States.[1, 2] The initial management has a profound effect on the neonates' survival and the handicaps they will have to cope with throughout their lives. Children born with these complex malformations need skilled and compassionate physicians familiar with their unique problems. Myelocystoceles are uncommon, closely related lesions that pose less of a problem in the initial neonatal period, but affected children need lifelong neurosurgical care.

TERMINOLOGY

Numerous, often confusing terms have been coined to describe the various defects that occur with failure of normal *neurulation*, the developmental process that describes the formation and closure of the neural tube. The term *neural tube defect* (NTD) includes improper development of both the anterior neuropore (anencephaly) and the posterior neuropore (spina bifida). *Spinal dysraphism* refers to all forms of *spina bifida. Spina bifida aperta* is a midline spinal lesion that communicates with the external environment. *Spina bifida cystica* is a more specific type of spina bifida aperta that denotes a myelomeningocele or meningocele. *Spina bifida occulta*, or occult spinal dysraphism, refers to skin-covered spina bifida lesions that may lead to occult neurological deterioration.

In children with *myelomeningocele*, the spinal cord fails to fuse dorsally during primary neurulation, leaving a flat plate of neural tissue called the *neural placode* (Fig. 203–1). In children with *meningocele*, the spinal cord forms normally, but the dura fails to fuse dorsally, creating a cystic lesion that does not directly involve neural tissue. Distinguishing between these two lesions is important, because myelomeningoceles are almost invariably associated with the Chiari II malformation and its cranial manifestations (Fig. 203–2) and are often associated with hydrocephalus. By contrast, the Chiari II malformation and hydrocephalus are not associated with meningoceles. Myelomeningoceles may occur as tandem lesions, with skin-covered occult spina bifida

lesions occurring more rostrally. Split cord malformations have been found in 36% to 50% of patients with myelomeningoceles.[3] In a *hemimyelomeningocele*, one of the hemicords is the neural placode, and the other hemicord often lies below the placode and an oblique septum.

Some forms of occult spina bifida have terms that misleadingly suggest an association with myelomeningocele. In a *lipomyelomeningocele*, the conus fuses into a lipoma that tethers the cord. A *terminal myelocystocele* is a skin-covered midline mass with a distal, trumpet-like dilatation of the distal spinal cord central canal into a posterior defect with a meningocele and lipoma.

MYELOMENINGOCELE

Anatomic Considerations

A myelomeningocele results from a failure of primary neurulation during days 18 to 27 of human embryogenesis. The groove in the center of the placode is the remnant of the central canal. The spinal roots exit from the anterior surface of the placode, such that the ventral roots lie medially and the dorsal roots lie laterally. The dura fuses with the defect in the fascia laterally. Functional neural tissue may be present caudal to the placode or in the nerve roots exiting from the placode.

Most myelomeningoceles (85%) are located in the caudal thoracolumbar spine or more distally. Ten percent are in the thorax, and the rest are cervical. Cervical myelomeningoceles are often very similar to meningoceles, without the associated Chiari II malformation and hydrocephalus.[3]

Almost all patients with myelomeningocele also have the Chiari II hindbrain malformation, a constellation of abnormalities that affects the entire CNS (see Fig. 203–2). Associated brainstem defects include medullary kinking, tectal beaking, and intrinsic nuclei abnormalities.[4] Supratentorial abnormalities include partial or complete dysgenesis of the corpus callosum, polymicrogyria, large massa intermedia, and gray matter heterotopias. The mesodermal development is also affected, with a small posterior fossa, short clivus, low-lying tentorium and torcular Herophili, wide incisura, and enlarged foramen magnum. Lückenschädel, or

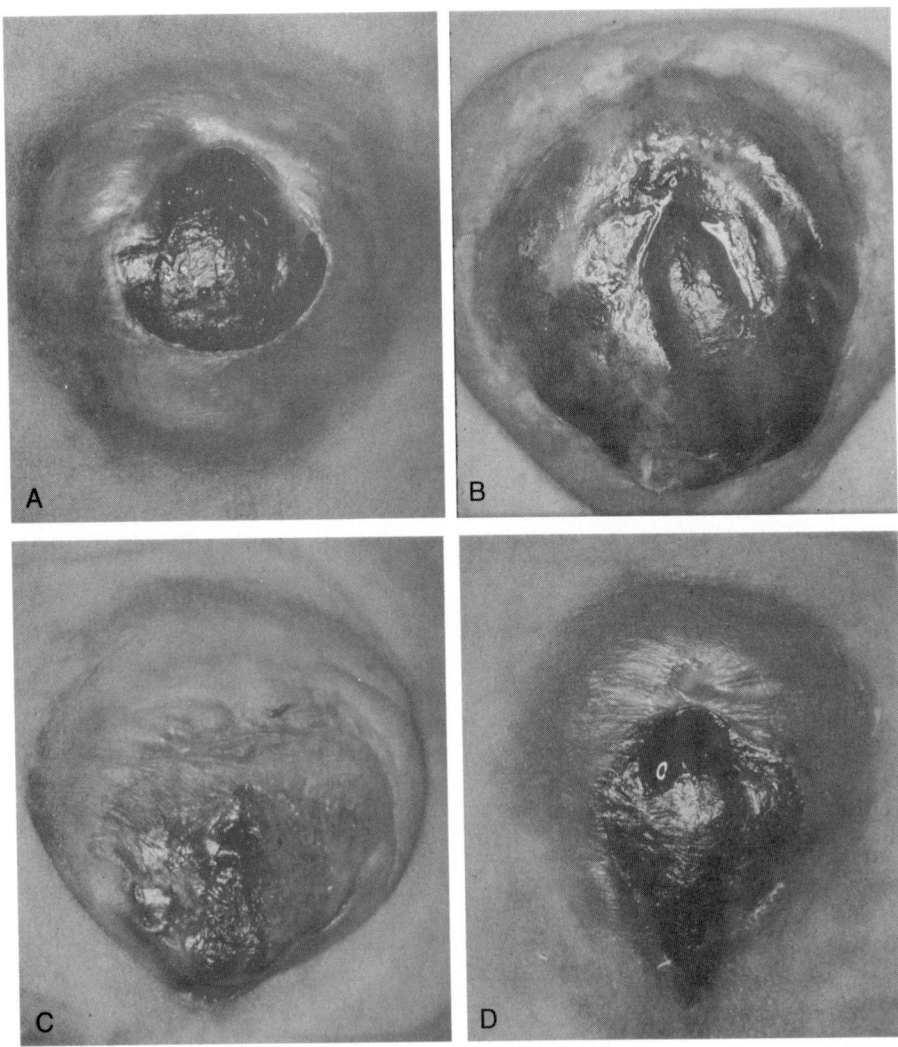

FIGURE 203–1. *A–D*, Examples of myelomeningoceles. In each photograph, rostral is superior.

craniolacunia, refers to the mesodermal skull abnormality of infants with myelodysplasia. These lesions are not due to increased intracranial pressure and usually resolve by 1 year of age.

The majority (80% to 90%) of patients with myelomeningocele have hydrocephalus that requires treatment. The hydrocephalus may result from both obstructive and communicating components. *Hydrosyringomyelia* occurs in 40% to 80% of patients with spina bifida and is usually nonprogressive.[5] In patients with spina bifida, neurological deterioration can result from symptomatic hydrocephalus or Chiari II malformation, hydrosyringomyelia, or retethering. Most often, the cause of neurological deterioration is hydrocephalus from a shunt malfunction.[5]

History

Spina bifida was described in ancient civilizations. Peter Van Forest first recorded a child with spina bifida in 1587,[6] and in 1610 he performed the first reported surgical resection of the myelomeningocele sac.[7] The first anatomic illustration was drawn by Tulp in 1641.[8] In 1761 Morgagni was the first to associate the clinical changes observed in spina bifida patients with the myelomeningocele.[9] The first theory to explain spina bifida was advanced by Lebedeff in 1881.[10] He attributed the myelomeningocele to failure of the neural tube to close. In 1886, von Recklinghausen described the types of spina bifida and reviewed the surgical treatment.[11] In Fraser's report of the first series of spina bifida patients treated with surgery, two thirds of the patients operated on between 1898 and 1923 survived until hospital discharge. Six years later, nearly one quarter (23%) of the patients were still alive.[12]

More aggressive surgical treatment for children with spina bifida was undertaken after the development of ventriculoperitoneal shunting for hydrocephalus in the 1950s. Because many patients developed delayed complications, some physicians suggested selective surgical treatment of neonates with spina bifida.[13, 14] The ethical debate about selective treatment ended in the early 1980s with reports demonstrating that patients in nonselected series did as well as or better than those in series with selection.[15] Now, unless there is an anomaly incompatible with life, almost all newborns with myelomeningocele are treated aggressively to optimize their quality of life.

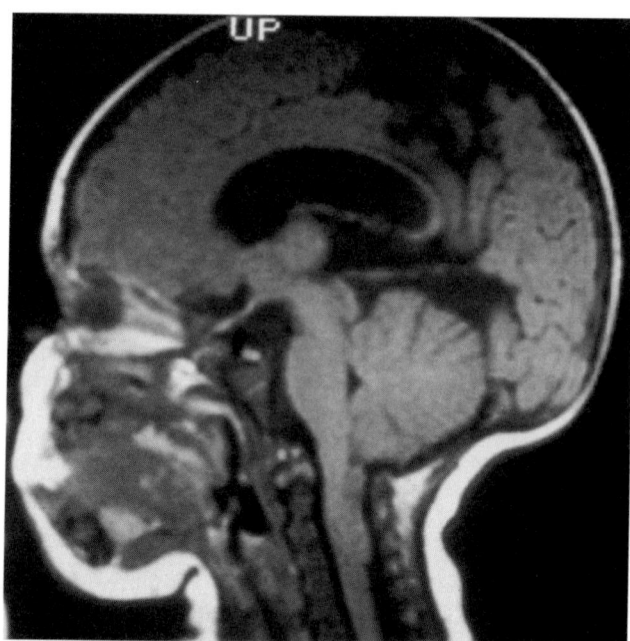

FIGURE 203–2. Midsagittal magnetic resonance imaging scan demonstrating a Chiari II malformation. Note the partial agenesis of the corpus callosum, occipital stenogyria, large massa intermedia, low-lying tentorium and torcular Herophili, extension of the elongated vermis to the C3 level, and elongated brainstem with medullary kinking.

Epidemiology

In the United States, the prevalence of myelomeningocele has declined owing to both prenatal folate supplementation and pregnancy termination. The prevalence began to decline before the widespread use of folate supplementation or the availability of prenatal diagnosis.[16] Before 1980, the prevalence of myelomeningocele in the United States was 1 to 2 per 1000 live births. More recently the prevalence has declined to 0.44 per 1000 live births.[16] Twenty percent to 30% of the decline can be attributed to pregnancy termination after prenatal diagnosis.[17–19] A slight (0.57% to 0.71%) female predominance exists.[20]

Geographic variation in the prevalence of spina bifida has been recognized for many years. The United Kingdom, particularly Ireland, has a higher prevalence of NTDs compared with continental Europe and the United States. The prevalence of spina bifida in the United Kingdom after 1980 was 0.74 to 2.5 per 1000 live births; the prevalence in the United States during the same period was 0.41 to 1.43 per 1000 live births.[21]

Racial and ethnic variation in the prevalence of spina bifida exists and persists after immigration. In the United States, the prevalence of NTDs is highest among Hispanics, followed by whites, then African Americans and Asians. The overall U.S. prevalence was 0.46 per 1000 live births, but Hispanics had a prevalence rate of 0.6 per 1000, and Asians 0.23 per 1000.[16] Internationally, the prevalence of spina bifida varies from a low among native Africans of 0.1 per 1000 live births to a high of 12.5 per 1000 among Celtics.[21] Pat-

terns of variation in the severity of the defect also exist among ethnic and racial groups.

Pathogenesis

Closure of the posterior neuropore occurs in human embryonic stage 12, at approximately 26 days of gestation. According to the most widely supported theory of spina bifida formation, the posterior neuropore fails to close completely during neurulation, and a myelomeningocele, Chiari II malformation, and hydrocephalus develop. The nonclosure theory has been substantiated by recent experimental evidence. Experimental studies using toxic agents and animal mutants provide insights into the pathogenesis of myelomeningocele. Toxic agents include cytochalasin, vinblastine, calcium-channel antagonists, phospholipase C, concanavalin A, retinoic acid, hydroxyurea, and mitomycin C. Folate and its pathophysiology have been the focus of the majority of recent investigations. Mutant mice, such as the splotch mouse with a homozygous mutation in the homeobox gene *Pax-3*, have been used to study the pathogenesis of NTDs.

A unified hypothesis to explain the sequential development of myelomeningocele and Chiari II hindbrain malformation has been proposed.[22] In normal development, during the period of rapid brain enlargement that occurs after closure of the posterior neuropore, the neurocele (primitive central canal) occludes transiently. If the posterior neuropore has failed to close, causing a myelomeningocele, the neurocele fails to occlude. Without appropriate neurocele occlusion, cerebrospinal fluid (CSF) flows out through the defect in the open posterior neuropore. With the lack of distention of the brain by CSF, formation of the cranium and its contents is disrupted. The posterior fossa is small, and both upward and downward herniation of the cerebellum occurs, resulting in the Chiari II malformation.[22] The unified hypothesis has been supported by experiments with chick embryos and with the homozygote splotch mouse.

Etiology

The cause of spina bifida is multifactorial. Because of the high prevalence of spina bifida among certain ethnic groups, a genetic predisposition has been suspected. The association with nutritional deficiencies, particularly folate and zinc, became evident in the mid-1980s.

FOLATE

The coenzyme folate is required for hematopoiesis, metabolism, and normal gastrointestinal and neurological function. The association between folate insufficiency and NTDs was suspected by Hibbard in 1964. A randomized, double-blind study in 1991 demonstrated that couples in the United States with a prior history of an infant with an NTD have a 2% to 3% chance of having a second child born with an NTD. If 4 mg of folic acid was consumed during the critical period (before and during pregnancy), the recurrence risk of having a second child born with spina bifida dropped 71%.[23] In 1991 the U.S. Public Health Service recommended that women with a prior pregnancy affected by an NTD ingest 4 mg/day of folic acid.[23] Currently, the recommendation is that women whose fetuses are at high risk for the development of NTDs consume 4 mg/day of folic acid from 1 month before pregnancy through the first trimester.[2] Women at high risk include those with an NTD or a partner with an NTD (2% to 3%), a close relative with an NTD (0.3% to 1%), diabetes mellitus type I (1%), and seizures treated with carbamazepine or valproic acid (1%).[2] Although obese women were not included in the recommendations, they also have a documented increased risk of having a child with an NTD and should have folate supplementation (Table 203–1).

Women who potentially could become pregnant should consume 0.4 mg/day of folic acid.[24] Many women remain unaware of the recommendations about folic acid ingestion during pregnancy (Table 203–2). Six years after the U.S. Public Health Service recommendations were released in 1992, a study found that only 30% of women aged 18 to 45 years were ingesting the recommended dose of folic acid.[25]

Folate can be consumed as natural compounds in food and as folic acid (pteroylmonoglutamic acid). Folic acid, a synthetic form of folate, has about twice the bioavailability compared with folate found in food.[26] The recommended daily allowances for folate are 0.4 mg for nonpregnant women, 0.6 mg for pregnant women, 0.5 mg for lactating women, and 4 mg/day for women at high risk for NTDs.[27] Smoking tobacco also decreases folate absorption significantly.[26] To safely achieve 4 mg/day, 1-mg folate tablets obtained by prescription are required. If several multivitamins are consumed to achieve 4 mg of folate per day, toxic levels

TABLE 203–2 ■ Recommendations for Daily Folate Supplementation

CIRCUMSTANCE	DOSE (MG)
Before Pregnancy	
Women with no known risk factor	0.4
Women at high risk	4
During Pregnancy	
Women with no known risk factor	0.6
Women at high risk	4
Post Partum while Breast-feeding	
Women with no known risk factor	0.5
Women at high risk	4

Adapted from Cohen AR, Robinson S: Myelomeningocele: Early management. In McLone DG (ed): Pediatric Neurosurgery, 4th ed. Philadelphia, WB Saunders, 2000, pp 241–259.

of other vitamins may be ingested, particularly vitamin A.[28] The erythrocyte folate level ranges from 160 to 640 ng/mL and provides a more accurate description of folate availability than does the serum folate level, which normally ranges from 6 to 20 ng/mL. A serum folate level less than 3 ng/mL, or an erythrocyte folate level less than 140 ng/mL, is the current definition of folate deficiency. A minimal serum level of 6.6 ng/mL may be more appropriate for pregnant women.[26]

Some insights into the potential abnormalities in folate metabolism that may predispose to the development of NTDs have been found in recent investigations. Mutations in the folate receptor alpha gene do not cause the majority of NTDs.[29] The rate-limiting step of folate metabolism in some women may be a low methionine synthase level. Excess folate through supplementation can compensate for this deficiency. Folate bioavailability is lowered by phenytoin, carbamazepine, primidone, phenobarbital, valproic acid, and other medications.[26] During pregnancy, women with seizures should try to minimize the use of multiple anticonvulsants, because these medications compound the reduction in the folate level. Oral contraceptives may also decrease the bioavailability of folate.[26] The risk of NTDs can be reduced only by 70% with adequate folate supplementation, suggesting that not all NTDs are related to abnormal folate metabolism.[28] The cause of the NTDs that are not prevented by folate supplementation is not known.

TABLE 203–1 ■ Risk Factors for Neural Tube Defects

RISK FACTORS	RISK (%)
Medical	
History of pregnancy with NTD	2–3
Partner with NTD	2–3
Diabetes mellitus type I	1
Seizure disorder (valproic acid or carbamazepine)	1
Close relative with NTD	0.3–1
Prepregnancy obesity (>110 kg)	0.2
Nonmedical	
Agricultural pesticides and chemicals	
Cleaning solvents and disinfectants	
Nursing	
Radiation	
Anesthetic agents	
Hot tubs, saunas, and fever (hyperthermia)	
Lead	
Tobacco smoke	

NTD, neural tube defect.
Adapted from Cohen AR, Robinson S: Myelomeningocele: Early management. In McLone DG (ed): Pediatric Neurosurgery, 4th ed. Philadelphia, WB Saunders, 2000, pp 241–259.

ANTICONVULSANTS

NTDs are associated with antiepileptic medications taken during pregnancy. The risk of having a child with spina bifida or anencephaly for a mother treated with carbamazepine or valproic acid is 1% or 1% to 2%, respectively.[26]

DIABETES MELLITUS

Type I diabetes mellitus places woman at a higher risk (1%) for a pregnancy complicated by spina bifida. This elevated risk appears to be independent from the increased risk of an NTD due to prepregnancy obesity.

OBESITY

Prepregnancy obesity is an independent risk factor for NTDs.[30, 31] Compared with nonobese women, the odds ratio of having a pregnancy complicated by an NTD was 1.9 for women with a body mass index greater than 29 kg/m² and 2.6 for women with a body mass index greater than 38 kg/m².[30]

Prenatal Diagnosis

DIAGNOSTIC STUDIES

Maternal Serum Alpha Fetoprotein

Maternal serum alpha fetoprotein (MSAFP) obtained in the early part of the second trimester is the initial screen for NTDs. In the amniotic fluid, the AFP concentration is 100-fold less than in the fetal CSF.[32] The optimal time for sampling MSAFP is at 16 to 18 weeks, although MSAFP levels can be determined between 14 and 21 weeks' gestation. Seventy-nine percent of open NTDs and 3% of normal singleton pregnancies have an MSAFP level 2.5 multiples of the median (MoM) at 16 to 18 weeks' gestation.[33] Based on the adjusted MoM MSAFP level for the patient's age and population, the MSAFP level at a specific gestational age provides a patient-specific risk of NTD. For example, an MSAFP level of 1.5 MoM predicts a risk of 1:2317 of an open NTD, and an MSAFP level of 2.5 MoM predicts a risk of 1:98. The estimated risk is adjusted based on the prevalence of NTDs in the population. The diagnostic accuracy of a single MSAFP level is limited to 60% to 70%. If the risk of spina bifida predicted by MSAFP is more than 1:500, further testing with high-resolution ultrasonography is recommended.

If the screening MSAFP level is elevated, the test can be repeated. A constant or decreasing MSAFP level is not consistent with a pregnancy with an NTD. In 40% of cases, the repeat level is normal.[34] Instead of repeating the test, high-resolution fetal ultrasonography can be performed. Ultrasonography can identify false-positive MSAFP levels due to incorrect estimated gestational age, multiple pregnancy, or fetal demise. If the initial and repeat MSAFP levels are elevated more than 3 MoM and the first fetal ultrasound study is normal, a second ultrasound study is recommended.

Ultrasonography

The sensitivity of high-resolution fetal ultrasonography is near 100% in prenatal screening for NTDs. An accurate prediction of the anatomic level of the spinal cord defect can be obtained in 64% of cases and is within one level of the defect in 79%.[35] High-resolution ultrasonography can also visualize two cranial abnormalities that are characteristic for hydrocephalus and the Chiari II malformation associated with spina bifida. The first, consisting of scalloping of the frontal bones on the biparietal view, is called the lemon sign.[36, 37] The

second, consisting of the abnormally shaped midbrain, elongated cerebellum, and obliteration of the cisterna magna characteristic of the Chiari II malformation, is referred to as the banana sign. The lemon sign was present in 80% of fetuses with myelomeningocele, and the banana sign was present in 93%.[36, 37]

The correlation among the findings of prenatal ultrasonography, level of spina bifida, degree of posterior fossa deformity, and degree of hydrocephalus has been examined.[38] No correlation was found between the ventricular diameter and the level of the spinal defect.[39] The posterior fossa deformity did not progress on serial ultrasound examinations.[38] If ultrasonography is nondiagnostic, amniocentesis may be indicated.

Amniocentesis

Amniocentesis is indicated if the MSAFP level and ultrasound study suggest the presence of an NTD. The amniotic acetylcholinesterase (AChE) level is used to increase the diagnostic accuracy of the amniotic AFP level because the latter can have a high false-positive rate in a population at low risk for NTDs.[40] If an NTD is present, neural AChE from the CSF leaks into the amniotic fluid. Other anomalies such as an omphalocele or Turner's syndrome can elevate the amniotic AChE level.[41] The amniotic fluid AFP and AChE levels had an accuracy of 99% and a false-positive rate of 0.34% in a large study of singleton pregnancies.[42]

DIFFERENTIAL DIAGNOSIS

At least 22 other fetal abnormalities besides myelomeningocele increase the MSAFP.[32] Abdominal abnormalities such as omphalocele, cloacal exstrophy, esophageal atresia, annular pancreas, duodenal atresia, and gastroschisis and urologic abnormalities such as congenital nephrosis, polycystic kidneys, urinary tract obstruction, and renal agenesis can also elevate the MSAFP.[33, 40] Elevated MSAFP and elevated amniotic fluid AFP and AChE can be caused by a sacrococcygeal cystic teratoma, but the teratoma can usually be distinguished from a myelomeningocele by fetal ultrasonography.

CHROMOSOMAL ABNORMALITIES

Trisomy 13 and 18 are associated with myelomeningoceles, but the fetuses rarely survive to term. Of the fetuses with NTDs diagnosed at or before the first half of the second trimester, 14% have trisomy 13 or 18 or another chromosomal error.[21]

Prenatal Counseling

PROGNOSIS

The present 2-year survival of neonates born with myelomeningocele is greater than 95%. Ten percent to 15% of children with spina bifida die before age 6 years, even with aggressive treatment.[1, 43] Hydrocephalus that requires treatment occurs in most (90% to 98%) of the patients.[1, 43]

The motor level determines the ambulatory status

of a patient. The motor level may or may not correspond to the anatomic level of the myelomeningocele. The prenatal anatomic level determined by ultrasonography accurately predicts the motor function level at the age of 3 to 4 years better than does the neonatal motor level from examination.[44] L3 function allows one to stand erect, and L4 and L5 function allows ambulation.[45] During the first decade, approximately 60% of children with spina bifida are community ambulators, without or with assistive devices; 26% are nonambulatory, and 15% are household ambulators.[46] The percentage of community ambulators decreases by about 17% during adolescence. As teenagers, many patients with spina bifida have to increase the level of assistance provided by devices. Normal urinary continence is present in only a small portion (6% to 17%) of these children.[47] Most (85%) are socially continent using a combination of clean intermittent catheterization and medications, and most (86%) have social fecal continence.[47]

The majority (75% to 80%) of children with spina bifida can have normal intelligence with aggressive management of hydrocephalus and infections. A correlation between a higher myelomeningocele level or severe ventricular enlargement on prenatal ultrasonography and lower intelligence has been found in some studies.[15, 48, 49] The intelligence quotient (IQ) remained normal if the CNS was not infected, but only about one third (31%) of the patients with a history of CNS infection had a normal IQ.[50] It remains controversial whether the number of shunt revisions affects IQ.[48, 51] Although complex learning disabilities are not unusual in children with spina bifida, more than half (58%) of children with spina bifida perform at their grade level.[47] Because of severe cognitive impairment, 10% to 15% require custodial care.[1] Only a small portion (<10%) of patients with spina bifida become economically independent. The majority (>80%) of patients with spina bifida need psychiatric care or counseling to help them cope with their disabilities.

A significantly better prognosis can be expected with cervical myelomeningoceles, which are often similar to meningoceles. The majority of patients with cervical myelomeningoceles have hydrocephalus and require a shunt.

SIBLING RISK

Parents of a child with a myelomeningocele may seek counseling about the chance of having another child with an NTD. The risk of a sibling having an NTD is estimated at 2.8% in the United States.[52] If the parents have had two previous pregnancies with NTDs, the risk increases to 4.8%.[53] If a parent has an NTD, the risk of his or her child having spina bifida is 3%.[54] Monozygotic twins have a low concordance rate.[55] Autosomal-dominant, autosomal-recessive, and X-linked inheritance patterns have been described.

FETAL MANAGEMENT OF SPINA BIFIDA AND HYDROCEPHALUS

A role for intrauterine surgery to minimize the neurological deficits of patients with myelomeningoceles has been suggested but remains highly controversial. According to some proponents of intrauterine myelomeningocele repair, a portion of the neurological deficit present in children with myelomeningoceles is acquired from persistent exposure of the dysplastic spinal cord to amniotic fluid.[56] In experimental animal models, intrauterine repair to cover the exposed spinal cord restored normal development.[57–60] Other experiments with rodents have shown that the dysplasia of the dorsal spinal cord results from the lack of normal afferent input from aberrant dorsal roots, rather than deterioration of normal tissue from exposure to amniotic fluid.[61]

Recent studies have not shown that intrauterine myelomeningocele repair improves the motor deficit, but it may minimize the degree of cerebellar herniation in the Chiari II malformation. In a nonrandomized observational study, patients who underwent intrauterine myelomeningocele repair were compared with patients who underwent standard neonatal repair.[62] The infants undergoing intrauterine repair were less likely to require a shunt for symptomatic hydrocephalus during the first 6 months than were the control infants (59% versus 90%), and they demonstrated less hindbrain herniation (38% versus 95%). The infants who underwent intrauterine repair were born significantly earlier than were the control infants (33 versus 37 weeks' gestation). The long-term effects on the cognitive development of these children have yet to be assessed. More progress and refinement of the procedure are needed before intrauterine repair of myelomeningocele can be routinely advocated, and randomized, prospective, controlled trials are needed to demonstrate that the benefits outweigh the risks.

Perinatal Management

LABOR AND DELIVERY

No difference in outcome between infants delivered vaginally or by cesarean section, with or without labor, was found in two retrospective studies.[63, 64] A prospective study found a difference in outcome depending on the type of delivery and the presence or absence of labor. The risk of neurological injury rose 2.2-fold if labor occurred.[65] The evidence from these and other studies is not conclusive, but it suggests that the exposed neural placode may suffer trauma during labor. The neurological outcome may be improved by performing an elective cesarean section after lung maturity but before the onset of labor. The exceptions are infants who are not expected to survive due to other fatal anomalies or chromosomal abnormalities.

PREOPERATIVE EVALUATION AND MANAGEMENT

A newborn with a myelomeningocele should receive treatment from an experienced multidisciplinary team. Delivery of the infant by cesarean section is scheduled with neonatologists and a neurosurgeon available, if possible. After delivery, the cardiac and respiratory status of the infant is stabilized. A sterile, saline-moistened gauze dressing can be used to cover the neural placode. The infant is positioned prone or on the side to avoid pressure on the neural placode. Latex precautions are used from birth.

General

The initial goal is to stabilize the neonate and prepare it for myelomeningocele repair. This includes maintaining normothermia and euvolemia and observing latex precautions. To minimize the risk of fecal contamination of the open neural placode, enteral feeding is avoided. Prophylactic antibiotics are recommended before repair to minimize the risk of meningitis. To diagnose any additional malformations that may delay the myelomeningocele repair or affect the infant's survival, an initial evaluation is performed. Less than 1% of infants have major anomalies of the cardiopulmonary, gastrointestinal, and genitourinary systems that might delay the myelomeningocele closure.

For parents who received a prenatal diagnosis of spina bifida and have had time to prepare themselves, the initial postnatal period may be manageable. Parents with no prior warning of the defect may be overwhelmed. Most parents grasp the need to proceed urgently with the myelomeningocele repair to prevent meningitis. It may be more difficult for parents to conceptualize the less obvious abnormalities such as hydrocephalus, Chiari II malformation, and urologic and orthopedic problems. The myelomeningocele repair and possible ventriculoperitoneal shunt placement should not be delayed solely to allow the family time to adjust to the defect. To encourage the parents to bond with the infant and to maximize their participation in the infant's care, an organized, empathetic, multidisciplinary team approach is important.

Neurosurgical

During the initial neurological examination, the spinal level of the defect and the severity of hydrocephalus, if present, are determined. Care in interpreting abnormal reflexes is important, because these reflexes may not reflect volitional function. For example, perineal stimulation may induce a contraction and spreading response that should not be mistaken for voluntary anal contraction. About two thirds of affected neonates show signs of myelopathy, including hyperreflexia and clonus, because they often have an incomplete functional spinal cord transection.[66] To determine the sensory level, a stimulus is applied to the lower extremities from distal to proximal until the infant grimaces. To determine the motor level, a stimulus is applied above the sensory level, and the distalmost voluntary motion is noted. With an L1-3 level, the infant has hip flexion with extended knees and clubfeet. Intact hip adduction, hip flexion, and knee extension with inverted feet are indicative of an L2-4 level. With an L5-S2 level, the infant has hip adduction, knee extension, and knee flexion with dorsiflexed feet. Infants with a sacral level may appear intact except for plantarflexion with rocker-bottom feet. A flaccid pelvic floor and pat-

ulous anus are often present. The future anal sphincter function is not accurately predicted by the presence of an anal wink or sphincter tone.[45] An underlying split cord malformation may cause a kyphoscoliosis or significant asymmetry between the lower extremities.[66] Other stigmata of occult spinal bifida such as hypertrichosis, hemangioma, or hyperpigmented areas may suggest the presence of a tandem lesion.

To determine the ventricular size, a cranial ultrasound study is obtained. Until the spinal defect is closed, relative microcephaly with small ventricles may be present. Computed tomography or magnetic resonance imaging is usually not necessary before myelomeningocele repair. If a severe kyphosis is present, plain radiographs of the spine are indicated.

Although neonates usually are not symptomatic from the Chiari II malformation, the patient should be observed for central or obstructive apnea, stridor, and opisthotonos. If the infant has stridor, inspection of the vocal cords by direct laryngoscopy is necessary to document their function.

Renal

To establish the importance of aggressive urologic management, the pediatric urology team is consulted early. Most children with spina bifida (90%) have a neurogenic bladder, and about one third have lower motoneuron dysfunction. A program of clean intermittent catheterization is initiated if the neonate fails to void regularly. If the infant voids, a postvoid residual volume is indicated to confirm adequate emptying of the bladder. All neonates with spina bifida should have renal ultrasonography to confirm the presence of a kidney and to identify any severe anomalies in the genitourinary system.

MYELOMENINGOCELE REPAIR

Timing

Myelomeningocele repair can be performed safely up to 72 hours after birth. This allows time for evaluation of the cardiopulmonary and genitourinary systems to be initiated and for cranial ultrasonography to be performed.[1] The morbidity after delayed repair is high. Ventriculitis occurs five times more frequently in infants that undergo delayed closure.[1] In patients with delayed repair, about 75% developed shunt infection, and the mortality was 13%.[67] Cultures from the neural placode should be obtained and shown to have no growth before the myelomeningocele repair if it is delayed beyond 72 hours after birth. If the cultures confirm infection, the neonate is treated with external ventricular drainage and appropriate antibiotics until the infection clears. Patients who undergo shunt placement before a delayed repair have a very high risk of shunt infection. Intellectual development is negatively affected by meningitis in the neonatal period.[50]

Preparation

Intraoperatively, precautions are taken to avoid hypothermia, hypovolemia, and hypoglycemia. A doughnut-shaped sponge can be used to protect the myelomeningocele while the infant is positioned supine for intubation.

Hydrocephalus

Immediate ventriculoperitoneal shunt placement is required in a small portion (15%) of patients with spina bifida and severe hydrocephalus. Ventriculoperitoneal shunt placement before myelomeningocele closure is recommended if the patient has evidence of hydrocephalus at birth, to minimize the pressure on the myelomeningocele dural closure. A standard ventriculoperitoneal shunt insertion is performed with the patient supine and the myelomeningocele protected in a doughnut-shaped sponge support. During the same anesthesia, the patient is repositioned prone for the myelomeningocele repair. The risk of shunt infection with simultaneous shunt placement rises significantly if the myelomeningocele repair is delayed. A significant difference in the shunt infection rate between a single-stage repair and shunt insertion (5/17, 29%) and a two-stage repair and shunt insertion (3/14, 21%) was not found in a retrospective study.[67]

Positioning

The patient is positioned prone for the myelomeningocele repair. The entire back and flanks are prepared and draped to facilitate an extensive closure if it is needed. Contact of povidone-iodine solution with the neural placode should be minimized.

Operative Technique

The purpose of myelomeningocele repair is to protect the functional tissue in the neural placode, prevent loss of CSF, and minimize the risk of meningitis by reconstructing the neural tube and its coverings (Fig. 203–3). The margin between the arachnoid of the neural placode and the dystrophic epidermis, the junctional zone, is the site of the initial incision. The goal is to free the neural placode from the surrounding junctional zone circumferentially. An effort is made to preserve all neural tissue. If indicated, any tandem spina bifida lesions such as dermoid, lipoma, neuroenteric cyst, myelomeningocele manqué (dorsal roots exiting from the cord or neural placode and aberrantly entering the dura), or split notochord syndrome (with loops of bowel present in the spine) are addressed. To minimize the risk of a dermoid or lipoma developing later, any residual epidermal or dermal elements are resected from the neural placode periphery.[1] Using a 7–0 monofilament suture, the pia is closed to re-form the neural placode into a tube. The dura requires mobilization before closure of the pia in some cases. Pial closure lowers the incidence of retethering. At the rostral end of the defect, just below the last intact lamina, the normal intact dura is identified. The dura is dissected free from the surrounding tissue by developing a plane in the epidural space from rostral to caudal bilaterally. To reconstruct the thecal sac, the dura is closed in the midline with nonabsorbable 5–0 suture.

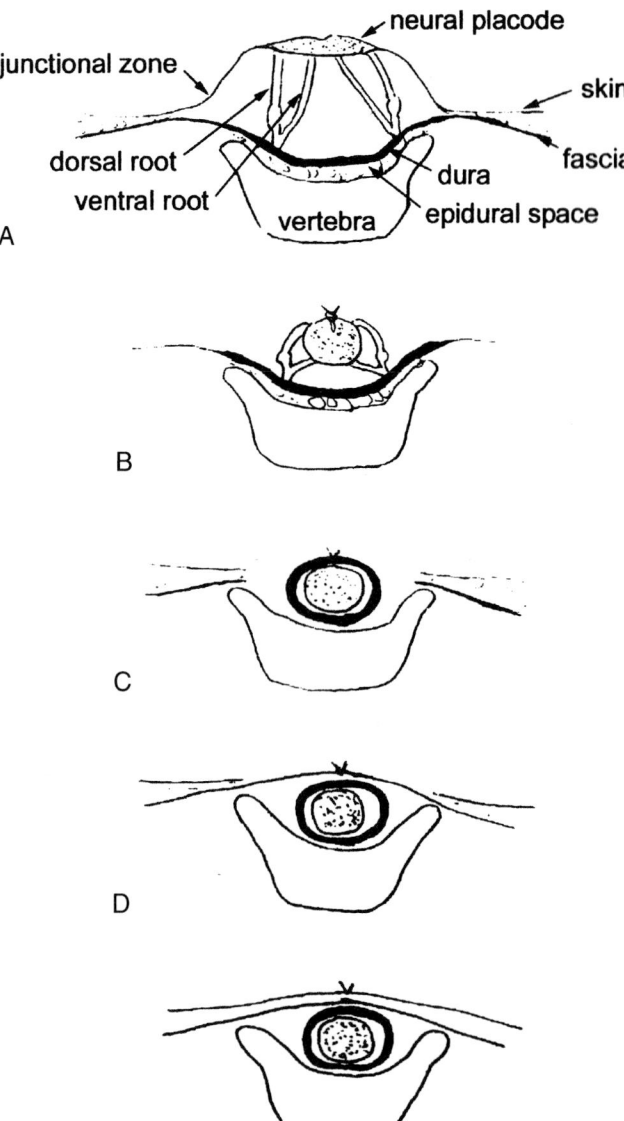

FIGURE 203–3. Drawing depicting the conceptual steps in surgical repair of myelomeningocele. *A,* Axial cross section of the myelomeningocele. Note that the placode mimics an open book, with the ventral roots lying medially and the dorsal roots lying laterally. *B,* Reconstruction of the neural tube. The placode is dissected from the surrounding tissue by incising the junctional zone. All dermal remnants are resected, and the neural tube is reconstituted by closing the pia with a 7–0 monofilament suture. *C,* Reconstruction of the thecal sac. The dura is dissected free from its junction with the fascia and skin. The goal is a watertight closure without causing constriction of the closed neural placode. *D,* Midline fascial closure. Relaxing incisions may be necessary to mobilize an adequate amount of fascia. *E,* Midline skin closure. (From Cohen AR, Robinson S: Myelomeningocele: Early management. In McLone DG [ed]: Pediatric Neurosurgery, 4th ed. Philadelphia, WB Saunders, 2000, pp 241–259.)

Neural placode ischemia should be prevented as the dura is closed. Duraplasty with thoracolumbar fascia or bovine pericardium is performed, if necessary, to optimize the closure and prevent CSF leak. The thoracolumbar fascia is reapproximated in the midline. To obtain a closure without tension, releasing incisions in the fascia laterally away from the defect may be necessary. Absorbable sutures are used to close the subcutaneous tissue in the midline. The skin is closed with nonabsorbable sutures that are left in place for about 2 weeks.

Large Defects

The closure of large spina bifida defects is controversial. Wheelchair- or crutch-dependent patients depend on the muscles of the upper torso for locomotion, and disruption of the musculature may contribute to the progression of scoliosis and kyphosis. Several types of cutaneous and musculocutaneous flaps have been suggested, reflecting the limited success of any specific procedure. A vertical midline closure that facilitates detethering is an important goal.

Kyphosis

Patients with thoracic spina bifida are prone to develop kyphosis. About 15% of spina bifida patients have a kyphosis at birth. If possible, spinal reconstruction for the kyphosis is delayed until the infant is older. Occasionally, kyphectomy is necessary to successfully complete the myelomeningocele repair.[68] After kyphectomy, the child requires an orthosis from 3 months to 2 years of age.[69]

POSTOPERATIVE MANAGEMENT

To minimize infection, perioperative antibiotics are usually given for 1 day. The infant is positioned with the lumbar area above the level of the head to minimize CSF leakage for 3 days. The child may be held in the reverse Trendelenburg position for short periods to allow oral feedings. The infant may be positioned supine, prone, or on the side after the repair. A plastic barrier drape is placed between the myelomeningocele wound and the anus to minimize wound soilage. The infant is closely monitored for central apnea and other signs of brainstem dysfunction that may be indicative of a symptomatic Chiari II malformation. Supplemental nutrition should be administered to the infant if necessary. The infant is transferred to a regular patient floor as soon as it is medically possibly. There, the parents have a better bonding experience and can learn clean intermittent catheterization, a bowel regimen, and a physical therapy program.

Complications

EARLY COMPLICATIONS OF MYELOMENINGOCELE REPAIR

The most common complication after myelomeningocele repair is superficial wound dehiscence.[69] Particularly if the infant does not yet have a shunt, daily examination of the head circumference, fontanelle fullness, and back wound for CSF leakage should be performed. An external ventricular drain should be placed until CSF cultures show no growth if the repair has already developed a leak before shunt placement.[69] Superficial wound infections usually occur about 1

week after the myelomeningocele is closed. The infant often has systemic symptoms such as mild fever, ileus, and mild leukocytosis. Dressing changes and intravenous antibiotics are the recommended treatment.

More serious infections with meningitis and sepsis pose a significant threat to the neonate. Owing to frequent fecal contamination of the myelomeningocele defect and an immature immune system, neonates have an elevated risk of enteric bacterial infection. Neonatal sepsis usually progresses over a day and is signaled by poor feeding, lethargy, livedo reticularis (ashen and blotchy skin), hypothermia, and leukopenia (<4000 cells/mm^3) with a left shift. A higher incidence of necrotizing enterocolitis occurs in full-term infants with spina bifida than in full-term infants without spina bifida. In neonates with a thoracic cord level from spina bifida, the diagnosis may be more difficult to recognize because the infants may lack typical abdominal findings. A subdural abscess may also form at the repair site and be visualized on magnetic resonance imaging. CSF must be obtained for culture from a shunt tap or a percutaneous ventricular tap. Broad-spectrum intravenous antibiotics with effective CNS penetration should be given. If the shunt is infected, temporary conversion to an externalized drain is necessary.

HYDROCEPHALUS

Most neonates with spina bifida develop symptomatic hydrocephalus within the first 6 weeks of life. Signs of increased intracranial pressure, including an increase in head circumference, full fontanelle, split sutures, and bulging myelomeningocele repair, should be sought daily. Increased intracranial pressure from hydrocephalus in spina bifida patients can also cause brainstem signs suggestive of a symptomatic Chiari II malformation. A shunt is indicated at the first sign of increased intracranial pressure to minimize the strain on the myelomeningocele repair.

Children with spina bifida often develop shunt malfunction. At least one shunt revision is required in the first year in almost half the shunted patients with spina bifida.[70] More shunt complications occurred in children with higher spinal lesions and more severe hydrocephalus. An alternative to CSF diversion with a shunt in some spina bifida patients is endoscopic third ventriculostomy.[71] Endoscopic third ventriculostomy is generally not recommended for infants with spina bifida because the outcome is poor, but it can be considered as an alternative to a shunt revision if a child with spina bifida presents with a shunt malfunction later in life. Among children with spina bifida who present with shunt malfunction and appropriate ventricular anatomy, endoscopic third ventriculostomy is successful in the majority of patients.[71]

CHIARI II MALFORMATION

Although a symptomatic Chiari II malformation rarely occurs in infants, it is associated with a relatively high (34% to 38%) mortality.[72] The degree of caudal herniation of the cerebellum does not correlate well with the severity of the symptoms and signs of brainstem dysfunction.[69] Intermittent obstructive or central apnea, cyanosis, bradycardia, dysphagia, nystagmus, stridor, vocal cord paralysis, torticollis, opisthotonos, hypotonia, upper extremity weakness, and spasticity are signs of a symptomatic Chiari II malformation. Twenty-three percent of children with spina bifida were symptomatic from the Chiari II malformation at some point, but only 17% required hindbrain decompression.[43] The average age at decompression was 14 months.

The presentation of a symptomatic Chiari II malformation may vary, depending on the child's age. Within the first 3 months of life, less than 20% of patients with spina bifida develop a symptomatic Chiari II malformation.[69, 73] Infants with a symptomatic Chiari II malformation can present with swallowing difficulties (69%), apnea (58%), stridor (56%), aspiration (40%), arm weakness (27%), and opisthotonos (18%).[72] With a rapid diagnosis and decompression, the majority (69%) of infants become asymptomatic within 2 days.[73]

Hindbrain decompression should be performed early for a symptomatic Chiari II malformation to achieve the best outcome.[73] Because the symptoms can be due to increased intracranial pressure, proper function of the shunt should be confirmed. If there is no shunt, an external ventriculostomy or shunt should be placed. If, after 48 hours, the symptoms are not relieved by lowering the intracranial pressure, hindbrain decompression should be performed.[69] Urgent hindbrain decompression is indicated if a child has a functioning shunt and life-threatening symptoms. A poor prognosis is associated with preoperative bilateral vocal cord paralysis, severe neurogenic dysphagia, and prolonged apnea.

For planning the extent of the hindbrain decompression, magnetic resonance imaging of the craniovertebral junction and cervical spine is helpful. Narrow cervical laminectomies are performed at the levels that overlie the cerebellar peg to minimize the development of cervical kyphosis. The torcular Herophili often lies quite low near the foramen magnum as part of the Chiari II malformation. Because of the risk of hemorrhage associated with a complete dural opening in infants with a Chiari II malformation, some surgeons have advocated only lysis of the compressive dural band and no duraplasty. Intraoperative ultrasonography is used to confirm the caudal extent of the cerebellum and adequate decompression of the brainstem.

ORTHOPEDICS

Involvement of the pediatric orthopedic team begins in the neonatal period to assess the need for initiating therapy and establish a relationship with the family. Treatment for hip dislocation or clubfeet may be initiated before the infant's discharge.

LATEX ALLERGY

Many spina bifida patients develop an allergy to latex, which can have life-threatening consequences if they experience a severe anaphylactic reaction. A 3.4% mortality has been reported with severe intraoperative complications from a type I hypersensitivity response (anaphylaxis) to latex.[74] Latex antibodies can be detected in the serum in up to half (36% to 51%) of spina bifida patients.[75, 76] A correlation has been found between the number of surgeries a patient has experienced and the incidence of latex allergy.[75] In particular, a higher incidence of latex allergy was found among patients who had undergone more ventriculoperitoneal shunt revisions. More than one third (36%) of patients with a ventriculoperitoneal shunt were sensitized to latex in one study.[75]

Latex precautions are recommended for all patients with spina bifida. The first allergic reaction can be anaphylaxis. The incidence of latex reactions can be lowered to almost zero (0% to 0.3%) with appropriate precautions.[77] Food allergies are also common among patients with latex allergy. Foods that can induce an allergic reaction, presumably by cross-reaction with the latex antibodies, include avocados, bananas, celery, chestnuts, kiwi, papaya, peaches, pears, and tomatoes.

Spina Bifida Clinic

Children with spina bifida have complex medical problems that can best be addressed by the coordination of services provided by a well-organized, experienced, multidisciplinary spina bifida clinic. The spina bifida clinic helps ensure that these children receive routine follow-up in multiple disciplines, as well as screening for potential problems.

Children with spina bifida are born with a neurological deficit that should remain fixed after the neonatal period. If there is progression of neurological, orthopedic, or urologic deficits, an evaluation of possible causes is recommended. For example, a tethered cord may present with subtle changes, such as an increase in the frequency of urinary tract infections or progression of a foot deformity. In some infants, urologic deficits do not manifest initially. In one study, half of children with myelomeningocele and normal bladder function near birth had developed abnormal function at 4 months.[78] Continual urologic follow-up is recommended for almost all patients with spina bifida, even those with no perceptible neurological deficit in the lower extremities. Abnormal urination occurs in the vast majority (>90%) of patients with normal neurological function.[79]

In addition to addressing neurological, orthopedic, and urologic problems, a spina bifida clinic can screen for other problems, such as pulmonary and sleep disorders, endocrine abnormalities, and neuropsychological issues. The importance of latex precautions can be reinforced. Learning disabilities, behavioral problems, and excessive weight gain can be addressed promptly to maximize the child's cognitive, psychological, and social development.

MYELOCYSTOCELE

Terminal myelocystoceles are skin-covered midline masses that occur in the lumbosacral area and are

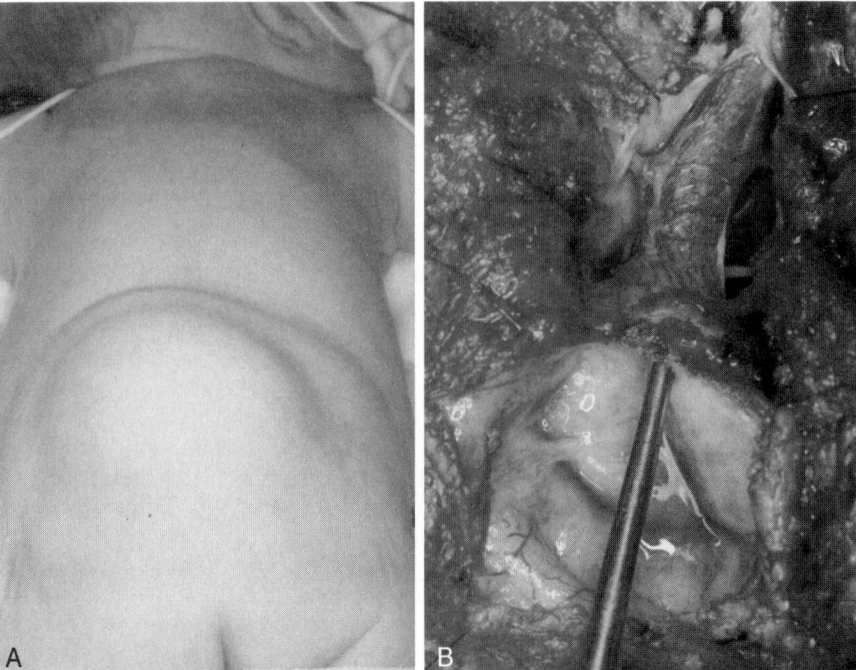

FIGURE 203–4. Myelocystocele. *A*, Skin-covered lumbar mass. *B*, Intraoperative dissection with probe entering from the terminal myelocystocele into the hydromyelic central canal.

distinct from myelomeningoceles (Fig. 203–4). Myelocystoceles account for 5% of skin-covered masses and most likely represent one end of a spectrum of lesions, with lipomyelomeningoceles at the other end. Alternative terms for myelocystocele are *syringocele, syringomyelocele,* and *lipomeningomyelocystocele.* The terminal myelocystocele is composed of a low-lying conus medullaris with cystic dilatation of the caudal central canal, a surrounding meningocele, and a lipoma that extends from the conus to a subcutaneous fat collection. The terminal cyst is lined with ependyma and dysplastic glia and does not communicate with the subarachnoid space. The meningocele communicates with the subarachnoid space and may lie dorsal or ventral to or circumferentially around the terminal cyst. The overlying skin may have a cutaneous signature typical of occult spina bifida, such as hemangioma, nevus, and hypertrichosis.

Myelocystoceles are often associated with hydromyelia and cloacal exstrophy. Cloacal exstrophy, also called *vesicointestinal fissure,* is a severe malformation of the abdomen and pelvis with an omphalocele, bladder exstrophy, ambiguous genitalia, imperforate anus, and pelvic abnormalities. When all these abnormalities are present, the defect is called the *OEIS complex* (for *o*mphalocele, bladder *e*xstrophy, *i*mperforate anus, and *s*pinal defect). Almost two thirds (62%) of patients with cloacal exstrophy have myelodysplasia.[80]

Anatomic Considerations

The myelocystocele is due to a defect in secondary neurulation. The caudal neural tube forms via canalization and regression, beginning at day 48. Normally, atrophy of the caudal neural tube forms the filum terminale (terminal thread) that joins the conus to the coccygeal medullary vestige. If an insult disrupts retrogressive differentiation, regression fails to occur, and an abnormally low conus results.

Myelocystoceles are not associated with hydrocephalus or the Chiari II malformation, and children with myelocystoceles can be expected to have normal intelligence. Infants may be neurologically normal, or they may have deficits in the lower extremities and associated orthopedic abnormalities.

History

Although cloacal exstrophy and an associated myelocystocele was first described in 1709 by Littre, the first successful closure was not reported until the 1960s by Rickham.[81] One of four patients survived. A literature review in 1976 showed that the survival rate remained at 22%. With recent advances in surgical technique, most children survive, and a few even have urinary continence.[80]

Epidemiology

Myelocystoceles are extremely rare lesions. Cloacal exstrophy occurs sporadically, with an incidence of 1 in 200,000 to 400,000 live births.[80] The change in prevalence that occurred with myelomeningoceles has not been noted with myelocystoceles, most likely reflecting the different causes of these lesions. No sibling risk has been identified,[82] although one case of two siblings with OEIS complex has been reported.[83]

Pathogenesis

Myelocystoceles are often associated with cloacal exstrophy. During embryogenesis, the cloaca is an endoderm-lined chamber that receives the hindgut (colon anlage) and allantois (bladder anlage). The cloacal membrane, a bilaminar veil of ectoderm and endoderm, divides the cloaca. Cloacal exstrophy occurs from rupture of the cloacal membrane and failure of the lateral abdominal wall to close. According to one theory, herniation of the lower abdomen and pelvis disturbs the notochord secretion of inductive factors that regulate development of the neural tube and retrogressive differentiation.[84] An alternative theory suggests that the CSF is unable to exit from the early neural tube as it should, and it distends the distal terminal ventricle after canalization. The terminal ventricle distends the surrounding dorsal membrane and arachnoid, causing the surrounding meningocele.[85] Neither of these theories has been tested experimentally. Teratogens that cause spina bifida aperta in hamsters, such as retinoic acid, also cause lesions resembling myelocystoceles. Most likely the pathogenesis reflects both mechanical disruption of normal development and a lack of appropriate induction of differentiation factors.

Etiology

In contrast to the strong association between folate and myelomeningoceles, no such association with myelocystoceles is known. This may reflect the rarity of these lesions. Loperamide hydrochloride, diphenylhydantoin, and retinoic acid have been associated with myelocystoceles. The influenza vaccine has been associated with OEIS complex. No genetic association has been identified.[82]

Prenatal Diagnosis

The AFP level is usually not elevated with myelocystocele because it is a skin-covered lesion. If there is a concurrent omphalocele, the AFP is frequently elevated. A myelocystocele can be diagnosed with high-resolution fetal ultrasonography. The primary lesion in the differential diagnosis is sacrococcygeal teratoma, which has polyhydramnios and intact vertebrae. By contrast, with a myelocystocele associated with OEIS complex, other abnormalities are often visualized, including hemivertebrae, sacral agenesis, small pelvic cavity, flared iliac bone, and no bladder.[82] Prenatal diagnosis allows the family to prepare, if necessary, for a scheduled cesarean section and for the multiple issues that must be addressed if cloacal exstrophy is present.

Perinatal Management

If the infant has an omphalocele or a large myelocystocele, it may lessen the trauma to the neural tissue if the fetus does not experience labor. No studies have been performed comparing vaginal and cesarean delivery, as has been done for myelomeningoceles. The infant often requires other surgeries to correct more life-threatening problems. Latex precautions are recommended for patients with cloacal exstrophy and myelocystocele because of the multiple operations they undergo. Once the infant is medically stable, magnetic resonance imaging scans of the brain and spine should be obtained to clarify the anatomy of the abnormalities.

Operative Repair

In contrast to the priority that myelomeningocele repair receives at birth, myelocystoceles are addressed after cloacal exstrophy is repaired, if it is present. Myelocystocele repair can be performed after the infant recovers from any other perinatal surgeries, has adequate nutrition, and is free of infection. Ideally, the repair is performed within the first 6 months to minimize neurological losses from spinal cord tethering. With smaller lesions, the subcutaneous lipoma and underlying spinal cord abnormality may not be recognized until several months after birth.

The same general principles are used for myelocystocele repair as for the repair of other myelodysplasias. The patient is positioned prone, and electrodes for electromyography should be placed if intraoperative monitoring is desired. Through a midline incision, the most caudal intact lamina is identified and removed to localize the normal thecal sac. Debulking of the subcutaneous lipoma is reserved until after the neural elements have been identified. Typically, a fibrous band that is adherent to the thecal sac is present just caudal to the last intact neural arch, at the level of the most rostral bifid lamina. After the fibrous band is divided, the dura is opened in the midline to open the meningocele and expose the conus and nerve roots. The conus blends into a lipoma that disrupts the dorsal dura and is contiguous with the subcutaneous lipoma. The terminal cyst in the distal conus is identified and drained, exposing the connection between the lumen of the cyst and the dilated distal central canal. Using microdissection, the neural elements are separated from the lipoma. The pial edges of the terminal cyst are reapproximated to reconstruct the conus, with elimination of any lipoma remnants that may predispose the patient to retethering. The dura is closed in a watertight manner. The remainder of the subcutaneous lipoma is debulked, and the wound is closed in layers, keeping in mind that the primary goal of the surgery is detethering and not cosmesis.

Outcome

A child with a repaired terminal myelocystocele must be followed throughout life for symptoms and signs of retethering. The infant may have a fixed deficit after the repair or a moderate improvement. When the child has stabilized after the surgery, a progressive neurological deficit or orthotic deformity should prompt an evaluation for retethering.

REFERENCES

1. McLone D: Care of the neonate with a myelomeningocele. Neurosurg Clin N Am 9:111–120, 1998.
2. American Academy of Pediatrics Committee on Genetics: Folic acid for the prevention of neural tube defects. Pediatrics 104: 325–327, 1999.

3. Dias M, Walker M: The embryogenesis of complex dysraphic malformations: A disorder of gastrulation. Pediatr Neurosurg 18: 229–253, 1992.

4. Gilbert J, Jones K, Rorke L, et al: Central nervous system anomalies associated with meningomyelocele, hydrocephalus, and the Arnold-Chiari malformation: Reappraisal of theories regarding the pathogenesis of posterior neural tube closure defects. Neurosurgery 18:559–564, 1986.

5. LaMarca F, Hermen M, Grant SA, McLone DG: Presentation and management of hydromyelia in children with Chiari type-II malformation. Pediatr Neurosurg 26:57–67, 1997.

6. Forestus P: De capitis et cerebre morbis ac symptomatis. Observationum Medicinalium, libri III. Leiden, Ex Off Plantiniana, 1587.

7. Forestus P: Observation chir, libri V, lib III, obs VII1610.

8. Tulpius N: Cum atieis figuris. Observationum Medicinalium, libra III, vol cap XXIX, XXX. Amsterdam, Apud Ludovican Elzevirium, 1641.

9. Morgagni J-B: De sedubis et causis morborum per anatomen indigatis, libri V. Venice, Ex Typographia Remondiona, 1761.

10. Lebedeff A: Uber che Enstehurg der Anencephalie und Spina Bifida dei Vogelin und Menschen. Virchows Arch Pathol Anat Physiol 86:263, 1881.

11. Von Recklinghausen F: Untersuchungen ubev che Spina Bifida. Arch Pathol Anat 105:243, 1886.

12. Fraser J: Spina bifida. Edinb Med J 36:284, 1929.

13. Lorber J: Results of treatment of myelomeningocele: An analysis of 524 unselected cases with special references to possible selection of treatment. Dev Med Child Neurol 13:279–303, 1971.

14. Lorber J, Salfield S: Results of selective treatment of spina bifida cystica. Arch Dis Child 56:822–830, 1981.

15. McLone D: Results of treatment of children born with a myelomeningocele. Clin Neurosurg 30:407–412, 1983.

16. Lary J, Edmonds L: Prevalence of spina bifida at birth—United States, 1983–1990: A comparison of two surveillance systems. MMWR Morb Mortal Wkly Rep 45:15–26, 1996.

17. Cragan J, Roberts H, Edmonds L, et al: Surveillance for anencephaly and spina bifida and the impact of prenatal diagnosis—United States, 1985–1994. MMWR Morb Mortal Wkly Rep 44(SS-4):1–13, 1995.

18. Roberts H, Moore C, Cragan J, et al: Impact of prenatal diagnosis on the birth prevalence of neural tube defects, Atlanta, 1990–1991. Pediatrics 96:880–883, 1995.

19. VanDorsten J, Hulsey T, Newman R, et al: Fetal anomaly detection by second-trimester ultrasonography in a tertiary center. Am J Obstet Gynecol 178:742–749, 1998.

20. Greene W, Terry R, DeMasi R, et al: Effect of race and gender on neurological level in myelomeningocele. Dev Med Child Neurol 33:110, 1991.

21. Shurtleff D, Lemire R: Epidemiology, etiologic factors, and prenatal diagnosis of open spinal dysraphism. Neurosurg Clin N Am 6:183–193, 1995.

22. McLone D: The cause of Chiari II malformation: A unified theory. Pediatr Neurosci 15:1–12, 1989.

23. Prevention CfDCa: Use of folic acid for prevention of spina bifida and other neural tube defects. MMWR Morb Mortal Wkly Rep 40:513–516, 1991.

24. Prevention CfDCa: Recommendations for the use of folic acid to reduce the number of cases of spina bifida and other neural tube defects. MMWR Morb Mortal Wkly Rep 41:1–8, 1992.

25. Prevention CfDCa: Knowledge and use of folic acid by women of childbearing age—United States 1995 and 1998. MMWR Morb Mortal Wkly Rep 48:325–327, 1999.

26. Lewis D, Van Dyke D, Stumbo P, et al: Drug and environmental factors associated with adverse pregnancy outcomes. Part I. Antiepileptic drugs, contraceptives, smoking, and folate. Ann Pharmacother 32:802–817, 1998.

27. Institute of Medicine, Committee on the Scientific Evaluation of Dietary Reference Intakes, Food and Nutrition Board: Dietary Reference Intakes for Thiamin, Riboflavin, Niacin, Vitamin B$_6$, Folate, Vitamin B$_{12}$, Pantothenic Acid, Biotin, and Choline. Washington, DC, National Academy Press, 1998.

28. Lewis D, Van Dyke D, Stumbo P, et al: Drug and environmental factors associated with adverse pregnancy outcomes. Part III. Folic acid: Pharmacology, therapeutic recommendations, and economics. Ann Pharmacother 32:1087–1095, 1998.

29. Barber R, Shaw G, Lammer E, et al: Lack of association between mutations in the folate receptor-alpha gene and spina bifida. Am J Med Genet 76:310–317, 1998.

30. Shaw G, Velie E, Schaffer S: Risk of neural tube defect—affected pregnancies among obese women. JAMA 275:1093–1096, 1996.

31. Werler M, Louik C, Shapiro S, et al: Prepregnant weight in relation to risk of neural tube defects. JAMA 275:1089–1092, 1996.

32. Main D, Mennuti M: Neural tube defects: Issues in prenatal diagnosis and counseling. Obstet Gynecol 67:1–16, 1986.

33. Wald N, Cuckle H, Brock J, et al: Maternal serum-alpha-fetoprotein measurement in antenatal screening for anencephaly and spina bifida in early pregnancy: Report of UK collaborative study on alpha-fetoprotein in relation to neural-tube defects. Lancet 1: 1323–1332, 1977.

34. Park T: Myelomeningocele. In Albright L, Pollack I, Adelson D (eds): Principles and Practice of Pediatric Neurosurgery. New York, Thieme Medical, 1999, pp 291–320.

35. Kollias S, Goldstein R, Cogen P, et al: Prenatally detected myelomeningoceles: Sonographic accuracy in estimation of the spinal level. Radiology 185:109–112, 1992.

36. Nicolaides K, Campbell S, Gabbe S, et al: Ultrasound screening for spina bifida: Cranial and cerebellar signs. Lancet 2:72–74, 1986.

37. Nyberg D, Mack L, Hirsch J, et al: Abnormalities of fetal contour in sonographic detection of spina bifida: Evaluation of the "lemon sign." Radiology 167:387–392, 1988.

38. Babook C, Goldstein R, Barth R, et al: Prevalence of ventriculomegaly in association with myelomeningocele: Correlation with gestational age and severity of posterior fossa deformity. Radiology 190:703–707, 1994.

39. Babook C, Drake C, Goldstein R: Spinal level of fetal myelomeningocele: Does it influence ventricular size. AJR Am J Roentgenol 169:207–210, 1997.

40. Loft A, Hogdall E, Larsen S, et al: A comparison of amniotic fluid alpha-fetoprotein and acetylcholinesterase in the prenatal diagnosis of open neural tube defects and anterior abdominal wall defects. Prenat Diagn 13:93–109, 1993.

41. Aitken D, Morrison N, Ferguson-Smith M: Predictive value of amniotic acetylcholinesterase analysis in the diagnosis of fetal abnormality in 3700 pregnancies. Prenat Diagn 4:329–340, 1984.

42. Wald N, Cuckle H, Nanchahal K: Amniotic fluid acetylcholinesterase measurement in the prenatal diagnosis of open neural tube defects: Second report of the Collaborative Acetylcholinesterase Study. Prenat Diagn 9:813–829, 1989.

43. Worley G, Schuster J, Oakes W: Survival at 5 years of a cohort of newborn infants with myelomeningocele. Dev Med Child Neurol 38:816–822, 1996.

44. Coniglio S, Anderson S, Ferguson J: Functional motor outcome in children with myelomeningocele: Correlation with anatomic level on prenatal ultrasound. Dev Med Child Neurol 38:675–680, 1996.

45. Hahn Y: Open myelomeningocele. Neurosurg Clin N Am 6: 231–241, 1995.

46. Swank M, Dias L: Myelomeningocele: A review of the orthopaedic aspects of 206 patients treated from birth with no selection criteria. Dev Med Child Neurol 34:1047–1052, 1992.

47. Steinbok P, Irvine B, Cochrane D, et al: Long-term outcome and complications of children born with meningomyelocele. Childs Nerv Syst 8:92–96, 1992.

48. Bier J, Morales Y, Liebling J, et al: Medical and social factors associated with cognitive outcome in individuals with myelomeningocele. Dev Med Child Neurol 39:263–266, 1997.

49. Coniglio S, Anderson S, Ferguson J: Developmental outcomes of children with myelomeningocele: Prenatal predictors. Am J Obstet Gynecol 177:319–326, 1997.

50. McLone D, Czyzewsky D, Raimondi A: Central nervous system infections as a limiting factor in the intelligence of children with myelomeningocele. Pediatrics 70:338–342, 1980.

51. Jensen P: Psychological aspects of myelomeningocele—a longitudinal study. Scand J Psychol 28:313–321, 1987.

52. Toriello H, Higgins J: Occurrence of neural tube defects among first-, second-, and third-degree relatives of probands: Results of a United States study. Am J Med Genet 15:601–606, 1983.

53. McBride M: Sib risk of anencephaly and spina bifida in British Columbia. Am J Med Genet 3:377–387, 1979.

54. Carter C, Evans K: Children of adult survivors with spina bifida cystica. Lancet 2:924–926, 1973.

55. Myriathopolous N, Melnick M: Studies in neural tube defects. I. Epidemiologic and etiologic aspects. Am J Med Genet 26:783–796, 1987.

56. Meuli M, Meuli-Simmen C, Hutchins G, et al: The spinal cord defect in human fetuses with myelomeningocele: Implications for fetal surgery. J Pediatr Surg 32:448–452, 1997.

57. Michejda M: Intrauterine treatment of spina bifida: Primate model. Z Kinderchir 39:259–261, 1984.

58. Heffez D, Aryanpur J, Hutchins G, et al: The paralysis associated with myelomeningocele: Clinical and experimental data implicating a preventable spinal cord injury. Neurosurgery 26:987–992, 1990.

59. Heffez D, Aryanpur J, Cuello-Rotellini N, et al: Intrauterine repair of experimental surgically created dysraphism. Neurosurgery 32:1005–1010, 1993.

60. Meuli M, Meuli-Simmen C, Yingling C, et al: Creation of myelomeningocele in utero: A model of functional damage from spinal cord exposure in fetal sheep. J Pediatr Surg 30:1028–1033, 1995.

61. McLone D, Dias M, Goosens W, et al: Pathological changes in exposed neural tissue of fetal delayed splotch (Spd) mice. Childs Nerv Syst 13:1–7, 1997.

62. Bruner J, Tulipan N, Paschall R, et al: Fetal surgery for myelomeningocele and the incidence of shunt-dependent hydrocephalus. JAMA 282:1819–1825, 1999.

63. Bensen J, Dillard R, Burton B: Open spina bifida: Does cesarean section delivery improve prognosis? Obstet Gynecol 71:532–534, 1988.

64. Cochrane D, Aronyk K, Sawatzky B, et al: The effects of labor and delivery on spinal cord function and ambulation in patients with meningomyelocele. Childs Nerv Syst 7:312–315, 1991.

65. Luthy D, Wardinsky T, Shurtleff D, et al: Cesarean section before the onset of labor and subsequent motor function in infants with meningomyelocele diagnosed antenatally. N Engl J Med 324:662–666, 1991.

66. Stark G: Neonatal assessment of the child with a myelomeningocele. Arch Dis Child 46:539–548, 1971.

67. Gamache F: Treatment of hydrocephalus in patients with meningomyelocele or encephalocele: A recent series. Childs Nerv Syst 11:487–488, 1995.

68. Reigel D: Kyphectomy and myelomeningocele repair. In Ransohoff J (ed): Modern Techniques in Surgery, vol 13, Neurosurgery. Mount Kisco, NY, Futura, 1979, pp 1–9.

69. Pang D: Surgical complications of open spinal dysraphism. Neurosurg Clin N Am 6:243–257, 1995.

70. Caldarelli M, DiRocco C, LaMarca F: Shunt complications in the first postoperative year in children with meningomyelocele. Childs Nerv Syst 12:748–754, 1996.

71. Cohen AR, Perneczky A: Endoscopy and the management of third ventricular lesions. In Apuzzo M (ed): Surgery of the Third Ventricle. Baltimore, Williams & Wilkins, 1998, pp 889–936.

72. Park T, Hoffman H, Hendrick E, et al: Experience with surgical decompression of the Arnold-Chiari malformation in young infants with myelomeningocele. Neurosurgery 13:147–152, 1983.

73. Pollack I, Kinnunen D, Albright A: The effect of early craniocervical decompression on functional outcome in neonates and young infants with myelodysplasia and symptomatic Chiari II malformations: Results from a prospective series. Neurosurgery 38:703–710, 1996.

74. Mazagri R, Ventureyra E: Latex allergy in neurosurgical practice. Childs Nerv Syst 15:404–407, 1999.

75. Nieto A, Estornell F, Mazon A, et al: Allergy to latex in spina bifida: A multivariate study of associated risk factors in 100 consecutive patients. J Allergy Clin Immunol 98:501–507, 1996.

76. Cremer R: The role of shunted hydrocephalus in the development of allergy to latex in patients with spina bifida [letter]. J Allergy Clin Immunol 100:719, 1997.

77. Holzman R: Clinical management of latex-allergic children. Anesth Analg 85:529–533, 1997.

78. Sillen U, Hansson E, Hermansson G, et al: Development of the urodynamic pattern in infants with myelomeningocele. Br J Urol 78:596–601, 1996.

79. Mevorach R, Bogaert G, Baskin L, et al: Lower urinary tract function in ambulatory children with spina bifida. Br J Urol 77:593–596, 1996.

80. Davidoff A, Hebra A, Balmer D, et al: Management of the gastrointestinal tract and nutrition in patients with cloacal exstrophy. J Pediatr Surg 31:771–773, 1996.

81. Rickham P: Vesico-intestinal fissure. Arch Dis Child 35:97–102, 1960.

82. Chen C-P, Shih S-L, Liu F-F, et al: Perinatal features of omphalocele–exstrophy–imperforate anus–spinal defects (OEIS complex) associated with large meningomyeloceles and severe limb defects. Am J Perinatol 14:275–279, 1997.

83. Smith N, Chambers H, Furness M, et al: The OEIS complex (omphalocele–exstrophy–imperforate anus–spinal defects): Recurrence in sibs. J Med Genet 29:730–732, 1992.

84. Cohen A: The mermaid malformation: Cloacal exstrophy and occult spinal dysraphism. Neurosurgery 28:834–843, 1991.

85. McLone D, Naidich T: Terminal myelocystocele. Neurosurgery 16:36–43, 1985.

CHAPTER 204

Lipomyelomeningocele

JOHN W. WALSH ■ RENATTA J. OSTERDOCK

Lipomas of the lumbosacral spine account for the majority of cases of occult spinal dysraphism and cause progressive impairment of lower extremity, bladder, or bowel function through spinal cord tethering and compression.[1-3] These malformations arise as a defect in embryogenesis and are often evident at birth. With surgical intervention for alleviation of the tethering and compression, the development of neurological deficits or progression of existing deficits can be prevented, and preexisting deficits can frequently be diminished.

The term *lipomyelomeningocele* is used by many neurosurgeons to address all occult spinal dysraphisms in which the spinal cord is tethered by a lipoma. However, strictly speaking, it does not apply to all lipomas of the lumbosacral spine. The term is widely used for all variants because lipomyelomeningocele is the most common one and tethers the spinal cord by a fibrous, subcutaneous lipoma, and because it shares the following significant characteristics with myelomeningoceles: (1) At the site of lipoma attachment, the spinal cord exhibits a partial dorsal myeloschisis and resembles a placode; (2) the unfused lipoma-cord interface is often distracted out of the spinal canal by traction created by tethering and the presence of an underlying or contralateral meningocele; and (3) there are similarities in their clinical presentation, radiologic diagnosis, and operative management. However, *lipomyelomeningocele* is not sufficiently inclusive, because it does not apply to lipomas with a lipoma-cord interface that is not distracted out of the spinal canal, whether that attachment is to a myeloschisis on the dorsal cord surface or to the conus or filum terminale. The terms *lipomyelocele* and *lipomas of the conus medullaris and filum terminale* have been proposed for the latter.[4] *Lipomyelomeningocele* is more properly reserved for lipomas with lipoma-cord interfaces posteriorly distracted out of the spinal canal and is used here in that more narrow and specific sense. For clarity, we use *congenital lumbosacral lipoma* as the general term for lipomatous malformations associated with spinal dysraphism.

Until about 20 years ago, little surgery was performed for congenital lumbosacral lipomas because the anatomy, embryogenesis, and pathophysiology were only poorly understood, and the procedure was considered risky. Referral for surgery of an asymptomatic infant with a subcutaneous lipoma was uncommon, and corrective surgery was almost never performed early, when the basic anatomy was least distorted by tethering or compression and the surgical outcome was most likely to be satisfactory. Patients were usually referred for surgery only after long periods of observation and hesitation, if at all, and unfortunately, only after the basic anatomy had become more distorted, the pathophysiology had become more complex, and multiple, severe, and often irreversible neurological deficits had occurred. The procedure was always difficult, and the outcome was likely to be disappointing. Only a few very experienced pediatric neurosurgeons were undertaking the task at all.[5-7] Taken together, these factors created a climate in which physicians were reluctant to refer these patients for surgery and in which most neurosurgeons were reluctant to undertake the necessary operative procedures.[3]

Today, the surgery is far more safe and effective, and the outcome is far better. We have a much larger fund of knowledge about the anatomy and embryogenesis of these lesions and about the pathophysiology of spinal cord tethering. We have the benefit of significant advances in surgical instrumentation—including the surgical microscope, the carbon dioxide (CO_2) laser, and intraoperative neurophysiologic monitoring—and in pediatric anesthesia. The natural history of these lipomas is one of inexorable and progressive development of neurological deficits, but early, prophylactic surgery can prevent them. It has become standard and commonplace among pediatric neurosurgeons to perform the surgery before the patient is 6 months old whenever possible so that the tethering can be alleviated before the often irreversible neurological deficits become established.[1, 2, 5, 8-10] It is also possible to perform the surgery with almost the same safety and efficacy in children, adolescents, and adults who already have deficits, stabilizing their neurological state and often restoring neurological function.

In patients who have not undergone corrective surgery, the patient's age and the level of lipoma-cord interface correlate with the anatomic features of the malformation, clinical presentation, radiographic findings, surgical management, and long-term outcome.

Age is related to the natural history of the condition. Infants are often born with a diagnosis suggesting subcutaneous lipoma or cutaneous anomaly but with no neurological deficits. As they pass through childhood and adolescence, they inevitably experience neurological deterioration until, as adults, they become incapacitated with severe lower extremity weakness and atrophy, urinary and fecal incontinence, scoliosis, and dysesthetic pain and undergo multiple orthopedic surgical procedures and urinary diversion. The level of lipoma-cord interface also determines the initial neurological deficit. Thus, when the upper border of lipoma attachment is at spinal cord level L3 or L4, patients most often present with proximal leg and hip weakness and perhaps scoliosis. When the upper border of the attachment is at the L5 or S1 level, patients are often first seen in clubfoot or other orthopedic clinics, with equinovarus or other foot deformities. When the lipoma attaches intradurally to the conus, patients most often present with urinary or fecal incontinence or with enuresis and are seen by pediatricians or in urology clinics. When the lipoma arises along the filum terminale, patients are usually asymptomatic when first seen, except for the presence of the subcutaneous lipoma and cutaneous anomalies.

ANATOMY

Congenital lumbosacral lipomas are hamartomas composed of fat and a large amount of connective tissue, which combine to impart a tough, fibrofatty consistency to the mass. They are partially encapsulated. They can be divided into three types, based on their anatomy: dorsal (type I; Fig. 204–1), intermediate or transitional (type II; Fig. 204–2), and caudal or terminal (type III; Fig. 204–3). These categories are based on the persistence or absence of a posterior duroschisis and myeloschisis at the site of lipoma attachment and on whether they are attached directly or by a fibrolipomatous stalk to the resulting placode at this spinal cord cleft or to the conus medullaris or filum terminale, or both.[11, 12]

A type I lipoma tethers the spinal cord to the posterior lumbosacral epidermis and subcutaneous tissue. It prevents the normal ascent of the cord with growth by an attachment to the posterior spinal cord surface, usually at the middle to lower lumbar or lumbosacral level. Characteristically, there is a yellow, fibrous, subcutaneous lipoma that tapers to a paler, smooth, tenacious, fibrolipomatous stalk. This stalk varies considerably in thickness and length. It passes through a defect in the deep lumbosacral fascia and lamina (spina bifida) and attaches directly to the underlying spinal cord. The posterior half of the lower spinal cord at this site is unfused (a partial dorsal myeloschisis is present), and the stalk attaches directly to the exposed alar and basal cord regions, just posterior and medial to the posterior columns and above the central canal. The lipoma may extend into the central canal for a variable distance and expand it. The dura and pia-arachnoid that surround ventral aspects of the cord in a normal manner together attach circumferentially to the lateral

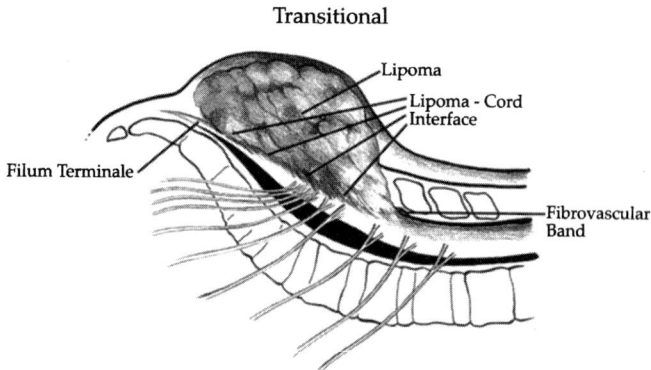

FIGURE 204–2. Type II (transitional) lipoma with a lipoma-cord interface that extends from the rostral end of the myeloschisis to the conus. Rostrally, the lipoma-cord interface is dorsal to the dorsal root entry zones, but as the attachment is followed caudally, the dorsal roots enter at or above the interface, often within lipoma. A thickened filum terminale is present.

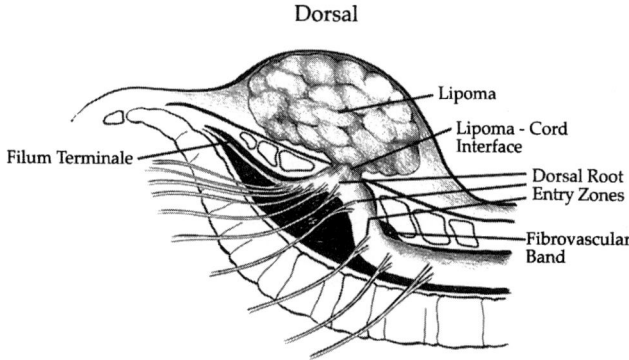

FIGURE 204–1. Type I (dorsal) lipoma with lumbar spinal cord distracted out of the spinal canal (lipomyelomeningocele). A transverse fibrovascular band, situated above the dura and just caudal to the lowest intact laminar edge, compresses the dorsal surface of the spinal cord as it passes through the spina bifida to the subcutaneous lipoma. The lipoma-cord interface is posterior to the dorsal root entry zones. The spinal cord caudal to the interface is normal, and a thickened filum terminale is present.

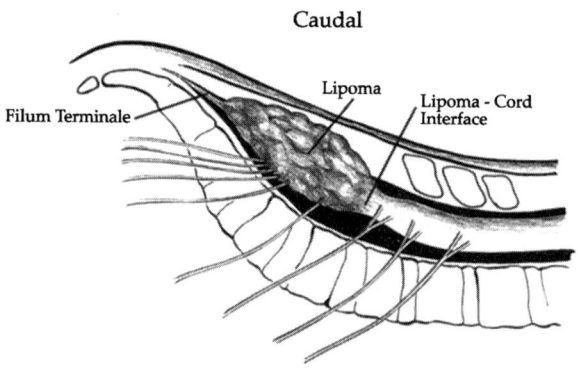

FIGURE 204–3. Type III (caudal) lipoma of the conus medullaris. The lipoma-cord interface is diffuse and vertically oriented, and the lipoma is largely or completely intradural. A thickened filum can be seen at the termination of the lipoma.

edge of the myeloschisis just above the dorsal root entry zones. This gives rise to an elliptical dural defect and an extradural location of the unfused posterior spinal cord, thereby creating an exposed and ideal site for attachment of the lipoma. Because the myeloschisis and site of fibrolipomatous stalk attachment are often limited to one or two vertebral levels, and because there is a relatively distinct plane between cord and lipoma, surgical separation of the stalk and dura from the dorsal cord surface should be possible. Spinal cord, pia-arachnoid, and dura caudal to the myeloschisis are usually normal, but the conus tapers more gradually than normal and typically ends at an abnormally low vertebral level attached to a thickened filum terminale (Fig. 204–4). These type I lipomas can be separated into two groups, based on whether the lipoma or fibrolipomatous stalk is attached to the spinal cord inside or outside the spinal canal. When it is attached within the spinal canal, the anatomy closely resembles that of a meningocele or myelocele, especially when the lipoma-cord interface is small, the conus ends at a low level, and the subarachnoid space develops a marked meningocele-like distention. These are referred to as *lipomyeloceles*.[4] In most of these cases, both the lipoma tissue and the fibrolipomatous stalk are within the spinal canal; occasionally, this intraspinal lipomatous component is so large that the spinal cord becomes displaced ventrally, and the nerve rootlets may course posteromedially and inferiorly and sometimes even through the

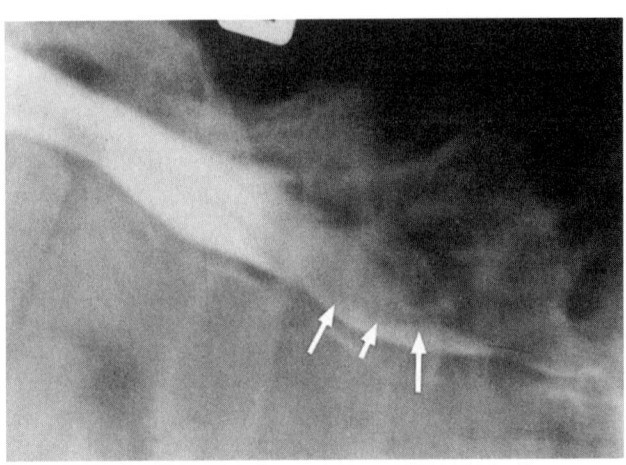

FIGURE 204–5. Metrizamide myelography of a type I lipoma (lipomyelocele) showing the spinal cord *(arrows)* ventrally displaced by a large intradural and attached lipoma.

lipoma (Fig. 204–5). When the lipoma-cord interface is outside the spinal canal, the dorsally displaced spinal cord, along with the lipoma-cord interface and its attached dura and pia-arachnoid, has been directed out of the spinal canal through the laminar defect (spina bifida) and sometimes through the deep fascia into the subcutaneous portion of the lipoma. These lesions are properly referred to as *lipomyelomeningoceles*.[4] The displacement may be caused either by traction exerted by the lipoma (tethering) or by pressure from a meningocele-like cerebrospinal fluid (CSF) expansion ventral to the cord. As the spinal cord leaves the spinal canal, it is frequently kinked by the posterior laminar edge of the lowest intact vertebra above the spina bifida and by a transverse thickened band of periosteum just beneath and caudal to it. The resulting compression can be an additional source of tethering and of present or future neurological deficits.

These lipomas may be situated in the midline (68%) or eccentrically (32%), regardless of whether the lipoma-cord interface is outside the spinal canal.[10] If they lie in the midline, nerve roots given off at the level of the myeloschisis may pass to their respective foramina transversely or even slightly rostrally because the spinal cord itself is so tethered that the cord-vertebra relationship has become similar to that of early fetal development, when spinal cord and vertebral segments were at the same levels (Fig. 204–6). If they are positioned eccentrically, surgical release of the tethering and decompression become more difficult. The lateralized attachment of the fibrolipomatous stalk to the spinal cord causes the stalk to be displaced laterally and rotated. The ipsilateral roots become shortened and displaced ventrally and act as a source of tethering. The contralateral roots become elongated and posteriorly displaced just under the dura, which makes them particularly vulnerable to injury during dural opening. Ipsilaterally, local arachnoiditis develops, causing the spinal cord and shortened nerve roots to become firmly adherent to dura. All this greatly increases the risk of injury to them during neurolysis and surgical decom-

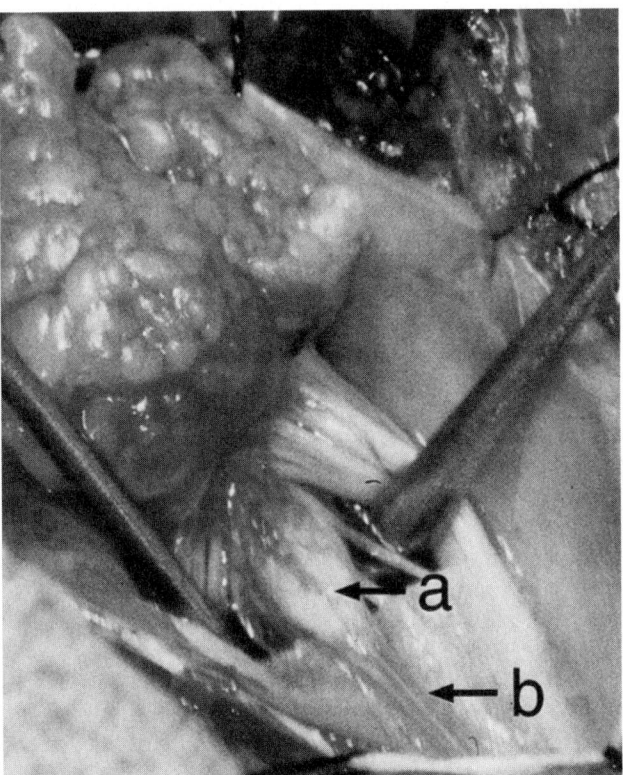

FIGURE 204–4. Intraoperative photomicrograph showing type I lipoma during resection. The normal conus (a) with attached thickened filum terminale (b) can be seen between nerve roots of the cauda equina extending caudal to a remnant of the lipoma.

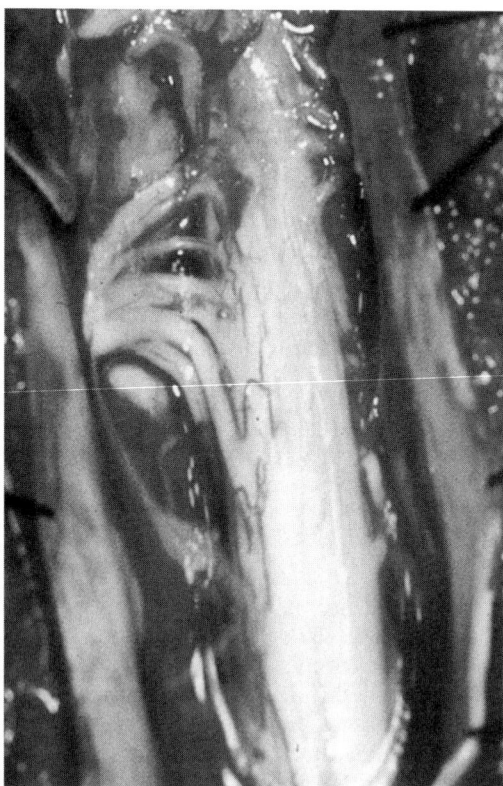

FIGURE 204–6. Intraoperative photomicrograph showing nerve roots passing horizontally from a low conus with a type III lipoma caudal to it.

pression. Asymmetric, contralateral projection of a meningocele dorsally into the subcutaneous lipoma compounds this rotation and displacement, even further increasing vulnerability to injury.

Type II lipomas share some of the anatomic features of type I and type III lipomas. Like type I, they have a fibrolipomatous stalk that attaches rostral to a dorsal cord myeloschisis. However, unlike type I, caudally this attachment continues beyond the myeloschisis to the conus medullaris. At the conus, the attachment resembles that of a type III lipoma (described later). Unlike type I lipomas, there is no normal spinal cord caudal or distal to the myeloschisis. In addition, the relationship between the lipoma-cord interface and the dorsal root entry zones is not always readily apparent. Rostrally, the relationship originates, as with type I, with a lipoma-cord interface immediately above and parallel to the dorsal root entry zones. However, as the lipoma-cord interface is followed caudally, the line of attachment of the fibrolipomatous stalk to the placode becomes increasingly oblique and more ventral, until it lies at or below the dorsal root entry zones and posterior roots, which then frequently become enmeshed within the lipoma. At the conus, the lipoma-cord interface becomes almost vertical in orientation and caudal to all but a few small sensory or rudimentary nerve roots. A dorsal myeloschisis is not seen at the cord termination; the conus appears normally developed, but a thickened filum terminale may be present. The duroschisis seen with type I lipomas is

present, with dura and leptomeninges attached to the lateral edges of the lipoma-cord interface, even though it may follow an oblique direction under some of the posterior roots. Type II lipomas tend to develop asymmetrically, with the lipoma extending ventrally to one side or the other, greatly increasing the difficulty of radiologic assessment and surgical management.

Although these lipomas are classified as a distinct group and are referred to as type II or transitional, they may in fact simply represent the continuum between types I and III.[8, 11, 13] They may be type I lesions in which the myeloschisis extends to the homologue of the posterior neuropore but in which the lipoma extends even further. Formation of a lipoma caudal to the posterior neuropore occurs as part of an abnormal secondary neurulation during the period when formation of the conus (the S2-coccygeal cord segment) takes place.

Type III lipomas arise directly from the conus medullaris or filum terminale. They are largely or completely intradural and can vary in size from small, locally attached nodules to large lipomas that extend caudally and fill the entire lower spinal canal, displacing or engulfing nerve roots of the cauda equina and, at times, extending through a caudal duroschisis to form a subcutaneous lipoma just above the intergluteal fold. When the lipoma arises from the conus, the lipoma-cord interface lies at the termination of, and perpendicular to, the long axis of the spinal cord; therefore, like the caudal part of type II lipomas, the interface is caudal rather than dorsal to the dorsal root entry zones. In contrast to the discrete lipoma-cord interface of type I and the variable interface of type II lipomas, the lipoma-cord interface in type III lipomas is always diffuse (Fig. 204–7). Individual roots arising ventral and rostral to the lipoma-cord interface may be firmly adherent to or pass through the lipoma. Such roots are often, but not always, rudimentary and nonfunctional. The lipoma-cord interface may be asymmet-

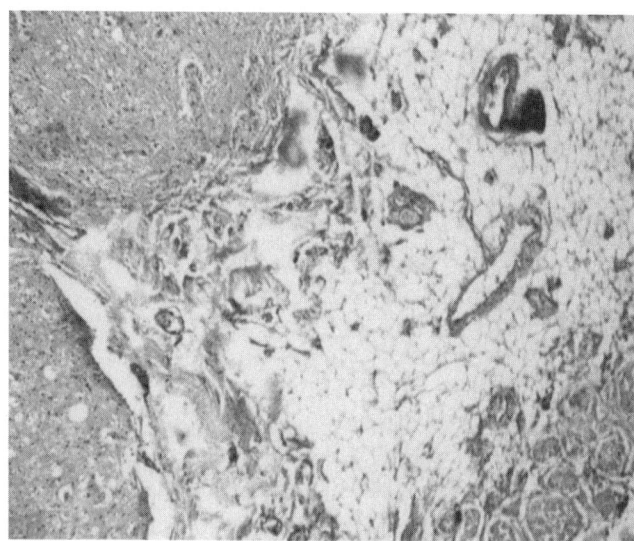

FIGURE 204–7. Photomicrograph of lipoma-cord interface of a type III lipoma showing the diffuse nature of the attachment.

ric, involving more of the cord and nerve roots on one side than on the other; this may make terminal nerve root identification and functional assessment more difficult. Leptomeninges and pia mater fuse and attach circumferentially at the lipoma-cord interface, beyond normal-appearing conus medullaris tissue and caudal to the dorsal root entry zones. The dura extends to about the S4 vertebral level and, along with surrounding myofascial layers, usually appears normal. The filum terminale may be surrounded by lipoma at the conus, or it may be replaced by lipoma and therefore not visible; it may be short and thickened and may arise from the lipoma at the termination of the dural sac (Fig. 204–8). At times, the filum terminale even passes through sacrococcygeal subcutaneous tissues to attach to, and pull on, epidermis and thus produce a sacral dimple.

A patient with any lipoma that attaches directly to the spinal cord may have lipoma extending rostrally up the central canal for several segments to form an intramedullary mass.[14, 15] With growth of the patient or unusual weight gain, this intramedullary mass may significantly increase in size, causing central spinal cord compression and related neurological deficits. Surgical management of this development requires the addition of a dorsal myelotomy and subtotal decompression of the intracanalicular fat, which is usually effective.

Lipomas arising from the filum may contribute to spinal cord tethering by causing fibrolipomatous thickening of all or part of the filum itself. Lipomas seen as a defined fatty mass can vary markedly in size and be single or multiple in number. They may become large enough to cause cauda equina compression, with accompanying neurological impairment. Even if small, the filum from which they arise is frequently, and independently, thickened. If a thickened filum is found, there is usually intrafilar fibrolipomatous tissue. An accessory filum may also be present, and lipomas may

arise from it. Lipomas that appear to arise from both the conus and the proximal filum are common.

Filum lipomas can develop without tethering or cauda equina compression, as has been established by long-term radiologic follow-up. They are usually small and may be multiple. They have been reported, as incidental findings, in 4% to 6% of normal adults.[4]

Occasionally, patients who have developed abnormalities of the central canal or terminal ventricle (terminal syringomyelia[14] or myelocystocele[16] or one of the various forms of caudal regression syndrome[17, 18]) may have a congenital lumbosacral lipoma with tethering and require appropriate neuroimaging and surgery. They may have typical dorsal as well as conus and filum lipomas, and a variety of other highly unusual tethering mechanisms have been reported.

EMBRYOLOGY

Congenital lumbosacral lipomas are the result of a disturbance in the embryologic sequence of events that occurs principally between the 25th and 48th postovulatory day (POD) (Fig. 204–9). This includes the period of primary neurulation, the process of normal neural tube closure during which closure of the caudal end of the neural tube and formation of the posterior neuropore at S2 take place.[19–21] This process is followed by secondary neurulation, during which the caudal eminence, a mass of poorly differentiated cells derived from the primitive streak, is formed caudal to, and attached to, the neuropore at S2 (condensation), and a secondary neural tube with a central lumen forms from it (canalization). It has also been proposed that secondary neurulation includes the subsequent period during which differentiation and reduction of the caudal eminence occur to form the conus medullaris (spinal cord extension from S2 to coccygeal level), associated dorsal root ganglia, terminal ventricle, filum terminale, and a sacrococcygeal medullary vestige (retrogressive differentiation).[13] There now is good information on the events that occur during primary neurulation,[19, 20] but unfortunately, secondary neurulation is still not well understood.

In the human fetus, primary neurulation is thought to occur bidirectionally in a stepwise but zipper-like manner, beginning at primitive rhombencephalon levels.[22] In this process, the neuroectoderm separates from the neural crest and cutaneous ectoderm, and the lateral ends of the primitive neural plate (neuroectoderm) fuse to each other posteriorly to form the neural tube or primitive spinal cord. At the same time, the cutaneous ectoderm fuses posterior to the cord in the midline, and the neural crest migrates ventrolaterally. The caudal part of this closure takes place in a rostral-caudal direction and ends during POD 25 to 27 with formation of the posterior neuropore.[23] The now tubular spinal cord ends at somites 30/31, which corresponds to spinal ganglion and vertebral level S2. Once the neuroectoderm and overlying cutaneous ectoderm close, paraxial mesenchyme migrates to form the intervening subcutaneous tissue, deep fascia, paravertebral muscu-

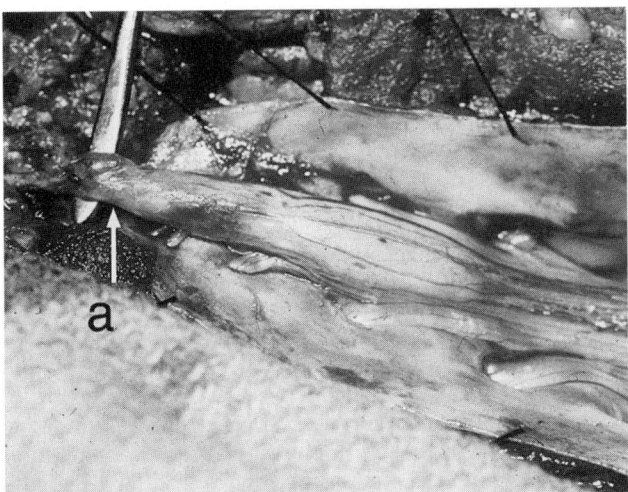

FIGURE 204–8. Type III lipoma extending from a markedly tapered conus. A thickened filum terminale (a) passes from the caudal end of the lipoma to the termination of the dura and spinal canal.

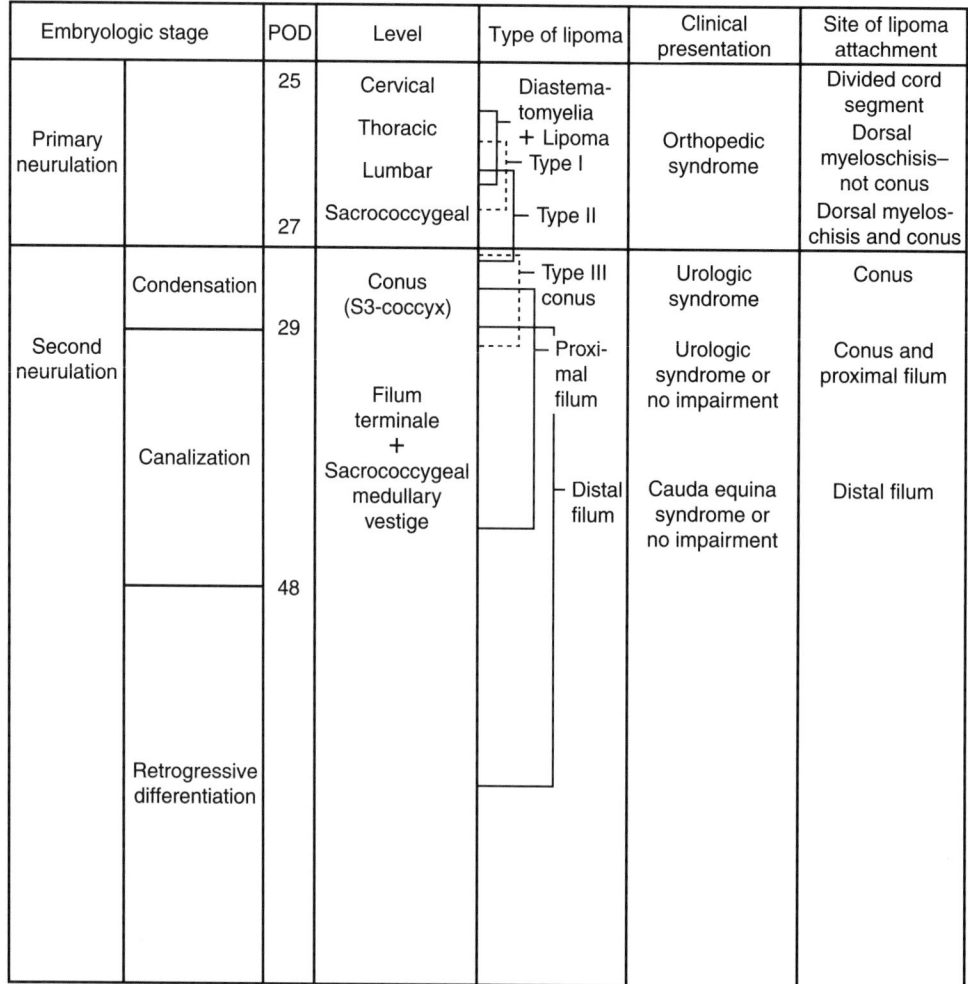

Embryologic stage		POD	Level	Type of lipoma	Clinical presentation	Site of lipoma attachment
Primary neurulation		25	Cervical	Diastema-tomyelia + Lipoma Type I	Orthopedic syndrome	Divided cord segment Dorsal myeloschisis– not conus
		27	Thoracic Lumbar Sacrococcygeal	Type II		Dorsal myelos-chisis and conus
Second neurulation	Condensation	29	Conus (S3-coccyx)	Type III conus	Urologic syndrome	Conus
	Canalization		Filum terminale + Sacrococcygeal medullary vestige	Proxi-mal filum	Urologic syndrome or no impairment	Conus and proximal filum
		48		Distal filum	Cauda equina syndrome or no impairment	Distal filum
	Retrogressive differentiation					

FIGURE 204–9. Representation of the close relationship between type of lipoma, anatomic level of spinal cord attachment, proposed embryologic stage of formation, and pattern of clinical presentation. POD, postovulatory day.

lature, and laminae and posterior spinous processes. The neural crest divides into two groups of cells, one of which migrates dorsally, just under the ectoderm, to become melanocytes, and the other of which migrates ventrolaterally to become dorsal root ganglia, Schwann cells, and sympathetic and adrenal ganglia.

Secondary neurulation follows these events. After primary neurulation and closure of the overlying ectoderm, the caudal eminence, a remnant that contains neurons, neural crest, glial cells, and ependymal cells, forms and fills the space from the posterior neuropore to the cloacal membrane.[24] This process begins with the laying down of neural tissue to form a solid neural cord, probably in direct continuity with the primary neural tube (condensation). Next, a dense outer cell layer with a central lumen that is in continuity with the central canal of the neural tube forms, and a sacro-coccygeal mesenchyme and primitive hindgut remain at the caudal end of the spinal canal (canalization). These two events occur between PODs 27 and 29.[25] Finally, the caudal eminence–derived neural cord undergoes retrogressive differentiation, and only the conus medullaris, lower sacral nerve roots, terminal

ventricle, filum terminale, and sacrococcygeal remnant remain.[19, 21, 24] This process is thought to be completed by POD 48 to 52.[25, 26] Further maturation of all these structures continues into the early postnatal period.

Congenital lumbosacral lipomas form because the separation of primitive ectoderm into neuroectoderm, neural crest, and cutaneous ectoderm and the simultaneous fusion posteriorly of the resulting neural plate edges and of the overlying edges of cutaneous ectoderm do not take place normally. A brief disjunction in timing occurs. Cutaneous ectoderm closes slightly before the neural tube, and a gap is left transiently through which paraxial mesenchyme can migrate. This mesenchyme becomes primarily fat under inductive influences from the inner ependymal surface of the placode,[27] although tissue of mixed embryonic origin, such as bone, cartilage, smooth and striated muscle, collagen, renal epithelium, and gastric mucosa, may also persist within these lipomas.[12, 28, 29] This process can occur unilaterally or bilaterally, which may account for the midline location of many lipomas and the marked eccentricity of others. It can occur over a varying period and at any lumbosacral level and, therefore, can lead to the development of lipomas at any level of the lumbosacral spine. It can give rise to lipomas whose fibrolipomatous stalk attachment to the persistently open neural plate (myeloschisis) is limited to a single vertebral level, with normal cord and conus caudal to it (type I), or whose attachment extends from the middle or upper lumbar level to the conus, with no normal cord caudal to the attachment (type II). Subsequent secondary neurulation and retrogressive differentiation are also affected, at least to the extent that a thickened filum is almost always found; occasionally, and more severely, a myelocystocele or one of the various forms of caudal regression syndrome may occur.[25]

The processes leading to the formation of the caudal part of type II lipomas and to the formation of type III lipomas are poorly understood. Anatomically, the lipoma-cord interfaces are similar. For type II lipomas, it has not been determined (1) whether the dorsal myeloschisis and the lipoma-cord interface extend fully to the termination of the cord, (2) whether the spinal cord at that level is a homologue of the posterior neuropore or is the S2-coccygeal cord segment added during secondary neurulation, and (3) whether this caudal portion of lipoma, like its more rostral part, is derived from paraxial mesenchyme, that is, from products of faulty canalization or retrogressive differentiation, or both. Thus, it is not established that the more rostral parts of type II lipomas develop as an expression of faulty primary neurulation and the more caudal parts as the consequence of faulty secondary neurulation, but at least one published report suggests that this is the case.[13]

Type III lipomas probably arise during canalization and retrogressive differentiation on the basis of the following observations: Lumbar and upper sacral cord segments are never involved; a dorsal myeloschisis or duroschisis is never found; the lipoma either is part of a thickened filum or replaces it altogether; terminal ventricle-like fluid spaces are frequently observed within the lipomatous mass, as are scattered nests of ependymal cells, glial cells, neurons, and ganglion cells; and large accumulations of fat are frequently found in the thickened filum.[13, 30] There are still many unanswered questions as well. We do not know why differentiation of some caudal eminence cells in these patients leads to a proliferation of fat rather than to the normal process of involution. It has been proposed that in patients with type III lipomas, mesenchymal precursor cells[26, 30] were present in excessive numbers and generated the inductive factors that cause differentiation of other mesenchymal cells into fat. We do not know why some conus lipomas are only small, circumscribed masses, whereas others fill the entire caudal spinal canal, sometimes passing out the end of the canal to the sacrococcygeal subcutaneous tissue, or why some merely displace nerve roots of the cauda equina, whereas others engulf them. We do not know why some lipomas replace the filum and others develop proximal to or alongside it. It may be that lipomas of the conus arise earlier, during canalization, and those of the distal filum arise later, during retrogressive differentiation.

As with other forms of spinal dysraphism, a congenital lumbosacral lipoma that tethers the spinal cord at the upper lumbar or thoracolumbar level must have formed at a slightly earlier embryologic stage than one that tethers the cord at a lower lumbar, lumbosacral, or sacral level. It is also more likely to develop concomitantly with other dysraphic malformations and malformations at other sites. This certainly is the case for myelomeningoceles.[5] In patients with thoracolumbar diastematomyelia,[31–33] it is not uncommon to find aberrant fibrous bands, anomalous nerve fibers, or a thickened filum terminale, in addition to a lipoma attached to one cord segment. Clinically, patients with thoracolumbar lipomas are more often found to have paralysis, kyphoscoliosis, and spastic bowel and bladder dysfunction; patients with lumbosacral or sacral lipomas most often have neurological deficits limited to the distal parts of the lower extremities or to flaccid bowel and bladder function. Obviously, this markedly influences management and prognosis.

Patients with congenital lumbosacral lipomas only rarely develop hydrocephalus, Arnold-Chiari malformations, or other brain anomalies that typically accompany development of a myelomeningocele,[25, 34] nor do they develop the intellectual impairment that accompanies it.[35] However, they do occasionally develop other serious malformations such as caudal dysgenesis syndrome, which may include a duplicated vagina, bifid uterus, cloaca, failure of fusion of the genital tubercle, or imperforate anus or anal agenesis, all of which are disturbances of secondary neurulation.[17, 36] In addition, they characteristically exhibit a more rapid and early deterioration associated with the lipoma and its tethering effect.[15]

PATHOPHYSIOLOGY

The neurological deficits produced by congenital lumbosacral lipomas are the result of spinal cord tethering or direct compression of the spinal cord or cauda equina structures, or both. When the cord is tethered to any firm structure, the normal ascent relative to the surrounding vertebral column that occurs naturally with growth of the patient is hindered or arrested. In the case of lumbosacral lipomas, this tethering is caused by the lipoma and secondarily by other dysraphic elements, such as a thickened filum terminale, aberrant nerve roots and fibrous bands, or dermal sinus, all formed coincident with, or as a consequence of, the development of the lipoma. The tethering can vary from slight, giving rise to stretching but no change in anatomic position of the conus, to such severe traction as to cause the conus to be retained at a low lumbar, lumbosacral, or even sacral vertebral level. It is this stretching or traction (along with compression) that generates the spectrum of neurological deficits that characterizes congenital lumbosacral lipomas.

Normally, spinal cord formation is completed by POD 48, with the conus at the level corresponding to the S2 vertebra and retrogressive differentiation still in progress.[19, 20, 30] At that point, the spinal cord and vertebral column are matched segment for segment. However, because the vertebrae grow much faster than the spinal cord, and because the spinal cord is continuous with the relatively immobile brain, the conus gradually ascends. The continued retrogressive differentiation, which leads to maturation of the conus and reduction in its size, adds to this effect.[30] At term, the normally developing spinal cord ends at the L3 vertebral level; by the first or second year of life, this has risen to the L1-2 level, the level usually found in adults.[37-39] Therefore, in a patient older than age 2 in whom the conus ends at L3 or below, the presence of tethering must be given serious consideration, and an assessment made for the presence of a congenital lumbosacral lipoma or thickened filum terminale, or both.

With all this taken together, one might expect neurological deficits to develop at the periods of most rapid growth of the spine—just before birth or during adolescence—and that is often the case. However, although progressive neurological deficits can be seen with rapid growth in adolescence, most deficits first appear during infancy and preadolescence, when growth is much slower. This apparent contradiction was resolved when it was established that these neurological deficits most often occur as the result of repeated sudden traction events on an already chronically stretched cord.[40] It has been shown that deficits sustained with chronic traction are caused primarily by cord ischemia, whereas those superimposed more acutely by repeated sudden cord stretching are caused by accelerated and irreversible neuronal damage.[41] In laboratory studies using reflection spectrophotometry and a feline model, sustained traction on the conus was found to favor the maintenance of cytochrome aa3, a terminal marker of mitochondrial respiration, in its reduced state, and this activity contributes to diminished adenosine triphosphate production, impaired oxidative metabolism and ionic transport, and ischemia.[42] It also leads to hypoglycemia[40] and reduced blood flow[43, 44] at the spinal cord region nearest the site of tethering. Additionally, the chronic traction produces stretching of blood vessels in the conus and adjacent cord, with accompanying reduction of regional blood flow and development of cord and nerve root swelling. This, in turn, results in lower cord segment ischemia, with characteristic neurological deficits.[45] The neuronal damage from superimposed sudden cord stretching was observed histologically, electrophysiologically, and ultrastructurally. The entire process has been demonstrated to occur similarly in humans.[46] Tethered cord stretching also leads to peripheral nerve changes with decreased axonal transport of cholinergic enzymes.[4]

With congenital lumbosacral lipomas, tethering is generated through attachment of the lipoma directly to the cord or through a fibrolipomatous stalk, and the degree of tethering is affected by the anatomic level of the lipoma, the size of the lipoma-cord interface, and the firmness of the lipoma or the fibrolipomatous stalk. Clearly, a lipoma that is subcutaneous and adherent to the overlying ectoderm, fibrous and therefore inelastic or inflexible, and firmly adherent to the cord will hinder normal spinal cord ascent. Unfortunately, little is known about what makes one lipoma, such as the lipomyelomeningocele, tether the spinal cord so severely that it displaces the involved cord segment dorsally, completely out of the spinal canal and through the deep lumbar fascia, whereas another, such as the lipomyelocele, barely displaces the cord segment at all or fills the spinal canal, displacing the cord ventrally. It may simply be a matter of growth, but other factors, such as the relative amount of lipoma located subcutaneously versus within the spinal canal, the thickness of the stalk and the extent to which it is fibrous, and the degree of growth factor stimulation of fibrous or collagen proliferation within the lipoma, may play important roles.

CLINICAL PRESENTATION

These congenital lesions have been found to develop in 1 of every 4000 births[16] and to occur more often in girls,[2, 10, 15, 19, 47, 48] but the occurrence of congenital lumbosacral lipomas among multiple family members is rare.[49]

Patients with congenital lumbosacral lipomas are frequently identified at birth even when there are no neurological deficits because they have subcutaneous fatty masses or one or more cutaneous anomalies in the dorsal lumbosacral region. As toddlers or preadolescent children, they present with muscular underdevelopment or wasting, weakness, trophic changes or sensory loss in the lower sacral distribution and in one or both lower extremities (orthopedic syndrome), bladder or bowel incontinence (urologic syndrome), scoliosis, or any combination of these; as adolescents or adults, they may additionally develop severe back, pelvic, perineal, and lower extremity pain.

More than 80% of patients, especially those with type I or type II lipoma, present with a dorsal, midline, or eccentric soft, fatty, subcutaneous mass of varying size over the lumbosacral spine.[1, 3] It is usually present at birth and enlarges as the patient grows in size and weight. There may also be a palpable CSF-containing sac (meningocele) of varying size, often laterally situated, within the lipoma. This subcutaneous mass is the earliest and most reliable indicator that the patient has a congenital lumbosacral lipoma, and its presence justifies neuroimaging studies. It generally overlies the area of cord involvement, but the stalk may occasionally pass one to two levels intradurally before attaching to the spinal cord. If the subcutaneous mass is situated in the sacrococcygeal region, just above the intergluteal cleft, the cleft may be deflected laterally or divided around its base.

Certain cutaneous anomalies that flag dysraphism are also seen dorsally over the lumbosacral spine in up to 50% of such patients.[1, 3] They are present whether or not an underlying subcutaneous mass is present and are therefore helpful for the early identification of type III lipomas. These lesions include a tuft of hair (hypertrichosis), capillary hemangioma or telangiectasia, hypo- or hyperpigmented area, cutis aplasia, dermal pit or sinus, and atretic meningocele. The tuft of hair is more common and more luxuriant in patients with other forms of spinal dysraphism, such as diastematomyelia; however, when present in a patient with a subcutaneous lumbosacral mass, it adds further weight to the need for neuroimaging. With lipomas, the hair is usually sparse and appears as only one of several cutaneous anomalies. A capillary hemangioma is usually small, may be midline or lateral in location, and may be raised above the level of the skin. It is frequently found over the subcutaneous lipomatous mass. A dermal pit may be the only cutaneous expression of a dermal sinus or a cutaneous retraction caused by extension of a thickened filum or other dysraphic abnormality. The appearance of a dermal sinus or an atretic meningocele is much less common and usually indicates a more complex dysraphic disorder. The sinus opening or meningocele may be very small and can be located anywhere between the upper border of the lipoma and the sacrum. The underlying epithelial tract typically courses upward to dura, may pass intradurally to the spinal cord, and may be associated with an intraspinal or intramedullary dermoid cyst or tumor or with the lipoma itself.

Children with congenital lumbosacral lipomas who do not undergo surgical intervention develop neurological deficits slowly and progressively. These usually begin by the first or second year of life and gradually increase in severity. As previously mentioned, the type of deficit—sensorimotor, orthopedic, or urologic—varies according to the site of attachment of the lipoma or fibrolipomatous stalk and the child's age. Thus, attachment between L3 and S1 usually first manifests between years 1 and 6 and favors orthopedic or neurological deficits, such as lower extremity sensorimotor loss and structural foot deformities. Attachment at sacral levels produces deficits after age 3 to 4 and most often leads to urologic disorders, such as bladder or bowel incontinence or enuresis. After puberty, scoliosis or impairment of sexual function can develop, and severe dysesthetic low back, pelvic, perineal, or lower extremity radicular pain usually begins and becomes the most disabling symptom.

Throughout this period, the patient is at risk for a precipitous deterioration in neurological function due to sudden increased traction superimposed on the chronically stretched cord. This usually occurs after an abrupt flexion movement, such as with knee-chest exercises, gymnastics, ballet, automobile accidents, examination in the lithotomy position, or sudden full flexion of the head.[3, 48, 50, 51] All these actions produce traction on an already stretched spinal cord, which leads to added ischemia and often irreversible neuronal damage.

The orthopedic syndrome first manifests by involvement of one or both feet and lower extremities. In infants, the initial manifestations are subtle and sometimes difficult to appreciate because of the child's overall pudginess and limited sensorimotor development. One foot or leg may be shorter or smaller than the other, and the child may not use it as well. In toddlers, motor development milestones associated with lower extremity function may be so delayed that the child drags the foot and an overall clumsiness is noted. Hammer toes (flexed interphalangeal and extended metatarsophalangeal joints), high pedal arches, and equino- or calcaneovarus or valgus foot deformities may be seen, and there may be atrophy of the buttocks, calves, and hollows of the feet unilaterally or bilaterally. Deep tendon reflexes are usually absent, and sensation to pinprick, including perineal, and the anal wink may be diminished. In preadolescents, the muscular wasting, weakness, and foot deformities are more striking, and scoliosis may develop. All these symptoms progress with age and increased tethering until, in the adult, there is marked distal lower extremity atrophy and weakness and severe trophic changes are manifested.

The urologic syndrome appears slightly later. Before toilet training, this is often difficult to recognize, but occasionally, incontinence can be suspected by the absence of normal dry periods between diaper changes or by visualizing an abnormally forceful urination. Usually, incontinence or enuresis is first noted during or just after toilet training, or there is only a general delay or lack of success with the toilet training process. When there is enuresis, a neurogenic bladder (and tethered cord) is suspected when the incontinence occurs both during the day and at night. If these signs are discovered, both urodynamic and neuroimaging studies are indicated. As the child grows, symptoms and signs of more extensive impairment (urgency, frequency, urge or stress incontinence, poor voluntary control of urination, and postvoid dribbling) become evident, and frequent urinary tract infections may occur. Finally, in later childhood or adolescence, persistent constipation or bowel incontinence can develop. Patients who initially present with disturbances of urinary function in early childhood most often have type III lipomas. Their lower extremity structure and function may be normal, because traction occurs mainly on the conus. With growth and the resultant additional chronic traction, adjacent higher cord levels become ischemic, and lower extremity impairments are added. With type I and type II lipomas, structural abnormalities and neurological impairments of leg function occur first; with increased traction affecting sacrococcygeal cord segments, urinary and eventually bowel incontinence also appears. The more rostral the myeloschisis and lipoma-cord interface, the more intense the tethering has to be to cause disturbances in bladder and bowel function.

With mild sacrococcygeal tethering, postvoid dribbling and stress incontinence are usually the only neurological deficits seen. They are the result of interference with the sympathetic innervation that affects internal urethral sphincter competence. With increased tethering, the disruption of urinary function is compounded. Detrusor muscle activity is weakened by bladder hypotonia and areflexia, and this leads to incomplete bladder emptying. This occurs in addition to the incontinence resulting from urethral sphincter incompetence. Finally, when the synchrony of contractile activity between detrusor and external urethral sphincter muscles becomes disturbed (detrusor-sphincter dyssynergia), severe hydronephrosis may develop secondary to the high intravesicular pressure and uncontrolled external urethral sphincter contractions.

Scoliosis may develop in some children or adolescents with congenital lumbrosacral lipomas. However, if the lipoma along with the tethering is removed in infancy, this complication usually is not seen. When it does become manifest, surgical correction or stabilization of the spine may be needed, but before this can safely be performed, any tethering being generated by the lipoma or other secondary dysraphic abnormalities must be released. This measure is necessary because permanent, catastrophic intra- or postoperative neurological deterioration can occur when the corrective spinal instrumentation and fusion are carried out before the tethering is released and sudden traction of the lower spinal cord is superimposed on the chronic traction.[13] The causes and mechanisms for the development of scoliosis and the extent to which it is produced or aggravated by the lipoma and the tethering are not yet established.

The initial presentation of congenital lumbosacral lipoma in adults is, unfortunately, not uncommon. Only about half these patients have a cutaneous or subcutaneous anomaly that would have signaled the possibility of a dysraphic malformation earlier, and the patterns of clinical presentation discussed previously were not appreciated. Therefore, the malformation was never surgically corrected, and the patient has developed, one after the other, the multiple, mostly irreversible, neurological deficits described here. Others suffer a precipitous onset of symptoms. What generally brings them to the attention of a neurosurgeon is severe, unrelenting, often incapacitating back, pelvic, perineal, and radicular leg pain. This is often dysesthetic and responds poorly to analgesics. It is the most common presenting symptom in adults and is the one most likely to be relieved with surgical decompression and release of tethering.[52]

NEUROIMAGING AND OTHER DIAGNOSTIC STUDIES

Radiographs of the Spine

These studies are no longer obtained as part of the initial workup in most pediatric neurosurgery centers. The information needed for diagnosis and preparation for surgery is more effectively provided by magnetic resonance imaging (MRI) and computed tomography–myelography (CTM), and the resolution of x-ray images in children is frequently inadequate because of insufficient calcification or overlying gas and fecal shadows. However, they can provide valuable information in particular circumstances. They are useful for demonstrating sacral agenesis and segmentation anomalies, anomalous bone malformations, laminar defects, hemivertebrae, and the bony spur of diastematomyelia.

Standard radiographs may also be helpful in planning for surgery. Preoperative visualization of the extent and configuration of the spina bifida, of other vertebral defects, and of the location of the lowest normal lamina above the spina bifida (using a small radiography opaque marker) can help guide and limit the extent of surgical exposure.

Ultrasonography

This is an especially useful diagnostic tool for infants younger than 6 months because lipoma, CSF, and spinal cord each have different echogenic properties, and ultrasonography makes it possible to identify the lipoma and define its attachment to the spinal cord.[53, 54] In the infant, with its poorly calcified, immature bone, the echogenic ultrasound waves can pass easily through the spine. In many cases, it is a useful screening method to demonstrate tethering and the presence of a low conus with a thickened filum terminale. Spinal cord motion can also be displayed so that decreased motion, which signals tethering, can be detected. Ultrasonography is most useful for imaging when the neurological examination is normal but a subcutaneous lipoma or other cutaneous malformation that raises concern about the presence of a congenital lumbosacral lipoma is present. It can even be used diagnostically for imaging in a pregnant woman when the fetus has a dorsal lumbosacral mass.[49] The procedure is safe, easy to use, and relatively inexpensive, but it does not provide the information necessary for the operative procedure that is regularly obtained with MRI or CTM.

Magnetic Resonance Imaging

Now widely recognized to be the procedure of choice, MRI provides both a clear diagnosis and valuable preoperative information in the majority of cases.[55–57] The lipoma generates a high-intensity signal on T1-weighted images and thereby stands out prominently against spinal cord tissue and CSF; the signal on T2-weighted images is slightly less bright than that of CSF. On sagittal views, the fibrolipomatous stalk, the lipoma-cord interface, and the normal cord caudal to the interface are well demonstrated for type I lipomas; for type II lipomas, the interface is less well visualized, particularly at its intermediate and caudal end. On axial views, the lateral position and rotation of the spinal cord associated with type I or II lipomas and the contralateral meningocele are well displayed. With type II lipomas, the more oblique lipoma-cord interface is also better visualized on axial than on sagittal views, especially when the lipoma attachment is asymmetric. For type III lipomas, the terminal lipoma and low-lying conus and filum are well demonstrated on both sagittal and axial views.[58] Fat within a thickened filum terminale and the thickness of the filum can be readily appreciated. Contrast enhancement is only occasionally useful.

Computed Tomographic Scanning and Computed Tomography-Myelography

Computed tomographic scanning alone is of limited use because the spinal cord and other intraspinal contents are better visualized with MRI. However, computed tomographic scanning with three-dimensional reconstruction can be of considerable value in preoperative planning, because the relevant bony anatomy is displayed in exquisite detail. Precise configuration of the spina bifida is well shown, and other vertebral anomalies are seen in considerable detail. CTM is used to reveal complex structural details that even MRI fails to demonstrate adequately, such as the lipoma-cord interface in type II and type III lipomas when the interface is asymmetric. Using thin-slice, contiguous, axial CTM images and bone algorithms, nerve roots exiting the cord can be especially well displayed; it can frequently be determined whether they exit rostral to the lipoma, as would be anticipated with type III lesions. MRI sagittal views are more useful for this than is CTM, but CTM often provides more information than MRI on axial views. Obtaining studies using MRI, computed tomography (CT) with three-dimensional reconstruction, and CTM would provide the greatest amount of information, but this is costly and, with some exceptions, redundant.

Urodynamics and Other Studies of Urinary Tract Function

The evaluation of any child who exhibits one or more clinical signs of occult spinal dysraphism and, in particular, of any child who presents with bladder dysfunction should include urinalysis, blood chemistry panels, renal and bladder ultrasonography, cystogram, and urodynamics.

Urodynamic studies provide quantitative measurements of the processes that occur in the bladder and urethra during urinary storage and release, both pre- and postoperatively.[59] This is especially useful for neurogenic voiding dysfunction and therefore for patients with congenital lumbosacral lipomas and tethered spinal cords. These studies most often include cystometry, uroflowmetry, and electromyography (EMG). Cystometry records pressure changes during progressive bladder filling and subsequent emptying, and the relationship between detrusor muscle–generated pressure and bladder volume is demonstrated. Bladder contractility, compliance, sensation, and capacity can also be examined with this procedure. Uroflowmetry measures the volume of urine emptied over a given time and provides a graphic characterization of the patient's voiding pattern. EMG assesses the external urethral activity by direct needle electrode recording or recording after surface electrode placement over pelvic floor musculature. In response to spinal cord tethering, these studies usually demonstrate detrusor areflexia or hyperreflexia, and this often improves after surgery. Detrusor–external sphincter dyssynergia can also be identified and treated.

Somatosensory Evoked Potentials and Other Electrophysiologic Studies

Posterior tibial, peroneal, and pudendal somatosensory evoked potential (SSEP) studies can occasionally be useful in preoperative planning as part of an assessment of the extent and laterality of tethering produced by a congenital lumbosacral lipoma or an associated thickened filum.[60] The degree of reduction, unilaterally or bilaterally, in the cauda equina evoked potential (N11) or the first lumbar level potential (N14), in comparison to those recorded at higher levels, provides this information. A return of these N11 and N14 potentials to more normal values after surgery corresponds with successful release of tethering (lipoma removal and filum sectioning).[61, 62]

INDICATIONS FOR SURGERY

Indications for surgical treatment are (1) presence of a subcutaneous lipoma or characteristic cutaneous anomaly posteriorly over the lumbosacral spine in an otherwise asymptomatic infant older than 2 months with a lipoma-cord attachment demonstrated by neuroimaging; (2) development of neurological, orthopedic, or urologic impairment in a patient with congenital lumbosacral lipoma, particularly if that impairment is progressive; (3) congenital lumbosacral lipoma and likely tethering in a patient with progressive scoliosis who is being considered for corrective or stabilizing surgery with spinal instrumentation and fusion; and (4) severe and unrelenting dysesthetic low back, pelvic, perineal, or lower extremity pain in an adolescent or adult with congenital lumbosacral lipoma and spinal cord tethering.

OPERATIVE PROCEDURE

Surgical goals are to (1) detach spinal cord tethering structures by transection and excision of the lipoma and by division of all other tethering anomalies (e.g., thickened filum terminale, aberrant fibrous bands, anomalous nerve roots); (2) remove as much lipomatous mass as possible to relieve spinal cord or cauda equina compression, foster dorsal spinal cord reconstruction, and improve the patient's cosmetic appearance; (3) close the myeloschisis and reconstruct the posterior half of the spinal cord to obtain complete coverage of the neural tube with pia-arachnoid and thereby reduce the risk of postoperative spinal cord retethering; (4) prevent the development of new deficits and possibly recover previously lost function; (5) alleviate severe and unrelenting pain associated with the lipoma; and (6) make future corrective or stabilizing surgery for scoliosis or other orthopedic impairments safer by prophylactically removing any coincident lipoma and spinal cord tethering.

General anesthesia is administered without long-acting muscle relaxants so that a nerve stimulator or EMG, bladder, or anal monitoring can be used during the procedure. Measures are taken to provide for intra-operative EMG, SSEP, and sacral nerve function assessment using bladder or anal sphincter manometry. The patient is placed prone on horizontally positioned rolls, leaving the abdomen free to prevent epidural vein distention. The surgery is best performed using a surgical microscope with CO_2 laser attachment[63] and microinstrumentation. A Cavitron ultrasonic aspirator is also occasionally helpful, as is a monopolar nerve stimulator for intraoperatively distinguishing nerve root from fibrous band.

For type I lipomas, a midline linear vertical skin incision is made over the subcutaneous lipoma and is extended one to two vertebral levels rostral and caudal to it. A plane is established circumferentially around or through the relatively well-encapsulated edge of lipoma to the underlying deep lumbosacral fascia. The fascia-lipoma plane is then developed medially until the defect in the deep fascia, through which the lipomatous stalk passes, is identified and fully exposed and the stalk itself is well visualized. At this point, if preoperative neuroimaging studies do not show herniation of the lipoma-cord interface dorsal to the plane of the lumbosacral fascia, the stalk can be cautiously transected to improve access to the spine and visualization of the lipoma-cord interface. In an infant or young child, transection of the stalk in usually unnecessary, but in an adolescent or adult, when the subcutaneous lipoma is large, transection can helpful. Next, the opening one to two levels rostral to the stalk is extended down to normal dura and spinal cord, and the dura is opened in the midline or slightly toward the side of the stalk. This is carried out because it is essential to enter the area of the malformation from a site where the anatomy is normal so that the surgeon can establish and maintain proper anatomic orientation when entering more caudally into the more complex area of lipoma attachment and tethering. The dural opening is then further extended caudally until a thick, fibrovascular periosteal band passing transversely between the lateral edges of the first widely bifid lamina is encountered and, along with underlying dura, divided. Because it tightly compresses the dorsal surface of an already posteriorly displaced and tethered spinal cord, division of this band produces an immediate and substantial release of focal spinal cord compression and tethering and is therefore critical.[34] The dural opening is then further extended to the dura–stalk–spinal cord junction.

At this point, it important to pause and study the position of the spinal cord, the lipoma-cord interface, and all the structures related to them in order to plan the next step—the safe and complete detachment of the dura circumferentially from the lipoma-cord interface. It must be determined whether the lipoma-cord interface is within the spinal canal (ventrally or laterally displaced or rotated) or outside it and to locate the dorsal root entry zones. Once these anatomic relationships are delineated, the dura can be safely separated from the lipoma-cord interface. With lipomyeloceles, in which the lipoma-cord interface is within the spinal canal, this can be performed without difficulty. How-

ever, with lipomyelomeningoceles, in which the spinal cord is distracted out of the spinal canal along with dura and dorsal root entry zones, special care must be taken to protect the dorsal root entry zones and roots. This requires exposing the dura-stalk-cord junction by first removing lipoma and fascia around it until it is entirely exposed and the underlying dorsal root entry zones are well visualized. The dural incision is then continued below the lipoma-cord interface, with midline extension caudally as far as necessary to establish whether there is a thickened filum terminale (surgical division of the thickened filum is covered later in this section). The dural edges are then retracted bilaterally with stay sutures, maximizing the exposure and identification of all intradural structures.

The stalk (and subcutaneous portion of lipoma, if it has not already been removed) can now be divided just peripheral to its attachment to the cord, either sharply or with the CO_2 laser,[63] and the lipoma can be removed. This is performed as completely as possible, but without placing the underlying spinal cord tissue or nerve roots at high risk for injury. With lipomyeloceles, a thorough removal of lipoma and release of tethering of the underlying cord are performed, sharply or with the CO_2 laser, usually without difficulty. The stalk is divided just above the lipoma-cord interface, and because these lipomas are hamartomas rather than tumors, and recurrence is therefore unlikely, a small margin of lipoma is left to prevent any damage to the cord. Occasionally, it is difficult or impossible to achieve stalk transection and lipoma removal. This is the case when an intradural lipoma compresses the spinal cord and displaces it ventrally, and the nerve roots exiting at the lipoma-cord interface pass dorsally and caudally through it. In such a situation, it may be impossible to accomplish anything safely, and the surgery must be concluded. However, in many cases, a significant decompression can be achieved, and the patient's neurological status can be stabilized or even improved. With lipomyelomeningoceles, once the lipoma-cord interface and dorsal root entry zones have been thoroughly exposed, transection of the stalk becomes an easier task and is carried out sharply or with the CO_2 laser.

If the spinal cord is rotated and laterally displaced either intradurally or extradurally, the same approach is followed, but there are additional concerns to address. A focal arachnoiditis that binds the ipsilateral cord surface, roots, and fibrolipomatous stalk to leptomeninges and dura is usually encountered and must be systematically taken down, and all tethering fibers must be lysed before cord-lipoma detachment. The ipsilateral roots are shorter, more ventrally situated, and buried in scar and can be a source of persistent tethering. The contralateral roots are longer and more dorsally displaced, just under the dura, where they can easily be injured during initial dural opening. A contralateral dorsal protrusion of a meningocele further compounds the risk of nerve root injury. Therefore, the attachment of arachnoid as well as dura above the dorsal root entry zones must be well visualized so that the roots are protected during dural and arachnoid opening. If any additional lipoma remains that can be safely removed, this is now resected or evaporated using the laser. For all these type I lipomas, any extension of the lipoma into the central canal causing spinal cord expansion, similar to that seen with intramedullary tumors, can also be resected now. This is carried out subtotally but extensively enough to provide an adequate decompression.

Once all resectable lipoma has been removed, the lateral edges of the myeloschisis are brought together dorsally in the midline to reconstruct the tubular shape of the spinal cord and are held together with 7–0 nonabsorbable sutures through the pia mater. This is performed to reduce the risk of postoperative retethering. If the filum is thickened (diameter >2 mm),[64] it is now divided. This is carried out even if it does not appear tense, because the patient's prone position on the table may mask any tension that is present, especially with flexion. It may be particularly difficult to locate the filum when there is lateral cord displacement and arachnoiditis, but a meticulous search for it is essential, because recurrent tethering years later is not uncommon (Fig. 204–10). The release of tethering is completed with a thorough search for any other dysraphic anomalies, aberrant nerve roots, or fibrous bands that can be divided or lysed. Once hemostasis is achieved, the dura is closed. Preservative-free morphine sulfate (Duramorph) may be instilled intradurally or epidurally to reduce postoperative pain. A dural closure using a continuous, nonabsorbable suture is performed if this can be accomplished without restricting the surrounding subarachnoid space. Otherwise, it is essential to impose autologous fascia, lyophilized dura, bovine pericardium, or other graft material between the tight dural edges. A watertight closure is essential.

Type II lipomas are more difficult to remove because the relationship between the lipoma-cord interface and the dorsal root entry zones becomes less predictable as the lipoma removal extends caudally; therefore, the risk of injury to exiting nerve roots increases substantially. The same general approach described earlier is

followed, but as the lipoma-cord interface becomes more ventral and caudal, the dorsal root entry zones frequently lie dorsal to it, and the exiting roots become enmeshed in lipoma. Therefore, the line of lipomatous stalk detachment must pass through the lipoma above the exiting dorsal roots until the conus is reached, at which point the lipoma can be separated from the conus just caudal to it and to the lowest functioning roots. In these cases, the relationship between the lipoma-cord interface and dorsal root entry zones is variable and unpredictable, and the interface itself is more diffuse (see Fig. 204–7). Therefore, complete removal of the lipoma is dangerous and should not be attempted, because it can easily cause injury to the conus and leave the patient with urinary and fecal incontinence. This is especially true when the lipoma attachment is asymmetric and the relationship between the lipoma-cord interface and dorsal root entry zones is even more difficult to follow. A small cuff of lipoma should be left. Occasionally, small nerve roots that pass through the lipoma are encountered. It is helpful to assess, with SSEP or EMG recording[60, 61, 65] or with direct nerve stimulation and bladder or anal monitoring,[8, 66, 67] whether these are actively functioning ventral or motor nerve roots that, if divided, would cause weakness in a lower extremity or sacral muscle, or whether they are sensory or nonfunctional and can safely be divided.

With type III lipomas arising from the conus, the same procedure is followed, with a similarly conservative lipoma detachment. This is easier to carry out than with type II lipomas because the dura is not attached to the lipoma-cord interface but passes to the S4 level, where it normally terminates. The lipoma is divided just caudal to the last exiting functional nerve roots. As with type II lipomas, and for the same reasons, complete removal should not be attempted; here, too, a small cuff of lipoma should be left. Sometimes, the nerve roots of the cauda equina have merely been displaced by the lipoma and can be separated from it, allowing the main body of the lipoma to be removed.

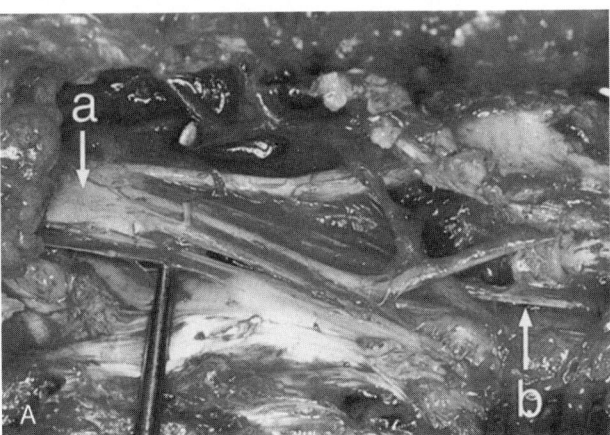
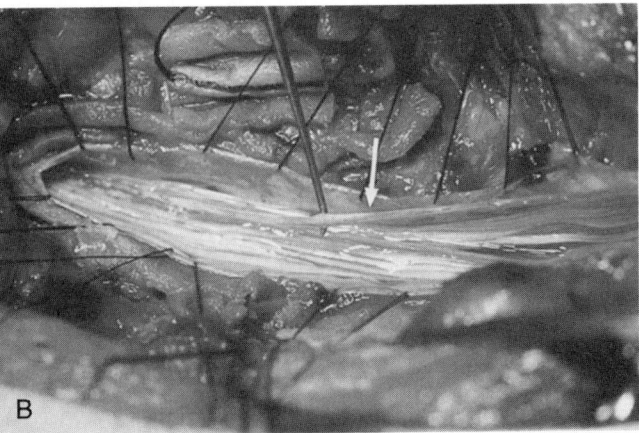

FIGURE 204–10. *A,* Intraoperative photomicrograph of an eccentric type I lipoma during resection. The conus (a) and nerve roots of the cauda equina are displaced laterally and enmeshed by scarring from arachnoiditis. A probable thickened filum terminale (b) was not identified or divided. *B,* Six years later, after new symptoms developed, the now markedly tight filum terminale is evident.

When this is not the case, when the nerve roots are not separable or are engulfed within the lipoma, it is not possible to remove the bulk of the lipoma. Separation of the lipoma from the conus without removal may nevertheless be possible and may release tethering of the cord. Occasionally, even that may not be possible.

The next step is to follow the laminectomy and dural opening caudally until it can be determined whether there is a defect in the dura at its termination through which the lipoma passes to become a subcutaneous mass or a thickened filum. If a filum is identified, it is divided intradurally, just rostral to the termination of the dural sac. The conus may be markedly enlarged secondary to development of a terminal syringohydromyelia.[68, 69] In that case, a needle is passed into the latter for drainage just before dural closure, or a midline dorsal myelotomy is performed.[69]

Lipomas of the filum terminale, those that do not extend to the conus, are removed through a small laminectomy based over the lesion. The filum terminale proximal and distal to the lipoma is identified and, if necessary, can frequently be distinguished from surrounding nerve roots by intraoperative nerve stimulation. Any adherent nerve roots are separated from the lipoma. The filum is then divided, and the lipoma is removed. If the nerve roots cannot safely be separated from the lipoma, the filum is divided caudal to the lipoma and roots to at least release the tethering produced by it.

Once the dura has been closed, primarily or with the aid of a suitable graft, meticulous hemostasis is obtained, and the paravertebral musculature, deep fascia, and subcutaneous tissue are closed in anatomic layers. Large fascial or myocutaneous flaps are sometimes necessary to fill the cavity left after subcutaneous lipoma removal. Excess skin can be trimmed, and a subcuticular closure of the skin with sterile adhesive strips (Steri-Strips) or a closure with running nylon suture is performed. A pressure dressing is applied, and the patient is kept prone or on the side for at least 72 hours. If fluid accumulates subcutaneously, it can be tapped and a new pressure dressing placed. If this fails, re-exploration of the wound for repair of a dural CSF leak or placement of a cyst-peritoneal shunt usually suffices.

Postoperatively, careful, regular follow-up assessments must be carried out, including detailed musculoskeletal evaluations and routine urologic studies. If any deterioration in neurological function is detected, an MRI scan is obtained. Although ascent of the conus after the first surgery usually is not fully achieved, retethering of the spinal cord and hydromyelia is not unusual, and a previously missed source of tethering is sometimes found.

COMPLICATIONS

The presence of new neurological deficits in the postoperative period has become much less common since the 1980s as new information about the anatomy, embryology, and physiology of congenital lumbosacral lipomas has become available and surgical techniques and instrumentation have improved. In recent studies, no mortality and only a 1.6% rate of neurological injury were reported.[47] However, complications associated with wound closure continue to be a problem.[70] Synthetic graft material for dural closure is useful for reducing retethering, but it is difficult to obtain a lasting watertight closure with it, and CSF in the large subcutaneous pocket left after lipoma removal is common. Wound dehiscence and meningitis are not uncommon.

Retethering is clearly the most significant long-term complication, but it is seen in only 10% to 20.2% of reported cases, depending on the length of follow-up after the initial surgery. It is seen most often in patients previously operated on for lumbosacral lipomas, with those having type II lipomas constituting the largest group. Children with retethering generally become symptomatic between ages 3 and 8, 11 to 22 months after their first surgery. The most common symptoms are low back and leg pain, lower extremity weakness, foot deformities, and urinary incontinence.[47, 48, 71, 72] Determining whether retethering has occurred is difficult. MRI or other neuroimaging is not helpful, because termination of the conus at an abnormally low level almost always persists, to some degree, after the initial surgery. Therefore, decision-making regarding the need for a second surgical procedure must be based primarily on clinical findings, with neuroimaging used only to confirm that the conus ends at a low level. After reoperation and release of all tethering, the patient's neurological deficits are generally stabilized and often improved. Pain is the most successfully alleviated symptom. A small subset of patients requires repeated operations for retethering, and each subsequent operation becomes more difficult because of the development of extensive postoperative arachnoiditis.[72] To date, tight closure of the dural sac and incomplete release of all tethering structures are the only identified, statistically significant causes of retethering.[72]

OUTCOME

Surgical excision of congenital lumbosacral lipomas and release of tethering generally provide a superior clinical outcome. In a series of eight studies that addressed this issue, lipomas arising from the spinal cord were considered separately from those arising from the filum terminale, and the clinical outcome of asymptomatic patients operated on prophylactically was considered separately from the outcome of those who were symptomatic at the time of surgery. Nearly all the neurologically normal children (95%) retained normal motor, sensory, and bladder function postoperatively for up to 20 years. In contrast, among children with preoperative motor, sensory, or bladder deficits, only about half (51%) experienced improvement in function; slightly fewer (46%) were stabilized. Recovery of bladder continence was the most difficult outcome to achieve and was obtained in only 13%, and then only partially. Recovery of complete bladder function was never achieved.[2, 32, 47, 48, 73–75]

In another long-term (6.6 years) study of patients

with lipomas arising from the spinal cord, only 5 of 71 initially normal patients lost function after surgery; the rest (66) remained clinically normal. Nine of 71 required subsequent surgery, after which 4 regained normal clinical function. In the same study, 87 patients who had already developed deficits fared much worse. A significant number (23%) deteriorated, and half (51%) remained at their preoperative clinical state. A large number (41%) required subsequent surgery, and a small number of those (26%) improved or returned to their preoperative clinical status.[76, 77]

Surgical management of patients with lipomas arising from the filum terminale offers a better outcome. In the same study, all patients who were clinically normal at the time of surgery remained so, and more than half of the patients with preoperative deficits (5 of 9) returned to normal clinical status. None deteriorated.[76, 77]

Studies that focused on bladder function further emphasize the importance of early, prophylactic surgery. In those studies, all infants younger than 18 months with normal bladder function preoperatively retained that normal function after surgery, and most of those (75% to 83%) with preoperatively abnormal urodynamic studies regained normal urologic function. However, in patients older than 18 months, surgery was much less successful. Only 38% of those who were normal before surgery remained normal after surgery, and none who had deficits preoperatively regained normal bladder function.[73, 74, 78]

CONCLUSIONS

The surgical management of congenital lumbosacral lipoma is now remarkably safe and effective. This is because we have greatly enhanced our understanding of the embryology and the resulting distorted anatomy and physiology of these lesions and their patterns of clinical presentation. It is the integration of all this information, along with major advancements in imaging and intraoperative technology, that has allowed us to formulate the optimal surgical approach and more regularly provide a good surgical outcome. We can operate prophylactically in neurologically normal infants and prevent the inevitable appearance of neurological deficits rather than struggle, often fruitlessly, to retrieve lost neurological function.

In contrast to the earlier reluctance to intervene surgically when the patient was neurologically normal, everything now known about congenital lumbosacral lipoma points to the fact that children born with this malformation require surgical intervention to relieve both compression and tethering as early as possible, before the appearance of any neurological deficits.

For a long time, the outlook for a normal life in patients born with congenital lumbrosacral lipoma was bleak, but today, it is enormously improved. Most patients operated on prophylactically can have the malformation corrected and thereby look forward to a normal life, and those operated on later can look forward to a substantial improvement in the quality of life.

REFERENCES

1. Bruce D, Schut L: Spinal lipomas in infancy and childhood. Childs Brain 5:192–203, 1979.
2. Hoffman HJ, Taecholarn C, Hendrick EB, et al: Management of lipomyelomeningoceles: Experience at the Hospital for Sick Children, Toronto. J Neurosurg 62:1–8, 1985.
3. Schut L, Bruce D, Sutton L: The management of the child with a lipomyelomeningocele. Clin Neurosurg 30:464–476, 1983.
4. Reigel DH, McLone DG: Tethered spinal cord. In Cheek WR, Marlin AE, McLone DG, et al (eds): Pediatric Neurosurgery: Surgery of the Developing Nervous System. Philadelphia, WB Saunders, 1994, pp 77–95.
5. Dubowitz V, Lorber J, Zachary RB: Lipoma of the cauda equina. Arch Dis Child 40:207–213, 1969.
6. Matson DD: Neurosurgery of infancy and childhood, 2nd ed. Springfield, Ill, Charles C. Thomas, 1969, p 46.
7. Till K: Spinal dysraphism: A study of congenital malformations of the back. Dev Med Child Neurol 10:470–477, 1968.
8. Chapman PH, Beyerl B: The tethered spinal cord, with particular reference to spinal lipoma and diastematomyelia. In Hoffman HJ, Epstein F (eds): Disorders of the Developing Nervous System: Diagnosis and Treatment. Boston, Blackwell Scientific, 1986, pp 109–131.
9. Lassman LP, James CCM: Lumbosacral lipomas: Critical surgery of 26 cases submitted to laminectomy. J Neurol Neurosurg Psychiatry 30:174–181, 1967.
10. McLone DG, Mutluer S, Naidich TP: Lipomeningoceles of the conus medullaris. In Raimondi AJ (ed): Concepts in Pediatric Neurosurgery, vol 3. Basel, Karger, 1983, pp 170–177.
11. Chapman PH: Congenital intraspinal lipomas: Anatomic considerations and surgical treatment. Childs Brain 9:37–47, 1982.
12. Chapman PH, Davis KR: Surgical treatment of spinal lipomas in childhood. In Raimondi AJ (ed): Concepts in Pediatric Neurosurgery, vol 3. Basel, Karger, 1983, pp 178–190.
13. Pang D: Tethered cord syndrome. In Wilkins RH, Rengachary SS (eds): Neurosurgery, 2nd ed. New York, McGraw-Hill, 1996, pp 3465–3496.
14. Iskandar BJ, Oakes WJ, McLaughlin C, et al: Terminal syringohydromyelia and occult spinal dysraphism. J Neurosurg 81:513–519, 1994.
15. Oakes WJ: Management of spinal cord lipomas and lipomyelomeningoceles. In Wilkins R, Rengachary S (eds): Neurosurgery Update II: Vascular, Spinal, Pediatric and Functional Neurosurgery. New York, McGraw-Hill, 1991, pp 345–352.
16. Kanev PM, Berger MS: Lipomyelomeningocele and myelocystocele. In Youmans JR (ed): Neurological Surgery, 4th ed. Philadelphia, WB Saunders, 1996, pp 861–872.
17. Pang D, Hoffman H: Sacral agenesis with progressive neurological deficits. Neurosurgery 7:118–126, 1980.
18. Warf BC, Scott RM, Barnes PD: Tethered spinal cord in patients with anorectal and urogenital malformations. Pediatr Neurosurg 19:25–30, 1993.
19. Lemire RJ, Loeser JD, Alvord EC Jr, et al: Normal and Abnormal Development of the Human Nervous System. Hagerstown, Md, Harper & Row, 1975, pp 71–83.
20. McLone DG, Diaz MS: Normal and abnormal early development of the nervous system. In Cheek WR, Marlin AE, McLone DG, et al (eds): Pediatric Neurosurgery: Surgery of the Developing Nervous System, 3rd ed. Philadelphia, WB Saunders, 1994, pp 3–39.
21. Schoenwolf GC: Histological and ultrastructural studies of secondary neurulation in mouse embryos. Am J Anat 169:361–376, 1984.
22. Van Allen ML, Kalousek DK, Chernoff GF, et al: Evidence for multi-site closure of the neural tube in humans. Am J Med Genet 47:723–743, 1993.
23. O'Rahilly R, Meyer DB: The timing and sequence of events in the development of the human vertebral column during the embryonic period proper. Anat Embryol (Berl) 157:167–176, 1979.
24. Muller F, O'Rahilly R: The development of the human brain, the closure of the caudal neuropore, and the beginning of secondary neurulation at stage 12. Anat Embryol (Berl) 176:413–430, 1987.
25. Sutton LN: Lipomyelomeningocele. Neurosurg Clin N Am 6:325–338, 1995.

26. French BN: The embryology of spinal dysraphism. Clin Neurosurg 30:295–365, 1983.

27. McLone DG, Naidich TP: Spinal dysraphism: Experimental and clinical. In Holzmann RN, Stein BM (eds): The Tethered Spinal Cord. New York, Thieme-Stratton, 1985, pp 3–15.

28. Alston SR, Fuller GN, Boyko OB, et al: Ectopic renal tissue in a lumbosacral lipoma: Pathologic and radiologic findings. Pediatr Neurosci 15:100–103, 1989.

29. Walsh JW, Markesbery WR: Histological features of congenital lipomas of the lower spinal cord. J Neurosurg 52:564–569, 1980.

30. French BN: Embryological aspects of the tethered cord syndrome and its relationship to spinal dysraphism. In Yamada S (ed): Tethered Cord Syndrome. Park Ridge, Ill, American Association of Neurological Surgeons, 1996, pp 5–20.

31. Emery JL, Lendon RG: Lipomas of the cauda equina and other fatty tumours related to neurospinal dysraphism. Dev Med Child Neurol Suppl 20:62–70, 1969.

32. Hakuba A, Fujitani K, Hoda K, et al: Lumbo-sacral lipoma, the timing of the operation and morphological classification. Neuro-orthopedics 2:34–42, 1986.

33. Walsh JW: Surgical management of congenital lumbosacral lipoma. Contemp Neurosurg 7:1–8, 1985.

34. Naidich TP, McLone DG, Mutluer S: A new understanding of dorsal dysraphism with lipoma (lipomyeloschisis): Radiologic evaluation and surgical correction. AJR Am J Roentgenol 140:1065–1078, 1984.

35. Friedrich W, Shurtleff D, Shaffer J: Cognitive abilities and lipomyelomeningocele. Psychol Rep 73:467–470, 1993.

36. Estin D, Cohen AR: Caudal agenesis and associated caudal spinal cord malformations. Surg Clin North Am 6:377–391, 1995.

37. Barson AJ: The vertebral level of termination of the spinal cord during normal and abnormal development. J Anat 106:489–497, 1970.

38. Kunitomo K: The development and reduction of the tail and caudal end of the spinal cord. Contrib Embryol 8:161–198, 1918.

39. Streeter GL: Factors involved in the formation of the filum terminale. Am J Anat 25:1–12, 1919.

40. Yamada S, Iacono R, Andrade T, et al: Pathophysiology of tethered cord syndrome. Neurosurg Clin N Am 6:311–323, 1995.

41. Yamada S, Schneider S, Ashwall S, et al: Pathophysiologic mechanisms in the tethered spinal cord syndrome. In Holtzman RN, Stein BM (eds): The Tethered Spinal Cord. New York, Thieme-Stratton, 1985, pp 29–40.

42. Yamada S, Zinke DE, Sanders D: Pathophysiology of "tethered cord syndrome." J Neurosurg 54:494–503, 1981.

43. Kang JK, Kim MC, King DS, et al: Effects of tethering on regional spinal cord blood flow and sensory-evoked potentials in growing cats. Childs Nerv Syst 3:35–39, 1987.

44. Schneider SJ, Rosenthal AD, Greenberg BM, et al: A preliminary report on the use of laser-Doppler flowmetry during tethered spinal cord release. Neurosurgery 32:214–217, 1993.

45. Yamada S, Iacono RP, Yamada BS: Pathophysiology of the tethered spinal cord. In Yamada S (ed): Tethered Spinal Cord. Park Ridge, Ill, American Association of Neurological Surgeons, 1996, pp 29–48.

46. Yamada S, Knierim D, Yonekura M: Tethered cord syndrome. J Am Paraplegia Soc 6:58–61, 1983.

47. Kanev PM, Lemire RJ, Loeser JD, et al: Management and long-term follow-up review of children with lipomyelomeningocele, 1952–1987. J Neurosurg 73:48–52, 1990.

48. Pierre-Kahn A, Lacombe J, Pichon J, et al: Intraspinal lipomas with spina bifida: Prognosis and treatment in 73 cases. J Neurosurg 65:756–761, 1986.

49. Seeds J, Powers S: Early prenatal diagnosis of familial lipomyelomeningocele. Obstet Gynecol 72:469–471, 1988.

50. Loeser JD, Lewin RJ: Lumbosacral lipoma in an adult (case report). J Neurosurg 29:405–409, 1968.

51. Lunardi P, Missori P, Ferrante L, et al: Long-term results of surgical treatment of spinal lipomas: Report of 18 cases. Acta Neurochir (Wien) 104:64–68, 1990.

52. Pang D, Wilberger JE: Tethered cord syndrome in adults. J Neurosurg 57:32–47, 1982.

53. Naidich TP, Fernbach SK, McLone DG, et al: John Caffey Award. Sonography of the caudal spine and back: Congenital anomalies in children. AJNR Am J Neuroradiol 5:221–234, 1984.

54. Naidich TP, McLone DG: Ultrasonography versus computer tomography. In Holtzman R, Stein B (eds): The Tethered Spinal Cord. New York, Thieme-Stratton, 1985, pp 47–58.

55. Brophy J, Sutton L, Zimmerman R, et al: Magnetic resonance imaging of lipomyelomeningocele surgery. Neurosurgery 25:336–340, 1989.

56. Komiyama M, Hakuba A, Inoue Y, et al: Magnetic resonance imaging: Lumbosacral lipoma. Surg Neurol 28:259–264, 1987.

57. Lantos G, Epstein R, Kory LA: Magnetic resonance imaging of intradural spinal lipoma. Neurosurgery 20:469–472, 1987.

58. Wippold GJ, Citrin C, Barkovich AJ, et al: Evaluation of MR in spinal dysraphism with lipoma: Comparison with metrizamide computed tomography. Pediatr Radiol 17:184–188, 1987.

59. Hadley R, Holevas RE: Lower urinary tract dysfunction in tethered cord syndrome. In Yamada S (ed): Tethered Cord Syndrome. Park Ridge, Ill, American Association of Neurological Surgeons, 1993, pp 79–88.

60. Pang D: Intraoperative neurophysiological monitoring of the lower sacral nerve roots and spinal cord. In Yamada S (ed): Tethered Cord Syndrome. Park Ridge, Ill, American Association of Neurological Surgeons, 1993, pp 135–147.

61. Gilmore RL, Walsh J: The clinical neurophysiology of tethered cord syndrome and other dysraphic syndromes. In Yamada S (ed): Tethered Cord Syndrome. Park Ridge, Ill, American Association of Neurological Surgeons, 1996, pp 167–182.

62. Roy MW, Gilmore R, Walsh JW: Evaluation of children and young adults with tethered cord syndrome. Surg Neurol 26:241–248, 1986.

63. McLone DG, Naidich TP: Laser resection of fifty spinal lipomas. Neurosurgery 18:611–615, 1986.

64. Naidich TP, McLone DG: Congenital pathology of the spine and spinal cord. In Taveras JD, Ferrucci JT (eds): Radiology. Philadelphia, JB Lippincott, 1986, pp 1–23.

65. Phillips LH, Park TS: Electrophysiological monitoring during lipomyelomeningocele resection. Muscle Nerve 13:127–132, 1990.

66. James HE, Mulcahy JJ, Walsh JW, et al: Use of anal sphincter electromyography during operations on the conus medullaris and sacral nerve roots. Neurosurgery 4:521–523, 1979.

67. Pang D, Casey K: Use of an anal sphincter pressure monitor during operations on the sacral spinal cord and nerve roots. Neurosurgery 13:562–568. 1983.

68. McLone DG, Naidich TP: Terminal myelocystocele. Neurosurgery 16:36–43, 1985.

69. Oakes WJ: Tethered spinal cord, intramedullary spinal lipoma, and lipomyelomeningocele. In Rengachary SS, Wilkins RH (eds): Neurosurgical Operative Atlas, 1st ed. Chicago, American Association of Neurological Surgeons, 1992, pp 133–141.

70. Zide BM: How to reduce the morbidity of wound closure following extensive and complicated laminectomy and tethered cord surgery. Pediatr Neurosurg 18:157–166, 1992.

71. Herman JM, McLone DG, Storrs BB, et al: Analysis of 153 patients with myelomeningocele or spinal lipoma reoperated upon for a tethered cord. Pediatr Neurosurg 19:243–249, 1993.

72. Colak A, Pollack IF, Albright AL: Recurrent tethering: A common long-term problem after lipomyelomeningocele repair. Pediatr Neurosurg 29:184–190, 1998.

73. Atala A, Bauer SB, Dyro FM, et al: Bladder functional changes resulting from lipomyelomeningocele repair. J Urol 148:592–594, 1992.

74. Foster LS, Kogan BA, Cogen PH, et al: Bladder function in patients with lipomyelomeningocele. J Urol 143:984–986, 1990.

75. Harrison MJ, Mitnick RJ, Rosenbluth BR, et al: Leptomyelolipoma: Analysis of 20 cases. J Neurosurg 73:360–367, 1990.

76. Byrne RW, Hayes EA, George TM, et al: Operative resection of 100 spinal lipomas in infants less than 1 year of age. Pediatr Neurosurg 23:182–187, 1995.

77. LaMarca F, Grant JA, Tomita T, et al: Spinal lipomas in children—outcome of 270 procedures. Pediatr Neurosurg 26:8–16, 1997.

78. Sathi S, Madsen JR, Bauer S, et al: Effect of surgical repair on neurological function in infants with lipomeningocele. Pediatr Neurosurg 19:256–259, 1993.

CHAPTER 205

Tethered Spinal Cord

BENJAMIN C. WARF

After Virchow coined the term *spina bifida occulta* in 1875, the awareness that this entity could be associated with progressive neurological deficits and orthopedic deformities developed only gradually. Observers in the early 20th century disputed whether the two phenomena were even related. Brickner, in 1918, reported attempts at removing intraspinal lipomas in three patients and was an early advocate of prophylactic surgery, but it was not until the middle of the 20th century that series reporting the operative repair of specific congenital anomalies that tethered the spinal cord were published. Operative series of diastematomyelia, lipomyelomeningocele, and tight filum terminale were first reported by Matson, Bassett, and Garceau, respectively, within 3 years of one another. The idea that the progressive deficit was caused by spinal cord stretching was a recurrent theme in these and subsequent reports, but it was not until the 1980s that scientific investigation began to elucidate the pathophysiology.

This chapter reviews the history, embryology, pathophysiology, clinical presentation, and management of tethering of the spinal cord by a "tight" or thickened, fatty filum terminale.

HISTORY

The concept that the spinal cord can be congenitally fixed, or tethered, at one point, leading to progressive neurological and urologic dysfunction and orthopedic abnormalities, has been in the process of development for almost 150 years.

Although Brickner once suggested that "the satyrs of the ancients may well have been suggested by instances of spina bifida occulta with short sacral 'tails' and club-feet,"[1] the first description in the medical literature appears to have been in 1857, when Johnson published *Fatty Tumor from the Sacrum of a Child Connected with the Spinal Membranes.*[2] In 1875, Virchow coined the term *spina bifida occulta* to delineate the skin-covered variety as opposed to the open defect.[3] Recklinghausen, in 1886, described a subcutaneous lipoma extending into the intradural space and connecting with the conus.[4] In 1892, Virchow and Maas related

the coexistence of hypertrichosis and occult spina bifida in *The Woman with the Horse's Mane,* who was reportedly a sideshow attraction[5]; however, Brickner credits Recklinghausen with being the first to suggest this association.[1] Such descriptions of what were considered curiosities initiated what was to become a growing literature on the subject over the next century.

In 1891, what may well have been the first successful surgery for spinal cord untethering was performed. Jones, in Manchester, England, published a report in the *British Medical Journal* from the Manchester Royal Infirmary entitled *Spina Bifida Occulta: No Paralytic Symptoms until Seventeen Years of Age: Spine Trephined to Relieve Pressure on the Cauda Equina: Recovery.*[6] It is, however, difficult to determine the exact pathologic anatomy of the dysraphism from the brief operative description.

In 1909, Fuchs described the association of enuresis, reflex and sensory abnormalities, and foot deformities with spina bifida occulta as determined by x-rays under the term *myelodysplasia,* which he coined.[7] Anything more than a chance association between spina bifida occulta and these neurological abnormalities was disputed at the time.[8] But Peritz, in 1911, supported the notion that the two were indeed related.[9] In 1916, Spiller suggested that sacral root stretching in patients with spina bifida occulta might be responsible.[8]

In 1918, Brickner, a surgeon at Mt. Sinai Hospital in New York, reported the attempted removal of intraspinal lipomas in three patients with spina bifida occulta who had presented with unrelenting trophic ulcerations of the feet and "sensory paralysis" involving the lower extremities.[1] Based on his experience, he advocated surgery in "infants and children [with] spina bifida occulta with congenital lipoma or hypertrichosis, even though without any symptoms . . . in the hope of obviating the development of symptoms during adolescence." He ascribed the symptoms, in part, to stretching of herniated nerves with the ascent of the spinal cord during development.

In 1928, de Vries published *Spina Bifida Occulta and Myelodysplasia with Unilateral Clubfoot Beginning in Adult Life* from the Peking Union Medical College.[10] The 30-year-old man described in the report had a history of urinary incontinence and kyphoscoliosis and developed progressive equinovarus deformity at age 27. On presentation, he also manifested unilateral wasting of the lower leg musculature. In the operation described, laminectomies were performed, but the dura was not opened. No outcome was mentioned, and no explanation of the symptoms was given; however, surgery was advocated "in every progressive case."

Lichtenstein, at the University of Illinois, apparently first used the term *spinal dysraphism* in a publication in 1940.[11] He then published *Distant Neuroanatomic Complications of Spina Bifida (Spinal Dysraphism)* in 1942, in which he suggested that a congenitally short cauda equina would cause retention of the infantile position of the conus medullaris, subsequently leading to development of the Arnold-Chiari malformation secondary to caudal fixation of the spinal cord and its resulting traction on the hindbrain.[12]

In 1943, Ingraham and Lowrey reported on 65 patients with spina bifida occulta, 22 of whom underwent intraspinal exploration.[13] Of these, five had intra- and extradural lipomas, two had intradural lipomas, and two had bifid spinal cords. Ingraham held to the idea that these lesions prevented "the normal movement of the caudal end of the spinal cord with growth." He advocated surgery only in those cases in which there was a definite history of "progressive difficulty" and stated that "it seems justifiable to consider a result as good . . . if no further progression of symptoms occurs."

It was not until 1950 that significant series of surgical experience with specific types of occult dysraphic anomalies began to appear in the literature. Hilal and coauthors cite Ollivier as having coined the term *diastematomyelia* in 1837[14]; however, it was Matson and coauthors who reported the first surgical series of 11 patients with diastematomyelia in 1950.[15] They cited seven previous case reports in the literature; in only one of those cases (that reported by Pickles[16]) had a preoperative diagnosis been made and subsequent surgery undertaken. It was also in 1950 that Bassett, at the University of Michigan, wrote, "not a rare type of anomaly seems to have been by-passed since little concerning its specific management and troublesome sequelae is apparent in the literature."[17] He was describing the lipomyelomeningocele, although he did not use this term, which would not appear for some 20 years, when coined by Rogers and coauthors in 1971.[18]

In 1952, Garceau of Indiana University Medical School reported to the Joint Meeting of the Orthopedic Associations in London on what he regarded as a previously unreported entity, the filum terminale syndrome or cord-traction syndrome. His report was published the following year.[19] He described three patients being followed for spinal curves (one congenital scoliosis, one idiopathic scoliosis, one kyphosis secondary to spinal tuberculosis) who experienced neurological deterioration that was ascribed to a thick filum terminale discovered at surgical exploration. No imaging studies were described that directed the diagnosis. All patients experienced recovery after sectioning of the filum. One patient was noted to have a low-lying conus (S2), but the conus level was not known in the others.

In another patient, the cut ends of the filum separated by 1 cm on severing. Oddly, the symptoms of one of these patients included nausea, vomiting, dizziness, headaches, pain and weakness in the upper extremities with absent reflexes, and spastic weakness in the lower extremities. "Almost complete recovery" was reported after sectioning the thick filum terminale. Citing the work by Lichtenstein mentioned earlier,[12] Garceau believed the tight filum to have distant effects on the rostral cord and hindbrain. "A tight filum terminale may cause the cord-traction symptoms known as the Arnold-Chiari syndrome. . . . The tight filum terminale may cause spinal-cord compression over an angulated spine. It may also cause cord traction, pulling the hind brain into the foramen magnum. . . . Decompression of the foramen magnum could have given the same result." This proposed relationship between the tight filum and "hindbrain herniation" was, however, disproved by further investigation.

Four years later, in 1956, Jones and Love at the Mayo Clinic published *Tight Filum Terminale*, describing improvement in lower extremity and urologic dysfunction after sectioning of a tight filum based on the clinical picture and spina bifida occulta seen on radiographs.[20] They also noted a separation of the cut ends of the filum, suggesting that it had been under tension. In contrast to the pathophysiology proposed by Garceau,[19] these authors suggested that an intrinsic failure of the filum terminale to elongate produced tension on the caudal spinal cord. They described spinal cords removed at necropsy in which "pulling on the filum terminale with the proximal end of the spinal cord fixed produces an elongation and narrowing in all transverse directions of the conus medullaris and, to a less extent, the lumbar enlargement." They also observed narrowing of the surface vessels with this maneuver. Thus, with failure of the filum to elongate properly with spinal growth and development of lumbar lordosis, as the conus-to-sacrum distance increases, "any fixation of the lower end of the cord will produce disturbances of function by increasing tension on the cord." The authors hypothesized that continued traction would produce "degenerative changes in the cells and fibers in the lower part of the spinal cord." In terms of management of congenital spinal anomalies, they suggested that Boettcher's[21] recommendation that exploration be done prophylactically was "an extreme view and is not held today." The authors cited Katzenstein[22] as advocating the delay of surgical management until "the onset of secondary changes." They stated, "Any patient with symptoms and signs of a progressive lesion should be given the benefit of surgical exploration." The association in children of pes cavus and tight filum terminale was reported in 1964 by Schlegel.[23]

In a classic paper published in 1976, Hoffman and colleagues in Toronto coined the term *tethered spinal cord* to specifically apply to a low conus with a thickened filum terminale measuring 2 mm or more in diameter.[24] The use of this term has broadened with time to include a spinal cord that is tethered by a variety of lesions, although these authors specifically excluded lipomyelomeningocele, meningocele, myelo-meningocele, diastematomyelia, and "intraspinal space occupying dysraphic conditions." The authors pointed out the evolution of the use of this term in a later article.[25] This series of 31 patients was a clear and definitive presentation of the clinical and radiographic presentation, operative findings, and outcome.

EMBRYOLOGY AND PATHOLOGY

Development of a tight filum terminale may arise from defective retrogressive differentiation of the caudal neural tube. The filum terminale and caudal portion of the conus develop from the embryonic caudal eminence after completion of primary neurulation and closure of the caudal neuropore by 28 days' gestation. During secondary neurulation, the caudal cell mass undergoes differentiation into the caudal neural tube between 4 and 7 weeks' gestation.[26] The portion rostral to the second coccygeal cord segment joins that portion of the cord formed by primary neurulation, giving rise to the distal conus. The caudal portion of the caudal neural tube regresses during the process of retrogressive differentiation to form the filum terminale.[27] Perversion of or interference with these events may give rise to dysraphic anomalies involving the conus and filum, including a thickened, fatty, or "tight" filum terminale.

Tethering of the conus by a tight filum is usually associated with the conus terminating at an abnormally caudal position, presumably secondary to restriction of the normal developmental ascent of the conus. The normal spinal level of conus termination in children and adults had been a point of some confusion in the older literature. Interestingly, in the two seminal papers by Bassett[17] and Matson and colleagues[15] describing the surgical anatomy and treatment of lipomyelomeningocele and diastematomyelia, respectively, the authors held that the normal conus position at birth was the fourth lumbar vertebra, subsequently ascending to its adult position over the course of development. In neither paper did the authors cite any studies to support this assertion. The normal adult conus level had been reported as L1-2 as early as 1894 by Thomson[28] and was later confirmed by McCotter in 1915,[29] Needles in 1935,[30] and Reimann and Anson in 1944.[31] Oddly, the conus in the newborn was reported to already be at the adult level by Ballantyne in 1892.[32] It is not apparent why Bassett and Matson located it at L4. In 1962, James and Lassman reported that the adult level was achieved by age 5 years, based on a study of autopsy specimens; they noted that there was no published information about the level of the conus between birth and adulthood.[33] Barson, in 1970, reported the newborn conus at L2, with a subsequent shift to the adult level by age 2 months.[34] An autopsy study by Govender and colleagues[35] in 1988 identified the normal conus position at term as L1, thus coming full circle back to Ballantyne's report in the previous century.[32] Since then, Wilson and Prince demonstrated the conus at L1-2 in newborns by magnetic resonance im-

aging (MRI),[36] and Wolf and coauthors demonstrated ascendance of the conus to L1-2 by the 40th postmenstrual week using ultrasonography.[37]

Symptomatic tethering of the spinal cord by an abnormal filum is not always associated with a low-lying conus. Warder and Oakes, in 1993 and 1994, reported patients with symptomatic tethered spinal cords, spina bifida occulta, and abnormal fila in whom the conus lies at a normal level.[38,39]

As an understanding of the normal limits of conus termination is essential to determining whether the conus is low lying, so knowledge of the normal thickness of the filum terminale is necessary to identifying an abnormally thickened filum. Hoffman and colleagues reported the upper limit of filum thickness on myelography to be 2 mm.[24] More recently, Yundt and coworkers performed in vivo measurements of the filum terminale in 31 children aged 2 to 14 years undergoing dorsal rhizotomy.[40] The mean thickness measured 1.21 and 1.16 mm at 10 and 15 mm caudal to the conus, respectively. Thus, the authors concluded that fila greater than 2 mm in diameter in children are abnormally thick.

The thickened, tethering filum usually contains fat, ranging from fatty infiltration of the filum to overt lipomatous expansions at its terminus. It has been suggested that some of the pluripotential cells of the caudal cell mass committed to differentiation into adipose cells may become trapped in the developing filum as an embryologic inclusion.[41] Incidental lipomas of the filum terminale were found in 4% to 6% of otherwise normal spinal cords in one postmortem study and in 4% on an MRI study.[41] Thus, fat in the filum terminale in the absence of any other findings may be incidental and of no clinical significance.

All observations taken together help determine whether a tethered spinal cord is present. Fat in the filum on MRI in the absence of spina bifida occulta or a low-lying conus may have no clinical significance, whereas a symptomatic patient with the conus terminating at a normal spinal level who has a thickened, fatty filum and spina bifida occulta may require untethering. One report made the controversial suggestion that symptomatic "tethering" of the cord can occur in the absence of any apparent intraspinal abnormality, with improvement reported after cutting an apparently normal filum.[42]

Dysraphic anomalies of the distal conus and filum, including a tight filum, can be associated with other congenital anomalies. An association between distal cord anomalies and anorectal and urogenital anomalies is well established.[43,44] This is not surprising, given that the caudal eminence gives rise to anorectal and urogenital structures as well as to the distal conus and filum. Between 4 and 7 weeks' gestation, concurrent with the secondary neurulation process, the cloaca is divided by the urorectal septum into a dorsal hindgut and a ventral urogenital sinus. The cloacal membrane is bisected to form the anal and urogenital membranes when the septum fuses with this structure at 7 weeks' gestation. Imperforate anus, rectovaginal fistula, bladder or cloacal exstrophy, persistent cloaca, and genital

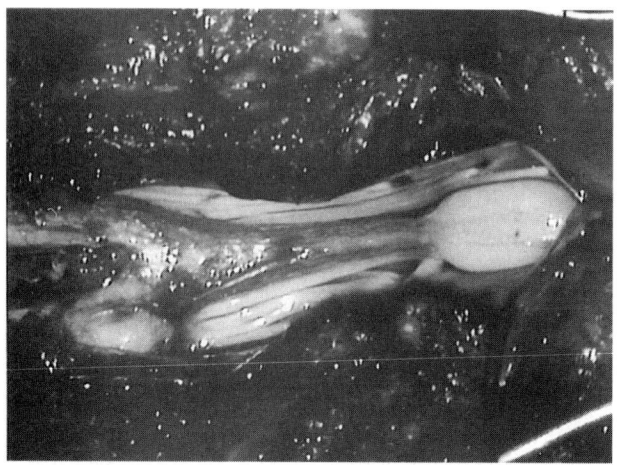

FIGURE 205–1. Intraoperative photograph of split cord malformation associated with a filum lipoma.

anomalies result from disturbed developmental events involving the cloaca, urorectal septum, and urogenital membranes. A thickened or fatty filum has been associated with cloacal exstrophy and other cloacal malformations, the VATER (vertebral defects, imperforate anus, tracheoesophageal fistula, and radial and renal dysplasia) association, and imperforate anus.[43,44]

The sacrum below S2 also arises from the embryonic caudal eminence, and sacral agenesis is associated with caudal spinal cord malformations, including tight filum terminale.[45] More severe sacral anomalies involving agenesis at high sacral levels are more likely to be associated with a blunt or wedge-shaped conus; less severe anomalies involving agenesis at lower sacral levels are more likely to have a conus tethered by a fatty filum. In addition, a thickened, fatty filum may be associated with other dysraphic states, including split cord malformations and myelomeningoceles (Fig. 205–1). Because these last two dysraphic conditions have embryologic origins that differ from that presumed for filum anomalies, these associations are not intuitive.

PATHOPHYSIOLOGY

Although the observation of neurological phenomena in association with congenital lesions that anchor the spinal cord have come to be accepted, the mechanism by which neurological symptoms come about has only recently been demonstrated. However, since these observations began to be made, there has been no shortage of speculation.

Brickner, in 1918, thought that symptoms associated with spina bifida occulta could be attributed to spinal cord stretching.[1] Ingraham and Lowrey, in 1943, thought of these lesions as interfering with the normal ascent of the spinal cord during development.[13] Likewise Matson and colleagues in 1950 (regarding diastematomyelia) and Bassett in the same year (regarding lipomyelomeningocele) ascribed the impaired function

to fixation, distortion, or traction on the neural elements that worsened with growth.[15,17]

Garceau,[19] in 1953, wrote that, in accordance with Lichtenstein's[12] explanation, a distally fixed spinal cord placed traction on distant rostral elements of the neuraxis, including downward herniation of the hindbrain through the foramen magnum, resulting in the Arnold-Chiari syndrome. However, Russell and Donald had reported in 1935 that the hindbrain was normal in patients with spina bifida occulta.[46] Thereafter, myelographic studies in patients with occult dysraphic lesions demonstrated no associated Arnold-Chiari malformation, as reported by Gryspeerdt in 1963,[47] Yashon and Beatty in 1966,[48] and Burrows in 1968.[49]

The experiments reported by Jones and Love in 1956 on spinal cords removed at necropsy and subjected to conus traction demonstrated local stretching and thinning of the conus with narrowing of the pial vessels, leading them to interpret the effect of the tight filum as being a local one at the distal cord.[20] They suggested a process of degeneration in the neurons and tracts of the affected cord. The following year, Barry and colleagues demonstrated that the mechanical effect of traction dissipates within five segments rostral to the point of tethering.[50] James and Lassman, in a 1962 publication, classified the mechanisms by which the cord is injured in occult dysraphism as pressure or traction, or a combination of the two.[33] In 1968, Burrows stated, "it is possible that in some instances an element of traction was responsible, perhaps causing ischemic changes in the cord."[49] However, Anderson proposed a slightly different idea in 1975, stating, "Tight filum terminale may actually be due to malconstruction and poor tolerance of the conus medullaris to the traction forces of growth and activity."[51]

It was not until the 1980s that further investigation began to offer insight into the pathophysiology of this phenomenon, which had spawned speculation over nearly a century. In 1981, Yamada and coauthors demonstrated impairment of mitochondrial oxidative metabolism under constant or intermittent cord stretching both in humans and in animal models.[52] Sarwar and colleagues demonstrated that distal cord traction produced maximal elongation in the lumbar region, with little or no elongation in the cervical cord.[53] A publication in 1987 by Tani and associates described the filum as having the greatest distensibility of the neural elements and functioning as a "buffer" in preventing cord stretching.[54] They demonstrated that the cord stretches only below the lowest dentate ligament attachment and that the lower the cord segment, the greater the stretch and the greater the impairment in oxidative metabolism. Fujita and Yamamoto demonstrated decreased somatosensory evoked potential amplitudes with increased cord traction in 1989.[55] In 1993, Schneider and coauthors demonstrated improved distal spinal cord blood flow after tethered cord release using intraoperative laser Doppler.[56] Thus, Brickner's[1] spinal cord stretching hypothesis of 1918, the observation by Jones and Love[20] in 1956 of a local stretch effect on the conus with thinning of pial vessels, and the suggestion by Burrows[49] in 1968 that the cause might be ischemic have now gained experimental support. Improvement in spinal cord blood flow on untethering correlates with clinical improvement; however, neurological deficits may be irreversible in some instances. This has been postulated to correspond to tissue damage noted at the ultrastructural level, including loss of axonal integrity, demyelination, and loss of organelles and mitochondrial damage within neurons.[57,58]

CLINICAL PRESENTATION

With the increased awareness of occult spinal dysraphism and tethered spinal cord among those providing medical care for children, the diagnosis of tethered cord is being made more often in infancy before the onset of clinical symptoms. This often comes about because one of the cutaneous stigmata, or "signatures," of occult dysraphism is recognized.[59] These include a lumbar or sacral dimple (which is much more likely to be associated with an intraspinal anomaly than the common intragluteal dimple positioned over the coccyx which rarely, if ever, shares this association), midline lumbar hemangioma, or asymmetric gluteal cleft. Hypertrichosis is most often associated with the split cord malformation, and subcutaneous lipoma suggests an underlying lipomyelomeningocele. The parchment-like skin of the meningocele manqué suggests an underlying attachment of sinus tract or aberrant nerve that tethers the cord dorsally (Figs. 205–2 to 205–5).

The clinical presentation of tethered cord syndrome falls into categories of neurological, urologic, and orthopedic presentations, as well as pain. Pain seems to be a more common presenting symptom in adults, but it is certainly seen in children. Pain in the lower back, often with radiation into one or both legs, is common. Forward flexion to touch the toes may be limited.

Neurological presentations include weakness or sensory loss in the lower extremities. Motor findings most typically involve the ankles, sparing the proximal musculature. A change in a child's gait may be reported, with more frequent falls being a common complaint.

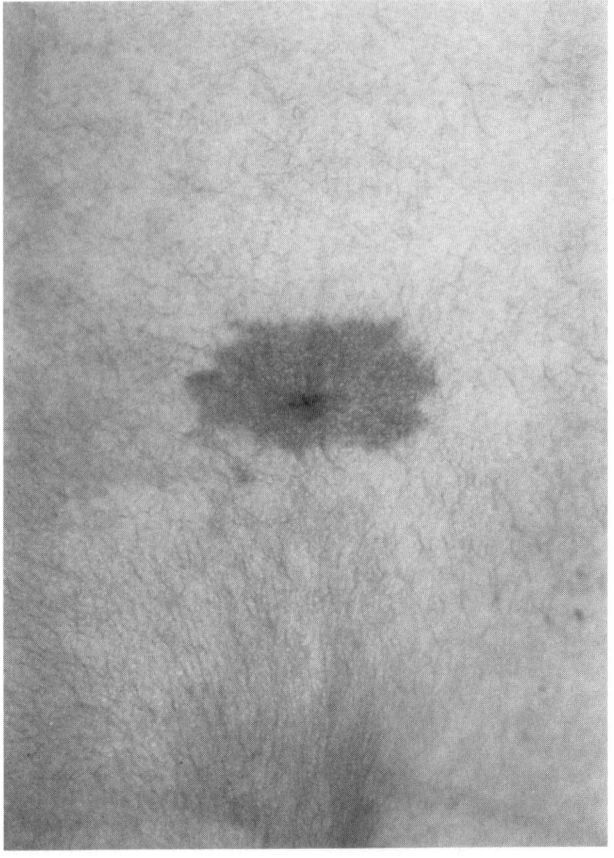

FIGURE 205–3. Midline lumbar hemangioma with a central dimple.

Reflex changes may be asymmetric and may suggest either an upper or a lower motor neuron process, being exaggerated or depressed, respectively. Muscle hypoplasia and asymmetry may be evident. A combination of both upper and lower motor neuron findings is common.

Urologic complaints are most commonly related to urinary incontinence or frequent urinary tract infections. In these cases, urodynamic studies often demon-

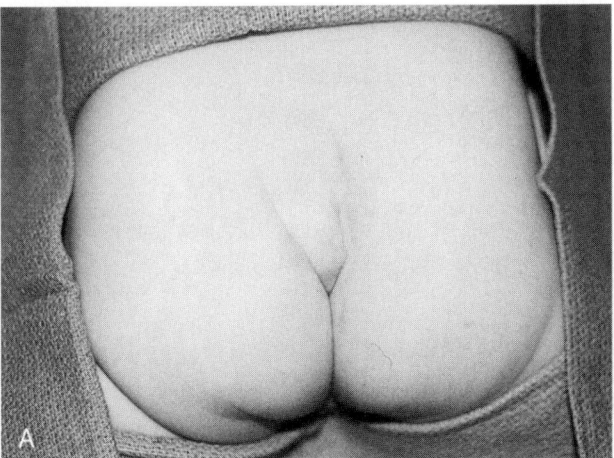
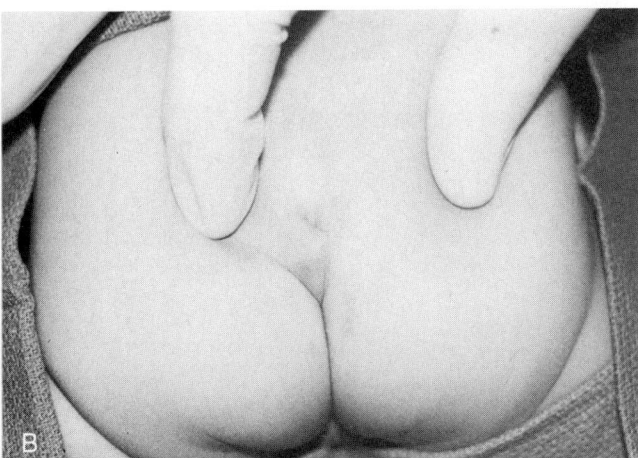

FIGURE 205–2. Infant with forked gluteal cleft *(A)* and dimple *(B)*.

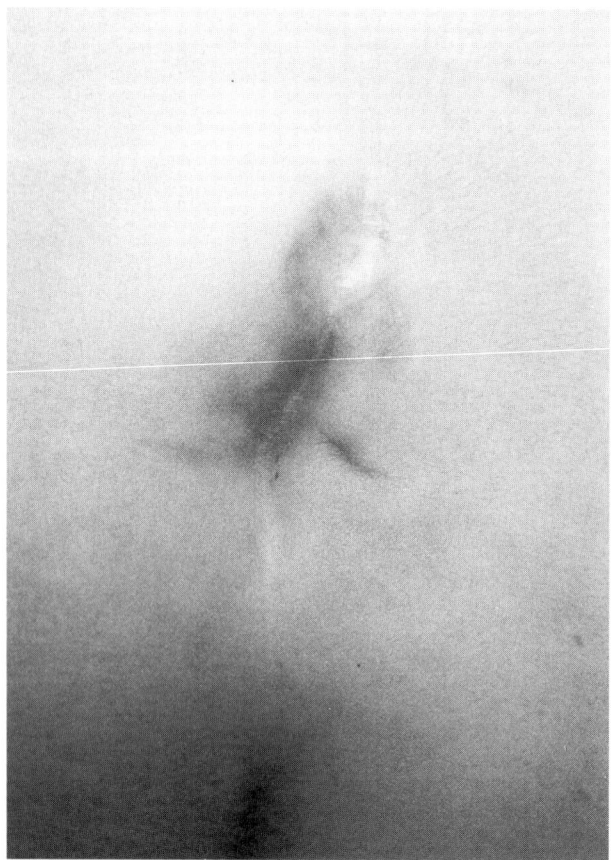

FIGURE 205–4. Area of "parchment" skin just above the gluteal cleft.

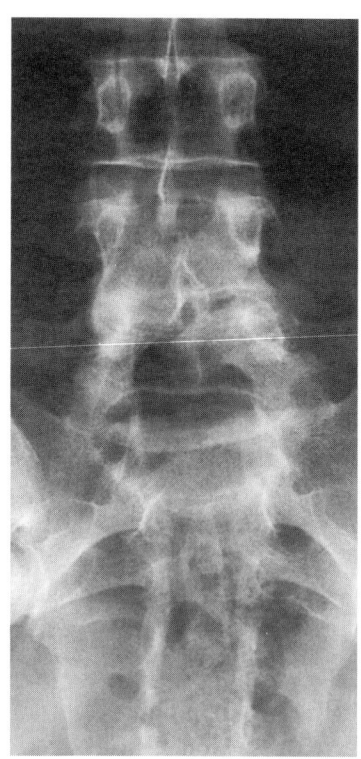

FIGURE 205–6. Anteroposterior spine radiograph demonstrating spina bifida occulta in a young adult.

strate detrusor hyperreflexia and abnormal compliance.[60]

The most common orthopedic presentations are foot deformities (e.g., asymmetry, claw toes, varus, valgus, cavovarus). Scoliosis is a less common presenting feature of tethered filum.

DIAGNOSIS

The history of the diagnosis of occult dysraphisms, as is generally true of many other clinical entities, parallels that of the development of diagnostic imaging modalities. With the case of Jones in 1891, the diagnosis rested solely on the clinical examination.[6] By 1909, Fuchs reported the association of enuresis and foot deformities with spina bifida occulta, as noted by "Roentgen rays"[7] (Fig. 205–6). Little changed until mid-century. In 1950, Matson and coauthors demonstrated

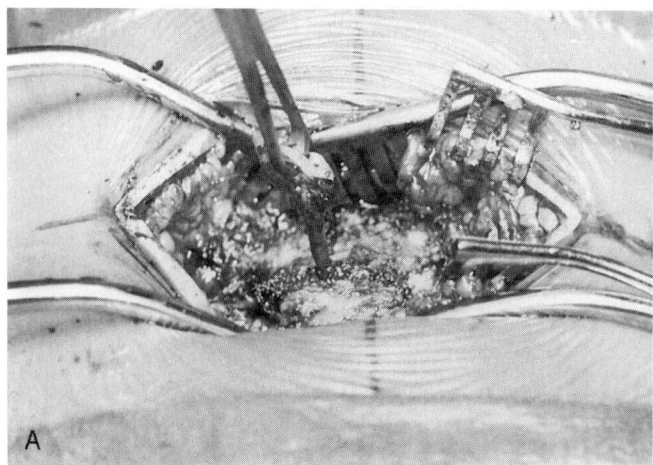
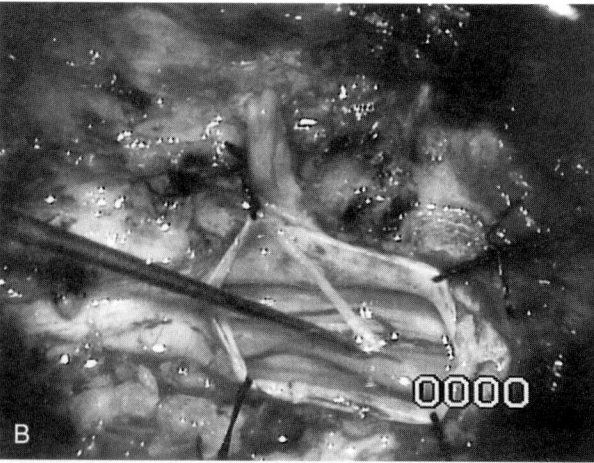

FIGURE 205–5. Intraoperative photograph of cutaneous sinus tract in the lumbar region *(A)* that leads to a dural attachment with an underlying intradural dorsal tethering band *(B)*.

the utility of pantopaque myelography in the diagnosis of diastematomyelia.[15] However, in 1956, Jones and Love based their surgical explorations on clinical grounds and plain radiographs.[20] In the discussion that followed the presentation of their paper, they stated that myelography was "of great value" but that it had been normal in their cases, and the diagnosis could "be made clinically." In 1962, James and Lassman stated, "Myelography is essential. The lesion may not be demonstrable by this technique, but if it is, its site is indicated."[33] Gryspeerdt enhanced the utility of myelography in these cases when, in 1963, he stressed the value of supine myelography to identify the conus level or prone myelography to identify a low-lying anterior spinal artery.[47] Yashon and Beatty, in a 1966 paper, demonstrated the findings of an enlarged thecal sac, cephalad-directed nerve roots, and low-lying conus by myelography.[48] In 1968, Burrows reported on 67 operated cases of occult dysraphism that had been studied preoperatively by myelography.[49] In 62 of these, the operative findings correlated with the myelogram, thus demonstrating its reliability as a diagnostic technique in occult spinal dysraphism.

Computed tomographic scans became a useful adjunct in the 1970s. The value of computed tomography (CT) in the imaging of diastematomyelia was reported by Weinstein and coauthors in 1975.[61] Its utility in spinal dysraphism in general was reported in 1977 by both James and Oliff[62] and Wolpert and coworkers.[63] Resjo and coauthors reported the superiority of computed tomographic myelography over plain myelography in 1978.[64]

The usefulness of ultrasonography in the diagnosis of spinal dysraphism in infants was reported in 1983 by Raghavendra and coauthors,[65] as well as by Naidich and coauthors[66] the following year. This is a useful screening examination in the newborn when posterior element development has not yet closed the sonographic window (Fig. 205–7).

MRI has become the most useful modality for detailed imaging of the anatomy of these lesions. This was reported as the imaging study of choice in spinal dysraphism by Roos and colleagues[67] in 1986 and Altman and Altman[68] in 1987. Levy and associates reported on the use of phase MRI to actually image spinal cord motion in tethering lesions.[69]

The typical MRI appearance of a cord tethered by a tight filum is that of a low-lying conus medullaris with an abnormally gradual taper and a thickened filum terminale that may contain fat signal (Fig. 205–8). The filum may even terminate in a discrete, expansile lipoma.

TREATMENT

Ingraham and Lowrey stated in 1943, "Probably too few of these patients have been given the benefit of local exploration, but it is only by careful study and selection that operation can be offered to the proper group."[13] Since that statement, it has become the consensus among many authors that children with teth-

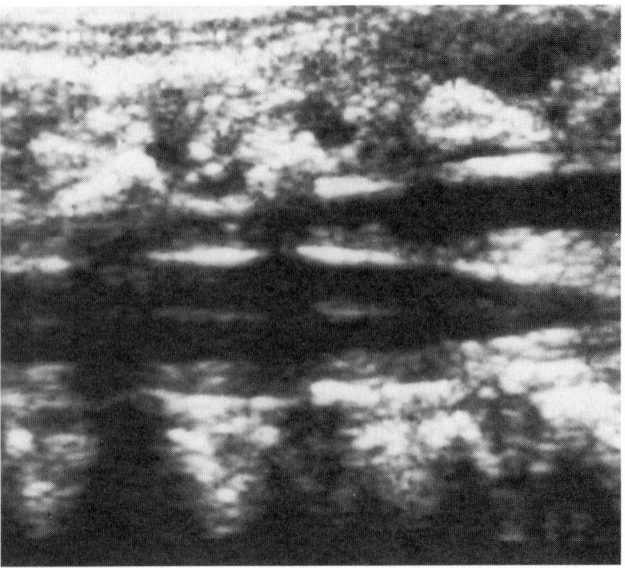

FIGURE 205–7. Normal spinal ultrasonogram in an infant demonstrating a hypoechoic conus surrounded by hyperechoic roots of the cauda equina.

ering dysraphic lesions should undergo preventive surgery for spinal cord untethering. As attested by the experience of many of the authors cited in the foregoing review as well as numerous others, the apparent natural history of these lesions seems compelling enough to warrant prophylactic treatment. For this reason, randomized, controlled trials of surgery versus observation in asymptomatic infants are lacking.

That operative intervention in a patient with symptomatic spinal cord tethering is indicated is not subject to debate. However, there is still disagreement whether asymptomatic patients should be operated on.[70] For instance, Liptak, in an analysis of the existing literature, concluded that no valid studies exist that answer critical questions about issues such as natural history and the benefit of prophylactic surgery.[71] He stated, "Virtually all the studies published in English on TSC [tethered spinal cord] have been case series using samples of convenience." Jamil and Bannister reported on a group of 12 children with occult dysraphic lesions whom they had followed for 2 to 10 years or more.[72] None developed new symptoms or signs, and there was no progression of existing neurological deficits. These authors concluded that "it cannot be accepted that the opinion that surgery is mandatory to prevent progressive neurological deficit is correct until it is proven to be so by controlled trials." Cornette and coauthors reported that 10 of 22 newborns diagnosed with occult dysraphism and followed for a mean of 67 months were stable without operative intervention, and those who developed new upper motor neuron symptoms improved with surgery.[73] They recommended a program of vigilant follow-up, including periodic screening urodynamic studies, with surgery indicated only by the onset of upper motor neuron signs. The difficulty lies in the observation that neurological, urologic, and orthopedic changes can be so

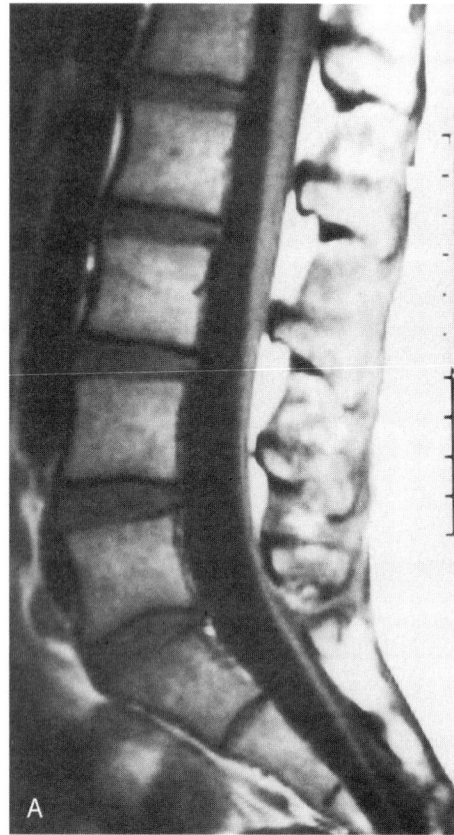

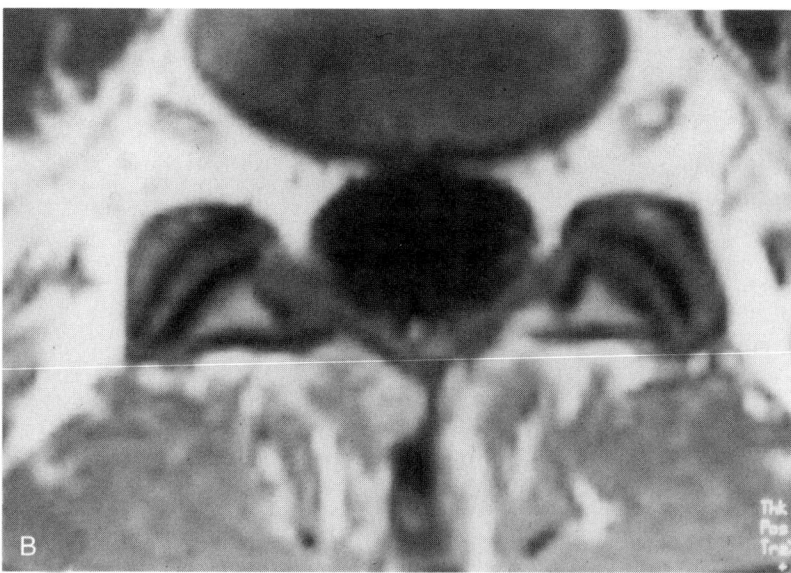

FIGURE 205–8. *A,* Sagittal T1-weighted lumbosacral magnetic resonance imaging (MRI) scan demonstrating a low-lying, abnormally tapered conus with a thick filum terminale. *B,* Axial T1-weighted image demonstrating the increased signal of fat in the filum terminale.

insidiously progressive that a few years' follow-up in a limited number of patients may not clearly demonstrate the true natural history. In addition, acute deterioration in patients with tethered cord, even in previously undiagnosed adults, can occur secondary to a traumatic event that acutely stretches the conus.[58,74] In patients with lipomyelomeningocele, it has been noted that infants are much more likely than older children to have intact neurological function, suggesting progressive deterioration as the natural history.[75] The case

for prophylactic surgery in an infant with tethered spinal cord from a simple thickened, fatty filum is particularly compelling because the procedure has such a low morbidity, with little risk to neurological or urologic function.

The goal of surgery is simply to release the conus from the abnormal filum terminale that anchors it. Other sources of tethering, such as dorsal tethering bands, should also be addressed if encountered. Other associated anomalies, such as a split spinal cord mal-

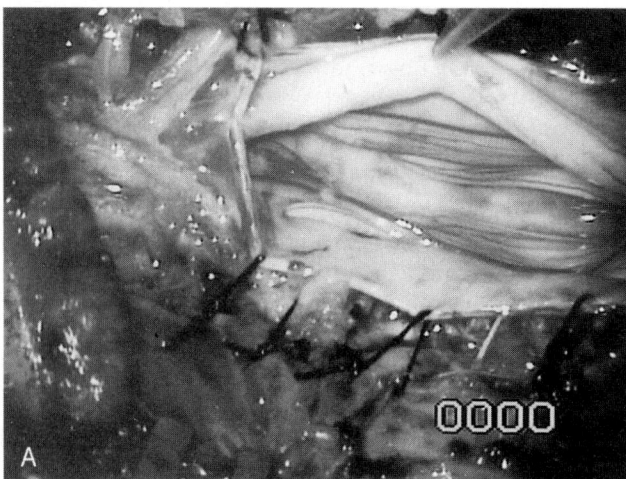

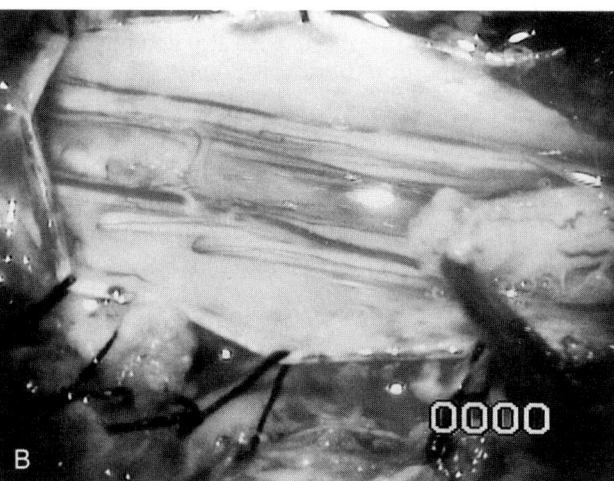

FIGURE 205–9. Intraoperative photograph of thickened, fatty filum (lifted up), surrounded by exiting lower sacral roots, before *(A)* and after *(B)* sectioning.

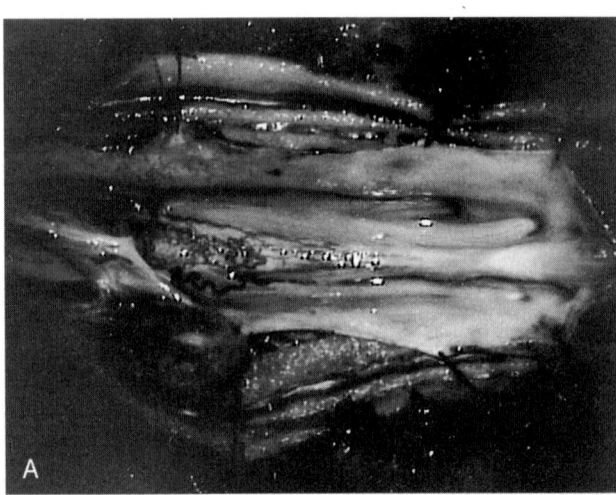
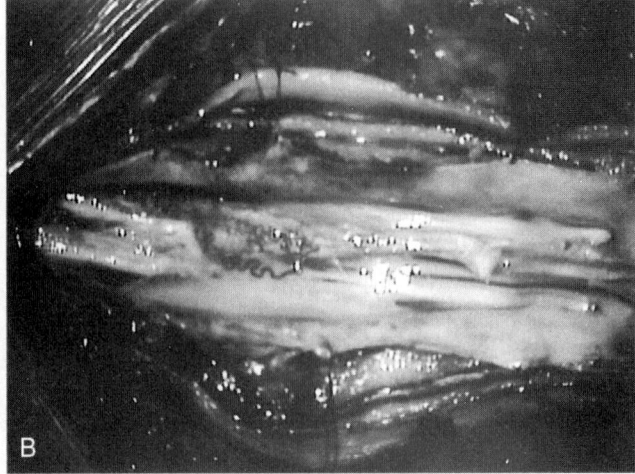

FIGURE 205–10. Intraoperative photograph of a low-lying conus *(left)* with a tight filum terminating in a bulbous lipoma before *(A)* and after *(B)* sectioning. Note that the filum is relaxed and retracted rostrally after sectioning.

formation, should have been satisfactorily ruled out before surgery by MRI. The procedure is accomplished through a limited sacral laminectomy over the thecal cul-de-sac. On opening the dura, the filum is identified and inspected under the microscope. It is easily distinguished from the sacral nerve roots by its slightly different coloration and vascular pattern and its midline exit at the terminus of the thecal sac. The abnormal filum is thickened and may contain obvious fatty tissue or even terminate in an expansile lipoma. Anal sphincter electrodes can be useful to monitor responses to electrical stimulation. However, this does not circumvent the need to inspect the circumference of the filum carefully to ensure that there are no small, clinging

lower sacral roots in jeopardy of being divided with the filum. The lower sacral roots are easily identified as they exit their respective foramina, and a clear segment of filum can be identified for sectioning. Having done this, the filum is coagulated and sharply divided, after which the proximal end may be noted to ascend rostrally. A segment may be sent for pathologic examination (Figs. 205–9 and 205–10).

OUTCOME

Untethering of the filum is an effective procedure associated with low morbidity,[24,25] and it prevents the con-

FIGURE 205–11. *A,* Lumbosacral T1-weighted sagittal MRI scan of a young woman presenting with symptomatic tethered filum terminale. Note the low-lying, abnormally tapered conus and thick filum. *B,* Similar study in the same patient with recurrent symptoms of tethered spinal cord approximately 1 year postoperatively. Note the anteriorly attached distal cord. At reoperation, the previously sectioned free end of the filum was bound in dense arachnoid scar.

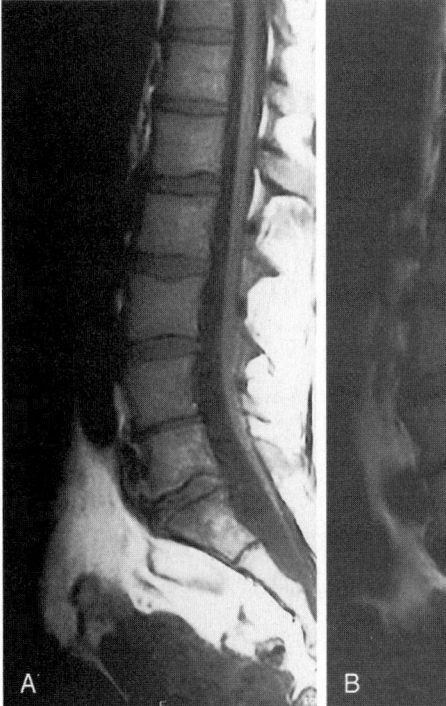
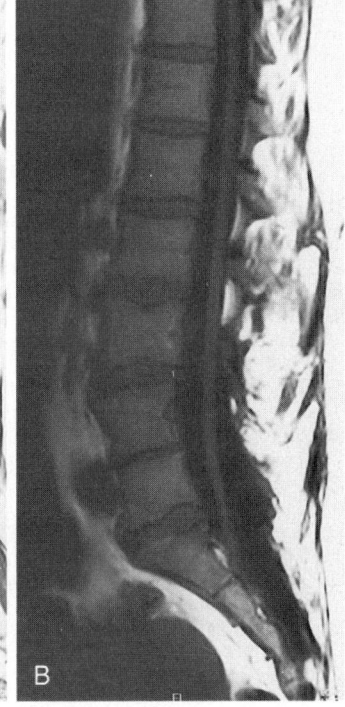

sequences of the natural history when performed prophylactically. Although recurrent tethering is common in the postrepair lipomyelomeningocele and myelomeningocele populations, the occurrence of symptomatic retethering after tethered filum sectioning is unusual, but it has been reported[76] and has been encountered by me (Fig. 205–11). Pain relief is usually achieved. Motor deficits are less reliably improved, but progression in deterioration should be arrested. The symptoms of neurogenic bladder may improve, especially when the urologic dysfunction was not long-standing.[60]

REFERENCES

1. Brickner WM: Spina bifida occulta: (1) with external signs, with symptoms; (2) with external signs, without symptoms; (3) without external signs, with symptoms; (4) without external signs, without symptoms. Am J Med Sci 155:473–502, 1918.
2. Johnson A: Fatty tumor from the sacrum of a child connected with the spinal membranes. Trans Pathol Soc Lond 8:16–18, 1857.
3. Virchow R: Ein fall von hypertrichosis circumscripta mediana, kombiniert mit spina bifida. Ztschr F Ethnologie 7:279, 1875.
4. Recklinghausen F v: Untersuchungen uber die spina bifida. Berlin, Ruiner, 1886.
5. Virchow, Maass: Die dame mit der pferdemahne. Ztschr F Ethnologie, 1892.
6. Jones: Reports on medical and surgical practice in the hospitals and asylums of Great Britain, Ireland, and the colonies, Manchester Royal Infirmary. Spina bifida occulta: No paralytic symptoms until seventeen years of age: Spine trephined to relieve pressure on the cauda equina: Recovery. BMJ 1:173–174, 1891.
7. Fuchs A: Ueber den klinischen nachweis kongenitaler defektbildungen in den unteren ruckenmarksabschnitten ("myelodysplasie"). Wien Med Wochenschr 37:2141, 1909.
8. Spiller WG: Congenital and acquired enuresis from spinal lesion: a) myelodysplasia, b) stretching of the cauda equina. Am J Med Sci 151:469–475, 1916.
9. Peritz: Enuresis nocturna und spina bifida occulta (myelodysplasie). Dtsch Med Wochenschr 27:1256, 1911.
10. de Vries E: Spina bifida occulta and myelodysplasia with unilateral clubfoot beginning in adult life. Am J Med Sci 175:365–371, 1928.
11. Lichtenstein BW: "Spinal dysraphism": Spina bifida and myelodysplasia. Arch Neurol Psych 44:792–809, 1940.
12. Lichtenstein BW: Distant neuroanatomic complications of spina bifida (spinal dysraphism): Hydrocephalus, Arnold-Chiari deformity, stenosis of the aqueduct of Sylvius, etc.; pathogenesis and pathology. Arch Neurol Psych 47:195–214, 1942.
13. Ingraham FD, Lowrey JJ: Spina bifida and cranium bifidum. III. Occult spinal disorders. N Engl J Med 228:745, 1943.
14. Hilal SK, Marton D, Pollack E: Diastematomyelia in children. Neuroradiology 112:609–621, 1974.
15. Matson DD, Woods RP, Campbell JB, Ingraham FD: Diastematomyelia (congenital clefts of the spinal cord): Diagnosis and surgical treatments. Pediatrics 6:98–112, 1950.
16. Pickles W: Duplication of spinal cord (diplomyelia): Account of clinical example with consideration of other reports. J Neurosurg 6:324, 1949.
17. Bassett RC: The neurological deficit associated with lipomas of the cauda equina. Ann Surg 131:109–116, 1950.
18. Rogers HM, Long DM, Chou SN, French LA: Lipomas of the spinal cord and cauda equina. J Neurosurg 34:349–354, 1971.
19. Garceau GJ: The filum terminale syndrome. J Bone Joint Surg 35:711–716, 1953.
20. Jones PH, Love JG: Tight filum terminale. Arch Surg 73:556–566, 1956.
21. Boettcher T: Die prognose der operation der spina bifida. Beitr Klin Chir 53:519–565, 1907.
22. Katzenstein M: Beitrag zur pathologie und therapie der spina bifida occulta. Arch Klin Chir 64:607–629, 1901.
23. Schlegel KF: Spina bifida occulta und klauenhohlfuss. Ergebn Chir Ortho 46:268–320, 1964.
24. Hoffman HJ, Hendrick EB, Humphreys RP: The tethered spinal cord: Its protean manifestations, diagnosis and surgical correction. Childs Brain 2:145–155, 1976.
25. Hendrick EB, Hoffman HJ, Humphreys RP: The tethered spinal cord. Clin Neurosurg 30:457–463, 1983.
26. Lemire RJ: Variations in development of the caudal neural tube in human embryos (horizons XIV–XXI). Teratology 2:361–370, 1969.
27. Streeter GL: Factors involved in the formation of the filum terminale. Am J Anat 25:1–11, 1919.
28. Thomson A: Fifth annual report of the committee of collective investigation of the Anatomical Society of Great Britain and Ireland for the year 1893–1894. J Anat Physiol Lond 29:35–60, 1894.
29. McCotter RE: Regarding the length and extent of the human medulla spinalis. Anat Rec 10:559–564, 1915.
30. Needles JH: The caudal level of termination of the spinal cord in American whites and American Negroes. Anat Rec 63:417–424, 1935.
31. Reimann AF, Anson BJ: Vertebral level of termination of the spinal cord with report of a case of sacral cord. Anat Rec 88:127–138, 1944.
32. Ballantyne JW: The spinal column in the infant. Edinb Med J 37:913–922, 1892.
33. James CCM, Lassman LP: Spinal dysraphism: The diagnosis and treatment of progressive lesions in spina bifida occulta. J Bone Joint Surg 44:828–840, 1962.
34. Barson AJ: The vertebral level of termination of the spinal cord during normal and abnormal development. J Anat 106:489–497, 1970.
35. Govender S, Charles RW, Haffejee MR: Level of termination of the spinal cord during normal and abnormal fetal development. S Afr Med J 75:484–487, 1989.
36. Wilson DA, Prince JR: MR imaging determination of the location of the normal conus medullaris throughout childhood. AJR Am J Roentgenol 152:1029–1032, 1989.
37. Wolf S, Schneble F, Troger J: The conus medullaris: Time of ascendence to normal level. Pediatr Radiol 22:590–592, 1992.
38. Warder DE, Oakes WJ: Tethered cord syndrome and the conus in a normal position. Neurosurgery 33:374–378, 1993.
39. Warder DE, Oakes WJ: Tethered cord syndrome: The low-lying and normally positioned conus. Neurosurgery 34:597–600, 1994.
40. Yundt KD, Park TS, Kaufman BA: Normal diameter of filum terminale in children: In vivo measurement. Pediatr Neurosurg 27:257–259, 1997.
41. Brown E, Matthes JC, Bazan C, Jinkins JR: Prevalence of incidental intraspinal lipoma of the lumbosacral spine as determined by MRI. Spine 19:833–836, 1994.
42. Nazar GB, Casale AJ, Roberts JG, Linden RD: Occult filum terminale syndrome. Pediatr Neurosurg 23:228–235, 1995.
43. Warf BC, Scott RM, Barnes PD, Hendron WH III: Tethered spinal cord in patients with anorectal and urogenital malformations. Pediatr Neurosurg 19:25–30, 1993.
44. Warf BC, Scott RM: Anorectal and urogenital anomalies associated with spinal cord tethering. In Albright L, Pollack I, Adelson D (eds): Principles and Practice of Pediatric Neurosurgery. New York, Thieme, 1999, pp 353–362.
45. Pang D: Sacral agenesis and caudal spinal cord malformations. Neurosurgery 32:755–778, 1993.
46. Russell DS, Donald C: The mechanism of internal hydrocephalus in spina bifida. Brain 58:203–215, 1935.
47. Gryspeerdt GL: Myelographic assessment of occult forms of spinal dysraphism. Acta Radiol Diagn (Stockh) 1:702–717, 1963.
48. Yashon D, Beatty RA: Tethering of the conus medullaris within the sacrum. J Neurol Neurosurg Psychiatry 29:244–250, 1966.
49. Burrows FGO: Some aspects of occult spinal dysraphism: A study of 90 cases. Br J Radiol 41:496–507, 1968.
50. Barry A, Patten BM, Stewart BH: Possible factors in the development of the Arnold-Chiari malformation. J Neurosurg 14:285–301, 1957.
51. Anderson FM: Occult spinal dysraphism: A series of 73 cases. Pediatrics 55:826–835, 1975.
52. Yamada S, Zinke DE, Sanders DS: Pathophysiology of "tethered cord syndrome." J Neurosurg 54:494–503, 1981.
53. Sarwar M, Crelin ES, Kier EL, Virapongse C: Experimental cord stretchability and the tethered cord syndrome. AJNR Am J Neuroradiol 4:641–643, 1983.

54. Tani S, Yamada S, Knighton RS: Extensibility of the lumbar and sacral cord. J Neurosurg 66:116–123, 1987.
55. Fujita Y, Yamamoto H: An experimental study on spinal cord traction effect. Spine 14:698–705, 1989.
56. Schneider SJ, Rosenthal AD, Greenberg BM, Danto J: A preliminary report on the use of laser-Doppler flowmetry during tethered spinal cord release. Neurosurgery 32:214–218, 1993.
57. Kocak A, Kilic A, Gulay N, et al: A new model for tethered cord syndrome: A biochemical, electrophysiological, and electron microscopic study. Pediatr Neurosurg 26:120–126, 1997.
58. Yamada S, Iacono RP, Andrade T, et al: Pathophysiology of tethered cord syndrome. Neurosurg Clin N Am 6:311–323, 1995.
59. Humphreys RP: Clinical evaluation of cutaneous lesions of the back: Spinal signatures that do not go away. Clin Neurosurg 43:175–187, 1996.
60. Fone PD, Vapnek JM, Litwiller SE, et al: Urodynamic findings in the tethered spinal cord syndrome: Does surgical release improve bladder function? J Urol 157:604–609, 1997.
61. Weinstein MA, Rothner AD, Duchesneau P, Dohn DF: Computed tomography in diastematomyelia. Radiology 117:609–611, 1975.
62. James HE, Oliff M: Computed tomography in spinal dysraphism. J Comput Assist Tomogr 1:391–397, 1977.
63. Wolpert SM, Scott RM, Carter BL: Computed tomography in spinal dysraphism. Surg Neurol 8:199–206, 1977.
64. Resjo IM, Harwood-Nash DC, Fitz CR, Chuang S: Computed tomographic metrizamide myelography in spinal dysraphism in infants and children. J Comput Assist Tomogr 2:549–558, 1978.
65. Raghavendra BN, Epstein FJ, Pinto RS, et al: The tethered spinal cord: Diagnosis by high-resolution real-time ultrasound. Radiology 149:123–128, 1983.
66. Naidich TP, Fernbach SK, McLone DG, Shkolnik A: Sonography of the caudal spine and back: Congenital anomalies in children. AJR Am J Roentgenol 142:1229–1242, 1984.
67. Roos RAC, Vielvoye GJ, Voormolen JHC, Peters ACB: Magnetic resonance imaging in occult spinal dysraphism. Pediatr Radiol 16:412–416, 1986.
68. Altman NR, Altman D: MR imaging of spinal dysraphism. AJNR Am J Neuroradiol 8:533–538, 1987.
69. Levy LM, Di Chiro G, McCullough DC, et al: Fixed spinal cord: Diagnosis with MR imaging. Radiology 169:773–778, 1988.
70. Bodensteiner J: Standard of care: The blind leading the blind? Clin Pediatr 34:655–656, 1995.
71. Liptak GS: Tethered spinal cord: An analysis of clinical research. Eur J Pediatr Surg 2:12–17, 1992.
72. Jamil M, Bannister CM: A report of children with spinal dysraphism managed conservatively. Eur J Pediatr Surg 2:26–28, 1992.
73. Cornette L, Verpoorten C, Lagae L, et al: Tethered cord syndrome in occult spinal dysraphism. Neurology 50:1761–1765, 1998.
74. Iskandar BJ, Fulmer BB, Hadley MN, Oakes WJ: Congenital tethered spinal cord syndrome in adults. J Neurosurg 88:958–961, 1998.
75. Kanev PM, Bierbrauer KS: Reflections on the natural history of lipomyelomeningocele. Pediatr Neurosurg 22:137–140, 1995.
76. Souweidane MM, Drake JM: Retethering of sectioned fibrolipomatous filum terminales: Report of two cases. Neurosurgery 42:1390–1393, 1998.

Occult Spinal Dysraphism and the Tethered Spinal Cord

R. F. KEATING ■ J. MULTANI ■ P. H. COGEN

Spinal dysraphism is defined as the incomplete fusion of dorsal midline structures during embryogenesis. It may variably involve the spinal cord, meninges, spine, and overlying integument. *Occult spinal dysraphism* represents a subset of spinal dysraphism in which the congenital spinal defects are covered by intact skin. Such anomalies are numerous and include lipomyelomeningocele, hypertrophic and lipomatous filum terminales, anterior and posterior meningoceles, myelocystocele, split cord malformations, neurenteric cysts, dermal inclusions, and terminal syringomyelia in addition to the ubiquitous sacral dimple (Table 206–1). These examples constitute a separate entity from the open defects known as spina bifida aperta, which is best characterized by the myelomeningocele.

Before the advent of sophisticated neuroimaging techniques, such anomalies often remained occult unless the patient developed signs or symptoms of a tethered cord. Magnetic resonance imaging (MRI) has opened a new arena of neuroanatomic definition, permitting appreciation of potentially deleterious congenital deformities that may compromise neurological states long before they are clinically evident.

The *tethered spinal cord* represents an altered range of normal physiologic movement of the spinal cord within the thecal sac, which over time may lead to ischemic changes within the cord that may produce various degrees of neurological compromise. Signs and symptoms of a tethered cord include back pain; lower extremity pain or cramping; changes in strength, stamina, or sensation; and bowel and bladder dysfunction. Scoliosis may develop with an increase in lower extremity tone and subsequent asymmetry. It is also important to appreciate the role of occult spinal lesions in the pathogenesis of spinal cord tethering. A patient with a tethered cord may present later with neurological compromise, which is frequently irreversible despite surgical intervention. Because of decreasing intraoperative morbidity and frequent recognition of this condition before the advent of neurological symptoms, prophylactic detethering is commonly recommended.

In this chapter, we hope to offer greater insight into several occult dysraphic states: hypertrophic and lipomatous filum terminale, split cord malformation, neurenteric cyst, dermal sinus tracts and inclusion cysts, meningocele, myelocystocele, and terminal syringohydromyelia.

EPIDEMIOLOGY

The incidence of occult spinal dysraphism in the general population is not completely known. The radiographic incidence among children younger than 8 years of age is as high as 49% at the S1 level, 13.5% at L5, 9.1% at L5, and 9.1% at S1.[1] Between 20% and 30% of the general population may have incidental findings on plain radiographs but fail to demonstrate any spinal cord or dural involvement.[2] There is a 2:1 female preponderance.[3]

The role of folic acid deficiency in contributing to open neural tube defects has become increasingly clear over the past decade,[4] but its responsibility as a causative agent in the development of closed neural tube anomalies remains to be elucidated. Dietary supplementation with folic acid (400 µg/day) before conception is strongly recommended for women of childbearing age, and it has been credited with reduction in the rate of open neural tube defects in South Carolina from 1.89 to 0.95 cases per 1000 live births.[5] In England, folic acid (4000 µg/day) given to women during the periconceptional period in a subsequent pregnancy, after a previous child was born with open neural tube defects, reduced the incidence of additional dysraphic states by 72%.[6] The use of folic acid in primipara mothers has also demonstrated a 60% decrease in the incidence of open neural tube defects in children born in the Boston, Philadelphia, and Toronto metropolitan regions.[7] A 30% reduction was demonstrated in Australia during a 4-year period,[8] and in Hungary, 800 µg of folate per day also significantly reduced the likelihood of spina bifida.[9] The association between folic acid and closed neural tube defects remains unclear.

There appears to be a genetic predisposition for various types of spinal dysraphism. When infants with siblings with occult spinal dysraphism were evaluated

TABLE 206-1 ■ **Spinal Dysraphic States**

LESION	SUSPECTED EMBRYOLOGIC ORIGIN	MRI APPEARANCE
Fatty filum terminale	Defective retrogressive differentiation	Filum lipoma > 2 mm thick Low or dorsally positioned conus (below L2–3)
Lipomyelomeningocele	Incomplete separation of neural tube from ectoderm	Intramedullary or extramedullary lipoma, low, dorsal conus
Split cord malformations, types I and II	Persistent neurenteric canal	Duplicated cord, with or without septum
Inclusion lesions (dermoid, dermal sinus tract)	Incomplete separation of neuroectoderm	Sinus tract isointense lesion, minimal enhancement
Neurenteric cyst	Persistent neurenteric canal	Isointense cyst (CSF); cord displacement
Terminal syringohydromyelia	Persistent ventriculus terminale (?)	Syrinx or expanded central canal cephalad to dysraphic state (split cord or tight filum)
Myelocystocele	Open neural tube defect in conjunction with hydromyelia	Myelo/lipomyelomeningocele, with cystic component

for open neural tube defects, the incidence of myelomeningocele or anencephaly was 4.12%, compared with an incidence of 0.8% in the general population.[3]

EMBRYOGENESIS

Any attempt to understand the origin of spinal dysraphism depends on an appreciation of the fundamentals of normal neuroembryogenesis. Development of the spine and spinal cord occurs in three distinct stages. Between days 18 and 28, neurulation proceeds, with the spinal cord forming into the neural tube. Canalization of the tail bud proceeds between days 28 and 40, and retrogressive differentiation ensues from day 41 onward. *Neurulation* involves an orderly sequence of cell migration leading to separation of the neural plate from the neuroectoderm to subsequently infold into the neural tube. Incomplete closure of the dural tube may lead to the development of myelomeningocele, meningocele, or myelocystocele. Separation of the notochord ensues after closure of the neural tube. At the same time, the cutaneous portion of the neuroectoderm separates and fuses in the midline to form the overlying integument (Fig. 206–1). Disorders of this process may lead to midline dermal anomalies such as dermal sinus tracts and inclusion cysts. The lateral mesoderm eventually migrates between the lateral portions of ectoderm to form the posterior vertebral arch and associated muscle and subcutaneous structures.

The caudal portion of the spinal cord is formed by a process of secondary neurulation or canalization and retrogressive differentiation. *Canalization* is a process by which the caudal ends of the neural tube and the notochord develop into a large collection of undifferentiated cells known as the caudal mass. This mass subsequently differentiates into the genitourinary, notochordal, and neural structures within the tail fold and is responsible for the occurrence of numerous developmental anomalies simultaneously affecting the genitourinary, vertebral, renal, anorectal, and neural systems. Within this caudal mass, several vacuoles eventually form, coalescing and ultimately fusing with the central canal of the spinal cord, allowing the distal spinal cord and central canal to extend into the tail fold (Fig. 206–2).

Retrogressive differentiation is the process by which

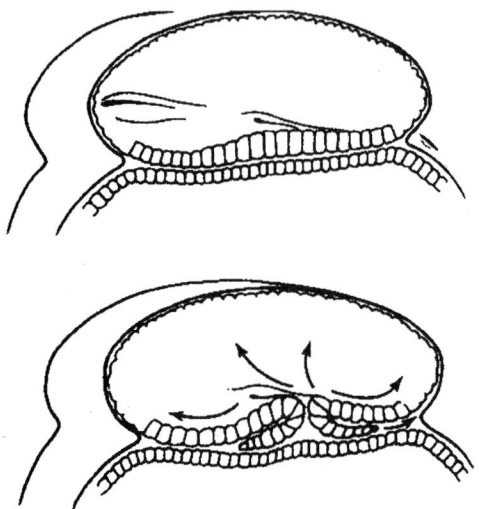

FIGURE 206–1. Neurulation involves separation of the neural plate from the ectoderm, which subsequently infolds to form the neural tube. Incomplete closure of the neural tube leads to open dysraphic states, whereas incomplete separation between the ectoderm and neural plate may promote variable occult dysraphic disorders.

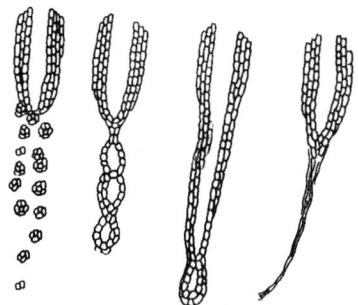

FIGURE 206–2. The caudal mass develops into numerous vacuoles distal to the terminal spinal cord that coalesce and form the cauda equina and conus. In time, retrogressive differentiation leads to involution of the distal thecal sac into a glial-ependymal strand, known as the filum terminale.

TABLE 206-2 ■ Manifestations of Occult Spinal Dysraphism

CUTANEOUS STIGMATA	ORTHOPEDIC DEFORMITIES	UROLOGIC PROBLEMS
Asymmetrical gluteal cleft	Foot or leg deformities	Neurogenic bladder
Capillary hemangioma	Scoliosis	Urinary tract infection
Subcutaneous lipomas	Sacral agenesis	Incontinence
Hypertrichosis		Delay in toilet training
Dermal sinus tract		
Cutis aplasia		

most of the newly formed spinal cord, with the exception of the conus, involutes into a glial-ependymal strand known as the filum terminale (see Fig. 206–2). Differential growth between the vertebral column and the spinal cord, as well as conus medullaris, results in the position of the conus at the level of L2-3 vertebral elements at birth, and they ascend to the final position of L1-2 by 3 months of age.[10] Errors during the process of retrogressive differentiation may lead to defects at the terminal cord or distal canal and can contribute to a tethered cord in the setting of a hypertrophic or lipomatous filum terminale.

CLINICAL PRESENTATION

Patients with occult spinal dysraphism may present with cutaneous, orthopedic, urologic, and neurological manifestations, as outlined in Tables 206–2 and 206–3.

Incontinence

Clinical presentation varies according to the child's age and the degree of neurological compromise in the setting of possible cord tethering. Visualization may be suboptimal during routine prenatal screening. Ultrasonography has become increasingly valuable,[11–18] with the efficacy of prenatal fetal MRI (Fig. 206–3) to be determined.

Cutaneous Lesions

The incidence of cutaneous stigmata in the healthy neonatal population is 4.8%, and most lesions are simple, superficial dimples in the sacral region.[19] The inci-

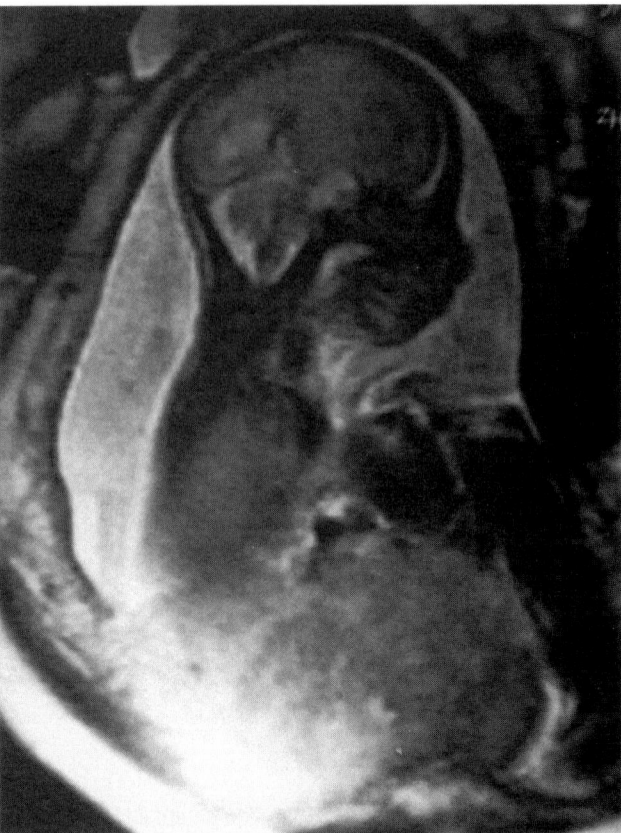

FIGURE 206–3. Magnetic resonance imaging has rapidly become a valuable adjunct in the prenatal evaluation of a child with suspected congenital deformities, which often are originally seen on routine prenatal ultrasound studies. Excellent definition of neural structures helps to define small, occult dysraphic lesions.

dence of significant cutaneous lesions of the craniospinal axis in the general population is 3%.[20] Nevertheless, any midline posterior cutaneous anomaly is often the first indication of an underlying dysraphic spinal state and warrants further clinical investigation. Two or more types of cutaneous lesion can coexist.

Several cutaneous lesions are associated with occult spinal dysraphism.[21–25] They may occur at any point along the spinal axis but are most frequently seen in the lumbosacral region. Atypical dimples (Fig. 206–4), particularly those that are larger than 3 to 5 mm in diameter; lesions above the gluteal cleft; or those appearing with other associated skin lesions such as capillary hemangiomas (Fig. 206–5), subcutaneous lipo-

TABLE 206-3 ■ Neurological Signs and Symptoms of Occult Spinal Dysraphism

INFANTS	TODDLER	OLDER CHILDREN	YOUNG ADULTS
Decreased spontaneous leg movement	Developmental delay (e.g., walking)	Asymmetrical motor or sensory development	Back pain
Absent reflexes	Abnormal gait	Painless ulcerations	Leg cramping or pain
Leg atrophy		Back or leg pain	Spasticity
Foot asymmetry		Upper motoneuron signs	Hyperreflexia
Decreased urinary stream			Bowel or bladder incontinence

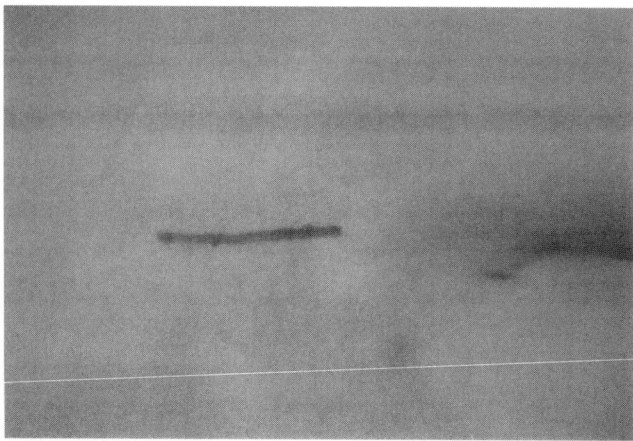

FIGURE 206–4. This paramedian sacral dermal sinus tract communicated directly with the spinal cord and was continuous with a filum lipoma, which was subsequently transected to detether the spinal cord.

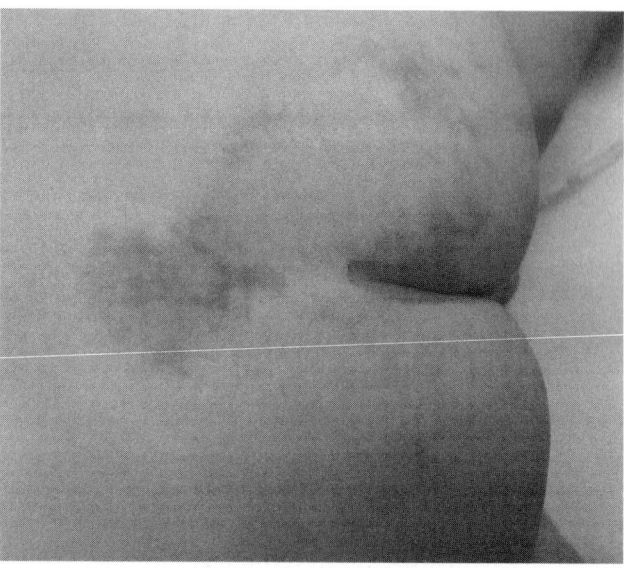

FIGURE 206–5. Midline capillary hemangiomas often herald an underlying spinal dysraphism. This 9-month-old infant had an associated split cord malformation with ventral adhesions that was found at the time of tethered cord release.

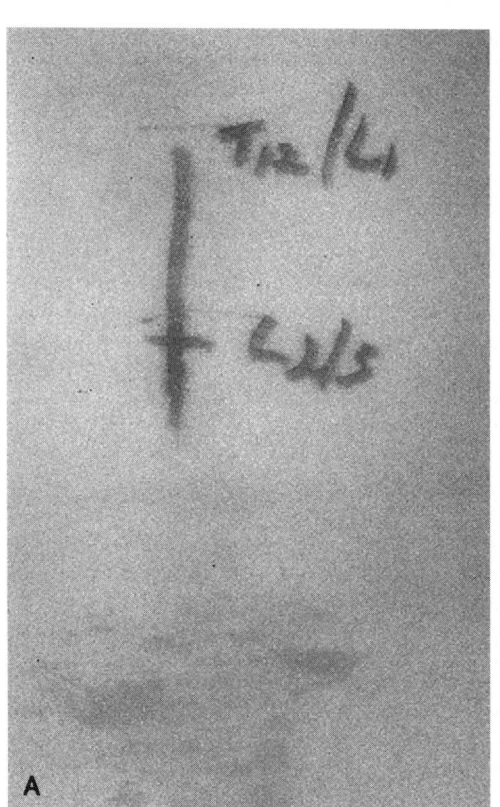

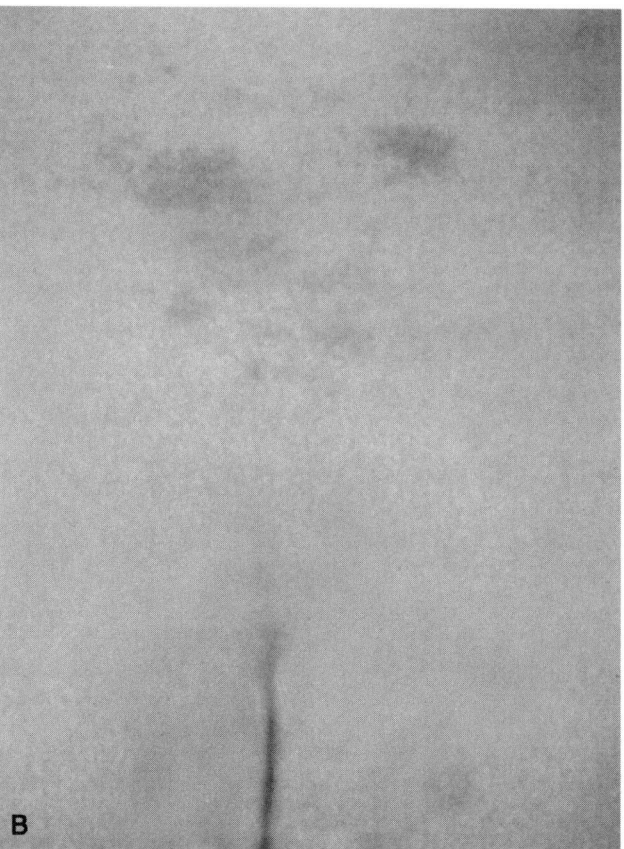

FIGURE 206–6. *A,* This 3-year-old boy had increasing external rotation of his right foot and underwent radiographic evaluation, which demonstrated a terminal syrinx and hypertrophic filum. His symptoms resolved after the filum was transected and after undergoing a syringostomy. *B,* A 6-month-old girl was evaluated for her midline capillary hemangioma and found to have a transitional lipoma, with her cord terminating at L4. She subsequently had the lipoma resected and remained neurologically intact.

mas, hairy patches, or dermal appendages (e.g., tails) often indicate underlying spinal dysraphism. The more common, innocuous recesses may be visualized within the gluteal cleft. These more caudal lesions often remain superficial and fail to connect to the underlying spinal canal, but there is a paucity of information regarding the overall incidence and the likelihood of spinal cord tethering. Although rare, it is possible for such lesions to be a manifestation of a dermal sinus tract or be connected to various examples of intradural filum dysgenesis.

Infants seen before 6 months of age may benefit from an ultrasound evaluation to reveal the position of the conus and to exclude intradural pathology. Children observed after the age of 6 months need MRI to rule out any intradural pathology. Any child presenting with associated skin lesions, lower extremity asymmetry, or neurological changes must undergo satisfactory radiologic workup with MRI to look for a tethered cord.

Hypertrichosis and capillary hemangiomas (Fig. 206–6) frequently herald an underlying split cord malformation. Up to two thirds of patients with diastematomyelia (i.e., type I split cord malformations) may have luxuriant hair growth (Fig. 206–7) over the defect.[26, 27] Such lesions mandate radiologic investigation of the entire spine. Although uncommon, the presence of multiple lesions, whether split cord malformations or other manifestations of spinal dysraphism, may occur and require careful evaluation of the entire neuraxis.[28, 29]

A *dermal sinus tract* is an opening in the skin connecting a subcutaneous tract lined by epithelium that extends in a cephalad direction directly to the dura or the underlying cord (Fig. 206–8). More than one half of these lesions may end in a dermoid cyst or other type of inclusion cyst.[30–32] Although the incidence of meningitis resulting from dermal sinus tracts is unknown, a dermal sinus tract often is discovered during evaluation of a patient who has had recurrent meningitis. Numerous organisms may be isolated; the most com-

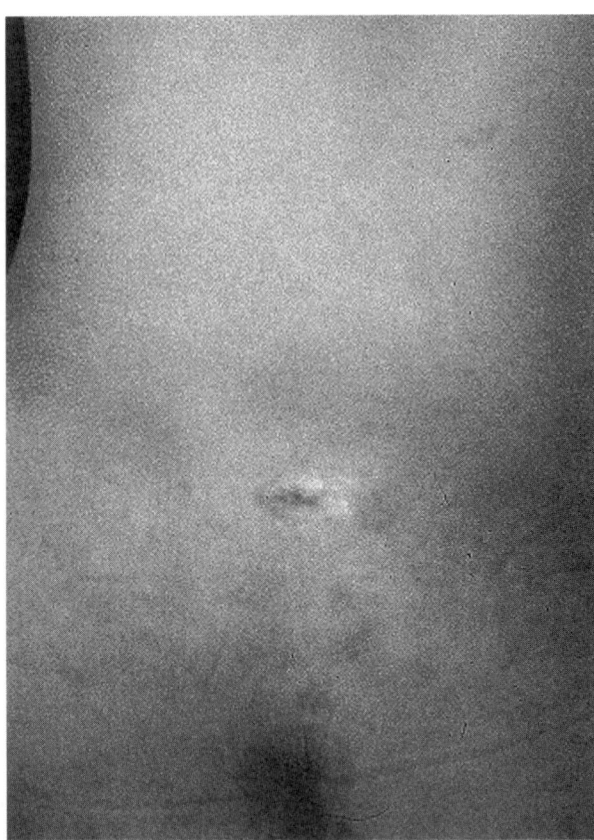

FIGURE 206–8. Dermal sinus tracts are usually in the midline and commonly extend to the intradural space. Large dimples above the lumbosacral junction warrant evaluation with magnetic resonance imaging to define the level of the conus and presence of any dysraphic elements.

mon are *Staphylococcus* and *Streptococcus* variants. Gram-negative organisms, including *Proteus mirabilis*, have also been identified.[33] Dermal sinus tracts often manifest at the lumbosacral region, frequently in conjunction with an asymmetrical gluteal crease (Fig. 206–9); however, they may appear anywhere in the midline from the coccygeal region to the nasion (Fig. 206–10). It is therefore critical to inspect the entire midline closely in the suspected patient with a history of recurrent meningitis.

Orthopedic Manifestations

Numerous orthopedic abnormalities may be associated with occult spinal dysraphism. Scoliosis is a common manifestation of the dysraphic state. It may occur in up to 90% of patients with a split cord malformation and is seen in nearly 25% of individuals with a tight filum terminale and tethered cord.[34] Any child with significantly progressive scoliosis should undergo clinical and radiologic evaluation for an intradural dysraphic lesion. Scoliosis accompanied by back or lower extremity pain, paresthesias in the legs or feet, and gait changes or abnormal tone in the lower extremities should alert the clinician to consider a neurogenic cause for the scoliosis. In the absence of vertebral

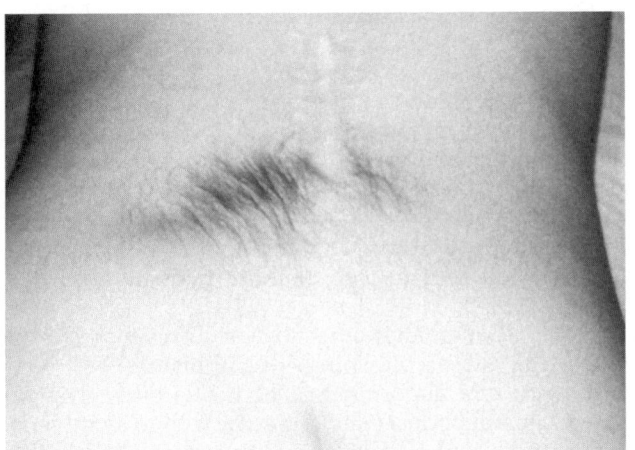

FIGURE 206–7. Focal regions of midline luxuriant hair growth typically occur with spinal dysraphism and often are the first indication of an underlying split cord malformation.

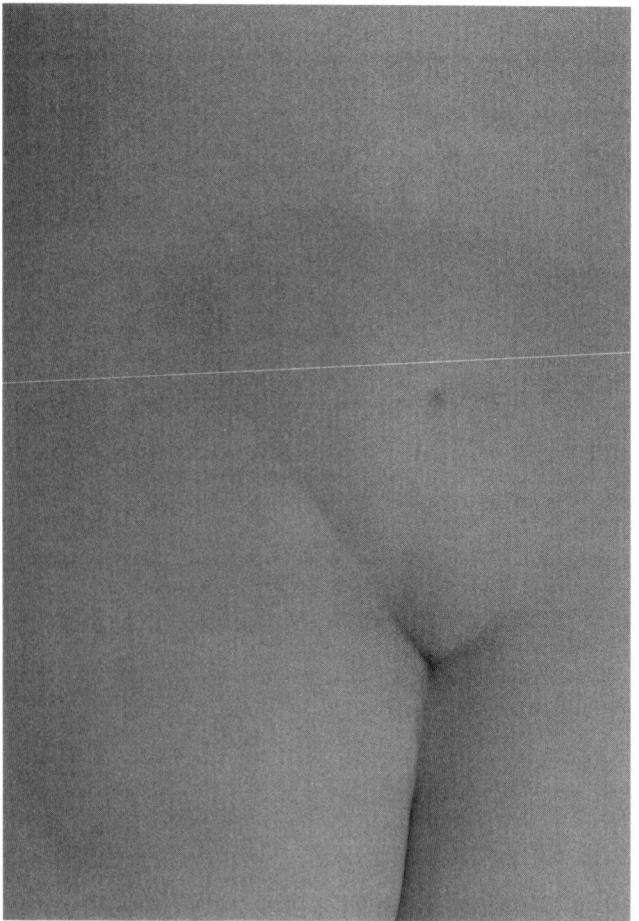

FIGURE 206–9. The dermal sinus tract is associated with an asymmetrical gluteal cleft. This 8-month-old infant demonstrated a low-lying cord resulting from an intradural dermoid in continuity with intradural and extradural fibrous tracts.

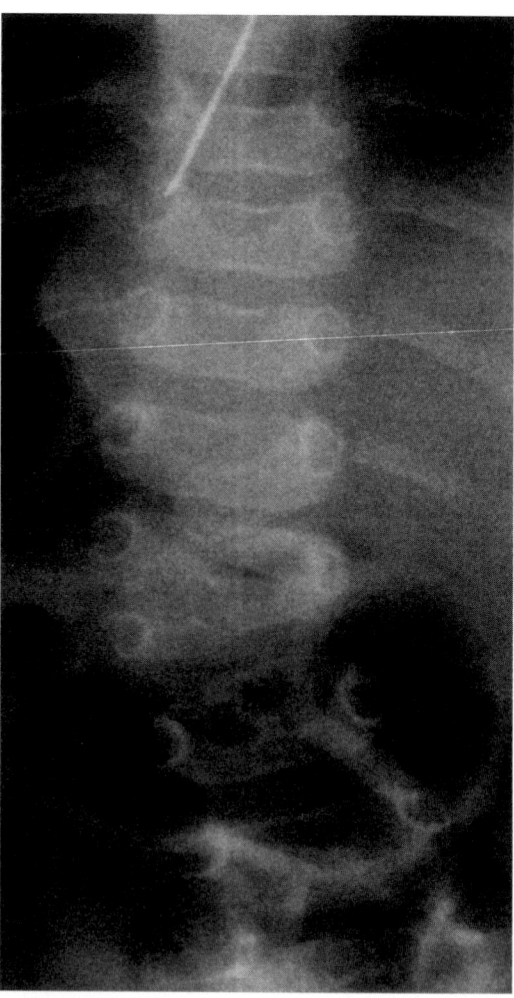

FIGURE 206–11. Scoliosis seen in conjunction with spinal dysraphism, which in this example involves a hemivertebra of L2 and dysmorphic changes at L1.

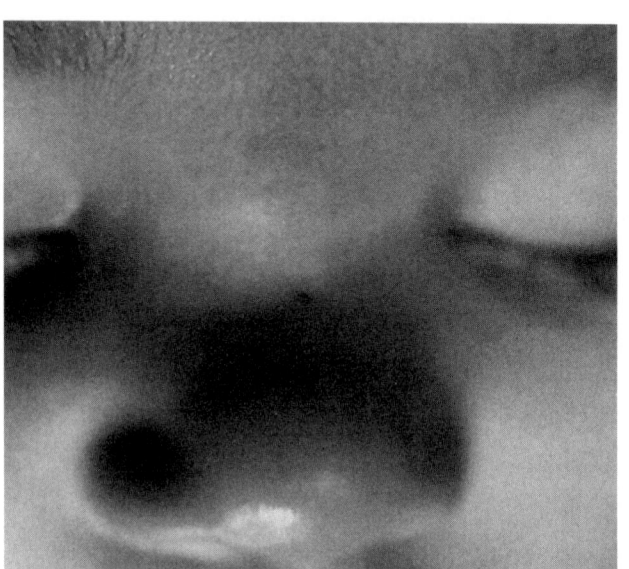

FIGURE 206–10. Dermal sinus tracts may occur anywhere in the midline over the entire neuraxis, including the nasion, as seen in this example. This sinus tract communicated with the cribriform plate and ended with an intracranial dermoid.

anomalies, additional factors increase the likelihood of a neurogenic cause for scoliosis. Thoracic curves to the left, patients younger than 11 years of age, rapidly progressive curves, and curves in excess of 50 to 55 degrees should alert the clinician to the possibility of an underlying intraspinal anomaly and require MRI investigation. The use of MRI has contributed to an increasing awareness of neurogenic causes for scoliosis. Previous studies involving plain radiographs (Table 206–4) and myelography demonstrated a 5% to 18% incidence of occult spinal dysraphism in conjunction with congenital scoliosis[35] (Fig. 206–11), whereas later studies incorporating MRI demonstrated intraspinal pathology in 15% to 58% of these patients (Fig. 206–12).[36–38]

Vertebral anomalies other than scoliosis may exist in the setting of occult spinal dysraphism. They commonly include abnormalities of the lamina, dysmorphic vertebral bodies (e.g., butterfly, wedge, hemivertebrae, unilateral and bilateral vertebral bars) (Fig. 206–13), deformities of the pedicles and disk space, and variants of sacral dysgenesis.

In addition to spinal anomalies, evaluation of the

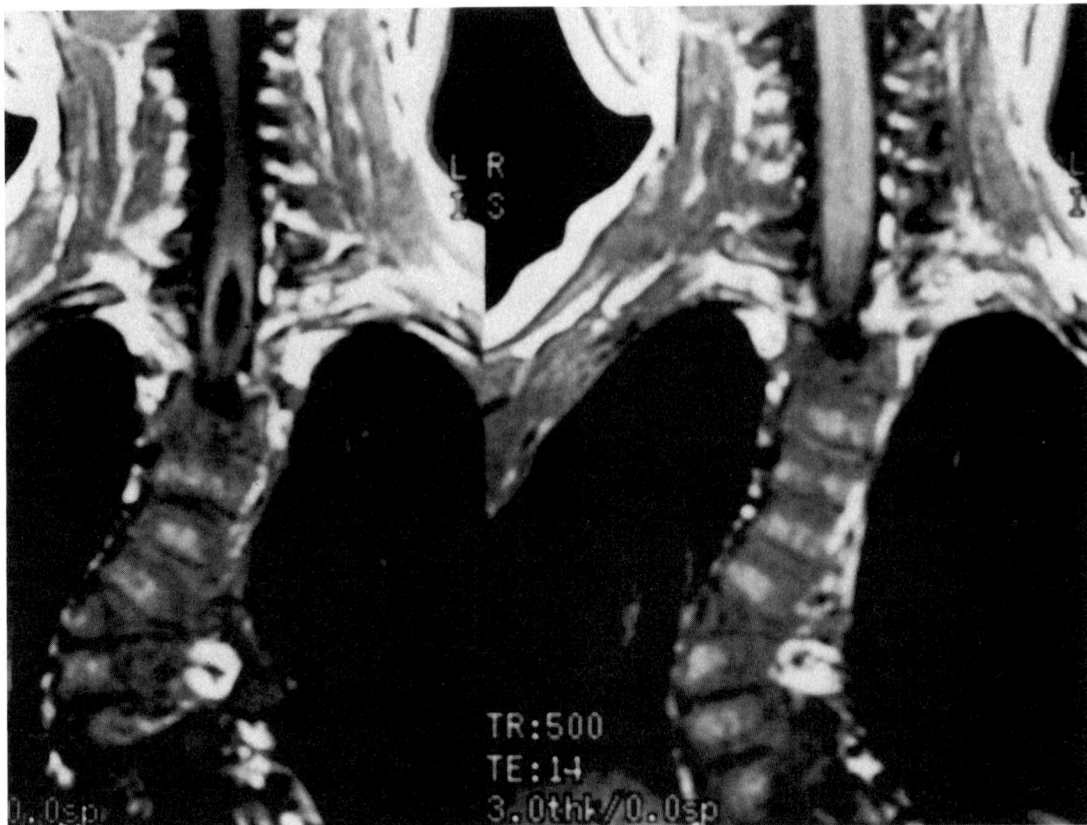

FIGURE 206–12. This example of scoliosis demonstrated a prominent syrinx at the cervicothoracic junction after magnetic resonance imaging (MRI) also depicted a split cord malformation distal to the syrinx. This child eventually underwent a tethered cord release and syringosubarachnoid shunt before spinal instrumentation. The syrinx remains collapsed 4 years after surgery, as confirmed on follow-up MRI.

TABLE 206–4 ■ **Plain Radiographic Findings of Occult Spinal Dysraphism**

Lamina
    Fusion defects
    Midline defects
    Abnormal spinous processes
Vertebral bodies
    Hemivertebrae
    Butterfly vertebrae
    Block vertebrae
    Midline cleft defects
    Canal stenosis
Disk space
    Congenital narrowing
Pedicles
    Flattening
    Thinning
Widening of spinal canal
    Interpedicular widening
    Scalloping of posterior border
    Midline bony spur
Failure of development
    Reduced number of vertebral bodies
    Absence of part of vertebrae
    Dysgenesis of sacrum
Spinal curvature
    Scoliosis
    Kyphosis
    Lordosis

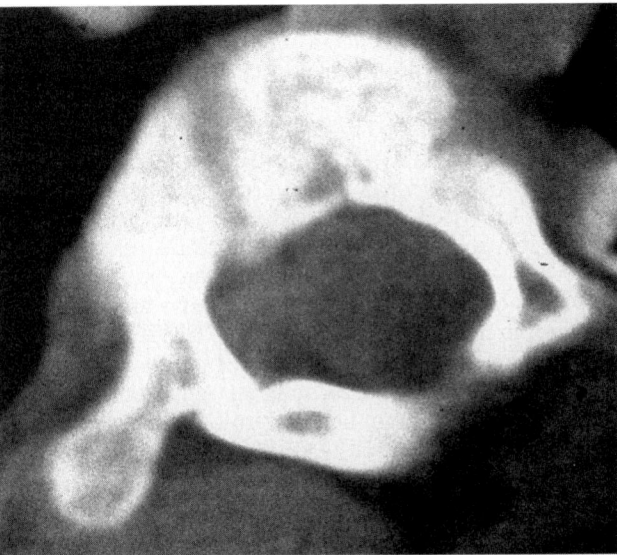

FIGURE 206–13. Other vertebral anomalies may be seen in occult spinal dysraphism. In this example, the vertebral body has an asymmetrical cleft and was associated with a split cord (type II) malformation.

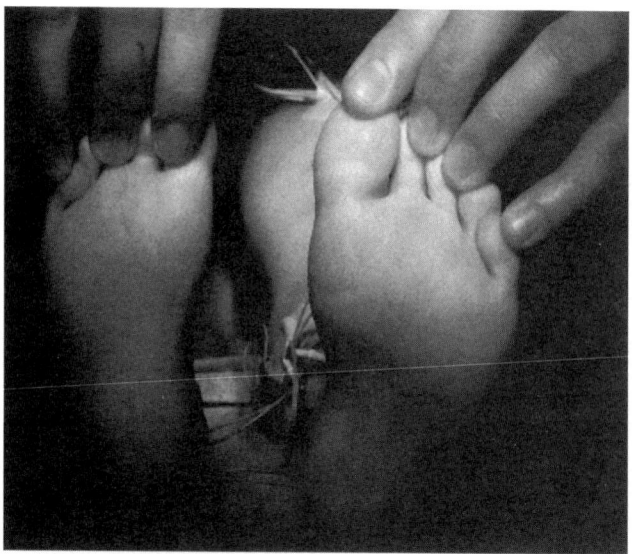

FIGURE 206–14. Lower extremity asymmetry is common in occult dysraphic spinal conditions and may be an indication of cord tethering. This patient had a split cord malformation with a small right hemicord.

lower extremities is critical in assessing for occult spinal dysraphism. Lower limb discrepancy (Fig. 206–14) may be related to an imbalance of muscle tone caused by a tethered cord and may include limb-length differences, asymmetrical changes, and foot deformities.[39, 40] Foot deformities are common, and patients may present with clubfeet, equinovarus, or valgus in addition to trophic ulceration.[41] The examiner must differentiate primary orthopedic deformities in the spine and lower extremities from neurogenic causes to offer appropriate therapeutic options.

Urologic Anomalies

The advent of accurate, noninvasive neuroradiology has promoted early detection of occult spinal dysraphism and potential tethering in certain individuals and led to the recognition of bowel and bladder dysfunction in asymptomatic patients. Prenatal recognition of concomitant urinary tract anomalies in association with occult dysraphism has become routine, whereas older patients may demonstrate delay in toilet training, enuresis, recurrent urinary tract infections, or new-onset incontinence or retention. In one study encompassing all spinal dysraphic states, 81% of individuals had normal upper genitourinary tracts, and 94% had normal renal function.[42] The remaining 19% had mild abnormalities, most often consisting of enlargement of the renal pelvis or ureters. Lower genitourinary abnormalities were more common overall, leaving only 29% with normal continence. Bowel and bladder difficulties are common with open dysraphic states, but they remain unlikely in patients with occult dysraphism. When they do occur, they often take an insidious course and may prove difficult to reverse.

Numerous studies[43–45] have demonstrated that development or progression of bowel and bladder diffi-

culties often remains irreversible despite surgical intervention for a tethered cord, especially in older patients. Younger patients fare somewhat better if the abnormal urologic function is diagnosed in the early years. Among patients younger than 3 years old with abnormal urologic findings identified in a preoperative workup, 60% had reversal of their findings to normal, 30% had some improvement, and 10% had further deterioration.[46, 47]

It is critical to evaluate bowel and bladder function carefully in patients suspected of having occult spinal dysraphism, and this is best accomplished by a thorough history and physical examination and by urodynamic studies and renal ultrasound, as needed. Urinary dysfunction is often easily discerned in the early course of cord tethering, but fecal incontinence may be more difficult to appreciate in the socially conscious older patient. Nevertheless, fecal incontinence is invariably accompanied by urinary involvement.

CLINICAL MANIFESTATIONS AND THERAPEUTIC APPROACHES

Filum Terminale Dysgenesis

Controversy continues to surround the origin and purpose of the filum terminale. Abnormal development of this remnant of caudal regression may lead to difficulty with spinal cord tethering. Frequently associated with sacral or gluteal cleft dimples, the presence of an enlarged or thickened filum is known as a *hypertrophic filum terminale*. However, almost 50% of such patients do not manifest any external cutaneous markings, and it is critical to consider the possibility of a tethered cord in the growing patient presenting with back or leg pain in addition to lower extremity weakness, numbness, and bowel or bladder changes. Such patients are found to have a conus ending below the level of L2-3[48] on MRI and have a filum thicker than 2 mm.[49] The filum may be predominantly thickened by fibrotic infiltration or, more commonly, by significant involvement by a lipoma, or it may be affected by both conditions (Fig. 206–15).

Several congenital conditions are associated with abnormalities in the filum. As many as 38% of patients presenting with VATER association (i.e., *v*ertebral, *a*nal, *t*racheal, *e*sophageal, and *r*adius or *r*enal problems or anomalies) or variants of anorectal malformations have had lipomatous filum terminale.[50–56] Other congenital variants, such as arthrogryposis, may be associated with filum terminale.

Therapeutic approaches principally involve division of the filum. The surgical approach generally involves exposure of the filum through a limited laminectomy at L5 to S1, although 15% of fila may fuse above S1, and 11% fuse off the midline.[57] A more generous exposure may be accomplished by a laminoplasty from L3 to L5 (Fig. 206–16). Advantages of a more generous exposure include greater visualization when a dermal sinus tract is suspected or when it is necessary to evaluate the conus for a terminal syrinx. Laminoplasty permits normalization of preexisting anatomy at the

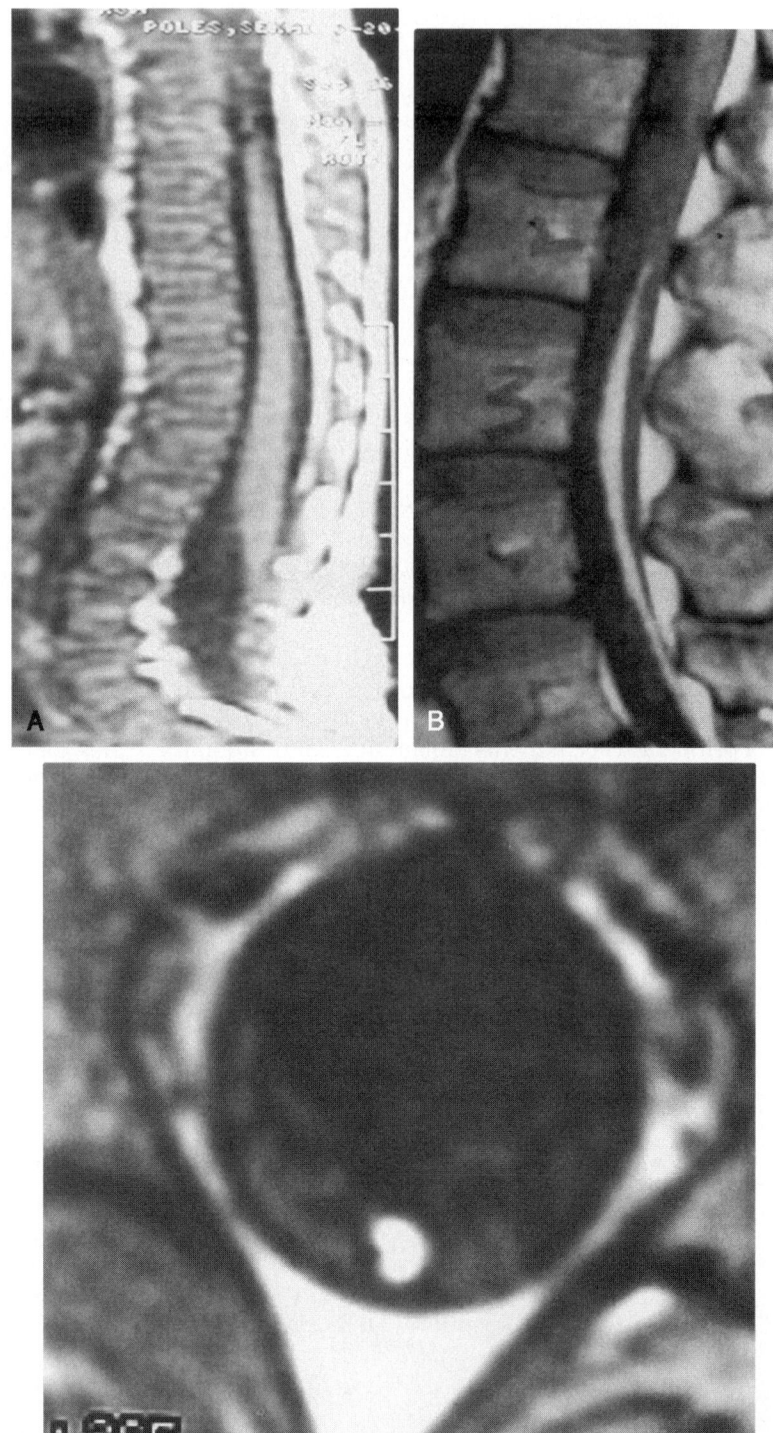

FIGURE 206–15. *A,* This 2-year-old boy had an anorectal malformation and was found on magnetic resonance imaging (MRI) to have a low cord resulting from a hypertrophic filum. *B,* This 5-year-old girl had a history of imperforate anus and developed back pain and lower extremity weakness. She was found to have a conus ending at the lower border of L2 with large and prominent filum lipomas. Her symptoms resolved after transection of the filum lipomas. *C,* An axial MRI view of the same patient as in *B* demonstrates the large (>2 mm) lipoma of the filum terminale.

surgical conclusion, thought by some surgeons to reduce the likelihood of postsurgical scoliosis. After exposure of the cauda equina, the filum is often easily identified and separated from the surrounding nerve roots. It may help to place the filum terminale on a cottonoid to separate it from the ubiquitous cauda equina (Fig. 206–17). The surgeon must ensure that the filum is completely free from any commonly conjoined small sacral roots and must test its distal outflow by means of a nerve stimulator. The filum may be transected at a single location or at two separate points with a laser (e.g., neodymium:yttrium-aluminum-garnet [Nd:YAG]) or directly with microscissors after ensuring that adequate coagulation of the ventral vein has occurred. If the filum retracts after transection, any incompletely coagulated vessels may be difficult to retrieve through such a limited exposure. The dura is closed in a watertight fashion and the laminoplasty

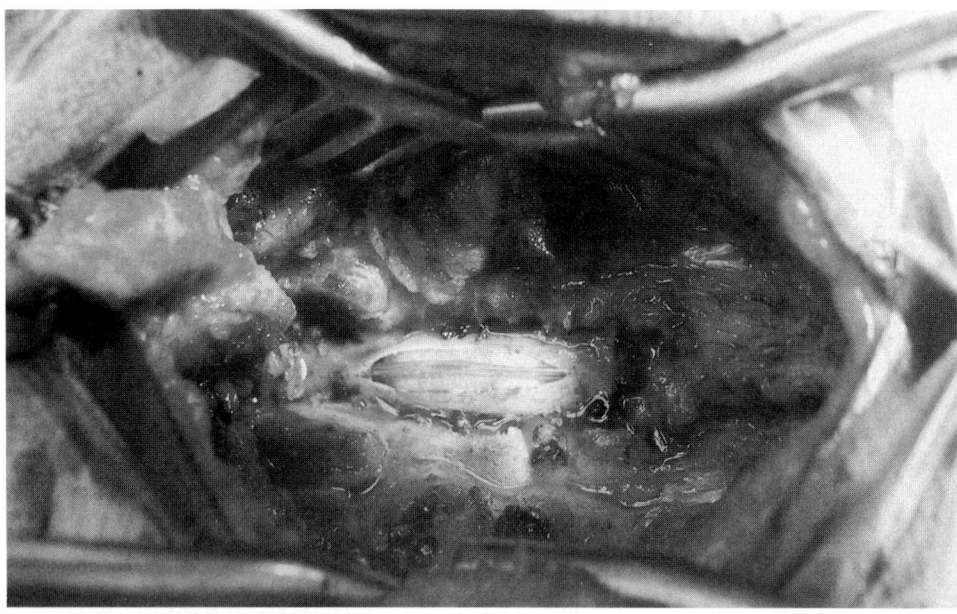

FIGURE 206–16. Exposure of the thecal sac from L3 to L5 was achieved by a laminoplasty, with the L2-3 interspinous ligament left intact to allow replacement of the posterior elements at the conclusion of surgery. The laminoplasty is retracted with a small towel clamp in a cephalad direction.

returned to its normal anatomic position. Resorbable sutures are used in the subcutaneous layer and skin.

Postoperatively, patients remain in a flat position for 24 to 48 hours, and most patients are ready for discharge by the third day. This operation is well tolerated, has minimal morbidity, and detethers the cord in most cases.

Retethering is uncommon but has been seen by us and has been reported in the literature.[58] Most patients have an improved clinical course, particularly those who presented with bowel and bladder difficulties.[40, 59–63] Although debate continues regarding the value of prophylactic sectioning of a thickened or lipomatous filum with a low-lying conus, numerous clinical examples have delineated neurological conditions deteriorating because of dysraphic fila, and this approach is now commonly employed.[64, 65] Although tethered cord symptoms most frequently manifest during periods of rapid growth, similar manifestations may be seen in adult patients.[66–70] An increasing body of literature[71–73] details tethered cord pathophysiology in the setting of a normally positioned conus accompanied by an abnormal filum or terminal cord. These patients may also benefit from sectioning of the filum.

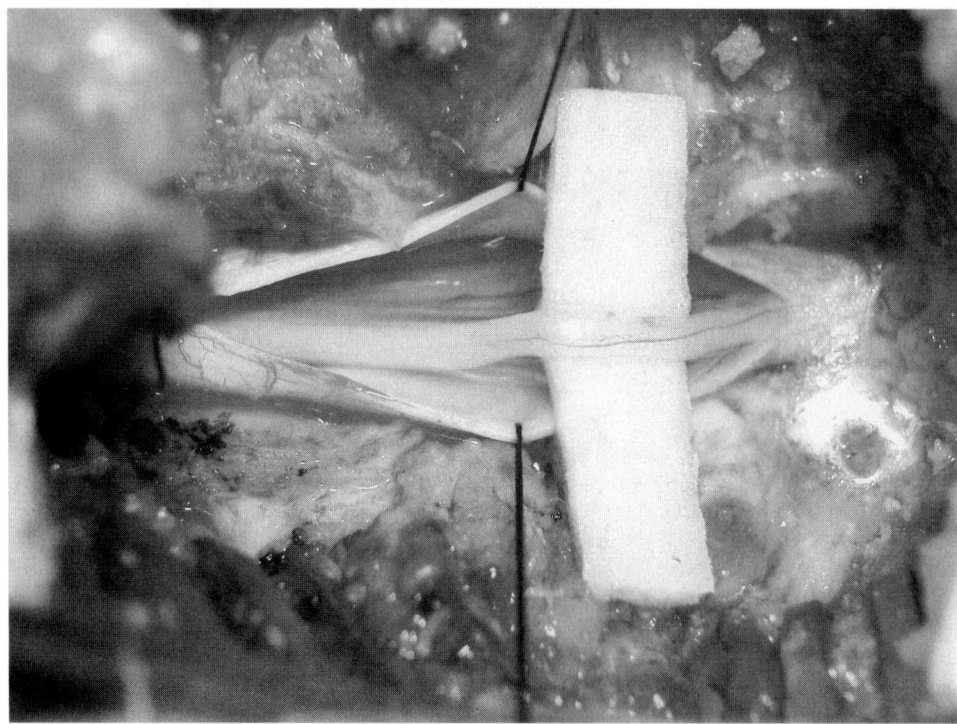

FIGURE 206–17. Exposure of the filum terminale and associated lipoma supported on a cottonoid. The filum is examined closely for any contiguous roots and evaluated by electrophysiologic testing before transection.

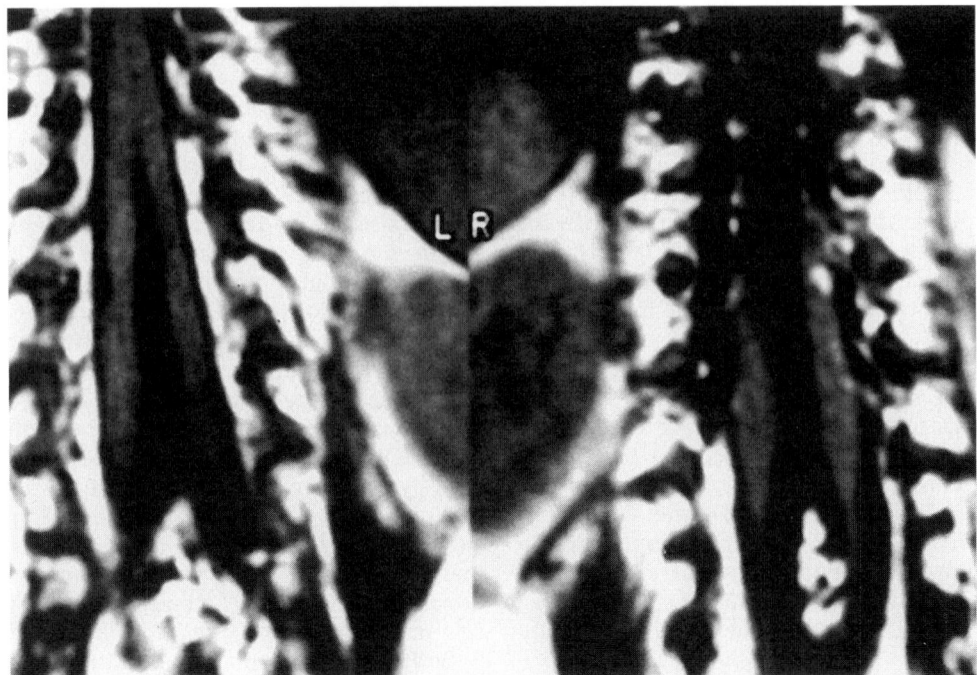

FIGURE 206–18. Magnetic resonance imaging demonstrates a type I split cord malformation (i.e., diastematomyelia) with a midline spur at the caudal end. Midline spurs may consist of bone, cartilage, fibrous elements, or a combination of these components.

Split Cord Malformations

Split cord malformations represent a continuum of spinal dysraphic disorders that encompass conditions previously known as *diastematomyelia* (Fig. 206–18), whereas the rare *diplomyelia* represents a true duplica-

tion of the cord with two sets of motor and sensory roots. Relatively uncommon, diastematomyelia was first described in 1837 by Ollivier, and the term was derived from the Greek words *diastema*, meaning cleft, and *myelos*, referring to the spinal cord. Split cord malformations may involve a longitudinal split over one

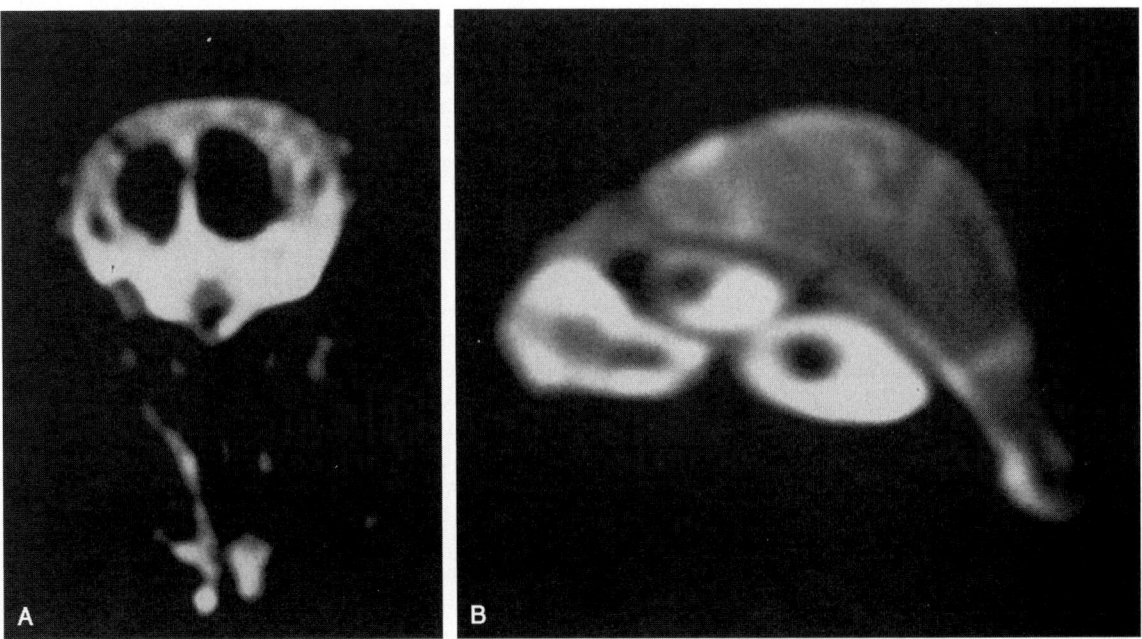

FIGURE 206–19. *A,* Axial magnetic resonance imaging (MRI) of a type II split cord malformation demonstrates a single dural compartment with two separate hemicords. *B,* Axial MRI of a type I split cord demonstrates two distinct dural tubes with their respective hemicords. The midline spur, separating the hemicords, is at a lower level.

or more vertebral levels with a fibrocartilaginous or bony septum producing two hemicords within two separate dural compartments, or the malformation may be composed of two hemicords, often split by fibrotic bands but positioned within a single dural tube (Fig. 206–19). Numerous variations may occur in which the cord splits and rejoins at a lower level (Fig. 206–20). Both types of split cord malformations can occur in the same patient at different locations (Fig. 206–21), and some individuals may have partial split cord malformations. All have tethered spinal cords that require surgical attention.

Before the era of ubiquitous MRI scans, antemortem diagnosis of split cord malformations was difficult. Commonly presenting during periods of accelerated growth with tethered cord symptoms (i.e., back pain, scoliosis, lower extremity weakness or numbness, and bowel or bladder difficulties), such patients were diagnosed in a delayed fashion after examination with myelography or computed tomography (CT) (Fig. 206–22). As associated signature cutaneous manifestations (e.g., focal hirsutism, midline capillary hemangiomas) were correlated with MRI findings, routine diagnosis became commonplace before symptoms manifested (Fig. 206–23).

Although type I and type II split cord malformations have distinguishing features, it is believed that their embryogenesis is similar. Initially proposed by Bremer[74] and further developed by Pang and others,[75–78] the persistence of the accessory neurenteric canal between the yolk sac and amnion acts to divide the neural canal and notochord, leaving behind an endomesenchymal tract. Depending on the timing of formation of this endomesenchymal tract and subsequent mesenchymal infiltration, the neural tube may split into two separate entities with an intervening fibrocartilaginous or bony septum (i.e., type I split cord malformations) or remain a single dural sleeve with a split cord by fibrous elements (i.e., type II split cord malformations) (Fig. 206–24). Various ectodermal or, rarely, endodermal remnants may persist, leading to development of dermal sinus tracts, lipomas, dermoids, or neurenteric cysts.[79, 80] A meningocele or myelomeningocele may also form.[81, 82]

Split cord malformations are three times more common in female than male patients[83–86] and may manifest within the first few weeks of life to the eighth decade, but the average age at presentation is 4 to 6.5 years.[76, 77, 87, 88] Hereditary influences appear to be rare, although one of the authors has treated identical twins who both presented with split cord malformations, with type I occurring in one individual and type II occurring in the other at a different spinal level. Diagnosis of the asymptomatic patient is promoted by various cutaneous stigmata and orthopedic deformities. Cutaneous lesions, such as the commonly visible focal hirsutism (i.e., hairy patch) (see Fig. 206–7), midline hemangioma, dimple, dermal sinus tract, or lipomas, are seen in as many as 71% of the patients with split cord malformations.[89] Orthopedic deformities, including scoliosis, are commonly seen in cases of lower extremity abnormalities. The scoliosis usually results from vertebral anomalies and may be exacerbated over time by eventual tethering of the spinal cord. Pang[75] observed that significant vertebral anomalies were demonstrated in 89% of diastematomyelia patients with a midline septum, whereas patients without a septum had 33% incidence of vertebral abnormalities. Lower extremity findings include asymmetry in foot or leg length, cavovarus feet, and clawed toes. The smaller limb often has a correspondingly smaller hemicord, which can be visualized on radiologic evaluation and may manifest initially with focal tethering symptoms in the symptomatic patient. Patients with split cord malformations whose cords become tethered have clinical courses similar to those of patients with tethered cords and other occult types of spinal dysraphism.

Radiologic evaluation of the suspected patient with a split cord malformation should include both CT and MRI. MRI can provide extraordinary detail regarding the type of split (i.e., type I versus type II) and often depicts the fibrocartilaginous bands that tether the cord and other intradural lesions, such as dermoids or filum lipomas. It has been reported[90] that the conus is abnor-

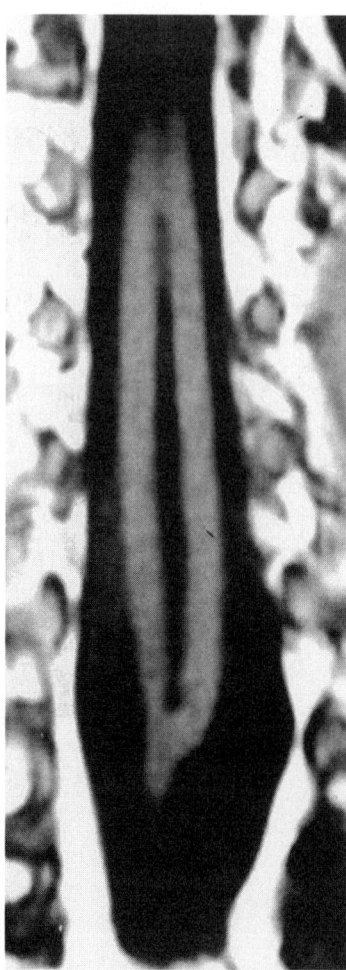

FIGURE 206–20. This patient had a type II split cord malformation that appeared to reconstitute at a lower level. At the time of tethered cord release, the split cords were found to have significant arachnoid adhesions in the ventral compartment over the region of the split.

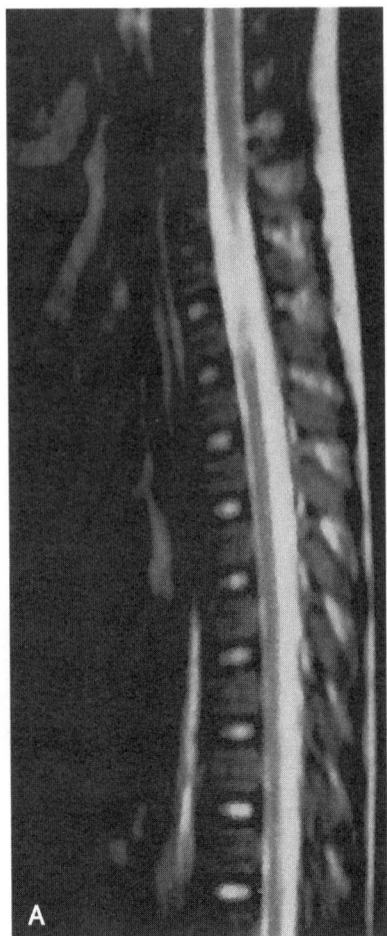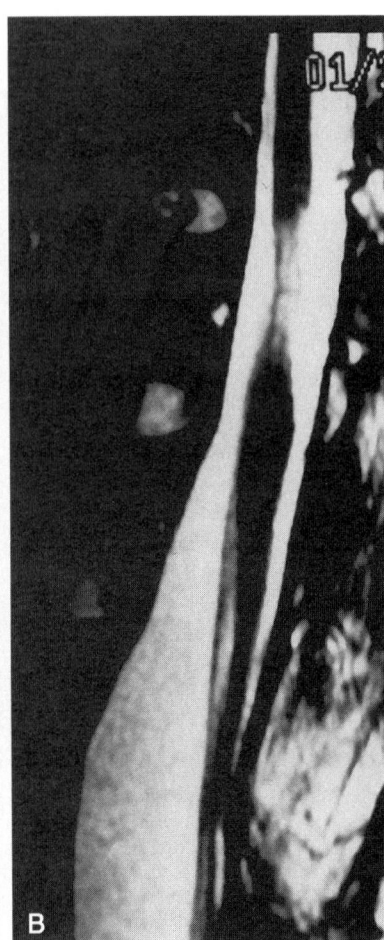

FIGURE 206–21. *A,* Cervical magnetic resonance imaging (MRI) of a 15-year-old girl with low back pain, increased lower extremity stiffness, and occasional bladder incontinence. This patient had an upper cervical split cord malformation and a lumbosacral split cord. *B,* Lumbosacral MRI of a 15-year-old girl who had a cervical split cord malformation. The patient presented with lower cord symptoms resulting from tethering of the lumbosacral split cord malformation. The cervical split cord malformation remained asymptomatic.

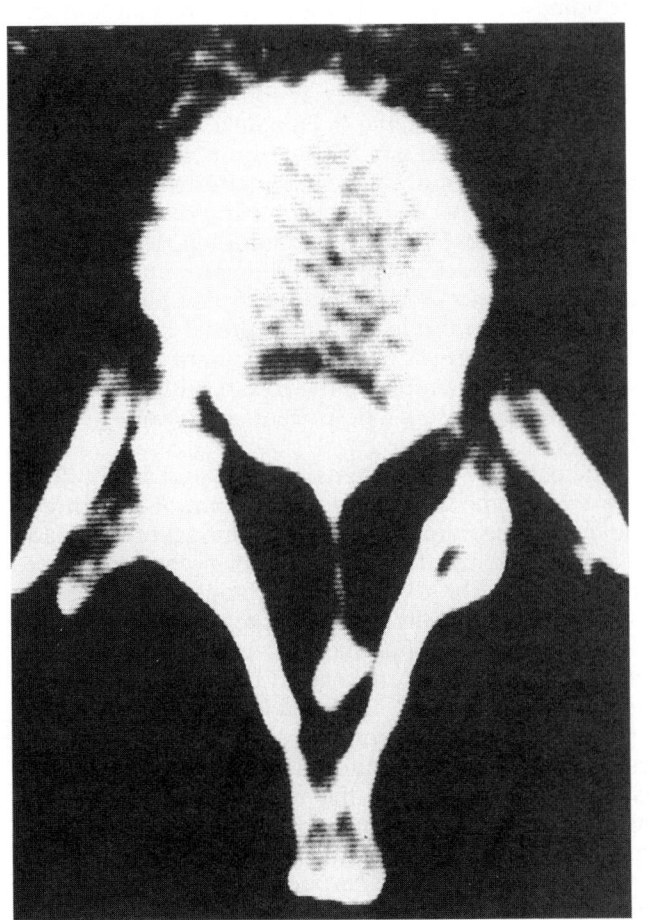

FIGURE 206–22. Computed tomography of an adolescent patient who presented with back pain and lower extremity weakness. Notice the midline bony septum extending from the vertebral body to the spinous process in this patient with a type I split cord malformation.

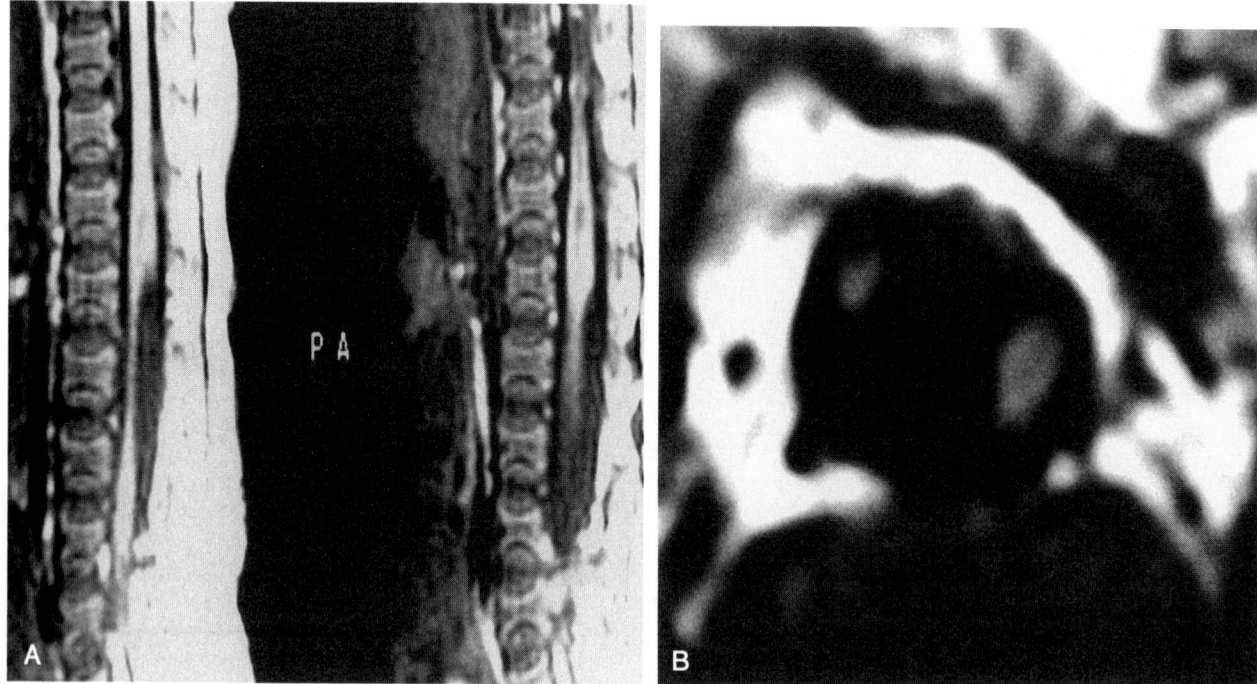

FIGURE 206–23. On magnetic resonance imaging, sagittal and axial views show the distal cord. The dysmorphic appearance of the cord is shown on the sagittal view, with a characteristic smaller hemicord seen on cross section. It is not uncommon for patients with monoparesis or atrophy to have a smaller hemicord on the same side.

mally low in as many as 83% of patients with diastematomyelia and is often associated with an abnormally thickened or lipomatous filum terminale. A hydromyelic cavity is often present just cephalad to the split in the cord, but it may also be distal to the fissure. Patients presenting with tethered cord symptoms may also have clinical exacerbation related to the syrinx. Additional dysraphic changes may occur and require MRI visualization of the entire cord. Routine CT and three-dimensional reconstruction may offer considerable insight into the type and number of vertebral anomalies. CT can demonstrate with considerable detail the location of any bony or fibrocartilaginous midline septum. The midline septum may originate from the ventral body, occur in the posterior elements, or more commonly, traverse the entire spinal canal. The location of the cleft[80] is solely lumbar in 47% of patients with diastematomyelia, thoracolumbar in 27%, exclusively thoracic in 23%, and sacral or cervical in 1.5%. In addition to CT and MRI, the workup should include plain spinal radiographs to demonstrate the site of diastematomyelia and provide an excellent overview of vertebral anomalies and associated scoliosis.

Treatment involves prophylactic detethering as a result of the work of Guthkelch in 1974.[91] Guthkelch, who followed 17 children presenting with diastematomyelia and associated septum, found that 14 developed neurological symptoms later, whereas only 1 of 22 patients treated with prophylactic detethering had later deterioration resulting from progressive scoliosis. Numerous investigators[76, 77, 81, 92–95] recommend prophylactic detethering for pediatric patients with diastematomyelia,

including children presenting with solitary dural tubes (type II), who have been shown by Pang[74] and by James and Lassman[81] to possess numerous intrathecal fibrous bands and to be at risk for cord tethering.

The surgical objective is complete release of all intrathecal bands and any midline spurs to effect detethering. Both types of split cord malformations require similar approaches but also have individual differences in the intraoperative setting. In addition to detethering affected cords, attention to additional pathologic entities is critical to prevent long-term neurological compromise. Individuals with intrathecal lipomas, dermoids, neurenteric cysts, and syrinxes require additional effort in freeing the cord. Multiple split cord malformations in a single patient may need detethering.

The patient with diastematomyelia and a split dural sleeve (i.e., type I) has an obvious point of tethering at the midline septum (Fig. 206–25). This septum is made of bone, cartilage, fibrous tissue, or a combination of these tissues. The dural sleeve is split by the septum and may remain split or rejoin at a lower level. Dorsal bony elements are often incomplete or abnormally developed and may be attached to the dorsal dural tube and underlying cord. Removal of the dorsal lamina and spinous processes should be undertaken with great care to avoid injury to underlying neural elements. It is necessary to remove the midline septum (with a rongeur or drill) to the ventral surface along with the medial walls of the split dural tube. Exposure of the involved region must incorporate proximal and distal areas of the septum to adequately view other potential

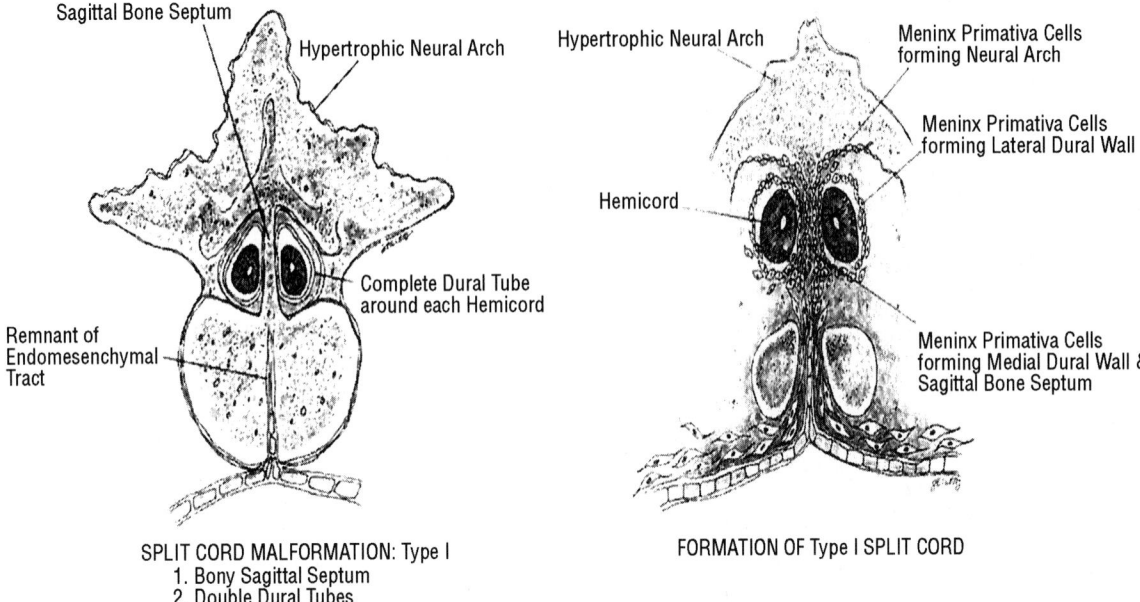

SPLIT CORD MALFORMATION: Type I
1. Bony Sagittal Septum
2. Double Dural Tubes
   ("Diastematomyelia")

FORMATION OF Type I SPLIT CORD

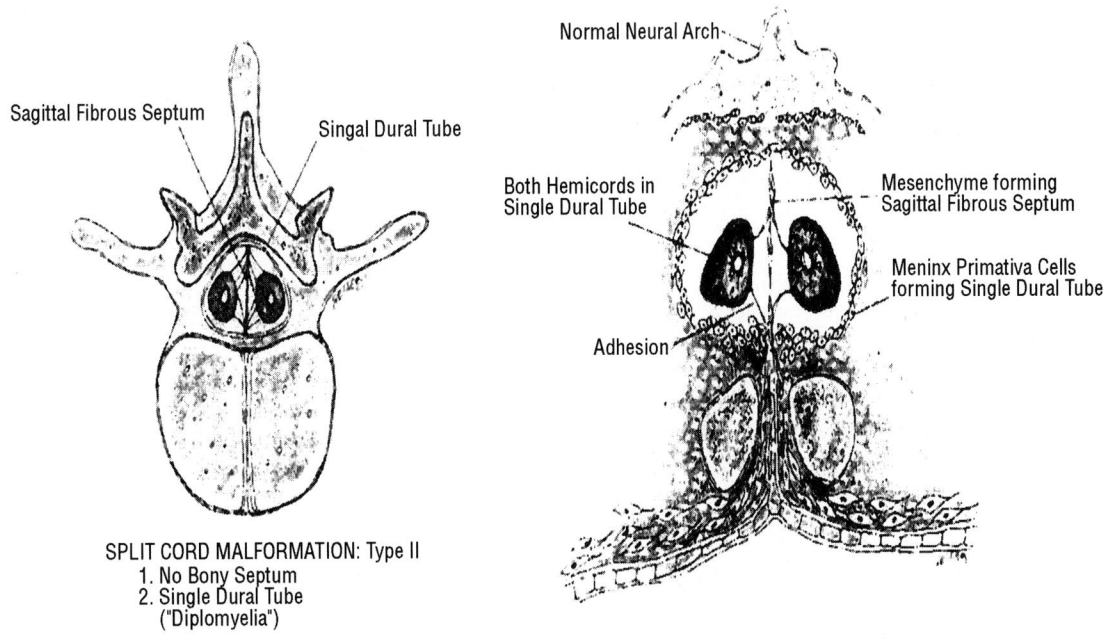

SPLIT CORD MALFORMATION: Type II
1. No Bony Septum
2. Single Dural Tube
   ("Diplomyelia")

FORMATION OF Type II SPLIT CORD

FIGURE 206–24. Embryogenesis of type I and II split cord malformations. A persistent accessory neurenteric canal leads to a remnant of an endomesenchymal tract, which leads to the development of two separate neural tubes. Depending on the timing, the patient develops an intervening septum resulting in diastematomyelia or formation of two separate neural tubes within a singular dural tube. (From Pang D, Dias MS, Ahab-Barmada M: Split cord malformation. Part I. A unified theory of embryogenesis for double spinal cord malformations. Neurosurgery 31:451–480, 1992.)

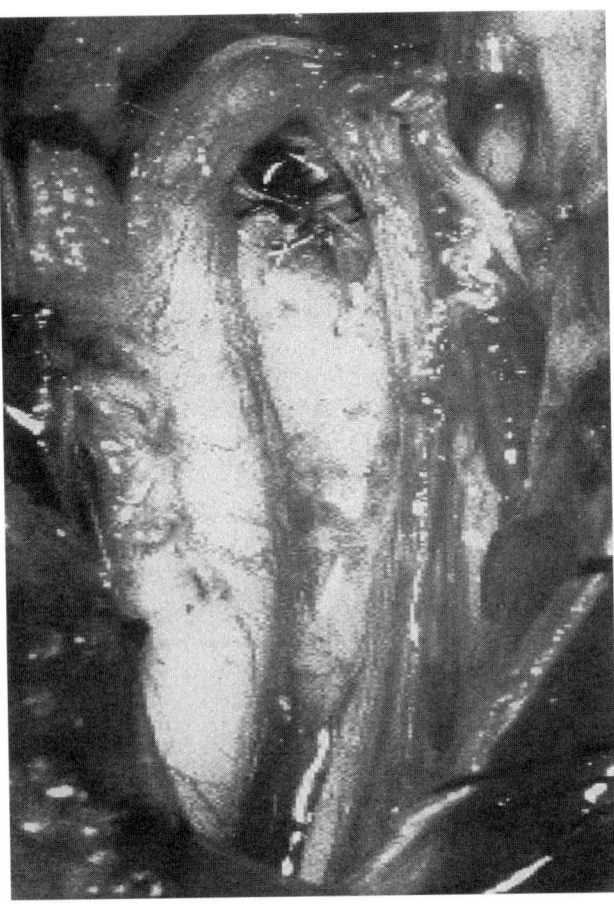

FIGURE 206–25. Intraoperative photograph of a patient with a type I split cord malformation. Notice the difference in the size of the hemicords and the location of the ventral spur, which has been surgically removed. The anterior dura has been repaired with 4–0 Neurolon suture.

sources of tethering. A syrinx proximal to the septum is frequently observed and may require drainage by means of syringostomy or shunt for adequate decompression or detethering of the cord. Considerable caution is needed during removal of the midline spur to protect the closely associated dural tubes and associated arachnoid adhesions and to avoid the blood vessels in the midline septum emanating or draining from the midline. Interruption of these vessels may lead to difficulty in controlling bleeding when they retract into the ventral bony surface. In addition to division of the arachnoid adhesions that are commonly present, evaluation of the distal conus and fila must be thorough. These patients typically have two separate filum terminales, and adequate detethering requires sectioning of both fila. It has been our experience that patients with split cord malformations whose cords retether may have had inadequate sectioning of all the fila and warrant re-exploration. Closure of the dural tube requires ventral and dorsal repairs, although incomplete closure of the anterior dura rarely leads to subsequent cerebrospinal fluid (CSF) leak.

Detethering of the split cord malformation within a single dural sleeve (i.e., type II) or any other variation, such as a partial split, requires a similar approach.[96]

Although it is not necessary to remove a midline septum, great care must be taken during exposure of the septal split and subsequent dissection of arachnoid adhesions and bands (Fig. 206–26). Such arachnoid reflections may be dense at the ventral surface, especially at the cleft, and may require division of the lateral dentate ligaments to provide sufficient exposure by rotating the cord. Extreme caution must be exercised when approaching the ventral adhesions. These patients frequently present with neurological compromise and tolerate minimal cord movement during dissection. They frequently have exacerbations of their neurological states. The surgeon must also evaluate the conus and section all fila.

After detethering, the outcomes of patients with split cord malformations are generally excellent, but outcomes vary for patients undergoing re-exploration for retethering. In Guthkelch's study in 1974,[84] prophylactic surgery offered significant protection against later neurological deterioration with minimal morbidity. Neurological improvement was demonstrated in 73% of patients in Kennedy's study[85] of 60 patients with diastematomyelia. In the same study, 14% of the patients remained unchanged, but 13 had subsequent deterioration. Gower and associates[76] found similar results and observed that a stable neurological state was sustained for as long as 28 years in a series of 21 patients who had undergone surgical treatment.

Neurenteric Cysts

The uncommon neurenteric cyst originates from a persistent neurenteric canal communicating between the yolk sac and the amniotic cavity through the developing notochord. This transient passageway permits the development of mucosa-lined tracts from the mediastinum (respiratory) or abdominal viscera to form intradural, extramedullary cysts within the thecal canal. Vertebral anomalies commonly coexist with split cord malformations and dermal sinus tracts.[79, 80, 97]

Neurenteric cysts occur most commonly in males and are most frequently encountered in the ventral, cervicothoracic region,[98–101] although they may develop dorsally[102] or anywhere along the remainder of neuraxis. The cysts usually manifest with cord compression and infrequently correlate with tethered cord symptoms. The patient presenting typically is 50 to 60 years old, and the cyst may be confused with disk herniation, schwannoma, meningioma, or a metastatic lesion. When encountered in the pediatric population, the neurenteric cyst may be accompanied by an abdominal mass or anorectal malformation.

Radiologic evaluation may reveal vertebral body anomalies, and block vertebrae or hemivertebrae are common.[103] Although most vertebral defects are ventral, posterior abnormalities and diastematomyelia may also be visualized. CT can demonstrate non–contrast-enhancing intradural extramedullary cysts, with occasional communication demonstrated between the mediastinum and abdominal viscera along with spinal body findings.[104] MRI, the study of choice, can define the non–contrast-enhancing intradural cyst from the

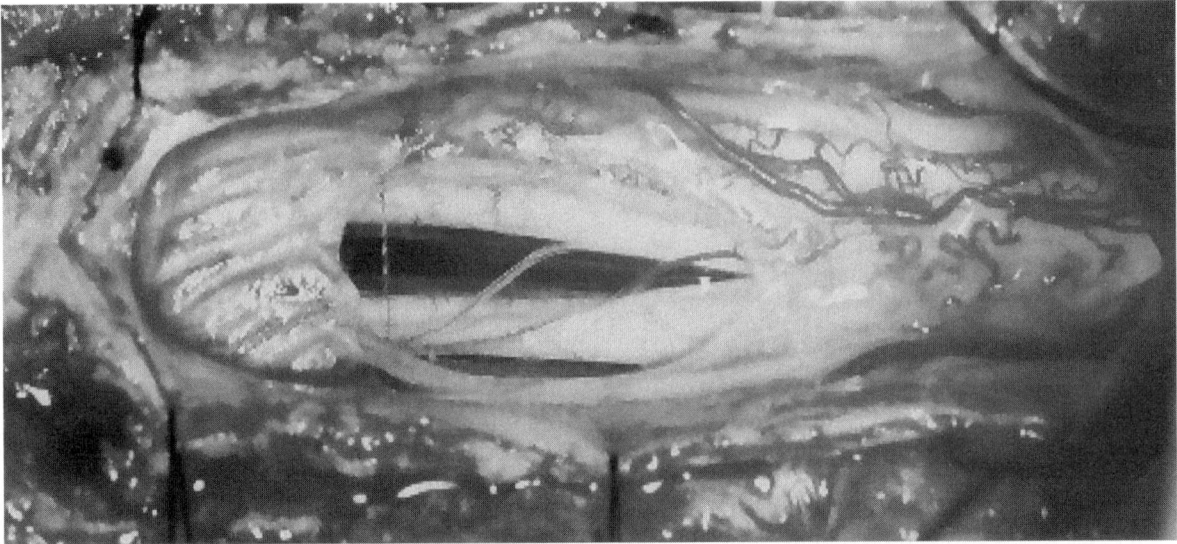

FIGURE 206–26. This 7-year-old patient presented with back pain and scoliosis. Magnetic resonance imaging showed a tethered cord resulting from a type II split cord malformation. This intraoperative photograph depicts the equal-sized hemicords but fails to demonstrate well the presence of numerous arachnoid granulations and adhesions, commonly found at the anterior surface.

spinal cord, which may be isointense or slightly hyperintense on T1-weighted images and slightly hyperintense on T2-weighted images, helping to separate this entity from an arachnoid cyst.

The goal of treatment remains complete excision of the cyst to avoid recurrence. Although the cyst often is ventral to the cord, a posterior-lateral approach usually provides the most direct avenue to resection. The cord is often displaced from the mass and may be dissected free from the cord after sectioning the dentate ligaments and aspirating the cyst contents. Because of the viscous, mucinous contents, this procedure may provide only partial collapse of the cystic mass, but this often allows sufficient room to maneuver safely around the spinal cord. Complete excision of the cyst and its wall is often associated with an improved neurological status and an excellent long-term prognosis. Incomplete resection necessitates close long-term follow-up to rule out recurrence. Anterior defects identified at the time of surgery may be occluded with muscle, fascia, or bone chips in addition to direct dural closure. Other associated lesions, such as dermal sinus tracts or diastematomyelia, may require separate attention and corroborate the need for complete neuraxis evaluation before planning eventual surgical therapeutics.

Terminal Syringomyelia

Long known to represent a pathophysiologic state in the spinal cord, syringomyelia may have a number of causes, such as Chiari malformations, tethered cord, tumor, and post-traumatic states. A dilated central canal at the terminus of the spinal cord (Fig. 206–27) appears to represent a different entity and remains problematic, especially in the era of increasingly sensitive MRI scans.[105] Patients may have other associated birth anomalies, such as anorectal malformations, sa-

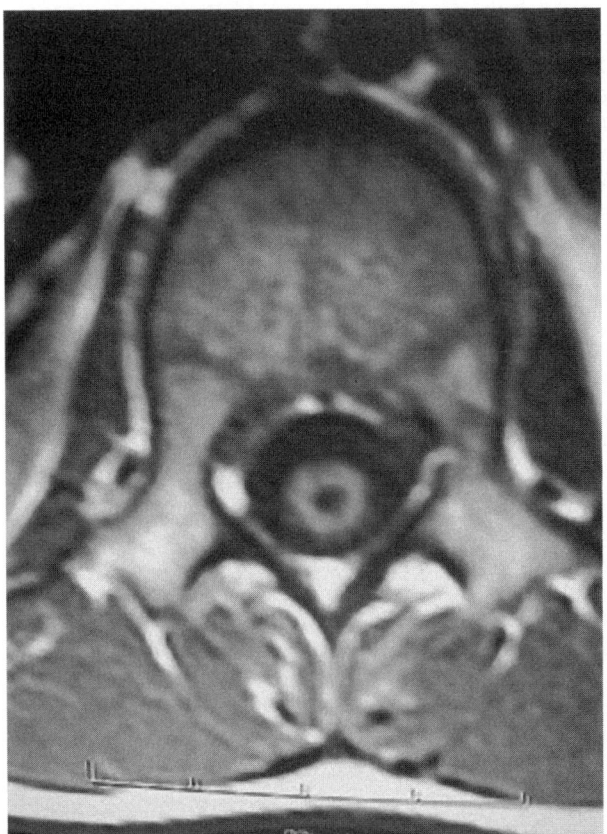

FIGURE 206–27. Terminal syringomyelia manifests with an expanded terminal central canal in the distal third of the cord. This may be seen without any other associated dysraphic conditions but is commonly seen in the setting of anorectal malformations and a hypertrophic or lipomatous filum terminale or in conjunction with a split cord malformation or meningocele manqué. It may represent an early sign of cord tethering or may be an incidental finding. Clinical correlation is imperative with this manifestation of occult spinal dysraphism.

cral dysgenesis, meningocele manqué, anterior meningoceles, and split cord malformations. An expanded terminal central canal is most commonly associated with a hypertrophic or lipomatous filum terminale in conjunction with anorectal malformations (67% of cases), meningocele manqué (54%), or split cord malformations (38%) and, to a lesser degree, with other types of spinal dysraphism.[105] A dilated terminal central canal may be identified during an evaluation for scoliosis and raises the issue of cord tethering. In the absence of other developmental or cord abnormalities, it may be difficult to ascribe any pathologic significance to a focal terminal syrinx. In the setting of other dysraphic states, terminal hydromyelia may indicate ongoing tethering and warrant closer scrutiny. Patients with suspected cord tethering should be followed closely for any evidence of symptoms or progression in their neurological or radiologic examination findings. A patient's scoliosis may demonstrate significant deterioration despite the absence of other causative factors, such as vertebral anomalies.

In these patients, detethering the cord frequently reduces the size of the terminal syrinx over time, and the progress can be monitored by serial MRI evaluations. The decision to drain the cavity must be considered in light of potential morbidity from the myelotomy and long-term issues arising from complications of syringosubarachnoid, syringoperitoneal, or syringopleural shunts. Patients presenting predominantly with tethered cord symptoms and who have small to moderately sized terminal dilatations are best served by release of the tethered cord only. For individuals with large or equivocally sized syringomyelic cavities and questionable contributions to their symptoms, a direct syringostomy or syringosubarachnoid shunt at the cord's thinnest location may be undertaken during the detethering. If the spinal cord is adequately released and the syrinx decompressed at the time of surgery, postoperative radiologic evaluation may demonstrate continued decompression of the syrinx. If the terminal syrinx reappears later, it is possible that the cord has retethered and may require another operation. Placement of a syringoperitoneal or syringopleural shunt should be reserved for patients with large, persistent syringohydromyelia despite adequate attempts to detether the cord and exclusion of other possible causes (e.g., Chiari malformation, hydrocephalus). Although shunt placement is often successful in decreasing the size of the syrinx, the long-term efficacy is unclear, and the course may be complicated by the development of myelomalacia, pain, and traction injury to the underlying cord.

Dermal Sinus Tracts

Congenital dermal sinus tracts have been long recognized as potential sites for the entry of bacteria into the intraspinal compartment, contributing to the development of meningitis.[106–112] The clinical connection between a dermal sinus tract and tethered cord has only recently been appreciated. These midline defects (see Figs. 206–4, 206–8, and 206–9) often appear innocuous and may be accompanied by hair and other cutaneous manifestations of spinal dysraphism. Most commonly found at the lumbosacral border, they may occur anywhere in the midline along the entire neuraxis, from the nasion (see Fig. 206–10) to the coccygeal terminus.[30, 113, 114] Approximately 13% of dermal sinus tracts occur below the sacrococcygeal junction, with 35% occurring at the lumbosacral junction, 41% in the lumbar region, 10% in the thoracic area, and 1% in the cervical segment.[115] The sinus tract terminates dorsal to the spinal elements in 6% to 7% of patients, ends in the epidural space in 10% to 20%, and terminates within the thecal canal in 58% to 60%. The tract is lined with epithelium and potentially represents a void in the normally impenetrable barrier to the thecal sac, but approximately one half of the tracts terminates in a dermoid (83%) or epidermoid (13%) cyst or a teratoma (4%).[116] These inclusion bodies may rest at the termination of the dermal sinus tract or may be remote, and they may sometimes be multiple (Fig. 206–28). Recurrent meningitis or the presence of atypical organisms should prompt a search for midline dermal defects over the entire neuraxis. *Escherichia coli* and *Streptococcus aureus* are the most commonly encountered organisms, and almost one half of the cases of meningitis are caused by gram-negative organisms.[113, 115]

The incidence of dermal sinus tracts is approximately 1 case per 2500 live births,[108, 117] although the sacrococcygeal dimples are seen in approximately 2% to 4% of newborns and are infrequently associated with underlying pathology. Nevertheless, because of the occasional association with dysraphic conditions and tethering, it is common practice to obtain a lumbosacral ultrasound scan within the first 4 to 6 months to delineate the level of the conus and exclude any intraspinal pathology. Prospective studies defining the overall incidence of a low-positioned conus (i.e., spinal cord tethering) and associated sacral dimples are lacking. Patients older than 4 to 6 months (i.e., beyond the ultrasound window) should undergo evaluation for lower extremity, spinal, or neurological findings to exclude possible dysraphic states associated with a higher risk for underlying tethering. For this subset of patients or any individual for whom there is clinical suspicion of occult dysraphism, MRI can demonstrate the level of the conus and rule out intraspinal pathology.

Clinical presentation varies according to the patient's age and the presence of infection. Meningitis resulting from dermal sinus tracts may occur at any age and is seen in infants and elderly patients. Inclusion tumors related to sinus tracts may often remain asymptomatic unless they contribute to cord tethering or cause cord or cauda equina compression. The slow growth rate of these tumors often masks their presentation for years, although there are numerous examples of patients with acute neurological deterioration (Fig. 206–29). Patients may present with concomitant infections of the dermal sinus tract and underlying inclusion cysts.

Radiologic investigation relies on ultrasonography and MRI for definitive documentation of the level of the

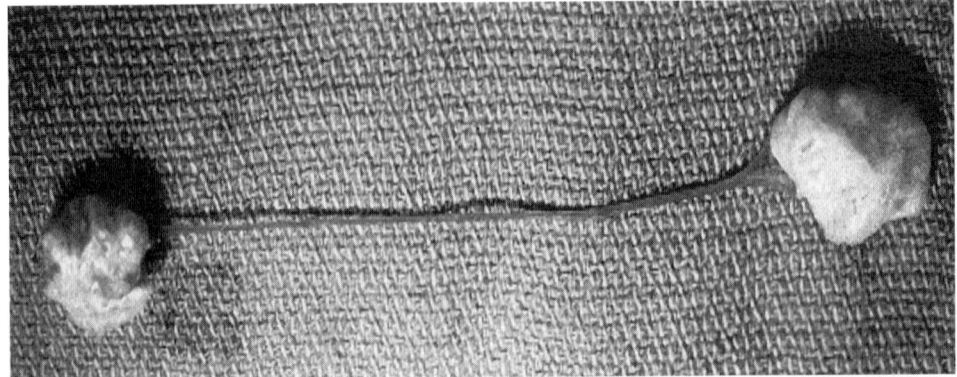

FIGURE 206–28. A 14-year-old boy presented with fluid emanating from his back and with back and leg pain. He was found to have a thoracolumbar dermal sinus tract. Magnetic resonance imaging (MRI) demonstrated a contiguous tract from his dermal sinus to the tip of the conus, ending in a likely dermoid. A secondary lesion was thought to be present at a more cephalad location, which was confirmed at the time of surgical exploration. The two dermoids shown here are attached by a fibrotic strand. It is critical to examine the entire spinal cord during MRI evaluation to exclude associated lesions.

conus, intraspinal extension of the tract (Fig. 206–30), and presence of inclusion cysts (i.e., epidermoid or dermoid). Infants have sufficient space between the interspinous processes for adequate delineation of intraspinal structures until approximately 4 to 6 months of age. MRI has become the reference study because of its ability to accurately depict the extraspinal and intraspinal portions of the sinus tract. MRI is able to define most intraspinal tumors at the site of the tract and the remainder of the neuraxis. Additional intraspinal pathology may be present elsewhere in the canal, and the entire spine should be evaluated before undertaking surgical planning. Plain radiographs of the spine may reveal associated dysraphic findings, but normal findings do not preclude underlying intraspinal pathology. CT-myelography was at one time commonly employed but has been supplanted by MRI.[30] When it is difficult to clearly ascertain the presence of a dermoid lesion on MRI, CT-myelography may be helpful.

In view of the risk of meningitis and associated difficulty in the setting of intraspinal inclusion cysts and possible spinal tethering, all dermal sinus tracts should be completely excised. The timing should allow for complete resolution of any associated infection and should proceed any time after 6 months of age once a diagnosis has been made. Although there is some controversy regarding the choice of prophylactic antibiotics for patients with dermal sinus tracts, most clinicians recommend using gram-positive and gram-negative coverage. Almost one half of the meningitis cases encountered before diagnosis demonstrates gram-negative organisms, and it is common to find gram-negative organisms in the lumbosacral region in infants.

Removal of the tract may be accomplished directly by an elliptical excision at the skin surface or from below in the subcutaneous plane. It may be difficult to sterilize deep-seated organisms within the sinus tract during the preoperative skin preparation, and this may

FIGURE 206–29. Intraspinal dermoids occur more commonly as congenital anomalies but may develop after routine spinal taps. The intraoperative photograph shows an 8-year-old boy who presented with acute back pain and new-onset bladder incontinence. Magnetic resonance imaging demonstrated a normally positioned conus with an intrathecal mass consistent with a dermoid. Closer scrutiny revealed a history of a spinal tap when the patient was a neonate undergoing a workup for fever. Complete resection of the dermoid led to resolution of his symptoms.

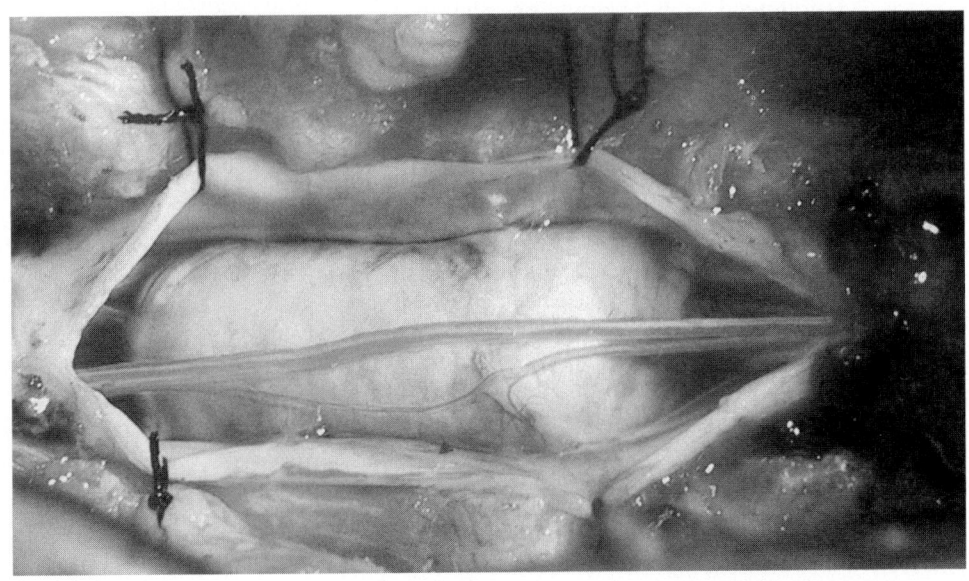

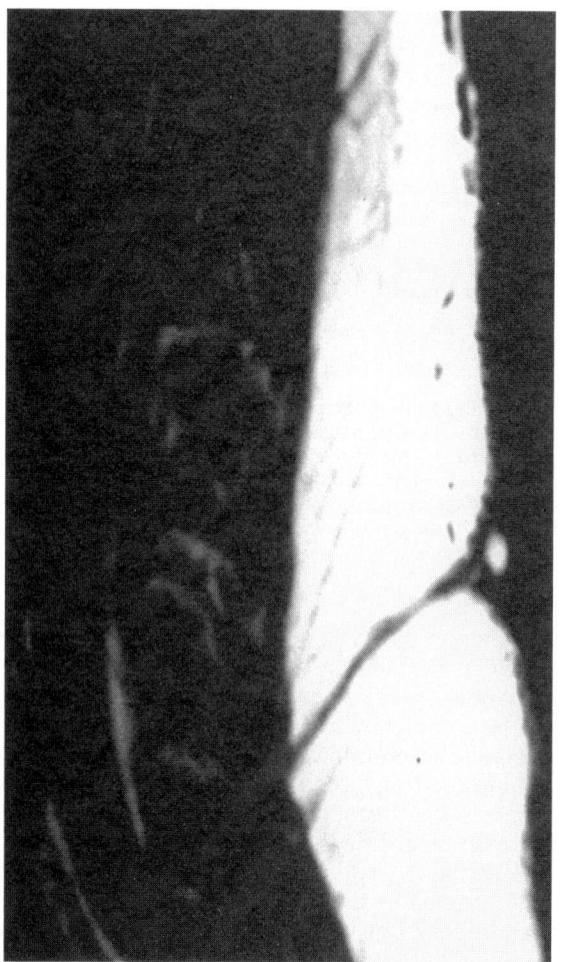

FIGURE 206–30. Magnetic resonance imaging of a 6-year-old boy with an obvious cutaneous dermal sinus tract. The tract is marked by a vitamin E tablet and ends at a low conus with prominent filum lipomas.

place the patient at some risk for development of a postoperative infection despite prophylactic antibiotics. After the tract has been disconnected from the skin surface, it is followed to its termination. Slightly more than one half end within the thecal sac, and it is recommended that the dura be opened unless radiologic studies and direct visualization show without any doubt that the lesion is solely extraspinal. Frequently, the tract continues through a defect at the lumbosacral fascia and posterior spinal elements. During the laminectomy or laminoplasty, care should be taken at the tract's insertion to the dural tube. The normal epidural fat and tissue planes may be anomalous and can include significant variations in vascular anatomy. Exposure of the thecal sac should allow adequate visualization of the entire area of cord involvement, including any associated intraspinal tumors. It is important to have complete radiologic visualization of the entire spinal cord to accurately ascertain all intraspinal pathology. After complete excision of the dermal sinus tract and associated intraspinal pathology, patients are kept prone for 48 hours and maintained on gram-positive and gram-negative antibiotic coverage for 48

hours. Surgical morbidity is minimal except for infection, and patients are usually ready for discharge within 3 to 4 days.

Meningoceles

POSTERIOR MENINGOCELES

Anterior and posterior meningoceles represent a herniation of meninges and CSF through a dural defect. Posterior involvement is often appreciated during prenatal evaluation with ultrasonography and may be confused with a myelomeningocele. The absence of hydrocephalus, Chiari malformation, or lower extremity abnormalities often helps to determine the diagnosis of a posterior meningocele. Found most commonly in the lumbosacral region, posterior meningoceles are covered with full- or partial-thickness, overlying integument (Fig. 206–31). Neurocutaneous lesions, such as hemangiomas, dermal sinus tracts, or lipomas, may be associated with a posterior meningocele. One study found the position of the conus below the level of L3 in all 28 patients with a dorsal meningocele evaluated by whole-spine MRI.[118] Frequently, children born with meningoceles have normal findings on neurological examinations, normal lower extremity architecture, and normal underlying cord anatomy without evidence for tethering. In the setting of concomitant dysraphic conditions (e.g., lipomas, split cord malformations, dermal sinus tract and inclusion cysts), such patients are likely to be at risk for cord tethering. Patients with posterior meningoceles also may have arachnoid adhesions that place them at risk for possible tethering. Consequently, all patients born with meningoceles require thorough MRI evaluation (Fig. 206–32) during the preoperative workup to exclude the presence of other associated dysraphic conditions[119] and dural and arachnoid adhesions. These patients must be followed over time to identify any evidence of tethering.

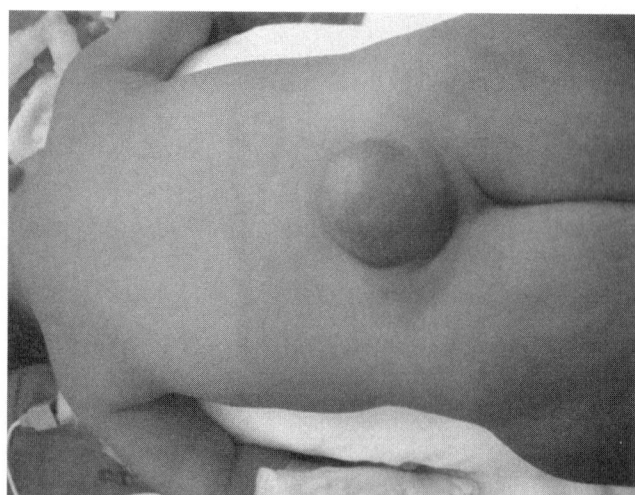

FIGURE 206–31. Lateral view of a lumbosacral meningocele in a patient with otherwise normal neurological examination findings. Preoperative magnetic resonance imaging demonstrated a low-lying cord and probable arachnoid adhesions.

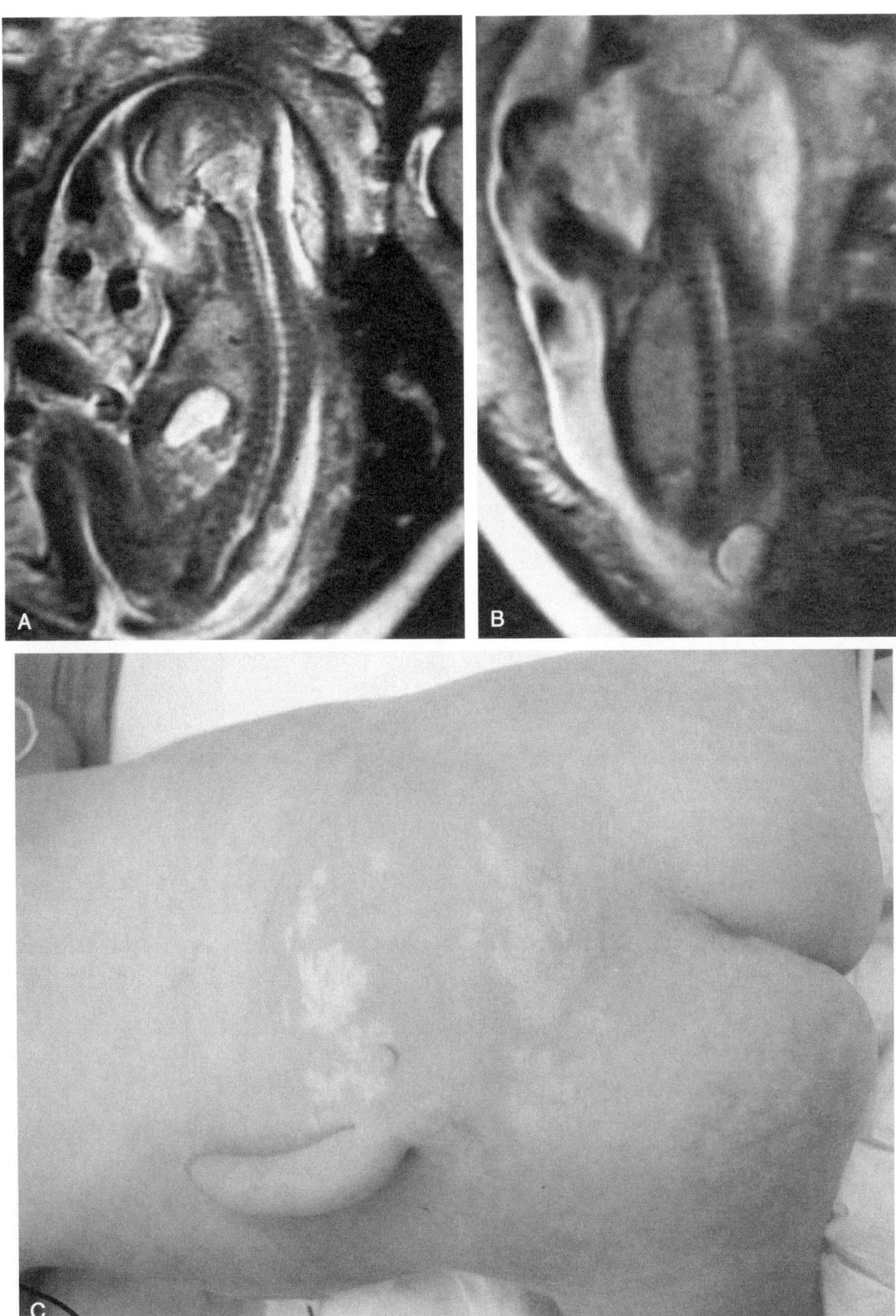

FIGURE 206–32. *A,* Prenatal, sagittal-view magnetic resonance imaging (MRI) demonstrates a lumbo-sacral sac with mixed signal characteristics consistent with a meningocele or a combined lipoma-meningocele. The brain is normal, and there is no evidence for any other associated spinal abnormali-ties. *B,* Coronal MRI of the lesion during the prenatal workup. This view appeared more consistent with a meningocele. *C,* At the time of birth, the patient had a moderate-sized lipoma with an associated tail and numerous areas of hypopigmentation. Notice the accessory, smaller tail medial to the primary appendage. The tail was removed initially for cosmetic purposes. The patient returned at 3 months for a second MRI scan and underwent detethering at 5 months. The initial MRI depicted a low-lying cord resulting from an extensive intradural lipoma.

Surgical repair should be undertaken in the immediate postnatal period if there is any likelihood of imminent rupture of the sac. A tenuous skin covering is best served by direct repair and closure of the defect during the first week of life. Although uncommon, hydrocephalus should be ruled out with CT or MRI before repair of the defect. For most patients, the skin covering provides sufficient protection to the underlying neural elements until the patient is 3 to 6 months old. Delaying surgery until a later time allows better radiologic definition of underlying structures and possible associated dysraphic conditions and arachnoid adhesions. It permits greater maturation of the immunologic system. During this time, the patient should be followed closely for any signs of tethering. Although extremely uncommon, it has been our experience that patients may present before the age of 6 months with evidence of tethering. In this situation, the patient should proceed directly to exploration and detethering.

The defects in most patients are repaired at 3 to 6 months of age. At the time of surgery, the children undergo gram-positive and gram-negative antibiotic prophylaxis. A midline incision is made in an elliptical fashion around the neck of the meningocele for small to moderately sized lesions (Fig. 206–33A). Larger lesions may be more easily approached through a transverse incision. Dissection is carried down to the fascial plane, isolating the neck and contents of the meningocele (see Fig. 206–33B). The sac is opened for direct exploration of the intradural compartment and release of any associated tethering from dural or arachnoid bands or other dysraphic elements, such as lipomas or dermoids (see Fig. 206–33C). After confirmation of free and unencumbered cord and roots, the dura is closed in a watertight fashion. Repair of the lumbosacral fascia and subcutaneous layer is completed, and the skin is closed with absorbable suture in two layers (see Fig. 206–33D).

ANTERIOR MENINGOCELES

Anterior meningoceles are defects in the dural envelope that permit herniation of meninges and CSF in a

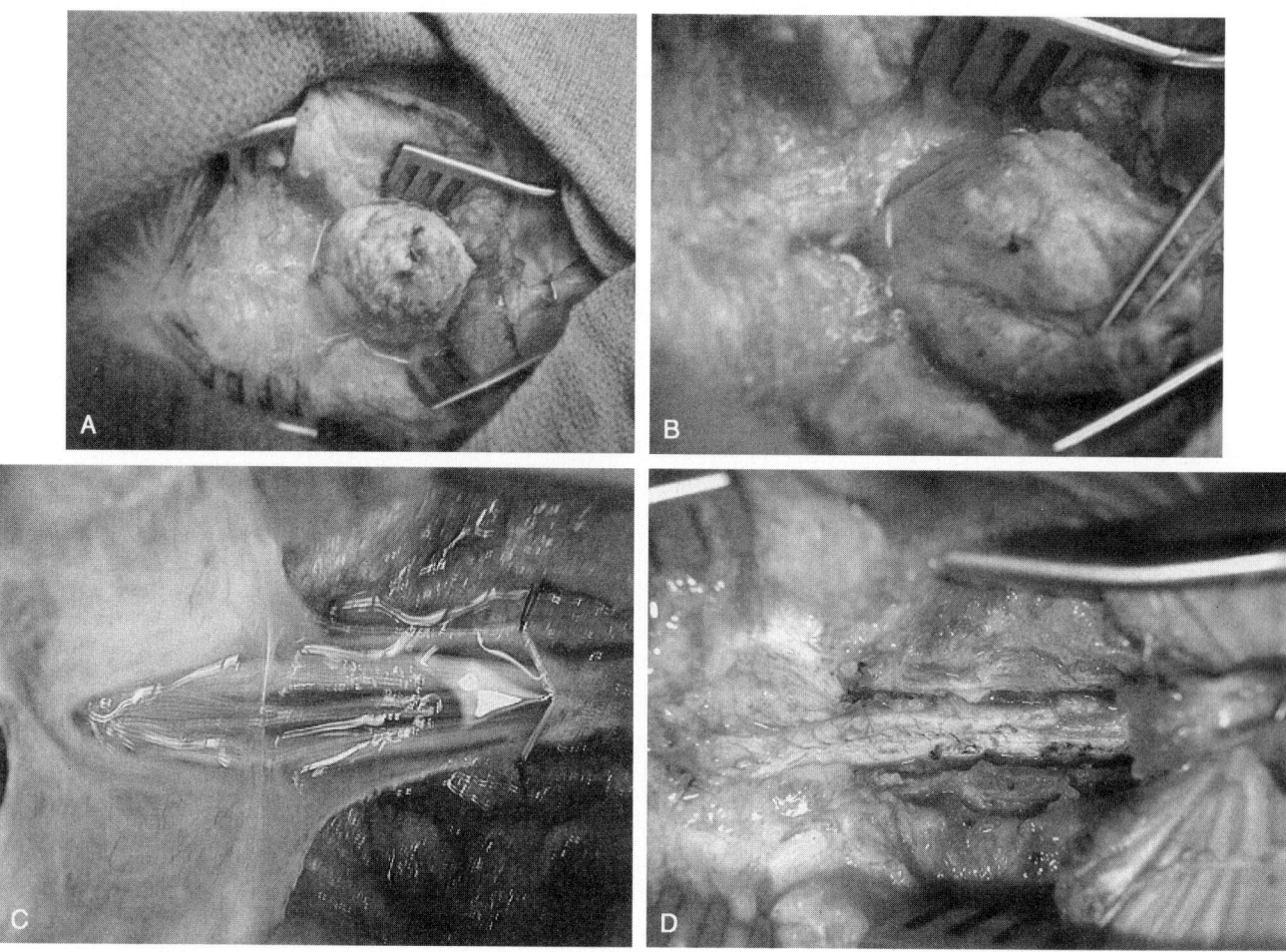

FIGURE 206–33. *A,* Intraoperative exposure of the meningocele seen in Figure 206–31. The superficial dermis has been carefully dissected to maintain the intact meningocele sac. *B,* The meningocele sac is separated from the fascial defect and is found to communicate with the dural tube. *C,* Opening the meningocele sac exposes a normal cauda equina except for the presence of numerous arachnoid adhesions and bands, which were lysed. There were no other associated lesions seen on magnetic resonance imaging or during the operative exposure. *D,* Resection of the meningocele sac and reapproximation of the dural edges.

ventral location, most commonly in the presacral or lumbosacral region. A strong female predominance (9: 1) and familial occurrence are characteristic. In 1981, Currarino and colleagues[120] described the triad of anorectal malformations, sacral bony abnormalities, and a presacral mass. The older child who presents with Currarino triad frequently has a long history of constipation, vague abdominal discomfort, progressive abdominal distention, recurrent urinary tract infections, and dysmenorrhea.[121] The older patient may also have tethered cord symptoms, bringing to light a low-lying spinal cord associated with sacral dysgenesis and a presacral mass. The initial diagnosis may be made by routine pelvic ultrasonography during pregnancy. The infant or toddler may present at an early age because of significant anorectal malformations that may involve rectal atresia, stenosis, or more involved cloacal disruptions. Although such individuals often have normal findings on neurological examinations, they are at significant risk for potential tethering and require resection of the presacral masses. The presacral tumors may consist of germ cell tumors such as dermoid cysts, epidermoid cysts,[122] or teratomas (40%) or may be lipomas or primarily simple meningoceles (47%).[123] In addition to potential growth and uncertain pathology, anterior sacral masses may provide a direct source for meningitis. Patients with recurrent meningitis or who present with unusual organisms without a clear source should undergo radiologic evaluation of the sacral bony architecture and MRI investigation of the presacral or lumbar regions.

Plain radiographs may demonstrate sacral abnormalities, particularly the scimitar sign, a unilateral, sickle-shaped, bony sacral defect (Fig. 206–34). CT may help to define bony landmarks and their relationship

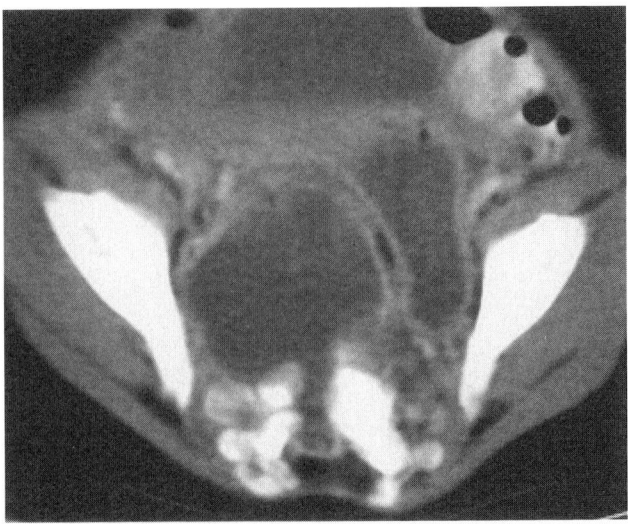

FIGURE 206–35. For the patient described in Figure 206–34, a computed tomographic scan of the pelvis demonstrates the anterior and posterior spinal defects associated with a large presacral cystic mass. There appears to be a direct communication with the thecal sac. The differential diagnosis included teratoma, dermoid, epidermoid, and probable meningocele.

with the anterior sacral defect (Fig. 206–35). MRI imaging[124-126] provides a three-dimensional overview of the anterior sacral mass relative to the surrounding intra-abdominal anatomy and may offer insight into tissue pathology and reveal other types of associated spinal dysraphism (Fig. 206–36).

Treatment approaches are directed by the age and presentation of the patient with the anterior meningocele. Patients presenting during the prenatal period are best served by elective delivery by means of cesarean section. This prevents inadvertent rupture of the sac and minimizes subsequent infection. Anterior sacral meningoceles discovered at birth or in the immediate postnatal period are best approached by direct surgical excision in the first 3 to 6 months. If the radiologic evaluation unequivocally demonstrates a CSF-filled sac consistent with a meningocele, it may be approached through a posterior, intraspinal procedure to repair the defect in the floor of the ventral dura. This operation also allows direct visualization of the terminal cord and cauda equina, including the filum, which may be tethered by lipomas or other dysraphic conditions and may be amenable to direct repair at the time of closure of the dural fistula. When uncertainty exists regarding the cause of the anterior sacral mass (e.g., Currarino triad) and resection is indicated, the best approach is surgery using a posterior sagittal approach for adequate exposure.[127, 128] This approach also permits surgical correction, if necessary, of associated anorectal malformations. Unfortunately, visualization of the spinal cord and filum must be undertaken separately. Children with tethered cord symptoms from associated dysraphic conditions in conjunction with an anterior meningocele need to have the cord detethered with simultaneous repair of the dural defect. Transabdominal surgery in this group is reserved for patients with

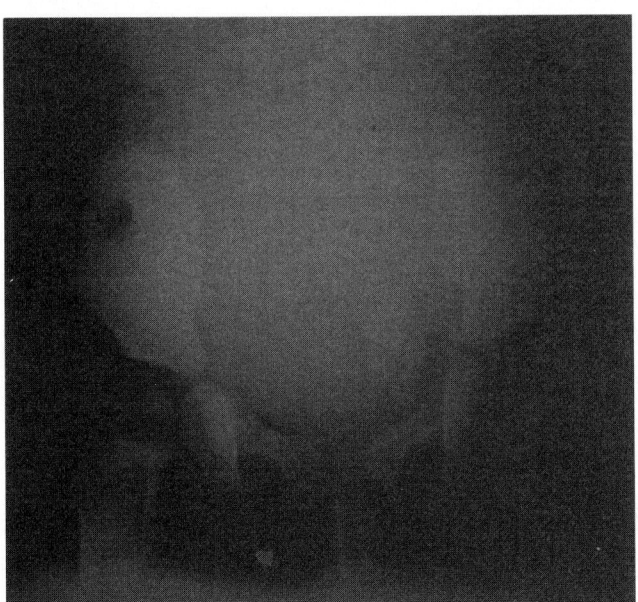

FIGURE 206–34. Plain, sacral radiographs of the pelvis in a 2-year-old girl with a history of atypical meningitis. There were no cutaneous markers of spina bifida occulta. Notice the scimitar-shaped defect over the patient's left side.

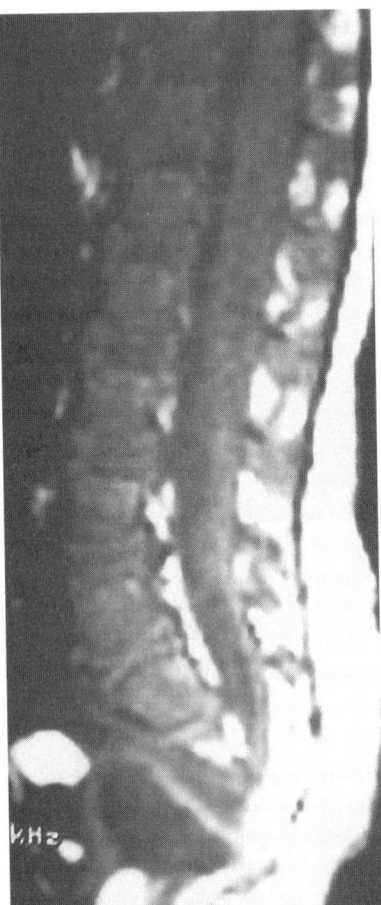

FIGURE 206–36. Sagittal magnetic resonance imaging of the patient in Figures 206–34 and 206–35 identifies the low-lying cord and presacral mass at the tip of the sacrum. The patient eventually was found to have filum lipomas, which required detethering.

undiagnosed presacral masses. The long-term prognosis for the patient with an anterior sacral meningocele with timely, focused general and neurological surgery is excellent. Patients discovered before the advent of meningitis generally do well but need to be followed over time for potential retethering.

MENINGOCELE MANQUÉ

Frequently associated with split cord malformations, a meningocele manqué represents an incompletely developed meningocele.[129, 130] It is a meningocele that partially formed in utero but failed to reach full form because of spontaneous healing or scarring. The meningocele manqué often is composed of dorsal bands (i.e., meningeal structures), and neural elements may be missing within the dysraphic region but may be present at the neck of the meningocele. The dorsal bands may tether the underlying cord or neural elements and must be differentiated from surrounding neural components. In addition to potentially tethering the cord, the dorsal bands may complicate removal of the overlying lamina when exposing the spinal cord for other dysraphic conditions, particularly split cord mal-

formations. Ventral adhesions may contribute to anterior regions of tethering and must be addressed to adequately detether the cord.

Myelocystocele

A myelocystocele is a terminal dilatation of the central canal that herniates through defective posterior elements, carrying some combination of an expanded spinal cord, CSF, fibrous bands, meninges, and lipomatous elements within a herniated, arachnoid-lined meningocele.[131–133] This herniated collection of neural elements may be continuous with a syrinx or may be intimately involved with lipomatous components (Fig. 206–37). It most likely results from the interruption of secondary neurulation and regression of the caudal cell mass. Consequently, there is a high incidence of associated anomalies of the anorectal system, lower genitourinary tract, and spinal column. Anal atresia, lumbar lordosis, kyphoscoliosis, and sacral dysgenesis are commonly seen in conjunction with myelocystoceles.

Radiologic diagnosis often is initiated by prenatal ultrasound studies[134, 135] that demonstrate variable-sized, extra-axial fluid collections consistent with a meningocele or myelomeningocele. The meningeal cysts often have a funnel-shaped appearance and may be accompanied by additional brain or spinal cord anomalies such as hydromyelia or hydrocephalus. Chiari malformations also may occur, especially in the setting of a cervical myelocystocele.[136, 137] MRI[138, 139] may disclose a cystic lesion over the back surrounded by two layers of membrane, representing the dural and arachnoid layers, and a tethered cord. Vertebral segmentation disorders are also common and may be best visualized on CT.

Frequently, extravasation of neural elements into a dorsal sac in the lumbosacral region ensures the likelihood of a tethered cord and requires eventual surgical intervention. An enlarged, trumpet-shaped conus within the terminal cyst often adheres to the superficial

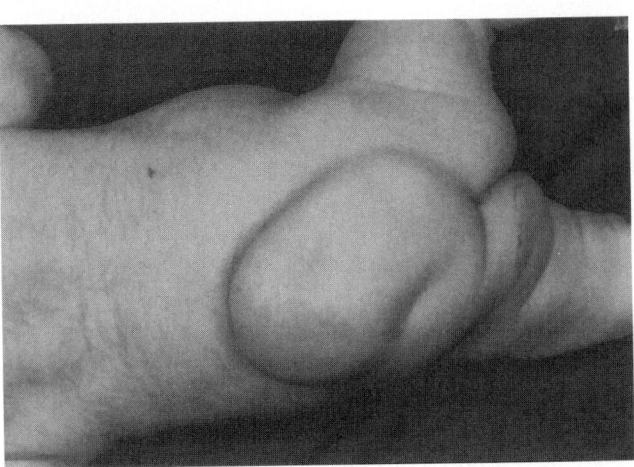

FIGURE 206–37. A newborn presented with a large, cystic lumbosacral mass, which magnetic resonance imaging showed to be a myelocystocele. The patient eventually underwent detethering without complication.

subcutaneous fat and may be difficult to detether adequately without risk of neurological compromise. Similar to the repair of a myelomeningocele, the pial edges of the distended conus may be retubulated with 6–0 Prolene suture before a watertight dural closure.

The long-term prognosis was determined to be fair by Choi and McComb,[140] who followed nine patients over a 63-month period. Although all of their patients had concomitant anorectal malformations, all patients had stable neurological function. All patients had no significant bowel or bladder control, but some were ambulatory. Nevertheless, all patients required numerous surgical interventions and extended hospital stays, demonstrating the need for coordinated, comprehensive, multidisciplinary care.

CONCLUSIONS

The range of disorders that constitute occult spinal dysraphism continues to expand because of a greater awareness of cutaneous stigmata in conjunction with increasingly sophisticated radiologic evaluation. Accordingly, examples of disordered embryogenesis have come to the forefront of neurosurgical therapeutics and have prompted more efficacious means of treatment at earlier ages, including prophylactic management. It has become the standard of care to offer prophylactic release of a tethered cord in many dysraphic conditions because of decreasing perioperative morbidity in the setting of improved surgical technique employing microsurgical approaches with laser and intraoperative monitoring. Earlier diagnosis and improved surgical therapeutics have contributed to improved outcomes for the patient with a tethered cord. Goals include increased diagnostic sensitivity, greater insight into the role of dysembryogenesis, and potential molecular and fetal therapies to prevent neurologic compromise.

REFERENCES

1. Sutow WW, Pyrde AW: Incidence of spina bifida occulta in relation to age. J Dis Child 91:211–217, 1956.
2. Iskander BJ, Oakes WJ: Occult spinal dysraphism. In Albright L, Pollack I, Adelson D (eds): Principles and Practice of Pediatric Neurosurgery. New York, Thieme Publishers, 1999, pp 321–351.
3. Carter CO, Evans KA, Till K: Spinal dysraphism. Genetic relationship to neural tube formations. J Med Genet 13:343–350, 1976.
4. Botto LD, Moore CA, Khoury MJ, et al: Neural tube defects. N Engl J Med 346:1509–1519, 1999.
5. Stevenson RE, Allen WP, Pai GS, et al: Decline in prevalence of neural tube defects in a high-risk region of the United States. Pediatrics 106:677–683, 2000.
6. Medical Research Council Vitamin Study Research Group: Prevention of neural tube defects: Results of the Medical Research Council Vitamin Study. Lancet 338:131–137, 1991.
7. Werler MM, Shapiro S, Mitchell AA: Periconceptional folic acid exposure and risk of occurrent neural tube defects. JAMA 269:1257–1261, 1993.
8. Bower C, Ryan A, Rudy E, et al: Trends in neural tube defects in Western Australia. Aust N Z J Public Health 26:150–151, 2002.
9. Czeizal AE, Dudas I: Prevention of the first occurrence of neural-tube defects by periconceptional vitamin supplementation. N Engl J Med 327:1832–1835, 1992.
10. Langman J: Medical Embryology: Human Development—Normal and Abnormal. Baltimore, Wilkins & Wilkins, 1995.
11. Boulot P, Ferran JL, Charlier C, et al: Prenatal diagnosis of diastematomyelia. Pediatr Radiol 23:67–68, 1993.
12. Sattar TS, Bannister CN, Russell SA, et al: Prenatal diagnosis of occult spinal dysraphism by ultrasonography and postnatal evaluation by MR scanning. Eur J Pediatr Surg 8(Suppl 1):31–33, 1998.
13. Achiron R, Lipitz S, Grisaru D, et al: Second trimester ultrasonographic diagnosis of segmental vertebral abnormalities associated with neurological deficit: A possible new variant of occult spinal dysraphism. Prenat Diagn 16:760–763, 1996.
14. Babcook CJ: Ultrasound evaluation of prenatal and neonatal spina bifida. Neurosurg Clin N Am 6:203–218, 1995.
15. Rypens F, Avni EF, Matos C, et al: Atypical and equivocal sonographic features of the spinal cord in neonates. Pediatr Radiol 25:429–442, 1995.
16. Kriss VM, Desai NS: Occult spinal dysraphism in neonates: Assessment of high risk cutaneous stigmata on sonography. Am J Radiol 171:1687–1692, 1998.
17. Korsvik HE: Ultrasound assessment of congenital spinal anomalies presenting in infancy. Semin Ultrasound CT MRI 15:264–274, 1994.
18. Korsvik HE, Keller SM: Sonography of occult dysraphism in neonates and infants with MR imaging correlation. J Radiogr 12:297–308, 1992.
19. McAtee-Smith J, Hebert AA, Rapini RP, et al: Skin lesions of the spinal axis and spinal dysraphism. Arch Pediatr Adolesc Med 148:740–748, 1994.
20. Powell KR, Cherry JD, Hougen TJ, et al: A prospective search for congenital dermal abnormalities of the craniospinal axis. J Pediatr 87:744–750, 1975.
21. Davis AS, Cohen PR, George RE: Cutaneous stigmata of occult spinal dysraphism. J Am Acad Dermatol 31:892–896, 1994.
22. Gibson PJ, Britton J, Hall DMB, et al: Lumbosacral skin markers and indentification of occult spinal dysraphism in neonates. Acata Pediatr 84:208–209, 1995.
23. Sattar TM, Bannister CM, Turnbull IW: Occult spinal dysraphism—the common combination of lesions and the clinical manifestations in 50 patients. Eur J Pediatr Surg 6(Suppl 1):10–14, 1996.
24. Serna MJ, Vazquez-Doval J, Vanaclocha V, et al: Occult spinal dysraphism: A neurosurgical problem with a dermatologic hallmark. Pediatr Dermatol 10:149–152, 1993.
25. Tavafoghi V, Ghandchi A, Hambrick GW, et al: Cutaneous signs of spinal dysraphism: Report of patient with tail-like lipomas and review of 200 cases in the literature. Arch Dermatol 114:573–577, 1978.
26. James CC, Lassman LP: Spinal dysraphism and treatment of progressive lesions in spina bifida occulta. J Bone Joint Surg Br 44:828–840, 1962.
27. Kennedy PR: New data on diastematomyelia. J Neurosurg 51:355–361, 1979.
28. Pang D, Dias MS, Ahab-Barmada M: Split cord malformations. Part 1. A unified theory of embryogenesis for double spinal cord malformations. Neurosurgery 31:451–480, 1992.
29. Pang D: Split cord malformations. Part II. Clinical syndrome. Neurosurgery 31:481–500, 1992.
30. Barkovitch AJ, Edwards MSB, Cogen PH: MR evaluation of spinal dermal sinus tracts in children. AJNR Am J Neuroradiol 12:123–129, 1990.
31. Hattori H, Higuchi Y, Tashiro Y: Dorsal dermal sinus and dermoid cysts in occult spinal dysraphism. Pediatrics 134:793, 1999.
32. Misago N, Abe M, Kohda H: Intradermal dermoid cyst associated with occult spinal dysraphism. J Dermatol 23:275–278, 1996.
33. Eder HG, Leber KA, Gruber W: Proteus meningitis in a child with occult spinal dysraphism. J Child Neurol 13:47–48, 1998.
34. McMaster JG: Occult intraspinal anomalies and congenital scoliosis. J Bone Joint Surg Am 66:588–601, 1984.
35. McMaster MJ: Occult intraspinal anomalies and congenital scoliosis. J Bone Joint Surg Am 66:588–601, 1984.
36. Schwend RM, Hennrikus W, Hall JE, et al: Childhood scoliosis: Clinical indications for magnetic resonance imaging. J Bone Joint Surg Am 77:46–53, 1995.
37. Bradford DS, Heithoff KB, Cohen M: Intraspinal abnormalities and congenital spine deformities: A radiographic and MRI study. J Pediatr Orthop 11:36–41, 1991.

38. Nokes SR, Murtagh FR, Jones JD 3rd, et al: Childhood scoliosis MR imaging. Radiology 164:791–797, 1987.

39. Peter JC: Occult dysraphism of the spine, a retrospective analysis of 88 operative cases. S Afr Med J 81:351–354, 1992.

40. Ward PJ, Clarke NP, Fairhurst JJ: The role of magnetic resonance imaging in the investigation of spinal dysraphism in the child with lower limb abnormality. J Pediatr Orthop 7(Pt B):141–143, 1998.

41. Rasool MN, Govender S, Naidoo KS, et al: Foot deformities and occult spinal abnormalities in children: A review of 16 cases. J Pediatr Othop 12:94–99, 1992.

42. Buffa P, Granata C, Di Rovensendra E, et al: Urological assessment in spinal dysraphism: Clinical review of 346 cases. Eur J Pediatr Surg 6(Suppl 1):25–26, 1996.

43. Kothari MJ, Bauer SB: Urodynamic and neuropsychologic evaluation of patients with diastematomyelia. J Child Urol 12:97–100, 1997.

44. Louis MA, Shaw J, Sattar TM, et al: Spectrum of spinal cord dysraphism and bladder neuropathy in children. Eur J Pediatr Surg 7(Suppl 1):35–37, 1997.

45. Keating MA, Rink RC, Bauer SB, et al: Neurological implications of the changing approach in the management of occult spinal lesions. J Urol 140:1299–1301, 1988.

46. Khouri AE, Hendrick EB, McLorie A, et al: Occult spinal dysraphism: Clinical and urodynamic outcome after division of the filum terminale. J Urol 144:426–428, 1990.

47. Silveri M, Capitanucci ML, Capozza N, et al: Occult spinal dysraphism: Neurogenic voiding dysfunction and long term follow-up. Pediatr Surg Int 12:148–150, 1997.

48. Govender S, Charles RW, Haffejee MR: Level of termination of the spinal cord during normal and abnormal fetal development. S Afr Med J 75:484–487, 1989.

49. Yundt KD, Park TS, Kaufman BA: Normal diameter of filum terminale in children: In vivo measurement. Pediatr Neurosurg 27:257–259, 1997.

50. Golonka NR, Haga LJ, Keating RF, et al: Routine MRI evaluation of low imperforate anus reveals unexpected high incidence of tethered cord. J Pediatr Surg (in press).

51. Chestnut R, James HE, Jones KL: VATER association and spinal dysraphism. Pediatr Neurosurg 18:144–148, 1992.

52. Davidoff AM, Thompson CV, Grimm JK, et al: Occult spinal dysraphism in patients with anal agenesis. J Pediatr Surg 26:1001–1005, 1991.

53. De Gennaro M, Rivosecchi M, Lucchetti MC, et al: Incidence of occult spinal dysraphisms and the onset of nervous cycle dysfunction in children with anal rectal anomalies. Eur J Pediatr Surg 4(Suppl 1):12–14, 1994.

54. Long FR, Hunter JV, Mahboubi S, et al: Tethered cord and associated vertebral anomalies in children and infants with imperforate anus: Evaluation with MR imaging and plain radiography. Radiology 200:377–382, 1996.

55. Sato S, Shirane R, Yoshimoto T: Evaluation of tethered cord syndrome associated with anal rectal malformations. Neurosurgery 32:1025–1028, 1993.

56. Tsakayannis DE, Shamberger RC: Association of imperforated anus with occult spinal dysraphism. J Pediatr Surg 13:110–112, 1995.

57. Hansasuta A, Tubbs RS, Oakes WJ: Filum terminale fusion and dural sac termination: Study in 27 cadavers. Pediatr Neurosurg 30:176–179, 1999.

58. Souweidane MM, Drake JM: Retethering of sectioned fibrolipomatous filum terminales: Report of two cases. Neurosurgery 42:1390–1393, 1998.

59. Balkan E, Kilic N, Avsar I, et al: Urodynamic findings in the tethered spinal cord: The effect of tethered cord division on lower urinary tract functions. Eur J Pediatr Surg 11:116–119, 2001.

60. Selcuki M, Unlu A, Ugur HC, et al: Patients with urinary incontinence often benefit from surgical detethering of tight filum terminale. Childs Nerv Syst 16:150–154, 2000.

61. Hawnaur JM, Hughes D, Jenkins JP, et al: Investigation of children with suspected spinal dysraphism by magnetic imaging. Eur J Pediatr Surg 1(Suppl 1):18–19, 1991.

62. De Gennaro M, Lais A, Fariello G, et al: Early diagnosis and treatment of spinal dysraphism to prevent urinary incontinence. Eur Urol 20:140–145, 1991.

63. Sharif S, Allcutt D, Marks C, et al: Tethered cord syndrome—recent clinical experience. Br J Neurosurg 11:49–51, 1997.

64. Koyanagi I, Iwasaki Y, Hida K, et al: Surgical treatment and supposed natural history of the tethered cord with occult spinal dysraphism. Childs Nerv Syst 13:268–274, 1997.

65. Satar N, Bauer SB, Shefner J, et al: The effects of delayed diagnosis and treatment in patients with an occult dysraphism. J Urol 145:754–758, 1995.

66. Klekamp J, Raimondi AJ, Samii M: Occult dysraphisms in adulthood: Clinical course and management. Childs Nerv Sys 10:312–320, 1994.

67. Maiuri F, Gamardella A, Trinchillo G: Congenital lumbosacral lesions with late onset in adult life. Neurol Res 11:238–244, 1989.

68. Akay KM, Ersahin Y, Cakir Y: Tethered cord syndrome in adults. Acta Neurochir (Wien) 142:1111–1115, 2001.

69. Iskander BJ, Fulmer BB, Hadley MN, Oakes WJ: Congenital tethered spinal cord syndrome in adults. J Neurosurg 88:958–961, 1998.

70. Pang D, Wilberger JE: Tethered cord syndrome in adults. J Neurosurg 57:32–47, 1982.

71. Warder DE, Oakes WJ: Tethered cord syndrome and the conus in a normal position. Neurosurgery 33:374–378, 1993.

72. Warder DE, Oakes WJ: Tethered cord syndrome: The low-lying and normally positioned conus. Neurosurgery 34:597–600, 1994.

73. Selcuki M, Coskun K: Management of tight filum terminale syndrome with special emphasis on normal level conus medullaris. Surg Neurol 50:318–322, 1998.

74. Hori A, Fischer G, Dietrich-Schott B, et al: Dimyelia, diplomyelia, and diastematomyelia. Clin Neuropathol 1:23–30, 1982.

75. Pang D, Dias MS, Ahab-Barmada M: Split cord malformation. Part I. A unified theory of embryogenesis for double spinal cord malformations. Neurosurgery 31:451–480, 1992.

76. Pang D: Split cord malformation. Part II. Clinical syndrome. Neurosurgery 31:481–500, 1992.

77. Dias MS, Pang D: Split cord malformations. Neurosurg Clin N Am 6:339–358, 1995.

78. Emura T, Asashima M, Furue M, et al: Experimental split cord malformations. Pediatr Neurosurg 36:229–235, 2002.

79. Muthukumar N, Arunthathi J, Sundar V: Split cord malformation and neurenteric cyst—case report and a theory of embryogenesis. Br J Neurosurg 14:488–492, 2000.

80. Birch BD, McCormick PC: High cervical split cord malformation and neurenteric cyst associated with congenital mirror movements: Case report. Neurosurgery 38:813–815, discussion 815-816, 1996.

81. Kumar R, Bansal KK, Chhabra DK: Occurrence of split cord malformation in myelomeningocele: Complex spina bifida. Pediatr Neurosurg 36:119–127, 2002.

82. Iskander BJ, McLaughlin C, Oakes WJ: Split cord malformations in myelomeningocele patients. Br J Neurosurg 14:200–203, 2000.

83. Gower DJ, Del Curling O, Kelly DL, et al: Diastematomyelia: A 40-year experience. Pediatr Neurosci 14:90–96, 1988.

84. Humphreys RP, Hendrick EB, Hoffman HJ: Diastematomyelia. Clin Neurosurg 30:436–456, 1983.

85. Kennedy PR: New data on diastematomyelia. J Neurosurg 51:355–361, 1979.

86. Schlesinger AE, Naidich TP, Quencer RM: Concurrent hydromyelia and diastematomyelia. AJNR Am J Neuroradiol 7:473–477, 1986.

87. Russell NA, Benoit BG, Joaquin AJ: Diastematomyelia in adults. Pediatr Neurosurg 16:252–257, 1990.

88. Scotti G, Musgrave MA, Harwood-Nash DC, et al: Diastematomyelia in children: Metrizamide and CT metrizamide myelography. Am J Radiol 135:1225–1232, 1980.

89. James CC, Lassman LP: Diastematomyelia: A critical survey of 24 cases submitted to laminectomy. Arch Dis Child 39:125–130, 1964.

90. Harwood-Nash DC, McHugh K: Diastematomyelia in 172 children: The impact of modern neuroradiology. Pediatr Neurosurg 16:247–251, 1990.

91. Guthkelch AN: Diastematomyelia with median septum. Brain 97:729–742, 1974.

92. Park TS, Kanev PM, Hennegar MM, et al: Occult spinal dysraphism. In Youmans JR (ed): Neurological Surgery, 4th ed. Philadelphia, WB Saunders, 1996, pp 873–889.

93. Jindal A, Mahapatra AK: Split cord malformations—a clinical study of 48 cases. Indian Pediatr 37:603–607, 2000.
94. Ersahin Y, Mutluer S, Koaman S, et al: Split cord malformations in children. J Neurosurg 88:57–65, 1998.
95. Andar UB, Harkness WF, Hayward RD: Split cord malformations of the lumbar region. A model for the neurosurgical management of all types of "occult" spinal dysraphism? Pediatr Neurosurg 26:17–24, 1997.
96. Keating RF, Goodrich JT: Tethered cord syndrome: Management of myelomeningocele, diastematomyelia, and hypertrophied filum terminale. In Rengachary SS, Wilkins RH (eds): Neurosurgical Operative Atlas, vol 7. Park Ridge, IL, AANS Publishers, 1998, pp 214–215.
97. Mann KS, Khosla VK, Gulati DR, et al: Spinal neurenteric cyst: Association with vertebral anomalies, diastematomyelia, dorsal fistula, and lipomas. Surg Neurol 21:358–362, 1984.
98. Agnoli AL, Laun A, Schonmayr R: Enterogenous intraspinal cysts. J Neurosurg 61:834–840, 1984.
99. D'Almeida AC, Stewart DH: Neurenteric cyst: Case report and literature review. Neurosurgery 8:596–599, 1981.
100. Miyagi K, Mukawa J, Merkaru S, et al: Enterogenous cyst in the cervical spinal canal: Case report. J Neurosurg 68:292–296, 1988.
101. Alrabeeah A, Gillis DA, Giacomantonio M, et al: Neurenteric cysts: A spectrum. J Pediatr Surg 23:752–754, 1988.
102. Macdonald RL, Schwartz ML, Lewis AJ: Neurenteric cyst located dorsal to the cervical spine: Case report. Neurosurgery 28:583–588, 1991.
103. Brooks BS, Duvall ER, el Gammal T, et al: Neuroimaging features of neurenteric cysts: Analysis of nine cases and review of the literature. AJNR Am J Neuroradiol 14:735–746, 1993.
104. Hoffman CH, Dietrich RB, Pais MJ, et al: The split notochord syndrome with dorsal enteric fistula. AJNR Am J Neuroradiol 14:622–627, 1993.
105. Iskandar BJ, Oakes WJ, McLaughlin C, et al: Terminal syringohydromyelia and occult spinal dysraphism. J Neurosurg 81:513–519, 1994.
106. Moise TS: *Staphylococcus* meningitis secondary to a congenital sacral sinus: With remarks on the pathogenesis of sacrococcygeal fistula. Surg Gynecol Obstet 42:394–397, 1926.
107. Powell KR, Cherry JD, Hougen TJ, et al: A prospective search for congenital dermal abnormalities of the craniospinal axis. J Pediatr 87:744–750, 1975.
108. Cheek WR, Laurent JP: Dermal sinus tracts. Concepts Pediatr Neurosurg 6:63–75, 1985.
109. Gindi SE, Fairburn B: Case reports and technical notes: Intramedullary spinal abscess as a complication of a congenital dermal sinus: Case report. J Neurosurg 30:494–497, 1969.
110. Haworth JC, Zachary RB: Congenital dermal sinuses in children: Their relation to pilonidal sinuses. Lancet 2:10–14, 1955.
111. Patey DH, Scarff RW: Pathology of postanal pilonidal sinus: Its bearing on treatment. Lancet 2:484–486, 1946.
112. Walker AE, Bucy PC: Congenital dermal sinuses: A source of spinal meningeal infection and subdural abscesses. Brain 57:401–421, 1934.
113. Wright RL: Congenital dermal sinuses. Progr Neurol Surg 4:175–191, 1971.
114. Venger B, Laurent JP, Cheek WR, et al: Congenital thoracic dermal sinus tracts. Concepts Pediatr Neurosurg 9:161–172, 1989.
115. French BN: Midline fusion defects and defects of formation. In Youmans JR (ed): Neurological Surgery, 3rd ed. Philadelphia, WB Saunders, 1990, pp 1081–1235.
116. Bale PM: Sacrococcygeal developmental abnormalities and tumors in children. Perspect Pediatr Pathol 1:9–56, 1984.
117. McIntosh R, Merritt K, Richards MR, et al: The incidence of congenital malformations: A study of 5,964 pregnancies. Pediatrics 14:505–521, 1954.
118. Ersahin Y, Barcin E, Mutluer S: Is meningocele really an isolated lesion? Childs Nerv Syst 17:487–490, 2001.
119. Sakai K, Sakamoto K, Kobayashi N, et al: Dermoid cyst within an upper thoracic meningocele. Surg Neurol 45:287–292, 1996.
120. Currarino G, Coln D, Votteler T: Triad of anorectal, sacral, and presacral anomalies. AJR Am J Neuroradiol 137:395–398, 1981.
121. Lee SC, Chun YS, Jung SE, et al: Currarino triad: Anorectal malformation, sacral bony abnormality, and presacral mass—a review of 11 cases. J Pediatr Surg 32:58–61, 1997.
122. Shamoto H, Yoshida Y, Shirane R, et al: Anterior sacral meningoceles completely occupied by an epidermoid tumor. Childs Nerv Syst 15:209–211, 1999.
123. Kochling J, Pistor G, Marzhauser Brands S, et al: The Currarino syndrome—hereditary transmitted syndrome of anorectal, sacral, and presacral anomalies: Case report and review of the literature. Eur J Pediatr Surg 6:114–119, 1996.
124. Riebel T, Maurer J, Teichgraber UK, et al: The spectrum of imaging in Currarino triad. Eur Radiol 9:1348–1353, 1999.
125. Gudinchet F, Maeder P, Laurent T, et al: Magnetic resonance detection of myelodysplasia in children with Currarino triad. Pediatr Radiol 27:903–907, 1997.
126. Pfluger T, Czekalla R, Koletzka S, et al: MRI and radiographic findings in Currarino's triad. Pediatr Radiol 26:524–527, 1996.
127. Samuel M, Hosie G, Holmes K: Currarino triad—diagnostic dilemma and a combined surgical approach. J Pediatr Surg 35:1790–1794, 2000.
128. Otagiri N, Matsumoto Y, Yoshida Y: Posterior sagittal approach for Currarino syndrome with anterior sacral meningoceles: A case report. J Pediatr Surg 35:1112–1114, 2000.
129. Kaffenberger DA, Heinz ER, Oakes JW, et al: Meningocele manqué: Radiological findings with clinical correlation. AJNR Am J Neuroradiol 13:1083–1088, 1992.
130. Lassman LP, James CCM: Meningocele manqué. Childs Brain 3:1–11, 1977.
131. McLone DG, Naidich TP: Terminal myelocystocele. Neurosurgery 16:36–43, 1985.
132. Sim K, Wang K, Cho BK: Terminal myelocystocele. J Korean Med Sci 11:197–202, 1996.
133. Cartmill M, Jaspan T, Punt J: Terminal myelocystocele: An unusual presentation. Pediatr Neurosurg 32:83–85, 2000.
134. Midrio P, Siberstein HJ, Bilaniuk LT: Prenatal diagnosis of terminal myelocystocele in the fetal sugery era: Case report. Neurosurgery 50:1152–1155, 2002.
135. Kolble N, Huisman TA, Stallmach T, et al: Prenatal diagnosis of a fetus with lumbar myelocystocele. Ultrasound Obstet Gynecol 18:536–539, 2001.
136. Nishino A, Shirane R, So K, et al: Cervical myelocystocele with Chiari II malformation: Magnetic resonance imaging and surgical treatment. Surg Neurol 49:269–273, 1998.
137. Sun JC, Steinbok P, Cochrane DD: Cervical myelocystoceles and meningoceles: Long-term follow-up. Pediatr Neurosurg 33:118–122, 2000.
138. Byrd SE, Harvey C, McLone DG, et al: Imaging of terminal myelocystocele. J Natl Med Assoc 88:510–516, 1996.
139. Peacock WJ, Murovic JA: Magnetic resonance imaging in myelocystoceles: Report of two cases. J Neurosurg 70:804–807, 1989.
140. Choi S, McComb JG: Long-term outcome of terminal myelocystocele patients. Pediatr Neurosurg 32:86–91, 2000.

CHAPTER 207

Dandy-Walker Syndrome

JEFFREY R. LEONARD ■ JEFFREY G. OJEMANN

Dandy-Walker syndrome (DWS) is determined by three findings: cystic dilation of the fourth ventricle, total or partial aplasia of the cerebellar vermis, and supratentorial hydrocephalus, although hydrocephalus is not necessary for the diagnosis of DWS. Multiple terms have been used to describe posterior fossa cystic lesions. For the purposes of this chapter, *Dandy-Walker variant* (DWV) is a term used to describe cases in which the floor and lateral walls of the fourth ventricle are visible and the vermis is hypoplastic. When comparing DWS and DWV, the anterior rotation of the hypoplastic vermis is more severe in cases of DWS.[1] Since the initial descriptions of DWS, more than 500 cases have been reported, leading to an extensive body of literature describing its clinical characteristics along with associated central nervous system (CNS) abnormalities, developmental origins of this disorder, and surgical treatment.[2-9] Improvement in the morbidity associated with treatments of DWS has been accomplished with the use of computed tomography and magnetic resonance imaging (MRI) and development of CNS shunting procedures.

HISTORICAL PERSPECTIVE AND PATHOGENESIS

The first description of hydrocephalus associated with cystic dilation of the fourth ventricle was published in 1887 by Sutton and colleagues.[10] In 1914, Dandy[11] described a 13-month-old girl with severe hydrocephalus and cystic dilation of the fourth ventricle. He was the first to associate these two pathologic findings. Explanations for the developmental origins of DWS began with Dandy. After a pathologic study of nine cases, he concluded that DWS was a result of a failure of the foramina of Magendie and Luschka to develop in utero or an inflammatory process causing obstruction after birth, or both.[12] In 1941, Sahs[13] reported a case of congenital abnormality of the cerebellum without hydrocephalus with a patent foramen Luschka. In 1954, Brenda[14] advanced the theory that is now the most widely accepted. He performed an autopsy study of six patients and suggested that congenital malformation of the fourth ventricle was related to the pathogenesis of

DWS. He postulated that the main abnormality consisted of a cleft of the cerebellum associated with malformations of the meningocele-like sac in place of the posterior medullary velum.[14] In 1959, other investigators used mice with congenital hydrocephalus and defective development of the cerebellar vermis to demonstrate that anomalies of the fourth ventricle occur at an earlier fetal stage than the formation of the foramina of Luschka and Magendie. This suggests the anomalies develop earlier than the opening of these foramina.[15] The association of facial and cardiovascular anomalies further localizes the event to approximately the fourth gestational week.[16] Because of the non-CNS abnormalities and the genetic disorders associated with DWS, much remains unknown about the cause of this disorder.

CLINICAL CHARACTERISTICS

Incidence of Dandy-Walker Syndrome

The incidence of DWS is approximately one case in 25,000 to 35,000 births. In most series, DWS is diagnosed before 1 year of age.[2-9, 17] Pascual-Castroviejo and coworkers[4] found that almost 80% of their patients were diagnosed before 1 year of life, but the diagnosis can be delayed until adolescence and even into adulthood.[18, 19] Freeman and Jones[18] described DWS manifesting as late as 75 years of age with the sudden onset of sensorineural hearing loss and episodic vertigo. Most studies have found a slight female prevalence (1.2:1 to 1.3:1) in the largest series, but not all studies have confirmed this finding.[3]

Incidence of Hydrocephalus

Most physicians consider hydrocephalus to be a common complication but not necessarily part of the disease entity.[2-9] Others have shown that, in several series of patients with hydrocephalus, DWS has an incidence of 2.2% to 4%.[3] Some estimate the incidence of hydrocephalus among patients with DWS to be approximately 90%, but this may be an overestimation because the only patients who come to the attention of a neurosurgical service are those who require treatment of the hydrocephalus.[4]

Associated Anomalies

Some series have found that associated CNS abnormalities can occur in up to 68% of DWS cases.[20] The most common abnormality in DWS is agenesis of the corpus callosum, which occurs in 7.5% to 40% of cases.[6, 9, 17, 20] Some have also found that agenesis of the corpus callosum is associated with a worse prognosis.[20] Other CNS abnormalities include occipital encephaloceles or meningoceles (found in 17% of cases), cerebral and cerebellar heterotopias, and aqueductal stenosis.[17,20] Systemic anomalies can be found in up to 25% of cases, based on an autopsy series.[20]

The most common non-CNS anomalies are cardiac defects, which include ventricular septal defects, patent ductus arteriosus, and arterial septal defects.[2, 21] Other anomalies are detectable because of their external dysmorphic appearance. The most common external anomalies are capillary hemangiomas.[3] Examples of other external anomalies include hexadactyly in cases of Ellis-van Creveld syndrome, arthrogrypotic lower limbs, hypoplasia of the upper limb, and Klippel-Feil syndrome; rare anomalies include cleft lip and palate, abnormalities of the ear, and abnormalities of the perineal region affecting the anus or genitalia, or both.[3, 4, 20]

When there are numerous external abnormalities, there is often a genetic disorder or syndrome associated with DWS. Chromosomal abnormalities, specifically trisomies 18, 21, and 13 and triploidy, occur in up to 55% of fetuses diagnosed with DWS prenatally.[22] In the largest autopsy series, Murray and associates[23] found that 7 (6%) of 113 of cases were associated with a syndrome. The familial risk of DWS was evaluated by examining 44 siblings from 106 index cases; the study found only one case of DWS, giving a recurrence risk of 2%.[23] Burton and coworkers[24] also studied 54 siblings in their 26 cases and were able to demonstrate no cases of DWS among the siblings, further illustrating the extremely low recurrence risk. Despite the low incidence of familial cases, experimental studies suggest that some genetic factor may be involved. Mice fed with a riboflavin-deficient diet had a strain-dependent incidence of DWS ranging from 5% to 80%.[15]

Symptoms at Presentation

Macrosomia is the most common presenting sign of DWS in patients younger than 1 year of age. Pascual-Castroviejo and colleagues[4] found that macrosomia necessitated a cesarian section at birth in 26% of cases. Most patients presenting after 1 year of age show delayed psychomotor development or symptoms of elevated intracranial pressure. The incidence of focal motor findings and cranial nerve palsies is low. Osenbach and Menezes[2] found that spasticity occurred in 15 (41%) of 37, cranial nerve palsies occurred in 7 (19%) of 37, and ocular abnormalities occurred in 11 (46%) of 37 patients. Despite DWS being a pathologic process involving the cerebellum, the incidence of cerebellar dysfunction is extremely low.[3] Mental retardation has been shown to be a feature of DWS. In postnatal series, the incidence of mental retardation found in several studies ranges from 41% to 71%.[4, 6, 8] Some investigators have suggested, however, that subnormal intelligence may be related to the presence of associated anomalies.

SURGICAL TREATMENT AND OUTCOME

The surgical treatment of DWS has generated considerable debate. Initially, Dandy and Walker advocated cystectomies to create a communication between the ventricles and the subarachnoid space. The success of this treatment was based on the belief that atresia of

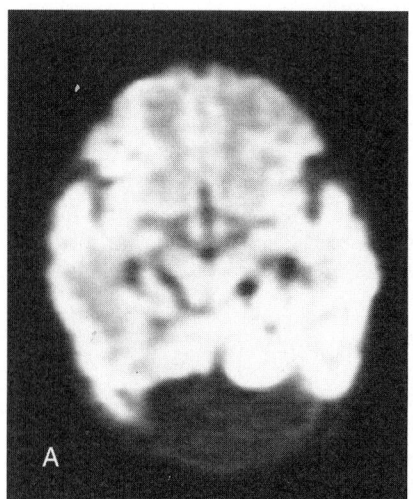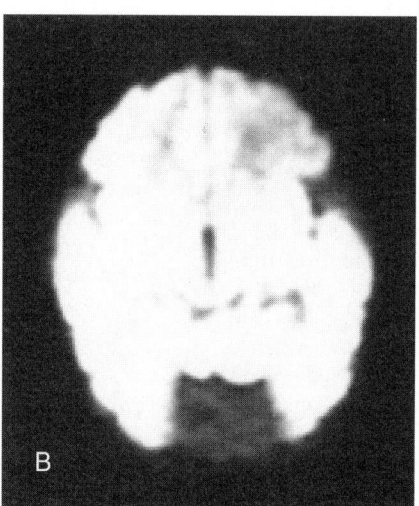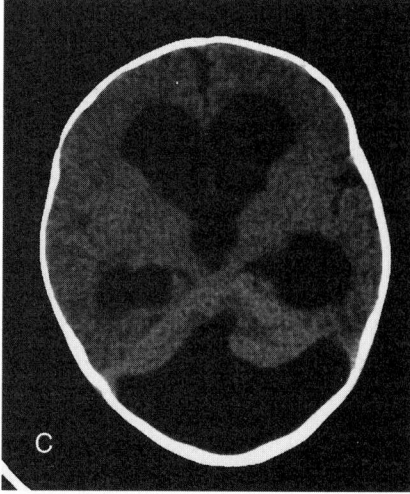

FIGURE 207–1. Magnetic resonance images of a 1-month-old girl who presented with Dandy-Walker syndrome. The initial image demonstrated a posterior fossa cyst of the fourth ventricle *(A)* without evidence of hydrocephalus *(B)*. Within 2 months, she developed severe hydrocephalus *(C)* and underwent placement of a ventriculoperitoneal shunt.

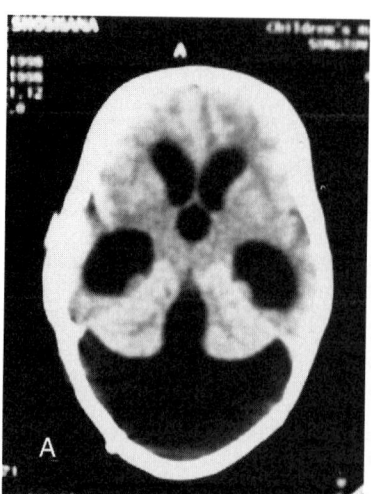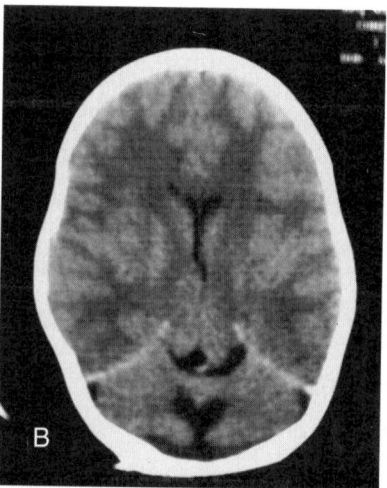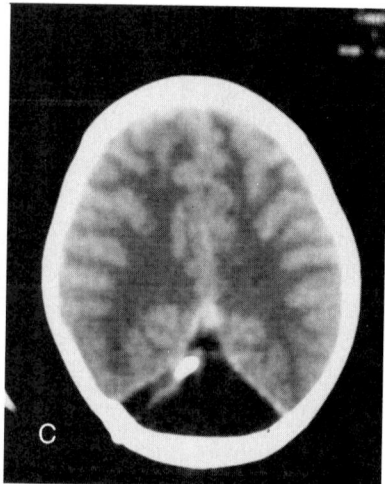

FIGURE 207–2. A 4-day-old infant presented with hydrocephalus and Dandy-Walker syndrome, which was diagnosed by antenatal ultrasonography. Computed tomography *(A)* shows the hydrocephalus and the cystic posterior fossa lesion. She underwent placement of a cystoperitoneal shunt, which resulted in resolution of the hydrocephalus *(B)* and decreased size of the cyst (C).

the foramina of Luschka and Magendie constituted the pathogenesis of this disorder. Later investigators showed that cystectomies did not control hydrocephalus and that they contributed to the initially high morbidity and mortality rates associated with treatment of DWS. The morbidity rate for series that included a number of patients treated before 1970 and that involved exploration of the posterior fossa was 26% to 50%.[6, 9, 25] Osenbach and Menezes[2] found that, of their eight patients who underwent resection of the posterior fossa cyst, only one achieved adequate control of hydrocephalus. A larger review of published cases by Hirsch and coworkers[3] of 48 cases showed failure in 36 cases (75%). The surgical treatment of DWS since then has evolved to shunting of the cyst or lateral ventricle, or both (Fig. 207–1). Later series demonstrated a mortality rate of about 10%.[2–9] Bindal and colleagues,[8] in a series of 50 patients with DWS, used a cystoperitoneal shunt in 21 (42%) cases, a ventriculoperitoneal shunt in 13 (26%) cases, and a dual shunt in 7 (14%) cases. Nine of their patients did not require any procedure. They found no statistically significant difference between the cystoperitoneal and ventriculoperitoneal shunts in complication or malfunction rates. In patients with dual shunts, the component that malfunctioned was more often the cystoperitoneal shunt. They did, however, find that 42% of the cystoperitoneal shunts required conversion to a dual shunt, compared with a 30% conversion rate for ventriculoperitoneal shunts. This suggests that the initial shunt should be a ventriculoperitoneal shunt or a combined one. Osenbach and Menezes[2] found that a dual shunt controlled hydrocephalus and alleviated posterior fossa symptoms in 92% of cases. In contrast, Asai and coworkers,[5] in a review of 35 patients, advocated cystoperitoneal shunting as the treatment choice for patients with DWS. They treated 21 patients with ventriculoperitoneal or ventricular-atrial shunting and found 9 (43%) of 23 patients developed secondary aqueductal stenosis

and required placement of a cystoperitoneal shunt. Ten patients were treated with cystoperitoneal shunts, and only one required placement of an additional ventriculoperitoneal shunt.[5] The success of the cystoperitoneal shunt presumably depends on the patency of the cerebral aqueduct (Fig. 207–2).

CONCLUSIONS

DWS results from maldevelopment of the inferior cerebellar vermis along with cystic dilation of the fourth ventricle. The advent of MRI and the evolution of surgical treatment have improved the overall mortality rate for these patients. Review of the literature shows that a ventriculoperitoneal or cystoperitoneal shunt, or both, is acceptable in the treatment of DWS, although the preference for one cavity or another is still debated. DWS is a complicated disorder. It is associated with a number of other CNS and non-CNS anomalies. The overall prognosis and development of normal intelligence may be related to adequate treatment of DWS and to the presence of associated anomalies.

REFERENCES

1. Harwood-Nash DC, Fitz CR: Neuroradiology in Infants and Children. St. Louis, CV Mosby, 1976, pp 461–504.
2. Osenbach RK, Menezes AH: Diagnosis and management of the Dandy-Walker malformation: 30 years of experience. Pediatr Neurosurg 18:179–189, 1992.
3. Hirsch JF, Pierre-Kahn A, Renier D, et al: The Dandy-Walker malformation: A review of 40 cases. J Neurosurg 61:515–522, 1984.
4. Pascual-Castroviejo I, Velez A, Pascual-Pascual SI, et al: Dandy-Walker malformation: Analysis of 38 cases. Childs Nerv Syst 7: 88–97, 1991.
5. Asai A, Hoffman HJ, Hendrick EB, Humphreys RP: Dandy-Walker syndrome: Experience at the Hospital for Sick Children, Toronto. Pediatr Neurosci 15:66–73, 1989.
6. Sawaya R, McLaurin RL: Dandy-Walker syndrome: Clinical analysis of 23 cases. J Neurosurg 55:89–98, 1981.

7. Kumar R, Jain MK, Chhabra DK: Dandy-Walker syndrome: Different modalities of treatment and outcome in 42 cases. Childs Nerv Syst 17:348–352, 2001.

8. Bindal AK, Storrs BB, McLone DG: Management of the Dandy-Walker syndrome. Pediatr Neurosurg 16:163–169, 1990.

9. Tal Y, Freigang B, Dunn HG, et al: Dandy-Walker syndrome: An analysis of 21 cases. Dev Med Child Neurol 22:189–201, 1980.

10. Sutton JB: The lateral recesses of the fourth ventricle: Their relation to certain cysts and tumors of the cerebellum and to occipital meningocele. Brain 9:352–361, 1887.

11. Dandy WE, Blackfan KD: Internal hydrocephalus. An experimental, clinical and pathological study. Am J Dis Child 8:406–482, 1914.

12. Dandy WE: The diagnosis and treatment of hydrocephalus due to occlusions of the foramina of Magendie and Luschka. Surg Gynecol Ostet 32:113–124, 1921.

13. Sahs AL: Cogenital anomalies of cerebellar vermis. Arch Pathol 32:52–63, 1941.

14. Brenda CE: The Dandy-Walker syndrome or so-called atresia of the foramen Magendie. J Neuropath Exp Neurol 13:14–29, 1954.

15. Kalter H, Warkany J: Congenital malformations in inbred strains of mice induced by riboflavin-deficient, galactoflavin-containing diets. J Exp Zool 136:531–565, 1957.

16. Le Dourarin N: The Neural Crest. Cambridge: Cambridge University Press, 1982, pp 9–259.

17. Raimondi AJ, Sato K, Shimoji T: The Dandy-Walker Syndrome. Basel, S Karger, 1984, pp 21–45.

18. Freeman SR, Jones PH: Old age presentation of the Dandy-Walker syndrome associated with unilateral sudden sensorineural deafness and vertigo. J Laryngol Otol 116:127–131, 2002.

19. Lipton HL, Preziosi TJ, Moses H: Adult onset of the Dandy-Walker syndrome. Arch Neurol 35:672–674, 1978.

20. Hart MN, Malamud N, Ellis WG: The Dandy-Walker syndrome: A clinicopathological study based on 28 cases. Neurology 22: 771–780, 1980.

21. Olson GS, Halpe DCE, Kaplan AM: Dandy-Walker malformation and associated cardiac abnormalities. Childs Brain 8:173–180, 1981.

22. Pilu G, Falco P, Perlono A, Visentin A: Ultrasound evaluation of the fetal neural axis. In Callen PW (ed): Ultrasonography in Obstetrics and Gynecology, 4th ed. Philadelphia, WB Saunders, 2000, pp 277–306.

23. Murray JC, Johnson JA, Bird TD: Dandy-Walker malformations: Etiologic heterogeneity and empiric recurrence risks. Clin Genet 28:272–283, 1985.

24. Burton BK: Recurrence risks for hydrocephalus. Clin Genet 16: 47–53, 1979.

25. Fischer EG: Dandy-Walker syndrome: An evaluation of surgical treatment. J Neurosurg 39:615–621, 1973.

CHAPTER 208

Arachnoid Cysts

PAUL M. KANEV

Arachnoid cysts are congenital fluid-filled compartments within the cerebrospinal fluid (CSF) cisterns and major cerebral fissures, intimately bordered by the arachnoid membrane. The cysts are filled with clear, colorless fluid nearly identical to CSF. Computed tomographic scanning and magnetic resonance imaging (MRI) readily facilitate the noninvasive diagnosis of arachnoid cysts with multiplanar visualization. Surgical management is based on the anatomy and clinical presentation of these collections. Surgical repair is recommended in symptomatic patients of all ages at the time of diagnosis. Optimal management of children with arachnoid cysts may require close cooperation between a pediatric neurosurgeon and multiple specialists dealing with congenital defects. This chapter reviews the pathology, clinical presentation, radiology, and surgical management of arachnoid cysts.

EMBRYOLOGY

During fetal development, arachnoid is the last of the meninges to differentiate.[1] Early in embryonic development, the perimedullary mesh is a fine mesodermal layer surrounding the inner aspect of the dura and the neural tube. Upon rupture of the rhombic roof, CSF invaginates into the layers of this mesh, guiding the differentiation of the subarachnoid from the subdural space; pia mater develops from the inner layer of the mesh. This separation sequence appears to begin when the embryo reaches 180 mm crown-rump length, at approximately 15 weeks of gestation. Cranial separation begins before differentiation of the spinal subarachnoid spaces, and incomplete separation of the mesh leads to septations within the subarachnoid space.

Arachnoid cysts may develop when alterations of CSF flow during the early phase of subarachnoid space formation lead to rupture of the developing webbed arachnoid.[1] A diverticulum may invaginate, entrapping spinal fluid in a compartment. An alternative hypothesis involves splitting of the arachnoid membrane during delamination from the overlying dura. Arachnoid cysts may be associated with agenesis of the corpus callosum and anomalies of the cerebral venous architecture.

Choi and Kim reviewed 90 cases of arachnoid cysts, focusing on traumatic origins.[2] Arachnoid cysts in seven patients appeared to develop following minor closed-head injuries in infancy; all but one occurred in the suprasellar region. The mean latent interval from trauma to clinical presentation was 2.2 years, with a range of 10 months to 6.2 years. The authors argued that trauma may create arachnoid splitting within incomplete cisterns during infancy, allowing entrapped spinal fluid diverticula. Fox and Al-Mefty also described a suprasellar arachnoid cyst that developed after closed-head injury in a young child.[3]

PATHOLOGY

The wall of an arachnoid cyst resembles normal arachnoid membranes and consists of lamellar collagen bundles.[4] The membrane may contain prominent veins and foci of capillaries, ependyma, or cuboidal epithelium. Rests of choroid plexus are encountered within the wall of posterior fossa cysts and neuroglia similar to that found on the floor of the third ventricle lines many suprasellar and prepontine cysts. In many cases, the arachnoid is split or duplicated at the margins of the cyst wall. Inflammatory cells or hemosiderin deposits are rarely encountered, even in suprasellar cysts thought to be of traumatic origin.[2] When studied at autopsy, cerebral cortex adjacent to arachnoid cysts is essentially normal. Subpial and subcortical gliosis has been observed in some patients with arachnoid cysts accompanied by neocortical epilepsy arising from adjacent cortex.

Although most arachnoid cysts are static fluid compartments throughout life, some enlarge under pressure, exerting a mass effect on adjacent neural structures. There may be active secretion of CSF from the cyst membrane by rests of choroid plexus, arachnoid granulation, or subdural neuroepithelium. This hypothesis is supported by ultrastructural evidence of neurosecretory epithelium, including basal lamina, microvilli, and desmosomal tight junctions.[5] The fluid within some arachnoid cysts has a higher protein content than CSF; an osmotic gradient with normal spinal fluid promotes bulk flow and expansion of the cyst.

Higher T2-sequence MRI attenuation of cyst fluid in some cases supports this hypothesis. In other cases in which the cyst contents communicate with the sub-arachnoid space, a ball-valve action may entrap spinal fluid during the Valsalva maneuver or transient episodes of increased intracranial pressure. This one-way pulsatile flow of spinal fluid has been demonstrated by cine-phase contrast-enhanced MRI sequences.[6] Caemaert and colleagues[7] and Schroeder and Gaab[8] endoscopically visualized an arachnoid slit-valve mechanism during fenestration of a suprasellar cyst. In each case, arachnoid membrane surrounded the basilar artery. In the first case, spinal fluid entered the cyst during inspiration, and the valve action closed during expiration. In the second case, valve action was synchronous with arterial pulsations, and the CSF propelled into the cyst was of vascular origin. Arterial pulsations and slit-valve communication within suprasellar arachnoid cysts were also observed by Choi and Kim[2] and Santamarta and coworkers.[6]

Additional evidence for one-way flow of spinal fluid into cysts is gathered following contrast cisternography. In some cases, there is progressive penetration of metrizamide into cysts and delayed emptying, even many hours after the loss of contrast enhancement of the subarachnoid space.

Okumura and associates reported the postnatal evolution of a large middle cranial fossa arachnoid cyst.[9] The authors speculated that the arachnoid cyst was formed during fetal development and that secondary cortical hypoplasia occurred during infancy, leading to cyst expansion.

CLINICAL PRESENTATION

The population incidence of arachnoid cysts is low, and autopsy estimates range from 0.1% to 0.7%. Arachnoid cysts account for about 1% of intracranial mass lesions.[10] Parsch and colleagues reviewed 11,847 cranial MRI studies completed at their institution between 1988 and 1994.[11] Previously untreated arachnoid cysts

were demonstrated in 89 patients (0.75%). Many cysts are incidental findings detected during diagnostic neuroimaging after head injury. With the increasing use of prenatal ultrasonography and the widespread availability of computed tomography (CT) and MRI, cysts are being detected at earlier ages.

Many arachnoid cysts are recognized during the first 2 decades of life, and nearly three quarters become symptomatic in children. The overall male-to-female predominance exceeds 2:1. Multiple or bilateral arachnoid cysts are unusual, and familial occurrence has been reported in only a few cases.[12] An association between bilateral sylvian fissure arachnoid cysts and glutaricaciduria type I has been demonstrated.[13]

The natural history of arachnoid cysts is not well understood. The majority of cysts are dormant fluid compartments that remain static during many years of serial neuroimaging. Some cysts, however, progressively enlarge, exerting increasing mass effect on adjacent neural structures; rarely a cyst involutes and disappears over time.[14] Arachnoid cysts can rupture after seemingly mild trauma, producing subdural hygroma and raised intracranial hypertension,[10] and they are associated with traumatic acute and chronic subdural hematomas.[13]

Arachnoid cysts can develop anywhere within the subarachnoid space, intimately related to arachnoid cisterns. In adults and children, nearly half of cysts occur within the sylvian fissure,[5, 15] and supratentorial cysts far outnumber those below the tentorium. Less common sites include the interhemispheric fissure and clival region (Table 208-l). Cysts of the suprasellar region are more commonly encountered in children than in adults.[16]

The optimal clinical management of arachnoid cysts remains controversial. Conservative management with serial neuroimaging studies is warranted for patients with asymptomatic or incidental arachnoid cysts. Surgical treatment is recommended in patients of any age with focal neurological signs or symptoms of elevated intracranial pressure. Intervention is warranted in children with head enlargement and should be considered

T A B L E   2 0 8 – 1 ■ **Distribution of Intracranial Arachnoid Cysts in Adults and Children**

LOCATION	ADULTS		CHILDREN	
	No. of Cases	%	No. of Cases	%
Supratentorial	161	77	366	77
Sylvian fissure	103	50	162	34
Parasellar	18	9	73	15
Cerebral convexity	9	4	70	15
Interhemispheric fissure	10	5	36	8
Quadrigeminal plate	21	10	25	5
Infratentorial	47	23	112	23
Cerebellopontine angle	22	11	86	17.5
Vermian	19	9	24	5
Retroclival	6	3	2	0.5

Data from Di Rocco C, Caldarelli M, Ceddia A: Incidence, anatomical distribution, and classification of arachnoidal cysts. In Raimondi A, Choux M, Di Rocco C (eds): Intracranial Cyst Lesions. New York, Springer-Verlag, 1993, pp 101–111; Rengachary S, Watanabe I, Brackett C: Pathogenesis of intracranial arachnoid cysts. Surg Neurol 9: 139–144, 1978.

in patients with seizure disorders linked to the presence of the cyst. The goal of surgical treatment is reduction of the pressure exerted by the arachnoid cyst on adjacent brain structures. The techniques for cyst surgery include craniotomy and cyst wall excision, stereotactic cyst aspiration, shunting of cystic fluid to the peritoneal cavity, and endoscopic fenestration of cysts to the subarachnoid space or the ventricles. Each procedure has distinct advantages and limitations.

The advantages of cyst-operitoneal (CP) shunt placement include the relative simplicity of the procedure and the low morbidity associated with fluid diversion. Disadvantages include the numerous complications of CSF shunts—infection, overdrainage, hindbrain herniation,[17] low-pressure headache syndromes, and shunt failure. After craniotomy, dense adherence of an arachnoid cyst to cortical and vascular structures may limit complete excision of the walls. The occurrence of cyst reaccumulation approaches nearly 25% in some patient series.[18, 19] With the refinement of endoscopy equipment and surgical technique, endoscopic fenestration is likely to become the treatment of choice.[8, 20]

Arachnoid cysts manifest unique clinical signs and symptoms according to their size and location within the subarachnoid space. The management of individual cysts is discussed later by anatomic site.

NEUROIMAGING

Conventional radiographs of the skull may demonstrate focal enlargement of the skull adjacent to an arachnoid cyst. There may be expansion of the middle cranial fossa or elevation and displacement of the sphenoid bone by cysts of the sylvian fissure. Thinning of the skull overlying large convexity cysts or posterior fossa cysts is common. Indirect effects of hydrocephalus accompanying suprasellar or quadrigeminal cysts may include suture diastasis and thinning of the dorsum sella and calvaria. Ultrasonography through the open fontanelle of a young infant readily demonstrates arachnoid cysts, hydrocephalus, and displacement of or mass effect on cortical tissue. Arachnoid cysts have been visualized as early as 26 weeks' gestation during prenatal ultrasonography (Fig. 208–1).

MRI facilitates diagnosis of these lesions with multiplanar visualization and has greater sensitivity to associated malformations than does contrast-enhanced CT. Arachnoid cysts are smooth-bordered, fluid-filled lesions on computed tomographic scans. Cyst fluid attenuation is nearly identical to CSF, and the walls do not enhance after the administration of intravenous contrast. The changes to the calvaria and skull base are demonstrated by bone window algorithm images. CT after intrathecal contrast demonstrates isolation or communication with normal CSF pathways (Fig. 208–2).

MRI is the preferred imaging study for arachnoid cysts.[21] The extra-axial location of cysts and their relationship to adjacent neural and vascular structures are best visualized by T1-weighted sequences. Cyst fluid has low attenuation on T1 images and a high signal on

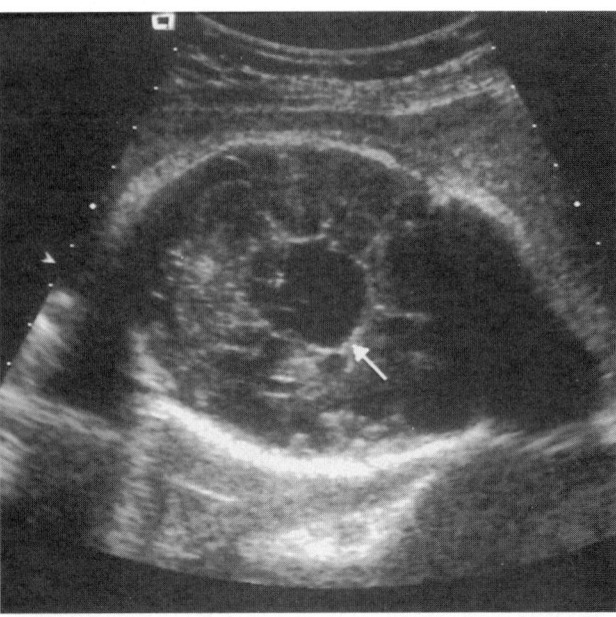

FIGURE 208–1. Transabdominal ultrasonographic study at 26 weeks' gestation. There is a 3-cm arachnoid cyst *(small arrow)* in the center of the fetus' brain. No hydrocephalus is demonstrated.

T2 sequences and is nearly identical to CSF (Fig. 208–3). Previous hemorrhage or stagnant spinal fluid circulation within a cyst may change the attenuation values in all image sequences. The signal characteristics with gadolinium contrast enhancement, FLAIR, T1, and pro-

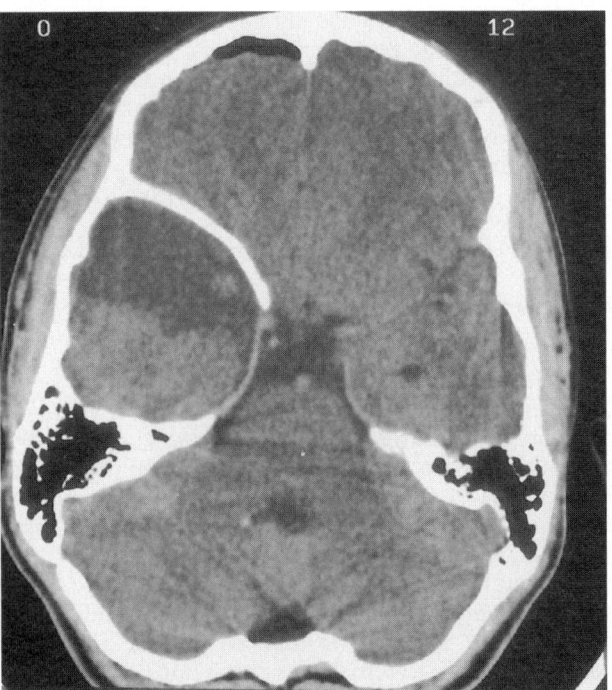

FIGURE 208–2. Axial noncontrast computed tomographic scan in a 14-year-old boy. The right middle cranial fossa is expanded, with displacement and elevation of the sphenoid wing. A type I right sylvian fissure arachnoid cyst is seen adjacent to the temporal tip.

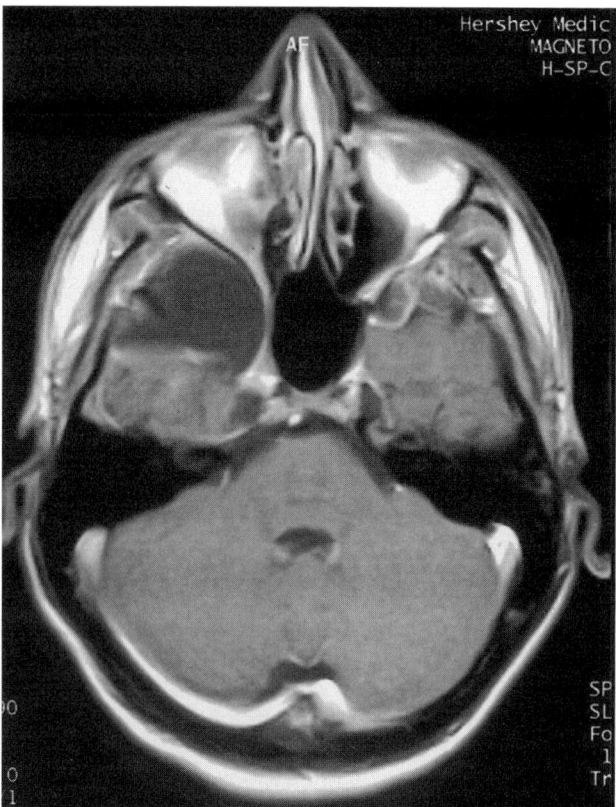

FIGURE 208–3. Axial T1-weighted magnetic resonance imaging (MRI) scan of the same teenager as in Figure 208–2. There is enlargement of the right middle fossa and temporal polar displacement by a sylvian fissure arachnoid cyst.

ton density sequences usually allow arachnoid cysts to be differentiated from other lesions, including cystic tumors; dermoid, ependymal, or epidermoid cysts; and lipomas. MRI readily demonstrates any associated malformations, such as agenesis of the corpus callosum[22] or holoprosencephaly.

SUPRATENTORIAL ARACHNOID CYSTS

Sylvian Fissure Cysts

Nearly half of all arachnoid cysts in adults, and about one-third in children, are located in the sylvian fissure. There is a wide range of cyst size, from small lenticular collections at the temporal tip to large volume collections that separate and displace the opercular cortex. The largest cysts compress the insular and temporal polar cortex and exert contralateral shift on the cerebral midline. Bilateral cysts are unusual.[23]

Although sylvian fissure cysts may become symptomatic at any age, presentation is more common in children and adolescents than in adults. There is a nearly 3:1 male-to-female predominance, and the left hemisphere is affected more often than the right. The most common symptom is unilateral headache, typically in the supraorbital and temporal region. Focal, complex-partial, or generalized seizures are the next most frequent symptom and may occur in up to one

fourth of patients. The cause of seizures in patients with arachnoid cysts is unknown, but it may be linked to compression of adjacent temporal cortex or to cortical dysplasia and subpial gliosis.

Some adolescents describe exacerbation of headache with chewing and increased pain during exercise and physical exertion. Other symptoms include mild proptosis, nausea, vomiting, mild contralateral hand weakness, or hemiparesis. Developmental delays or learning difficulties are uncommon in patients with even large cysts of the sylvian fissure. Handa and colleagues, however, reported two children with bilateral sylvian arachnoid cysts and severe psychomotor retardation; one child had hemiparesis.[12] Neurological milestones and learning failed to improve in these patients after CP shunt placement. Sylvian fissure arachnoid cysts are an unusual cause of facial pain syndromes.[24]

Large sylvian cysts lead to macrocrania and suture splitting in young children. A localized temporal skull bulge is encountered in many patients, and skull radiographs demonstrate thinning of the temporal squama and displacement of the wings of the sphenoid bone. CT shows the non–contrast-enhancing CSF density collections at the temporal tip and within the sylvian fissure. Galassi and colleagues classified three subgroups of sylvian fissure cysts.[23, 25] Type I cysts are lenticular, biconvex collections at the temporal tip linked with little remodeling of the middle fossa (see Figs. 208–2 and 208–3). These cysts freely communicate with CSF in the subarachnoid space. Type II cysts are larger quadrilateral cysts exerting moderate mass effect on adjacent neural and osseous structures. There is delayed uptake of iodine contrast after cisternography. Type III cysts are large, rounded collections causing severe compression of the operculum and insular cortices and midline shift with distortion of the lateral ventricles (Fig. 208–4). These cysts are isolated from spinal fluid communication within the subarachnoid spaces. It is unknown whether there is progression of type I cysts into larger mass lesions.

The three-dimensional relationships of sylvian arachnoid cysts are best visualized with MRI. The collections are nonenhancing and isointense with CSF in all sequences. The mass effect on the branches of the middle cerebral and cortical veins stretched by the cyst can be seen with magnetic resonance arteriography and venography. These veins may be easily injured during even mild closed-head injury and are likely the source of hemorrhage into the cysts or extension into the subdural space. In one clinical series, arachnoid cysts were detected in 2.43% of 658 patients with chronic subdural hematomas.[11]

Management decisions balance the neuroimaging findings and the clinical symptoms. Type I cysts are typically asymptomatic and require no surgical intervention. Conservative management with annual follow-up neuroimaging is recommended in these patients for 1 to 2 years; in children, scans are completed every 6 months for 18 months. Adults and children who harbor large and symptomatic type III cysts exerting significant mass effect require surgical intervention. Surgery is also recommended for intermediate

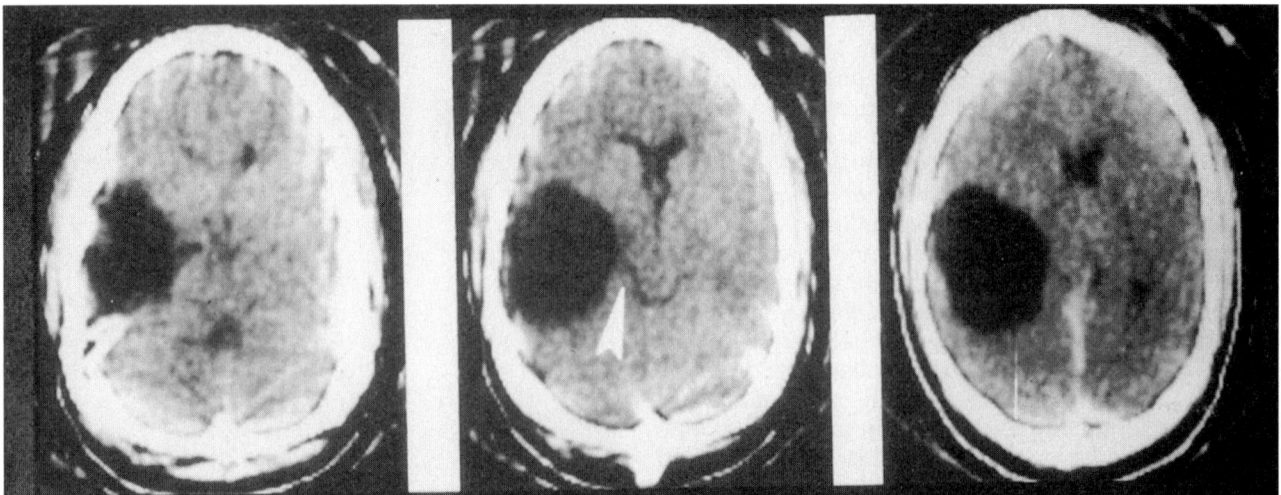

FIGURE 208–4. Serial axial noncontrast computed tomographic scans of a type III sylvian fissure arachnoid cyst. The large, round cyst compresses the operculum and insular cortices.

type II cysts when clinical symptoms are severe and out of proportion to the cyst volume.

In a symptomatic patient, the surgeon is challenged to select the appropriate drainage technique. CP shunting offers many advantages.[18] The technique is usually straightforward in patients of all ages, and catheter insertion can be guided by the use of intraoperative ultrasonography or frameless localization. Extra holes enhance long-term catheter patency and promote flow within any intracyst septations. Low-pressure valves are recommended. After shunt placement, displaced cortex and midline shift may realign rapidly. The complications of cyst shunt placement include the spectrum of difficulties with CSF drainage systems. Bridging veins stretched along the cyst walls may be injured during catheter placement, leading to intracyst or subdural hemorrhage. Other risks include infection, cyst reaccumulation, and low-pressure headaches. Several patients have developed slit-cyst syndrome (similar to slit-ventricle syndrome), with transient episodes of increased intracranial pressure. Shunt revision rates approach 30%.[18, 26]

In contrast to shunting, craniotomy overlying the cyst allows excision of the lateral cyst walls and fenestration of the cyst into the basal cisterns.[19, 26] Limited bone exposure can be assisted with frameless stereotactic localization. Bur holes should be made with a high-speed drill, because bone may be thin from underlying cyst pressure. The large pool of entrapped CSF transmits a blue color to the overlying dura. Stretched veins in the cyst wall can be easily coagulated. The lateral cyst walls readily separate from the cortex, exposing the insula and branches of the middle cerebral artery. With escape of spinal fluid, the mesial walls of the cyst become mobile and pulsatile. The operative microscope is used to visualize the tentorium, vessels of the circle of Willis, and cranial nerves at the skull base. Multiple fenestrations between the deep cyst wall and the basal cisterns are opened with microsurgical technique. After craniotomy, patients experience rapid relief of head-

aches; however, the postoperative computed tomographic or MRI scan may not demonstrate significant re-expansion of the displaced cortex. Headaches may return in 5% to 25% of patients because of cyst reaccumulation.[18, 19, 26] Raffel and McComb suggested that failure of cyst fenestration may be linked to the technical skill of the surgeon in the fastidious removal of cyst wall adherence to neural and vascular structures.[19]

Excellent outcomes have been reported after endoscopic cyst fenestration.[8, 20, 27] Schroeder and colleagues used a rigid endoscope technique for drainage of sylvian cysts.[8] They introduced the endoscope into the cyst along a tangential trajectory selected by computed tomographic or MRI scans and coagulated the outer cyst membrane. A wide cystocisternostomy was dilated with a balloon catheter, and a ventricular catheter was advanced into the basal cisterns. Significant bleeding within the cyst occurred during a single case in which the endoscopic procedure was aborted and a craniotomy was performed. In each patient, cyst size diminished on postoperative neuroimaging, and clinical symptoms resolved with long-term follow-up of 15 to 30 months. The authors highlight the importance of coagulation of all fragile vessels in the outer cyst wall to minimize intraoperative bleeding.

In another series of patients reported by Hopf and Perneczky,[28] the neuroendoscope was used for fenestration of small sylvian cysts and to supplement open microsurgical fenestration of large sylvian cysts. Although cyst size and clinical symptoms improved in 5 of 10 patients, subdural hemorrhage occurred in 2 patients. With more widespread experience with endoscopic cyst fenestration, minimally invasive cyst drainage may become the surgical technique of choice for sylvian arachnoid cysts.

Suprasellar Cysts

The most common parasellar region cysts occur within the suprasellar cistern. Nearly 50% of cases are diagnosed in children younger than 5 years,[29] and almost 20% present in children younger than 1 year. The most common symptoms include hydrocephalus, vision impairment, and endocrinologic dysfunction. Focal neurological signs including gait ataxia and opisthotonos may be encountered in patients with large suprasellar cysts that elevate and displace the midbrain posteriorly. There is a 2:1 male-to-female predominance.

Hydrocephalus develops in infancy when the cyst balloons superiorly, elevating the third ventricle and distorting the foramen of Monro and the internal circulation of CSF. This may progress to macrocephaly with suture splitting; some children may have the dull percussion note, or Macewen sign, in cases of medulloblastoma. Ophthalmic examination may reveal optic atrophy, papilledema, decreased acuity in one or both eyes, and the spectrum of visual field cuts. The bobblehead doll syndrome of to-and-fro head oscillation in patients with suprasellar arachnoid cysts was first described in two patients in 1966.[30] Among the 106 cases reviewed by Pierre-Kahn and colleagues, this unusual neurological symptom occurred in 10% of patients.[31] In a case reported by Albright,[32] bobble-head doll movements in a 9-year-old boy were accompanied by headaches and memory and learning difficulties. The pathogenesis of this bobbing movement may reflect cyst pressure exerted on the dorsomedial nucleus of the thalamus.[33] Developmental or intelligence quotient (IQ) testing among seven of nine children reported by Pierre-Kahn and colleagues was between 80 and 100.[23] Endocrinologic dysfunction may include isosexual precocious puberty and short stature. Static and provocative hormone studies demonstrated growth hormone and adrenocorticotropin deficiency and, rarely, panhypopituitarism. Dysfunction of the hypothalamic-pituitary axis was present in 60% of 15 patients reported by Pierre-Kahn and colleagues; however, endocrine recovery did not occur following cyst management in their patients.[31]

Ultrasonographic or computed tomographic scans identify a cystic mass filling and engulfing the suprasellar cistern, with distortion of the third ventricle. The borders of the sella may be expanded and sculptured by cyst pressure. Associated hydrocephalus or brainstem displacement is readily apparent. Sagittal and coronal MRI sequences better visualize the extra-axial nature of the cystic collection and the elevation of the floor of the third ventricle (Figs. 208–5 and 208–6). The attenuation signals on all image sequences allow differentiation from craniopharyngioma, dermoid or epidermoid inclusion cysts, and Rathke's cleft cysts.

Many procedures have been advocated for the surgical management of suprasellar cysts. CP shunt placement is straightforward in patients without hydrocephalus (Fig. 208-7). Catheter placement may be assisted by ultrasonography or frameless stereotactic trajectory guidance. Ventriculoperitoneal (VP) shunting of the lateral ventricles controls hydrocephalus, but progression of cyst size may occur in nearly 40% of patients. This complication can be avoided by Y-linking proximal cyst and ventricular catheters into a common low-

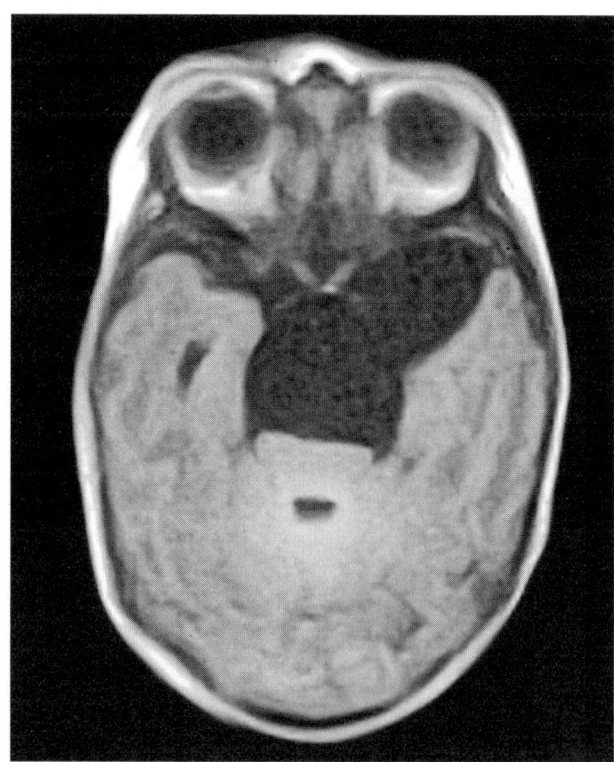

FIGURE 208–5. Axial T1-weighted MRI scan in a 3-day-old infant with in utero diagnosis of an arachnoid cyst (see Fig. 208–1). There is a large retrochiasmatic suprasellar arachnoid cyst with extension toward the left sylvian fissure and retroclival region and brainstem displacement.

pressure shunt system to achieve drainage of each fluid compartment. In the series of patients reported by Hoffman and coworkers,[29] eight patients underwent subfrontal craniotomy with cyst fenestration into the

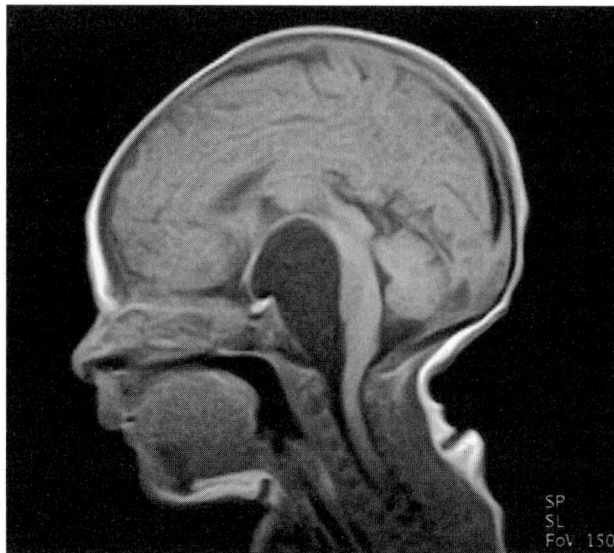

FIGURE 208–6. Sagittal T1-weighted MRI scan of the same child as in Figure 208–5. The retrochiasmatic arachnoid cyst is elevating the floor of the third ventricle and displacing the midbrain and pons posteriorly. The ventricles are normal size.

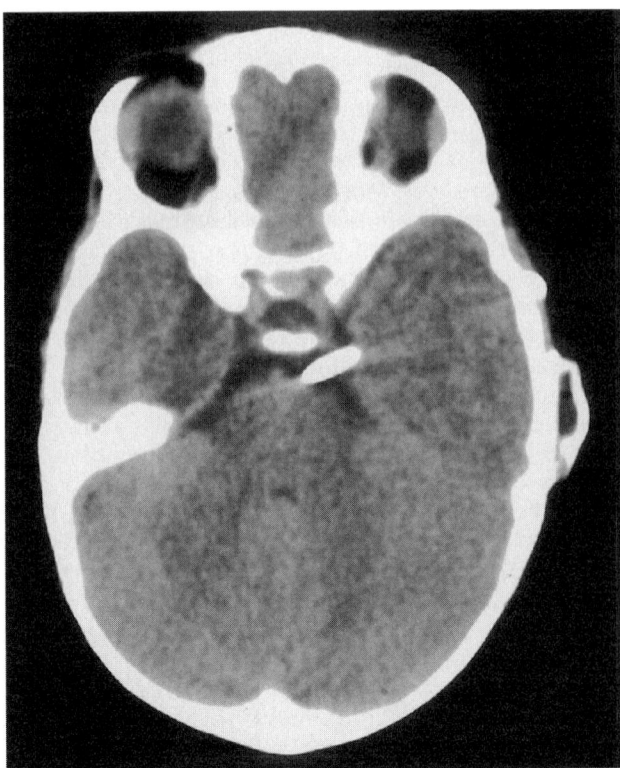

FIGURE 208-7. Axial noncontrast computed tomographic scan in the same child as in Figures 208-5 and 208-6. A shunt was introduced into the large suprasellar arachnoid cyst and directed 4 cm toward the midline. There is postoperative drainage of the retroclival and sellar region arachnoid cyst, with normal alignment of the brainstem.

basal cisterns. Five additional patients completed unilateral VP shunt placement, followed by transcallosal communication of the cyst into the ventricular system. After completing transcallosal fenestration and incomplete cyst wall resection, Albright reported improved memory function in a 9-year-old child.[32] Raffel and McComb selected cyst fenestration in 31 patients with arachnoid cysts, including five cysts that were suprasellar.[19] Thirteen of 24 patients whose cysts had not been previously shunted had complete resolution of their symptoms and required no additional surgery. Four patients required a VP shunt, and five patients needed a CP shunt after craniotomy because of continued symptoms. The overall success of fenestration was 73% in patients without hydrocephalus and 75% in 12 patients with arachnoid cysts accompanied by hydrocephalus.[19]

Pierre-Kahn and colleagues advocate percutaneous ventriculocystostomy.[31] In their patient series, this radiographically guided technique was successfully completed in 12 children, with improved postoperative IQ and ventricle and cyst size. An increasing number of suprasellar cysts have been treated with bur hole endoscopic neurosurgery. In a patient series reported by Hopf and Perneczky,[28] six patients with suprasellar cysts and hydrocephalus or neurological deficits underwent endoscopic ventriculocystostomy. The patients had uniform improvement in clinical symptoms and

ventricle size. Direct cyst visualization aided the coagulation and perforation of the cyst wall, which may be toughened by fusion of the arachnoid, neuroglia, and ependymal membranes.

Primary intrasellar cysts are unusual collections that typically become symptomatic in the fourth or fifth decade of life, although there was a case of a 9-year-old patient with a large hemorrhagic intrasellar cyst (Fig. 208-8). The most common symptom in patients of all ages is headache. These cysts develop within the sella turcica, compressing the pituitary gland and elevating the shelf of the diaphragma sellae upward. Most intrasellar cysts are discovered incidentally during skull x-rays or CT scans after closed-head injury. In contrast to suprasellar collections, visual disturbances and endocrinopathy are unusual. Treatment consists of transsphenoidal drainage of the cyst and packing of the residual cavity with muscle or fat.[34]

Cerebral Convexity Cysts

As in other locations, arachnoid cysts along the lateral cerebral convexity vary considerably in size and in the degree of compression on adjacent cortex. Small and medium-sized collections focally compress the underlying brain, whereas larger cysts lead to asymmetric calvaria expansion and distortion of the entire cerebral cortex. Unlike most cysts, however, these collections are more common in females than in males.

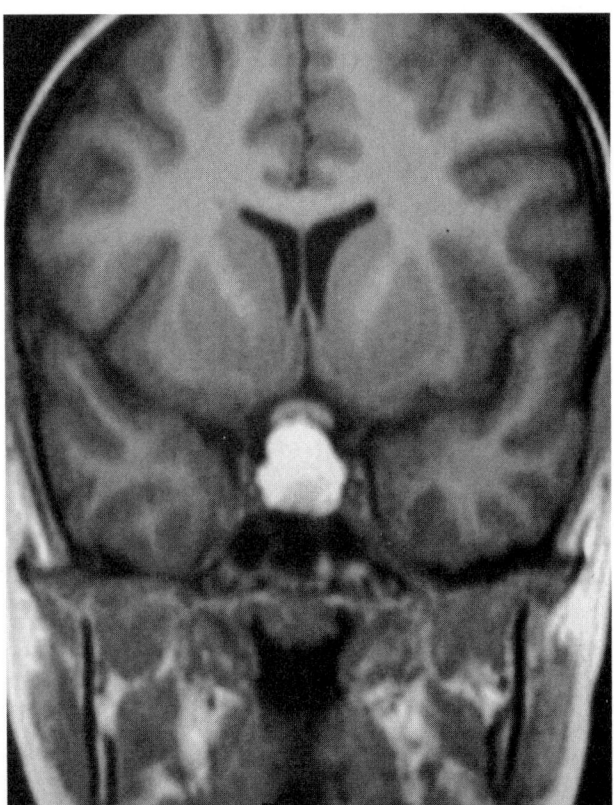

FIGURE 208-8. Coronal T1-weighted MRI scan of a hemorrhagic intrasellar arachnoid cyst in a 9-year-old boy who presented with severe headaches. There is elevation of the optic chiasm and enlargement of the sella turcica.

Hemispheric cysts are massive collections that lie across the entire hemisphere and displace the midline contralaterally. Many appear to be in continuity with large sylvian collections (Fig. 208-9). These cysts lead to rapidly expanding macrocrania and cranial asymmetry in young children, accompanied by full fontanelles and suture diastasis. Focal convexity cysts, however, apply only local compression on adjacent cortex and may thin and distort the overlying bone. Despite the magnitude of the cyst, affected children have a paucity of neurological symptoms, whereas in adults, the cysts are often symptomatic, causing headache, retro-orbital pain, hemiparesis, or seizures.

CT confirms the bone remodeling overlying focal and large cysts, and both CT and MRI reveal the extra-axial CSF collections compressing the cortex. Large collections may initially be confused with chronic subdural collections in young children, but their different clinical presentation and fluid attenuation signals that are higher than those of CSF allow their distinction from arachnoid cysts.

Many hemispheric cysts are treated with CP shunt placement. At craniotomy, the entire cyst is exposed, and membranes are excised (Fig. 208-10); if the deep cyst wall is adjacent to a basal cistern, fenestrations are completed. Rampini and colleagues described their experience with a stereotactic-guided endoscopic fenestration of a convexity cyst into the lateral ventricle in a 1-year-old girl.[35]

Interhemispheric Cysts

Cysts within the interhemispheric fissure are rare collections, accounting for about 5% to 8% of arachnoid cysts.[15, 16] These collections may present with a paucity of clinical signs and symptoms, despite the considerable size of the cyst. Most patients present with macrocrania or nonspecific headache. Hydrocephalus frequently accompanies cysts linked with partial or complete agenesis of the corpus callosum.[21] MRI in these cases reveals the typical bat-wing ventricular configuration, hypoplasia of the falx, and horizontal bundles of crossing fibers within the cingulum.

Contrast-enhanced MRI readily demonstrates the mass effect the cyst exerts on the falx and the displacement of parasagittal cortex. The attenuation on all MRI sequences is helpful in differentiating arachnoid cysts from other midline lesions, including ependymal and neoplastic cysts. Parasagittal cysts are frequently wedge-shaped, although in one case, a large, round collection was encountered, with midline shift and mass effect on the corpus callosum and anterior cerebral vessels (Fig. 208–11).

No single surgical technique has proved universally successful in the management of interhemispheric cysts. As in other locations, CP shunt placement reduces cyst size and relieves symptoms; however, drainage malfunction is common. Craniotomy and excision of the cyst wall have proved successful and may avoid

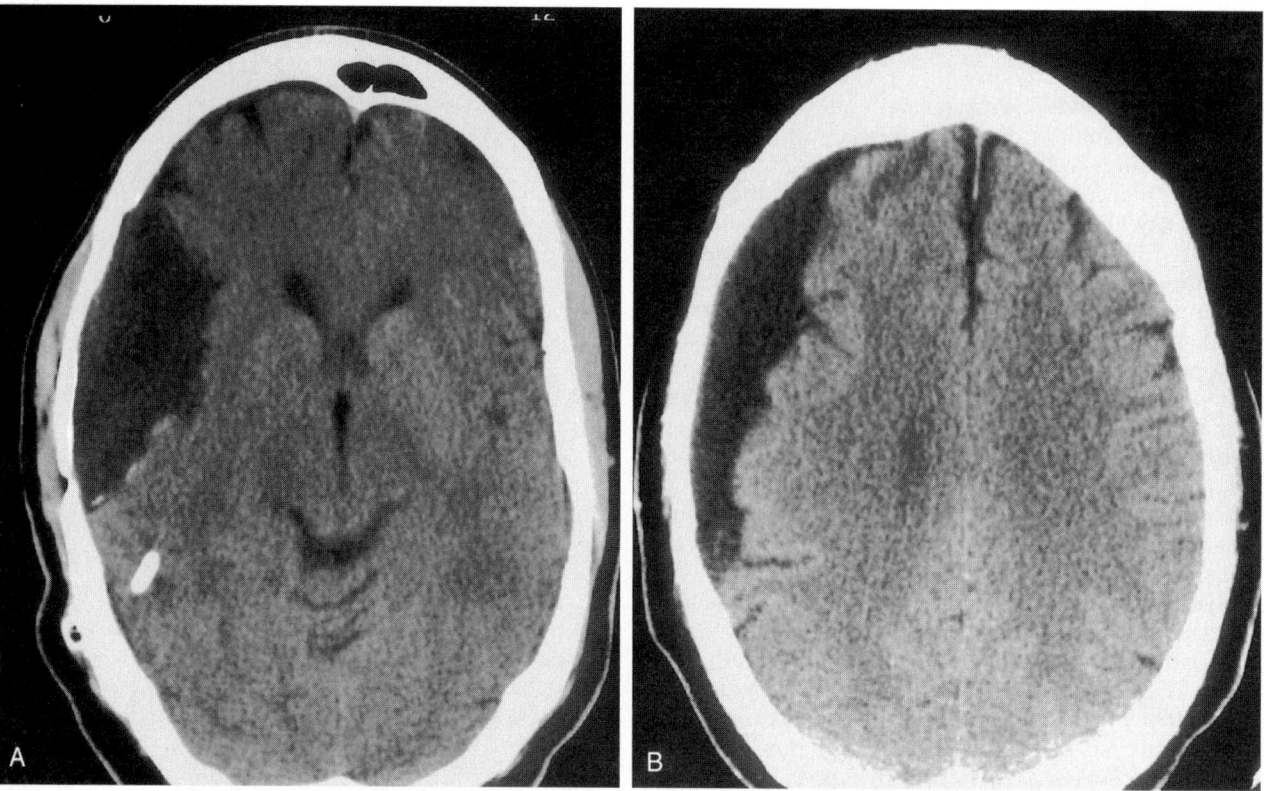

FIGURE 208–9. *A,* Axial noncontrast computed tomographic scan of a large right sylvian fissure arachnoid cyst causing wide displacement of the frontal and temporal operculum. *B,* Axial noncontrast computed tomographic scan in the same patient showing extension of the sylvian fissure cyst along the convexity, with broad mass effect on the right frontal cortex.

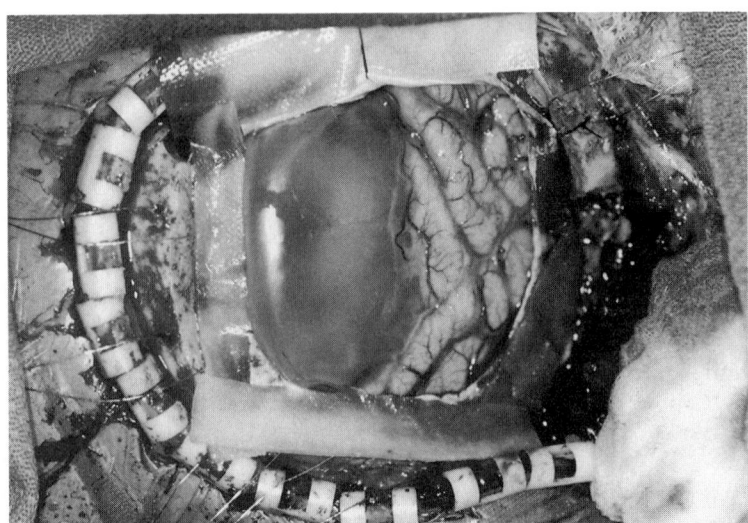

FIGURE 208–10. Operative photograph of a left cerebral convexity arachnoid cyst. In contrast to sylvian fissure cysts, there are few vessels within the cyst wall, which bridges the compressed frontal lobe.

shunt dependence. In their series of 27 arachnoid cysts treated endoscopically, Hopf and Perneczky drained a frontal interhemispheric cyst, resulting in improvement in symptoms and reduction in cyst size.[28] A postoperative subdural-peritoneal shunt was necessary for long-term drainage of a subdural hygroma.

Quadrigeminal Cysts

Arachnoid cysts within the quadrigeminal cistern and posterior third ventricle mimic the clinical symptoms of pineal region masses. Clinical presentation syndromes include macrocephaly with suture splitting, headache, and the spectrum of signs and symptoms associated with hydrocephalus and increased intra-

cranial pressure. With compression of the tectal plate, there may be paresis of up-gaze and pupillary dysfunction. Eccentric expansion of the cyst may compress the geniculate body or the medial parieto-occipital lobe, leading to visual field changes. Other symptoms may include ataxia, tremor, or seizures.

MRI is the neuroimaging method of choice. The three-dimensional relationships of quadrigeminal cysts with the posterior third ventricle, brainstem, and tributaries of the vein of Galen are readily apparent (Fig. 208–12). Most midline collections are ovoid, whereas eccentric displacement may compress and distort the atria of the ventricle.

CP shunt placement is successful in reducing cyst

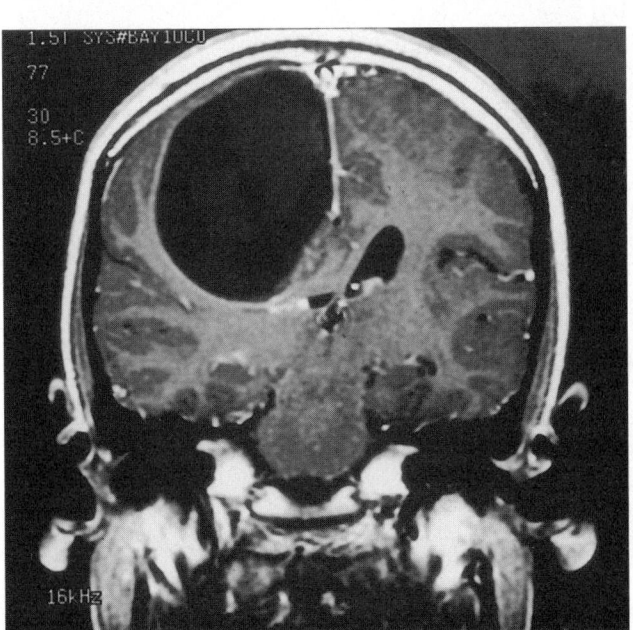

FIGURE 208–11. Coronal T1-weighted MRI scan in an 11-year-old boy with a large, round interhemispheric arachnoid cyst exerting mass effect on the corpus callosum and anterior cerebral vessels, with midline shift.

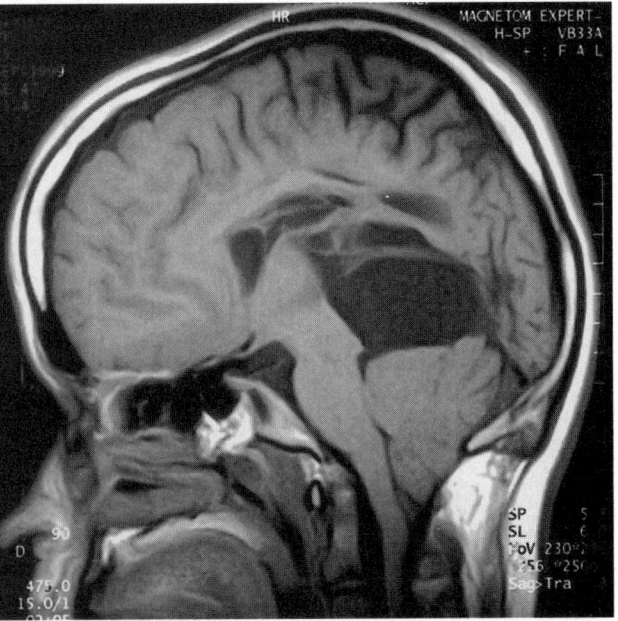

FIGURE 208–12. Sagittal T1-weighted MRI scan in a 12-year-old boy with myelomeningocele and ventriculoperitoneal-shunted hydrocephalus. There is a large quadrigeminal arachnoid cyst compressing the quadrigeminal plate and the superior cerebellar vermis.

size and controlling clinical symptoms.[18, 19, 26] Ultrasonographic or frameless stereotactic guidance may assist catheter placement within the cyst. Most quadrigeminal cysts can be approached via the supracerebellar, infratentorial route, with microsurgical cyst fenestration into the posterior third ventricle or the superior medullary velum.[36, 37] Open exposure and direct fenestration of cyst membranes are advocated by Raffel and McComb,[19] whereas Hopf and Perneczky recommend endoscopically controlled or assisted microsurgery.[28] These authors have used the endoscope for illumination and video control of microsurgical instruments and completed successful drainage of quadrigeminal cysts in two patients through limited craniotomies. Regardless of which drainage technique is used, cyst reaccumulation is common, and postoperative management includes frequent serial neuroimaging.

INFRATENTORIAL ARACHNOID CYSTS

Arachnoid cysts of the posterior fossa are much less common than those above the tentorium. Although the cyst of the Dandy-Walker syndrome accompanies vermis hypoplasia and freely communicates with the posterior fossa, arachnoid cysts remain extra-axial, isolated from CSF circulation within the subarachnoid spaces. Cystic collections in the midline compress the vermis and separate the cerebellar hemispheres (Fig. 208–13). In adults and children, the predominant clinical symptom is headache, accompanied by hydrocephalus secondary to compression of the fourth ventricle. There may be macrocrania, asymmetry of the skull

base, and truncal ataxia. Teenagers frequently describe suboccipital headache that intensifies during sports activity, similar to the symptoms of a Chiari I malformation. Collections that also compress the lateral cerebellar hemisphere may lead to tremor, incoordination, or dysmetria.

Cysts of the cerebellopontine angle are unusual, and fewer than 50 have been reported in the literature. The mean age of these patients was nearly 32 years; in the five patients reported by Jallo and colleagues, however, the age at diagnosis was much younger, ranging from 14 months to 18 years.[38] The most common presenting symptoms are ataxia, tinnitus, and headache; less common cranial nerve symptoms included trigeminal neuralgia and hemifacial spasm. MRI demonstrates a sharp-walled, nonenhancing CSF collection within the cerebellopontine angle. The attenuation of image sequences allows differentiation from cholesteatomas and hemangioblastomas.

Shunting of midline or lateral cysts may reduce cyst size sufficiently so that hydrocephalus will resolve on restoration of normal CSF circulation. Catheter placement is straightforward from a midline or lateral bur hole, and ultrasonographic guidance assists a trajectory into the widest segment of the cyst. Suboccipital craniotomy and cyst excision are recommended for the treatment of cerebellopontine angle collections. Jallo and colleagues resect the lateral and posterior cyst walls widely and microsurgically fenestrate the anterior membranes into the cisterns surrounding the adjacent cranial nerves.[38] Endoscopically controlled microsurgical fenestration has been used, but McComb considers open exposure to be superior to the commu-

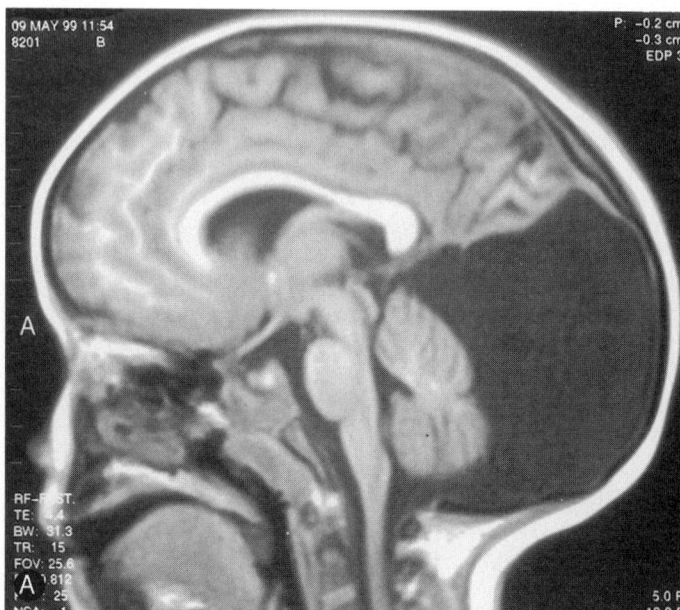
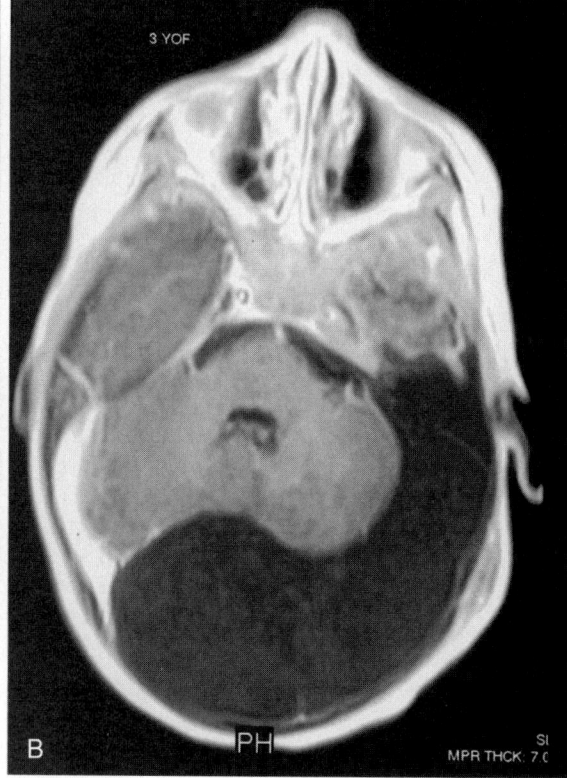

FIGURE 208–13. *A*, Sagittal T1-weighted MRI scan of a large arachnoid cyst of the posterior fossa in a 3-year-old girl. There is bulging of the bone overlying the arachnoid cyst, which compresses the cerebellar hemispheres. *B*, Enhanced axial T1-weighted MRI scan of the same patient. The arachnoid cyst compresses the cerebellar hemispheres and distorts the fourth ventricle.

nication with the subarachnoid spaces achieved through a neuroendoscope.[39]

CONCLUSIONS

With the universal availability of CT and MRI, arachnoid cysts are being diagnosed with increasing frequency. Many collections are asymptomatic and are managed conservatively with observation. Patients with cysts that cause headaches or focal neurological signs or significant distortion of adjacent cerebral cortex or the midline are candidates for drainage. Regardless of the site of the arachnoid cyst, surgical techniques include shunting, craniotomy or endoscopic membrane excision, and fenestration. With refinements in neuroendoscope optics and surgical techniques since the early 1990s, minimally invasive drainage may be the preferred initial decompression procedure. Long-term follow-up and serial imaging studies are necessary in patients of all ages.

REFERENCES

1. Lemire RJ, Loeser JD, Leech RW, et al: Normal and Abnormal Development of the Human Nervous System. New York, Harper & Row, 1975, pp 1–421.
2. Choi J, Kim D: Pathogenesis of arachnoid cyst: Congenital or traumatic? Pediatr Neurosurg 29:260–266, 1998.
3. Fox J, Al-Mefty O: Suprasellar arachnoid cysts: An extension of the membrane of Liliequest. Neurosurgery 7:615–618, 1980.
4. Go K, Simpson D, North J: Arachnoid cysts: A critical review of 41 cases. Childs Nerv Syst 4:92–96, 1988.
5. Rengachary S, Watanabe T: Ultrastructure and pathogenesis of intracranial arachnoid cysts. J Neuropathol Exp Neurol 40:616–663, 1981.
6. Santamarta D, Arguas J, Ferrer E: The natural history of arachnoid cysts: Endoscopic and cine-mode MRI evidence of a slit-valve mechanism. Minim Invasive Neurosurg 38:133–137, 1995.
7. Caemaert J, Abdullah J, Calliauw L, et al: Endoscopic treatment of suprasellar arachnoid cysts. Acta Neurochir (Wien) 119:68–73, 1992.
8. Schroeder H, Gaab M: Endoscopic observation of a slit-valve mechanism in suprasellar prepontine arachnoid cyst: Case report. Neurosurgery 40:198–200, 1997.
9. Okumura Y, Sakaki T, Hirabayashi H: Middle cranial fossa arachnoid cyst developing in infancy: Case report. J Neurosurg 82:1075–1077, 1995.
10. Albuquerque F, Giannotta S: Arachnoid cyst rupture producing subdural hygroma and intracranial hypertension: Case reports. Neurosurgery 41:951–954, 1997.
11. Parsch C, Kraub J, Hofman E, et al: Arachnoid cysts associated with subdural hematomas: Analysis of 16 cases, long-term follow-up, and review of the literature. Neurosurgery 40:483–490, 1997.
12. Handa J, Okamoto K, Sato M: Arachnoid cyst of the middle cranial fossa: Report of bilateral cysts in siblings. Surg Neurol 16:127–130, 1981.
13. Jamjoon Z, Okamoto E, Jamjoon A, et al: Bilateral arachnoid cysts of the sylvian region in female siblings with glutaric aciduria type I. J Neurosurg 82:1078–1081, 1995.
14. Yamanouchi Y, Someda K, Oka N: Spontaneous disappearance of middle fossa arachnoid cyst after head injury. Childs Nerv Syst 2:40–43, 1986.
15. Di Rocco C, Caldarelli M, Ceddia A: Incidence, anatomical distribution, and classification of arachnoidal cysts. In Raimondi A, Choux M, Di Rocco C (eds): Intracranial Cyst Lesions. New York, Springer-Verlag, 1993, pp 101–111.
16. Rengachary S, Watanabe I, Brackett C: Pathogenesis of intracranial arachnoid cysts. Surg Neurol 9:139–144, 1978.
17. Hassounah M, Rahm B: Hindbrain herniation: An unusual occurrence after shunting an intracranial arachnoid cyst. J Neurosurg 81:126–129, 1994.
18. Stein S: Intracranial developmental cysts in children: Treatment by cystoperitoneal shunting. Neurosurgery 8:647–650, 1981.
19. Raffel C, McComb J: To shunt or to fenestrate: Which is best surgical treatment for arachnoid cysts in pediatric patients? Neurosurgery 23:338–342, 1988.
20. Shroeder H, Gaab M, Niendorf W: Neuroendoscopic approach to arachnoid cysts. J Neurosurg 85:293–298, 1996.
21. Heier L, Zimmerman R, Amster J, et al: Magnetic resonance imaging of arachnoid cysts. Clin Imaging 13:281–291, 1989.
22. Zingesser L, Schechter M, Gonatas N, et al: Agenesis of the corpus callosum associated with an inter-hemispheric arachnoid cyst. Br J Radiol 37:905–909, 1964.
23. Galassi E, Piazza G: Arachnoid cysts of the middle cranial fossa: A clinical and radiological study of 25 cases treated surgically. Surg Neurol 14:211–219, 1980.
24. Martuzza R, Ojemann R, Shillito J, et al: Facial pain associated with a middle fossa arachnoid cyst. Neurosurgery 8:712–716, 1981.
25. Galassi E, Gaist G, Giulani G, et al: Arachnoid cysts of the middle cranial fossa: Experience with 77 cases treated surgically. Acta Neurochir 42:201–207, 1988.
26. Harsh G, Edwards M, Wilson C: Intracranial arachnoid cysts in children. J Neurosurg 64:835–842, 1986.
27. Walker M, Petronio J, Carey C: Ventriculoscopy. In Cheek W, Marlin A, McLone D, et al (eds): Pediatric Neurosurgery, 3rd ed. Philadelphia, WB Saunders, 1994, pp 572–581.
28. Hopf N, Perneczky A: Endoscopic neurosurgery and endoscope-assisted microneurosurgery for the treatment of intracranial cysts. Neurosurgery 43:1330–1336, 1998.
29. Hoffman H, Hendrick E, Humphreys R, et al: Investigation and management of suprasellar arachnoid cysts. J Neurosurg 57:597–602, 1982.
30. Benton J, Neilhaus G, Huttencocker P, et al: The bobble-head doll syndrome. Neurology 16:725–769, 1966.
31. Pierre-Kahn A, Capelle L, Brauner R, et al: Presentation and management of suprasellar arachnoid cysts: Review of 20 cases. J Neurosurg 73:355–359, 1990.
32. Albright L: Treatment of bobble-head doll syndrome by transcallosal cystectomy. Neurosurgery 8:593–595, 1981.
33. Russo R, Kindt G: A neuroanatomical basis for the bobble-head syndrome. J Neurol 41:720–723, 1974.
34. Baskin D, Wilson C: Transphenoidal treatment of non-neoplastic intrasellar cysts. J Neurosurg 60:8–13, 1984.
35. Rampini P, Zavanone M, Orsi M, et al: Stereotactically guided endoscopy for the treatment of arachnoid cysts. Pediatr Neurosurg 29:102–104, 1998.
36. Hayahi T, Kuratomi A, Kuramoto S: Arachnoid cyst of the quadrigeminal cistern. Surg Neurol 14:267–273, 1980.
37. Huckman M, Davis D, Coxe W: Arachnoid cyst of the quadrigeminal plate. J Neurosurg 32:367–370, 1970.
38. Jallo G, Woo H, Meshki C, et al: Arachnoid cysts of the cerebellopontine angle: Diagnosis and surgery. Neurosurgery 40:31–37, 1997.
39. McComb J: Review of Jallo G, Woo H, Meshki C, et al: Arachnoid cysts of the cerebellopontine angle: Diagnosis and surgery. Neurosurgery 40:31–37, 1997. Neurosurgery 40:38, 1997.

CHAPTER **209**

Nonsyndromic Craniosynostosis and Abnormalities of Head Shape

MARION L. WALKER ■ JOHN J. COLLINS

INITIAL ASSESSMENT OF ABNORMAL HEAD SHAPE

Abnormal head shape as the presenting problem prompts a large number of referrals to pediatric neurosurgeons for outpatient evaluation. As a symptom, abnormal head shape has many possible underlying causes and several different treatment options, both surgical and nonsurgical. Optimal outcomes require clarity of thought during assessment to ensure appropriate treatment selection.

The first issue to resolve is whether the abnormality arises from structures within the skull (e.g., hydrocephalus, intracranial cyst, intracranial tumor) or structures outside the skull (e.g., cephalohematoma), or whether it involves the skull bones and their suture interfaces. The perinatal and developmental history, neurologic examination, and physical examination—including occipitofrontal circumference measurement and palpation of fontanelles, skull bones, and sutures—generally give a reliable initial impression.

When bony or suture abnormalities cause abnormalities of head shape, clinicians should have three concerns about the potential implications of this finding: Does the abnormality (1) cause focal brain compression, (2) induce global intracranial pressure elevation, or (3) have the potential to cause cosmetic deformity of sufficient magnitude to risk healthy psychosocial development? Evidence in support of any one of these three possibilities justifies a more detailed assessment and therapeutic intervention. Abnormalities along a single suture line do not usually elevate intracranial pressure, but this may occur when multiple skull bones and suture lines are involved. Any clinical evidence of elevated intracranial pressure should prompt a more expeditious workup and more urgent intervention. Concern about cosmesis is not urgent, but some procedures have better outcomes when performed at a younger age, so early assessment is advisable.

Having decided that the magnitude of the problem warrants some type of therapeutic intervention, the next concern is whether noninvasive treatments such as positional therapy or cranial orthosis are likely to help. Three sets of circumstances may predict the inefficacy of such mechanical treatments:

- Underlying systemic or metabolic conditions that require primary treatment, such as rickets, hypophosphatemia, hyperthyroidism, severe anemia, or mucopolysaccharidosis
- Persistent mechanical factors that cause abnormal deforming forces against the head or skull base, such as torticollis, prolonged bedridden state, hemivertebra, or Klippel-Feil syndrome
- A fixed structural impediment, such as a truly ossified cranial suture (referred to as *craniosynostosis*) or a nonfused suture subjected to such protracted misshaping forces that *irreversible* secondary bony changes have occurred

Most of the controversy surrounding management of a child with abnormal head shape has focused on the distinction between reversible conditions responsive to the changing of deforming forces applied to the cranial vault and irreversible or progressive conditions that involve fusion of suture interfaces. A review of the knowledge that has emerged from this sometimes difficult distinction should provide clarity and help guide clinical decisions.

DIFFERENTIATION BETWEEN SKULL MOLDING AND PRIMARY SYNOSTOSIS

The neonatal skull has a natural design that allows considerable anatomic flexibility.[1] As early as the second month of gestation, intramembranous ossification begins to form the skull bones at centers of osteogenesis within the epidural mesenchymal tissue.[2-7] Cancellous bone then forms by appositional growth that extends radially from the ossification centers.[3] Eventually the cancellous bone condenses into compact bone, and the expansions of intramembranous bone articulate with one another along suture lines.[8] Each suture, or syndesmosis, between two adjacent bones contains osteogenic cells, which promote further bony growth. A process of apoptosis, by which cells undergo an orderly process of cellular death, appears to prevent the fusion of these sutures until later in development.[5, 9] The metopic suture, for example, generally ossifies during the second year of life, whereas the coronal sutures normally do not fuse until much later, generally around 24 years of age.[8] The sutures provide hingelike connections that allow adjacent skull plates to move relative to one another, thereby permitting the head to change shape in response to applied forces that may occur in utero, during birth, or postnatally.[10] The typically rounded head shape of an older infant or child results from the symmetrical forces from within the skull. These forces are caused by steady brain growth against the plates of skull bone, unrestricted by any points of premature suture fusion or by any persistent asymmetrical external forces applied to the head.[11]

Given the inherent flexibility of the developing skull, it is no surprise that a variety of craniofacial anomalies have been reported as a consequence of in utero compressive forces against the fetal head.[12-15] Obstetric conditions that predispose to craniofacial abnormalities include primiparity, early descent into the maternal pelvis, aberrant fetal lies, and fetal head constraint due to a bicornuate uterus or the presence of twins or triplets. The infant head may also undergo molding of shape during descent through the pelvis at the time of birth. The vast majority of these abnormalities, however, resolve spontaneously during the first few months after delivery as a result of the reshaping force of rapid brain growth. The infant's brain mass normally doubles during the first 6 months of life and triples by 2.5 years.[16]

Assessment of Anterior Plagiocephaly

The most common cause of anterior plagiocephaly is deformation, usually from obstetric causes. During spontaneous vaginal delivery, most vertex presentations are in the left occipital anterior position. This correlates with the fact that 73% of deformational frontal plagiocephaly is left-sided.[17, 18] Engagement of the head in the pelvis at a much earlier date than usual is associated with an increased incidence of significant deformational plagiocephaly.[19]

Deformational anterior plagiocephaly presents with frontal flatness and an ipsilateral narrow palpebral fissure. The ipsilateral eyebrow and ear may be displaced downward. The chin may deviate toward the affected side. A vertex view reveals a parallelogram shape to the head, with the ipsilateral malar eminence and ear pushed back. The ipsilateral posterior parietal region may show compensatory bossing. The nasal root, however, shows no deviation or angulation.[20]

True premature bony fusion of one coronal suture produces a type of anterior plagiocephaly distinct from that produced by head molding within the pelvis. The ipsilateral palpebral fissure is widened instead of narrowed. The supraorbital rim and eyebrow are displaced superiorly and posteriorly instead of inferiorly. The ipsilateral ear may be higher than the contralateral ear. The chin may point to the contralateral side instead of the ipsilateral side. The nasal root deviates toward the flattened side (Figs. 209–1 and 209–2; Table 209–1).[17, 20]

Assessment of Dolichocephaly

External deformational forces can also occur after birth, most commonly as a consequence of the force of gravity on an infant's head lying in a single preferred position (positional molding).[21] A well-recognized syndrome of positional molding that occurs in neonatal intensive care units is dolichocephaly (long head shape) caused by intubated neonates persistently lying on one side of the head.[22] This can easily be prevented by frequent head turning and is rarely confused with the characteristic scaphocephaly (boat-shaped head) with sagittal ridging and frontal bossing of primary sagittal synostosis.

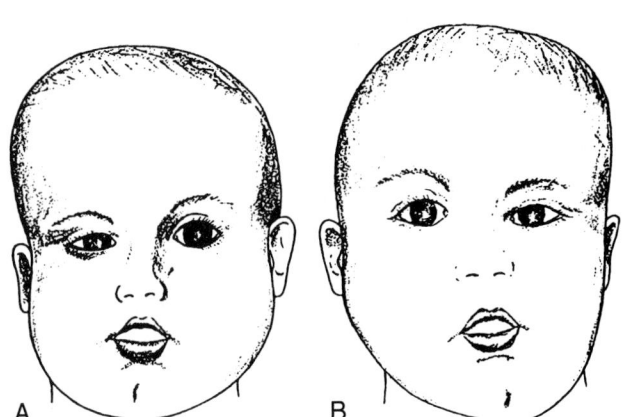

FIGURE 209–1. Composite drawing of left coronal synostosis *(A)* and left deformational frontal plagiocephaly *(B)*. The affected forehead is flattened in both conditions; however, the position and shape of the ipsilateral eye, position of the ears, and deviation of the chin point are opposite. The nasal root is deviated toward the affected side in synostotic frontal plagiocephaly; it is usually straight in deformational frontal plagiocephaly. (From Bruneteau RJ, Mulliken JB: Frontal plagiocephaly: Synostotic, compensational or deformational. Plast Reconstr Surg 89:25, 1992.)

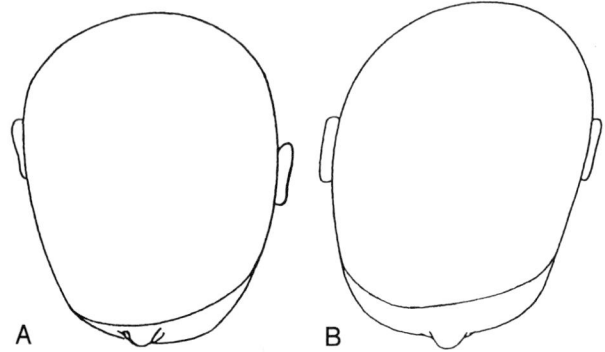

FIGURE 209–2. Drawings from the vertex view, illustrating the differences between left synostotic *(A)* and left deformational *(B)* frontal plagiocephaly. Note the opposite configuration of the left malar eminence and the opposite position of the ears. (From Bruneteau RJ, Mulliken JB: Frontal plagiocephaly: Synostotic, compensational or deformational. Plast Reconstr Surg 89:25, 1992.)

Assessment of Posterior Plagiocephaly

Most common and controversial is the problem of posterior plagiocephaly of infancy. Various studies have identified increasing numbers of cases, perhaps coincident with the trend to encourage a supine sleeping position for infants to reduce the incidence of sudden infant death syndrome (SIDS).[23–25] Posterior plagiocephaly refers to an asymmetrical appearance of the occipital region. This generally presents as a flatness of one side of the occiput relative to the other, best appreciated from the vertex view. The clinician should first determine whether the pattern of findings suggests the rare occurrence of true primary lambdoid suture synostosis or the vastly more common pattern of deformational plagiocephaly. Huang and colleagues provided a set of unambiguous criteria that help establish this distinction (Figs. 209–3 and 209–4; Table 209–2).[26]

True primary unilateral lambdoid suture synostosis

TABLE 209–1 ■ **Differential Diagnosis of Anterior Plagiocephaly**

ANATOMIC FEATURES	DEFORMATIONAL	UNICORONAL SYNOSTOSIS
Ipsilateral superior orbital rim	Down	Up
Ipsilateral ear	Posterior and low	Anterior and high
Nasal root	Midline	Ipsilateral
Ipsilateral cheek	Backward	Forward
Chin deviation	Ipsilateral	Contralateral
Ipsilateral palpebral fissure	Narrow and high	Wide and low
Anterior fontanelle deviation	None	Contralateral

creates an ipsilateral occipitomastoid bossing and a thick external ridge over the affected fused suture that results in posterior and inferior displacement of the ipsilateral ear, with contralateral compensatory frontal and parietal bossing. From the vertex view, this causes the head to appear trapezium-shaped; from the posterior view, a tilt of the skull base axis creates the impression of a parallelogram-shaped head. Computed tomographic scans or skull radiographs reveal true bony fusion of the lambdoid suture ipsilateral to the flattened occipital bone (Fig. 209–5). By these criteria, in Huang and associates' series of 102 patients presenting with posterior plagiocephaly, only 4 had this pattern of primary lambdoid synostosis. All four had progressive worsening of head shape that prompted surgical synostectomy, and all had histologically proven complete bony fusion of the excised suture. These investigators estimated that true primary lambdoid synostosis constitutes only 3.1% of craniosynostosis cases.[26]

Deformational posterior plagiocephaly, in contrast, has no ipsilateral occipital mastoid bossing or prominent ipsilateral lambdoid suture ridging. Displacement of the ipsilateral ear is directed anteriorly, and compen-

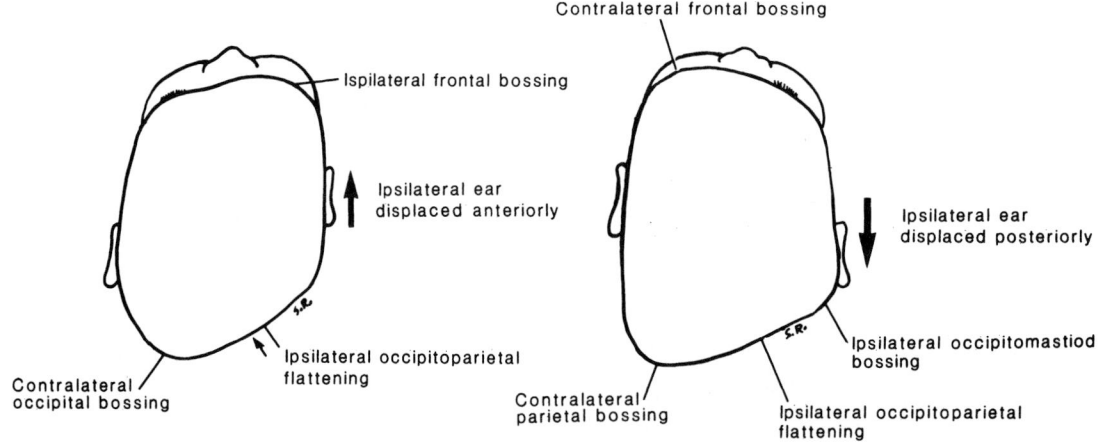

FIGURE 209–3. Diagrammatic summary of the differences between positional molding *(left)* and unilambdoid synostosis *(right)*. (From Huang MH, Gruss JS, Clarren SK, et al: The differential diagnosis of posterior plagiocephaly: True lambdoid synostosis versus positional molding. Plast Reconstr Surg 98:773, 1996.)

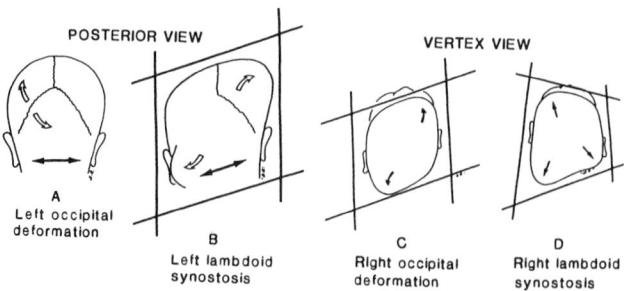

POSTERIOR VIEW

VERTEX VIEW

A
Left occipital
deformation

B
Left lambdoid
synostosis

C
Right occipital
deformation

D
Right lambdoid
synostosis

FIGURE 209–4. Head shape differences from the posterior view *(left)* and the vertex view *(right)* between occipital deformational posterior plagiocephaly *(A and C)* and true unilateral lambdoid synostosis *(B and D)*. Arrows indicate the directions of compensatory growth vectors. (From Huang MH, Gruss JS, Clarren SK, et al: The differential diagnosis of posterior plagiocephaly: True lambdoid synostosis versus positional molding. Plast Reconstr Surg 98:773, 1996.)

TABLE 209–2 ▪ **Differential Diagnosis of Posterior Plagiocephaly**

ANATOMIC FEATURES	DEFORMATIONAL	UNILAMBDOID SYNOSTOSIS
Contralateral posterior bossing	Occipital	Parietal
Frontal bossing	Ipsilateral	Contralateral
Ipsilateral occipitomastoid bossing	Absent	Present
Displacement of ipsilateral ear	Anterior	Posterior and inferior
Skull base and face	Not tilted	Ipsilateral inferior tilt
Ridging of lambdoid suture	Absent	Present
Head shape: vertex view	Parallelogram	Trapezium
Head shape: posterior view	Normal	Parallelogram
Status of lambdoid suture	No fusion or fibrous union	Bony union

satory bossing occurs in the ipsilateral frontal and contralateral occipital regions. From the vertex view, this causes the head to take the shape of a parallelogram. Because there is no tilt of the skull base axis, the head shape appears normal when viewed posteriorly. Computed tomographic scans or skull radiographs do not reveal true bony fusion of the lambdoid suture ipsilateral to the flattened occipital bone (Fig. 209–6). In Huang and colleagues' series, 98 of the 102 patients presented with this pattern, and only 3 of those 98 had sufficient persistence or severity of deformity to require surgery.[26] Operative findings and histologic appearance in these three cases confirmed patency of the excised lambdoid sutures.

After identifying the more common pattern of deformational posterior plagiocephaly, the next distinction the clinician should make is whether the condition may respond to interventions that either remove existing

deformational forces or provide counterforces to the external skull. Posterior plagiocephaly may respond to a variety of management techniques. Simply allowing time for brain growth to occur may result in improvement. Spontaneous improvement may also become evident after the infant achieves sufficient strength to support the head and to sit up. Behavioral perseverance of the preferred head position while lying down can be countered by keeping the infant in a supported sitting position. Lying in a sling may also redistribute external forces on the head more evenly. Torticollis, if present, should be addressed with physical therapy or more invasive techniques if indicated.[27] The use of external orthotic skull molding helmets may help promote a more rapid resolution.[28–30] The relative efficacy of these techniques, however, remains a topic of de-

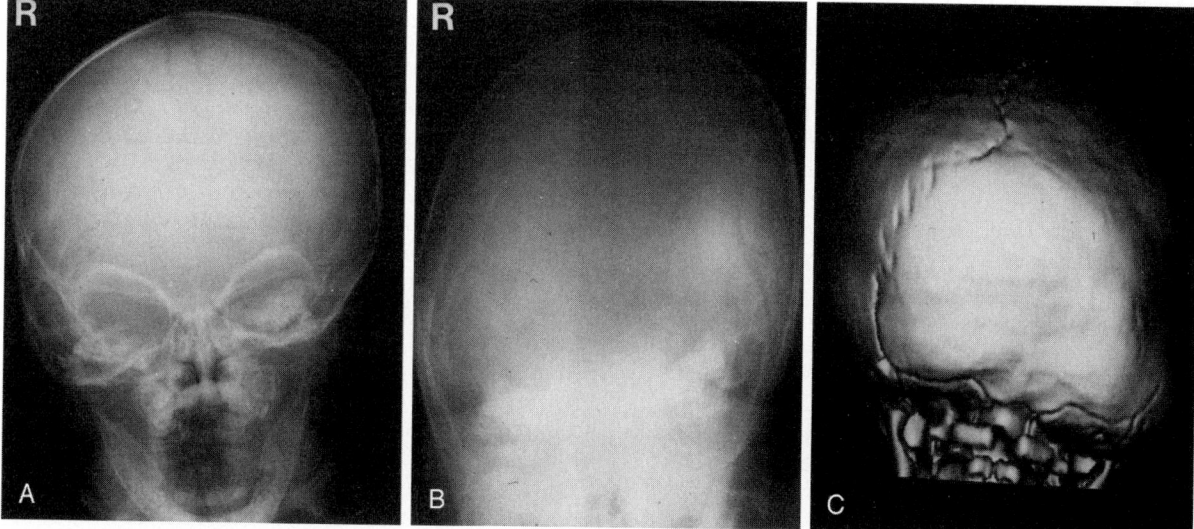

FIGURE 209–5. Radiographic features of true right lambdoid craniosynostosis. *A* and *B*, Plain radiographs. *C*, Three-dimensional computed tomographic scan, posterior view. Note the bony fusion of the right lambdoid suture, the ipsilateral occipitomastoid bossing, and the ipsilateral inferior tilt of the skull base.

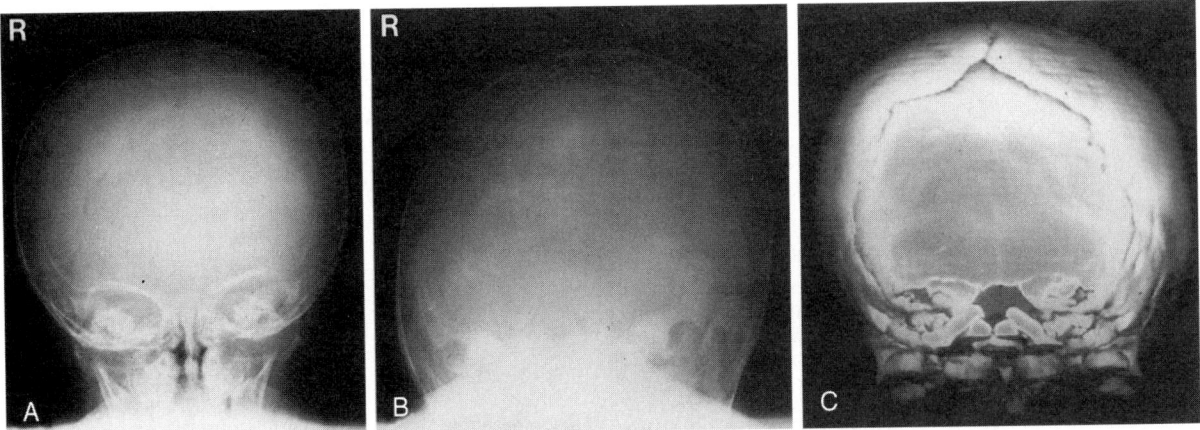

FIGURE 209–6. Radiographic features of deformational left posterior plagiocephaly. *A* and *B*, Plain radiographs. *C*, Three-dimensional computed tomographic scan, posterior view. Although the left lambdoid suture appears slightly less distinct, it does not exhibit bony fusion. There is no occipito-mastoid bossing and no ipsilateral inferior tilt of the skull base.

bate.[31] Dias and coworkers described computed tomographic measurements that quantitate the severity of deformational posterior plagiocephaly based on the geometry of the calvarial parallelogram shape and the acuity of the petrous angle.[32] These measurements, together with serial physical examinations of the head over time, can establish whether improvement occurs.

It is rare for patients to be unresponsive to the previously noted therapeutic options. However, a subset of patients with the deformational pattern of posterior plagiocephaly will be unresponsive to all these conservative measures over time (3% in Huang and associates' series of 102 patients).[26, 33] The skull deformity may become severe enough or sufficiently persistent that the patient becomes a candidate for surgical intervention. Such intervention might be particularly appropriate to correct a prominent compensatory frontal bossing that fails to resolve. Moderate occipital flatness is generally of less concern, because hair growth can hide the posterior head shape. Age is the most significant factor in whether spontaneous resolution of shape will occur, probably because the rate of increasing brain volume slows after age 1 to 2. An older child has less of an internal restorative force arising from brain growth. Actual bony union across the lambdoid suture is a rare histologic finding.[10, 34, 35] It has been postulated that a variety of secondary changes may occur along the ipsilateral lambdoid suture in the absence of true bone fusion of the lambdoid suture.[33, 36] Several such radiographic and histologic findings include sclerotic suture margins along the inner table, exaggerated and prolonged suture activity on radionucleotide bone scan, increased cellular proliferation at the suture line, increased sutural interdigitation, and small foci of bridging bone. Most patients with these features, however, still respond to conservative management,[37] and these features should not be used to predict unresponsiveness of posterior plagiocephaly. It is possible that secondary changes that create bony bridging in the posterolateral skull base or asterion region might contribute to persistent posterior plagiocephaly, but this pattern of secondary change is not common.[38]

The vast majority of posterior head shape anomalies seen in general clinical practice present with a pattern consistent with deformational causes rather than premature fusion of a cranial suture. A significant majority of these patients either improve spontaneously or respond to conservative management, including the various types of molding helmets. Surgical treatment should be reserved for the rare case of true lambdoid craniosynostosis or the few cases of deformational plagiocephaly that persist and exhibit progressive deformity that is unresponsive to conservative measures.

PRIMARY NONSYNDROMIC CRANIOSYNOSTOSIS

Although the world literature contains some earlier references to the association of premature closure of cranial suture lines with skull deformity, Otto in 1830[39] and Virchow in 1851[40] observed that when sutures fuse prematurely, skull growth decreases perpendicular to the suture's axis. Virchow added the observation that growth increases in the plane parallel to the fused suture. In the 1950s, Moss hypothesized that fusion at the cranial base occurred primarily, which secondarily altered the cranial vault.[41] Based on animal model experimentation, however, Persing and associates established that changes in the skull base in craniosynostosis develop secondarily to the cranial vault suture closure.[42, 43] Marsh and Vannier further observed that surgical correction of a single sutural abnormality could lead to restoration of a more normal head shape, including resolution of the associated cranial base abnormalities.[44] These principles underlie our current concept of primary nonsyndromic craniosynostosis. Premature bony fusion of a suture causes the adjacent cranial bones to act like a single bony plate, which promotes an abnormal and asymmetrical increase of bone deposition at open sutures distant from this plate.

TABLE 209–3 ■ Patterns of Craniosynostosis

TYPE OF CRANIOSYNOSTOSIS	CHARACTERISTIC HEAD SHAPE
Single-Suture Synostosis	
Sagittal	Scaphocephaly
Coronal	Anterior plagiocephaly
Metopic	Trigonocephaly
Lambdoid	Posterior plagiocephaly
Double-Suture Synostosis	
Bicoronal	Anterior brachycephaly
Bilambdoid	Posterior brachycephaly
Sagittal plus metopic	Scaphocephaly
Complex Multisuture Synostosis	
Bicoronal, sagittal, metopic	Turribrachycephaly
Multisuture	Kleeblattschädel

Such compensatory bone deposition occurs to a greater extent at patent sutures near the fused plate compared with the bone growth that occurs symmetrically at more distant patent sutures.[45] Characteristic abnormalities of head shape therefore occur (Table 209–3).

Epidemiologic studies indicate that there are about 5 to 6 cases of craniosynostosis per 10,000 live births.[46, 47] Earlier estimates based on surgical series data suggested a higher incidence,[48] but differences in diagnostic criteria and sample bias probably account for these variations. In the late 1980s, reports of an increasing incidence of craniosynostosis in Colorado created the impression of an epidemic of the disorder. A subsequent population-based birth prevalence study with independent review of diagnostic criteria, however, revealed that excessively low diagnostic thresholds had created a semblance of increased rates of disease.[49]

GENETIC FACTORS IN PRIMARY CRANIOSYNOSTOSIS

Familial Patterns of Occurrence

The majority of primary craniosynostosis cases that present without associated anomalies appear to occur sporadically. Over the years, however, reports have accumulated that reveal occasional familial patterns of nonsyndromic sagittal,[50–53] metopic,[54–56] and coronal[57, 58] craniosynostosis. The predominant pattern of inheritance suggested by these reports is autosomal dominant with variable penetrance. Lajeunie and colleagues' broad study of 260 probands of nonsyndromic coronal craniosynostosis discovered 26 of 180 pedigrees (14.4%) with a high degree of familial aggregation. This suggested transmission as a dominant disorder with 0.60 penetrance and 61% sporadic incidence.[58] Few reports exist, however, that claim familial inheritance of lambdoid craniosynostosis. Fryburg and associates' report of recurrent lambdoid synostosis in two families described a deformational pattern of posterior plagiocephaly in all but one case. None of these patients who received surgical treatment had histologic evidence of true bony fusion along the excised lambdoid sutures at the time of pathologic examination.[59]

Chromosomal Anomalies

The observation of familial patterns in primary nonsyndromic craniosynostosis has prompted an intensive search for molecular biologic correlates that could account for aberrations in cranial suture development. This search began at the chromosomal level. Various forms of nonsyndromic double-suture or complex-suture fusion pattern phenotypes combined with several accompanying deformities occur in association with specific chromosomal deletions. Deletions of the terminal short arm of chromosome 7 (particularly in the region of 7p21) results in coronal, sagittal, and metopic multisuture synostosis that causes turribrachycephaly.[60–63] Partial deletion of 15q has resulted in sagittal, metopic, and bilateral lambdoid fusion that produces a kleeblattschädel appearance.[64, 65] A more focal deletion of 15q15 was associated with a less extensive double-suture pattern involving only metopic and sagittal synostosis.[66] Fryburg and Golden reported a case of true bilateral lambdoid craniosynostosis with distinct lambdoid ridging and radiographic confirmation of bony sutural fusion in a patient with deletion at 8q13.3-22.1.[67] Muller and colleagues described a complex multisuture pattern of craniosynostosis in a patient with deletion of the terminal portion of 5q.[68]

Focal Gene Mapping in Craniosynostosis

Rapid advances in molecular genetic technology and a computer-based method to number and catalogue genes have greatly facilitated the discovery of specific genes responsible for certain types of craniosynostosis.[69] The initial successes in this endeavor occurred in the investigation of several well-known autosomal dominant craniofacial syndromes. It is now known that the Boston-type craniosynostosis gene *MSX2* (OMIN 123101) on chromosome 5p codes for a protein that regulates apoptosis of neural crest cell–derived tissue.[70–72] The fibroblastic growth factor receptor (FGFR) genes (a family that produces four tyrosine kinase cell surface receptors for fibroblast growth factors) have been implicated in Pfeiffer's syndrome type I (*FGFR-1* [OMIM 136350] on locus 8p12) and Apert's, Crouzon's, and Pfeiffer's syndromes types I to III, and Jackson-Weis syndrome (*FGFR-2* [OMIM 176943] on locus 10q26).[70, 73] New evidence has begun to accumulate that identifies specific gene foci that correlate to nonsyndromic, single-suture fusion patterns of phenotype. Reardon reported two sporadic cases of unilateral coronal synostosis that presented with neonatal anterior plagiocephaly, without any other syndromic features, that had a specific pro250arg mutation of *FGFR-3*.[74] Moloney went on to determine that the C749G (pro250arg) mutation in the gene for FGFR-3 was present in 31% of 26 patients studied with nonsyndromic coronal synostosis. In two of these cases, transmission was autosomal dominant. Six cases were sporadic.[75] Models to explain the pathogenesis of premature suture fusion must now incorporate this new molecular biologic data. Abnormalities of biochemical intercellular signaling and genetic control of apoptosis probably underlie all forms of craniosynostosis in which the head shape abnormality results from primary premature suture fusion rather than external deformational forces.[76, 77] The distinction between syndromic and nonsyndromic craniosynostosis may simply reflect differences in the offending genetic foci.

SAGITTAL CRANIOSYNOSTOSIS

Clinical Assessment

The hallmark of sagittal craniosynostosis is the long scaphocephalic (boat-shaped) head with associated bifrontal and suboccipital compensatory bossing. A palpable ridge occurs along a portion or the entire length of the sagittal suture. These features are often present at birth. They always become increasingly evident with advancing age. This deformity eventually causes a significantly undesirable dysmorphism that places the child at high risk for psychosocial problems during development.[78, 79] For this reason, in most cases, surgical correction is the recommended treatment option. Parents who do not choose surgical correction often experience anger or ambivalence later with progression of the deformity.[78] Sagittal craniosynostosis is the most common form of craniosynostosis and appears to occur more frequently in males than in females by a ratio of 4:1.[80]

Skull radiographs can provide diagnostic confirmation (Fig. 209–7). CT generally is not required to establish the diagnosis but may provide useful information concerning the extent of the disorder, especially in the more advanced cases of older infants (Fig. 209–8). CT

may reveal or rule out synostosis at other sutures and indicate the presence of a large inner table keel beneath the fused sagittal suture. The clinician should look for additional abnormalities, including (but not limited to) the following associated findings: cleft lip and palate, shallow orbits, patent ductus arteriosus, atrial or ventricular septal defects, cardiac arrhythmia, tetralogy of Fallot, seizures, laryngomalacia, and developmental delay.[81]

Surgical Management

Although the published literature includes descriptions of many different surgical treatments for sagittal synostosis, all the proposed operations fall into one of two categories: cranial release or cranial reconstruction.

Cranial release procedures have in common excision of the fused suture longitudinally along the entire length of the parietal bone at a very early age.[82–84] Although now out of favor, in the past, interventions such as polymeric silicone (Silastic) strips were proposed to prevent suture refusion.[85, 86] Bone cuts of various extents or osteoclastic morcellation can be added to allow restoration of the dura's normal rounded shape.[81, 87] An alternative approach introduced by Jane in 1978 was to remove a pi-shaped piece of bone to create bony release adjacent to the fused sagittal suture and behind the coronal sutures, without actual sagittal synostectomy.[88] These techniques restore the normal vectors of skull growth and allow reossification during the months of rapid head size increase to spontaneously re-form the skull to a more normal-appearing shape. With these approaches, the younger the patient and the wider or more extensive the craniectomy, the better the cosmetic result. Blood loss, however, is a limiting factor that increases the risk with decreasing age. We favor operating when the patient is 8 weeks

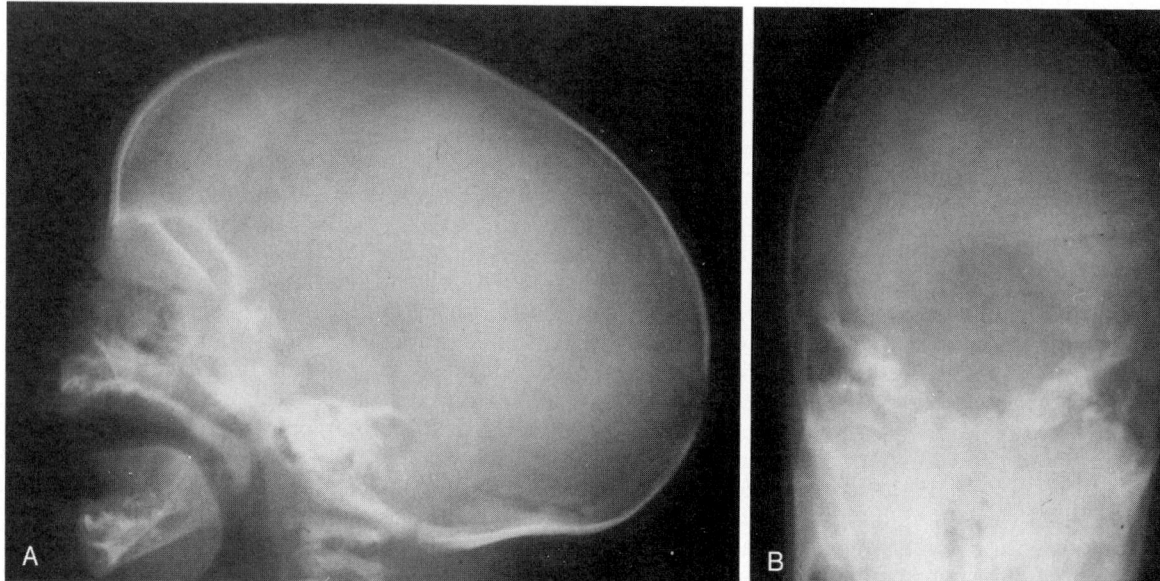

FIGURE 209–7. Features of sagittal craniosynostosis in an 8-week-old infant shown on plain radiographs, sagittal *(A)* and posteroanterior *(B)* views. Note the elongated head shape with occipital bossing and the bony fusion of the sagittal suture.

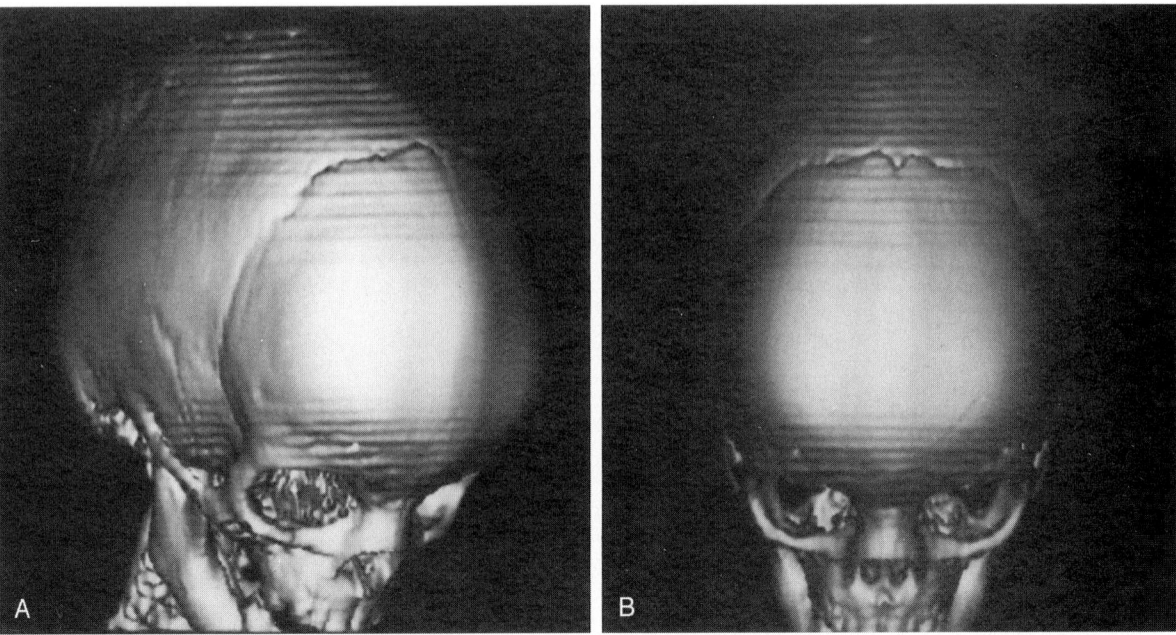

FIGURE 209–8. Features of sagittal craniosynostosis in a 22-month-old infant shown on three-dimensional computed tomographic scans, right anterior oblique view *(A)* and anterosuperior view *(B)*. Note the elongated head shape with frontal bossing, narrowed supraorbital rim, narrowed but prominent occiput, and bony fusion of the sagittal suture.

to perform a 5-cm-wide midsagittal craniectomy that extends from the coronal sutures to beyond the lambdoid sutures, with partial bilateral lambdoid suture excision and bilateral barrel stave osteotomies (Fig. 209–9).

Cranial vault reconstruction procedures attempt to alter the skull shape immediately by directly reducing the anterior-posterior axis of the skull and increasing the biparietal width. Older infants with more advanced deformity may require total calvarectomies (bilateral removal of frontal, parietal, and occipital bones), followed by reshaping and reconfiguring of these bones (Fig. 209–10).[80] The underlying principle in all such reconstruction procedures is that spontaneous head growth and reossification cannot be relied on to recreate normal head shape, because the deformity has become too advanced or the rate of head growth has slowed because of the infant's age.

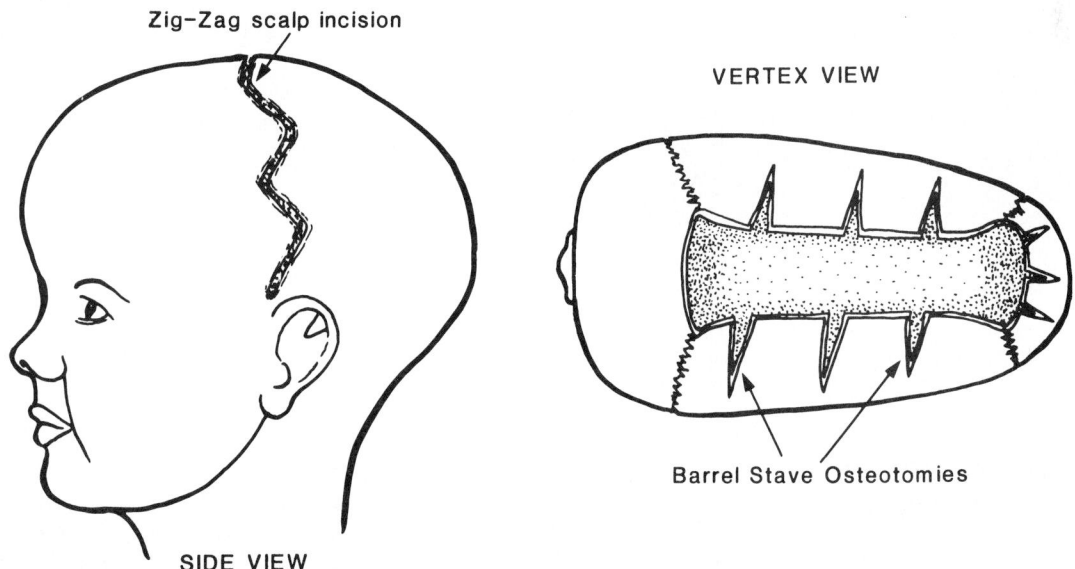

FIGURE 209–9. Diagram depicting the cosmetic zigzag scalp incision *(left)* and the midsagittal craniectomy with barrel stave osteotomies *(right)* performed in an 8-week-old infant to correct sagittal craniosynostosis.

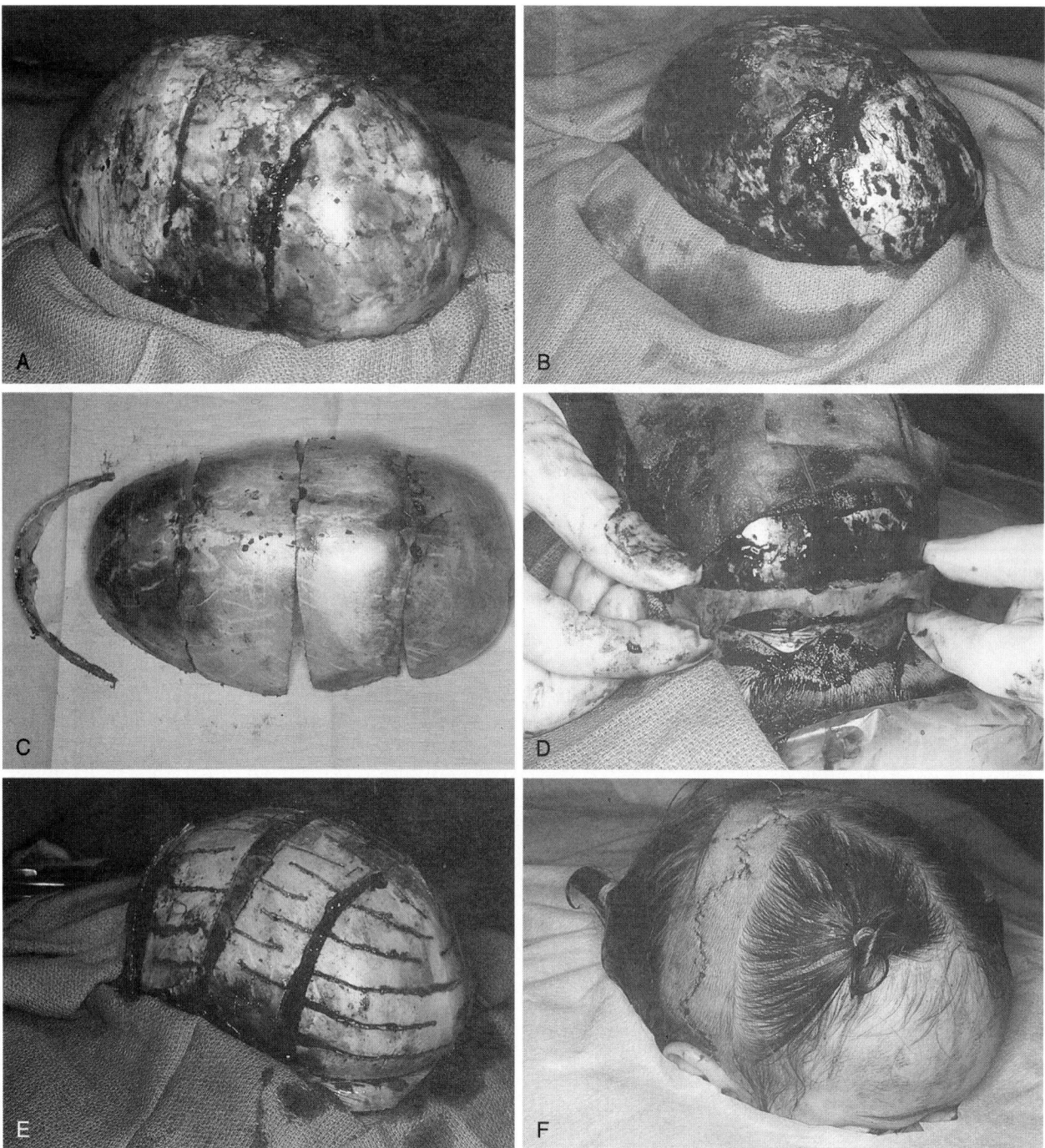

FIGURE 209–10. Intraoperative photograph of extensive cranial vault reconstruction to correct advanced sagittal craniosynostosis in a 22-month-old infant. *A*, Multiple strip craniotomy cuts in bilateral coronal planes. *B*, Dura is exposed after complete removal of the cranial vault. *C*, The segments of cranial vault are removed. Note the suboccipital band to the left. *D*, Removal of the supraorbital rim. *E*, Replacement of the remodeled cranial vault. *F*, Final appearance. Note the cosmetic zigzag scalp incision; it will not create an abnormal part in the hair later.

UNILATERAL CORONAL CRANIOSYNOSTOSIS

Clinical Assessment

Astute physical examination alone can establish the distinction between deformational anterior plagioceph-

aly and the frontal plagiocephaly of true unilateral coronal craniosynostosis. Skull radiographs may provide confirmatory information (Fig. 209–11). Unilateral coronal craniosynostosis creates a characteristic "harlequin mask" shape to the orbital region on the anteroposterior skull film because of superior displacement of the ipsilateral lesser sphenoid wing. Deviation of

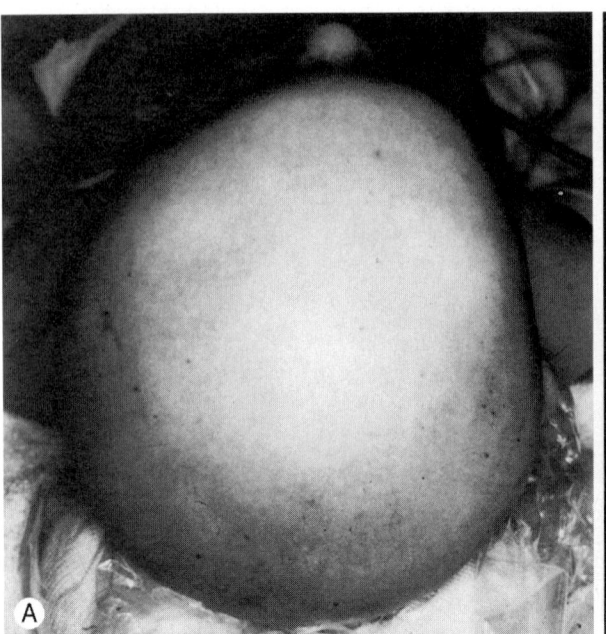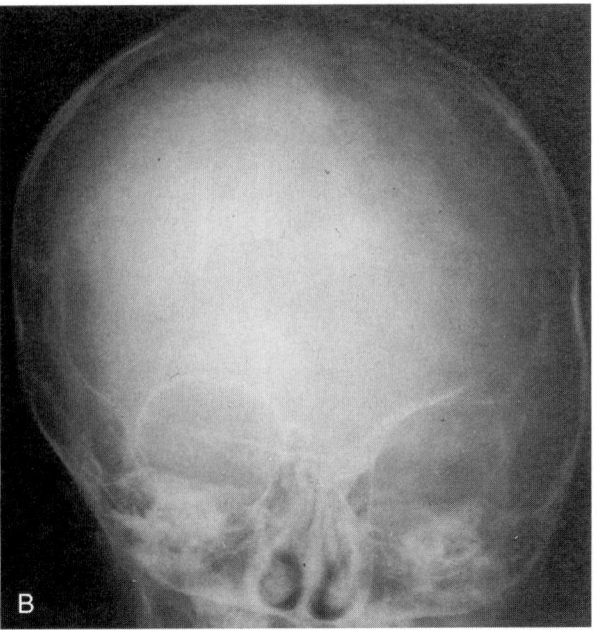

FIGURE 209–11. Morphologic and radiographic features of left coronal craniosynostosis. *A,* Preoperative photograph of the head from the vertex view. Note the flattened left forehead. *B,* Plain radiograph, anteroposterior view. Note the bony fusion of the left coronal suture and the left "harlequin eye" sign caused by superior displacement of the ipsilateral lesser sphenoid wing.

the nasal root toward the flattened side may also be evident. The lateral radiograph may indicate absence of one coronal suture.

Surgical Management

Coronal strip craniectomies do not reliably produce anterior craniofacial symmetry, even when performed in the first months of life and extended into the cranial base. For this reason, Hoffman and Mohr proposed frontal craniotomy combined with lateral canthal advancement in 1976.[89] This form of unilateral orbital advancement was given greater stability by a tongue-in-groove technique developed by Whitaker and colleagues that modeled the frontal bone to secure the repositioned supraorbital rim.[90] Today many centers use metallic or resorbable microplates and screws to provide additional stability of fixation.

METOPIC CRANIOSYNOSTOSIS

Clinical Assessment

Although metopic synostosis is relatively uncommon (<10% of all craniosynostosis cases),[47, 85, 91] it can result in an extremely conspicuous deformity. Ridging caused by increased bone formation at the prematurely fused suture creates a prominent keel in the middle of the forehead; it is generally most pronounced just above the nasion and less noticeable at the anterior fontanelle. In addition, trigonocephaly (Greek *trigonos* ["triangular"] and *kephale* ["head"]) occurs; this results in a narrow forehead and, in its more extreme form, may include ethmoidal hypoplasia and hypotelorism, often

accompanied by elevation of both lateral canthal angles. The lateral supraorbital rims may appear very deficient, with bitemporal excavation. Biparietal expansion may occur to compensate for the shortened, wedge-shaped anterior cranial fossa. Because the metopic suture may begin to fuse prematurely at any time from before birth to age 2, the extent of synostosis and the severity of the resultant deformity range from minor, almost imperceptible ridging to extreme aesthetic disruption. This variable expression necessitates individualized surgical management.

The clinical assessment of metopic craniosynostosis must determine the degree to which specific features occur: severity of the midline ridge, acuity of supraorbital rim angulation, degree of intercanthal distance foreshortening, severity of ethmoidal hypoplasia, and extent of bitemporal narrowness versus magnitude of biparietal flaring. Physical examination can measure only a few of these parameters. Plain radiographs add some information, but computed tomographic scans, including three-dimensional computed tomographic reconstructions, provide the most detailed assessment (Fig. 209–12). The presence or absence of various features influences the selection of specific surgical maneuvers.

Surgical Management

Adequate surgical correction of the mildest deformity, with midline ridging but without trigonocephaly, might be achieved by simply burring off the metopic suture with a shaping burr or performing a limited strip craniectomy.[92, 93] Correction of trigonocephaly, however, requires both frontal and supraorbital remod-

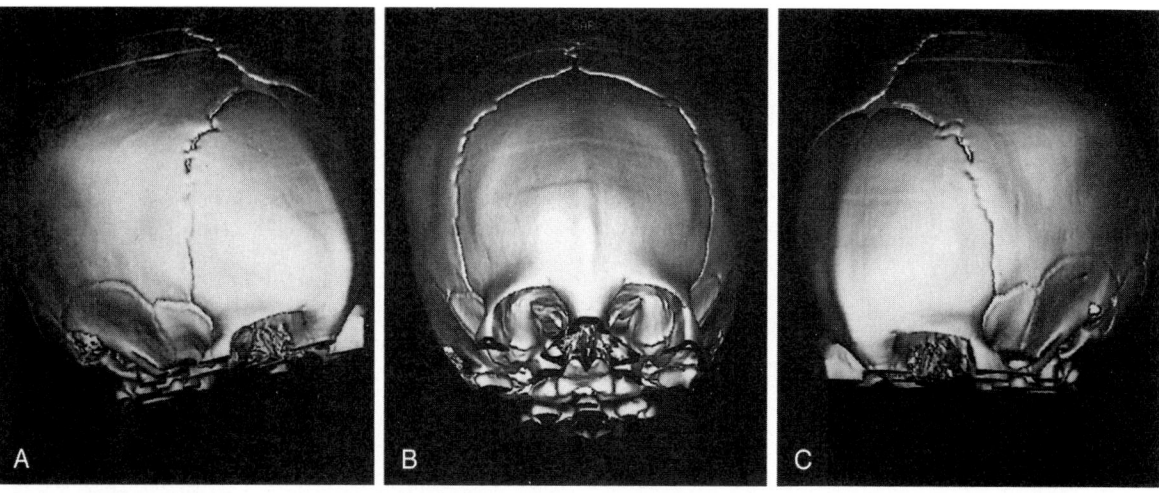

FIGURE 209–12. Radiographic features of metopic craniosynostosis. Three-dimensional computed tomographic scans of the frontal region from right anterior oblique *(A)*, straight anterior *(B)*, and left anterior oblique *(C)* views. Note the prominent midfrontal ridge overlying the fused metopic suture.

eling. Bifrontal craniotomy with the bone flap split into two pieces permits frontal reshaping.[85, 94] Extending this craniotomy behind the coronal sutures may facilitate correction of the narrow temporal regions.[94] If the supraorbital rims are thin, the lateral rims may be broken like a greenstick fracture forward to a sufficient extent.[92] A thicker supraorbital bar, however, requires complete removal and fracture at the midline to permit sufficient lateral canthal advancement. The left and right portions of the orbital band may require further scoring or wedging along its inner cortical surface to facilitate bending and shaping. The reconstructed forehead may then be rigidly fixed or attached only at the glabella to allow the growing brain to push and reshape the fronto-orbital segment.[95] Hypotelorism may require supraorbital bar expansion with a piece of calvarial bone interposed between the left and right segments.[96] Titanium microplates and screws provide significant rigidity to reconstructed bone segments, albeit with some concerns about screw migration and effects on long-term bone growth. Resorbable polymeric fixation plates now offer equivalent fixation without these risks.[96] Release and forward rotation of the temporalis muscle to fill the concavity can address the problem of persistent pterional deficiency.[92] With the introduction of osteogenic cement-like paste, however, it has become possible to fill the hollow temporal region with material that will eventually ossify.[97]

LAMBDOID CRANIOSYNOSTOSIS

Clinical Assessment

As stated earlier, the rare entity of true lambdoid suture craniosynostosis presents with characteristic defining morphologic features. Plain skull radiographs reveal bony fusion of the affected suture. Three-dimensional computed tomographic scans reveal lambdoid ridging plus the expected asymmetry and compensatory change.[98]

Surgical Management

In the past, linear craniectomy of the involved suture, extended to include the sagittal junction medially and the asterion region laterally, with or without resection of a few millimeters of petrous ridge, reportedly gave good cosmetic results.[35] The inclusion criteria at that time, however, allowed surgery for many cases of deformational posterior plagiocephaly. When the surgical indications restrict operative treatment to only those rare cases of true lambdoid craniosynostosis, the severity of the cranial deformities prevents simple strip craniectomy from achieving an adequate cosmetic outcome. The treatment, therefore, should involve reconstruction. The usual method of accomplishing this involves the release, rotation, and remodeling of a parieto-occipital bone flap, which contains the fused suture. Alternatively, left and right bilateral posterior free bone flaps can be transposed, rotated, remodeled, and then replaced. Kolk and Carson described a biparieto-occipital craniotomy composed of true transverse segments plus the removal of an occipital bar and the placement of suboccipital barrel stave osteotomies. Both transverse craniotomy sections are rotated 190 degrees, and their superior-inferior relationship is reversed. Microplates provide rigid fixation.[99]

BILATERAL CORONAL CRANIOSYNOSTOSIS

Clinical Assessment

Although often presenting as one feature in complex craniofacial deformities such as Apert's or Crouzon's syndrome, bilateral coronal craniosynostosis can also present as an isolated, nonsyndromic deformity. The skull shape appears shortened anteroposteriorly and widened mediolaterally (brachycephalic), often with vertical elongation as well (turribrachycephaly).[100] The anterior cranial base is shortened, the orbital rims are deficient, the occiput appears flat, and the superior frontal and squamous portions of the temporal bone show compensatory bulging. Evaluation should include plain skull radiographs (which may show the bilateral "harlequin eye" sign, indicating superior displacement of the lesser wings of both sphenoid bones) and a skull base computed tomographic scan. Lateral flexion and extension cervical radiographs should also be taken to rule out any instability or anomalies that would prevent safe positioning in a modified head-up prone position.[101]

Surgical Management

Persing and Jane described a comprehensive approach to cranial reconstruction for this condition, which requires bifrontal, biparieto-occipital, and separate bilateral temporal craniotomies.[100, 102] Barrel stave osteotomies in the parieto-occipital skull base, fractured outward, expand the posterior cranial vault. Radial osteotomies of the bifrontal and biparieto-occipital bone flaps permit remodeling of these segments. The parietal bone adjacent to the sagittal sinus remains in situ as a vaulted arch based on bilateral parietal struts. These struts are cut to shift that arch posteriorly 1 or 2 cm, and these struts are shortened the desired amount to reduce the vertex height. Intracranial pressure is monitored during the reconstruction. An orbital osteotomy is performed to advance the orbital rim.

Because the cranial reconstruction required to correct this condition involves such an extensive procedure, fronto-orbital advancement by gradual distraction at a very early age has been proposed as a less invasive way to achieve acceptable cosmetic results.[103] In this operation, the osteotomy cuts are nearly identical to those of conventional fronto-orbital advancement, but without the supraorbital cut or the lateral tongue-in-groove cuts. Both sphenoid ridges are removed through a wide resection. Internal distraction devices are then attached to the fronto-orbital plate and both parietal and temporal bones. The rods of the distraction device pierce the scalp. Five days after scalp closure, gradual distraction begins: twice daily, 0.5 mm at a time, over about 2 weeks. The devices remain in place another 3 weeks before removal. Long-term outcomes of this relatively new procedure have not yet been determined, but initial results are promising. Early age is essential, however, because the procedure does not alter the shape of the frontal bone. Distraction must take place before the onset of extreme bony deformity.

COMPLEX MULTISUTURE CRANIOSYNOSTOSIS

Complex patterns of multisuture craniosynostosis may occur early in life and fit a specific morphologic pattern, such as the kleeblattschädel, or cloverleaf, skull deformity, in which the craniofacial dysostosis results in a characteristic trilobar skull shape.[104] Direct compression on the brain and elevated intracranial pressure often pose the greatest threats to the very young infant. Multiple linear craniectomies along the fused sutures, skull morcellation techniques, or a posterior skull release procedure performed very early in life can allow sufficient decompression to restore essentially normal brain development and greatly reduce the cosmetic deformity. A second-stage reconstruction operation is usually required at a later age to achieve the best final appearance.[105–107]

A patient may present with complex multisuture craniosynostosis at a later age. Any abnormal head shape can occur, but it typically takes the form of either microcephaly or oxycephaly, in which the head elongates in the direction toward the vertex. This may result from progression of what initially appeared to be a single suture pattern of craniosynostosis, or it may develop primarily. In either case, the surgical treatment required is cranial vault reconstruction. This involves cutting the skull bone into segments that are removed, recontoured, and then fixed rigidly to create an immediate expansion and restored shape. Contour of the bone segments can be accomplished with a Tessier rib bender or may require grooving of the inner table.

SECONDARY CRANIOSYNOSTOSIS

Most cases of nonsyndromic craniosynostosis present as primary conditions. Some underlying systemic diseases, however, can promote premature cranial suture closure, usually in a pattern of pansynostosis. These diseases include inborn errors of metabolism causing storage disorders such as Hurler's or Morquio's syndrome, metabolic deficiencies such as rickets (vitamin D deficiency), endocrinologic abnormalities such as hyperthyroidism, hematologic disturbances such as thalassemia or polycythemia vera, and drug-related toxicities such as retinoic acid or diphenylhydantoin. A rare neurosurgical cause for secondary craniosynostosis is chronic ventriculoperitoneal shunt overdrainage. This unusual complication occurs in the context of shunt placement in a very young or premature infant. Cranial vault reconstruction may become necessary if this occurs to a significant degree.

OUTCOMES OF SURGERY FOR CRANIOSYNOSTOSIS AND LONG-TERM FOLLOW-UP

There is general consensus that with the evolving techniques in craniofacial surgery, the clinical outcomes of patients have improved. The vast majority of published reports describe "good results" using postoperative photographs or radiographs. These images provide objective outcome information, but they do not provide quantifiable outcome data or comparison to any control group. Some clinical investigators have begun to provide anthropomorphic measures as a method of quantifying the outcomes of different treatments for a given condition. Unfortunately, normative values often do not exist, and there are no natural history studies that use such measurements as parameters. The field of craniofacial surgery needs a more formal approach to outcome analysis. Cosmetic and functional improvement after intervention must be measured and compared to determine whether alternative treatment strategies yield better, worse, or similar results. Follow-up must also extend long term, throughout the child's entire development. This is essential because there are many reports of delayed secondary sequelae after surgery, sometimes necessitating reoperation. Statistical rates of all complications from craniofacial procedures must also be recorded and reported. The individual practitioner should continue to provide follow-up evaluations over several years to ensure that recurrent craniofacial problems or secondary complications do not occur.

REFERENCES

1. McPherson GK, Kriewall TJ: Fetal head molding: An investigation utilizing a finite element model of the fetal parietal bone. J Biomechan 13:17–28, 1980.
2. Mathijssen IMJ, Vaandrager JM, Van Der Meulen JC, et al: The role of bone centers in the pathogenesis of craniosynostosis: An embryologic approach using CT measurements in isolated craniosynostosis and Apert and Crouzon syndromes. Plast Reconstr Surg 98:17–26, 1996.
3. Inman VT, Saunders JB de CM: The ossification of the human frontal bone: With special reference to its presumed pre- and postfrontal elements. J Anat 71:383, 1937.
4. Mall EP: On ossification centers in human embryos less than one hundred days old. Am J Anat 5:433, 1906.
5. Vermeij-Keers C: Craniofacial embryology and morphogenesis: Normal and abnormal. In Stricker M, Van Der Meulen JC, Raphael B, et al (eds): Craniofacial Malformations. Edinburgh, Churchill-Livingstone, 1990.
6. Noback CR, Robertsom GG: Sequences of appearance of ossification centers in the human skeleton during the first five prenatal months. Am J Anat 89:1, 1951.
7. O'Rahilly R, Gardner E: The initial appearance of ossification in staged human embryos. Am J Anat 134:291, 1972.
8. Kokich VG: Biology of sutures. In Cohen MMJ (ed): Craniosynostosis: Diagnosis, Evaluation, and Management. New York, Raven Press, 1986.
9. Furtwangler JA, Hall SH, Koskinen-Moffet LK: Sutural morphogenesis in the mouse calvaria: The role of apoptosis. Acta Anat 124:74–80, 1985.
10. Cohen MM Jr: Sutural biology and the correlates of craniosynostosis. Am J Med Genet 47:581–616, 1993.
11. Keating RF: Craniosynostosis: Diagnosis and management in the new millennium. Pediatr Ann 26:600–612, 1997.
12. Graham JM Jr, Badura RJ, Smith DW: Coronal craniostenosis: Fetal head constraint as one possible cause. Pediatrics 65:995–999, 1980.
13. Graham JM Jr, Smith DW: Metopic craniostenosis as a consequence of fetal head constraint: Two interesting experiments of nature. Pediatrics 65:1000–1002, 1980.
14. Graham JM Jr, deSaxe M, Smith DW: Sagittal craniostenosis: Fetal head constraint as one possible cause. J Pediatr 95:747–750, 1979.
15. Higginbottom MC, Jones KL, James HE: Intrauterine constraint and craniosynostosis. Neurosurgery 6:39–44, 1980.
16. Boyd E: Organ weights from birth to maturity: Man, North American. In Altman PL, Dittmer DS (eds): Growing Including Reproduction and Morphological Development. Washington, DC, Federation of American Societies for Experimental Biology, 1962, p 364.
17. Bruneteau RJ, Mulliken JB: Frontal plagiocephaly: Synostotic, compensatory or deformational. Plast Reconstr Surg 89:21, 1992.
18. Watson GH: Relationship between side of plagiocephaly, dislocation of hip, scoliosis, bat ears and sternomastoid tumors. Arch Dis Child 46:203, 1971.
19. Danby PM: Plagiocephaly in some 10 year old children. Arch Dis Child 37:500, 1962.
20. Hansen M, Mulliken JB: Frontal plagiocephaly diagnosis and treatment. Clin Plast Surg 21:543–553, 1994.
21. Chadduck WM, Kast J, Donahue DJ: The enigma of lambdoid positional molding. Pediatr Neurosurg 26:304–311, 1997.
22. Huang MHS, Mouradian WE, Cohen SR, Gruss JS: The differential diagnosis of abnormal head shapes: Separating craniosynostosis from positional deformities and normal varients. Cleft Palate Craniofac J 35:204–211, 1998.
23. AAP Task Force on Infant Positioning and SIDS: Positioning and SIDS. Pediatrics 89:1120, 1992.
24. Argenta LC, David LR, Wilson JA, Bell WO: An increase in infant cranial deformity with supine sleeping position. J Craniofac Surg 7:5, 1996.
25. Turk AE, McCarthy JG, Thorne CH, Wisoff JH: The "back to sleep" campaign and deformational plagiocephaly: Is there cause for concern? Craniofac Surg 7:12, 1996.
26. Huang MH, Gruss JS, Clarren SK, et al: The differential diagnosis of posterior plagiocephaly: True lambdoid synostosis versus positional molding. Plast Reconstr Surg 98:765–774, 1996.
27. Golden KA, Beals SP, Littlefield TR, Pomatto JK: Sternocleidomastoid imbalance versus congenital muscular torticollis: Their relationship to positional plagiocephaly. Cleft Palate Craniofac J 36:256–261, 1999.
28. Clarren SK: Plagiocephaly and torticollis: Etiology, natural history, and helmet treatment. J Pediatr Neurosurg 98:92–95, 1982.
29. Pattisapu JV, Walker ML, Myers CG, et al: Use of helmets in positional molding. In Marlain AE (ed): Concepts of Pediatric Neurosurgery. Basel, Karger, 1989, pp 178–184.
30. Ripley CE, Pamatto J, Beals SP, et al: Treatment of positional plagiocephaly with dynamic orthotic cranioplasty. J Craniofac Surg 5:150–159, 1994.
31. Moss SD: Nonsurgical, nonorthotic treatment of occipital plagiocephaly: What is the natural history of the misshapen neonatal head? J Neurosurg 87:667–670, 1997.
32. Dias MS, Klein DM, Backstrom JW: Occipital plagiocephaly: Deformation or lambdoid synostosis? I. Morphometric analysis and results of unilateral lambdoid craniectomy. Pediatr Neurosurg 24:61–68, 1996.
33. Dias MS, Klein DM: Occipital plagiocephaly: Deformation or lambdoid synostosis? II. A unifying theory regarding pathogenesis. Pediatr Neurosurg 24:69–71, 1996.
34. Hinton DR, Becker LE, Muakkassa KF, Hoffman HJ: Lambdoid synostosis. Part 1. The lambdoid suture: Normal development and pathology of "synostosis." J Neurosurg 61:333–339, 1984.
35. Muakkassa KF, Hoffman HJ, Hinton DR, et al: Lambdoid synostosis. Part 2. Review of cases managed at the Hospital for Sick Children 1972–1982. J Neurosurg 61:340–347, 1984.
36. McComb JG: Treatment of functional lambdoid synostosis. Neurosurg Clin N Am 2:665–672, 1981.
37. Pollack IF, Losken HW, Fasick P: Diagnosis and management of posterior plagiocephaly. Pediatrics 99:180–185, 1997.
38. Jimenez DF, Barone CM, Argamaso RV, et al: Asterion region synostosis. Cleft Palate Craniofac J 31:136–141, 1994.
39. Otto AW: Lehrbook der pathologischen desmenschen und der thiere. Berlin, Rucker, 1830.
40. Virchow R: Uber den cretinismus, namentlich in Franken, und uber pathologische Shadelformen. Verh Phys Med Ges 2:230–270, 1851.
41. Moss ML: The pathogenesis of premature cranial synostosis in man. Acta Anat 37:351–370, 1959.
42. Babler WJ, Persing JA: Experimental alteration of cranial suture growth: Effects on neurocranium, basicranium, and midface. In Dixon AP, Sarnat BG (eds): Factors and Mechanisms Influencing Bone Growth. New York, Alan R. Liss, 1982, pp 333–345.
43. Francel PC, Persing JA: Evolving concepts in the pre-operative management and surgical treatment of craniosynostosis. Indian J Pediatr 58:183–190, 1991.
44. Marsh JL, Vannier MW: Cranial base changes following surgical treatment of craniosynostosis. Cleft Palate J 23:9–18, 1986.

45. Persing JA, Jane JA, Edgerton MT: Surgical treatment in craniosynostosis. In Persing JA, Edgerton MT, Jane J (eds): Scientific Foundations and Surgical Treatment of Craniosynostosis. Baltimore, Williams & Wilkins, 1989, pp 117–238.

46. Shuper A, Merlob P, Grunebaum M, Reisner SH: The incidence of isolated craniosynostosis in the newborn infant. Am J Dis Child 139:85–86, 1985.

47. Singer S, Bower C, Southall P, Goldblatt J: Craniosynostosis in western Australia, 1980–1994: A population-based study. Am J Med Genet 83:382–387, 1999.

48. Tessier P: Relationship of craniosynostosis to craniofacial dysostosis and to facial stenosis—a study with therapeutic implications. Plast Reconstr Surg 48:224–237, 1971.

49. Alderman BW, Fernbach SK, Greene C, et al: Diagnostic practice and the estimated prevalence of craniosynostosis in Colorado. Arch Pediatr Adolesc Med 151:159–164, 1997.

50. Duguid H: An incidence of familial scaphocephaly. J Mental Sci 75:704, 1929.

51. Murphy JW: Familial scaphocephaly in father and son. US Armed Forces Med J 4:1496, 1953.

52. Bell HS, Clare FB, Wentworth AF: Familial scaphocephaly. J Neurosurg 18:239, 1961.

53. Goebert HW Jr: Craniostenosis in one dizygotic twin. Hawaii Med J 28:286–287, 1969.

54. DeMyer W: Autosomal recessive phenotypes. In McKusick VA (ed): Mendelian Inheritance in Man, 3rd ed. Baltimore, Johns Hopkins Press, 1971, p 530.

55. Hunter AGW, Rudd NL, Hoffman HJ: Trigonocephaly and associated minor anomalies in mother and son. J Med Genet 13:77–79, 1976.

56. Hennekam RCM, Van den Boogaard M-J: Autosomal dominant craniosynostosis of the sutura metopica. Clin Genet 38:374–377, 1990.

57. Kosnick EJ, Gilbert G, Sayers MP: Familial inheritance of coronal craniosynostosis. Dev Med Child Neurol 17:630–633, 1975.

58. Lajeunie E, Le Merrer M, Bonaiti-Pellie C, et al: Genetic study of nonsyndromic coronal craniosynostosis. Am J Med Genet 55:500–504, 1995.

59. Fryburg JS, Hwang V, Lin KY: Recurrent lambdoid synostosis within two families. Am J Med Genet 58:262–266, 1995.

60. McPherson E, Hall JG, Hickman R: Chromosome 7 short arm deletion and craniosynostosis a 7p-syndrome. Hum Genet 35:117–123, 1976.

61. Dhadial RK, Smith MF: Terminal 7p deletion and 1;7 translocation associated with craniosynostosis. Hum Genet 50:285–289, 1979.

62. Motegi T, Ohuchi M, Ohtaki C, et al: A craniosynostosis in a boy with a del(7)(p15.3p21.3) assignment by deletion mapping of the critical segment for craniosynostosis to the mid-portion of 7p21. Hum Genet 71:160–162, 1985.

63. Schomig-Spingler M, Schmid M, Brosi W, Grimm T: Chromosome 7 short arm deletion, 7p21-pter. Hum Genet 74:323–325, 1986.

64. Pederson C: Partial trisomy 15 as a result of an unbalanced 12/15 translocation in a patient with a cloverleaf skull anomaly. Clin Genet 9:378–380, 1976.

65. Van Allen MI, Siegel-Bartelt J, Feigenbaum A, Teshima IE: Craniosynostosis associated with partial duplication of 15q and deletion of 2q. Am J Med Genet 43:688–692, 1992.

66. Fukushima Y, Wakui K, Nishida T, et al: Craniosynostosis in an infant with an interstitial deletion of 15q(46,xy, del(15) (q15q22.1)). Am J Med Genet 36:209–213, 1990.

67. Fryburg JS, Golden WL: Interstitial deletion of 8q13.3-22.1 associated with craniosynostosis. Am J Med Genet 45:638–641, 1993.

68. Muller U, Warman ML, Mulliken JB, Weber JL: Assignment of a gene locus involved in craniosynostosis to chromosome 5qter. Hum Mol Genet 2:119–122, 1993.

69. Anonymous: Online Mendelian Inheritance in Man (OMIM). Baltimore, Center for Medical Genetics, Johns Hopkins University; Bethesda, Md, National Center for Biotechnology Information, National Library of Medicine.

70. Robin NH: Molecular genetic advances in understanding craniosynostosis. Plast Reconstr Surg 103:1060–1070, 1999.

71. Liu YH, Kundu R, Wu L, et al: Premature suture closure and ectopic cranial bone in mice expressing Msx2 transgenes in the developing skull. Proc Natl Acad Sci 92:6137, 1995.

72. Jabs EW, Muller U, Li X, et al: A mutation in the homeodomain of the human MSX2 gene in a family affected with autosomal dominant craniosynostosis. Cell 75:443, 1993.

73. Malcolm S, Reardon W: Fibroblast growth factor receptor-2 mutations in craniosynostosis. Ann N Y Acad Sci 785:164–170, 1996.

74. Reardon W, Wilkes D, Rutland P, et al: Craniosynostosis associated with FGFR3 pro250arg mutation results in a range of clinical presentations including unisutural sporadic craniosynostosis. Med Genet 34:632–636, 1997.

75. Moloney DM, Wall SA, Ashworth GJ, et al: Prevalence of Pro250Arg mutation of fibroblast growth factor receptor 3 in coronal craniosynostosis. Lancet 349:1059–1062, 1997.

76. Wilkie AOM: Craniosynostosis: Genes and mechanisms. Hum Mol Genet 6:1647–1656, 1997.

77. Jabs EW: Toward understanding the pathogenesis of craniosynostosis through clinical and molecular correlates. Clin Genet 53:79–86, 1998.

78. Barritt J, Brooksbank M, Simpson D: Scaphocephaly: Aesthetic and psychosocial considerations. Dev Med Child Neurol 23:183–191, 1981.

79. Foltz EL, Loesser JD: Craniosynostosis. J Neurosurg 43:48–57, 1975.

80. Ocampo RV Jr, Persing JA: Sagittal synostosis. Clin Plast Surg 21:563–574, 1994.

81. Greene CSJ, Winston KB: Treatment of scaphocephaly with sagittal craniectomy and biparietal morcellation. Neurosurgery 23:196–202, 1988.

82. Shillito J: A plea for early operation for craniosynostosis. Surg Neurol 37:182–188, 1992.

83. Albright AL: Operative normalization of skull shape in sagittal synostosis. Neurosurgery 17:329–331, 1985.

84. Boop FA, Shewmake K, Chadduck WM: Synostectomy versus complex cranioplasty for the treatment of sagittal synostosis. Childs Nerv Syst 1996:371–375, 1988.

85. Anderson FM, Geiger LE: Craniosynostosis: A survey of 204 cases. J Neurosurg 22:229–240, 1965.

86. Ingraham FD, Alexander E, Matson DD: Clinical studies in craniosynostosis: Analysis of fifty cases and description of a method of surgical treatment. Surgery 24:518–541, 1948.

87. Hassler W, Zentner J: Radical osteoclastic craniectomy in sagittal synostosis. Neurosurgery 27:539–543, 1990.

88. Jane JA, Edgerton MT, Futrell JW, Park TS: Immediate correction of sagittal synostosis. J Neurosurg 49:705–710, 1978.

89. Hoffman HJ, Mohr G: Lateral canthal advancement of the supraorbital margin: A new corrective technique in coronal synostosis. J Neurosurg 45:376, 1976.

90. Whitaker LA, Schut L, Kerr LP: Early surgery for isolated craniofacial dysostosis. Plast Reconstr Surg 60:575, 1977.

91. Shillito J Jr, Matson DD: Craniosynostosis: A review of 519 surgical cases. Pediatrics 41:829, 1968.

92. Delashaw JB, Persing JA, Park TS, Jane JA: Surgical approaches for the correction of metopic synostosis. Neurosurgery 19:228–234, 1986.

93. Matson DD: Surgical treatment of congenital anomalies of the coronal and metopic sutures. J Neurosurg 17:413, 1960.

94. Albin RE, Hendee RW Jr, O'Donnell RS, Majure JA: Trigonocephaly: Refinements in reconstruction. Experience with 33 patients. Plast Reconstr Surg 76:202–211, 1985.

95. Marchac D: Radical forehead remodeling for craniostenosis. Plast Reconstr Surg 61:823, 1978.

96. Manson P: Commentary on "long-term effects of rigid fixation on the growing craniomaxillofacial skeleton." J Craniofac Surg 2:69, 1991.

97. Gossain AK: Hydroxyapatite cement paste cranioplasty for the treatment of temporal hollowing after cranial vault remodeling in a growing child. J Craniofac Surg 8:506–511, 1997.

98. Gul de Chauliac CMC, Montpellier CHR: Lambdoid craniosynostosis: A 3D computed tomographic approach. J Neuroradiol 20:24–33, 1993.

99. Kolk CAV, Carson BS: Lambdoid synostosis. Clin Plast Surg 21:575–584, 1994.

100. Persing JA, Jane JA, Delashaw JB: Treatment of bilateral coronal

synostosis in infancy: A holistic approach. J Neurosurg 72: 171–175, 1990.

101. Park TS, Haworth CS, Jane JA, et al: Modified prone position for cranial remodeling procedures in children with craniofacial dysmorphism: A technical note. Neurosurgery 16:212–224, 1985.

102. Persing JA, Jane JA: Treatment of syndromic and nonsyndromic bilateral coronal synostosis in infancy and childhood. Neurosurg Clin N Am 2:655–663, 1991.

103. Hirabayashi S, Sugawara Y, Sakurai A, et al: Frontoorbital ad-

vancement by gradual distraction. J Neurosurg 89:1058–1061, 1998.

104. Holtermuller K, Wiedemann HR: Kleeblattschädel syndrome. Med Monatsschr 14:439, 1960.

105. Muller PJ, Hoffman HJ: Cloverleaf skull syndrome: Case report. J Neurosurg 43:86, 1975.

106. Turner PT, Raynolds AF: Generous craniectomy for kleeblattschadel. Neurosurgery 6:555, 1980.

107. Zuletat A, Basauri L: Cloverleaf skull syndrome. Childs Brain 11:418, 1984.

CHAPTER 210

Craniofacial Syndromes

JOSEPH H. SHIN ■ JOHN A. PERSING

Although uncommon, syndromic craniosynostosis and craniofacial syndromes remain among the most challenging disorders that are routinely cared for by craniofacial surgeons and neurosurgeons. Concomitant advances in molecular genetics and surgical techniques have greatly altered our understanding as well as the treatment options for those affected with these congenital anomalies. Therapies to treat these disorders are continually being developed and modified.

Nonsyndromic craniosynostosis is seen more commonly, with a reported frequency of 0.4 to 1 case per 1000 live births.[1] By comparison, syndromic craniofacial anomalies associated with craniosynostosis are seen in 1 of 25,000 births for Crouzon's syndrome to 1 of 160,000 for Apert's syndrome.[2] Others, such as Pfeiffer's syndrome, Saethre-Chotzen syndrome, and Carpenter's syndrome, are even more unusual. Despite the variability of the phenotypic manifestation of these conditions, almost all have associated craniosynostosis, faciostenosis, and a variable pattern of limb abnormalities, which allow distinction among the individual diagnoses.

The development of craniofacial surgery over the past 30 years has been profound. Technologic advances and greater safety in the care of these patients has come from the development of the craniofacial team. In the care of these patients, the team incorporates the expertise of a multidisciplinary group, including the geneticist, neurosurgeon, plastic surgeon, pediatric anesthesiologist, ophthalmologist, otolaryngologist, orthodontist, speech and physical therapist, and psychologist.

The care of these patients may be complex, and coordination of care is required over an extended time. Treatment plans require long-range planning over the entire period of childhood and adolescence into adulthood. In the following sections, we describe our understanding and current options for treatment planning for patients with syndromic craniosynostosis.

HISTORY AND PATHOGENESIS

As many as 90 syndromes may have craniosynostosis as an associated feature.[3] Of these, five syndromic conditions (i.e., Apert's, Crouzon's, Pfeiffer's, Saethre-Chotzen, and Carpenter's syndromes) represent the more commonly seen diagnoses. The cause of these syndromes remains confusing because the physical manifestations may be protean. In 100 BC, Hippocrates recorded the variability of calvarial deformities and correlated these with a pattern of cranial suture fusion. In 1651, Harvey[4] postulated maternal posture and uterine abnormality as a cause of congenital anomalies. Sommerring,[5] however, reported in 1791 that bone growth and development in the skull occurred along suture lines, distortions of which may result in skull deformity. Virchow[6] reported in 1851 that premature fusion along the suture lines resulted in compensatory growth along a plane parallel to the fused suture and in decreased growth of the skull in relation to the perpendicular axis (Fig. 210–1). This hypothesis of skull maldevelopment remained unchanged for nearly 100 years, until Van der Klaauw[7] in 1946 and Moss[8] in 1959 proposed that the cranial base was the source of abnormal physical stress leading to dural abnormalities that then yielded premature sutural fusion; this was called the *functional matrix theory*. Subsequent animal studies[9–11] have, however, elucidated that, in normal laboratory animals, cranial vault abnormalities associated with synostosis can be reproduced with experimental fusion of developing cranial vault sutures. Moreover, cranial base deformities are secondarily induced by restrictions in growth of cranial vault sutures. In their congenital synostosis rabbit model, Mooney and colleagues[12] corroborated the importance of suture fusion in the development of cranial vault and cranial base changes.

Frequently, patients with craniosynostosis syndromes have additional physical disorders, which include primary cranial base defects and other hallmark features such as syndactyly. Molecular genetic techniques have identified mutations in the receptor genes for fibroblast growth factor (FGF) in several skeletal disorders, which are transmitted in an autosomal-dominant pattern. Mutations located on chromosome 8, 10q, and 4p in three of the four known FGF receptor genes have been identified in Apert's, Crouzon's, Pfeiffer's, and Jackson-Weiss syndromes and in achondroplasia.[13] Apert's syndrome and Crouzon's syndrome

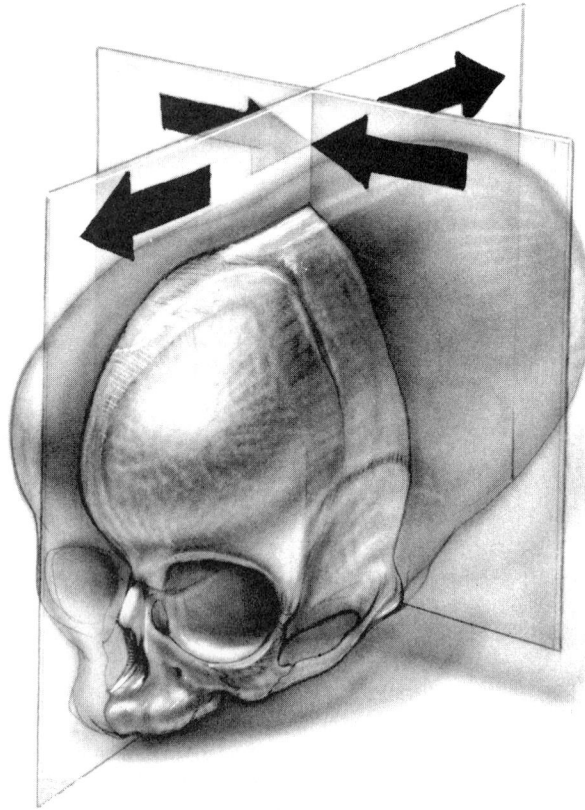

FIGURE 210–1. Schematic illustration of a child's skull with sagittal synostosis in which growth is restricted in a plane perpendicular to the fused suture and elongated in a plane parallel to that fused suture. (From Persing JA, Jane JA, Edgerton MT: Surgical treatment of craniosynostosis. In Persing JA, Jane JA, Edgerton MT [eds]: Scientific Foundations and Surgical Treatment of Craniosynostosis. Baltimore, Williams & Wilkins, 1989, p 118.)

appear to be linked with mutations in the FGF receptor-2 mutations, whereas Pfeiffer's syndrome appears to be linked with mutations on the FGF receptor-1 and receptor-2.[14, 15] Despite the heterogeneity of the presenting features of these syndromes, it appears the variability and presentation can be linked to these mutations.

Surgical treatment of craniosynostosis began with Lane (1892) and Lannelongue (1890).[16, 17] Both performed strip craniectomies for fused sutures in young infants. Such procedures had some temporary popularity but did not gain widespread interest due to operative procedures on misdiagnosed children. Of equal importance was the work of Rene Le Fort in his investigational work of facial fractures. Published in 1901 in the *Revue de Chirurgie*, his work elucidated the "three great lines of weakness" of the facial skeleton, lines along which the facial bones routinely break after trauma (Le Fort I, II, and III).[18] The first midfacial osteotomy to correct the facial deformities associated with syndromic craniosynostosis was reported by Gillies in 1950.[19] The published photographs and operative diagrams detail a subcranial Le Fort III osteotomy and midfacial advancement for probable Crouzon's syndrome. In 1964, Paul Tessier and Gerard Guiot,[20] with

knowledge of Gillies' and Le Fort's work, performed the first transcranial hypertelorism correction. This work ushered in the modern era of craniofacial surgery.

Tessier's recommendations include the use of wide exposure, the intracranial approach to correcting some forms of facial deformity, the liberal and exclusive use of autogenous bone grafting, and reliance on rigid bony fixation. Subsequent developments have included three-dimensional radiographic visualization and precise computer-guided modeling. Improved pediatric anesthesia, critical care, and monitoring have contributed to overall decreases in morbidity and mortality. Rigid microfixation and the development of resorbable plates and screws and bone substitutes have also greatly improved the efficacy of the surgical armamentarium. Development of the techniques of distraction osteogenesis applied to the cranial vault and the facial skeleton have radically altered and expanded surgical options for correction of these deformities.

PREOPERATIVE CONSIDERATIONS

Evaluation

The neurosurgeon or craniofacial surgeon who wishes to undertake care of this group of patients benefits from a multidisciplinary team approach. History-taking and delineation of the family history are essential features that may confirm diagnosis before determination of need for intervention. Genetic testing and counseling is highly desirable in confirming the diagnosis and assisting the patient and family to understand the full spectrum of associated current and future problems. Neuropsychological evaluation also is important to discern the adequacy of acquisition of developmental milestones. The neurological evaluation is instrumental in determining the possible role of increased intracranial pressure (i.e., anorexia, lethargy, or visual changes) among other complicating factors. A careful history of respiratory problems should be taken. In patients with significant midfacial retrusion, airway compromise and the presence of sleep apnea should be evaluated. Pulmonary and otolaryngologic evaluation may include fiberoptic laryngoscopy and sleep studies. Early intervention in such infants may include continuous positive airway pressure. In selected patients, tracheostomy may be required.

We have found that a sensitive and supportive psychological therapist may provide significant benefits to the patient and family. Additional evaluations by the orthodontist, otolaryngologist, and ophthalmologist are critical in patients with syndromic craniosynostosis. For patients undergoing extensive reconstruction, it is important to have the patient evaluated by the anesthesiologist and pediatric intensivists to anticipate potential complicating factors. Special attention and discussion should center on the best use of blood replacement products. Autologous blood products, if feasible, are preferred.

Physical examination should include assessment of suture ridging, evidence of sutural patency by manual palpation, skull defects, overall and regional descriptions of skull and facial configuration, fullness and patency of the anterior and posterior fontanelles, and an age-appropriate neurological examination. Definition of the position of the medial and lateral canthi and the presence of exophthalmos, orbital dystopia, or upper lid ptosis are desirable in making the diagnosis.

Visual acuity, diplopia, and papilledema are assessed by an ophthalmologist. Occlusal relationship and dental development are appropriately assessed by the orthodontist. For patients in the appropriate age range, cephalometric studies and dental models are very useful. Preoperative and postoperative photographs are required to document progress through all phases of treatment.

Radiographic Assessment

Although a wide variety of radiographic examinations may be useful, plain film radiographs (anteroposterior and lateral skull) may document "sclerosis," or closure of additional sutures, and possible widening of adjacent, compensating sutures. Lateral cephalometric radiographs and orthopantographic (Panorex) radiographs are frequently taken to document the occlusal and facial relationships. Computed tomography (CT) of the cranial vault, base, and facial structures through the mandible is a routine evaluation. Three-dimensional reconstruction of the cranium, orbits, and face is particularly useful in demonstrating the general volume relationships and overall shape of the underlying bony structures (Fig. 210–2). Refinements in computer-aided design are likely to be of additional benefit in the future for patients requiring primary or secondary correction. Computer-generated models can be manufactured and milled from three-dimensional CT data

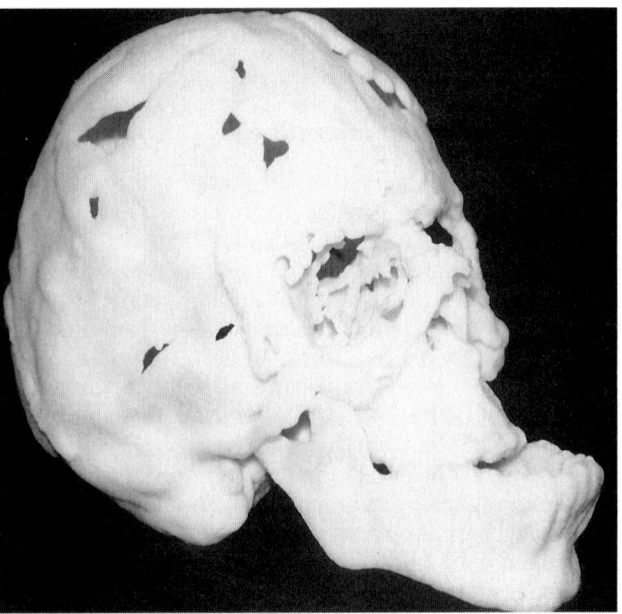

FIGURE 210–3. Computer-generated model of the skull and facial bones of a patient with Pfeiffer's syndrome.

and used preoperatively to assist in planning osteotomies (Fig. 210–3). Magnetic resonance imaging has limited applicability in the treatment of syndromic craniosynostosis, with the exception of ruling out suspected cases of tonsillar herniation in cases of Arnold-Chiari malformation.

Because we frequently use the modified prone position for optimal whole-vault exposure at the time of surgery, cervical spine radiographs are taken to exclude the presence of craniovertebral anomalies or instability that may lead to spinal cord or brainstem injury.[21]

Timing of Operation

In general, timing of the operation and the extent of possible correction depend in part on the age at presentation of the patient. Previous experimental and clinical data have demonstrated that surgical intervention performed in children at earlier ages may be associated with a better outcome in intelligence and subsequent markers for mental development, including IQ scores.[22]

Secondary corrections, generally with the exception of a planned reoperation, should not be performed until approximately 1 year to 18 months after the primary procedure. The rationale for such delay is to ensure that any correction be more stable and lasting. However, this is not always feasible, and for some patients, there may be some necessity in performing earlier reoperations. In such cases, we use a variety of techniques that are tailored to the unique, age-specific demands of the correction.[23] Techniques used for the older child, in whom skull growth has ceased and in whom the surgeon wishes to produce rigid and secure fixation restricting growth of the skull, may be counterproductive and potentially harmful in the younger child with further brain growth. Translocation of the fixation devices placed on the external skull in early

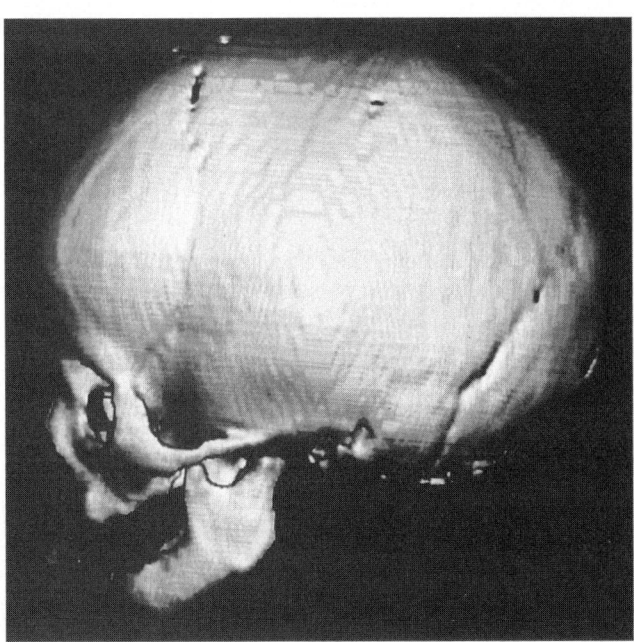

FIGURE 210–2. Three-dimensional computed tomographic scan of a patient with craniosynostosis.

infancy may result in the fixation hardwave migrating to the internal aspect of the skull.[24]

Psychological Considerations

Psychological evaluation of the patient and family is an important feature in the treatment of a child born with congenital anomaly. During birth and infancy, major stress is conferred on the parents, who are essentially mourning the loss of an anticipated healthy infant. Stages of parental reaction follow and may include shock, denial, sadness, anger, adaptation, and reorganization. Early counseling of parents during the first months of life is therefore critical to parental attachment and bonding with the child. Preoperative management should include thorough discussions with the family regarding surgery, in which realistic expectations of surgery are conveyed.

The sense of body image generally does not fully develop until the age of 4 to 5 years. This is a consideration in the timing of surgery; experience indicates that adaptation to physical changes is favorable at age 4. Physical properties of the bone, however, may argue for a later optimal date for surgery to achieve the best morphologic result. Decision making related to reoperative surgery relies on support from the family and physician, because they can assist the child in the coping process, which may expand the window of optimal timing for surgery.

SYNDROMES

Crouzon's Syndrome

Crouzon's syndrome is the most common of the craniofacial malformation syndromes associated with craniosynostosis. Originally described in 1912 by Crouzon, this syndrome is associated with bilateral coronal synostosis, midfacial retrusion, severe proptosis, and external strabismus (Fig. 210–4).[25] Additional forms of craniosynostosis leading to scaphocephaly and cloverleaf skull (i.e., kleeblattschädel) have been seen. Cranial base and maxillary synchondroses also account for the severe maxillary and midface hypoplasia resulting in characteristic features, such as severe proptosis and upper airway obstruction. It has an incidence of 1 case in 25,000 births and is transmitted in an autosomal-dominant pattern, although as many as one third of cases arise de novo. Molecular genetic testing has localized this syndrome to a mutation in the *FGFR2* gene, with a sensitivity of more than 50%.[13] Unlike the other FGFR-related syndromes, there are generally no associated limb abnormalities. Neurological manifestations may include hydrocephalus (approximately 30%), cervical spine abnormalities, and Chiari malformations, although their manifestations vary. Developmental delay is generally uncommon, and intelligence is often normal in these patients. Secondary facial deformities may result from the associated maxillary hypoplasia and may include mandibular hypoplasia, retrogenia,

and a class III malocclusion with pseudoprognathism. Airway concerns are paramount in this group because many are obligate oral breathers and have associated glossoptosis, choanal atresia, and sleep apnea. In more severe cases, tracheostomy may be required early in life. In some cases, severe proptosis may result in corneal exposure keratopathy and ulceration and hence temporary tarsorrhaphy and early management of exposure may be required. Approximately 5% of patients have associated acanthosis nigricans, which is associated specifically with a mutation in *FGFR3*.[13]

Apert's Syndrome

Apert's syndrome is characterized by bilateral coronal craniosynostosis with turribrachycephaly (other forms of craniosynostosis may be present as well), anterior cranial base synostosis, and maxillary synchondroses with severe midface hypoplasia (Fig. 210–5). Soft tissue and bony syndactyly of both hands (i.e., mitten hands) and feet (Fig. 210–6) may be seen, as well as ankylosis of elbows, hips, and knees. As with Crouzon's syndrome, secondary facial abnormalities develop, characteristically leading to a classic appearance with severe proptosis with hypertelorism, eyelid ptosis, beaked nose, and downward-slanting palpebral fissures. This syndrome was originally described by Wheaton in 1894 and later by Apert in 1906.[26, 27] The incidence of Apert's syndrome is approximately 1 in 100,000 births, and it has autosomal-dominant transmission, although, like Crouzon's syndrome, it also occurs sporadically. Molecular diagnosis can be confirmed genetically by a mutation in *FGFR2* with greater than 98% sensitivity.[13, 14] Neurological features of this syndrome also may include hydrocephalus (uncommon [2%]), Chiari malformation, and fused cervical vertebrae (C5, C6). Developmental delay is common, with mental retardation seen in 50% to 85% of patients. Secondary malformation includes pseudoprognathism, retrogenia, high-arched palate, cleft palate, class III malocclusion, and a large skeletal open-bite deformity with severe maxillary dental crowding. Hearing abnormalities, strabismus, and severe acne are often seen.

Pfeiffer's Syndrome

Pfeiffer's syndrome is heterogeneous in its presentation. Like Apert's syndrome, it is characterized by craniosynostosis and limb abnormalities. Originally described by Pfeiffer in 1964,[28] the syndrome was subsequently classified as types 1, 2, and 3. All types are associated with *FGFR1* and *FGFR2* mutations, and molecular genetic diagnosis is highly sensitive.[13, 15] The mode of inheritance is autosomal-dominant with complete penetrance. Expression can be variable and appears to be linked to subtype. In patients with Pfeiffer's syndrome type 1, bilateral coronal synostosis with associated turribrachycephaly is common. There is moderate-to-severe midface hypoplasia with associated proptosis and hypertelorism. Hydrocephalus is common, as is strabismus and hearing loss. Severe malocclusion (class III), retrogenia, and pseudoprognathism

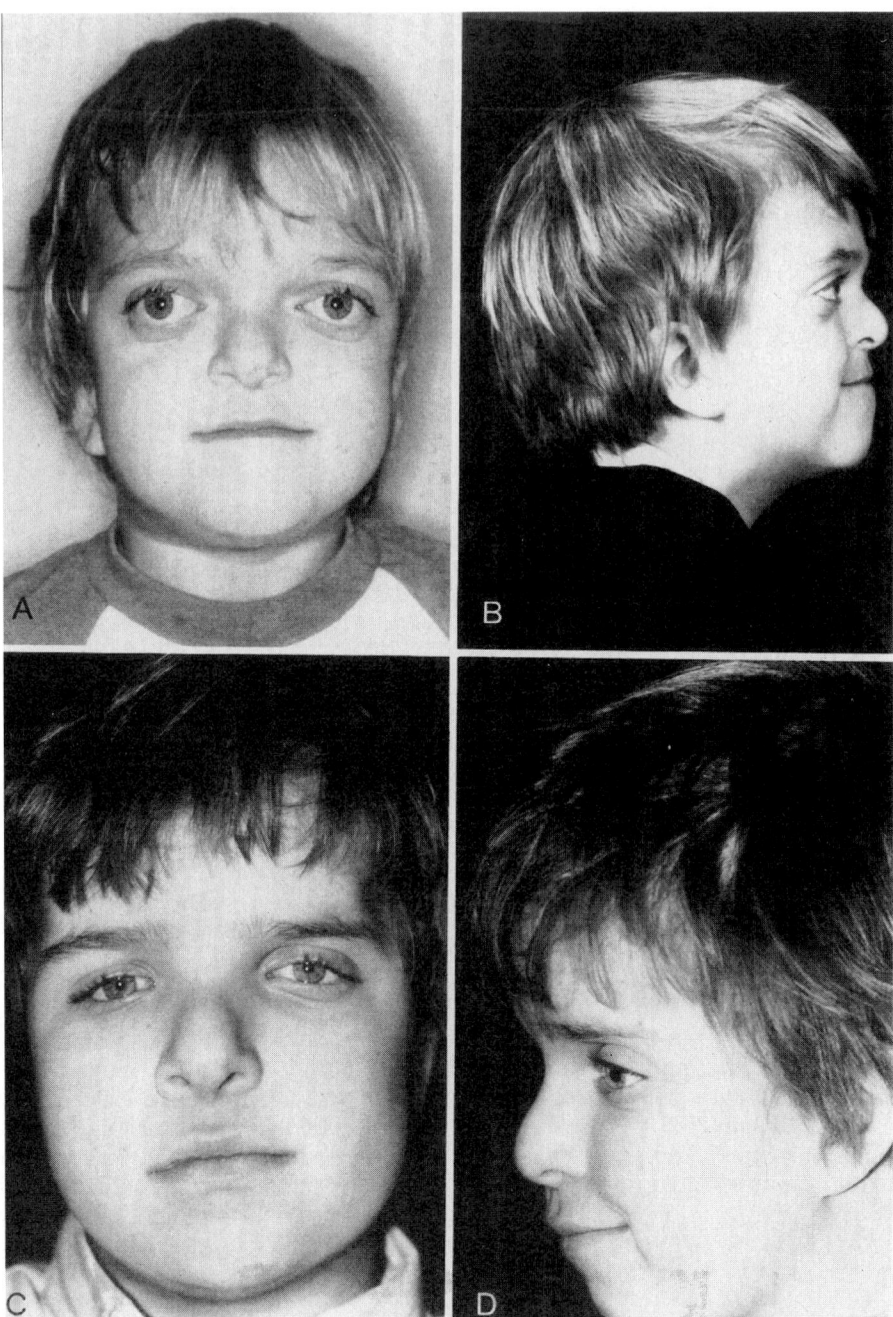

FIGURE 210–4. Photographs of a patient with Crouzon's syndrome. *A,* Preoperative anteroposterior view. *B,* Preoperative lateral view. *C,* Postoperative anteroposterior view. *D,* Postoperative lateral view. (From Persing JA, Jane JA, Edgerton MT: Surgical treatment of craniosynostosis. In Persing JA, Jane JA, Edgerton MT [eds]: Scientific Foundations and Surgical Treatment of Craniosynostosis. Baltimore, Williams & Wilkins, 1989, p 118.)

are also seen (Fig. 210–7). Broad and radially deviated thumbs and great toes, as well as complete or partial ankylosis of the shoulder, hip, knees, and elbows, are hallmarks of the axial skeletal malformations. Cervical and lumbar vertebrae may be fused. In patients with type 1 Pfeiffer's syndrome, development may be normal and the prognosis generally better than that in types 2 and 3.

Patients with Pfeiffer's syndrome type 2 and 3 appear to have a more severe expression of the phenotype. The skeletal abnormalities are similar to those of type 1 and include radially deviated thumbs and great toes and various forms of ankylosis, and the craniofacial abnormalities generally are more severe. Type 2 is

characterized by a cloverleaf skull, whereas type 3 is associated with a turribrachycephaly. Extreme midface hypoplasia and its attendant sequelae, such as severe proptosis and hypertelorism, are seen in all three subtypes. Types 2 and 3 are associated with choanal atresia or stenosis, laryngotracheal abnormalities, hydrocephalus, and seizures. Long-term prognosis for subtypes 2 and 3 is generally worse, and there is an increased risk for early death.

Saethre-Chotzen Syndrome

The Saethre-Chotzen syndrome was first reported by Saethre in 1931 and Chotzen in 1932.[29, 30] It is character-

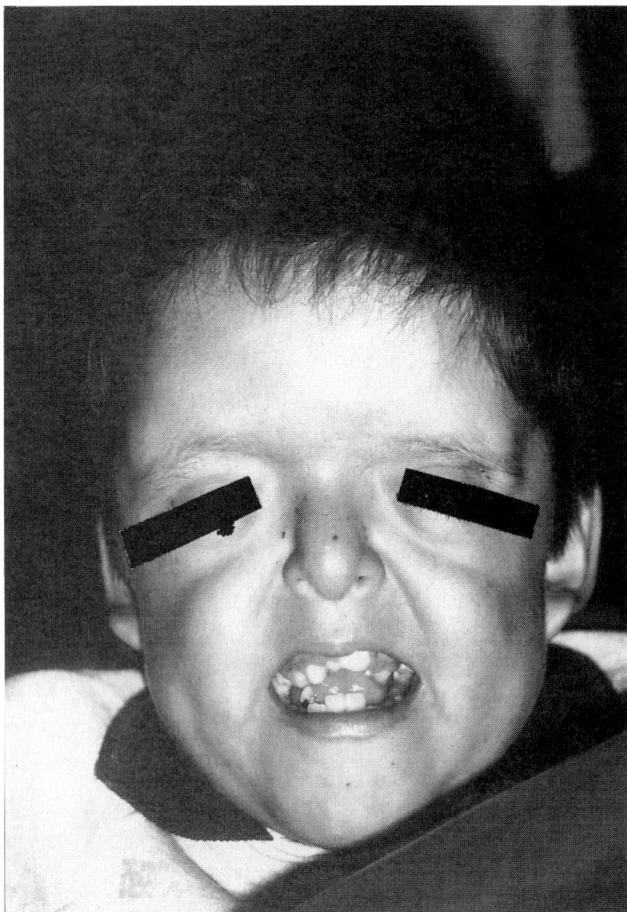

FIGURE 210–5. Patient with Apert's syndrome.

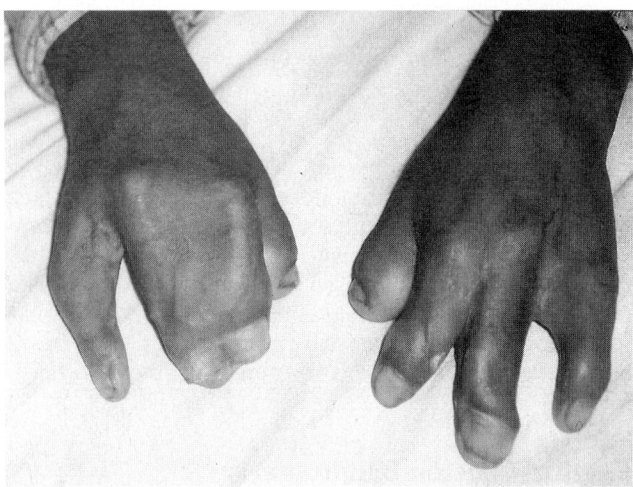

FIGURE 210–6. Hand syndactyly in a patient with Apert's syndrome.

ized by craniosynostosis and limb abnormalities similar to the FGFR family of syndromes but appears to be associated with a mutation in a separate and distinct gene, *TWIST*, in 75% of patients with the Saethre-Chotzen syndrome.[13] The autosomal-dominant inheritance pattern is associated with complete penetrance and

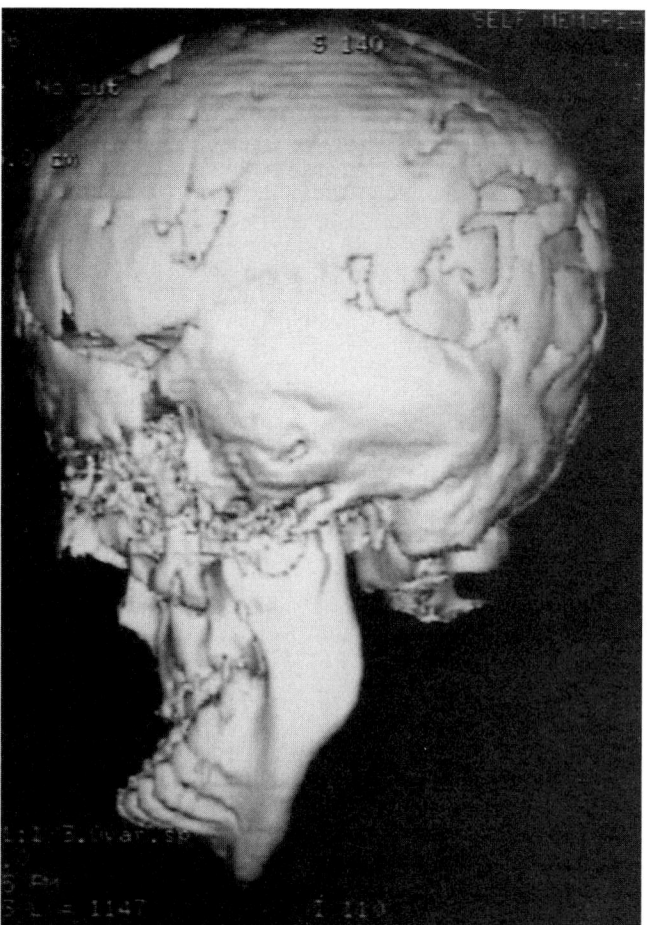

FIGURE 210–7. Three-dimensional computed tomographic scan of a patient with Pfeiffer's syndrome demonstrates severe malocclusion (class III) and midface hypoplasia.

variable expressivity. Despite the difference in genotype, the phenotypic expression is similar to patients with *FGFR* gene mutations. Features include coronal synostosis that in many instances is unilateral, leading to plagiocephaly. Turribrachycephaly may also be seen. A distinct but common feature is the presence of a low-set frontal hairline; long, prominent ear crura; and facial asymmetry. Hypertelorism, proptosis, strabismus, and beaked nose are characteristic sequelae of midfacial hypoplasia and restriction in the anterior cranial base. Associated limb abnormalities include broad and laterally deviated thumbs and great toes, brachydactyly, and partial cutaneous syndactyly of the index and middle fingers and the third and fourth toes. Mild-to-moderate developmental delay and hearing loss are associated with this syndrome.

Carpenter's Syndrome

Carpenter's syndrome is characterized by variable forms of craniosynostosis (i.e., sagittal and lambdoid), polysyndactyly of the feet, brachydactyly and clinodactyly, and various soft tissue syndactyly. The patients may often be short and obese. Associated cardiac abnormalities include ventricular or atrial septal defect, tetralogy of Fallot, pulmonary stenosis, transposition of the great vessels, and patent ductus arteriosus. This syndrome was first identified by Carpenter in 1901.[31] Unlike the FGFR family of syndromes or Saethre-Chotzen, Carpenter's syndrome has yet to be characterized to a specific gene locus. Its mode of transmission is autosomal-recessive, and it is considerably more uncommon than the previously described syndromes. Patients generally have significant developmental and cognitive delays. Early neurosurgical intervention may be beneficial in these patients, especially those with pansynostosis.

A variety of other uncommon syndromes exist that have craniosynostosis as an associated manifestation. Others in which there are FGFR-related abnormalities include Jackson-Weiss and Beare-Stevenson syndromes, which are extremely uncommon.[13] Boston-type craniosynostosis is a syndrome associated with craniosynostosis and limb abnormalities, and it appears to be linked to a mutation in the *MSX2* gene.[32] With heterogeneity of the genotype and phenotypic manifestations, there remains much flexibility in the timing and sequence of operative intervention, as well as a variety of newer modalities for treating the previously described conditions.

SURGICAL APPROACHES AND TREATMENTS

For the infant diagnosed with a craniofacial dysostosis malformation such as Crouzon's, Apert's, or Pfeiffer's syndrome, treatment options are usually planned as elective procedures that will require a number of procedures over the years of skeletal growth. Team management is beneficial in planning multiple surgeries staged to take advantage of ongoing morphologic development and the growth of the brain as an adjunct to surgical remodeling. Urgent conditions, however, may necessitate earlier intervention such as tracheostomy for airway management, tarrsorhaphy for exposure keratopathy and corneal ulceration, and ventricular shunting or urgent surgical decompression in patients with multiple suture closures and papilledema. There are numerous options in the treatment of children with syndromic craniosynostosis. We present a series of techniques that are useful in dealing with the various presentations and specific conditions common to this group of patients.

In the child with syndromic craniofacial dysostosis, bilateral coronal synostosis is the most commonly seen of the craniosynostoses. Variations may occur, but the resultant deformity usually yields classic turribrachycephaly. A similar approach is taken for most children with such syndromes. In these patients, factors such as the development of hydrocephalus and cervical spine abnormalities must be taken into account when deciding to proceed with surgery and may require special treatment such as ventriculoperitoneal shunting, modification of skull height reduction, or modification of the operative position because of the cervical spine abnormalities. These abnormalities may preclude the

use of the modified prone position for whole-vault cranioplasty, and in such cases, a two-stage procedure may be required.

Bilateral Coronal Synostosis

Bilateral coronal synostosis is characterized by ridging of the coronal suture, flattening of the caudal portion of the frontal bones and supraorbital ridges, and bulging of the cephalad portion of the frontal bones. The occiput is flattened, and the squamous portion of the temporal bones is unusually prominent. The vertex of the skull is more anteriorly situated than normal. Radiographically, bilateral harlequin abnormalities are present in the orbits, and basal CT demonstrates shortened anterior cranial fossae and bilaterally narrowed sphenopetrosal angles.

OPERATIVE TECHNIQUE IN CHILDREN YOUNGER THAN 1 YEAR OF AGE

Because the abnormalities of coronal synostosis are situated anteriorly and posteriorly within the skull, a different approach to intraoperative patient positioning is elected. The modified prone position, in which the anterior and posterior portions of the skull are exposed simultaneously, has proved optimal; however, to use this position, certain precautions should be taken. The presence of craniovertebral anomalies and the stability of the patient who may be at risk for neurological injury should be assessed. If anomalies such as the Arnold-Chiari malformation and instability of the cervical spine are identified, a two-stage approach with the patient alternately in a supine and then a prone position should be elected.

If no vertebral abnormalities exist, the patient's head is placed on a well-padded chin support (usually the combination of a beanbag and a well-cushioned anterior portion of a Philadelphia collar for stabilization) (Fig. 210–8). A coronal incision is performed, and anterior and posterior supraperiosteal dissection is done. The posterior limit is the foramen magnum, and the anterior limit is the lateral portion of the orbital rims at the level of the frontal zygomatic suture bilaterally. Frontal and parieto-occipital bone grafts are elevated, leaving bone over the vertex of the skull and two lateral struts of bone extending from the vertex to the base of the skull. Subperiosteal dissection is performed posteriorly in the occiput. Barrel stave osteotomies are performed in the occipital region, with the individual bone segments fractured posteriorly to increase the potential space in the posterior skull later in surgery for the repositioned brain and dural envelope (Fig. 210–9). The superior orbital rims are elevated bilaterally to the level of the frontal zygomatic suture, contoured, and fixed in the advanced position. The squamous portion of the temporal bone is elevated with the overlying temporalis muscle and advanced and attached to the superior orbital rims. The more basal temporal bone undergoes osteotomy and infracture to reduce the abnormal convexity in the region. Frequently, an intracranial pressure monitor is placed in

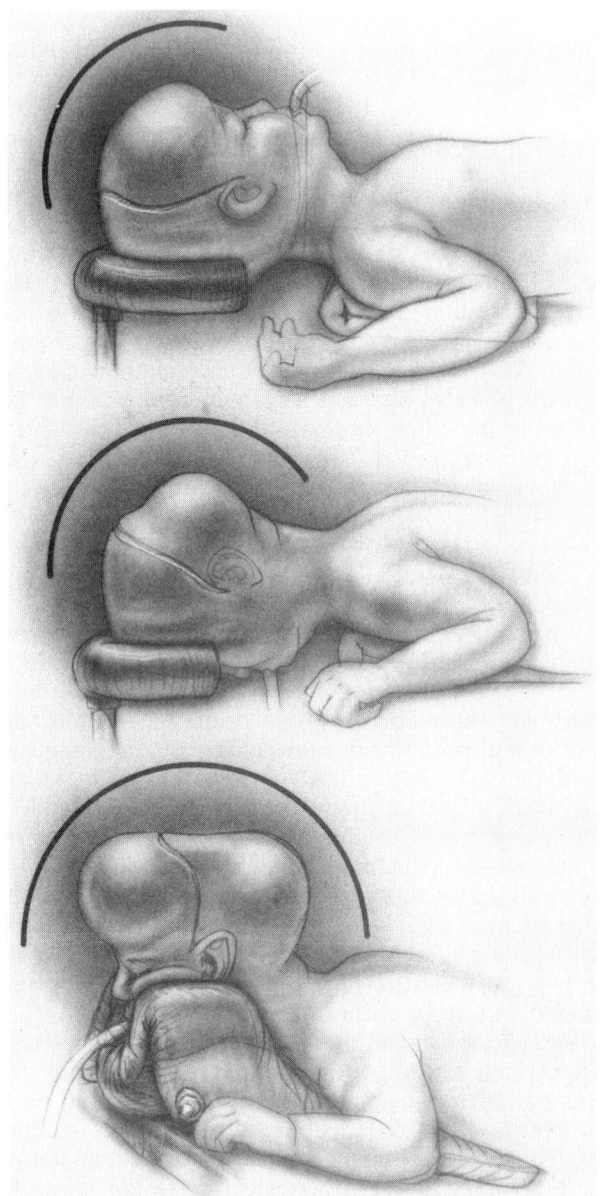

FIGURE 210–8. Schematic illustrations of various operative positions for surgery: supine on a padded "horseshoe" headrest *(top)*; prone on a padded headrest allowing access to the posterior half of the skull *(middle)*; and a modified prone position, with chin support in a padded beanbag to allow simultaneous access to the front and back of the skull *(bottom)*. (From Persing JA, Jane JA, Edgerton MT: Surgical Treatment of Craniosynostosis. In Persing JA, Jane JA, Edgerton MT [eds] Scientific Foundations and Surgical Treatment of Craniosynostosis. Baltimore, Williams & Wilkins, 1989, p 134.)

the right parietal bone, off the midline. The struts extending from the vertex of the skull in the parietal region to the basal temporal region are then divided, shifted posteriorly, and reduced in height (usually 1.0 to 1.5 cm) to change the position of the vertex of the skull, flatten the frontal contour, and reduce the height of the skull (Fig. 210–10).

Height reduction corrects the abnormal turret shape of the skull and encourages brain and dural shift to fill the space created in the occiput. This achieves the

desired elongation of the anteroposterior axis of the skull. Reduction in the height of the skull is achieved slowly, monitoring intracranial pressure under the conditions of normotension and normocapnia. Intracranial pressure should only be increased for brief periods, followed by rapid reduction to normal tension as the height of the skull is reduced.

The bifrontal bone graft undergoes radial osteotomy, reshaping to the desired effect and attachment to the superior orbital rim; however, the frontal bone is not attached to the anterior parietal region. A neocoronal suture bone defect approximately 1 cm wide is created at the site of the normal coronal suture. The posterior occipital bone is reshaped to achieve greater convexity, and a defect of approximately 1 cm is created between the reshaped bone graft and surrounding bone to allow for preferential expansion of the parieto-occipital region.

OPERATIVE TECHNIQUE IN CHILDREN OLDER THAN 3 YEARS OF AGE

In a child older than 3 years of age, a zigzag coronal incision and supraperiosteal dissection plane is carried out, similar to the technique used for the younger child. After elevation of the bifrontal and parietal occipital bone grafts, barrel stave osteotomies are performed in the occipital region. The orbital rims are elevated and advanced as a unit extending into the frontal process of the zygoma. The squamous temporal bone and temporalis muscle are elevated as a composite and advanced to attach to the posterior border of the advanced orbital rim. The height of the skull is again reduced, and the intracranial pressure may need to be monitored as in the younger child; however, patients older than 3 years of age may require a much more prolonged period of accommodation than the younger child, and less height reduction is ordinarily achieved. Correction of more than 1 cm is unusual in the child older than 3 years of age, whereas 1.0 to 1.5 cm of correction is quite common in a child younger than 1 year of age. The bifrontal and parietal occipital bone grafts are then remodeled by dividing the bone segments into vertical slats, weakened on the endocranial surface by kerfs and then reshaped with bone-molding instruments and microfracture (Fig. 210–11). Individual bone slats are reapproximated frontally to the superior orbital rim and proceed posteriorly to the occiput.

Hypertelorism

The operative correction of orbital hypertelorism and congenitally acquired hypercanthorum is usually performed between 5 and 6 years of age. Before age 5, craniofacial bones are thin and fragile, making surgical correction difficult. Surgery of the orbit during infancy may impair midface growth. For these reasons, operative manipulation of the orbits is not performed until the child is between 5 and 6 years of age, unless there are extenuating circumstances such as a large frontoethmoid encephalocele or dermoid tumor. Even un-

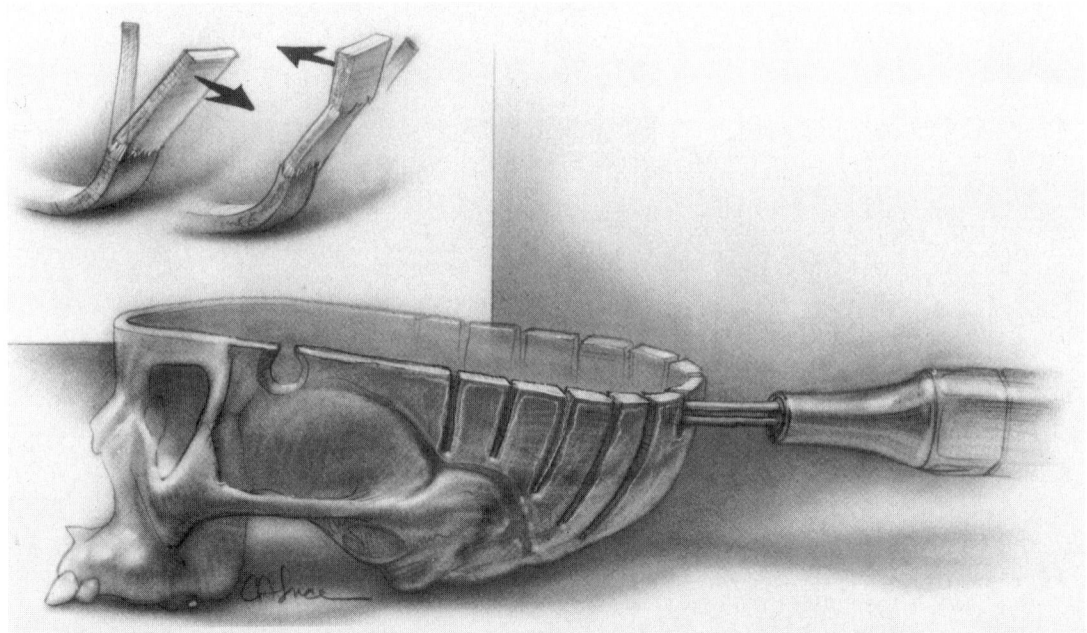

FIGURE 210–9. The schematic drawing demonstrates posterior barrel stave osteotomies that are used to increase bone projection locally. (Adapted from Persing JA, Jane JA, Edgerton MT: Surgical treatment of craniosynostosis. In Persing JA, Jane JA, Edgerton MT [eds]: Scientific Foundations and Surgical Treatment of Craniosynostosis. Baltimore, Williams & Wilkins, 1989, p 146.)

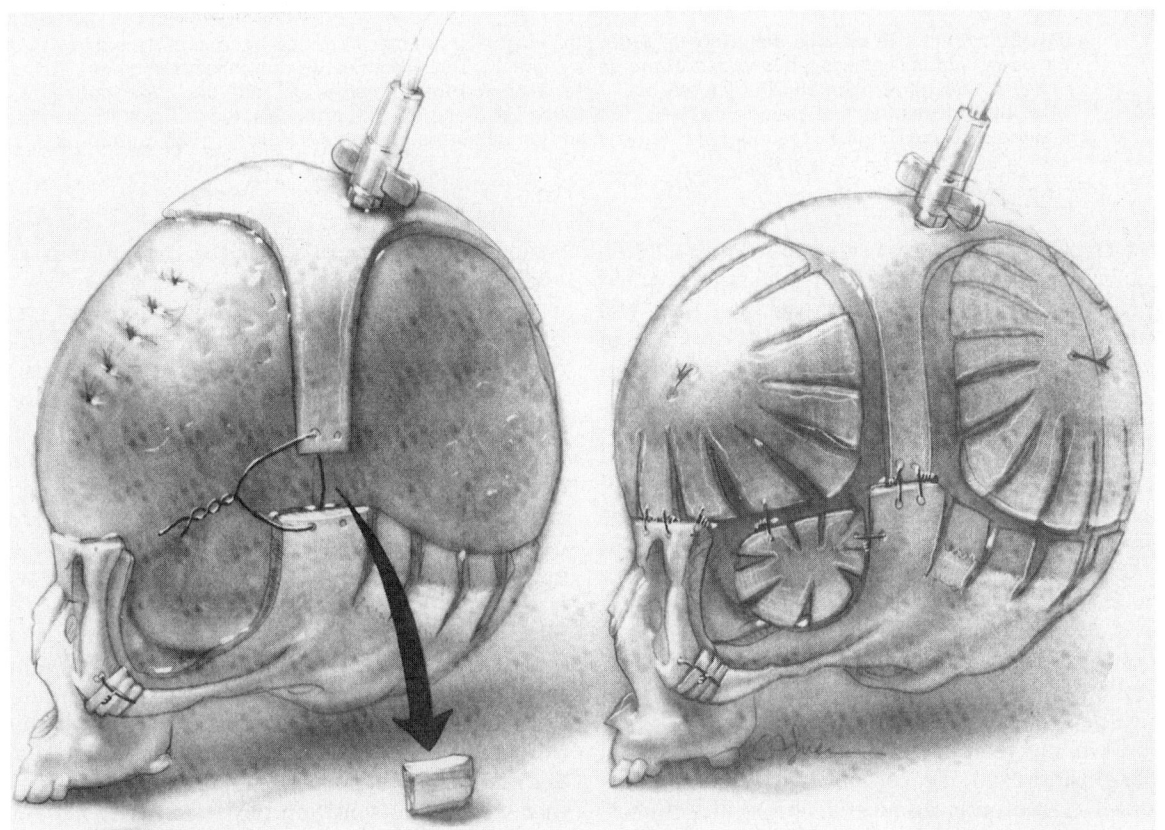

FIGURE 210–10. The height of the skull is reduced by removing a segment of parietal bone at the inferior portion of the parietal strut. The basal and parietal segments are cinched together while monitoring the intracranial pressure. (From Persing JA, Jane JA, Edgerton MT: Surgical treatment of craniosynostosis. In Persing JA, Jane JA, Edgerton MT [eds]: Scientific Foundations and Surgical Treatment of Craniosynostosis. Baltimore, William & Wilkins, 1989, p 183.)

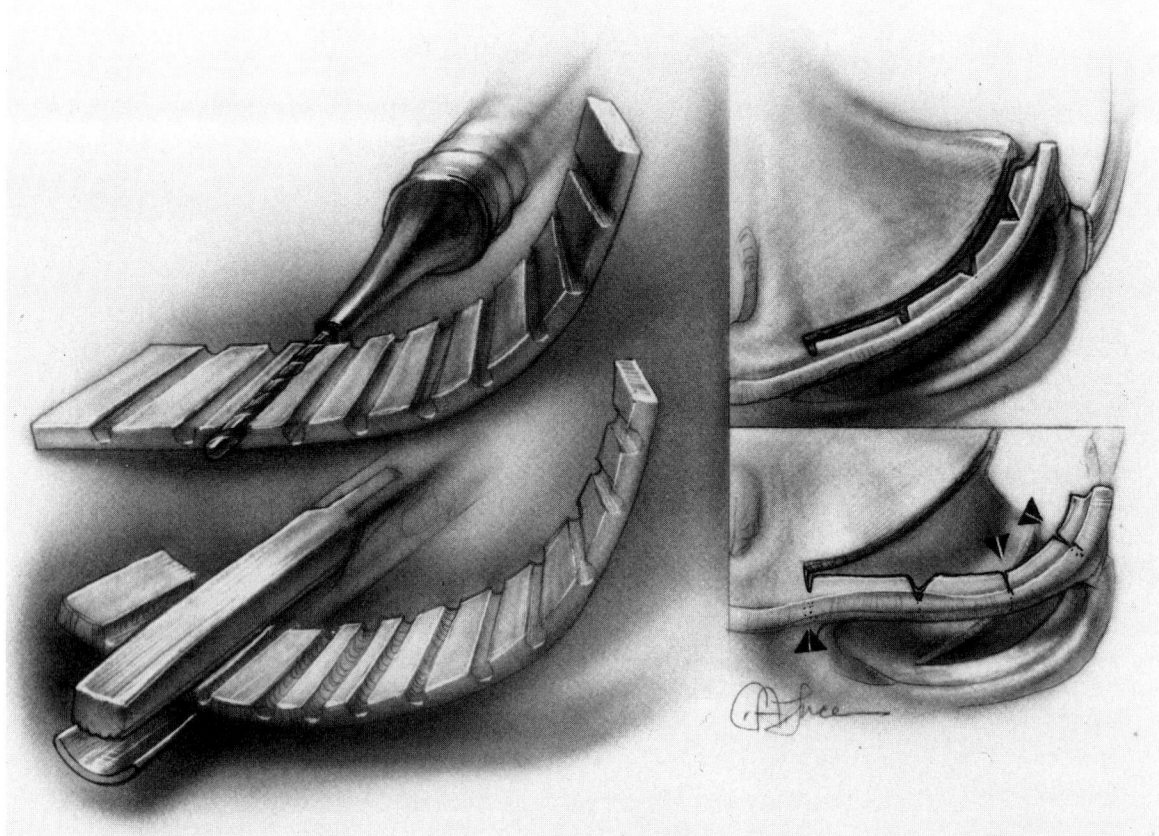

FIGURE 210–11. To reshape mature bone, kerfs (i.e., channels) are placed on the internal surface of the bone perpendicular to the long axis of the bone segment. This allows convex or concave shaping of the cranial vault bone and the supraorbital rims. (Adapted from Persing JA, Jane JA, Edgerton MT: Surgical treatment of craniosynostosis. In Persing JA, Jane JA, Edgerton MT [eds]: Scientific Foundations and Surgical Treatment of Craniosynostosis. Baltimore, Williams & Wilkins, 1989, p 145.)

der these circumstances, a two-stage procedure is often planned, in which reduction of the lesion is performed during infancy and orbitoplasty is delayed until the patient is approximately 5 to 6 years old. Correction at this age also addresses the psychosocial issues important in the child's early school-age years.

The operation begins with insertion of a cerebrospinal drain into the lumbar cistern. The rationale is that the drain allows reduction of cerebrospinal fluid (CSF) pressure, thereby reducing resistance to frontal lobe retraction required during the operative procedure. In certain circumstances, intravenous agents such as mannitol or furosemide (Lasix) may be used instead of lumbar cistern drainage. The patient is then placed supine on a horseshoe-shaped headrest. A coronal incision is followed by subperiosteal dissection of the anterior scalp flap. Bilateral bur holes in the lateral frontal region above the temporal crest and one parasagittal bur hole posterior to the coronal suture are placed. A bifrontal craniotomy, excluding temporalis muscle elevation, is performed. Osteotomies performed in the supraorbital bar are 1 cm wide at the level of the orbital rim apex. This supraorbital bar is then transversely bisected, except at the nasal midline, before orbital translocation. This approach results in formation of a 5-mm-wide supraorbital bar for fixation and a 5-mm-wide orbital rim superiorly.

After CSF drainage, the frontal lobes are gently retracted to allow an osteotomy in the orbital roof that extends posterior to the midpoint of the globe's anteroposterior axis. In a similar fashion, the anterior tip of the temporal lobe is carefully retracted, allowing a lateral orbital wall osteotomy posterior to the midpoint of the anteroposterior axis of the globe. The lateral cribriform plate is the medial limit of the roof osteotomy to avoid injury to the olfactory nerve fibers. However, the cribriform plate is characteristically widened and typically obstructs medial translocation of the orbital rim. The anterior olfactory fibers are usually divided, followed by oversewing of the proximal segments of the nerve fibers and the surrounding dura. This step is performed to prevent postoperative CSF rhinorrhea. The latter portions of the ethmoid air cells are removed using a rongeur to provide room for further medial translocation of the orbit.

The medial orbit osteotomy is performed using the sagittal or oscillating saw to avoid uncontrolled fracture of the nasal and lacrimal bones. If the nasal profile is acceptable, a 3-mm segment of midline bone may be left as the nasal bridge. Paramedian resection of excess bone responsible for the excess "medial width" is then resected. If the nasal profile is unacceptable, two approaches have been devised to address this defect. In the first, the midline bone is resected, and the medial orbital walls, when medially translocated, form a new nasal profile. In the second, more common case, a 2- to 3-mm midline segment of nasal bone is preserved as scaffolding for onlay bone graft augmentation of the nasal dorsum (Fig. 210–12).

Infraorbital dissection and osteotomy are performed thereafter. A lateral canthotomy, transconjunctival, or Caldwell-Luc incision may be necessary for adequate exposure. For the transconjunctival and lateral canthotomy approaches, preseptal dissection is performed for exposure of the inferior orbital rim. Horizontally oriented osteotomies are placed on the anterior maxillary wall at the level of the infraorbital foramen. The more cephalad osteotomy is performed to avoid injury to the developing tooth buds.

After the osteotomies are completed, the bony orbits are mobilized medially. The greatest resistance to movement is usually encountered in the deep nasomaxillary region. An osteotome is carefully used to "pry" the rim free from bony and soft tissue attachments. Great care must be taken during these maneuvers to avoid injury to the nasolacrimal duct. With medial translocation of the orbits, infolding of the nasal septal and upper lateral cartilages, as well as the nasal mucosa, usually occurs. This requires trimming of the excess tissue and subsequent closure of the mucosal openings to prevent air and bacterial contamination into the epidural space postoperatively. The medial orbital walls of nasal bone are trimmed with the air drill shaping bur such that the resulting distance between the bilateral dacryons measures approximately 10 mm or less. The nasal process of the maxilla at its medial inferior portion is aggressively contoured to avoid occlusion of the nasal airway during medial mobilization of the orbit. The orbital rims are placed in position but not secured at this point.

The medial canthi are assessed, and if they are positioned reasonably, the surgeon should dissect around the canthi, avoiding detachment from the dacryon to preserve optimal positioning and fixation postoperatively. However, the medial canthi may require repositioning. A transnasal medial canthopexy is performed

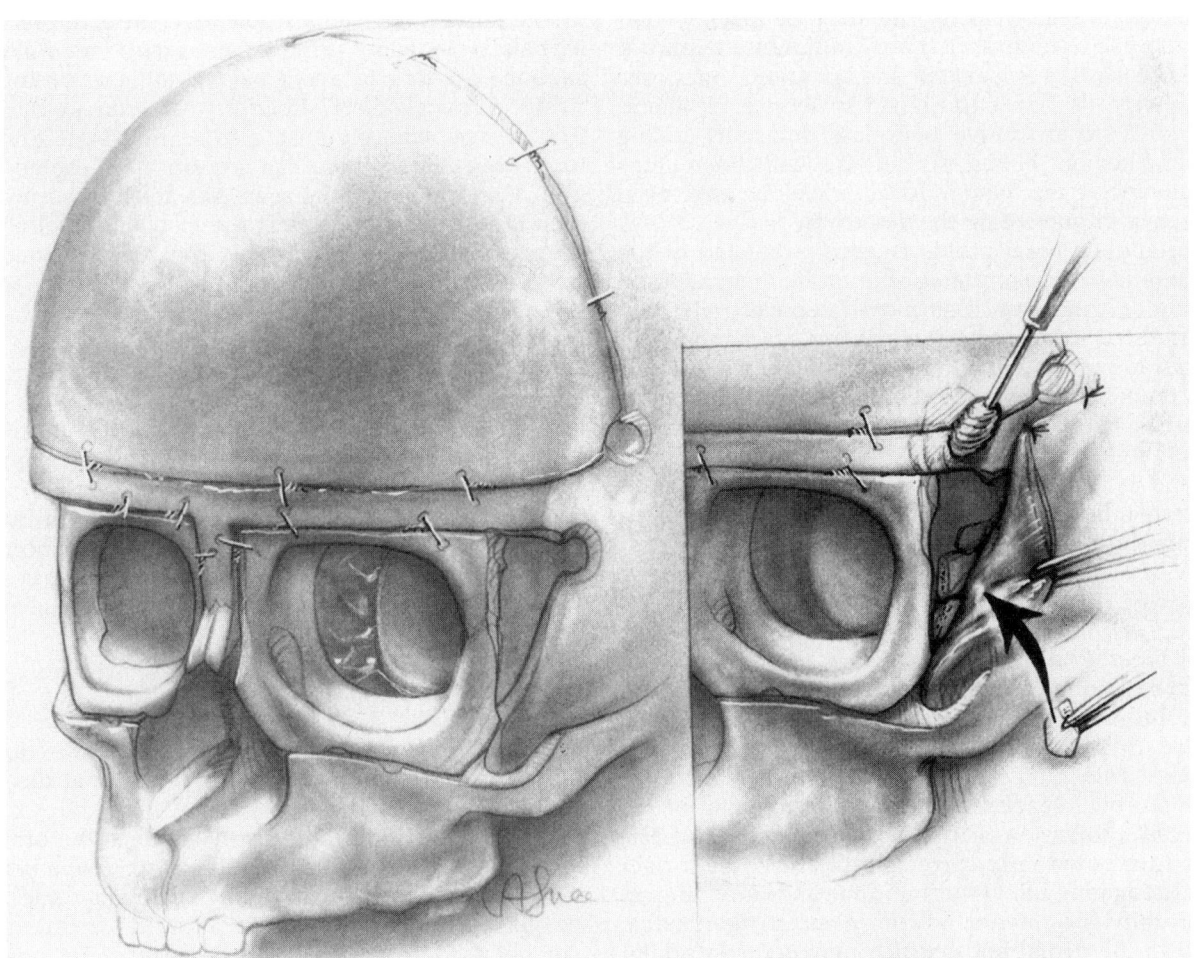

FIGURE 210–12. Telorbitism. The orbits are translocated medially. Bone grafts are inserted posterior to the orbital rim and positioned laterally for stability. (Adapted from Persing JA, Jane JA, Edgerton MT: Surgical treatment of craniosynostosis. In Persing JA, Jane JA, Edgerton MT [eds]: Scientific Foundations and Surgical Treatment of Craniosynostosis. Baltimore, Williams & Wilkins, 1989, p 219.)

before bony stabilization because of the greater exposure allowed by the mobile and easily separable bone fragments. An air drill is used to create an opening into the posterior superior lacrimal bone. The lacrimal bone, along with the rest of the medial orbital wall, is quite thin and prone to fracture with operative manipulation. If this occurs, a split calvarial bone graft from the parietal region is used to buttress the medial orbital wall. This effectively provides stabilization of the medial canthopexy and aids in preventing anterior and lateral migration of the canthus postoperatively. After this step is completed, the orbits are translocated medially and secured to each other and to the frontal supraorbital bar superiorly.

In patients with orbital hypertelorism, the lateral canthi frequently require repositioning. They are typically positioned at a level approximately 2 mm above the medial canthi. After translocation and fixation of the orbits, the lateral canthi are frequently attached to a point on the "internal" aspect of the zygomatic process of the frontal bone. However, if severe proptosis coexists, the lateral canthi are anchored to a point on the exterior surface of the eyelid. After lateral canthopexy, the temporal fossa is assessed. If, after translocation, there is a significant gap between the lateral orbit and temporal region (as is ordinarily the case), a composite muscle (temporalis) and squamous temporal myo-osseous flap is elevated and advanced anteriorly. This composite flap is designed to reduce the likelihood of a postoperative hourglass deformity in the temporal region. Filling in this area with bone chips and advancing the temporalis muscle alone have been ineffective in preventing the deformity.

The midline nasal profile is again evaluated. If the profile remains unacceptable after orbital medial translocation, a cantilever costochondral bone graft may be harvested to augment the existing nasal profile. In contrast to cortical membranous bone, a costochondral rib is the ideal graft material because the cartilaginous tip resists resorption quite well. Before closure, a pericranial or galeal flap is elevated from the anterior scalp flap and tacked over the ethmoid air cells on the anterior cranial base to decrease the potential for postoperative epidural infections.

Facial Bipartition

Facial bipartition may be applied to the correction of certain cases of congenital orbital hypertelorism. A single fronto-orbitomaxillary segment is created that is divided in the midline and mobilized medially and caudally. With medial rotation, there is narrowing of the interorbital space and effective lengthening of the "vertical" dimension of the paramedian maxilla. The procedure potentially corrects orbital hypertelorism while elongating the vertical midline and providing an opportunity for anterior advancement of the maxilla. Injury to the dental buds, which may occur in orbital translocation procedures that use transmaxillary osteotomies, may be prevented, particularly in patients with alveolar and palatal clefts in which the cuspid tooth buds are elevated. Facial bipartition may be indicated in cases of orbital hypertelorism resulting from midline, paramedian, and paranasal clefts and in certain cases of Apert's syndrome in which orbital hypertelorism is associated with palatal abnormalities, narrowed maxillary width, anterior open-bite deformity, and class III malocclusion.

The technique of facial bipartition involves the performance of osteotomies at the frontal, orbital, and pterygomaxillary levels. These osteotomy lines allow disimpaction of the "frontofacial" segment from the cranial base and pterygoid plates. Separation of the pterygoid process and maxillary tuberosity, as with the Le Fort III osteotomy, must be carefully performed to avoid injury to the molar buds. Midface vertical bony resection is then performed in a V-shaped manner at the midline and extended to the maxillary alveolar ridge. This results in the division of the frontofacial segment at its "midpoint," creating two "free" hemifacial segments. The segments can be mobilized medially, thereby correcting the orbital hypertelorism. With forward advancement and outward rotation of the segments at the palatal level, maxillary vertical lengthening and expansion are achieved, potentially leveling the occlusal plane in patients with an anterior open-bite deformity. If a cleft of the alveolus or palate exists preoperatively, the bipartition procedure is preceded by palatal widening using palatal expanders, followed by bone grafting to avoid palatal collapse postoperatively. A bone defect superiorly, as seen in cases of frontal encephalocele, may also require bone grafting to create a supraorbital bar necessary for orbital fixation. The two hemifacial segments are then secured to each other in the midline at the glabellar level and at the premaxillary level to achieve the desired correction.

Monobloc and Le Fort III Facial Advancement

After treatment of all the craniosynostosis associated with most of the previously described syndromes, midfacial osteotomies may be required to correct the midface hypoplasia that is seen with the associated conditions (i.e., Apert's, Crouzon's, or Pfeiffer's syndrome). Of the various procedures, the monobloc advancement and the Le Fort III procedures provide the necessary versatility in correcting the midface and orbital retrusion seen in these syndromes.

LE FORT III OSTEOTOMY

The Le Fort III procedure increases the projection of the midface medially at the nose, laterally at the inferior orbit, and inferiorly at the level of the occlusal arch in the maxilla. It effectively enlarges the orbit by advancing the orbital rim, decreasing globe prominence and proptosis. The timing of repair varies, but we generally perform the Le Fort III osteotomy in patients 4 to 5 years of age because of its positive psychological benefit. We recognize that the procedure may need to be performed later in life because the advanced midface does not always maintain commensurate growth in the postoperative period. The procedure may be required before this time, especially if exorbitism (particularly in patients with Crouzon's syndrome) results in corneal exposure or keratopathy. The Le Fort III procedure may be performed through subcranial or intracranial routes. Determination of the optimal route is based on the position of the cribriform plate, previous surgical procedures, and the need to advance the superolateral orbital rim to correct the frontal abnormalities.

If the subcranial route is elected, the patient is placed supine and intubated nasotracheally if possible. Tracheostomy or, if occlusion is less critical, oral intubation may be performed. Arch bars are applied to the teeth. An occlusal wafer constructed from preoperative dental models may be required postoperatively to secure fixation of the advanced maxilla.

A coronal incision is made, and subperiosteal dissection is carried out after orbital rim dissection is performed. Periorbital dissection is carried out posterior to the lacrimal system, and the medial canthus is left intact. If inferior osteotomies cannot be made from above, a transconjunctival inferior lid incision may be used to provide exposure of the orbital floor. Osteotomies are performed transversely through the nasal bone, caudal to the frontonasal suture, posterior to the lacrimal crest, and inferior to the inferior fissure. The lateral osteotomies are made through the zygoma at the level of the frontozygomatic suture or more superiorly along the orbital rim. The lateral orbital osteotomy is extended through the pterygomaxillary fissure with a curved osteotome. A finger is placed intraorally to gauge the depth and direction of the osteotome. The midline osteotomy is directed inferiorly and posteriorly through the perpendicular plate of the ethmoid. Care must be taken to avoid sectioning the endotracheal tube. A separate intraoral incision and sectioning of the pterygomaxillary fissure may be required to complete the osteotomy from above.

Rowe disimpaction forceps are used to down-fracture the maxilla. Hemorrhage may be brisk at this time and can be controlled by reimpaction of the maxilla. Branches of the internal maxillary artery often bleed heavily, but they rarely require direct control. After the maxilla is completely mobile, anterior and inferior displacement is performed. Bone grafts harvested from the ilium, cranium, or rib are then interposed in the gaps between the cranium and maxilla. An acrylic wafer is placed and intermaxillary fixation of the mandible performed, unless the child is young enough that occlusion is not critical. Miniplate fixation is carried out, stabilizing the bone grafts and the maxilla at the nasomaxillary, zygomaticomaxillary, nasofrontal, and frontozygomatic buttresses and junctions. The zygomatic arch is also plated or wired. The nasal bone may require onlay grafting using a costochondral graft, and the orbital floor usually requires additional bone grafts to reconstruct the new floor. Postoperatively, miniplate fixation is typically left in for 4 to 6 weeks, but if the fixation is rigid and secure, the intermaxillary fixation device may be removed considerably earlier.

The intracranial approach to the Le Fort III is essentially the same as that for the subcranial Le Fort III, except that a frontal craniotomy is performed to retract the frontal lobes and dura before performing the midline and lateral periorbital osteotomies. This approach provides greater safety in patients who have a low-lying cribriform plate; however, this risk is balanced by the inherent risk of a frontal craniotomy in a patient who probably has had previous surgery in this area.

MONOBLOC PROCEDURE

The monobloc procedure was developed by Ortiz Monasterio and colleagues[33] and represents an effort to simultaneously correct the fronto-orbital and anterior cranial base hypoplasia and to address the midface and maxillary retrusion in one operation. This procedure assumes that the length of the nasal profile is correct or will not be changed at surgery.

The patient is placed supine, and a lumbar drain may be required. A bifrontal craniotomy is performed, and a bifrontal bone graft with parietal "tongues" to secure the bifrontal segment are taken as a unit. A 5-mm segment of frontal bone is left above the apex of the superior orbital rim, which traverses the forehead. An orbital roof osteotomy is performed posterior to the midpoint of the globe, extending medially to the midline but with the anteriormost osteotomy line in front of the cribriform plate (Fig. 210–13). The remainder of the procedure is carried out as in the Le Fort III procedure. The frontal bone may be reshaped if necessary using vertically oriented slats to achieve a normal forehead contour. Elements of the bony fixation are similar, except that the anterior cranial base is covered by a large, pericranial flap that is secured to the surrounding cranial base bone. This tissue separates the nasal cavity from the dura and provides support for interpositional calvarial bone grafts, which are used for the cranial base between the cribriform and the posterior fronto-orbital segment.

This procedure is most beneficial in the young child with a growing brain. Retrofrontal dead space can be minimized by active brain growth. When used in the older child or adult, this procedure may be fraught with significant complications (e.g., infection) because retrofrontal dead space may persist and become infected.

Distraction Osteogenesis of the Cranial Base and Orbit

Technical advances in craniofacial surgery have included application of the techniques of distraction osteogenesis to the craniofacial skeleton. In 1992, following the work of Ilizarov,[34] McCarthy initiated distraction of the craniofacial skeleton by performing the first human mandibular distraction procedure with an external distraction device.[35] Since then, there have been rapid technical innovations resulting in distraction of the maxilla and the mandible. As previously demonstrated by Persing,[36] distraction of the cranial base as an adjunct to surgery for craniosynostosis syndromes is being developed. The techniques of distrac-

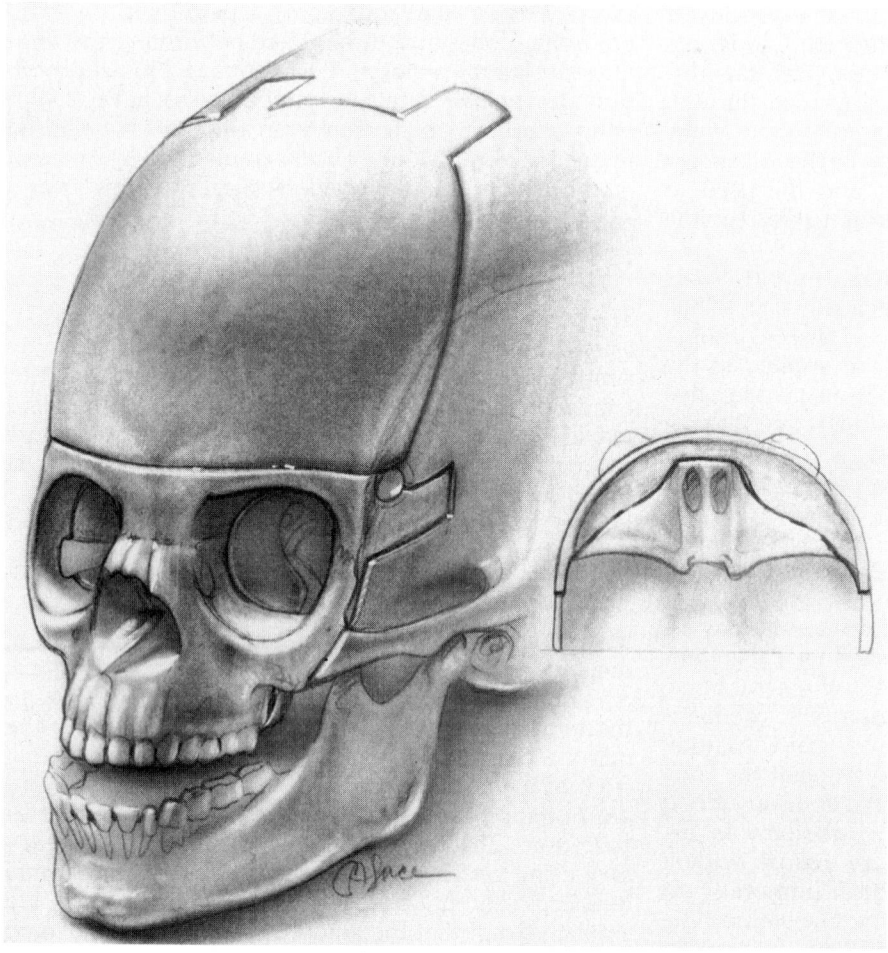

FIGURE 210–13. Schematic illustration of the monobloc osteotomy. The osteotomy is similar to the Le Fort III osteotomy, except that the frontal osteotomy is extended medially, transversely, and across the frontal bone approximately 5 mm above the apex of the superior rim. An osteotomy line extends across the cranial base floor anterior to the cribriform plate *(inset)*. (Adapted from Persing JA, Jane JA, Edgerton MT: Surgical treatment of craniosynostosis. In Persing JA, Jane JA, Edgerton MT [eds]: Scientific Foundations and Surgical Treatment of Craniosynostosis. Baltimore, Williams & Wilkins, 1989, p 233.)

tion osteogenesis as applied to the craniofacial skeleton have demonstrated several benefits. Gradual distraction of bone at a rate of 1 mm/day appears to create sufficient quantity and quality of bone without the need for bone grafting and associated donor morbidity. The distraction process as applied to bone also effects expansion of the soft tissue envelope, thereby reducing the constrictive component of the soft tissue, which may ameliorate the relapse seen with the use of bone grafting, despite of the use of rigid fixation. Research centers on the use of distraction in the frontal, maxillary, and mandibular regions. Maxillary distraction can be carried out in multiple planes and can be external or internal. Procedures such as the monobloc procedure and the Le Fort I and Le Fort III maxillary advancements may be performed.

COMPLICATIONS

Complications are relatively infrequent and may be divided into those that are acute or late. Acute complications include blood loss, air embolus, dural tear with CSF leak, and infectious and respiratory complications. Blood loss occurs nearly continuously intraoperatively; therefore, vigilant attention to accurate blood replacement is paramount to avoid coagulopathy caused by

dilution of clotting agents. Blood loss may also be rapid and hemodynamically significant with a tear of the venous sinus or major cortical vein. Abnormal transosseous veins in people with some syndromes (e.g., Carpenter's syndrome) in the region of the torcular may be torn during bone dissection and require immediate control. In the presence of sutural fusion, the dural connection to the underlying sinus is often attenuated, and the risk of a tear of the sinus is generally reduced. Air embolus has been documented in children undergoing cranioplasty and may occur with any operative position. It is appropriate to consider the placement of precordial Doppler monitors and use of end-tidal carbon dioxide monitors to ascertain entrainment of air into the venous system and central venous lines for large-volume blood and fluid replacement and air embolus evacuation. Blood loss may continue for 12 to 24 hours after cranioplasty, and intensive care unit monitoring is essential. Dural tears may lead to CSF leak with or without infection. Immediate repair is indicated in most cases. Postoperative CSF leak may be controlled with a lumbar drain but, if persistent, may require surgical closure. Loss of continuity of the osteogenic dura may result in thinning of the overlying bone and result in a cranial defect.

Among acute complications, infection represents an uncommon but potentially life-threatening problem.

Generally, infection is associated with persistent communication of the intracranial cavity with the nasal cavity or frontal sinus. Because the frontal sinus develops quite late in childhood, sinus infection is seen as a consequence of surgery in the older child or adolescent. Whitaker and colleagues[37] reported an infection rate of approximately 7% for patients undergoing craniofacial surgery. When undertaken in the adolescent patient, the monobloc procedure is considered to carry a greater risk of infectious complications because the capacity of the brain to expand into the retrofrontal dead space is limited. In patients younger than 14 years, Wolfe[38] reported excellent results with the monobloc procedure, with only one infection in a consecutive series of 32 patients.

Acute airway problems may be related to inadvertent transection of the nasotracheal tube during frontofacial advancement. This may require immediate change to an oral endotracheal tube or possibly tracheostomy. In a retrospective analysis of 542 patients undergoing 579 craniofacial procedures at the Hospital for Sick Children, Crysdale and coworkers[39] reported that 18% of patients required tracheostomy for management of the airway. Patients who were intubated for longer than 24 hours experienced considerably more complications. The use of small-caliber fiberoptic flexible bronchoscopy has greatly facilitated nasotracheal intubation in patients previously considered incapable of endotracheal intubation.

Late complications generally are associated with the sequelae of abnormal bone healing and impaired bone growth. Children older than 1 year of age have a decreased ability to fill cranial defects compared with younger patients. In a series of 592 patients after cranioplasty, Prevot and associates[40] reported that 5% of patients had inadequate ossification. Generally, defects larger than 2 cm in diameter in children older than 1 year should be filled with split calvarial bone grafts to prevent postoperative cranial defects. Significant bone loss requiring bone grafting may occur in the setting of infection and subsequent resorption.

The use of miniplate and microplate rigid fixation has greatly improved the outcome of craniofacial surgery from its inception. However, Persing and colleagues[24] reported significant transcranial plate migration in the growing child. Although no harmful effects have been reported, the potential for risk and difficulty posed for reoperative surgery have been noted. We use resorbable plating and suture fixation in the young child when this approach is feasible.

With complete and adequate cranioplasty, relapse and recrudescence to the original defect of the cranial vault is uncommon, assuming normal brain growth and development. However, in the region of the orbits and midface, if operated on at a very young age, bone contour may relapse significantly. The degree of relapse depends on the severity of the phenotype and on the continued effect of cranial base restriction. The constricting force of the soft tissue envelope and resorption of bone grafts may contribute to further relapse. The advent of distraction osteogenesis is of particular interest in the prevention of relapse because soft tissue expansion is combined with new bone development. Orthodontic occlusal management is also important in ensuring stability of the final result in the older patient.

Overall, the morbidity and mortality from the treatment of craniofacial syndromes is quite low. Mortality rates are between 1.5% and 2%. In 1979, Whitaker and coworkers[37] reported the experience of six craniofacial centers and reported 13 deaths, representing a 1.6% mortality rate. It is likely that ongoing advances in monitoring and anesthetic techniques, as well as refinements in surgical techniques, will continue to yield similar or better results.

Despite the significant problems that these children and their families face, the future continues to be bright, with technical advances providing a multiplicity of diagnostic and treatment alternatives that will affect our ability to provide care to these patients.

REFERENCES

1. Pyo D, Persing JA: Craniosynostosis. In Aston SJ, Beasley RW, Thorne CHM (eds): Grabb and Smith's Plastic Surgery. Philadelphia, Lippincott Raven, 1997, p 281.
2. Fink SC, Hardesty RA: Craniofacial syndromes. In Bentz M (ed): Pediatric Plastic Surgery. New York, McGraw-Hill, 1997, pp 1-37.
3. Cohen MM: Sutural biology and the correlates of craniosynostosis. Am J Genet 47:581–616, 1993.
4. Harvey W: Exercitationes de Generatione Animalium. London, Puleyn, 1651.
5. Sommering ST: Von Baue des mensd'lichen Korpers, 2nd ed. Leipzig, Voss, 1839.
6. Virchow R: Ueber den Cretisnismus, namentlich in Franken, und ueber pathologische Schadelformen. Verh Phys Med Ges Wurzburg 2:230–271, 1851.
7. Klaauw CJ: Cerebral skull and facial skull. Arch Neerl Zool 7: 16, 1946.
8. Moss ML: The pathogenesis of premature cranial synostosis in man. Acta Anat (Basel) 37:351–370, 1959.
9. Babler WJ, Persing JA: Alterations in cranial suture growth associated with premature closure of the sagittal suture in rabbits [abstract]. Anat Rec 211:14A, 1985.
10. Persing JA, Babler WJ, Jane JA, et al: Experimental unilateral coronal synostosis in rabbits. Plast Reconstr Surg 77:369–376, 1986.
11. Persson KM, Roy WA, Persing JA, et al: Craniofacial growth following experimental craniosynostosis and craniectomy in rabbits. J Neurosurg 50:187–197, 1979.
12. Mooney MP, Losken HW, Tschakaloff A, et al: Congenital bilateral coronal suture synostosis in a rabbit and craniofacial growth comparisons with experimental models. Cleft Palate Craniofac J 30:121–128, 1993.
13. Wilkie AOM: Molecular genetics of craniosynostosis. In Lin KY, Olge RC, Jane JA (eds): Craniofacial Surgery. Philadelphia, WB Saunders, 2002, p 41.
14. Wilkie AOM, Slaney SF, Oldridge M, et al: Apert syndrome results from localized mutation in FGFR2 and is allelic with Crouzon syndrome. Nat Genet 9:165, 1994.
15. Reardon W, Winter RM, Rutland P, et al: Mutations in the FGF receptor 2 gene cause Crouzon syndrome. Nat Genet 8:98–103, 1994.
16. Lane LC: Pioneer craniectomy for relief of imbecility due to premature sutural closure and microcephalus. JAMA 18:49, 1892.
17. Lannelongue OM: De la craniectomie dans la microcephalie. Compt-Rendu Acad Sci 110:1382–1385, 1890.
18. LeFort R: Etude experimental sur les fractures de la machoire superieure. Rev Chir Paris 23:280–360, 1901.
19. Gillies H, Harrison SH: Operative correction by osteotomy of recessed malar maxillary compound in a case of oxycephaly. Br J Plast Surg 3:123–127, 1950.
20. Tessier P, Guiot G, Rougerie J, et al: Hypertelorism: Cranionaso-orbito-facial and sub-ethmoid osteotomy. Ann Chir Plast 12:103, 1967.

21. Park TS, Haworth CS, Jane JA, et al: A modified prone position for cranial remodeling procedures in children with cranial dysmorphism. A technical note. Neurosurgery 16:212–214, 1985.
22. Renier D, Sainte-Rose C, Marchac D, et al: Intracranial pressure in craniosynostosis. J Neurosurg 57:370–377, 1982.
23. Shin JH, Persing JA: Secondary correction of nonsyndromic synostosis. Clin Plast Surg 24:415–428, 1997.
24. Persing JA, Posnick J, Magee S, et al: Cranial plate and screw fixation in infancy: An assessment of risk. J Craniofac Surg 7:267–270, 1996.
25. Crouzon O: Dysostose craniofaciale hereditaire. Bull Mem Soc Med Hosp (Paris) 33:545, 1912.
26. Wheaton SW: Two specimens of congenital cranial deformity in infants associated with fusion of the fingers and toes. Trans Pathol Soc Lond 45:238, 1894.
27. Apert E: De l'acrocephalosyndactylie. Bull Soc Med 23:1310, 1906.
28. Pfeiffer RA: Dominant erbliche acrocephalosyndactylie. Z Kinderheilkd 90:301, 1964.
29. Saethre H: Ein beitrag zum turmschaedelproblem (pathogenesis, erblichkeit und symptomatology). Z Nervenheilkd 117:533, 1931.
30. Chotzen F: Eine eigen familiare Entwicklungsstorung. (Akroocephalosyndactylie, dysostosis craniofacial und hypertelorismus.) Monatsschr Kinderheilkd 55:97, 1932.
31. Carpenter G: Two sisters showing malformations of the skull and other congenital abnormalities. Rep Soc Study Dis Child Lond 1:110, 1901.
32. Jabs EW, Muller U, Li X, et al: A mutation in the homeodomain of the human MSX2 gene in a family affected with the autosomal dominant craniosynostosis. Cell 75:443, 1993.
33. Ortiz-Monasterio F, Fuente del Campo A, Carillo A: Advancement of the orbits and the midface in one piece, combined with frontal repositioning for the correction of Crouzon's deformities. Plast Reconstr Surg 61:507, 1978.
34. Ilizarov GA: A new principle of osteosynthesis with the use of crossing pins and rings. In Collection of Scientific Works of the Kurgan Regional Scientific Medical Society. Kurgan, USSR, 1954, pp 145-160.
35. McCarthy JG, Schreiber J, Karp N, et al: Lengthening of the human mandible by gradual distraction. Plast Reconstr Surg 89:1–8, 1992.
36. Persing JA, Morgan EP, Cronin AJ, Wolcott WP: Skull base expansion: Craniofacial effects. Plast Reconstr Surg 187:1028–1033, 1991.
37. Whitaker LA, Bartlett SP, Schut L, et al: Craniosynostosis: An analysis of the timing, treatment and complications in 164 patients. Plast Reconstr Surg 80:195, 1987.
38. Wolfe SA, Morrison G, Page LK, Berkowitz S: The monobloc frontofacial advancement: Do the pluses outweigh the minuses? Plast Reconstr Surg 91:977–987, 1993.
39. Crysdale WS, Kohli-Dang N, Mullind GC, et al: Airway management in craniofacial surgery: Experience in 542 patients. J Otolaryngol 16:207–215, 1987.
40. Prevot M, Renier D, Marchac D: Lack of ossification after cranioplasty for craniosynostosis: A review of relevant factors in 592 consecutive patients. J Craniofac Surg 4:247–254, discussion 255–256, 1993.

CHAPTER 211

Developmental Abnormalities of the Craniovertebral Junction

ARNOLD H. MENEZES

The first anatomic description of "manifestations of occipital vertebrae" was attributed to Meckel in 1815 by Gladstone and Erickson-Powell.[1] The clinical significance became appreciated after the classic radiologic studies on basilar invagination by Chamberlain in 1939.[2]

The term *craniovertebral junction* refers to the occipital bone that surrounds the foramen magnum and the atlas and axis vertebrae. Into the 1970s, surgical treatment of conditions affecting the craniovertebral junction consisted of posterior decompression by enlargement of the foramen magnum and removal of the posterior arch of the atlas and axis vertebrae. However, the mortality and morbidity rates associated with this treatment were high for patients with irreducible lesions and cervicomedullary compression.[3] A physiologic approach based on an understanding of the craniovertebral dynamics, the site of encroachment, and the stability of the craniovertebral junction was adopted at the University of Iowa Hospitals and Clinics in 1977. Since then, 3600 patients with neurological symptoms and signs secondary to an abnormality of the craniovertebral region have been studied. Understanding the pathology of these abnormalities and their treatment is simplified if one has a knowledge of the bony anatomy, biomechanics, and embryology of the region.

ANATOMY

Bone-Ligament Complex

The atlantoaxial complex is unique among the intervertebral joints, in that it is horizontally oriented. The lateral facet joints are relatively flat and allow for a pivoting motion at the atlantodental articulation, which is permitted by the special ligamentous support. The second cervical nerve exits from the cervical canal immediately adjacent and dorsal to the joint capsules. The transverse atlantal ligament is a band 3 to 5 mm thick that originates from the tubercles and the inner aspect of the lateral masses of the atlas vertebra and is in close apposition to the odontoid, permitting axial rotation.

By itself, the geometry of the craniovertebral complex is meant to provide mobility at the cost of stability.[4] However, the complex is maintained in a clamplike vise by the craniovertebral musculature, which assists in stabilization of the spine, initiates movements within the joints, and maintains the fluidity of the motion complex.

Blood Supply

The blood supply to the odontoid process is from anterior and posterior ascending vessels from the vertebral arteries, with a contribution from the carotid arteries, which form an apical arcade around the alar ligament.[5] Thus, the odontoid process blood supply is vulnerable in type II odontoid fracture.[6]

Parke and coworkers demonstrated pharyngovertebral veins with frequent lymphovenous anastomoses.[7] This connection may provide an additional route for septic involvement of the craniovertebral complex, which can result in osteomyelitis of the bone as well as joint effusions.

Lymphatic Drainage

The lymphatic drainage of the occipitoatlantoaxial joint complex is primarily into the retropharyngeal lymph nodes and then into the upper deep jugular cervical chain.[3] These nodes also receive drainage from the nasopharynx, paranasal sinuses, and retropharyngeal area. A retrograde infection may affect the synovial lining of the craniovertebral joint complex, with a resultant inflammatory effusion, instability, and possible neurological deficit, contributing to the so-called Grisel's syndrome.[8]

EMBRYOLOGY AND DEVELOPMENT OF CRANIOVERTEBRAL JUNCTION DISORDERS

Congenital anomalies of the base of the skull and the atlanto-occipital region involve both the osseous structures and the nervous system. The frequent occurrence of patterns with various combinations suggests an interrelationship between, if not a common cause of, the origin and development of these structures.[3]

The bony cranial base is developed by the process of endochondral ossification in which a cartilaginous framework is first developed and subsequently resorbed with further deposition of bone, based on distorting forces such as brain and eye development.[9, 10] The clivus is elongated by sutural growth of the spheno-occipital synchondrosis and by further sutural growth along the lateral portion of the base.

The majority of the skull and facial bones develop by intramembranous ossification. This development bypasses the intermediate cartilaginous stage characteristic of the development of the bony cranial base.[10, 11]

The occipital sclerotomes correspond to the segmental nerves that group together to form the hypoglossal nerve, with a path through the individual foramina through the bone.[6, 10] The first two occipital sclerotomes ultimately form the basiocciput. The third sclerotome is responsible for the exoccipital center as it forms the jugular tubercles.[11, 12] The key to understanding the craniovertebral junction is the embryology of the fourth occipital sclerotome, which in lower animals is called the proatlas. The hypocentrum of the fourth occipital sclerotome forms the anterior tubercle of the clivus. The centrum of the proatlas itself forms the apical cap of the dens as well as the apical ligament. The neural arch component of the proatlas divides into a ventral-rostral component and a caudal-dorsal portion. The ventral portion forms the U-shaped anterior margin of the foramen magnum, as well as the occipital condyles and the midline occipital condyle. The cruciate ligament and the alar ligaments are condensations of the lateral portion of the proatlas. The caudal division of the neural arch of the proatlas forms the lateral atlantal masses of C1, as well as the superior portion of the posterior arch of the atlas.

The atlas vertebra is formed by the first spinal sclerotome. It is modified from the remaining spinal vertebrae, and the centrum is separated to fuse with the axis body, forming the odontoid process. The neural arch of the first spinal sclerotome forms the posterior and inferior portion of the atlas arch. The hypochordal bow of the proatlas itself may survive and join with the anterior arch of the atlas to form a variant such that an abnormal articulation may exist among the clivus, the anterior arch of the atlas, and the apical segment of the odontoid process.

During embryogenesis, the hypocentrum of the second spinal sclerotome disappears. The centrum forms the body of the axis vertebra, and the neural arches develop into facets and the posterior arch of the axis. Thus, the body of the dens appears from the first sclerotome, whereas a terminal portion of the odontoid process arises from the proatlas. The most inferior portion of the axis body is formed by the second spinal sclerotome. Thus, at birth, the odontoid process is separated from the body of the axis vertebra by a cartilaginous band that represents a vestigial disk and is referred to as the neural central synchondrosis.[6, 13] This

lies below the level of the superior articular facets of the axis and does not represent the anatomic base of the dens. This synchondrosis is present in most children younger than 3 to 4 years and disappears by age 8 years. In most instances the odontoid process is seen at birth but does not fuse to the base of the axis.[14] The tip of the odontoid is not ossified at birth and is not seen on lateral radiographs. It is represented by a separate ossification center, which is usually seen at age 3 years and fuses with the remainder of the dens by age 12 years.

Expansion in the posterior fossa occurs as a result of a combination of endochondral resorption, sutural growth, and bony accretion. Growth of the basion elongates the basiocciput and lowers the frontal margins of foramen magnum. There is a comparably matched resorptive drift downward and backward at the opisthion as a result of the cerebellar downward displacement, together with the rotation of the occipital and temporal lobes of the brain.

The stability of the craniovertebral articulation with the forward inclination of the top-heavy cranial end of the fetus must be maintained by the geometry of the articular surfaces of the craniovertebral junction, as well as by the ligamentous attachments and, more importantly, by the heavy development of the dorsal and lateral cervical musculature, which provides a clamping action on the craniovertebral region.[3, 4]

Significant advances have occurred with the discovery of developmental control genes.[9–11, 15, 16] Two families of regulatory genes have been implicated in the subsequent development of the sclerotomal parts of the somites during their resegmentation to form the vertebral primordia and in the specification of the identity of each vertebra. Common to all these genes are phylogenetically highly conserved DNA sequences termed *homeovox* (*HOX* genes) and *paired vox* (*PAX* genes) sequences. They promote proteins that modulate morphogenesis by influencing the transcription of specific downstream genes.

Teratogen-induced disturbance of *HOX* gene expression and mutations in *HOX* genes can cause alterations in both the number and the identity of cervical vertebrae forming at or near the limit of their expression domain. For example, inactivation of the *HOX-D3* gene results in mutant mice with atlas assimilation to the basiocciput.[17] The sensitivity of the occipitocervical junction to disturbances in *HOX* gene expression might prove to be the underlying cause of malformations in this region. *PAX* genes are expressed in diverse cell types and contribute to the development of the early nervous system. Control of resegmentation of the sclerotomes to establish the intervertebral boundaries seems to be independently controlled by two regulatory genes in the *PAX* family.[15, 18]

IMPLICATIONS OF CRANIOVERTEBRAL ABNORMALITIES

A wide variety of congenital anomalies of the craniovertebral junction exists, occurring singly or multiply in the same individual and involving both osseous and neural structures. An insult to both types of structures may occur between the fourth and seventh week of intrauterine life and result in a combination of anomalies consisting of failure of segmentation, failure of fusion of different components of each bone, hypoplasia, and ankylosis.

Congenital diseases involving connective tissue, such as Morquio's syndrome and other mucopolysaccharidoses as well as Down syndrome, can involve severe atlantoaxial subluxation.[3, 14] There is a high incidence of anterior and posterior spina bifida of C1 and also os odontoideum in these instances. It is possible that owing to abnormal, excessive head movements in the embryo between 50 and 53 days, the process of chondrification is impaired, resulting in anterior and later posterior spina bifida of C1.

Os odontoideum was previously thought to be congenital, described as a failure of fusion between the centrum component of C1 and that of C2. However, the radiographic abnormality always has a hypoplastic dens, and the neural central synchondrosis is a definite visible entity.[13] To be congenital, the defect would have to be below the superior slopes of the C2 facets.[6] Os odontoideum most likely originates as odontoid trauma that may predate birth but certainly occurs before age 4 years, with subsequent distraction and separation of the odontoid fragments.[19] The superior segment is distracted upward by the apical and alar ligaments and receives its blood supply from the descending branch of the occipital artery, which courses along the apical ligament. This subsequently leads to incompetence of the cruciate ligament and further abnormalities.

Spinal trauma in children younger than 8 years is mainly centered at the craniovertebral border owing to the high fulcrum of neck motion.[3] This results in ligamentous injuries more often than fractures. However, odontoid fractures in this age group are usually seen as avulsion injuries with separation of the neural central synchondrosis.

Anomalies and malformations of the caudal occipital sclerotomes are collectively called *manifestations of an occipital vertebra* and result in abnormal bony ridges and outgrowths of the ventral aspect of the foramen magnum.[1] At times, segmentation abnormalities of the clivus are recognized and represent a failure of the last occipital sclerotome to separate from the basiocciput and the clivus. Consequently, bone growth in the anterior aspect of foramen magnum indents the ventral cervicomedullary junction with age (as the clivus expands inferiorly and dorsally).

The ongoing growth of the posterior fossa from birth into late adolescence provides a rationale for the need to continue to observe children who have undergone dorsal occipitocervical stabilization or ventral craniovertebral decompression. The downward growth of the brain as well as elongation of the posterior fossa and clivus may re-create a ventral bony abnormality later in life, despite a previous ventral decompression at the craniovertebral junction performed during the first 2 decades of life.

BIOMECHANICS

The unique anatomic configuration of the craniovertebral junction creates a distinct biomechanical behavior that differs from that of other spinal joints. The motion characteristics of the different levels of the craniovertebral junction are due to the geometry of the opposing bones of the vertebrae and the skull base, the shape of the joints, and the arrangement of the ligaments.[4, 20-22] The intervertebral disk is absent between the occiput and C1 and C2. The ball-and-socket–shaped occiput-C1 joint allows slightly more flexion-extension than the other levels of the cervical spine, although it is quite rigid in axial rotation and lateral bending.

The biconvex articular surfaces of the C1-2 joints allow gliding and wide rotation of C1 around the dens. The atlantoaxial motion segment is the most flexible motion segment in the entire spine with respect to axial rotation, allowing a bilateral range of motion of 90 degrees. More than half of all cervical axial rotation occurs at the C1-2 motion segment, a point that should be kept in mind when considering atlantoaxial arthrodesis. In a child, the amount of anterior-posterior translation that occurs between the dens and the anterior ring of the atlas is up to 5 mm. When the transverse component of the cruciate ligament has been disrupted, the alar ligaments are still intact. Hence, the amount of displacement remains between 5 and 6 mm until the alar ligaments become incompetent. It is only when the alar ligaments and the transverse portion of the cruciate ligament are incompetent that a separation of more than 5 to 6 mm occurs. Beyond the age of 8 years, the excursion of the predental space must be limited to 3 mm.[23]

Failure of one alar ligament results in moderate rotary atlantoaxial instability.[24] Bilateral transection of the alar ligaments causes considerably more alterations in the craniovertebral motion, and the coupling action is disturbed. The transverse atlantal ligament is the strongest and thickest ligament of the entire spine. It is the predominant stabilizer of the atlas, constraining C1 around the dens. When torn, the transverse ligament is incapable of repair. Because this ligament injury renders C1 grossly unstable, C1-2 fusion is mandated. The largest degree of rotation occurs at the atlantoaxial joint. When rotation exceeds 40 to 50 degrees, an interlock of the lateral inferior facet of the atlas over the superior articular facet of the axis vertebra occurs. If the transverse ligament becomes deficient, the anterior arch will sublux forward, producing a unilateral dislocation and an interlock at less than 40 degrees.[23] Rotation of more than 30 to 35 degrees produces an angulation of the contralateral vertebral artery.[22, 25] With greater rotation there is stretching of the vertebral artery, and the ipsilateral vessel may demonstrate occlusion.[26] This phenomenon has an implication in wrestling and football injuries and in certain head rotation maneuvers performed under general anesthesia or forced chiropractic manipulations.[27, 28] There is a muscle clamping action that takes place in vivo that produces compressive forces across the cervical spine. This muscular action produces the "interlocking stiffening" that maintains alignment during rotation. When protective muscles are relaxed or inadequately developed, as in the case of a young child under general anesthesia, the craniovertebral junction becomes inherently less stable than in the adult.[3] As muscular development occurs, there is less tendency for instability at the craniovertebral junction.

BIOMECHANICAL COMPARISON OF CERVICAL ORTHOSES

An orthosis acts as a restraint to restrict spinal motion or immobilize the surrounding tissues. Orthoses are used as load-sharing devices to reduce the external loads applied to the spine while an injury or a fixation fusion is healing.

The halo brace is most effective at constraining cervical motion at all levels, and the control of spinal motion is related to the distance of the spinal segment from the region of the rigid skull fixation.[3, 24] The halo provides the best control of motion at the craniovertebral junction, intermediate control of midcervical motion, and the least control of motion at the cervicothoracic junction. This pattern reflects snaking movements of the spine.

The soft cervical collar provides little immobilization and only tends to remind the patient to restrict motion. Molded collars, four-poster braces, sternal-occipital-mandibular immobilization, and cervicothoracic braces have intermediate properties for controlling flexion and extension, lateral bending, and axial rotation.

CLASSIFICATION OF CRANIOVERTEBRAL JUNCTION ABNORMALITIES

A wide variety of congenital, developmental, and acquired abnormalities exist at the craniovertebral junction and may occur singly or multiply in the same individual. The pathology of these abnormalities is extensive. A working classification has been provided, but it must be appreciated that there are overlapping causes within this classification (Table 211–1).

EPIDEMIOLOGY

Abnormality of the craniovertebral junction must be suspected in infants with Goldenhar's syndrome, skeletal dysplasias, and Conradi's syndrome.[3] It should be suspected in infants who present with torticollis. Diseases such as Down syndrome have a 14% to 20% incidence of atlantoaxial dislocation. In Morquio's syndrome, a combination of atlantoaxial instability, os odontoideum, and cervicothoracic abnormalities occur in 30% to 50% of individuals.[3, 14, 29] The incidence of atlas assimilation is 0.25% in the general population. Many such patients have associated segmentation failures of the upper cervical spine.[30]

TABLE 211–1 ■ **Classification of Craniovertebral Junction Abnormalities**

I. Congenital anomalies and malformations of the craniovertebral junction
  A. Malformations of occipital bone
    1. Manifestations of occipital vertebra
      a. Clivus segmentations
      b. Remnants around foramen magnum
      c. Atlas variants
      d. Dens segmentation anomalies
    2. Basilar invagination
    3. Condylar hypoplasia
    4. Assimilation of atlas
  B. Malformations of atlas
    1. Assimilation of atlas
    2. Atlantoaxial fusion
    3. Aplasia of atlas arches
  C. Malformations of axis
    1. Irregular atlantoaxial segmentation
    2. Dens dysplasias
      a. Ossiculum terminale persistens
      b. Os odontoideum
      c. Hypoplasia-aplasia
    3. Segmentation failure of C2–3
II. Developmental and acquired abnormalities of the craniovertebral junction
  A. Abnormalities of foramen magnum
    1. Secondary basilar invagination (e.g., Paget's disease, osteomalacia, rheumatoid cranial settling, renal resistant rickets)
    2. Foraminal stenosis (e.g., achondroplasia)
  B. Atlantoaxial instability
    1. Errors of metabolism (e.g., Morquio's syndrome)
    2. Down syndrome
    3. Infections (e.g., Grisel's syndrome)
    4. Inflammatory (e.g., rheumatoid arthritis)
    5. Traumatic occipitoatlantal and atlantoaxial dislocation; os odontoideum
    6. Tumors (e.g., neurofibromatosis, syringomyelia)
    7. Miscellaneous (e.g., fetal warfarin syndrome, Conradi's syndrome)

Once the stage is set by congenital craniovertebral anomalies, the developmental and acquired phenomenon may supervene, producing atlantoaxial instability and subsequently basilar invagination. This is much more common in developing countries where heavy loads are carried on the head from childhood. Thus, the erroneous diagnosis of "congenital dislocations" has been reported. Likewise, upper respiratory tract infections that lead to stiff neck, torticollis, and ligamentous instability come to attention much later in developing countries than in places where medical attention is more readily available. For this reason, it appears that abnormalities of the craniovertebral junction are more frequently encountered in populous, less advantaged countries.

CLINICAL PRESENTATION

The most interesting feature of the clinical presentation of craniovertebral abnormalities is the diversity. This is due to the compromise of the lower brainstem, cervical spinal cord, cranial nerves, cervical roots, and vascular supply.[6] The symptoms of craniovertebral dysfunction may be insidious and may present as false localizing signs. Infrequently, a rapid neurological progression is followed by sudden death. More often than not, there is an antecedent history of minor trauma that sets off a pattern of symptoms and signs that may progress at a galloping pace.

Congenital abnormalities of the craniovertebral junction are often associated with an abnormal general physical appearance. The head may be cocked to one side, as in patients with rotary luxation of the atlas on the axis, or the classic triad of Klippel-Feil syndrome (abnormally low hairline posteriorly, limitation of neck motion, and short neck) may be noted. There may be facial asymmetry and webbing of the neck in conjunction with this syndrome. At times, scoliosis is present. It is not uncommon to see children with a small dysmorphic stature. There is an increased incidence of craniovertebral abnormalities with disease states such as achondroplasia, spondyloepiphyseal dysplasia, and related diseases of dwarfism. The most common neurological symptoms and signs are listed in Table 211–2.

The most common symptom is neck pain originating in the suboccipital region with radiation to the cranial vertex, occurring in 85% of patients. False localizing signs associated with abnormalities of the foramen magnum are usually motor and include monoparesis, hemiparesis, paraparesis, and quadriparesis. Central cord syndrome is often seen in children with basilar invagination in whom the myelopathy mimics a lower cervical spinal cord disturbance.

Sensory abnormalities usually manifest as neurological deficits related to posterior column dysfunction. Brainstem and cranial nerve deficits cause abnormalities such as dysphagia and sleep apnea. Not uncommonly, internuclear ophthalmoplegia is present, leading to a misdiagnosis of mesencephalic and upper pontine disturbance. Downbeat nystagmus is present in strictly compressive lesions of the craniovertebral border with or without an associated Chiari malformation.

The phenomenon of basilar migraine affects about 25% of children with basilar invagination and compression of the medulla. This usually involves compression

of the vertebrobasilar arterial system. The symptoms regress with decompression of the area and stabilization. The excessive mobility of an unstable craniovertebral junction may cause repeated trauma to the anterior spinal artery and the perforating vessels of the upper cervical cord and medulla oblongata, as well as the vertebral and basilar arteries. This may lead to spasm or occlusion and attendant neurological deficit.

The most common neurological deficit encountered in affected children is myelopathy, and the most common cranial nerve dysfunction is hearing loss, occurring in 25% of cases. There has been an increased incidence of this finding in Klippel-Feil syndrome. Unilateral or bilateral paralysis or dysfunction of the soft palate or pharynx may lead to repeated bouts of aspiration pneumonia, as well as poor feeding and inability to gain weight.

Vascular symptoms such as intermittent attacks of altered consciousness, transient loss of visual fields, confusion, and vertigo appear in 15% to 25% of patients with abnormalities of the craniovertebral junction. This may be provoked by extension or rotation of the head, as with manipulation of the head and neck.

NEURODIAGNOSTIC IMAGING

The diagnostic procedure of choice is magnetic resonance imaging (MRI), but plain cervical spine radiographs, with lateral flexion and extension views, are essential to gain a better understanding of the biomechanics. Numerous craniometric reference lines were described before the advent of computed tomography (CT) and MRI.[30–33] These were used to locate the position of the neural structures with the associated osseous abnormality (Fig. 211–1). Chamberlain's palato-occipital line joins the hard palate to the posterior edge of the foramen magnum.[2] In normal individuals, the tip of the dens should lie below this line or at most 3 to 5 mm above it. Basilar invagination occurs when the dens projects above this line. Wackenheim's clivus canal line is of greatest significance.[33] This line is drawn along the clivus and extrapolated into the cervical spinal canal. The odontoid process must be ventral to this line or tangential to it. The odontoid process transects this line in basilar invagination, atlantoaxial dislocation, and anterior occipitoatlantal dislocation. McRae's foramen magnum line joins the anterior and posterior edges of the foramen magnum.[30] The tip of the dens must be below this line. If the sagittal space for the cervicomedullary junction is less than 20 mm in a child older than 8 years, neurological deficit is usually present.

MRI is used to identify the neural abnormalities and osseous compression, as well as to recognize any instability if present. In this examination, flexion and extension dynamic views are obtained in the parasagittal dimension in both T1- and T2-weighted modes. Axial views supplement this. The effects of cervical traction are also documented with MRI to visualize the neural-osseous relationships. Magnetic resonance angiography and CT–angiography can provide a better

T A B L E   2 1 1 – 2 ■ **Signs and Symptoms of Craniovertebral Anomalies (Insidious or Rapid Onset)**

Head tilt
Short neck, low hairline, limitation of neck motion
Web neck
Scoliosis
Features of skeletal dysplasias
Neck pain and posterior occipital headache
Basilar migraine
Isolated weakness in hand or foot
Quadriparesis, paraparesis, monoparesis
Sensory abnormalities
Nystagmus (usually downbeat and lateral gaze)
Sleep apnea
Repeat aspiration pneumonia, dysphagia
Tinnitus and hearing loss
Vertigo

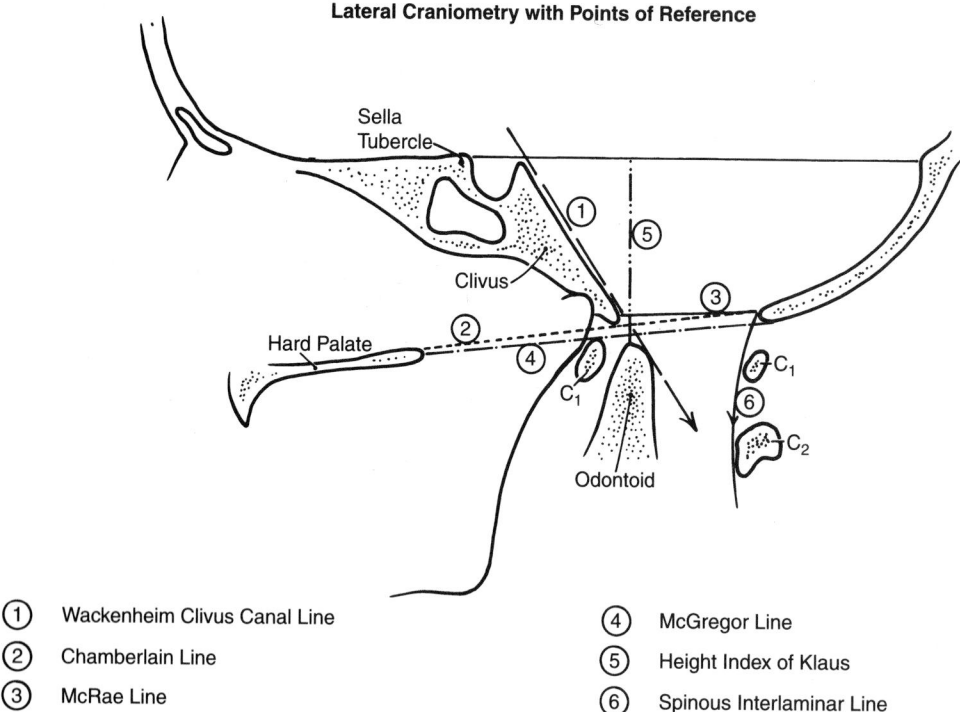

Lateral Craniometry with Points of Reference

① Wackenheim Clivus Canal Line

② Chamberlain Line

③ McRae Line

④ McGregor Line

⑤ Height Index of Klaus

⑥ Spinous Interlaminar Line (Posterior Canal Line)

FIGURE 211–1. Lateral craniometry with points of reference.

understanding of the vasculature as well as any vascular deformities that may occur with motion of the craniovertebral junction.

Three-dimensional CT is useful for defining the abnormality as well as allowing coronal and sagittal sectioning. I have found CT to be invaluable in recognizing the presence or absence of epiphyseal growth plates in toddlers and young children and for assessing the extent of fusion and segmentation defects as well as "missing" osseous components. Spondylolisthesis and spondylolysis are best appreciated with three-dimensional studies.

Each of these imaging modalities provides complementary information to define the craniovertebral deformity.

TREATMENT

The factors that influence the specific treatment of craniovertebral junction abnormalities are as follows[6]: (1) the reducibility of the bony lesion (i.e., the ability to restore anatomic alignment, thereby relieving compression on the neural structures); (2) the mechanics of compression and the direction of encroachment; (3) the cause of the pathologic process, as well as the presence of hindbrain herniation, syrinx, and vascular abnormalities; and (4) the presence of abnormal ossification centers and epiphyseal growth plates.

The primary aim of treatment is to relieve compression at the cervicomedullary junction. Stabilization is paramount in reducible lesions to maintain the neural decompression. Irreducible lesions require decompression at the site where the compression has occurred;

these can be subdivided into ventral and dorsal compression states. In the former, the operative procedure is ventral decompression through a transpalatopharyngeal route, Le Fort drop-down maxillotomy, or lateral extrapharyngeal route. In dorsal compression states, a posterolateral decompression is required. If instability is present after decompression, posterior fixation is mandated for stability. It is thus necessary to select the operation or combination of operations for each individual patient based on a clear understanding of the pathophysiology and the functional anatomy.

Disease states such as spondyloepiphyseal dysplasia, mucopolysaccharidosis, osteogenesis imperfecta, Goldenhar's syndrome, and allied situations in very young children present an interesting and difficult problem of instability at the craniovertebral junction. In such circumstances, it is essential that the treating physician be able to identify the potential for osseous development by recognizing the epiphyseal growth plates, which can be seen only on thin-section CT. When there is an absence of growth plates, development can be allowed to take place by supporting the occipitocervical region with custom-built cervical orthoses that are revised every few months. The toddler or young child is then re-evaluated periodically with diagnostic procedures aimed at identifying the status of the developing craniovertebral junction and the neural compromise. Once the child is 3 to 4 years old (when all components of the craniovertebral junction are present), surgical therapy may be attempted if the situation remains unchanged.

Skeletal traction should be performed using an MRI-compatible halo device. I prefer a crown halo rather than a complete ring, because distortion on MRI is minimal. In children younger than 2 years, 8- to 10-point skull fixation is used. The pin pressure is maintained with the thumb and forefinger. This generates no more than 1 to 2 pounds of torque. At 5 years of age, the maximal pin pressure needed is 4 pounds. Traction is initiated at a very low rate, starting at 3 to 4 pounds in a 5-year-old child and not exceeding 7 pounds. In an adult, traction should start at 7 pounds and should not exceed 15 pounds for the craniovertebral region. It is imperative that the crown of the halo be placed below the equator of the cranium so that the pins do not migrate and slip.

Reducible lesions that are the result of inflammatory states or recent trauma will respond to conservative management with external immobilization once reduction is achieved. The healing is usually ligamentous and may include bony reconstitution. If this does not occur, or if the condition is not the result of trauma or infection, bony fixation is mandated.

Atlantoaxial arthrodesis requires a minimum of 3 months of immobilization for fusion. I use halo vest immobilization for 5 to 6 months with fusions that extend to the occiput. Rates of fusion failure reach 50% when immobilization is inadequate. Wire fixation between the cervical vertebrae or between the skull and the cervical spine should be avoided.

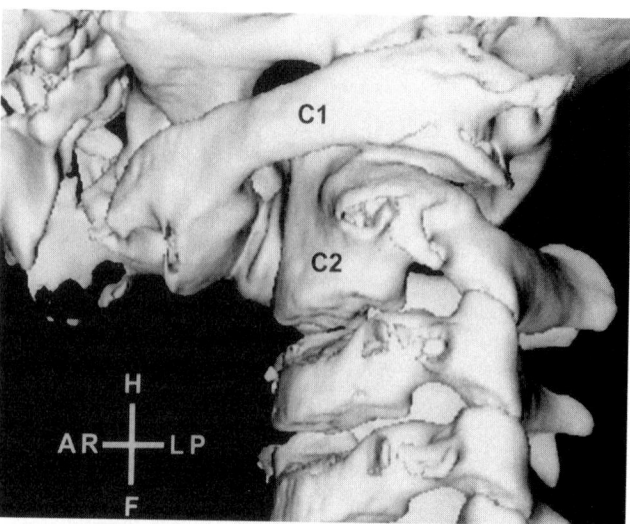

FIGURE 211–2. Three-dimensional computed tomographic scan of the craniovertebral junction and upper cervical spine in a 7-year-old with significant rotational abnormality of the occipitoatlantoaxial joints. Note the perching of the occipital condyle on the right lateral atlantal mass of C1. There is rotational luxation of C1 on C2 that is best visualized on the frontal, lateral, and upward view into the craniovertebral region. The patient had undergone tonsil and adenoid resection a few days earlier.

DEVELOPMENTAL ABNORMALITIES AFFECTING THE CRANIOVERTEBRAL REGION

Grisel's Syndrome

Grisel's syndrome is defined as an inflammatory, spontaneous subluxation that affects the atlantoaxial joints following parapharyngeal infection.[8] This may occur with tonsillitis, mastoiditis, retropharyngeal abscess, and otitis media. Most children affected are younger than 12 years. These children present with torticollis, neck pain, or neurological deficit.[34] The severe subluxation may produce symptoms and signs of cervical cord compression (Fig. 211–2).

In 1987, Wilson and coworkers reviewed 62 cases of Grisel's syndrome.[35] This included 14 children who developed subluxation after tonsillectomy, adenoidectomy, mastoiditis, and resection of a pharyngeal rhabdomyosarcoma. Twelve children had symptoms of pharyngitis or cervical adenitis, seven had tonsillitis, and seven harbored cervical abscesses. There were five children with acute rheumatic fever and four with acute mastoiditis. Several patients were assigned a diagnosis of nonspecific parapharyngeal infection.

The erythrocyte sedimentation rate is invariably elevated. MRI identifies parapharyngeal soft tissue masses, the presence of dislocation, and osteomyelitis or bone erosion. Needle biopsy of the prevertebral masses is essential to confirm the presence of a pyogenic focus and to obtain a specimen for bacterial culture. Appropriate antibiotics must be administered intravenously as quickly as possible for treatment of the primary infection. Reduction of the dislocation by

manipulation with cervical traction is reserved only for gross dislocations. Otherwise, immobilization in a sternal-occipital-mandibular immobilizer is sufficient. However, occipitocervical dislocation requires halo immobilization. It is only rarely necessary to perform fusion.

Down Syndrome

Down syndrome is easily recognized by the characteristic facial features, hypotonia, mental retardation, ligamentous laxity, and transverse palmar creases.[3] Almost every organ is involved. This syndrome is the most commonly recognized chromosomal abnormality in humans, with an incidence of 1 in 700 live births. Craniovertebral instability in Down syndrome has received increasing attention since the report by Spitzer and associates of occipitoatlantal (O-C1) dislocation in 9 of 26 patients investigated with Down syndrome. However, atlantoaxial instability in Down syndrome has been the most described since the initial publication by Tisher and Martel in 1965.[36] The incidence of atlantoaxial instability is 14% to 24% of patients, although the incidence of symptomatic atlantoaxial instability is believed to be less than 1% (Fig. 211–3). The prevalence of bony abnormalities such as os odontoideum, hypoplastic odontoid process, and rotary atlantoaxial luxation in patients with Down syndrome has caused concern about their participation in the Special Olympics, and it has been recommended that cervical spine radiographs be required for such participants.[37] An atlantodental interval greater than 4.5 mm was thought to require medical attention.[37]

The lack of attendant neurological symptoms and signs has resulted in the unfortunate belief that these

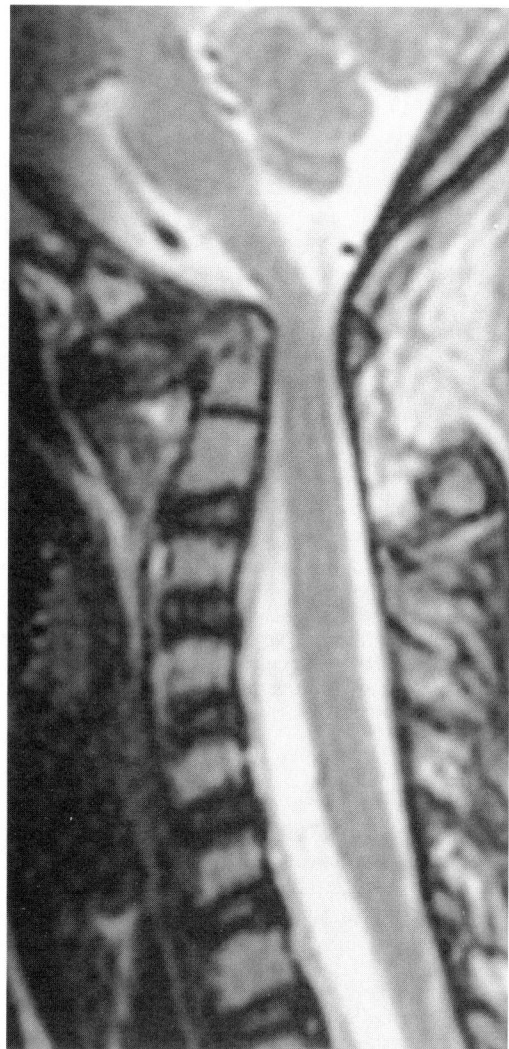

FIGURE 211–3. Midsagittal T2-weighted magnetic resonance imaging scan of the posterior fossa and upper cervical spine in a 13-year-old with Down syndrome. There is posterior displacement of the axis body, with marked constriction of the subarachnoid sac at the cervicomedullary junction. This patient presented with quadriparesis.

children do not require surgical attention. Minor trauma as well as upper respiratory infection has resulted in severe neurological deficits in children with previously recognized pathologic instability without any intervention.[4, 31, 38]

Burke and coworkers studied 32 individuals with Down syndrome and found that only one had atlantoaxial instability at the onset of examination.[31] However, at 13-year follow-up, seven children had developed a predental space of more than 5 mm. Two patients underwent atlantoaxial arthrodesis, and one succumbed to the disease before treatment. Three of the 32 individuals in this study developed an odontoid abnormality consistent with os odontoideum. Review of the initial radiographs showed that these abnormalities had not been present then.

In my experience between 1979 and 1996, 64 patients with Down syndrome and cervicomedullary compro-

mise were encountered.[6] A fixed atlantoaxial luxation was present in 30; in 18 of these patients, cervicomedullary compression developed precipitously. Occipitoatlantal instability was present in 40 of 64 patients, with an associated rotary luxation in 30. The average predental space was 8 mm in the neutral position in these 40 individuals. In four adolescents, a previously successful dorsal atlantoaxial arthrodesis led to subsequent basilar invagination caused by unrecognized occipitoatlantal instability. Os odontoideum was found in 12 of 64 patients. An irreducible invagination occurred in six and was treated with anterior decompression followed by dorsal occipitocervical fusion. The fusion rate for all 64 patients was 95% at the first attempt. Thus, the results of stabilization have been encouraging.

Atlantoaxial arthrodesis in Down syndrome is best accomplished with transarticular C1-2 screw fixation.[39] This is supplemented with bilateral interlaminar fusion using full-thickness rib grafts. Occipitoatlantoaxial instability is best treated using instrumentation with a threaded, contoured loop supplemented with bone graft and an attempt at atlantoaxial stabilization with a transarticular screw, if possible. This is necessary because postoperative maintenance of halo immobilization is problematic in such children.

Segmentation Failures, Fusions, and Remnants at the Foramen Magnum

Malformations and anomalies of the most caudal of the occipital sclerotomes are collectively called *manifestations of occipital vertebrae* and are due to proatlas segmentation failures. Failure of fusion of the first and second occipital sclerotomes produces a bipartite clivus. At times, the proatlas component of the dens may fail to separate from the portion that forms the basiocciput of the clivus. Thus, the anterior arch of the atlas comes to rest above the axis body. The proatlas segmentation abnormality is united with the clivus, grossly distorting the cervicomedullary junction ventrally. Variations of this may be seen in the ventral midline or ventrolaterally on either side, thus causing paramesial invagination (Fig. 211–4).

Failures of segmentation of the atlas result in abnormal articulations between the clivus, the atlas, and the odontoid process. Variations may consist of partial absence of the posterior arch of the atlas and fusions between the atlas and the axis. A bifid anterior and posterior atlas leads to significant neurological abnormality as a result of cranial settling, with the two halves of the atlas vertebra acting like a complex Jefferson fracture with lateral displacement. The condition of bifid anterior and posterior arch of the atlas should be considered grossly pathologic if it is present beyond the age of 3 years, and it must be addressed. I reviewed 160 normal computed tomographic scans of the cranioverbral junction in subjects between birth and 4 years old and concluded that the atlas should be a complete ring by age 3 years. Thus, these patients require operative intervention between 3 and 4 years of age if the atlas has not united.

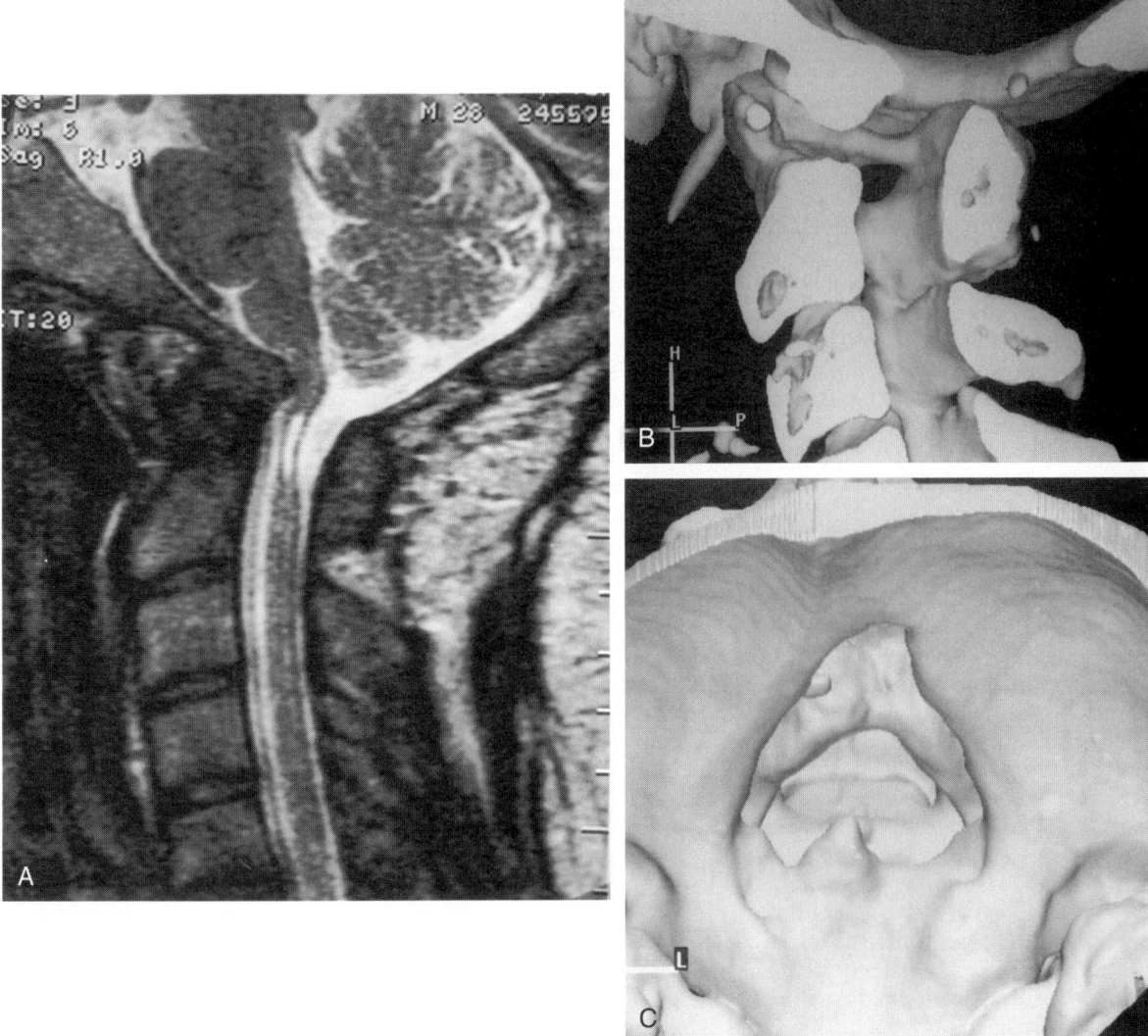

FIGURE 211–4. *A*, Midsagittal T2-weighted magnetic resonance imaging scan of the craniovertebral junction. This 28-year-old man had spastic quadriparesis with difficulty swallowing, hoarseness, and sleep apnea. He had undergone two previous transoral procedures to resect the odontoid process, as well as a C1-2 dorsal arthrodesis. There is a ventral bony mass extending from the clivus into the ventral cervicomedullary junction. Just below this, the uppermost cervical cord has atrophy, with an intramedullary high signal change representing myelomalacia. *B*, Composite midline section of a three-dimensional computed tomographic scan of the craniovertebral junction. *C*, Three-dimensional visualization of the craniovertebral junction from within the foramen magnum. The odontoid process apex never formed, because the proatlas component of the odontoid is still unsegmented from the midline clivus.

Assimilation of the Atlas and Klippel-Feil Syndrome

Atlas assimilation is defined as failure of segmentation between the fourth occipital sclerotome and the first spinal sclerotome. This anomaly occurs in 0.25% of the population and may be unilateral, segmental, focal, or bilateral.[30] In most instances, it occurs in conjunction with other abnormalities such as basilar invagination and Klippel-Feil syndrome. The finding of atlas assimilation was present in 400 of 3500 individuals who were evaluated for craniovertebral abnormalities. Hindbrain herniation was present in 152 of these 400 patients.[40] It is also fairly common to see segmentation failures of the second and third cervical vertebrae in association with atlas assimilation. This setup leads to an excessive load on the atlantoaxial motion segment, which subsequently becomes unstable. Initially, a reducible atlantoaxial instability was found in these individuals, but this subsequently led to a reducible basilar invagination. This is common in children younger than 14 years. As these children age, the lesion becomes an irreducible basilar invagination. During the phase of reducibility and partial reducibility, a prolific granulation tissue mass crowns the odontoid process in an effort to limit the excursion. This in turn compounds the compression of the cervicomedullary junction. In irreducible basilar invagination, there is an associated horizontally oriented clivus and the abnormal grooving that occurs behind the occipital condyles as a result of the upward migration of the axis vertebra onto the assimilated axis. Thus, these lesions are now completely irreducible. A child who comes for evaluation between 4 and 16 years of age has a better chance of having a reducible atlantoaxial dislocation or reducible basilar invagination than does a 25-year-old individual. Experience shows that a reduced posterior fossa volume reduction can lead to an acquired hindbrain herniation syndrome.[6, 41] The association of hindbrain herniation in this situation is 20% to 35%.[40] An operative procedure that relies strictly on posterior decompression without addressing the potential of instability thus leads to unfortunate results.

Unilateral atlas assimilation may present as torticollis in a young child. This is especially critical with head manipulation under general anesthesia, such as for myringotomy and placement of ear tubes, with the trunk staying in one position and the head being rotated 90 degrees to either side. Thus, it behooves the treating physician to be aware of these problems, especially in children with Klippel-Feil syndrome. A similar situation occurs in children who are prone to atlantoaxial dislocation, such as those with Down syndrome.[3]

The classic triad of Klippel-Feil syndrome consists of a low hairline, a short neck, and a webbed neck, with limitation of neck motion. The other congenital abnormalities described with Klippel-Feil syndrome include cleft face, deafness, high arch palate, and facial palsies.[38, 42–44] Cardiovascular abnormalities include mitral valve disease, ventricular septal defect, coarctation of the aorta, and patent ductus arteriosus; thoracic abnormalities can occur in the form of dysplasia or ectopic lung or rib fusions. Abnormalities of the genitourinary tract occur in 30% of individuals. The most common are unilateral kidney, horseshoe kidney, and ectopic kidney. Bicornuate uterus is a frequent occurrence. It is thus imperative that these abnormalities and the underlying state be recognized early to avoid surprises once surgical therapy has begun.

Basilar Invagination

This is a primary developmental defect implying prolapse of the vertebral column into the skull at the base. It is frequently associated with developmental anomalies of the region, such as occipitalization, assimilation, and blocked vertebra.[3, 13, 14, 30] The common manifestations of neurodysgenesis, such as Chiari I malformation and syringohydromyelia, occur in 25% to 30% of patients with basilar invagination (Fig. 211–5).

The term *basilar invagination* was used by Chamberlain in 1939 as a synonym for platybasia.[2] In addition, *basilar impression* has been used interchangeably with the latter. Basilar impression is an acquired form of basilar invagination secondary to softening of the skull and occurs in diseases such as osteogenesis imperfecta, rickets, hyperparathyroidism, Paget's disease, Hurler's syndrome, and acro-osteolysis (Hajdu-Cheney syn-

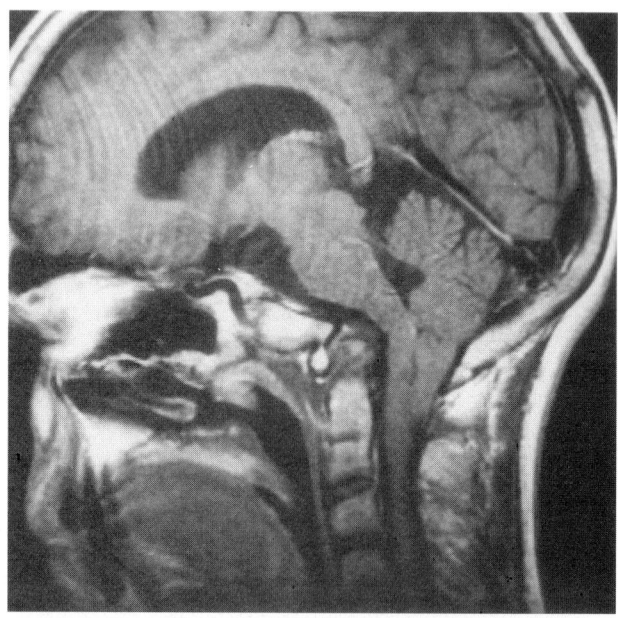

FIGURE 211–5. Midsagittal T1-weighted magnetic resonance imaging scan in 14-year-old boy with headaches, ataxic gait, spastic quadriparesis, and downbeat nystagmus. There is atlas assimilation with basilar invagination, a short clivus, and an abnormal clivus-C1-C2 articulation. The vertical height of the posterior fossa is markedly reduced, and the cerebellar tonsils extend down to the lower border of C2.

drome).[29, 45–51] *Platybasia* refers to an abnormal obtuse basal angle formed by the clivus and the anterior skull base. There are no symptoms or signs attributable to platybasia alone. It is not a measure of basilar invagination, although platybasia may be associated with invagination.[13]

There are two types of basilar invagination. In the ventral variety, there is shortening of the basiocciput so that the clivus is short and horizontally oriented, thus displacing the plane of the foramen magnum in an upward direction compared with the spinal column.[6] In the paramesial type, condylar hypoplasia may be present so that the clivus becomes dorsally displaced into the posterior fossa but may be of normal length.[3] The occipital hypoplasia may be unilateral and leads to torticollis. The distinction between these two types is not clinically rigid, because a mixture often occurs.

Basilar invagination is commonly associated with an abnormal odontoid process invaginating into the posterior fossa. Of significance is the fact that the axis body becomes elongated and the true odontoid process is small.[3, 14] Of greater significance is the abnormal clivus-odontoid articulation. The resultant abnormal clivus-canal angle produces an indentation on the pons, medulla, or cervicomedullary junction in a ventral manner.

The Chiari malformation is associated with basilar invagination in about 25% to 30% of individuals.[3, 40] In this situation, ventral compression of the cervicomedullary junction by the bony abnormality should be relieved by ventral decompression, which must be performed before any posterior surgical procedure. If a posterior procedure is done before relieving the ventral compression, 30% of individuals have an unfavorable outcome. The reason for this poor outcome is that the ventral abnormality acts like a peg, indenting into the pontomedullary or cervicomedullary junction when the patient is positioned for the posterior procedure. In addition, fusion in a flexed position compromises the ability to perform a satisfactory ventral decompression. The ability to reduce the invagination is age related, as previously described for atlas assimilation. The presence of syringohydromyelia with hindbrain herniation and basilar invagination should not sway the neurosurgeon to perform a posterior operative procedure. In most cases, syringohydromyelia disappears once the ventral abnormality has been corrected.

ANOMALIES OF THE ODONTOID PROCESS

Aplasia-Hypoplasia of the Dens

This anomaly has several degrees of expression, so that the rudimentary dens may be present or completely absent.[13] Theoretically, the cruciate ligament is incompetent, leading to atlantoaxial instability. This is quite common in patients with atlas assimilation with failure of segmentation of C2 and C3. In these individuals, the axis body is abnormal, but the dens itself may be hypoplastic. Significant vascular compromise from stretching and distortion of the vertebral arteries has been seen in such lesions.[3, 26] Chronic atlantoaxial dislocation in this situation may result in the formation of granulation tissue at the site of luxation, with compression of the cervicomedullary junction.

Os Odontoideum

Os odontoideum refers to an independent bone cranial to the axis, in the place of the dens. It is not an isolated dens but exists apart from a small hypoplastic dens. Radiographically, an os odontoideum has rounded, smooth cortical borders separated by a variable gap from a small odontoid process.[3, 13] It is usually located in the position of the normal odontoid tip or near the basiocciput in the area of the foramen magnum, where it may fuse with the clivus. The gap between the free ossicle and the axis usually extends above the level of the superior facets of the axis. This leads to incompetence of the cruciate ligament and, subsequently, atlantoaxial instability.

Fielding and Griffin described two types of os odontoideum: the orthotopic variety, in which the ossicle lies in the position of the normal dens and moves in unison with the atlas and the axis vertebrae, and the dystopic variety, in which the ossicle lies near the inferior end of the clivus and fuses with the occipital bone and moves in unison with the clivus (Fig. 211–6).[19]

Evidence favors an unrecognized fracture in the region of the base of the odontoid as the most common cause of os odontoideum.[4, 19] It has been seen in patients who had a recognized complete odontoid process in early childhood and subsequently developed an os

odontoideum, in one of identical twins who had cervical trauma, and in patients with gross ligamentous laxity such as those with Down or Morquio's syndrome.[14, 31]

The biomechanics of os odontoideum must be carefully studied, because it varies. The movement of os odontoideum is individual with each patient and cannot be extrapolated to another. In the dystopic variety, a dorsal compromise of the spinal cord may occur by the forward position of the posterior arch of the atlas in the flexed position, as well as ventral compromise by the odontoid ossicles. The axis may be displaced dorsally in extension and increase the ventral compromise. Thus, each patient should be carefully assessed by dynamic studies in the flexed, extended, and lateral positions. Lateral displacement of the atlantoaxial complex is a frequent finding at the time of operative fixation in such individuals.

Direct pathologic examination of the area at the time of ventral decompressive surgery has shown that an irreducible state may be caused by slippage of the transverse portion of the cruciate ligament beneath the ossicle or even in front of it. In addition, intense granulation proliferation may occur ventral to the bony defect due to repeated luxations. In severe, chronic dislocation, this may become fixed over several years, with severe basilar invagination. At its worst, os odontoideum has significant implications regarding compression of the cervicomedullary junction. It is not uncommon for children with asymptomatic os odontoideum to have severe neurological deficits after minor trauma, such as dental work or sports activities. Thus, all patients with recognizable instability at the craniovertebral junction and associated os odontoideum should undergo stabilization. If a fixed irreducible abnormality exists, decompression should be done first.

Basilar Impression and Bone Softening Syndromes

Basilar impression arises as a consequence of constitutive skeletal disease. These so-called bone softening disorders may be congenital, as in osteogenesis imperfecta, spondyloepiphyseal dysplasia, acro-osteolysis, Hurler's syndrome, and achondroplasia, or they may be associated with Paget's disease, osteomalacia, hyperparathyroidism, and renal rickets.[29, 45–49, 52–54]

In contrast to the acquired forms, in which the underlying metabolic or biochemical abnormalities may be corrected, congenital developmental basilar impression is characteristically relentless in its progression because of the irreversible nature of the genetically determined errors in bone composition. Thus, any therapeutic intervention must be considered palliative, because the fundamental pathology is not addressed. Anatomically and radiographically, there is infolding of the squamous-occipital bone; as a result, the posterior fossa floor becomes elevated, and the margin of foramen magnum curves upward. The basiocciput becomes foreshortened and elevated, with the clivus becoming thinned, truncated, and horizontally oriented,

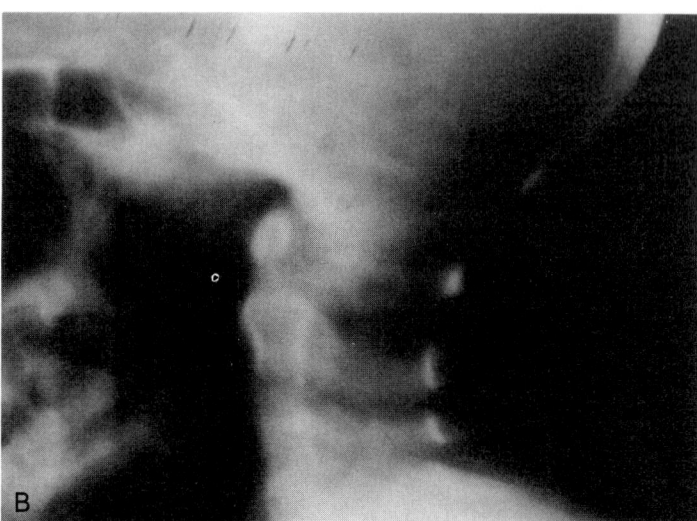

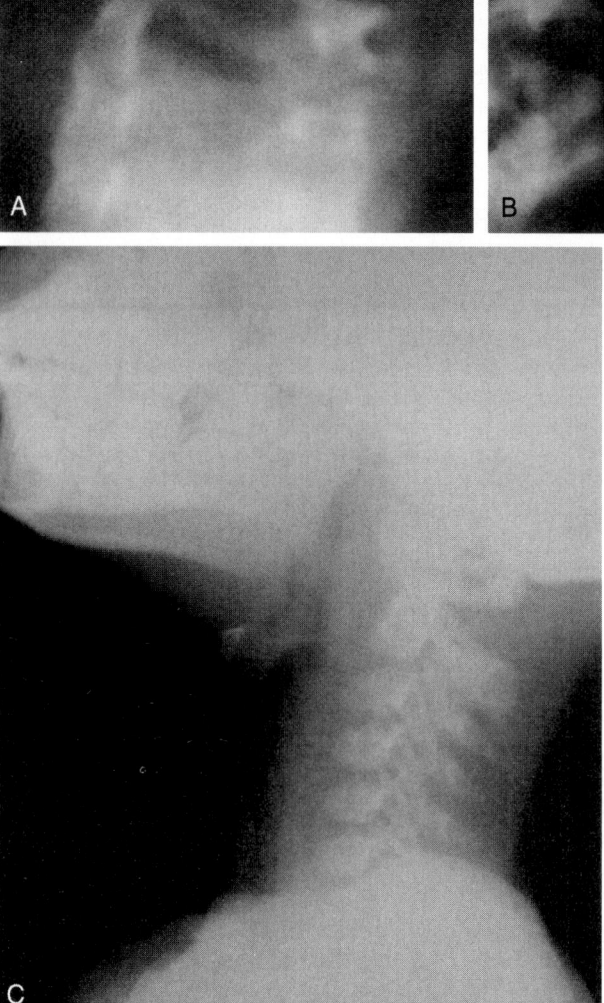

FIGURE 211–6. Composite of craniovertebral junction pluridirectional tomograms in the frontal plane *(A)* and midline sagittal plane *(B)*. This 13-year-old girl presented severely quadriparetic after a minor fall. There is a dystopic os odontoideum. The ossicle has smooth, rounded cortical borders, and there is a gap separating it from a small, hypoplastic dens. It is attached to the clivus. Lateral radiograph *(C)* of the same patient at age 4 years following a rear-ending motor vehicle accident. Note the atlantoaxial dislocation. She was treated with Minerva cast immobilization.

creating an obtuse basal and acute craniovertebral angle. Anteroposteriorly, the petrous portion of the temporal bone is also deformed. These changes ultimately permit the clivus-atlas-odontoid complex to assume an abnormally rostral location within the foramen magnum, further restricting the space within the posterior fossa (Fig. 211–7).

The rostral extent of invagination dictates the attendant neurological manifestations. The brainstem is elevated and splayed over the ventrally situated clivus-atlas-odontoid complex. In addition to causing mechanical compression, this acts as a fulcrum by which traction is applied to the caudal brainstem and the rostral cervical spinal cord, producing bulbar dysfunc-

tion and myelopathy.[6] The lower cranial nerves are stretched and distorted as the brainstem is forced upward, resulting in characteristic lower cranial nerve palsies.[50] Cerebellar involvement may be primary, caused by compression from the foramen magnum infolding, or secondary, caused by hindbrain herniation. This acquired form of hindbrain herniation may lead to syringohydromyelia formation. Neurological dysfunction may thus be coupled with hydrocephalus, syringohydromyelia, and hindbrain herniation.

The pathogenesis of secondary invagination and osteochondroplasias remains obscure.[53] Certainly there is inherent bone fragility, with the load-bearing chondrocranium unable to maintain the weight of the cranium

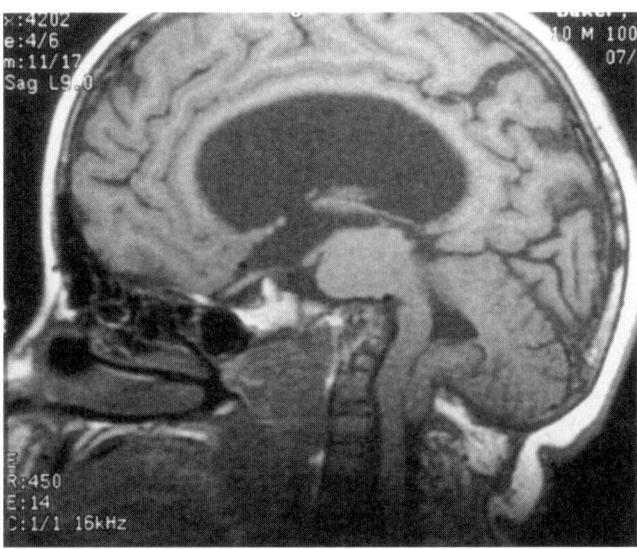

FIGURE 211–7. Midsagittal T1-weighted magnetic resonance imaging scan of the head and neck in an 11-year-old with osteogenesis imperfecta. There is severe basilar impression, secondary aqueductal stenosis with hydrocephalus, a horizontal clivus, and hindbrain herniation with marked diminution in the vertical height of the posterior fossa.

and its contents. Thus, there is deformation of both the skull base and the cranial vault. It is possible that recurrent microfractures in the region of the foramen magnum underlie the progressive infolding of the posterior skull base.[54] At surgery, it is not uncommon to find proliferation of bone composing the skull base, with a finding reminiscent of exuberant callus. The high metabolic activity of the reactive bone is confirmed by radioactive bone scanning and indicates chronic active bone remodeling. Osteogenesis imperfecta is noted for its wide clinical and genetic variability; it is surprising that, given the high tensile strength and load-bearing properties of bone in these syndromes, basilar impression is not more common. The various types of osteogenesis imperfecta show different clinical manifestations. Infants born with type II osteogenesis imperfecta have the most severe bone fragility and a high propensity to fracture because of reduction of type I collagen synthesis. Hence, neonates with this variant rarely survive past infancy. In the other subtypes, abnormalities of the atlas and axis region with upper cervical buckling lead to quadriparesis. In young individuals with basilar impression or upper cervical abnormalities, I recommend a custom-fitted modified Minerva brace to "shore up" the skull and prevent progression of the secondary invagination. This must be documented with MRI.

Surgical intervention, regardless of the approach, was well tolerated in my series, with a 100% fusion rate. Neural decompression was accomplished in 32 individuals. All these symptomatic patients improved with good fusion. However, although functional improvement persisted, basilar invagination progressed in 80% of patients according to imaging criteria, despite successful fusion. In all these patients, the entire fusion mass migrated rostrally as a result of further squa-

mous-occipital and petrous bone infolding.[3, 6] Additionally, the posterior fusion mass tends to act as a fulcrum on which the lever arm of the anterior skull base turns, thus exacerbating ventral compression. In all patients who were braced with a Minerva orthosis, the brace provided ventral cranial base stability, thus affording symptomatic relief and preventing further skeletal deformity.

Skeletal Dysplasias

Skeletal dysplasias are divided into five large categories: osteochondral dysplasias, dysostosis, idiopathic osteolysis, chromosomal aberrations, and primary metabolic abnormalities.[47, 54] The osteochondral dysplasias and dysostosis account for the largest and most complex entities.

Osteochondral dysplasias are defined as abnormalities of cartilage or bone growth in development. This category includes achondrogenesis, thanatophoric dysplasia, chondrodysplasia punctata (Conradi-Hünermann syndrome), achondroplasia, dystrophic dysplasia, metatrophic dysplasia, spondyloepiphyseal dysplasia, Kniest dysplasia, cleidocranial dysplasia, and multiple epiphyseal dysplasias.

The dysostoses are defined as malformations of individual bones singly or in combination. The category includes Crouzon's, Apert's, and Carpenter's syndromes with vertebral defects, as well as Sprengel's deformity and Klippel-Feil syndrome.

The subcategory of idiopathic osteolysis includes the diagnosis of spondyloepiphyseal dysplasia tarda, fibrous dysplasia, neurofibromatosis, osteogenesis imperfecta, and multicentric forms such as the Hajdu-Cheney type.

The primary metabolic and chromosomal abnormalities are numerous. Metabolic abnormalities include problems with calcium or phosphorus metabolism, such as rickets and pseudohypoparathyroidism. Abnormalities of calcium and phosphorus metabolism lead to bone softening and a secondary form of invagination. This may be paramesial, which is common with achondroplasia, in which case the sagittal diameter of the foramen magnum is preserved and the transverse diameter is markedly reduced (Fig. 211–8). In addition, an inward bending of the exoccipital bone results in further invagination and creation of a dural shelf, which compresses the dorsal cervicomedullary junction. Thus, in these syndromes, posterior decompression is necessary with a duraplasty.

Atlantoaxial instability occurs with increasing incidence in the skeletal dysplasias. Sleep apnea is a major symptom, as is progressive spastic quadriparesis. There is an inward bending of the posterior arch of the atlas, adding to the paramesial foramen magnum stenosis. Before embarking on therapy, one must ascertain that proper attention has been given to hydrocephalus, if present.

Spondyloepiphyseal dysplasia is a complex disorder when atlantoaxial instability is encountered in infancy. One approach is to brace the infant with a custom-built orthosis until definitive surgical treatment can be

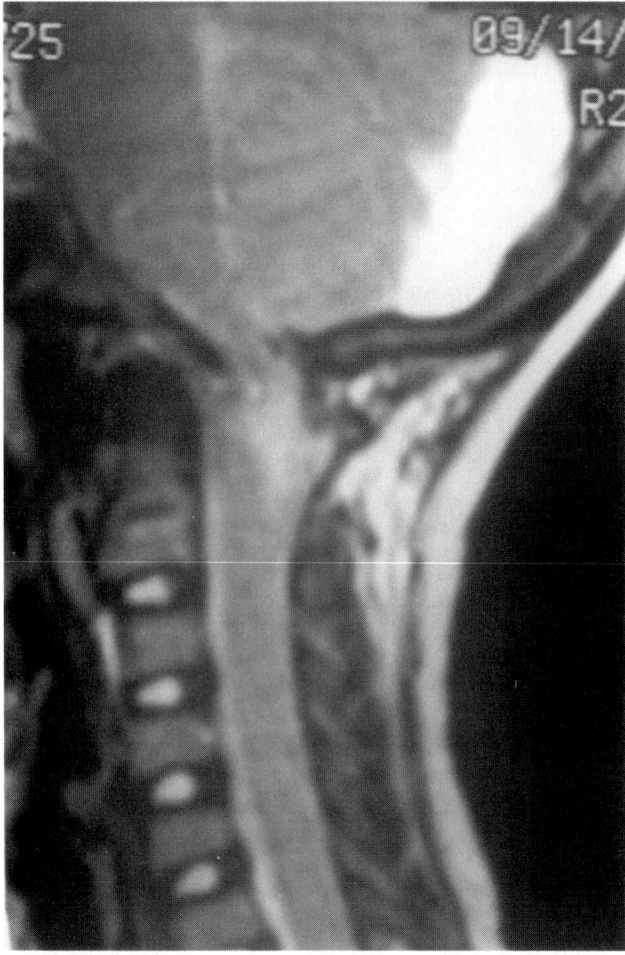

FIGURE 211–8. Midsagittal T2-weighted magnetic resonance imaging scan of the craniovertebral region in a 4-year-old with achondroplasia. There is stenosis at the foramen magnum with a dorsal bony and dural shelf indenting into the cervicomedullary junction.

performed sometime between age 2 and 4 years. When atlantoaxial instability occurs at a later age, the treatment is as previously outlined.

Mucopolysaccharidosis

The mucopolysaccharidoses are primary metabolic abnormalities of complex carbohydrate metabolism. These are inheritable storage diseases often manifested by dwarfism, mental retardation, macrocephaly, corneal clouding, and skeletal dysplasia. Generalized ligamentous laxity is thought to contribute to the atlantoaxial luxation described in a variety of mucopolysaccharidoses. Death commonly occurs from Morquio's syndrome (mucopolysaccharidosis type IV) by age 7, secondary to cervical myelopathy as well as respiratory system effects and resultant hypoxia. Holzgreve and coworkers described atlantoaxial instability in a review of 13 patients with type IV mucopolysaccharidosis.[51]

REFERENCES

1. Gladstone J, Erickson-Powell W: Manifestation of occipital vertebra and fusion of atlas with occipital bone. J Anat Physiol 49: 190–199, 1914–1915.
2. Chamberlain WE: Basilar impression (platybasia). Yale J Biol Med 11:487, 1938–1939.
3. Menezes AH: Congenital and acquired abnormalities of the craniovertebral junction. In Youmans JR (ed): Neurological Surgery, 4th ed. Philadelphia, WB Saunders, 1995, pp 1035–1089.
4. Goel VK, Clark CR, Gallaes K, et al: Movement-rotation relationships of the ligamentous occipito-atlanto-axial complex. J Biomech 21:678, 1988.
5. Schiff DCM, Parke WW: The arterial blood supply of the odontoid process (dens). Anat Rec 172:399–400, 1972.
6. Menezes AH: Developmental and acquired abnormalities of the craniovertebral junction. In Crockard A, Hayward R, Hoff J (eds): Neurosurgery: The Scientific Basis of Clinical Practice, 3rd ed. London, Blackwell Scientific, 2000, pp 1120–1145.
7. Parke WW, Rothman RH, Brown MD: The pharyngovertebral veins: An anatomical rationale for Grisel's syndrome. J Bone Joint Surg Am 66:568, 1984.
8. Grisel P: Enucleation de l'atlas et torticollis nasopharyngien. Presse Med 38:50–56, 1930.
9. Christ B, Wilting J: From somites to vertebral column. Ann Anat 174:23–32, 1992.
10. Dietrich S, Kessel M: The vertebral column. In Thorogood P (ed): Embryos, Genes and Birth Defects. Chichester, England, Wiley, 1997, pp 281–302.
11. Kessel M, Gruss P: Homeotic transformations of murine vertebrae and concomitant alteration of Hox codes induced by retinoic acid. Cell 67:89–104, 1991.
12. Keynes RJ, Stern C: Mechanisms of vertebrate segmentation. Development 103:413–429, 1988.
13. VonTorklus D, Gehle W: The upper cervical spine: Regional anatomy, pathology and traumatology. In Georg Thieme Verlag (ed): A Systemic Radiological Atlas and Textbook. New York, Grune & Stratton, 1972, pp 1–99.
14. Stevens JM, Chong WK, Barber C, et al: A new appraisal of abnormalities of the odontoid process associated with atlantoaxial subluxation and neurological disability. Brain 117(Pt 1):133–148, 1994.
15. Koseki H, Wallin J, Wilting J, et al: A role of Pax-1 as a mediator of notochordal signals during the dorsoventral specification of vertebrae. Development 119:649–660, 1993.
16. Lufkin T, Mark M, Hart CP, et al: Homeotic transformation of the occipital bones of the skull by ectopic expression of a homeobox gene. Nature 359:835–841, 1992.
17. Condie BG, Capecchi MR: Mice homozygous for a targeted disruption of Hoxd-3 (Hox-4.1) exhibit anterior transformations of the first and second cervical vertebrae, the atlas and the axis. Development 119:579–595, 1993.
18. Kimura Y, Matsunami H, Inoue T, et al: Cadherin-11 expressed in association with mesenchymal morphogenesis in the head, somite and limb bud of early mouse embryos. Dev Biol 169:347–358, 1995.
19. Fielding JW, Griffin PP: Os odontoideum: An acquired lesion. J Bone Joint Surg Am 56:187–190, 1974.
20. Panjabi MM, Dvorák J, Duranceau J, et al: Three-dimensional movements of the upper cervical spine. Spine 13:726–730, 1988.
21. Panjabi MM, Dvorák J, Crisco JJ III, et al: Flexion, extension and lateral bending of the upper cervical spine in response to alar ligament transections. J Spinal Disord 4:157–167, 1991.
22. Werne S: Studies in spontaneous atlas dislocation: The craniovertebral joints. Acta Orthop Scand Suppl 23:11–83, 1957.
23. Fielding JW, Cochron GB, Lawsing JF III, Hohl M: Tears of the transverse ligament of the atlas: A clinical and biomechanical study. J Bone Joint Surg Am 56:1683–1691, 1974.
24. Dickman CA, Crawford NR, Paramore CG: Biomechanical characteristics of C1-2 cable fixations. J Neurosurg 85:316–322, 1996.
25. Selecki BR: The effects of rotation of the atlas on the axis: Experimental work. Med J Aust 1:1012, 1969.
26. Bhatnagar M, Sponseller PD, Carroll C IV, et al: Pediatric atlantoaxial instability presenting as cerebral and cerebellar infarcts. J Pediatr Orthop 11:103–107, 1991.
27. Miyachi S, Okamura K, Watanabe M, et al: Cerebellar stroke due to vertebral artery occlusion after cervical spine trauma: Two case reports. Spine 19:83–88, 1994.
28. Okawara S, Nibbelink D: Vertebral artery occlusion following hyperextension and rotation of the head. Stroke 5:640–642, 1974.

29. Blaw ME, Langer LO: Spinal cord compression in Morquio-Brailsford's disease. J Pediatr 74:593–600, 1969.
30. McRae DL, Barnum AS: Occipitalization of the atlas. AJR Am J Roentgenol 70:23–46, 1953.
31. Burke SW, French HA, Roberts E: Chronic atlantoaxial instability in Down's syndrome. J Bone Joint Surg Am 67:1356–1360, 1985.
32. McGregor M: The significance of certain measurements of the skull in the diagnosis of basilar impression. Br J Radiol 21:171–181, 1948.
33. Wackenheim A: Radiologic diagnosis of congenital forms, intermittent forms and progressive forms of stenosis of the spinal canal of the level of the atlas. Acta Radiol Diagn (Stockh) 9:481–486, 1969.
34. Wetzel FT, LaRocca H: Grisel's syndrome: A review. Clin Orthop Rel Res 240:141–152, 1989.
35. Wilson BC, Jarvis BL, Handon RC: Nontraumatic subluxation of the atlantoaxial joint: Grisel's syndrome. Ann Otol Rhinol Laryngol 96:705, 1987.
36. Tisher J, Martel W: Dislocation of the atlas in mongolism. Radiology 84:904–906, 1965.
37. American Academy of Pediatrics Committee on Sports Medicine: Atlantoaxial instability in Down's syndrome. Pediatrics 74:152, 1984.
38. Msall ME, Reese ME, DiGaudio K, et al: Symptomatic atlantoaxial instability associated with medical and rehabilitative procedures in children with Down syndrome. Pediatrics 85:447–449, 1990.
39. Grob D, Crisco JJ III, Panjabi MM, et al: Biomechanical evaluation of four different posterior atlantoaxial fixation techniques. Spine 17:480–490, 1992.
40. Menezes AH: Primary craniovertebral anomalies and the hindbrain herniation syndrome (Chiari I): Data base analysis. Pediatr Neurosurg 23:260–269, 1995.
41. Marin-Padilla M, Marin-Padilla T: Morphogenesis of experimentally induced Arnold-Chiari malformation. J Neurol Sci 50:29–55, 1981.
42. Palant DI, Carter BL: Klippel-Feil syndrome and deafness. Am J Disabled Child 123:218–221, 1972.
43. Pueschel SM, Scola F: Atlantoaxial instability in individuals with Down's syndrome: Epidemiologic, radiographic and clinical studies. Pediatrics 80:555, 1987.
44. Müller F, O'Rahilly R: Occipitocervical segmentation in staged human embryos. J Anat 185:251–258, 1994.
45. Aryanpur J, Hurko O, Francomano C, et al: Craniocervical decompression for cervicomedullary compression in pediatric patients with achondroplasia. J Neurosurg 73:375, 1990.
46. Cheney WD: Acro-osteolysis. AJR Am J Roentgenol 94:595, 1965.
47. Dubousset J: Cervical abnormalities in osteochondroplasia. Basic Life Sci 48:207, 1988.
48. Gertner JM, Root L: Osteogenesis imperfecta. Orthop Clin North Am 21:151, 1990.
49. Hajdu N, Kauntze R: Cranioskeletal dysplasia. Br J Radiol 21:42, 1948.
50. Harkey HL, Crockard HA, Stevens JM, et al: The operative management of basilar impression in osteogenesis imperfecta. Neurosurgery 27:782, 1990.
51. Holzgreve W, Grope H, VonFigwrak E: Morquio syndrome: Clinical findings in 11 patients with mucopolysaccharidosis type IVA and two with mucopolysaccharidosis type IVP. Hum Genet 57:360–365, 1981.
52. Fremion AS, Garg BP, Kalsbeck J: Apnea as the sole manifestation of cord compression in achondroplasia. J Pediatr 104:398–401, 1984.
53. Hecht JT, Butler IJ: Neurological morbidity associated with achondroplasia. J Child Neurol 5:84, 1990.
54. Ryken TC, Menezes AH: Cervicomedullary compression in achondroplasia. J Neurosurg 81:43–48, 1994.

Chiari Malformations

W. JERRY OAKES ■ R. SHANE TUBBS

The four traditional types of Chiari malformations represent various clinical and anatomic processes that entail varying degrees of involvement of the rhombencephalon (hindbrain). Chiari types I, II, and III involve varying degrees of herniation of rhombencephalic derivatives out of the posterior fossa. Chiari type IV malformations involve cerebellar hypoplasia or aplasia, with no herniation of the hindbrain. At present, there is no consensus on how to define, treat, or label an etiologic process for the pathologic term *Chiari malformation*. Although the Chiari classification is helpful in categorizing patients, this scheme probably does not represent a precise continuum of the same disease and does not provide the classification needed to compartmentalize all forms of hindbrain hernias encountered.

HISTORY

Hans Chiari (1851–1916) was an Austrian professor of pathology at German University in Prague, Czechoslovakia. In 1891 and 1896 he published two reports in which he analyzed data collected from more than 40 postmortem examinations of patients with hindbrain malformations.[1, 2] Chiari malformations I, II, and III were coined in the earlier work, and Chiari IV malformations were added in the 1896 publication. Chiari defined his malformations as follows: Type I malformations have cerebellar tonsils that lie below the plane of the foramen magnum. Type I malformations are occasionally associated with mild degrees of fourth ventricular and medullary elongation. Type II malformations, also referred to as Arnold-Chiari malformations, are almost exclusively seen in patients with myelodysplasia and involve the caudal descent of the cerebellar vermis, brainstem, and fourth ventricle below the plane of the foramen magnum. Type III malformations are posterior fossa encephaloceles containing hindbrain structures that herniate through an upper cervical spina bifida. Type IV malformations are cerebellar hypoplasia or aplasia with tentorial hypoplasia.

Chiari is not the only person historically associated with these anomalies. In 1883, John Cleland (1835–1925), a professor of anatomy in Glasgow, Scotland, described hindbrain hernia in one postmortem examination of a patient with myelodysplasia.[3] In 1894, Julius A. Arnold (1835–1915), a professor of pathologic anatomy at Heidelberg, Germany, also described a single myelodysplastic patient with associated hindbrain herniation.[3] Another historical citing of hindbrain herniation in a myelodysplastic individual is found in *Observationes Medicae*, written by the famous Dutch physician and anatomist Nicholas Tulp (1593–1674).[3] Although the names Arnold and Cleland are occasionally added to Chiari's in describing what is currently termed a *Chiari II malformation*, it is more justified to use only Chiari's name and classification method, considering his more detailed analysis and larger group of patients. Table 212–1 summarizes the definitions of Chiari malformations I through IV.

FINDINGS

Chiari I

The Chiari I malformation was originally described as caudal displacement of the cerebellar tonsils to a level below the plane of the foramen magnum. Today, mi-

TABLE 212–1 ■ **Definitions of Chiari Malformations I–IV**

Chiari Type I

Caudal herniation of the cerebellar tonsils >5 mm below the foramen magnum
Generally not associated with caudal descent of the brainstem
Hydrocephalus is uncommon

Chiari Type II

Caudal herniation of the cerebellar vermis, brainstem, and fourth ventricle
Many other intracranial anomalies seen
Almost all have myelomeningocele and hydrocephalus
Many have syringohydromyelia

Chiari Type III

Occipital encephalocele with many of the same intracranial anomalies seen with the type II malformation

Chiari Type IV

Cerebellar aplasia or hypoplasia, with aplasia of the tentorium cerebelli

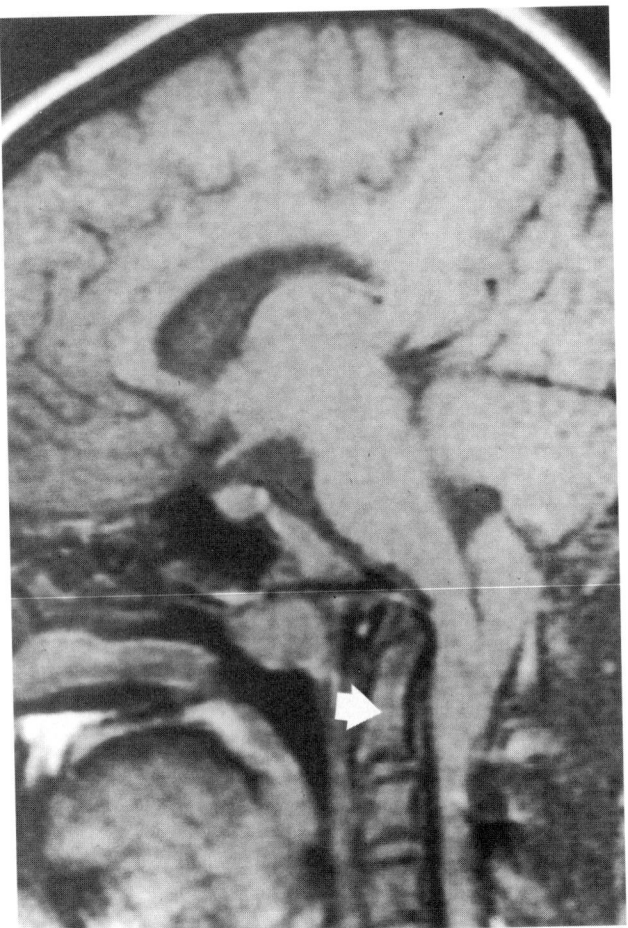

FIGURE 212–1. Midsagittal T1-weighted magnetic resonance imaging (MRI) scan illustrating a retroflexed odontoid process *(arrow).*

tal keels, and remnants of the proatlas, such as an accessory occipital condyle.[7]

SPINE

Klippel-Feil deformity and atlantoaxial assimilation are two of the more common spinal defects in type I malformations. Other occasional findings are retroflexion of the odontoid process (Fig. 212–1) and thickening of the ligamentum flavum. Another common entity seen in Chiari I malformations is scoliosis. This is usually due to an underlying syrinx and is most likely to be a single curve with its convexity to the left (Fig. 212–2). This levoscoliosis is contrasted to the right convexity seen in the most cases of idiopathic scoliosis.

VENTRICLE AND CISTERN

Ventricular anatomy, other than an occasionally elongated fourth ventricle, is relatively normal in type I malformations. Hydrocephalus has been described in 3% to 10% of this subgroup.[8, 9] It should be noted that

grations up to 7 mm may be considered within the normal range. Generally, more than 5 mm of caudal descent of the tonsils is considered suspicious for a Chiari type I malformation. There are other associated findings seen surgically, radiographically, and at postmortem in Chiari I patients. These findings are described and categorized here according to their anatomic location.

SKULL

Basilar skull and craniocervical junction anomalies are seen in approximately 50% of patients with Chiari I malformations.[4] It is now appreciated that the supraocciput and exocciput are underdeveloped in many patients with Chiari I malformations, and there is shortening of the supraocciput. The clivus is also shorter, with a larger than normal foramen magnum, although in some diseases involving Chiari I malformation, the foramen magnum may actually be smaller than normal.[5, 6] The posterior fossa is smaller and shallower in many patients with this type of malformation. Other basilar skull abnormalities are empty sellae, clival concavities, platybasia, basilar impression, midline occipi-

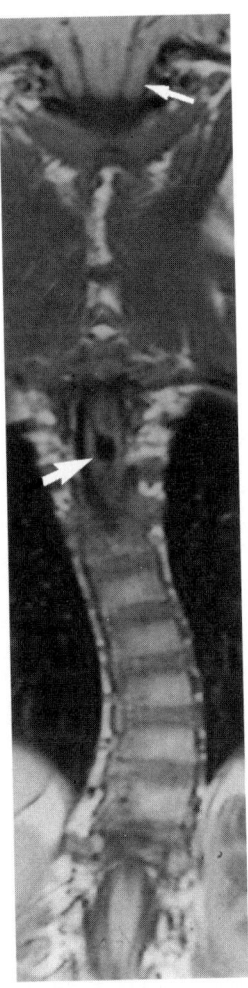

FIGURE 212–2. Coronal T1-weighted MRI scan demonstrating tonsillar herniation in a Chiari type I malformation *(small arrow).* One can also see a small cervicothoracic syrinx *(large arrow)* and a moderate degree of levoscoliosis.

in many of these patients, the retrocerebellar cerebro-spinal fluid (CSF) spaces are obliterated or diminished.

MENINGES

The slope of the tentorium cerebelli is elevated in type I malformations. In addition, one routinely sees thickening of the arachnoid at the level of the foramen magnum. This may be accompanied by a constricting dural band. Also described are veils of arachnoid that obstruct the fourth ventricular outlet. Another thickened and constricting band of dura is occasionally found at the level of the posterior arch of the atlas.

SPINAL CORD

The prominent spinal cord finding in type I malformations is a syrinx. The term *syrinx* was first used by Charles-Prosper Ollivier d'Angers (1796–1845). Previously, a colleague of d'Angers, Antoine Portal (1742–1832), had described postmortem specimens with a dilated cavity within the cord as "dans lequel on eût pu introduire une grosse plume à écrire," or a cavity in which a writing quill could have been introduced. Using magnetic resonance imaging (MRI), cavitation of the cord has been reported in 50% to 75% of patients.[4, 10–12] These syringes are usually found in the lower cervical and upper thoracic spinal cord. Holocord syringes are also found (Fig. 212–3). There is routinely a segment of cord that is spared from cavitation between the fourth ventricle and the beginning of the syrinx in the cervical cord. Sagittal images often demonstrate septations of the syrinx within the cord (see Fig. 212–3).

BRAIN

With Chiari I malformations, the brain is generally free from anomalies other than the tonsillar herniation. In rare instances, the midbrain, pons, and medulla have been noted to be elongated, with occasional medullary kinking or flattening. The herniated tonsils often lose their folial pattern and become atrophic from chronic compression. They are usually described as peglike or pointed and are often asymmetric (Fig 212–4).

Chiari II

The type II malformation involves vermian herniation with caudal descent of the brainstem and fourth ventricle. Unlike the Chiari I malformation, which has relatively few associated findings, the type II malformation has many anomalies that are commonly seen in conjuction with the hindbrain herniation. These anomalies also occur in various other pathologic conditions, but when seen in combination, they are highly indicative of a Chiari II malformation. Type II malformations are seen in almost all patients with myelomeningocele, although there are occasional references to type II deformities without myelodysplasia.[13]

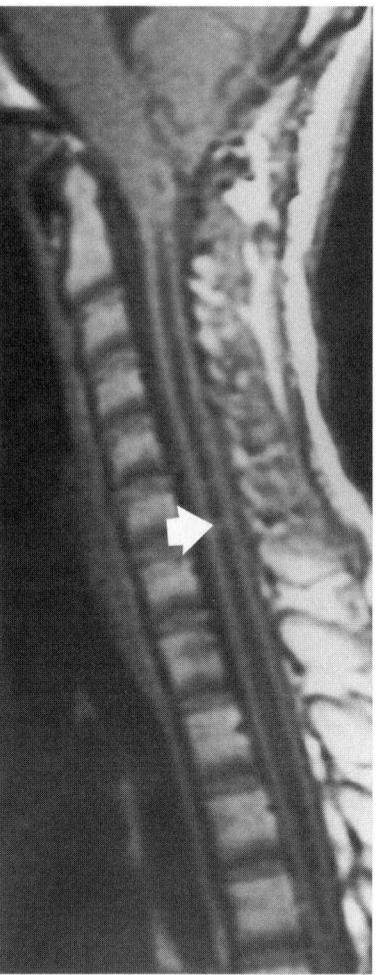

FIGURE 212–3. Midsagittal MRI scan showing a holocord syrinx in a patient with no myelomeningocele but caudal descent of the brainstem (Chiari type 1.5). Also note the septations or haustra, tending to compartmentalize the syrinx *(arrow)*.

SKULL

The calvaria of many patients with the type II malformation takes on a "beaten copper" appearance, termed *craniolacunia* or *lückenschädel*. This phenomenon decreases with age, and both the inner and outer tables may be affected. Lückenschädel, when present, is more prominent over the upper half of the calvaria (Fig. 212–5). When seen on ultrasonographic studies, the frontal bone may be scalloped anteriorly; this is termed the *lemon sign*.[14] Another scalloping phenomenon is seen on the posterior medial aspect of the petrous bones and jugular tubercles. This scalloping effect foreshortens the internal acoustic meatus. The type II malformation, like the type I, has an enlarged foramen magnum that opens superiorly into a flattened posterior fossa floor. The opisthion may be notched, and cranioschisis is occasionally seen. The posterior fossa also tends to be smaller. The basioccipital portion of the clivus is increased in its concavity, with partial or full obliteration of the diploic space. The inion is normally lower in patients with type II malformations. There may be a midline occipital keel. Finally, basilar

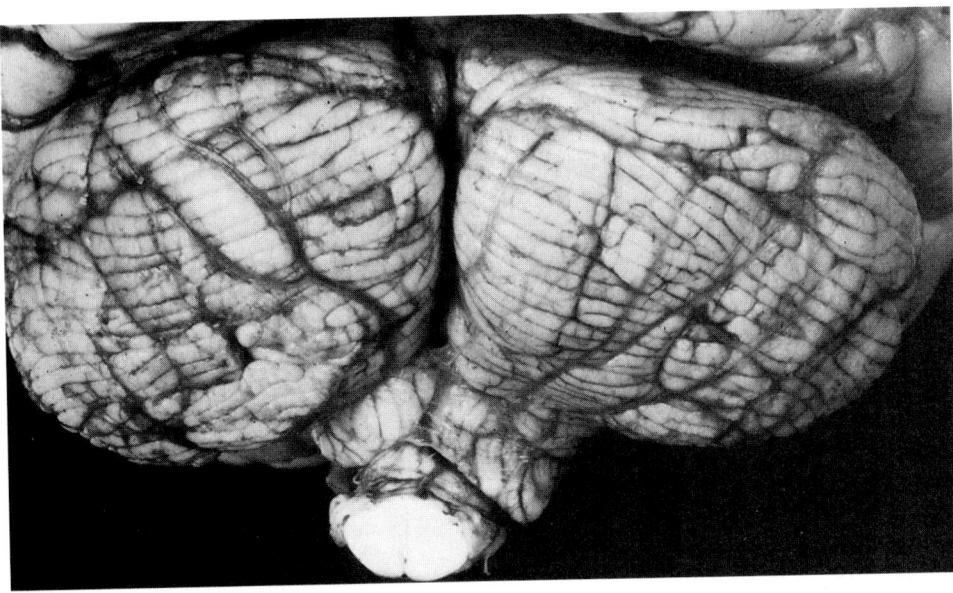

FIGURE 212–4. Posterior view of a postmortem specimen of a Chiari type I malformation. Notice the asymmetry of the tonsillar descent.

impression and assimilation of the atlas are sometimes encountered, but not as often as with type I malformations.

SPINE

Anomalies that may be seen in the spine, specifically the cervical spine, include an enlarged cervical canal, scalloping of the odontoid process, incomplete posterior arch of C1, and Klippel-Feil deformity.[15]

VENTRICLE AND CISTERN

Hydrocephalus is seen in approximately 90% of patients with Chiari II malformations.[16] Intrinsic malformations of the chambers may include lateral ventricles that are asymmetric between left and right sides and have pointed frontal horns. There may be medial pointing of the inferior margins of the floor of the lateral ventricles near the foramen of Monro. Also noted is lateral pointing of the frontal horns superior to the head of the caudate. Additional lateral pointing may be observed near the foramen of Monro and is directed toward the striothalamic groove posterior and inferior to the head of the caudate. The atria and occipital horns may be disproportionately enlarged; this is termed *colpocephaly.* The third ventricle is curious because of two possible diverticula—one anterior diverticulum known as the *shark tooth deformity,*[16] and one posterior diverticulum. The commissure of Meynert is occasionally seen bridging the floor of the third ventricle and connecting nonthalamic deep gray matter on either side.[17] The fourth ventricle is typically small, flat, and elongated, with lateral recesses that are not well defined (Fig. 212–6). The choroid plexus of the fourth ventricle usuallly maintains its embryologic location outside the ventricle near its caudal pole. The inferior medullary velum may be absent. Finally, the foramen of Magendie may be absent or have a cyst associated with it. The cisterns of a type II malformation may be enlarged around the cerebellum and anterolateral to the pons.

MENINGES

The tentorium cerebelli is usually widened, heart- or V-shaped, low-lying, and hypoplastic. There can be large venous lakes between its leaves, especially near the foramen magnum. The incisura is elongated in the sagittal plane. The low-lying tentorium results in a vertical straight sinus (see Fig. 212–6). The low tentorium also brings the torcular Herophili and lateral sinuses close to the foramen magnum. The falx cerebri may be fenestrated or hypoplastic. The less developed portion is generally found anteriorly. The leptomenin-

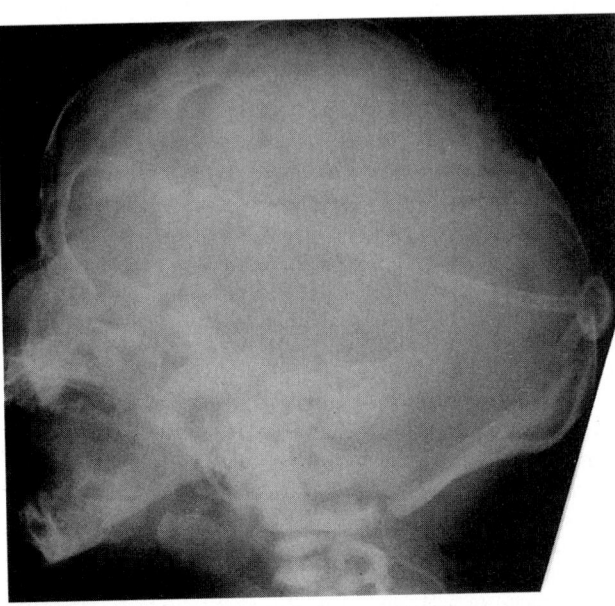

FIGURE 212–5. Lateral radiograph of the skull of a child with Chiari type II malformation demonstrating craniolacunia, which is more prominent in the frontal bone. Note the ventriculoperitoneal shunt in place.

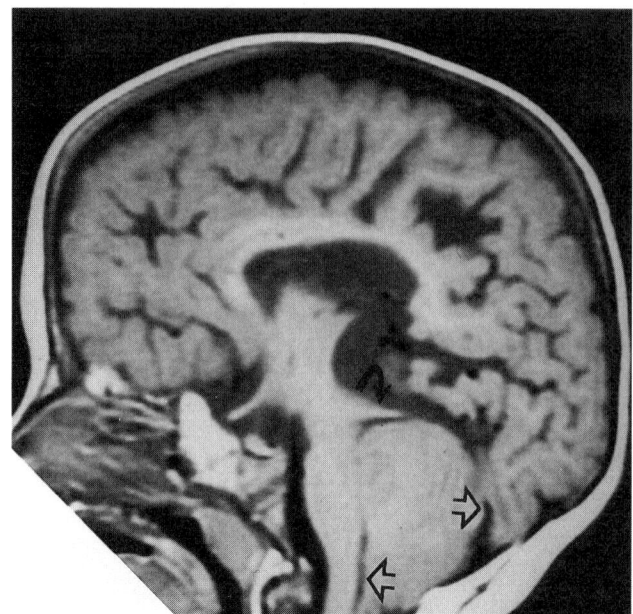

FIGURE 212–6. Midsagittal T1-weighted MRI scan demonstrating tectal beaking *(curved arrow)* and a vertically oriented straight sinus *(right facing arrow)*. An elongated and narrowed fourth ventricle is seen *(left facing arrow)*. A small cerebellum is also evident.

ges are thickened and vascular at the level of the foramen magnum. Occasionally, arachnoid cysts are seen anterior to the upper cervical cord. In addition, the most cephalad dentate ligaments may be thickened.

SPINAL CORD

Some aspects of the Chiari type II malformation are seen in almost all patients with myelomeningocele. In approximately 6%, there is an associated split cord anomaly.[18] The reported incidence of syringohydromyelia in type II malformations has a wide range of 20% to 95%.[19] Huge exophytic syringes may be found in association with the cord. These thin-walled structures have been confused with true arachnoid cysts.[20] Grossly, the cervical spinal cord is shortened and displaced caudally. Histologically, there are reduced neuronal counts in the upper cervical cord and a reduction in myelinization, especially in the corticospinal tracts.

TELENCEPHALON

There may be complete or partial agenesis of the corpus callosum and partial or complete absence of the septum pellucidum, especially anterior to the foramen of Monro. The anterior commissure is usually prominent. There is polygyria, with no anomalies of the histologic layering of the cerebral cortex.[21] There can be obliteration of the longitudinal fissure, allowing for interdigitation of the occipital and parietal lobes. Radiographically, this is termed *Chinese lettering* (Fig. 212–7). There may be partial or complete agenesis of the olfactory tract and bulb. The cingulate gyrus may be absent. The head of the caudate nucleus is generally prominent. Additionally, heterotopic gray matter con-

sisting of neurons separated from the cortex by bands of white matter and from the ventricle by ependyma may bulge into the ventricles. This can give the internal aspect of the ventricles a granular appearance.

DIENCEPHALON

Massa intermedia (interthalamic adhesion) is more frequently encountered in patients with type II malformations than in the general population. It is routinely enlarged in 75% to 90% of individuals with type II deformities.[17] The massa is also anteriorly displaced. The hypothalamus can be elevated. Both the pineal gland and the habenular commissure may be elongated.

MESENCEPHALON

The midbrain is typically elongated, with a shortened quadrigeminal plate. There can also be fusion of the colliculi to form a single peak. This is termed *tectal beaking* and is usually contributed to predominantly by the inferior colliculi (see Fig. 212–6). The aqueduct of Sylvius may be stenotic, stretched, posteriorly kinked, laterally compressed, or forked. Histologically, the mesencephalic tegmental nuclei may have varying degrees of dysgenesis. Cranial nerve nuclei can be malformed.

METENCEPHALON

The cerebellum is grossly smaller in the type II malformation and may tower above the tentorium (Fig. 212–8). This towered portion may appear bullet-shaped. The vermis, with or without the tonsil, is herniated

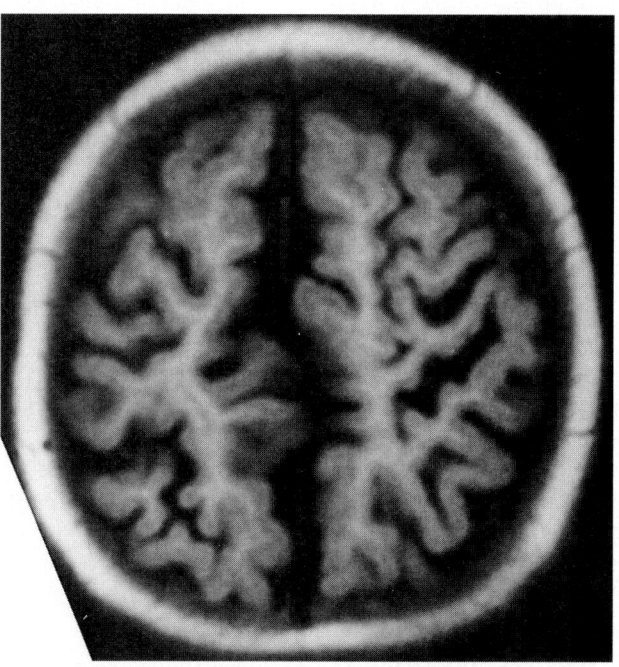

FIGURE 212–7. Axial MRI scan of a child with Chiari type II malformation and hypoplasia of the falx cerebri. Notice the interdigitation of the parietal lobes, known as *Chinese lettering*.

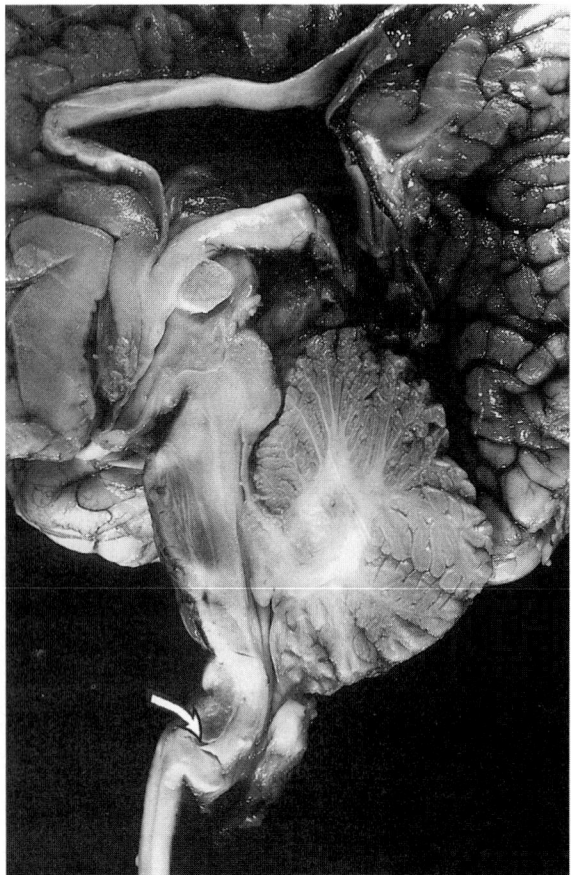

FIGURE 212–8. Postmortem specimen of a Chiari type II malformation illustrating the classic medullary kink *(arrow)*. The cerebellum can also be seen "towering" above the midbrain. The corpus callosum is hypoplastic posteriorly.

through the foramen magnum. There may be dysplasia with absent folia. The cerebellum is generally displaced laterally, and this can allow the lower cranial nerves to traverse its folia as they travel toward their respective foramina. The overall appearance of the cerebellum is curved, producing the banana sign, which is appreciated on ultrasonography.[14] The lateral cerebellar edges may touch anterior to the brainstem and basilar artery; this is known as cerebellar inversion (Fig. 212–9). Also noted are cerebellar heterotopias. Histologically, there may be reduced cell counts with dysplastic deep gray matter. The herniated tail of the cerebellum may be covered dorsally with ependyma.

The pons is elongated and flattened. There may also be indentations on the ventral pontine surface. This may be from a caudally displaced vertebral artery or from the anterior rim of the foramen magnum. The pontomedullary junction may be difficult to distinguish. Basal pontine nuclei may be dysplastic. Nuclei of the pontine tegmentum, along with cranial nerve nuclei, may also be dysplastic.

MYELENCEPHALON

The medulla oblongata may be elongated and flattened in the sagittal plane; this shape may be interpreted as

trumpet-like on imaging. A protuberance is usually seen just caudal to the gracile and cuneate tubercles in up to 70% of individuals. It usually occurs between C2 and C4. The protuberance is also known as the cervicomedullary kink, hump, spur, buckle, or knickung (see Fig. 212–8).[13, 22] In addition, the pyramidal decussation may occur more cephalad than normal.

OTHER

The Chiari II malformation is known for cranial and upper cervical nerves that pursue an upward or horizontal course. Upper cranial nerves also tend to have a longer intracranial course. The vertebrobasilar system and its branches may be caudally displaced. The vein of Galen tends to be elongated.

Chiari III

Chiari described only one case of his type III deformity, which is indicative of its rarity. The type III deformity is characterized by an occipital or cervical encephalocele, along with other anomalies commonly seen with the type II malformation. Chiari also originally described the type III deformity as having an enlarged foramen magnum.[23] The encephalocele contains varying amounts of neural elements. The tissue in the encephalocele is generally dysmorphic and ischemic.

Chiari IV

The type IV malformation described by Chiari has no hindbrain herniation. The only findings are cerebellar hypoplasia or aplasia, with possible tentorial hypoplasia.

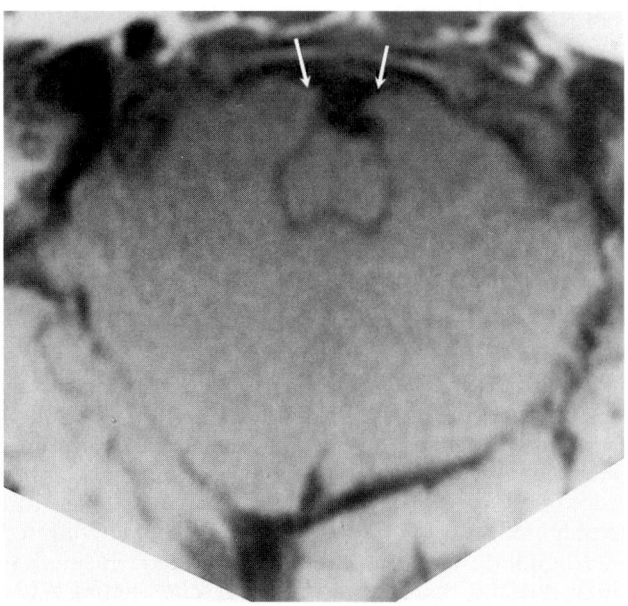

FIGURE 212–9. Axial MRI through the lower portion of the posterior fossa in a child with type II malformation. The lateral edges of the cerebellum course anterior to the brainstem and basilar artery *(arrows)*. This entity is known as cerebellar inversion.

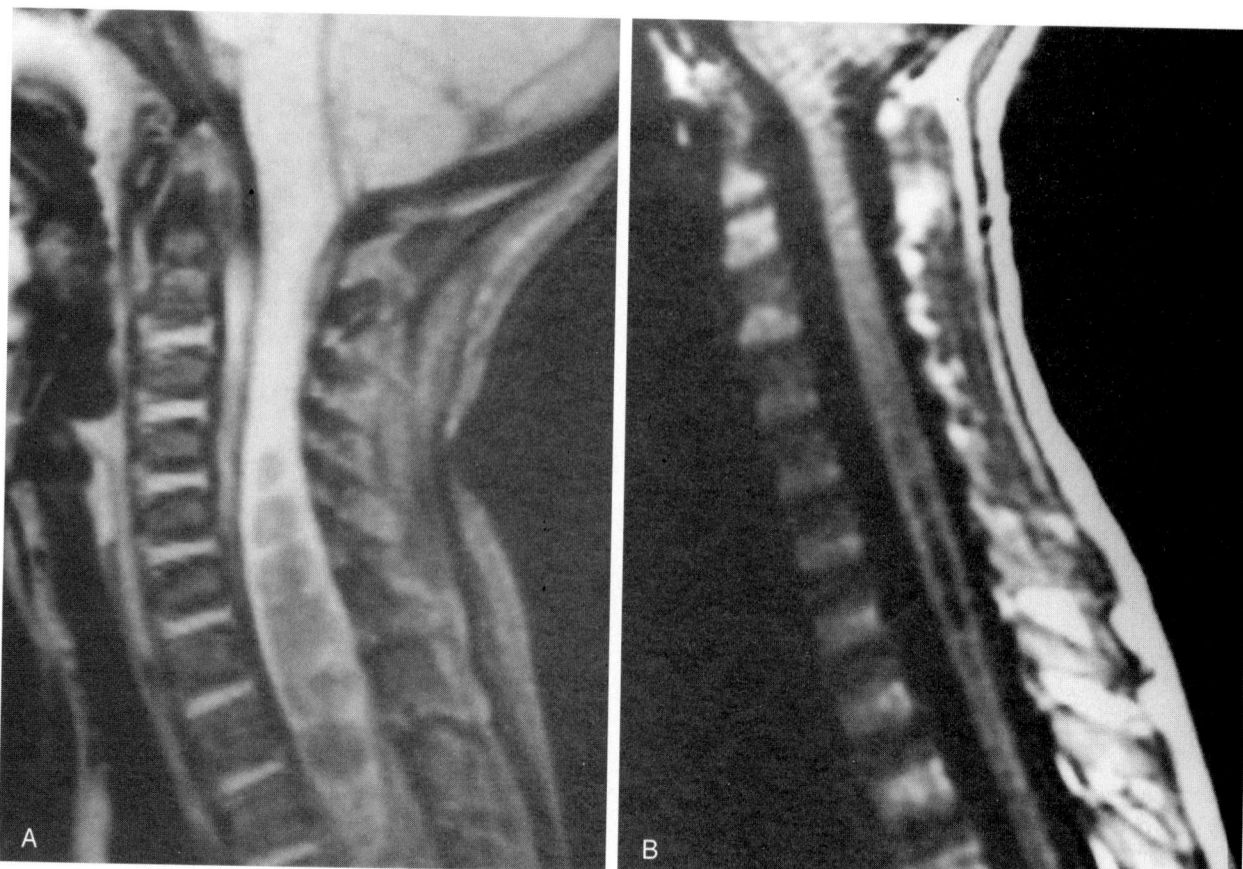

FIGURE 212–10. *A,* Midsagittal MRI scan of a young girl without a hindbrain hernia but with a large cervicothoracic syrinx with septations (Chiari type 0). *B,* The same patient several months after a Chiari decompression. The syrinx is much reduced in size.

Chiari 1.5

Chiari 1.5 specifically addresses patients with the tonsillar herniation seen in Chiari type I malformations but with the addition of an elongated brainstem and fourth ventricle.[19]

Chiari 0

A group of patients with CSF equilibrium changes at the craniocervical junction has been said to have the type 0 malformation. These patients have syringohydromyelia but minimal or no findings of hindbrain herniation (Fig. 212–10*A*). In these patients, posterior fossa decompression may result in a dramatic improvement, both clinically and radiographically, in the syrinx (see Fig. 212–10*B*).[24] Before recommending such a procedure, however, it is important to exclude other causes of syringomyelia. Many of the Chiari type 0 group have craniocervical anomalies such as those seen in the Chiari type I malformation. Operative findings include arachnoidal veils and adhesions obstructing the foramen of Magendie and crowding the tissue at the foramen magnum.

PATHOGENESIS

There is currently no universally accepted theory to explain the Chiari malformations involving hindbrain herniation. A single theoretical proposal would have to explain the many other anomalies associated with each specific Chiari entity as well as the hindbrain herniation. It is also not clear whether the malformations are always on an embryologic continuum or whether some hindbrain hernias occur as a consequence of other pathologic conditions. For example, type II malformations have been reported without an associated myelomeningocele. Acquired hindbrain hernias should also be considered, as they may occur outside of any embryologic influence. There seems to be a female predilection in type I and II malformations.[25] Genetic commonality is still unclear, but it may exist in some of the varieties of hindbrain herniation.[26, 27] The main theories that are currently available are those that consider anomalous mechanical forces and those that consider embryologic development that has gone awry.

The caudal traction theory poses that tethering at a myelomeningocele site elicits traction on the hindbrain, thus pulling it caudally.[28] This does not explain the upward movement of the cerebellum through the tentorium that is commonly seen in type II malformations, and it has been postulated that caudal tension of the spinal cord is dissipated over four spinal segments.[29]

Chiari originally proposed that herniation is due to chronic hydrocephalus. We now know that there are clearly cases in which hydrocephalus is absent and there is still hindbrain herniation. The hydrodynamic theory, based on Gardner's work,[30] states that pulsatile forces generated by CSF drive the development of the neutral tube by expanding it. Gardner believed that the equilibrium between pulsatile forces generated by the choroid plexus in the supratentorial ventricular spaces and fourth ventricular space directed brain growth differentially. If forces were greater supratentorially, the tentorium would be pushed caudally, and compaction of posterior fossa contents would occur. If the fourth ventricular pulsations were hyperactive, a Dandy-Walker malformation could occur. Regarding downward forces, this would not allow flow from the fourth ventricular outlets, and a subsequent syringohydromyelia could occur from fluid entering at the level of the obex into the central canal. Williams elaborated on Gardner's theory by proving that there are indeed pressure gradients between the cranium and the spine in patients with hindbrain herniation.[31] He demonstrated that with the Valsalva maneuver, intraspinal pressure was increased because of epidural venous congestion that created a pressure wave directed cephalad and caudally. Using a manometer, he demonstrated that the cephalad CSF wave enters the cranium with little resistance. However, flow out of the cranium is hindered by the hindbrain hernia when venous pressures normalize. This difference in pressure allows for greater herniation and the development of a syrinx as CSF is drawn into the more yielding areas of the spinal cord. The hydrodynamic theory, both original and revised, fails to explain why one routinely finds no communication between the fourth ventricle and the upper cervical syrinx. However, the idea that a gradient can be established lends credence to reports of acquired hindbrain herniation after procedures in which the spinal subarachnoid space is accessed and the intraspinal pressure lowered.[32, 33]

There are several theories that consider embryologic causes for the Chiari malformations. For example, Marin-Padilla and Marin-Padilla treated hamster embryos with vitamin A to induce a mesodermal insufficiency that led to underdevelopment of the occipital bone and a subsequent small posterior fossa.[34] This theory may help in our understanding of type I malformations, but it does not explain the many associated findings of type II malformations. The speculation that excessive loss of CSF from the myelomeningocele site could potentially create a pressure gradient that would encourage caudal displacement of the hindbrain is supported by the work of Osaka and colleagues.[35] They found that the neural tube insult predates the hindbrain hernia. McLone and Naidich elaborated on this idea with their unified theory.[36] This theory proposes that with excessive loss of CSF at the myelomeningocele site, there is not enough fluid to distend the developing ventricular system adequately. This theory supports several of the findings seen in type II malformations but cannot be applied to type I malformations, in which there is no associated myelomeningocele.

Other embryologic causes of hindbrain herniation include primary dysgenesis of the brainstem, introduced by Cleland,[37] and failure of the pontine flexure to occur, resulting in an elongated brainstem.

Another idea related more specifically to the type I malformation is whether anterior compression from a posteriorly directed dens may cause congestion around the foramen magnum, resulting in hydrocephalus that then causes secondary herniation of the tonsils.[38] This theory can be applied to many cases of Chiari type I malformations in which ventral compression is seen, but it does not address type II malformations and their many associated anomalies.

SIGNS AND SYMPTOMS

Chiari I

Historically, the type I malformation was an entity first demanding clinical attention in adulthood. With the advent of MRI, the type I malformation is increasingly being reported and treated in younger symptomatic patients (Table 212–2). The major difference in presentation between younger and older patients with type I malformations is that sleep apnea is more common in the younger group. In addition, younger children usually have a shorter history of symptoms before being diagnosed.

The most common presenting symptom is pain,[19] reported in 60% to 70% of patients. It is generally described in the occipital or cervical region and may be reproduced with a Valsalva maneuver. It is generally nondermatomal. In nonverbal children, pain may be manifested as irritability, opisthotonos, crying, or failure to thrive. Other symptoms include nonradicular pain in the shoulder, back, chest, and extremities that may be described as deep and burning; motor and

---

TABLE 212–2 ■ **Signs and Symptoms of Chiari Type I Malformations**

High cervical or occipital pain or dysesthesia
Upper extremity weakness or atrophy
Lower extremity spasticity
Scoliosis
Hemiparesis
Dissociated or suspended sensory loss (pain and temperature)
Clumsiness or truncal and appendicular ataxia
Dysphagia
Dysarthria
Hoarseness
Hiccoughs
Apnea
Nystagmus
Recurrent aspiration
Hyper- or hyporeflexia
Babinski response
Oscillopsia
Esotropia
Sinus bradycardia
Trigeminal or glossopharyngeal neuralgia
Opisthotonos
Severe snoring
Drop attacks
Glossal atrophy
Facial sensory loss

sensory alterations in the arms and legs; clumsiness; dysphagia; dysarthria; hiccoughs; severe snoring; drop attacks; and urinary incontinence. Cerebellovestibular problems have also been cited.

Signs seen in Chiari I malformation are variable but include upper motor neuron changes in the legs, with spasticity, exaggerated deep tendon reflexes, and upgoing toes. The upper extremities may have evidence of lower motor neuron injury, with loss of muscle bulk, diminished or absent reflexes, and fasciculations. Sensory loss is classically described as suspended and dissociated. This nondermatomal loss involves pain and temperature but spares light touch and proprioception. Ataxia, irregular respirations, and lower cranial nerve dysfunction may also be seen. The lower cranial nerve dysfunction may be manifested as vocal cord paralysis, dysarthria, soft palate weakness, glossal atrophy, cricopharyngeal achalasia, absent gag reflex, and facial sensory loss. Nystagmus is another presenting sign that is classically the downbeat type and increased on lateral gaze.[39] This variety of nystagmus is specific for pathologic conditions involving the cervicomedullary junction. Some type I malformations present with scoliosis because of underlying syrinx. This may be a levoscoliosis with a single curve. Other less common signs are esotropia, sinus bradycardia, oscillopsia, trigeminal and glossopharyngeal neuralgia, and sensorineural hearing loss.[40–45]

Chiari II

Almost all patients born with a myelomeningocele have some aspect of a Chiari II malformation. A typical sequence is that these children have their spinal lesions repaired soon after birth and then have their progressive hydrocephalus addressed with a ventriculoperitoneal shunt. On follow-up over the next few weeks, symptoms of hindbrain herniation are noted by the parents (Table 212–3). These symptoms may range from occasional irritability to episodes of apnea. This hindbrain anomaly is the leading cause of death in myelodysplastic patients. Approximately 33% of myelodysplastic patients develop some form of hindbrain symptoms before the age of 5, and the outcome is specifically worse for children who present at younger than age 3 months. Mortality is usually due to respiratory insufficiency.[19] Apnea may be the result of a stridor associated with inspiration that is prolonged, or it may originate from central events in the form of prolonged expiratory apnea with cyanosis.[16] Prolonged expiratory apnea with cyanosis can lead to an arching of the neck (opisthotonos), decreased heart rate, and even acute death. On examination, the child may have downbeat nystagmus that is increased on lateral gaze, a diminished gag reflex, and fixed retrocollis. Vocal cord examination may reveal intact adduction with paresis of abduction. Over time, long tract signs may develop with spasticity.

Symptom type and age of onset are closely correlated in the type II malformation. Newborns with type II malformations are generally without symptoms. Infants are more commonly symptomatic for brainstem dysfunctions such as dysphagia and dysarthria. Between infancy and young adulthood, symptoms are commonly those associated with cerebellar and spinal cord dysfunction, such as ataxia and upper extremity weakness. An array of symptoms are seen in adults, with ophthalmic problems being common; these include strabismus, nystagmus, defects of optokinetic movements, and defects of pursuit and convergence.[19, 46, 47]

It should be remembered that patients with Chiari type II malformations generally have stable neurological examinations. If this examination changes, it is usually due to tethering of the spinal cord at the myelomeningocele closure site, raised intracranial pressure, or symptoms caused by an underlying syrinx. New symptoms attributable to either brainstem or long tract dysfunction, such as stridor and spasticity, should alert the clinician to a possible symptomatic hindbrain herniation.

IMAGING

Our understanding of the anatomy and physiology of the Chiari malformations has greatly increased with the advent of MRI. Before its use, computed tomography and other techniques were less than adequate in visualizing the soft tissue anatomy around the foramen magnum, and many anomalies seen with Chiari malformations, such as syringomyelia, were missed. When MRI cannot be performed, computed tomographic myelography is an alternative, but visualization within the cord is limited. Ultrasonography cannot be used except in very young infants or intraoperatively, when it can be of some assistance.

Chiari I

In Chiari's original definition, the type I malformation was considered herniation of the tonsils below the plane of the foramen magnum. It has been noted, how-

T A B L E 2 1 2 – 3 ■ Signs and Symptoms of Chiari Type II Malformations

Apnea
Retrocollis or opisthotonos
Irritability
Aspiration pneumonia
Dysphagia
Dysarthria
Nystagmus
Strabismus
Inspiratory wheeze or stridor
Quadriparesis with hypotonia
Upper extremity spasticity
Ataxia
Hand weakness with atrophy
Scoliosis
Head and neck pain
Breathholding
Defects of pursuit movements and convergence
Defects of optokinetic movements

ever, that normal or asymptomatic patients may have tonsils that are more than 7 mm below the foramen magnum. Therefore, the precise definition of the type I malformation has been debated. Aboulezz and colleagues retrospectively examined 95 cases based on the clinical examination at the time of imaging.[48] It was found that in normal controls, the tonsils did not extend more than 3 mm below the plane of the foramen magnum. They also considered herniation below 5 mm to be pathologic. Barkovich and coworkers examined 200 normal patients and 25 patients with the diagnosis of type I malformation.[49] This study considered 2 mm of tonsillar herniation to be within normal limits. Using this criterion, symptomatic patients can be predicted with a sensitivity of 100% and a specificity of 98.5%. In addition, Mikulis and associates found that normal tonsils may prolapse up to 6 mm during the first 10 years of life and ascend gradually with increasing age.[50] In addition to defining an absolute for length of tonsillar descent, one should consider the morphologic appearance of the tonsillar tips. It is known that tips that are elongated and pointed are more likely to become symptomatic than are tips that are rounded and blunt. Associated pathology of the skull base and cervical spine is also frequently visualized on MRI.

It is now known that like type II malformations, type I malformations often have smaller than normal posterior fossa volumes.[51, 52] Using MRI, Badie and colleagues determined that Chiari patients with smaller posterior fossa volumes generally develop symptoms sooner than do Chiari patients with normal volumes, and the former group is more likely to respond to surgical decompression.[53] Indeed, small posterior fossa volumes and subsequent hindbrain herniation have been cited as the mechanism by which one sees type I malformations in craniosynostosis, Paget's disease, rickets, achondroplasia, and acromegaly.[54–57]

Dynamic MRI studies are now used to determine flow around the foramen magnum and its constituents. Cine-mode MRI demonstrates flow patterns during the cardiac cycle and can show flow anterior and posterior to the craniocervical junction, as well as whether there is obstruction by hindbrain herniation or the presence of a syrinx. Many use cine-mode MRI pre- and postoperatively to determine the adequacy of a decompression of the craniocervical junction. Armonda and coworkers evaluated eight patients pre- and postoperatively with cine-mode MRI.[58] They found flow obstruction, decreased velocities, shorter duration of flow, and preferential cranial flow in patients with greater than 5 mm of tonsillar herniation. Cine-mode MRI performed after operation was comparable to the scans of controls and showed correlation between syrinx reduction and symptoms. Although this technique is promising, it should be noted that it results in a significant number of false-positive as well as false-negative results.

Syringohydromyelia is easily demonstrable and evaluated on MRI. It has been shown using MRI that this condition is seen more often in the cervical cord and frequently does not communicate with the fourth ventricle via a radiographically identifiable central canal or other syringeal pathway. There is currently no consensus on the correlation between the extent of tonsillar herniation and the presence of a syrinx. Syringomyelia can occur throughout the spinal cord, but syringes that spare the cervical spinal cord should be evaluated for a non-Chiari origin.

Computed tomographic scans and plain radiographs are useful in evaluating bony anomalies associated with the type I malformation. In addition, computed tomography (CT) is cheaper and equally precise in the routine evaluation of hydrocephalus, which is frequently seen with this malformation.

Chiari II

MRI is the preferred imaging modality in evaluating type II malformations. In this malformation, one finds vermian herniation with caudal descent of the brainstem and fourth ventricle. Many other anomalies are associated with this malformation and have already been discussed. CT and plain radiographs are also useful for the same reasons as discussed earlier. In addition, in utero ultrasonography can be used to gather anatomic data on patients with this malformation. Nicolaides and colleagues described two in utero entities seen on ultrasonographic studies that suggest a type II malformation[14]: The banana sign describes cerebellar hemispheres that are curved anteriorly, with a small or absent cisterna magna; the lemon sign denotes a scalloping of the frontal bones.

MRI demonstrates the majority of the various anomalies associated with type II malformations. It should be mentioned that in contrast to type I malformations, type II malformations have a propensity for syrinx formation in the lower cervical and upper thoracic cord. This may be missed with routine craniocervical imaging, which frequently terminates by the third or fourth cervical vertebra.

SURGICAL INDICATIONS AND TECHNIQUE

Chiari I

There is currently no medical therapy for the Chiari I malformation, and there are many management algorithms and surgical procedures used in its treatment. The natural history of an asymptomatic type I malformation is not known. In patients with a Chiari I malformation who are asymptomatic, observation alone may be adequate. In symptomatic patients or in patients with a syrinx, intervention is warranted, depending on the degree of caudal herniation and the presence of a syrinx. The majority of symptomatic patients improve or stabilize with surgical intervention, although lost functions generally do not return postoperatively. Headache, scoliosis, and sleep apnea are three symptoms that predictably improve postoperatively. Surgical intervention in this group of patients carries a less than 2% chance of serious, irreversible injury.[19, 59]

The majority of neurosurgeons favor posterior fossa decompression with expansion duraplasty for Chiari

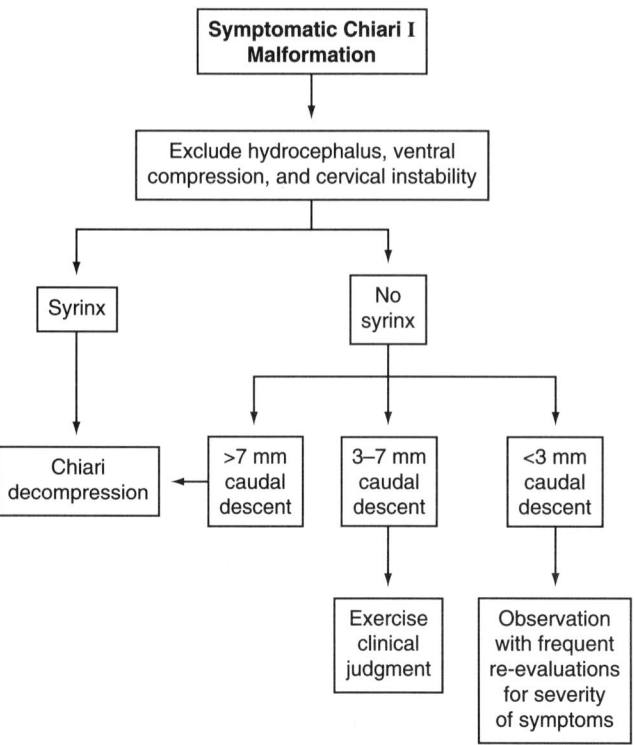

FIGURE 212–11. Algorithm for symptomatic Chiari I malformation.

malformations and syringohydromyelia. Our experience led to the development of algorithms that are applicable in the majority of patients with a defined Chiari I malformation (Figs. 212–11 and 212–12). Although seen in a minority of type I malformations,

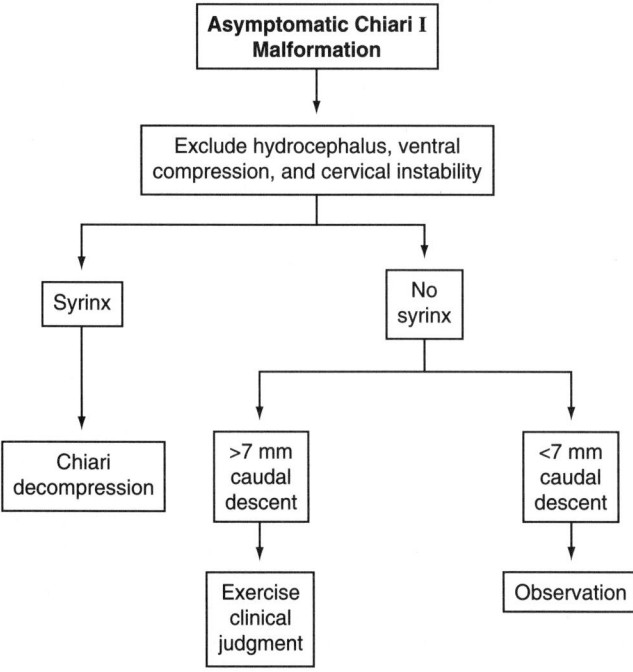

FIGURE 212–12. Algorithm for asymptomatic Chiari I malformation.

hydrocephalus must be addressed first. Hydrocephalus should be shunted, and the patient should be re-evaluated in several months. If symptoms persist and there is an associated syrinx with no severe ventral compression,[38] a posterior fossa decompression should be considered. Generally, with an adequate decompression, most symptoms abate postoperatively. Associated syringes generally resolve over the next few months. If a syrinx persists, re-exploration of the posterior fossa with additional opening of the foramen of Magendie should be considered. This can be accomplished by coagulating or resecting one or both cerebellar tonsils. In our experience, this second posterior fossa exploration has not failed in resolving a syrinx. If one initially finds significant ventral compression, this anomaly should be addressed before posterior fossa decompression is considered.

The technique for a Chiari I decompression is to begin with the patient prone and the head fixed in pins and flexed in order to flatten and flex the craniocervical juncture. The skin is opened from just below the inion down to the cephalad aspect of the axis. The midline is found by appreciating the fat-laden, avascular midline plane between the suboccipital musculature. Next, the soft tissue is dissected off the foramen magnum, and a subperiosteal dissection of the posterior arch of the atlas is performed. Dissections are carried laterally to expose the posterior ring of C1 and the foramen magnum. Minimizing muscle manipulation, especially below the atlas, helps decrease postoperative pain and reduces the chance of postoperative kyphosis,[60] multilevel fusion, or cervical instability.

A craniotomy is then performed in the exposed occipital bone. With bone rongeurs, the posterior rim of the foramen magnum and posterior arch of the atlas are removed. Care must be taken with the atlantal arch to avoid compromising its laterally placed vertebral artery segment. The pathologic condition is in the midline, and significant lateral exposure is not necessary. Bone edges are waxed, and further hemostasis is obtained. Constricting bands anterior to the posterior arch of C1 are looked for and cut, if present.

At this time, some surgeons elect to end the operation and consider bony decompression sufficient.[61] Others advocate merely opening the outer layer of the dura.[62] We routinely apply ultrasound to the intact dura and evaluate for tonsillar motion. If it is not present, the dura is opened in a vertical fashion. Once the dura is opened, the arachnoid is entered and clipped to the dura laterally. Next, the foramen of Magendie is inspected by gently separating the tonsils. Obstructive veils, vascular bands, and patency are assessed. Unilateral tonsillar coagulation is generally not carried out in the initial exploration.[63] Extreme care must be used with this technique so as not to harm the posterior inferior cerebral artery. The avascular floor of the fourth ventricle is visualized and noted for pathology. No plug is placed in the cephalad opening of the central canal; this is unnecessary and potentially hazardous.[59, 64] If the dura is opened, we routinely sew a patch in using the patient's own pericranium harvested from a separate site just cephalad to the original incision. Others have discussed alternative grafting materials, such as bovine pericardium, various synthetic materials, and other soft tissues harvested from the patient. The dural graft allows additional space for the herniated tonsils and protects the neural elements from overlying tissues and fluids. Hemostasis must be established before dural closure to minimize arachnoidal scarring and the prospensity for postoperative hydrocephalus. The operative sites are closed in standard, anatomic layers.

Chiari II

This malformation is a significant challenge with regard to both management and surgical technique. Our experience in managing the type II malformation is summarized in Figures 212–13 and 212–14. The type II malformation is the leading cause of death in children with myelodysplasia, and conflicting reports exist regarding surgical intervention. Many believe that the dysmorphism in the brainstem is the underlying problem and cannot be altered surgically. Others see the constricted herniated tissue as the surgical target and readily address it. Those who choose operative intervention generally do so for symptomatic patients. Symptoms warranting surgery include inspiratory stridor, aspiration pneumonia, central sleep apnea, opisthotonos, progressive spasticity, and progressive truncal and appendicular ataxia. Just as in the type I malformation, hydrocephalus or shunt patency should be evaluated first. Most shunted myelodysplastic patients with the type II malformation are difficult to evaluate for shunt malfunction, and if they are symptomatic, we do not hesitate to explore operatively and demonstrate shunt function (see Figs. 212–13 and 212–14). This point cannot be overemphasized. The intraoperative requirements for an adequately functioning shunt are both CSF flow from the intracranial catheter

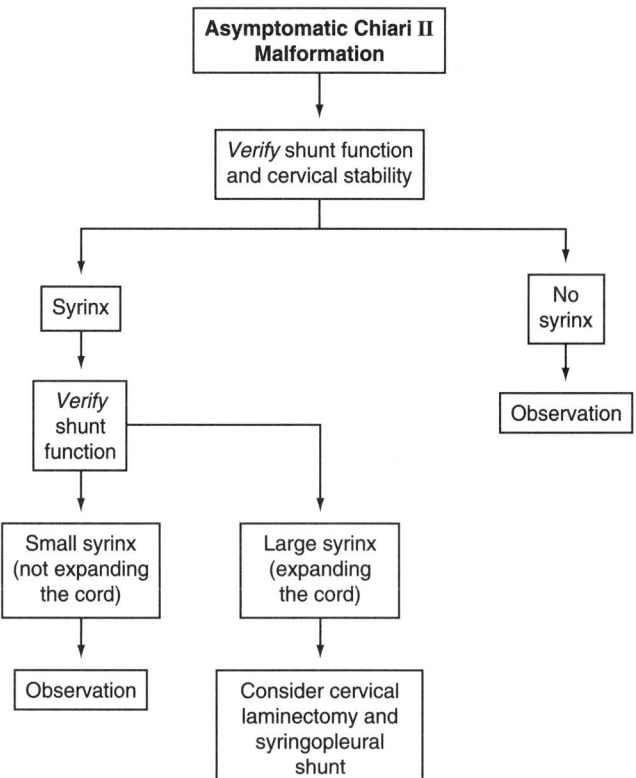

FIGURE 212–14. Algorithm for asymptomatic Chiari II malformation.

and lack of adherence of this catheter within the brain. If some flow is present but the ventricular catheter is fixed within the ventricle, it should be removed and repositioned so that there is no question that it lies within the ventricular cavity. This may be best performed with endoscopic control.

Once adequate shunt function is established, one can focus on whether surgical decompression is warranted. Several diagnostic studies may be useful. These include a swallow study, brainstem auditory evoked potentials, evaluation of vocal cord function by an otolaryngologist, and pulmonary function studies to differentiate between obstructive and centrally mediated sleep apnea.

The most recent advance in the treatment of the hindbrain hernia in myelodysplastic individuals is in utero repair of the myelomeningocele. Tulipan and colleagues had promising results demonstrating a decrease in hindbrain herniation after this procedure.[65] Athough they found no significant hindbrain hernia, other anomalies commonly seen in the type II malformation were noted, including polygyria, large massa intermedia, and small posterior fossa. These data seem to support the theories that advocate loss of fluid via the myelomeningocele as a reason for hindbrain herniation.

The surgical technique for a Chari II malformation begins with the patient in the prone position and fixated in pins. Soft tissue exposure is comparable to that performed for the type I malformation described earlier. One should be aware of bony defects as this

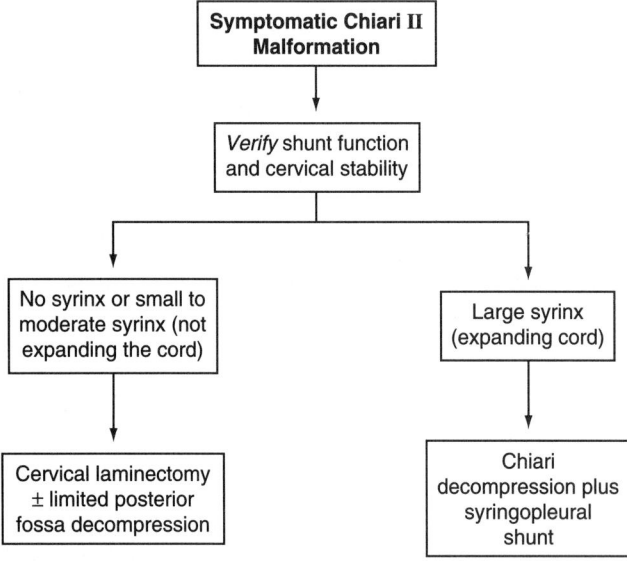

FIGURE 212–13. Algorithm for symptomatic Chiari II malformation.

dissection is performed. The cervical laminectomy should uncover the inferior margin of the herniated cerebellar tissue and need not include the cervicomedullary kink. A limited suboccipital craniectomy may be performed, but it is usually not needed owing to the enlarged foramen magnum and the propensity for venous insult. Bony removal should decompress only the underlying nervous tissue. Limited removal of bone decreases the chance of postoperative cervical instability. After the bony removal, constricting dural bands should be sought and cut, if present. The dura is opened in the midline up to the level of the foramen magnum. The arachnoid is clipped to the dura laterally, and adhesions are carefully sectioned. Frequently, the spinal cord is hypervascular below the constricted site. The next step is key—finding the outlet of the fourth ventricle. If one finds the normally extraventricular choroid plexus, it can be used as a guide into the ventricle. Obstructive vermian tissue may be coagulated to encourage CSF flow out of the ventricle. Occasionally, the opening is not obvious, and the vermis may be directly penetrated with bipolar cautery to gain ventricular access. Care must be used in differentiating the vermis from the medullary kink, so as not to inadvertently enter the brainstem with the dissection. We routinely use intraoperative ultrasonography and chest Doppler to better ascertain our orientation. Finally, an expansion duraplasty is performed, and anatomic layers are closed appropriately.

COMPLICATIONS

The most common non-neurological complication after a Chiari decompression is aseptic meningitis. Other subacute complications include wound dehiscence, pseudomeningocele formation, and CSF fistula. Long-term complications include cerebellar sag (ptosis),[64] kyphoscoliosis,[60] progressive neurological compromise, regeneration of the foramen magnum and other bony components,[66, 67] and failure of preoperative symptoms to resolve. Failure to improve postoperatively should alert the clinician to the possibility of ventral compression, recurrent syringohydromyelia, craniocervical instability, inadequate decompression, or another diagnosis. At each step, the clinician should remain aware of the possibility of shunt malfunction.

OUTCOME

Chiari I

The literature regarding outcome after a Chiari I decompression is conflicting and difficult to interpret, given our limited understanding of the pathophysiology of this disease process. Retrospective studies are not sufficient, because we know little about the natural history of this malformation. Although results from several large surgical series seem favorable, care should be exercised when applying these summations.

It has been shown that postoperative outcome is not based on age and that mild neurological deficits, when treated early, have the best outcome. Approximately 85% of patients are relieved of headache and neck pain postoperatively.[4, 68] Patients who fare the worst are those with symptoms produced from a syrinx. Milhorat and associates addressed this observation by stating that central cord lesions cause irreversible damage to nonglial neural tissues.[69, 70] Patients with brainstem compression fall in the middle with regard to outcome. Nagib found that the problems most likely to be improved are scoliosis less than 30 degrees, headache and neckache, and sleep apnea.[68] He also stated that motor and sensory deficits are least likely to improve. It has been demonstrated that patients with small posterior fossa volumes tend to do better postoperatively than do patients with normal volumes. Results after posterior fossa decompression are also skewed by the vast array of techniques used.

Chiari II

Although the natural history of this disease is not well understood, early surgical intervention for a symptomatic patient is widely accepted. Pollack and colleagues prospectively decompressed symptomatic type II malformations and concluded that early treatment provides the best chance of recovery.[71] Charney and coworkers grouped their symptomatic type II patients into those with stridor, those with stridor and apnea spells, and those with stridor, apnea, cyanotic spells, and dysphagia.[72] These were defined as groups 1, 2, and 3, respectively. Group 1 had the best chance of recovery. Group 2 had a 50% chance of recovery and a 75% chance of survival. Group 3 had a minimal chance of recovery and a 40% chance of survival.

We advocate syringopleural shunt insertion when a large syrinx exists, along with the Chiari decompression. There have been few instances of type II malformations in which a large syrinx resolves with just a decompressive procedure.

CONCLUSIONS

The hindbrain hernias known as the Chiari malformations represent a wide range of anatomy that may or may not have common embryologic origins. The types of Chiari malformations may actually represent various entities, with some being caused by other pathologic conditions and others merely representing milder degrees of the other types. Any theory proposed must address all findings seen in the spectrum of hindbrain herniation for each type. Neural anomalies associated with these malformations include hydrocephalus, myelomeningocele, and syringohydromyelia.

Time and prospective studies are needed to better ascertain the natural history of these processes. Better imaging and embryologic work have heightened our understanding of these anomalies. On the forefront of treatment is earlier detection and appreciation of these entities and earlier intervention, such as in utero repair of myelomeningoceles, with lessening of their hindbrain herniation.

REFERENCES

1. Chiari H: Uber Veranderungen des Kleinhirns infolge von Hydrocephalie des Grosshirns. Dtsch Med Wochenschr 17;1172–1175, 1891.
2. Chiari H: Uber Veranderungen des Kleinhirns, der Pons und der Medulla oblongata infolge von congenitaler Hydrocephalie des Grosshirns. Denkschr Akad Wiss (Wien) 63:71–115, 1895.
3. Koehler PJ: Chiari's description of cerebellar ectopy (1891): With a summary of Cleland's and Arnold's contributions and some early observations of neural-tube defects. J Neurosurg 75:823–826, 1991.
4. Menezes AH: Chiari I malformations and hydromyelia complications. Pediatr Neurosurg 17:146–154, 1991.
5. Nakai T, Asato R, Miki Y, et al: A case of achondroplasia with downward displacement of the brainstem. Neuroradiology 37:293–294, 1995.
6. Day R, Park T, Ojemann G, et al: Foramen magnum decompression for cervicomedullary encroachment in craniometaphyseal dysplasia: Case report. Neurosurgery 41:960–964, 1997.
7. Menezes A: Primary craniovertebral anomalies and the hindbrain herniation syndrome (Chiari I): Data base analysis. Pediatr Neurosurg 23:260–269, 1995.
8. Logue V, Edwards MR: Syringomyelia and its surgical treatment—an analysis of 75 patients. J Pediatr 118:567–569, 1991.
9. Oakes W: Chiari malformations and syringomyelia. In Rengachary S, Wilkins R (eds): Principles of Neurosurgery. London, Wolf Publishing, 1994, pp 9.1–9.18.
10. Batzdorf U: Chiari I malformation with syringomyelia: Evaluation of surgical therapy by magnetic resonance imaging. J Neurosurg 68:726–730, 1988.
11. Cahan LD, Bentson JR: Consideration in the diagnosis and treatment of syringomyelia and Chiari malformation. J Neurosurg 57:24–31, 1982.
12. Carmel PW, Markesbery W: Early descriptions of the Arnold-Chiari malformation: The contribution of John Cleland. J Neurosurg 37:543–547, 1972.
13. el Gammal T, Mark EK, Brooks BS: MR imaging of Chiari II malformation. AJR Am J Roentgenol 150:163–170, 1988.
14. Nicolaides KH, Campbell S, Gabbe SG, Guidetti R: Ultrasound screening for spina bifida: Cranial and cerebellar signs. Lancet 2:72–74, 1986.
15. Curnes JT, Oakes WJ, Boyko OB: MR imaging of hindbrain deformity in Chiari II patients with and without symptoms of brainstem compression [see comments]. AJNR Am J Neuroradiol 10:293–302, 1989.
16. Rauzzino M, Oakes WJ: Chiari II malformation and syringomyelia. Neurosurg Clin N Am 6:293–309, 1995.
17. Gooding CA, Carter A, Hoare RD: New ventriculographic aspects of the Arnold-Chiari malformation. Laryngoscope 73:85–92, 1963.
18. Emery JL, MacKenzie N: Medullo-cervical dislocation deformity (Chiari II deformity) related to neurospinal dysraphism (meningomyelocele). Brain 96:155–162, 1973.
19. Iskandar B, Oakes W: Chiari malformation and syringomyelia. In Albright L, Pollack I, Adelson P (eds): Principles and Practice of Pediatric Neurosurgery. New York, Thieme, 1999, pp 165–187.
20. Heinz R, Curnes J, Friedman A, et al: Exophytic syrinx, an extreme form of syringomyelia: CT, myelographic, and MR imaging features. Radiology 183:243–246, 1992.
21. McLendon RE, Crain BJ, Oakes WJ, Burger PC: Cerebral polygyria in the Chiari type II (Arnold-Chiari) malformation. Clin Neuropathol 4:200–205, 1985.
22. Peach B: The Arnold-Chiari malformation: Anatomic features of 20 cases. Arch Neurol 12:613–621, 1965.
23. Krutt E, Jetts R: Skull abnormalities associated with the Arnold-Chiari malformation. Acta Radiol Diagn 5:9–24, 1966.
24. lskandar BI, Hedlund GL, Grabb PA, Oakes WJ: The resolution of syringomyelia without hindbrain herniation after posterior fossa decompression. J Neurosurg 89:212–216, 1998.
25. Elster AD, Chen MY: Chiari I malformations: Clinical and radiological reappraisal. Radiology 183:347–353, 1992.
26. Cavender R, Schmidt J: Tonsillar ectopia and Chiari malformations: Monozygotic triplets. J Neurosurg 82:497–500, 1995.
27. Ishikawa M, Kikuchi H, Fujisawa I, Yonekawa Y: Tonsillar herniation on magnetic resonance imaging. Neurosurgery 22:77–81, 1988.
28. Lichtenstein BW: Distant neuroanatomic complications of spina bifida (spinal dysraphism): Hydrocephalus, Arnold-Chiari deformity, stenosis of the aqueduct of Sylvius, etc., pathogenesis and pathology. Arch Neurol Psychiatry 47:195–214, 1942.
29. Goldstein F, Kepes J: The role of traction in the development of the Arnold-Chiari malformation: An experimental study. J Neuropathol Exp Neurol 25:654–666, 1966.
30. Gardner WJ: Hydrodynamic factors in Dandy-Walker and Arnold-Chiari malformations. Childs Brain 3:200–212, 1977.
31. Williams B: Cerebrospinal fluid pressure-gradients in spina bifida cystica, with special reference to the Arnold-Chiari malformation and aqueductal stenosis. Dev Med Child Neurol Suppl 35:138–150, 1975.
32. Chumas PD, Armstrong DC, Drake JM, et al: Tonsillar herniation: The rule rather than the exception after lumboperitoneal shunting in the pediatric population [see comments]. J Neurosurg 78:568–573, 1993.
33. Sathi S, Stieg PE: "Acquired" Chiari I malformation after multiple lumbar punctures: Case report. Neurosurgery 32:306–309, 1993.
34. Marin-Padilla M, Marin-Padilla TM: Morphogenesis of experimentally induced Arnold-Chiari malformation. J Neurol Sci 50:29–55, 1981.
35. Osaka K, Tanimura T, Hirayama A, Matsumoto S: Myelomeningocele before birth. J Neurosurg 49:711–724, 1978.
36. McLone DG, Naidich TP: Developmental morphology of the subarachnoid space, brain vasculature, and contiguous structures, and the cause of the Chiari II malformation. Pediatr Neurosci 15:1–12, 1989.
37. Cleland J: Contribution to the study of spina bifida, encephalocele, and anencephalus. J Anat Physiol 17:257–292, 1883.
38. Grabb P, Mapstone T, Oakes W: Ventral brainstem compression in pediatric and young adult patients with Chiari I malformations. Neurosurgery 44:520–528, 1999.
39. Cogan DG: Downbeat nystagmus. Arch Ophthalmol 80:757–768, 1968.
40. Yglesias A, Narbona J, Vanaclocha V, Artieda J: Chiari malformation, glossopharyngeal neuralgia and central sleep apnea in a child. Dev Med Child Neurol 38:1126–1130, 1996.
41. Rosetti P, Taib N, Brotchi J, et al: Arnold Chiari type I malformation presents as a trigeminal neuralgia: Case report. Neurosurgery 44:1120–1124, 1999.
42. Gingold SI, Winfield JA: Oscillopsia and primary cerebellar ectopia: Case report and review of the literature. Neurosurgery 29:932–936, 1991.
43. Lewis AR, Kilne LB, Sharpe JA: Acquired esotropia due to Arnold-Chiari I malformation. J Neuroophthalmol 16:49–54, 1996.
44. Sclafani AP, DeDio RM, Hendrix RA: The Chiari-I malformation. Ear Nose Throat J 70:208–212, 1991.
45. Selmi F, Davies KG, Weeks RD: Type I Chiari deformity presenting with profound sinus bradycardia: Case report and literature review. Br J Neurosurg 9:543–545, 1995.
46. Bertrand RA: [Changes of the vestibular response in various cervical pathologies of intrinsic and extrinsic origin]. Acta Otorinolaryngol Iber Am 24:122–138, 1973.
47. Chait GE, Barber HO: Arnold-Chiari malformation—some otoneurological features. AJNR Am J Neuroradiol 13:107–113, 1992.
48. Aboulezz AO, Sartor K, Geyer CA, Gado MH: Position of cerebellar tonsils in the normal population and in patients with Chiari malformation: A quantitative approach with MR imaging. J Comput Assist Tomogr 9:1033–1036, 1985.
49. Barkovich AJ, Wippold FJ, Sherman JL, Citrin CM: Significance of cerebellar tonsillar position of MR. AJNR Am J Neuroradiol 7:795–799, 1986.
50. Mikulis DJ, Diaz O, Egglin TK, Sanchez R: Variance of the position of the cerebellar tonsils with age: Preliminary report. Radiology 183:725–728, 1992.
51. Schady W, Metcalfe RA, Butler P: The incidence of craniocervical body anomalies in the adult Chiari malformation. J Neurol Sci 82:193–203, 1987.

52. Stovner LJ, Bergan U, Nilsen G, Sjaastad O: Posterior cranial fossa dimensions in the Chiari I malformation: Relation to pathogenesis and clinical presentation. Neuroradiology 35:113–118, 1993.

53. Badie B, Mendoza D, Batzdorf U: Posterior fossa volume and response to suboccipital decompression in patients with Chiari I malformation. Neurosurgery 37:214–218, 1995.

54. Cinalli G. Renier D, Sebag G, et al: Chronic tonsillar herniation in Crouzon's and Apert's syndromes: The role of premature synostosis of the lambdoid suture. J Neurosurg 83:575–582, 1995.

55. Epstein BS, Epstein JA: The association of cerebellar tonsillar herniation with basilar impression incident to Paget's disease. Am J Roentgenol Radium Ther Nucl Med 107:535–542, 1969.

56. Lemar HJ Jr, Perloff JJ, Merenich JA: Symptomatic Chiari-I malformation in a patient with acromegaly. South Med J 87:284–285, 1994.

57. Nohria V, Oakes WJ: Chiari I malformation: A review of 43 patients. Pediatr Neurosurg 16:222–227, 1990.

58. Armonda RA, Citrin CM, Foley KT, Ellenbogen RG: Quantitative cine-mode magnetic resonance imaging of Chiari I malformations: An analysis of cerebrospinal fluid dynamics. Neurosurgery 35:214–223, 1994; discussion 223–224.

59. Cai C, Oakes W: Hindbrain herniation syndromes: The Chiari malformations (I and II). Semin Pediatr Neurol 4:179–191, 1997.

60. McLaughlin M, Wahlig J, Pollack I: Incidence of post laminectomy kyphosis after Chiari decompression. Spine 22:613–617, 1997.

61. Haines SJ, Berger M: Current treatment of Chiari malformations types I and II: A survey of the Pediatric Section of the American Association of Neurological Surgeons. Neurosurgery 28:353–357, 1991.

62. Isu T, Sasaki H, Takamura H, Kobayashi N: Foramen magnum decompression with removal of the outer layer of the dura as treatment of syringomyelia occurring with Chiari I malformation. Neurosurgery 33:844–849, 1993; discussion 849–850.

63. Won DJ, Nambiar U, Muszynski CA, Epstein FJ: Coagulation of herniated cerebellar tonsils for cerebrospinal fluid pathway restoration. Pediatr Neurosurg 27:272–275, 1997.

64. Batzdorf U: Chiari malformation and syringomyelia. In Apuzzo MLJ (ed): Brain Surgery: Complications, Avoidance, and Management, vol 2. New York, Churchill Livingstone, 1993, pp 985–2001.

65. Tulipan N, Hernanz-Schulman M, Bruner J: Reduced hindbrain herniation after intrauterine myelomeningocele repair. A report of four cases. Pediatr Neurosurg 29:274–278, 1998.

66. Aoki N, Oikawa A, Sakai T: Spontaneous regeneration of the foramen magnum after decompressive suboccipital craniectomy in Chiari malformation: Case report. Neurosurgery 37:340–342, 1995.

67. Hudgins RJ, Boydston WR: Bone regrowth and recurrence of symptoms following decompression in the infant with Chiari II malformation [see comments]. Pediatr Neurosurg 23:323–327, 1995.

68. Nagib MG: An approach to symptomatic children (ages 4–14 years) with Chiari type I malformation. Pediatr Neurosurg 21:31–35, 1994.

69. Milhorat TH, Capocelli AL Jr, Anzil AP, et al: Pathological basis of spinal cord cavitation in syringomyelia: Analysis of 105 autopsy cases. J Neurosurg 82:802–812, 1995.

70. Milhorat T, Chou M, Trinidad E, et al: Chiari I malformations redefined: Clinical and radiographic findings for 364 symptomatic patients. Neurosurgery 44:1005–1017, 1999.

71. Pollack IF, Pang D, Albright AL, Krieger D: Outcome following hindbrain decompression of symptomatic Chiari malformations in children previously treated with myelomeningocele closure and shunts. J Neurosurg 77:881–888, 1992.

72. Charney EB, Rorke LB, Sutton LN, Schut L: Management of Chiari II complications in infants with myelomeningocele. J Pediatr 111:364–371, 1987.

CHAPTER 213

Achondroplasia and Other Dwarfism

BENJAMIN S. CARSON, SR. ▪ DANIELE RIGAMONTI ▪ RAYMOND R. HAROUN

Hypochondroplasia, achondroplasia, and thanatophoric dysplasia are clinically related skeletal dysplasias caused by mutations of the fibroblast growth factor receptor 3 (*FGFR3*) gene. The phenotype, disproportionately short stature with rhizomelic shortening of the extremities, results from defective formation of endochondral bone.

Hypochondroplasia yields the mildest phenotype, which varies within and between families and frequently lacks the neurological complications often seen in achondroplasia, such as hydrocephalus, cervicomedullary compression, and spinal stenosis. Life expectancy in this group may approach normal. The pathologic features of micromelic short stature, reduced or unchanged interpedicular distances in the lumbar spine, disproportionately long fibulas, squared and shortened pelvic ilia, and reduced subischial leg length are significantly less in hypochondroplasia than in achondroplasia. Achondroplasia patients have increased age-specific mortality rates at all ages, with the highest increase occurring in childhood. Cervicomedullary compression likely accounts for the excess deaths in children; however, cardiovascular causes of death appear to be increased in adults. Individuals with thanatophoric dysplasia seldom survive to adulthood.

Given our present understanding of short-limb dysplasias, neurosurgical approaches to achondroplastic, thanatophoric, and hypochondroplastic patients are similar. Hydrocephalus and cervicomedullary compression are typically pediatric concerns, whereas spinal stenosis is seen primarily in adults. Presenting symptoms often do not have strictly neurosurgical resolutions; thus, a comprehensive treatment plan involving a multidisciplinary team of physicians is useful.[1] Patients referred to our institution are usually evaluated according to a standardized protocol that involves a team composed of a neurosurgeon, neurologist, pulmonary specialist, sleep specialist, geneticist, anesthesiologist, neuroradiologist, orthopedic surgeon, and otolaryngologist.[2,3] Because these patients are at risk for brainstem compression, comprehensive testing is directed toward the detection of central and obstructive apnea and cervicomedullary compression, all of which contribute to the risk of sudden death.

Several areas of research are leading to new initiatives in the management of skeletal dysplasias. First is the application of advanced diagnostic tools and imaging techniques. Second is an emphasis on outcome studies, a movement based on the well-supported assumption that different operative strategies can yield marked long-term differences in the patient's health.[4] Third, a better understanding of molecular biology has led to fresh ideas for gene therapy. A fourth area, the use of recombinant growth hormone to treat pediatric patients, is outside the scope of this chapter. Here we describe our current approach to the evaluation and management of short-limb dysplasias and summarize the molecular biology, diagnostic findings, and outcome studies that have been reported since 1995.

EPIDEMIOLOGY

Achondroplasia is an autosomal-dominant disorder that results from a guanine (G) to adenine (A) mutation at base 1138 (*G1138A*) in the *FGFR3* gene on chromosome 4, at 4p16.3.[5-7] The gene codes for a tyrosine kinase receptor expressed in developing bones. The nucleotide (missense) mutation results in an amino acid glycine (G) to arginine (R) substitution at amino acid 380 (*G380R*) in the transmembrane domain of the protein. Achondroplasia appears to be genetically homogeneous. No significant racial difference has been detected in North America, Spain, Korea, Japan, China, or Sweden.[8-13]

The *FGFR3* hypochondroplasia mutation pattern is more diverse than that for achondroplasia.[12,14-16] In many patients, a *C1620G* or *C1620A* mutation results in an asparagine to lysine substitution at amino acid 540 (*N450K*) in the *FGFR3* proximal tyrosine kinase domain. In a substantial number of patients who express a mild phenotype, the mutation has yet to be identified.[14] The phenotypic diversity confounds estimates of incidence data. Accurate prenatal ultrasonographic diagnosis is rare.[17] Before the identification of the specific nucleotide mutations, some achondroplasia case reports probably included patients with hypochondroplasia. The overlap should be considered in efforts to compare current and past case series.

An arginine to cysteine (*R248C*) substitution in the

extracellular domain of the receptor has been found in thanatophoric patients. Other mutations are likely because at least two phenotypes have been identified, TD type I and TD type II. Less is known about this dysplasia because the mutation is almost always lethal neonatally.[18]

Compound mutations for achondroplasia and hypochondroplasia have been reported in children whose achondroplastic father or mother had the *G380R* mutation, and the other parent had the hypochondroplasia *N450K* mutation.[19,20] The phenotypic expression of the compound mutation appears to be more severe than that of achondroplasia.[20]

New mutations account for about 80% of children born with achondroplasia. As in many autosomal-dominant conditions, a positive correlation exists between advanced paternal age and the occurrence of new mutations. Factors influencing DNA replication or repair during spermatogenesis, but not during oogenesis, may predispose to the occurrence of the *G1138A* mutation in the *FGFR3* gene.[21] Offspring of couples who are both affected by achondroplasia have a 25% chance of inheriting both parental achondroplasia alleles, resulting in homozygous achondroplasia, which is almost universally fatal within the first year of life.[22] The skeletal features of achondroplasia are highly exaggerated in the homozygous condition, resulting in significantly shorter limbs, a smaller chest size, and a smaller foramen magnum. A brief summary of medical complications by age is given in Table 213–1.

Approximately 150 skeletal dysplasias have been identified, a number of which manifest neurological symptoms.[23] Achondroplasia is the most common in clinical series. Although frequency estimates cluster between 1 in 25,000 and 1 in 35,000 live births, the true frequency must be recalculated, because these data were generated before the *FGFR3* mutations were identified.[5, 6,24] In addition to the short-limb dwarfism syndromes, some syndromic craniosynostoses have been associated with mutations in one or more of the *FGFR* genes: autosomal-dominant craniosynostosis and Jackson-Weiss, Saethre-Chotzen, Pfeiffer's, type 2 Antley-Bixler, Crouzon's, and Apert's syndromes.[25]

MEDICAL COMPLICATIONS

Most individuals with achondroplasia have normal intelligence. A cross-sectional survey (using self-reported SF-36 data) of the functional health status of adults with achondroplasia revealed that the Mental Component Summary scores did not differ significantly compared with scores from the general population. In contrast, the Physical Component Summary scores were significantly lower starting in the fourth decade of life.[26] In children, motor milestones are delayed, partly because of generalized hypotonia and partly because of the mechanical disadvantage imposed by short limbs.[1, 22,27–29] Psychosocial problems arising from short stature include lack of acceptance by peers and the tendency for adults, including parents and teachers, to treat children with achondroplasia appropriately for their height rather than their age.[30,31] Quality-of-life issues on which the patient's perceived status is suboptimal require special attention during adolescence.[32] Involvement with other families with children of short stature, in an organization such as the Little People of America, can improve self-esteem and can assist parents in guiding their achondroplastic children through the difficulties of growing up in a culture that often equates stature with status.

Reproductive difficulties have not been conclusively documented, but evidence of reduced fertility, frequent fibroid cysts, and early menopause has been reported. Women with achondroplasia must deliver their infants by cesarean section because of cephalopelvic disproportion, and administration of spinal anesthesia is strongly discouraged.

Obstructive sleep apnea, or sleep-disordered breathing secondary to a small upper airway, is common. Tonsillectomy and adenoidectomy decrease the degree of upper airway obstruction in most children. The ma-

TABLE 213–1 ■ Medical and Neurologic Complications of Achondroplasia

COMPLICATION	CUMULATIVE PERCENTAGE AFFECTED, BY AGE IN YEARS				
	<1	<5	<10	<20	>20
Otitis media	60	93	96		
Ventilation tubes	16	68	78		
Tonsillectomy		25	33	37	39
Hearing loss		17	24	28	38
Speech delay		17	19	19	19
Orthodontics			3	22	48
Shunt	2	6	9	11	11
Apnea	8		13	16	16
Cervicomedullary decompression	4		9	13	17
Cervical signs		4	7	8	15
Back pain		5		16	20
Spinal stenosis					
Surgery			1	3	7

Data from Hunter AGW, Bankier A, Rogers JG, et al: Medical complications of achondroplasia: A multicentre patient review. J Med Genet 35:705–712, 1998.

jority do not have significant obstructive or central apnea, but a significant minority are severely affected.[33–36] The cause of different patterns of sleep disorders may be related to localized alterations or chondrocranial development.[34] Many infants sleep with their necks in a hyperextended position, which functionally increases the size of the upper airway. Although the hyperextended neck position relieves intermittent obstruction, it also can exacerbate the neurological sequelae of cervicomedullary compression related to a small foramen magnum. Abnormal respiratory sinus arrhythmias may be present.[37] A small thoracic cage can result in restrictive pulmonary disease in infancy. Respiration may be further compromised by aspiration secondary to gastroesophageal reflux or swallowing dysfunction, or both, resulting in recurrent pneumonia. Anesthesia can be given safely to children, with special consideration for limited neck extension and appropriate endotracheal tube size.[35]

A relatively high rate (about 3%) of jugular bulb dehiscence—complete absence of the roof over the jugular bulb—was identified in a series of 126 achondroplastic children. This increased incidence may account for unexplained hearing loss, tinnitus, and self-audible bruits in these children and poses a risk of difficult-to-control bleeding at myringotomy.[38]

EVALUATION AND DIAGNOSIS

Cervicomedullary Compression

CLINICAL PATHOLOGY AND PRESENTATION

Cervicomedullary compression stems primarily from a reduction in the diameter of the foramen magnum in both the sagittal and coronal dimensions, a reduction that is sometimes more than 5 standard deviations less than normal.[39–44] Cervicomedullary compression warrants early and aggressive treatment because it results in high cervical myelopathy and increases the risk of sudden death by central respiratory failure.[45–47] A prospective evaluation of achondroplastic infants found radiographic evidence of craniocervical stenosis in 58% of the patients studied, and a diagnosis of cervicomedullary compression was made in 35%.[48] Although these figures are for a selected population and are therefore higher than for the general population, they are a strong argument for the careful evaluation and treatment of achondroplastic children. A retrospective study found increased mortality (compared with population standards) in achondroplastic children younger than 4 years, with sudden death resulting from brainstem compression identified as the cause of half the deaths. The same study also found a 7.5% risk of sudden death in the first year of life.[22]

Chronic medullary and upper cervical cord compression may exist as a neurologically asymptomatic lesion, exhibiting neither signs of root compression in the arms nor symptoms of cranial nerve impairment. Nonetheless, microcystic histopathologic changes, cervical syringomyelia, and necrosis and gliosis have been reported in autopsies of achondroplastic children who died unexpectedly. Presumably, lesions of this type interrupt neural respiratory pathways from the nucleus tractus solitarii to the phrenic nerve nucleus—arresting the muscles of inspiration and resulting in sudden death in some cases. We therefore consider infants with a history of sleep apnea or other severe respiratory or neurological abnormalities to be at increased risk for respiratory complications resulting from occult cervicomedullary compression. Some authors have recommended performing sleep and imaging studies on all children with achondroplasia.[49] We believe that a careful history and neurological examination should precede costlier and more uncomfortable diagnostics. A composite profile of the patient with cervicomedullary compression includes upper or lower extremity paresis, apnea or cyanosis, hyperreflexia or hypertonia, and delay in motor milestones beyond achondroplastic standards. These patients can present a striking contrast to the usual floppy, hypotonic achondroplastic infant.[50]

EVALUATION

Once a high-risk patient with respiratory or neurological symptoms or signs has been identified, we advise comprehensive testing. Parents should be carefully interviewed about the health and medical history of their child, with emphasis on respiratory symptoms. A general physical examination, including chest measurements, should be performed. Respiratory evaluation should include the evaluation of blood pH, a chest radiograph, and overnight polysomnography. Electrocardiograms and echocardiograms should be performed to see whether there is cardiac evidence of chronic oxygen deprivation during sleep. A neurological examination for signs of brainstem compression, such as hyperreflexia, hypertonia, paresis, asymmetry of movement or strength, or abnormal plantar responses, is essential. Brainstem auditory evoked potential and upper extremity somatosensory evoked potential evaluation should be considered as an adjunct, especially in patients with normal results on neurological examination. Imaging studies of the craniocervical junction are necessary, particularly magnetic resonance imaging (MRI) in the sagittal plane. We also strongly recommend cardiac-gated MRI flow studies of the cerebrospinal fluid (CSF) at the foramen magnum.

INDICATIONS FOR OPERATION

Concerns have been expressed about the indications for surgical decompression of the foramen magnum in this population.[51–53] Radiographic studies during the first years of life show some degree of compression at the foramen magnum level. MRI evidence of spinal cord compression with indentation or narrowing of the upper cervical cord is a common finding, which is usually graded as "marked" or "severe" in the MRI report.[51] In one report, myelomalacia was observed in 13 of 30 achondroplastic children.[43] Yet, other than the routinely observed generalized hypotonia seen in the achondroplastic population, the majority of these children are asymptomatic and outgrow their developmental delays.[52,54–56] Cervicomedullary decompression (CMD) as a routine prophylactic measure is therefore not warranted.

Several groups have published guidelines for surgical intervention.[54, 55,57] Our indications are based on lower limb symptoms, polysomnography, and MRI flow studies. The underlying principle must be to identify patients who are at risk for neurological damage or sudden death. We recommend that patients with cervicomedullary compression be identified and treated prophylactically, before abrupt and irreversible changes occur. For the purpose of diagnosis, we define clinically significant cervicomedullary compression to be (1) neurological evidence of upper cervical myelopathy; (2) evidence of stenosis on imaging studies, including the absence of flow above and below the foramen magnum; and frequently (3) an otherwise unexplained respiratory or developmental abnormality.

Hunter and coworkers conducted a multicenter review of 193 patients with chondrodysplasias. The study reported data on the rates of medical complications at specific age intervals (see Table 213–1). At age 4 the rate of CMD was 6.8%. The authors emphasized the important role of surgery, primarily because progressive neurological symptoms continue into adulthood. Ultimately, about 17% of the patients in the series underwent CMD.[58]

Hydrocephalus

CLINICAL PATHOLOGY AND PRESENTATION

Hydrocephalus in an achondroplastic patient is likely secondary to deformation of the cranial base. Constriction of the basal foramina, particularly the jugular foramina, is thought to reduce venous drainage and potentially raise intracranial venous pressure. In theory, absorption of CSF into the sagittal venous sinus is thus reduced, resulting in hydrocephalus.[44] Some investigators have reported that CSF dynamics are frequently abnormal. Identifying patients at high risk for hydrocephalus currently is not possible. Hydrocephalus may resolve in some patients with continued growth of the skull base during puberty.

It is easy to suspect hydrocephalus in a patient with achondroplasia, given that macrocrania is a morphologic hallmark of the disease. Concerns about hydrocephalus may also arise because of the enlarged ventricles and the delayed acquisition of gross motor skills. Although hydrocephalus is associated with enlarged ventricles in the achondroplastic population, it generally resolves through growth and maturation of the cranial bones.[59] The achondroplastic child typically displays transient hypotonia, but the papilledema that is expected with symptomatic hydrocephalus is rare. Radiographically, mild to moderate ventricular enlargement, prominent cortical sulci, and an increased frontal subarachnoid space are apparent. Hydrocephalus severe enough to require shunting is often discovered after craniocervical decompression, when CSF leaks often complicate wound healing.

EVALUATION

A degree of abnormal CSF dynamics is common in achondroplasia. We believe that routine surveillance of achondroplastic infants for hydrocephalus is best limited to noninvasive measures that are easily incorporated into the pediatric examination and should not require referral to special centers and complex diagnostic procedures. Longitudinally evaluating head circumference and tracking the acquisition of developmental milestones, with comparison to published standards, are usually sufficient. Imaging studies can be reserved for patients whose head circumference crosses percentiles on the achondroplastic chart or those who manifest unexplained neurological signs or developmental retardation.

INDICATIONS FOR OPERATION

Stenosis of the jugular foramina contributes to the altered CSF dynamics in achondroplasia.[44] Jugular foramen decompression is an option.[60] We believe that this option should be used only for a child with severe jugular stenosis and debilitating hydrocephalus for whom conventional ventriculoperitoneal shunting is contraindicated. Given the high percentage of complications, shunting is best reserved for those in whom symptoms are severe and threatening.[42] CSF pressure profiles can be determined with an external transducer attached to an open fontanelle, with an epidural pressure monitor, or with an intraventricular catheter in older patients. If no critical pressure elevations are detected during a 48-hour period, shunt placement is not required, ventriculomegaly notwithstanding. However, the presence of severe clinical stigmata for hydrocephalus obviates such demonstrations.

For patients who have undergone craniocervical decompression, we expect sustained intracranial pressure (ICP) to be less than 20 mm Hg during the immediate postoperative period. Transient increases above this level can be associated with activity or irritation in normal individuals. In situations in which ICP is abnormally elevated, we proceed with shunting. In situations in which the interpretation is equivocal, we extend the period of monitoring for 1 or 2 days. Occasionally, even when no elevation of ICP is documented, a persistent CSF leak or subgaleal collections of CSF develop soon after the ventriculostomy is removed. It is sometimes difficult to tell whether shunting should be carried out on the basis of a developing subgaleal CSF collection. One certainly does not want to place a shunt if the fluid collection is likely to resolve on its own. For this reason, we usually wait several days and observe for resolution or an increase in the amount of scalp swelling. We take a more aggressive approach to shunting, however, if subcutaneous collections develop over the site of craniocervical decompression. The dura in this area should have been closed in a watertight fashion and checked with a sustained Valsalva maneuver of 40 mm Hg intraoperatively; therefore, the development of a fluid collection in this area most likely represents elevated ICP. Collections in this region delay wound healing. Furthermore, because this is a high-contact area (i.e., an area with a significant risk of infection because of contact transmission of microbes), there is a proclivity toward subsequent infection. For these reasons, in situations in which postoperative cervicomedullary CSF collections occur, we generally proceed with shunting much more rapidly than for scalp collections.

Spinal Stenosis

CLINICAL PATHOLOGY AND PRESENTATION

Spinal stenosis is the most common complication of achondroplasia, usually becoming symptomatic in the third decade or later. The anatomy of the achondroplastic spine is distinctive in several respects, all of which contribute to spinal cord compromise and nerve root compression. The superior and inferior articular facets of the vertebral bodies are susceptible to hypertrophy, resulting in a "mushroom" shape that is clearly evident on a contrast myelogram. Abbreviated and thickened pedicles of the vertebral arches result from premature fusion. Intervertebral disks tend to bulge prominently, further aggravating neural encroachment by the enlarged vertebral body articular surfaces. The interpediculate distance decreases in the lumbar region of the spine, resulting in a canal that tapers caudally, the opposite of normal (the canal normally widens caudally). The overall picture is one of dramatic stenosis in every dimension of the spine.

Although the problems relating to hydrocephalus and cervicomedullary compression are frequently identified in infancy and childhood, neurological problems below the foramen magnum frequently present in late adolescence and adulthood. In one series of patients treated at our institution, however, 35% became symptomatic before reaching 15 years. Moreover, estimates of the incidence of symptomatic spinal stenosis range from 37% to 89%, suggesting that a significant proportion will eventually have this problem.[58] Because the achondroplastic spinal canal tends to have severe congenital constriction, more intensive early screening might reveal substantial numbers of young achondroplastic patients with occult symptoms of spinal stenosis. Thorough urologic and neurological testing plays a useful part in the prospective evaluation for occult stenosis.

In the management of the achondroplastic spine, it is possible to distinguish between the neurosurgical and orthopedic aspects of this disease. The hypotonia that an achondroplastic infant typically exhibits suggests that muscular tone may be insufficient for adequate protection of pediatric skeletal structures in weight-bearing postures. Achondroplastic children are in fact developmentally delayed in supporting their heads independently, as well as in upright sitting and walking. In our opinion, parents should not encourage early sitting because of the potential for aggravation of thoracolumbar kyphosis in this posture. Sitting and standing postures affect the curvature of the spine, and in achondroplastic children, muscular weakness, short vertebral pedicles, and lax spinal ligaments complicate these mechanics. Attention has also been drawn to the dynamic effect of a small chest and a globulus abdomen in the formation of a progressive kyphosis.[61] Moreover, delayed standing predisposes to development of a gibbus, with wedging of one or more vertebral elements. These wedged deformities are both debilitating and preventable. Because surgical repair has risks, effort is well spent on prevention. Orthopedic bracing is used prophylactically when formation of a wedged gibbus seems likely. Parents should also be urged not to use any infant carriers, strollers, or baby seats that exaggerate the thoracolumbar kyphosis.

In an adult, compromise can result from abnormalities such as hyperlordosis, minor disk bulging, hypertrophic osteoarthritis, or ligamentous hypertrophy. The presence of a thoracolumbar kyphosis is also positively correlated with symptomatic spinal stenosis.[61] Although low back pain is a common complaint among achondroplastic patients, those with severe stenosis can develop symptomatic neurogenic claudication. Prolonged walking produces first paresthesias and later weakness of the lower extremities, which is usually bilateral. These symptoms are promptly relieved by resting, squatting, or leaning forward, which straightens the lordosis and increases the transverse diameter of the lumbosacral canal.[62] With progressive stenosis, the distance walked before claudication ensues decreases, making this symptom a useful clinical parameter.

EVALUATION

In more advanced cases of stenosis, neurological abnormalities, such as weakness of the lower extremities (particularly dorsiflexors of the toes and feet) and hypoesthesia, often at a truncal level, persist at rest. Occasionally, a partial Brown-Séquard syndrome is seen. Spasticity and hyperreflexia of the legs typically indicate compression of the thoracic cord but may indicate coexistent cervical compression. The results of neurological examinations in patients with claudication often remain otherwise normal until late in the disease process. Straight leg raising and reverse straight leg raising test results are usually normal unless a superimposed disk problem is present. Therefore, the thoracolumbar spine must be evaluated in all symptomatic achondroplastic patients, even in the absence of neurological findings. The traditional study is myelography followed by computed tomographic scanning; however, MRI techniques are becoming increasingly reliable. Because of the stenotic lumbar canal, it is advisable to inject contrast via a lateral C1-C2 puncture. Lumbar puncture is less advisable, because the likelihood of herniation of the nerve roots is greater in the narrow lumbar canal. We reviewed our experience with MRI and computed tomographic myelography and found that there was good correlation between CSF block by computed tomographic myelography and loss of T2 signal on MRI. MRI more frequently demonstrated significant disk bulges and soft tissue hypertrophy than did computed tomographic myelography. MRI consistently predicts much more severe pathology in the lumbar spine among achondroplastic patients than does computed tomographic myelography. MRI has the advantage of revealing focal regions of compression secondary to soft tissue hypertrophy and providing information distal to the level of complete block. In our experience, therefore, both studies are valuable and complementary in the preoperative planning of these patients.

INDICATIONS FOR OPERATION

We recommend decompressive laminectomies for achondroplastic patients whose ambulation is severely limited by claudication, who show significant weakness (other than mild extensor hallucis longus weakness) at rest, or who have urinary incontinence or urgency that is attributable to compression of the cauda equina or spinal cord. There is a high incidence of urologic complications after laminectomy and a high correlation between preoperative urologic abnormalities and postoperative complaints. We therefore recommend thorough urologic testing as part of the preoperative evaluation for patients undergoing laminectomy.

OPERATIVE MANAGEMENT

At our institution, we use a common high-speed drill technique for both craniocervical and spinal decompressions. Although laminectomy is a widely practiced spinal procedure, we believe that modifications that address several of its shortcomings, including inadequate decompression and secondary spinal instability, are necessary for its use in achondroplastic patients.[63,64]

Cervicomedullary Compression

Craniocervical surgical decompression for cervicomedullary compression in children with achondroplasia has been used at several centers and yields generally good results.[45] Decompression of the cervicomedullary junction has been shown to bring about dramatic and sustained improvement in neurological and respiratory function when it is combined with other therapy as needed for respiratory compromise.[48,50] The procedure is not widespread, however, because its successful performance relies on careful management of the anatomic difficulties presented by the achondroplastic patient. Clinical evaluation, moreover, is frequently difficult because achondroplastic patients can have respiratory difficulties for many reasons, some of which are unrelated to neurological compromise. Long-term follow-up data that would allow a definitive assessment of craniocervical decompression have also been lacking.[51,65] As with any surgical procedure, detailed prior consultation must be conducted with the parents to inform them of the potential risks and expected benefits for their achondroplastic child.

A large operating room is used to accommodate all the equipment and personnel necessary to decompress the craniocervical junction. Before coming to the operating room, the patient is sedated, and antibiotics are administered. Patients also receive steroids preoperatively to protect the spinal cord and brainstem from local trauma. Patients are positioned prone on the operating table, with the head and neck carefully supported in slight flexion by use of a padded pediatric horseshoe headrest. Upper extremity somatosensory evoked potentials are assessed routinely during positioning as well as during the decompression procedure itself. The anesthesiologist is situated for easy access to the patient and is also in close proximity to the evoked potential monitoring equipment.

After some untoward experience with postoperative CSF leakage from the surgical wound, we began to perform a ventriculostomy before craniocervical decompression. We hypothesized that duraplasty and wound healing were compromised as a result of the raised ICP typically found in achondroplastic children. Nonetheless, not all these children's preoperative symptoms necessarily resulted from hydrocephalus. We implemented a solution, therefore, that would address the postoperative problem without necessitating permanent shunt placement. An external ventricular drain is inserted via a right frontal approach into the anterior horn of the right lateral ventricle. The external ventricular drain is left in place (closed) throughout the subsequent decompression and is opened postoperatively to allow continuous drainage at an ICP of greater than 10 cm H_2O. ICP is monitored for 48 hours, with drainage release pressure gradually increased to 15 to 20 cm H_2O. The standard protocol is to record ICP, mean arterial pressure, cerebral perfusion pressure, and the amount of CSF drainage, along with hourly vital signs. Ultimately, some of these patients will require shunting, and the ability to monitor ICP postoperatively yields important information for this determination. Thus, the benefits of perioperative ventriculostomy appear to outweigh the risks associated with this procedure in this group of patients. We have stopped placing ventriculostomies in all but the most obviously symptomatic hydrocephalic children. Instead, we use intraoperative ultrasonography to determine the adequacy of CSF flow once the bony decompression has been completed.

For the decompression, a midline suboccipital incision is made, and the ligaments and musculature are dissected subperiosteally to expose the occiput and the spinous processes and laminae of C1 and C2. The arch of C1 is then removed with a high-speed drill and small curettes. One frequently sees a thick, fibrous band or pannus above the level of C1 that should be left in place during the bony dissection to protect the underlying dura and cord from incidental injury. Compression of the cervical cord occasionally necessitates removal of the arch of C2 or extension of the decompression even farther in a caudal direction. The posterior rim of the foramen magnum is thinned gradually with a high-speed drill and removed with small, straight, and angled curettes. Invariably, the bone of the foramen magnum is thickened and oriented more horizontally than usual, severely indenting the underlying dura. The most delicate part of the dissection occurs as the drill approaches the posterior rim of the foramen magnum. Once the bony decompression is complete, the fibrous pannus is removed as well, often revealing a transverse dural channel that offers dramatic evidence of the extent of dural constriction; consequently, adequate attention must be paid to the soft tissue aspects of the decompression. Duraplasty, by opening the dura in the midline along the area of constriction, is performed to relieve any persistent dural constriction. Adequate cord pulsations and CSF flow can be confirmed, and a dural patch graft can be performed, using paraspinous fascia, pericranium, or commercially available human cadaveric dura. A watertight seal is confirmed, and the wound is copiously irrigated and closed in several layers; it is not drained, however, to avoid potentiating the development of a CSF fistula. Somatosensory evoked potentials are evaluated before the patient is undraped, in case it is necessary to re-explore the wound. Once movement is confirmed in all four extremities, the patient is sent to the pediatric intensive care unit. Extubation is often performed immediately postoperatively; however, in some cases, facial and laryngeal edema make this procedure inadvisable for 12 to 24 hours. After surgery, primary attention is directed toward monitoring ICP as a part of postoperative nursing care.

The surgeon should bear in mind several important pitfalls when undertaking CMD in achondroplastic patients. First, the patient's head must not be overflexed during positioning, because such a position often reduces the subarachnoid space at the cervicomedullary junction. Second, the surgeon should avoid placing any instruments beneath the posterior arch of C1 or beneath the rim of the foramen magnum, even though these patients are pretreated with steroids. The cervicomedullary junction is already under tremendous constrictive pressure, and even the brief introduction of instruments into the already compromised space can be disastrous. The spinal cord and brainstem of a child with achondroplasia are small; therefore, the decompression should be correspondingly small. To gain an accurate conception of the size of the spinal cord and brainstem to perform an appropriate decompression, the surgeon must study results of the preoperative MRI. Moreover, the decompression must be extended not only along the dorsal surface of the cervicomedullary junction but also sufficiently along the lateral dimensions of the medulla to decompress the stenosis at the level of the foramen magnum adequately.

Frequently, engorged veins exist beneath the ligamentum flavum, located dorsally and laterally, and sometimes insinuating through the ligamentum flavum. These can create enormous bleeding and must be controlled rapidly if they are compromised. The possibility of air embolization also exists through these veins, and the surgeon should ensure that the patient is not in any degree of reverse Trendelenburg's position. Finally, once the bony decompression is complete, the underlying dura, which in many cases is itself severely constricted, must be carefully checked. The dura is often fused with the ligamentum, and this soft tissue band serves to constrict the underlying neural tissues, even without the presence of the overlying bone. When

this situation occurs, the band must be divided and a dural patch placed. When the band is divided, a significantly engorged annular sinus is commonly present beneath the foramen magnum; therefore, the band should be slowly divided, and measures should be taken to control the annular sinus as it is encountered.

Spinal Stenosis

Decompression of the achondroplastic spinal canal is difficult because of the extent and severity of the stenosis. The quantitative magnitude of this stenosis has been well documented.[66] Moreover, poor postoperative results were relatively common for spinal decompressions in achondroplastic patients.[63, 64,67] Before the era of CT and MRI, the degree and extent of spinal compression were often not appreciated with conventional myelography because of the lack of adequate contrast medium diffusion. Insertion of bulky instruments under the laminae during the conventional techniques frequently traumatized neural tissue. Another source of poor results was postoperative instability resulting from overly wide laminectomies.

The following procedure has been used at our institution with good results. MRI obtains adequate anatomic delineation, and intrathecally enhanced computed tomographic scanning is used, but myelography is sometimes helpful as an adjunct. Based on the results of these studies, the surgeon can devise an operative plan for adequate decompression that includes at least three segments above the level of demonstrated block and three segments below (or to S2). The incision is midline, and dissection is carried subperiosteally to expose the spinous processes, laminae, and facet joints over the extent of the area to be decompressed. When adequate exposure is achieved, the laminae immediately medial to the facet joints are gradually thinned with a high-speed drill, forming a groove approximately parallel to the longitudinal axis of the spinal column. The drill head is held at an attitude of about 45 degrees to the laminal surface rather than 90 degrees; this angle offers the surgeon the control necessary to avoid accidental perforation of the laminae. The groove is deepened until the dura can be seen through the thinned laminal mantle. Drilling is then concluded in this area and is continued on the opposite side in a similar fashion. An opening is made at the caudal part of the groove on the first side, a thin surgical punch is inserted into the epidural space, and the laminectomy is carried along the groove. A small Leksell rongeur is inserted through this opening to complete the laminectomy by lifting off the laminae in a piecemeal fashion. This technique minimizes dural tearing, preserves the facet joints, and protects the neural structures from injury. If the facet joints are violated on both sides, spinal fusion is necessary. In our experience, because the primary compressive dimension in the achondroplastic spine is cephalocaudal, not lateral, undermining of the facets is not recommended.

Removal of the spinous processes and detachment of the paraspinal soft tissues create a large and deep void, particularly at the lumbosacral junction. To minimize the risk of pseudomeningocele formation, an overlapping closure using paraspinal muscle was developed, whereby muscle masses are brought in to fill the dead space. First, a paraspinal muscle encased in fascia is partially detached from the iliac spine and the lumbosacral laminae by use of a split-thickness incision, if necessary, to mobilize the required tissue, which is then reflected around its pedicle. The edge of the flap is brought down to the opposite lateral end of the lamina and is attached with heavy sutures to the inferior part of the paraspinal muscle mass on that side. The superior part of the muscle mass on that side is then retracted over the first flap, thereby completing the muscle closure and collapsing the void. As with craniocervical decompression, somatosensory evoked potentials are monitored intraoperatively. Postoperative care is generally routine, with the exception of a high incidence of transient urologic dysfunction. Staff should be advised to help the patient be prepared for this possibility.

A different viewpoint concerning the ideal strategy for spinal laminectomy recommends a wide decompression with foraminotomies and mandatory undermining of the facets.[68] The rationale for this strategy is that compression is lateral as well as longitudinal in the achondroplastic spinal canal. Our experience, however, does not bear this out, despite the hypothesized impact of small lateral recesses in the achondroplastic vertebral foramen. Moreover, the stabilization problems encountered with wide laminectomies can be more debilitating than the initial disease. In fact, there is no reason why every spinal level could not be subjected to the laminectomy we describe without the need for concomitant spinal stabilization. Therefore, in light of the results obtained at our institution with spinal decompressions, we believe that a narrow, extensive laminectomy is the spinal decompression of choice for achondroplastic patients. Some surgeons have adopted this operative technique for their nonachondroplastic patients as well. The goal is adequate decompression of neural elements and not simply enlargement of bony canals.

OUTCOME

Craniocervical Decompression

Concerns have been expressed about the morbidity accompanying the relatively high number of patients with cervicomedullary compression who undergo CMD and go on to require shunts.[52] In our opinion, however, this hydrocephalus is not a complication of the operation but rather is discovered as a result of the violation of the dural layer, a situation that allows a much more sensitive picture of the ICP dynamics than is otherwise possible. This view receives additional support from research that suggests a strong predisposition to hydrocephalus in achondroplastic children and a higher than normal ICP as a result of the bony anatomy. In light of these findings, the morbidity and mortality of our reported craniocervical decompression

series are not only low for a procedure of this delicacy but also low relative to the general morbidity and mortality of achondroplastic disease. This argument is strengthened by the fact that a large number of the patients we diagnose have a combination of severe respiratory and neurologic disease, and after their procedures, they go on to make developmental strides at a rapid pace, with resolution of their symptoms. Although we believe that our treatment of achondroplastic hydrocephalus is uncontroversial, our understanding of it does rest on some unproven assumptions. First, the current understanding of ICP dynamics is neither comprehensive nor general. Despite evidence strongly favoring the theory that raised ICP in achondroplastic patients is secondary to venous hypertension, this view has not been conclusively demonstrated. The balance of the evidence, however, both published and experiential, favors this view, and we will continue to use it as a working theory until a better understanding of ICP in general, and hydrocephalus in achondroplasia in particular, is available.

At present, there are no long-term outcome reports of large, well-followed cohorts with documented perspectives, management protocols, and neurosurgical techniques.[51,65] There is a need for this information so that we can identify specific patients requiring immediate CMD and address questions about children who will go on to require CMD and whether early surgery prevents subsequent morbidity.

Spinal Decompression

From 1980 to 1990 at our institution, Uematsu performed spinal decompressive laminectomies on 67 individuals who ranged in age from 10 to 66 years. The mean age at time of surgery was 37 years, and the mean duration of symptoms before operation was 5 years. Of these patients, 44 had laminectomies confined to the lower thoracic, lumbar, or sacral spine; others required laminectomies in the upper thoracic or cervical spine as well. In the former group, the average number of segments decompressed was 11. The most common extent of decompression was from T8 to S1. Outcome was judged by comparison of functional assessments performed preoperatively and at the time of the latest follow-up examination (mean follow-up, 29 months). Outcome was quantified by a functional rating scale that included consideration of arm strength, ambulation, urinary function, and pain. By this scale, 70% of patients with thoracolumbar decompressions improved, 22% deteriorated, and the remainder showed no change. The best predictor of improvement was the duration of symptoms before operation. Those who had been symptomatic for less than 1 year showed an average improvement of 40% on our functional ratings scale, whereas those who had been symptomatic for longer than 1 year had an average improvement of only 15%. The most common complication of surgery was urinary retention, which developed in 38% of patients; however, in most patients, this was a transient problem. Forty-three percent of patients experienced either single or multiple dural tears during the procedure, and 10% of patients developed a pseudo-meningocele that required repair. Wound infection developed in 13.5%. Three patients developed a gastrointestinal bleed or pseudomembranous colitis, and one patient had a deep venous thrombosis.

We also looked at the incidence of restenosis at previously operated levels.[69] From 1994 to 1996, eight patients required repeat spinal decompression. Preoperatively, they all had impaired motor function, 87% had sensory dysfunction, 50% had neurogenic claudication, 50% had severe radiating pain, 37.5% had bladder incontinence (one patient had additional bowel incontinence), and 50% had evidence of myelopathy. Six patients were improved at discharge. The long-term results show motor improvements in all but one patient, and bladder symptoms disappeared in two of three patients.

Spinal Restenosis in Achondroplasia

In a spine that has been previously decompressed, restenosis may occur because of accelerated facet hypertrophy, bony overgrowth, and scarring. This acceleration of facet hypertrophy may represent instability in the previously operated achondroplastic spine or some exaggerated response to normal motion that results

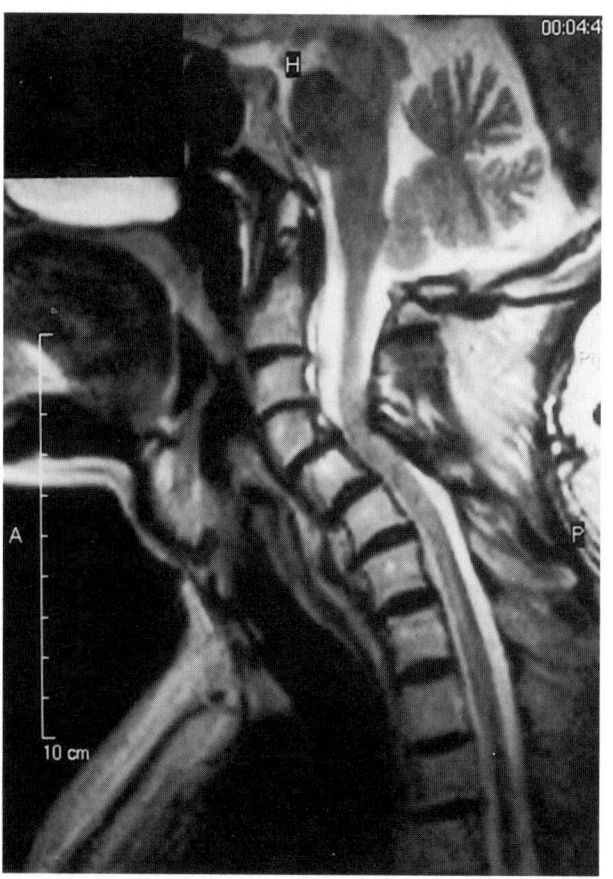

FIGURE 213–1. Sagittal T2-weighted MRI scan of the cervical spine in a patient with hypochondroplasia. Cord compression is the result of reverse lordosis at C5-7. Otherwise, canal diameter appears adequate.

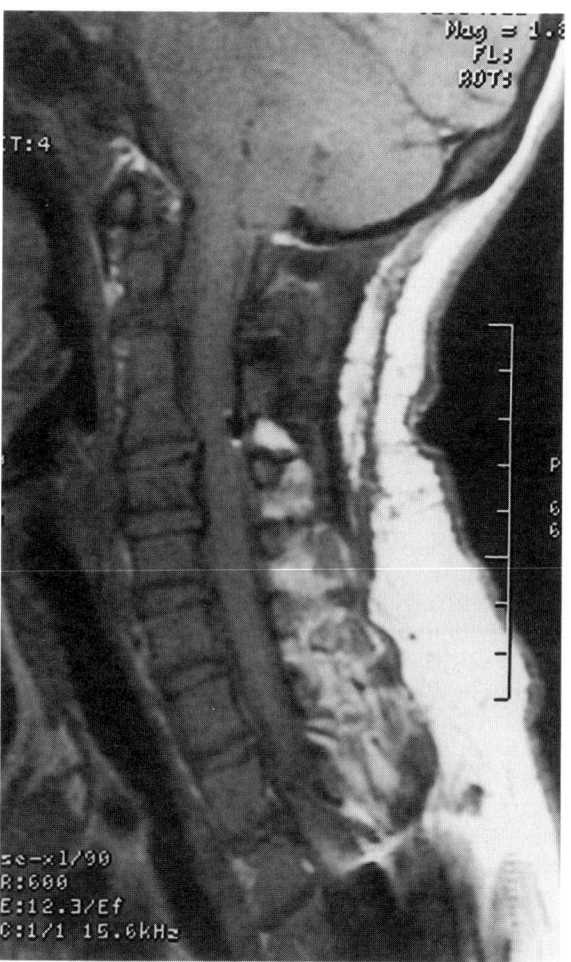

FIGURE 213–2. Sagittal T1-weighted MRI scan of the cervical spine in a previously operated patient with achondroplasia. Initially the patient underwent a laminectomy for cervical stenosis. However, fusion became necessary for delayed instability. At the time of our evaluation, a progressive myelopathy had developed. MRI suggests cord compression at C4-5 (note the presence of blocked vertebrae at C3-4) resulting from a sublaminar wire.

from the genetic defect in this disease. There are many reports documenting the efficacy of decompressive therapy in the treatment of achondroplastic spinal stenosis. In several of these series, reoperation was often necessary for achondroplastic spinal restenosis.[69]

We reviewed our series of eight patients who underwent reoperation for spinal restenosis in achondroplasia between 1994 and 1996. These eight patients represent 4.3% of all achondroplastic patients operated on for spinal stenosis at the Johns Hopkins Hospital since the early 1980s. There were five men and three women. Mean age was 43 years. The most common neurologic sign of recurrent stenosis was impaired motor function, which occurred in all eight (100%) patients. Seven (87.5%) of the patients had sensory dysfunction, four (50%) had neurogenic claudication, four (50%) had severe radicular pain, one (37.5%) had bladder incontinence (one also had bowel incontinence), and four (50%) had signs of myelopathy. Axial low back pain was present in all seven patients who had thoracolumbar stenosis. Two of the eight patients presented with abrupt deterioration of their neurologic condition. All other patients presented with gradual deterioration over a mean interval of 8.9 months. All seven patients who had thoracolumbar stenosis showed complete block on computed tomographic myelography. An incomplete block was observed in the patient with cervical stenosis. The most common cause of recurrent stenosis was facet hypertrophy in six (75%) patients (Fig. 213–1). Other causes included disk pathology in four (50%) patients, bony overgrowth in three (37%) patients, kyphosis in three (37.5%) patients, spur formation in two (25%) patients, and fusion construct (Figs. 213–2 and 213–3) in one (12.5%) patient. The mean interval between the most recent surgeries was 8.2 years; however, for surgery at the same level, the mean interval was 9.5 years. Complications included a dural tear and cerebellar hemorrhage in one patient and transient neurologic worsening in another patient. One patient died 24 hours after surgery when she developed acute respiratory insufficiency and a fatal cardiac arrest after extubation. The patient had been placed in halo stabilization after a repeat cervical laminectomy and lateral mass fusion for cervical subluxation and progressive quadriparesis.

Repeat surgery carries a higher risk of dural tear than do initial procedures, but the greater challenge in these cases is to balance the need for further decompression with the risk of destabilization of the spine. The difficulties of performing a fusion in a patient who has undergone previous multisegmental decompressive laminectomies can be great. If facetectomy or extensive foraminotomy is performed, instability is likely to occur. This situation was encountered in four (50%) of our cases. Two patients underwent transverse

process fusion and external orthosis. These patients had no preoperative kyphosis and appeared to be destabilized by the reoperative decompression. The other two patients required fusion with instrumentation. These two patients had kyphotic deformities preoperatively, and one required extensive facetectomies intraoperatively that were thought to be further destabilizing. Outcome assessment revealed that six of the patients (75%) had postoperative improvement in their strength. Bladder symptoms disappeared in two patients and remained unchanged in one patient. In summary, our retrospective review suggests that, in spite of its technical challenges, redecompression of the spinal canal can be successful in alleviating the majority of these patients' symptoms.

CONCLUSIONS

Skeletal dysplasias are complex diseases, and their treatment requires several disciplines and strategies. Although delicate procedures performed on children naturally involve risks, these risks can be minimized through knowledge, experience, and a well-trained support staff. Furthermore, the resilience of a child treated appropriately for his or her disease is one of the most satisfying events for a surgeon to witness.

Spinal stenosis is more frequently encountered than cervicomedullary compression, and a modified technique for laminectomy offers a better prospect for patients than does the conventional technique. Craniocervical decompression, however, is a potentially life-saving procedure that significantly improves the natural history of achondroplasia and allows these young patients to make developmental strides without debilitating neurologic impairment. The objective is always to identify more accurately the subpopulation of achondroplastic patients at risk. Craniocervical decompression is often associated with the discovery of hydrocephalus, but this is best viewed as a preexisting condition that surgical intervention reveals and renders treatable. Achondroplastic patients are generally predisposed to hydrocephalus as a result of their anatomy, but most of them tolerate their symptoms relatively well; accordingly, those who do not undergo craniocervical decompression can be treated by a more conservative protocol. Notwithstanding the relatively low frequency of achondroplasia, if the goal of the neurosurgeon is relief of debilitating symptoms, the high incidence of central nervous system disease in this population offers compelling opportunities to effect a satisfying and dramatic change in a patient's condition and prospects.

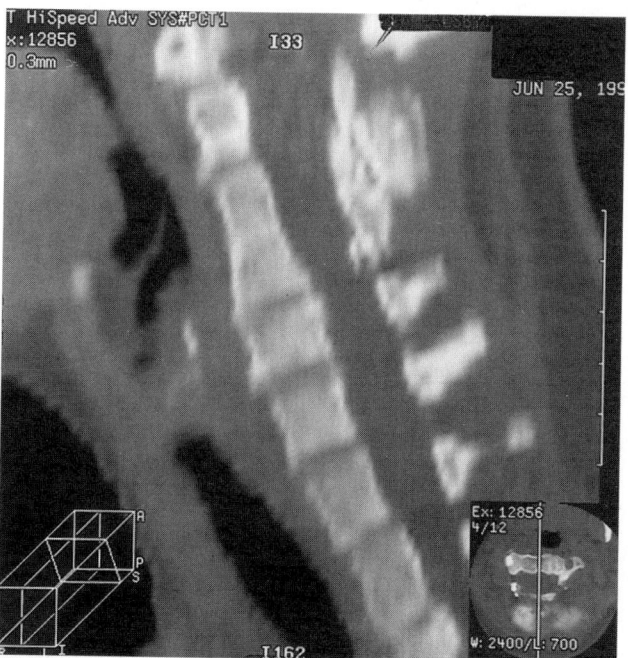

FIGURE 213–3. Computed tomographic image with sagittal reconstruction in the same patient as in Figure 213–2 highlights the bone fusion and posterior wire.

REFERENCES

1. Committee on Genetics: Health supervision for children with achondroplasia. Pediatrics 95:443–451, 1995.
2. Carson BS, Francomano C, Hurko O, et al: Management of achondroplasia and its neurosurgical complications. In Schmidek HH (ed): Operative Neurosurgical Techniques. Philadelphia, WB Saunders, 1999.
3. Carson BS, Sponseller PD, Guarnieri M: Congenital spine anoma-

lies. In Albright AL, Pollack IF, Adelson PD (eds): Principals and Practices of Pediatric Neurosurgery. New York, Thieme, 1998.

4. Clancy CM, Eisenberg JM: Outcomes research: Measuring the end results of health care. Science 282:245–246, 1998.

5. McKusick V, Amberger J, Francomano C: Progress in medical genetics. Am J Med Genet 63:98–105, 1996.

6. Francomano C: The genetic basis of dwarfism. N Engl J Med 332:58–59, 1995.

7. Cohen MM Jr: Achondroplasia, hypochondroplasia and thanatophoric dysplasia: Clinically related skeletal dysplasias that are also related at the molecular level. Int J Oral Maxillofac Surg 27:451–455, 1998.

8. Tanaka H: Achondroplasia: Recent advances in diagnosis and treatment. Acta Paediatr Jpn 39:514–520, 1997.

9. Climent C, Lorda-Sanchez I, Urioste M, et al: Achondroplasia: Molecular study of 28 patients. Med Clin (Barc) 110:492–494, 1998.

10. Yang SW, Kitoh H, Yamada Y, et al: Mutation in the gene encoding the fibroblast growth factor-3 in Korean children with achondroplasia. Acta Paediatr Jpn 40:324–327, 1998.

11. Zhao P, Ma H, Wang Y, et al: Mutations of the fibroblast growth factor receptor-3 gene in achondroplasia. Chung Hua I Hsueh I Chuan Hsueh Tsa Chih 16:16–18, 1999.

12. Zubicaray EB, Iguacel AO, Varela Junquera JM, et al: Gly380Arg and Asn540Lys mutations of fibroblast growth factor receptor 3 in achondroplasia and hypochondroplasia in the Spanish population. Med Clin (Barc) 112:290–293, 1999.

13. Alderborn A, Anvret M, Gustavson KH, et al: Achondroplasia in Sweden caused by the G1138A mutation on FGFR3. Acta Paediatr 85:1506–1507, 1996.

14. Ramaswami U, Rumsby G, Hindmarsh PC, et al: Genotype and phenotype in hypochondroplasia. J Pedatr 133:99–102, 1998.

15. Tsai FJ, Wu JY, Tsai CH, et al: Identification of a common N540K mutation in 8/18 Taiwanese hypochondroplasia patients: Further evidence for genetic heterogeneity. Clin Genet 55:279–280, 1999.

16. Matsui Y, Yasui N, Kimura T, et al: Genotype phenotype correlation in achondroplasia and hypochondroplasia. J Bone Joint Surg Br 80:1052–1056, 1998.

17. Lemyre E, Azouz EM, Teebi AS, et al: Bone dysplasia series. Achondroplasia, hypochondroplasia and thanatophoric dysplasia: Review and update. Can Assoc Radiol J 50:185–187, 1999.

18. Baker KM, Olsen DS, Harding CO, et al: Long-term survival in typical thanatophoric dysplasia type 1. Am J Med Genet 70:427–436, 1997.

19. Huggins MJ, Smith JR, Chun K, et al: Achondroplasia-hypochondroplasia complex in a newborn infant. Am J Med Genet 84:396–400, 1999.

20. Chitayat D, Fernandez B, Gardner A, et al: Compound heterozygosity for the achondroplasia-hypochondroplasia FGFR3 mutations: Prenatal diagnosis and postnatal outcome. Am J Med Genet 84:401–405, 1999.

21. Wilkin DJ, Szabo JK, Cameron R, et al: Mutations in fibroblast growth-factor receptor 3 in sporadic cases of achondroplasia occur exclusively on the paternally derived chromosome. Am J Hum Genet 63:711–716, 1998.

22. Hecht JT, Francomano CA, Horton WA, et al: Mortality in achondroplasia. Am J Hum Genet 41:454–464, 1987.

23. Lachman RS: Neurologic abnormalities in the skeletal dysplasias: A clinical and radiological perspective. Am J Med Genet 69:33–43, 1997.

24. Gardner RMJ: A new estimate of the achondroplasia rate. Clin Genet 11:31–38, 1977.

25. Passos-Bueno MR, Wilcox WR, Jabs EW, et al: Clinical spectrum of fibroblast growth factor receptor mutations. Hum Mutat 14:115–125, 1999.

26. Mahomed NN, Spellman M, Goldberg MJ: Functional health status of adults with achondroplasia. Am J Med Genet 78:30–35, 1998.

27. Thompson NM, Hecht JT, Bohan TP, et al: Neuroanatomic and neuropsychological outcome in school-age children with achondroplasia. Am J Med Genet 88:145–153, 1999.

28. Ruiz-Garcia M, Tovar-Baudin A, Del Castillo-Ruiz V, et al: Early detection of neurological manifestations in achondroplasia. Childs Nerv Syst 13:208–213, 1997.

29. Castiglia PT: Achondroplasia. J Pediatr Health Care 10:180–182, 1996.

30. Haverkamp F, Noeker M: Short stature in children—a questionnaire for parent's: A new instrument for growth disorder–specific psychosocial adaption in children. Qual Life Res 7:447–455, 1998.

31. Fowler ES, Gilinski LP, Reiser CA, et al: Biophysical basis for delayed and aberrant motor development in young children with achondroplasia. J Dev Behav Pediatr 18:143–150, 1997.

32. Apajasalo M, Sintonen H, Rautonen J, et al: Health-related quality of life of patients with genetic skeletal dysplasias. Eur J Pediatr 157:114–121, 1998.

33. Mogayzel PJ, Carroll JL, Loughlin GM, et al: Sleep-disordered breathing in children with achondroplasia. J Pediatr 131:667–671, 1998.

34. Tasker RC, Dundas I, Laverty A, et al: Distinct patterns of respiratory difficulty in young children with achondroplasia: A clinical, sleep, and lung function study. Arch Dis Child 79:99–108, 1998.

35. Sisk EA, Heatley DG, Borowski BJ, et al: Obstructive sleep apnea in children with achondroplasia: Surgical and anesthetic considerations. Otolaryngol Head Neck Surg 120:248–254, 1999.

36. Zucconi M, Weber G, Castronvo V, et al: Sleep and upper airway obstruction in children with achondroplasia. J Pediatr 129:743–749, 1996.

37. DiMario FJ, Bauer L, Baxter D: Respiratory sinus arrhythmia of brainstem lesions. J Child Neurol 14:229–232, 1999.

38. Pauli RM, Modaff P: Jugular bulb dehiscence in achondroplasia. Int J Pediatr Otorhinolaryngol 48:169–174, 1999.

39. Thomas IT, Frias JL, Williams JL, et al: Magnetic resonance imaging in the assessment of medullary compression in achondroplasia. Am J Dis Child 142:989–992, 1988.

40. Marin-Padilla M, Marin-Padilla TM: Developmental abnormalities of the occipital bone in human chondrodystrophies. Birth Defects 13:7–23, 1977.

41. Hecht JT, Nelson FW, Butler IJ, et al: Computerized tomography of foramen magnum: Achondroplastic values compared to normal standards. Am J Med Genet 20:355–360, 1985.

42. Hurko O, Pyeritz R, Uemastu S: Neurological considerations in achondroplasia. In Nicoletti B, Kopits SE, Ascani E, et al (eds): Human Achondroplasia. New York, Plenum Press, 1988, pp 153–162.

43. Boor R, Fricke G, Bruhl K, et al: Abnormal subcortical somatosensory evoked potentials indicate high cervical myelopathy in achondroplasia. Eur J Pediatr 158:662–667, 1999.

44. Steinbok P, Hall J, Flodmark O: Hydrocephalus in achondroplasia: The possible role of intracranial venous hypertension. J Neurosurg 71:42–48, 1989.

45. Colamaria V, Mazza C, Beltramello A, et al: Irreversible respiratory failure in an achondroplastic child: The importance of an early cervicomedullary decompression, and a review of the literature. Brain Dev 13:270–279, 1991.

46. Mador MJ, Tobin MJ: Apneustic breathing: A characteristic feature of brainstem compression in achondroplasia? Chest 97:877–883, 1990.

47. Wang H, Rosenbaum AE, Reid CS: Pediatric patients with achondroplasia: CT evaluation of the craniocervical junction. Radiology 164:515–519, 1987.

48. Reid CS, Pyeritz RE, Kopits SE: Cervicomedullary compression in young patients with achondroplasia: Value of comprehensive neurologic and respiratory evaluation. J Pediatr 110:522–530, 1987.

49. Thomas IT, Frias JL: The prospective management of cervicomedullary compression in achondroplasia. Birth Defects 25:83–90, 1990.

50. Aryanpur J, Hurko O, Francomano C, et al: Craniocervical decompression for cervicomedullary compression in pediatric patients with achondroplasia. J Neurosurg 73:375–382, 1990.

51. Rekate HL: Management of cervicomedullary compression [letter]. Childs Nerv Syst 13:359, 1997.

52. Wasserman ER, Rimoin DL: Cervicomedullary compression with achondroplasia [letter]. J Pediatr 113:411, 1988.

53. Larsen PD, Snyder EW, Matsuo F, et al: Achondroplasia associated with obstructive sleep apnea [letter]. Arch Neurol 40:769, 1983.

54. Rimoin DL: Cervicomedullary junction compression in infants with achondroplasia: When to perform neurosurgical decompression [editorial]. Am J Hum Genet 56:824–827, 1995.

55. Pauli RM, Horton VK, Glinski LP, et al: Prospective assessment of risks for cervicomedullary-junction compression in infants with achondroplasia. Am J Hum Genet 56:732–744, 1995.

56. Pauli RM: Surgical intervention in achondroplasia. Am J Hum Genet 56:1501–1502, 1995.

57. Yamada Y, Ito H, Otsubo Y, et al: Surgical management of cervicomedullary compression in achondroplasia. Childs Nerv Syst 12:737–741, 1996.

58. Hunter AGW, Bankier A, Rogers JG, et al: Medical complications of achondroplasia: A multicentre patient review. J Med Genet 35: 705–712, 1998.

59. Erdincler P, Dashti R, Kaynar MY, et al: Hydrocephalus and chronically increased intracranial pressure in achondroplasia. Childs Nerv Syst 13:345–348, 1997.

60. Lundar T, Bakke SJ, Nornes H: Hydrocephalus in an achondroplastic child treated by venous decompression at the jugular foramen. J Neurosurg 73:138–140, 1990.

61. Kopits SE: Thoracolumbar kyphosis and lumbosacral lordosis: In Nicoletti B, Kopits SE, Ascani E, et al (eds): Human Achondroplasia. New York, Plenum Press, 1988, pp 241–255.

62. Siebens AA, Hungerford DS, Kirby NA: Curves of the achondroplastic spine: A new hypothesis. Johns Hopkins Med J 142: 205–210, 1978.

63. Lutter LD, Langer LO: Neurological symptoms in achondroplastic dwarfs: Surgical treatment. J Bone Joint Surg Am 59A:87–92, 1977.

64. Morgan DF, Young RF: Spinal neurological complications of achondroplasia: Clinical variations and spinal stenosis. J Neurosurg 52:463–472, 1980.

65. Raimondi AJ: Editorial comment. Childs Nerv Syst 13:213, 1997.

66. Lutter LD, Lonstein JE, Winter RB, et al: Anatomy of the achondroplastic lumbar canal. Clin Orthop 26:139–142, 1977.

67. Shikata J, Yamamuro T, Lida H, et al: Surgical treatment of achondroplastic dwarfs with paraplegia. Surg Neurol 29:125–130, 1988.

68. Lonstein JE: Treatment of kyphosis and lumbar stenosis in achondroplasia. In Nicoletti B, Kopits SE, Ascani E, et al (eds): Human Achondroplasia. New York, Plenum Press, 1988, pp 283–292.

69. Ain MC, Elmaci I, Hurko O, et al: Reoperation for spinal restenosis in achondroplasia. J Spinal Disord 13:168–173, 2000.

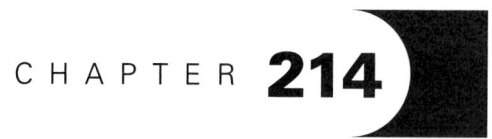

CHAPTER **214**

Physiology of Cerebrospinal Fluid Shunt Devices

HOWARD J. GINSBERG ■ JAMES M. DRAKE

The insertion of a cerebrospinal fluid (CSF) shunt is the most common procedure performed in most neurosurgical centers and accounts for the overwhelming majority of procedures in pediatric centers. Few topics generate as much discussion and controversy as the issue of which shunt system is best for a particular patient. There is often confusion about what a particular shunt device does or how it works. Much of what neurosurgeons know about shunts comes from advertisements or displays by vendors and also from ingenious neurosurgical inventors who believe strongly in the merits of their design. Knowledge of the principles of shunt function allows neurosurgeons to select intelligently among the myriad designs and understand some of the complications of these devices.

HISTORY

A mere half century ago, a diagnosis of hydrocephalus carried a terminal or intellectually devastating prognosis. Our earliest ancestors must have recognized the overt clinical manifestations of untreated infantile hydrocephalus, but early attempts at treatment were doomed owing to a lack of understanding of CSF physiology and the absence of sterile technique. It is possible that Hippocrates made the first attempt at treating hydrocephalus by ventricular puncture, although he may have actually drained the subdural space.[1] Ventricular puncture continued to be used into the 18th century. Head wrapping or binding was recorded as a treatment for hydrocephalus from the 16th century to the middle of the 19th century.[2] It was later recognized that to avoid infection, a closed system of ventricular drainage was required. Drainage of CSF into various intracranial and extracranial spaces has been investigated since the turn of the 20th century,[3] and virtually no imaginable site has not been tried (Table 214–1).

It was not until the development of compatible biomaterials and one-way valves that the modern era of shunt surgery began. Nulsen and Spitz were first to report the successful use of a ventriculojugular shunt with a spring and stainless steel ball valve.[4] In 1955, Pudenz introduced silicone as a shunt tubing material while investigating the feasibility of shunting CSF into the circulatory system of animals. The first child to receive a silicone ventriculoatrial shunt survived 2 years, only to die from shunt obstruction. Silicone has since become the material of choice for implanted shunts. Ventriculoatrial, ventriculoperitoneal, and lumboperitoneal shunting procedures became widespread in the 1970s, and the management of their complications became a major focus. The quest for the perfect shunt will continue well into this millennium.

All current ventricular CSF shunt systems contain a proximal ventricular catheter, a one-way valve, and a distal catheter terminating in the peritoneum, venous system or, less commonly, pleural space. Ventriculoperitoneal shunting, which was first reported in 1908 and subsequently fell out of favor,[5] is now the shunt proce-

TABLE 214–1 ■ Distal Sites Historically Used for Cerebrospinal Fluid Diversion

HEAD AND NECK REGION	ABDOMINAL REGION	THORACIC REGION
Subgaleal region	Peritoneal cavity	Thoracic duct
Superior sagittal sinus	Omental bursa	Spinal epidural space
Internal jugular vein	Stomach	
Common facial vein	Gallbladder	Bone marrow
Subdural space	Ileum	Pleural cavity
Subarachnoid space	Ureter	Right atrium
Mastoid antrum	Fallopian tube	Superior vena cava
Salivary gland ducts		

dure of choice in the initial treatment of obstructive hydrocephalus.

CEREBROSPINAL FLUID SHUNT HYDRODYNAMICS

Hydrodynamics is a branch of physics that deals with the motion of fluids and the forces acting on solid bodies in motion relative to them. The hydrodynamics of shunt systems is concerned with the flow of CSF in silicone tubing and valves or, more precisely, the resistance to flow and the driving pressure. The clinical importance of shunt hydrodynamics has been emphasized in numerous publications.[6-26] The transformation of the open-ended tube into today's modern shunt systems is a testament to our improved understanding of hydrodynamics.

An ideal shunt system would be one that mimics the normal brain's reabsorption of CSF into the venous system via the arachnoid granulations, controls intracranial pressure, and reconstitutes the cerebral mantle.[7] The fact that there are so many shunt products on the market and that new ones are continually being developed implies that the ideal shunt is far from realized.

Most cases of hydrocephalus are due to a pathologic increase in the hydrodynamic resistance to the outflow of CSF.[18] A shunt system provides a low-resistance pathway for CSF diversion. Resistance is therefore a particularly important concept.

Flow in shunt systems can be related to resistance and the pressure gradient by the following simple equation:

$$Q = \Delta P/R$$

where Q is the flow rate, R is the resistance to flow, and ΔP is the driving pressure. Shunt flow rates have been documented in vivo from 0.6 to 116 mL/hour,[27] although pumping a shunt valve can produce peak flow rates up to 2000 mL/hour.[28] R is made up of R_T, resistance from the shunt tubing, plus R_V, resistance from the valve components. R_T is dependent on a number of factors, including the length and inner diameter of the shunt tubing and the viscosity of the CSF, as described by Poiseuille's law:

$$R_T = \frac{8\eta L}{\pi r^4}$$

where η is the coefficient of absolute viscosity, L is the length of the shunt tubing, and r is the inner radius of the shunt tubing. It is important to note that viscosity is highly dependent on temperature. Any shunt testing should use fluid of 37°C, otherwise erroneous pressure-flow characteristics will be obtained (η_{water} at 37°C is 0.6915 cp, and at room temperature of 22°C, it is 0.9548 cp—a difference of 38%). The flow through shunt systems under normal physiologic conditions is usually laminar (Reynolds' number typically <1), even at

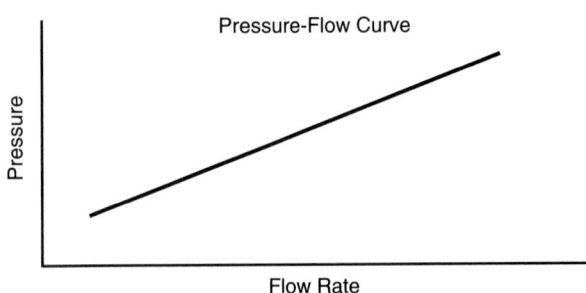

FIGURE 214–1. Linear pressure versus flow curve for valveless tubing with constant resistance.

sharp corners and through narrow valves, because of the relatively low flow rates. R_T remains constant at any flow rate, thus producing a linear pressure versus flow curve for the tubing (Fig. 214–1). R_V is much more complicated because of the complex geometry and moving parts. In many cases, the resistance is not constant in the range of physiologic flow rates, and a curved pressure versus flow relationship is seen. Studies in our laboratory and those by others show that a 90-cm-long distal catheter provides an additional resistance to flow that is roughly equivalent to the resistance provided by a differential pressure valve and may provide up to 94% of the total resistance of a shunt system.[7, 28] Care must therefore be taken when shortening a distal catheter, as this can significantly alter the shunt's pressure-flow characteristics.

The resistance of a shunt system ($R_T + R_V$) plays an important role in defining the intraventricular pressure with a given rate of CSF production and absorption and is therefore at least as important as the opening pressure. It is also important to note that the presence of air bubbles or particulate matter can drastically increase the resistance and thus alter the performance of the shunt or cause it to fail. Resistance to bulk flow of CSF across the arachnoid granulations, in the absence of hydrocephalus, is approximately 60 cm H_2O/mL per minute. Resistance of a typical low-pressure shunt system flowing at 25 mL/hour is approximately 8 cm H_2O/mL per minute, a much lower value.

The pressure gradient driving the flow in a ventriculoperitoneal shunt system is determined by[29]:

$$\Delta P = IVP + \rho gh - OPV - DCP$$

where IVP is the intraventricular pressure, ρgh (density × gravitational constant × vertical height difference between proximal and distal ends) is the hydrostatic pressure, OPV is the opening pressure of the valve, and DCP is the distal cavity pressure (Fig. 214–2). If the distal catheter is placed in the venous system, the DCP is obviously the venous pressure. If the catheter is placed in the peritoneal cavity, the DCP becomes the intra-abdominal pressure, which is usually zero relative to the atmosphere but can climb transiently during straining.

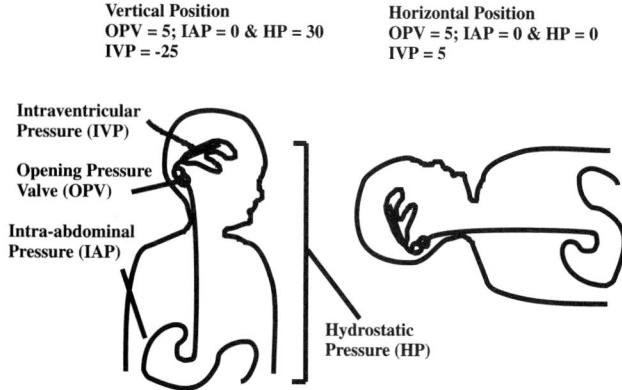

Vertical Position
OPV = 5; IAP = 0 & HP = 30
IVP = -25

Horizontal Position
OPV = 5; IAP = 0 & HP = 0
IVP = 5

Intraventricular
Pressure (IVP)

Opening Pressure
Valve (OPV)

Intra-abdominal
Pressure (IAP)

Hydrostatic
Pressure (HP)

FIGURE 214–2. Illustration of compartment pressures and the effect of position. Hydrostatic pressure predominates in the upright position. (From Drake JM, Sainte-Rose C: The Shunt Book. New York, Blackwell Science, 1995, p 23.)

SIPHONING

Siphoning occurs when there is a difference in the height of the ventricular catheter and that of the distal catheter. A rapid increase in flow rate occurs, due to a pressure differential equal to ρgh that is generated when the patient moves from the recumbent to the upright position.[2] A canine study revealed that on assuming the upright position, the flow rate rapidly increases and then progressively decreases until it becomes stabilized (Fig. 214–3).[19] Flow rates up to 170 times the normal rate of CSF production can be achieved in simulations.[25] This siphoning effect does not occur in the normal brain because there is no posture-related change in the CSF–sagittal sinus pressure gradient.[7] Because the head is not open to atmospheric pressure, fluid will flow until the intracranial pressure drops to negative ρgh to balance the siphon effect (Fig. 214–4). This can cause low-pressure symptoms,[30] tear bridging veins, cause a subdural hematoma,[31, 32] and prematurely close cranial sutures[33, 34] or cause slit-ventricle syndrome.[35] Low-pressure symptoms were reported by Pudenz and Foltz to occur in

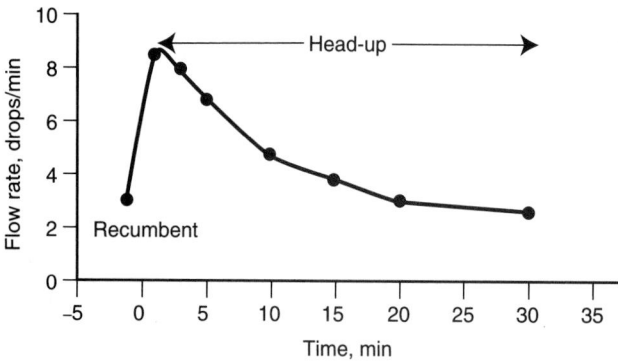

FIGURE 214–3. Change in cerebrospinal fluid flow rate when moving from supine to upright position in dogs. (Adapted from Yamada S: Dynamic changes of cerebrospinal fluid in upright and recumbent shunted experimental animals. Childs Brain 1: 187–192, 1975.)

10% to 12% of patients, indicating that many patients can tolerate this siphoning effect without malady.[35] It is important to understand that the hydrostatic pressure generated in the upright position (25 to 50 cm H_2O) is significantly higher than the opening pressure of a typical low-pressure (1 to 4 cm H_2O) or high-pressure (8 to 10 cm H_2O) valve. Raising the opening pressure of the valve by δ cm H_2O simply decreases the magnitude of the negative IVP generated from siphoning by δ cm H_2O. Thus, changing the shunt valve to one with a higher opening pressure may delay ventricular collapse but will not prevent it in those who are prone to slit-ventricle syndrome.[36, 37]

SHUNT VALVES

Although valved CSF shunts have been around since the 1950s,[4] and shunt design has improved to more closely match physiologic function, complications are still prevalent. This has led to the development of numerous ingenious shunt valves aimed at diminishing these complications. The valves currently used in practice include differential pressure regulators (static and programmable), flow regulators, siphon-resistive devices, and gravity-actuated valves.

Differential Pressure Valves

Numerous differential pressure one-way valves have been developed in four broad categories: slit valves, miter valves, diaphragm valves, and ball-in-cone valves.[2, 38] These devices all attempt to achieve the same goal of keeping the IVP from climbing too high or falling too low. Differential pressure valves are defined by their opening or closing pressure. As the IVP climbs above the valve opening pressure, the valve opens to allow egress of CSF at a rate determined by the resistance of the entire shunt system, until the pressure falls below the closing pressure and the flow of CSF ceases. Although it has not been demonstrated in vivo, it is possible that the valve opens and closes with each cardiac cycle. The opening pressure is not necessarily the same as the valve closing pressure, owing to the phenomenon of hysteresis.[2, 7] Hysteresis occurs because of a slight change in the mechanical properties of the valves, depending on whether they are opening or closing, and occurs most frequently with slit and miter valves. Most manufacturers provide differential pressure valves with various opening pressure ranges in three or four categories: very low (<1 cm H_2O), low (1 to 4 cm H_2O), medium (4 to 8 cm H_2O), and high (>8 cm H_2O). Two different differential pressure valves may have the same opening pressure and completely different resistance values and therefore behave differently.

Slit valves may be at the proximal end (Holter-Hausner valve) or at the distal end (Codman Unishunt, Codman, Randolph, Massachusetts) of a shunt. Simple distal slit valves offer the lowest resistance to flow, and in fact no significant difference in resistance can be

Siphoning

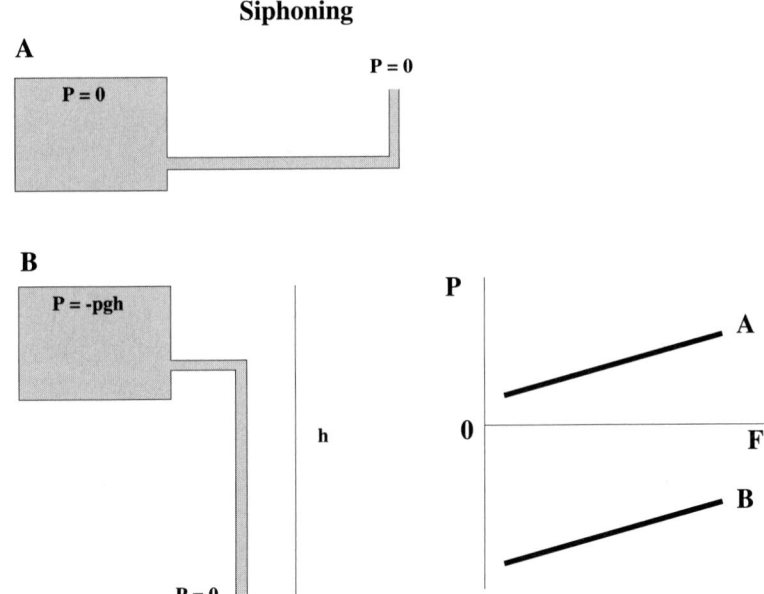

FIGURE 214–4. Changes in intraventricular pressure that occur with siphoning. Pressure (P) and flow (F) curves in horizontal *(A)* and vertical *(B)* position. (From Drake JM, Sainte-Rose C: The Shunt Book. New York, Blackwell Science, 1995, p 21.)

measured between a tube with a distal slit valve and an equally long open-ended tube.

The diaphragm valve is probably the most commonly produced type of differential pressure valve. Generally, these valves involve the deflection of a silicone membrane in response to pressure in order to allow flow of CSF.

Programmable Valves

Programmable valves are more appropriately called *externally adjustable differential pressure valves.* They act in the same fashion as nonadjustable differential pressure valves, except that the surgeon has the option of altering the opening pressure with an external device, obviating the need for surgical shunt revision.[39] This increases convenience and marginally decreases risk, but it is not clear that this benefit outweighs the increased cost of using these valves in all patients. Several authors have reported clinical success and complications associated with these devices.[39–44] It has been suggested that this type of shunt is well suited for difficult-to-manage cases of overdrainage (e.g., slit ventricles, subdural collections) or underdrainage (e.g., persistent symptoms of hydrocephalus). It has also been suggested that externally adjustable shunts are particularly useful in gradually decreasing the size of arachnoid cysts and the size of the ventricles in normal-pressure hydrocephalus.[41, 44, 45] It is important to note that these programmable valves are also susceptible to siphoning.

The Codman Medos programmable valve (Fig. 214–5) has an adjustable ball-spring mechanism. A cam and stepper motor assembly (akin to a spiral staircase) is used to adjust the tension on the spring. The opening pressure can be read from radiopaque markers printed on the valve and can be adjusted from 3 to 20 cm H_2O in 1-cm H_2O increments. The motor assembly is adjusted with an externally applied magnetic field from the valve programmer. In adjusting the pressure over the total range from 3 to 20 cm H_2O, the spring moves by less than 1 mm.[46] The Sophy programmable pressure valve (Sophysa, France) is also a ball-spring type of valve in which a semicircular spring can be adjusted for various tensions by rotation with magnets. This device has eight possible positions in the range of 5 to 17 cm H_2O opening pressure. Because both these valves contain magnets, they produce an artifact on magnetic resonance imaging scans and may possibly be reprogrammed by a magnetic field.[47–50]

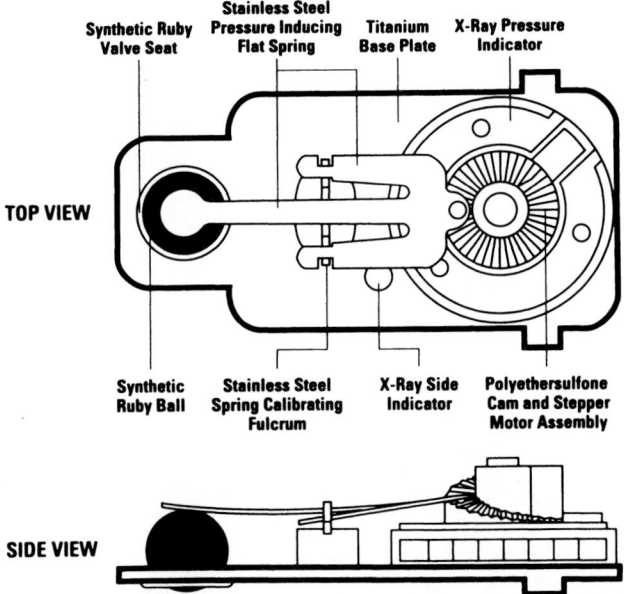

FIGURE 214–5. Schematic diagram of Codman Medos programmable valve. (From Drake JM, Sainte-Rose C: The Shunt Book. New York, Blackwell Science, 1995, pp 94–95.)

Orbis Sigma

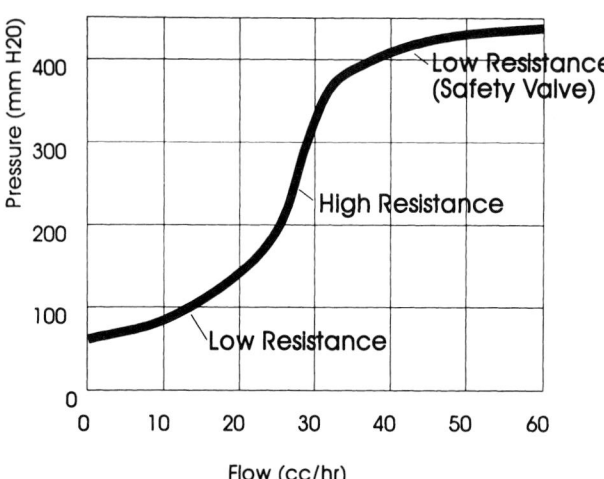

FIGURE 214–6. Pressure versus flow rate for Orbis Sigma valve. (From Drake JM, Sainte-Rose C: The Shunt Book. New York, Blackwell Science, 1995, p 98.)

Flow-Regulated Valves

Flow-regulating devices are designed to increase the hydrodynamic resistance as the pressure gradient increases, in an attempt to keep the flow rate constant.[2] It is in fact the differential pressure that controls the resistance, and perhaps these valves should be called pressure-controlled, variable-resistance, constant-flow valves. These devices produce pressure-flow curves with a sigmoid shape (Fig. 214–6). This is accomplished by the Orbis Sigma valve (NMT Medical, Inc., Boston, Mass.) with a contoured synthetic ruby flow-control pin that fits inside a movable synthetic ruby ring (Fig. 214–7). As the pressure increases, the ruby ring is deflected downward, and because the ruby pin is tapered,

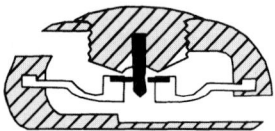

Low Resistance

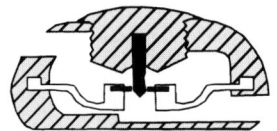

High Resistance

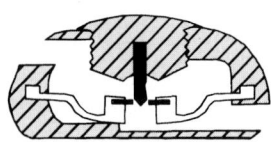

Low Resistance at High Pressure
(safety pressure release)

FIGURE 214–7. Schematic diagram of Orbis Sigma valve. (From Drake JM, Sainte-Rose C: The Shunt Book. New York, Blackwell Science, 1995, p 98.)

the flow aperture decreases, which increases resistance and reduces flow. If the pressure increases further, beyond a predetermined threshold, the ruby ring is deflected further downward until resistance is lowered to allow a rapid increase in flow rate. Sainte-Rose and coworkers described three stages: The first stage consists of a medium-pressure low-resistance valve that operates as a conventional differential pressure valve until the flow through the shunt reaches a mean value of 20 mL/hour. A second stage consists of a variable-resistance flow regulator that maintains flow between 20 and 30 mL/hour at differential pressures of 8 to 35 cm H₂O. The third stage is a safety device that operates at differential pressures above 35 cm H₂O (inducing a rapid increase in CSF flow rate) and therefore prevents excessive intracranial pressure. Flow-regulating valves are less likely to be associated with siphoning and overdrainage and have been shown to improve symptomatic low intracranial pressure in shunted individuals.[30] However, flow-regulated valves typically have very small orifices, which makes the valve itself a likely site of obstruction.[51] In addition, the high resistance has a propensity to cause fluid collections under the scalp in young children unless they are nursed upright with a compressive dressing.

Antisiphon Devices

One strategy developed to avoid the complication of overdrainage is the siphon-resistive or antisiphon device (ASD). This device, which is typically placed under the scalp, has a small diaphragm that reduces flow of CSF when the pressure inside the shunt falls below atmospheric pressure (Fig. 214–8). The PS Medical siphon control device (Medtronic PS Medical, Goleta, California), which contains two membranes, is designed to be closed in its resting position and can be forced open only when the internal shunt pressure exceeds atmospheric pressure. The PS Medical Delta valve consists of a siphon-control device just distal to a differential pressure valve. The ASD can theoretically be placed anywhere along the length of the shunt, giving the surgeon some control over the ventricular pressure at which the ASD closes.[52, 53] The more distally the ASD is placed, the more negative pressure is re-

Antisiphon Device

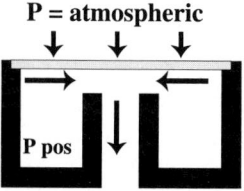
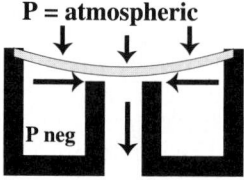

FIGURE 214–8. Schematic mechanism of siphon-resistive devices. As pressure inside the container falls, atmospheric pressure pushes the membrane toward the orifice, narrowing it and increasing resistance. Ppos, positive pressure; Pneg, negative pressure. (From Drake JM, Sainte-Rose C: The Shunt Book. New York, Blackwell Science, 1995, p 27.)

quired inside the ventricle to reduce flow by the same degree. An ASD placed at the distal end of a peritoneal catheter has no effect. Portnoy and colleagues were the first to report successful obliteration of symptomatic low intracranial pressure using an ASD in 11 of 13 patients, although 6 patients developed subdural hematoma.[31] Gruber and associates reported the results of placing ASDs in 41 children (31 previously shunted and 10 primary shunts).[54] They reported a marked decrease in slit-ventricle syndrome and patient complaints about low-pressure symptoms during the daytime or after excessive activity. Four cases of severe neurological deterioration after ASD implantation, in the absence of shunt obstruction, have been reported.[55] Symptoms resolved with removal of the ASD. The fact that these four patients suffered from signs of intracranial hypertension suggests that the ASDs in those cases either remained closed or failed to open once siphoning ceased, or did not open at all. Drake and coworkers demonstrated that raised tissue compartment pressure from scar tissue overlying an ASD can lead to functional obstruction and was the likely cause in those cases.[56]

Gravity-Actuated Valves

Gravity-actuated valves attempt to prohibit or reduce siphoning by increasing opening pressure with the assistance of gravity when a patient sits or stands. The Cordis horizontal-vertical valve is one such device designed for use with lumboperitoneal shunts (Fig. 214–9). This device has an inlet valve and an outlet valve. The inlet valve is a ball-spring valve and does not markedly change resistance with position. The outlet valve has a synthetic ruby ball that sits in a conical seat, and there are three stainless steel balls that sit on top of the ruby ball. In the upright position, the weight of the steel balls weighs down the ruby ball in its seat, thus creating high resistance. In the recumbent position, the balls fall away from the seat to allow flow at a low resistance. It is therefore extremely important to ensure that gravity-actuated valves are secure and in the proper position.

VALVE DESIGN TRIALS

It is impossible to sort through the merits of various shunt valve designs by attempting to evaluate uncontrolled case series. These series are frequently reported by proponents of the devices, who sometimes have financial or other incentive interests. A multicenter randomized trial of CSF shunt valve design in pediatric hydrocephalus failed to demonstrate any difference among valves in cases of shunt failure resulting from shunt obstruction, overdrainage, loculations of the cerebral ventricles, or infection over a minimal 1-year period of follow-up.[51, 57, 58] In this trial, 344 hydrocephalic children (age birth to 18 years) undergoing their first CSF shunt insertion were randomized at 12 North American or European pediatric neurosurgical centers. These patients received one of three valves: a standard differential pressure valve; a Delta valve that contains a siphon-control component designed to reduce siphoning in the upright position; or an Orbis-Sigma valve (Cordis, Miami, Florida), with a variable-resistance, flow-limiting component. A randomized trial comparing a conventional valve and a Codman Hakim programmable valve with respect to shunt failure and valve explantation also did not demonstrate any significant difference between valves.[59] These studies compared different valve types, with completely different hydrodynamic profiles, with respect to mechanical and infectious complications. There is, however, no longitudinal study comparing the impact that these different valve types may have on intellectual outcome.

PROXIMAL AND DISTAL CATHETERS

All ventricular and distal catheters currently in use are made from synthetic silicone rubber. Most of these catheters are impregnated with barium along their entire length or have separated tantalum markers for radiographic visualization. Ventricular catheters are designed to be stiff enough to be kink resistant and compliant enough to prevent brain injury if the ventricles collapse onto the catheter. Various lengths, shapes, inner and outer diameters, and wall thicknesses are available. Inner diameters from 1.0 to 1.6 mm are available, the smallest being designed for neonates. It is important to note that changing the diameter of tubing from 1.3 to 1.0 mm results in a nearly threefold increase in resistance. Straight catheters, angled catheters, and catheters with flanges and recessed holes have been produced (Fig. 214–10). Flanged catheters were designed to keep the choroid plexus away from the draining holes to diminish the likelihood of mechanical obstruction from the choroid plexus.[60] However, they do not decrease the incidence of ventricular catheter occlu-

Horizontal-Vertical Valve

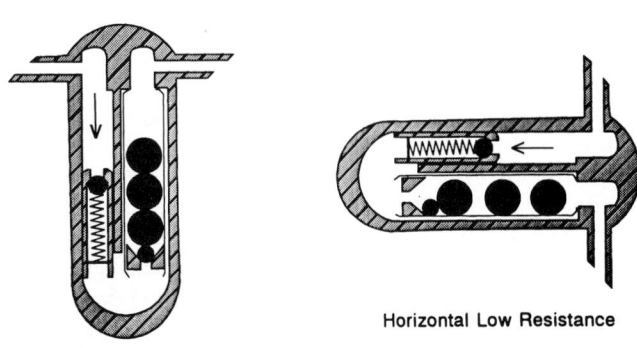

Horizontal Low Resistance

Vertical High Resistance

FIGURE 214–9. Schematic of horizontal-vertical valve. (From Drake JM, Sainte-Rose C: The Shunt Book. New York, Blackwell Science, 1995, p 103.)

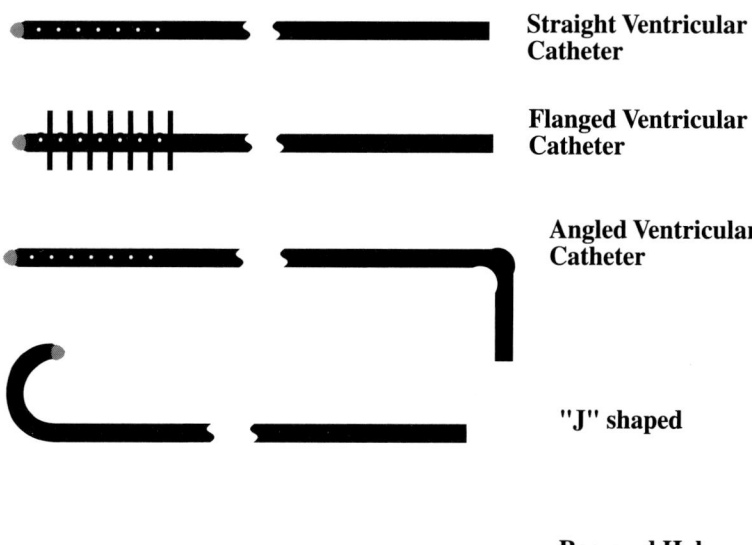

Straight Ventricular Catheter

Flanged Ventricular Catheter

Angled Ventricular Catheter

"J" shaped

Recessed Holes

FIGURE 214–10. Various ventricular catheter designs. (From Drake JM, Sainte-Rose C: The Shunt Book. New York, Blackwell Science, 1995, p 72.)

sion.[61] In fact, close inspection of explanted flanged catheters demonstrates that the flanges can act like scaffolding for the choroid plexus to attach to. The size and number of drainage holes in a ventricular catheter are variable, although most of the holes are redundant. There is some resistance to flow from the ventricular catheter and its holes, and this resistance increases as the number of holes decreases due to partial obstruction. We have shown in our laboratory that there is no significant increase in the total resistance of a shunt system even if only a single 500-μm hole allows CSF to flow.

Distal shunt tubing is either open-ended or closed at the tip, with slit valves near the distal end. Some have both open ends and slits; in the event that the open-ended tip becomes obstructed, the slits provide an alternative pathway for CSF flow. With the exception of the distal ends of these catheters, they are simply silicone rubber tubes.

IN VITRO SHUNT TESTING

In vitro testing of shunt systems allows the determination of their hydrodynamic performance under various conditions. Several laboratories have performed in vitro shunt testing to obtain additional and independent performance information about shunt systems beyond that provided by manufacturers and to confirm whether a valve performs according to its specifications.[7, 9, 12, 15, 17, 18, 23, 26, 62, 63] The hydrodynamic characteristics that are usually measured are opening and closing pressure, pressure-flow response, resistance, and retrograde flow.[2] Shunt valves can be tested in two basic ways: by generating a pressure gradient across the valve and measuring the resultant flow, or by allowing a known flow rate and measuring the backpressure produced by the resistance to flow across the valve. In the first method, a differential pressure must be generated across the valve being tested. The simplest way to

generate a constant differential pressure is to use two water-filled beakers at different heights. The shunt valve is connected to both beakers, and the differential pressure is determined by the difference in water levels. For short-term testing, the water level in the beakers is not likely to change significantly. The resultant fluid flow can then be determined with various pressure gradients by measuring the timed increase in mass or volume flowing into the lower beaker. Opening pressure can be measured with this technique by starting with no pressure gradient and slowly increasing it until flow is initiated. Closing pressure can be determined by gradually decreasing the pressure gradient until flow stops. It is useful to use both ascending and descending pressures to determine the presence of hysteresis, which has been most frequently observed with slit and miter valves. Hysteresis is likely caused by minute differences in the precise forces acting on valves, depending on whether the pressure is increasing or decreasing.

The second method requires a calibrated pump (typically a syringe pump) placed proximal to the shunt valve and either a manometer or a pressure transducer to measure the pressure generated. Flow rate then becomes the independent variable, and pressure is recorded over a wide range of flow rates. The American Society for Testing Materials requires shunts to be tested in the range of 5 to 50 mL/hour, although in vivo measurements have demonstrated flow rates greater than 100 mL/hour.[27] Both methods can be used to determine hydrodynamic resistance and generate pressure versus flow curves. Retrograde testing is performed in the same manner, with the valve simply reversed to evaluate reflux potential. It is important that the fluid used in the test closely match the properties of CSF in vivo. Water or saline at 37°C is sufficient, because CSF is 99% water and has a nearly identical viscosity and surface tension.[59, 64, 65] It is also critical to use deaerated water and to remove bubbles from the shunt system being tested. This can be facilitated by perfusing the shunt for several hours and placing it in a liquid-filled vacuum to allow smaller bubbles to expand; they can then be easily removed. It is important to know whether the shunt tubing is included in the test, noting its length and internal diameter, because it can make up a significant amount of the total resistance. A computerized system for recording from transducers and driving pumps is a useful tool for tedious data collection, reducing human error and facilitating long-term testing.

Once the basic setup is in place, the shunts can be tested to determine their performance in various simulated clinical scenarios, such as siphoning. Watts and Keith introduced pulsatile flow to shunt testing and determined that opening and closing pressures were significantly different when pulsed flow was compared with steady-state testing.[15] This effect disappeared with increasing compliance in the proximal chamber, which probably acted to dampen the pulsations. The United Kingdom Shunt Evaluation Laboratory uses superimposed pulsed and static pressures to more closely mimic intracranial physiology.[7] This laboratory also examined the effects of injecting microscopic particles into valves, as well as the tolerance to 200 mm Hg shock waves, simulating the rapid increase in intracranial pressure experienced during coughing. The majority of the shunts tested in this laboratory appear to provide nonphysiologically low hydrodynamic resistance; the clinical significance of this is not clear. Aschoff and colleagues focused on accuracy, long-term drift, valve distortion, effects of protein concentration, and air bubbles.[46] They showed that bending a valve to fit the curvature of a neonatal skull causes it to become distorted and can alter hydrodynamic properties by up to 500%. A greater than 1000% increase in resistance can occur when patients rest their heads on their valves in 50% of those tested. ASDs are especially prone to this phenomenon. This fact should be kept in mind when deciding on the location of the valve.

In vitro shunt testing has demonstrated that different valve designs produce widely varying pressure-flow characteristics, nonphysiologic pressures are frequently observed, long-term variability is common, and manufacturers' specifications are often inaccurate. It is difficult to determine the clinical significance of in vitro testing, because it is not yet possible to measure thoroughly pressure and flow characteristics of a shunt system in vivo. As newer and more sophisticated methods of testing are implemented, more light will be shed on the reasons for mechanical shunt failure and the relevance of in vitro testing.

MEASURING IN VIVO SHUNT PERFORMANCE

Although numerous experimental techniques have been developed, there is currently no practical way to clinically measure detailed shunt performance (e.g., flow rate) in vivo. The current commonly used techniques for assessing shunt function include computed tomography and magnetic resonance imaging, radioisotope injection,[66–68] and plain radiographs. These methods provide qualitative information about shunt function but no significant quantitative information. An implantable telemetric pressure sensor can provide useful information about IVP and has been used to help understand changes that occur with third ventriculostomy and ventriculopleural shunting.[64, 65] Plain radiographs, or the so-called shunt series, are an invaluable tool for diagnosing shunt fracture, migration, or disconnection. Radiographs can also be used to read the manufacturers' radiopaque markers and determine the type of shunt when medical records are lacking. Computed tomography is the test of choice for assessing ventricular size. Although it does not definitively determine shunt patency, comparison with previous images taken during normal shunt function may show an increase in ventricular size, which, when combined with appropriate clinical signs and symptoms, indicates shunt failure. This point emphasizes the importance of obtaining a computed tomographic scan in the absence of shunt malfunction. Magnetic resonance imaging can be used to determine shunt patency,[69, 70] although at this time, it is not a cost-effective test for this purpose.

Quantitative methods that have been investigated but have not gained widespread popularity include radioisotope injection,[71, 72] contrast material injection,[73] a thermal conduction technique,[74] and an implanted bubble-generating device using electrolysis.[75]

A promising technique under investigation in our laboratory uses Doppler ultrasonography to determine noninvasively not only shunt patency but also quantitative information about shunt performance. CSF contains no natural ultrasound scatterers and does not produce a signal when a Doppler probe is applied to a shunt. However, this technique creates short-lived microbubbles inside the shunt using low-frequency ultrasonic cavitation applied through the tissue overlying the shunt.[76, 77] The bubbles flow along the shunt with the CSF, and their scattered Doppler signal can be used to determine flow velocity. This method has proved successful with in vivo testing on externalized shunts but has not yet been applied to implanted shunts.

BRAIN BIOMECHANICAL MODEL

Behind every shunt design is some concept of a mathematical model of CSF production, absorption, and intracranial pressure. Several mathematical and computer biomechanical models applicable to the hydrocephalic brain have been developed, with varying degrees of sophistication. These models give us a better understanding of the pathophysiology of hydrocephalus and can be used to improve the design of CSF shunts. It is extremely difficult to test the performance of implanted shunts in terms of flow, pressure, ventricular size, rate of CSF production, and postural changes. Models, by their very nature, allow us to test numerous hypotheses for the design of new valves to see how they would perform in various clinical scenarios. A theoretical prototype of a new valve design can be tested before an actual device is produced. The usefulness of the model depends on how closely it mimics the real situation. Most neurosurgeons are familiar with the foundation of these models, which stems from the original work done by Munro[78] in 1783 and modified by Kellie[79] in 1824. The Munro-Kellie doctrine describes the intracranial pressure–volume relationship with a three-compartment model (brain, arteries, and veins) and has been used for decades to help explain the pathophysiology of increased intracranial pressure. Modern models are typically multicompartmental and use computational methods to solve differential equations and thus determine time-varying behavior. An excellent critical review of several models was compiled by Tenti and colleagues.[80] Guinane developed an equivalent circuit analysis of CSF hydrodynamics in which absorption is modeled by resistance, elastic properties of adjacent tissue by parallel capacitance, and CSF formation by a constant current.[81] This model does not take into account pulsations of CSF, assumes a constant compliance, and produces a linear pressure versus volume curve. The best known modern mathematical model is the pressure-volume index of Marmarou and coworkers.[82–84] This model modified previous compartment models by assuming that intracranial compliance is not constant but decreases linearly with increasing pressure. Close agreement was shown between theoretical and experimental studies. The pressure-volume index can be obtained by plotting intracranial pressure logarithmically against volume and using its slope to determine the volume needed to raise intracranial pressure by a factor of 10. Pressure-volume index is a measure of intracranial volume buffering capacity, with higher slopes indicating a larger increase in intracranial pressure for a given increase in volume. Pressure-volume index has been used extensively to examine intracranial physiology, for therapy of intracranial hypertension,[85] and to model CSF shunting and the effects of siphoning. A more accurate computer model of siphoning that allows for negative pressure-volume relationships, which is where the pressure-volume index fails, was subsequently developed.[86] This technique closely matches the data from the precise dog experiments performed by Yamada.[19]

More sophisticated mathematical models take into account the spongelike consistency of the brain proposed by Hakim and associates[87, 88] and further developed by Nagashima and colleagues.[89, 90] The brain is modeled as a porous, deformable solid matrix that allows CSF to percolate through the pores. This provides a model for transependymal absorption of CSF, which more closely matches the pathophysiology of hydrocephalus, but it requires much more sophisticated mathematical formulations. By assuming that the brain is a spherical viscoelastic shell, it is possible to model the change in ventricular size produced by a transient elevation in IVP.[91]

Mathematical modeling of hydrocephalus and CSF shunts is still in its infancy. With the collaborative efforts of neurosurgeons, engineers, and mathematicians, and with rapidly increasing computational power, this area of research has the potential to greatly improve our understanding and our ability to deliver quality care to patients with hydrocephalus.

UNBLOCKING SHUNTS

Mechanical obstruction is the most common cause of shunt failure,[51, 92] and the ventricular catheter is the most likely site of obstruction. In the pediatric population, the ventricular catheter is obstructed in up to 90% of mechanical shunt failures.[93] The catheters are most commonly blocked by ingrowth of the choroid plexus, due to flow of CSF drawing the plexus in, and by glial tissue from astrocyte proliferation.[94] Less commonly, ventricular catheters are obstructed with connective tissue, clotted blood, ependymal cells, necrotic brain tissue, lymphocytes, multinucleated giant cells, neutrophils, and foreign material (e.g., hair, fiber). Despite modifications in ventricular catheter position[61, 95, 96] and design,[60] including changes in shape and material, no significant improvement has been shown. The current treatment for mechanical shunt failure is surgical replacement of the obstructed shunt components. A 31% risk of visible hemorrhage has been reported for shunt revision surgery, visualized during surgery or diagnosed by postoperative computed tomographic scan.[97] Although most of these hemorrhages are not clinically significant, they can reduce the time to subsequent shunt revision by 70%.[97] It may therefore be advantageous to leave the ventricular catheter in situ and simply recanalize it. Additional advantages of this procedure include avoiding the replacement of ventricular catheters when the ventricles are small and reducing the incidence of intraventricular hemorrhage caused by removal of an adherent catheter.

In 1988, Chambi and Hendrick reported on the use of electrocautery to remove adherent ventricular catheters, which is probably a routine part of shunt revision in most centers.[98] It has since been shown that electrocautery can be used inside a ventricular catheter to reestablish flow during open shunt revision[99] or percutaneously via a Rickham reservoir.[100] Pattisapu inserts a wire and fiberoptic endoscope through a Rickham reservoir and into the ventricular catheter. He cauterizes the obstructing tissue under direct endoscopic vision. Eighty-five percent of patients maintained a patent shunt with a mean follow-up of 20 months in this study.[100]

The use of fiberoptic delivery of laser energy to remove occlusions has been investigated experimentally.[101] A 300-msec pulse of a 2.09-fm wavelength laser was used to create short-lived vapor bubbles at the fiber tip to expel tissue blocking the inflow holes. Our group is currently investigating the use of percutaneous ultrasonic cavitation to recanalize blocked ventricular catheters. Ultrasound waves are passed down a wire that is placed inside the ventricular catheter, and bubbles are formed at the tip. These bubbles subsequently collapse and create minute shock waves that act locally to break up the debris. This system can effectively clean explanted ventricular catheters but has not yet been subjected to clinical trials. Ultrasound energy cleans more quickly and thoroughly than electrocautery and does not damage silicone the way a laser system may. We have also shown that only a single hole need be reopened to restore appropriate hydrodynamics to most shunt systems. At this point, it is not clear whether ventricular catheter cleaning will offer any short- or long-term benefits to patients over traditional shunt revision, but it clearly deserves further investigation.

THE FUTURE

The art and science of CSF shunting have advanced significantly since the 1950s with the development of an ever-increasing body of knowledge. Biocompatible materials and one-way valves are arguably the two most important steps to date. Ingenious new valve designs seem to offer advantages to select groups of patients, but it has yet to be shown conclusively in clinical trials that they are significantly better than conventional designs.

Improvements in mathematical and computer models of CSF hydrodynamics, along with sophisticated in vitro testing techniques, may prove to be the keys in further refining shunt design. The ideal shunt, which mimics the normal process of CSF absorption, has not yet been built. To achieve this ideal, it will probably be necessary to incorporate a sensor into a shunt system with servofeedback to the valve; this idea was first alluded to by Hakim in 1973.[102] It is conceivable that a shunt, with the aid of miniature embedded microprocessors, could constantly control the intracranial pressure by adjusting the valve. With the aid of nanotechnology, it is now possible to design and build microscopic machines and switches that can be manipulated electronically. The increased sophistication and cost should be offset by a decreased incidence of complications. It is also possible that a more physiologic shunt could have a positive impact on the developing brain, although this would require a carefully designed long-term outcome study.

Another future direction in the treatment of hydrocephalus is aimed at reducing the morbidity of the overall management of shunt complications. With the advent of noninvasive techniques for diagnosing shunt patency in difficult cases and determining shunt performance, patients will no longer be subjected to invasive tests and unnecessary operations. No matter how sophisticated the shunt system is, shunt failure will always remain a problem in some cases. The treatment of shunt occlusion by minimally invasive means is currently being explored and promises an overall improvement in the care of shunt patients and a decrease in the cost of that care.

We envision a future in which a patient receives only one shunt in his or her lifetime that is sophisticated enough to control intracranial pressure within normal physiologic limits, can be adjusted and monitored noninvasively, and is amenable to minimally invasive treatment for shunt obstruction.

REFERENCES

1. Davidoff LE: Treatment of hydrocephalus. Arch Surg 18:1737–1762, 1929.
2. Drake JM, Sainte-Rose C: The Shunt Book. New York, Blackwell Science, 1995.
3. Pudenz RH: The surgical treatment of hydrocephalus—an historical review. Surg Neurol 15:15–26, 1981.
4. Nulsen FE, Spitz EB: Treatment of hydrocephalus by direct shunt from ventricle to jugular vein. Surg Forum 2:399–403, 1952.
5. Kausch W: Die Behandlung des Hydrocephalus der kleinen Kinder. Arch Klin Chir 87:709–796, 1908.
6. Miyake H, Ohta T, Kajimoto Y, et al: The evaluation of various flow control valves in VP shunt system. In Nagai H, Kamiya K, Ishikawa Y (eds): Intracranial Pressure, IX. Berlin, Springer-Verlag, 1994, pp 579–580.
7. Czosnyka M, Czosnyka Z, Whitehouse H, et al: Hydrodynamic properties of hydrocephalus shunts: United Kingdom Shunt Evaluation Laboratory. Neurol Neurosurg Psychiatry 62:43–50, 1997.
8. Czosnyka M, Maksymowicz W, Batorski L, et al: Comparison between classic-differential and automatic shunt functioning on the basis of infusion tests. Acta Neurochir (Wien) 106:1–8, 1990.
9. Sainte-Rose C, Hooven MD, Hirsch JF: A new approach in the treatment of hydrocephalus. Childs Nerv Syst 66:213–226, 1987.
10. Sainte-Rose C, Piatt JH, Renier D, et al: Mechanical complications in shunts. Pediatr Neurosurg 17:2–9, 1991.
11. Fox JL, McCullough DC, Green RC: Effect of cerebrospinal fluid shunts on intracranial pressure and on cerebrospinal fluid dynamics. 2. A new technique of pressure measurements: Results and concepts. 3. A concept of hydrocephalus. J Neurol Neurosurg Psychiatry 36:302–312, 1973.
12. Fox JL, Portnoy HD, Shulte RR: Cerebrospinal fluid shunts: An experimental evaluation of flow rates and pressure values in the anti-siphon valve. Surg Neurol 1:299–302, 1973.
13. Hoffman HJ: Technical problems in shunts. Monogr Neural Sci 8:158–169, 1982.
14. Portnoy HD: Hydrodynamics of shunts. Monogr Neural Sci 8:179–183, 1982.
15. Watts C, Keith HD: Testing the hydrocephalus shunt valve. Childs Brain 10:217–228, 1983.
16. Kadowaki C, Hara M, Numoto M, et al: CSF shunt physics: Factors influencing shunt CSF flow. Childs Nerv Syst 11:203–206, 1995.
17. Trost HA, Heissler HE, Claussen G, et al: Testing the hydrocephalus shunt valve: Long-term bench test results of various new and explanted valves. The need for models for testing valves under physiological conditions. Eur J Pediatr Surg 1:38–40, 1991.
18. Andersson H, Logren J: Hydrodynamic evaluation of shunt performance in hydrocephalus. Dev Med Child Neurol Suppl 4:30–34, 1968.
19. Yamada S: Dynamic changes of cerebralspinal fluid in upright and recumbent shunted experimental animals. Childs Brain 1:187–192, 1975.
20. Shapiro K, Fried A: The theoretical requirements of shunt design as determined by biomechanical testing in pediatric hydrocephalus. Childs Nerv Syst 4:348–353, 1998.
21. Martins AN: Resistance to drainage of cerebrospinal fluid: Clinical measurement and significance. J Neurosurg Psychiatry 36:313–318, 1973.
22. Portnoy HD, Croissant PD: A practical method for measuring hydrodynamics of cerebrospinal fluid. Surg Neurol 5:273–277, 1976.
23. Portnoy HD, Tripp L, Croissant PD: Hydrodynamics of shunt valves. Childs Brain 2:242–256, 1976.
24. Hakim S: Flow through CSF shunts. Childs Nerv Syst 39:127–128, 1973.
25. Aschoff A: Overdrainage and shunt technology: A critical comparison of programmable, hydrostatic and variable-resistance valves and flow-reducing devices. Childs Nerv Syst 11:193–202, 1995.
26. Rayport M, Reiss J: Hydrodynamic properties of certain shunt assemblies for the treatment of hydrocephalus. 1. Report of a case of communicating hydrocephalus with increased cerebrospinal fluid production treated by duplication of shunting de-

vice. 2. Pressure-flow characteristics of the Spitz-Holter, Pudenz-Heyer, and Cordis-Hakim shunt systems. J Neurosurg 30:455–467, 1969.

27. Kadowaki C, Hara M, Numoto M, et al: Factors affecting cerebrospinal fluid flow in a shunt. Br J Neurosurg 1:467–475, 1987.
28. Aschoff A, Benesch C, Kremer P, et al: The solved and unsolved problems of hydrocephalus valves: A critical comment. In Lorenz R, Klinger M, Brack M (eds): Advances in Neurosurgery, vol 21. Berlin and New York, Springer-Verlag, 1993, pp 103–114.
29. Portnoy HD: Treatment of hydrocephalus. In section of Pediatric Neurosurgery of the American Association of Neurological Surgeons (eds): Pediatric Neurosurgery: Surgery of the Developing Nervous System. New York, Grune & Stratton, 1982, pp 211–227.
30. Foltz EL, Blanks J: Symptomatic low intracranial pressure in shunted hydrocephalus. Childs Nerv Syst 68:401–408, 1988.
31. Portnoy HD, Schulte RR, Fox JL, et al: Anti-siphon and reversible occlusion valves for shunting in hydrocephalus and preventing post-shunt subdural hematomas. Childs Nerv Syst 38:729–738, 1973.
32. McCullough DC, Fox JL: Negative intracranial pressure hydrocephalus in adults with shunts and its relationship to the production of subdural hematoma. Childs Nerv Syst 40:372–375, 1974.
33. Kaufman B, Weiss MH, Young HF, et al: Effects of prolonged cerebrospinal fluid shunting on the skull and brain. Childs Nerv Syst 38:288–297, 1973.
34. Loop JE, Foltz EL: Craniostenosis and diploic lamination following operation for hydrocephalus. Acta Radiol 13:8–13, 1972.
35. Pudenz RH, Foltz EL: Hydrocephalus: Overdrainage by ventricular shunts: A review and recommendations. Surg Neurol 35:200–212, 1991.
36. Holness RO, Hoffman HJ, Hendrick EB: Subtemporal decompression for the slit-ventricle syndrome after shunting in hydrocephalic children. Childs Brain 5:137–144, 1979.
37. Hyde-Rowan MD, Rekate H, Nulsen FE: Reexpansion of previously collapsed ventricles: The slit ventricle syndrome. Childs Nerv Syst 56:536–539, 1982.
38. Post EM: Currently available shunt systems: A review. Neurosurgery 16:257–260, 1985.
39. Lumenta CB, Roosen N, Dietrich U: Clinical experience with a pressure-adjustable valve Sophy in the management of hydrocephalus. Childs Nerv Syst 6:270–274, 1990.
40. Reinprecht A, Dietrich W, Bertalanffy A, et al: The Medos Hakim programmable valve in the treatment of pediatric hydrocephalus. Childs Nerv Syst 13:588–593, 1997.
41. Belliard H, Roux FX, Turak B, et al: The Codman Medos programmable shunt valve: Evaluation of 53 implantations in 50 patients. Neurochirurgie 42:139–145, 1996.
42. Aihara N, Takagi T, Hashimoto N, et al: Breakage of shunt devices (Sophy programmable pressure valve) following implantation in the hypochondriac region. Childs Nerv Syst 13:636–638, 1997.
43. O'Reilly G, Williams B: The Sophy valve and the el-Shafei shunt system for adult hydrocephalus. J Neurol Neurosurg Psychiatry 59:621–624, 1995.
44. Chidiac A, Pelissou-Guyotat I, Sindou M: Practical value of transcutaneous pressure adjustable valves (Sophy SU 8) in the treatment of hydrocephalus and arachnoid cysts in adults (75 cases). Neurochirurgie 38:291–296, 1992.
45. Black PM, Hakim R, Bailey NO: The use of the Codman-Medos programmable Hakim valve in the management of patients with hydrocephalus: Illustrative cases. Neurosurgery 34:1110–1113, 1994.
46. Aschoff A, Benesch C, Kremer P, et al: 44 "Programmable" valves in bench-test [abstract]. Childs Nerv Syst 12:503, 1996.
47. Benesch C, Friese M, Aschoff A: Four year follow up study of 146 patients with programmable Medos Hakim valve shunt system. Childs Nerv Syst 10:475, 1994.
48. Will BE, Müller-Korbsch U, Bucholz R: Experience with the programmable Sophy SU-8 valve. Childs Nerv Syst 10:476, 1994.
49. Ortler M, Kostron H, Felber S: Transcutaneous pressure-adjustable valves and magnetic resonance imaging: An ex vivo examination of the Codman-Medos programmable valve and the Sophy adjustable pressure valve [see comments]. Neurosurgery 40:1050–1057, 1997.
50. Fuse T, Takagi T, Fukushima T, et al: Problems encountered with a programmable pressure valve (Sophy) positioned in the chest wall. No Shinkei Geka 24:41–45, 1996.
51. Drake JM, Kestle J, Milner R, et al: Randomized trial of cerebrospinal fluid shunt valve design in pediatric hydrocephalus. Neurosurgery 43:294–305, 1998.
52. Tokoro K, Chiba Y: Optimum position for an anti-siphon device in a cerebrospinal fluid shunt system. Neurosurgery 29:519–525, 1991.
53. Kremer P, Aschoff A, Kunze S: Therapeutic risks of anti-siphon devices. Eur J Pediatr Surg 1(Suppl 1):47–48, 1991.
54. Gruber R, Jenny P, Herzog B: Experiences with the anti-siphon device (ASD) in shunt therapy of pediatric hydrocephalus. J Neurosurg 61:156–162, 1984.
55. McCullough DC: Symptomatic progressive ventriculomegaly in hydrocephalics with patent shunts and antisiphon devices. Neurosurgery 19:617–621, 1986.
56. Drake JM, da Silva MC, Rutka JT: Functional obstruction of an antisiphon device by raised tissue capsule pressure. Neurosurgery 32:137–139, 1993.
57. Drake JM, Kestle J: Determining the best cerebrospinal fluid shunt valve design: The pediatric valve design trial. Neurosurgery 38:604–607, 1996.
58. Drake JM, Kestle J: Rationale and methodology of the multicenter pediatric cerebrospinal fluid shunt design trial: Pediatric Hydrocephalus Treatment Evaluation Group. Childs Nerv Syst 12:434–447, 1996.
59. Pollack IF, Albright AL, Adelson PD, et al: A randomized, controlled study of a programmable shunt valve versus a conventional valve for patients with hydrocephalus. Neurosurgery 45:1399–1408, 1999.
60. Haase J, Weeth R: Multiflanged ventricular catheter for hydrocephalic shunts. Acta Neurochir (Wien) 33:213–218, 1976.
61. Sainte-Rose C, Piatt JH, Renier D, et al: Mechanical complications in shunts. Pediatr Neurosurg 17:2–9, 1991.
62. Aschoff A, Kremer P, Benesch C, et al: Overdrainage and shunt technology: A critical comparison of programmable, hydrostatic and variable-resistance valves and flow-reducing devices. Childs Nerv Syst 11:193–202, 1995.
63. Sparrow OC: Laboratory performance of single-piece ventriculoperitoneal shunts with distal slit-valve control. Childs Nerv Syst 70:946–953, 1989.
64. Frim DM, Goumnerova LC: Telemetric intraventricular pressure measurements after third ventriculocisternostomy in a patient with noncommunicating hydrocephalus. Neurosurgery 41:1425–1428, 1997.
65. Munshi I, Lathrop D, Madsen JR, et al: Intraventricular pressure dynamics in patients with ventriculopleural shunts: A telemetric study. Pediatr Neurosurg 28:67–69, 1998.
66. Harbert JC, McCullough DC: Radionuclide tests of cerebral fluid shunt patency. J Nucl Med 25:112–114, 1984.
67. Graham P, Howman-Giles R, Johnston I, et al: Evaluation of CSF shunt patency by means of technetium-99m DTPA. Childs Nerv Syst 57:262–266, 1982.
68. Harbert JC: Radionuclide techniques in the evaluation of cerebrospinal fluid shunts. Crit Rev Diagn Imaging 9:207–228, 1977.
69. Drake JM, Martin AJ, Henkleman RM: Determination of cerebrospinal fluid shunt obstruction with magnetic resonance phase imaging. Childs Nerv Syst 75:535–554, 1991.
70. Frank E, Buonocore M, Hein L: Magnetic resonance imaging analysis of extremely slow flow in a model shunt system. Childs Nerv Syst 8:73–75, 1992.
71. Howman-Giles R, McLaughlin A, Johnston I, et al: A radionuclide method of evaluating shunt function and CSF circulation in hydrocephalus: Technical note. Childs Nerv Syst 61:604–605, 1984.
72. Harbert J, Haddad D, McCullough D: Quantitation of cerebrospinal fluid shunt flow. Radiology 112:379–387, 1974.
73. Seppanen U, Serlo W, Saukkonen AL: Valvography in the assessment of hydrocephalus shunt function in children. Neuroradiology 29:53–57, 1987.
74. Chiba Y, Ishiwata Y, Suzuki N, et al: Thermosensitive determination of obstructed sites in ventriculoperitoneal shunts. Childs Nerv Syst 62:363–366, 1985.

75. Hara M, Kadowaki C, Konishi Y, et al: A new method for measuring cerebrospinal fluid flow in shunts. Childs Nerv Syst 58:557–561, 1983.
76. Lam K, Drake JM, Cobbold RSC: Noninvasive cerebrospinal fluid shunt measurement by Doppler ultrasound using ultrasonically excited bubbles: A feasibility study. Ultrasound Med Biol 25:371–389, 1999.
77. Lam K, Drake JM, Cobbold RSC: Generation and maintenance of bubbles in small tubes by low-frequency ultrasound. J Acoust Soc Am 1999.
78. Munro A: Observations on the Structure and Functions of the Nervous System. Edinburgh, 1783.
79. Kellie G: An account . . . with some reflections on the pathology of the brain. Edin Med Chir Soc Trans 1:84–169, 1824.
80. Tenti G, Drake JM, Sivaloganathan S: Brain biomechanics: Mathematical modeling of hydrocephalus. Neurol Res 22:19–24, 2000.
81. Guinane JE: An equivalent circuit analysis of cerebrospinal fluid hydrodynamics. Am J Physiol 223:425–430, 1972.
82. Marmarou A, Shulman K, Rosende RM: A nonlinear analysis of the cerebrospinal fluid system and intracranial pressure dynamics. Childs Nerv Syst 48:332–344, 1978.
83. Shulman K, Marmarou A: Pressure-volume considerations in infantile hydrocephalus. Dev Med Child Neurol 13(Suppl 25): 90–95, 1971.
84. Shapiro K, Marmarou A, Shulman K: Characterization of clinical CSF dynamics and neural axis compliance using the pressure-volume index. I. The normal pressure-volume index. Ann Neurol 7:508–514, 1979.
85. Shapiro K, Marmarou A: Clinical applications of the pressure-volume index in treatment of pediatric head injuries. Childs Nerv Syst 56:819–825, 1982.
86. Drake JM, Tenti G, Sivaloganathan S: Computer modeling of siphoning for CSF shunt design evaluation. Pediatr Neurosurg 21:6–15, 1994.
87. Hakim S, Venegas JG, Burton JD: The physics of the cranial cavity, hydrocephalus and normal pressure hydrocephalus: Mechanical interpretation and mathematical model. Surg Neurol 5: 187–210, 1976.
88. Hakim S, Hakim C: A biomechanical model of hydrocephalus and its relationship to treatment. In Shapiro K, Marmarou A, Portnoy HD (eds): Hydrocephalus. New York, Raven, 1984.
89. Nagashima T, Tanaki N, Matsumoto S, et al: Biomechanics of hydrocephalus. Neurosurgery 21:898–904, 1987.
90. Pena A, Bolton MD, Whitehouse H, et al: Effects of brain ventricular shape on periventricular biomechanics: A finite-element analysis. Neurosurgery 45:107–116, 1999.
91. Spertell RB: The response of brain to transient elevations in intraventricular pressure. J Neurol Sci 48:343–352, 1980.
92. Sainte-Rose C: Shunt obstruction: A preventable complication? Pediatr Neurosurg 19:156–164, 1993.
93. Ventureyra EC, Higgins MJ: A new ventricular catheter for the prevention and treatment of proximal obstruction in cerebrospinal fluid shunts. Neurosurgery 34:924–926, 1994.
94. Collins P, Hockley AD, Woollam DHM: Surface ultrastructure of tissues occluding ventricular catheters. Childs Nerv Syst 48: 609–613, 1978.
95. Bierbauer KS, Storrs BB, McLone DG, et al: A prospective, randomized study of shunt function and infections as a function of shunt placement. Pediatr Neurosurg 16:287–291, 1990.
96. Albright AL, Haines SJ, Taylor FH: Function of parietal and frontal shunts in childhood hydrocephalus. Childs Nerv Syst 69:883–886, 1988.
97. Brownlee RD, Dold ON, Myles ST: Intraventricular hemorrhage complicating ventricular catheter revision: Incidence and effect on shunt survival. Pediatr Neurosurg 22:315–320, 1995.
98. Chambi I, Hendrick EB: A technique for removal of an adherent ventricular catheter. Pediatr Neurosci 14:216–217, 1988.
99. Hudgins RJ, Boydston WR: Shunt revision by coagulation with retention of the ventricular catheter. Pediatr Neurosurg 29:57–59, 1998.
100. Pattisapu JV, Trumble ER, Taylor KR, et al: Percutaneous endoscopic recanalization of catheter: A new technique of proximal shunt revision. Neurosurgery 45:1361–1366, 1999.
101. Christens-Barry WA, Guarnieri M, Carson BS: Fiberoptic delivery of laser energy to remove occlusions from ventricular shunts: Technical report. Neurosurgery 44:345–350, 1999.
102. Hakim S: Hydraulic and mechanical mis-matching of valve shunts in the treatment of hydrocephalus: The need for a servo-valve shunt. Dev Med Child Neurol 15:646–653, 1973.

CHAPTER 215

Hydrocephalus in Children

HAROLD L. REKATE

In hydrocephalus, an excess of cerebrospinal fluid (CSF) accumulates within the ventricular system of the brain, and intracranial pressure (ICP) increases as a result. The condition is not a disease but results from various conditions that affect the fetus, infant, and child. Nor is it an "all-or-none" phenomenon. Some children can be managed with observation if the hydrocephalus is mild,[1] and some cases may resolve without treatment.[2]

Adequate treatment for hydrocephalus did not exist before the valve-regulated shunt was developed in the early 1950s. Before then, most children who were born with or acquired hydrocephalus died, and the condition of the survivors was poor.[3] At that time, the diagnosis of hydrocephalus depended on angiography or the injection of air into the ventricular system; a significant percentage of patients now seen by neurosurgeons would not even have been diagnosed. They also would not have been captured in natural history studies of patients with hydrocephalus from that era. The natural history of children with stable, moderately enlarged ventricles with large heads is still unknown.

In 1973, the first computed tomography scanner was installed in the United States. About the same time, real-time cranial ultrasonography began to be performed routinely in neonatal intensive care units. The diagnosis of hydrocephalus no longer depended on invasive and dangerous tests, and milder forms of hydrocephalus were discovered. In the mid-1980s, the development of magnetic resonance imaging (MRI) allowed neurosurgeons not only to diagnose hydrocephalus but also to determine the actual site of obstruction to the flow of CSF that caused it. Consequently, the ability to diagnose the underlying condition leading to hydrocephalus has improved, and new treatment paradigms have been developed to manage many of these infants and children.

This chapter discusses the pathophysiology of hydrocephalus as a guide to establishing the cause of the condition and thus improve our ability to select the best treatment and predict outcomes. It also discusses the options for managing the various forms of hydrocephalus and the potential complications associated with the condition itself and the treatment chosen.

PATHOPHYSIOLOGY

To understand the pathophysiology of hydrocephalus, one must first understand the normal dynamics of CSF flow (Fig. 215–1), the interaction of CSF flow with the viscoelastic properties of the brain, and how both relate to cerebral blood flow. CSF is produced at a rate of about 0.33 mL/minute by two distinct processes. First, CSF is produced by an energy-requiring process performed by the choroid plexuses in the lateral, third, and fourth ventricles. This process depends on the enzyme carbonic anhydrase and can be blocked by the carbonic anhydrase inhibitor acetazolamide (Diamox). Originally, the choroid plexuses were thought to be the sole source of CSF production,[4-6] but CSF production returns to normal after the choroid plexuses have been removed.[7] The remainder of the CSF is produced as a by-product of cerebral and white matter metabolism. The brain and spinal cord extracellular fluid flows into the ventricular system and central canal of the spinal cord by bulk flow. In normal circumstances, choroidal CSF production constitutes 50% to 80% of the total CSF production.[8]

After its production, the ventricular CSF flows through a series of narrowings from one compartment to the next. The compartments begin with the lateral ventricles through the foramina of Monro to the third ventricle. From there it flows through the aqueduct of Sylvius into the fourth ventricle. From there it exits the outlet foramina of the fourth ventricle (Luschka and Magendie) and flows into the cisterna magna, where it mixes with the CSF from the spinal subarachnoid space (SSAS). Finally, the CSF flows through the cortical subarachnoid space (CSAS) to be absorbed through specialized organs, the arachnoid villi, into the sagittal sinus (Fig. 215–2).

The energy for the circulation of CSF is generated by the pumping of arterial blood into the choroid plexus by the left ventricle of the heart. A parallel circuit involves cerebral blood flow, the total of which is about 1 L/minute, in contrast to the 0.33 mL/minute associated with CSF. Arterial blood is pumped into the choroid plexuses and the parenchymal arterioles at the mean arterial pressure. In both locations, the mean arterial pressure immediately drops to the level of the ICP within the ventricles and the brain parenchyma. The channels between the compartments within both the CSF and the flowing blood pathways can be thought of as resistors in a circuit. Each channel can also be obstructed by some pathologic processes that lead to abnormal CSF and ICP dynamics.

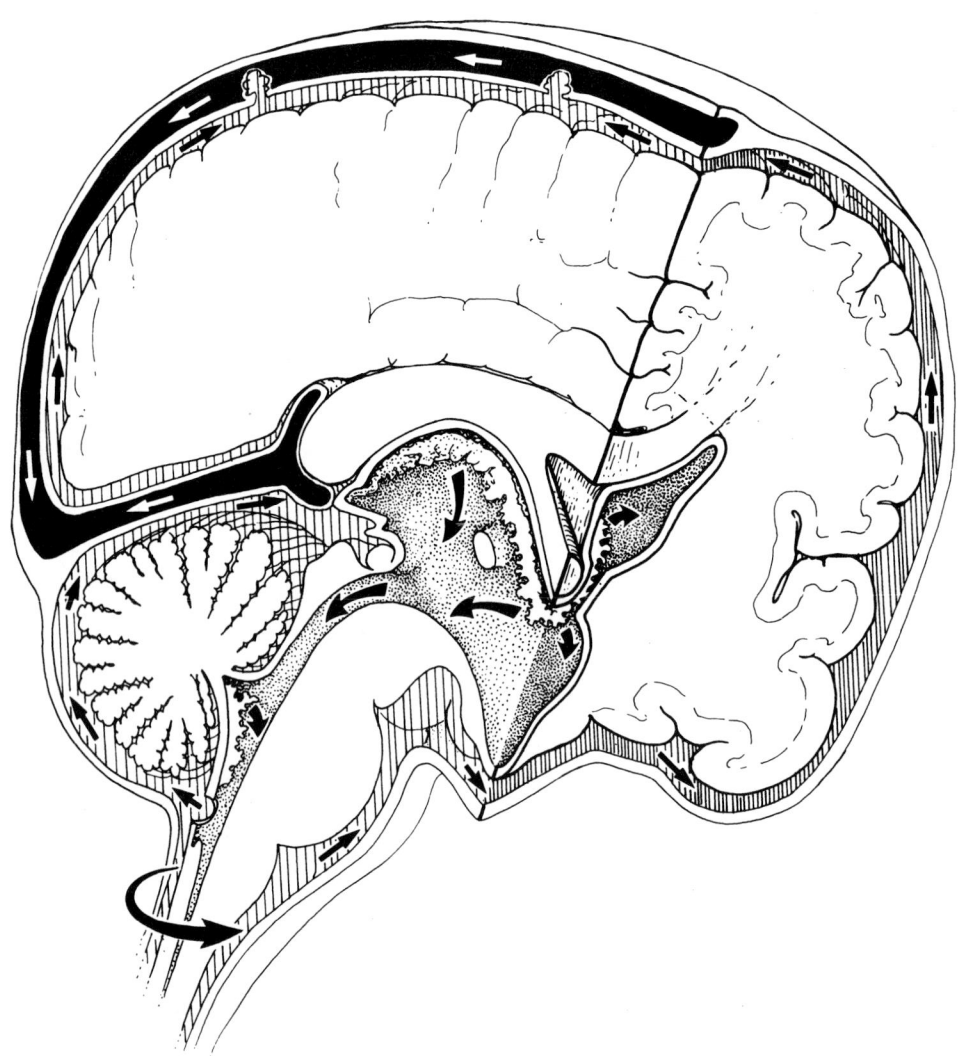

FIGURE 215–1. Schematic diagram of the anatomy of the cerebrospinal fluid pathways. (Courtesy of Barrow Neurological Institute, Phoenix, AZ.)

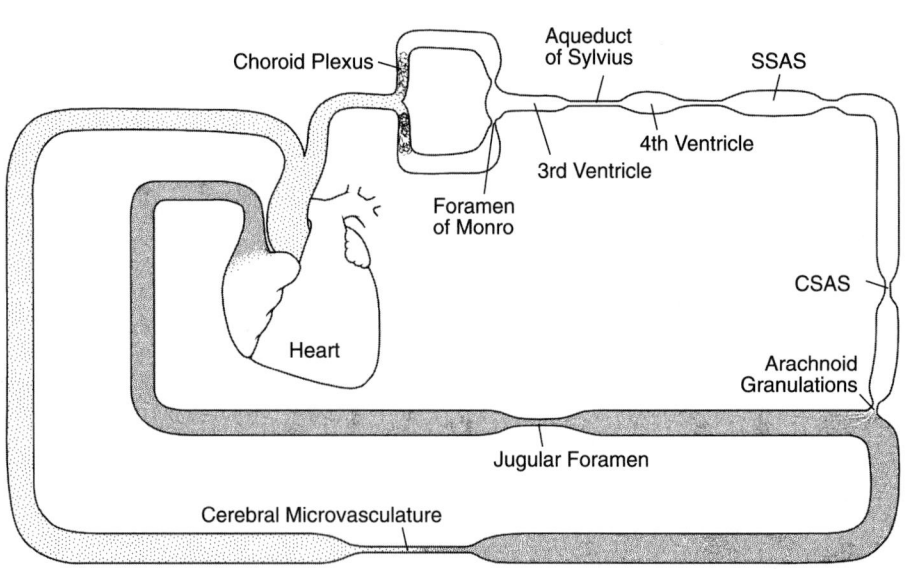

FIGURE 215–2. Schematic diagram of the circulation of cerebrospinal fluid (CSF) as a hydraulic circuit. The left ventricle of the heart functions as the power source for CSF flow. CSAS, cortical subarachnoid space; SSAS, spinal subarachnoid space. (Adapted from Rekate HL: Circuit diagram of the circulation of cerebrospinal fluid. Pediatr Neurosurg 21: 248–253, 1994.)

The physical properties of the hydraulic circuit (see Fig. 215–2) have been studied extensively in our laboratory, primarily in animals, but occasionally in human patients when it was possible to measure pressures in several compartments simultaneously. During these studies, ICP differentials could be recorded in only two conditions. In all cases, a pressure differential could be measured between the CSAS and the sagittal sinuses,[9, 10] supporting an earlier report by Ransohoff and coworkers.[11] In both laboratory animals and humans, the usual pressure differential across the arachnoid villi is between 5 and 7 mm Hg. These findings agree with the work of Cutler and colleagues,[12] who defined an "opening" pressure of about 70 mm H_2O (about 5 mm Hg), below which no absorption occurred. This opening pressure associated with the normal CSF absorptive process is due to the valvular mechanism of the arachnoid villi. A valvular mechanism of the same magnitude also exists between the cortical veins and the sagittal sinus, and the cortical veins are in equilibrium with the ICP.[13, 14]

The only other condition in which pressure differentials could be measured within the intracranial compartment occurred in the context of artificial drainage of CSF from smaller than normal ventricles. In this situation, the intact septum pellucidum is distorted or pulled over against the head of the caudate nucleus, creating an obstruction to flow in a retrograde fashion across the obstructed foramen of Monro.[15]

In other situations, pressure differentials cannot be measured in living animals for two reasons, even if CSF is completely obstructed. First, the rate of CSF production and therefore CSF flow is very slow (0.33 mL/minute, or 20 mL/hour). Pressure sensors upstream and downstream from the point of constriction or obstruction that are far more sensitive than those currently used in routine laboratory studies would be needed to measure such a slow rate of flow. The second and probably more important reason involves the general nature of the brain as a viscoelastic substance. As a pressure sump develops in one location, the brain tends to shift into that area rapidly, and the pressure differential is dissipated instantaneously.[16, 17]

With the biophysics of the formation, absorption, and flow of CSF as a backdrop, the study of hydrocephalus is simplified by reference to Figure 215–2. Depending on which point along the circuit an obstruction occurs, the differential diagnosis of the cause of the hydrocephalus, the treatment options, and the probable outcome of treatment vary.[10, 18] It is not always possible to determine the point of obstruction at presentation without subjecting a patient to unjustifiable risk or discomfort. However, with MRI, particularly with CSF flow studies, considerable information can be obtained about the physics of the CSF system in an individual patient. Occasionally, a radiographic dye must be injected into the CSF pathways to determine the actual point of obstruction. Further, CSF may be obstructed at more than one point along the pathway. In particular, Chiari II malformations can cause as many as four different sites of obstruction to CSF flow.[19] Severe meningitis can also cause multiple sites of obstruction.

CLASSIFICATION BASED ON SITE OF CEREBROSPINAL FLUID FLOW OBSTRUCTION

In the earliest studies of the pathophysiology of hydrocephalus, Dandy and Blackfan[4] classified hydrocephalus into two types: communicating and noncommunicating. This classification was based on the injection of a supravital dye into the lateral ventricle and its collection in the SSAS after a spinal tap.[5] Because shunting devices were unavailable then, they attempted several operations to treat obstructive hydrocephalus, including an open third ventriculostomy, originally sacrificing an optic nerve and removing the choroid plexuses of the lateral ventricles, which they believed were the source of all CSF production. Probably owing to the extreme nature of hydrocephalus in the era when transillumination was the standard diagnostic test, the mortality rate associated with these operations was high, and the success rate was extremely low.

In 1960, Ransohoff and coworkers[11] recognized the basically obstructive nature of all hydrocephalus and proposed a new classification using the terms *intraventricular obstructive* (noncommunicating) and *extraventricular obstructive* (communicating) *hydrocephalus*. Obstruction at the foramen of Monro, aqueduct of Sylvius, and outlet foramina of the fourth ventricle leads to intraventricular obstructive hydrocephalus, and obstruction at the basal cisterns (CSAS to SSAS), arachnoid villi, or venous outflow creates extraventricular obstructive hydrocephalus (see Fig. 215–2). Using the imaging modalities now available to neurosurgeons, the classification of hydrocephalus should reflect the actual anatomic site of obstruction, because each site is associated with different causes and clinical syndromes.

The following discussion focuses on the possible sites of obstruction in the CSF pathway in terms of the potential causative pathologies, the available treatment options, the likely clinical picture at the time of shunt failure, and the long-term results of treatment.

Obstruction of One Foramen of Monro

Like most other forms of hydrocephalus, unilateral monoventricular hydrocephalus can be congenital or acquired. The congenital absence or constriction of the foramen of Monro is a rare birth defect. Even when severe, it is often missed in infancy because the child is perceived to be normal. The condition is often diagnosed when a disproportionately rapid increase in head circumference occurs. At this point, neuroimaging studies usually reveal a markedly enlarged lateral ventricle on the side of the occlusion. Uniquely in this condition, the calvaria on the side of the enlarged ventricle is greatly expanded, and the falx encases the normal hemisphere far from the midline. Careful neurological assessment often reveals increased tone of the contralateral upper and lower extremities, a finding that can become more obvious later in life.

Acquired obstruction of the foramen of Monro is

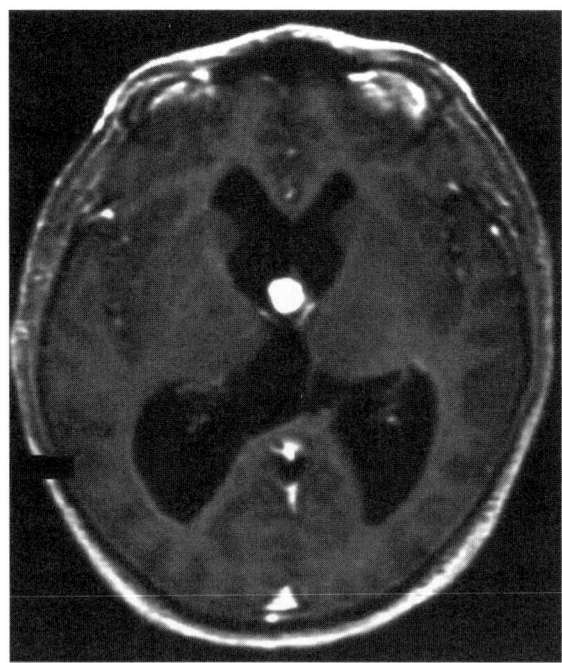

FIGURE 215–3. Magnetic resonance imaging scan showing biventricular hydrocephalus in a patient with an anterior third ventricular colloid cyst.

caused by mass lesions in the region or by inflammatory processes (usually bacterial ventriculitis). When obstruction of the foramen of Monro is due to ventriculitis, it is usually part of a more global compartmentalization of the ventricular system involving multiple sites of obstruction. Very complex treatment strategies are required. Tumors in this location are most common in children and typically arise below or within the anterior third ventricle. Tumors that tend to obstruct the foramen of Monro in children include craniopharyngiomas, opticohypothalamic astrocytomas, choroid plexus papillomas, and germinomas. In a few older children and adults, colloid cysts are important causes of obstruction at this location. In such cases, the foraminal obstruction is usually bilateral, yielding the picture of biventricular hydrocephalus (Fig. 215–3).

Probably the most common tumors leading to unilateral obstruction of the foramen of Monro are subependymal giant cell astrocytomas. Although these rare tumors may be the presenting sign of this condition, they are found only in the context of tuberous sclerosis (Fig. 215–4). The tumors arise in the region of the foramen of Monro and are very small and asymptomatic in these patients. Like so many of the tumors associated with the phakomatoses, their natural history is unpredictable. They can, however, grow and cause severe symptoms very rapidly.

TREATMENT OPTIONS AT PRESENTATION

At diagnosis, patients with a congenital absence of one foramen of Monro usually have severe unilateral dilatation of one lateral ventricle and a very thin ipsi-

lateral cortical mantle. The pathophysiology of this condition is clear. Because the ipsilateral brain has been chronically subjected to severe thinning, it is unlikely that the cerebral mantle will be reconstituted significantly on that side by simple perforation of the septum pellucidum. Most neurosurgeons would elect to shunt the affected ventricle, with or without performing an endoscopic septum pellucidotomy at the same time. This approach gives the cortical mantle the best chance to reconstitute significantly and maintains the option of enabling the patient to do without the shunt when it fails.

When biventricular hydrocephalus is caused by an anterior third ventricular mass, several treatment options are available. Which form of treatment to pursue depends on many factors, including the patient's clinical condition and surgeon's previous experience. If a patient with biventricular hydrocephalus is severely ill, shunting one lateral ventricle may be insufficient to alleviate the signs of increased ICP and may even worsen the patient's clinical condition. Either both lateral ventricles need shunt tubes, or an endoscopic septum pellucidotomy must be performed at the time of insertion.

When a tumor obstructs the foramina of Monro, removal or debulking of the lesion often unblocks the points of obstruction, and no shunt is needed after surgical treatment of the tumor itself. Treating hydrocephalus by unblocking the foramen is an important strategy in the case of subependymal giant cell astrocytomas. Uniquely in this case, it is difficult to maintain a working shunt. The tumor tends to block the ventricular catheter, and its protein content upstream from the point of obstruction is very high. Gross total resection of the tumor is probably essential because it is so difficult to maintain a working shunt in this context.

PRESENTATION AND OUTCOME AT SHUNT FAILURE

When the shunt of a patient with congenital obstruction of the foramen of Monro fails and the ventricles have remained large, the failure may lead to subtle symptoms, if any. If the patient is old enough to assess his or her neurological condition easily and the shunt failure is discovered incidentally, there may be no compelling reason to revise the shunt, depending on the surgeon's judgment and the family's desires.

The most likely presentation associated with shunt failure is progressive severe headache. The size of the already enlarged ventricles may or may not increase, and the diagnosis may be made presumptively or by placing a small needle in the reservoir incorporated in the shunt system and testing for proximal obstruction or by physically measuring the ICP. Patients with congenital atresia of the foramen of Monro and ventricular dilatation at the time of shunt failure should be considered candidates for endoscopic septum pellucidotomy, because their CSF absorptive capacity is unaffected.

The prognosis for patients with hydrocephalus related to obstruction of the foramen of Monro by an

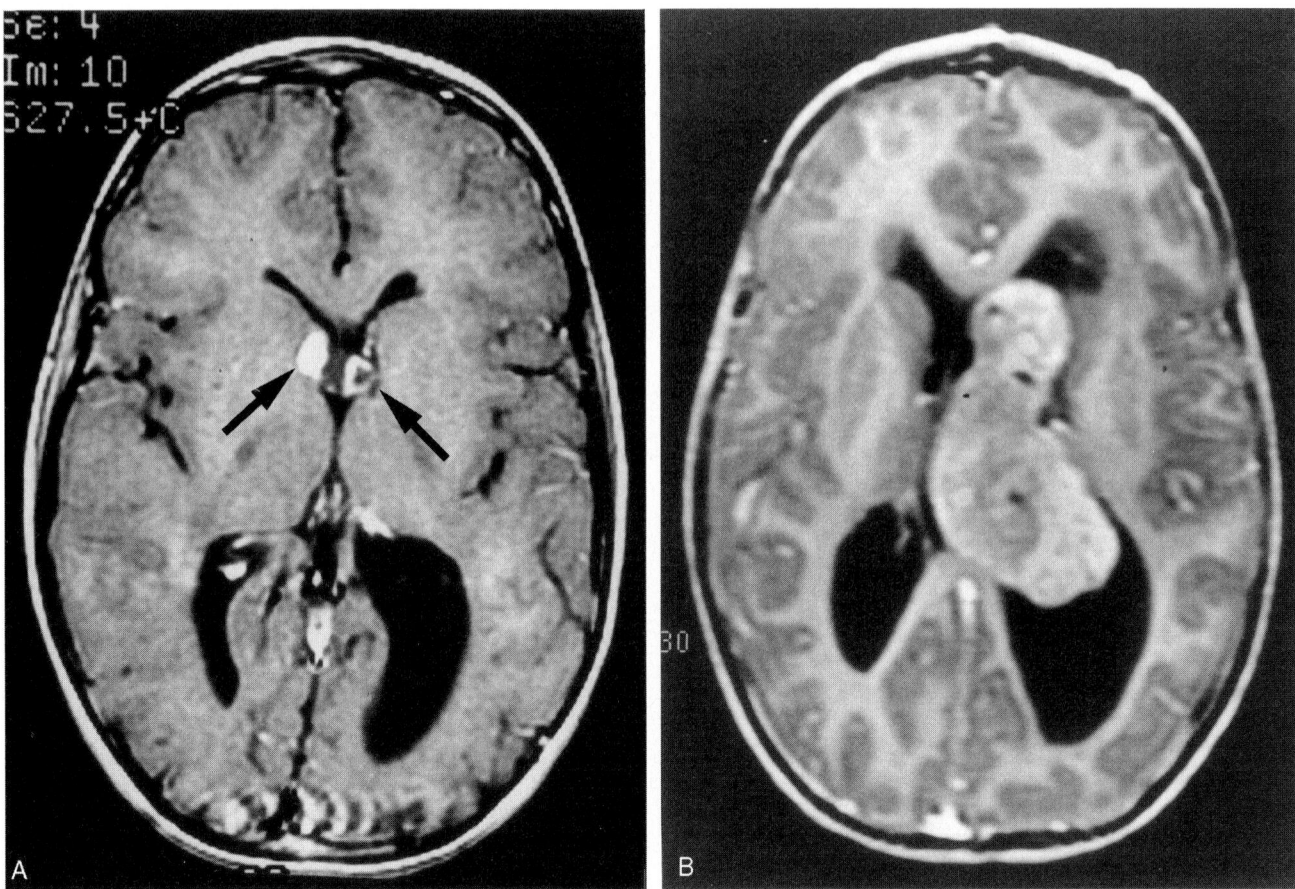

FIGURE 215–4. Monoventricular hydrocephalus related to a subependymal giant cell astrocytoma of the foramen of Monro, seen exclusively in patients with tuberous sclerosis. *A*, Magnetic resonance imaging (MRI) scan of the brain obtained during the patient's initial screening. Two subependymal giant cell astrocytomas are present *(arrows)*, neither of which is causing significant hydrocephalus. *B*, MRI scan obtained when the child acutely became symptomatic, showing marked enlargement of the tumor and isolated lateral ventricle hydrocephalus.

anterior third ventricular mass depends mostly on tumor management. Removal of a colloid cyst, either endoscopically or via a transcallosal route, should arrest the hydrocephalus permanently, without the need for a shunt.

Obstruction of the Aqueduct of Sylvius

The cause of constriction or occlusion of the aqueduct of Sylvius can be either congenital or acquired. After hydrocephalus associated with spina bifida, the congenital form is the second most common diagnosis of hydrocephalus in utero. In this context, it is usually an isolated and unexpected finding. It can occur in families as a sex-linked condition found only in boys. It is also found in many animal models of hydrocephalus. Pathologically, the usual postmortem description is of a "forked" aqueduct, analogous to attempting to create a tunnel by beginning to dig through the mountain from either end but missing in the center. In both animal models and human studies, hydrocephalus itself has been found to cause further hydrocephalus by constricting the upper midbrain as the temporal horns of the lateral ventricles expand.[20]

Acquired aqueductal stenosis may result from an infectious process and may even be caused by chronic overdrainage of spinal fluid by a lateral ventricle shunt. This shunt-related complication is extremely rare, except in the context of secondary ventriculitis. When it occurs later in life, most cases of aqueductal obstruction are due to tumorous occlusion along the length of the aqueduct. A typical example of this phenomenon is occlusion of the aqueduct by intrinsic astrocytic tumors of the tectal plate. Characteristically, these tumors are associated with triventricular hydrocephalus. MRI shows an expanding lesion of the midbrain with no contrast enhancement and often with high signal intensity on T2-weighted images (Fig. 215–5). Although histologically the tumors are clearly astrocytic, they rarely progress, and management involves treatment of the hydrocephalus and surveillance of the tumor. Tumors of the pineal region tend to manifest with triventricular hydrocephalus due to downward pressure on and obstruction of the aqueduct. Finally and most important in the management of childhood hydrocephalus, posterior fossa brain tumors (medulloblastomas, cerebellar astrocytomas, ependymomas, and choroid plexus tumors) are often very large and grow into the aqueduct.

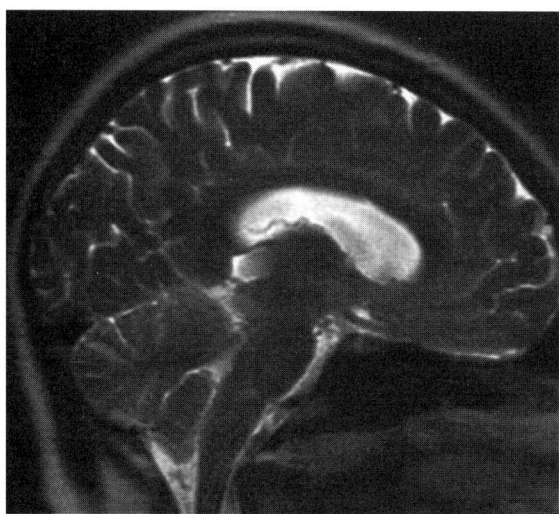

FIGURE 215–5. Aqueductal stenosis caused by a tumor of the tectal plate, usually seen only on T2-weighted images.

TREATMENT OPTIONS AT PRESENTATION

Three different epochs (prenatal, birth to 1 year, and beyond 1 year) must be considered relative to the management of aqueductal stenosis that causes severe hydrocephalus. First are those children who are found to have significant hydrocephalus on routine prenatal ultrasonographic examinations. A thorough discussion of all aspects of the decision-making process for these babies is beyond the scope of this chapter. Much of the decision-making process involves the perinatologist and mother, either with or without the involvement of a pediatric neurosurgeon. The ethical issues and religious arguments regarding the management of children at high risk for significant neurological disability is not discussed here. At the beginning of the process, the role of the pediatric neurosurgeon is to help predict the severity of the condition and counsel the family and perinatologist about the child's overall management.

Next, whether the hydrocephalus is associated with other life- or function-threatening abnormalities is evaluated. Usually serial high-definition ultrasonograms are obtained to follow the progression of the hydrocephalus and its "attack" on the brain. Maternal serum studies include alpha fetoprotein. Usually, amniocentesis is performed for chemical assessment and chromosomal studies. If all studies are negative, the child is categorized as having "hydrocephalus overt at birth." The available data on these children predate the routine use of abdominal ultrasonography and the general availability of computed tomography. Typically, hydrocephalus overt at birth is associated with unpredictable outcomes. One third of such infants are essentially vegetative, a third have significant developmental delays, and a third are essentially normal after treatment of the hydrocephalus.[21, 22] If a decision is made to deliver the baby, the questions become when? and how? If hydrocephalus is severe enough for long enough, a "point of no return" can be reached after which treat-

ment in terms of cognitive outcome is futile.[23] Some evidence suggests that this point of no return tends to occur as the brain mantle becomes thinner than 1 cm.[24]

In the mid-1980s, there was considerable enthusiasm for in utero management of prenatally diagnosed hydrocephalus.[25, 26] Owing to the high percentage of fetal loss and poor cognitive outcomes, a voluntary moratorium was placed on this intervention. Recently, enthusiasm for prenatal management of hydrocephalus has resurged. Either a transabdominal drainage from the resurfaced ventricle to an extraventricular drainage system[27] or ventriculoamniotic shunts can be used (S. Cavalheiri, personal communication, 1998). The outcomes have been good, but the procedures have not gained widespread acceptance. Tulipan and Bruner[28] and others at Vanderbilt and Sutton and colleagues[29] at the University of Pennsylvania have shown that it is possible to remove a child from the womb to repair a myelomeningocele. The possibility of performing open surgery on a fetus reopens the entire question of prenatal surgery for other birth defects.[30, 31] If fine detail of the neuroanatomy of the child's brain is needed to determine when a child should be delivered or by what method, this information can be obtained from prenatal MRI, which is proving increasingly useful in prenatal diagnosis.[32, 33]

Regarding the need for ventilator support or visual loss, the overall prognosis for babies born at 34 weeks does not differ significantly from that of babies delivered at term. If the mother is treated with systemic steroids before delivery, fetal lung maturity may be reached at about 32 weeks. Therefore, whereas in utero management is highly controversial, elective delivery for management of hydrocephalus is used regularly.

For the babies discussed previously and for those born with large heads and severe ventriculomegaly (epoch 2), the only treatment option is to insert a ventriculoperitoneal (VP) shunt. The shunt can lower intraventricular pressure to subatmospheric levels and is the only way to reduce the size of severely dilated ventricles in neonates. In older children with a more subtle degree of hydrocephalus, the option of performing an endoscopic third ventriculostomy (ETV) becomes more realistic. Pediatric neurosurgeons who perform ETVs agree that this treatment is unlikely to resolve the hydrocephalus from birth to about age 1 year. This belief, however, is by no means universal. Buxton and colleagues[34] demonstrated that although the success rate for the procedure performed in children younger than 1 year is only about 25%, the complication rate is low. They recommend that families be given the opportunity to decide whether the procedure should be attempted.

To explain the poor success rate of ETV in infants and newborns, it is necessary to review the physics of CSF circulation. Even when the aqueduct is completely obstructed, most infants have a form of normal-pressure hydrocephalus (NPH). ICP must be 5 mm Hg above sagittal sinus pressure for CSF to be absorbed. When the fontanelle is open and the sutures are unfused, ICP cannot reach levels significantly above atmospheric pressure so that CSF can be absorbed. The size of the head grows instead. In the first year of life, the smaller the fontanelle and the older the child, the more likely it is that the procedure will be successful.

Management with ETV should be seriously considered in patients who develop hydrocephalus related to obstruction of the aqueduct of Sylvius beyond the first year of life (epoch 3). The success rate in this group of patients is at least 70%, with a permanent complication rate of about 1% and a temporary complication rate of about 3%.[35] In experienced hands, this complication rate is about the same as that associated with placement of a ventricular shunt, and it is definitely lower than the complication rate associated with lifetime shunt dependency.

The role of ETV in the preoperative management of patients whose treatment includes the removal of a pineal or fourth ventricular tumor is controversial and yet to be defined. My practice is to place an external drain at surgery, remove as much of the tumor as possible for both oncologic reasons and treatment of the hydrocephalus, and attempt to remove the external ventriculostomy a few days after surgery.

PRESENTATION AND OUTCOME AT SHUNT FAILURE

Patients who are treated for aqueductal stenosis with VP shunts are likely to need treatment for increased ICP soon after occlusion, especially if the size of the ventricles is subnormal, as would be expected. This phenomenon is purely a matter of physics. The post-treatment ventricular volume may be as small as 3 mL of CSF proximal to the occlusion, while the body is producing 20 mL of new CSF each hour. The ventricles expand quickly, and rapid intervention is necessary to prevent deterioration and even death. An ideal candidate for ETV is one whose system can respond in a timely manner or whose obstruction does not involve the proximal catheter so that the patient can be kept comfortable and safe until the system responds. This option should be discussed when the patient is stable so that the decision to revise the shunt or to attempt ventriculostomy can be made in advance.

Chronically shunted patients with hydrocephalus related to aqueductal stenosis have at least an 80% chance of shunt-independent arrest of their hydrocephalus after ETV. They are also at significant risk for death or serious neurological injury if they cannot obtain timely and responsive medical care. Almost half these patients have had an episode of coma during a shunt failure. Therefore, independent living is dangerous unless a system can be established to check on the patient periodically (Hydrocephalus Association, unpublished data, 1997).

Obstruction of the Outlet Foramina of the Fourth Ventricle

There are three distinct pathways for the exit of CSF from the fourth ventricle: the one foramen of Magendie and the two foramina of Luschka. For hydrocephalus to result from occlusion of these outlet foramina, all three must be involved in the same process. The most common cause is infection, but it is also associated with severe forms of Chiari I and II malformations. In these situations, the foramen of Magendie is encased in densely scarred arachnoid, and the brainstem has descended far enough into the area of the foramen magnum to occlude the lateral exiting foramina of the fourth ventricle. This scarring effect is a well-recognized cause of obstruction of the outlet foramina of the fourth ventricle. The presence of a Chiari I malformation and a strong history of traumatic delivery are highly correlated. At surgery, a dense, adhesive arachnoiditis is often found around the foramen of Magendie, which is routinely opened as part of the procedure. A history of a traumatic birth and particularly of dense, adhesive arachnoiditis is especially prominent in cases of Chiari I malformation associated with syringomyelia.

Obstruction of CSF outflow as a cause of hydrocephalus and syringomyelia has long been recognized. Hall and colleagues[36] recognized the relationship between shunt failure and scoliosis in patients with spina bifida who had no overt signs of intracranial hypertension. I saw an adolescent with a midlumbar myelomeningocele who presented with subacute paraplegia as the only sign of shunt failure. The cause of the hydrocephalus was obstruction of the outlet foramina of the fourth ventricle. The CSF produced within the lateral ventricles was forced into the central canal of the spinal cord, causing distention of the central canal and then neurological deterioration. The condition improved slightly after shunt revision.

Perhaps the most dramatic case of hydrocephalus related to obstruction of the outlet foramina of the fourth ventricle occurs in the context of a Dandy-Walker malformation. In this condition, agenesis or partial agenesis of the cerebellar vermis is associated with failure of the outlet foramina of the fourth ventricle to open. The brainstem is displaced anteriorly, and the tentorium is pushed upward on the calvaria, displacing the encased torcula (Fig. 215–6).

Another form of outlet foraminal obstruction occurs in the context of the "trapped" fourth ventricle. This condition is almost always a complication of a severe shunt infection. The infection leads not only to occlusion of the outlet foramina but also to occlusion of the aqueduct of Sylvius. The fourth ventricle becomes isolated and distended because CSF is still being produced within it.[37–40] Infants with this condition are already under observation for their supratentorial shunts. They progress slowly and exhibit low overall body tone, poor feeding, drooling, and significantly abnormal coordinated eye movements.[37–40]

TREATMENT OPTIONS AT PRESENTATION

It is often difficult if not impossible to diagnose occlusion of the outlet foramina of the fourth ventricle as the overall cause of hydrocephalus. Findings on MRI suggest that occlusion of these foramina are associated with marked enlargement of the fourth ventricle, moderate enlargement of the lateral ventricles, and

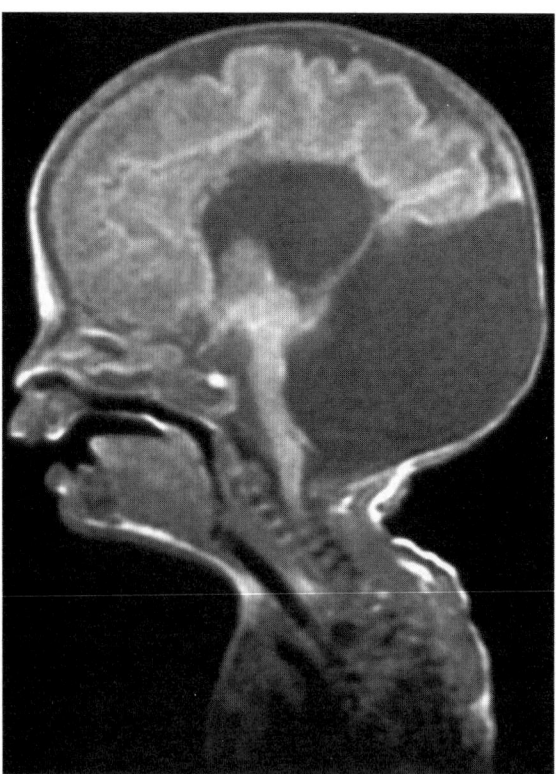

FIGURE 215–6. Magnetic resonance imaging scan of a patient showing the classic radiographic appearance of a Dandy-Walker malformation.

the coexistence of syringomyelia. Based on Dandy's classification, this form of hydrocephalus is noncommunicating, and the decision-making process is similar to that for aqueductal stenosis. Theoretically, it would be ideal to shunt the CSF from the fourth ventricle to prevent the coaptation of the aqueduct from creating an isolated fourth ventricle. In practical terms, however, it is both easier and safer to shunt the lateral ventricles. As long as the aqueduct is open, the symptoms and the size of the fourth ventricle on imaging studies will improve rapidly. In an interesting study, syringomyelia associated with obstruction of the outlet foramina of the fourth ventricle was treated by performing an ETV. Afterward, the syrinx and the hydrocephalus resolved completely.[41]

Both the Dandy-Walker malformation and the pathophysiologically related isolated fourth ventricle fall into the category of multiloculated hydrocephalus.[42, 43] The compelling principle in managing these complicated cases is that the pressure within the various compartments must be balanced, or the same. In the case of the Dandy-Walker malformation, the aqueduct of Sylvius is often open; shunting either the lateral ventricle or the cyst itself may be all that is needed. If, however, the aqueduct is or becomes closed, herniation inferiorly from the posterior fossa or superiorly across the tentorium may occur. Therefore, it is essential to balance the pressure above and below the tentorium.

Before neuroendoscopic techniques were used routinely, I recommended that ventricular catheters be placed above and below the tentorium in the isolated compartments and spliced together proximal to the valve to balance the pressure in each compartment (Fig. 215–7).[42] Alternatively, a stent can be placed in the aqueduct either through an open craniotomy from below or endoscopically through the third ventricle.

PRESENTATION AND OUTCOME AT SHUNT FAILURE

Shunt failure in the context of obstruction of the outlet foramina of the fourth ventricle often leads to insidious signs and symptoms. Headaches are often mild and suboccipital. Snoring, drooling, diplopia, or increased clumsiness may occur. Shunt failure can re-exacerbate syringomyelia, increasing scoliosis[36] or even causing rapidly progressive paraplegia. Imaging studies usually reveal either distention of the isolated fourth ventricle or dilatation of the fourth ventricle associated with distention of the supratentorial ventricular system. The former implies that the ventricular catheter in the fourth ventricle is occluded. When all the ventricles are dilated, either a single shunt has failed or the valve or distal drainage catheter has failed in a complex shunt with two ventricular catheters. At this point, it may be reasonable to attempt to create communication among the various compartments through endoscopic or open surgical approaches. Although rarely leading to a life completely free of shunt-related problems, a posterior fossa craniotomy with stenting of the aqueduct and communication between the encysted fourth ventricle and the CSAS and SSAS may simplify these children's management. Open posterior fossa craniotomy with stenting of the third ventricle into the fourth may open the entire CSF pathway so that it can be managed with lumboperitoneal shunting (W. B. Cherny, K. Manwaring, and H. L. Rekate, unpublished data).

Obstruction between the Spinal and Cortical Subarachnoid Spaces: The Basal Cisterns

After CSF exits from the fourth ventricle, it mixes with CSF in the CSAS in the cisterna magna. A number of pathologic processes can impede this mixing and therefore impede the flow of CSF from the SSAS to the CSAS. Hydrocephalus associated with neonatal intraventricular hemorrhage, aneurysmal subarachnoid hemorrhage, trauma, and bacterial meningitis is caused by marked thickening of the arachnoid at the base of the brain. This form of hydrocephalus makes it critical for neurosurgeons to think beyond the Dandy classification of communicating and noncommunicating hydrocephalus. According to Dandy's classification, this form of hydrocephalus is, by definition, communicating; however, it is also clearly obstructive. This point is important, because this form of hydrocephalus may be amenable to treatment using ETV. When the circulation of CSF is seen as a circuit, the point of obstruction is clearly proximal to the cisterns of the CSAS (especially the interpeduncular cistern), where CSF is deliv-

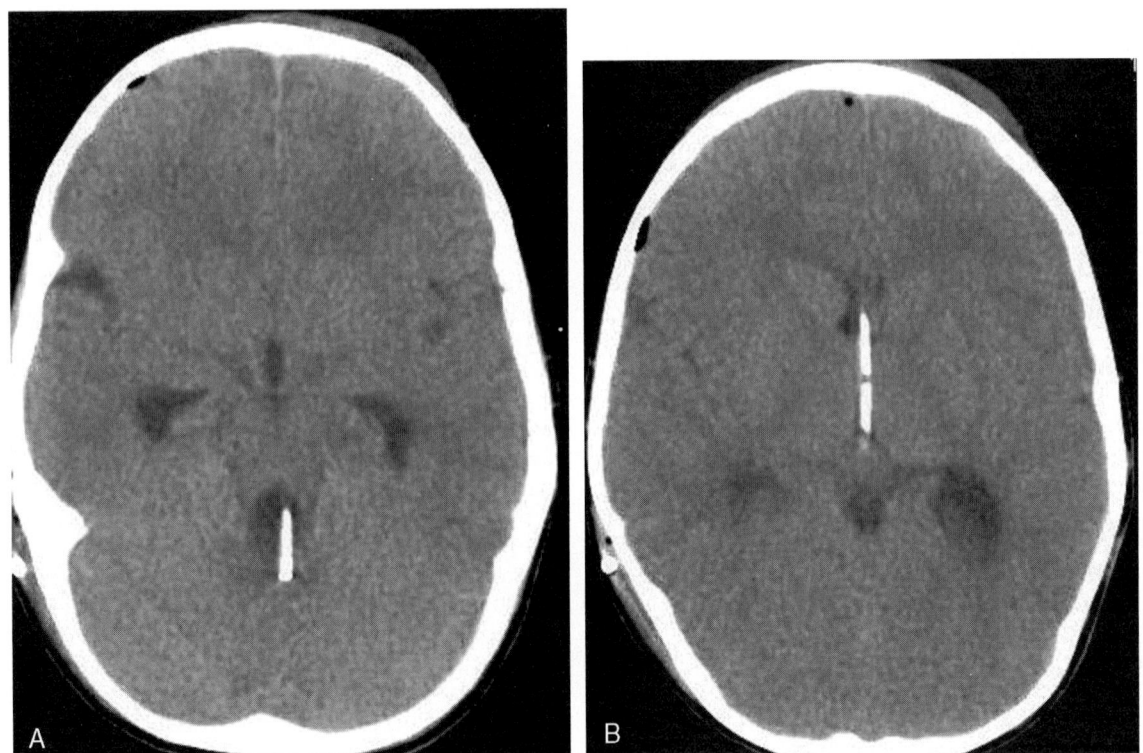

FIGURE 215–7. Computed tomographic scan of a patient with an isolated encysted fourth ventricle managed by placing a stent from the posterior fossa *(A)* into the third ventricle *(B)* via a posterior fossa craniotomy to balance the pressure above and below the tentorium.

ered after the internal bypass created by ETV (Fig. 215–8).

Such an obstruction is never complete; it is only a constriction. Based on a hydraulic analog of Ohm's law, only an increase in ICP is needed to increase the rate of CSF flow across this point of obstruction.[10, 44] Epstein and colleagues[45] exploited this characteristic when they treated this form of hydrocephalus by wrapping an infant's head with an Ace bandage. Such hy-

drocephalus in premature newborns may stabilize or resolve on its own in about 4 weeks, and half the infants do not need a shunt.[46] In a study of the potential for shunt-independent arrest of hydrocephalus, over time, at least half the patients with posthemorrhagic or late postmeningitic hydrocephalus survived safely without shunts.[47]

Failure of CSF flow between the SSAS and CSAS is a characteristic pathophysiologic mechanism of both

FIGURE 215–8. Schematic diagram showing obstruction to the flow of cerebrospinal fluid at the level of the basal cisterns (between the spinal subarachnoid space [SSAS] and the cortical subarachnoid space [CSAS]). (Adapted from Rekate HL: Circuit diagram of the circulation of cerebrospinal fluid. Pediatr Neurosurg 21:248–253, 1994.)

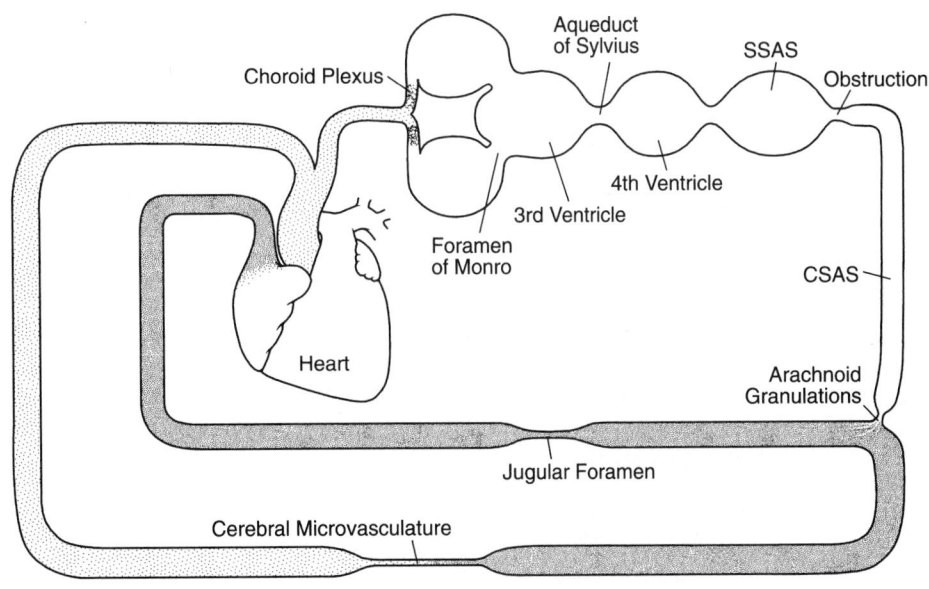

Chiari I and II malformations. Especially in the context of Chiari I malformations, it is often difficult to determine whether the hydrocephalus led to the hindbrain herniation or the hindbrain herniation caused the hydrocephalus. This distinction is crucial, because decompression of the Chiari I malformation may or may not be adequate treatment for hydrocephalus.

From autopsy studies, a commonality among elderly patients who have responded to shunting for NPH is marked thickening of the arachnoid membranes in the area of the basal cisterns.[48, 49] Radioisotope cisternography has been advocated for the diagnosis of NPH. A protein-bound radioactive tracer is injected into the SSAS via lumbar puncture, and multiple scans are obtained over 3 days. In a positive response, which suggests the potential for shunt responsiveness, the dye enters the ventricular system rapidly, but its emptying is greatly delayed. Flow of the tracer is blocked at the region of the basal cisterns, and flow over the convexity is poor despite the large amount of CSF external to the brain.[50–52] This result would be expected in patients with hydrocephalus related to obstruction at the basal cisterns. Therefore, this form of hydrocephalus is the most likely root cause of NPH when combined with the normal softening of the brain associated with aging.[44, 53, 54] We are left with significant concerns about the shunt-independent patients described earlier: Will they later develop NPH?

TREATMENT OPTIONS AT PRESENTATION

For patients with hydrocephalus related to obstruction of CSF flow from the SSAS to the CSAS, many of the management decisions depend on how sick the patient is and why. Many of the conditions that lead to CSF absorptive problems increase the resistance to CSF outflow only transiently. Although it is relatively easy to place a shunt, it may be impossible to remove it, even if the pathologic process that led to its implantation resolves. Even in patients with signs and symptoms of hydrocephalus, it is often to the patient's benefit to delay definitive treatment to determine whether the condition is self-limited. In the case of posthemorrhagic hydrocephalus of the premature newborn, such temporizing can simply mean following the infant with serial ultrasonography, performing lumbar punctures, or placing a ventricular access device for the intermittent withdrawal of CSF.[55–58]

After aneurysmal subarachnoid hemorrhage or severe head injury, it is often impossible to tell whether a patient's condition reflects intervening hydrocephalus or the primary insult to the central nervous system. Placing a shunt is occasionally required so that the patient's treatment can proceed without excessive delay. In such patients, the reason for shunting may be the inability to wean the patient from external ventricular drainage quickly enough.

Multiple options exist for the treatment of these conditions. The most common method is placement of a VP shunt to make certain that everything possible has been done to prevent secondary injury in severely injured individuals. Lumboperitoneal (LP) shunting may be the

ideal method for managing this condition. This form of treatment significantly lowers morbidity and mortality rates compared with VP shunts.[59] It also maintains circulation within the intact ventricular system and therefore is associated with a lower incidence of ventricular coaptation than are VP shunts, resulting in a higher likelihood of later shunt independence.[37, 39, 40] Except in elderly patients being treated for NPH, all adults and children should have a valve incorporated into their shunt systems to prevent overdrainage and possibly hindbrain herniation.[60–62]

Because these patients have "communicating" hydrocephalus, neurosurgeons have considered them inappropriate candidates for ETV or have been reluctant to perform the procedure because of their fragile condition. It is difficult to discern the success rate of ETV for managing this form of communicating hydrocephalus.

Because the obstruction to CSF flow in NPH is at the level of the basal cisterns, patients with this condition theoretically should respond to ETV (F. Epstein, personal communication, 1998). A single series reported the successful treatment of NPH with ETV; three of the four patients in whom it was attempted showed positive responses.[63] NPH can be treated using either VP or LP shunting. The former is associated with significant risks of infection and subdural hematoma but is more reliable over years. Its function is also more easily assessed than is that of LP shunting. In contrast, LP shunting is effective and considerably safer than ventricular shunting but tends to fail early and be difficult to assess. At this time, theoretically, the patient and family should be given options to choose from. If evidence for NPH is compelling, I tend to provide both options to the patient and family but recommend that the patient undergo VP shunting using either a Level 1 Delta Valve (Medtronic–PS Medical, Santa Barbara, CA) or the Hakim Programmable Valve (Codman Corporation, Randolph, MA). In a number of studies, lower valve opening pressures have led to a higher likelihood of clinical success with shunting.[64, 65] In patients whose clinical picture is not as likely to be associated with a positive response to treatment, the less dangerous LP shunt is placed as both treatment and a chronic diagnostic test.

PRESENTATION AND OUTCOME AT SHUNT FAILURE

Patients who have been shunted for hydrocephalus related to obstruction between the SSAS and CSAS often have nonworking shunts at the time of shunt surveillance and are asymptomatic. If this situation occurs, subtle signs of neurological compromise should be sought, and neuropsychological studies should be performed, if indicated. Except for patients with concurrent spina bifida (Chiari II malformation) and the elderly, patients who have communicating hydrocephalus but no symptoms can be considered shunt independent.[47] If patients with this form of hydrocephalus exhibit signs and symptoms consistent with increased ICP, including significant enlargement of the lateral and third ventricles, an attempt should be made to remove the shunt by performing an ETV. When ETV was used to treat slit-ventricle syndrome, more than 80% of the patients achieved shunt independence.[66] In fact, one patient who had undergone almost 50 shunt revisions over a 25-year period did very well after ETV when his shunt was removed.

Agenesis or Occlusion of the Arachnoid Villi

Many neurologists and neurosurgeons assume that hydrocephalus associated with subarachnoid hemorrhage or meningitis is due to occlusion of the arachnoid villi. Usually, such hydrocephalus manifests as an obstruction between the SSAS and CSAS. This distinction is important, because obstruction at the level of the arachnoid villi is an absolute contraindication to ETV—the procedure adds nothing but risk. There is no impediment to CSF flow from the lateral ventricles to the interpeduncular cistern, which would be the terminus of CSF flow after ETV.

The clinical syndrome most associated with failure of the arachnoid villi results from the congenital absence of these structures.[67, 68] This abnormality tends to run in families and is presumably the pathophysiologic substrate for the condition called benign familial megalencephaly. The child's head circumference is either near or above the 98th percentile of the head circumfer-

ence curve and in most circumstances follows that curve (Fig. 215–9). MRI usually shows mildly enlarged ventricles and distended subarachnoid spaces (Fig. 215–10A), leading to use of the descriptive term *external hydrocephalus* to characterize this condition.[69]

A similar condition of external hydrocephalus can result from the traumatic subarachnoid hemorrhage associated with the whiplash shake syndrome. In this situation, the child is born with a normal-sized head. After injury, the head begins to grow too rapidly as blood filtrates through the arachnoid villi. The same situation—mildly increased ventricular size and markedly enlarged subarachnoid spaces—results (see Figs. 215–9 and 215–10B). In this case, the child's head circumference crosses the percentile lines abruptly. From a forensic perspective, if the heads of both parents are of normal size and the child's head growth curve suddenly crosses the percentile lines, nonaccidental trauma should be suspected. In either of its forms, this condition is difficult to diagnose from ultrasound studies, the resolution of which decreases as the area of interest becomes closer to the probe.

Clinically, these babies are likely to have large fontanelles and larger-than-normal heads compared with control babies. In the familial form, the head circumference of one parent is almost always above average. On developmental screening, these children have normal fine motor and personal social assessments but may

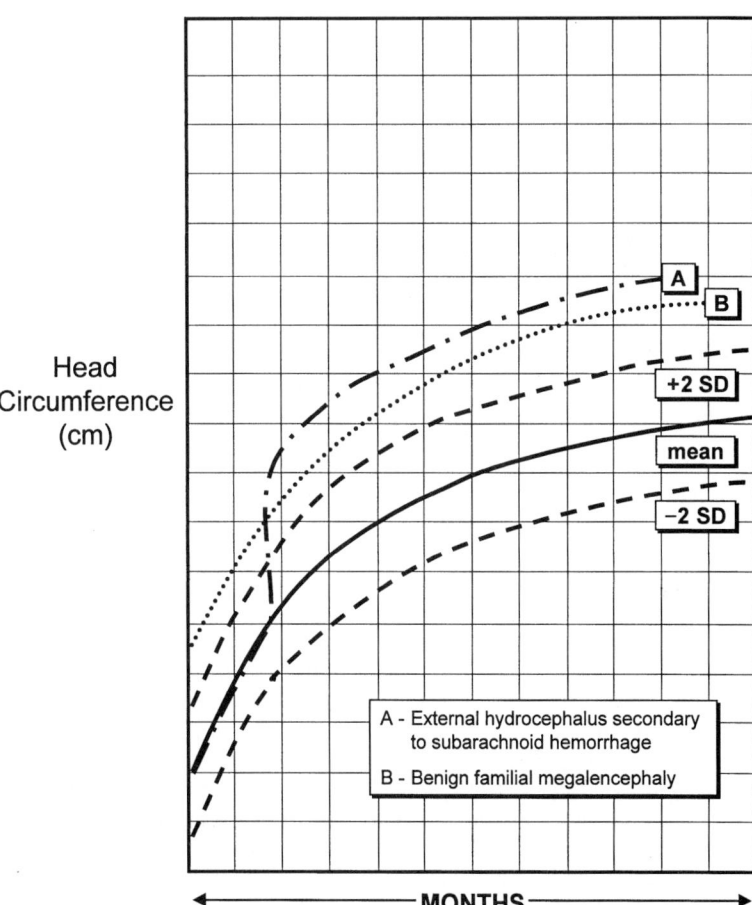

FIGURE 215–9. Head circumference curves in patients with external hydrocephalus in the context of benign familial megalencephaly and in a patient with extracerebral cerebrospinal fluid collections caused by violent shaking. (Courtesy of Barrow Neurological Institute, Phoenix, AZ.)

Head Circumference (cm)

A
B
+2 SD
mean
−2 SD

A - External hydrocephalus secondary to subarachnoid hemorrhage
B - Benign familial megalencephaly

◄——— **MONTHS** ———►

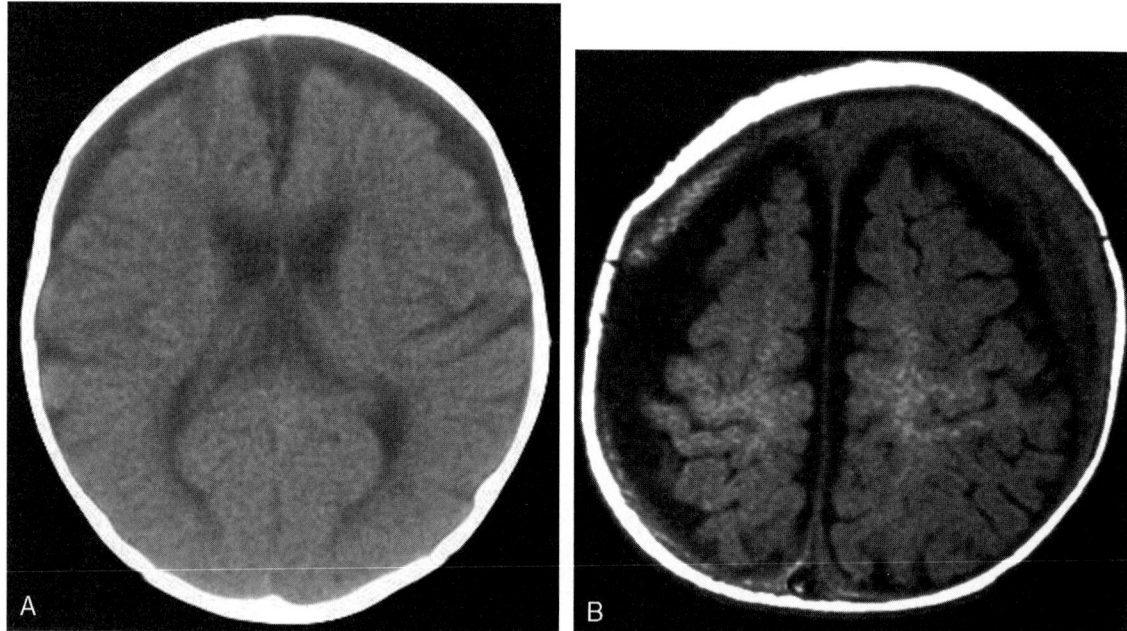

FIGURE 215–10.   *A*, Magnetic resonance imaging (MRI) scan of the brain of a child with typical physical and radiographic familial external hydrocephalus. Note the abnormally distended cerebrospinal fluid spaces anteriorly and the generous ventricles. *B*, MRI scan of the brain of a patient with extracerebral fluid collections associated with acute bleeding. The resolving subdural hematoma suggests that the patient's external hydrocephalus was related to a shaking event.

show significant gross motor delays between age 6 and 18 months, primarily due to the significant enlargement of the head. Almost all these children catch up with their peers and siblings by age 2 years.[69, 70]

TREATMENT OPTIONS AT PRESENTATION

This condition is completely benign. It requires no treatment, with the exception of reassuring the family. Parents are usually most reassured when shown a projection of their child's head circumference compared with that of the parent with the larger head. This common condition leads to two or three referrals to my office each week. Over the last 15 years of practice, I have shunted only one little girl for this condition. The shunt was placed to decrease the overall size of her head, which was becoming noticeably much larger than normal.

PRESENTATION AND OUTCOME AT SHUNT FAILURE

My personal experience with this situation is limited; I have shunted only one individual with obstruction at the level of the arachnoid villi. As far as I can tell, the shunt is working. When the fontanelle finally closes (later than normal) and the sutures close, MRI reveals that the fluid outside the brain has resolved and the size of the ventricles has decreased. Skull growth continues to increase along the same curve seen in infancy (see Fig. 215–9).

Hydrocephalus Due to Increased Sagittal Sinus Pressure

Recently, the role of venous hypertension in the pathogenesis of hydrocephalus has been the subject of intense study.[71–74] Generally, venous hypertension causes and is the universal mechanism of pseudotumor cerebri.[75] Rising venous pressure inhibits the absorption of CSF, because for CSF to be absorbed, ICP must exceed sagittal sinus pressure by 5 to 7 mm Hg.[9, 44, 76] If, however, the fontanelle and sutures are closed, ICP will increase until CSF can be absorbed at a rate sufficient to prevent the enlargement of the ventricles. This condition is pseudotumor cerebri. If the sutures and fontanelles are open, the brain is in communication with atmospheric pressure, and the size of the head increases due to increases in both extracerebral and intraventricular CSF. In the case of craniofacial syndromes such as Crouzon's syndrome, this effect may not become apparent until an opening of the closed sutures allows the ventricles to enlarge.[74] In an elegant study of achondroplastic dwarfs with ventriculomegaly, Steinbok and coworkers[73] demonstrated marked stenosis at the level of the jugular foramen and a pressure differential. Sainte-Rose and colleagues[71] took the idea significantly further, successfully treating hydrocephalus in Crouzon's syndrome with a venous bypass from the transverse sinus to the jugular vein.

For venous hypertension to cause hydrocephalus, it must be severe and present before the fontanelle closes, when the skull still has the ability to distend without dramatically increasing ICP. This effect occurs in achondroplasia and multiple craniofacial syndromes,

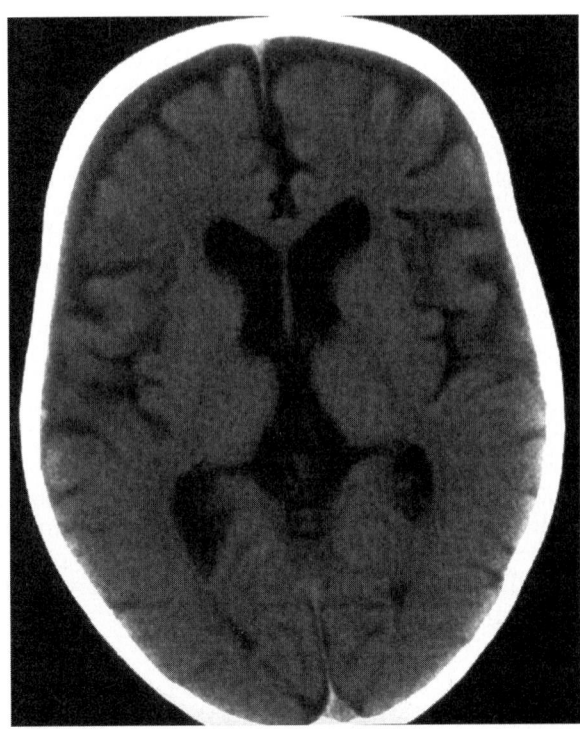

FIGURE 215–11. Magnetic resonance imaging scan of the brain of a child who was developing normally. His head circumference was two standard deviations above the 98th percentile, the result of external hydrocephalus caused by occlusion of the superior vena cava. He remained neurologically and cognitively normal and never received a shunt.

including Crouzon's, Pfeiffer's, and unnamed syndromes involving fibroblast growth factor receptor genes. It is also a complication of venous hypertension related to congenital heart disease, a diaphragmatic hernia, and any form of superior vena cava syndrome (Fig. 215–11). Occasionally, it occurs in premature neonates with chronic invasive lines. This form of hydrocephalus occurs in about 20% of children with hydrocephalus related to spina bifida (H. L. Rekate, unpublished data).

TREATMENT OPTIONS AT PRESENTATION

Except in the contexts of achondroplasia and craniofacial syndromes, venous hypertension is rarely recognized as the cause of hydrocephalus at initial presentation. The child has a full and often bulging fontanelle as well as prominent scalp veins, which can also be associated with other forms of hydrocephalus. It is important to recognize that venous hypertension may be the cause of the hydrocephalus; shunting should be avoided as long as the cortical mantle exceeds 3.5 cm and the child has no overt signs of increased ICP.[77] If venous hypertension is the cause of the hydrocephalus, the outlook for intellectual development with or without a shunt is significantly better than it is with other forms of hydrocephalus. If shunting becomes unavoidable, it is essential to use the highest-resistance valve that the child can tolerate. When this diagnosis is obvious, I recommend using two valves in series, because

the average time to the first proximal failure in the context of achondroplasia is 9 months (H. L. Rekate, unpublished data).

PRESENTATION AND OUTCOME AT SHUNT FAILURE

Usually, this form of hydrocephalus cannot be distinguished from other forms of extraventricular obstructive hydrocephalus, and standard shunt systems are used for the initial management of the condition. These children often (but not always) begin their lives of recurrent shunt failure while still in infancy. They present because of intermittent or permanent obstruction of the proximal shunt. Headache is the universal symptom for either complete occlusion or intermittent obstruction of the ventricular catheter. In infants, this manifests as extreme irritability. The child is described as being not herself or himself. Imaging studies show ventricles that are either normal or smaller than normal. The parents are reassured that the shunt cannot be failing, and the child is either admitted for observation or sent home. The child repeatedly returns for care. Those whose shunts have totally failed become increasingly bradycardic and somnolent. A manometric shunt tap is usually difficult to interpret, because sufficient CSF cannot be obtained to load the manometric column. If the column is loaded, however, artificial CSF often flows freely. Exploration of the shunt system reveals complete occlusion of the ventricular catheter and the presence of small ventricles. The ventricular catheter is removed and replaced with a new, slightly longer catheter down the already established track. Because the ventricles are so small, it may be difficult to replace the shunt in another position.

Occlusion of the ventricular catheter is a sign of shunt overdrainage and implicates the valve in the process of the failure. When a ventricular catheter is replaced, the valve should be replaced as well. A high-resistance or high-pressure valve with a device to retard siphoning should be used in an attempt to prevent this complication in the future. A growing number of these valves, designed to prevent the extreme negativity that usually occurs in patients with standard differential pressure valves, are becoming available.[78, 79]

The occlusion of the ventricular catheter is often temporary. After blockage, the ventricle begins to distend imperceptibly, finally allowing CSF to egress again through one of the holes in the ventricular catheter. This situation is frustrating for the patient and family, because the headache eventually subsides, giving credence to the false diagnosis of a working shunt when the imaged ventricles are small. When monitored, ICP has been as high as 60 mm Hg in these children. During a discussion of headaches and shunts at a recent convention of the Hydrocephalus Association, 400 participants were polled about whether their ventricles had expanded at the time of shunt failure. In 20%, their ventricles had not expanded at shunt failure. All had been sent from emergency rooms and neurosurgeons' offices reassured that their shunts were working, only to find later that their shunts had failed and their ventricles could not expand. The condition described here has many names, including that bestowed at its first recognition, normal-volume hydrocephalus.[1] It has also been called stiff slit-ventricle syndrome, severe slit-ventricle syndrome, and shunt-related pseudotumor.[79]

What causes this condition, and how should it be treated? Regardless of whether it can be detected when hydrocephalus is originally treated, pseudotumor cerebri results from the high venous pressure that caused the hydrocephalus in the first place. The nonresponsive ventricles are thought to reflect the chronic changes in the brain associated with chronic shunting. After treatment with a ventricular shunt, the ventricles rapidly shrink, the fontanelles and sutures close, and pressure in the superior sagittal sinuses remains very high (Fig. 215–12). Hydrocephalus has now been converted to pseudotumor cerebri.

Unless the opening pressure of the valve exceeds the pressure in the sagittal sinus, all CSF must drain through the valve system. The opening pressure of the valvular mechanism in the arachnoid villi will not be exceeded, and CSF must flow in a retrograde fashion through the CSF pathways through the shunt. As the ventricles shrink, the retrograde pathway becomes increasingly difficult to access. Drainage of a lateral ventricle may lead to partial obstruction of the foramen of Monro, because the distorted septum pellucidum rests on the head of the caudate nucleus (Fig. 215–13). The CSF in the CSAS cannot be absorbed into the superior sagittal sinuses, and it cannot pass out through the shunt.[15] The volume of the CSAS increases, exerting an inward pressure on the brain, which tends to cause the brain to collapse around the ventricular catheter.

Strategies that prevent the brain's collapse around the ventricular catheter require the ability to drain the CSF through the shunt. If the strategy involves manipulation of a ventricular shunt, the opening pressure and resistance in the valve mechanism must be as high as the patient can tolerate. For the most part, this means using more than one valve mechanism in series, both with very high pressure settings, and a device to retard siphoning.[79] If this strategy fails, it probably means that the superior sagittal sinus pressure is too high for the valve strategies to work. Both the CSAS and the ventricle must then be accessed. T2-weighted images typically show a significant amount of CSF in the frontal CSAS. It is often possible to place a ventricular catheter in the frontal CSAS to relieve the problem. If neither strategy is successful, the condition must be treated with a shunt from the cisterna magna[80] or with an LP shunt with high-resistance valves to prevent the potential problem of hindbrain herniation.

COMPLICATIONS

A thorough description of the potential mechanical and infectious complications associated with shunts is beyond the scope of this chapter. Complications specific to different pathophysiologies were discussed previously. This section concentrates on general problems that patients with shunts confront. Hard data on the

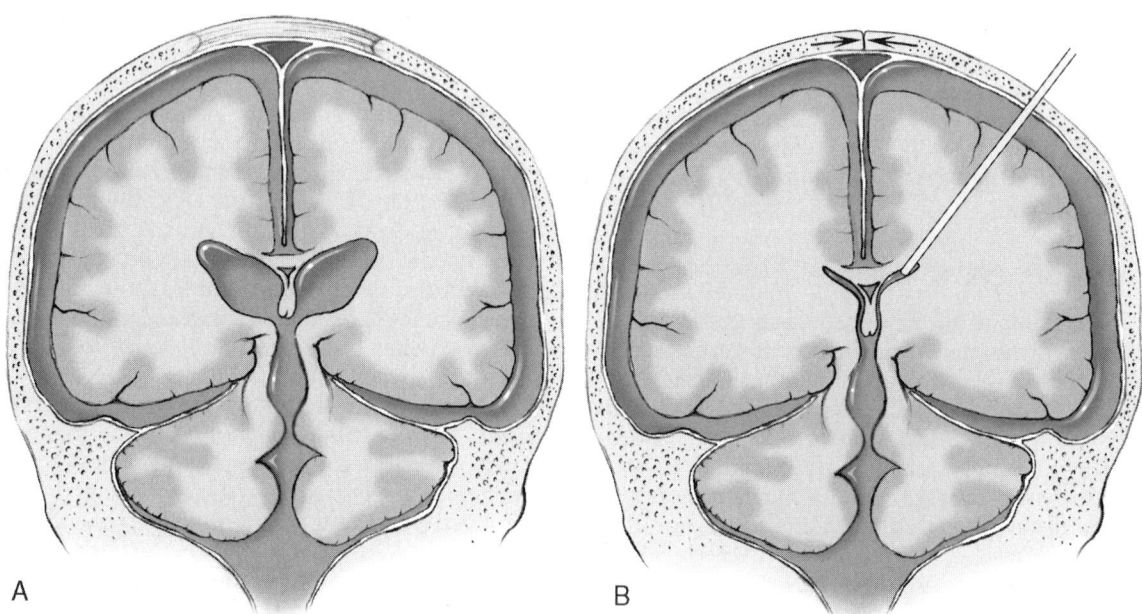

A   B

FIGURE 215–12. Schematic diagram showing what happens when patients with pseudotumor-like syndromes receive ventricular shunts. *A,* An increase in cerebrospinal fluid in both the ventricles and especially the cortical subarachnoid space is demonstrated. The ventricles quickly collapse around the ventricular catheter. Because of the high sagittal sinus pressure, the cerebrospinal fluid in the cortical subarachnoid space cannot escape from the intracranial compartment, except retrogradely through the ventricular catheter. *B,* Permanent or intermittent proximal shunt obstruction without enlargement of the ventricles results. (Courtesy of Barrow Neurological Institute, Phoenix, AZ.)

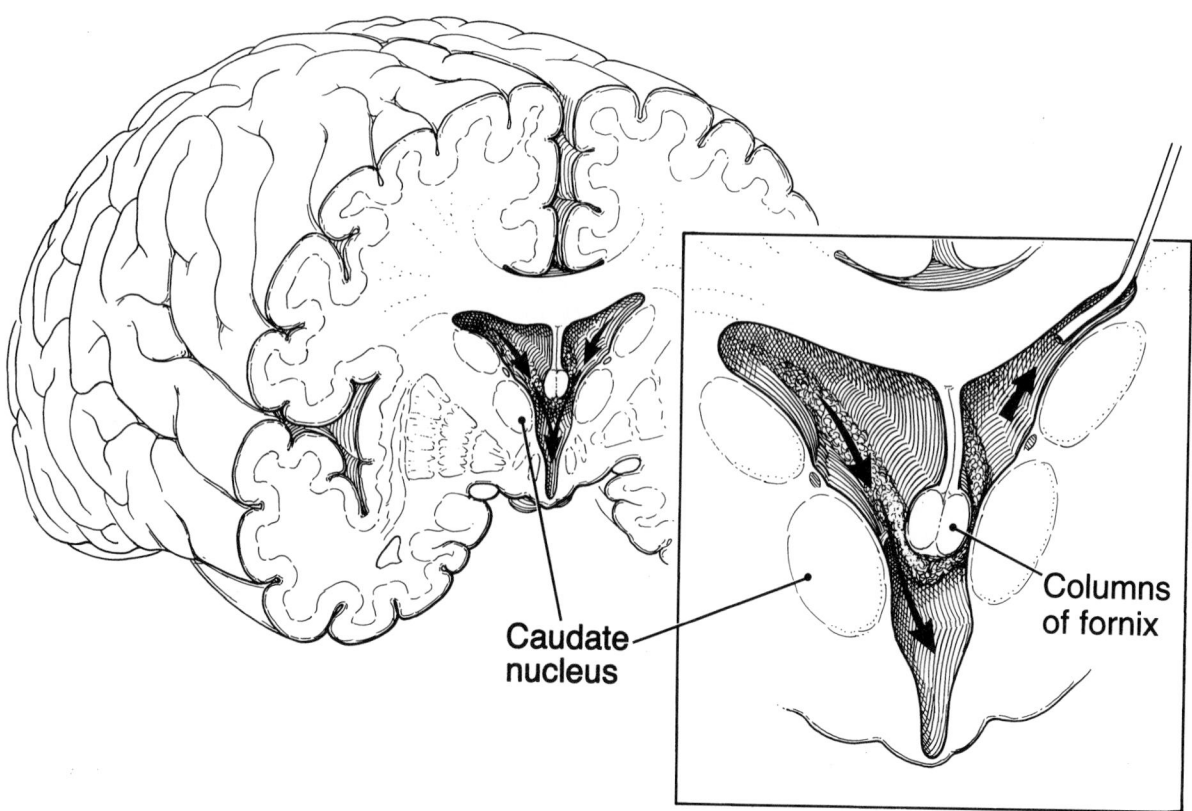

FIGURE 215–13. Schematic diagram of the cause of asymmetrical ventricles after successful shunt surgery. With successful drainage from the lateral ventricles, the ventricles shrink, and the septum pellucidum rests on the head of the ipsilateral caudate nucleus. Consequently, the cerebrospinal fluid from the other compartments is unable to drain out through the shunt. (Courtesy of Barrow Neurological Institute, Phoenix, AZ.)

rates of shunt failure and complications are difficult to obtain. A multicenter study of first shunt implantation in children found that an 8% infection rate was associated with placement of the first shunt. Among children with newly implanted shunts, 40% of shunts failed in the first year, and 50% failed by the end of the second year.[81] Most of these patients were infants; data related to shunts placed later in life may not be the same. This careful study also showed that the complication rates were the same regardless of the center and regardless of the shunt system used. Patients with shunts are likely to need shunt revisions as they age.

How long do patients with shunts survive? Do they live as long as patients without shunts? Theoretically, they may live into old age. The first successful valve-regulated shunts were reported in the early 1950s. Therefore, the oldest patients shunted in infancy are now middle-aged. For infantile hydrocephalus, the mortality rate associated with shunt dependency is thought to be 1% per year, or a 20% mortality rate before adulthood is reached.[82] This frightening statistic is not spread across all diagnoses equally. Patients with spina bifida (Chiari II malformation) are at high risk owing to the potential for respiratory compromise. Shunt-dependent patients who do not have spina bifida and are otherwise doing well may die or suffer permanent neurological deterioration because they are unable to access medical care in time to intervene when their shunts fail.[83] Shunt-dependent individuals must be aware that their shunts might fail at any time. Such individuals must seek care for severe headaches if their symptoms might be related to shunt failure.

Perhaps the most common complication associated with shunt dependency is the so-called slit-ventricle syndrome. This name is applied generically to patients who have small ventricles on imaging studies and chronic headaches. When asked, at least four of five adolescents and adults with shunts complain of chronic headache. These headaches reflect a variety of historical differences and causes. Not all such patients need surgical intervention. My personal threshold for suggesting intervention is when headaches interfere with the patient's ability to enjoy life in a significant way (e.g., leaving school or going to the nurse's station two to four times a month). Intervention usually begins with a valve upgrade to a system that contains a device to retard siphoning. This intervention resolves the symptoms in at least 80% of these patients, who represent only 15% of the total population of shunted patients.[79] The remaining patients often require a large number of shunt revisions, which interrupt their general functioning.

In one study, patients who failed simple valve upgrades were subjected to chronic ICP monitoring, which revealed four different variants of severe headache disorders.[79] The headaches were caused by severe intracranial hypotension, intermittent proximal shunt obstruction, or severe intracranial hypertension without ventricular distention, with or without a working shunt. Some patients also had severe migraines independent of ICP. These data and the finding that shunts can be removed in a significant number of chronically shunted individuals with or without ETV[66] led to an overall algorithm for the management of intractable headaches in patients with shunts (Fig. 215–14). For one reason or another, all patients whose ventricles

did not expand had venous hypertension. Injection of iohexol showed free CSF communication in 24 of the 27 patients. The three patients whose CSF did not communicate freely between the ventricles and the interpeduncular cistern had had severe ventriculitis that complicated the treatment of their hydrocephalus. The 24 patients were treated with a number of strategies, but most underwent placement of a valve-regulated LP shunt. Patients whose ventricles did enlarge were subjected to third ventriculostomy, resulting in the ability to remove the shunts permanently in at least two thirds.[66]

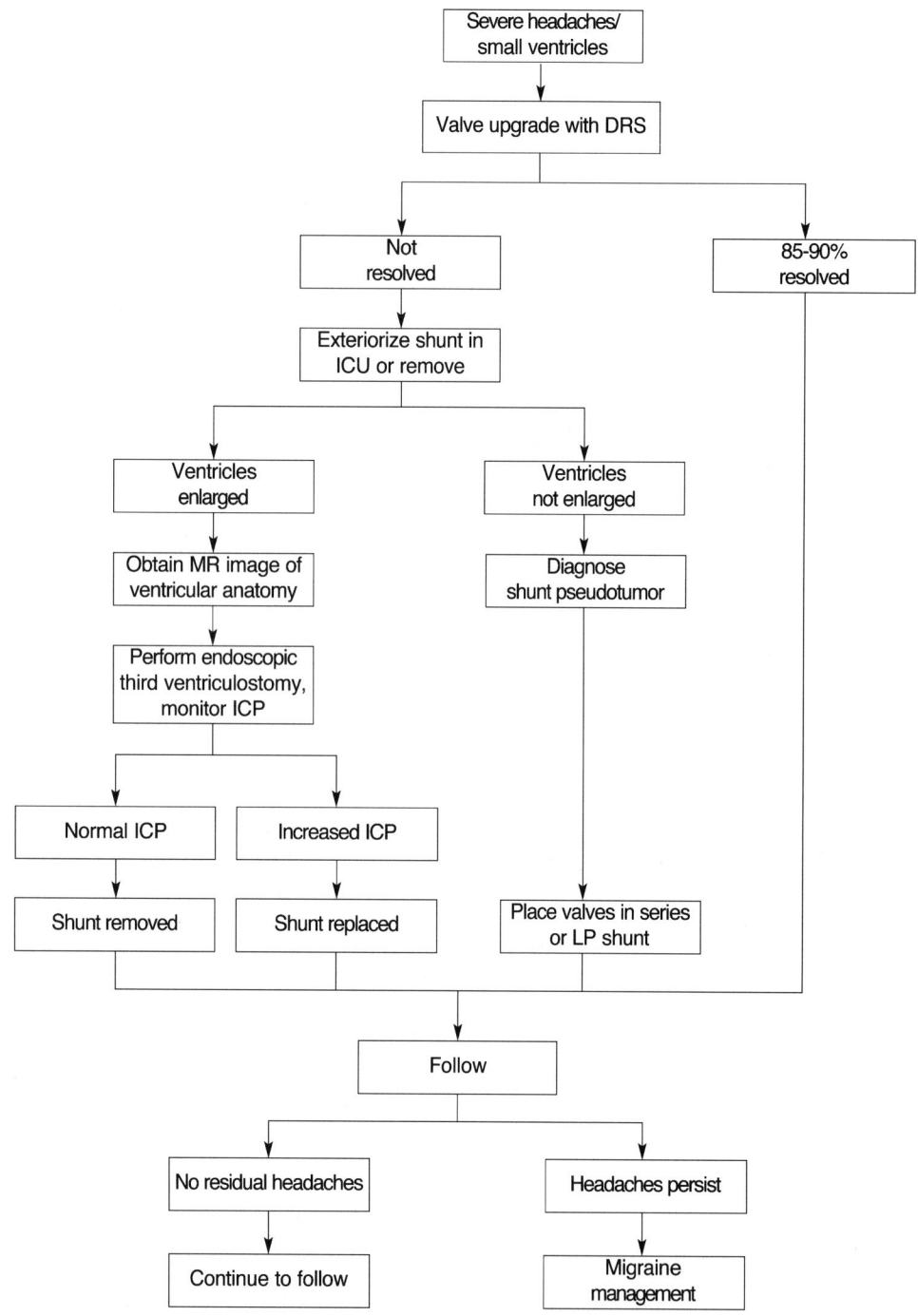

FIGURE 215–14. Algorithm for the management of headaches in children and adults with long-standing shunts. DRS, device to retard siphoning; ICP, intracranial pressure; ICU, intensive care unit; LP, lumboperitoneal; MR, magnetic resonance. (Courtesy of Barrow Neurological Institute, Phoenix, AZ.)

CONCLUSION

Hydrocephalus is not a single entity but results from many different pathophysiologies, all of which obstruct CSF flow and increase the size of the ventricular system proximal to the point of obstruction. To understand and intelligently manage individuals with hydrocephalus, physicians must evaluate each patient as an individual and plan interventions specific to his or her problems.

ACKNOWLEDGMENTS

The view that hydrocephalus results from a point of obstruction to CSF flow evolved from a long-term collaboration with Professors Wen Ko and Howard Chizeck in the School of Engineering at Case Western Reserve University in Cleveland, Ohio. This work was supported by a grant from the National Institutes of Health (R01-NS22901).

REFERENCES

1. Engel M, Carmel PW, Chutorian AM: Increased intraventricular pressure without ventriculomegaly in children with shunts: "Normal volume" hydrocephalus. Neurosurgery 5:549–552, 1979.
2. Volpe JJ: Intraventricular hemorrhage in the premature infant—current concepts. Part II. Ann Neurol 25:109–116, 1989.
3. Laurence KM, Coates S: The natural history of hydrocephalus: Detailed analysis of 182 unoperated cases. Arch Dis Child 37:345–362, 1962.
4. Dandy WE, Blackfan KD: An experimental and clinical study of internal hydrocephalus. JAMA 61:2216–2217, 1913.
5. Dandy WE, Blackfan KD: Internal hydrocephalus: An experimental, clinical and pathological study. Am J Dis Child 8:406–482, 1914.
6. Bering EA Jr: Circulation of the cerebrospinal fluid: Demonstration of the choroid plexuses as the generator of the force for flow of fluid and ventricular enlargement. J Neurosurg 19:405–413, 1962.
7. Milhorat TH: Failure of choroid plexectomy as treatment for hydrocephalus. Surg Gynecol Obstet 139:505–508, 1974.
8. Milhorat TH, Hammock MK, Fenstermacher JD, et al: Cerebrospinal fluid production by the choroid plexus and brain. Science 173:330–332, 1971.
9. Olivero WC, Rekate HL, Chizeck HJ, et al: Relationship between intracranial and sagittal sinus pressure in normal and hydrocephalic dogs. Pediatr Neurosci 14:196–201, 1988.
10. Rekate HL: Circuit diagram of the circulation of cerebrospinal fluid. Pediatr Neurosurg 21:248–252, 1994.
11. Ransohoff J, Shulman K, Fishman RA: Hydrocephalus: A review of etiology and treatment. J Pediatr 56:399–411, 1960.
12. Cutler RW, Page L, Galicich J, et al: Formation and absorption of cerebrospinal fluid in man. Brain 91:707–720, 1968.
13. Castro ME, Portnoy HD, Maesaka J: Elevated cortical venous pressure in hydrocephalus. Neurosurgery 29:232–238, 1991.
14. Portnoy HD, Branch C, Castro ME: The relationship of intracranial venous pressure to hydrocephalus. Childs Nerv Syst 10:29–35, 1994.
15. Rekate HL, Williams FC Jr, Brodkey JA, et al: Resistance of the foramen of Monro. Pediatr Neurosci 14:85–89, 1988.
16. Rekate HL, McCormick JM: Failure to demonstrate a brain transmissibility factor. In Marlin AE (ed): Concepts in Pediatric Neurosurgery. Zurich, Karger, 1990, pp 235–242.
17. Rekate HL: Brain turgor (Kb): Intrinsic property of the brain to resist distortion. Pediatr Neurosurg 18:257–262, 1992.
18. Rekate HL: Cerebrospinal fluid circulation. In Guthkelch CN (ed): Scientific Foundations of Neurology. Cambridge, Mass, Blackwell Scientific, 1996, pp 323–336.
19. Rekate HL: Neurosurgical management of the newborn with spina bifida. In Rekate HL (ed): Comprehensive Management of Spina Bifida. Boca Raton, Fla, CRC, 1991, pp 1–26.
20. Nugent GR, Al-Mefty O, Chou S: Communicating hydrocephalus as a cause of aqueductal stenosis. J Neurosurg 51:812–818, 1979.
21. McCullough DC, Balzer-Martin LA: Current prognosis in overt neonatal hydrocephalus. J Neurosurg 57:378–383, 1982.
22. Mealey JJ, Gilmor RL, Bubb MP: The prognosis of hydrocephalus overt at birth. J Neurosurg 39:348–355, 1973.
23. Young HF, Nulsen FE, Weiss MH, et al: The relationship of intelligence and cerebral mantle in treated infantile hydrocephalus (IQ potential in hydrocephalic children). Pediatrics 52:38–44, 1973.
24. Rosseau GL, McCullough DC, Joseph AL: Current prognosis in fetal ventriculomegaly. J Neurosurg 77:551–555, 1992.
25. Clewell WH, Johnson ML, Meier PR, et al: A surgical approach to the treatment of fetal hydrocephalus. N Engl J Med 306:1320–1325, 1982.
26. Clewell WH: Intra-uterine shunting procedures. Br J Hosp Med 34:149–153, 1985.
27. Ammar A, Al-Jama F, Rahman S, et al: Prolonged intrauterine transabdominal ventricular external drainage: A method to decompress dilated fetal ventricles. Minim Invasive Neurosurg 39:1–3, 1996.
28. Tulipan N, Bruner JP: Fetal surgery for spina bifida [letter; comment]. Lancet 353:406, 1999.
29. Sutton LN, Adzick NS, Bilaniuk LT, et al: Improvement in hindbrain herniation demonstrated by serial fetal magnetic resonance imaging following fetal surgery for myelomeningocele. JAMA 282:1826–1831, 1999; see comments.
30. Bruner JP, Tulipan N, Paschall RL, et al: Fetal surgery for myelomeningocele and the incidence of shunt-dependent hydrocephalus. JAMA 282:1819–1825, 1999.
31. Adzick NS, Sutton LN, Crombleholme TM, et al: Successful fetal surgery for spina bifida [letter]. Lancet 352:1675–1676, 1998; see comments.
32. D'Ercole C, Girard N, Boubli L, et al: Prenatal diagnosis of fetal cerebral abnormalities by ultrasonography and magnetic resonance imaging. Eur J Obstet Gynecol Reprod Biol 50:177–184, 1993.
33. Girard N, Raybaud C, Dercole C, et al: In vivo MRI of the fetal brain. Neuroradiology 35:431–436, 1993.
34. Buxton N, Macarthur D, Mallucci C, et al: Neuroendoscopic third ventriculostomy in patients less than 1 year old. Pediatr Neurosurg 29:73–76, 1998.
35. Teo C, Rahman S, Boop FA, et al: Complications of endoscopic neurosurgery. Childs Nerv Syst 12:248–253, 1996.
36. Hall P, Lindseth R, Campbell R, et al: Scoliosis and hydrocephalus in myelocele patients: The effects of ventricular shunting. J Neurosurg 50:174–178, 1979.
37. Hawkins JC, Hoffman HJ, Humphreys RP: Isolated fourth ventricle as a complication of ventricular shunting: Report of three cases. J Neurosurg 49:910–913, 1978.
38. Foltz EL, Shurtleff DB: Conversion of communicating hydrocephalus to stenosis or occlusion of the aqueduct during ventricular shunt. J Neurosurg 24:520–529, 1966.
39. Foltz EL, DeFeo DR: Double compartment hydrocephalus—a new clinical entity. Neurosurgery 7:551–559, 1980.
40. Lourie H, Shende MC, Krawchenko J, et al: Trapped fourth ventricle: A report of two unusual cases. Neurosurgery 7:279–282, 1980.
41. Nishihara T, Hara T, Suzuki I, et al: Third ventriculostomy for symptomatic syringomyelia using flexible endoscope: Case report. Minim Invasive Neurosurg 39:130–132, 1996.
42. Rekate HL: Treatment of hydrocephalus. In Cheek W (ed): Pediatric Neurosurgery: Surgery of the Developing Nervous System. Philadelphia, WB Saunders, 1994, pp 362–377.
43. Rekate H: Multiloculated compartments of cerebrospinal fluid: Pathophysiology and management. Crit Rev Neurosurg 1:309–318, 1991.
44. Rekate HL, Brodkey JA, Chizeck HJ, et al: Ventricular volume regulation: A mathematical model and computer simulation. Pediatr Neurosci 14:77–84, 1988.
45. Epstein F, Hochwald GM, Ransohoff J: Neonatal hydrocephalus treated by compressive head wrapping. Lancet 1:634–636, 1973.
46. Tarby TJ, Volpe JJ: Intraventricular hemorrhage in the premature infant. Pediatr Clin North Am 29:1077–1104, 1982.

47. Rekate H, Nulsen FE, Mack H, et al: Establishing the diagnosis of shunt independence. Monogr Neural Sci 8:223–226, 1982.

48. Di Rocco C, Di Trapani G, Maira G, et al: Anatomo-clinical correlations in normotensive hydrocephalus: Reports on three cases. J Neurol Sci 33:437–452, 1977.

49. Jellinger K: Neuropathological aspects of dementias resulting from abnormal blood and cerebrospinal fluid dynamics. Acta Neurol Belg 76:83–102, 1976.

50. Wolinsky JS, Barnes BD, Margolis MT: Diagnostic tests in normal pressure hydrocephalus. Neurology 23:706–713, 1973.

51. Adapon BD, Braunstein P, Lin JP, et al: Radiologic investigations of normal pressure hydrocephalus. Radiol Clin North Am 12:353–369, 1974.

52. Black PM: Normal-pressure hydrocephalus: Current understanding of diagnostic tests and shunting. Postgrad Med 71:57–67, 1982.

53. Chimowitz MI, Estes ML, Furlan AJ, et al: Further observations on the pathology of subcortical lesions identified on magnetic resonance imaging. Arch Neurol 49:747–752, 1992.

54. Awad IA, Johnson PC, Spetzler RF, et al: Incidental subcortical lesions identified on magnetic resonance imaging in the elderly. II. Postmortem pathological correlations. Stroke 17:1090–1097, 1986.

55. Kreusser KL, Tarby TJ, Kovnar E, et al: Serial lumbar punctures for at least temporary amelioration of neonatal posthemorrhagic hydrocephalus. Pediatrics 75:719–724, 1985.

56. Manwaring K, Pittman HW, Tarby TJ: New techniques in the investigation and management of post-hemorrhagic hydrocephalus. BNI Q 1:24–28, 1985.

57. McComb JG, Ramos AD, Platzker AC, et al: Management of hydrocephalus secondary to intraventricular hemorrhage in the preterm infant with a subcutaneous ventricular catheter reservoir. Neurosurgery 13:295–300, 1983.

58. Marlin AE: Protection of the cortical mantle in premature infants with posthemorrhagic hydrocephalus. Neurosurgery 7:464–468, 1980.

59. Selman WR, Spetzler RF, Wilson CB, et al: Percutaneous lumboperitoneal shunt: Review of 130 cases. Neurosurgery 6:255–257, 1980.

60. Chumas PD, Drake JM, Del Bigio MR: Death from chronic tonsillar herniation in a patient with lumboperitoneal shunt and Crouzon's disease. Br J Neurosurg 6:595–599, 1992.

61. Chumas PD, Kulkarni AV, Drake JM, et al: Lumboperitoneal shunting: A retrospective study in the pediatric population. Neurosurgery 32:376–383, 1993.

62. Chumas PD, Armstrong DC, Drake JM, et al: Tonsillar herniation: The rule rather than the exception after lumboperitoneal shunting in the pediatric population. J Neurosurg 78:568–573, 1993.

63. Mitchell P, Mathew B: Third ventriculostomy in normal pressure hydrocephalus. Br J Neurosurg 13:382–385, 1999.

64. Black PM, Ojemann RG, Tzouras A: CSF shunts for dementia, incontinence, and gait disturbance. Clin Neurosurg 32:632–651, 1985.

65. Boon AJ, Tans JT, Delwel EJ, et al: Dutch normal-pressure hydrocephalus study: Randomized comparison of low- and medium-pressure shunts. J Neurosurg 88:490–495, 1998.

66. Baskin JJ, Manwaring KH, Rekate HL: Ventricular shunt removal: The ultimate treatment of the slit ventricle syndrome. J Neurosurg 88:478–484, 1998.

67. Gilles FH, Davidson RI: Communicating hydrocephalus associated with deficient dysplastic parasagittal arachnoidal granulations. J Neurosurg 35:421–426, 1971.

68. Gutierrez Y, Friede RI, Kaliney WJ: Agenesis of arachnoid granulations and its relationship to communicating hydrocephalus. J Neurosurg 43:553–558, 1975.

69. Rekate H: External hydrocephalus. Crit Rev Neurosurg 3:372–378, 1999.

70. Andersson H, Elfverson J, Svendsen P: External hydrocephalus in infants. Childs Brain 11:398–402, 1984.

71. Sainte-Rose C, LaCombe J, Pierre-Kahn A, et al: Intracranial venous sinus hypertension: Cause or consequence of hydrocephalus in infants? J Neurosurg 60:727–736, 1984.

72. Pierre-Kahn A, Hirsch JF, Renier D, et al: Hydrocephalus and achondroplasia: A study of 25 observations. Childs Brain 7:205–219, 1980.

73. Steinbok P, Hall J, Flodmark O: Hydrocephalus in achondroplasia: The possible role of intracranial venous hypertension. J Neurosurg 71:42–48, 1989.

74. Rekate H: Hydrocephalus and chronic tonsillar herniation in patients with Crouzon's syndrome. BNI Q 8:29–34, 1992.

75. Karahalios DG, Rekate HL, Khayata MH, et al: Elevated intracranial venous pressure as a universal mechanism in pseudotumor cerebri of varying etiologies. Neurology 46:198–202, 1996.

76. Shulman K, Ransohoff J: Sagittal sinus venous pressure in hydrocephalus. J Neurosurg 23:169–173, 1965.

77. Rekate HL: To shunt or not to shunt: Hydrocephalus and dysraphism. Clin Neurosurg 32:593–607, 1985.

78. Rekate HL, Fleming D, Leung A, et al: Chronic monitoring of intraventricular pressure in children using telemetry: Engineering and physiologic aspects. In Ishii S, Nagal H, Brock M (eds): Intracranial Pressure V. Berlin, Springer-Verlag, 1983, pp 127–130.

79. Rekate HL: Classification of slit-ventricle syndromes using intracranial pressure monitoring. Pediatr Neurosurg 19:15–20, 1993.

80. Johnston IH, Sheridan MM: CSF shunting from the cisterna magna: A report of 16 cases. Br J Neurosurg 7:39–43, 1993.

81. Drake JM, Kestle JR, Milner R, et al: Randomized trial of cerebrospinal fluid shunt valve design in pediatric hydrocephalus. Neurosurgery 43:294–303, 1998.

82. Iskandar BJ, Tubbs S, Mapstone TB, et al: Death in shunted hydrocephalic children in the 1990s. Pediatr Neurosurg 28:173–176, 1998.

83. Sgouros S, Mallucci C, Walsh AR, et al: Long-term complications of hydrocephalus. Pediatr Neurosurg 23:127–132, 1995.

CHAPTER 216

Infantile Posthemorrhagic Hydrocephalus

MARK LUCIANO ■ JOGI V. PATTISAPU ■ AGADHA WICKREMESEKERA

Congenital anomaly is the most common cause of hydrocephalus in infants born at full term. For infants born prematurely, 90% of hydrocephalus is acquired, resulting from a germinal matrix–intraventricular hemorrhage (GM-IVH).[1] Infantile posthemorrhagic hydrocephalus (IPHH) can be defined as perinatal ventricular distention in the premature infant after GM-IVH, in which the intraventricular hemorrhage impairs cerebrospinal fluid (CSF) flow.

Historically, IPHH was an ominous diagnosis because treatment was difficult, and the outcome was associated with a high occurrence of neurodevelopmental disability.[2] Because of advances in neonatal care over the past 20 years, more infants now survive and develop normally.[3] Although controversial, aggressive intervention in preterm infants has been an acceptable course of action since the 1970s, increasing the number of IPHH cases.[4] At most institutions, the pediatric neurosurgeon is called on to assist in the treatment of these preterm infants, hoping to improve their neurodevelopmental outcome.

In this chapter, we discuss the epidemiology, pathophysiology, diagnostic evaluation, clinical course, treatment, and the outcomes in patients with IPHH. Because this condition is associated with prematurity, the following discussion excludes full-term and post-term infants with hydrocephalus after IVH. Because IPHH is acquired and progresses in a hospital setting, understanding its pathophysiology is essential to assist neonatal colleagues and determine the limitations of effective treatment.

EPIDEMIOLOGY

The incidence of IPHH depends on the occurrence and survival of the premature infant and the frequency of GM-IVH in the premature population. Premature infants are defined as those born before 37 weeks' gestation and can be further subdivided by gestational age or birth weight, or both (Table 216–1). In recent years, improved survival of these extremely premature infants has led to an increased occurrence of GM-IVH.

Approximately 50,000 infants weighing less than 1500 g are born each year in the United States. Because of advances in neonatal care, approximately 85% of these infants survive the neonatal period. As a result of preventative measures, the rate of GM-IVH among the premature decreased from 40% to 44% (1970) to 20% (1987).[5] In low-birth-weight infants, the rate of GM-IVH declined from 11.5% (1986) to 5.5% (1995), and the mortality decreased by 30%.[6]

Over the past decade, the number of preterm infants has increased and infant mortality has decreased, and more neonates are surviving the neonatal period. In contrast, the incidence of GM-IVH has declined, leading to a reduction in the percentage of infants that develop IPHH.

PATHOPHYSIOLOGY

The initial event leading to IPPH is hemorrhage into the subependymal germinal matrix (GM) from immature vasculature. In approximately 80% of cases, GM hemorrhage spreads into the ventricular system. Central nervous system (CNS) damage results from IVH and sequelae related to the hemorrhage, and some of these injuries may not improve with CSF drainage.

Germinal Matrix Embryology

The GM is the subventricular zone where active glial proliferation occurs during cerebral hemisphere development. During the last 12 weeks of gestation, the GM is highly cellular, richly vascularized, and gelatinous.

TABLE 216–1 ■ **Subgroups of Premature Infants**

PRETERM GROUP	GESTATIONAL AGE	WEIGHT GROUP	BIRTH WEIGHT
Moderately	<37–32 wk	Low	<2500–1500 g
Very	<32–28 wk	Very low	<1500–700 g
Extremely	<28 wk	Ultra low	<700 g

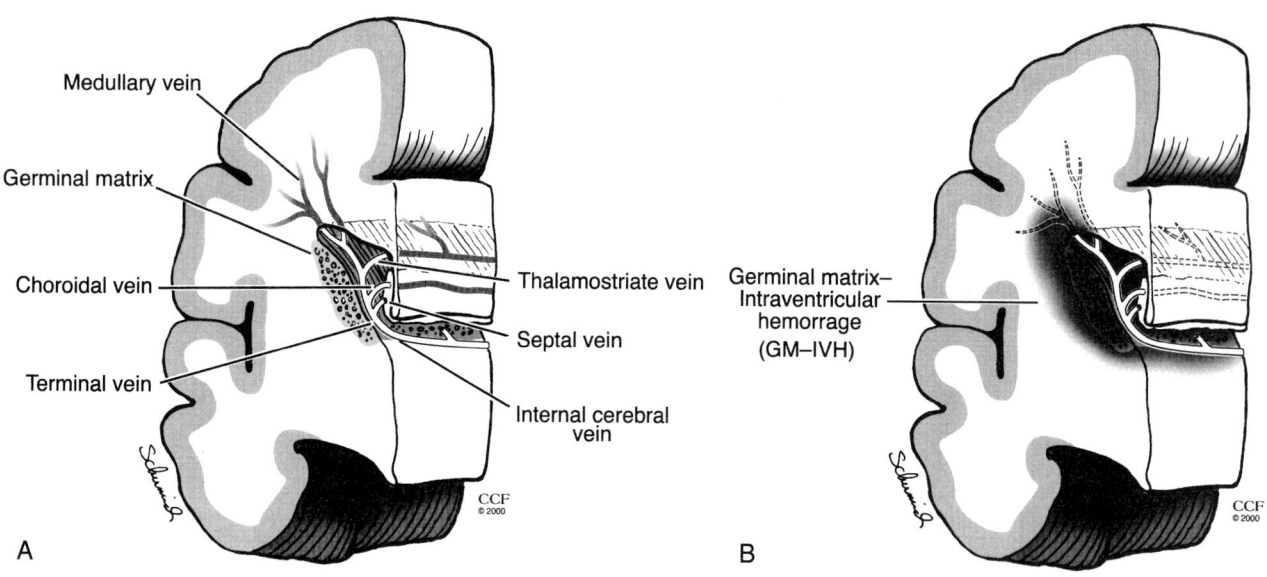

FIGURE 216–1. *A,* Germinal matrix. *B,* Germinal matrix hemorrhage.

It is nourished by a capillary bed, receiving blood supply from the anterior cerebral artery (i.e., Heubner's artery), the middle cerebral artery (i.e., lateral striate arteries), and the anterior choroidal artery.[7] The capillary bed is composed of large, endothelium-lined channels, which, along with medullary, choroidal, and thalamostriate veins, drains into the terminal vein. This vessel subsequently drains into the vein of Galen through the internal cerebral veins (Fig. 216–1A). In the seventh month, there is a transition from immature GM vessels to cortical vessels. From the sixth month of gestation and continuing into the last trimester, these channels begin to disappear and remodel into vessels resembling cortical vessels.[8] Near the end of this period, the GM gradually becomes less active, becoming fastigial at term.[9]

FACTORS ASSOCIATED WITH THE PATHOGENESIS OF GM–IVH

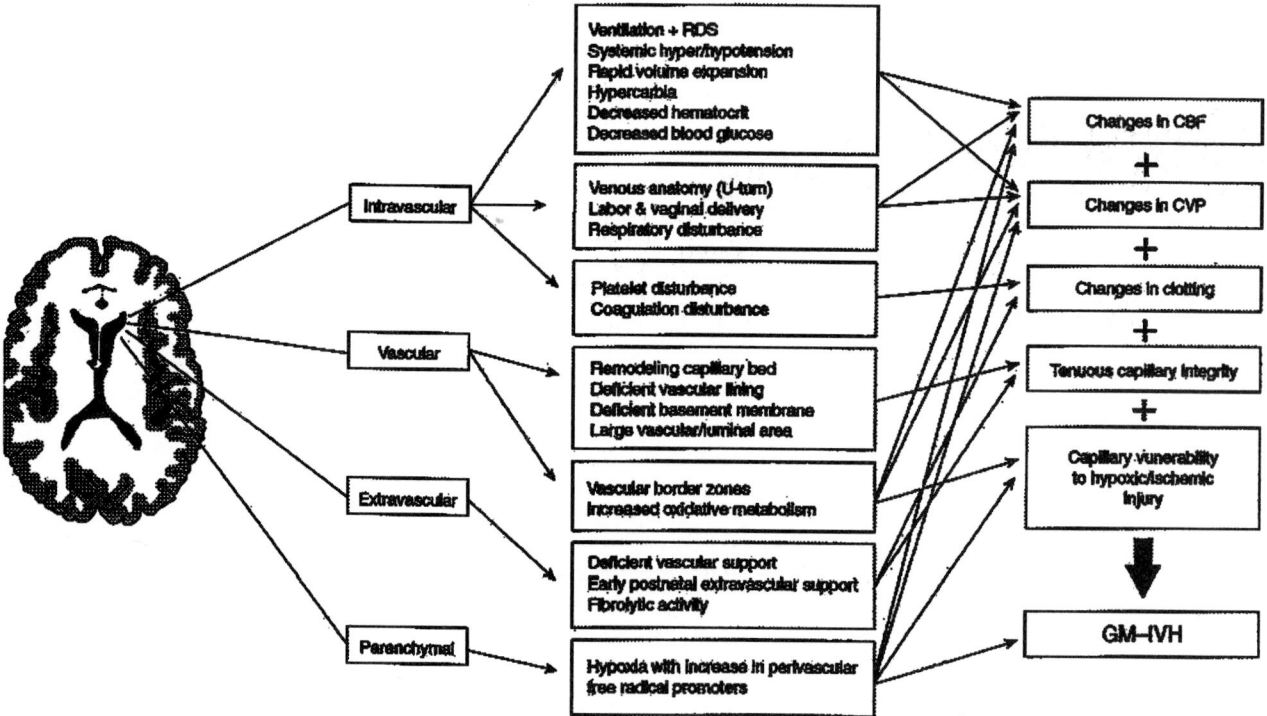

FIGURE 216–2. Factors associated with the pathogenesis of germinal matrix–intraventricular hemorrhage. CBF, cerebral blood flow; CVP, central venous pressure.

Pathogenesis of Germinal Matrix–Intraventricular Hemorrhage

In preterm infants, there is a predisposition for GM-IVH, because immature vessels are unable to tolerate cerebral blood flow (CBF) fluctuations. Because structural support develops rapidly, the risk period for this hemorrhage is the initial 3 to 4 postnatal days, especially the first 24 hours. The usual site of the GM bleed is at the confluence of draining veins, where the direction of blood flow is reversed abruptly (see Fig. 216–1B). Microscopically, the site of GM-IVH seems to be the venous endothelial cell–lined channels and, less commonly, the proximal capillary-venule junctions.[10] Ghazzi-Berri and colleagues[11] found that hemorrhage dissected along the perivascular spaces, collapsing the offending vein and rupturing the tethered connecting tributaries. Macroscopically, the most common site of

GM-IVH is at the head of the caudate nucleus, just posterior to the foramen of Monro.[12] Less commonly, hemorrhage may occur in the body of caudate nucleus and the choroid plexus.[13]

As Volpe[14, 15] describes, the pathogenesis of GM-IVH is multifactorial and can be considered in terms of vascular, intravascular, and extravascular factors, and various parenchymal factors (Fig. 216–2).

Neuropathology Resulting from Germinal Matrix–Intraventricular Hemorrhage

Periventricular hemorrhagic infarction (PHI) and hydrocephalus are the direct result of GM hemorrhage. PHI refers to hemorrhagic necrosis of the periventricular white matter in the region immediately lateral and superior to the ventricles (Fig. 216–3A). This condition occurs in 15% of infants with GM hemorrhage, and

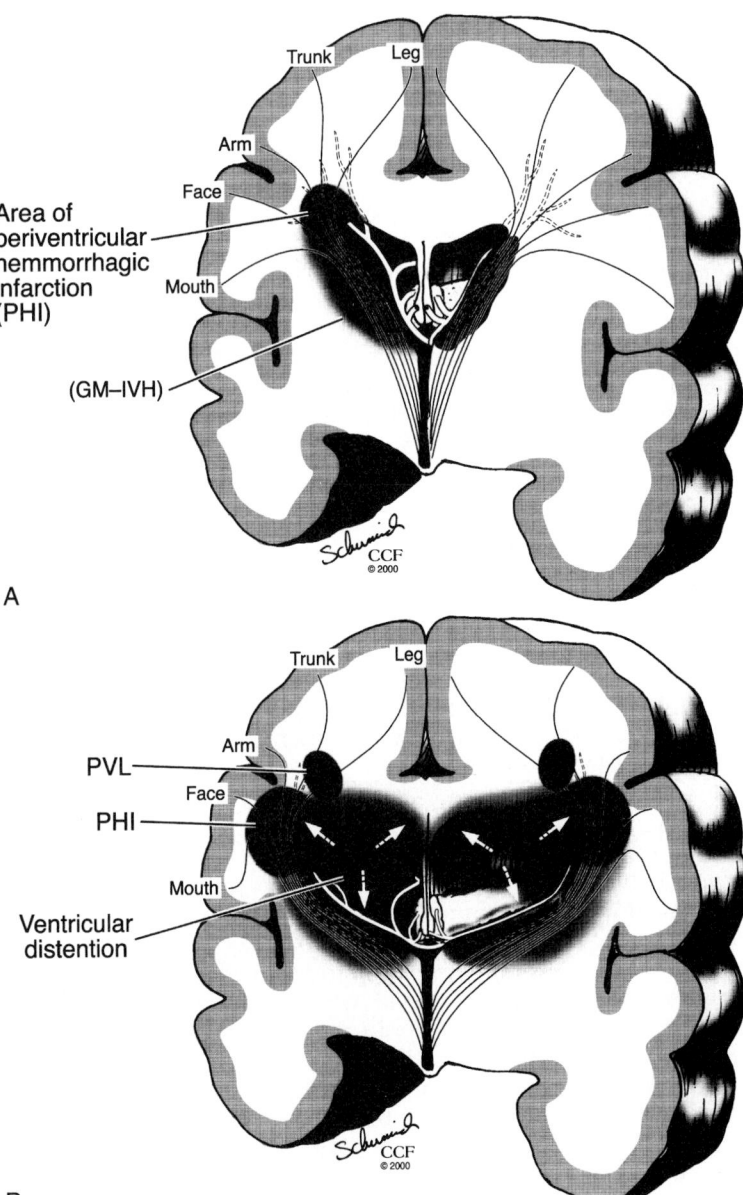

FIGURE 216–3. Pattern of injury in germinal matrix–intraventricular hemorrhage. *A,* Periventricular hemorrhagic infarction (PHI). *B,* Combined injury: PHI, periventricular leukomalacia (PVL), and hydrocephalus. (Adapted from Volpe JJ: Intraventricular hemorrhage and brain injury in the premature infant: Neuropathology and pathogenesis. Clin Perinatol 16:361–386, 1989.)

TABLE 216–2 ■ **Severity of Germinal Matrix – Intraventricular Hemorrhage**

SEVERITY	DESCRIPTION	MORTALITY (%)	PROGRESSIVE VENTRICULAR DISTENTION (% OF SURVIVORS)
I	GM hemorrhage with small IVH (<10% of ventricular area on parasagittal view)	5	5
II	GM hemorrhage with moderate IVH (10–50% of ventricular area on parasagittal view)	10	20
III	GM hemorrhage with large IVH and lateral ventricular distention (>50% of ventricular area on parasagittal view)	20	55
IV	GM hemorrhage with periventricular echodensity indicating infarction (grade III + PHI)	50	80

GM, germinal matrix; IVH, intraventricular hemorrhage; PHI, periventricular hemorrhagic infarction.

approximately 70% of the lesions are unilateral. The peak incidence of PHI is the fourth postnatal day, whereas most GM hemorrhage occurs within the first 24 hours. Toxic substances within the perivascular spaces or vasospasm are possible contributing factors.

IPHH is considered to be a direct consequence of GM-IVH (see Fig. 216–3B). Ventriculomegaly seen on imaging studies may reflect progressive hydrocephalus with ventricular distention, ventriculomegaly ex vacuo from loss of developing white matter, or a combination of both.[16] The distinction between progressive IPHH and hydrocephalus ex vacuo ventricular distention is often difficult because of the delayed clinical features of progressive hydrocephalus, and the various individual clinical courses in infants.[17]

The mortality and development of ventricular distention depends on the severity of the GM-IVH (Table 216–2).[18] IPHH develops in approximately 13% of preterm infants with GM hemorrhage, and 6% ultimately require a ventriculoperitoneal shunt.[19] The timing of posthemorrhagic hydrocephalus is a function of the quantity of IVH and may occur early. Severe IVH causes early obstructive (noncommunicating) hydrocephalus within the first week, with an associated mortality of 40%.[13] Communicating hydrocephalus occurs later, mostly caused by cisternal arachnoiditis obstructing CSF flow at the tentorial hiatus or the foramina of Magendie and Luschka. In some cases, delayed obstructive hydrocephalus occurs at the aqueduct of Sylvius, with outflow blockage by hematoma, ependymal tear, or periaqueductal gliosis.[20, 21]

Brain Injury in Hydrocephalus

Hydrocephalus results in CNS injury through fiber stretch and vessel compression with secondary hypoxia. Compression of the venous system may decrease perfusion pressure and impair parenchymal oxygen delivery. The immature arterial vessels do not have a muscularis layer and therefore are unresponsive to increased CBF.[22] These alterations may occur with early ventricular distention, before clinical or radiologic evidence of raised intracranial pressure. As IPHH progresses, the intracranial pressure may increase, further impairing CBF and causing hypoxic-ischemic injury in periventricular white matter.[23]

There is only indirect evidence that ventricular distention causes secondary hypoxia-ischemia in humans. Doppler ultrasonography in cases of IPHH show that a decrease in the mean CBF velocity and an increase in the cerebral vascular resistance occur in hydrocephalus.[24] Changes in CBF velocity correlate more closely with the degree of ventricular distention rather than ICP.[25] Biochemical CSF markers in IPHH show increased levels of hypoxanthine[26] and eicosanoids,[27] reflecting cerebral hypoxia-ischemia. Hypoxanthine is absent in the CSF of normal infants.[26]

In vivo studies of infants with IPHH demonstrate that abnormalities in visual evoked potentials[28] and brainstem auditory evoked potentials[29] are reversible with CSF drainage. However, the rapid reversibility of these electrophysiologic abnormalities suggests axonal distortion, rather than reversible hypoxic-ischemic injury.[28]

Ex vacuo ventriculomegaly is associated with loss of white matter due to the effects of hypoxic-ischemic injury and not related to hemorrhage or CSF flow obstruction. In contrast, the intraventricular blood causes secondary injury by acute ventricular distention in hydrocephalic infants. Neuropathologic changes, such as disruption of the ependymal lining, subependymal rosette formation, lipid-laden microglia, reduction of myelinated axons, and hemosiderin deposits associated with ballooning axonal injury,[30, 31] have been demonstrated in animal[32] and human studies.[33] The pathologic consequence of early hydrocephalus is unknown, and some animal studies indicate decreased dendritic arborization and lower levels of catecholamines with prolonged ventricular dilatation.[34] Early CSF drainage has shown benefit in some animal models, with improved structural and behavioral outcomes.[34]

CLINICAL PRESENTATION AND DIAGNOSTIC STUDIES

Premature infants are primarily treated in a neonatal intensive care unit (NICU), and the neurosurgeon is consulted after a hemorrhage is recognized. These infants are usually lethargic, intubated, and sedated, making the neurological assessment very difficult.

Clinical criteria indicative of IPHH include measurement of changes in head circumference (i.e., growth of more than 2 cm per week), bulging of the anterior fontanelle, separation of skull sutures, episodes of apnea or bradycardia, and a reduced level of alertness.

Diagnostic evaluations that can be performed at the bedside are the most practical in IPHH. More complex studies that require transporting the infant out of the NICU are more difficult to use routinely. Imaging studies available for evaluating infants with IPHH include cranial ultrasonography, Doppler ultrasound measurement of CBF velocities, near-infrared spectroscopy, computed tomography (CT), magnetic resonance imaging (MRI), and magnetic resonance spectroscopy (MRS). Of these, cranial ultrasonography and CT are most frequently used.

Weekly studies are often performed to document resolution of IVH and observe for the progression or resolution of hydrocephalus. Loculations and trapped ventricles are identified, and the degree of periventricular leukomalacia is evaluated.

CT and MRI scans can denote the extent of GM-IVH and the size of the ventricles. These studies may be used initially to evaluate the anatomy, especially of the posterior fossa, cystic changes, loculations, and other abnormalities; considering the proposed pathology of GM-IVH and hydrocephalus, MRS may be of clinical value in early ventricular distention.

GM-IVH specifically refers to hemorrhage seen in preterm infants and is graded according to severity on the basis of ultrasound studies.[35] The ultrasound features can be correlated with the gross pathologic and CT findings (see Table 216–2).

Doppler ultrasound measurement of cerebral arterial flow has been used to determine the optimal timing of CSF drainage in IPHH.[36] Doppler ultrasonography is performed by insonating a major artery through the anterior fontanelle (i.e., pericallosal artery) or temporal window (i.e., proximal middle cerebral artery) and then calculating the resistive index (i.e., [mean systolic-diastolic velocity]/mean systolic velocity). Drainage of CSF in cases of ventricular distention tends to decrease the resistive index toward normal, whereas in infants with ventriculomegaly ex vacuo CSF, drainage has no effect on the resistive index.[37]

PREVENTION

Because IPHH is a chronic condition that often begins and evolves under medical care, the opportunity for intervention includes prevention, control of progression, and long-term stabilization. Palliation of early ventricular distention is frequently included in various treatment protocols, but it is unclear whether these interventions have altered the need for ventriculoperitoneal shunt insertion, or the overall neurological outcome. A management algorithm for IPHH, progressing from diagnosis to a ventriculoperitoneal shunt implantation, includes several modes of medical and surgical treatments (Fig. 216–4).

With advances in prenatal, antenatal, and neonatal intensive care, the prevention of GM-IVH in preterm infants has been relatively successful. Based on a greater understanding of the cause of the hemorrhage, several treatments have been useful in decreasing the incidence of this devastating condition. Tocolytic agents such as β-adrenergic agonists can delay labor for about 48 hours, but treatment is associated with a greater risk of GM-IVH.[38] Prostaglandin inhibitors (e.g., indomethacin) are also effective in inhibiting labor, but they are associated with increased GM-IVH and necrotizing enterocolitis.[39]

Antenatal phenobarbital reduces the occurrence of severe GM-IVH; however, this benefit may be offset by an increased incidence of respiratory distress syndrome and a greater need for ventilatory support in these infants.[40] The use of antenatal phenobarbital and vitamin K has not gained universal acceptance, because some studies failed to show a significant benefit.[41, 42] Steroid administration before onset of labor has shown a consistent beneficial effect in reducing the incidence of GM-IVH in preterm infants. The mode of action may be by improving the airway and GM vasculature architecture.[43] Because prolonged labor and delivery may cause skull deformation and venous obstruction, semi-elective cesarean section is often suggested as an option to reduce stress on the newborn infant and decrease the severity of IVH.[44] Postnatal measures to prevent GM-IVH are aimed at minimizing rapid changes in venous pressure, CBF, coagulation, and improving parenchymal tissue perfusion.

In the newborn infant, it is critical to establish an adequate airway and to avoid hypoxia and hypercapnia, two conditions that favor a pressure-passive cerebral circulation.[45] To prevent hypertension, rapid infusion of volume expanders or hypertonic solutions such as sodium bicarbonate, tracheal suctioning, exchange transfusions, apneic episodes, seizures, and pneumothorax should be avoided. The use of muscle relaxants to minimize respiratory effort in ventilated preterm infants has been proved to minimize the incidence and severity of GM-IVH by decreasing CBF fluctuations.[46] The use of high-frequency jet ventilation has also been shown to stabilize the CBF variations, decreasing the incidence of GM-IVH.

Medications such as opiates assist in synchronizing the infant and the mechanical ventilator, which reduces fluctuations in CBF.[47, 48] Muscle relaxants aid in maintaining normotension and decrease stress-induced vital sign changes, such as during tracheal suctioning. The administration of fresh-frozen plasma and factor XIII reduces the incidence of GM-IVH, although the mechanism is unclear.[49, 50] Postnatal drug interventions with phenobarbital, indomethacin, ethamsylate, and vitamin E have not been consistently beneficial in preventing GM-IVH, and their use is not routinely recommended.[18] Evidence suggests that free radical scavenging agents, such as vitamin E, prevent the toxic effects on the vulnerable periventricular oligodendrocytes.[51]

CLINICAL COURSE

The natural clinical course of IPHH varies among patients. The short-term course of GM-IVH is often re-

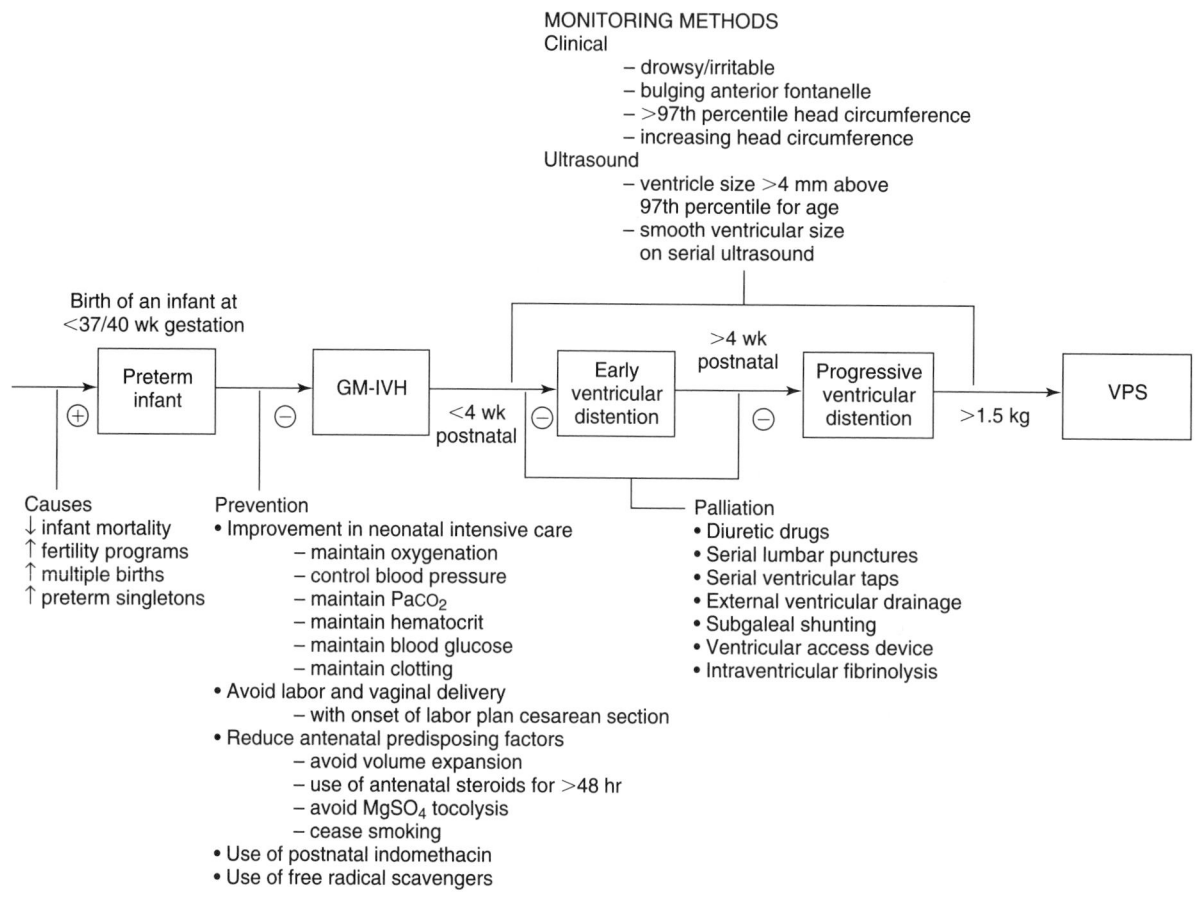

MONITORING METHODS
Clinical
  – drowsy/irritable
  – bulging anterior fontanelle
  – >97th percentile head circumference
  – increasing head circumference
Ultrasound
  – ventricle size >4 mm above
    97th percentile for age
  – smooth ventricular size
    on serial ultrasound

Causes
↓ infant mortality
↑ fertility programs
↑ multiple births
↑ preterm singletons

Prevention
• Improvement in neonatal intensive care
  – maintain oxygenation
  – control blood pressure
  – maintain PaCO₂
  – maintain hematocrit
  – maintain blood glucose
  – maintain clotting
• Avoid labor and vaginal delivery
  – with onset of labor plan cesarean section
• Reduce antenatal predisposing factors
  – avoid volume expansion
  – use of antenatal steroids for >48 hr
  – avoid MgSO₄ tocolysis
  – cease smoking
• Use of postnatal indomethacin
• Use of free radical scavengers

Palliation
• Diuretic drugs
• Serial lumbar punctures
• Serial ventricular taps
• External ventricular drainage
• Subgaleal shunting
• Ventricular access device
• Intraventricular fibrinolysis

FIGURE 216–4. Monitoring and intervention for postventricular hydrocephalus.

lated to the severity of the hemorrhage and is evident over the initial 4 to 6 weeks (see Table 216–2).[18, 21] Approximately 5% of GM-IVH cases suffer a rapidly progressive phase within days of the bleeding episode.[19] Immediate ventricular distention can develop in infants with severe hemorrhages due to blockage of CSF flow within the structures, and it usually requires urgent treatment. Delayed hydrocephalus may lead to spontaneous arrest in 65% of cases after a brief period of progressive ventricular distention. In another 30% of cases, an initial period of slow progression is followed by an accelerated phase, usually after 4 weeks. The variable clinical course during the first month after GM-IVH frequently requires the clinician's vigilant involvement. IPHH progression can be defined in stages, which may help in guiding an intervention protocol (see Fig. 216–4). Infants destined for a ventricular-peritoneal shunt include those who continue to have progressive ventricular distention after 4 weeks despite measures for prevention and palliation.[52]

TREATMENT

Observation

Because many infants do not have progressive ventriculomegaly, a conservative approach is often consid-

ered an appropriate initial course. Although this initial step seems reasonable in many cases, it may be controversial because we lack knowledge about permanent secondary injury resulting from ventricular distention.

During this time (usually 3 to 4 weeks), the infant is observed for increased respiratory requirements and vital sign instability (e.g., oxygen desaturation, apnea, bradycardia). Physical findings, including increasing head circumference (>1.5 cm/week), full or tense fontanelle with splitting sutures, and sunset eye phenomenon, are documented. Neurological signs are assessed, including increased irritability, lethargy, seizure frequency, and increased tone. Weekly cranial head ultrasound studies are used to monitor the ventricular size during this period.

Brain compliance in the premature infant is increased, because progressive ventriculomegaly may occur without outward clinical findings of increased pressure. Anterior fontanelle pressures are normally between 50 and 80 mm H₂O and can increase to 120 mm H₂O before significant intracranial changes and brain compression occur.[51]

Medical Management

The aim of medical management is to maintain appropriate intracranial homeostasis and prevent secondary damage related to hydrocephalus. This approach also allows the infant to improve CSF absorption or stabilize medically until more aggressive interventions can be used. Medical treatment of IPHH has been attempted for over 50 years with minimal and transient benefit. Osmotic diuretics such as isosorbide and glycerol have limited efficacy and may cause severe dehydration and electrolyte abnormalities, and they have not been included in the management strategy for IPHH.[53, 54]

Acetazolamide (i.e., carbonic anhydrase inhibitor) has been used in clinical trials for IPHH and has demonstrated a temporary decrease in intracranial pressure.[55] A suggested dosage regimen is furosemide (1 mg/kg daily) and acetazolamide (20 mg/kg daily, increasing gradually up to 100 mg/kg daily), administered intravenously or orally.[56] Side effects of these diuretics include electrolyte disturbance with metabolic acidosis (requiring bicarbonate replacement), dehydration, nephrocalcinosis, diarrhea, appetite suppression, and hypocalcemia.

The limited benefit and significant complication rate of current medical therapy restrict its use in the management of IPHH.

A large, multi-institution study questions the efficacy of acetazolamide. The international Posthemorrhagic Ventricular Dilatation (PHVD) drug trial group found acetazolamide and furosemide to be ineffective in the prevention of progressive ventricular distention or the need for shunting in IPHH.[57] Standard treatment group required CSF drainage alone, and the drug treatment group also received acetazolamide and furosemide. Shunting or infant death was seen in 65% of the drug therapy group and 46% of the standard therapy group, and diuretics therefore could not be recommended for the treatment of IPHH.

Treatment of Early Ventricular Distention

Early ventricular distention, seen before symptoms or certainty of progression, has been treated in the hope of reducing secondary injury and halting the progression of ventricular enlargement and permanent shunting. Physiologic control and pharmacologic agents have been tried with limited success. Serial lumbar punctures (SLPs) and ventricular infusions of streptokinase or urokinase have also been studied.

LUMBAR PUNCTURE

Early studies of SLPs failed to demonstrate a positive benefit in the reduction rate of subsequent shunting (Fig. 216–5A).[20, 58] Lumbar punctures were commenced at postnatal day 11 ($\pm$5) and continued for 20 ($\pm$16) days in grade III and IV infants, with removal of approximately 60 mL of CSF in 4 to 28 punctures. Lumbar punctures resulted in no difference in the rate of shunting compared with controls obtaining supportive care only.

Although the benefit of SLP for palliation of progressive ventricular distention has been questioned in several studies,[20, 58–62] it is possible that an early and more

rigorous protocol of lumbar drainage may reduce subsequent hydrocephalus. If SLP is started immediately after grade 3 and 4 GM-IVH without a 7- to 10-day delay, a benefit may be seen.[63, 64] The incidence of subsequent shunting was only 10% and 29% for grades 3 and 4, respectively.

INTRAVENTRICULAR FIBRINOLYSIS

Intraventricular fibrinolysis has been advocated to expedite intraventricular clot resorption, restore CSF pathways, and reduce the rate of ventricular-peritoneal shunting (VPS).[65, 66] Agents used include streptokinase,[67] urokinase,[68] and human recombinant plasminogen activator.[69] Commencement of treatment well before a median age of 30 days[70] has theoretical potential to change the rate of VPS, but it may increase the risk of further hemorrhage. However, there is insufficient evidence to justify the claim that intraventricular fibrinolytic agents are safe and effective in the treatment of IPHH.[71]

Palliation

With progressive ventricular distention, the goals of palliative treatments are to stabilize ventricular size and pressure until definitive treatment can be performed based on the weight of the infant and general medical condition. Palliative intervention may be initiated at any time (early or later) based on symptoms, signs, and head ultrasound results. These interventions continue until not needed or until a shunt is implanted. It is hoped that, after 4 to 6 weeks, the blood clot resolves, and the proteinaceous debris and other blood products are partially resorbed, which may minimize the need for more invasive interventions or decrease the risk of shunt malfunction if one is eventually needed.

Palliative measures include drug administration, SLPs, ventricular puncture, placement of an external ventriculostomy for continuous drainage, and insertion of a ventricular access device or subgaleal shunt.

The use of acetazolamide and early lumbar punctures has already been mentioned in the context of early treatment to avoid progressive hydrocephalus. In the case of diuretic therapy, it appears to be ineffective in reducing the need for shunting; however, the treatment may allow postponement of the definitive shunt procedure until the infant is clinically stable. This drug regimen may be useful as a palliative measure, rather than a treatment cure.

Serial Lumbar Puncture

SLP has long been used as a palliative measure to stabilize the ventricles and delay the need for shunting. Unfortunately, it is often difficult to obtain a sufficient amount of CSF regularly enough to rely on it as the sole means of palliation. Possible complications of SLP, including meningitis[72] and epidural abscess,[73] have also caused some reservation about the use of SLP for palliation of IPHH. Overall, however, it remains useful as

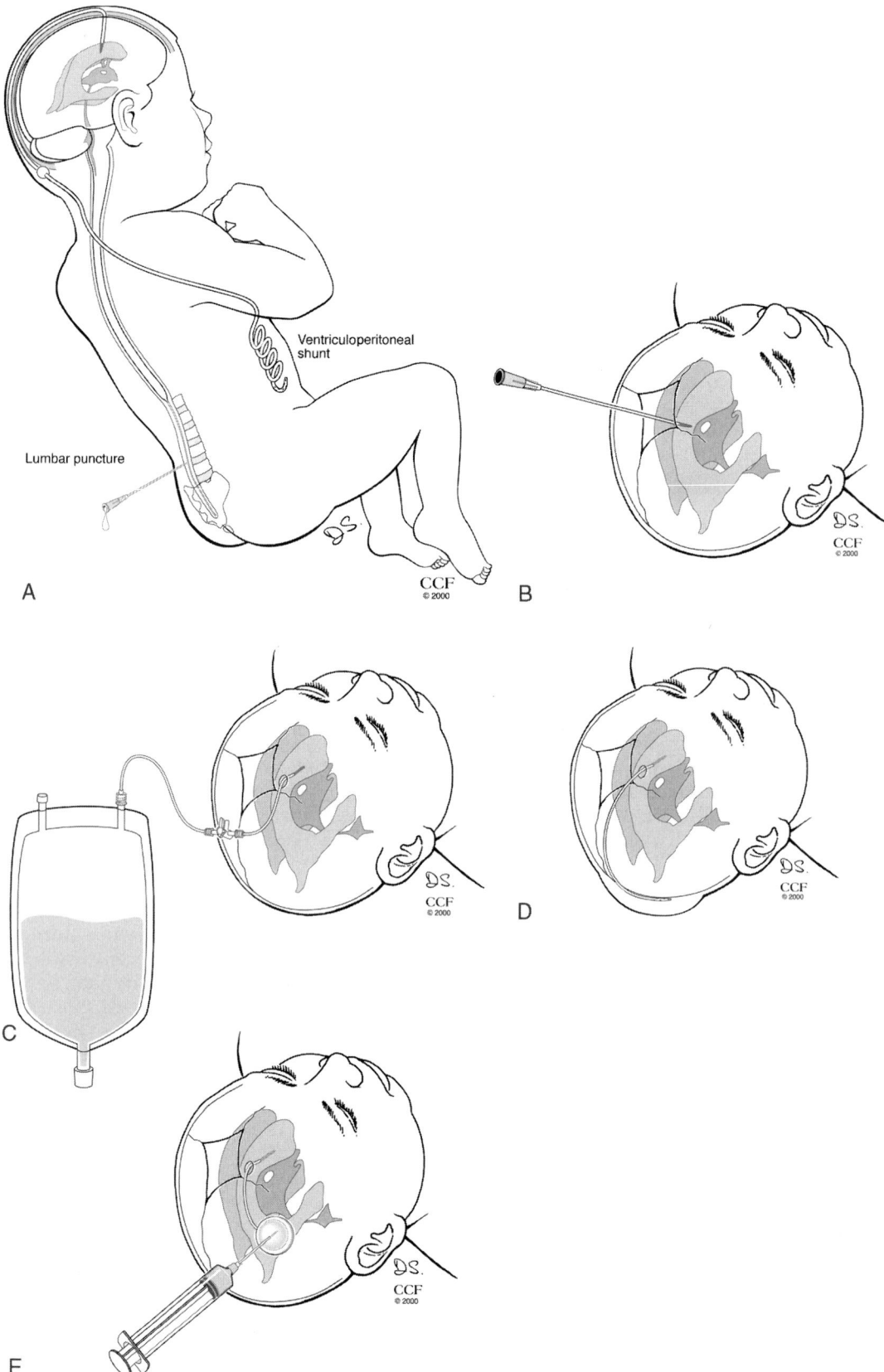

FIGURE 216–5.   Methods of cerebrospinal fluid removal. *A,* Lumbar puncture (i.e., palliation) and shunting (i.e., definitive treatment). *B,* Ventricular tap. *C,* External ventricular drainage. *D,* Ventricular subgaleal shunt. *E,* Ventricular access device.

an initial, interim treatment before shunting can be performed.

Ventricular Taps

Ventricular taps have been in use for the treatment of IPHH, performed free hand[74, 75] or with ultrasound guidance[76–78] (see Fig. 216–5B). The procedure may be undertaken at the bedside in the NICU. Using aseptic technique, an angiocatheter may be inserted into the region of the frontal horn, piercing the scalp at the lateral angle of the anterior fontanelle in line with the coronal suture. After the needle passes through the scalp, the skin is retracted, and the trajectory is altered so that the needle enters the dura at a point away from the puncture site in the scalp, reducing the likelihood of CSF leakage. The needle is then withdrawn, and 20 to 30 mL may drain freely through the plastic catheter. The procedure holds less risk of complications with the aid of ultrasonogrpahy.[76] Drainage of CSF by ventricular taps may result in diminished ventricular size in up to 50% of infants with IPHH, and this approach therefore may be of value in palliation. However, hemorrhage and neural injury occur with repeated taps. If repeated taps are considered likely, an implanted device, which requires only a single traumatic insertion, should be considered.

External Ventricular Drainage

External ventricular drainage (EVD) has been in use for some time as a temporizing measure for the treatment of IPHH[79–82] (see Fig. 216–5C). However, a retrospective study reports an unacceptable incidence of morbidity, particularly infection, requiring a change of practice to implantation of a ventricular access device to reduce morbidity.[83] Other studies suggest EVD as a safe and effective method of palliation for IPHH[84, 85] and as more effective than SLP.[86]

The EVD system may be placed in the NICU, where infants are often ventilated and have multiple invasive catheters for monitoring and support.[87] Under sterile conditions, local anesthetic is injected subcutaneously (1% Xylocaine with 1:200,000 epinephrine), and a twist drill opening is made at or just anterior to the coronal suture, approximately 2 cm lateral to the midline. With the dura incised, a ventricular catheter is placed in the frontal horn, tunneled within the scalp, and connected to a drainage system. The height of the EVD system is set so that the mean daily drainage approximates 20 mL. The ventricular catheter may be placed for 3 to 10 weeks.[84, 86] The rate of meningitis or ventriculitis was 0% to 5%, and the rate of permanent shunt dependence was 30% to 65%.[85, 86] Although EVD may not alter the frequency of later shunting, it appears to be an effective means of temporizing progressive ventricular distention.

Ventriculosubgaleal Shunting Procedures

Ventriculosubgaleal shunting was suggested as a form of treatment for hydrocephalus in the late 1920s (see Fig. 216–5D). Later, ventriculosubgaleal shunting was advocated for temporary decompression of obstructive hydrocephalus through a parietal[88] or frontal approach[89] and was shown to be useful in head injury for control of ICP[90] and in high-pressure hydrocephalus.[91] A role for ventriculosubgaleal shunting in treating IPHH has become evident in the past 10 years.[92] Ventriculosubgaleal shunting has a role in palliation of progressive ventricular distention to temporarily divert CSF in a more physiologic and closed system, particularly for infants who weigh less than 1500 g and may not tolerate VPS. The procedure may be performed at the bedside in the NICU, with the ventricular catheter placed as previously described. As the catheter exits the dura, the elbow bend is fixed to the pericranium in addition to ensuring free drainage of CSF into the subgaleal space. The result is often a large subgaleal fluid collection and scalp expansion that later resolves after full ventricular-peritoneal shunting. This entirely internal CSF diversion probably reduces the risk of infection seen with repeated lumbar punctures or external drainage, although the large overall accumulation of subgaleal fluid may negate this advantage. Subgaleal shunting provides an adequate CSF diversion with minimal complications and should be considered for the palliation of IPHH.[93]

Ventricular Access Devices

The ventricular access device (VAD) or ventricular reservoir was introduced for palliation of progressive ventricular distention and IPHH in the early 1980s and has proved to be a safe alternative temporizing method (see Fig. 216–5E). In the 1980s, a low-profile, subcutaneous ventricular catheter reservoir, specially designed by McComb and colleagues,[94] was placed by the 12th day of life in 20 preterm neonates. A VAD may be placed at the bedside in the NICU under aseptic conditions or placed in the operating room. The reservoir can be repeatedly aspirated with little morbidity such as CSF infection, reservoir obstruction, or skin breakdown overlying the reservoir. The system can then be converted to a VPS.[94] Although criteria for the intervals and volumes of drainage through a VAD are not clear and depend on clinical signs of increased ICP and changes on cranial ultrasonogrpahy,[95] some have changed the method of palliation at their institution from EVD to VAD based on the significant reduction in morbidity and mortality.[83] Although the reported infection rates associated with the reservoir are consistently low,[94, 96, 97] the shunt- or reservoir-related infection rate may be as high as 32%, and the shunt revision rate is in the vicinity of 60% in the first year of life.[95, 98]

Evidence substantiates the place of VADs in the palliation of IPHH. One hundred forty-nine preterm infants were temporized with a VAD and serial CSF drainage to control ICP and ventricular size. Ninety-three percent of the infants had grade III or IV GM-IVH. For all the infants with VADs, complications included VAD occlusion (10%), VAD infection (8%), subgaleal collection (9%), and CSF leak (3%). Six percent required placement of a contralateral VAD for a trapped ventricle. Slightly less than one half the VAD infections were treated successfully with a combination of systemic and intra-VAD antibiotic therapy without removal of the VAD. The VAD may also be used for administration of intraventricular thrombolytic agents. In this group of infants, among the survivors, the rate of shunt placement was 88%. VAD is a safe alternative for palliation of progressive ventricular distention and IPHH, with an acceptable rate of morbidity.[97]

Surgical Treatment: Ventricular-peritoneal Shunting

Development of valve mechanisms for surgical treatment of hydrocephalus heralded the modern era of CSF shunting, and the current technique for VPS has been described in detail elsewhere.[99, 100] In the premature infant, surgical hazards are related to poor wound healing and CSF leakage, which may lead to infection. These problems may be compounded by bulky shunt hardware with a high profile. Although a frontal placement may avoid pressure on the skin in the supine position, we prefer a right occipital approach. The occipital catheter is in line with the long axis of the lateral ventricle, which allows brain growth to occur without pulling the catheter out of the ventricle. In general, incisions should be planned to avoid crossing underlying hardware or tubing. The choice of shunt depends on available pressure settings, device profile, ease of handling, and surgeon familiarity. In general, infants may require a low pressure for adequate drainage, although such a pressure may allow overdrainage in later years when the child is upright.

The decision to perform VPS is based on the treatment algorithm previously described. Practically, the end point of palliation is the continuation of progressive ventricular enlargement, confirmed on serial ultrasonography, despite intervention and extending beyond the first 4 weeks of life. However, several additional factors have to be considered before proceeding with VPS. Infants weighing 1500 g or less may be unable to reabsorb peritoneal CSF, presumably because of the inadequate available absorptive surface area.[83] Children below this weight are also at risk for necrotizing enterocolitis, which may lead to devastating gram-negative meningitis. Ventricular-peritoneal shunts are placed in infants weighing 1500 g or more at our institution. A popular notion exists that a high CSF protein level increases risk of shunt complications; however, this has been questioned in a prospective study by Brydon and colleagues.[101] Ninety-five patients were enrolled in the study and had 116 shunt operations over 15 months. Shunt complications occurred in 24.6% within 2 months, but the distribution was not significant compared with CSF protein content. It was concluded that increased CSF protein did not increase the risk of shunt complications. Protein adsorption by catheters, initially thought to be related to obstruction,[102] may be advantageous in improving the biocompatibility of silicone rubber and inhibiting bacterial adhesion.[103] Blood cells do adversely affect shunt flow characteristics, and a perfusate of more than 0.25%

blood suspension (10,000 red blood cells/μL) gave erratic results, partly blocking the valves sometimes and, at other times, making valves unable to properly close.[101] At the Cleveland Clinic Foundation, a level of 2000 red blood cells/μL is used as a safe margin. A single dose of preoperative antibiotics (e.g., ceftriaxone) is used with continuation for 24 hours in an attempt to limit overgrowth of resistant bacteria. Others have found more aggressive protocols with perioperative broad-spectrum antibiotics[104] or intrathecal injection useful.[105] A low-pressure valve with a low profile has been used, but a programmable valve has been used more recently; it starts at a low-pressure setting in anticipation of changing drainage requirements over time. As the infant grows and assumes a more upright posture and depending on the situation at follow-up, the drainage pressure may be increased.

To reduce infection, the VPS surgery is done in two steps. The first step is the opening of the cranium and abdominal cavity. The surgical areas are re-draped and gloves are changed. The second step includes shunt placement and closure. A small curvilinear incision is made in the occipital region, and a small bur hole 2.5 cm superior to the inion and 2.5 cm lateral to the occipital midline[106] is made with a curet. Care is taken to avoid trauma or cautery to the skin edges. The abdominal incision is made just above the umbilicus in the linea alba. Gloves are changed, all exposed skin edges are covered with antibiotic-soaked sponges, and sterile towels are draped around the wound before shunt insertion. The trajectory of the catheter is aimed at a point just lateral to midline and above the orbital ridge. The optimal position for the shunt catheter tip is in the frontal horn, just lateral to and beyond the foramen of Monro, avoiding the choroid plexus. A bur hole reservoir is useful to anchor the catheter in position, and we leave ample length of distal catheter in the abdomen to allow for growth. Other surgeons report using catheter lengths of up to 120 cm without complication.[107] Shunt placement is documented with a plain radiograph shunt series, and neonates are observed with six weekly cranial ultrasound studies.

OUTCOME

Approximately 40 years ago, a report of the natural history of untreated congenital hydrocephalus depicted a poor outcome. Of 182 children, 46% survived infancy, and of these infants who survived, 38% were deemed to have normal intelligence. The actuarial rate for survival to adult life was only 20% to 23%.[108]

The outcome of children with IPHH depends on the extent and treatment course of their hydrocephalus and on the extent of associated neurological injuries and other system problems. Infants in whom IPHH develops have a mortality rate reaching 34%, mainly resulting from non-neurological complications. Among the survivors, up to 70% to 95% have some neurological impairment,[109] and approximately 60% may require a VPS.[58] In some studies, extensive or diffuse intraparenchymal echodensity suggests a high mortality rate (up to 80%), and most shunted infants have abnormal results on delayed neurological examinations.[83] Posthemorrhagic infarction results in intellectual deficits and spasticity. The major long-term effect of periventricular leukomalacia is spastic diplegia, which is usually more severe in the lower than the upper limbs. Infants who have greater upper limb involvement tend to have more associated neuropsychological deficits.[110]

These data suggest that current treatment strategies achieve a greater number of survivors but do not always prevent the adverse neurological sequelae that may be reversible. Such injury occurs primarily at the time of the GM-IVH, but ongoing injury associated with progressive ventricular distention continues before definitive treatment to control intracranial hypertension. Neurological deficits may be reduced by neonatal intensive care aimed at preventing and avoiding the progression of GM-IVH in addition to appropriate early treatment of developing hydrocephalus.

The outcome of preterm infants with IPHH remains less favorable than that for other forms of hydrocephalus. The infants who are fortunate to experience spontaneous resolution of ventricular distention have a better outcome than infants in whom ventricular distention develops, requiring palliation and probable shunt placement.[111] In a study of 61 preterm infants born from 1967 to 1982, 26% died before the age of 2 years. Among the survivors, 47% had cerebral palsy, 51% had mental retardation, and 33% had epilepsy. Gestational age of less than 28 weeks was found to be a poor prognostic factor.[112] As expected, infants with more severe hemorrhage (grades 3 and 4) more often require shunting and have a worse functional outcome when evaluated in early or late childhood.[19, 113–116]

How much additional morbidity is caused by hydrocephalus, rather than differences in prematurity, bleed severity, or the treatment of shunting, is still uncertain. Although prematurity itself may result in little dysfunction on physiologic testing, the occurrence of hydrocephalus and need for shunting are predictors of worsening function.[111] Outcome data suggest that severity and progression of hydrocephalus, rather than prematurity or shunt complications, are important in functional outcome.[111] This supports efforts in hydrocephalus prevention and early treatment.

CONCLUSIONS

The occurrence of IPHH has been influenced by improvements in neonatal care, which has increased survival of the most vulnerable premature infants while reducing the risk of hemorrhage through better physiologic control. An understanding of the basic pathophysiology is needed to guide medical prevention and control. Treatment ranges from preventive and palliative to acute and chronic. Although most gains have been made in reducing the frequency of hemorrhage, interruption of the process between hemorrhage and hydrocephalus is an important area of active investigation. Unfortunately, secondary pathologic events after GM hemorrhage, such as PHI and periventricular leu-komalacia, limit the response to treatment of hydrocephalus and the overall outcome.

ACKNOWLEDGMENTS

The authors are grateful for the assistance of Sarel J. Vorster, MD, in the preparation of this chapter.

REFERENCES

1. Fernell E, Hagberg G, Hagberg B: Infantile hydrocephalus epidemiology: An indicator of enhanced survival. Arch Dis Child Fetal Neonatal Ed 70:F123–F128, 1994.
2. Papile LA, Munsick-Bruno G, Schaefer A: Relationship of cerebral intraventricular hemorrhage and early childhood neurologic handicaps. J Pediatr 103:273–277, 1983.
3. Stjernqvist K, Svenningsen NW: Extremely low-birth-weight infants less than 901 g. Growth and development after one year of life. Acta Paediatr 82:40–44, 1993.
4. Fernell E, Hagberg G: Infantile hydrocephalus: Declining prevalence in preterm infants. Acta Paediatr 87:392–396, 1998.
5. Philip AG, Allan WC, Tito AM, Wheeler LR: Intraventricular hemorrhage in preterm infants: Declining incidence in the 1980s. Pediatrics 84:797–801, 1989.
6. Sheth RD: Frequency of neurologic disorders in the neonatal intensive care unit. J Child Neurol 13:424–428, 1998.
7. Hambleton G, Wigglesworth JS: Origin of intraventricular haemorrhage in the preterm infant. Arch Dis Child 51:651–659, 1976.
8. Takashima S, Tanaka K: Microangiography and vascular permeability of the subependymal matrix in the premature infant. Can J Neurol Sci 5:45–50, 1978.
9. Kedzia A: Characteristics of periventricular matrix vascularization in image computer transformation system. Folia Neuropathol 33:267–270, 1995.
10. Moody DM, Brown WR, Challa VR, Block SM: Alkaline phosphatase histochemical staining in the study of germinal matrix hemorrhage and brain vascular morphology in a very-low-birth-weight neonate. Pediatr Res 35:424–430, 1994.
11. Ghazi Birry HS, Brown WR, Moody DM, et al: Human germinal matrix: Venous origin of hemorrhage and vascular characteristics. AJNR Am J Neuroradiol 18:219–229, 1997.
12. Leech RW, Kohnen P: Subependymal and intraventricular hemorrhages in the newborn. Am J Pathol 77:465–475, 1974.
13. Armstrong DL, Sauls CD, Goddard-Finegold J: Neuropathologic findings in short-term survivors of intraventricular hemorrhage. Am J Dis Child 141:617–621, 1987.
14. Volpe JJ: Intraventricular hemorrhage and brain injury in the premature infant: Neuropathology and pathogenesis. Clin Perinatol 16:361–386, 1989.
15. Volpe JJ: Brain injury in the premature infant: Neuropathology, clinical aspects, pathogenesis, and prevention. Clin Perinatol 24: 567–587, 1997.
16. Leviton A, Gilles F: Ventriculomegaly, delayed myelination, white matter hypoplasia, and "periventricular" leukomalacia: How are they related? Pediatr Neurol 15:127–136, 1996.
17. Roland EH, Hill A: Intraventricular hemorrhage and posthemorrhagic hydrocephalus. Current and potential future interventions. Clin Perinatol 24:589–605, 1997.
18. Volpe JJ: Neurology of the Newborn. Philadelphia, WB Saunders, 1995.
19. Dykes FD, Dunbar B, Lazarra A, Ahmann PA: Posthemorrhagic hydrocephalus in high-risk preterm infants: Natural history, management, and long-term outcome. J Pediatr 114:611–618, 1989.
20. Ventriculomegaly Trial Group: Randomized trial of early tapping in neonatal posthaemorrhagic ventricular dilatation. Arch Dis Child 65:3–10, 1990.
21. Larroche JC: Post-haemorrhagic hydrocephalus in infancy: Anatomical study. Biol Neonate 20:287–299, 1972.
22. Kuban KC, Gilles FH: Human telencephalic angiogenesis. Ann Neurol 17:539–548, 1985.
23. Shirane R, Sato S, Kameyama M, et al: Cerebral blood flow and

oxygen metabolism in infants with hydrocephalus. Child Nerv Syst 8:118–123, 1992.

24. Goh D, Minns RA: Intracranial pressure and cerebral arterial flow velocity indices in childhood hydrocephalus: Current review. Childs Nerv Syst 11:392–396, 1995.

25. Goh D, Minns RA, Hendry GM, et al: Cerebrovascular resistive index assessed by duplex Doppler sonography and its relationship to intracranial pressure in infantile hydrocephalus. Pediatr Radiol 22:246–250, 1992.

26. Bejer R, Saugstad OD, James H, Gluck L: Increased hypoxanthine concentrations in cerebrospinal fluid of infants with hydrocephalus. J Pediatr 103:44, 1983.

27. White R, Leffler CW, Bada HS: Eicosanoid levels in CSF of premature infants with posthemorrhagic hydrocephalus. Am J Med Sci 299:230–235, 1990.

28. McSherry JW, Walters CL, Horbar JD: Acute visual evoked potential changes in hydrocephalus. Electroencephalogr Clin Neurophysiol 53:331–333, 1982.

29. Walker M, MacDonald J, Wright LC: The history of ventriculoscopy: Where do we go from here? Pediatr Neurosurg 18:218–223, 1992.

30. Del Bigio MR: Neuropathological changes caused by hydrocephalus. Acta Neuropathol (Berl) 85:573–585, 1993.

31. Rowlatt U: The microscopic effects of ventricular dilatation without increase in head size. J Neurosurg 48:957–961, 1978.

32. Wright LC, McAllister JP, Katz SD, et al: Cytological and cytoarchitectural changes in the feline cerebral cortex during experimental infantile hydrocephalus. Pediatr Neurosurg 16:139–155, 1990.

33. Fukumizu M, Takashima S, Becker LE: Neonatal posthemorrhagic hydrocephalus: Neuropathologic and immunohistochemical studies. Pediatr Neurol 13:230–234, 1995.

34. Harris NG, McAllister JP 2nd, Jones HC: The effect of untreated and shunt-treated hydrocephalus on copyramidal neurone morphology in the H-Tx rat. Eur J Pediatr Surg 3:31–32, 1993.

35. Papile LA, Burstein J, Burstein R, Koffler H: Incidence and evolution of subependymal and intraventricular hemorrhage: A study of infants with birth weights less than 1,500 gm. J Pediatr 92:529–534, 1978.

36. Kempley ST, Gamsu HR: Changes in cerebral artery blood flow velocity after intermittent cerebrospinal fluid drainage. Arch Dis Child 69:74–76, 1993.

37. Hanlo PW, Gooskens RH, Nijhuis IJ, et al: Value of transcranial Doppler indices in predicting raised ICP in infantile hydrocephalus. A study with review of the literature. Childs Nerv Syst 11:595–603, 1995.

38. Higby K, Xenakis EM, Pauerstein CJ: Do tocolytic agents stop preterm labor? A critical and comprehensive review of efficacy and safety. Am J Obstet Gynecol 168:1247–1256, 1993.

39. Major CA, Lewis DF, Harding JA, et al: Tocolysis with indomethacin increases the incidence of necrotizing enterocolitis in the low-birth-weight neonate. Am J Obstet Gynecol 170:102–106, 1994.

40. Kaempf JW, Porreco R, Molina R, et al: Antenatal phenobarbital for the prevention of periventricular and intraventricular hemorrhage: A double-blind, randomized, placebo-controlled, multihospital trial. J Pediatr 117:933–938, 1990.

41. Morales WJ, Angel JL, O'Brien WF, et al: The use of antenatal vitamin K in the prevention of early neonatal intraventricular hemorrhage. Am J Obstet Gynecol 159:774–779, 1988.

42. Thorp JA, Parriott J, Ferrette-Smith D, et al: Antepartum vitamin K and phenobarbital for preventing intraventricular hemorrhage in the premature newborn: A randomized, double-blind, placebo-controlled trial. Obstet Gynecol 83:70–76, 1994.

43. Leviton A, Kuban KC, Pagano M, et al: Antenatal corticosteroids appear to reduce the risk of postnatal germinal matrix hemorrhage in intubated low birth weight newborns. Pediatrics 91:1083–1088, 1993.

44. Leviton A, Fenton T, Kuban KC, Pagano M: Labor and delivery characteristics and the risk of germinal matrix hemorrhage in low birth weight infants. J Child Neurol 6:35–40, 1991.

45. Pryds O: Control of cerebral circulation in the high-risk neonate. Ann Neurol 30:321–329, 1991.

46. Perlman JM, Goodman S, Kreusser KL, Volpe JJ: Reduction in intraventricular hemorrhage by elimination of fluctuating cerebral blood-flow velocity in preterm infants with respiratory distress syndrome. N Engl J Med 312:21,1353–1357, 1985.

47. Miall-Allen VM, De Vries LS, Whitelaw AG: Mean arterial blood pressure and neonatal cerebral lesions. Arch Dis Child 62:1068–1069, 1987.

48. Shaw NJ, Cooke RW, Gill AB, et al: Randomised trial of routine versus selective paralysis during ventilation for neonatal respiratory distress syndrome. Arch Dis Child 69:479–482, 1993.

49. Beverley DW, Pitts-Tucker TJ, Congdon PJ, et al: Prevention of intraventricular haemorrhage by fresh frozen plasma. Arch Dis Child 60:710–713, 1985.

50. Shirahata A, Nakamura T, Shimono M, et al: Blood coagulation findings and the efficacy of factor XIII concentrate in premature infants with intracranial hemorrhages. Thromb Res 57:755–763, 1990.

51. Volpe JJ: Brain injury in the premature infant—from pathogenesis to prevention. Brain Dev 19:519–534, 1997.

52. du Plessis A, André J: Posthemorrhagic hydrocephalus and brain injury in the preterm infant: Dilemmas in diagnosis and management. Semin Pediatr Neurol 5:161–179, 1998.

53. Liptak G, Gellerstedt ME, Klionsky N: Isosorbide in the medical management of hydrocephalus in children with myelodysplasia. Dev Med Child Neurol 34:150–154, 1992.

54. Lorber J, Salfield S, Lonton T: Isosorbide in the management of infantile hydrocephalus. Dev Med Child Neurol 25:502–511, 1983.

55. Libenson MH, Kaye EM, Rosman NP, Gilmore HE: Acetazolamide and furosemide for posthemorrhagic hydrocephalus of the newborn. Pediatr Neurol 20:185–191, 1999.

56. Shinnar S, Gammon K, Bergman EW, et al: Management of hydrocephalus in infancy: Use of acetazolamide and furosemide to avoid cerebrospinal fluid shunts. J Pediatr 107:31–37, 1985.

57. International PHVD Drug Trial Group: International randomised controlled trial of acetazolamide and furosemide in posthaemorrhagic ventricular dilatation in infancy. Lancet 352:433–440, 1998.

58. Ventriculomegaly Group: Randomized trial of early tapping in neonatal posthaemorrhagic ventricular dilatation: Results at 30 months. Arch Dis Child Fetal Neonatal Ed 70:F129–136, 1994.

59. Anwar M, Kadam S, Hiatt IM, Hegyi T: Serial lumbar punctures in prevention of post-hemorrhagic hydrocephalus in preterm infants. J Pediatr 107:446–450, 1985.

60. Kreusser KL, Tarby TJ, Kovnar E, et al: Serial lumbar punctures for at least temporary amelioration of neonatal posthemorrhagic hydrocephalus. Pediatrics 75:719–724, 1985.

61. Papile LA, Burstein J, Burstein R, et al: Posthemorrhagic hydrocephalus in low-birth-weight infants: Treatment by serial lumbar punctures. J Pediatr 97:273–277, 1980.

62. Mantovani JF, Pasternak JF, Mathew OP, et al: Failure of daily lumbar punctures to prevent the development of hydrocephalus following intraventricular hemorrhage. J Pediatr 97:278–281, 1980.

63. Müller W, Urlesberger B, Naurer U, et al: Serial lumbar tapping to prevent posthaemorrhagic hydrocephalus after intracranial haemorrhage in preterm infants. Wien Klin Wochenschr 110:631–634, 1998.

64. Goldstein GW, Chaplin ER, Maitland J, Norman D: Transient hydrocephalus in premature infants: Treatment by lumbar punctures. Lancet 1:512–514, 1976.

65. Whitelaw A, Rivers P, Creighton L, Gaffney P: Low dose intraventricular fibrinolytic treatment to prevent posthaemorrhagic hydrocephalus. Arch Dis Child 67:12–14, 1992.

66. Pang D, Sclabassi RJ, Horton JA: Lysis of intraventricular blood clot with urokinase in a canine model: Part 3. Effects of intraventricular urokinase on clot lysis and posthemorrhagic hydrocephalus. Neurosurgery 19:553–572, 1986.

67. Luciano R, Tortorolo L, Chiaretti A, et al: Intraventricular streptokinase infusion in acute post-haemorrhagic hydrocephalus. Intensive Care Med 24:526–529, 1998.

68. Hudgins RJ, Boydston WR, Hudgins PA, Adler SR: Treatment of intraventricular hemorrhage in the premature infant with urokinase: A preliminary report. Pediatr Neurosurg 20:190–197, 1994.

69. Nowak S, Rudecka M, Polis L: Intraventricular administration of human recombinant plasminogen activator for posthemor-

rhagic hydrocephalus of the newborn. Acta Paeditr 88:348–349, 1999.

70. Hansen AR, Volpe JJ, Goumnerova LC, Madsen JR: Intraventricular urokinase for the treatment of posthemorrhagic hydrocephalus. Pediatr Neurol 17:213–217, 1997.

71. Haines SJ, Lapointe M: Fibrinolytic agents in the management of posthemorrhagic hydrocephalus in preterm infants: The evidence. Childs Nerv Syst 15:226–234, 1999.

72. Smith KM, Deddish RB, Ogata ES: Meningitis associated with serial lumbar punctures and post-hemorrhagic hydrocephalus. J Pediatr 109:1057–1060, 1986.

73. Bergman I, Wald ER, Meyer JD, Painter MJ: Epidural abscess and vertebral osteomyelitis following serial lumbar punctures. Pediatrics 72:476–480, 1983.

74. Gyorgy I: Neonatal intracranial haemorrhage: Aspiration through anterior fontanel in 23 cases. Acta Paediatr Acad Sci Hung 22:347–352, 1981.

75. Simon G: Neonatal ventricular haemorrhage: Treatment by puncture. Acta Paediatr Hung 26:281–287, 1985.

76. Levene MI: Ventricular tap under direct ultrasound control. Arch Dis Child 57:873–875, 1982.

77. Fleischer AC, Bundy AL, Hutchison AA, et al: Sonographic depiction of changes in ventricular size associated with repeated ventricular aspirations. J Ultrasound Med 2:499–504, 1983.

78. Afschrift M, Jeannin P, de Praeter C, et al: Ventricular taps in the neonate under ultrasonic guidance: Technical note. J Neurosurg 59:1100–1101, 1983.

79. Haraugh RE, Saunders RL, Edwards WH: External ventricular drainage for control of posthemorrhagic hydrocephalus in premature infants. J Neurosurg 55:766–770, 1981.

80. Kreusser KL, Tarby TJ, Taylor D, et al: Rapidly progressive posthemorrhagic hydrocephalus. Treatment with external ventricular drainage. Am J Dis Child 138:633–637, 1984.

81. Amato M, Guggisberg C, Kaiser G: Treatment of progressive posthemorrhagic hydrocephalus with temporary external ventricular drainage. Preliminary results. Helv Paediatr Acta 41:317–324, 1986.

82. Rhodes TT, Edwards WH, Saunders RL, et al: External ventricular drainage for initial treatment of neonatal posthemorrhagic hydrocephalus: Surgical and neurodevelopmental outcome. Pediatr Neurosci 13:255–262, 1987.

83. Gurtner P, Bass T, Gudeman SK, et al: Surgical management of posthemorrhagic hydrocephalus in 22 low-birth-weight infants. Childs Nerv Syst 8:198–202, 1992.

84. Weninger M, Salzer HR, Pollak A, et al: External ventricular drainage for treatment of rapidly progressive posthemorrhagic hydrocephalus. Neurosurgery 31:52–57, 1992.

85. Massone ML, Cama A, Leone D, et al: Results of early external ventricular diversion in posthemorrhagic ventricular dilatation in the newborn (in Italian). Minerva Anesthesiol 60:663–668, 1994.

86. Cornips E, Van Calenbergh F, Plets C, et al: Use of external drainage for posthemorrhagic hydrocephalus in very low birth weight premature infants. Childs Nerv Syst 13:369–374, 1997.

87. Finer NN, Woo BC, Hayashi A, Hayes B: Neonatal surgery: Intensive care unit versus operating room. J Pediatr Surg 28:645–649, 1993.

88. Perret GE, Graf CJ: Subgaleal shunt for temporary ventricle decompression and subdural drainage. J Neurosurg 47:590–595, 1977.

89. Drapkin AJ, Levine ME, Yang WC: Ventriculo-subgaleal shunt; evaluation by computed tomography. Acta Neurochir (Wien) 55:107–115, 1980.

90. Savitz MH, Katz SS: Ventriculosubgaleal shunting for acute head trauma. Crit Care Med 11:290–292, 1983.

91. Savitz MH: Another look at ventriculosubgaleal shunting procedures. Mt Sinai J Med 64:189–193, 1997.

92. Sklar F, Adegbite A, Shapiro K, Miller K: Ventriculosubgaleal shunts: Management of posthemorrhagic hydrocephalus in premature infants. Pediatr Neurosurg 18:263–265, 1992.

93. Rahman S, Teo C, Morris W, et al: Ventriculosubgaleal shunt: A treatment option for progressive posthemorrhagic hydrocephalus. Childs Nerv Syst 11:650–654, 1995.

94. McComb JG, Ramos AD, Platzker AC, et al: Management of hydrocephalus secondary to intraventricular hemorrhage in the preterm infant with a subcutaneous ventricular catheter reservoir. Neurosurgery 13:295–300, 1983.

95. Gaskill SJ, Marlin AE, Rivera S: The subcutaneous ventricular reservoir: An effective treatment for posthemorrhagic hydrocephalus. Childs Nerv Syst 4:291–295, 1988.

96. Leonhardt A, Steiner HH, Linderkamp O: Management of posthaemorrhagic hydrocephalus with a subcutaneous ventricular catheter reservoir in premature infants. Arch Dis Child 64:24–28, 1989.

97. Hudgins RJ, Boydston WR, Gilreath CL: Treatment of posthemorrhagic hydrocephalus in the preterm infant with a ventricular access device. Pediatr Neurosurg 29:309–313, 1998.

98. Benzel EC, Reeves JP, Nguyen PK, Hadden TA: The treatment of hydrocephalus in preterm infants with intraventricular haemorrhage. Acta Neurochir (Wien) 122:200–203, 1993.

99. Nulsen FE, Spitz EB: Treatment of hydrocephalus by direct shunt from ventricle to jugular vein. Surg Forum 2:399, 1952.

100. McComb JG: Techniques for CSF diversion. Concepts Neurosurg 47–66, 1990.

101. Brydon HL, Bayston R, Hayward R, Harkness W: The effect of protein and blood cells on the flow-pressure characteristics of shunts. Neurosurgery 38:498–504, discussion 505, 1996.

102. Scarff TB, Anderson DE, Anderson CL, et al: Complications of ventriculo-peritoneal shunts in premature infants. Concepts Pediatr Neurosurg 4:81–89, 1983.

103. Brydon HL, Keir G, Thompson EJ, et al: Protein adsorption to hydrocephalus shunt catheters: CSF protein adsorption. J Neurol Neurosurg Psychiatry 64:643–647, 1998.

104. Porter RW, Detwiler PW, Rekate HL: Hydrocephalus in children. In Kay AH, Black P (eds): Operative Neurosurgery. New York, Churchill Livingstone, 2000, pp 1215–1233.

105. Frim DM, Scott RM, Madsen JR: Surgical management of neonatal hydrocephalus. Neurosurg Clin North Am 9:105–110, 1998.

106. Keskil SI, Ceviker N, Baykaner K, Alp H: Index for optimum ventricular catheter length: Technical note. J Neurosurg 75:152–153, 1991.

107. Couldwell WT, LeMay DR, McComb JG: Experience with use of extended length peritoneal shunt catheters. J Neurosurg 85:425–427, 1996.

108. Laurence KM: Natural history of hydrocephalus. Detailed analysis of 182 unoperated cases. Arch Dis Child 37:345–362, 1962.

109. Resch B, Gedermann A, Maurer U, et al: Neurodevelopmental outcome of hydrocephalus following intra-/periventricular hemorrhage in preterm infants: Short- and long-term results. Childs Nerv Syst 12:27–33, 1996.

110. Fazzi E, Lanzi G, Gerardo A, et al: Neurodevelopmental outcome in very-low-birth-weight infants with or without periventricular haemorrhage and/or leucomalacia. Acta Paediatr 81:808–811, 1992.

111. Fletcher JM, Landry SH, Bohan TP, et al: Effects of intraventricular hemorrhage and hydrocephalus on the long-term neurobehavioral development of preterm very-low-birthweight infants. Dev Med Child Neurol 39:596–606, 1997.

112. Fernell E, Hagberg B, Hagberg G, et al: Epidemiology of infantile hydrocephalus in Sweden. Current aspects of the outcome in preterm infants. Neuropediatrics 19:143–145, 1988.

113. Landry SH, Fletcher JM, Denson SE, Chapieski ML: Longitudinal outcome for low birth weight infants: Effects of intraventricular hemorrhage and bronchopulmonary dysplasia. J Clin Exp Neuropsychol 15:205–218, 1993.

114. McCallum JE, Turbeville D: Cost and outcome in a series of shunted premature infants with intraventricular hemorrhage. Pediatr Neurosurg 20:63–67, 1994.

115. Sostek AM: Prematurity as well as intraventricular hemorrhage influence developmental outcome at 5 years. In Friedman SL, Sigman MD (eds): The Psychological Development of Low-Birthweight Children: Annual Advances in Applied Developmental Psychology. Norwood, NJ: Ablex, 1992, pp 259–274.

116. Selzer SC, Lindgren SD, Blackman JA: Long-term neuropsychological outcome of high risk infants with intracranial hemorrhage. J Pediatr Psychol 17(4):407–422, 1992.

CHAPTER 217

Shunt Infection

ELIZABETH B. CLAUS ■ CHARLES DUNCAN

Ventricular shunt catheter placement is a relatively common neurosurgical procedure performed for the treatment of hydrocephalus as well as for associated conditions in which the natural flow of cerebrospinal fluid (CSF) is obstructed. Approximately 125,000 individuals (or approximately 40 per 100,000 population) in the United States have shunts in place, the majority of whom are children.[1-3] The overall cost of surgical care for shunt procedures in 1991, excluding hospitalization, was estimated at $94 million.[1,2] One of the principal complications associated with the use of these devices is infection, with reported rates ranging from 1.5% to as high as 38%.[4-10] Age seems to be an important risk factor, with neonates and young children most frequently affected. The development of a shunt infection in a pediatric patient represents a particularly morbid condition; extended hospital stays and the loss or delay of educational and developmental milestones are common. Of even greater concern is the infection-related mortality among children, with rates up to 20% reported in the literature.[11] This high infection rate associated with a relatively common medical device predicts a large cost to individual patients, as well as to the health care system as a whole. These costs have led researchers to focus their efforts on isolating clinical covariates associated with shunt infection and developing treatment guidelines that attempt to lower the overall rate of infection. Despite the high prevalence of infection among shunted pediatric patients, greater numbers of these children are surviving into adulthood, making the study of health-related quality of life and long-term medical outcomes for these patients an exciting avenue of research in the field of neurosurgery. This chapter summarizes the clinical and epidemiologic risk factors, preventive measures, treatments, and long-term medical outcomes associated with the development of shunt infections in the pediatric population.

INFECTION RATE

Numerous researchers have attempted to estimate the overall rate of infection using a wide variety of sample sizes, study designs, and patient populations. The majority of these research efforts consist of a retrospective review of patient records, generally using data collected before 1990. In the largest of these investigations, Walters and colleagues[11] reviewed a population of almost 1500 patients who were treated with CSF shunting at the Hospital for Sick Children in Toronto over the 20-year period from 1960 to 1979. They found that 18% of shunted patients became infected at some time during the study period. When examining the infection rate per surgical procedure (rather than per patient) over the same period, the authors reported a value of 5%. Using a similar study design, Ammirati and Raimondi[4] reviewed the medical records of 431 children who were shunted between 1973 and 1982 at Children's Memorial Hospital in Chicago and found infection rates of 22% per patient and 6% per procedure over the 10-year period. More recently, Borgbjerg and associates[5] studied 884 individuals (440 of whom were younger than age 14) who underwent placement of a new shunt in Copenhagen from 1958 to 1989. The patient infection rate in this group was 6.2% for the first postoperative month, with an overall rate of 7.4%. In a study with relatively good follow-up data, Casey and colleagues[6] reviewed the 10-year course of 155 children with shunted hydrocephalus. These authors found that by 6 months, 9% of patients had suffered shunt infections; by 10 years, 19% had suffered infections.

In 1994, the general lack of consensus regarding the incidence of infection among patients undergoing shunt placement led the Education Committee of the International Society of Pediatric Neurosurgeons to sponsor a cooperative study to evaluate the issue.[12] This multicenter effort, which included data from 38 neurosurgical centers around the world, examined the risk of first complication (including infection) in newly implanted CSF devices for the treatment of hydrocephalus. The patients (children and adults) included in the analysis were operated on for the first time in 1991 and followed for at least 1 year. At the end of that time, 50 of 773, or approximately 6.5% of patients, had developed a shunt infection.

TIME TO INFECTION

Among pediatric patients, the majority of shunt infections occur relatively soon after placement of the shunt catheter.[6, 7] In one of the larger series of pediatric patients with extended follow-up, Casey and colleagues[6] reported that among children with shunted hydrocephalus who underwent a first shunt revision for infection, 92% of infections occurred within 3 months of the initial shunt placement. A second study of 81 children younger than 6 months old at the time of initial shunt placement noted similar patterns of shunt infection, with the majority of infections (11 of 14) occurring in the first 3 months after surgery.[7] This finding that shunt infection occurs soon after surgery is generally confirmed by the majority of researchers who have examined the subject.[5-7]

RISK FACTORS

In an effort to modify or reduce the rate of infection associated with the use of shunt devices, many investigators have attempted to identify risk factors. Despite such efforts, few clinical covariates have been consistently related to variations in infection rate. In general, the factor most frequently associated with an increased rate of shunt infection is the age of the patient,[4, 6, 11-13] with neonates and very young children at greatest risk. In their cohort study, Casey and colleagues[6] reported that children aged 6 months or younger had a 19% rate of infection, versus a rate of 7% among older children, a finding that is similar to the reports of other groups.[13]

A variety of potential explanations exist for the increased CSF shunt infection rate in very young children, including the presence of age-related changes in the density and identity of bacterial populations on the skin of neonates, as well as increased susceptibility to pathogens due to the relative deficiency of the neonatal immune system. In particular, children younger than 6 months have immunoglobulin G levels that are approximately half that of normal adults. Although maternal breast-feeding has been associated with the maintenance of immunoglobulin G levels in neonates, no data exist to explore the potential role of breast-feeding in reducing the risk of shunt infection. In addition to immunologic theories, intriguing data suggest that more highly adherent strains of coagulase-negative *Staphylococcus*, the most prevalent organism in shunt infections, occur among children younger than 6 months than among older children.[13]

Along with age, numerous other factors have been examined for their role in shunt infection, including time period, educational level of the surgeon, length and time of surgery, use of antibiotics before and after surgery, surgical method for placement of the distal catheter, type of shunt, reason for shunt (e.g., posthemorrhagic versus congenital hydrocephalus), previous shunt history, spinal dysraphism, number of early revisions, and concurrent infection. Among these variables, only reason for shunt placement,[6, 7] type of shunt,[5, 11] educational level of the surgeon,[3] and presence of spinal dysraphism[4] have been associated with increased rates of infection; it should be noted that these findings are not universal across studies. Two studies reported that patients with congenital hydrocephalus had lower rates of infection than did patients with either postinfectious or posthemorrhagic hydrocephalus. Dallacasa and associates[7] reported that half the children in the postinfectious-posthemorrhagic hydrocephalus group had at least one episode of shunt infection by the end of 1 year. With respect to type of shunt, two of the larger reviews of shunt infections reported that ventriculoperitoneal shunts had the highest rates of infection, although the increase was not statistically tested in the first[11] or significant in the second.[5] There is evidence that children with myelomeningocele may be at greater risk for infection than those with only congenital hydrocephalus.[4]

Few studies have the statistical power to test for potential interactions between or among risk factors or to perform subgroup analyses. One of the few investigations to do so identified a subgroup at particularly high risk, resulting in an important change in the clinical management of these children. In a study of 431 children with new shunt placements, Ammirati and Raimondi[4] found that children with myelomeningocele who were shunted in the first week of life had a two-fold increase in the incidence of infection relative to those shunted at 2 weeks of age or older. Almost 50% of the children with myelomeningocele who were shunted within 1 week of birth developed a shunt infection, versus 24% of those who underwent shunt placement between 2 and 8 weeks of life and 16% of those shunted between 9 and 52 weeks of life. Thus, clinically stable children with myelomeningocele might benefit from a delay in shunt placement.

PRESENTATION

The presenting symptoms of shunt infection are variable and age dependent but frequently include headache and lethargy, as well as nausea and vomiting. Infants may present with increased irritability or, in more severe cases, apnea and bradycardia. Additional complaints include fever; gait disturbances; seizures (particularly in patients with a baseline seizure disorder, although new-onset seizures are possible); visual disturbances, including upward gaze palsy and papilledema; abdominal pain; erythema or edema along the shunt tubing; fluid collection; and pseudocyst. The clinical presentation often varies by type of infecting organism. For example, patients with shunt infection caused by gram-negative bacilli such as *Escherichia coli* frequently present in a relatively acute fashion with severe abdominal pain or septicemia, whereas shunt infections caused by skin organisms such as *Staphylococcus epidermidis* tend to be more indolent in nature. *Staphylococcus aureus* infections may be associated with erythema along the shunt tract. Individuals with ventricular-vascular shunts may present with subacute bacterial endocarditis as well as shunt nephritis, an immune-complex disorder of the kidneys that is similar to glomerulonephritis.

EVALUATION AND DIAGNOSIS

As with all medical complaints, a complete history should be obtained and a physical examination per-

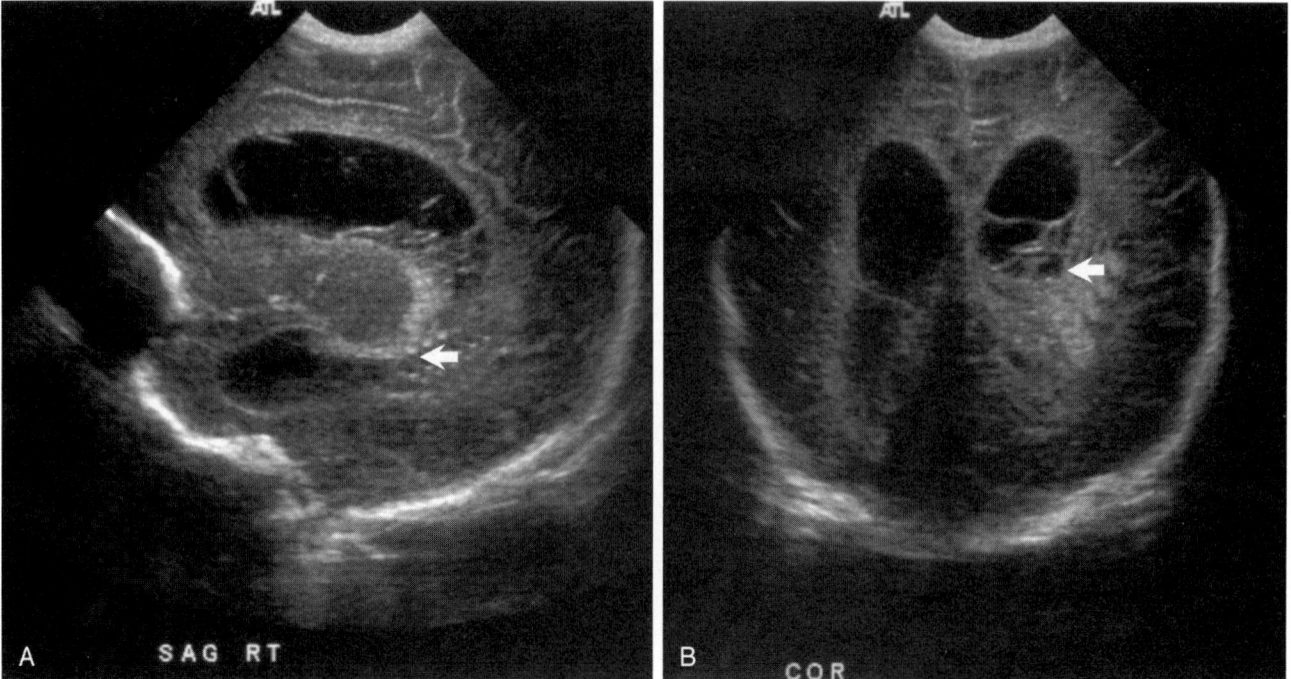

FIGURE 217-1. Sagittal *(A)* and coronal *(B)* ultrasographic views of the ventricular system and surrounding brain of a shunted newborn with sepsis and ventriculitis *(arrows)* after infection with *Serratia*.

formed in all patients with suspected shunt infections, with additional laboratory and imaging data collected as necessary. This is particularly important for infants and young children, in whom it may be difficult to distinguish between a shunt infection and syndromes such as viral infections; gastroenteritis, with its associated fever, nausea, and vomiting; urinary tract infections; upper respiratory tract infections; pneumonia; and even appendicitis. In general, a serum white blood cell count with differential, urinalysis, and blood cultures may be helpful. A thorough inspection of the skin overlying the shunt tubing is necessary; infection can occur along any aspect of the device.

Imaging is obtained to determine whether a shunt device is malfunctioning. In particular, plain x-ray films may reveal disruptions or disconnections in the shunt tubing. Such films can also elucidate a fluid collection, such as an abdominal abscess, or movement of the distal catheter out of the peritoneal space, as sometimes occurs with growth of the child. Although computed tomographic scans and ultrasonographic examinations are not specifically diagnostic of shunt infection—the exception being the ependymal enhancement that is characteristic of ventriculitis (Fig. 217–1)—these imaging modalities may be extremely helpful in defining generalized shunt malfunction when they are used to determine whether there is an enlargement of the ventricular space. Scans such as these are particularly useful when preexisting films are available for comparison, but they can be difficult to use in children with slit ventricles or in new patients with unusual baseline ventricular anatomy. In patients in whom distal catheter dysfunction is suspected or in

whom the abdomen is tender or distended, an abdominal ultrasonographic study helps define fluid collections (Fig. 217–2), as well as identify the location of the distal portion of the catheter.

If the previously mentioned analyses prove nondiagnostic but suspicion of a shunt infection remains high, a tap of the shunt can be performed under sterile

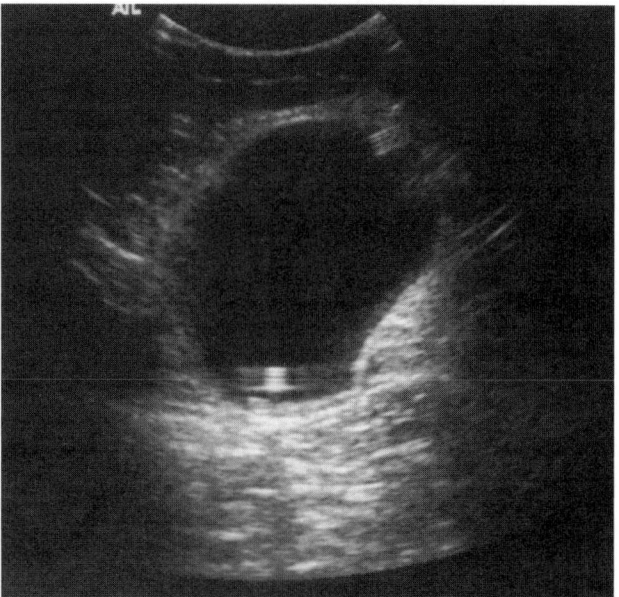

FIGURE 217-2. Sagittal ultrasonographic view of an abdominal fluid collection in a 7-year-old child with a ventriculoperitoneal shunt infected with methicillin-resistant *Staphylococcus aureus*.

conditions using a 22-gauge (or smaller) needle and manometer set. If the clinical suspicion of a shunt infection is low, the patient can be observed overnight in the hospital to avoid introducing infections into the shunt via a tap. If a tap is needed, the appropriate scalp area is prepared with an iodine solution. The initial insertion of the needle into the reservoir portion of the device provides evidence for or against function in the proximal (ventricular) portion of the device by the presence or absence of spontaneous flow of CSF. The opening pressure is also obtained at this time and is a measure of device function, with high pressure indicative of shunt malfunction. A rise in the opening pressure after the valve is manually occluded is indicative of at least partial valve function. To check distal catheter function, a column of sterile saline is raised (above the expected pressure level of the valve) in the manometer. Forward flow is indicative of distal function. To check for infection, CSF is tested for glucose, protein, cell counts, and microbiologic features, with low glucose, high protein, and high nucleated cell counts indicative of infection. CSF cultures may also be positive for infectious organisms, although this generally occurs in less than 50% of patients tested; hence, negative cultures cannot be used as a reliable indicator of shunt infection.

PREVENTION

Given the high medical, social, and economic costs associated with the occurrence of shunt infection, many investigators have attempted to identify preventive measures to reduce the rate of infection. In addition to the implementation of sterile surgical technique, perioperative antibiotic use has been intensely studied as a means of reducing infection rates. When one examines the various studies on their own, the conclusions are not consistent, with some providing evidence of a positive association and others reporting a negative association or none at all.[11, 14–16] In general, the reported risk ratio across studies ranged from approximately 0.40 to 0.60, corresponding to a 50% reduction in infection risk; unfortunately, all the studies were characterized by small sample sizes—with most including fewer than 75 individuals in both the treatment and the control arms—and thus had insufficient statistical power to declare this reduction significant.

Despite the limitations posed by small samples and low statistical power, the similarity in risk estimates led several investigators to attempt to circumvent this difficulty by combining information across studies in the form of a meta-analysis.[17, 18] In 1993, Langley and coworkers[18] identified 37 trials from the literature that examined the use of antibacterial drugs in shunt placement and selected 12 of them for more detailed evaluation based on a standardized set of selection criteria. In this meta-analysis of 1359 patients, the authors concluded that the perioperative use of antimicrobial agents in CSF shunt placement significantly reduced the rate of infection by approximately 50% (risk ratio [RR] = 0.52; 95% confidence interval [CI]: 0.37, 0.73).

Haines and Walters[17] performed a similar analysis but included data from eight randomized trials of antibiotic prophylaxis for shunt surgery using the selection criteria of Chalmers and associates.[19] Once again, the authors found that the use of prophylactic antibiotics before the placement of a shunt was associated with a 50% reduction in the infection rate relative to a control population (RR = 0.48; 95% CI: 0.31, 0.73). However, this effect was strongly related to the baseline infection rate and disappeared when the institution's baseline rate was less than or equal to 15%. Furthermore, although there was no significant modification in effect in the pooled results based on duration of antibiotic use or patient age, the studies included in the meta-analysis differed with respect to the specific type, duration, and dosage of antibiotic used, as well as the timing of first administration of the drug (although most investigators administered antibiotics either at the time of anesthesia induction or 1 to 2 hours before surgery). This lack of uniformity makes the development of a specific prophylactic treatment regimen difficult, despite the overall inference that the prophylactic use of antibiotics around the time of shunt placement reduces the rate of infectious complications.

In addition to prophylactic antibiotic use at the time of surgery, several other preventive measures have been suggested, including the administration of antibiotics before dental procedures, the use of a surgical isolation bubble system during surgery, the use of shunt tubing with polymeric silicone (Silastic) impregnated with antimicrobial agents, the use of one-piece systems (rather than two- or three-piece systems), annual or biannual screening examinations,[20] and the use of hypothermia at the time of surgery.[21] There is little evidence that any of these measures are associated with reduced infection rates, although many have been examined in samples that are too small to have any sort of statistical power.

ORGANISMS

CSF ventricular shunt catheter infections occur via three routes: the bloodstream, along the shunt tubing from an abdominal source (generally associated with bowel perforation, although in some instances, no gross disruption of the bowel is observed), and contamination of the shunt material with skin organisms at the time of surgery. The most common organisms found in shunt infections are typical skin flora. In most series, the predominant organism is the coagulase-negative *Staphylococcus epidermidis*,[6, 7, 9, 11, 12] followed, in roughly a 2:1 ratio, by *Staphylococcus aureus*. Interestingly, data suggest that in addition to its easy access to shunt material by virtue of being a skin contaminant, *Staphylococcus epidermidis* secretes a mucoid material that enhances its ability to adhere to foreign bodies such as shunt material.[22] Shunt infections in which enteric organisms are isolated are also frequently seen, including gram-negative bacteria such as *Escherichia coli*, *Proteus*, and *Klebsiella*. Delayed infections with anaerobic diphtheroids such as *Propionibacterium* are particularly difficult to assess and treat, as cultures may remain negative for more than a week. Fungal infections are reported but are less common than bacterial infections.

Infection can be defined as the presence of a positive CSF culture or, alternatively, as a positive culture from shunt hardware. The two are not necessarily highly correlated; in fact, in most instances of shunt infection, only the shunt hardware tests positive for bacterial or other growth, and the fluid itself remains negative. This finding is illustrated by Vanaclocha and colleagues,[23] who examined a series of 54 patients who had ventriculoperitoneal shunts removed because of malfunction and found that CSF cultures were positive in only 9% of cases, whereas 59% of the hardware (e.g., valve, tubing) cultures were positive, primarily for coagulase-negative organisms. A number of hypotheses exist to explain this finding; the primary one relates to the suggestion that bacteria and other microorganisms favor adhesion to foreign material over CSF, leading to a greater density on hardware and thus a positive culture test.

TREATMENT

Although the specifics may differ slightly among surgeons and institutions, the majority of shunt infections are currently treated by surgical removal of the infected shunt. A new shunt is then placed (if the patient still needs such a device) either at the time of removal of the infected device or at a later date. In many instances, shunt replacement is delayed until an interval of antibiotic use, with treatment given until CSF cultures are determined to be negative for bacterial growth. The recommended interval between shunt removal and reinsertion averages approximately 10 to 14 days, with at least 48 hours between the final negative CSF culture and reinsertion. In the interval between shunt removal and reinsertion, a variety of methods can be used to support shunt-dependent patients, including shunt externalization or placement of external ventricular or lumbar drainage catheters. In patients for whom temporary external drainage systems are not appropriate, intermittent lumbar punctures or ventricular taps can be performed. Patients who might require these methods include those with high CSF protein levels, and hence an increased propensity for valve malfunction, and those with repeated shunt infections, for whom the temporary removal of all foreign material may be necessary to clear material from the CSF. Replacement shunts are frequently placed at a new, contralateral location relative to the old shunt. In the case of infections associated with abdominal pseudocysts or abscesses, drainage of the abdominal wound must also be performed, and the shunt tubing removed.

CSF culture results are used to guide the selection of antibiotics during the interval between removal of the infected shunt and replacement of a new shunt. Given the preponderance of skin organisms such as *Staphylococcus epidermidis* and *Staphylococcus aureus* that are identified as infectious agents, intravenous vanco-

mycin is frequently used initially; rifampin may be added for increased coverage. Once the cultures have returned, antibiotics can be selected based on the identified organism and drug sensitivities. For example, in the absence of methicillin-resistant *S. aureus* organisms or penicillin-allergic patients, both *Staphylococcus epidermidis* and *Staphylococcus aureus* can be treated with oxacillin or nafcillin with good results.

An alternative to surgical replacement of the infected shunt is the use of antibiotics alone. Although there have been instances of eradication of shunt infection by this method,[10, 16, 24, 25] in general, purely medical treatment, administered either intravenously or via a joint intravenous-intrathecal protocol, appears to be less effective than surgical treatment with respect to patient morbidity and mortality.[11, 14] A number of authors have presented data from case series of patients with shunt infections treated with some combination of oral, intravenous, and intrathecal antibiotic therapy.[16, 25, 26] In general, these series report high rates of cure from the use of antibiotics alone; however, the sample sizes are small and are not from randomized trials. There is some evidence that the rates of success with medical treatment alone may vary by organism, although, again, the data are sparse, and the organisms for which this form of treatment may be more successful are not frequently implicated in shunt infection.[24] If the treatment regimen for a shunt infection is to be only antibiotics, the method of administration is extremely important, with the addition of intrathecal antibiotics associated with increased rates of cure and survival.[11] The use of intrathecal antibiotics is a necessary supplement to systemic treatment, given the known failure of most antibiotics to penetrate the blood-CSF barrier. Furthermore, frequent monitoring of the antibiotic level within the CSF is necessary to ascertain that the minimal inhibitory, bactericidal concentrations of these drugs are obtained.[25]

In the largest retrospective study comparing medical treatment with surgical treatment of shunt infections, Walters and colleagues[11] reviewed the medical records of 222 patients with infected CSF shunts treated at the Hospital for Sick Children in Toronto. They reported that only 14% of patients treated medically were cured of infection, versus approximately 60% of patients who received surgical treatment. Although the authors did not test the hypothesis statistically, their data suggest that cure rates obtained via purely medical treatment do not differ from those obtained when no treatment is offered. It should be noted that the majority of patients (85 of 92) treated medically in this study received only systemic antibiotics, with an associated cure rate of 9%. The small number of patients (7 of 92) who received systemic as well as intraventricular antibiotics had a cure rate of 43%, which, although less than that achieved in surgically treated patients, was much greater than for patients treated solely with systemic antibiotics. This highlights the need for appropriate administration of medication in patients for whom only medical intervention is possible.

In the sole randomized trial to compare medical versus surgical treatment of shunt infection, Frame and McLaurin[16] randomized 30 patients with ventriculoperitoneal shunts to one of three treatment arms: (1) removal of the shunt accompanied by the use of systemic antibiotics and an interim period of external ventricular drainage or ventricular taps, (2) immediate surgical replacement of the infected shunt along with antibiotic treatment, and (3) use of antibiotics only. To ensure that patients received the maximal benefit from the antibiotics, all the study subjects were given both intravenous and intraventricular antibiotics. The cure rates, as measured by negative CSF cultures 48 hours and 1 to 4 months after treatment, were 100%, 90%, and 30% for the three groups, respectively. In addition to lower rates of cure, medically treated patients had a mean hospital stay of 47 days, versus 33 and 25 days for the two surgical groups, respectively. These findings are confirmed by Walters and colleagues,[11] who noted that patients receiving medical treatment had longer hospital stays and higher rates of morbidity and mortality than did patients receiving surgical treatment.

In general, because of the relatively low reported rates of success in treating shunt infections with purely medical means, this form of management is usually reserved for patients who are poor surgical or anesthesia candidates or whose cerebral anatomy (e.g., slit ventricles) makes replacement of a ventricular catheter technically difficult.

OUTCOMES

It is of great interest to determine whether patients with shunt infections and hence repeated surgical procedures for shunt replacement have a poorer health-related quality of life as well as higher overall medical morbidity and mortality. Although some studies report no increase in the rate of death in infected versus noninfected children with shunts,[6] the data from many studies suggest an increased mortality risk.[8, 11] In a series of 108 infants presenting with hydrocephalus at birth and operated on from 1971 to 1981, Renier and associates[8] reported a 10-year survival rate of 71% in noninfected children, versus 51% in infected children. Similarly, Walters and colleagues[11] reported a mortality rate of 34% among infected patients, versus 18% in a group of shunted patients without infection.

Few studies include data on the long-term outcomes for patients with shunts, and the data that do exist provide conflicting results. Casey and colleagues[6] followed 155 shunted hydrocephalic children for 10 years and found no evidence that the number of infection-related episodes affected final intellectual outcome, with a good outcome defined as the child's being able to attend school. The statistics provided by others are more pessimistic.[7, 27] McLone and coworkers[27] found that shunted children with infections had a significantly lower average IQ (73 ± 26) than did shunted children without a history of infection (95 ± 19). Renier and associates[8] found similar results when reporting on 108 shunted infants followed for approximately 7 years and evaluated for intellectual performance, academic level, and psychological status. In this report, shunt infections were associated with poor functional

results; the mean "late" postoperative IQ was 40 among children who had had at least one shunt infection, versus an IQ of 60 among children without infection. Less than 5% of infected children had an IQ greater than 80, whereas approximately 36% of noninfected children had an IQ greater than 80. There has been no examination of the possible correlation between intellectual outcome and clinical or demographic patient characteristics, such as severity of infection or the age at which a child suffers an infection. Future studies need to examine these relationships in greater detail.

CONCLUSIONS

Infection remains a life-threatening and costly complication of ventricular shunt catheter placement. Costs for the care of individuals with shunts are high. In Canada, the average cost of one hospitalization in 1996 for shunt treatment of a hydrocephalic patient was approximately $17,500. A 1985 study in New York estimated that the average cost for the placement of a shunt was approximately $27,600.[3] Although an extensive literature exists on the topic, few preventable risk factors have been elucidated, and no consensus exists regarding the true annualized rate of infection, making it difficult to develop and implement standardized guidelines for shunt placement associated with reduced infection rates. Despite these limitations, the prevalence of shunt infections appears to have decreased since the 1970s, and several straightforward means of preventing shunt infections exist. In particular, strict adherence to sterile surgical technique and the use of prophylactic antibiotics at the time of surgery are two effective methods of reducing the rate of infection. In addition, among clinically stable neonates with both hydrocephalus and myelomeningocele, a delay in the placement of a shunt until the child is several weeks of age appears to reduce the rate of infection significantly.

The need for additional prospective studies of patients with ventricular shunt catheters is obvious, given the large number of individuals with such devices in place and the fact that the majority of these individuals will undergo at least one revision in their lifetime owing to infection. Furthermore, future studies need to define the long-term outcomes and quality-of-life issues associated with the development of infection so that the needs of this population can be addressed and the full intellectual potential of these children realized.

REFERENCES

1. Moss A, Hamburger S, Moore R, et al: Use of Selected Medical Device Implants in the United States, 1988. Vital and Health Statistics no. 191. Hyattsville, Md, National Center for Health Statistics, 1990.
2. Bondurant CP, Jimenez DF: Epidemiology of cerebrospinal fluid shunting. Pediatr Neurosurg 23:254–259, 1995.
3. Del Bigio MR: Epidemiology and direct economic impact of hydrocephalus: A community based study. Can J Neurol Sci 25: 123–126, 1998.
4. Ammirati M, Raimondi AJ: Cerebrospinal fluid infections in children: A study on the relationship between the etiology of hydro-

cephalus, age at the time of shunt placement, and infection rate. Childs Nerv Syst 3:106–109, 1987.

5. Borgbjerg BM, Gjerris F, Albeck MJ, et al: Risk of infection after cerebrospinal fluid shunt: An analysis of 884 first-time shunts. Acta Neurochir 136:1–7, 1995.

6. Casey ATH, Kimmings EJ, Kleinlugtebeld AD, et al: The long-term outlook for hydrocephalus in children: A ten-year cohort study of 155 patients. Pediatr Neurosurg 27:63–70, 1997.

7. Dallacasa P, Dappozza A, Galassi E, et al: Cerebrospinal fluid shunt infections in infants. Childs Nerv Syst 11:643–649, 1995.

8. Renier D, Sainte-Rose C, Pierre-Kahn A, et al: Prenatal hydrocephalus: Outcome and prognosis. Childs Nerv Syst 4:213–222, 1988.

9. Rotim K, Miklic P, Paladino J, et al: Reducing the incidence of infection in pediatric cerebrospinal fluid shunt operations. Childs Nerv Syst 13:584–587, 1997.

10. Caldarelli M, DiRocco C, LaMarca F: Shunt complications in the first postoperative year in children with meningomyelocele. Childs Nerv Syst 12:748–754, 1996.

11. Walters BC, Hoffman HJ, Hendrick EB, et al: Cerebrospinal fluid shunt infection: Influences on initial management and subsequent outcome. J Neurosurg 60:1014–1021, 1984.

12. Di Rocco C, Marchese E, Velardi F: A survey of the first complication of newly implanted CSF shunt devices for the treatment of nontumoral hydrocephalus. Cooperative Study of the 1991–1992 Education Committee of the ISPN. Childs Nerv Syst 10:321–327, 1994.

13. Pople IK, Bayston R, Hayward RD: Infection of cerebrospinal fluid shunts in infants: A study of etiological factors. J Neurosurg 77:29–36, 1992.

14. James HE, Walsh JW, Wilson HD, et al: Prospective randomized study of therapy in cerebrospinal fluid shunt infection. Neurosurgery 7:459–463, 1980.

15. Schmidt K, Gjerris F, Osgaard O, et al: Antibiotic prophylaxis in cerebrospinal fluid shunting: A prospective randomized trial in 152 hydrocephalic patients. Neurosurgery 17:1–5, 1985.

16. Frame PT, McLaurin RL: Treatment of CSF shunt infections with intrashunt plus oral antibiotic therapy. J Neurosurg 60:354–360, 1984.

17. Haines SJ, Walters BC: Antibiotic prophylaxis for cerebrospinal fluid shunts: A meta-analysis. Neurosurgery 34:87–93, 1994.

18. Langley JM, LeBlanc JC, Drake J, et al: Efficacy of antimicrobial prophylaxis in placement of cerebrospinal fluid shunts: Meta-analysis. Clin Infect Dis 17:98–103, 1993.

19. Chalmers TC, Smith H Jr, Blackburn B, et al: A method for assessing the quality of a randomized clinical trial. Control Clin Trials 2:31–49, 1981.

20. Colak A, Albright AL, Pollack IF: Follow-up of children with shunted hydrocephalus. Pediatr Neurosurg 27:208–210, 1997.

21. Gerszten PC, Albright AL, Pollack IF, et al: Intraoperative hypothermia and ventricular shunt infections. Acta Neurochir 140:591–594, 1998.

22. Bayston R, Penny SR: Excessive production of mucoid substance in *Staphylococcus* SIIA: A possible factor in colonization of Holter shunts. Dev Med Child Neurol 14(suppl 24):25, 1972.

23. Vanaclocha V, Saiz-Sapena N, Leiva J: Shunt malfunction in relation to shunt infection. Acta Neurochir 138:829–834, 1996.

24. Lerman SJ: *Haemophilus influenzae* infections of cerebrospinal fluid shunts: Report of two cases. J Neurosurg 54:261–263, 1981.

25. Wald SL, McLaurin RL: Cerebrospinal fluid antibiotic levels during treatment of shunt infections. J Neurosurg 52:41–46, 1980.

26. Mates S, Glaser J, Shapiro K: Treatment of cerebrospinal fluid shunt infections with medical therapy alone. Neurosurgery 11:781–783, 1982.

27. McLone DG, Czyewski D, Raimondi AJ, et al: Central nervous system infections as a limiting factor in the intelligence of children with myelomeningocele. Pediatrics 70:338, 1992.

CHAPTER 218

Neuroendoscopy

KERRY R. CRONE

Current trends in surgical disciplines have been toward the use of minimally invasive forms of diagnosis and treatment. Endoscopy represents one modality in the spectrum of minimally invasive techniques. Although interest in this modality is great, the use of endoscopic surgery for the treatment of neurosurgical disorders is not new.

HISTORICAL PERSPECTIVE

During the first part of the 20th century, attempts were made to use endoscopy for the diagnosis and treatment of hydrocephalus. In 1910, L'Espinase inserted a cystoscope designed for the adult bladder into the cerebral ventricles of two infants with hydrocephalus.[1] Although fulguration of the choroid plexus was successful in both patients, one infant died immediately; the second infant survived for at least 5 years. In 1922, Dandy was the second to report on this procedure, again attempting to fulgurate the choroid plexus of infants with hydrocephalus; these attempts failed because of the primitive instrumentation available.[2]

Despite the limited effectiveness of these early procedures, other attempts were made to treat hydrocephalus using fenestration techniques. In 1923, Fay and Grant failed in their attempt to create a fistula in the corpus callosum between the ventricles and the subarachnoid spaces.[3] The same year, Mixter performed the first successful third ventriculostomy in a 9-month-old infant with noncommunicating hydrocephalus.[4] As a result, the infant's head circumference decreased and the fontanelle softened. All these reports discussed the inspection of enlarged ventricles and the attempted endoscopic treatment of hydrocephalus, a condition for which no alternative method of treatment existed.

During the next several decades, two investigators tried to treat hydrocephalus by obliterating the choroid plexus. In 1943, Putnum reported that among 23 patients treated, 6 improved and 4 died.[5] In 1970, Scarff observed that among 39 patients treated, 26 had arrested hydrocephalus and 4 died.[6] However, with the development of the Spitz-Holter valve and diversionary shunt systems to control hydrocephalus, interest in endoscopic surgery for the treatment of hydrocephalus

decreased. In 1960, the development of the rod-lens scope by Hopkins provided superior optics and improved illumination, leading to renewed interest in endoscopy.[7]

ENDOSCOPIC TECHNOLOGY

The general components of the instruments used for neurosurgical endoscopy are identical to those used in other surgical disciplines, except for the small size of the neurosurgical endoscope. Presently, two general types of endoscopes are available: rod-lens scopes and fiberscopes.

Rigid endoscopes transmit images through a series of lenses, whereas fiberscopes transmit images through carefully sorted and arranged fiber-optic threads. Rigid systems give clearer images than fiberscopes do (Fig. 218–1; see color section in this volume), but fiberscopes can be maneuvered without image distortion. In addition to the basic elements for viewing, other ports or working channels may be available for instrumentation, including energy delivery systems (e.g., laser fibers, electrocautery systems) and irrigation apparatuses (with or without suction). The diameter of the working channel limits the type of endoscopic instrumentation that can be developed. Rigid endoscopes that offer an assortment of viewing angles are available but are useful only for viewing. The appropriate endoscope for a particular procedure is selected dudring preoperative planning.

Although the procedure can be viewed directly through the endoscope, I prefer to operate with the aid of a viewing system comprising a camera, monitor, and light source. The light source, which is connected to the endoscope via a fiber-optic cable, must be bright enough to illuminate the operative field without transmitting excessive heat to the tip of the scope. Halogen, mercury vapor, and xenon light sources are available. The camera, which is connected to the endoscope via an adapter, transmits the image to a video monitor for viewing by the surgical team.

Irrigation is essential during the operative procedure to clear the lens of debris, clear the operative field of any blood, help prevent the collapse of the fluid-filled

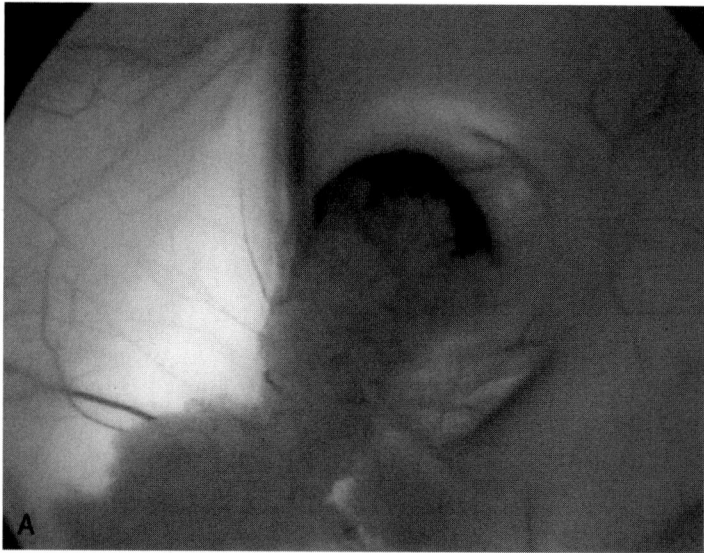
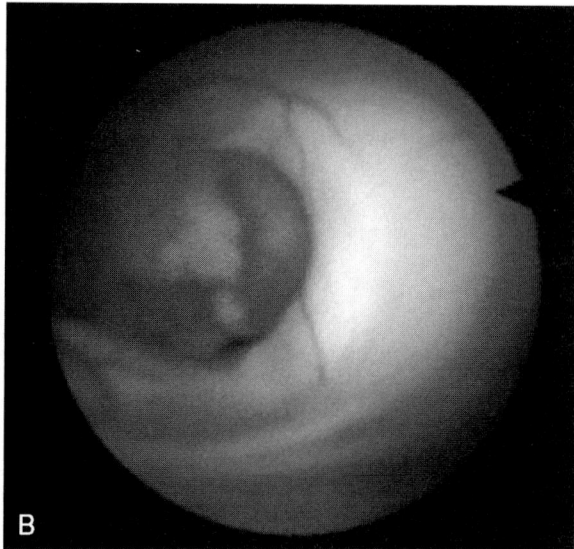

FIGURE 218–1. View of the foramen of Monro though the lateral ventricle using a rod-lens (rigid) endoscope *(A)* and a 4-mm steerable fiberscope *(B)* (see color section in this volume). (Courtesy of Mayfield Clinic, Cincinnati, OH.)

ventricular system, and avoid thermal injury. Lactated Ringer's solution is preferred over 0.9% sodium chloride because it is more physiologically accurate.

APPLICATIONS

Endoscopy has both diagnostic and therapeutic applications. The endoscope can be used as a diagnostic tool for anatomic surveillance. Therapeutically, it can be used to take biopsy samples or resect tumors, optimally position the ventricular catheter in diversionary shunts, or fenestrate membranes between isolated compartments to establish cerebrospinal fluid flow or communication. The endoscope can be used as either the principal operative tool or an adjunct to conventional craniospinal procedures.

Ventricular Shunts

The most common causes of shunt malfunction include infection, disconnection, and proximal or distal catheter obstruction.[8] During the first year after shunting, expected malfunction rates approximate 31%; proximal catheter obstruction is the most common cause of malfunction.[8]

Techniques for optimal positioning of the ventricular catheter during shunting procedures offer several advantages, such as reducing ventricular catheter obstruction from cannulation of the temporal horn or parenchyma and reducing the growth of the choroid plexus into the catheter holes.[9] These techniques include checking the position of the catheter with plain radiographs or air cisternography and using ultrasound-guided catheter placement, stereotactic frames, or frameless stereotactic technology. Although these techniques increase the precision for optimal placement

compared with blind cannulation of the ventricle, each technique has distinct disadvantages. Plain radiographs or air cisternography cannot always identify the position of the catheter, and radiographs only indirectly guide the surgeon to reposition the catheter if the trajectory or depth is believed to be incorrect. Ultrasound guidance requires a craniectomy if the child does not have an open fontanelle. Framed and frameless stereotactic technology requires additional preoperative imaging and immobilization of the head, which may not be feasible for shunting procedures.

The best technique should be safe, simple, and easy to use. Current endoscopes used for positioning the ventricular catheter are thin fiber-optic scopes that are passed through the lumen of the shunt catheter. The endoscope is passed through a small slit in the tip of the catheter to permit guidance through the ventricular system (Fig. 218–2). The catheter tip is positioned above the choroid plexus through a coronal approach, or anterior to the choroid plexus through a parieto-occipital approach. Using this technique, Taha and Crone reported a 98% accuracy as confirmed by postoperative computed tomographic scans.[10]

Endoscopy has been used successfully in the management of proximal shunt revision. When the catheter appears densely adherent to the choroid plexus or ventricular ependyma, intraventricular hemorrhage may result from vigorous attempts to dislodge the catheter.[11] Although several techniques have been described to remove an adherent ventricular catheter, they do not provide direct visualization of the site of catheter adherence.[11, 12] Therefore, the potential for intraventricular hemorrhage is unchanged if these techniques are used. A maneuverable fiberscope, with a laser fiber or monopolar electrode to coagulate the choroid plexus, greatly reduces the risk of hemorrhage because the obstruction can be dissected and coagulated with precision.

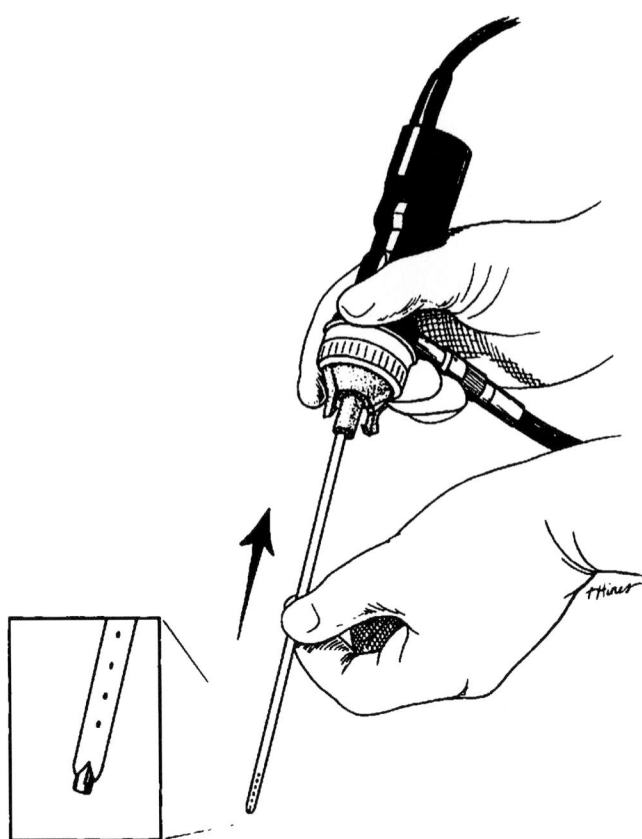

FIGURE 218–2. Disposable fiberscope placed through a proximal shunt catheter for accurate placement of the shunt tip. (Courtesy of Mayfield Clinic, Cincinnati, OH.)

Membrane Fenestration

The possibility of managing hydrocephalus without implanting shunt systems has attracted the greatest interest in neuroendoscopy. The ability to bring into communication previously loculated compartments within the ventricular system with minimal cortical disruption has many advantages over the use of complex shunt systems or conventional craniotomy. Despite the interest in this endoscopic method for treating compartmentalized or loculated hydrocephalus, until recently, little information was available regarding its success.

Indications for endoscopy in the management of hydrocephalus are divided into four categories: (1) compartmentalized hydrocephalus arising from intraventricular septations, (2) unilateral hydrocephalus comprising an isolated lateral ventricle, (3) noncolloid neuroepithelial cysts, and (4) obstructive hydrocephalus treated with third ventriculostomy.

Compartmentalized hydrocephalus can be either uniloculated or multiloculated. This distinction is important, because the pathogenesis of these cysts and the chance of their successful treatment differ markedly. Multiloculated cysts usually occur after an episode of meningitis or germinal matrix hemorrhage, whereas most cases of uniloculated hydrocephalus result from noncolloid neuroepithelial cysts. The man-

agement goals for both types of hydrocephalus are the same: control the hydrocephalus, avoid implanting a diversionary shunt if possible, and reduce the operative morbidity. Powers reported on the endoscopic treatment of two patients with loculated ventricular cysts.[13, 14] Heilman and Cohen described the endoscopic treatment of three patients with ventricular obstructions.[15] Although both reports demonstrated favorable outcomes, the series were too small to be conclusive.[16] Lewis and colleagues reported a significant reduction in the shunt revision rate of patients with loculated hydrocephalus who underwent endoscopic fenestration.[17] Patients with posthemorrhagic or postmeningeal multiloculated hydrocephalus and patients with uniloculated hydrocephalus who have indwelling shunt systems often require repeat endoscopic procedures.

Unilateral hydrocephalus may result from any condition that produces an asymmetrical gradient across the foramen of Monro. Common causes include congenital atresia of the foramen of Monro, tumors situated in the anterior third ventricle, and after-shunting ventricle syndrome. Endoscopic fenestration of the septum pellucidum provides a safe and effective form of treatment to allow communication between the lateral ventricles. A diversionary shunt system can be avoided in cases of congenital foraminal atresia, whereas a simplified shunt system can be used in tumor obstruction (Fig. 218–3; see color section in this volume).

Neuroendoscopy has provided a safe, effective method for the management of intraventricular and paraventricular noncolloid neuroepithelial cysts. Suprasellar arachnoid cysts can be fenestrated into the ventricular system, and in most instances, an indwelling diversionary shunt system can be avoided.[18] Pineal cysts that cause obstructive hydrocephalus can be fenestrated to relieve the obstruction, permitting the return of normal flow through the aqueduct of Sylvius.[19]

Third ventriculostomy has attracted the most atten-

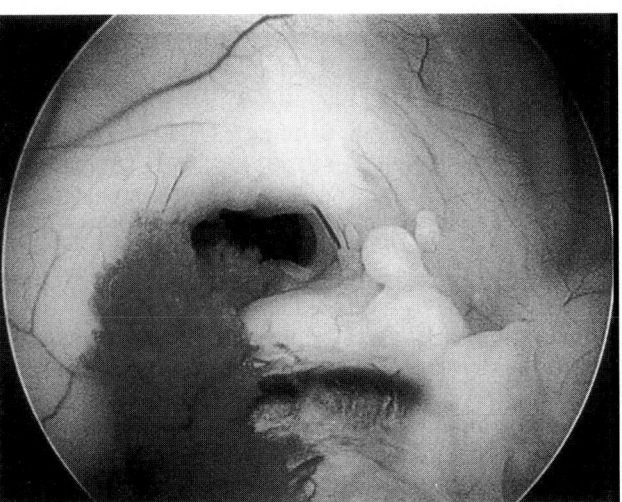

FIGURE 218–3. Endoscopic view of a thalamic tumor protruding through the ventricular wall at the time of shunt placement. The endoscopic biopsy determined it to be a low-grade glioma (see color section in this volume). (Courtesy of Mayfield Clinic, Cincinnati, OH.)

tion among all neuroendoscopic procedures. In 1923, Mixter performed the first endoscopic third ventriculostomy using a urethroscope directed into the ventricle; a flexible sound was used for fenestration.[4] The procedure never became popular because of poor illumination and the cumbersome size of the instrumentation. During the next several decades, additional reports of third ventriculostomy yielded inconsistent results with unacceptable morbidity. This fact, coupled with the development of valve-regulated shunts, resulted in loss of interest in third ventriculostomy. Diversionary shunt systems appeared to offer a simplistic approach to the treatment of hydrocephalus without the risks associated with an endoscopic procedure. Neurosurgeons soon realized, however, that diversionary shunt systems posed new lifelong problems for patients, including shunt obstruction, disconnection, and infection. The development of computed tomography, which aided in the understanding of hydrocephalus, coupled with improvements in endoscopic technology sparked a renewed interest in third ventriculostomy that continues to the present.

The major challenge in endoscopic third ventriculostomy is selection of those patients who are the best candidates for the procedure. Whereas Grant and McLone[16] proposed managing both communicating and noncommunicating forms of hydrocephalus with third ventriculostomy, indicating success in communicating hydrocephalus, most reports have focused on the application of third ventriculostomy for noncommunicating or obstructive forms of hydrocephalus.[7, 20–26] Previous radiation treatment and meningeal infection have been reported to decrease the success rate of the procedure in obstructive forms of hydrocephalus; likewise, reports have detailed the failure of third ventriculostomy in patients with congenital aqueductal stenosis.[27] The highest success rates (patency 8% to 90%) have been achieved in adolescents with late-onset aqueductal stenosis.[15, 28]

Tumor Biopsy and Resection

The use of endoscopy for the biopsy and removal of intraventricular lesions has proved to be effective. An early report by Fukishima demonstrated the benefits of endoscopic biopsy.[29] Despite its accuracy rate of only 50% in establishing the diagnosis, lesions smaller than 2 to 3 cm in diameter were removed easily without complication.[30]

Currently, the colloid cyst is the lesion most commonly removed by endoscopic methods (Fig. 218–4; see color section in this volume). Several reports detail the successful endoscopic management of third ventricular colloid cysts.[31, 32] Although the initial results are comparable or superior to those of conventional craniotomy with regard to operative morbidity, considerable uncertainty remains concerning the potential long-term recurrence rate of colloid cysts removed through this minimally invasive approach. No long-term studies have reported on recurrence rates because few procedures have been performed, and the duration of follow-up is quite short. Since 1992, 30 patients have

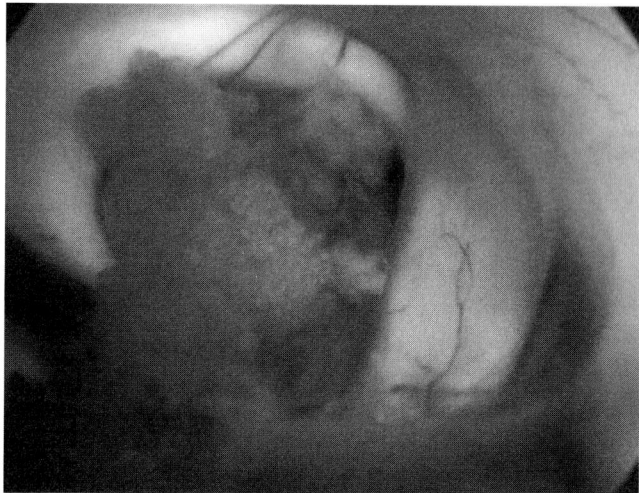

FIGURE 218–4. Endoscopic approach through the lateral ventricle to a third ventricular colloid cyst sitting just inside the foramen magnum, viewed through a rod-lens endoscope (see color section in this volume). (Courtesy of Mayfield Clinic, Cincinnati, OH.)

undergone endoscopic removal of colloid cysts at the University of Cincinnati Medical Center. To date, only one patient developed a recurrent colloid cyst during the follow-up period (mean, 4 years); this suggests that recurrence is infrequent.

Endoscope-Assisted Microsurgery

The use of neuroendoscopy as an operative adjunct to conventional craniotomy has been reported.[33–35] Hopf and coworkers demonstrated the effectiveness of endoscopy in the management of various intracranial conditions (e.g., vascular anomalies, tumors, arachnoid cysts).[22, 36] The endoscope may be used to evaluate clip placement in cerebral aneurysms by inspecting the backside of the aneurysm to be certain that perforating vessels have been excluded from the occlusive vascular clip. Similarly, a rigid endoscope with varying viewing-angle lenses has been used to inspect tumor resections in cranial skull base procedures. Further advances in endoscopic technology may someday supplant the need for a large microscope in many of these procedures.

Spinal Applications

Spinal endoscopic procedures were performed in cadavers by Burman[37] in 1931 and Stern[38] in 1936 and were first performed in patients in 1938. Pool's primitive instrumentation enabled visualization of the intradural contents and the diagnosis of arachnoiditis and spinal neoplasms.[39] Despite significant advances in endoscope technology, few references exist between these early reports and later ones that describe the application of endoscopy to the spinal axis.

Huewel and colleagues described the use of a fiberscope to inspect intramedullary cavities in syringomyelia.[28] After a myelotomy was performed, a small-diameter fiberscope inserted into the spinal cord syrinx was used to visualize the many septations traversing the cavity and, in rare instances, the compartmentalization of the syrinx.

Perhaps the greatest challenge in neurosurgical applications of endoscopy has involved endoscopic diskectomy, including the thoracoscopic removal of thoracic disks, posterolateral approaches for the removal of L4-5 disks, and laparoscopic approaches for the removal of L5-S1 disks.[40, 41] Paraspinal tumors in the thoracic and lumbar regions may also be approached with thoracoscopic and laparoscopic techniques, respectively.

Surgical management for lumbar disk disease currently consists of microsurgical diskectomy—a safe and effective procedure that requires a short hospital stay. Although percutaneous lumbar diskectomy encompasses many techniques, the goal is removal of the herniated nucleus pulposus in the dorsal portion of the disk space. However, if an endoscope is not used, most percutaneous techniques are limited to removal of the central disk contents. If subligamentous prolapse is included in the spectrum of indications, then endoscopic control is necessary. Single and biportal approaches, as well as transforaminal diskectomy with small fiberscopes, have been described.[40, 41] Presently, the indications for these approaches are few; the essential surgical instrumentation has not yet been perfected, and extensive comparisons of these approaches versus microdiskectomy are not available. Despite these limitations, efforts to perfect percutaneous dorsolateral diskectomy, laparoscopic lumbar diskectomy with fusion, and thoracoscopic diskectomy are continuing. Certainly these procedures will evolve and become the techniques of choice for spinal surgery in various clinical situations.

COMPLICATIONS

Expected complications associated with endoscopic surgery are similar to those of conventional neurosurgical procedures and include hemorrhage, infection, and neurological deficit. To date, few complications have been reported with endoscopic techniques. In a 1988 report by Auer and coworkers on a series of 109 endoscopic procedures, no patient developed intraoperative bleeding, and two patients experienced postoperative intracranial hemorrhage.[33] In 1994, Jones and colleagues reported two major complications and two minor complications in 24 patients undergoing third ventriculostomy.[23] The two major complications were related to bleeding: one patient who had undergone previous radiotherapy experienced significant bleeding before the third ventricular floor was perforated, and the second patient developed a subdural hematoma and improved. The two minor complications were scalp abscess and ataxia. Two cases of hemorrhage were reported by Powers in seven patients undergoing intraventricular cyst fenestration.[13] Zamarano and colleagues reported on one patient who had an intraoperative seizure that resulted in irreversible cerebral hypoxia.[42] More recent reports have described additional complications associated with neuroendoscopic surgery.[43]

SUMMARY

Minimally invasive surgery has generated enthusiasm in all surgical disciplines. Although limited experience precludes firm conclusions regarding the potential benefits of neurosurgical applications, most reports demonstrate that many procedures can be performed safely with minimal risk to patients. Questions regarding the impact on health care costs remain unanswered. The true benefits and applications of endoscopy may not be fully appreciated until image-guided systems are coupled with endoscopes and more technically precise instruments are developed for performing more complex procedures. At that time, the role of endoscopy in neurosurgical practice may be more clearly defined.

REFERENCES

1. Davis L: Neurological Surgery. Philadelphia, Lea & Febiger, 1939, p 405.
2. Dandy WE: Treatment of non-encapsulated brain tumors by extensive resection of contiguous brain tissue. Johns Hopkins Hosp Bull 33:118–190, 1922.
3. Fay T, Grant FC: Ventriculoscopy and intraventricular photography in internal hydrocephalus. JAMA 80:461–463, 1923.
4. Mixter WJ: Ventriculostomy and puncture of the floor of the third ventricle. Boston Med Surg J 188:277–278, 1923.
5. Putnum TJ: The surgical treatment of infantile hydrocephalus. Surg Gynecol Obstet 76:171–182, 1943.
6. Scarff JE: The treatment of nonobstructive hydrocephalus by endoscopic cauterization of the choroid plexus. J Neurosurg 33:1–18, 1970.
7. Gans SL: Principles of optics and illumination. In Gans SL (ed): Pediatric Endoscopy. Philadelphia, Grune & Stratton, 1983, pp 1–8.
8. Sainte-Rose C, Piatt JH, Renier D, et al: Mechanical complications in shunts. Pediatr Neurosurg 17:2–9, 1991–1992.
9. Vries JK: Endoscopy as an adjunct to shunting for hydrocephalus. Surg Neurol 13:69–72, 1980.
10. Taha JM, Crone KR: Endoscopically guided shunt placement. In Techniques in Neurosurgery, vol 1. Philadelphia, Lippincott Raven, 1996, pp 159–167.
11. Aoki N, Sakai T: Avulsion of the choroid plexus during revision of ventricular shunting: Its high incidence and predictive value on computed tomography scan. Surg Neurol 33:256–260, 1990.
12. Chehrazi B, Duncan C: Removal of retained ventricular shunt catheters without craniotomy: Technical note. J Neurosurg 56:160–161, 1982.
13. Powers SK: Fenestration of intraventricular cysts using a flexible, steerable endoscope. Acta Neurochir Suppl (Wien) 54:42–46, 1992.
14. Powers SK: Fenestration of intraventricular cysts using a flexible, steerable endoscope and argon laser. Neurosurgery 18:637–641, 1986.
15. Heilman CB, Cohen A: Endoscopic ventricular fenestration using a "saline torch." J Neurosurg 74:224–229, 1991.
16. Grant J, McLone D: Third ventriculostomy: A review. Surg Neurol 47:210–212, 1997.
17. Lewis AI, Keiper GL, Crone KR: Endoscopic treatment of loculated hydrocephalus. J Neurosurg 82:780–785, 1995.
18. Caemaert J, Absullah J, Calliauw L: Endoscopic diagnosis of and treatment of para- and intraventricular cystic lesions. Acta Neurochir (Wien) 61:69–75, 1994.
19. Ruge J, Johnson R, Bauer J: Burr hole neuroendoscopic fenestration of quadrigeminal cistern arachnoid cyst: Technical case report. Neurosurgery 38:830–837, 1996.

20. Baskin J, Manwaring K, Rekate H: Ventricular shunt removal: The ultimate treatment of the slit ventricle syndrome. J Neurosurg 88:478–484, 1998.

21. Cinalli G, Salazar C, Mallucci C, et al: The role of endoscopic third ventriculostomy in the management of shunt malfunction. Neurosurgery 43:1323–1329, 1998.

22. Hopf N, Grunert P, Fries G, et al: Endoscopic third ventriculostomy: Outcome analysis of 100 consecutive procedures. Neurosurgery 44:795–805, 1999.

23. Jones RFC, Kwok BCT, Stening WA: Neuroendoscopic third ventriculostomy: A practical alternative to extracranial shunt in noncommunicating hydrocephalus. Acta Neurochir Suppl (Wien) 61: 79–83, 1994.

24. Jones RFC, Stening WA, Brydon M: Endoscopic third ventriculostomy. Neurosurgery 26:86–92, 1990.

25. Schwartz T, Yoon S, Cutruzzola F, Goodman R: Third ventriculostomy: Post-operative ventricular size and outcome. Minim Invasive Neurosurg 39:122–129, 1996.

26. Torrens M: Endoscopic neurosurgery. Neurosurg Q 5:18–33, 1995.

27. Cinalli G, Sainte-Rose C, Chumas P, et al: Failure of third ventriculostomy in the treatment of aqueductal stenosis in kids. J Neurosurg 90:448–454, 1999.

28. Huewel N, Perneczky A, Urban V, Fries G: Neuroendoscopic techniques for the operative treatment of septated syringomyelia. Acta Neurochir Suppl (Wien) 54:59–62, 1982.

29. Fukishima T: Endoscopic biopsy of intraventricular tumors with the use of a ventriculofiberscope. Neurosurgery 2:110–113, 1976.

30. Gaab MR, Schroeder WS: Neuroendoscopic approach to intraventricular lesions. J Neurosurg 88:496–505, 1998.

31. Abdou M, Cohen M: Endoscopic treatment of colloid cysts of the third ventricle. J Neurosurg 89:1062–1068, 1998.

32. Lewis AI, Crone KR, Taha JM, et al: Surgical resection of third ventricle colloid cysts: Preliminary results comparing transcallosal microsurgery with endoscopy. J Neurosurg 81:171–178, 1994.

33. Auer LM, Holzer P, Ascher PW, Heppner F: Endoscopic neurosurgery. Acta Neurochir (Wien) 90:1–14, 1988.

34. Frazee JG, King WA: Endoscopic-assisted craniotomy and microsurgery. In Jimenez D (ed): Intracranial Endoscopic Neurosurgery. Park Ridge, IL, AANS Publications, 1998, pp 147–158.

35. Cohen AR, Perneczky A, Rodziewicz GS, Gingold SI: Endoscope-assisted craniotomy: Approach to the rostral brainstem. Neurosurgery 36:1128–1130, 1995.

36. Hopf N, Perneczky A: Endoscopic neurosurgery and endoscopic-assisted microsurgery for the treatment of intracranial cysts. Neurosurgery 43:1330–1337, 1998.

37. Burman MD: Myeloscopy of the directed visualization of the spinal canal and its contents. J Bone Joint Surg 13:695, 1931.

38. Stern EL: The spinal scope: New instrument for visualizing spinal canal and its contents. Med Rec 143:31–32, 1936.

39. Pool JL: Direct visualization of dorsal roots of the cauda equina by means of a myeloscope. Arch Neurol Psychiatry 39:1308–1312, 1938.

40. Mayer HM, Brock M: Percutaneous endoscopic discectomy: Surgical technique and preliminary results compared to microsurgical discectomy. J Neurosurg 78:216–225, 1993.

41. Mayer HM, Brock M, Berlien HP, Weber B: Percutaneous endoscopic laser discectomy (PELD): A new surgical technique for non-sequestrated lumbar disc. Acta Neurochir Suppl (Wien) 54: 53–58, 1992.

42. Zamarano L, Chavantes C, Dujovny M, et al: Stereotactic endoscopic intervention in cystic and intraventricular brain lesions. Acta Neurochir Suppl (Wien) 54:69–76, 1992.

43. McLaughin MR, Wahlig JB, Kaufman AM, Albright AL: Traumatic basilar aneurysm after endoscopic third ventriculostomy: Case report. Neurosurgery 41:1400–1404, 1997.

CHAPTER **219**

Vein of Galen Malformations

J. PARKER MICKLE ■ ROBERT A. MERICLE ■ MATTHEW V. BURRY ■
LORNA SOHN WILLIAMS

The modern treatment of vein of Galen malformations involves a multidisciplinary approach with transvenous[1, 2] and transarterial embolization[3] as the cornerstone of early and effective therapy.[4] When undertaking the treatment of vein of Galen malformations, the neurosurgeon strives to rid the patient of this lesion in a staged fashion while maintaining somatic and neurological integrity. This relatively simple therapeutic goal can be achieved in most patients presenting with the various syndromes associated with vein of Galen malformations. Also, there is an opportunity for cure when this multidisciplinary approach is adopted by an experienced treatment team.[5]

Before 1980, these malformations were treated principally with an open surgical approach. Even though the mortality and morbidity of surgery were very high, open surgical techniques were believed to provide better outcomes than no treatment.[6] Since 1980, with the explosion of endovascular techniques, open surgery is generally reserved for patients with hydrocephalus and for exposure of vein of Galen malformations not accessible by endovascular approaches.[4] In rare cases, surgical exposure of this deep-seated midline lesion can be curative in the final stages of treatment.

Vein of Galen malformations are rare lesions, and patients harboring these malformations present with well-defined syndromes not easily confused with other disease processes.[2] About 1% of vascular malformations in the central nervous system involve the vein of Galen.[6] Because of the paucity of cases, our knowledge base for treatment and outcome remains limited.[4] Also, because this lesion is difficult to obliterate, multiple therapies are often used in each patient; therefore, clear-cut therapeutic benefit is difficult to ascertain for any one modality.[7]

Before 1984, we operated on most patients presenting with vein of Galen aneurysms with a direct surgical approach to clip the feeders and treat hydrocephalus. The few neonates who survived this procedure were often left with persistent fistulas and significant morbidity. With the rapid development of endovascular and neuroimaging technologies came the impetus to develop new therapies for this complex and threatening condition. There is no more frustrating exercise in clinical neurosurgery than the attempted microsurgical obliteration of one of these deep, complex vascular malformations in a neonate suffering from high-output cardiac failure with acidosis and the anatomic substrate of poorly myelinated brain. We believe that the elegant and precise endovascular approaches available today at most tertiary care centers are superior to open surgical obliteration approaches.[4, 8, 9]

This chapter discusses two primary principles of modern therapy of vein of Galen malformations: (1) treatment is better than conservative management, and (2) combined endovascular and surgical approaches offer the best chance for a good outcome and possible cure.[5, 8]

HISTORY AND VENOUS ANATOMY

A description of the deep venous system in lower animals is ascribed to Galen in the second century AD. The anatomic correlate in human beings became better defined over the years and was named the vein of Galen, where the paired basal veins of Rosenthal and the paired internal cerebral veins converge with the inferior sagittal sinus and straight sinus (Fig. 219–1). The vein of Galen is located in the quadrigeminal cistern just under the splenium of the corpus callosum. It drains the thalamus, occipital lobes, medial temporal lobes, and superior cerebellar vermis. Bedford[10] reported a detailed study of this vascular structure in the monkey in 1934. Steinheil[11] in 1895 described the first malformation of this venous complex, and Jaeger and associates,[12] Oscherwitz and Davidoff,[13] and Boldrey

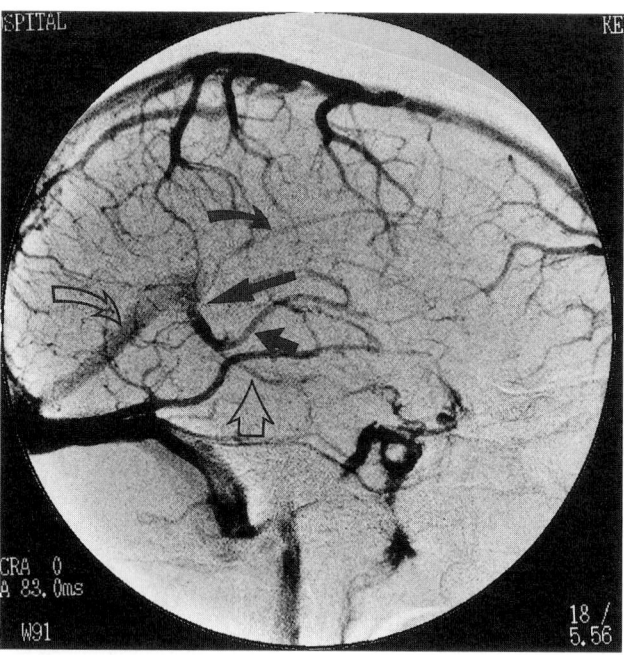

FIGURE 219–1. Lateral-projection digital subtraction angiography of a normal subject in the late venous phase. Many of the important venous structures are easily identified. The basal vein of Rosenthal *(open arrow)* joins the internal cerebral veins *(small black arrow)* and the inferior sagittal sinus *(curved black arrow)* to form the vein of Galen *(large black arrow)*. This system then drains through the straight sinus *(open curved arrow)*.

and Miller[14] defined the first clinical and surgical attempts at treatment of these lesions. Gold and co-workers[15] in 1964 and Amacher and Shillito[16] in 1973 developed the first clinical classification for patients presenting with vein of Galen aneurysms. Norman and Becker[17] in 1974 reported that significant cerebral damage resulted from the high-flow central shunt in these patients in the neonatal period. Hoffman and colleagues[18] reported on the treatment of 29 patients at the Toronto Hospital for Sick Children and compiled all the data available in the literature on a total of 128 patients. Their conclusions from this review were that children with vein of Galen malformations who were treated did better than those who were not treated, and that infants and older children did far better than neonates presenting with heart failure from vein of Galen malformations. A similar review by Johnston and coworkers[19] in 1987 expanded these conclusions with a review of 232 cases.

A major advance in understanding and planning the treatment of vein of Galen malformations came with the efforts of Litvak and associates[20] and Yasargil[21] to classify these malformations based on angiographic findings. These authors showed that prognosis was connected to the angiographic classification of these lesions. Next, Lasjaunias and colleagues[22] developed a simple classification system with just two general categories: true vein of Galen malformations and secondary vein of Galen malformations. The secondary lesions are shunts with compensatory dilatation of the vein of Galen complex secondary to an adjacent dural or parenchymal arteriovenous (AV) malformation. The true vein of Galen malformations can be subdivided into several types, as described by Yasargil,[21] based on the predominant arterial supply to these lesions.

These classification schemes set the stage for improved treatment planning. Before 1980, therapeutic goals entailed aggressive medical therapy and attempted surgical obliteration of these lesions. Hydrocephalus, a common accompaniment of this symptom complex, was treated in a standard fashion, often with devastating complications. The pivotal turning point in the 1980s was the appreciation by many that these lesions are best treated with endovascular therapy.[23, 24] Although these patients continue to present great challenges to even the most experienced teams, the prognosis is far better today than at any time in the past. Advances in technology and a better understanding of the pathophysiology of these various syndromes have contributed to improved survival with low morbidity.

EMBRYOLOGY

The anatomic correlate of the vein of Galen aneurysm is found in the embryo as a median prosencephalic vein, which normally involutes between the fifth and seventh weeks of development.[25] It is believed that direct fistulous connections in this primitive vascular bed represent a substrate for persistent shunting throughout fetal development and in the neonatal period. The persistent fistulas and the vein of Galen itself are abnormal remnants of the prosencephalic vein and result in true vein of Galen malformations.[26] Secondary vein of Galen malformations result from persistent adjacent dural and parenchymal AV shunts leading to secondary dilatation of a normally developed vein of Galen. Angiographically, these lesions are easily differentiated, which is essential, because therapeutic options differ among the various types of vein of Galen malformations.

PATHOPHYSIOLOGY

The presence of these AV shunts in utero can result in major anatomic and physiologic injury to the child. In neonates, the high-flow central AV shunt can cause high-output cardiac failure with associated central and somatic hypoperfusion and acidosis. The shunt can also produce cerebral and pulmonary venous hypertension, which can result in major permanent parenchymal damage to the brain and lungs. At birth, severe cerebral venous hypertension can result in hydrocephalus, chronic cerebral ischemia, and risk of cerebral hemorrhage.[27, 28] The degree of injury and the clinical presentation of these patients are age related.[9, 15, 16] The clinical course, long-term outcome, and most efficacious mode of therapy are all predicted by the clinical subgroups based on age at presentation.

A fetus harboring one of these malformations is not protected from injury, although the effects of the high-flow central shunt are somewhat blunted by the presence of the low-resistance placental circulation, effectively reducing the central shunt in the head.[29] Some of these malformations are being diagnosed prenatally with ultrasonography,[30, 31] and the effects of these lesions on the heart and brain can be appreciated even at this early time.

Some neonates are born with major injury to the brain, as evidenced by dystrophic calcifications within the parenchyma and massive ventricular enlargement with atrophy. The prognosis is extremely poor, and most patients in this group are not treated.[9] At birth, if the central shunt is high, the cardiac demands can become overwhelming. The neonate develops progressive high-output cardiac failure with pulmonary hypertension and progressive acidosis unresponsive to medical therapy. Such patients rapidly succumb unless urgent reduction of the shunt is accomplished.

An infant who presents slightly later in life with a vein of Galen malformation has a smaller central shunt compared with a neonate. The infant typically presents with mild to moderate intracranial venous hypertension with enlargement of the head and occasionally mild heart failure. The heart failure in this age group generally responds well to medical management.[16]

An older child or young adult harboring one of these congenital lesions may present with headaches, learning disability, increasing spasticity, seizures, and occasionally subarachnoid hemorrhage. Pathophysiologically, virtually all these lesions are progressive; therefore, reduction or elimination of the AV shunt nearly always improves the outcome of these patients. Rarely, a completely asymptomatic malformation is found in an older child or young adult, and these patients have the best prognosis among all the groups.[32]

CLASSIFICATION

Clinical Classification

The clinical presentation of vein of Galen malformations is age dependent, and the outcome of patients with these lesions can be predicted based on the age at presentation.[16, 33] Gold and associates[15] were the first to classify vein of Galen malformations clinically, and their classification system was refined by Amacher and Shillito.[16] In 1990, Wisoff and coworkers[33] defined another group consisting of those rare individuals with complete spontaneous thrombosis of their malformations.[34, 35] The current clinical classification scheme divides patients according to age into three groups: (1) neonate, (2) infant, and (3) older child and adult.

If a neonate is symptomatic, he or she is born with a hyperactive precordium, which over the first 24 hours rapidly deteriorates to high-output cardiac failure resistant to all medical therapies. A chest radiograph reveals signs of heart failure such as cardiomegaly (Fig. 219–2). Untreated, the neonate becomes progressively acidotic, with decreasing urinary output, progressive pulmonary deterioration, and certain death. There is a very loud, machine-like bruit over the head and chest. The venous and arterial pulsations in the neck are hyperdynamic, demonstrative of the catastrophic flow abnormalities in these babies. We have had the oppor-

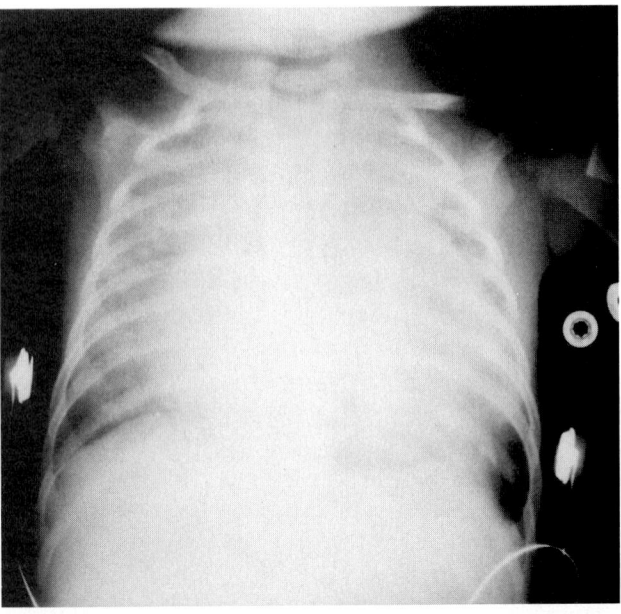

FIGURE 219–2. Posteroanterior projection of a chest radiograph in a neonate with a high-flow vein of Galen malformation. The patient had clinical signs of heart failure, and the chest film shows severe cardiomegaly. If left untreated, this will progress to severe bilateral pulmonary edema and certain eventual death.

tunity to follow several of these patients before birth and noted that cardiac ventricular dilatation before delivery predicts early deterioration from high-output cardiac failure, necessitating early, aggressive endovascular embolization for survival. The cardiac ischemia present in such high-output cardiac failure can result in myocardial infarction. If this occurs, the patient could suffer medically resistant heart failure even if the shunt is successfully eliminated.

An infant who is symptomatic from a vein of Galen aneurysm usually presents with progressive enlargement of the head and an intracranial bruit during the first 6 months of life. Because of drainage of some of these lesions through the facial venous system, dilated supraorbital veins can be seen in this age group. Some of the patients in this clinical category can have mild heart failure, which is frequently responsive to standard medical therapies. The enlarged head is a result of mild hydrocephalus, often with a capacious subarachnoid space and mild to moderate ventricular enlargement.[36] Occasionally, these patients can deteriorate quickly because of massive and rapidly progressive hydrocephalus. This can be dangerous, because early cerebrospinal fluid (CSF) diversion procedures are associated with an unusually high risk of intracranial hemorrhage. Infants who present with vein of Galen malformations have a favorable clinical prognosis compared with neonates, regardless of which mode of therapy is chosen.[9]

An older child or young adult with a true vein of Galen malformation has a more subtle injury to the central nervous system than do younger age groups. However, even these patients are often impaired by progressive syndromes, including learning disabilities, severe and incapacitating headaches, progressive spas-

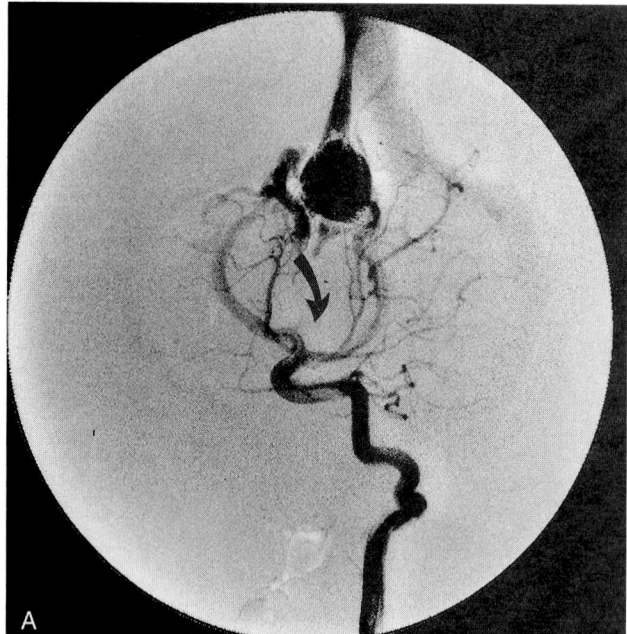

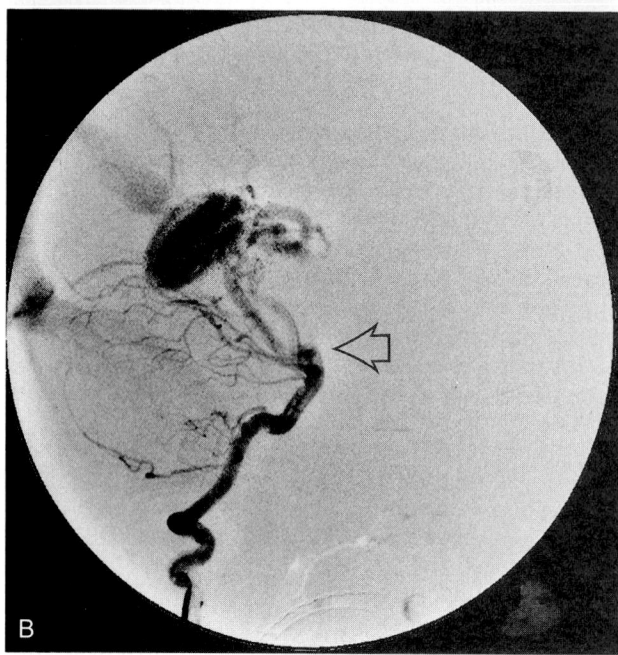

FIGURE 219–3. *A,* Anteroposterior-projection digital subtraction angiogram of the left vertebral artery in a patient with a Yasargil type I vein of Galen malformation. There are only a few feeders from the main trunks of the bilateral posterior cerebral arteries (PCAs). Note that there are no thalamoperforating feeders to the lesion *(curved arrow). B,* Lateral projection of the same angiogram. Note the absence of feeders from the basilar apex *(open arrow).* This patient also had a feeder from the left pericallosal artery from the left internal carotid artery injection (not shown).

ticity, and occasionally subarachnoid hemorrhage or seizures. This group of older children and young adults responds very well to endovascular treatment.

The subgroup of patients with completely asymptomatic occult lesions can be followed expectantly. In this situation, we believe that the natural history is less

threatening to the patient, and the risk-benefit ratio of endovascular surgery may not be favorable.

Angiographic Classification

Vein of Galen malformations were first classified angiographically by Lasjaunias and colleagues[22] as mural, choroidal, and secondary types.[22] This classification system was later refined into four types by Yasargil.[21] The Yasargil type I lesion has few feeders, which are principally from the pericallosal and posterior cerebral arteries (Fig. 219–3). Yasargil type II lesions are supplied principally by thalamoperforating branches and posterior cerebral arteries (Fig. 219–4). The Yasargil type III mixed variety is, unfortunately, the most common type of lesion. These malformations have a mixed pattern of supply from pericallosal, thalamoperforating, and posterior cerebral arteries (Fig. 219–5). The Yasargil type IV lesion is the secondary type of shunt proposed by Lasjaunias and colleagues. These aneurysms result from shunting of an adjacent parenchymal or dural true AV malformation into an otherwise normal vein of Galen system (Fig. 219–6). This venous drainage pattern causes high-pressure, arterialized blood to dilate the otherwise normal vein of Galen into a venous aneurysm. This angiographic classification is important therapeutically and can often be correlated with clinical presentation.

The most common type of vein of Galen malformation is the type III, or choroidal type. Generally, the more complex the lesion, the higher the flow in the AV shunt. Therefore, patients with more complex lesions

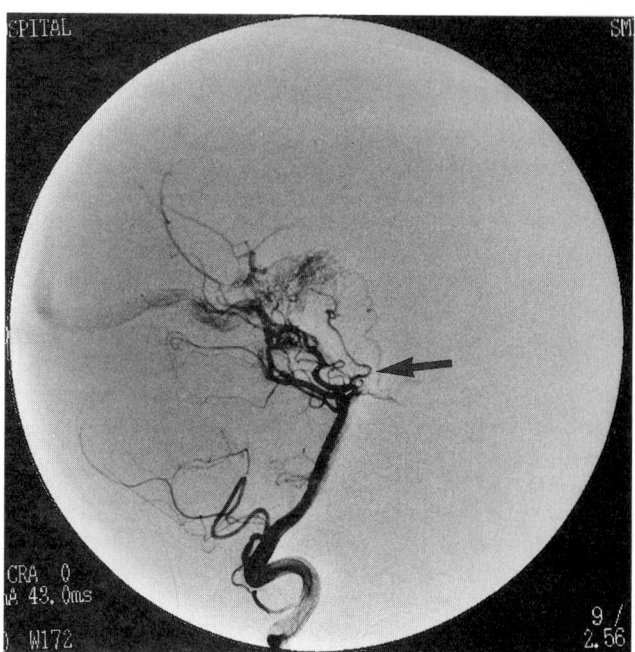

FIGURE 219–4. Lateral-projection digital subtraction angiogram of the right vertebral artery demonstrating a Yasargil type II vein of Galen malformation. Most of the feeders from the bilateral posterior cerebral arteries (PCAs) have been embolized, which improves visualization of several thalamoperforating feeders *(arrow).* There were no feeders from the anterior circulation.

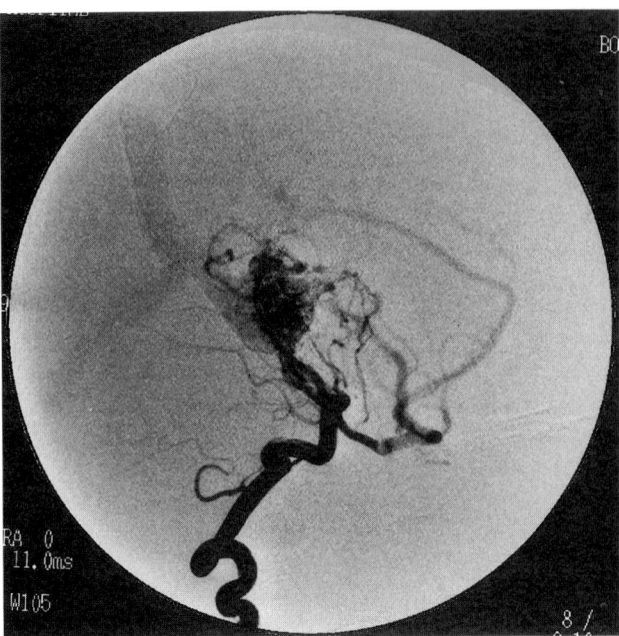

FIGURE 219–5. Lateral-projection digital subtraction angiogram of the left vertebral artery demonstrating a Yasargil type III vein of Galen malformation. Note the mixed pattern of posterior cerebral arteries (PCAs), thalamoperforators, and pericallosal artery feeders.

tend to present as neonates. Also, patients with higher shunting usually present in the most severe medical condition. However, we have seen early heart failure in several neonates with simple type I vein of Galen

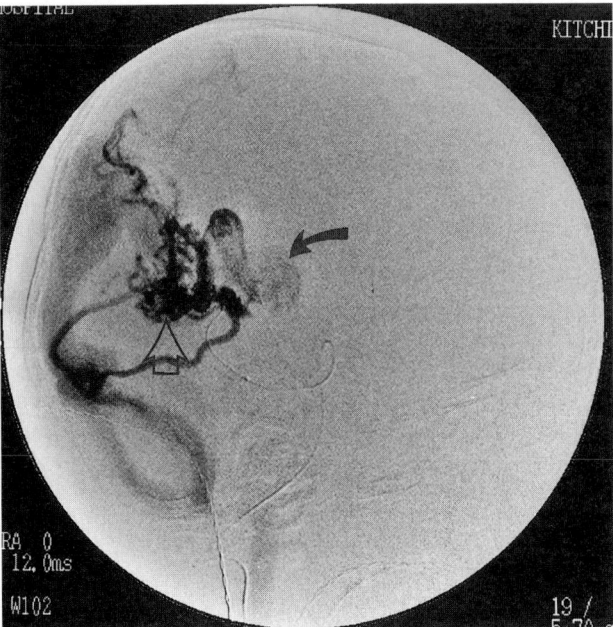

FIGURE 219–6. Lateral-projection digital subtraction superselective angiogram of the right posterior cerebral artery (PCA) demonstrating an arteriovenous malformation (AVM) adjacent to a secondarily dilated vein of Galen aneurysm (Yasargil type IV). The nidus of the AVM *(open arrow)* is slightly lateral and posterior to the dilated vein of Galen *(curved arrow).*

malformations that were obliterated with one or two endovascular procedures.[5, 31]

Another imaging method for classifying vein of Galen malformations is based on the venous outflow pattern in these lesions.[37, 38] In grade 1, the vein of Galen and straight sinus are minimally enlarged. Grade 2 lesions occur when the vein of Galen is dilated more than the venous outlet and both are moderately increased in size. Grade 3 lesions demonstrate huge dilatation of structures, and grade 4 shunts have significant enlargement of the vein of Galen with stenotic or absent straight sinuses. Patients harboring a shunt with significant stenosis of outflow rarely have heart failure. Often a falcine sinus is present.

DIAGNOSIS

Clinically, the diagnosis of a patient with a vein of Galen malformation is fairly straightforward. A neonate suffering from high-output cardiac failure has a central shunt of the vein of Galen or dural variety or has a primary cardiac cause. Rarely, vascular tumors, peripheral or central, can cause a similar problem in neonates. High on the list of differential possibilities is a vein of Galen aneurysm in a neonate with high-output cardiac failure, hyperdynamic precordium, dilated cervical and cranial veins, and arteries with a loud, machine-like bruit heard over the head and neck.

These lesions are more subtle in infants and older children but should be suspected in patients with hydrocephalus, seizures, subarachnoid hemorrhage, progressive spasticity, headaches, and learning disabilities.

Transcranial ultrasonography is an excellent way to diagnose a vein of Galen lesion in a neonate or infant with an open fontanelle (Fig. 219–7). These lesions can even be seen in utero with transvaginal ultrasonography.[30, 31] Color flow Doppler has been used to define the basic makeup of a vein of Galen malformation complex and is particularly useful in following therapy as changes in flow patterns occur.[2, 31, 39] Computed tomography is the most common imaging modality used for the early diagnosis of vein of Galen malformations (Fig. 219–8). When combined with contrast material, computed tomography defines with great accuracy the presence of a vein of Galen malformation and the effects the lesion has had on the brain and CSF pathways (see Fig. 219–8A). Magnetic resonance imaging (MRI) is useful in patients in all categories to better define the lesion's effects on the brain (Fig. 219–9). MRI shows the general health of the brain and demonstrates the effects of venous hypertension, ischemia, and hydrocephalus on the brain parenchyma. Dystrophic calcifications are not demonstrated well with MRI but are easily seen with computed tomographic scanning (see Fig. 219–8B). Magnetic resonance angiography is helpful in defining the general type of vein of Galen malformation.

The gold standard for diagnosis and for planning therapy is catheter cerebral angiography. The general type of lesion is easily defined, and therapy can be instituted at the same setting with transarterial emboli-

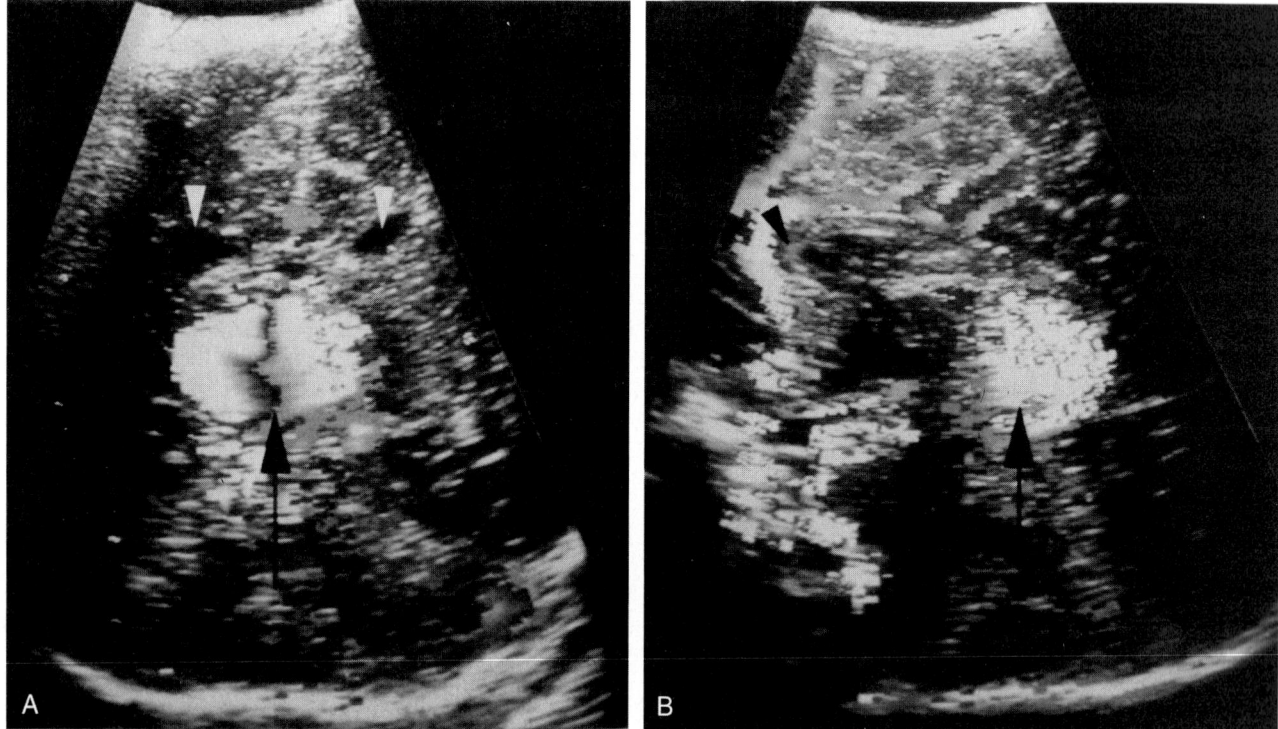

FIGURE 219–7. Transcranial Doppler ultrasonography. *A,* Coronal ultrasonography through the anterior fontanelle demonstrates a vein of Galen malformation *(black arrow)* with turbulent flow and minimally dilated lateral ventricles *(white arrowheads). B,* Ultrasonography through the anterior fontanelle in the same patient shows the vein of Galen malformation *(black arrow)* in sagittal orientation. The genu of the corpus callosum is noted *(black arrowhead).* (Courtesy of William Cumming, MD.)

zation using materials such as glue, silk, coils, or polyvinyl alcohol particles. However, the angiogram itself can be a great challenge in some neonates and infants because the femoral arteries are very small, and the patient does not tolerate large volumes of saline flush or radiographic contrast. Angiography and subsequent endovascular embolization are usually best performed in a staged fashion, if the patient can tolerate it. This typically avoids contrast overload, fluid overload, and sudden dramatic changes in cerebral circulation.

Transfemoral or transtorcular venography and embolization are often useful for rapidly reducing AV shunting and therefore achieving an optimal outcome. We have treated multiple neonates with high-output heart failure without angiography in an effort to establish a resistance basket within the venous aneurysm to reduce flow through the malformation. This is a quick and effective technique and is discussed in more detail later. Although we have used single photon emission computed tomography scanning in several patients, we have not found this to be particularly useful in predicting cerebral blood flow and outcome.

NATURAL HISTORY

Because the natural history of patients with vein of Galen malformations is usually progressive neurological decline, treatment of the lesion with a reduction in

AV shunting appears to provide a better outcome than conservative management alone. Some absolutes are apparent in treating certain categories of patients, especially neonates suffering from progressive heart failure. In this situation, medical treatment will fail and the patient will succumb without significant urgent reduction in the shunt.[9] Multiple studies have demonstrated that the natural history of vein of Galen malformations in infants and older children is progressive, but appropriate treatment can effectively interrupt the neurological syndromes.[18, 19] With the most current therapies, up to 80% of these individuals can have a good prognosis.

We now see many patients who are stable clinically but, after multiple endovascular procedures, still harbor small residual or partially treated malformations (Fig. 219–10). The natural history of these partially treated but persistent lesions is unclear. The most common scenario for persistent feeders is when only small thalamoperforators exist, because these tiny arteries are difficult to catheterize and carry a high risk of postembolization morbidity. We have investigated stereotactic radiosurgery as a mode of treatment for residual compact thalamoperforating feeders, but the results have been inconclusive. We have followed a number of children with partially treated vein of Galen malformations. Some of these children should be periodically re-evaluated to assess the severity of their disease and the progressive nature of the shunt or venous hypertension. If the disease is found to be progressive, fur-

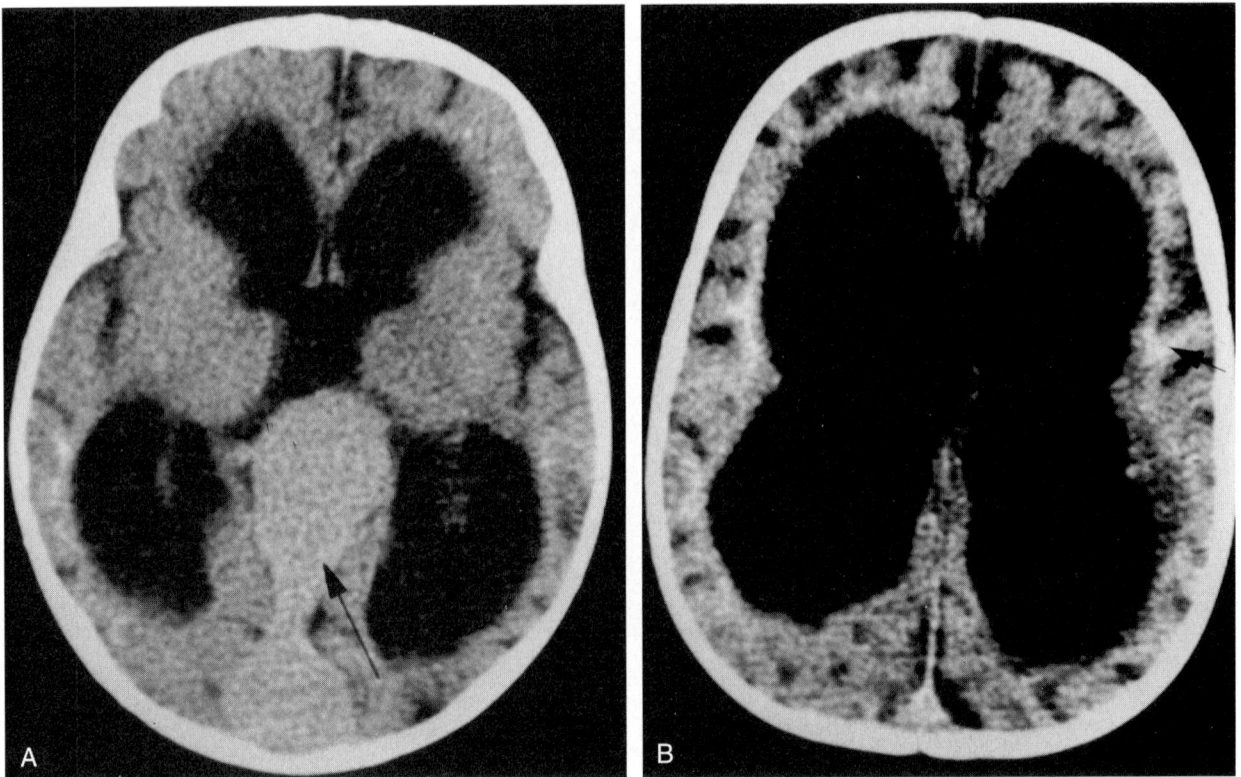

FIGURE 219–8. Computed tomography. *A*, Noncontrast axial computed tomographic scan demonstrates a large vein of Galen malformation *(black arrow)* with a moderate to severe degree of hydrocephalus in this 8-month-old infant who presented with macrocephaly. *B*, Noncontrast axial computed tomographic scan in the same patient shows dystrophic calcification *(black arrow)* within the white matter secondary to chronic venous hypertension.

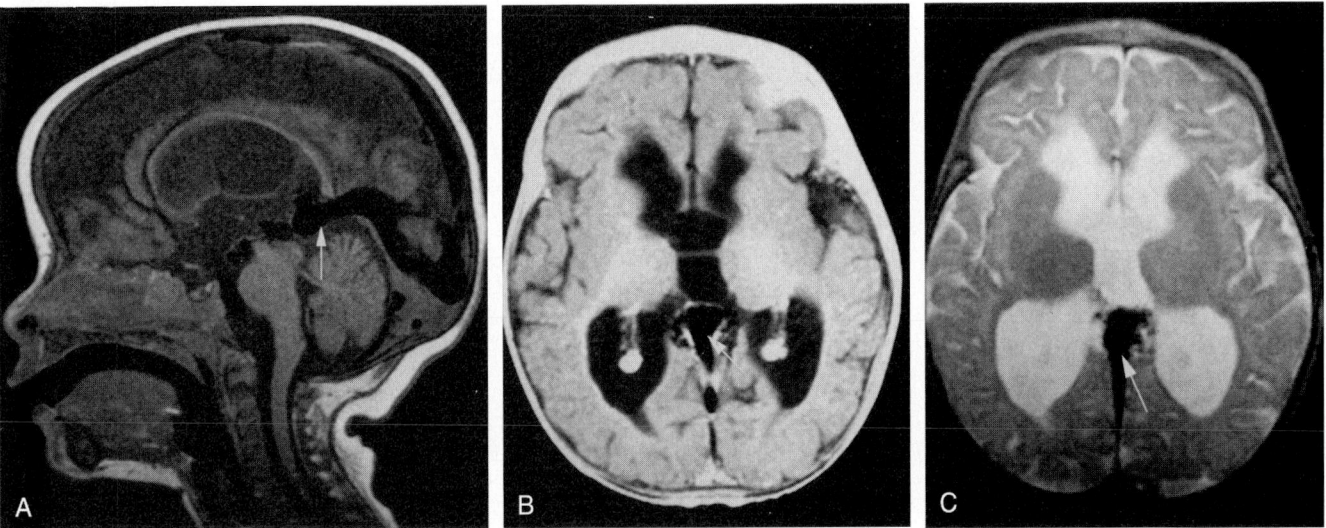

FIGURE 219–9. Magnetic resonance imaging (MRI). *A*, Sagittal T1-weighted MRI scan without contrast depicts a vein of Galen malformation *(white arrow)* in a neonate with drainage into the straight sinus. *B*, Axial T1-weighted MRI scan in the same patient shows moderate hydrocephalus. The lesion *(white arrow)* is markedly hypointense, representing a flow void of signal. *C*, Axial T2-weighted MRI scan in the same patient demonstrates the lesion *(white arrow)*. A minimal degree of transependymal flow of cerebral spinal fluid (CSF) is seen into the periventricular white matter adjacent to the frontal and occipital horns of the lateral ventricles, caused by the moderate hydrocephalus.

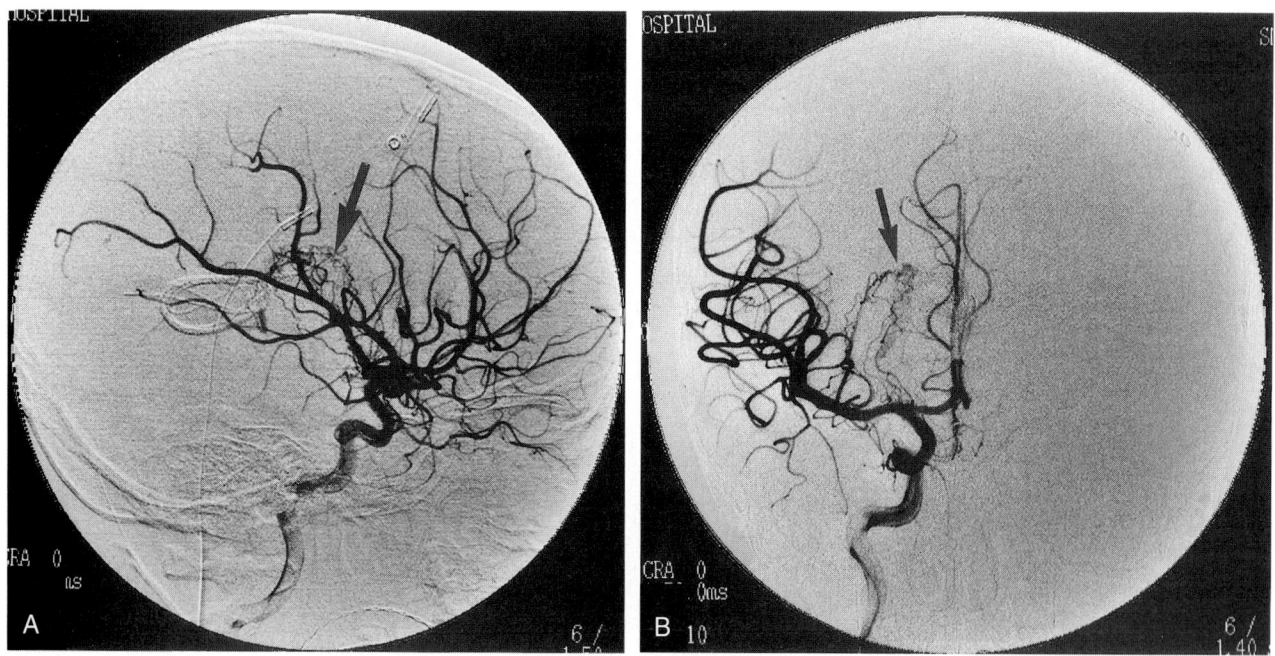

FIGURE 219–10. *A,* Lateral-projection digital subtraction angiogram of the right internal carotid artery (ICA) after transtorcular embolization of the venous pouch, followed by multiple transarterial embolizations. There are a few tiny perforating feeders remaining that are impossible to selectively catheterize *(black arrow).* *B,* Anteroposterior projection of the same angiogram injection showing a small residual lesion *(black arrow).*

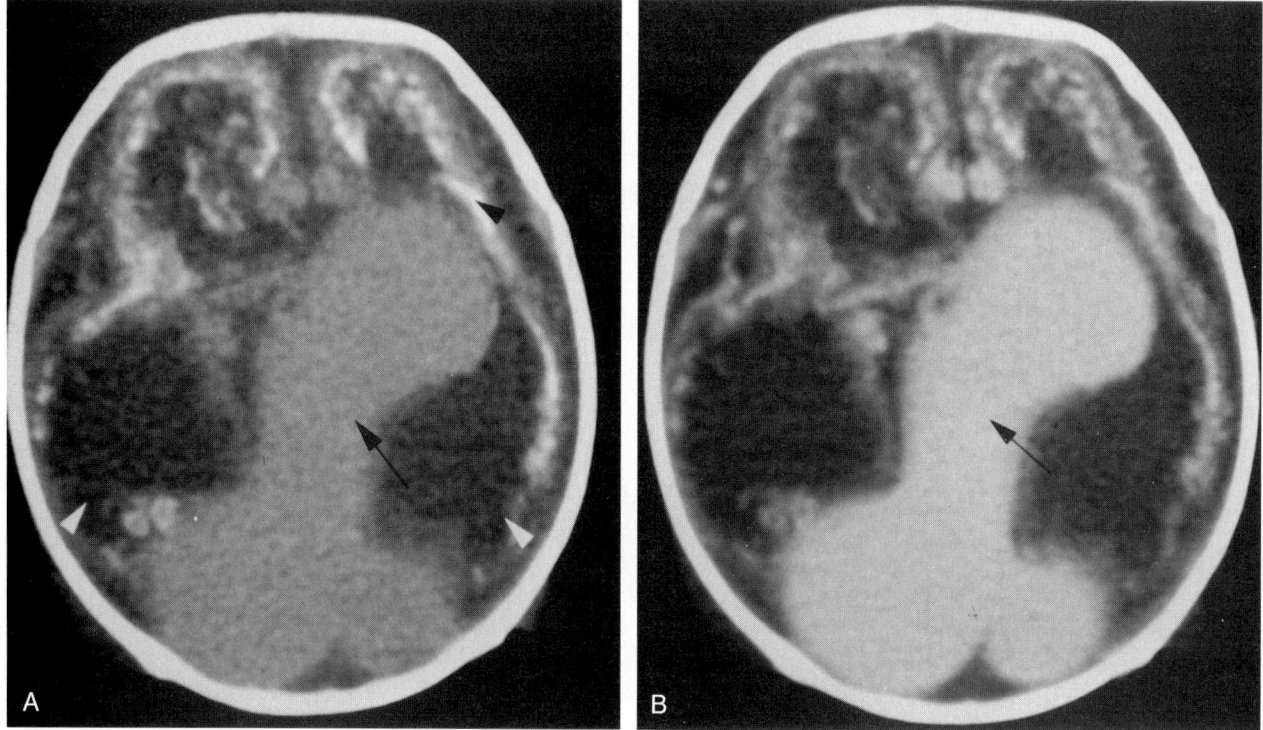

FIGURE 219–11. Computed tomography in a neonate with severe parenchymal injury as a result of a vein of Galen malformation. *A,* Noncontrast axial computed tomographic scan shows a large vein of Galen malformation *(black arrow)* that has produced severe hydrocephalus, with marked dilatation of the lateral ventricle *(white arrowheads)* and severe dystrophic parenchymal calcification *(black arrowhead).* *B,* Contrast-enhanced computed tomographic scan shows enhancement of the lesion *(black arrow),* implying that the lesion is patent. Such a degree of parenchymal injury has a poor prognosis, and this child died 2 days after birth.

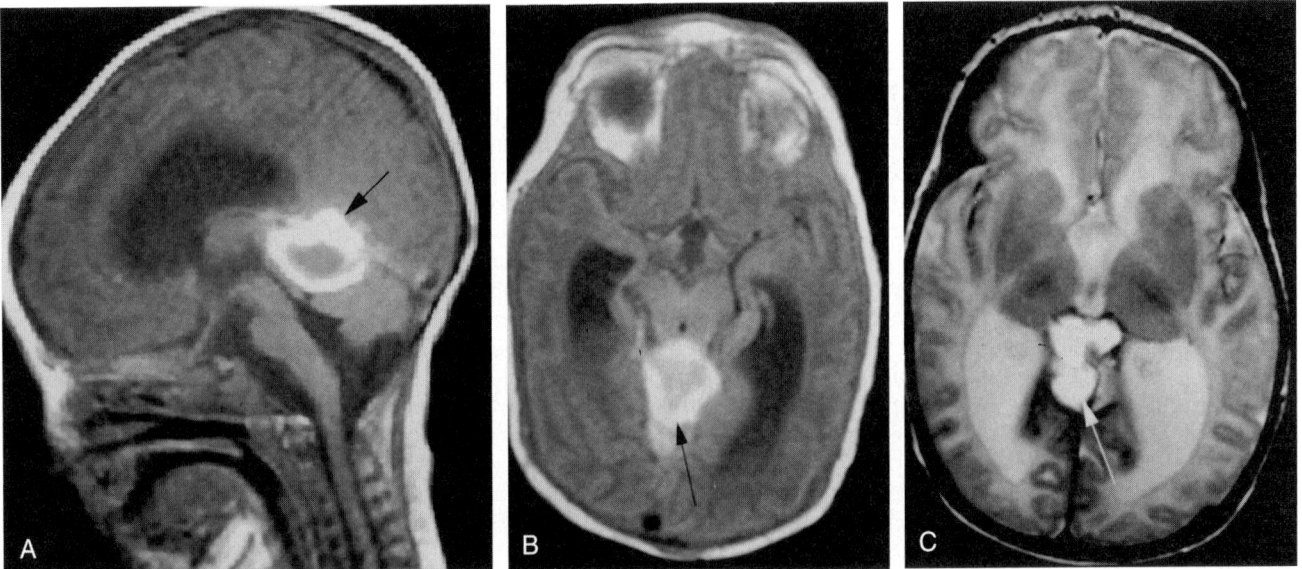

FIGURE 219–12. Magnetic resonance imaging (MRI) of a spontaneously thrombosed vein of Galen malformation. *A*, Sagittal T1-weighted MRI scan without contrast depicts a thrombosed vein of Galen malformation *(black arrow)* in a neonate. The high signal intensity with the lesion represents subacute blood products. *B*, Axial T1-weighted MRI scan without contrast in the same patient shows the lesion *(black arrow)* and moderate hydrocephalus. *C*, Axial T2-weighted MRI scan in the same patient demonstrates the lesion *(white arrow)* with a ring of marked hypointensity, representing chronic blood products.

ther endovascular surgery can be helpful. The decision to re-evaluate is generally based on clinical information such as headaches, cognitive changes, psychological changes, neurological deficits, or physical examination findings such as increasing dilatation of the facial veins. Currently, an arteriogram is the standard method of re-evaluating a child with a vein of Galen malformation. MRI perfusion studies show promise as a noninvasive alternative to evaluate cerebral perfusion in these patients. An increasing shunt would be expected to cause venous hypertension, which might result in perfusion abnormalities that could be detected as MRI perfusion defects. In the future, the evaluation of these patients with computed tomography–angiography or MRI perfusion studies may obviate the need for follow-up invasive angiography to evaluate the shunt or venous hypertension. Of course, care would have to be taken to ensure that all materials (such as coils) used in these patients are MRI compatible if follow-up MRI is being considered.

Patients at the two extremes of neurological function and prognosis should sometimes be given no treatment. The unfortunate neonate with severe cerebral atrophy and dystrophic calcifications of the brain has a very poor prognosis if salvaged (Fig. 219–11). Even with maximal treatment, there is a high mortality rate, and those who survive are frequently left in a vegetative state. Therefore, withdrawal of care should be carefully considered. At the other end of the spectrum, a slow-flow asymptomatic lesion that is not easily approached by routine endovascular or open surgical techniques may be better managed with close observation rather than risky attempts at complete obliteration.

There are a few rare cases of documented spontaneous thrombosis of vein of Galen malformations that do not require treatment (Fig. 219–12).

Aside from these general categories of individuals who probably should not be treated aggressively, the remaining patients with vein of Galen malformations have a serious disease with a poor natural history but good treatment options. If the Spetzler-Martin grading system for AV malformations were applied to vein of Galen malformations, practically all these lesions would be assigned a minimum of grade 4.[19, 32, 40, 41] This connotes a dangerous, progressive lesion for which open surgical resection carries a high risk and can result in a poor outcome. This appreciation leads to a recommendation of staged endovascular surgery. Certainly, most progressive clinical syndromes should be treated aggressively, and recent advances in endovascular techniques have made this a safe and effective treatment strategy.[4, 8]

TREATMENT

The options available for treatment of vein of Galen malformations are varied and depend on the clinical presentation and the experience of the treatment team. The general guidelines for treatment of vein of Galen malformations that we use at the University of Florida are summarized here. In neonates, craniotomy with attempted direct obliteration of the AV fistula is fraught with technical difficulty and rarely results in a good outcome. Combined transvenous and transarterial endovascular surgery offers the best chance for a good outcome in this age group.[2, 4, 8, 9, 31] The concept is to first eliminate the high-flow shunt and then decrease the size and flow through the malformation with graded endovascular embolizations. This approach occasionally leads to an angiographically complete obliteration but most often converts a neonate in high-output cardiac failure to an infant with a persistent fistula, which is tolerated very well.

Of course, all patients suffering from heart failure should receive aggressive medical treatment in addition to endovascular surgery. In an infant with mild heart failure, this is essential to provide the optimal environment in which to eliminate the lesion with endovascular or open surgical techniques. Once the fistula is eliminated or the flow is greatly reduced, the medical treatment can gradually be weaned.

In an older child or young adult with a symptomatic shunt from a vein of Galen malformation, the philosophy remains a gradual and graded elimination of the shunt with endovascular surgery, usually from a transarterial approach. The persistence of a small fistula after multiple embolizations provides an opportunity for other therapies such as open surgery or possibly stereotactic radiosurgery.

The treatment of hydrocephalus in a patient with a vein of Galen malformation can be treacherous. It has been suggested by several studies that the most common cause of hydrocephalus in these patients is severe venous hypertension resulting in a situation suggestive of external hydrocephalus.[27, 42] This type of hydrocephalus often resolves after treatment, once the CSF pressure versus venous pressure discrepancy has returned to normal (Fig. 219–13). The routine treatment of hydrocephalus with a standard ventriculoperitoneal shunt in these children has an unusually high incidence of acute subdural hematoma formation. These are frequently associated with mass effect and often require surgical evacuation and removal of the shunt to save the child's life.

Craniotomy for open microsurgical obliteration of a vein of Galen malformation can be extensive or relatively simple. A Yasargil type I or II lesion in an infant or older child can be eliminated by an open surgical approach with minimal risk to the patient.[16, 21, 32] If direct open surgery is chosen in a patient with a vein of Galen malformation, it is usually performed in the three-quarter prone position with a suboccipital transtentorial approach. Depending on the vascular anatomy, a supracerebellar or even a subtemporal approach can be chosen. We have used the suboccipital approach most often and describe the basic steps here.

The patient is placed in the three-quarter prone position with the side of interest slightly down so that gravity can help in the exposure, minimizing retraction. The brains of neonates and very young children are resistant to retraction in any form, and positioning

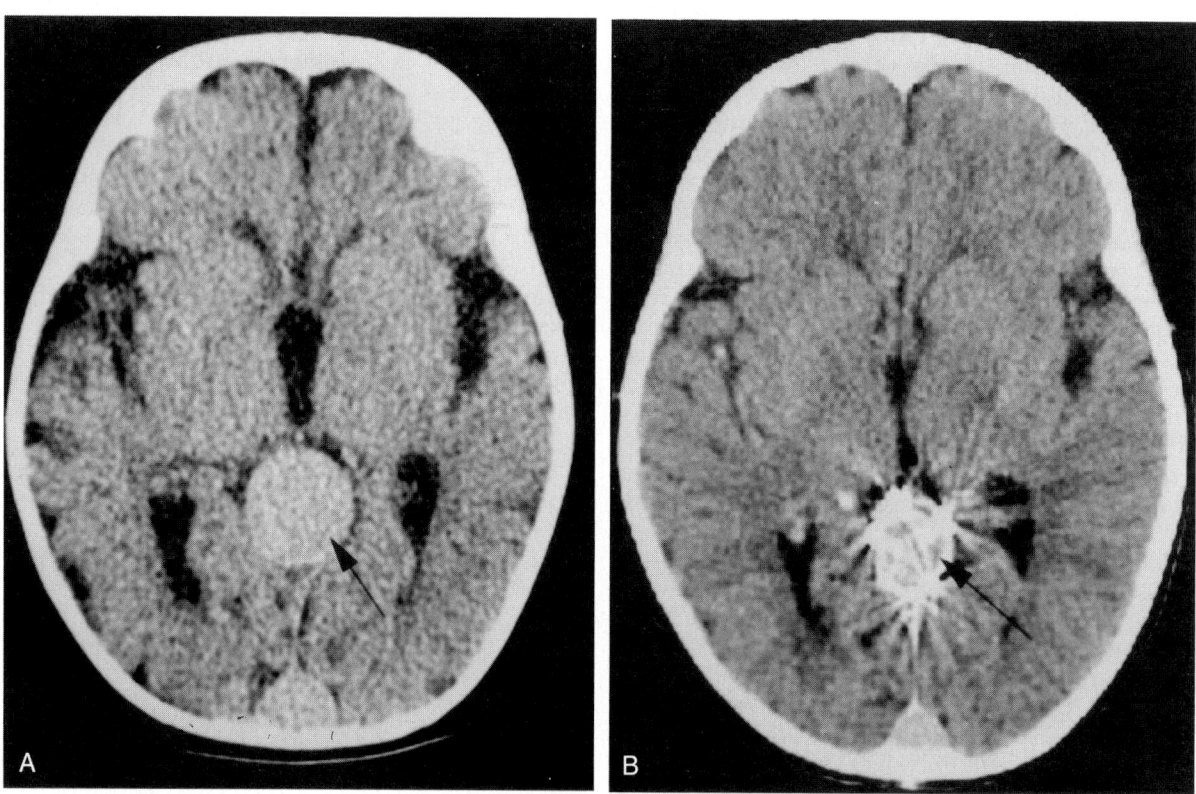

FIGURE 219–13. Computed tomography. *A*, Noncontrast computed tomographic scan in an infant with a vein of Galen malformation *(black arrow)* and mild hydrocephalus. *B*, Noncontrast computed tomographic scan in the same patient following transtorcular placement of a wire lattice *(black arrow)* and resolution of the hydrocephalus.

is critical to accomplish adequate exposure. The vein of Galen malformation is approached like a pineal region lesion. Feeders into the tough, dura-like, dilated vein of Galen can be approached directly, and the superior (pericallosal) lateral and posterior feeders can easily be taken at the time of the initial exposure. Feeders are taken in turn, and the more difficult anterior and inferior feeders from the medial choroidals are eliminated last, if possible. The thickened aneurysmal venous sac can be gently deflated and retracted to reach these more anterior feeders. At this point, it is usually safer to deposit thrombogenic material within the partially deflated sac to eliminate the remaining anterior feeders.[43, 44] The contralateral choroidal feeders can be reached after opening the tentorium or resecting the most posterior component of the corpus callosum. Drainage of CSF via a ventriculostomy is helpful in exposing these more distant feeders.

Less than 50% of our patients required CSF diversion procedures for the control of progressive hydrocephalus. Some cases of mild hydrocephalus resolve after significantly decreasing the high-flow shunt with transtorcular coil placement in the vein of Galen aneurysm. If hydrocephalus is a persistent problem, we prefer to use a ventriculoperitoneal shunt with an antisiphon programmable valve. This approach minimizes the risk of subdural hematoma and associated complications.

The endovascular approaches to vein of Galen malformations are diverse and still evolving. In our opinion, these techniques offer the patient a better chance at a good outcome and potential cure. Today, the most common approach to vein of Galen aneurysms in multispecialty centers entails transarterial embolization with n-butyl-cyanoacrylate (NBCA) glue at the arterial side of the fistula. Other materials such as silk, coils, polyvinyl alcohol, or even balloons have been used in the past, with some degree of success. In Yasargil type III lesions, transarterial embolization must be performed multiple times and graded to significantly reduce the shunt with minimal complications. Transvenous embolization is more effective at reducing the AV shunt after one procedure.[1] We prefer to significantly decrease the AV shunt at the initial procedure with a transvenous transtorcular deposition of a wire lattice (0.035-inch demandeled coil guide wire).[43, 44] After the urgent high-flow heart failure has stabilized, we perform staged, graduated transarterial NBCA embolizations. The initial transvenous transtorcular embolization quickly reverses neonatal heart failure and establishes an aneurysmal lattice that assists with future transarterial procedures and helps reduce excessive transarterial glue penetration into the venous system. The advantages of the transtorcular approach over a transfemoral venous approach include lower cost, simplicity, ease, and speed at reducing the AV shunt.

Transarterial treatment can be administered at the time of diagnostic angiography, if tolerated by the child. Neonates and infants tolerate only the smallest volumes of contrast material.[9] In the case of a Yasargil type I or II lesion with few feeders, the small arterial feeders are taken in turn, with a high likelihood of eliminating the lesion completely. In more complex

vascular lesions, multiple procedures are usually necessary to eliminate the lesion. This can be difficult in very young children with small femoral arteries and tortuous vessels caused by the AV shunt. The transvenous approach can be accomplished through the femoral vein or the jugular vein or through a transtorcular route.[1] We prefer the more direct, simple transtorcular route, which can be performed in a neonate with a simple needle-stick through the "paper-thin" skull overlying the torcular. The torcular is entered with a standard Seldinger needle to identify a brisk arterial flow.[45] The rest of the procedure is performed through the blunt outer Seldinger needle without the inner sharp stylet. The torcular, straight sinus, and vein of Galen aneurysm are easily identified with transcranial ultrasonography or intraoperative angiography at the time of the surgery. A soft, demandelized guide wire is carefully placed through the blunt Seldinger needle into the vein of Galen. Intra-aneurysmal pressures can be obtained before and after treatment to guide the amount of coil placed in the venous aneurysm. Usually, 100 to 200 cm can be folded in the vein of Galen aneurysm in less than 5 to 10 minutes. This usually results in a discernible and significant change in flow pattern and in intra-aneurysmal pressures measured before termination of the procedure. In neonates, an adequate volume of coil must be placed to obtain a significant reduction in intra-aneurysmal pressure, or the improvement in the cardiac status of these patients will be short-lived.

Venograms are performed during the embolization, and we have used transtorcular therapy in some critically ill neonates as the initial step, without catheter angiography, to immediately and dramatically reduce shunting and heart failure (Fig. 219–14). Standard catheter angiography with transarterial or transfemoral transvenous embolization requires more time, is more expensive, and has a less dramatic immediate result compared with the transtorcular approach. This is because the transtorcular approach allows placement of 200 cm of coil in the vein of Galen aneurysm in a single step, usually taking less than 1 hour from the time of needle-stick to the end of the procedure. The transfemoral transvenous approach usually includes directing a catheter through the femoral vein, iliac vein, inferior vena cava, right atrium of the heart, superior vena cava, subclavian vein, and jugular vein. This guiding catheter is then connected to a rotating hemostatic valve with a continuous saline flush. Only the slowest-rate microdrip chamber is tolerated by neonates and most infants. A microcatheter is then advanced through the guiding catheter up to the sigmoid sinus, followed by the transverse sinus and ultimately the torcular, straight sinus, and vein of Galen. Because of size and length limitations, Guglielmi detachable coils are usually not the best option. These coils are hundreds of times more expensive, require slower placement with individual detachments, and usually require more than 10 coils (costing approximately $7000) to equal a similar volume achieved with one demandelized 200-cm, 0.035-inch guide wire (costing approximately $20) placed through a direct torcular

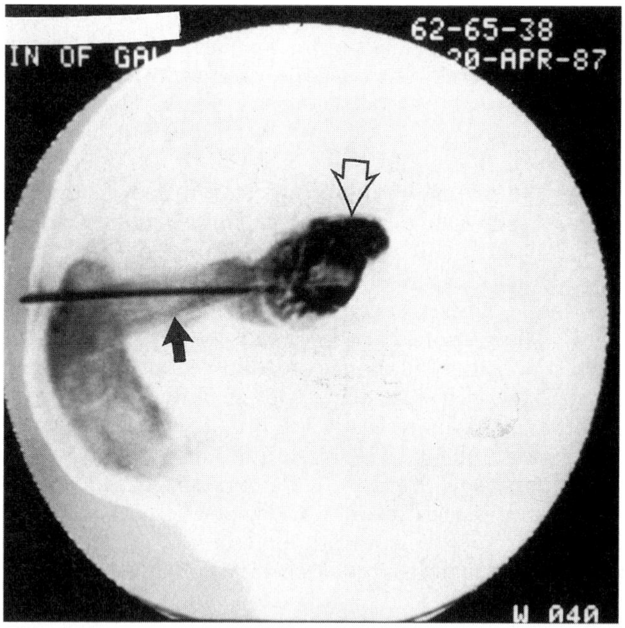

FIGURE 219–14. Lateral-projection transtorcular venogram during transtorcular embolization of a vein of Galen aneurysm. The vein of Galen aneurysm *(open arrow)* and the draining straight sinus *(black arrow)* are easily identified. This patient was a critically ill neonate who was deteriorating rapidly from heart failure. Ultrasonography and computed tomography confirmed the vein of Galen malformation, but diagnostic cerebral angiography was initially skipped because of the urgency of the case. The transtorcular approach is more rapid and achieves a more dramatic result than either the transarterial or transfemoral transvenous approach, and it allows the placement of up to 200 cm of coils within the vein of Galen aneurysm in only a few minutes. This provides a rapid reduction in flow through the shunt and a rapid decrease in intra-aneurysmal pressure.

stick. A transfemoral vein approach often takes many more hours than a direct transtorcular stick and is more likely to require multiple procedures.

Once a significant change in the flow pattern and pressure is obtained after transtorcular embolization, the blunt Seldinger needle is removed and a piece of Gelfoam is placed over the exit site in the torcular and held for 5 minutes. If a small incision was made in the scalp, it is closed in two layers. One should not attempt a suture closure of the exit hole in the torcular, because this will lead to significant bleeding, and simple pressure with Gelfoam is very effective. Risks to the patient with this venous approach include perforation of the thin anteroinferior portion of the sac with a wire or catheter, venous outlet obstruction with acute thrombosis, and an increased incidence of hydrocephalus. Rosenberg and Nazar[46] reported a severe coagulopathy after the transtorcular procedure in a neonate.

A recurring theme in this chapter has been the necessity of treating patients with vein of Galen malformations. Today, endovascular approaches are usually the best treatments initially, but in some patients, open surgery has a role.[47] Hydrocephalus should be treated carefully and conservatively in these patients, only after the process has been defined as chronic and progressive.

OUTCOME

The various series in the literature consist of mixed therapies, making it impossible to clearly evaluate any one type of therapy on an outcome basis.[1, 2, 4–6, 16, 18, 19, 45, 47–50] Some general statements can be made, however. A neonate with significant heart failure will die if untreated or if treated primarily with medical therapies. Direct open surgical therapy in a neonatal patient carries excessive risks and limited benefits. On average, approximately 50% of neonates with vein of Galen malformations can be salvaged with aggressive transarterial-transvenous endovascular treatment.

Ninety percent of patients who present as infants or children can look forward to survival with a good quality of life if they are treated aggressively with multiple interventional approaches (transarterial-transvenous). Direct open surgery is reserved for lesions no longer treatable with endovascular surgery or for the exposure of the lesion to deposit more embolic material for final elimination.[8] Surgery is also used in the treatment of hydrocephalus in those patients with progressive hydrocephalus.

A risk-benefit analysis should be included in any discussion with families concerning therapy in these patients. Today, depending on age, patients have a significant chance of survival with a good quality of life if the initial computed tomographic scan or MRI demonstrates a healthy central nervous system.

CONCLUSION

Vein of Galen malformations are a group of deep-seated, central, high-flow vascular shunts. The clinical presentation and prognosis of these patients are age dependent, and they remain a significant challenge to neurosurgeons. A neonate with high-output cardiac failure will die quickly if untreated, and medical therapy will only temporarily stabilize such an acutely ill patient. An infant or older child has a much less ominous prognosis and can be treated with direct surgery or endovascular approaches.[8] Most multispecialty centers use combined transarterial and transvenous embolization to eliminate these lesions in a gradual, staged fashion. The transtorcular approach has many clear advantages when transvenous embolization is considered.

REFERENCES

1. Dowd CF, Halbach VV, Barnwell SL, et al: Transfemoral venous embolization of vein of Galen malformations. AJNR Am J Neuroradiol 11:643–648, 1990.
2. Ciricillo SF, Edwards MSB, Schmidt KG, et al: Interventional neuroradiological management of vein of Galen malformation in the neonate. Neurosurgery 27:22–28, 1990.
3. Casasco A, Lylyk P, Hodes JE, et al: Percutaneous transvenous catheterization and embolization of vein of Galen aneurysms. Neurosurgery 28:260–266, 1991.
4. Lasjaunias P, Hui F, Zerah M, et al: Cerebral arteriovenous malformations in children: Management of 179 consecutive cases and review of the literature. Childs Nerv Syst 11:66–79, 1995.
5. Mericle RA, Mickle JP, Quisling RG: Vein of Galen malformation. Pediatr Neurosurg 31:279–280, 1999.

6. Drake CG: Cerebral arteriovenous malformations: Considerations for and experience with surgical treatment in 166 cases. Clin Neurosurg 26:145–208, 1979.

7. Hanner JS, Quisling RG, Mickle JP, et al: Gianturco coil embolization of vein of Galen aneurysms: Technical aspects. Radiographics 8:935–946, 1988.

8. Halbach VV, Dowd CF, Higashida RT, et al: Endovascular treatment of mural-type vein of Galen malformations. J Neurosurg 88:74–80, 1998.

9. Mitchell PJ, Rosenfeld JV, Dargaville P, et al: Endovascular management of vein of Galen aneurysmal malformations presenting in the neonatal period. AJNR Am J Neuroradiol 22:1403–1409, 2001.

10. Bedford THB: The venous system of the velum interpositum of the rhesus monkey and the effect of experimental occlusion of the great vein of Galen. Brain 57:255–265, 1934.

11. Steinheil SO: Ueber einen Fall von Varix aneurysmaticusim Bereich der Gehirngefoesse. Inaug diss, Würzburg, 1895. Cited in Dandy WE: Arteriovenous aneurysm of the brain. Arch Surg 17:190–243, 1928.

12. Jaeger JR, Forbes RP, Dandy WE: Bilateral congenital cerebral arteriovenous communications aneurysm. Trans Am Neurol Assoc 63:173, 1937.

13. Oscherwitz D, Davidoff LM: Midline calcified intracranial aneurysm between occipital lobes: Report of a case. J Neurosurg 4:539–541, 1947.

14. Boldrey E, Miller ER: Arteriovenous fistula (aneurysm) of the great cerebral vein (of Galen) and the circle of Willis. Arch Neurol Psychiatry 62:778–783, 1949.

15. Gold AP, Ransohoff JR, Carter S: Vein of Galen malformation. Acta Neurol Scand 40:5–31, 1964.

16. Amacher AL, Shillito J Jr: The syndromes and surgical treatment of aneurysms of the great vein of Galen. J Neurosurg 39:89–98, 1973.

17. Norman MG, Becker LE: Cerebral damage in neonates resulting from arteriovenous malformation of the vein of Galen. J Neurol Neurosurg Psychiatry 37:257–258, 1974.

18. Hoffman HJ, Chuang S, Hendrick EB, et al: Aneurysms of the vein of Galen: Experience at the Hospital for Sick Children, Toronto. J Neurosurg 57:316–322, 1982.

19. Johnston IH, Whittle IR, Besser M, et al: Vein of Galen malformation: Diagnosis and management. Neurosurgery 20:747–758, 1987.

20. Litvak J, Yahr MD, Ransohoff J: Aneurysms of the great vein of Galen and midline cerebral arteriovenous anomalies. J Neurosurg 17:945–954, 1960.

21. Yasargil MG: Microneurosurgery: IIIB. AVM of the Brain, Clinical Considerations, General and Special Operative Techniques, Surgical Results, Non-operated Cases, Cavernous and Venous Angiomas, Neuroanesthesia. New York, Thieme, 1988, pp 323–357.

22. Lasjaunias P, Terbrugge K, Piske R, et al: Vein of Galen dilatation: Anatomo-clinical forms and endovascular treatment. Fourteen cases explored and/or treated between 1983 and 1986. Neurochirurgie 33:315, 1987.

23. Lasjaunias P, Rodesch G, Pruvost P, et al: Treatment of vein of Galen aneurysmal malformation. J Neurosurg 70:746–750, 1989.

24. Lasjaunias P, Garcia-Monaco R, Rodesch G, et al: Vein of Galen malformation: Endovascular management of 43 cases. Childs Nerv Syst 7:360–367, 1991.

25. Raybaud CA, Strother CM, Hald JK: Aneurysms of the vein of Galen: Embryonic considerations and anatomical features relating to the pathogenesis of the malformation. Neuroradiology 31:109–128, 1989.

26. Garcia-Monaco R, Rodesch G, Terbrugge K, et al: Multifocal dural arteriovenous shunts in children. Childs Nerv Syst 7:425–431, 1991.

27. Andeweg J: Intracranial venous pressures, hydrocephalus and effects of cerebrospinal fluid shunts. Childs Nerv Syst 5:318–323, 1989.

28. Askenasy HM, Herzberger EE, Wijsenbeek HS: Hydrocephalus with vascular malformations of the brain: A preliminary report. Neurology 3:213–220, 1953.

29. Cumming GR: Circulation in neonates with intracranial arteriovenous fistula and cardiac failure. Am J Cardiol 45:1019–1024, 1980.

30. Sanders RC: Prenatal ultrasonic detection of anomalies with a lethal or disastrous outcome. Radiol Clin North Am 28:163–177, 1990.

31. Yamashita Y, Abe T, Ohara N, et al: Successful treatment of neonatal aneurysmal dilatation of the vein of Galen: The role of prenatal diagnosis and trans-arterial embolization. Neuroradiology 34:457–459, 1992.

32. Herman JM, Hamilton MG, Spetzler RF: Vein of Galen malformations: Surgical indications and techniques. In Carter LP, Spetzler RF (eds): Neurovascular Surgery. New York, McGraw-Hill, 1994, pp 1041–1047.

33. Wisoff JH, Berenstein A, Choi IS, et al: Management of vein of Galen malformations. Concepts Pediatr Neurosurg 10:137, 1990.

34. Nikas DC, Proctor MR, Scott RM: Spontaneous thrombosis of vein of Galen aneurysmal malformation. Pediatr Neurosurg 31:33–39, 1999.

35. Beltramello A, Perini S, Mazza C: Spontaneously healed vein of Galen aneurysms: Clinical radiological features. Childs Nerv Syst 7:129–134, 1991.

36. De Lange SA, De Vilieger M: Hydrocephalus associated with raised venous pressure. Dev Med Child Neurol 12:28–32, 1970.

37. Quisling RG, Mickle JP: Venous pressure measurements in vein of Galen aneurysms. AJNR Am J Neuroradiol 10:411–417, 1989.

38. Viñuela F, Drake CG, Fox AJ, et al: Giant intracranial varices secondary to high-flow arteriovenous fistulae. J Neurosurg 66:198–203, 1987.

39. Westra SJ, Curran JG, Duckwiler GR, et al: Pediatric intracranial vascular malformations: Evaluation of treatment results with color Doppler US. Work in progress. Radiology 186:775–783, 1993.

40. Spetzler RF, Martin NA: A proposed grading system for arteriovenous malformations. J Neurosurg 65:476–483, 1986.

41. Hamilton MG, Herman JM, Khazata MH: Aneurysms of the vein of Galen. In Youmans JR (ed): Neurological Surgery, 4th ed. Philadelphia, WB Saunders, 1996, pp 1491–1510.

42. Zerah M, Garcia-Monaco R, Rodesch G, et al: Hydrodynamics in vein of Galen malformations. Childs Nerv Syst 8:111–117, 1998.

43. Mickle JP, Quisling R, Ryan P: Transtorcular approach to vein of Galen aneurysms. Pediatr Neurosurg 20:163–168, 1994.

44. Mickle JP, Quisling RG: The transtorcular embolization of vein of Galen aneurysms. J Neurosurg 64:731–735, 1986.

45. Halbach VV, Higashida RT, Hieshima GB, et al: Transvenous embolization of dural fistulas involving the transverse and sigmoid sinuses. AJNR Am J Neuroradiol 10:385–392, 1989.

46. Rosenberg EM, Nazar GB: Neonatal vein of Galen aneurysms: Severe coagulopathy associated with transtorcular embolization. Crit Care Med 19:441–443, 1991.

47. King WA, Wackym PA, Viñuela F, et al: Management of vein of Galen aneurysms: Combined surgical and endovascular approach. Childs Nerv Syst 5:208–211, 1989.

48. Garcia-Monaco R, Lasjaunias P, Berenstein A: Therapeutic management of vein of Galen aneurysmal malformations. In Viñuela F, Halbach VV, Dion JE (eds): Interventional Neuroradiology: Endovascular Therapy of the Central Nervous System. New York, Raven Press, 1992, pp 113–127.

49. Glasser RS, Mickle JP, Quisling R, et al: The transvenous treatment of the vein of Galen aneurysms: A review of 40 cases. Paper presented at the meeting of the American Association of Neurological Surgeons, 1994, San Diego, CA.

50. Lylyk P, Viñeula F, Dion JE, et al: Therapeutic alternatives for vein of Galen vascular malformations. J Neurosurg 78:438–445, 1993.

CHAPTER 220

Arteriovenous Malformations and Intracranial Aneurysms in Children

ROBIN P. HUMPHREYS ■ FARHAD PIROUZMAND

When evaluating pediatric cerebrovascular disease, whether of ischemic or hemorrhagic origin, one must resist scaling down adult disease information to fit the pediatric mode. Children are not small adults. Since the 1970s, a number of causes of both ischemic and hemorrhagic stroke events in children have been studied. Not unexpectedly, many of the causes of pediatric stroke were found to be unique to that age group and thus differ dramatically from stroke insults that occur in adults.[1]

There has been considerable expansion of our knowledge about pediatric stroke because of improved diagnostic technology, and novel therapies are now being administered to children. Although it is true that pediatric hemorrhagic stroke in particular often has a devastating presentation that demands early intervention, it is now much easier to define the primary cause of the brain hemorrhage. This, in turn, allows one to map a treatment plan best suited for the specific cause and its attendant phenomena. The operative evacuation of a cerebral clot should no longer be the *only* strategy to rescue a child's impaired neurological functions. Clot removal may be only one component of the therapy. Spiral computed tomographic angiography, fine-cut magnetic resonance imaging (MRI) with angiography, stereotactic mapping of a vascular nidus, and superselective contrast arteriography are all diagnostic advances that can detail the geography, number, and idiosyncratic details of the offending vascular lesion. Further, endovascular embolization techniques for aneurysms or vascular malformations and the application of radiosurgery for some malformations are now legitimate adjuncts or alternatives to traditional treatments. These multimodal advances have resulted in improved morbidity and mortality outcomes with respect to cerebral hemorrhages in children. For example, with the advent of computed tomographic scanning alone, the early and rapid triage of patients with cerebral hemorrhage from arteriovenous malformation (AVM) has resulted in a 50% decline in mortality in children.[2] Similarly, MRI can precisely define the cavernous angioma occurring at one or more sites in the cerebral tissue of adults and children. Such information allows the neurosurgeon to respond intelligently to the symptomatic lesion and determine its appropriate treatment.

These exciting advances, along with those in neuroanesthesia and critical care, have improved survival and its quality for children struck by spontaneous cerebral hemorrhage.

SPONTANEOUS CEREBRAL HEMORRHAGE OF STRUCTURAL ORIGIN

Intracranial arterial aneurysms and AVMs are collectively the most common causes of spontaneous subarachnoid hemorrhage (SAH) and intraventricular hemorrhage (IVH). Matson declared the AVM "the most frequent abnormality of intracranial circulation in childhood" and reported on his experience with 34 patients.[3] In adults, a ruptured saccular aneurysm would be 6.5 times more likely than an AVM to account for hemorrhage.[4] It is moot whether the ratio is reversed in children. Hourihan and associates,[5] in a review of 167 patients aged 20 years and younger, noted that in twice as many patients SAH was caused by aneurysm rather than by AVM. Their paper included the work of other authors studying pediatric SAH.[4, 6, 7] In a total review of 478 such patients, ruptured aneurysm accounted for 40% of children's SAH and AVM for 26%; no lesion was defined in 31%. This cumulative experience might appear to be at odds with the results of the Cooperative Study, in which 33% of AVMs associated with hemorrhage occurred before age 20. This finding contrasts with the finding that only 1.5% of intracranial aneurysms became symptomatic in the same period.[4, 8]

The material reviewed in this chapter is taken from the experience at the Hospital for Sick Children (HSC) in Toronto, which serves as a widespread referral base exclusively for the care of children up to age 18 years. With regard to SAH as the presenting symptom, 33 of 46 children with aneurysm presented with SAH or IVH, whereas 160 children presented with AVM during the same interval. This contrasts with 128 children who bled from their AVMs and presented with brain hemorrhage. Hence, rupture of an AVM in a child is almost four times as likely to be the cause of hemorrhage than is a ruptured aneurysm.

If each of these structural lesions is thought to represent a developmental fault in the cerebral vasculature, one might expect them to be detected not only in symptomatic children but also incidentally. This is rarely the case. With the exception of a post-traumatic aneurysm discovered on a computed tomographic scan performed as a follow-up to head injury treatment, in our experience, no incidental aneurysm or AVM has been defined by cerebral arteriography or computed tomography (CT) performed for other reasons.[9]

There have been few children identified with a conglomerate of vascular problems. The Cooperative Study contains 37 patients with coexisting angioma malformations and one or more aneurysms.[8] Hayashi and coworkers reviewed 73 patients with AVM associated with aneurysm and noted that only two patients were younger than age 10.[10] Ostergaard added two more children with saccular aneurysms attendant to an AVM.[11] In the HSC series, there was one child with a left internal carotid aneurysm who bled and died from a ruptured sylvian AVM. A small aneurysmal dilatation may be noted adjacent to the AVM nidus or on a feeding vessel; however, when these are explored operatively, they are often difficult to find. In one personal instance, the involved vessel did not show any aneurysmal formation when the excised tissue was analyzed.

Most series of AVMs note a common age of presentation between 20 and 40 years.[12–16] The fact that most lesions become symptomatic during this time suggests a latency in the malformation's usual evolution.[8]

INTRACRANIAL ANEURYSMS IN CHILDREN

Pediatric cerebral aneurysms are uncommon. The Cooperative Study of 6368 patients reported that 41 (0.6%) occurred in patients younger than 19 years.[4] This is remarkably similar to our experience at the University of Toronto. At the HSC, the incidence of newly diagnosed intracranial aneurysm is 1.1 per year. This constitutes 0.7% of all the intracranial aneurysms treated in our adult university hospitals. The information in this section is based on our study of 46 consecutive patients younger than 18 years with intracranial aneurysm who were treated at the HSC.

Developmental Features and Pathology

The genesis of an intracranial aneurysm is thought to be a consequence of congenital and acquired influences. If diabetes, hypertension, obesity, hypercholesterolemia, and other known factors responsible for SAH in adults are virtually nonexistent in children, is the development of an aneurysm in a child related *only* to congenital causes? The logical expectation for childhood aneurysms to arise at arterial bifurcations

from the remnants of small, rudimentary vascular trunks has not been confirmed. Moreover, the lack of incidental aneurysms detected in children either by angiography or in pediatric autopsies,[17] as well as the relative rarity of neonatal and early childhood cases, suggests that factors other than purely developmental anomalies are involved. Stehbens, in his critical review of the histology of documented cases of aneurysm in pediatric patients, concluded that inadequate pathologic examinations or atypical histologic features provide little support for an inborn developmental defect as the underlying cause of aneurysm.[18, 19] He also noted that the presence of a few true congenital aneurysms does not mean that all aneurysms are secondary to a developmental defect. Instead, he favors degenerative changes at the arterial bifurcation caused by axial blood flow as the main predisposing factor in aneurysm creation.

Pathologic studies of pediatric aneurysms are limited. The majority of reported cases, however, indicate that they are characterized by common wall features—absence of the internal elastic lamina and the muscularis layer of the media—that also occur in adults. There are a few underlying pathologic conditions that may promote aneurysmal formation and SAH in childhood,[20] such as infection and trauma (Fig. 220–1), which may cause a relatively greater number of aneurysms in children than in adults. Mycotic aneurysm has an increased preponderance in children and accounted for three of our cases. Karsner indicated that infectious aneurysms may occur secondary to bacterial endocarditis (the most common form) or by direct extension from an adjacent focus of infection.[21] All three of our cases had septicemia at the time of admission, and two of them suffered from SAH. Head or neck trauma is also a fairly common culprit in the evolution of pediatric aneurysm and subsequent SAH.[22] Typically, the traumatic aneurysm occurs at junctures where

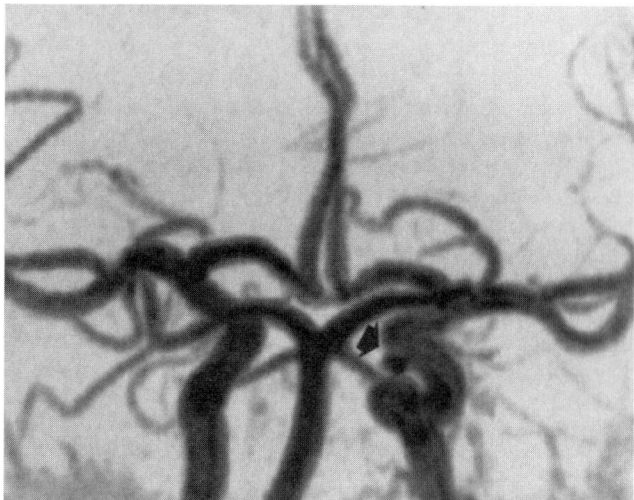

FIGURE 220–1. As a result of multiple sharp penetrating wounds to his left temporal region, this 10-year-old boy suffered a post-traumatic aneurysm *(arrow)* on the ipsilateral internal carotid artery at the takeoff of the ophthalmic artery. The lesion has not been treated and remains unchanged in size.

surface cerebral vessels may be vulnerable to adjacent fixed tissues, such as the anterior and posterior cerebral arteries and the adjacent falx and tentorial edge, respectively, and the middle cerebral artery juxtaposed to the lesser sphenoid wing. There were six of these cases in our series, occurring in both the anterior and the posterior circulation. Most of these patients presented within the first month after trauma.

A number of disorders may be associated with an intracranial aneurysm in a child.[23] Many are extraordinarily uncommon, but a few can be considered somewhat idiosyncratic to childhood. These include coarctation of the aorta, polycystic kidney disease, tuberous sclerosis, and human immunodeficiency virus infection (Fig. 220–2). Notwithstanding our active cardiovascular service, we have not encountered an aneurysm in a child with aortic coarctation, nor among our patients with tuberous sclerosis. We had one child with polycystic renal disease who died of her aneurysmal SAH.

The majority of our patients (72%) had aneurysms that were idiopathic in nature. The incidence of multiple aneurysms was 10% (less than the incidence reported in adults). This may further weaken the possibility of an inherited defect in cerebral vasculature as the sole basis for aneurysmal formation.

The distribution of aneurysms in children demonstrates a strong predilection for the region of the internal carotid artery (ICA) bifurcation. It has been shown that the angle of the bifurcation of the ICA gradually changes in adults, by increasing to a more horizontal direction. Theoretically, in children, the more acute angle creates a more concentrated vector of blood-

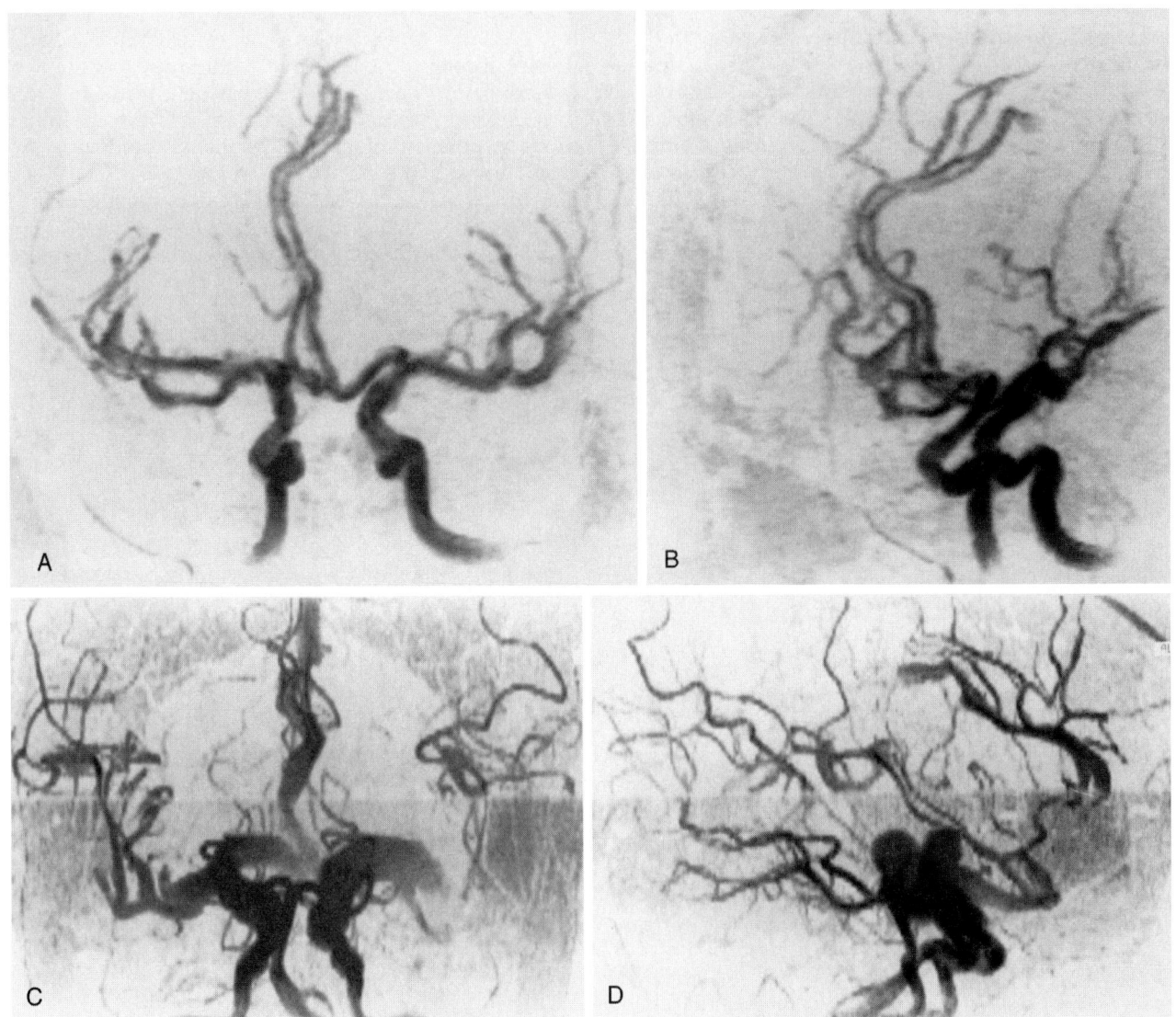

FIGURE 220–2. This 14-year-old girl had acquired immunodeficiency syndrome. In the 18 months before her death, she demonstrated on magnetic resonance angiography progressive fusiform aneurysmal dilatation of the internal carotid and middle cerebral arteries. *A,* Anteroposterior (AP) view. *B,* Lateral view. *C* and *D,* AP and lateral views 9 months later. The bilateral anterior cerebral arteries and pericallosal complex subsequently became involved, and an isolated pericallosal aneurysm developed. She did not suffer subarachnoid hemorrhage.

stream forces within the ICA, which acts on the apex of the distal bifurcation. This explains the prevalence of ICA bifurcation aneurysms in children. Conversely, in adults, the more horizontal alignment of the anterior and middle cerebral arteries with the carotid termination downloads the impact of blood flow onto the next immediate bifurcation (at the anterior communicating region). This accounts for the higher incidence of aneurysms in this region in adults. Posterior circulation aneurysms are reportedly three times more prevalent in children than in adults (there were seven in our series), especially among cases occurring in the first 2 years of life.[24–26] This is also the case for giant aneurysms; there were 13 such cases in our series, with 4 found in the posterior circulation. The reason for this predilection in the pediatric age group is not clear.

Natural History

There is not an extensive clinical experience with these uncommon lesions in children.[9, 19, 23, 27–30] The cumulative evidence, however, shows differences between children and adults in a variety of aspects of intracranial aneurysms. These include the sex ratio (with the exception of our own series, a bias toward male cases in children),[23] size, location, underlying cause, and clinical presentation. A child's vulnerability to SAH from a ruptured aneurysm is difficult to predict, given the

small number of cases available for study. Khoo and Levy, basing their calculation on the average annual incidence of aneurysmal SAH in Western countries being 10 per 100,000 population, provide a formula for children based on a "crude estimate of one to three cases of childhood aneurysm (productive of subarachnoid hemorrhage) per 1 million population."[23] There is also a paucity of data regarding the management outcome for these patients.[31] Aneurysmal SAH appears to be devastating to the developing brain and results in high pediatric mortality and morbidity. It seems that just as advanced age in adults is a recognized risk factor for poor outcome from SAH, young children are also more vulnerable to the deleterious effects of hemorrhage.

Initial Clinical Assessment

The management strategies for a child's aneurysm follow the same general rules as those for adults, although more complex or innovative techniques are often required. SAH, characterized by sudden headache, vomiting, seizures, coma, or meningism, is the predominant mode of presentation of a ruptured aneurysm in a child, occurring in 52% to 74% of cases.[23, 28, 31–33] It was present in 33 (72%) of our cases. In this group, 17 children presented with a poor prognostic grade (i.e., IV or V), often the result of a secondary bleed. Rebleed-

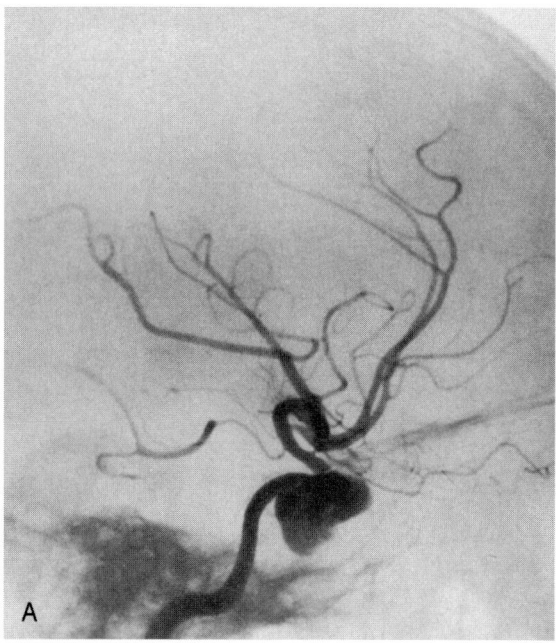
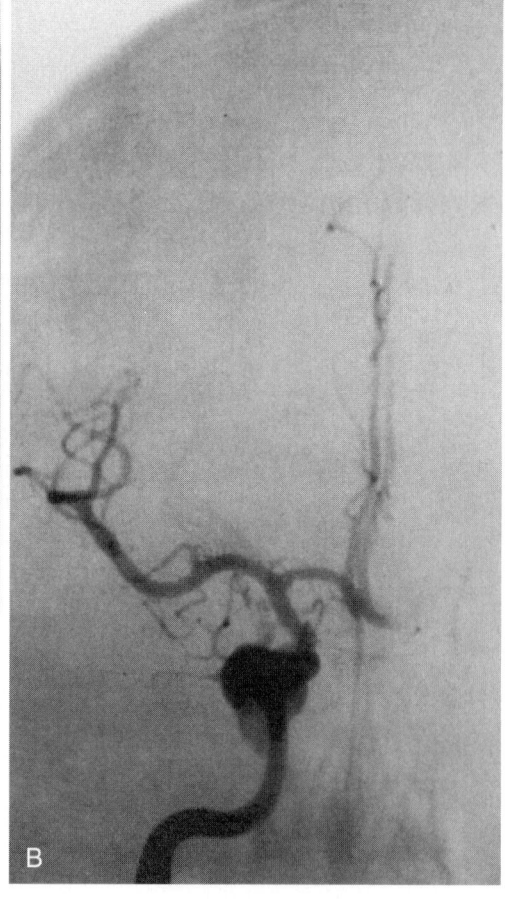

FIGURE 220–3. A sudden painless right ophthalmoplegia was the presenting feature in this 9-year-old girl. An intracavernous carotid aneurysm was apparent on computed tomographic imaging and was confirmed on the carotid angiogram. *A*, Right lateral view. *B*, AP view. Both anterior cerebral arteries fill, a fairly common and reassuring feature of pediatric cerebral angiography. The lesion was trapped.

ing is common in all SAH grades and was seen in 57% of our cases, half of whom rebled in the first 24 hours (significantly more common than in the adult population).[34] The occurrence of rebleeding usually led to clinical deterioration.

Focal neurological deficits, usually representing expansion of the aneurysm, may occur, particularly with ophthalmic manifestations (Fig. 220–3). Ten percent of our group presented with some ocular finding. Associated preretinal or subhyaloid hemorrhage was detected in 21% of patients presenting with SAH, more frequently in higher grade SAH. This is similar to the experience in adults.

Seizures, which are a common ictal event of cerebral insult in children, may be part of the presenting symptom complex at the time of SAH. Focal or generalized seizures may occur in 7% to 25% of children.[23, 35] Characteristic features of intracranial hypertension may relate to the presence of a giant aneurysm, probably unruptured; more than likely, however, they are associated with cerebral hemorrhage or IVH, with or without obstruction of the cerebrospinal fluid pathways. In children, the mortality increases with intracerebral hemorrhage, a morbid phenomenon more common with middle cerebral artery aneurysms than those in other locations.[36]

The impact of cerebral vasospasm in a child after SAH is difficult to predict. Ostergaard and Voldby documented severe angiographic spasm in 25% of their cases, and an additional 25% showed milder features.[36] This does not necessarily translate into an increase in morbidity or mortality in children, presumably because of their abundant collateral circulation.[32, 37]

Investigations

The sudden and dramatic presentation of a child's SAH should not be confused with an infectious process, which would demand a lumbar puncture.[38] In the vast majority of children with subarachnoid blood from any source, it will show up on a computed tomographic scan performed within 2 days of the provoking incident.[39] The hyperinfused images can outline larger aneurysms, especially in the anterior circulation. Hematoma, edema, infarction, and hydrocephalus may also be detected. Either computed tomographic or MRI scans obtained for reasons other than spontaneous hemorrhage may reveal an unanticipated aneurysm (Fig. 220–4). Thereafter, traditional four-vessel angiograms are obtained and studied for the idiosyncrasies of pediatric aneurysm collections. These include the aneurysm's location (typical or distal, and at nonbranching points), size, and, if more than one aneurysm is found, some overt feature indicating which one bled. If the study is negative, it must be repeated after an arbitrary interval.

Definitive Management

Few other circumstances in pediatric neurosurgery call for the collaborative effort that is required for a child with SAH from a ruptured intracranial aneurysm. It is

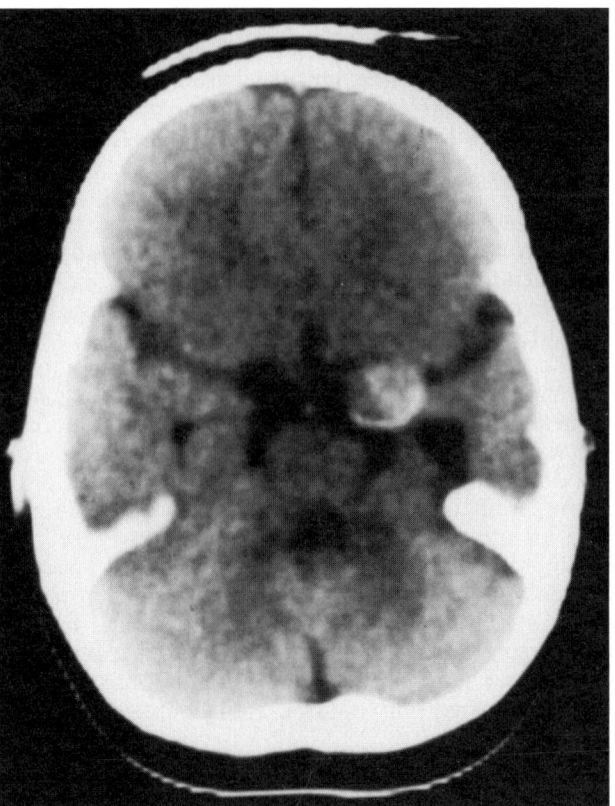

FIGURE 220–4. This 9-month-old girl suffered a severe closed-head injury as a result of nonaccidental trauma. In this surveillance follow-up computed tomographic scan, a giant left internal carotid artery aneurysm is suspected and was subsequently confirmed with cerebral angiography. The aneurysm was operatively trapped.

in the best interests of the child that he or she be cared for in a tertiary pediatric facility with skilled staff. The preoperative medical management requires delicate titration of fluids and electrolytes, blood pressure management, analgesia and sedation, seizure control, and ventilation (if required) by critical care intensivists who are familiar with the biologic nuances of pediatric patients. An on-site pediatric neurosurgeon will be able to structure a timetable of care and advise about the need to control cerebral vasospasm and release obstructed spinal fluid or hematoma, as well as provide surveillance for repeat hemorrhage.

A cerebrovascular surgeon who is experienced with adults should consult and assist with the operative procedure, for reasons of experience and technology. As a simple example, it is unlikely that a children's hospital will have a full array of aneurysm clips, including one that is ideal for obliteration of a child's aneurysm. The more experienced aneurysm surgeon should determine the timing of the operation and, having defined its architecture, plan the route to the lesion. The pediatric neurosurgeon, in addition to recognizing the importance of temperature control and avoidance of substantial blood loss and appreciating the more delicate nature of children's cerebral tissues, realizes that each child may require customized and innovative care. This surgeon also appreciates the deceptive features of some pediatric aneurysms in terms of their size, intraluminal thrombosis, and absence of a crotch from which the aneurysm has arisen. It is also a fact that children are far more tolerant of proximal vessel ligation, should that be the only solution.

Although all patients are managed by traditional methods of supportive and surgical therapy, with the notable exception of antifibrinolytic therapy, the general trend is toward a delayed (i.e., after 48 hours) approach to definitive surgical treatment. In our group, only two patients had an aneurysm operation in the first 3 days after the hemorrhage.

The experience with aneurysm obliteration by endovascular techniques is sparse, given the relative rarity of pediatric intracranial aneurysms. On the one hand, the bizarre character of some children's aneurysms and the desire to minimize manipulation of the still developing brain argue in favor of alternative therapies, such as intravascular embolization. On the other hand, the interventional radiologist may be handicapped by anomalous, tortuous, or small arteries that preclude catheter placement in close proximity to the targeted aneurysm. Lasjaunias successfully embolized seven children's aneurysms.[40] Our experience consists of six children treated with balloon occlusion or coils.[41]

Postoperative Care and Results

There is a direct relationship between a child's initial grade at presentation with an aneurysmal SAH and outcome. Death from SAH or its complications occurred in 17 patients (52%) in our series. Rebleeding occurred in 57%. We examined all the patients with SAH according to the time of their presentation (i.e., before or after 1975, the landmark year for CT availability and the operating diploscope in our hospital). A comparison of the outcomes in early (before 1975) versus later (after 1975) groups confirmed the *same* trend for both groups. Despite advances in both the medical and the surgical management of these patients, the overall prognosis remains guarded. Fifty-four percent of *all* the patients who were subject to some type of invasive intervention for their aneurysms returned to their premorbid functional status; only 43% of those who had SAH did so. These outcome figures are comparable to those in adults after SAH.

Considering the high risk of rebleeding, especially in the early stages, and the uniformly poor prognosis of these patients, regardless of the type of treatment, we believe that surgical intervention in the first 24 hours might improve the long-term outcome for these children. Increased awareness by primary care physicians of the early symptoms of an aneurysm's warning leak, which occurred in 57% of our patients, is needed. Associated ophthalmic and ischemic symptoms should also lead to timely diagnostic intervention and treatment.

ARTERIOVENOUS MALFORMATIONS OF THE BRAIN

Developmental Features and Pathology

The classic AVM is presumed to represent a structural defect in the formation of the primitive arteriolar-capillary network normally interposed between brain arteries and veins. The stimulus, timing, and early architectural deficiencies for such malformations are not entirely clear. Padget believed that most of the malformations occur before the achievement of 40 mm embryonal length; that is, they occur before the arterial walls thicken, notwithstanding that it is after this time that the late histologic changes in the vessel walls convert them into the final adult form.[42]

The pathologic analysis of resected AVM specimens does not provide much additional information about the causes of AVMs. The tangled arteriovenous communications attract exaggerated blood flow because of their low resistance. Given enough time, the malformations have the capacity to expand their bulk by enlarging and increasing the tortuosity of the feeding and draining channels. The number of fistulous connections, however, probably does not change, and some lesions, such as those of the brainstem, may always remain small.[43]

The conglomeration of turgid, tortuous vessels covered by opacified and thickened arachnoid on the brain's surface is easily recognized as the classic AVM. Sometimes in a child, however, the malformation is hidden in a sulcus or the subcortical tissues and is served by a straightened, dilated, anomalous artery that acts as its only superficial hallmark. The nearby cerebral convolutions show variable degrees of atrophy, and there may be local rusty staining from a previous hemorrhage. The tough texture of the adjacent gray and white matter is due to gliosis, inert tissue that permits circumferential dissection of the lesion.

Although some malformations have a globular shape, most describe a course to the subjacent ventricle in an inverted wedge-shaped fashion. The component vessels show variation in their number, caliber, and wall thickness. Venous tortuosity, intimal thickening, arteriolization of veins, and evidence of hemorrhage and neuronal loss are indicative of the long-standing hemodynamic consequences within and around the malformation. In almost all circumstances, there is microscopic evidence of previous hemorrhage by hemosiderin-laden macrophages.[44, 45] Elastic and muscle fibers in the arteries are altered; the media varies in thickness, and substantial thinning of some vessels can result in aneurysmal dilatation of the structure.[45–47] Those vessels with dramatic saccular dilatations are usually venous in origin.[44]

An interesting theory has been proposed by Sonstein and colleagues concerning the role of vascular endothelial growth factor as a possible general mediator of angiogenesis in AVM development.[48] The immunocytochemical expression of vascular endothelial growth factor in AVM tissue was analyzed in four children and may be related to the "regrowth" or reappearance of AVMs that were thought to have been totally excised.

Although ruptured AVM is the most common cause of hemorrhagic stroke in children, most of these lesions become symptomatic after age 20. It is therefore tempting to believe that whatever the early embryologic fault, there may be substantial postnatal and delayed factors that influence the development and declaration of cerebral AVMs.

Natural History

Because of improvements in diagnostic and therapeutic technologies, the patient selection criteria for treatment of cerebral AVMs are not as controversial as they once were. It is now recognized that technologic advances have broadened the indications for intervention and improved the rate of success, whatever the type of intervention. Contemporary AVM literature also analyzes the long-term outcomes in adults and children treated for cerebral AVMs by alternative therapies such as radiosurgery and embolization.

The natural history of AVMs in the pediatric population is not well known. In our series, 80% of the lesions presented with hemorrhage, a rate that is higher than that reported for adults.[7, 13] By defining our pediatric population as patients up to age 18, we do not mean to imply that there are differences between AVMs in patients age 17 versus those age 20; rather, there is a difference between the *populations* of children and adults. Celli and associates reported a hemorrhage rate in children of more than 80% for AVMs less than 2 cm in diameter.[49] Mori and coworkers concluded that the prognosis was less favorable in children with AVMs than in adults, and they described a higher mortality rate in younger patients because of hemorrhage.[50] Gerosa and colleagues reported that the primary hemorrhage was fatal in 5.4% of their patients; rebleeding occurred in 29% and carried a grim prognosis.[51]

The higher mortality rate from AVM hemorrhage in children (21% for our entire series) may be due to several factors. First, in children, there is a higher incidence of AVMs located in the posterior cranial fossa, where the effects of hemorrhage are more critical. A substantial difference was found between the number of posterior fossa AVMs in our pediatric series (36 of 160) and the number in the general adult series of Jomin and coworkers (8 of 150).[2, 16] Similarly, infratentorial AVMs were present in only 32 of 453 patients in the Cooperative Study[8]; again, this difference was significant. We believe that the hemodynamic compressive or hemorrhagic effects of a critically located infratentorial AVM lead to an earlier onset of symptoms when compared with most supratentorial malformations. Second, hemorrhage from an AVM may be more severe in children than in adults. Celli and associates stated that cerebral hemorrhages in children show more violent and massive bleeding, as demonstrated by a higher frequency of intraparenchymal hemorrhage *and* IVH.[49] There is no evidence, however, that the vessels of a "younger" AVM are more fragile than those in an adult. The Cooperative Study reported an adult mortality rate from hemorrhage between 6% and 10%.[8] Finally, there is some evidence that a smaller AVM is more inclined to bleed than is a larger one.[12, 52] It is also our observation that children's vascular malformations tend to be small rather than large and are secreted in unusual or awkward locations.

A number of reports of adult patients with AVMs

indicated that the risk of rehemorrhage is 2% to 4% per year, independent of previous hemorrhage.[12, 53-56] Risk estimates were provided by large series of patients managed conservatively. The lack of large pediatric AVM series and the small number of patients *without* resection in our series prohibit a reasonable estimate of the rebleeding risk in children.

Initial Clinical Assessment

The symptoms of a cerebral AVM, whenever they appear, are representative of the structural defects in the vessels of the malformation and the sump effect of the direct arteriovenous shunting. A greater percentage of children than adults experience hemorrhage as their first symptom. It is not always clear at operation or on histopathologic examination of excised tissues just where the hemorrhage originated. Certainly, there are deficiencies in some vessel walls, possibly making them liable to rupture, yet other abnormal channels are thickened.[45] It appears to be true that smaller AVMs have a greater tendency to bleed and that there is generally less violent parenchymal disruption after AVM hemorrhage than after ruptured aneurysm. Characteristically, the hemorrhage tends to dissect fiber bundles within the centrum semiovale rather than destroying these bundles outright. In many instances, the hemorrhage tends to vent itself to the adjacent ventricle, which is not surprising, given the almost uniform extension of the malformation to the ventricular wall and perhaps even to the choroid.

A child's AVM declares itself most frequently with cerebral or ventricular hemorrhage, or both. In our review, 128 of 160 patients (80%) experienced spontaneous intracranial hemorrhage, as determined by the syndrome of headache and bloody spinal fluid or blood clot recognized on CT or recovered at operation or autopsy. The ictus is often explosive, with a previously well child screaming out because of sudden headache. Although one might expect hemorrhagic cerebrovascular events to occur during periods of exercise or similiar activity, we noted that a surprising number of children's AVMs bled during periods of quietude (e.g., while watching television or even during sleep).[4] Not surprisingly, therefore, the subarachnoid grading reflects the critical nature of the child's condition at the time of first assessment. Altered consciousness, meningism, and appropriate lateralized motor and sensory signs are present.

Epilepsy, which presumably results from gliosis of brain because of chronic ischemia adjacent to the arteriovenous shunt, occurs as a presenting symptom in 20% to 67% of adult patients with AVM.[57, 58] Twenty-two children had chronic seizure disturbances in our series, the symptoms of which were infrequent in most. The proper management for a patient who has had one or two seizures from an AVM, exclusive of a frank hemorrhage, is challenging. Recent reports indicate that more than 70% of patients with epilepsy related to an AVM will remain seizure free (or nearly so) when the associated epileptogenic tissue is excised.[57]

Of the remaining 10 children in our series, 4 were

infants with congestive heart failure, 3 presented with developmental delay, 2 with chronic headache, and 1 with evidence of cerebral ischemia.

Investigations

A certain number of children will, without warning, experience the onset of a severe, generalized headache that is not representative of any organic pathology within the cranium. Perhaps they are suffering their first migraine events. The ready availability of CT usually sorts out these cases at the primary referral level. CT may, however, document the cerebral hemorrhage suffered after a child has ruptured an AVM. In many such instances, the explosive nature of the event, the severity of the headache, and the altered consciousness with a neurological deficit underscore the presence of a vascular brain lesion.

The computed tomographic head scan outlines the blood clot and calcification, if present; an enhanced study may detail the dilated feeding and draining vascular channels and large blood-containing varices (Fig. 220–5). Similarly, MRI scans are capable of defining the nature of the hemorrhage as well as the involved vasculature. In reality, however, the urgent nature of the child's condition often makes it unfeasible to take the time necessary to perform an MRI scan. Additionally, the surgeon should not rely on the MRI scan to

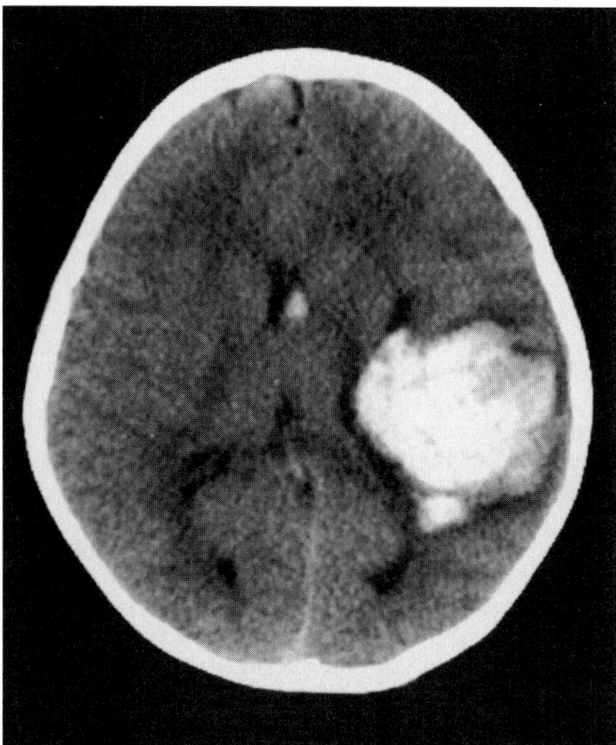

FIGURE 220–5. The intake computed tomographic scan of a child who sustained a sudden cerebral hemorrhage outlines the generous intracerebral clot, with a venting extension into the lateral ventricle and midline tissue shifts. The decision was whether an urgent craniotomy for clot evacuation *alone* should be planned without angiography.

identify all the vascular abnormalities (Fig. 220–6). It has already been indicated that most AVMs that bleed are small, and this is especially true in children. The tiny feeding and draining vessels associated with a nidus of varying size may be completely obscured on an MRI scan, particularly when there is also a blood clot. MRI is a valuable adjunct in elective situations, especially for small lesions adjacent to the ventricular wall or within the diencephalon or brainstem. The valuable information obtained from this imaging technique could change the type of therapy chosen.

Selective carotid and vertebral arteriography, with superselective views, if necessary, remains the standard of investigation for a child's AVM. The number and location of arterial feeders can be examined by films processed with subtraction and magnified techniques. Seldom is a malformation served by only one arterial channel. There may be only one major artery contributing to the lesion, but the surgeon should anticipate any number of minor vessels coming from pial or deep perforating sources, especially in relation to the underlying ventricle. Conversely, the major venous drainage from a child's AVM is frequently through a solitary large cortical vein, or one ending in the deep venous system. This venous outflow is usually precisely defined on arteriography.

Some vascular malformations are angiographically cryptic and thus are not demonstrated on arteriography.[59] These lesions, often in the distribution of the middle cerebral artery, are usually small, and there is evidence of a recent or old hemorrhagic history. Meticulous processing of the pathologic material uncovers the vascular malformation. There were five such cases in our series. Close follow-up must be maintained for all children with an intracerebral hemorrhage small enough to be treated nonoperatively; these patients may harbor an occult malformation.

As a rule, 90% of AVMs are supratentorial, most frequently within the distribution of the middle cerebral artery.[8, 47] Any intracranial artery can be associated with a malformation, however, and in the HSC study, 22% of the lesions were found below the tentorium.

Definitive Management

Inasmuch as the presenting symptom in children is spontaneous intracranial hemorrhage in 80% of cases, urgent neurodiagnostic assessment and operative care must be undertaken to identify and release the associated clot. However, because AVM surgery can be tedious and protracted, it is desirable, whenever circumstances permit, to schedule the malformation excision as an elective procedure. Thus, if only IVH has occurred, or if the intracerebral hemorrhage is small and the patient's condition is stable, interval surgery may be staged after a few days' wait. During that time, the child is monitored appropriately. Cerebral vasospasm is seldom a problem in children with AVMs, but rebleeding may be. If the operation can possibly be delayed for 3 to 7 days after the hemorrhage, the surgeon will be rewarded with a properly prepared patient whose relaxed brain contains a partially liquefying he-

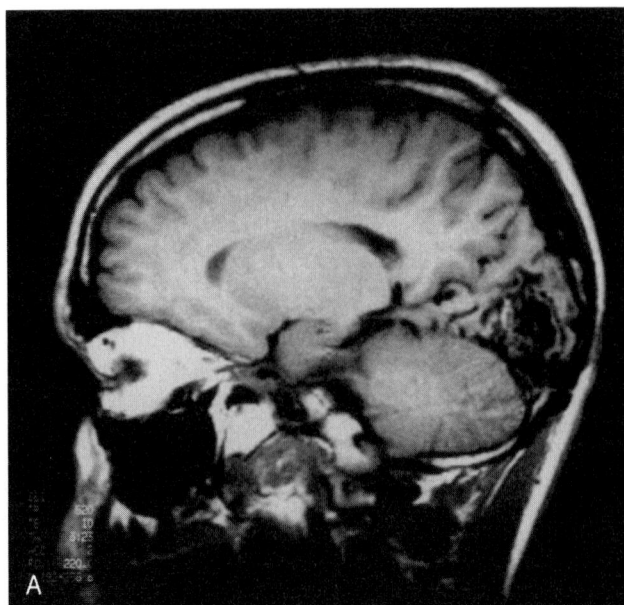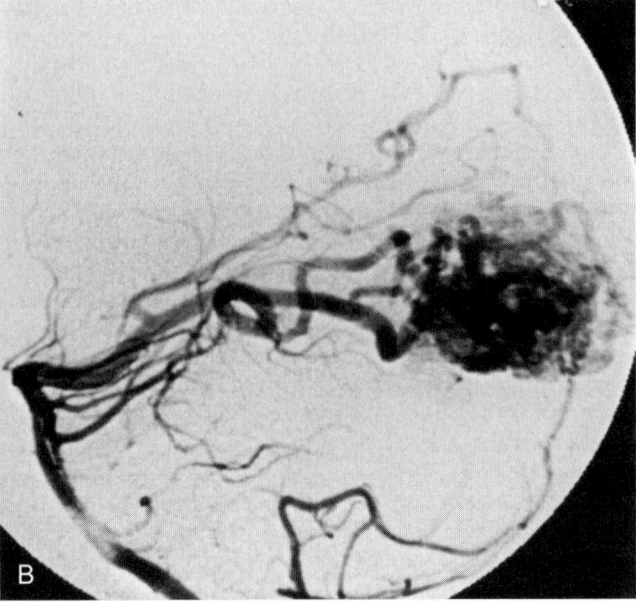

FIGURE 220–6. *A,* MRI scan of this right occipital pole arteriovenous malformation provides anatomic information with respect to its neighboring boundaries. This is useful information for operative planning, but surgery should not proceed without detailed angiography. *B,* Angiography shows the lesion to be fed exclusively by the posterior cerebral artery.

matoma. This does not deny that a certain percentage of patients will arrive in a precarious condition because of the size and location of the brain hematoma. Under these circumstances, the surgeon has no option but to perform a craniotomy for clot removal. Once the brain compression is alleviated, the stage is properly set for an interval elective arteriogram.

There is not the same urgency in the 20% of patients whose presenting symptom is not spontaneous hemorrhage. This group has been investigated in a traditional fashion, and the clinical challenge is to determine in advance whether surgical obliteration of the malformation will influence the seizure events, headaches, or developmental problems and whether it should even be undertaken.[60]

The ideal treatment for brain AVM is total excision.[3, 43, 60] Such excision has now been achieved in almost all eloquent regions of brain (motor, basal ganglia, brainstem), as well as in less critical areas.[61] Thus, except for lesions that penetrate the brainstem or basal ganglia, it is not so much the anatomic location of the lesion that restrains the surgeon as it is the lesion's size. Large, lush, and thirsty AVMs are not common in children, and it is usually the small malformations that produce hemorrhage. Paradoxically, it may be the small, awkwardly positioned AVM that presents the greatest challenge to the surgeon. Lesions that are about 1 cm across and located adjacent to or within a ventricle or are positioned deeply along the medial face of the hemisphere can be difficult to isolate, particularly if the malformation lies between the surgical approach and the hemorrhage.

Moreover, the lateral hemispheric AVM may not always be found classically curled on the cortex. Instead, it may be hidden subcortically, and its only surface landmark may be an unusually straightened feeding artery running a nonanatomic course or a red draining vein that is striking out toward an adjacent venous sinus. The most reliable surface markings are the veins, because regardless of their origin, all cross the brain's surface at some point.[61] Some form of stereotactic guidance may be necessary to isolate these covert malformations. This is particularly true in regions of eloquent cortex, where the malformation target and its depth below the brain's surface can be accurately mapped and the route and cortical incision planned accordingly. Stereotactic localization is especially valuable for lesions within the motor or speech cortex or for small, residual malformations that escaped attention during the first operation.

Surgical management of a child with an AVM requires all the major anesthetic and pharmacologic techniques available. The operative and microvascular techniques have been described elsewhere.[62] Once the malformation dissection is completed, bleeding ceases in its bed, and the brain is considerably relaxed. If operation has been decided on, the surgeon should be satisfied with nothing less than total excision, even if two stages are necessary to achieve it. Proximal vessel ligation can be dangerous and is an inadequate solution; subtotal excision is messy, and the shunt remains served by the newly recruited contributors.

Intravascular Embolization

Knowledge is expanding with regard to the use of absorbable embolic agents, nonabsorbable solids and liquids, and other opacifying agents for the endovascular obliteration of a variety of pediatric brain and spinal cord lesions.[63, 64] Most pediatric experience that has been reported to date concerns endovascular treatment of the galenic malformation and other direct arteriovenus fistulas, both intra- and extracranial, that may involve the dura. Wisoff and Berenstein, in relating their experience with this technique for children's brain AVMs, acknowledged that "a cure is seldom obtained with embolization alone," but staged embolizations "are extremely useful in managing large lesions."[63] They also noted that although partial obliteration of an AVM may ameliorate symptoms, there is no evidence that it will protect against hemorrhage. Frizzel and Fisher analyzed published reports of 1246 patients treated with embolization of brain AVMs.[65] Such treatment resulted in cure of only 5% of the malformations. Wikholm and colleagues reported on a series of 192 patients with AVMs, most of which were regarded as unsuitable for surgical excision. With embolization techniques alone, they were able to occlude only 13% of the lesions in these patients.[66]

Although staged embolization followed by resection has been reported to be beneficial for large AVMs,[67] few children in our series had such large malformations. Only four of our patients had intravascular embolization—one for reduction of AVM size so that it could then be subjected to radiosurgery and two as a prelude to operative excision. The fourth child, a 2-day-old neonate, had an unsuccessful embolization attempt in an effort to control her severe congestive heart failure. The experience with this infant, who is still alive, highlights some of the unique difficulties associated with pediatric endovascular techniques for traditional brain AVMs. Most children's AVMs are small rather than large, so the anomalous, tortuous vessels may be extremely difficult to cannulate, and their small branches defy invasion by even the finest of contemporary microcatheters. Children who have larger malformations may be relatively asymptomatic, so the risk-benefit ratio often favors no intervention of any sort. Obviously, the decision to use embolization techniques has to be made with as much care as the decision to perform surgery.

Radiosurgery

The role of radiosurgery for treating AVMs in children remains to be precisely defined. Until recently, there was little information available on the use of this technology in children, but early encouraging results in carefully selected patients have been reported.[68–70] Altschuler and coworkers reported on 15 patients younger than age 18 and noted that of the seven lesions subjected to arteriography, at 1 year, three were completely obliterated and three were smaller.[68] Levy and associates, using Bragg peak radiosurgery in 25 children and adolescents, stated that 14 of 18 had total obliteration of their AVMs by 2 years after treatment.[69] Our limited experience supports the literature with respect to the length of time between radiosurgery and obliteration of the malformation (Fig. 220–7).

Postoperative Care and Results

As previously indicated, 80% of children who suffer from cerebral AVMs require an operation to salvage life or prevent further neurological harm. If a deliberate decision has been made to stage the procedure, with a second attempt planned after an interval, the surgeon should discontinue the first procedure when the operative region is neither bleeding nor swelling. Whether one or two procedures are required to obliterate the lesion, the surgeon cannot be satisfied that total excision has been achieved until postoperative arteriography confirms it. The study should also show a diminished size of the proximal contributing arteries. If there is residual malformation, reoperation may be necessary to excise the remaining lesion, although at this stage, it is not the only strategy. A recurrent cerebral AVM may appear, even when postoperative arteriograms were deemed negative.

With regard to the postoperative arteriogram, it must first be determined when it is appropriate to obtain the study. There are some arguments in favor of completing it during the patient's first hospital admission so that if a residual malformation is identified, it can be removed during a second procedure at this time. The contrary argument is that early arteriography may, by virtue of residual tissue swelling or brain manipulation, overlook a small vascular remnant, especially if the lesion is small. Kader and colleagues reported on five patients with recurrent AVMs after negative postoperative arteriography.[71] The patients ranged in age from 5 to 13 years, and they had hemispheric AVMs that presented initially with hemorrhage. Recurrence was noted 1 to 9 years later. Four patients underwent arteriography that showed recurrence of the AVM at or adjacent to the original site. The fifth patient died from a large intracerebral hemorrhage and IVH originating in the previous location of the AVM. The initial negative arteriograms obtained postoperatively in these five children can be explained by postoperative spasm or thrombosis of a small residual malformation. However, in these authors' cumulative experience with 808 patients who had undergone complete surgical removal of AVMs, no case of recurrent AVM had been observed in 667 patients who were older than 18 years. It is postulated that actual regrowth of an AVM may occur in children and might be a consequence of their relatively immature cerebral vasculature. Hence, the Kader study lends weight to the recommendation for a delayed postoperative arteriogram after a child's brain AVM has been resected.[71]

The child's convalescence depends only on rehabilitation needs, if any. The degree of motor, speech, and cerebellar recovery can be remarkable. Prophylactic anticonvulsant medication is usually required for 6 to 24 months after surgery.

In the HSC series, nonoperative management was the treatment for 29 children (18%), either because the terminal hemorrhage produced coma and subsequent death or because the children had extensive malformations in eloquent regions of brain that were associated with infrequent headache or convulsive episodes.[72] One hundred thirty-one children received operative intervention, which in 88 (67%) resulted in the complete resection of the malformation at the first or a subsequent procedure. Sixty-nine children (55%) returned to

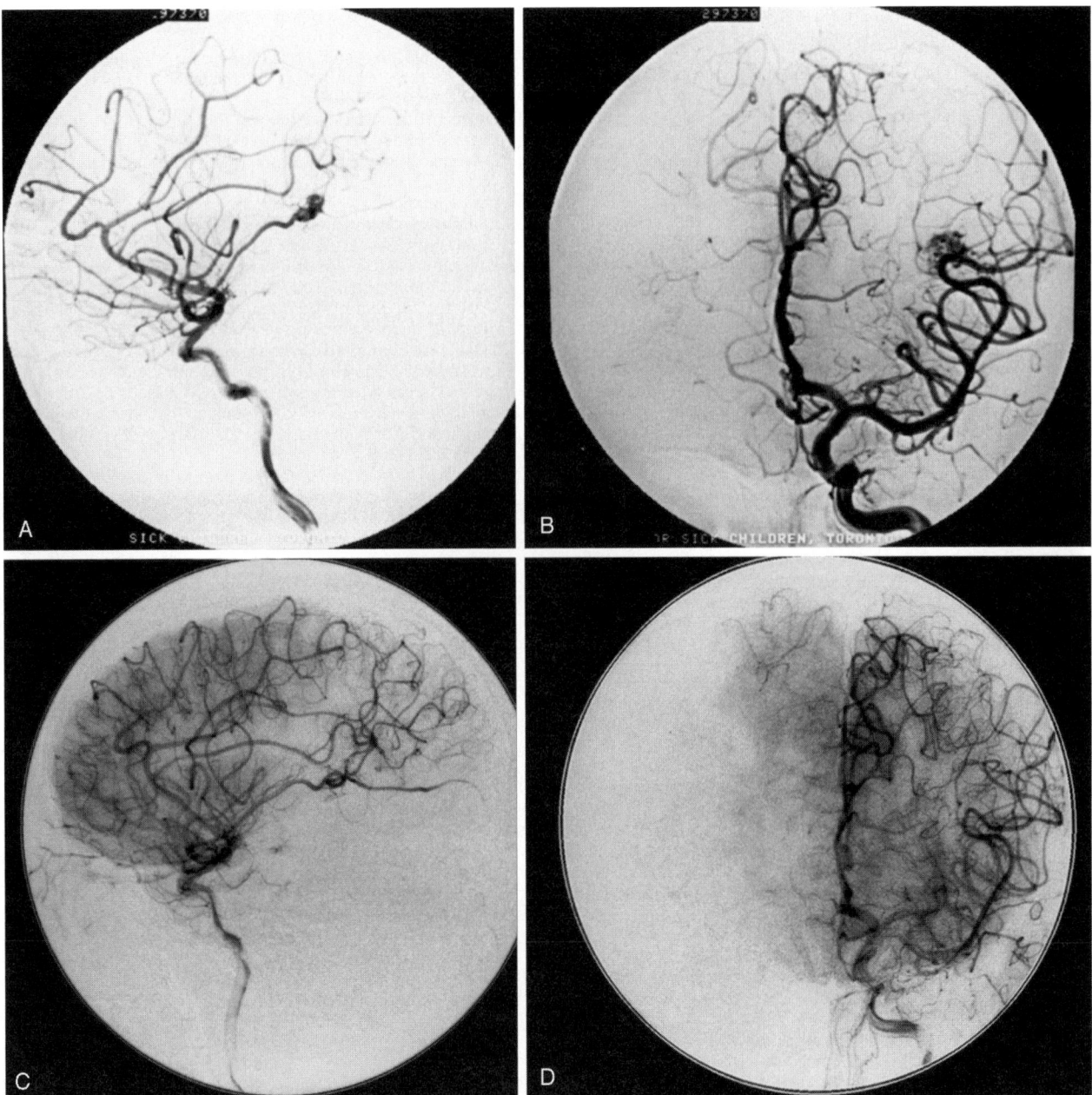

FIGURE 220–7. *A,* Left lateral view. *B,* AP view. Nine months after operative resection of this left temporal arteriovenous malformation, a small remnant remains. It was subject to radiosurgery and subsequent surveillance angiography. It disappeared by the end of the third year after treatment. *C,* Left lateral view. *D,* AP view.

normal performance, and 30 (24%) had a neurological deficit. Twenty-seven children (21%) who bled perished from their hemorrhage. Chronic epilepsy, once thought to be the predominant syndrome of pediatric AVMs, is now known to play a much smaller role in comparison to hemorrhage. In 22 of our patients who had surgical resection procedures, 13 (59%) became seizure free and are no longer taking anticonvulsant medication. Some of these convulsive occurrences were acute ictal events in which a large parenchymal hematoma was present. This is a long-term adverse factor with regard to either seizures or persistent neurological deficit.

REFERENCES

1. Gold AP, Challenor YB, Gilles FH, et al: Report of the Joint Committee for Stroke Facilities. IX. Strokes in children (part 1). Stroke 4:835–858, 1973.
2. Kondziolka D, Humphreys RP, Hoffman HJ, et al: Arteriovenous malformations of the brain in children: A forty year experience. Can J Neurol Sci 19:40–45, 1992.
3. Matson DD: Neurosurgery of Infancy and Childhood. Springfield, Ill, Charles C Thomas, 1969, p 749.
4. Locksley HB: Report on the Cooperative Study of Intracranial Aneurysms and Subarachnoid Hemorrhage. Section V, part I. Natural history of subarachnoid hemorrhage, intracranial aneurysms and arteriovenous malformations: Based on 6368 cases in the Cooperative Study. J Neurosurg 25:219–239, 1966.

5. Hourihan M, Gates PC, McAllister VL: Subarachnoid hemorrhage in childhood and adolescence. J Neurosurg 60:1163–1166, 1984.
6. Laitinen L: Arteriella aneuryusm med subarachnoidal-blodning hos barn. Nord Med 71:329, 1964.
7. Sedzimir CB, Robinson J: Intracranial hemorrhage in children and adolescents. J Neurosurg 38:269–281, 1973.
8. Perret G, Nishioka H: Report on the Cooperative Study of Intracranial Aneurysms and Subarachnoid Hemorrhage. Section VI. Arteriovenous malformations: An analysis of 545 cases of craniocerebral arteriovenous malformations and fistulae reported to the Cooperative Study. J Neurosurg 25:467–490, 1966.
9. Becker DH, Silverberg GD, Nelson DH, et al: Saccular aneurysm of infancy and early childhood. Neurosurgery 2:1–7, 1978.
10. Hayashi S, Arimoto T, Itakura T, et al: The association of intracranial aneurysms and arteriovenous malformations of the brain: Case report. J Neurosurg 55:971–975, 1981.
11. Ostergaard JR: Association of intracranial aneurysm and arteriovenous malformation in childhood. Neurosurgery 14:358–362, 1984.
12. Graf CJ, Perret GE, Torner JC: Bleeding from cerebral arteriovenous malformations as part of their natural history. J Neurosurg 58:331–337, 1983.
13. Guidetti B, Delitala A: Intracranial arteriovenous malformations: Conservative and surgical treatment. J Neurosurg 53:149–152, 1980.
14. Heros RC, Korosue K, Diebold PM: Surgical excision of cerebral arteriovenous malformations: Late results. Neurosurgery 26:578–579, 1990.
15. Itoyama Y, Uemura S, Ushio Y, et al: Natural course of unoperated intracranial arteriovenous malformations: Study of 50 cases. J Neurosurg 71:805–809, 1989.
16. Jomin M, Lesoin F, Lozes G: Prognosis for arteriovenous malformations of the brain in adults based on 150 cases. Surg Neurol 23:362–366, 1985.
17. Housepian EM, Pool JL: Systematic analysis of intracranial aneurysms from the autopsy file of the Presbyterian Hospital 1914–1956. J Neuropathol Exp Neurol 17:409–429, 1958.
18. Stehbens WE: Ultrastructure of aneurysms. Arch Neurol 32:798–807, 1975.
19. Stehbens WE: Intracranial berry aneurysm in infancy. Surg Neurol 18:58, 1982.
20. Stehbens WE: Etiology of intracranial berry aneurysms. J Neurosurg 70:823–831, 1989.
21. Karsner HT: Acute Inflammation of Arteries. Springfield, Ill, Charles C Thomas, 1947, p 16.
22. Ventureyra EC, Higgins MJ: Traumatic intracranial aneurysm in childhood and adolescence: Case reports and review of the literature. Childs Nerv Syst 10:369–379, 1994.
23. Khoo LT, Levy ML: Intracerebral aneurysms. In Albright AL, Pollack IF, Adelson PD (eds): Principles and Practice of Pediatric Neurosurgery. New York, Thieme, 1999, pp 973–1002.
24. Choux M, Lena G, Genitori L: Intracranial aneurysms in children. In Raimondi AJ, Choux M, Di Rocco CD (eds): Cerebrovascular Disease in Children. New York, Springer-Verlag, 1991.
25. Roach ES, Riela AR (eds): Intracranial aneurysms. In Pediatric Cerebrovascular Disorders. Armonk, NY, Futura, 1995.
26. Shucart WA, Wolpert SM: Intracranial arterial aneurysms in childhood. Am J Dis Child 127:288–293, 1974.
27. Humphreys RP, Hendrick EB, Hoffman HJ, et al: Childhood aneurysms—atypical features, atypical management. Concepts Pediatr Neurosurg 6:213–229, 1985.
28. Meyer FB, Sundt TM Jr, Fode NC, et al: Cerebral aneurysm in childhood and adolescence. J Neurosurg 70:420–425, 1989.
29. Patel AN, Richardson AE: Ruptured intracranial aneurysms in the first two decades of life: A study of 58 patients. J Neurosurg 35:571–576, 1971.
30. Storrs BB, Humphreys RP, Hendrick EB, et al: Intracranial aneurysms in the pediatric age-group. Childs Brain 9:358–361, 1982.
31. Amacher AL, Drake CG: The result of operating on cerebral aneurysms and angioma in children and adolescents. I. Cerebral aneurysms. Childs Brain 5:151–165, 1979.
32. Gerosa M, Licata C, Fiore DL, et al: Intracranial aneurysms of childhood. Childs Brain 6:295–302, 1980.
33. Herman JM, Rekate HL, Spetzler RF: Pediatric intracranial aneu-
34. Jakobsson K, Saveland H, Hillman J: Warning leak and management outcome in aneurysmal subarachnoid hemorrhage. J Neurosurg 85:995–999, 1996.
35. Orozco M, Trigueros F, Quintana F, et al: Intracranial aneurysms in early childhood. Surg Neurol 9:287–291, 1978.
36. Ostergaard JR, Voldby B: Intracranial arterial aneurysms in children and adolescents. J Neurosurg 58:832–837, 1983.
37. Pasqualin A, Mazza C, Cavazzani P, et al: Intracranial aneurysms and subarachnoid hemorrhage in children and adolescents. Childs Nerv Syst 2:185–190, 1986.
38. Humphreys RP: Is lumbar puncture alive and well [editorial]? Pediatr Neurosurg 17:114, 1991.
39. Kopitnik TA, Samson DS: Management of subarachnoid hemorrhage. J Neurol Neurosurg Psychiatry 56:947–959, 1993.
40. Lasjaunias PL, Campi A, Rodesch G, et al: Aneurysmal disease in children: Review of 20 cases with intracranial arterial localisations. Interv Neuroradiol 3:215–229, 1997.
41. Laughlin S, terBrugge KG, Willinsky RA, et al: Endovascular management of pediatric intracranial aneurysms. Interv Neuroradiol 3:205–214, 1997.
42. Padget DH: The cranial venous system in man in reference to development, adult configuration and relation to the arteries. Am J Anat 98:307, 1956.
43. Drake CG: Cerebral arteriovenous malformations: Considerations for and experience with surgical treatment in 166 cases. Clin Neurosurg 26:145–208, 1979.
44. McCormick WE: Pathology of vascular malformations of the brain. In Wilson C, Stein B (eds): Intracranial Arteriovenous Malformations. Baltimore, Williams & Wilkins, 1984, pp 44–63.
45. Takashima S, Becker LE: Neuropathology of cerebral arteriovenous malformations in children. J Neurol Neurosurg Psychiatry 43:385, 1980.
46. Northfield DWC: The Surgery of the Central Nervous System: A Textbook: For Postgraduate Students. Oxford, Blackwell Scientific, 1973, p 402.
47. Russell DS, Rubinstein LJ: Pathology of Tumors of the Nervous System, 4th ed. London, Edward Arnold, 1977, p 136.
48. Sonstein WJ, Kader A, Michelsen WJ, et al: Expression of vascular endothelial growth factor in pediatric and adult cerebral arteriovenous malformations: An immunocytochemical study. J Neurosurg 85:838–845, 1996.
49. Celli P, Ferrante L, Palma L, et al: Cerebral arteriovenous malformations in children: Clinical features and outcome of treatment in children and in adults. Surg Neurol 22:43–49, 1984.
50. Mori K, Murata T, Hashimoto N, et al: Clinical analysis of arteriovenous malformations in children. Childs Brain 6:13–25, 1980.
51. Gerosa MA, Cappelloto P, Licata C, et al: Cerebral arteriovenous malformations in children (56 cases). Childs Brain 8:356–371, 1981.
52. Waltimo O: The relationship of size, density and localization of intracranial arteriovenous malformations to the type of initial symptom. J Neurol Sci 19:13–19, 1973.
53. Fults D, Kelly DL: Natural history of arteriovenous malformations of the brain: A clinical study. Neurosurgery 15:658–662, 1984.
54. Crawford PM, West CR, Chadwick DW, et al: Arteriovenous malformations of the brain: Natural history in unoperated patients. J Neurol Neurosurg Psychiatry 49:1–10, 1986.
55. Ondra SL, Troupp H, George ED, et al: The natural history of symptomatic arteriovenous malformations of the brain: A 24-year follow-up assessment. J Neurosurg 73:387–391, 1990.
56. Wilkins RH: Natural history of intracranial vascular malformations: A review. Neurosurgery 16:421–430, 1985.
57. Leblanc R, Feindel W, Ethier R: Epilepsy from cerebral arteriovenous malformations. Can J Neurol Sci 10:91–95, 1983.
58. Mohr JP: Neurological manifestations and factors related to the therapeutic decisions. In Wilson CB, Stein BM (eds): Intracranial Arteriovenous Malformations. Baltimore, Williams & Wilkins, 1984, pp 1–11.
59. Cohen HCM, Tucker WS, Humphreys RP, et al: Angiographically occult histologically verified cerebrovascular malformations. Neurosurgery 10:704–714, 1982.
60. Wilson CB, Sang UH, Dominque J: Microsurgical treatment of

intracranial vascular malformations. J Neurosurg 51:446–454, 1979.

61. Stein BM: General techniques for the removal of arteriovenous malformations. In Wilson CB, Stein BM (eds): Intracranial Arteriovenous Malformations. Baltimore, Williams & Wilkins, 1984, pp 143–155.

62. Humphreys RP: Vascular malformations: Surgical treatment. In Albright AL, Pollack IF, Adelson PD (eds): Operative Techniques of Pediatric Neurosurgery. New York, Thieme, 2000, pp 229–237.

63. Wisoff JH, Berenstein A: Interventional neuroradiology. In Edwards MSB, Hoffman HJ (eds): Cerebral Vascular Disease in Children and Adolescents. Baltimore, Williams & Wilkins, 1989, pp 139–157.

64. terBrugge KG: Neurointerventional procedures in the pediatric age group. Childs Nerv Syst 15:751–754, 1999.

65. Frizzel RT, Fisher WS III: Cure, morbidity, and mortality associated with embolization of brain arteriovenous malformations: A review of 1246 patients in 32 series over a 35-year period. Neurosurgery 37:1031–1040, 1995.

66. Wikholm G, Lundqvist C, Svendsen P: Embolization of cerebral arteriovenous malformations. Part I. Technique, morphology, and complications. Neurosurgery 39:448–459, 1996.

67. Spetzler RF, Martin NA, Carter LP, et al: Surgical management of large AVMs by staged embolization and operative excision. J Neurosurg 67:17–28, 1987.

68. Altschuler EM, Lunsford LD, Coffey RJ, et al: Gamma knife radiosurgery for intracranial arteriovenous malformations in childhood and adolescence. Pediatr Neurosci 15:53–61, 1989.

69. Levy RP, Fabrikant JI, Frankel KA, et al: Stereotactic heavy-charged-particle Bragg peak radiosurgery for the treatment of intracranial arteriovenous malformations in childhood and adolescence. Neurosurgery 24:841–852, 1989.

70. Lunsford D, Kondziolka DS, Pollock BE: Modern stereotactic management of arteriovenous malformations. In Tamaki N (ed): Cerebrospinal Vascular Diseases. Tokyo, Springer-Verlag, 1994, pp 179–194.

71. Kader A, Goodrich JT, Sonstein WJ, et al: Recurrent cerebral arteriovenous malformations after negative postoperative angiograms. J Neurosurg 85:14–18, 1996.

72. Humphreys RP, Hoffman HJ, Drake JM: Choices in the 90s for the management of pediatric cerebrovascular malformations. Pediatr Neurosurg 25:277–285, 1996.

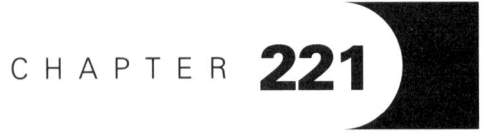

CHAPTER 221

Mild Brain Injury in Children, Including Skull Fractures and Growing Fractures

PAUL C. FRANCEL ■ JOHN HONEYCUTT

Minor brain injury in children is very common. In the pediatric population, the mechanism of brain injury, response of the skull and cranial contents, and long-term prognosis are dissimilar to those in the adult population. The child's nervous system is undergoing maturation and accelerated learning, and the immature skull has different mechanical properties. The brain of an infant or child reacts differently to trauma, and there is substantial variation in the typical cause of head trauma. In this chapter we review mild brain injury and skull fractures in children and discuss differences compared with adults.

MILD BRAIN INJURY WITHOUT SKULL FRACTURE

Epidemiology

Trauma is the major cause of death in children between the ages of 1 and 14 years, with brain injury accounting for 40% of fatal childhood injuries (Fig. 221–1).[1–8] Brain injury accounts for 100,000 pediatric hospitalizations per year in the United States.[9] The incidence of pediatric brain injury is approximately 200 per 100,000, with an ensuing mortality rate of 10%.[10] Boys are twice as likely as girls to suffer brain injury, and their injuries are more likely to be severe or fatal.[4, 11, 12] Despite this gender dichotomy in the overall frequency of pediatric head injuries, the difference is minimal for children younger than 5 years. Brain-injured children may show a higher incidence of premorbid hyperactive or aggressive personalities and often share certain socioeconomic characteristics; for example, more patients come from lower income families.[12, 13]

There are numerous mechanisms of injury in the pediatric age group that are distinct from those seen in adult injury. The highest incidence of injury occurs in motor vehicle, pedestrian, and bicycle accidents and falls.[9, 12–16] Child abuse is the most common cause of head injury in infants younger than 2 years.[17] Falls are the major cause of pediatric brain trauma, particularly in children 4 years old and younger. As children get older, falls become less common than vehicle-related accidents, such as those involving bicycles and other recreational activities. Recreational injuries continue to increase in later years as children become more involved in contact athletics.

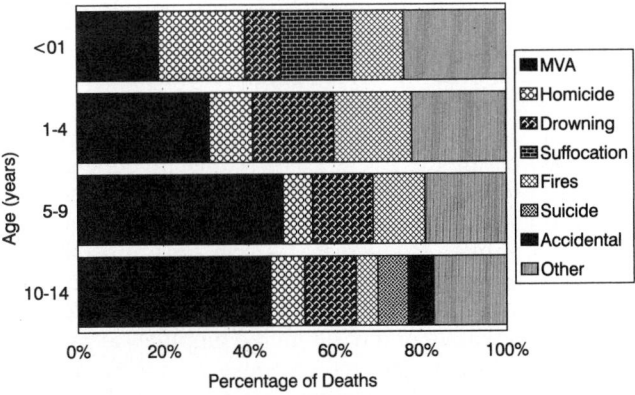

FIGURE 221–1. Major causes of death in children between the ages of 1 month and 14 years. Note that the incidence of trauma as the cause of death increases as the child's age increases. Motor vehicle accidents are the cause of a significant percentage of deaths in the adolescent age group.

Unique Attributes of the Pediatric Brain and Skull

The newborn's brain is encased in a skull that can significantly deform, possessing calvarial bone plates with open sutures that can override during the birth process. This pliable, thin skull also can expand markedly to avoid compression or expansion of the brain. However, the pliability of the immature skull makes the brain more vulnerable to injury. In addition, the orbital roof and floor of the middle fossa lack the prominent ridging seen in the adult skull and offer little resistance to the shifting brain during the first years of life. The subarachnoid space and the distance from the skull to the underlying brain are significantly narrower in newborns than in older children or adults. It has been postulated that the smaller subarachnoid space in infancy reduces the buffering capacity for externally applied impact. It has been noted that in newborn trauma there is only a 10% frequency of contrecoup injury in fatal head injuries, compared with 85% to 95% in older children and adults. It has been suggested that the incidence of contrecoup lesions increases rapidly between infancy and 3 years of age and remains stable thereafter.[18] The smooth inner skull of infancy may contribute to this phenomenon, along with smaller subarachnoid spaces.

The size of the head in relation to the size of the body differs among infants, children, and adults.[19] A newborn's body weight is approximately 5% of an adult's; however, a newborn's brain constitutes 15% of total body weight, compared with 3% in an adult. The rate of new growth in the neonatal brain increases during the first several months and reaches its maximal rate. Then at approximately 1 year of age, deceleration occurs, and the growth rate reaches a plateau. The infant's brain is 75% of its adult size by the end of the second year and 90% of adult size by the sixth year.[20] The skull shows parallel growth, and its character changes quickly during this time. The very soft, pliable bone that is present until 1 year of age changes to a much harder and more brittle consistency. In addition, sutural fusion begins at this time and reduces some of the pliability and vulnerability of the skull.

The chemical composition of the brain varies significantly during childhood because of sequential changes that occur in myelination, biochemical composition, and neuronal development.[20–22] Although myelination continues until the end of the second decade, the majority of the brain has become myelinated by the second year of life. Compared with that of the cerebral cortex, the relative water content of the white matter continues to decrease as one ages and reaches adulthood.[22] This is attributable to the increased myelination and fat content of the brain. The resultant decrease in water content alters the biophysical properties of the brain and its response to injury. In the developing brain, the proliferation of glial cells, vascular channels, and dendritic arborization results in increased brain growth. This arborization of neural dendrites and dendritic spines, combined with increased myelination, is responsible for children's achievement

of developmental milestones. If this development is interrupted by a focal or global mechanical insult, children can show significant impairment in subsequent global cognitive and performance potential that is not seen in adults with equivalent trauma.

At birth, cerebral perfusion appears to be fairly homogeneous, but regional patterns later emerge that reflect the ongoing sequence of functional maturation of the brain. Cerebral blood flow changes are linked to changes in metabolism. Regional variation in blood flow may explain altered susceptibility of certain areas of the developing brain to head trauma. However, the immature brain appears to tolerate anoxia and hypoxia better than the adult brain.[23] In fact, there is a significant retardation of brain growth when increased ambient oxygen is administered, particularly during the first week of life.[24] It is not known if this relative hypoxic tolerance reflects lower metabolic requirements.[25] The cerebral perfusion pressure appears to be lower in children than in adults. A minimal cerebral perfusion pressure of 50 mm Hg is required in adults to maintain adequate blood flow to the brain. The mean systemic blood pressure in children is lower; the cerebral perfusion pressure in normal children may already be below 50 mm Hg. The actual minimal cerebral perfusion pressure for the immature brain has not been determined and may vary with the child's age.[26]

The blood-brain barrier also appears to act differently in experimental trauma studies.[27] It has been noted that immature animals have less brain edema than older animals, and some researchers attribute this to differences in the blood-brain barrier.[28] Others ascribe it to the lower mean arterial blood pressure seen in younger animals.[29] It has also been noted in experimental animals that brain edema clears more rapidly in immature brains.[30] It is likely that the pediatric brain accumulates less edema and can clear it more rapidly than the adult brain.

Neuroplasticity has also generated much interest.[31, 32] Experimental and clinical studies have shown that younger animals have distinct patterns of recovery after brain injury. A specific brain injury that produces a typical hemiparesis in a mature animal may not produce the same motor deficit in an infant animal.[32] This sparing of function after brain injury may depend on the specialization of a specific area of brain at the time of injury. Some evidence suggests that this plasticity is secondary to the degree of myelination of cortical neurons and that as myelination increases, the amount of plasticity decreases.[31] The strongest clinical example of an age-dependent difference in neuroplasticity relates to language function.[33–35] In children younger than 5 years, injury to the left hemisphere is much less likely to result in severe dysphasia than is the same injury in an older child.[35]

Younger children may suffer greater damage from diffuse brain injury than their older counterparts. Although the immaturity of the brain may protect against loss of more focal functions, it may result in a more significant decrease in overall cognitive function. In equivalent injuries, the residual neuropsychological defects are often more profound in infants and young children than in adolescents and adults.[33, 34] Histopathologic studies following blunt trauma have shown that developing brains and older brains respond differently. In contrast to the frequent contusions observed in mature brains, similar trauma to infants' brains usually produces macroscopic tears in the cerebral white matter, which are parallel to the surface, and microscopic tears in the superficial cortical layers.[36] These tears can extend through the cortex and the ventricular wall. Traumatic tears occur only in infants younger than 5 months; older children show the pattern of contusion and necrosis seen in the mature brain.

Pathophysiology

After trauma, there can be both primary and secondary injury. The primary injury is the immediate central nervous system damage incurred at the time of impact. Examples include skull fracture, scalp damage, concussion, contusion, brain laceration, and neuronal and vascular disruption from the impact. Secondary injuries are those processes that affect the brain after the primary insult. These include hypoxia, hypotension, brain edema, delayed intracerebral hemorrhage, dysautoregulation of cerebral vasculature, seizure, and deleterious endogenous cascade.

Concussion is a clinical syndrome characterized by immediate and transient post-traumatic impairment of neurological function, such as alteration of consciousness and disturbances of vision or equilibrium caused by brainstem involvement. This injury can be subdivided into three levels: mild concussion, with no loss of consciousness; moderate concussion, with mild impairment of consciousness and retrograde amnesia; and severe concussion, with unconsciousness lasting more than 5 minutes.[37] Pathologically, concussion is probably secondary to shearing stresses within the brain substance.[37, 38] Linear acceleration does not produce concussion; rotational acceleration does. It is likely that white matter axons and gray matter nerve cell bodies are damaged in both the cerebral or cerebellar hemispheres and the brainstem.[39, 40]

Contusions are focal lesions that are due to direct impact. These lesions may "blossom" or have more mass effect after 24 to 48 hours. They can cause delayed deterioration and occasionally need to be removed to control intracranial pressure. Special attention is needed for contusions in the mesial temporal lobe or posterior fossa, because swelling can quickly cause herniation.

In diffuse axonal injury there is distortion and transient dysfunction of axons, followed by myelin sheath disruption.[37, 41, 42] Prolonged unconsciousness in children is not necessarily caused by brainstem injury but may be related to a combination stretch and shearing injury to the axons and myelin of white matter and either transient or permanent neuron cell body dysfunction.[43] Injury can produce axotomy of some axons; in other cases, it causes internal axonal damage without a frank axotomy. This disruption causes an accumulation of assorted metabolites carried down the axon by axoplasmic transport, resulting in axonal swelling. The injured axon can repair itself and ultimately regain a normal appearance. Frequently, a secondary axotomy occurs more than 12 hours after the injury, and one sees the production of retraction balls. By 2 to 3 weeks after the injury, the number of axon retraction balls diminishes. Astrocytosis, microgliosis, and demyelination occur at the site of injury.[44]

Diffuse axonal injury is diagnosed on computed tomography (CT) by the presence of small hemorrhages, particularly in the corpus callosum, deep white matter of the hemispheres, dorsolateral pons, and superior cerebellar peduncle. These areas are the most obvious sites of injury because they are the points of fixation at which shearing forces are maximal. A magnetic resonance imaging scan is more sensitive in picking up these lesions.

Subarachnoid and intraventricular hemorrhage can occur in brain injury. Complaints are consistent with meningeal irritation, such as photophobia, headache, and meningismus. If diffuse subarachnoid hemorrhage is seen, cervico-occipital distraction injury needs to be ruled out.[44, 45] The use of calcium channel blockers or other prophylactic treatments for vasospasm is controversial in adults, and the effects are unknown in children. For both subarachnoid and intraventricular hemorrhage, the physician needs to watch for the development of hydrocephalus and anticipate the possible need for ventriculostomy or even shunt placement.[46]

Assessment

HISTORY

The history is an integral part of the evaluation of a child with a mild brain injury. Details about the mechanism of injury should be sought, such as the height of the fall, the shape and velocity of the striking objects, and whether anyone else was injured and how severely. Special attention should be devoted to the patient's immediate post-traumatic neurological status. Was there loss of consciousness, and if so, how long did it last? Was there any evidence of seizures or vomiting? The child may be able to voice complaints (if old enough), and all of these should be investigated thoroughly. In addition, the child should specifically be asked about neck and head pain, visual disturbances, paresthesias, amnesia, and weakness. If the child is old enough, the use of alcohol or other drug use should be ascertained. If the parents or caregivers are available, the child's complete medical history should be obtained. Finally, the physician should always be aware of the possibility of child abuse and be alert for any discrepancies or unlikely circumstances obtained in the history from the child or caregivers.

PHYSICAL EXAMINATION

A general physical examination is undertaken, with special attention to the head and scalp. Lacerations, abrasions, and hematomas in the scalp should be carefully inspected. Direct palpation of the skull can sometimes reveal fractures and can also alert the physician to painful areas. The presence or absence of periauricular and periorbital ecchymoses, hemotympanum, and cerebrospinal fluid (CSF) otorrhea or rhinorrhea should be documented. The neurological examination should be thorough, including the evaluation of cranial nerves, motor and sensory systems, and deep tendon reflexes, as well as a cerebellar examination. Finally, a Glasgow Coma Scale (GCS) score should be documented. The GCS works well for children 2 years or older but is a poor measure for younger children. Several scales have been proposed for infants. With young children, we admit and observe them and obtain a computed tomographic scan if there is any decreased level of consciousness.

RADIOGRAPHIC ANALYSIS

The use of skull radiographs in the evaluation of brain injury in children remains a controversial issue. Skull radiographs are still the most sensitive method of detecting a skull fracture but are not useful in detecting brain injury. Although head CT may miss some linear skull fractures, it allows adequate assessment of the more important issue of brain injury. If a child is found to have a skull fracture by plain radiography, it is necessary to perform CT owing to the 100-fold increased incidence of intracranial hematoma in patients with new skull fractures compared with injured patients without skull fractures.[47] Studies have shown that if there is concern about brain injury, head CT is the preferred screening examination.[48] However, in cases of suspected abuse, skull films are warranted as part of a radiographic bone survey.

Although head CT has become the screening tool of choice, it has some limitations. In the adult population, both observation without computed tomographic scanning and mandatory computed tomographic scanning have been recommended.[49–55] Rivara and colleagues[56] retrospectively reviewed 98 children with head injury who had CT performed. In 51 patients with GCS scores of 13 or better, 31% had abnormal findings on CT. They concluded that clinical status does not adequately predict brain injury seen on CT. Another retrospective review looked at children with GCS scores of 15 on arrival and a brief loss of consciousness.[57] Intracranial hemorrhage was noted in 7.5% of patients, and 8% had depressed or basilar skull fractures by clinical examination. Interestingly, among 17 patients with ventriculoperitoneal shunts in place, 12% had intracranial hemorrhage by CT. Those children with GCS scores of 15, normal neurological examinations, no clinical evidence of skull fracture, and no shunt in place had a 0% incidence of intracranial hemorrhage. They concluded that children with normal examinations and no evidence of fracture or shunt did not require CT and could be discharged home. In a study of pediatric patients, the authors recommended that computed tomographic scans be obtained in children with GCS scores of 14 or less.[58] They also considered CT warranted in patients with GCS scores of 15 if they have the following clinical features: loss of consciousness,

amnesia for the event, vomiting, seizures, headache, or focal neurological deficit. Those children with GCS scores of 15 and normal computed tomographic scans can be discharged home with informed caregivers.

Treatment

The major thrust of treatment for mild brain injury is identifying those patients who are at risk of neurological deterioration. The syndrome of the child who "talks and dies" has been well described.[59–62] Snoek and colleagues[62] reported 42 pediatric patients with trivial injuries who deteriorated. Of these, 40% had no loss of consciousness, and 31% deteriorated secondary to seizure activity. Among the 29 children whose deterioration was not attributable to seizures, cerebral dysfunction was the cause, as none of these children had mass lesions identified on CT. Humphreys and associates[61] described four children who had lucid intervals and then deteriorated and died, but all four had GCS scores of 12 or less at initial evaluation in the emergency room. The pathophysiologic causes of delayed deterioration can be varied. Seizures and mass lesions need to be ruled out. The physician must also be aware that the history may be wrong, and the patient may have sustained a more significant injury. The possibility of child abuse also needs to be considered, especially in younger children. Finally, the patient may have the "pediatric concussion syndrome," which is seen more commonly in patients younger than 1 year. The child becomes pale, sweaty, irritable, nauseated, and lethargic. The patient requires symptomatic support, and the syndrome is usually self-limited. In an older child, however, this can progress to coma. Occasionally, more intensive management is required, and surgical intervention may be needed (e.g., intracranial pressure monitoring, ventriculostomy).[59]

Fortunately, if a patient has a GCS score of 15 and a normal computed tomographic scan, the likelihood of delayed deterioration is exceedingly rare, and if it occurs, it is usually mild and limited. Those patients with GCS scores of 13 or 14 or with abnormal computed tomographic scans need to be admitted and observed for delayed deterioration. Davis and coworkers[57] performed a retrospective review of children who were discharged home after normal computed tomographic scans. Of the 400 children reviewed, only 4 required readmission. Of these, one had a symptomatic subdural hematoma that had to be evacuated; complicating this case was the fact that the child was taking warfarin (Coumadin) for a heart condition. One child developed a hemorrhagic contusion that required observation. Two were readmitted for concussive symptoms and were discharged home after brief observation.

If the child meets the previously stated criteria for admission, management entails close observation with frequent neurological assessment, medications for headache, and intravenous hydration for those patients with emesis. Emesis is more common in mild brain injury than in more severe injury. Vomiting may be seen in up to 50% of mildly brain injured children, but fortunately, it is not protracted in the majority of cases.[63] The parents or caregivers need to be taught about the possible delayed complications of brain injury but should be reassured that in the majority of cases there are no long-term sequelae of mild head injury.

Outcome

Mild head injury in the pediatric population is extremely common, but fortunately, the outcome is usually complete recovery. Mortality is exceedingly uncommon. Morbidity is low, with headaches being the most common complaint (in 7% of patients).[64] Physical morbidity is rare; more common is neurobehavioral morbidity. School absenteeism may be high, with Casey and colleagues[64] showing that 40% of 5- to 14-year-olds missed at least 1 day of school within 1 month of injury (compared with 10% for grade schools and 19% for middle schools in the control group). Another concern is parental anxiety. Even with extensive counseling in the emergency room, 85% of parents were still anxious about their children's injuries 1 month later. This may negatively affect the child by causing school absenteeism and "overprotection."[65] Overall, children make exceptional recoveries, and except for unusual cases, a full recovery can be expected.

MILD BRAIN INJURY IN CHILDREN WITH ACCOMPANYING SKULL FRACTURE

Skull fractures are common in children, with approximately 20% of children admitted for brain injury harboring some sort of fracture.[1, 48] The majority of these fractures are simple linear fractures that require no operative intervention. However, the importance of diagnosing a fracture lies in identifying those children who are at risk for brain injury. It has been well documented that children and adults with skull fractures have an increased incidence of underlying brain injury or hematoma.[47, 48, 66–68] If a patient is suspected of having a fracture or one is evident by plain radiography, CT is indicated not only to evaluate the fracture but also to assess for hematoma or underlying brain injury.

Biomechanical studies of the skull indicate that fracture characteristics are related to the energy imparted to the skull, the geometry and thickness of the skull, and the presence and proximity of cranial sutures.[69] The location of the fracture does not necessarily correlate with the area of impact or compression.[70] The skull fractures at the site that allows energy dissipation to occur.[71] Fractures are more commonly seen in infants because of their thinner skulls.[1]

Linear Skull Fractures

Linear skull fractures are the most common fractures seen in children, accounting for more than two thirds of fractures. The parietal bone is the most common site

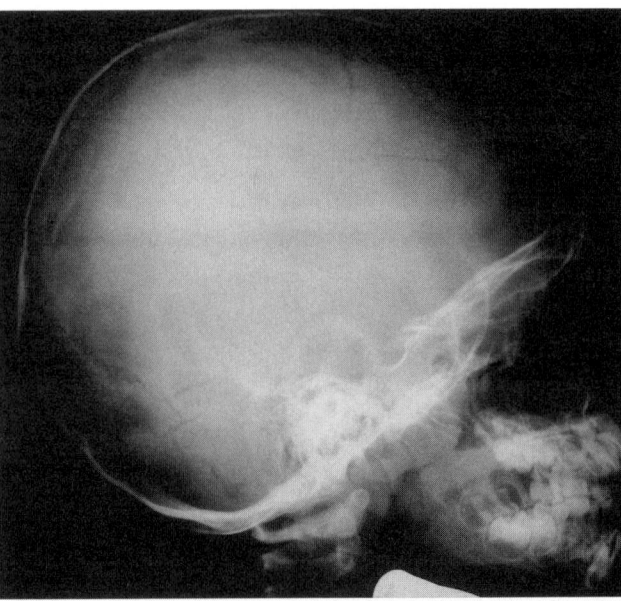

FIGURE 221–2. Linear skull fractures frequently involve the parietal bone. Particular attention should be paid to fractures that cross the vascular pattern of the middle meningeal artery.

of fracture (Fig. 221–2). The fracture involves more than one cranial bone in up to 48% of patients.[1] The most common sign is pain and swelling at the impact site. Approximately 15% of fractures are contralateral to the external scalp lesion.[1] Thirty percent of children show no evidence of external trauma.[64] Subgaleal or subperiosteal hematomas can occur in conjunction with fractures and can be quite large in young children (Fig. 221–3); in neonates and infants, they may be large enough to require transfusion. However, these do not need to be treated surgically. They will spontaneously resolve, and surgical intervention only risks infection.

Treatment of linear skull fractures is nonsurgical, with reassurances to the parents that these fractures will heal in time. Late complications of growing skull fractures are rare and are discussed later in the chapter. Once again, the importance of diagnosing fractures is to recognize the increased risk of underlying brain injury. If the head computed tomographic scan is normal, as it usually is in these cases, expectant management is indicated. We routinely send such patients home with close observation but would not hesitate to admit a child for observation if he or she lived several hours away or if there was concern about the caregivers' reliability. A follow-up visit is scheduled in 1 month; this includes radiographs only if there is concern about proper healing.

Depressed Skull Fractures

Depressed skull fractures occur in roughly one quarter of all fractures. Once again, the parietal bone is the most common site. Compound fractures are more commonly seen in this group, with nearly half being contaminated. Epidural hematomas (3%) and subdural hematomas (1%) are uncommon.[1] Most of these fractures

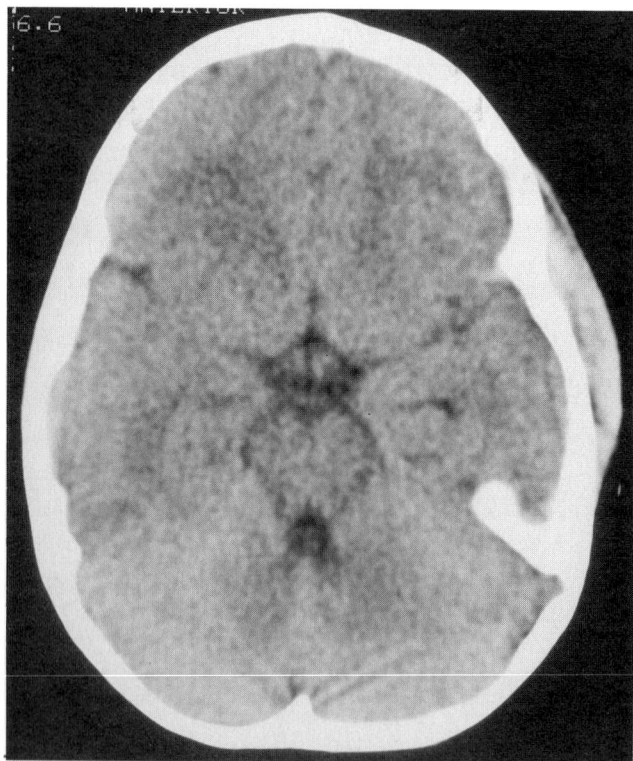

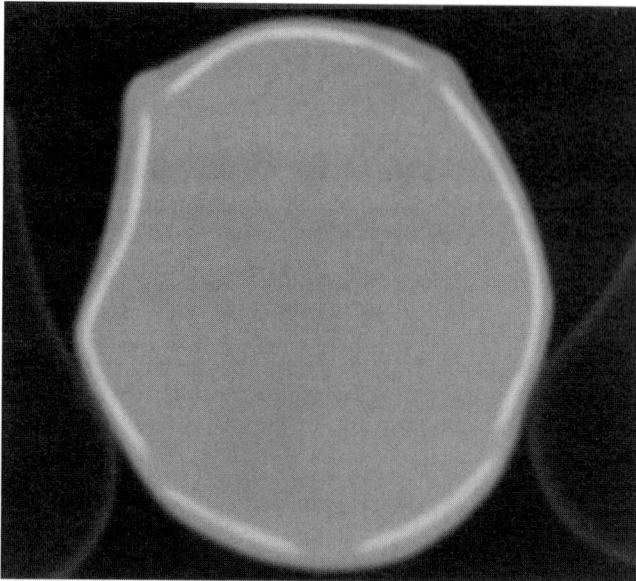

FIGURE 221–4. Ping-pong fracture. In a sense, this is actually a "greenstick" type of fracture, and a distinct fracture line is not visualized. The abnormality is readily apparent on visual inspection and usually repairs itself gradually without surgical intervention.

FIGURE 221–3. Subgaleal hematomas are noted by the bright signal of blood below either the galea or the subperiosteal layer. Although these are dramatic in appearance, they are usually of little consequence and resolve spontaneously in most cases.

are "greenstick" fractures, with the "ping-pong" type in neonates being an excellent example. Only 15% of depressed skull fractures involve fragments that are separated from the skull.[71] Dural lacerations are also uncommon, seen in 10% of cases.[72]

Signs of depressed skull fracture are swelling and abrasions at the impact site. The swelling may be large enough to hide the fracture from an examiner. Pain can also limit the examination. If a fracture is suspected, CT is warranted.

The ping-pong fracture was once thought to result from the application of forceps, but it is probably caused by compression of the infant's head against the mother's sacral promontory (Fig. 221–4). It is usually seen after prolonged labor but does not require passage through the birth canal. These fractures are frequently seen in infants delivered by cesarean section, suggesting that uterine contractions are the cause.[73] Newborn ping-pong fractures are initially treated conservatively, because significant remodeling can occur over time, even with large fractures. However, if there is evidence of cortical injury or dural laceration, exploration is necessary. Historically, these fractures have also been treated nonoperatively with manual bedside manipulation with vacuum devices.[74, 75] If the fracture does not remodel, delayed operative intervention can be undertaken. Several techniques can be used. A small craniotomy can be performed, with levering of the fracture with a blunt instrument. A larger craniotomy can also be made around the fracture, with the remod-

eling being performed at the table with replacement and fixation (our preference is absorbable plates).

Depressed skull fractures in older children are more problematic, owing to the lesser degree of remodeling. The rule of thumb has been that if the fracture is depressed to a depth greater than the thickness of the skull, surgical intervention is warranted. It used to be axiomatic that a depressed skull fracture should be elevated to reduce the possibility of pulsations of the growing brain against the depressed calvarial segment, which would cause cortical damage. It was presumed that these pulsations would lead to an epileptogenic focus in the underlying brain. However, there is no clinical support for this supposition. There have been several studies of whether neurological outcome was improved with operative intervention, but none of these showed any benefit of surgery.[76–78] This is not surprising, because most of the neurological problems are related to the contusion rather than the compression from the fracture. Another factor to consider is cosmesis. A cosmetic repair of a depressed fracture in the frontal region is entirely justifiable (Fig. 221–5). It is usually advisable to refrain from operative correction of depressed skull fractures that overlie major dural sinuses. Removal of these bony fragments should be considered only if the depressed fracture occludes a sinus and is causing neurological deterioration.

Absolute indications for immediate elevation of depressed fractures include evidence of a dural tear, gross contamination of the wound, and evidence of significant underlying intracerebral hematoma. Our approach to cosmetic repair is to individualize each case.

Comminuted and Complex Fractures

Comminuted and complex fractures are seen with higher impact injuries, such as high falls and motor

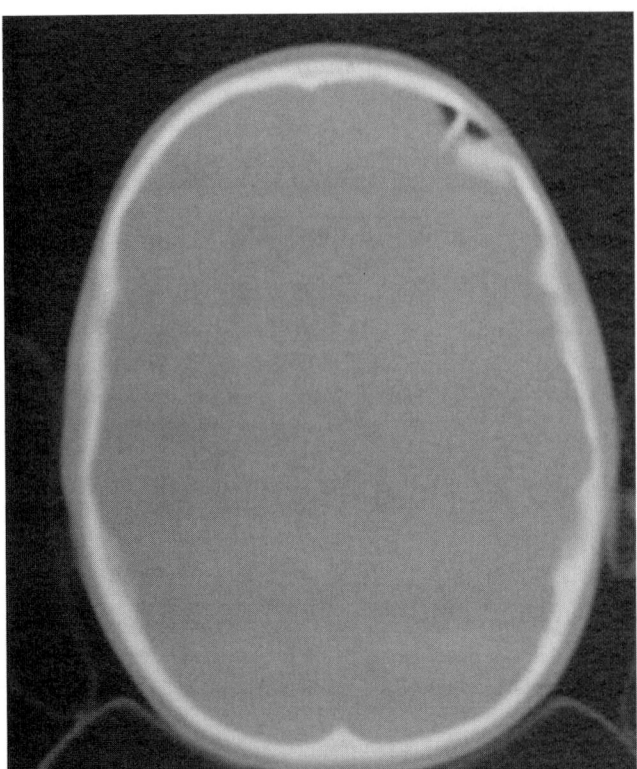

FIGURE 221–5. Depressed skull fracture in the frontal area. This fracture needs to be repaired purely for cosmetic reasons. If the dura is torn and there is clear evidence of cerebrospinal fluid leak, or if there is evidence of gross contamination or intracerebral hemorrhage, operative intervention is necessary. Fracture elevation is not done purely to correct neurological deficits, because these usually occur secondary to the underlying brain contusion rather than the depressed fracture itself.

vehicle accidents. These fractures are associated with greater brain injury, and management is first directed at treatment of the brain injury. These fractures more commonly require repair, but only after the brain injury and swelling are under control. Fragments that maintain alignment will eventually heal, as long as the dura is not violated.

Compound Skull Fractures

Compound fractures have communication with the environment, which requires some sort of scalp penetration or laceration, or communication with the cranial sinuses. These can be seen in up to 20% of childhood skull fractures.[71] Besides the usual causes of injury such as falls, assaults, and motor vehicle accidents, we see a fair number of injuries from accidental golf club strikes and horse kicks. The concern with open fractures is contamination and subsequent infection. In linear skull fractures, we routinely clean and close the wound at the bedside, as long as there is no evidence of dural laceration, CSF leak, or pneumocephalus. In these latter instances, the child is taken to the operating room for a craniotomy and débridement of the wound. In comminuted or complex fractures, operative débridement is required.

Basilar Skull Fractures

Basilar skull fractures should be suspected when the clinical findings include CSF otorrhea or rhinorrhea, periorbital ecchymoses (raccoon eyes), periauricular ecchymoses (Battle's sign), and hemotympanum. Radiographic diagnosis can be difficult, and special imaging may be required to detect the fracture. However, even if the fracture cannot be found radiographically, this does not change the management of presumed basilar skull fracture. This type of fracture is found more commonly in adults than in children, accounting for less than 10% of childhood fractures.[79, 80] CSF rhinorrhea is seen in only 10% of basilar skull fractures in children.[81]

After the treatment of any underlying brain injuries, the focus is management of CSF fistulas and cranial nerve palsies. The timing of CSF leak can be quite variable. In one series, 80% of patients developed a CSF leak within 48 hours of injury.[82] In other series, only half the patients developed CSF leak within 48 hours.[83] Whatever the true timing is, some children will develop a leak after being discharged home. Parents must be told to watch for the signs of CSF leak and meningitis and to return promptly if they occur. Fortunately, the natural history of childhood post-traumatic CSF leaks is that the vast majority stop spontaneously. Persistent CSF leaks in children are extremely rare[80, 84] and are usually associated with more complex fractures.[85] It does not appear that a CSF leak puts the patient at higher risk for meningitis.[83, 86, 87]

There is debate about the use of antibiotics in patients with CSF leak, and numerous articles have recommended prophylactic antibiotic treatment in these cases.[88–91] Others suggest antibiotic treatment only for anterior fossa fractures.[92] However, several papers have recommended no antibiotic treatment, citing a lack of benefit.[80, 86, 93, 94] In our practice, we do not give prophylactic antibiotics to patients with CSF leak; we treat only when there is a documented infection by CSF analysis.

CSF rhinorrhea has different implications than otorrhea does. Rhinorrhea is more frequently prolonged, carries a greater chance of intracranial infection, and resolves less often. If the leak does not stop within 7 days, multiple spinal punctures or the placement of a lumbar drain may be beneficial. If CSF diversion is unsuccessful, operative intervention is necessary, with identification of dural and bony defects and closure of the dural tear. One should also be alert to a possible leak in patients with no obvious evidence of CSF leakage but recurrent bouts of meningitis after sustaining a head injury.

The other concern with basilar skull fractures is cranial nerve palsies. Post-traumatic cranial nerve palsies have been described for all the cranial nerves. The mechanism can be direct shear injury to the nerve, which should cause immediate symptoms and signs. More commonly, the cranial nerve palsy occurs several days after the injury; this is most likely the result of nerve edema and should be transient. The most commonly injured nerve is the olfactory nerve, reportedly involved in up to 7% of all head injuries,[95] but the true incidence is unknown owing to the lack of routine testing. Sixth nerve palsies are also common. These usually are not due to direct trauma from the fracture; rather, the long intracranial course of the nerve predisposes it to damage from swelling.

Several specific cranial nerve palsies deserve special attention, owing to their frequency of occurrence and their relationship to the skull base. These include optic neuropathy, facial neuropathy, and auditory and vestibular dysfunction.

TRAUMATIC OPTIC NEUROPATHY

Traumatic optic neuropathy is not uncommon, with up to 28% of head-injured children showing some sort of ocular dysfunction.[96] Specifically, in one study, optic neuropathy was seen in about 6% of head-injured children.[95] The initial complaint is visual loss that usually occurs immediately, but in up to 10% of patients it can have a delayed onset.[97] Surprisingly, the majority of children with post-traumatic optic neuropathy did not have a fracture involving the optic canal (14%), but half did have a fracture elsewhere (Fig. 221–6).[97]

The natural history of traumatic optic neuropathy is encouraging, with up to 40% of patients recovering.[98] It has also been shown that high-dose corticosteroids improve the rate of recovery.[98, 99] Surgical intervention may be indicated to decompress the optic canal, but most authorities recommend surgical decompression only if there is documented optic canal compromise by bony fracture or fragments. Because most fractures do not involve the optic canal, the need for surgery is rare.

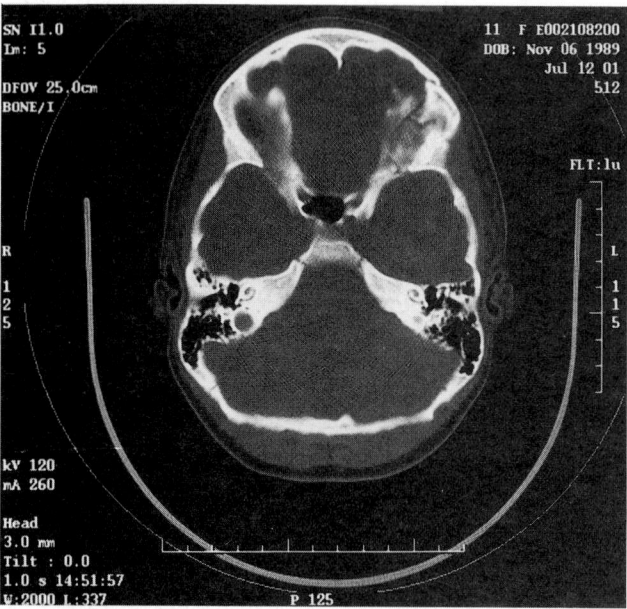

FIGURE 221–6. Patients presenting with basilar skull fractures should undergo evaluation of cranial nerve function. Clear evidence of the fracture through the orbital roof should prompt a careful examination of visual function, even if the fracture does not directly involve the optic canal.

TRAUMATIC FACIAL NEUROPATHY

Fractures through the petrous bone can injure either the seventh or eighth cranial nerve or both. Transverse fractures are more likely to injure these nerves, with up to half of patients having some sort of facial or vestibulocochlear neuropathy.[100] Complete facial paralysis present at the time of injury often suggests transection of the facial nerve by fractured bone fragments. In this situation, evaluation of the petrous bone is mandatory and is usually done with the help of an otolaryngologist. Facial electromyography recordings are used in instances of complete facial muscle weakness. The more common longitudinal fractures usually spare these nerves, but if they are affected, it is usually due to perineural swelling that resolves spontaneously.[100] At this time, there is no indication for steroid treatment in longitudinal petrous fractures.

AUDITORY AND VESTIBULAR DYSFUNCTION

Auditory and vestibular dysfunction after head injury is common. Patients complain of hearing loss, tinnitus, and vertigo. Hearing loss can be from damage to the ossicles or hemotympanum, causing conductive hearing loss, or from sensorineural hearing loss, which unfortunately is more common and has a worse prognosis for recovery.[71] Steroids have not been helpful, and currently no acute surgical intervention is indicated. If the hearing loss persists for at least a month, referral to an otolaryngologist is warranted.

Growing Skull Fractures

Growing skull fractures are a rare entity, complicating less than 1% of all fractures. Howship first described this fracture in 1816. Since then, it has been given several different names: spurious meningocele, cephalhydrocele, traumatic ventricular cyst, leptomeningeal cyst, cerebrocranial erosion, craniocerebral erosion, "Die Wachsende Schadelfraktur," fibrosing osteitis, growing fracture of the skull, cranial malacia, and expanding skull fracture.[101] The most common names are growing skull fracture and craniocerebral erosion. As in linear skull fractures, the most common site of a craniocerebral erosion is the parietal bone (Fig. 221–7). Most cases are seen in patients younger than 1 year. Neurological deficit is seen more commonly than in patients with routine linear fractures. In a series of 60 patients, Tandon and coworkers[101] reported that two thirds of the patients had hemiparesis, and nearly half had seizures, with 79% being intractable. Craniocerebral erosion can occur several weeks to several years after the initial injury. The fracture must be separated at least 2 to 3 mm at the time of injury for the process to occur.

The pathophysiology requires a fracture with enough force to cause an underlying tear in the dura and an outward driving force such as a growing brain, leptomeningeal cyst, hydrocephalus, or porencephaly. Analyzing the pathology of 17 cases, Roy and colleagues[102] described constant features at the time of

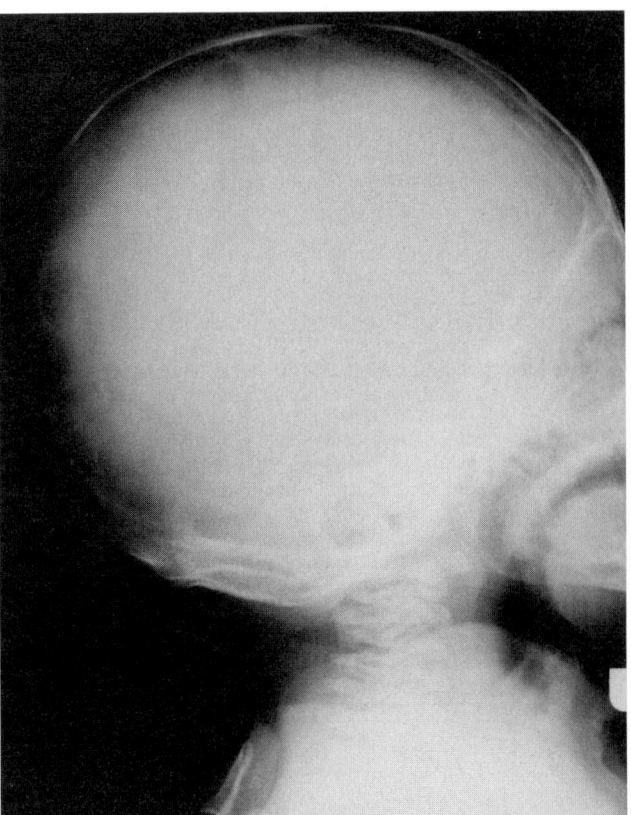

FIGURE 221–7. Skull radiograph of a patient with a growing skull fracture (leptomeningeal cyst, craniocerebral erosion). Although they often look benign on examination, growing skull fractures carry a significant risk of neurological deficit. The most common site is the parietal bone.

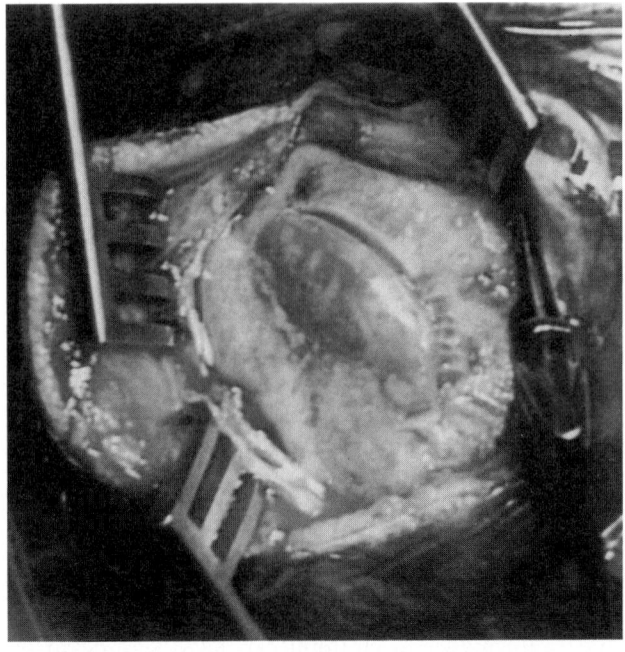

FIGURE 221–8. Operative exposure of a growing skull fracture. Notice the pulsatile mass located between scalloped bony edges. At surgery, the dural defect is always noted to be larger than the bony defect. The underlying brain is osseous and gliotic, with adhesions between the dura and the pia-arachnoid space. Brain that has extruded between the bony defects is potentially epileptogenic (see color section in this volume).

surgery. These included a linear fracture with irregular margins and separation of at least 2 to 8 mm, with scalloped edges and an inner table that was ragged, pitted, and irregular (Fig. 221–8 shows our own operative example; see color section in this volume). The dural defect was always larger than the bony defect. The underlying brain was noted to be osseous and gliotic, with adhesions between the dura and the pia-arachnoid space. The brain was abnormal until it was past the dural edge. The gap between the dural defect and the brain was filled with fibrogliotic scar that sometimes contained loculated fluid. Inconstant features included pseudomeningocele; brain herniation; migration of the dilated lateral ventricle toward the defect, with occasional ventricular herniation; and intradiploic cyst. In six of nine cases, microscopic examination of the brain showed what appeared to be active and ongoing degeneration and necrosis of deeper parts of the brain (Fig. 221–9). The cause of this is unknown, but two theories have been advanced. There may be ongoing brain damage due to brain herniation and pulsations of the brain against the bone edges. Alternatively, there may be vascular compromise of vessels at the bony edges.[102] It is emphasized that brain injury has to occur for craniocerebral erosion to develop.

Surgical treatment is indicated because these types of fractures never heal spontaneously, and late neuro-

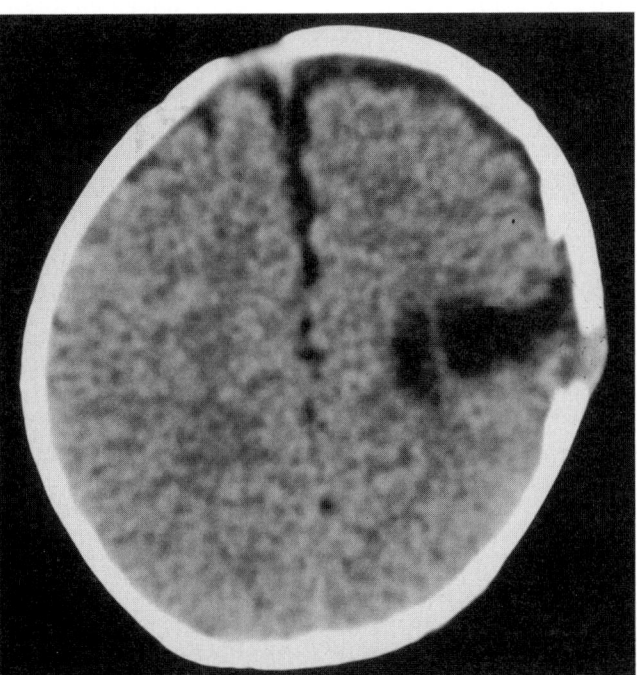

FIGURE 221–9. Microscopic examination often reveals necrosis of deeper portions of the brain. This is well illustrated by a computed tomographic scan showing necrosis of the brain extending from the osseous defect centrally.

logical deficits can occur. Surgery must be carefully planned, because in addition to correction of the fracture site with a cranioplasty, the dural defect must be repaired with a duraplasty. Because the dural edges are located underneath the skull edges, we prefer to perform a craniotomy encompassing the fracture so that the dural edges are easily identified. The duraplasty must free the gliotic tissue from the edges of the dura. There are a number of techniques for performing the cranioplasty. If the defect is large, we prefer a split calvarial graft to cover the site. However, if there is a smaller fracture site, we prefer to use hydroxyapatite cement or some other form of bone cement to cover the defect. We always use an absorbable plate to cover the bone cement; this keeps it in place while healing occurs. If this is not done, brain pulsations can lift the bone cement off the defect and cause reabsorption of the bone cement.

CONCLUSION

Mild brain injury in children can have significant effects during their growing years and into adulthood. The child's skull and brain respond differently to injuries compared with those of the adult, and this affects long-term prognosis. Although a child who has traumatic brain injury is less likely to show focal neurological deficits, he or she is more likely to develop global deficits because the brain is in the process of maturation and accelerated learning.

Given that the pathophysiology is somewhat different in children compared with adults, the history, physical examination, and radiographic analysis can all vary to some degree. The pathophysiology of brain injury accompanied by fracture is particularly interesting. A significant percentage of patients with skull fracture have mild brain injury and fracture findings either by skull film or by CT of the head, and the type of fracture plays a role in determining patient care and management.

REFERENCES

1. Harwood-Nash DC, Hendrick EB, Hudson AR: The significance of skull fractures in children. Radiology 101:151–155, 1971.
2. Annegers JF: The epidemiology of head trauma in children. In Shapiro K (ed): Pediatric Head Trauma. New York, Futura, 1983, pp 1–10.
3. Bruce DA: Scope of the problem: Early assessment and management. In Rosenthal M, Griffith ER, Bond M, et al (eds): Rehabilitation of the Adult and Child with Traumatic Brain Injury. Philadelphia, FA Davis, 1983, pp 521–537.
4. Filley DM, Cranberg LD, Alexander MP, et al: Neurobehavioral outcome after closed head injury in childhood and adolescence. Arch Neurol 44:194–198, 1987.
5. Kalsbeek ED, McLaurin RL, Harris BSH, et al: The national head and spinal cord injury survey: Major findings. J Neurosurg 53:519–531, 1980.
6. McLaurin RL, Towbin RB: Diagnosis and treatment of head injury in infants and children. In Youmans JR (ed): Neurological Surgery. Philadelphia, WB Saunders, 1990, pp 2149–2193.
7. Sharples PM, Storey A, Aynsley-Green A, et al: Causes of fatal childhood accidents involving head injury in northern region, 1979–1986. BMJ 301:1193–1197, 1990.
8. Waller AE, Baker SP, Syocha A: Childhood injury deaths, national analysis and geographical variations. Am J Public Health 79:310–315, 1989.
9. Kraus JF, Fife D, Conroy C: Pediatric brain injuries: The nature, clinical course, and early outcomes in a defined United States population. Pediatrics 79:501–507, 1987.
10. Goetting MG, Preston G: Jugular bulb catheterization: Experience with 123 patients. Crit Care Med 18:1220–1223, 1990.
11. Berger MS, Pitts LH, Lovely M, et al: Outcome from severe head injury in children and adolescents. J Neurosurg 62:194–199, 1985.
12. Goldstein FC, Levin HS: Epidemiology of pediatric closed head injury: Incidence, clinical characteristics and risk factors. J Learn Disabil 20:518–525, 1987.
13. Cardia E, Zaccone C, Molina D, et al: Outcome of craniocerebral trauma in infants and children. Childs Nerv Syst 6:23–26, 1990.
14. Alberico AM, Ward JD, Choi SC, et al: Outcome after severe head injury, relationship to mass lesions, diffuse injury, and ICP course in pediatric and adult patients. J Neurosurg 67:648–656, 1987.
15. Bijur PE, Haslum M, Golding J: Cognitive and behavioral sequelae of mild head injury in children. Pediatrics 86:337–344, 1990.
16. Kissoon N, Dreyer J, Walia M: Pediatric trauma: Differences in pathophysiology, injury patterns and treatment compared with adult trauma. J Can Med Assoc 142:27–34, 1990.
17. McClelland CQ, Rekate H, Kaufman B, et al: Cerebral injury in child abuse: A changing profile. Childs Brain 7:225–235, 1980.
18. Courville CB: Contrecoup injuries of the brain in infancy. Arch Surg 90:157–165, 1965.
19. Friede R: Developmental Neuropathology. New York, Springer-Verlag, 1975.
20. McLennan JR, Gilles F: A growth model for the total weight of the prenatal human brain. Trans Am Neurol Assoc 101:271–272, 1976.
21. Katzman R, Pappius HM: Brain Electrolytes and Fluid Metabolism. Baltimore, Williams & Wilkins, 1973.
22. Norton W: Formation, structure and biochemistry of myelin. In Siegel GJ, et al (eds): Basic Neurochemistry. Boston, Little, Brown, 1972, pp 74–99.
23. Duffy TE, Vannucci RC: Metabolic aspects of cerebral anoxia in the fetus and newborn. In Berenberg SR (ed): Brain, Fetal and Infant. The Hague, Martinus-Nijhoff, 1976, pp 216–232.
24. Sokoloff L: Toxic effects of elevated oxygen tension on brain maturation. In Berenberg SR (ed): Brain, Fetal and Infant. The Hague, Martinus-Nijhoff, 1976, pp 178–183.
25. Rapoport SI, Ohata M, London ED: Cerebral blood flow and glucose utilization following opening of the blood-brain barrier and during maturation of the brain. Fed Proc 40:2322–2325, 1981.
26. Shapiro K, Smith LP: Special considerations for the pediatric age group. In Cooper PR (ed): Head Injury, 3rd ed. Baltimore, Williams & Wilkins, 1993, pp 427–457.
27. Bradbury MD: The blood-brain barrier during the development of the individual and the evolution of the phylum. In Bradbury MD (ed): The Concept of a Blood-Brain Barrier. Toronto, John Wiley & Sons, 1979, pp 289–322.
28. Lkatzo I, Wisniewski H, Steinwall O, et al: Dynamics of cold injury edema. In Klatzo I, Seiterlberg F (eds): Brain Edema. New York, Springer-Verlag, 1967, pp 554–563.
29. Go KG, Ebels EJ, Van Woudenberg F, et al: The development of oedema in the immature brain. Psychiatr Neurol Neurochir 76:427–437, 1973.
30. Bass NH, Lundborg P: Cerebral edema: The effect of dexamethasone during brain maturation in the rat. Arch Neurol 29:151–157, 1973.
31. Bishop DMV: Plasticity and specificity of language localization in the developing brain. Dev Med Child Neurol 23:251–255, 1981.
32. Goldman PD: An alternative to developmental plasticity: Heterology of CNS structures in infants and adults. In Stein DG, Rosen JJ, Butters N, et al (eds): Plasticity and Recovery of Function in the Central Nervous System. New York, Academic Press, 1974, pp 149–174.
33. Brink JD, Garrett AL, Hale WR, et al: Recovery of motor and intellectual function in children sustaining severe head injuries. Dev Med Child Neurol 12:565–571, 1970.

34. Kriel RL, Krach LE, Panser LA: Closed head injury: Comparison of children younger and older than 6 years of age. Pediatr Neurol 5:296–300, 1989.
35. Levin HS, Eisenberg HM, Miner ME: Neuropsychologic findings in head injured children. In Shapiro K (ed): Pediatric Head Trauma. New York, Raven Press, 1983, pp 223–240.
36. Lindenberg R, Freytag E: The mechanism of cerebral contusion. Arch Pathol 69:440–469, 1960.
37. Ommaya AK, Gennarelli TA: Cerebral concussion and traumatic unconsciousness: Correlation of experimental and clinical observations on blunt head injuries. Brain 97:633–654, 1974.
38. Ghajar J, Hairi RJ: Management of pediatric head injury. Pediatr Clin North Am 39:1093–1125, 1992.
39. Symonds C: Concussion and its sequelae. Lancet 1:1–5, 1962.
40. Winckle WF, Groat RA: Disappearance of nerve cells after concussion. Anat Rec 93:201–209, 1945.
41. Gennarelli TA, Thibault LF, Adams TH, et al: Diffuse axonal injury and traumatic coma in the primate. Ann Neurol 12:564–568, 1982.
42. Graham DI, Adams JH, Gennarelli TA: Head injury (neuropathology). In Head and Neck Injury Criteria: A Consensus Workshop. Washington, DC, National Transportation Safety Board, 1981, p 26.
43. Adams JH, Mitchell DE, Graham DI, et al: Diffuse brain damage of immediate impact type: Its relationship to primary brain stem damage in head injury. Brain 100:489–502, 1977.
44. Erb DC, Povlishock JT: Axonal damage in severe traumatic brain injury: An experimental study in the cat. Acta Neuropathol (Berl) 76:347–358, 1988.
45. Duhaime AC, Eppley M, Marguile S, et al: Crush injuries to the head in children. Neurosurgery 37:401–407, 1995.
46. Cardoso ER, Galbraith S: Posttraumatic hydrocephalus—a retrospective review. Surg Neurol 23:261–264, 1985.
47. Teasdale GM, Murray G, Anderson E, et al: Risks of acute traumatic intracranial haematoma in children and adults: Implications for managing head injuries. BMJ 300:363–365, 1990.
48. Lloyd DA, Carty H, Patterson M, et al: Predictive value of skull radiography for intracranial injury in children with blunt head injury. Lancet 349:821–824, 1997.
49. Harad FT, Kerstein MD: Inadequacy of bedside clinical indicators in identifying significant intracranial injury in trauma patients. J Trauma 32:359–363, 1992.
50. Stein SC, Ross SE: Mild head injury: A plea for routine early CT scanning. J Trauma 33:11–13, 1992.
51. Mohanty SK, Thompson W, Rakower S: Are CT scans for head injury patients always necessary? J Trauma 31:801–805, 1991.
52. Stein SC, Ross SE: The value of computed tomographic scans in patients with low-risk head injuries. Neurosurgery 26:638–640, 1990.
53. Jeret JS, Mandell M, Anziska B, et al: Clinical predictors of abnormality disclosed by computed tomography after mild head trauma. Neurosurgery 32:9–16, 1993.
54. Miller EC, Derlet RW, Kinser D: Minor head trauma: Is computed tomography always necessary? Ann Emerg Med 27:290–294, 1996.
55. Shackford SR, Wald SL, Ross SE, et al: The clinical utility of computed tomographic scanning and neurological examination in the management of patients with minor head injuries. J Trauma 33:385–394, 1992.
56. Rivara FR, Tanaguchi D, Parish RA, et al: Poor prediction of positive computed tomographic scans by clinical criteria in symptomatic pediatric head injury. Pediatrics 80:579–584, 1987.
57. Davis RL, Mullen N, Makela M, et al: Cranial computed tomography scans in children after minimal head injury with loss of consciousness. Ann Emerg Med 24:640–645, 1994.
58. Dietrich AM, Bowman MJ, Ginn-Pease ME, et al: Pediatric head injuries: Can clinical factors reliably predict an abnormality on computed tomography? Ann Emerg Med 22:1535–1540, 1993.
59. Bruce DA: Delayed deterioration of consciousness after trivial head injury in childhood. BMJ 289:715–716, 1984.
60. Dacey RG, Alves WM, Rimel RW, et al: Neurosurgical complications after apparently minor head injury: Assessment of risk in a series of 610 patients. J Neurosurg 65:203–210, 1986.
61. Humphreys RP, Hendrick EB, Hoffman HJ: The head-injured child who "talks and dies": A report of 4 cases. Childs Nerv Syst 6:139–142, 1990.
62. Snoek JW, Minderhoud JM, Wilmink JT: Delayed deterioration following mild head injury in children. Brain 107:15–36, 1984.
63. Hugenholtz H, Izukawa D, Shear P, et al: Vomiting in children following head injury. Childs Nerv Syst 3:266–270, 1987.
64. Casey R, Ludwig S, McCormick MC: Morbidity following minor head trauma in children. Pediatrics 78:497–502, 1986.
65. Casey R, Ludwig S, McCormick MC: Minor head trauma in children: An intervention to decrease functional morbidity. Pediatrics 80:159–164, 1987.
66. Levi L, Guilburd JN, Linn S, et al: The association between skull fracture, intracranial pathology and outcome in pediatric head injury. Br J Neurosurg 5:617–625, 1991.
67. Chan KH, Mann KS, Yue CP, et al: The significance of skull fracture in acute traumatic intracranial hematomas in adolescents: A prospective study. J Neurosurg 72:189–194, 1990.
68. Hsiang JNK, Yeung T, Yu ALM, et al: High risk mild head injury. J Neurosurg 87:234–238, 1997.
69. Bandak FA, Vander Vorst MJ, Stuhmiller LM, et al: An imaging-based computational and experimental study of skull fracture: Finite element model development. J Neurotrauma 12:679–688, 1995.
70. Yoganandan N, Pintar FA, Sances A, et al: Biomechanics of skull fracture. J Neurotrauma 12:669–678, 1995.
71. Luerssen TG: Skull fractures after closed head injury. In Albright L, Pollack I, Adelson PD (eds): Principles and Practice of Pediatric Neurosurgery. New York, Thieme Medical, 1999, pp 813–829.
72. Steinbok P, Flodmark O, Martens D, et al: Management of simple depressed skull fractures in children. J Neurosurg 66:506–510, 1987.
73. Ingram MD, Hamilton WM: Cephalohematoma in the newborn. Radiology 55:503–507, 1950.
74. Schrager GO: Elevation of a depressed skull fracture with a breast pump. J Pediatr 77:512–514, 1979.
75. Saunders BS, Lazonitz S, McArtor RD: Depressed skull fracture in the neonate. J Neurosurg 50:512–514, 1979.
76. Braakman R: Depressed skull fracture: Data, treatment, and follow up in 225 consecutive cases. N Neurol Neurosurg Psychiatry 35:395–402, 1972.
77. Jennett B, Miller JD, Braakman R: Epilepsy after nonmissile depressed skull fracture. J Neurosurg 41:208–216, 1974.
78. Van den Heever CM, van der Merwe DJ: Management of depressed skull fractures: Selective conservative management of nonmissile injuries. J Neurosurg 71:186–190, 1989.
79. Hendrick EB, Harwood-Nash, DCF, Hudson AR: Head injuries in children: A survey of 4465 consecutive cases at the Hospital for Sick Children, Toronto, Canada. Clin Neurosurg 11:46–65, 1964.
80. Einhorn A, Mizrahi EM: Basilar skull fractures in children: The incidence of CNS infection and the use on antibiotics. Am J Dis Child 132:1121–1124, 1978.
81. Cooper PR: Cerebrospinal fluid fistulas and pneumocephalus. In Barrow DI (ed): Complications and Sequelae of Head Injury. Park Ridge, Ill, American Association of Neurological Surgeons, 1992, pp 1–12.
82. Park J-I, Strezlow VV, Freidman WH: Current management of cerebrospinal fluid rhinorrhea. Laryngoscope 93:1294–1300, 1983.
83. Westmore GA, Whittam DE: Cerebrospinal fluid rhinorrhea and its management. Br J Surg 69:489–492, 1982.
84. Kadish HA, Schunk JE: Pediatric basilar skull fracture: Do children with normal neurological findings and no intracranial injury require hospitalization? Ann Emerg Med 26:37–41, 1995.
85. Talamonti G, Fontana R, Villa F, et al: "High risk" anterior basal skull fractures: Surgical treatment of 64 consecutive cases. J Neurosurg Sci 39:191–197, 1995.
86. Rathore MH: Do prophylactic antibiotics prevent meningitis after basilar skull fracture? Pediatr Infect Dis J 10:87–88, 1991.
87. Brown E: Antimicrobial prophylaxis for cerebrospinal fluid fistula. Br J Neurosurg 4:367–371, 1990.
88. Dagi TF, Meyer FB, Poletti CA: The incidence and prevention of meningitis after basilar skull fracture. Am J Emerg Med 3:295–298, 1983.
89. Glarner H, Meuli M, Hof E, et al: Management of petrous bone fractures in children: Analysis of 127 cases. J Trauma 36:198–210, 1994.

90. MacGee EE, Cauthen JC, Brackett CE: Meningitis following acute traumatic cerebrospinal fluid fistula. J Neurosurg 33:312–316, 1970.

91. Leech PJ, Paterson A: Conservative and operative management for cerebrospinal fluid leakage after closed head injury. Lancet 1:1013–1016, 1973.

92. Ash GJ, Peter J, Bass DH: Antimicrobial prophylaxis for fractured base of skull in children. Brain Inj 6:521–527, 1992.

93. Klastersky J, Sadeghi M, Brihaye J: Antimicrobial prophylaxis in patients with rhinorrhea or ottorrhea: A double-blind study. Surg Neurol 6:111–114, 1976.

94. Ignelzi RJ, VanderArk GE: Analysis of the treatment of basilar skull fractures with and without antibiotics. J Neurosurg 43:721–726, 1975.

95. Murali R, Rovit RL: Injuries of the cranial nerves. In Barrow DL (ed): Complications and Sequelae of Head Injury. Park Ridge, Ill, American Association of Neurological Surgeons, 1992, pp 109–126.

96. Shokunbi T, Agbeja A: Ocular complications of head injury in children. Childs Nerv Syst 7:147–149, 1991.

97. Mahapatra AK, Tandon DA: Traumatic optic neuropathy in children: A prospective study. Pediatr Neurosurg 19:34–39, 1993.

98. Cook MW, Levin lA, Joseph MP, et al: Traumatic optic neuropathy: A metaanalysis. Arch Otolaryngol Head Neck Surg 122:389–392, 1996.

99. Kline LB, Morawetz RB, Swaid SN: Indirect injury of the optic nerve. Neurosurgery 14:756–764, 1984.

100. Healy GB: Hearing loss and vertigo secondary to head injury. N Engl J Med 306:1029–1031, 1982.

101. Tandon PN, Banerji AK, Bhatia R, et al: Cranio-cerebral erosion (growing fracture of the skull in children). Part II. Clinical and radiological observations. Acta Neurochir (Wien) 88:1–9, 1987.

102. Roy S, Sarkar C, Tandon PN, et al: Cranio-cerebral erosion (growing fracture of the skull in children). Part I. Pathology. Acta Neurochir (Wien) 87:112–118, 1987.

CHAPTER 222

Pediatric Head Injury

EGON M. R. DOPPENBERG ■ JOHN D. WARD

Accidents are the leading cause of death in children younger than 15 years of age. In this group, head injury is the most common cause of mortality.[1, 2] It is twice as common as cancer and congenital diseases combined. Because of the frequency of this condition in the pediatric population, it is important that it be handled appropriately and effectively. The outcome in head injury, in many cases, is directly related not only to the severity of injury, but also to how well the injury is managed.[3, 4] Because children have many years ahead of them, it is crucial that children be given the best care possible.

This chapter deals with moderate and severe head injuries, which include closed head injuries with and without mass lesions. We define moderate head injuries as a Glasgow Coma Scale score (GCS) of 9 to 12 and a severe head injury as a GCS of 8 or less. Most of what we discuss is applicable to moderate and severe head injury. If something is specific to one or the other, it is indicated.[5–7]

EPIDEMIOLOGY

When head injuries in children are classified in the categories of mild, moderate, and severe, mild injuries are far more common than moderate or severe injuries.[8] Head trauma is one of the most common childhood injuries, annually accounting for more than 500,000 emergency department visits, 95,000 hospital admissions, 7000 deaths, and 29,000 permanent disabilities; hospital care costs alone exceed $1 billion annually.[9] The mildly brain-injured child accounts for most of the hospital days consumed. Most instances of death occur in the severe brain-injured child with a GCS of 8 or less. The annual brain injury rate per 100,000 children is approximately 185, with boys being twice as likely to be injured as girls. Common causes of injuries are falls (35%), recreational activities (29%), and motor vehicle accidents (24%).[9–11]

If minor head injuries are excluded, the major causes for moderate and severe brain injury are motor vehicle accidents, bicycle accidents, and falls.

If the brain injuries are grouped based on age of occurrence, different patterns emerge. For children younger than 36 months, the most common cause of a brain injury is a fall (75%). For children between 0 and 4 years of age, only 23% of the head injuries were caused by traffic injuries. For children 5 to 9 years of age, traffic injuries accounted for 47% of cases, and for children 10 to 14 years old, traffic injuries accounted for 65% of cases of brain injury. For adolescents 15 to 19 years of age, the rate of brain injury due to traffic accidents was 82%. Bicycle injuries were also more common in the 5- to 9-year-old and 9- to 14-year-old age group.[8–11]

There are also mechanisms of injury that are more specific to the pediatric age group. These include bicycles, walkers, all-terrain vehicles, and car seats. One significant factor that seems to be identified with disturbing frequency in all of these cases is that many of these injuries are preventable.

PATHOPHYSIOLOGY

One of the unique characteristics of the pediatric brain is that it is undergoing a process of maturation and development. Because of this process, the brain of the child reacts differently to similar injuries depending on the age of the child when the injury occurs. There is a variation in the amount of white and gray matter, brain water content, and the consistency and size of the skull. As a child ages, the gray matter expands due to dendritic expansion and branching of the astrocytes until the second year of life. Maturation and differentiation of the white matter occur at a slower rate, with myelination occurring rapidly in the first 2 years of life and then spreading more slowly through the first decade.[12]

The skull is initially a one-layered structure in infants and neonates with open sutures and small diploic spaces. However, by the age of 4 years, it has become a rigid, closed system.[12] Because of the more compressible brain and pliability of the calvarium in the younger child, there are fewer mass lesions, with more white matter shear injuries.[1, 13, 14] As the child ages, the incidence of mass lesions becomes more like that of the adult.[2, 13, 15] Another unique aspect is the relationship of the size of the head of the infant to the body, which changes with age. In the newborn, the brain constitutes 15% of the total body weight, compared with 3% in the adult. In looking at a head growth chart, it is easy to see that the brain and head growth are maximal in the first 2 years.

The physiology of the young child's cerebral vasculature is also different than that of the adult. It is thought that the cerebral perfusion pressure is lower in the child because mean arterial blood pressure is lower in children.[16]

EVALUATION OF PATIENTS WITH MODERATE AND SEVERE HEAD INJURIES

When a child sustains a moderate or severe head injury, it must be decided where to take the child for care. There is a tendency to take the child to the closest available hospital. However, there is evidence that children tend to do better if taken to a facility that has experience in caring for children with significant and severe injuries, especially brain injuries.[17] This is a judgment made at the scene of the accident, but deterioration has been documented due to delay in initiating appropriate treatment.

Many of the basic principles involved with the workup and evaluation of children with moderate and severe head injuries are similar to those for the adult. Initial attempts are directed at stabilization of the patient's vital signs, ensuring an adequate airway, good venous access, a normal blood pressure, and evaluation of life-threatening injuries. After the vital signs have been ascertained, and there is an adequate airway, a complete neurological examination is performed, the minimal components of which are the GCS, assessment of pupillary reaction, determination of the presence or absence of the oculocephalic response, and some assessment of motor power bilaterally. The core of the neurological assessment of the patient is the GCS. Although this is adequate for children older than 5 years and probably older than 3 years, in children younger than 3 years it is difficult to apply the adult coma score. Several pediatric coma scores have been devised to take into account a young child's maturation process. All of these scales tend to be related to the GCS but supply specific areas of evaluation that can be accessed in the young child[18] (Tables 222–1 and 222–2). All patients with severe head injury must have an established and secure airway. Often, this means that the patient must be paralyzed and then intubated. This significantly affects the neurological examination, and it is of utmost importance that those initially assessing the patient perform an adequate neurological evaluation.

After the vital signs are stabilized, the airway is secure, and there are no life-threatening injuries, the next determination is whether there is a mass lesion. This is accomplished with computed tomography (CT). Magnetic resonance imaging (MRI) has been used with increased frequency, but MRI still has no significant

role to play in the emergency department evaluation of the patient with a severe head injury.

Although the patient with a moderate head injury does not require such emergent workup, the steps are similar. Evaluation is done to ensure adequacy of the patient's vital signs. An accurate neurological examination is performed, and CT should be done on all patients with moderate head injuries. If the computed tomographic scan results are negative, the patient is taken to the intensive care unit. If the patient has a mass lesion, mannitol is given in a dose of 1 to 2 g/kg, and the patient is taken immediately to the operating room. If at any time it is suspected that the patient may be harboring a mass lesion (i.e., if focal neurological deficits develop or there is a decrease in the patient's neurological function), mannitol should be given if the blood pressure is stable.

The issue of hyperventilation is one of moderate controversy. There is overwhelming evidence that hyperventilation in the presence of ischemia worsens is-

T A B L E 2 2 2 – 1 ■ **Modified Glasgow Coma Score for Pediatric Patients**

CHARACTERISTIC	SCORE
Eye Opening	
Spontaneously	4
To speech	3
To pain	2
No response	1
Verbal Response	
Oriented	5
Words	4
Vocal sounds	3
Cries	2
No response	1
Motor Response	
Obeys commands	5
Localizes	4
Abnormal flexion	3
Abnormal extension	2
No response	1

From Reilly PL, Simpson DA, Sprod R, et al: Assessing the conscious level in infants and young children: A paediatric version of the Glasgow Coma Scale. Childs Nerv Syst 4:30–33, 1988.

T A B L E 2 2 2 – 2 ■ **Best Possible Glasgow Coma Score Adjusted for Age**

AGE	BEST MOTOR	BEST VERBAL	BEST OVERALL
0–6 mo	2–3	2	9
6–12 mo	4	3	11
12–24 mo	4	4	12
2–5 yr	4–5	4	13
>5 yr	5	5	14

From Reilly PL, Simpson DA, Sprod R, et al: Assessing the conscious level in infants and young children: A paediatric version of the Glasgow Coma Scale. Childs Nerv Syst 4:30–33, 1988.

chemia and causes a lack of adequate blood flow to the brain.[19–27] Recommendations have been made by the Brain Trauma Foundation regarding this matter for adult head-injured patients.[21] However, there are no conclusive studies done to provide answers for the pediatric patient. Probably the best course of action is to prevent significant hyperventilation and to maintain the $PaCO_2$ above 30 mm Hg.

MASS LESIONS

A significant factor in producing intracranial mass lesions in the neonate is birth trauma. However, this topic is not addressed because it is described in another chapter.

Mass lesions, including subdural hematomas, epidural hematomas, and intracerebral hemorrhages, account for a fairly small portion of intracranial pathology in childhood trauma (Figs. 222–1 and 222-2). The incidence of mass lesions in pediatric head injuries increases with age.[28] Epidural hematomas occur in 1% to 2.5% of neonates and infants and occur in 1.5% to 5% of older children and adolescents.[28] Subdural hematomas in the pediatric population vary from 3.5% to 10.8%, whereas the risk of sustaining an intracerebral hemorrhage is less than 1% to approximately 4%.[29]

Extradural Hematoma

There are many reasons why extradural hematomas are relatively uncommon in neonates. The dura is attached tightly to the periosteum, preventing formation of epi-

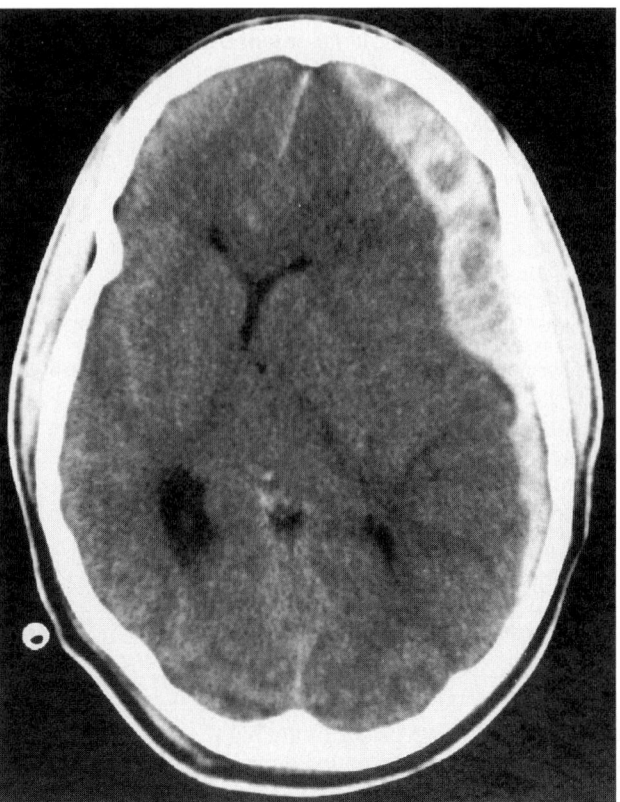

FIGURE 222–2. Large left subdural hematoma with mass effect in a 12-year-old boy.

dural fluid collections. The middle meningeal artery groove is shallow, and the artery is not encased in bone; it is therefore less susceptible to tearing during a fracture of the soft cranium, which also dissipates energy. The most common cause of epidural hematoma in neonates is bleeding due to birth trauma.[29, 30] Injury can be located anywhere in the cranium but most commonly is in the temporoparietal and frontal regions. Between 25% and 40% of all lesions in the posterior fossa have been documented as epidural hematomas.[31] Extradural hematomas are usually associated with a fracture.[29]

Treatment of extradural hematomas can frequently be accomplished by needle aspiration. If this is not successful, a craniotomy is necessary.[30, 32, 33] As children age, they become more susceptible to the classic extradural hematoma resulting from middle meningeal artery bleeding. The most common location is the parietal temporal region; however, posterior fossa hematomas also can be observed in this population.[31, 34, 35] Most epidural hematomas are treated with surgical evacuation (see Fig. 222-1). Generally speaking, epidural hematomas are usually removed when documented. If the patient shows any sort of neurological findings or deterioration, the epidural hematoma should be removed immediately. Some series in the literature show that these hematomas can be observed while they spontaneously regress.[36] However, if the physician anticipates observing an epidural hematoma, the patient must have a GCS of 15 and be essentially neurologi-

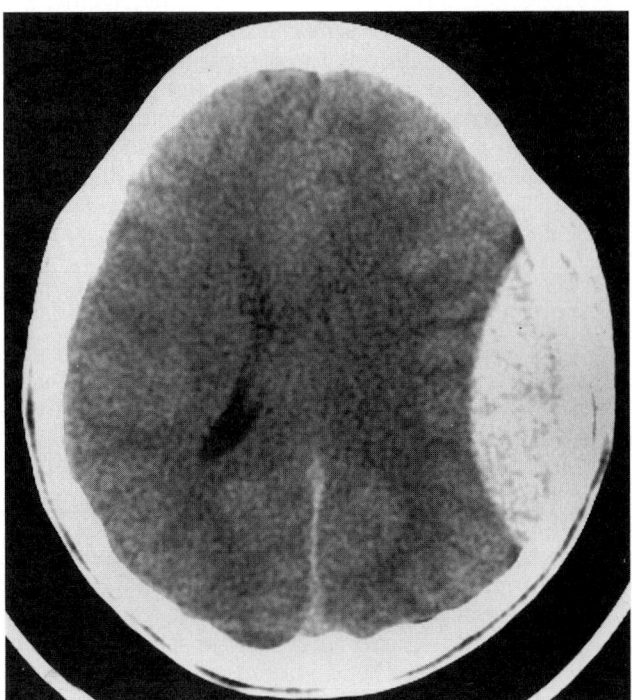

FIGURE 222–1. Left epidural hematoma in a 13-year-old boy after a motor vehicle accident.

T A B L E 2 2 2 - 3 ■ **Surgical and Nonsurgical Management of Epidural Hematomas**

Surgical Indications

1. Focal, neurological examination, cranial nerve III palsy, increasing drowsiness
2. Focal, significant cortical compression, seen with clots > 15 mm in diameter
3. Brainstem herniation
4. Epidural clot volume > 30 mL
5. Midline shift or uncal herniation, with temporal lobe clot
6. Concomitant intraparenchymal or subdural hematoma with mass effect
7. Associated fracture transversing a major dural vessel with neurological impairment

Indications for Observation

1. Neurologically intact, with only headache, nausea, vomiting, and irritability (cranial nerve VI palsy without posterior fossa clot may be accepted)
2. Clot in frontal, parietal, or occipital region
3. Small posterior fossa clot without compression of cortex, fourth ventricle, or brainstem

Data from references 37 and 61.

cally normal. The patient can have headaches, but if there are any signs of neurological impairment or deterioration, the epidural hematoma must be removed emergently (Table 222–3). The procedure is fairly benign, and if there is any hint of a problem, the epidural hematoma should be removed at once. Large hematomas associated with significant midline shift or those in a comatose or deteriorating patient require immediate craniotomy.

Subdural Hematoma

Subdural hematomas are uncommon in the neonate, but they occur with increased frequency during the following years (see Fig. 222-2).[37–41] Subdural hematomas can occur in the supratentorial space or in the posterior fossa. Radiographically, posterior fossa hematomas are usually located near the falx and tentorium cerebri. Posterior fossa subdural hematomas, especially those on the surfaces of the cerebellum under the falx, are usually treated conservatively if there are no signs of brainstem compression or obstructive hydrocephalus.[42, 43] Supratentorially, the hematomas can occur over the hemisphere or in the interhemispheric fissure. Posterior interhemispheric subdural hematomas usually do not require surgery and can be closely observed. Any acute subdural hematoma with large displacement of the midline in the patient who is comatose or who has a focal neurological deficit requires an emergency open craniotomy. However, the child with minimal neurological deficits and a small subdural hematoma can be observed. The child with neurological impairment who has a significant amount of shift; a small, thin rim of subdural hematoma; and fairly significant brain swelling presents a problem. It can be difficult to decide whether to operate on these children. In general, it is probably wise to at least operate on the child and

open the dura a small amount to allow evacuation of the hematoma. Many of these hematomas can be larger than indicated on CT. Multiple small openings in the dura can be accomplished in a slitlike fashion, and the subdural hematoma can be at least partly decompressed. In this way, the surgeon avoids the terrible situation of a tremendously swollen brain herniating through a large dural opening, preventing adequate closure of the scalp. In most cases, the bone flap is left out.

Intraparenchymal Hematoma

Intracerebral hematomas in the neonate are discussed elsewhere. In the older child, these hematomas are frequently caused by acceleration or deceleration injuries, resulting in hemorrhagic contusions, as in the adult. Most common sites are the subfrontal and temporal lobes. Contrecoup injuries occur in increasing frequency as the child gets older.

Little concluding literature exists about management of these lesions. Overall, the same rules apply as for the previously described subdural hematomas. If the child is neurologically intact and there is only minimal mass effect from a small intraparenchymal hematoma, close observation in an intensive care unit setting may be appropriate. Otherwise, a craniotomy should be performed for lesion removal.[1]

Traumatic Subarachnoid Hemorrhage

Traumatic subarachnoid hemorrhage is relatively common in the postnatal child after significant head trauma (Fig. 222-3). If imaging studies reveal a significant amount of blood in the subarachnoid spaces in a child who fails to improve after aggressive management, a cerebral angiogram is warranted to exclude a traumatic arterial aneurysm. Traumatic aneurysms typically arise at the skull base or from distal anterior or middle cerebral arteries or branches after direct mural injury or acceleration-induced shear. Pediatric traumatic cerebral aneurysms may manifest early or late. Once diagnosed, these aneurysms should be treated immediately with a surgical or endovascular approach.[44]

MODERATE HEAD INJURY

Little has been studied regarding the moderately head-injured pediatric patient, even though they constitute a substantial portion of the head-injured population. The moderately injured child, based on the initial GCS score, requires close monitoring, especially if any abnormalities were seen on initial computed tomographic studies. If the patient fails to improve over the next 24 hours, repeat head CT should be performed. If further deterioration occurs to a point at which the GCS is 8 or less, the child should undergo the same aggressive therapy as a severely head-injured child. This includes intracranial pressure monitoring and, if necessary, aggressive intracranial pressure management with measures such as mannitol, respiratory support, sedation

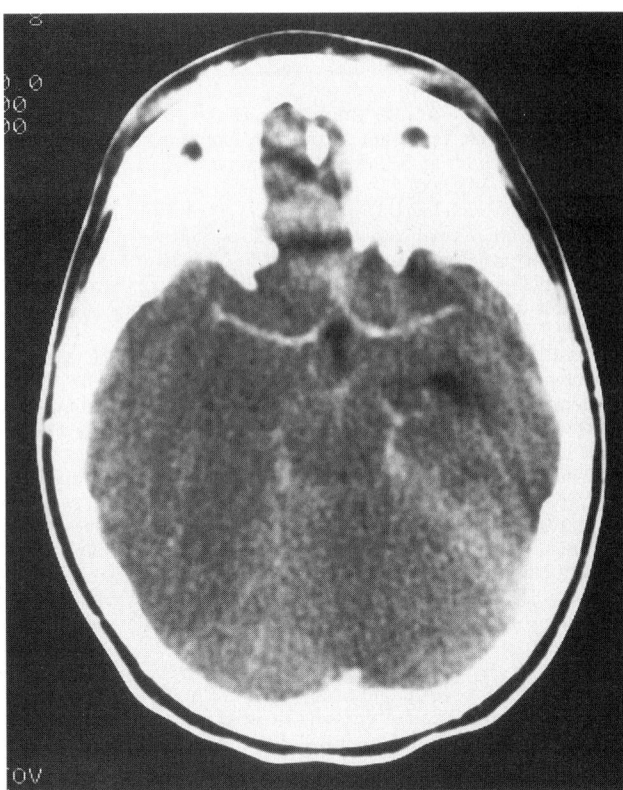

FIGURE 222–3. Extensive, traumatic subarachnoid hemorrhage in a 14-year-old girl. A subsequent angiogram revealed no evidence of an aneurysm.

and paralytics, mild hyperventilation, and hypothermia. However, these children often fail to show any significant mass lesion or brain swelling on CT, but on further imaging such as MRI, the examiner may find punctate hemorrhages in the corpus callosum, pons, or gray-white matter junction suggestive of diffuse axonal injury. These imaging studies often do not change the acute therapy but may help in predicting recovery and may provide information to the physician and parents about what to expect.[45–48]

OUTCOMES

Traumatic brain injury in the United States is one of the leading causes of death and disability of children. Unfortunately, a myth exists that the pediatric population has a much better outcome than adults. However, studies have shown that children involved in motor vehicle accidents are just as likely to die of severe head injury as adults.[49]

Many of the poor outcomes observed are best prevented by preventing the initial impact or the second insults that typically occur after traumatic brain injury. Very young and preschool children have worse outcomes in terms of mortality and long-term disability than older children and adolescents. The deficits observed are often persistent and severe in the long term, even with aggressive management.[50]

In an animal model, diffuse traumatic brain injury in the immature rat creates a consistent, marked, but reversible motor deficit up to 10 days after injury. However, the effect on performance is a long-term, sustained deficit in cognitive skills up to 3 months after trauma. At the same time, diffuse injury affects body and brain weight gain in the developing rat for 3 months after injury.[51]

Evidence is available that the immature brain is far more vulnerable to apoptotic neurodegeneration and therefore contributes in an age-dependent fashion to neuropathologic outcome after head trauma. This explains the unfavorable outcomes of very young pediatric head trauma patients.[52]

Even more so than in the adult population, many factors influence prognosis in the head-injured pediatric population. The age at injury, disproportionate cranial size to trunk in infancy, mechanism of injury, injury severity (e.g., GCS score), multiple trauma, second insults, early childhood injury, and the extent of secondary injury can all impact the final outcome.[53] Other risk factors that worsen outcome include brain edema, midline shift, intracranial hemorrhage, hyperglycemia, hypokalemia, coagulopathy, and focal neurological deficits.[54–58]

The outcome is in part related to the nature of mass lesions. Epidural hematomas in the pediatric population have a relatively good outcome, with an overall mortality rate between 9% and 17%.[29, 34, 59, 60] Subdural hematomas have a better prognosis in the child compared with the adult population, with a morbidity and mortality rate of approximately 8% in operative cases.[61] These numbers, however, do not include the "nonaccidental" injuries, which appear to have a much higher incidence of poor recovery.

Post-traumatic hydrocephalus due to traumatic subarachnoid hemorrhage is a common phenomenon with a clearly adverse outcome. It can develop as late as 2 to 3 years after the initial injury, and previously head-injured children who arrest or regress in their recovery should always be evaluated for increased intracranial pressure due to hydrocephalus. A careful evaluation should be made with imaging studies to differentiate post-traumatic hydrocephalus from ex vacuo hydrocephalus due to brain atrophy.[62–64]

Children treated at pediatric trauma centers have significantly better outcomes compared with those treated at adult trauma centers. This difference in outcome may in part be explained by the approach to operative and nonoperative management of head, liver, and spleen injuries.[65, 66]

The initial therapy given to the head-injured patient is important in improving the survival chances and overall outcome. It is known from adults with severe head injuries that low cerebral perfusion pressure due to hypotension or high intracranial pressure has proved to adversely affect outcome in the pediatric population.[66–69] A significant percentage of (severely) head-injured children sustain hypoxemia or hypotension in the prehospital setting. Evidence shows that patients with severe head injury who are intubated in the prehospital setting have better outcomes.[70]

More advanced tools have been used to monitor

the head-injured adult. They include microdialysis to monitor the changes in contents of the extracellular fluid such as glutamate aspartate, glucose, and lactate. This may help in therapeutic interventions and to predict outcome. However, only few studies are available for the pediatric head-injured population. In one study, increased CSF glutamate and glycine levels were associated with poor outcome. A trend toward an association between high glutamate concentration and ischemic blood flow was observed. Young age and child abuse are associated with extremely high CSF glutamate concentrations after traumatic brain injury.[71]

Other tools to better assess prognosis include intraparenchymal brain oxygen, carbon dioxide tension, and pH monitoring, as well as imaging studies such as proton magnetic resonance spectroscopy (MRS). With use of proton MRS, lactate was evident in 91% of infants and 80% of children with poor outcomes; none of the patients with a good outcome had evidence of lactate.[72–74]

Until recently, the Kennard principle (i.e., assumption that recovery after similar lesions is greater in children than in adults) was supposed to be always true. However, if the lesions are diffuse, recovery is not better in children than adults or in younger children than older children. The prognosis depends on the remaining ability to learn new practices. Normal IQ does not mean absence of sequelae. The cognitive deficits are very similar to those found in adults during the acute phase. For instance, visuospatial neglect often is identified when systematically looked for.

Another study showed that only 28% of the group of surviving adolescent brain-injured victims functioned within normal limits. The most crucial disabling component was poor social integration.[75, 76]

One study showed that, 1 year after injury, the performance of moderately and severely injured children was worse than their controls on 40 of 53 variables from the same neuropsychological test battery. This result shows the persistent and comprehensive nature of neuropsychological deficits in children and adolescents with moderate and severe traumatic brain injury.[77] Reduced fine motor performance, neurological status, self-care, and school or academic performance are significantly impaired after severe head injury.[78] The severity of impairment is related to premorbid psychosocial variables.[79, 80]

In conclusion, sophisticated end-point measurements are available to study the head-injured child during the critical phase and during the later recovery period. These studies show more clearly that the simple myth that children do better than adults needs to be revised. There is too much at stake in treating this population for the patient and the parents, as well as from a socioeconomic standpoint.

REFERENCES

1. Hahn YS, Chyung C, Barthel MJ, et al: Head injuries in children under 36 months of age. Demography and outcome. Childs Nerv Syst 4:34–40, 1988.
2. Luerssen TG, Klauber MR, Marshall LF: Outcome from head injury related to patient's age. A longitudinal prospective study of adult and pediatric head injury. J Neurosurg 68:409–416, 1988.
3. Adelson PD: Pediatric trauma made simple. Clin Neurosurg 47:319–335, 2000.
4. Kochanek PM, Clark RS, Ruppel RA, et al: Cerebral resuscitation after traumatic brain injury and cardiopulmonary arrest in infants and children in the new millennium. Pediatr Clin North Am 48:661–681, 2001.
5. Kohi YM, Mendelow AD, Teasdale GM, et al: Extracranial insults and outcome in patients with acute head injury—relationship to the Glasgow Coma Scale. Injury 16:25–29, 1984.
6. Levin HS, Grossman RG, Rose JE, et al: Long-term neuropsychological outcome of closed head injury. J Neurosurg 50:412–422, 1979.
7. Teasdale G, Murray G, Parker L, et al: Adding up the Glasgow Coma Score. Acta Neurochir Suppl (Wien) 28:13–16, 1979.
8. Henry PC, Hauber RP, Rice M: Factors associated with closed head injury in a pediatric population. J Neurosci Nurs 24:311–316, 1992.
9. Schutzman SA, Greenes DS: Pediatric minor head trauma. Ann Emerg Med 37:65–74, 2001.
10. Kraus JF, Fife D, Conroy C: Pediatric brain injuries: The nature, clinical course, and early outcomes in a defined United States' population. Pediatrics 79:501–507, 1987.
11. Kraus JF, Fife D, Cox P, et al: Incidence, severity, and external causes of pediatric brain injury. Am J Dis Child 140:687–693, 1986.
12. Friede R: Developmental Neuropathology. New York, Springer-Verlag, 1975, pp 1–76.
13. Zimmerman R, Bilaniuk L: Pediatric head trauma. In Neuroimaging Clinics of North America. Philadelphia, WB Saunders, 1994 349–366.
14. Bruce DA, Raphaely RC, Goldberg AI, et al: Pathophysiology, treatment and outcome following severe head injury in children. Childs Brain 5:174–191, 1979.
15. Luerssen T: Head injuries in children. In Neurosurgery Clinics of North America. Philadelphia, WB Saunders, 1991, pp 399–410.
16. Downard C, Hulka F, Mullins RJ, et al: Relationship of cerebral perfusion pressure and survival in pediatric brain-injured patients. J Trauma 49:654–658, 2000.
17. Potoka DA, Schall LC, Gardner MJ, et al: Impact of pediatric trauma centers on mortality in a statewide system. J Trauma 49:237–451, 2000.
18. Reilly PL, Simpson DA, Sprod R, et al: Assessing the conscious level in infants and young children: A paediatric version of the Glasgow Coma Scale. Childs Nerv Syst 4:30–33, 1988.
19. Zwienenberg M, Muizelaar JP: Severe pediatric head injury: The role of hyperemia revisited. J Neurotrauma 16:937–943, 1999.
20. Skippen P, Seear M, Poskitt K, et al: Effect of hyperventilation on regional cerebral blood flow in head-injured children. Crit Care Med 25:1402–1409, 1997.
21. The Brain Trauma Foundation, The American Association of Neurological Surgeons: The Joint Section on Neurotrauma and Critical Care: Hyperventilation. J Neurotrauma 17:513–520, 2000.
22. Letarte PB, Puccio AM, Brown SD, et al: Effect of hypocapnia on CBF and extracellular intermediates of secondary brain injury. Acta Neurochir Suppl (Wien) 75:45–47, 1999.
23. Gopinath SP, Valadka AB, Uzura M, et al: Comparison of jugular venous oxygen saturation and brain tissue P_{O_2} as monitors of cerebral ischemia after head injury. Crit Care Med 27:2337–2345, 1999.
24. Robertson CS, Valadka AB, Hannay HJ, et al: Prevention of secondary ischemic insults after severe head injury. Crit Care Med 27:2086–2095, 1999.
25. Ausina A, Baguena M, Nadal M, et al: Cerebral hemodynamic changes during sustained hypocapnia in severe head injury: Can hyperventilation cause cerebral ischemia? Acta Neurochir Suppl (Wien) 71:1–4, 1998.
26. Zauner A, Doppenberg E, Woodward JJ, et al: Multiparametric continuous monitoring of brain metabolism and substrate delivery in neurosurgical patients. Neurol Res 19:265–273, 1997.
27. Dings J, Meixensberger J, Amschler J, et al: Continuous monitoring of brain tissue P_{O_2}: A new tool to minimize the risk of ischemia caused by hyperventilation therapy. Zentralbl Neurochir 57:177–183, 1996.

28. Alberico AM, Ward JD, Choi SC, et al: Outcome after severe head injury. Relationship to mass lesions, diffuse injury, and ICP course in pediatric and adult patients. J Neurosurg 67:648–656, 1987.
29. Leggate JR, Lopez-Ramos N, Genitori L, et al: Extradural haematoma in infants. Br J Neurosurg 3:533–539, 1989.
30. Negishi H, Lee Y, Itoh K, et al: Nonsurgical management of epidural hematoma in neonates. Pediatr Neurol 5:253–256, 1989.
31. Ammirati M, Tomita T: Posterior fossa epidural hematoma during childhood. Neurosurgery 14:541–544, 1984.
32. Aoki N: Epidural haematoma in the newborn infants: Therapeutic consequences from the correlation between haematoma content and computed tomography features: A review. Acta Neurochir (Wien) 106:65–67, 1990.
33. Aoki N: Epidural hematoma communicating with cephalohematoma in a neonate. Neurosurgery 13:55–57, 1983.
34. Mohanty A, Kolluri VR, Subbakrishna DK, et al: Prognosis of extradural haematomas in children. Pediatr Neurosurg 23:57–63, 1995.
35. Mazza C, Pasqualin A, Feriotti G, et al: Traumatic extradural haematomas in children: Experience with 62 cases. Acta Neurochir (Wien) 65:67–80, 1982.
36. Pang D, Horton JA, Herron JM, et al: Nonsurgical management of extradural hematomas in children. J Neurosurg 59:958–971, 1983.
37. Herrera EJ, Viano JC, Aznar IL, et al: Postraumatic intracranial hematomas in infancy. A 16-year experience. Childs Nerv Syst 16:585–589, 2000.
38. Jayawant S, Rawlinson A, Gibbon F, et al: Subdural haemorrhages in infants: Population based study. BMJ 5:1558–1561, 1998.
39. Tzioumi D, Oates RK: Subdural hematomas in children under 2 years. Accidental or inflicted? A 10-year experience. Child Abuse Negl 22:1105–1112, 1998.
40. Matsuzaka T, Yoshinaga M, Tsuji Y, et al: Incidence and causes of intracranial hemorrhage in infancy: A prospective surveillance study after vitamin K prophylaxis. Brain Dev 11:384–388, 1989.
41. Romodanov AP, Brodsky YS: Subdural hematomas in the newborn. Surgical treatment and results. Surg Neurol 28:253–258, 1987.
42. Hayashi T, Hashimoto T, Fukuda S, et al: Neonatal subdural hematoma secondary to birth injury. Clinical analysis of 48 survivors. Childs Nerv Syst 3:23–29, 1987.
43. Fishman MA, Percy AK, Cheek WR, et al: Successful conservative management of cerebellar hematomas in term neonates. J Pediatr 98:466–468, 1981.
44. Ventureyra EC, Higgins MJ: Traumatic intracranial aneurysms in childhood and adolescence: Case reports and review of the literature. Childs Nerv Syst 10:361–379, 1994.
45. Murgio A, Patrick PD, Andrade FA, et al: International study of emergency department care for pediatric traumatic brain injury and the role of CT scanning. Childs Nerv Syst 17:257–262, 2001.
46. Tabori U, Kornecki A, Sofer S, et al: Repeat computed tomographic scan within 24–48 hours of admission in children with moderate and severe head trauma. Crit Care Med 28:840–844, 2000.
47. Jaffe KM, Fay GC, Polissar NL, et al: Severity of pediatric traumatic brain injury and neurobehavioral recovery at one year—a cohort study. Arch Phys Med Rehabil 74:587–595, 1993.
48. Barzilay Z, Augarten A, Sagy M, et al: Variables affecting outcome from severe brain injury in children. Intensive Care Med 14:417–421, 1988.
49. Johnson DL, Krishnamurthy S: Severe pediatric head injury: Myth, magic, and actual fact. Pediatr Neurosurg 28:167–172, 1998; comment in Pediatr Neurosurg 30:55–61, 1999.
50. Adelson PD: Pediatric trauma made simple. Clin Neurosurg 47:319–335, 2000.
51. Adelson PD, Dixon CE, Kochanek PM: Long-term dysfunction following diffuse traumatic brain injury in the immature rat. J Neurotrauma 17:273–282, 2000.
52. Bittigau P, Sifringer M, Pohl D, et al: Apoptotic neurodegeneration following trauma is markedly enhanced in the immature brain. Ann Neurol 45:724–735, 1999.
53. Chiaretti A, De Benedictis R, Polidori G, et al: Early post-traumatic seizures in children with head injury. Nerv Syst 16:862–866, 2000.
54. Paret G, Ben Abraham R, Berman S, et al: Head injuries in children—clinical characteristics as prognostic factors. Harefuah 136:677–681, 755, 1999.
55. Ben Abraham R, Lahat E, Sheinman G, et al: Metabolic and clinical markers of prognosis in the era of CT imaging in children, with acute epidural hematomas. Pediatr Neurosurg 33:70–75, 2000.
56. Paret G, Tirosh R, Lotan D, et al: Early prediction of neurological outcome after falls in children: Metabolic and clinical markers. J Accid Emerg Med 16:186–188, 1999.
57. Ong L, Selladurai BM, Dhillon MK, et al: The prognostic value of the Glasgow Coma Scale, hypoxia and computerised tomography in outcome prediction of pediatric head injury. Pediatr Neurosurg 24:285–291, 1996.
58. Chiaretti A, Pezzotti P, Mestrovic J, et al: The influence of hemocoagulative disorders on the outcome of children with head injury. Pediatr Neurosurg 34:131–137, 2001.
59. Raimondi AJ, Hirschauer J: Head injury in the infant and toddler: Coma scoring and outcome scale. Childs Brain 11:12–35, 1984.
60. Knuckey NW, Gelbard S, Epstein MH: The management of "asymptomatic" epidural hematomas: A prospective study. J Neurosurg 70:392–396, 1989.
61. Aoki N, Masuzawa H: Infantile acute subdural hematoma. Clinical analysis of 26 cases. J Neurosurg 61:273–280, 1984.
62. Gudeman SK, Kishore PR, Becker DP, et al: Computed tomography in the evaluation of incidence and significance of posttraumatic hydrocephalus. Radiology 141:397–402, 1981.
63. Kishore PR, Lipper MH, Domingues da Silva AA, et al: Delayed sequelae of head injury. J Comput Tomogr 4:287–295, 1980.
64. Kishore PR, Lipper MH, Miller JD, et al: Post-traumatic hydrocephalus in patients with severe head injury. Neuroradiology 16:261–265, 1978.
65. Potoka DA, Schall LC, Gardner MJ, et al: Impact of pediatric trauma centers on mortality in a statewide system. J Trauma 49:237–251, 2000.
66. Downard C, Hulka F, Mullins RJ, et al: Relationship of cerebral perfusion pressure and survival in pediatric brain-injured patients. J Trauma 49:654–658, discussion 658–659, 2000.
67. Kokoska ER, Smith GS, Pittman T, et al: Early hypotension worsens neurological outcome in pediatric patients the moderately severe head trauma. J Pediatr Surg 33:333–338, 1998.
68. Pigula FA, Wald SL, Shackford SR, et al: J Pediatr Surg 28:310–314, discussion 315–316, 1993.
69. Downard C, Hulka F, Mullins RJ, et al: Relationship of cerebral perfusion pressure and survival in pediatric brain-injured patients. J Trauma 49:654–658, discussion 658–659, 2000.
70. Gausche M, Lewis RJ, Stratton SJ, et al: Resuscitation of blood pressure and oxygenation. J Neurotrauma 17:471–478, 2000.
71. Ruppel RA, Kochanek PM, Adelson PD, et al: Excitatory amino acid concentrations in ventricular cerebrospinal fluid after severe traumatic brain injury in infants and children: The role of child abuse. J Pediatr 138:18–25, 2001; comment in J Pediatr 138:1–3, 2001.
72. Ashwal S, Holshouser BA, Shu SK, et al: Predictive value of proton magnetic resonance spectroscopy in pediatric closed head injury. Pediatr Neurol 23:114–125, 2000.
73. Ashwal S, Holshouser BA, Tomasi LG, et al: ¹H-magnetic resonance spectroscopy-determined cerebral lactate and poor neurological outcomes in children with central nervous system disease. Pediatr Neurosurg 30:127–311, 1999.
74. Holshouser BA, Ashwal S, Luh GY, et al: Proton MR spectroscopy after acute central nervous system injury: Outcome prediction in neonates, infants, and children. Radiology 202:487–496, 1997.
75. Emanuelson I, von Wendt L, Beckung E, et al: Outcome after severe traumatic brain injury in children and adolescents. Pediatr Rehabil 2:65–70, 1998.
76. Laurent-Vannier A, Brugel DG, De Agostini M: Rehabilitation of brain-injured children. Childs Nerv Syst 16:760–764, 2000.
77. Fay GC, Jaffe KM, Polissar NL, et al: Outcome of pediatric traumatic brain injury at three years: A cohort study. Arch Phys Med Rehabil 75:733–741, 1994.
78. O'Flaherty SJ, Chivers A, Hannan TJ, et al: The Westmead Pediatric TBI Multidisciplinary Outcome study: Use of functional out-

comes data to determine resource prioritization. Arch Phys Med Rehabil 81:723–729, 2000.

79. Massagli TL, Jaffe KM, Fay GC, et al: Neurobehavioral sequelae of severe pediatric traumatic brain injury: A cohort study. Arch Phys Med Rehabil 77:223–231, 1996.

80. Woodward H, Winterhalther K, Donders J, et al: Prediction of neurobehavioral outcome 1–5 years post pediatric traumatic head injury. Head Trauma Rehabil 14:351–359, 1999.

81. Ritter AM, Ward JD: Mass lesions after head injury in the pediatric population. In Albright L, Pollack I, Adelson D (eds): Principles and Practice of Pediatric Neurosurgery. New York, Thieme, pp 848–859, 1999.

CHAPTER **223**

Birth Head Trauma

ROBIN BOWMAN ■ TADANORI TOMITA

Traumatic head injuries in newborns result from the mechanical forces involved in the birthing process. This chapter does not discuss brain injuries secondary to hypoxic or ischemic events. Although the impact of hypoxic-ischemic encephalopathy on children with birth trauma cannot be taken lightly, our main focus is the mechanical factors associated with birth that affect the child.

INCIDENCE AND RISK FACTORS

The incidence of major birth trauma such as fractures, paralysis, and lacerations is between 1 and 11.7 in every 1000 to 2000 live births.[1–3] Perinatal death secondary to birth trauma alone is a rare event, occurring in 1 in 1000 to 2000 births.[1] Many factors related to the fetus, the mother, and the birthing process have been correlated with an increased incidence of traumatic birth. Such factors include macrosomia, growth retardation, preterm labor, breech presentation, and multiparity.[1, 2, 4–7]

The mode of delivery has also been implicated in birth trauma. There is much debate in the obstetric literature regarding the efficacy and safety of vaginal delivery assistive devices, such as forceps and vacuum extractors.[8–11] As with all medical instruments, these instruments are safe when used in the appropriate manner by trained physicians. The indications for assisted vaginal delivery are delay, malrotation, or fetal distress in the second stage of labor. The cervix should be fully dilated, and the fetal head should be at the level of the ischial spines or below. There is, however, an increased risk of certain types of birth trauma associated with their use (discussed later).[12–17] One would assume that having a lower threshold to proceed with cesarean section would lower the rate of birth trauma in vaginally delivered newborns. An extensive study conducted by Puza and colleagues showed that this assumption was not true.[3] Although they were able to

decrease the incidence of traumatic injury in neonates born by cesarean section, there was no impact on birth trauma experienced by children delivered vaginally.

SCALP INJURY

The scalp consists of five layers. From the outside inward, they are the skin, connective tissue, aponeurosis galea, loose connective tissue, and pericranium. The outer three layers are tightly apposed, whereas the pericranium adheres firmly to the bone. When one turns a skin flap, it is the loose connective tissue that gives way, allowing the outer three layers to peel away from the periosteum and skull.

In a newborn, scalp injury occurs in three distinct areas: the outer layers, the potential subgaleal space, and the subperiosteal plane. The most common scalp injury is a caput succedaneum.[4] This occurs in virtually all children, normally at the vertex. Rather than being a true injury, it is edema of the outer layers of the scalp, usually collecting in the portion of the scalp that leads the way down the birth canal. To the obstetrician, it is known as chignon and is commonly associated with use of vacuum extraction.[4] It is usually noted immediately after birth and resolves within 24 hours. Rarely, it may have associated skin ecchymoses, abrasions, or lacerations.[18] Soft cups used for vacuum extraction cause scalp injury less frequently than do rigid cups.[8]

Although rare, the most life-threatening scalp injury is a hematoma in the subgaleal plane.[12, 16, 19] Plauche reported a mortality of 22.8% associated with this neonatal emergency.[16] The aponeurosis galea extends from the supraorbital rims to the hairline posteriorly and laterally to the level of the ears. This sizable potential space can easily accommodate the entire blood volume of a neonate.

Three conditions put newborns at risk for developing a subgaleal hematoma.[12] A coagulation defect or a vitamin K deficiency after a routine or complicated delivery increases the risk of subgaleal hematoma. The third condition, and the most common, is a difficult delivery in which vacuum extraction is used. In Plauche's review of 123 patients with subgaleal hematomas, vacuum extraction was used in 49% of the cases, and forceps in 14%.[16]

Clinical diagnosis of this lesion relies on identifying a fluctuant scalp mass that extends beyond cranial sutures and is more sizable than a caput succedaneum. A computed tomographic scan easily identifies the massive extent of the hematoma. Treatment consists of emergent transfusion of blood and coagulation factors, as needed, with hemodynamic support of the newborn.

The last type of scalp injury is a cephalohematoma, which occurs in 1% to 2% of all births.[20, 21] It is an accumulation of blood between the periosteum and bone; therefore, the cranial sutures limit its expansion. The hemorrhage is thought to occur when the forces of labor acting on the neonatal head shear the periosteum away from the bone.[20] Both the bone and the undersurface of the periosteum bleed, and a collection forms. The most common location is in the parietal region, but it can occur anywhere over the skull.

Usually, cephalohematomas are of no clinical significance and resolve spontaneously within a few weeks to months. Rarely, the child develops hyperbilirubinemia, anemia, or hemodynamic instability. There are a few reported cases of cephalohematomas that became infected.[21–24] Infection may occur spontaneously, as a complication of fetal monitoring, or after sepsis or meningitis. Infection of a cephalohematoma can also lead to osteomyelitis, meningitis, and sepsis in the newborn. The most common infecting organism is *Escherichia coli*, and the infection usually occurs within 3 weeks. In this situation, a diagnostic tap or open irrigation and drainage are indicated.[21] However, drainage of the hematoma is not generally advised because of the risk of introducing bacteria. In less than 5% of patients, the cephalohematoma calcifies. If it is large or cosmetically unpleasant, the parents may opt to have it removed. To do so, one merely burs the calcified lesion down to the outer layer of the skull. All bleeding should be judiciously controlled with bone wax and electrocautery.

SKULL FRACTURES

Three types of skull fractures can occur in newborns: linear; depressed or "ping-pong"; and occipital osteodiastasis. The cause of skull fracture is a narrow pelvic passage or pressure against the promontory of the sacrum by forceps and vacuum extractors. The exact incidence in newborns is difficult to determine. Although skull fractures are demonstrable on plain radiographs and computed tomographic scan bone windows, linear fractures can be difficult to visualize. It has been reported that linear skull fractures occur in as many as 10% of all births.[20] Most linear skull fractures occur in the parietal bone, although they can occur in the occipital and frontal bones as well. They usually heal within 2 to 3 months and require only a

follow-up skull radiograph to rule out a growing skull fracture.[13–15] Growing fractures are associated with underlying dural laceration and brain injury. Growing fractures associated with birth trauma are rare and have been reported in only a few cases.[13] Vacuum extraction can rupture suture lines, resulting in a growing fracture.[25]

Anywhere from 5.4% to 25% of linear skull fractures have an associated cephalohematoma.[4, 26, 27] In such patients, a computed tomographic scan should be obtained to rule out an epidural hematoma. Blood can easily seep back and forth through the bone fracture and create a collection external (cephalohematoma) or internal (epidural hematoma) to the bone. Some epidural hematomas require surgical removal (discussed in the next section).

Depressed skull fractures are unique to the newborn period. Owing to the thin, pliable nature of a newborn's skull, the bone cortex indents or buckles inward. True indentation is rare, however, and skull fracture is often observed by computed tomographic scans or at surgical repair of a depressed fracture (Fig. 223–1). As with linear fractures, the parietal bone is the most common location.

For all children with such lesions, a computed tomographic scan of the head should be obtained to rule out an associated intracranial hemorrhage. There is debate whether these lesions need to be surgically elevated in an otherwise asymptomatic child. There are case reports in the literature of a breast pump, digital pressure, and a vacuum extractor being used to elevate these frac-

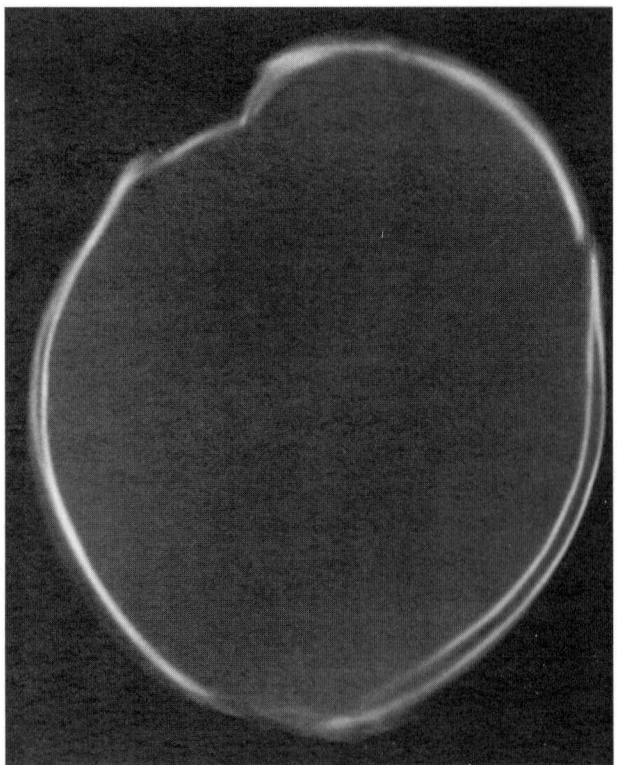

FIGURE 223–1. Axial computed tomographic scan of a bone window showing a depressed fracture caused by forceps.

tures.[28–31] However, depressed fractures in newborns often improve and elevate spontaneously. Loeser and co-workers recommend surgical intervention only for children who have bone fragments in the cerebrum, neurological deficits with or without increased intracranial pressure, or an associated dural tear with leakage of cerebrospinal fluid beneath the galea.[32] They would also consider surgical elevation in neonates who failed conservative management, had poor cosmetic results, or had unreliable long-term follow-up.

Most depressed fractures can be elevated by sliding a periosteal elevator from a bur hole or the nearest coronal or lambdoid suture line to directly under the most concave portion of the indentation. One should then apply steady upward pressure to elevate the fracture. Care must be taken to completely strip the dura away from the suture line and under the fracture. When elevating the fracture, one should never use the intact skull as a fulcrum. For fractures that do not elevate easily, one should proceed immediately to an open craniotomy for elevation of the depressed fracture.

During a difficult delivery, particularly after a forceps breech delivery, it is theorized that the synchondrosis opens between the squamous and condylar portions of the occipital bone.[12, 33, 34] In this manner, the squamous bone is able to slide anteriorly, thereby allowing excessive vertical molding of the skull. This separation of the occipital bones is known as *occipital osteodiastasis*. Although it allows the fetal head to pass more easily through the birth canal, it is stressful on the intracranial contents, often resulting in tentorial and falcial tears, with damage to draining venous structures. In some cases, the squamous portion may undergo vertical fracture resulting from compression at breech delivery (Fig. 223–2).

INTRACRANIAL HEMORRHAGE

Hemorrhage may occur in the epidural, subdural, subarachnoid, or intraparenchymal space. These hemorrhages can occur both above and below the tentorium. They are the most serious complications related to birth trauma. The presenting symptoms are usually secondary to mass effect, especially for lesions in the posterior fossa. Perinatal seizures also commonly herald an intracranial hemorrhage. A computed tomographic scan is the imaging modality of choice for determining the location and extent of the hemorrhage. It also demonstrates any associated soft tissue or skull injury.

An epidural hematoma may occur without an associated skull fracture in 30% to 40% of cases.[28] Owing to its pliable nature, the skull may distort without fracturing, thereby tearing the dura away from the undersurface of the cranium. Bleeding may occur from torn emissary dural veins or, less likely, from branches of the middle meningeal artery.[28, 35] Because of the expansibility of the skull and the compliance of the brain of newborns, an epidural hematoma may initially go undetected (Fig. 223–3). Only after it has reached a

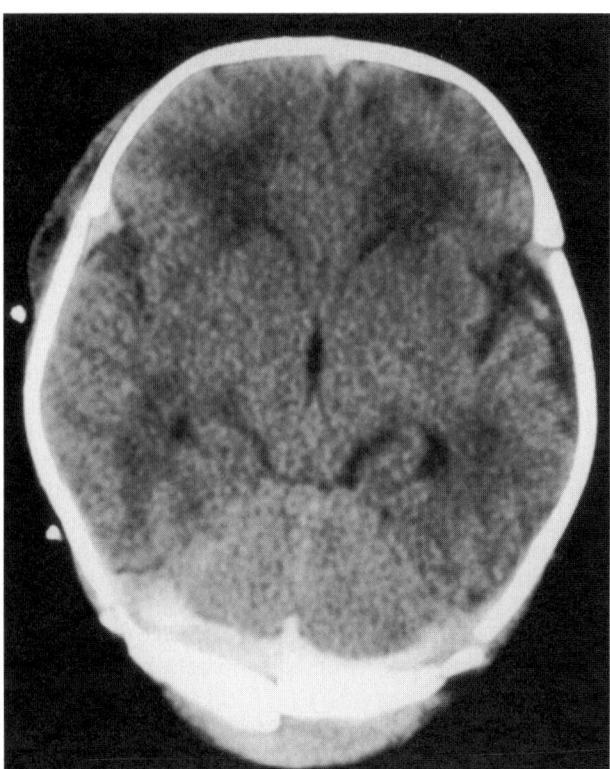

FIGURE 223–2. Axial computed tomographic scan showing a vertical fracture in the occipital bone caused by a difficult breech delivery. Note an associated posterior fossa subdural hematoma.

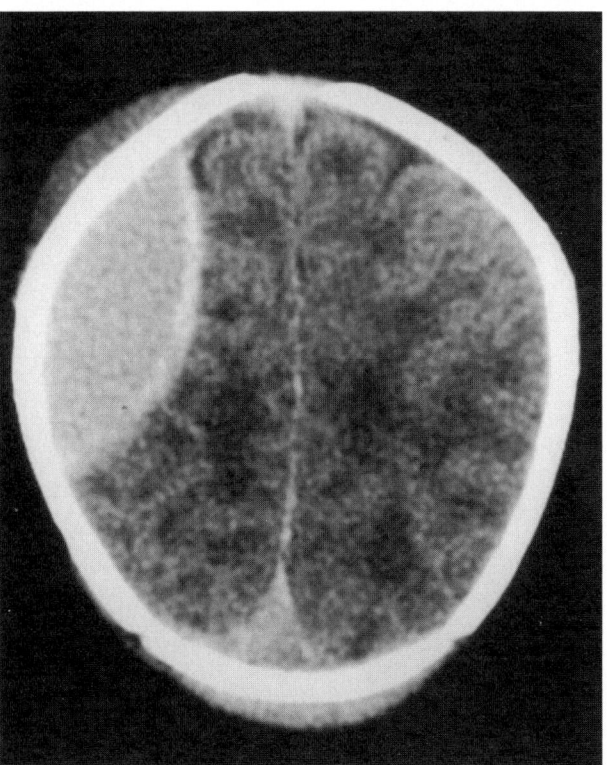

FIGURE 223–3. Axial computed tomographic scan showing a large epidural hematoma over the cerebral convexity in a neonate.

significant size do neonates develop signs of increased intracranial pressure. Initially, they may have irritability with a full fontanelle and increasing head circumference. Later, they may develop signs of brain or brainstem compression with pupillary changes.

A small epidural hematoma less than 1 cm thick can be treated conservatively with serial surveillance computed tomographic scans. Surgical treatment consists of an open craniotomy with evacuation of the hematoma. The dura is then tacked up to the cranium to prevent reaccumulation of blood. Long-term residual deficits from these lesions are rare.

Subdural hematomas in newborns may occur over the convexity or adjacent to the tentorium. Hemorrhages overlying the convexity are usually secondary to rupture of cortical veins; those above or below the tentorium are the result of a torn tentorium, falx, or dural sinus.[28, 36] All such hemorrhages are thought to be caused by excessive vertical molding of the head, and infrequently there is associated occipital osteodiastasis.[37] Elongation and distortion of the head, which are part of the physiologic process of parturition, can cause excessive stress during the descent through the birth canal.

In the cerebral convexity, excessive cranial molding causes stretching of the bridging veins and may tear them. Cerebral convexity subdural hematomas are often minimal and subclinical. At times, however, these

hemorrhages may be sizable, making it difficult to distinguish between a large subdural hematoma and an intraparenchymal hemorrhage (Fig. 223–4). These lesions are rare in premature newborns because of underdeveloped bridging veins.[36]

During passage through the birth canal, the head undergoes compressive fronto-occipital foreshortening. As a result, the distance between the skull base and the vertex increases. Excessive vertical cranial molding causes stretching of the tentorium at the junction of the falx and the tentorium, near the vein of Galen. This skull molding is often aggravated by suction delivery. This excessive vertical skull molding and stretching of the tentorium and posterior falx may result in tentorial laceration. The tentorial laceration may extend into the vein of Galen or the straight sinus, resulting in posterior fossa subdural hematoma (PFSH). Some hemorrhage may originate from injured cerebellar bridging veins or tentorial leaflets at the attachment to the lateral sinus.[33] Most posterior fossa hemorrhages are of venous origin. Rarely, the deformation to the region of the incisura causes a disruption of the posterior cerebellar artery, the superior cerebellar artery, or their branches. This causes not only hemorrhage but also post-traumatic arterial aneurysm.[38] PFSHs can occur in both term and premature newborns.[36]

Neonates with PFSHs usually develop symptoms within 24 hours of birth. In the study by Perrin and

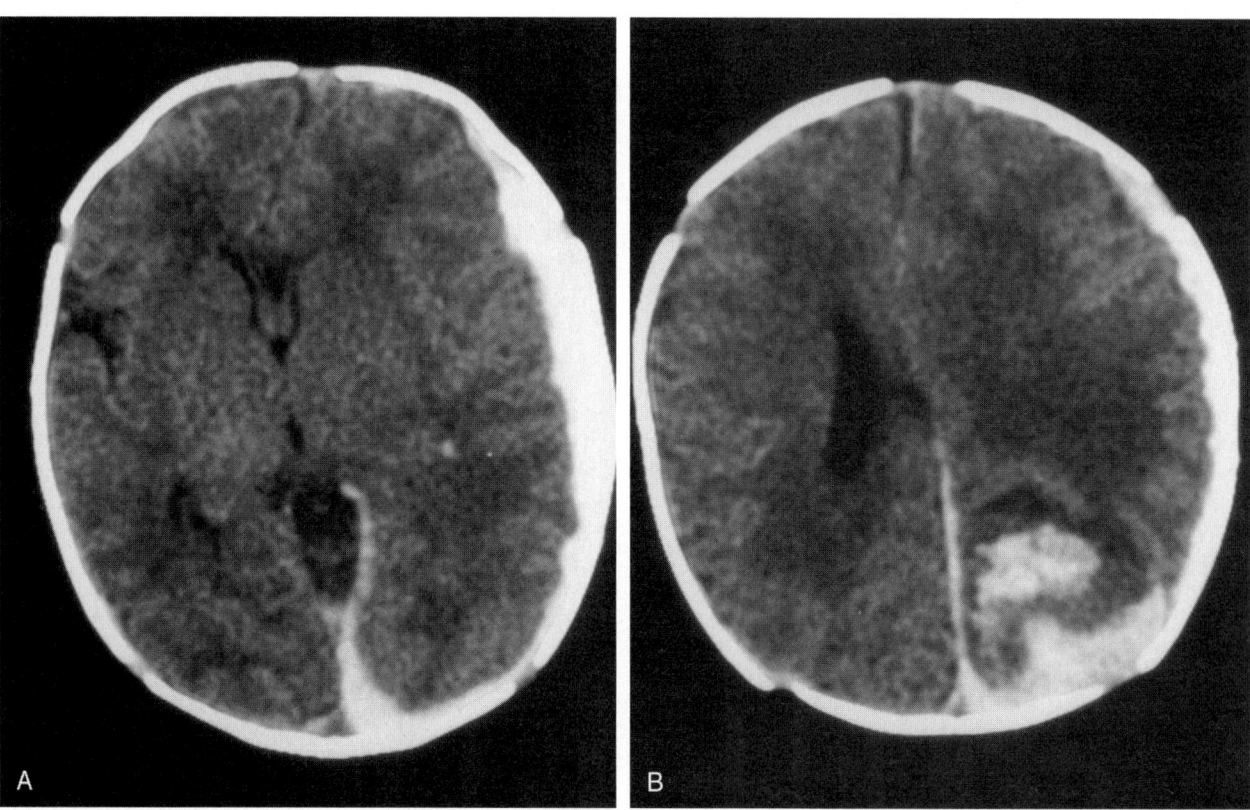

FIGURE 223–4. *A,* Axial computed tomographic scan showing a diffuse, acute subdural hematoma extending from the cerebral convexity to the posterior interhemispheric fissure. *B,* Axial computed tomographic scan of a higher section showing an associated intracerebral hematoma in the posterior parietal lobe.

associates, 14 of 15 neonates presented within 24 hours of birth; only one child presented in a delayed fashion at 41 days of age.[37] The most common presenting symptoms are irritability, lethargy, full fontanelle, hypotonia, poor oral intake, and unstable vital signs. Perinatal seizures may also be associated with PFSH.

The imaging modality of choice is a computed tomographic scan of the head. Although an ultrasonographic scan is easier to obtain and involves no radiation, it is less reliable in demonstrating the posterior fossa lesion. Ultrasonography does, however, demonstrate the ventriculomegaly that is often associated with posterior fossa hemorrhages and may be used to follow the ventricular size. Magnetic resonance imaging provides much better delineation of the posterior fossa anatomy. The sagittal projection in particular shows the precise location and size of the hematoma and the degree of brainstem compression.

There is much debate among pediatric neurosurgeons regarding the appropriate management of PFSHs in neonates.[37] One group advocates aggressive surgical drainage of any subdural hematoma causing signs of increased intracranial pressure or brainstem compression.[39, 40] Drainage may consist of needle aspiration through the lambdoid suture, bur hole placement, or open craniotomy with clot evacuation. It is often difficult to gain access to a newborn baby's small posterior fossa and to control intraoperative hemorrhage, because its source and location are invariably at the region of the superior vermis and tentorial hiatus. Others strongly believe that the friable nature of the neonatal brain is not amenable to surgical intervention and should be avoided.[12, 37] PFSHs often dissolve spontaneously over time (Fig. 223–5). Aggressive intervention is recommended only when signs of serious brainstem compression, such as apnea and bradycardia, develop. Hydrocephalus is common in association with PFSHs. An external ventricular drain or cerebrospinal fluid reservoir may be used to manage this obstructive hydrocephalus, which usually resolves within a few weeks of birth (Fig. 223–6). Only rarely do these children develop progressive hydrocephalus requiring permanent cerebrospinal fluid diversion.[41] Most neonates with PFSH have a good outcome when attended to promptly. Those children with poorer outcomes have been shown, in retrospect, to have had more extensive traumatic injury, especially of the cerebral hemisphere.

Intraparenchymal hemorrhages usually occur in conjunction with subdural hematomas. Intracerebellar hematomas may be due to mechanical deformation of the intraoccipital synchondrosis during delivery when the lower lip of the squamous portion of the occipital bone is depressed, causing cerebellar contusion or laceration. They are associated with forceps or breech delivery.[17] Neonates have symptoms similar to those of a subdural hematoma alone. They may initially be irritable with a full fontanelle, which may progress to lethargy, seizures, hemiparesis, or bradycardia. An ultrasonographic or computed tomographic scan demonstrates the lesion. Small clots causing few or no symptoms can be treated conservatively; larger ones causing signs of brain or brainstem compression require surgical evacuation. As with all surgical intervention in newborns, an experienced surgical and anesthesia team is mandatory, with careful attention to hemostasis and blood replacement.

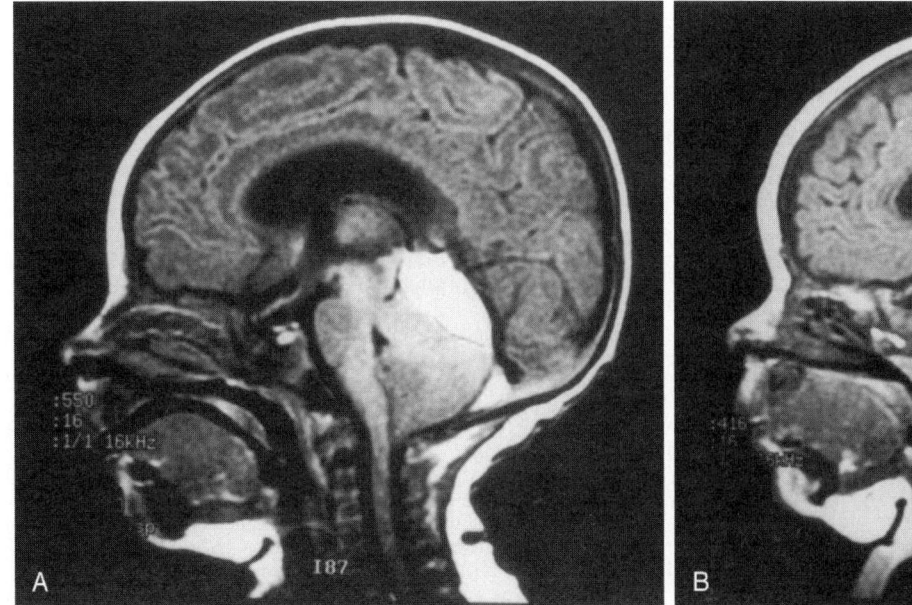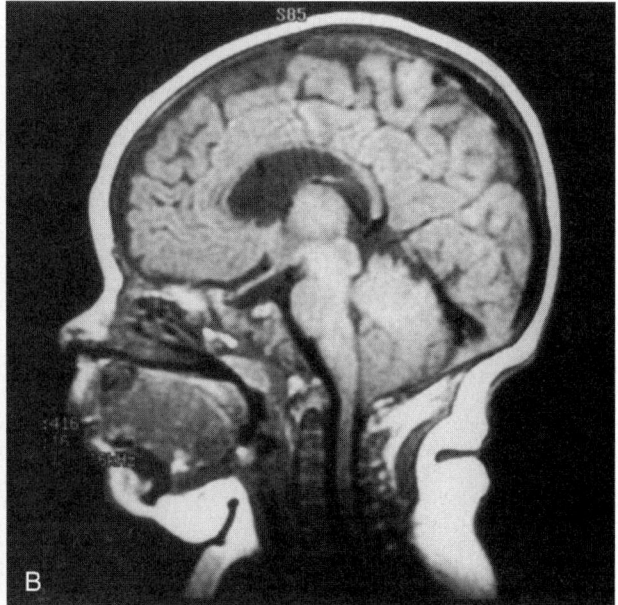

FIGURE 223–5. *A,* Midsagittal magnetic resonance imaging (MRI) scan showing a posterior fossa subdural hematoma at the region of the superior vermis and the tentorial hiatus. There is also hydrocephalus and a cerebellar tonsillar herniation. *B,* Midsagittal MRI scan obtained 2 weeks later showing spontaneous resolution of the posterior fossa subdural hematoma and hydrocephalus. Note the persistent tonsillar herniation.

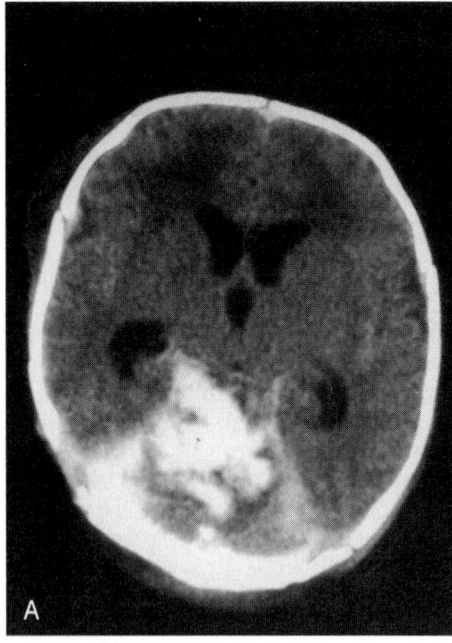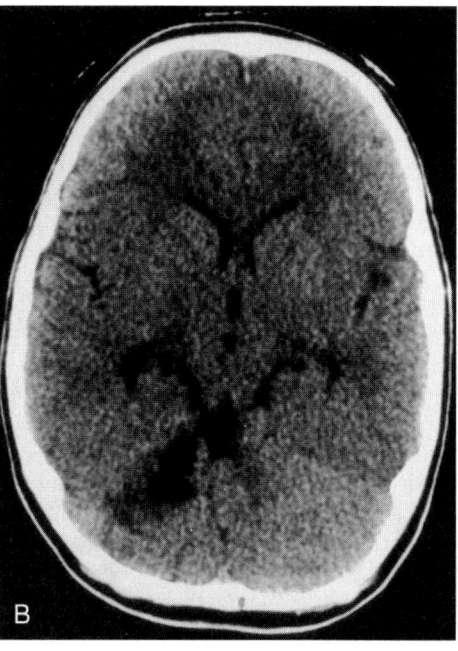

FIGURE 223-6. *A,* Axial computed tomographic scan showing the typical appearance of a posterior fossa subdural hematoma with hydrocephalus. This newborn was treated with intermittent cerebrospinal fluid drainage through a ventricular access device without clot evacuation. *B,* Axial computed tomographic scan 3 weeks later showing total resolution of the hematoma and hydrocephalus.

REFERENCES

1. Geirsson RT: Birth trauma and brain damage. Baillieres Clin Obstet Gynecol 2:195–212, 1988.
2. Perlow JH, Wigton T, Hart J, et al: Birth trauma: A five-year review of incidence and associated perinatal factors. J Reprod Med 41:754–760, 1996.
3. Puza S, Roth N, Macones OA, et al: Does cesarean section decrease the incidence of major birth trauma? J Perinatol 18:9–12, 1998.
4. Curran JS: Birth-associated injury. Clin Perinatol 8:111–129, 1981.
5. Kolderup LB, Laros RY Jr, Musei TJ: Incidence of persistent birth injury in macrosomic infants: Association with mode of delivery. Am J Obstet Gynecol 177:37–41, 1997.
6. Koo MR, Dekker GA, van Geijn HP: Perinatal outcome of singleton term breech deliveries. Eur J Obstet Gynecol Reprod Biol 78:19–24, 1998.
7. Mikulandra F, Stojnic E, Perisa M, et al: Fetal macrosomia—pregnancy and delivery. Zentralbl Gynakol 115:553–561, 1993.
8. Kuit JA, Eppinga HG, Wallenburg HCS, et al: A randomized comparison of vacuum extraction delivery with a rigid and a pliable cup. Obstet Gynecol 82:280–284, 1993.
9. Thompson JP: Forceps deliveries. Clin Perinatol 22:953–972, 1995.
10. Williams MC: Vacuum-assisted delivery. Clin Perinatol 22:933–952, 1995.
11. Williams MC, Knuppel RA, O'Brien WF, et al: A randomized comparison of assisted vaginal delivery by obstetric forceps and polyethylene vacuum cup. Obstet Gynecol 78:789–794, 1991.
12. Govaert P, Vanhaesebrouck P, De Praeter C, et al: Vacuum extraction, bone injury and neonatal subgaleal bleeding. Eur J Pediatr 151:532–535, 1992.
13. Hes R, de Jong TH, Pazy Geuze DH, et al: Rapid evolution of a growing skull fracture after vacuum extraction in case of fetal hydrocephalus. Pediatr Neurosurg 26:269–274, 1997.
14. Hickey K, McKenna P: Skull fracture caused by vacuum extraction. Obstet Gynecol 88:671–673, 1996.
15. Papaefthymiou G, Oberbauer R, Pendl O: Craniocerebral birth trauma caused by vacuum extraction: A case of growing skull fracture as a perinatal complication. Childs Nerv Syst 12:117–120, 1996.
16. Plauche WC: Subgaleal hematoma: A complication of instrumental delivery. JAMA 244:1597–1598, 1980.
17. Riihsinghani A, Belsare TJ: Neonatal intracerebellar hemorrhage after forceps delivery: Report of a case without neurological damage. J Reprod Med 42:127–130, 1997.
18. Matheson GW, Davajan V, Mischell DR Jr: The use of the vacuum extractor: A reappraisal. Acta Obstet Gynecol Scand 47:155, 1968.
19. Benaron DA: Subgaleal hematoma causing hypovolemic shock during delivery after failed vacuum extraction: A case report. J Perinatol 13:228–231, 1993.
20. Hovind KH: Traumatic birth injuries. In Raimondi AJ, Choux M, Di Rocco C (eds): Head Injuries in the Newborn and Infant. New York, Springer Verlag, 1985, pp 87–109.
21. LeBlanc CM, Allen UD, Ventureyra E: Cephalhematomas revisited. Clin Pediatr 34:86–89, 1995.
22. Blom NA, Vreede WB: Infected cephalohematomas associated with osteomyelitis, sepsis, and meningitis. Pediatr Infect Dis J 12:1015–1017, 1993.
23. Ellis SS, Montgomery JR, Wagner ME, et al: Osteomyelitis complicating neonatal cephalhematoma. Am J Dis Child 127:100–102, 1974.
24. Miedema CJ, Ruige M, Kimpen JLL: Primarily infected cephalhematoma and osteomyelitis in a newborn. Eur J Med Res 22:8–10, 1999.
25. Hansen KN, Pedersen H, Petersen MB: Growing skull fracture: Rupture of the coronal suture caused by vacuum extraction. Neuroradiology 29:502, 1987.
26. Kendall N, Woloshin H: Cephalohematoma associated with fracture of the skull. J Pediatr 41:125, 1952.
27. Zelson C, Pearl M: The incidence of skull fractures underlying cephalohematomas in newborn infants. J Pediatr 85:371, 1974.
28. Faix RG, Donn SM: Immediate management of the traumatized infant. Clin Perinatol 10:487–505, 1983.
29. Raynor R, Parsa M: Nonsurgical elevation of depressed skull fracture in an infant. J Pediatr 72:262, 1968.
30. Schrager GO: Elevation of depressed skull fracture with a breast pump. J Pediatr 77:300, 1970.
31. Tan KL: Elevation of congenital depressed fractures of the skull by the vacuum extractor. Acta Paediatr Scand 63:562–564, 1974.
32. Loeser JD, Kilburn HL, Jolley T: Management of depressed skull fracture in the newborn. J Neurosurg 44:62–64, 1976.
33. Govaert P, Calliauw L, Vanhaesebrouck P, et al: On the management of neonatal tentorial damage: Eight case reports and a review of the literature. Acta Neurochir 106:52–64, 1990.
34. Hemsath FA: Birth injury of the occipital bone with a report of thirty-two cases. Am J Obstet Gynecol 27:194–203, 1934.
35. Takagi T, Nagai R, Wakabayashi S: Extradural hemorrhage in the newborn as a result of birth trauma. Childs Brain 4:306, 1978.

36. Towbin A: Central nervous system damage in the human fetus and newborn infant. Am J Dis Child 119:529–542, 1970.
37. Perrin RG, Rutka JT, Drake JM, et al: Management and outcomes of posterior fossa subdural hematomas in neonates. Neurosurgery 40:1190–1200, 1997.
38. Piatt JH, Clunie DA: Intracranial arterial aneurysm due to birth trauma: Case report. J Neurosurg 77:799–803, 1992.
39. Ravenel SD: Posterior fossa hemorrhage in the term newborn: Report of two cases. Pediatrics 64:39–42, 1979.
40. Serfontein GL, Rom S, Stein S: Posterior fossa subdural hemorrhage in the newborn. Pediatrics 65:40–43, 1980.
41. Tanaka Y, Sakamoto K, Kobayashi S, et al: Biphasic ventricular dilatation following posterior fossa subdural hematoma in the full-term neonate. J Neurosurg 68:211–216, 1988.

CHAPTER 224

Birth Brachial Plexus Injury

T. S. PARK ■ STUART S. KAPLAN

Pediatric obstetric brachial plexus injuries have been attributed to traction injuries at the time of birth, with an incidence of 0.19 to 2.5 per 1000 live births.[1-8] This incidence has declined significantly in the 1900s as a result of early recognition of risk factors, improved obstetric technique, and an increased rate of cesarean section.[1-3, 9, 10] However, the incidence has remained stable since the 1980s, with palsies said to be less severe than previously.[1] Those injuries that do occur generally improve with conservative management in approximately 80% to 92% of cases.[1, 3, 7, 11] In the past, injuries that failed to improve were thought to be unamenable to surgical treatment. Although many controversies remain, it is clear that with proper patient selection, timing of surgical intervention, and implementation of microsurgical techniques, pediatric brachial plexus palsies are surgically treatable.

It is important to realize, however, that the long-term goals of surgery are to improve motor functions of the affected upper extremity and that this functional return will be less than perfect. Only a few hundred axons seem to be sufficient to reinnervate poorly differentiated muscles such as the biceps; however, thousands are required to restore the delicate balance of the intrinsic muscles of the hand.[12] It is thus unlikely that the hand will regain complete motor function after severe brachial plexus injury.

HISTORY AND PATHOGENESIS

Smellie, a London obstetrician, is credited with the first medical description of a brachial plexus injury in 1768.[13] In 1872, Duchenne, in his book *Traité de l'électrisation localisée*, described traction during birth as the mechanism of injury.[14] Erb in 1874 reported that weakness of the deltoid, biceps, coracobrachialis, and brachioradialis muscles was caused by a disruption of the C5 and C6 nerve roots.[15] The location where the C5 and C6 nerve roots join to form the upper trunk is thus called Erb's point. Description of the much less common lower brachial plexus palsy (C8-T1) came in 1885 by Klumpke.[16]

Surgery for obstetric brachial plexus injury was introduced in 1903 by Kennedy, who reported on three patients. At 2 months of age, his patients underwent resection of C5-6 neuromas with direct suturing of the ends, with favorable results.[17] Additional reports during the early 1900s resulted in many surgeons advocating early brachial plexus surgery in children who did not improve spontaneously.[18-20] However, in 1925, Sever reported on 1100 cases of obstetric brachial plexus palsy and concluded that there was no difference in outcome between surgically treated and conservatively managed patients.[21] The results of Sever's series, coupled with the relatively high morbidity and mortality rates associated with surgery during the first part of the 20th century, led to an almost complete abandonment of brachial plexus surgery for nearly 5 decades.

With the advent of microsurgical technique, the operating microscope, and modern pediatric anesthesia, a resurgence of interest in the surgical treatment of brachial plexus injuries ensued in the 1970s. The reports of Gilbert and Tassin,[22, 23] demonstrating favorable outcomes after direct repair of obstetric brachial plexus injury, are largely responsible for the increasing use of surgical treatment in the past 2 decades.[24-45]

PATHOPHYSIOLOGY

The acquired, traumatic origin of birth brachial plexus lesions is generally accepted, with the position of the arm at the time of injury of paramount importance. Damage to the upper roots of the brachial plexus usually occurs during vertex delivery when shoulder dystocia necessitates excessive lateral flexion of the neck, with the arm in adduction, to free the shoulder from the pubic arch (Fig. 224-1). The right arm is involved more frequently because of the more common left occipitoanterior position of the descending fetus.[10, 46-48] During breech deliveries, the upper roots are also more commonly affected.

Although birth trauma is responsible for the majority of cases, the possibility has been raised of a prenatal origin in rare cases.[49-56] Evidence for this possibility is the occurrence of plexus injuries after cesarean section and uncomplicated vaginal deliveries of infants with smaller than average birth weights.[57, 58] There are also

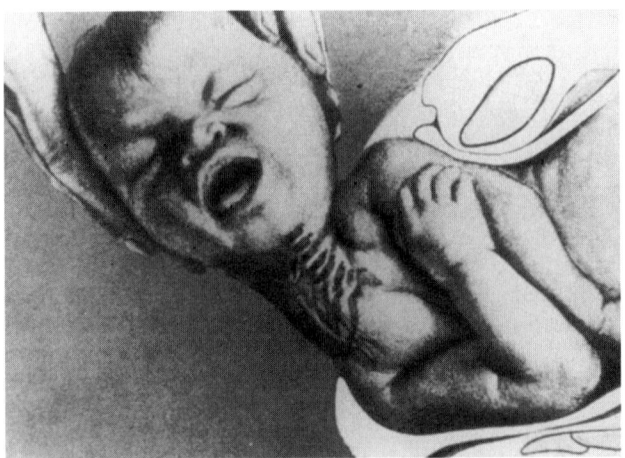

FIGURE 224–1. The most common mechanism of brachial plexus injury during vertex delivery, with lateral flexion of neck to free the shoulder from the pubic arch. (From Brown KLB: Review of obstetrical palsies: Nonoperative treatment. Clin Plast Surg 11: 182, 1984.)

case reports of isolated nerve palsies that predate delivery, suggesting the antenatal development of brachial plexus palsy.[59]

Recognized obstetric risk factors for these injuries include high birth weight (>4 kg), shoulder dystocia, prolonged labor, primiparity, grand multiparity, instrument deliveries, breech presentation, siblings with obstetric palsy, and maternal gestational diabetes. Bilateral injuries are relatively rare (4%) and occur more commonly with breech presentation.[24, 46] Brachial plexus injuries are associated with clavicle and humerus fractures, facial nerve injury, cephalohematoma, and torticollis,[1, 3, 4, 7, 60] but these conditions do not appear to portend a worse prognosis.[61]

NATURAL HISTORY

In early reports, spontaneous recovery from birth brachial plexus injury occurred in less than 40% of cases.[5, 62] However, later studies indicate a good prognosis for these patients, with 65% to 100% achieving complete spontaneous recovery[1, 3, 6, 7, 11, 24, 63–65] (Table 224–1). The rate of spontaneous recovery has been used as a guide to predict which patients will have full spontaneous recovery and which will have incomplete recovery and

thus could benefit from surgical reconstruction of the brachial plexus.

In infants who completely recover motor function, improvement of strength begins as early as age 2 weeks and is complete by 12 to 18 months.[66] In contrast, infants with no signs of recovery by age 2 months have suffered severe total brachial plexus palsy, and their long-term outcome is poor.[19, 23, 27, 28, 44] If infants show some recovery but do not flex the elbow against gravity by 3 months, limited shoulder movements are a likely consequence.[67] Some investigators, however, have noted that if an infant is to have functional use of an extremity, some recovery must be seen by 4, 5, 6, or 12 months.[6, 7, 11, 20, 24, 29, 62, 66] Similarly, we have noted in our own patients that strength testing at age 3 to 6 months was an excellent predictor of outcome, and patients who displayed greater than antigravity strength at 3 months had no disabilities later; however, infants with less than antigravity strength of the biceps at 6 months had unsatisfactory outcomes.[64] All patients who had complete spontaneous recovery made the recovery by age 3 months. We thus recommend surgery for patients with less than antigravity strength of the biceps, triceps, or deltoid muscles at age 6 months.

The most important indicator of recovery appears to be biceps muscle function at the end of the third month, as shown in Tassin's prospective, randomized study of conservatively treated infants who were followed from birth to 5 years.[67] Likewise, Michelow and colleagues reported that favorable outcome was correctly predicted by biceps function at age 3 months in 87% of their patients.[63] The prediction rate improved to 95% if biceps function along with extensor function of the elbow, wrist, thumb, or finger was used in the clinical assessment.

CLINICAL PRESENTATION

Brachial plexus injury patterns vary, and anatomic classification of the injury assists in localizing the lesion and in surgical planning. The injury may be supraclavicular, involving the roots or trunks, or both, or infraclavicular, with injury distal to the level of the cords. In general, postganglionic rupture of the roots and trunks is more common in the upper spinal roots, and preganglionic avulsions are more common in the lower spinal roots.

In avulsion injuries, motor fibers are separated from

TABLE 224–1 ■ Reported Rates of Spontaneous Recovery

| AUTHOR | PERCENTAGE RECOVERED, BY AGE | | | | | PERCENTAGE WITH WEAKNESS |
	1 (mo)	2 (mo)	3 (mo)	4 (mo)	12 (mo)	
Tan[65]	46		69			11
Hardy[7]	17			63	80	11
Greenwald et al[1]	37	58		74	79	15.8
Jackson et al[6]	66		92		95	3
Laurent and Lee[24]				100	100	0

the cell bodies, and all musculature supplied by the injured root is denervated, with resultant weakness. An elevated ipsilateral hemidiaphragm is present with C3-5 root injury. T1 root avulsion produces Horner's syndrome. Sensory fibers remain connected to cell bodies in the dorsal root ganglion, so nerve conduction is normal.

Rupture-type injuries demonstrate sensory conduction delay and paralysis of muscles receiving innervation from the trunk level and beyond. The only trunk branch that lends itself to clinical testing is the supraclavicular nerve supplying the supra- and infraspinatus muscles.

Injuries at or distal to the level of the cords are classified as infraclavicular. Cord-level branches include the lateral and medial pectoral, thoracodorsal, and subscapular nerves. Therefore, if the most proximal weakness is noted in the pectoralis major, a lateral cord injury should be suspected. Weakness of internal rotation driven by the latissimus dorsi denotes a posterior cord injury. Medial cord injury is clinically detectable only by forearm sensory loss.

There are four major patterns of injury. The first is a purely upper brachial plexus lesion involving only C5 and C6, resulting in weakness of the deltoid and biceps, with sparing of the triceps and distal musculature. It has been suggested that such patients typically demonstrate good spontaneous recovery.[68] The second and most common form of presentation is the classic Erb's palsy involving C5-7. This is manifested by an extended arm, internally rotated shoulder, volarflexed wrist, and extended fingers, resulting in the "waiter's tip" posture. The third type of injury is a total plexopathy involving C5 to T1, which is reported in 9% to 26% of obstetric palsies.[1, 27, 45] In this lesion, the arm lies flaccid, and the skin may be marbled owing to vasomotor disturbance. Damage to the spinal cord may have occurred. The last type of injury pattern seen is Klumpke's palsy, indicating involvement of only the lower (C8 to T1) brachial plexus. Clinically, this is manifested by an inability to pronate the forearm, hand paralysis with a "claw-hand" posture, and Horner's syndrome. Isolated lower brachial plexus injury is rare and reportedly constitutes less than 2% of obstetric palsies.[1, 27, 45, 69] We have not encountered such a case among our own patients. Patients with injury to the lower brachial plexus are less likely to recover useful function of the arm with conservative management than are those who suffer upper brachial plexus injury.

Other causes of arm immobility or paralysis, both reversible and irreversible, should be considered in the differential diagnosis. These include epiphyseal separation of the humeral head, fracture of the clavicle or humerus, and septic arthritis of the upper limb, as well as possible birth injury to the spinal cord itself.[70]

PATIENT EVALUATION

Since 1991 at our institution, evaluation of patients with obstetric brachial plexus palsy has been performed in a multidisciplinary brachial plexus clinic staffed by a pediatric neurosurgeon, pediatric neurologist, orthopedic surgeon, physical and occupational therapists, electrophysiologist, and nurse coordinator. Detailed obstetric and birth histories are taken, with attention to the predisposing factors discussed previously. Associated injuries such as rib, transverse process, clavicle, or humeral fractures are noted on plain radiographs. Clinically observed asymmetry of chest wall expansion and chest radiographic evidence of an elevated hemidiaphragm denote phrenic nerve injury. The patient is assessed for evidence of facial paresis or Horner's syndrome. Passive range of motion of the involved arm, especially the shoulder, is noted. Motor strength is assessed using the simplified British Medical Council scale for muscle testing (0 to 5 scale). The Mallet score,[71] which documents functional changes in the shoulder and arm, requires patient cooperation and is used in patients older than 2 years. Sensory examination is difficult, although reaction to pinch is helpful. Sensory loss is sometimes evidenced by self-mutilation (i.e., biting) of fingers.

Some palsies may resolve within days. It is not unusual for an arm to be entirely flaccid at birth, with rapid improvement revealing an upper palsy. After a few weeks, when the initial traumatic neuritis has resolved, physical therapy can be instituted for persistent weakness. This entails passive range of motion exercises performed by a family member under the guidance of a physical therapist.

The infant is re-examined at about 4 weeks of age. Often, recovery is complete or nearly complete, signifying a neurapraxic injury. At this point, if there is still total palsy associated with Horner's sign, the outlook is poor, and parents are informed of the possible need for surgical intervention. If hand function is improving without evidence of shoulder recovery, the patient is managed conservatively, as there is still some chance for recovery.[34] Patients should be followed on a monthly basis. Infants who make progressive recovery and have antigravity or greater than antigravity strength in the biceps, triceps, or deltoid muscles by age 3 to 4 months continue to be followed expectantly.[64] Infants displaying less than antigravity strength in each of these muscles are referred for neuroimaging and electrophysiologic studies. If the deltoid, biceps, or triceps muscle still has less than antigravity strength at age 6 months, we recommend brachial plexus surgery. Braces are no longer advocated because of the propensity for contracture.[46]

When surgery is being considered, electromyography (EMG) with nerve conduction studies is delayed until the third month. If an intrauterine lesion is suspected, EMG is performed within a week after delivery to document denervation.[53, 72] At our center, we always perform EMG before surgery. EMG can provide useful information concerning the extent and distribution of brachial plexus injury and the recovery pattern. Also, nerve root avulsion can be confirmed by normal sensory conduction in the presence of severe motor weakness. The usefulness of EMG in postoperative follow-up of patients remains to be determined. In infants, it takes only a small number of intact axons to provoke an electrical response, which may not be associated with clinical recovery.

Preoperative computed tomographic myelography is a useful tool in the evaluation of nerve root avulsion.[73] The presence of pseudomeningoceles has been associated with nerve root avulsion; however, this finding is not pathognomonic and should be considered a sign of root damage, as 15% of pseudomeningoceles are not associated with complete nerve root avulsion.[74] In addition, 20% of avulsed nerve roots may not have an associated pseudomeningocele.[75] Although computed tomographic myelography is 85% to 91% accurate in diagnosing nerve root avulsion confirmed by operative exploration or by somatosensory evoked potentials,[74, 75] it is unable to detect nerve root avulsion in the absence of a pseudomeningocele. The correlation coefficient of computed tomographic myelography's prediction of nerve root avulsion has been reported to be as low as 0.5.[45] Magnetic resonance imaging (MRI) has been used to study nerve root avulsion in infants with birth-related brachial plexus injuries.[76–79] Our group uses fast spin-echo MRI for preoperative neuroimaging because it is less invasive and provides data comparable to those of computed tomographic myelography for operative planning (Fig. 224–2).[76] MRI appears to detect pseudomeningoceles as accurately as does computed tomographic myelography, but it does not clearly delineate nerve roots within the pseudomeningocele. In cases of total palsy, MRI would rule out any associated spinal cord injury.

SURGICAL TREATMENT

Exposure of Brachial Plexus

Under general anesthesia with a short-acting neuromuscular agent, the patient is placed supine using a shoulder roll to elevate the clavicular region. The head is turned to the contralateral side. The neck, chest, affected upper extremity, and both lower extremities are prepared, the incision is marked, and drapes are applied. An arm board usually is not necessary in an infant. The entire affected upper extremity is kept available for visual inspection of muscle contraction in response to electrical stimulation during surgery. The supraclavicular portion of the incision begins two finger breadths beneath the mastoid tip and courses along the posterior border of the sternocleidomastoid muscle to the clavicle. For infraclavicular exposure, the incision then turns in a lateral direction along the superior border of the clavicle to reach the deltopectoral groove. At this point, it curves inferiorly along the groove and anterior axillary fold (Fig. 224–3). Additional incisions are made on the anterior chest wall if intercostal nerve exposure is needed. Repair of the upper roots is performed through a supraclavicular approach, whereas treatment of a total palsy requires a combined approach.

The supraclavicular exposure is begun with an incision through the skin and platysma muscle along the posterior border of the sternocleidomastoid. The skin flaps are raised, followed by a second flap of fibrofatty tissue overlying the brachial plexus. The omohyoid muscle is divided. The transverse cervical vessels are spared, if possible, and retracted. Dissection is extended down to expose the clavicle; the subclavius muscle and periosteum of the clavicle are divided. When a neuroma extends beyond the divisions of the brachial plexus, it is necessary to free the clavicle off the clavicular portion of the pectoralis major muscle and to expose the cords of the brachial plexus. A pectoral nerve arising from the anterior division of the upper trunk is identified and spared.

The initial dissection is directed to expose the C5 and C6 nerve roots and upper trunk. While exposing the upper trunk, it is important to identify the phrenic nerve along the anterior scalene muscle and the spinal accessory nerve arising from C4. The accessory nerve emerges from the posterior part of the sternocleidomastoid muscle at the junction of its upper and middle thirds and continues toward the trapezius muscle. Direct electrical stimulation helps identify the phrenic and accessory nerves.

A neuroma involving the upper trunk is readily identified. The C5 nerve root is identified by following the most superficial portion of the upper trunk toward the neural foramen. In order to expose the C6-T1 nerve roots, the anterior scalene muscle must be divided and

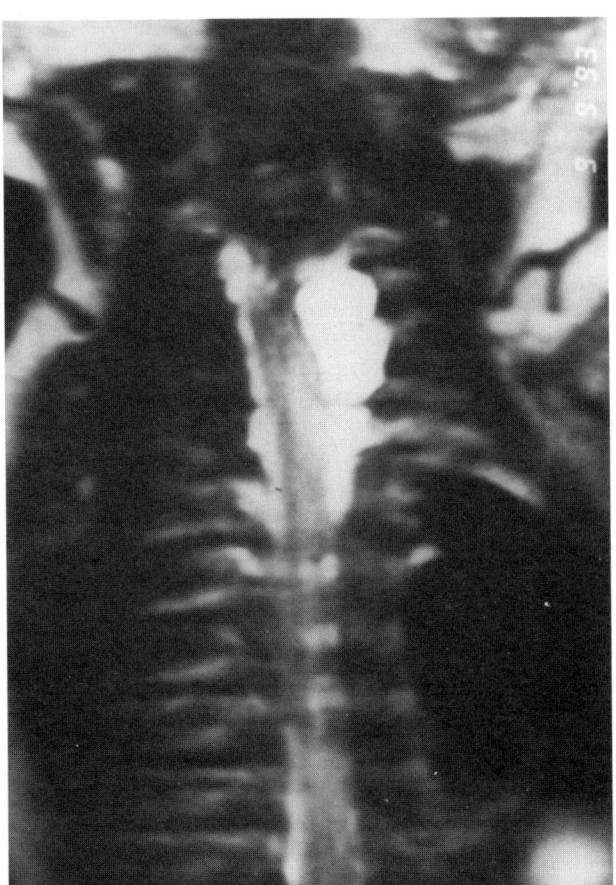

FIGURE 224–2. Fast spin-echo magnetic resonance image. Note pseudomeningocele on the left.

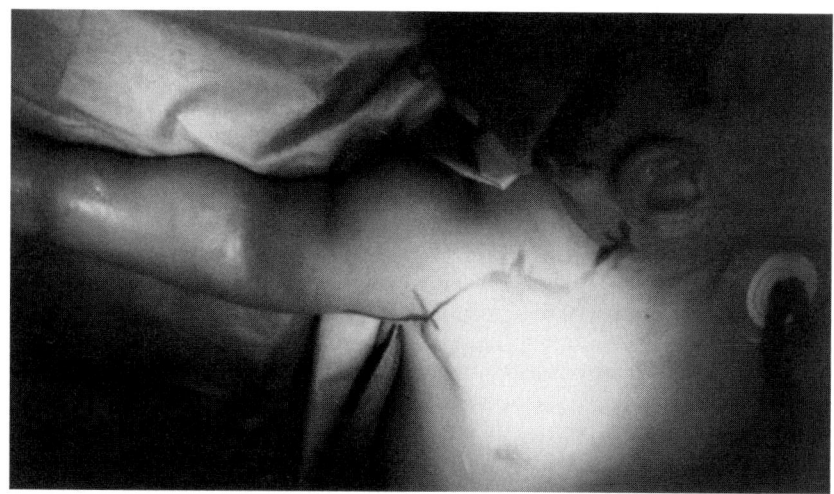

FIGURE 224–3. Operating room positioning and incision for complete exposure of the brachial plexus.

removed. The T1 nerve root is adjacent to the pleura and subclavian vessels, and care is taken to avoid injury to these structures. One can recognize the varying thickness of the nerve roots. In cases of nerve root avulsion, the nerve root is replaced by thin fibrotic tissue; neuroma in the nerve roots thickens the affected roots. Soft polymeric silicone (Silastic) vessel loops are placed around the roots for identification and traction. The three trunks are identified close to the clavicle. When a neuroma at the level of the nerve roots and trunk is extensive, it is necessary first to identify the trunks and divisions of the brachial plexus and continue dissection toward the roots. One should keep in mind that the lower trunk is also immediately adjacent to the pleura and subclavian vessels. The upper trunk gives rise to the supraclavicular nerve, which is found above the clavicle. It is common to encounter trunks surrounded by fibrotic tissues and scarred medial scalene muscle. In order to free the trunks, it is necessary to remove the fibrotic tissue. At this point, one should look for the long thoracic and dorsal scapular nerves, which are located under the upper trunk and above the medial scalene muscle, and spare them. Infraclavicular exposure is obtained by extending the incision as previously described with dissection along the deltopectoral groove. The cephalic vein should be spared. Marking sutures are applied to the pectoralis major before dividing its insertion onto the humerus, and a cuff of tendon should be left at each end for later approximation. The pectoralis minor is divided, and repair is not essential at closure. A clavicular osteotomy is not needed. After division of the pectoralis muscles, the cords of the brachial plexus, median nerve, ulnar nerve, musculocutaneous nerve, and axillary nerve are identified.

Although the sural nerve is generally used for grafting, donor nerves can also be obtained from parts of the plexus where reconstruction is unlikely to succeed, such as the medial cord, ulnar nerve, or medial cutaneous nerve of the forearm. We harvest sural nerve grafts via an open posterior lower leg incision, but they can also be obtained by an endoscopic technique, with the

proposed advantages of shorter incisions and scar, as well as decreased postoperative pain and shorter recovery time.[80]

Resection of Neuromas

Surgical techniques used in birth brachial plexus injury include neurolysis, neurotization, and nerve grafting, either alone or in combination. External neurolysis alone is performed, albeit rarely, when resection of neuroma is deemed unnecessary. We do not perform internal neurolysis because of its unproven efficacy. A critical issue is the indications for resection of neuromas. The use of intraoperative nerve action potential as a prognostic study has been determined in the adult population[81, 82] but not in the obstetrically injured patient. Laurent and colleagues use the compound muscle action potential in response to stimulation both proximal and distal to the neuroma to determine whether to perform a neurolysis or a grafting procedure. Neuromas are resected and a graft is performed if the amplitude of the compound muscle action potential drops more than 50% across the neuroma. Conversely, neurolysis is performed if there is a decrease of less than 50%.[24, 29, 45, 83] The validity of this approach remains to be determined. Alternatively, other authors advocate a more aggressive approach, with resection of all neuromas in continuity regardless of the presence of conducting fibers.[27, 28, 41, 44, 84] We currently base our decisions about the resection of neuromas on intraoperative inspection, semiquantitative assessment of muscle contraction in response to electrical stimulation of the nerve root proximal to the neuroma, preoperative muscle strength, EMG results, and MRI findings. If a ruptured root or trunk is present and electrical stimulation (up to 10 mA) elicits no or weak muscle contraction, neuromas are resected. If nerve root avulsion is present and there is minimal conduction through the remaining nerve root—as assessed by degree of muscle contraction in response to electrical stimulation of the proximal nerve root, somatosensory evoked potential, preoperative MRI scan, and EMG—the remaining nerve root sheath is divided. If the brachial plexus is in continuity but elicited muscle contraction is weak, neuromas are resected. If the brachial plexus is in continuity, strong muscle contraction is elicited, and neuromas are not extensive, no resection is performed. If the infant has some hand and wrist functions, C8-T1 roots and the lower trunk are left alone.

Repair Procedures

Various grafting and neurotization procedures are needed to repair the brachial plexus. The main goal of surgery for primarily upper palsy is to restore shoulder and biceps muscle functions. This goal can be achieved by nerve grafting to all or part of the upper trunk, supraclavicular nerve, or axillary nerve arising from the posterior cord. The accessory nerve; stumps of the C5 or C6 roots, or both; or the C7 nerve root can be used for grafting (Fig. 224–4). In cases of total plexus injury, various combinations of nerve grafting are needed. If two or three nerve root stumps are found, the nerve roots are divided and used for grafting all trunks or cords of the brachial plexus. If only one nerve root stump is available, it is grafted to the musculocutaneous nerve, and three to four intercostal nerves are connected to the ulnar nerve. When intercostal neurotization is selected, the third and fourth intercostal nerves are approached through a separate incision over the fourth rib. The space between the third, fourth, and fifth ribs is exposed posterior to the midaxillary line. The intercostal muscle is incised, and the parietal

pleura is exposed. The third, fourth, and fifth intercostal nerves are identified, mobilized, and transected as distally as possible. The cut ends are then anastomosed to the recipient nerve. Nerve grafts 10% to 15% longer than the measured length should be prepared to account for later contraction. Anastomosis can be completed with 9–0 Prolene epineural sutures or fibrin glue. We prefer to combine suture with fibrin glue, because the results of repair using glue are equivalent to or slightly better than those obtained using suture alone. The pectoralis major is reinserted with nonabsorbable suture, and the wound is closed in layers, including the platysma muscle, in routine fashion. The shoulder is held in an adducted position over the trunk with a large elastic bandage.

Neurotization is required in avulsion injuries. It implies nerve crossover or nerve transfer such that an uninjured neighboring donor nerve is connected directly or by grafts to a distal portion of a nonfunctioning nerve. Spinal accessory, phrenic, intercostal, medial pectoral, thoracodorsal, long thoracic, and subscapular nerves have been used for neurotization. When the spinal accessory nerve is used, one should use the nerve distal to the first branch to the trapezius muscle to avoid massive denervation of the trapezius. Partial denervation of the trapezius does not result in another deficit, as it usually alleviates the elevated shoulder, which most adult patients consider an aesthetic benefit.[12, 85] Although phrenic nerve transfer is safe in adult patients with normal diaphragmatic function, it is not recommended in infants because of their immature

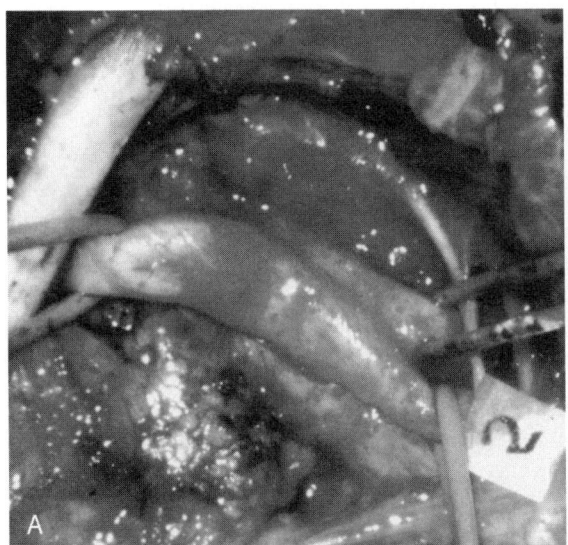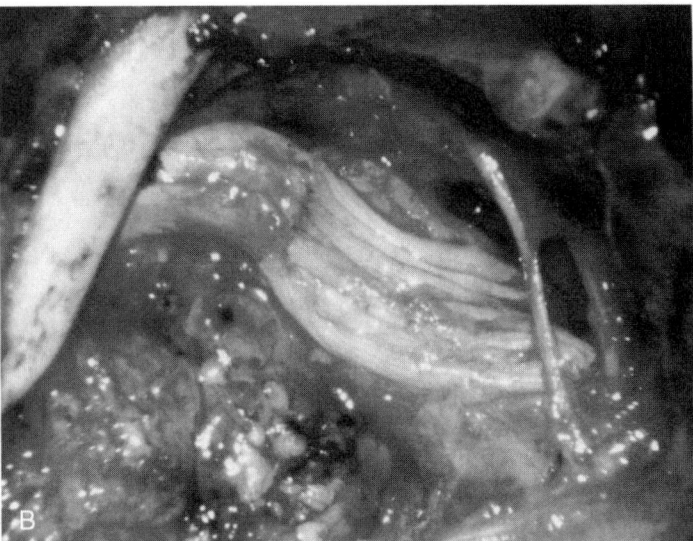

FIGURE 224–4. Operative photographs of brachial plexus reconstruction and grafting in a 7-month-old girl with a right-sided birth brachial plexus injury that failed to improve with conservative therapy. Magnetic resonance imaging revealed no evidence of nerve root avulsion. Electromyography revealed an incomplete brachial plexus injury with the most prominent findings involving the upper trunk. Preoperatively, the patient had 0/5 deltoid, 2/5 biceps, and 4/5 triceps strength. At surgery, a neuroma was found involving primarily C5 and extending into the upper trunk *(A)*. Intraoperative nerve testing revealed poor conduction through C5 and C6 into the upper trunk. C7 was normal. The neuroma was excised and sural nerve interposition grafts placed from C5 and C6 to the upper trunk *(B)*. At 7 months postoperatively (14 months of age), the patient showed marked improvement in her upper extremity function (deltoid 3/5, biceps 4/5, triceps 4/5).

respiratory systems and increased risk of fatal pulmonary complications. The efficacy of neurotization of the long thoracic nerve and the thoracodorsal, subscapular, and pectoral nerves in infants is unknown.

COMPLICATIONS

Potential complications include pseudarthrosis of the clavicle associated with osteotomy of the clavicle, loss of motor function, phrenic nerve injury, cerebrospinal fluid leakage, pneumothorax, thoracic duct injury (left side), vascular injury to the carotid artery or the jugular or subclavian vein, and wound infection. Edema of the neck with airway compromise is a potential problem. The infant's ability to clear secretions and maintain adequate airway exchange should be monitored. The ability to swallow and the presence of a gag reflex should be ascertained, as vagal and laryngeal nerve function may be altered after manipulation.[86]

POSTOPERATIVE CARE

The average postoperative hospitalization is 2 to 3 days. The patient's arm is immobilized in a sling for 3 weeks. Pain is generally well controlled with acetaminophen. After wound healing and immobilization, patients are started on a rigorous physical therapy regimen to prevent joint stiffness or contractures and are followed in the clinic at regular intervals (every 3 months). EMG is performed every 6 months.

SURGICAL OUTCOME

Surgical reinnervation is advocated to avoid permanent changes in the denervated muscle and developing skeletal system that result in long-term orthopedic sequelae.[87, 88] Surgical treatment aims to achieve stabilization of the shoulder by reactivation of the supraspinatus and deltoid; establish elbow flexion with reactivation of the biceps; and, in cases of a nonfunctional hand, restore median nerve sensory function for future secondary reconstruction procedures.[40] Some surgeons believe that primary reinnervation should be considered when the patient is age 18 months or younger, after which time secondary procedures should be performed.[83] For infants who are appropriate surgical candidates, surgery offers a chance for better long-term functional recovery. A number of authors have shown that neurological improvement occurs in 75% to 95% of patients undergoing surgical reconstruction of the brachial plexus,[22, 24, 25, 27–29, 31–35, 40–42, 44, 45] with the majority attaining antigravity strength in the shoulder or elbow or both. Boome and Kaye reported that greater than 95% of the deltoid and

T A B L E 2 2 4 – 2 ■ **Reported Surgical Results in Obstetric Brachial Plexus Palsy**

AUTHOR	LOCATION	NUMBER OF CASES	PROCEDURE	RESULTS*	FOLLOW-UP (Yr)
Birch et al[35]	C5, C6	6	Graft	IV or V shoulder: 100%	2.5
	C5, C6, C7	25	Graft	III shoulder: 32% IV shoulder: 44% V shoulder: 24%	2.5
	C5–T1	34	Graft	III shoulder: 38% IV shoulder: 24% V shoulder: 18%	2.5
Gilbert and Whitaker[31]	C5, C6	135	Graft/neurotization	III, IV or V shoulder: 81%	2
	C5, C6, C7	84	Graft/neurotization	III, IV, or V shoulder: 76%	2
	C5–T1	71	Graft/neurotization	III, IV, or V shoulder: 65%	2
Kawabata et al[42]	C5, C6 ± C7	5	Neurotization	Grade IV or V: biceps 100%, triceps 25%, deltoid 76%	5.8
	C5–T1	8	Neurotization		
Boome and Kaye[28]	C5, C6	15	Graft	At least 3/5 strength: biceps 80%, deltoid 96%; at least 4/5 strength: biceps 55%, deltoid 80%	1.8
	C5, C6, C7	5	Graft		
Clarke et al[41]	C5, C6	2	Neurolysis	At least 3/5 strength: biceps 89%, triceps 56%, deltoid 78%	1
	C5, C6, C7	7	Neurolysis		
	C5–T1	7	Neurolysis	At least 3/5 strength: biceps 43%, triceps 29%, deltoid 14%	1
Sherburn et al[33]	C5, C6 ± C7	13	Neurotization, neurolysis, or graft	At least 3/5 strength: biceps 75%, triceps 75%, deltoid 50%	2
	Others	3			
Laurent and Lee[24]	C5, C6 ± C7	45	Neurolysis or graft	> Antigravity: biceps 95%, deltoid 86%	1.5
	C5–T1	7 (?)	Neurolysis or graft	> Antigravity: biceps and deltoid 87%	1.5

*Modified Mallet classification of the shoulder: grade III, 30–90 degrees active abduction; grade IV, >90 degrees; grade V, normal. British Medical Council scale for individual muscle testing: 3/5, movement against gravity; 4/5, movement against resistance.

80% of the biceps muscles attained antigravity strength after surgery.[28] Laurent and colleagues found that 85% to 95% of patients recover antigravity strength above the elbow, and 50% to 70% recover antigravity strength below the elbow.[24, 45, 83] In our series, the biceps and triceps fared better, with 75% of patients attaining antigravity strength, compared with the deltoid, in which 50% attained antigravity strength (Table 224–2).[33]

Recovery begins at approximately 4 to 10 months and continues for 2 years for upper root lesions and 3 to 4 years for complete lesions. It is generally slower in grafted nerves than in sutured or directly repaired nerves. Clinical and electrophysiologic recovery in sensory nerve fibers is poor.

SECONDARY RECONSTRUCTION

Secondary reconstructions are performed in patients with chronic obstetric brachial plexus lesions that are not amenable, or fail to respond, to microsurgical reconstruction. These reconstructions are required because of the muscle imbalance and abnormal stresses placed on the bones and joints of the upper limb, with the resultant progressive bony deformities of the shoulder and elbow and dislocations of the radial head, as well as joint contractures. These procedures include arthrodesis, tenodesis, muscle releases, muscle-tendon transfers, and free neurovascular tissue transfers; they are reviewed elsewhere.[35, 40, 83, 89–94]

CONCLUSIONS

The incidence of birth brachial plexus injury has remained constant in recent years, but there has been a resurgence of interest in the surgical management of this disorder. Patients should be given a trial of conservative therapy. Motor strength examination at age 3 to 6 months is predictive of good outcome if antigravity strength of the deltoid, biceps, and triceps is present. Strength testing at age 6 months is predictive of poor outcome if antigravity strength in these muscles has not been attained; surgical treatment is then recommended. Operative planning requires a thorough clinical examination and a detailed understanding of the anatomy of the brachial plexus. MRI is recommended over computed tomographic myelography for preoperative evaluation. Intraoperative electrophysiology can help determine repair strategies, and knowledge of historically successful donor graft sites is important in determining surgical repair options. Each operation must be tailored to the individual patient's needs.

Results of surgical exploration and reconstruction are promising, with the majority of patients making functional gains. Outcome is determined after several years of recovery; secondary operations may be required. However, results of surgical intervention can be difficult to interpret without a universally applied system of evaluation. Future advancements may allow for the direct anastomosis of roots to the spinal cord,[95–97] as well as enhanced environments to potentiate nerve regeneration.[96]

REFERENCES

1. Greenwald AG, Schute PC, Shiveley JL: Brachial plexus birth palsy: A 10 year report on the incidence and prognosis. J Pediatr Orthop 4:689–692, 1984.
2. Painter MJ, Bergman I: Obstetrical trauma to the neonatal central and peripheral nervous system. Semin Perinatol 6:89–104, 1982.
3. Specht EE: Brachial plexus palsy in the newborn. Clin Orthop 110:32–34, 1975.
4. Levine MG, Holroyde J, Woods JR, et al: Birth trauma: Incidence and predisposing factors. Obstet Gynecol 63:792–795, 1984.
5. Sjoberg I, Erichs K, Bjerre I: Cause and effect of obstetric (neonatal) brachial plexus palsy. Acta Paediatr Scand 77:357–364, 1988.
6. Jackson ST, Hoffer MM, Parrish N: Brachial-plexus palsy in the newborn. J Bone Joint Surg 70A:1217–1220, 1988.
7. Hardy AE: Birth injuries of the brachial plexus. J Bone Joint Surg 63B:98–101, 1981.
8. Salonen IS, Uusitalo R: Birth injuries: Incidence and predisposing factors. Z Kinderchir 45:133–135, 1990.
9. Adler JB, Patterson RL: Erb's palsy. J Bone Joint Surg 49A:1052–1064, 1967.
10. Brown KL: Review of obstetrical palsies: Nonoperative treatment. Clin Plast Surg 11:181–187, 1984.
11. Gordon M, Rich H, Deutschberger J, et al: The immediate and long-term outcome of obstetric birth trauma. Am J Obstet Gynecol 117:51–56, 1973.
12. Narakas A: Surgical treatment of traction injuries of the brachial plexus. Clin Orthop Rel Res 133:71–90, 1978.
13. Smellie WJ: Collection of Cases and Observations in Mid Wifery, vol 2, 4th ed. 1768, pp 504–505.
14. Duchenne GBA: Traité de l'électrisation localisée et de son application à la pathologie et à la thérapeutique, 3rd ed. Paris, Ballière, 1872.
15. Erb W: Über eine eigentümliche localisation von lähmungen im plexus brachialis. Verh Naturhist-Med Heidelberg 2:130, 1874.
16. Klumpke A: Contribution à l'étude des paralysies radiculaires du plexus brachial. Rev Med Paris 5:591, 1885.
17. Kennedy R: Suture of the brachial plexus in birth paralysis of the upper extremity. BMJ 11:298–301, 1903.
18. Clark LP, Taylor AS, Prout TP: A study on brachial birth palsy. BMJ 130:670–707, 1905.
19. Wyeth JA, Sharpe W: The field of neurological surgery in a general hospital. Surg Gynecol Obstet 24:29–36, 1917.
20. Taylor AS: Brachial birth palsy and injuries of similar type in adults. Surg Gynecol Obstet 30:494–502, 1920.
21. Sever JW: Obstetric paralysis: Report of eleven hundred cases. JAMA 85:1862–1870, 1925.
22. Gilbert A, Tassin JL: Reparation chirurgicale du plexus brachial dans la paralysie obstetricale. Chirurgie 110:70–85, 1984.
23. Gilbert A, Tassin JL: Obstetrical palsy: A clinical pathologic and surgical review. In Terzis JK (ed): Microreconstruction of Nerve Injuries. Philadelphia, WB Saunders, 1987, pp 529–533.
24. Laurent JP, Lee RT: Birth-related upper brachial plexus injuries in infants: Operative and non-operative approaches. J Child Neurol 9:111–117, 1994.
25. Piatt JH, Hudson AR, Hoffman HJ: Preliminary experiences with brachial plexus exploration in children: Birth injury and vehicular trauma. Neurosurgery 22:715–723, 1988.
26. Piatt JH: Neurosurgical management of birth injuries of the brachial plexus. Neurosurg Clin N Am 1:175–185, 1991.
27. Gilbert A, Brockman R, Carlioz H: Surgical treatment of brachial plexus birth palsy. Clin Orthop Rel Res 264:39–47, 1991.
28. Boome RS, Kaye JC: Obstetric traction injuries of the brachial plexus: Natural history, indications for surgical repair and results. J Bone Joint Surg 70B:571–576, 1988.
29. Laurent JP, Lee R, Shenaq S, et al: Neurosurgical correction of upper brachial plexus birth injuries. J Neurosurg 79:197–203, 1993.
30. Slooff ACJ: Obstetric brachial plexus lesions and their neurosurgical treatment. Microsurgery 16:30–34, 1995.
31. Gilbert A, Whitaker I: Obstetrical brachial plexus lesions. J Hand Surg 16B:489–491, 1991.

32. Kawabata H, Masada K, Tsuyuguchi Y, et al: Early microsurgical reconstruction in birth palsy. Clin Orthop Rel Res 215:233–242, 1987.

33. Sherburn EW, Kaplan SS, Kaufman BA, et al: Outcome of surgically treated birth-related brachial plexus injuries in twenty cases. Pediatr Neurosurg 27:19–27, 1997.

34. Hentz VR, Meyer RD: Brachial plexus microsurgery in children. Microsurgery 12:175–185, 1991.

35. Birch R, Bonney G, Wynn Parry CB: Birth lesions of the brachial plexus. In Birch R, Bonney G, Wynn Parry CB (eds): Surgical Disorders of the Peripheral Nerves. Edinburgh, Churchill Livingstone, 1998, pp 209–233.

36. Meyer RD: Treatment of adult and obstetrical brachial plexus injuries. Orthopedics 9:899–903, 1986.

37. Hunt D: Surgical management of brachial plexus birth injuries. Dev Med Child Neurol 30:821–828, 1988.

38. Hentz VR: Congenital anomalies—looking ahead. Clin Plast Surg 13:175–189, 1986.

39. Narakas AO: The treatment of brachial plexus injuries. Int Orthop 9:29–36, 1985.

40. Terzis JK, Liberson WT, Levine R: Obstetric brachial plexus palsy. Hand Clin 2:273–286, 1986.

41. Clarke HM, Al-Qattan MM, Curtis CG, et al: Obstetrical brachial plexus palsy: Results following neurolysis of conducting neuromas-in-continuity. Plast Reconstr Surg 97:974–982, 1996.

42. Kawabata H, Kawai H, Masatomi T, et al: Accessory nerve neurotization in infants with brachial plexus birth palsy. Microsurgery 15:768–772, 1994.

43. Alanen M, Halonen JP, Viikki KP: Early surgical exploration and epineural repair in birth brachial palsy. Z Kinderchir 411:335–337, 1986.

44. Gilbert A, Razaboni R, Amar-Khodja S: Indications and results of brachial plexus surgery in obstetrical palsy. Orthop Clin North Am 19:91–105, 1988.

45. Laurent JP: Neurosurgical intervention for birth related brachial plexus injuries. Neurosurg Q 7:69–75, 1997.

46. Eng GD, Koch B, Smokvina MD: Brachial plexus palsy in neonates and children. Arch Phys Med Rehabil 59:458–464, 1978.

47. Burr C: Spinal birth palsies: A study of nine cases of obstetric paralysis. Boston Med Surg J 127:235–238, 1892.

48. Eng G: Brachial plexus palsy in newborn infants. Pediatrics 48:18–28, 1971.

49. Gherman RB, Ouzounian JG, Miller DA, et al: Spontaneous vaginal delivery: A risk factor for Erb's palsy? Am J Obstet Gynecol 178:423–427, 1998.

50. Jennett RJ, Tarby TJ, Kreinick CJ: Brachial plexus palsy: An old problem revisited. Am J Obstet Gynecol 166:1673–1677, 1992.

51. Dunn DW, Engle WA: Brachial plexus palsy: Intrauterine onset. Pediatr Neurol 1:367–369, 1985.

52. Gherman RB, Goodwin TM: Shoulder dystocia. Curr Opin Obstet Gynecol 10:459–463, 1998.

53. Koenigsberger MR: Brachial plexus palsy at birth intrauterine or due to delivery trauma. Ann Neurol 8:228, 1980.

54. Peterson GW, Bohr TW: Neonatal obstetric palsy a preexisting condition: Two case reports. Muscle Nerve 18:1031, 1995.

55. Paradiso G, Granana N, Maza E: Prenatal brachial plexus paralysis. Neurology 49:261–262, 1997.

56. Ouzounian JG, Korst LM, Phelan JP: Permanent Erb palsy: A traction-related injury? Obstet Gynecol 89:139–141, 1997.

57. Nocon JJ, McKenzie DK, Thomas LJ, et al: Shoulder dystocia an analysis of risks and obstetric maneuvers. Am J Obstet Gynecol 168:1732–1737, 1993.

58. Al-Qattan MM, el-Sayed AA, al-Kharfy TM, et al: Obstetrical brachial plexus injury in newborn babies delivered by caesarean section. J Hand Surg 21B:263–265, 1996.

59. Ross D, Jones RJ, Fisher J, et al: Isolated radial nerve lesion in the newborn. Neurology 33:1354–1356, 1983.

60. de Chalain TM, Clarke HM, Curtis CG: Case report: Unilateral combined facial nerve and brachial plexus palsies in a neonate following a midlevel forceps delivery. Ann Plast Surg 38:187–190, 1997.

61. Al-Qattan MM, Clarke HM, Curtis CG: The prognostic value of concurrent phrenic nerve palsy in newborn children with Erb's palsy. J Hand Surg 23B:225, 1998.

62. Gjorup L: Obstetrical lesion of the brachial plexus. Acta Neurol Scand Suppl 42:8–38, 1966.

63. Michelow BJ, Clarke HM, Curtis CG, et al: The natural history of obstetrical brachial plexus palsy. Plast Reconstr Surg 93:675–680, 1994.

64. Noetzel MJ, Day RA, Pillet S, et al: A prospective analysis of recovery following brachial plexus injury. Ann Neurol 40:321, 1996.

65. Tan KL: Brachial palsy. J Obstet Gynecol Br Commonwlth 80:60–62, 1973.

66. Bennet GC, Harrold AJ: Prognosis and early management of birth injuries to the brachial plexus. BMJ 1:1520–1521, 1976.

67. Tassin JL: Paralysies obstetricales du plexus brachial. Evolution spontanée resultats des interventions reparatrices precoces [thesis]. Paris, Université Paris, 1984.

68. Hoffer HM: Assessment and natural history of brachial plexus injury in children. In Gelberman RH (ed): Operative Nerve Repair and Reconstruction. Philadelphia, JB Lippincott, 1991, pp 1361–1368.

69. Al-Qattan MM, Clarke HM, Curtis CG: Klumpke's birth palsy: Does it really exist. J Hand Surg 20B:19–23, 1995.

70. Morota N, Sakamoto K, Kobayashi N: Traumatic cervical syringomyelia related to birth injury. Childs Nerv Syst 8:234–236, 1992.

71. Mallet J: Paralysie obstétricale du plexus brachial. Traitement des séquelles. Primauté du traitement de l'épaule—Méthode d'expression des résultats. Rev Chir Orthop 58(Suppl):166, 1972.

72. Mancias P, Slopis JM, Yeakley JW, et al: Combined brachial plexus injury and root avulsion after complicated delivery. Muscle Nerve 17:1237–1238, 1994.

73. Walker AT, Chaloupka JC, de Lotbiniere AC, et al: Detection of nerve rootlet avulsion on CT myelography in patients with birth palsy and brachial plexus injury after trauma. AJR 167:1283–1287, 1996.

74. Carvalho GA, Nikkhah G, Matthies C, et al: Diagnosis of root avulsions in traumatic brachial plexus injuries: Value of computerized tomography myelography and magnetic resonance imaging. J Neurosurg 86:69–76, 1997.

75. Hashimoto T, Mitomo M, Hirabuki N, et al: Nerve root avulsion of birth palsy: Comparison of myelography with CT myelography and somatosensory evoked potential. Radiology 178:841–845, 1991.

76. Francel PC, Koby M, Park TS, et al: Fast spin-echo magnetic resonance imaging for radiological assessment of neonatal brachial plexus injury. J Neurosurg 83:461–466, 1995.

77. Popovich MJ, Taylor FC, Helmer E: MR imaging of birth-related brachial plexus avulsion. AJNR 10:S98, 1989.

78. Miller SF, Glasier CM, Griebel ML, et al: Brachial plexopathy in infants after traumatic delivery: Evaluation with MR imaging. Radiology 189:481–484, 1993.

79. Urabe F, Matsuishi T, Kojima K, et al: MR imaging of birth brachial palsy in a two-month-old infant. Brain Dev 13:130–131, 1991.

80. Capek L, Clarke HM, Zuker RM: Endoscopic sural nerve harvest in the pediatric patient. Plast Reconstr Surg 98:884–888, 1996.

81. Tiel RL, Happel LT, Kline DG: Nerve action potential recording and equipment. Neurosurgery 39:103–108, 1996.

82. Kline DG, Judice DJ: Operative management of selected brachial plexus lesions. J Neurosurg 58:631–649, 1983.

83. Shenaq SM, Berzin E, Lee R, et al: Brachial plexus birth injuries and current management. Clin Plast Surg 25:527–536, 1998.

84. Capek L, Clarke HM, Curtis CG: Neuroma in continuity resection: Early outcome in obstetrical brachial plexus palsy. Plast Reconstr Surg 102:1555–1564, 1998.

85. Allieu Y, Cenac P: Is surgical intervention justifiable for total paralysis secondary to multiple avulsion injuries of the brachial plexus? Hand Clin 4:609–618, 1988.

86. Brucker J, Laurent JP, Lee R, et al: Brachial plexus birth injury. J Neurosci Nurs 23:374–380, 1991.

87. Pollock AN, Reed MH: Shoulder deformities from obstetrical brachial plexus paralysis. Skeletal Radiol 18:295–297, 1989.

88. Jahnke AH Jr, Bovill DF, McCarroll HR Jr, et al: Persistent brachial plexus birth palsies. J Pediatr Orthop 11:533–537, 1991.

89. Akasaka Y, Hara T, Takahashi M: Free muscle transplantation combined with intercostal nerve crossing for reconstruction of elbow flexion and wrist extension in brachial plexus injuries. Microsurgery 12:346–351, 1991.

90. Berger A, Becker MH: Brachial plexus surgery: Our concept of the last twelve years. Microsurgery 15:760–767, 1994.
91. Berger A, Brenner P: Secondary surgery following brachial plexus injuries. Microsurgery 16:43–47, 1995.
92. Berger A, Flory PJ, Schaller E: Muscle transfers in brachial plexus lesions. J Reconstr Microsurg 6:113–116, 1990.
93. Berger A, Schaller E, Mailander P: Brachial plexus injuries: An integrated treatment concept. Ann Plast Surg 26:70–76, 1991.
94. Richards RR: Operative treatment for irreparable lesions of the brachial plexus. In Gelberman RH (ed): Operative Nerve Repair and Reconstruction. Philadelphia, JB Lippincott, 1991, pp 1303–1327.
95. Carlstedt T, Noren G: Repair of ruptured spinal nerve roots in a brachial plexus lesion. J Neurosurg 82:661–663, 1995.
96. Glasby MA, Hems TE: Repairing spinal roots after brachial plexus injuries. Paraplegia 33:359–361, 1995.
97. Bertelli JA, Mira JC: Brachial plexus repair by peripheral nerve grafts directly into the spinal cord in rats: Behavioral and anatomical evidence of functional recovery. J Neurosurg 81:107–114, 1994.

CHAPTER 225

Child Abuse

ANN-CHRISTINE DUHAIME ■ CINDY CHRISTIAN

Child abuse is now recognized as a major cause of serious head injury in children and is second only to motor vehicle–related injuries as a cause of traumatic mortality in the pediatric population.[1-3] For the purposes of this chapter, *child abuse* refers to deliberate, inflicted injury, rather than to accidental injury occurring in the setting of neglect or inadequate supervision. Because of its nature, the true incidence of inflicted injury remains unknown; many cases are unrecognized as such by health care providers and go unreported. Nonetheless, it has been estimated that nearly one fourth of all hospital admissions for head injury in children younger than 2 years of age are the result of deliberate inflicted trauma, and these patients suffer disproportionately severe injuries.[2, 4] Many children with less severe injuries may not receive acute medical attention, adding to the difficulties in epidemiologic assessment. It has been postulated that many cases of unexplained developmental delay and retardation are related to head injuries inflicted in infancy.[5] The costs of acute and chronic care related to child abuse, and of the loss of potential from brain damage suffered so early in life and with such high frequency, are enormous and have only recently begun to be recognized.

As our understanding of the biomechanics of head injury in young children has increased, it has become clear that neurologically serious head injuries rarely result from common household falls; the only major exception is epidural hematoma.[2, 6–9] Familiarity with traumatic mechanisms of injury in children and with the presentation and evaluation of nonaccidental injury is important for practicing neurosurgeons, because a missed diagnosis frequently results in recurrent injury.[10] Jenny and colleagues found that the correct diagnosis was missed in nearly one third of children with head injuries caused by abuse who presented for medical attention, and this failure resulted in medical complications, reinjury, and fatality.[11] Furthermore, a neurosurgeon's opinion as to the presumptive mechanism of injury necessary to cause a specific clinical picture is often given a great deal of weight in medicolegal determinations. These decisions affect the patient, siblings, parents, and caretakers in profound ways, and a responsible neurosurgeon must be careful to separate what is known and understood from what is conjecture. The role of the physician as witness is discussed in more detail later.

In many institutions, a team approach to cases of suspected nonaccidental injury provides an organized means of addressing the frequently complex, disturbing, and time-consuming issues involved in caring for these patients. The goal of this chapter is to provide an overview and reference for neurosurgeons, including recognition of common child abuse syndromes, management of acute injuries, outcome prediction, medicolegal responsibilities and consequences, and prevention efforts.

EVALUATION OF CHILD ABUSE SYNDROMES

Battered Child Syndrome

This syndrome, which was described by Kempe and coworkers in 1962, was the first child abuse syndrome to become widely recognized, and its description brought the problem of inflicted injury into focus.[12] Battered child syndrome can be seen in infants through adolescents but is most common in children younger than 3 years of age. Children with this syndrome are brought to medical attention for an unrelated problem or in the setting of a particular acute injury. When evaluated, they are noted to have signs of chronic abuse, which may include poor hygiene, malnutrition, growth retardation, multiple cutaneous bruises of different ages, pattern injuries, burn marks, and skeletal injuries at different stages of healing (Fig. 225–1). Typically, caretakers blame these visible traumatic injuries on various accidental mechanisms, often of a relatively trivial nature. On questioning, parents may characterize infants as fussy or stubborn and older children as clumsy, hyperactive, or accident prone. Chronically abused children may appear passive and withdrawn but often show strong attachment to the parent, even when he or she is the perpetrator.

The diagnosis of the "classic" battered child is usually straightforward from the history and physical examination. Although readily available computed tomographic scans enable us to rapidly characterize a

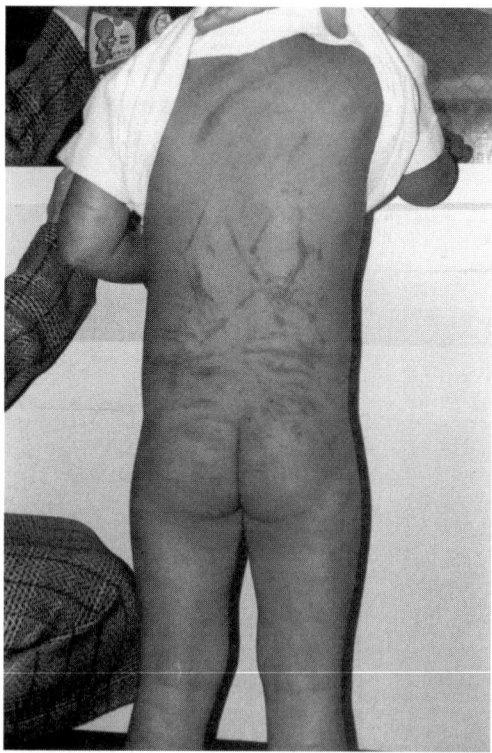

FIGURE 225–1. Extensive cutaneous bruising of the trunk in a child with "battered baby syndrome."

patient's head injury, a thorough physical examination of the rest of the body, with removal of the clothes, is the best tool for diagnosing a battered child. The history itself is often sketchy and elusive, and it is not uncommon that the adult accompanying the child is not the patient's regular or exclusive caretaker. Members of the child protection team can be invaluable at this juncture; pediatricians, social workers, and others experienced in dealing with families in which child abuse is suspected are skilled at interviewing and piecing together the known sequence of events. Their involvement is also particularly useful as the evaluation progresses and the possibility of child abuse is broached with family members, who often respond with adamant denial and even frank hostility. The physician's role in these exchanges is discussed in more detail later.

Central to Kempe's early description of the battered child was the idea that episodes of physical trauma are recurrent rather than isolated events. This principle has been widely supported by subsequent clinical experience, making early diagnosis of the syndrome imperative. However, obvious evidence of chronic abuse may not be readily apparent in all children. Therefore, certain types of injuries that occur with greater frequency in the setting of physical abuse should raise the physician's level of suspicion for nonaccidental causation. These include spiral fractures of the humerus, spiral fractures of the femur in infants, metaphyseal fractures in infants, duodenal hematomas, "tin ear," frenulum tears in nonambulatory infants, immersion burns, patterned bruises, and retinal hemorrhages.[13–16] In addi-

tion, children with preexisting disabilities or prematurity may be at particular risk.[17] "Coin rubbing," seen in Southeast Asian children, and similar therapeutic maneuvers resulting in pattern marks should not be confused with abuse. With respect to neurological trauma, "red flag" injuries include stellate skull fractures, bilateral or multiple skull fractures, and subdural hematomas outside the setting of motor vehicle trauma.[1, 18] Additionally, the entire range of soft tissue contusions, cephalohematomas (sometimes from severe hair-pulling), skull fractures, and intracranial hemorrhages can occur in the setting of inflicted injury.

A skeletal survey is a mandatory part of the evaluation of suspected nonaccidental injury in infants and young children, and a bone scan may be useful when plain films are equivocal. Anemia, thrombocytopenia, or other hematologic abnormalities are evaluated by standard laboratory tests. Toxicology screening is sometimes unexpectedly positive because of forced ingestions. The question of osteogenesis imperfecta predisposing to multiple fractures is sometimes raised, but in most forms of this condition, patients are distinguished by other radiographic and clinical features (such as blue sclera), a history of consistent and well-described mechanisms of injury, and the seeking of prompt and appropriate medical care.

It may be useful to obtain a baseline computed tomographic or magnetic resonance imaging (MRI) scan in patients with battered child syndrome, even if an acute head injury is not part of the presenting clinical picture. Such a study can both ascertain evidence of previous brain injury and provide a comparison in the event of future injuries.

Shaking-Impact Syndrome

The term *shaken baby syndrome* was originally coined by Caffey in 1972 to describe infants with acute subdural and subarachnoid hemorrhages, retinal hemorrhages, and periosteal new bone formation at the epiphyseal regions of the long bones.[19] Some authors include infants with more chronic extra-axial collections in this category, but for purposes of this discussion, such cases are considered separately. Although the diagnosis of shaken baby syndrome rests on clinical and radiographic features, the name implies a specific mechanism of injury and was derived in part from the case of a nursemaid who admitted shaking several infants injured in her care in an attempt to burp them.[19] At about the same time that this syndrome was described, clinical and laboratory evidence for the damaging effects of angular acceleration on the brain was being reported.[20–22] Thus, the mechanism of the injuries commonly found in abused infants was postulated to result from "whiplash-shaking" as a form of discipline, and the term *shaken baby syndrome* became widely accepted as both a diagnosis and a mechanistic description. Support for the validity of the term was found in the observation that many infants with the intracranial findings of the syndrome had little if any evidence of blunt impact to the head on the initial physical examination. In addition, infants' relatively large heads, weak neck muscles, and watery brain consistency were thought to render them particularly vulnerable to severe injury from being shaken back and forth by a caretaker.[23] The long bone findings, which can be seen in accidental injuries in which the limbs are jerked or pulled, were also thought to occur from violent shaking. Central to the concept of shaken baby syndrome was the idea that caretakers might inflict these injuries unwittingly in the course of a generally acceptable means of discipline, during choking, or even during play.[5]

Controversy about the mechanism of these injuries arose because of the paucity of reliable history typically available to the evaluating physician. When a history of trauma is offered, it is usually that of a relatively minor blunt impact, and only rarely is an unsolicited history of shaking obtained. More recently, the term *shaken baby syndrome* has been questioned because clinical series, autopsies, and biomechanical and radiographic analyses have suggested that many if not most of these infants do, in fact, have evidence of blunt impact to the head and that the deceleration forces generated by shaking alone are insignificant compared with those caused by impact, even when it is against a padded object.[24-26] The frequent lack of dramatic cutaneous bruising can be explained by the dissipation of angular deceleration forces across a relatively wide and soft surface.[27] It seems likely both from these studies and from careful questioning of perpetrators that although an infant may be shaken, the final thrust involves the head striking a surface, resulting in the high deceleration forces required to cause subdural hemorrhage and frequently severe parenchymal damage. For these reasons, some authors prefer the term *shaking-impact syndrome* to distinguish the mechanism of shaking in child abuse from shaking during play, shaking to resuscitate, or other less violent scenarios sometimes postulated as being responsible for injuries.[28, 29] In addition, the frequent findings of long bone injuries, rib fractures, cutaneous bruises, skull fractures, subgaleal and subperiosteal hemorrhages, and focal contusions of the brain parenchyma belie a simple nonimpact cause. Still, the question of whether shaking alone is ever sufficient to cause the brain injuries commonly seen in abused infants remains controversial, and battered child syndrome and shaking-impact syndrome result in a spectrum of overlapping injury types and chronicities seen in patients of varying ages.[30]

Regardless of the exact mechanism of injury, the clinical scenario in shaking-impact syndrome is often remarkably similar from case to case. Affected children are nearly always 2 years old or younger, and most are younger than 6 months old. They are brought to medical attention because of irritability, poor feeding, or lethargy in mild cases and because of seizures, apnea, or unresponsiveness in more severe cases. The history is often vague, and it is common that those accompanying the child are not the exclusive caretakers. In many cases, no history of trauma is offered, and the diagnosis may come to light when a lumbar puncture done as part of a sepsis evaluation shows bloody spinal fluid. In other cases, a history of relatively trivial

trauma is given. Sometimes, on questioning, a history of shaking to resuscitate is obtained.

The child abuse evaluation team, if available, is notified, and specific histories from all caretakers involved with the child should be obtained as soon as possible. Although these types of injuries occur in families of all sorts, they present most commonly in more fragmented family situations; typically, the infant has multiple caretakers, the parents are young, there are few resources, or other stressful conditions are present. Drugs or alcohol may be involved. One commonly encountered scenario involves a fussy baby being watched by an inexperienced caretaker, such as the mother's boyfriend. Starling and colleagues found that perpetrators were fathers, boyfriends, female baby sitters, and mothers, in descending order of frequency.[31]

On physical examination, a range of neurological abnormalities may be found, from mild irritability and lethargy to flaccid coma. Some children with seizures may show "bicycling" movements, which can be mistaken for normal spontaneous activity. Even severely injured young infants often show nonspecific withdrawal to noxious stimulation and may even have spontaneous eye opening, but they can usually be identified by a paucity of normal, spontaneous motor activity and by a distinct lack of crying or of vigorous grimacing to pain. The fontanelle may be full. Careful inspection often reveals mild bruising, most often in the parieto-occipital region or, less commonly, in the frontal area, which may be more apparent after several days. Retinal hemorrhages are usually found. Computed tomographic scans show subdural or subarachnoid hemorrhage, ranging from barely perceptible to sizable collections with mass effect requiring emergent surgery (Figs. 225–2 and 225–3). Hemorrhage may be unilateral or bilateral and has a particular propensity for the posterior interhemispheric space.[32] This may result from impact to the back of the head and bony displacement across the lambdoid sutures, resulting in strains to the underlying venous sinuses and deep veins. MRI is frequently superior to computed tomography in demonstrating small subdural hemorrhages and parenchymal contusions; this is particularly helpful when the diagnosis is equivocal, such as when trauma is denied by the caretakers (Fig. 225–4).[33] MRI is also a useful screening test for arteriovenous malformations or other vascular anomalies that could cause subarachnoid hemorrhage, particularly when all other tests for associated injuries are unrevealing and the cause of the hemorrhage remains unclear. In rare cases, arteriography may be considered to rule out vascular abnormalities when there is no history or radiographic evidence clearly pointing to trauma and the child presents with an ictal intracranial hemorrhage.[34]

In severe cases of shaking-impact syndrome, the brain may lose its normal gray-white differentiation and have the appearance of a large unilateral or bilateral supratentorial infarction. This finding may be visible on the initial scan or may develop 1 to 2 days after injury.[35, 36] Children with this finding are usually unresponsive on admission and have a dismal prognosis for neurological recovery. The pathophysiology of

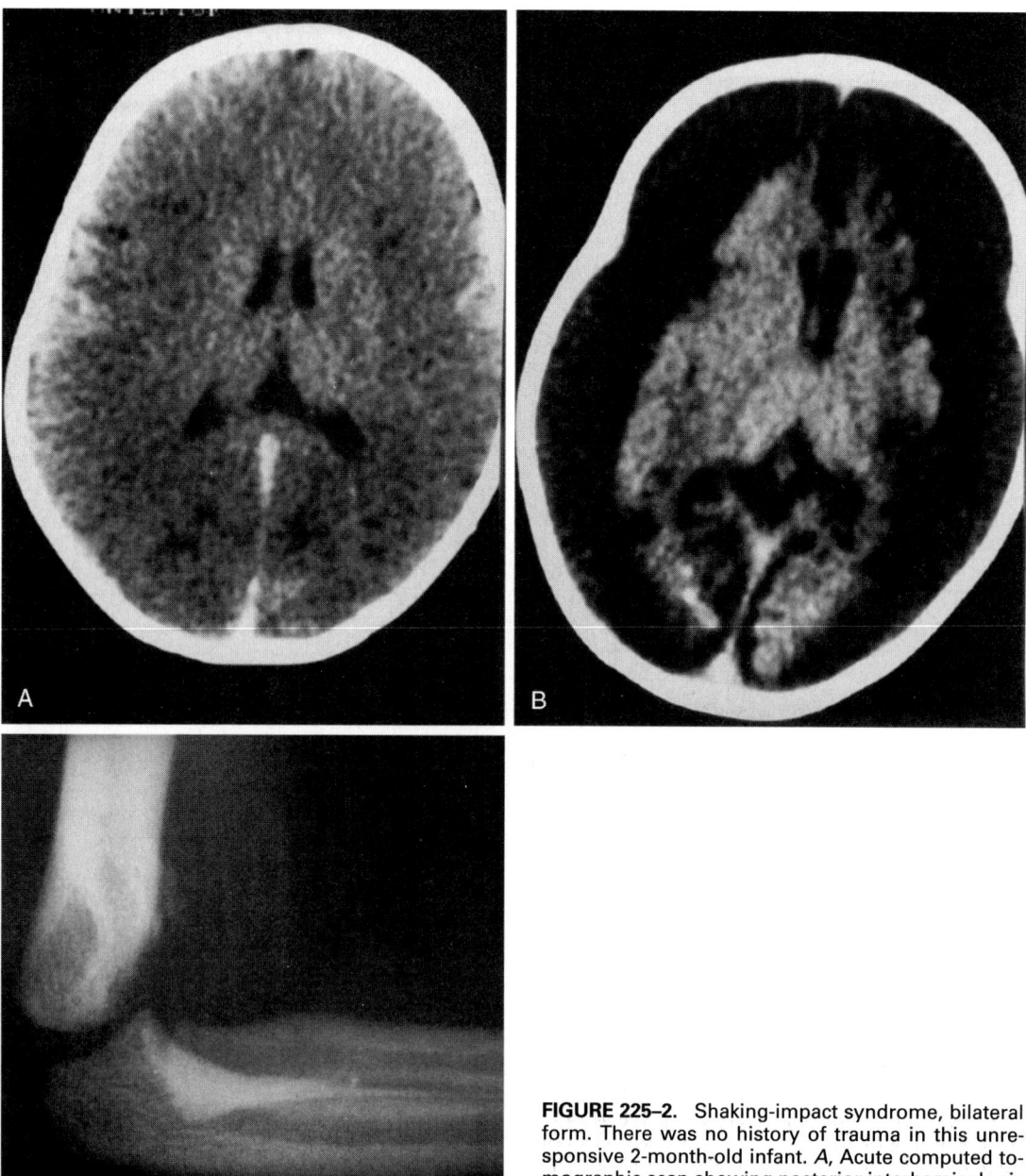

FIGURE 225–2. Shaking-impact syndrome, bilateral form. There was no history of trauma in this unresponsive 2-month-old infant. *A,* Acute computed tomographic scan showing posterior interhemispheric blood. *B,* Severe diffuse brain atrophy seen 2 months after injury. *C,* Typical long bone injury, humerus.

the so-called black brain seen in these children is incompletely understood but may be due to the synergistic effects of hypoxia, mechanical trauma, and subdural hemorrhage.[37–40] In some children, evidence of a high spinal cord injury can be found, and this may contribute to the apnea and poor outcome seen in some cases.[41] Spinal injuries in child abuse are discussed in more detail later.

Once the acute management issues have been attended to, as outlined later, a diagnostic evaluation for associated injuries and causes should be pursued. A general screening for other occult injuries should be performed, preferably by the pediatric trauma team. Routine laboratory studies for anemia, thrombocyto-

penia, visceral injury, and coagulopathy are part of the workup; it should be kept in mind that coagulopathy can occur as a result of severe brain injury and does not necessarily imply a preexisting condition.[42]

As in a battered child, a skeletal survey is mandatory, and a bone scan is sometimes helpful in equivocal cases. A repeat skeletal survey in 2 weeks may increase the yield of diagnosed injuries because of more visible changes with healing.[43] A formal ophthalmic consultation with mydriatics, when clinically suitable, should be obtained to document retinal hemorrhages. Although these have been reported in 65% to 95% of patients with shaking-impact syndrome, they are not always present and, conversely, may be found in occa-

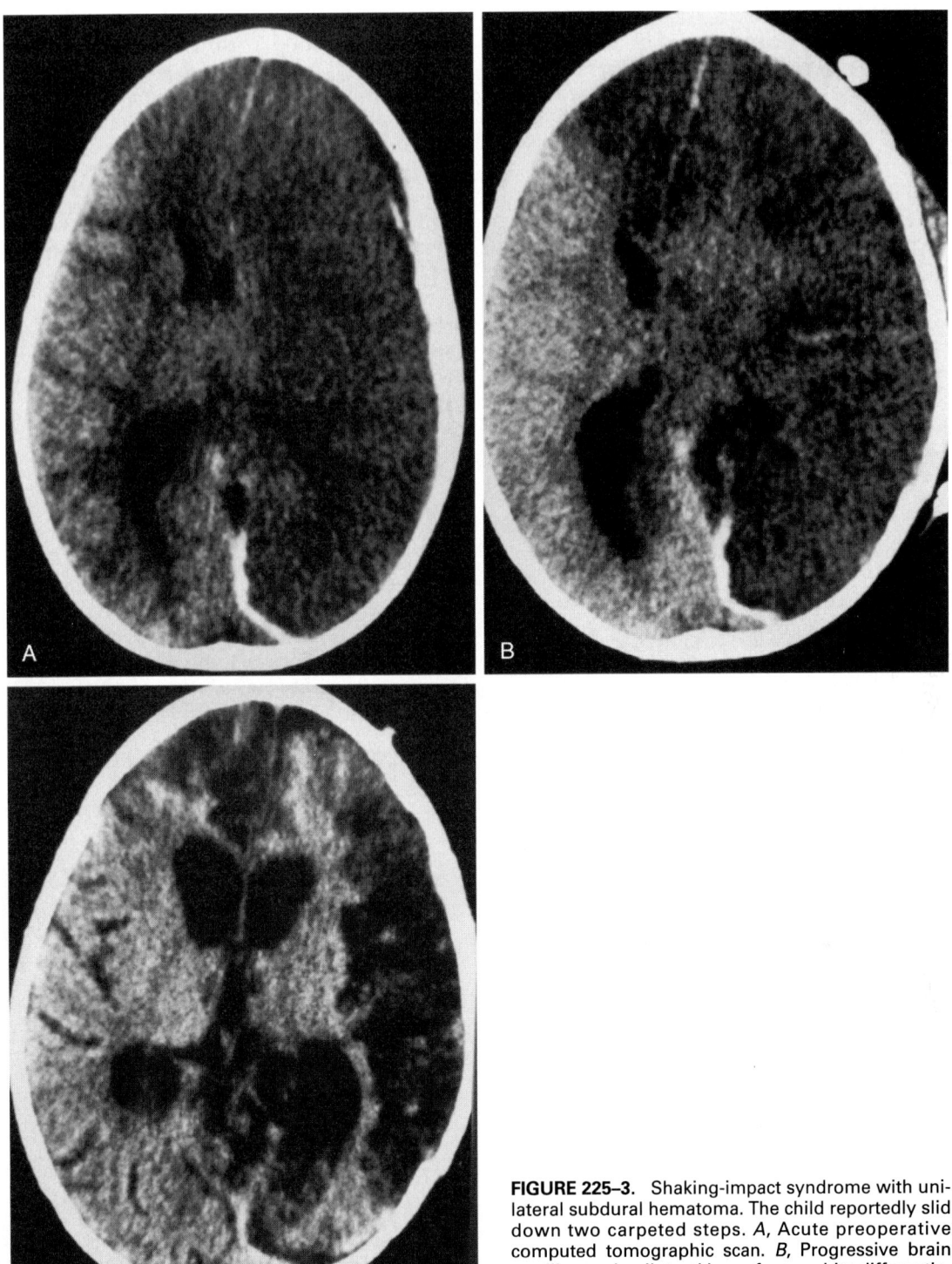

FIGURE 225–3. Shaking-impact syndrome with unilateral subdural hematoma. The child reportedly slid down two carpeted steps. *A,* Acute preoperative computed tomographic scan. *B,* Progressive brain swelling and unilateral loss of gray-white differentiation. *C,* Scan 1 year after injury. The child remains severely impaired.

sional head injuries from accidental causes and, rarely, after resuscitation.[1, 2, 15, 41, 44–48] Nonetheless, the presence of retinal hemorrhages adds greatly to the suspicion of nonaccidental injury, especially when they are bilateral and severe.[49]

No other medical condition fully mimics all the features of full-blown shaking-impact syndrome, but certain features can occur in other conditions. Coagulopa-

thies, vascular anomalies, and anatomic abnormalities such as arachnoid cysts can be associated with subdural hemorrhage.[50–52] Osteogenesis imperfecta can be associated with fractures and, rarely, subdural collections, but not with the other features of shaking-impact syndrome.[53] Glutaricaciduria can cause progressive neurological decline and subdural collections, sometimes triggered by a viral illness or injury, but it does

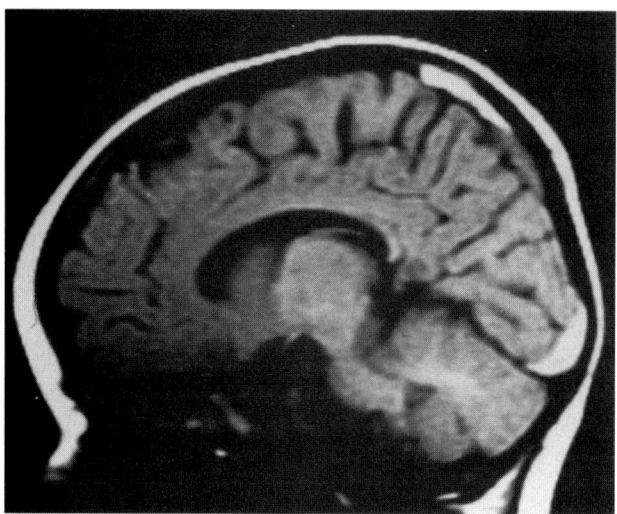

FIGURE 225–4. Magnetic resonance imaging scan of an infant with shaking-impact syndrome. Note the thin subdural hemorrhages and focal intraparenchymal contusion.

not feature bony abnormalities or retinal hemorrhage.[54] The single most common diagnosis mimicking nonaccidental trauma is accidental injury. In these cases, small epidural hemorrhages or traumatic subarachnoid hemorrhages can be mistaken for subdural bleeding, and unusual subdural hemorrhages can occur when the requisite biomechanics are present in settings not usually associated with this injury; such cases occasionally exhibit retinal hemorrhages as well.[47, 55] However, in these cases, the history is clear and consistent, and the clinical status is concordant with the forces involved in the injury, without unexplained skeletal or soft tissue injuries.

In many cases, such as those in which there is no history of trauma but the infant has skull fractures and unexplained long bone trauma, the diagnosis is quite clear. In other cases, in spite of careful evaluation, the mechanism of injury remains obscure. An algorithm has been developed that matches the patient's injury type with associated findings and best history in an attempt to more objectively classify infant head injuries as accidental or inflicted.[2] However, until more is understood about the injury thresholds for children of different ages, the pathophysiology of retinal hemorrhages and "black brain," and the effects of chronic, repeated trauma on the immature nervous system, efforts to assign a definitive mechanism to every suspicious injury will be unsuccessful.

Two additional issues that arise frequently and on which the neurosurgeon may be asked to comment involve the timing of injury and the possibility of multiple, sublethal accidental injuries that might behave synergistically. With respect to the first issue, Willman and colleagues reported on a series of 95 fatal accidental head injuries in children; in all but one patient, there was an immediate onset of neurological symptoms and decreased level of consciousness. The one exception was a child with an expanding epidural hematoma.[56] Although this study included only a small number of infants, it suggests that a prolonged lucid interval is unlikely in a child with a fatal primary brain injury. This conclusion is in accord with data from accidental trauma in adults and from animal models.[27] It should also be kept in mind that care must be taken when attempting to time an injury based on radiographic findings, as these may include a spectrum of abnormalities.[36] With respect to the possibility of "second impact syndrome" mimicking child abuse, such rare events have been reported in older children and adults and usually involve well-documented concussive sports injuries resulting in acute subdural or subarachnoid bleeding and brain swelling.[57, 58] At present, there is no evidence to support the notion that fatal acute traumatic subdural hematoma in otherwise healthy infants occurs from multiple trivial impacts.

Physical Abuse in Older Children

Most physically abused older children brought to medical attention suffer from soft tissue or visceral injuries from direct blows, although intracranial injuries sometimes occur and can be serious or even fatal. The setting is usually that of a biologic or foster family in which deviations from rigid codes of behavior are dealt with by physical punishment and beating, sometimes in an attempt to "save" the child (Fig. 225–5). The parents of both older and younger abused children may have been the victims of child abuse themselves. Occasionally the perpetrator is psychiatrically impaired, but this is the exception.

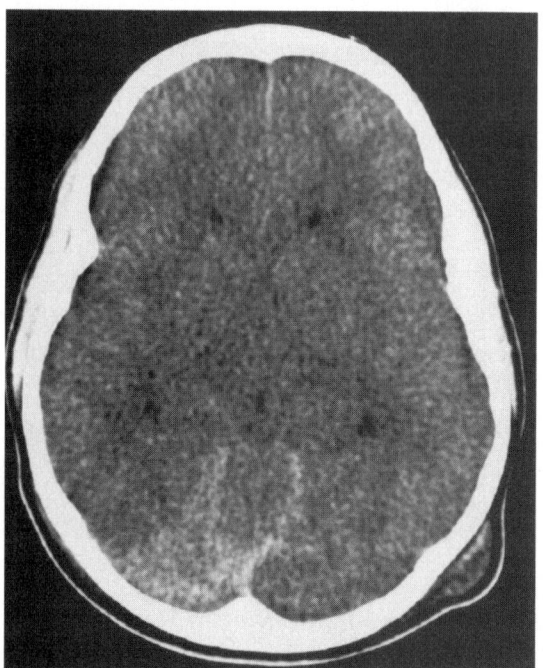

FIGURE 225–5. Computed tomographic scan of a 9-year-old boy who was beaten by his foster mother and forced to drink water as a means of discipline. He became unconscious and was found to be profoundly hyponatremic; he succumbed from diffuse brain swelling. Autopsy showed only minor superficial contusions of the brain and subarachnoid hemorrhage.

Evaluation includes a careful history, and the child should be questioned apart from the parent, once some degree of trust has been attained. A general trauma evaluation is done, including routine studies such as urinalysis for hematuria or myoglobinuria. A skeletal survey is usually of limited use in an older child because the typical occult injuries (e.g., metaphyseal and rib fractures) seen in infants do not occur in this age group, and remote skeletal injuries have usually healed to the point of being undetectable. A careful history of previous trauma, including fractures, and the physical examination are usually more helpful in detecting suspicious findings in this age group.

Head injuries may include soft tissue lesions; linear, depressed, or basilar fractures; and the range of intracranial lesions seen in trauma in general. Management is guided by the specific injury. Counseling is often in order, and a neuropsychological evaluation may be useful in an older child with acute or chronic brain involvement or behavioral disturbances to help with appropriate school placement.

MANAGEMENT OF HEAD INJURIES FROM CHILD ABUSE

Acute Subdural Hematoma

Some subdural hematomas resulting from inflicted injury appear identical to those from accidental injury and clearly have mass effect; these require emergency evacuation in the standard fashion. Even with prompt evacuation, however, changes to the underlying brain often persist or progress, having the appearance of widespread infarction (see Fig. 225–3*A* and *B*). More commonly, subdural and subarachnoid blood is quite diffuse in child abuse injuries and appears as a thin layer without marked compression of the underlying hemisphere. These "smear" collections are generally managed nonoperatively; although aggressive surgical evacuation and decompression have been reported, this strategy has not been strictly compared with medical management.[59] Often, the processes leading to the widespread parenchymal loss commonly seen in severely affected infants have already been initiated at the time of arrival at the hospital and may be the result of local compression, apnea, hypoxia, mechanical trauma, or seizures.[36, 60] Conversely, infants who do not appear critically ill at presentation often remain alert and regain a normal level of consciousness quite promptly, in spite of their acute subdural collections, and do not go on to suffer large delayed infarctions.

In children in whom gray-white differentiation is lost, brain swelling may be amenable to standard or even extraordinary medical management for increased intracranial pressure, but conventional therapy rarely if ever prevents the swollen brain from going on to severe atrophy (see Fig. 225–3). In very young infants, brain swelling may not present a life-threatening problem, as the skull simply expands to accommodate the swelling; these infants survive, but in a devastated state (see Fig. 225–2*B*). Because of this dismal outlook,

the role of more aggressive measures, including intracranial pressure monitoring, is controversial in this population.[61, 62]

Chronic Extracerebral Fluid Collection

Large, bilateral, chronic extracerebral fluid collections composed of old blood products or proteinaceous cerebrospinal fluid are sometimes discovered in infants. The term *chronic subdural hematoma* is often applied to these collections, although the content of the accumulation may vary from thin, watery fluid resembling cerebrospinal fluid to the thick "motor oil" often associated with adult chronic subdural hematomas. Even modern, sophisticated imaging techniques such as MRI may not be able to distinguish fluid in the subdural space from that in the subarachnoid space, and the term *chronic extracerebral fluid collection* is probably more accurate.[63] A definite history of antecedent trauma may not be obtained, and the question of child abuse often arises.

Guthkelch[23] pointed out that sudden acceleration and deceleration of the head, even without direct impact, can result in the tearing of cortical bridging veins in adults. Chronic subdural hemorrhage resulting from relatively small forces occurs most commonly in elderly individuals in whom the bridging veins cross a widened subarachnoid space and are "on stretch" at baseline. Another example of this phenomenon occurs in children or adults with ventricular shunts in whom the extracerebral space enlarges as the ventricles become smaller; these patients are well known to be prone to subdural hemorrhage from relatively trivial trauma. Whether a similar mechanism may be at work in infants with enlarged extracerebral spaces, perhaps due to so-called external hydrocephalus or atrophy, is not entirely clear, although this phenomenon is occasionally witnessed (Fig. 225–6). In this situation, tearing of bridging veins and arachnoid from relatively mild trauma, such as might occur accidentally, could theoretically result in a mixed collection of blood and cerebrospinal fluid in both the subdural and the subarachnoid spaces.

With respect to the issue of whether chronic subdural collections represent a manifestation of child abuse, several key questions remain unanswered. First, what are the mechanical thresholds for hemorrhage in a child with enlarged extracerebral spaces? Second, do some infants with shaking-impact syndrome escape acute medical attention, presenting in a delayed fashion with chronic collections? Finally, what is the effect of repeated injuries, either inflicted or accidental?[10] Such a situation could produce atrophy, thus lowering the mechanical threshold for subdural hemorrhage, as it does in the elderly, and result in recurrent hemorrhage with each new injury. Ultrastructural evaluation of the membranes that often develop around chronic bloody collections reveals abnormal capillary fragility, and repeated hemorrhage into established extracerebral fluid collections is now believed to account for their enlargement.[64] Perhaps in these situations, when the anatomy of the brain and extracerebral space is no longer "normal," the biomechanical threshold for in-

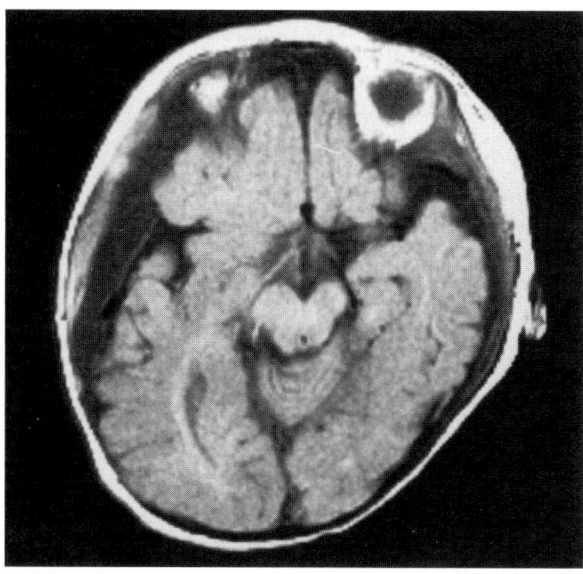

FIGURE 225–6. Magnetic resonance imaging scan of a 5-month-old baby with a prolonged hospitalization for meningitis, who developed proteinaceous effusions with hemorrhage while in the hospital. This illustrates the difficulty of assigning a mechanism of injury in children with hemorrhage into enlarged extra-axial spaces, because the mechanical threshold for hemorrhage in this situation is unknown. A presumption of child abuse in this setting must rely on other findings.

jury is sufficiently lowered that either shaking without impact or trivial accidental trauma could result in subdural hemorrhage.

Infantile chronic extracerebral collections are most frequently detected between 1 and 14 months of age, with a preponderance toward the younger age group.[23, 65, 66] For reasons that are not clear, most series report a higher incidence in male infants. In some instances, a specific cause can be established by history or laboratory analysis. Accidental trauma, coagulopathy, and postshunt cerebral collapse account for about 33% of cases, and documented or suspected child abuse accounted for an additional 44% in one series.[65] Documented birth trauma accounts for a relatively small number of cases. An extremely rare cause of subdural hematoma in infancy is a form of osteogenesis imperfecta, a genetic condition affecting collagen metabolism and resulting in fragile bones.[53] Despite its rarity, this condition is occasionally invoked to defend an alleged perpetrator of child abuse in criminal proceedings. The condition is sporadic in about two thirds of cases, and absence of a family history does not rule out the disease. Nonetheless, as mentioned previously, in most forms of osteogenesis imperfecta there are specific clinical signs, such as blue sclera, hypoplastic teeth, and hearing abnormalities, that point to the diagnosis, and biochemical abnormalities of type I collagen may be demonstrated.[67] Glutaricaciduria has also been associated with chronic extracerebral collections and neurological decline in infancy.[54]

In most instances of chronic subdural collections, however, no specific cause is found. Although it is reasonable to assume that some form of trauma pre-

ceded the development of the collection, it is not possible to presume child abuse in the absence of other supporting evidence. Until more is understood about the biomechanical questions raised earlier, the diagnosis of child abuse as the cause of chronic collections must rest on other findings indicative of child abuse, such as unexplained long bone fractures or characteristic soft tissue injuries, because the presence of collections alone is insufficient to presume a deliberate, violent traumatic event. Whether retinal hemorrhage qualifies as corroborating evidence remains controversial; it should probably be considered supportive rather than unequivocally diagnostic of inflicted injury.

The principal clinical features of extracerebral fluid collections in infancy arise from chronic intracranial hypertension. These consist of macrocephaly, fullness of the fontanelle, "sunsetting," vomiting, sleepiness, and irritability. The child's clinical appearance often suggests hydrocephalus, and only the imaging studies reveal the true nature of the problem. Seizures may occur from cortical irritation. Anemia may also accompany large fluid collections, probably arising from nutritional deficiency rather than blood loss into the extracerebral spaces.[66]

Diagnosis is by transfontanelle ultrasonography, computed tomography, or MRI examination of the head. An extra-axial fluid collection is seen, usually with imaging characteristics consistent with protein-rich fluid or chronic blood. There may be multiple laminations, composed of blood of varying ages.[65] Skull radiographs and long bone films should be obtained to search for evidence of fracture, and a child abuse evaluation should be initiated. MRI readily distinguishes high-protein or bloody extra-axial collections from the extra-axial cerebrospinal fluid collections that are commonly seen in asymptomatic but sometimes macrocephalic infants with benign external hydrocephalus, which requires no treatment. Whether such enlarged extra-axial cerebrospinal fluid spaces predispose to hemorrhage after minor trauma remains unclear, but it does not seem to be a common occurrence.

Therapy for chronic hemorrhagic extracerebral collections of infancy has undergone a significant evolution over the last 5 decades. Although small, asymptomatic collections can sometimes be followed conservatively, large collections with mass effect, neurological symptoms, or cranial enlargement require intervention. Historically, such collections were treated by large craniotomies with attempted resection of the investing membranes and, more recently, by reduction cranioplasty and lowering of the sagittal sinus in an attempt to treat the craniocerebral disproportion that may accompany the condition.[68, 69] Current practice is to manage symptomatic collections initially by intermittent fontanelle taps and to insert a shunt to the pleural or peritoneal space if the collections do not resolve in 2 or 3 weeks.[65] Other authors favor proceeding directly to shunting once the diagnosis is established (Fig. 225–7).[70] A unilateral shunt is usually sufficient, although there have been cases in which bilateral collections had poor communication, requiring bilateral shunts.[70, 71] It has been suggested that

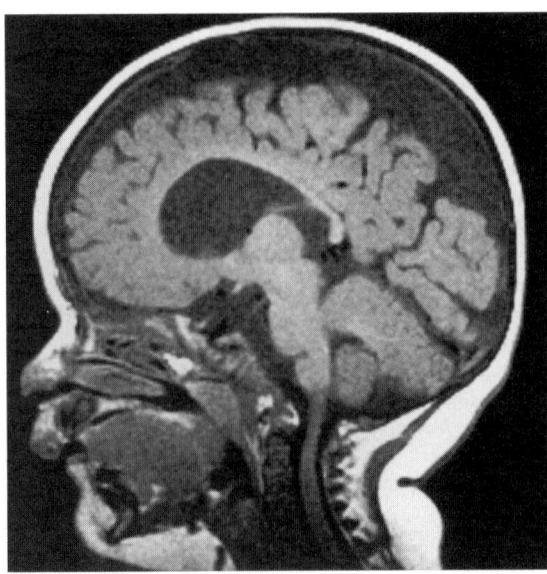

FIGURE 225–7. Extra-axial collections in an infant with a rapidly enlarging head. A subdural-peritoneal shunt was placed.

computed tomography–subdurography, in which contrast dye is instilled via the fontanelle into the collection, could predict the need for bilateral shunts.[72] An alternative is simply to place bilateral shunts routinely.

The outcome of children with treated chronic extracerebral collections is highly variable. Approximately 50% can be expected to have normal development, but 30% will be moderately disabled, and 13% will be severely disabled.[72] Child abuse as the cause of the collection is a particularly poor prognostic factor, presumably because of underlying brain parenchymal damage that occurred at the time of the original injury. Series that include abused children probably include a certain number of children with brain atrophy as a contributing cause of delayed extracerebral collections, which would tend to increase the number of poorer outcomes.

Ex Vacuo Cerebrospinal Fluid Collection

Young children who have suffered documented severe closed head injuries due to child abuse and develop extracerebral collections weeks or months afterward pose a special problem. The pathophysiology of this condition remains poorly understood, but as discussed earlier, large areas of low-density "black brain" evolve to frank infarction in most instances.[25, 37] Serial computed tomographic or MRI scans performed some months after the initial injury show severe atrophy with a prominent sulcal pattern, loss of white matter, and massive extracerebral collections of slightly proteinaceous or cerebrospinal fluid density (see Fig. 225–2B). These are the result of brain dissolution and shrinkage and are invariably accompanied by severe neurological damage. The head circumference may increase somewhat but tends to plateau over time. In general, surgical drainage of this sort of post-traumatic

collection does not result in clinical improvement. In rare cases, drainage can be considered if there is clinical deterioration consistent with the time course of the collection's appearance or overt signs or symptoms of intracranial hypertension.

SPINAL INJURY DUE TO CHILD ABUSE

In view of the commonly assumed "whiplash" pathophysiology of child abuse, surprisingly little attention has been paid to the spine in clinical and autopsy series. Several aspects of the infant and child spine render it particularly vulnerable to damage due to flexion-extension forces: (1) the interspinous ligaments, posterior joint capsule, and cartilaginous end plates are elastic; (2) the facet joints are horizontally oriented; (3) the anterior portion of the vertebral bodies is wedged; (4) the uncinate processes are flat and therefore ineffective in withstanding flexion-rotation forces; (5) the head of an infant is relatively large compared with the underdeveloped neck musculature; and (6) the atlanto-occipital joint of an infant is inherently unstable, and weak supporting ligaments allow the arch of C1 to invert within the foramen magnum during extension, compressing the vertebral arteries.[73–76] Furthermore, it is now clear that devastating neurological injury can occur in children without bony fractures or other radiographic abnormalities, making spinal cord injury difficult to detect without sophisticated radiographic imaging procedures.[77] The incidence of spinal injury in the setting of child abuse is probably underappreciated, because overwhelming brain injury may mask an associated injury to the cervical spinal cord. Even at autopsy, the brain is often removed at the cervicomedullary junction, and the spinal cord is not examined at all.

There is evidence, however, that a significant percentage of fatally injured abused infants have autopsy findings of subdural and epidural hemorrhage and contusion of the high cervical cord, which may contribute to morbidity and mortality.[41] Because most of the information regarding spinal injuries in child abuse has come from autopsy series, it may be that these injuries are usually fatal and that survivors are unlikely to be affected. Indeed, it is rare to have a clinically detected spinal cord injury in a child with a recoverable brain injury. Nonetheless, it is conceivable that apnea from transient spinal cord compression in association with a shaking-impact injury might significantly contribute to the cerebral insult that is so prominent in child abuse cases. Vascular compression of the vertebral arteries has also been considered, although the posterior circulation distribution is usually spared in child abuse cases with widespread infarction.

Spinal fracture and overt spinal instability appear to be uncommon aspects of nonaccidental trauma to infants but might be underrecognized.[78] Nevertheless, it is appropriate to immobilize the neck and obtain screening radiographs of the spine as part of the evaluation of suspected child abuse. If MRI of the brain is performed, a screening study of the upper cervical region can also be obtained, although findings in survi-

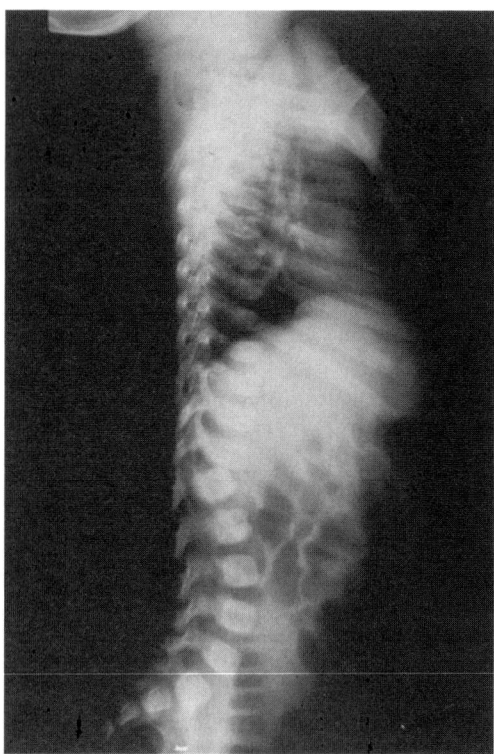

FIGURE 225–8. Thoracic spine injury in a previously healthy 1-year-old girl whose caretaker said he "bounced" her during rough play. She also had bite marks on her hands.

vors are unusual. Occasionally, spinal injuries are seen in "battered" children and appear to occur from extreme hyperflexion or hyperextension forces applied to the immature spine (Fig. 225–8).[79]

The principles of management that apply to adults and older children with spinal injury apply to infants, and fusion may be required for unstable injuries. The treatment of spinal instability in an infant may pose special challenges. In the cervical region, standard methods of skeletal traction and halo fixation cannot be used, owing to the thinness of the infant skull. The use of a Minerva jacket cast may be all that is possible during the acute phase. Spinal instrumentation may require modification because of size constraints and the relative paucity of suitable autologous bone available for fusion.

OUTCOME OF HEAD INJURIES FROM CHILD ABUSE

It has been recognized in large series of pediatric head injury that severely head-injured infants have a worse prognosis than do older children, probably because of the preponderance of inflicted injuries in this age group.[80, 81] Mortality among abused children with head injuries ranges between 10% and 27% in various series, although exact figures are difficult to compile because of differences in the definition of child abuse and in referral populations.[2, 24, 26, 44, 82] Nonetheless, it is clear

that this cause of head injury correlates with a high mortality.

Morbidity in survivors of inflicted injury is uncertain, because long-term follow-up of patients injured in infancy is, by nature, difficult, and outcome may depend on factors other than the brain injury itself. Nonetheless, it is obvious that children with infarction and severe brain atrophy remain severely disabled; children with bilateral diffuse hypodensity who survive are blind, nonverbal, nonambulatory, and severely developmentally delayed.[62] The long-term deficits of children who are more mildly injured are less well studied, but it appears that the majority of children suffer persistent deficits, with less than one third approaching age-appropriate functioning.[60–62, 83]

With respect to visual problems, retinal hemorrhages resolve over time, but amblyopia may develop if the macula is obscured by hemorrhage for a prolonged period, and close follow-up is recommended. Retinal detachments frequently result in marked visual compromise and may require repair to optimize recovery. Retinal folds may also adversely affect visual outcome.[84]

Another relevant outcome measure is risk of recurrence of physical abuse. In one series, more than half of abused children had radiographic or autopsy evidence of prior physical abuse.[10] In a group of children in whom the diagnosis of abusive head injury was missed at medical contact, 27.8% were reinjured before the diagnosis was made.[11] Other series found even higher rates of reinjury.[83] These data suggest that a child who is returned to the caretakers responsible for the injury is at high risk for repeated trauma, and for this reason, child welfare agencies commonly place a child in protective custody when abuse is suspected.

MEDICOLEGAL CONSIDERATIONS IN CHILD ABUSE

The recognition of child physical abuse as a theoretically preventable problem has led to the development of child abuse legislation. In 1963 the U.S. Department of Health, Education, and Welfare's Children's Bureau developed principles and suggested language for states to use in generating child abuse statutes.[85] Within a few years, all states in the country had developed child physical abuse reporting laws. In 1974 the Federal Child Abuse Prevention and Treatment Act required states to expand reporting laws to include other forms of abuse and provided grants to states meeting the new standards. Over the last 30 years, each state has developed criminal and civil laws to define child abuse. Although each state's law differs, they are all intended to identify and protect children who are victims of child abuse.

Physician Responsibility and Liability

Each state's child abuse law identifies individuals who are required to report suspected abuse. These *mandated reporters* generally include all adults who come in contact with children in some professional capacity, including physicians, teachers, librarians, dentists, and so forth. Mandated reporters are required to identify children, based on reasonable knowledge and experience, who may be the victims of abuse. Reporting laws require only a suspicion of abuse, not proof that abuse has occurred. Although anyone can report suspected cases, professionals tend to report more true cases of abuse than does the general public.[86] Physicians are not exempt from filing reports of suspected abuse based on principles of doctor-patient confidentiality.

All reporting statutes protect mandated reporters from civil liabilities, assuming such reports are made "in good faith" and not as a malicious attack against an individual. Although challenges to reporting immunity have been made in recent years, the past protection of mandated reporters has been almost complete. Physicians who report clinically sound concerns should continue to be afforded protection. Relatively mild criminal laws, primarily misdemeanors, exist for failing to report suspected abuse cases. In actuality, civil liability for not reporting is a greater threat for physicians. Failure to diagnose child abuse and failure to report cases of suspected abuse are recognized grounds for civil liability, and malpractice suits against physicians have been successful in this regard. Ultimately, the physician's concern for the safety and protection of a child, and not a fear of civil lawsuits, should be the impetus for reporting suspicious cases.

Reports regarding child abuse are made to child protective services (CPS), law enforcement, or both, depending on the circumstances of the case. It is the responsibility of CPS to investigate abuse that occurs in the child's home or by a caretaker of the child. Abuse committed by an individual who is not a caretaker (e.g., a stranger) requires a police investigation and not a CPS referral. The majority of inflicted head injury is perpetrated by caretakers, requiring almost universal involvement of CPS agencies. CPS agencies are responsible for ensuring the ongoing safety of the child and determining safe placement of the child after hospital discharge. CPS workers continue to work with the family and child in an attempt to prevent further abuse and improve parenting. Unfortunately, with the explosion of child abuse reports made over the last decade, the focus of CPS has shifted from prevention and treatment to investigation.

Law enforcement's responsibility is in investigating crime. Although not all cases of child physical abuse are reported to the police, severe head trauma and injuries extensive enough to warrant neurosurgical intervention usually meet the threshold for police involvement.

The actual method by which a report of suspected child abuse is filed with the CPS agency or the police varies among states and institutions, but it usually involves filling out appropriate forms and notifying CPS by telephone. Large medical centers and most children's hospitals have child protection teams that are involved with the treatment of abused children and can contact the appropriate social and law enforcement agencies. In smaller hospitals, a social worker or the hospital's lawyer can aid the physician with the mechanics of reporting suspected abuse.

One of the more daunting tasks for a physician treating an abused child is informing the family of the suspicion and the need to report the suspected abuse. Although this is difficult to do, not sharing this information only fosters mistrust and may have negative consequences for the ongoing doctor-patient relationship. Unless the parents seem seriously psychologically disturbed or dangerous, their right to be informed about their child's condition requires honesty on the part of the treating physician. In discussing the case with the parents, the physician should remain objective and nonaccusatory. The doctor should not attempt to assign blame or determine the guilt or innocence of the parents; rather, the focus should be on the need to treat the child and ensure his or her future protection. It is helpful to present this information using a team approach that includes the treating physician, child abuse team members, and the primary nurse; this avoids the family's receiving different versions of the ongoing evaluation and treatment plan from different sources.

Once a report is filed, CPS (and law enforcement, when appropriate) must begin the investigation within 24 to 48 hours, although the full investigation may last weeks or months. Parents should be told to expect to hear from the CPS agency or the police. The involvement of a social worker is often invaluable to both the physician and the family. The social worker can serve as a liaison between the physician and CPS and law enforcement and can provide ongoing information and support to the family.

Civil and Criminal Judicial Intervention

In an effort to protect children from abuse, laws have been enacted to allow governmental intervention in a child's life without parental consent. Both the circumstances and the severity of the abuse determine the involvement of the civil and criminal court systems. Although civil intervention can occur in any situation of alleged abuse, the criminal court system is involved in more severe cases of maltreatment.

The civil system is responsible for (1) child protective legislation that defines child abuse, establishes reporting procedures, and imposes regulations on the way the state investigates and documents allegations of abuse; (2) the juvenile court laws, which govern the way the state obtains the authority to intervene in the family and ensure the ongoing protection of the child; and (3) federal funding laws regarding the abuse of children. Although the civil courts can become involved in any case of alleged child abuse, not all cases reach the court system. If an investigation fails to identify any abuse or neglect, the report is expunged and the case closed. If there is reason to believe that the child is at risk, CPS can offer services to the family on a voluntary basis. If the parents refuse services or are unable to protect the child, the case can be brought to court by the CPS agency to secure the child's ongoing safety. A civil proceeding, referred to as an *adjudicatory hearing*, involves the presentation of evidence to a

TABLE 225–1 ■ **Comparison of Civil and Criminal Child Abuse Proceedings**

	CIVIL	CRIMINAL
Laws	State child protection laws	State criminal codes for specific crimes
Focus	Child protection	Offender accountability
Need to prove	Child was injured by nonaccidental means	Defendant injured child at specific time
Fact finder	Judge	Judge, or judge and jury
Maximum penalty	Removal of child from home	Incarceration
Rules of evidence	Lenient	Strict
Burden of proof	Predominance of the evidence	Beyond a reasonable doubt

Adapted from Ludwig S, Kornberg A (eds): Child Abuse and Neglect: A Medical Reference. New York, Churchill Livingstone, 1991, p 424.

judge that indicates the child's need for ongoing protection. Physicians may be asked to testify at adjudicatory hearings as fact or expert witnesses; this distinction is discussed in more detail later. In general, the physician is asked to present the medical findings to the judge and may be asked to offer an opinion whether the injuries were accidental, consistent with the explanation provided, or inflicted. Based on the evidence presented, the judge weighs the right of the parents to raise their child against the right of the child to be protected from harm. At the *dispositional hearing* (akin to sentencing in a criminal trial), the judge may find that there is not enough evidence to authorize ongoing involvement by the court, in which case all intervention is stopped. If the judge finds that the child is at risk, a variety of options may be ordered, such as foster care placement, in-home social work services, or ongoing psychological counseling for the parents, the child, or both.

State laws define intentional or reckless acts that cause harm to a child as crimes. The criminal system addresses whether an individual is responsible for a child's injuries. The decision to prosecute is made by a prosecuting attorney (working on behalf of the state) after an investigation by law enforcement. The purpose of a criminal trial is to determine whether a crime has been committed and whether the defendant was the perpetrator of that crime. The rules of evidence and the formality of the proceedings are stricter in a criminal trial than in a civil hearing (Table 225–1). In general, severe cases of physical abuse, including inflicted head trauma, are brought to criminal trial. The charges against the defendant are determined by the prosecutor and depend on the facts of the case. The guilt of the defendant is determined by either a jury or a judge and a jury, at the option of the defendant. The penalties for guilt depend on the charges filed, the past criminal record of the defendant, and other circumstances regarding the case; they can range from probation to lifetime incarceration.

The Physician as Witness

Physician testimony is often needed in civil and criminal trials. The principles that apply to child abuse cases may be familiar to neurosurgeons from other medicolegal realms, such as medical malpractice, but they bear repeating in the present context. To begin with, the physician can testify as either a *fact witness* or an *expert witness*. This legal distinction is designed to prevent witnesses of fact, who are asked only to report their actions or observations, from expressing personal opinions based on conjecture or bias, which might unfairly influence a jury. A treating physician may be subpoenaed to provide information regarding only the child's treatment or care, thus serving as a fact witness. Whereas fact witnesses are not permitted to offer opinions or conclusions derived from the facts of a case, an expert witness is expected to do just that. An expert witness is an individual who, by training, education, and clinical experience, has knowledge in a particular field that goes beyond what a layperson would know. After hearing the credentials of the witness, the judge determines whether the witness qualifies as an expert, allowing him or her to offer opinions and conclusions. Based on this broad definition, most neurosurgeons would be considered experts with respect to head injuries and their causes. Unfortunately, the concept of "expert" as it applies to this sort of case poses some practical problems. First, the court's definition of an expert differs from that of the medical community, legally allowing for expert testimony from medical scientists who have advanced degrees but no true expertise on the subject in question. Second, an expert witness should be thought of as someone who can educate the judge and jury; the facts and opinions of the expert should assist them in determining the guilt or innocence of the defendant. Although many clinicians in various specialties, including neurosurgery, have some familiarity with inflicted head injuries, it is often tempting to infuse facts with opinions in an area in which considerable uncertainty exists. Brent reviews the problem of irresponsible expert witness testimony and outlines the qualities of a responsible expert, who should be a nonpartisan scholar with publications in the field in question and an active clinician for whom legal activities constitute only a minor part of professional activities.[87]

Preparing for Court Testimony

Physician involvement in a court proceeding is usually heralded by a served subpoena. The first step in preparing to testify in court is to determine who has sent the subpoena and for what purpose. This is accomplished by calling the court or law office that served the subpoena. In cases of child abuse, the state, or the prosecuting attorney, is most likely to request the participation of the patient's physician. The physician should find out who the lawyer represents, the setting of the hearing (civil versus criminal proceeding), and the extent of his or her expected participation (fact versus expert witness). The medical records should be available to the physician when discussing the case with attorneys. Opposing counsel sometimes calls to discuss the case as well, and given the expert physician's role as a nonpartisan educator, it is usually best to cooperate with both sides. It is important to be careful and specific when answering questions and not to volunteer information that is not asked.

A physician who serves as an expert witness is often asked to provide a written report before the court date. This report will likely be shared with opposing counsel. In preparing this report, the physician should list the documents reviewed (including police reports, statements, and other documents provided), summarize the facts of the case, and offer an expert opinion and an explanation of the basis for those conclusions. When preparing the report, care should be taken to be factual and precise. Information contained in the report may be questioned during the court proceeding.

If the physician is called as an expert witness in a trial, the judge first hears the physician's qualifications and determines whether the physician meets the criteria of an expert. The direct examination of the witness, which is done by the attorney requesting the physician's presence, follows. The purpose of the direct examination is to present all the information pertinent to the case. The witness often reviews the questions with the lawyer beforehand, to be sure that all the necessary information is included. Any information covered during direct examination is subject to cross-examination by opposing counsel. When testifying in court, it is important that the physician understand the question, avoid guessing or speculating, not go beyond his or her area of expertise, be honest and concise, and avoid offering information not requested.

Involvement in a civil or criminal case can be frustrating for physicians. The procedures, language, and adversarial flavor of the courtroom are foreign to physicians, and despite an attempt to protect a child or hold the perpetrator responsible, the outcome may not be favorable. Fortunately, the majority of reported cases of child abuse do not require court involvement, and only a minority of abuse cases are severe enough to warrant criminal prosecution.[88]

Legal and Social Outcomes of Child Physical Abuse

Few studies have examined the legal outcome of physical abuse cases. Showers and Apolo studied the legal disposition of 72 cases of fatal child abuse that occurred in Columbus, Ohio, from 1965 to 1984.[89] Of the 72 deaths, the majority were the result of severe head trauma. In 51% of cases, insufficient evidence existed to file charges against the suspected perpetrator. Of the 27 suspects charged with a crime, 5 were acquitted, 1 case resulted in a hung jury and the charges were dismissed, and 21 were convicted of a crime. Of the 21 convictions, 9 pleaded guilty. The sentences ranged from 6 months' probation to 15 years to life in prison. Fourteen percent of the convicted individuals served no prison sentence, and 19% served less than 1 year. Females were less likely than males to be charged, convicted, or imprisoned. The number of suspects charged and convicted varied greatly between the first and second decades studied, probably owing to increased awareness of the problem of child abuse and improved identification and investigation of physical abuse. The study suggests that the criminal consequences of murdering a child have not been great in the past but may be increasing.

Few parents or caretakers have been convicted of first-degree murder (premeditated, deliberate murder) in child homicide cases. Many perpetrators do not appear to deliberately murder the child, and because abuse occurs in the privacy of the home and usually without a "weapon," it is difficult to prove that the parent or caretaker intended to kill the child. As a result, the penalties for killing children tend to be less severe than those for killing adults. As a response to this state of affairs, several states have modified their definitions of first-degree murder to include child abuse homicides, known as "homicide by abuse" statutes.[90] These statutes eliminate the "intent to kill" requirement in cases of child death due to abuse. They allow for first-degree murder charges to be filed in child homicide cases if the prosecutor can show that the defendant abused the child and the abuse caused the child's death. These statutes were first developed in the mid-1980s, and their effect has not yet been fully evaluated.

Despite the research done in the last 30 years, there has been little focus on the long-term effects of physical abuse. This is partly due to the relatively recent professional recognition of child abuse. Widom carefully studied the effects of physical abuse on subsequent delinquent and adult criminal and violent behavior.[91] In this study, Widom identified a large sample of validated cases of child abuse from the 1960s, matched them with nonabused children, and analyzed the subsequent criminal records for both groups. Although the majority of the abused children did not become delinquents or adult criminals, being abused as a child increased the risk for juvenile delinquency, adult criminal behavior, and violent criminal behavior.

Martin and Elmer describe the social functioning of a small group of adults who were severely battered as children in the 1960s.[92] Although children who sustained head trauma were included in the group, these subjects were not analyzed separately. Owing to both the small sample size and the complexity of factors that determine adult social skills, no clear relationship developed between a history of severe abuse and adult functioning. The adult victims of abuse tended to be resentful and suspicious but not overtly aggressive.

Some exhibited limited autonomy, and others were competently raising families and holding jobs. Overall, the outcomes for the individuals studied were extremely variable, supporting the need for further investigation in this field.

There are no studies that specifically address the long-term social outcome of infants and toddlers who were victims of inflicted head trauma. This is primarily due to the relatively recent recognition of abusive head injury as a medical diagnosis. As the recognition of abused children improves and the management of these patients advances, more older children and adults will become available for study.

PREVENTION OF CHILD ABUSE

The importance of eliminating child abuse seems obvious, yet it is premature to consider the primary prevention of abuse an attainable goal. The factors related to the cause of child abuse are varied and complex. Poverty, societal violence, inadequate pediatric health care, family isolation, domestic violence, unrealistic parental expectations, and the temperament and behaviors of children all contribute to abuse and neglect. Much of what we currently consider prevention is actually reactive: high-risk families are identified and monitored; counseling and psychotherapy are provided when available; and when the danger is too great, children are placed in foster care, and the criminal justice system assists in an effort to modify behavior.

Much of the recent effort in prevention has focused on identifying child, parent, and caretaker factors that increase the risk of abuse. Thus, although child abuse occurs in a wide variety of situations, particular risk factors have been identified; these include young parents, low socioeconomic status, unstable family situations, disability or prematurity of the child, and male caretakers.[17, 31, 93] Efforts to target future or current high-risk caretakers for specific interventions, including education in parenting skills, stress management, and appropriate choices in surrogate child care, might best direct prevention resources toward those most likely to benefit.

Prevention of all forms of abuse and neglect would require the elimination of poverty and violence from society, the development of comprehensive support systems for both new parents and nuclear families, and improved education of the children and young adults who represent the next generation of parents. Comprehensive health care reform is needed to provide adequate medical insurance to millions of children who are currently uninsured. Studies have shown that a public health nurse or a layperson acting as a home visitor can prevent abuse.[94, 95] Many school districts have incorporated child abuse prevention into education curricula.[96] Finally, specific campaigns against "shaking" injuries have been developed to educate parents about the dangers of shaking infants.[97] To date, these programs have examined participant learning about the purported dangers of shaking, but they have not been evaluated for effectiveness in preventing inflicted head trauma.

Research into prevention has not kept pace with progress in the diagnosis, pathophysiology, and management of inflicted head injury, and more work is needed to study the efficacy of specific interventions. Because of financial constraints, there has been a significant trend for CPS efforts to shift from prevention and therapeutic services toward investigation. As in many medical and social problems, in child abuse, prevention is the ultimate goal, on both an individual and a public health level. It is incumbent on neurosurgeons who treat children to recognize abuse when it occurs and to participate in public and professional education when possible so that these potentially devastating injuries might be prevented.

REFERENCES

1. Billmire ME, Myers PA: Serious head injury in infants: Accident or abuse? Pediatrics 75:340–342, 1985.
2. Duhaime AC, Alario AJ, Lewander WJ, et al: Head injury in very young children: Mechanism, injury types, and ophthalmologic findings in 100 hospitalized patients younger than 2 years of age. Pediatrics 90:179–185, 1992.
3. Gotschall CS: Epidemiology of childhood injury. In Eichenberger MR (ed): Pediatric Trauma: Prevention, Acute Care, Rehabilitation. St. Louis, Mosby Year Book, 1993, pp 16–19.
4. Ewing-Cobbs L, Kramer L, Prasad M, et al: Neuroimaging, physical, and developmental findings after inflicted and noninflicted traumatic brain injury in young children. Pediatrics 102(Pt 1): 300–307, 1998.
5. Caffey J: The whiplash shaken infant syndrome: Manual shaking by the extremities with whiplash-induced intracranial and intraocular bleedings, linked with residual permanent brain damage and mental retardation. Pediatrics 54:396–403, 1974.
6. Helfer RE, Slovis TL, Black MB: Injuries resulting when small children fall out of bed. Pediatrics 60:533–535, 1977.
7. Joffe M, Ludwig S: Stairway injuries in children. Pediatrics 82(Pt 2):457–461, 1988.
8. Nimityongskul P, Anderson L: The likelihood of injuries when children fall out of bed. J Pediatr Orthop 7:184–186, 1987.
9. Shugerman RP, Paez A, Grossman DC, et al: Epidural hemorrhage: Is it abuse? Pediatrics 97:664–668, 1996.
10. Alexander R, Crabbe L, Sato Y, et al: Serial abuse in children who are shaken. Am J Dis Child 144:58–60, 1990.
11. Jenny C, Hymel KP, Ritzen A, et al: Analysis of missed cases of abusive head trauma. JAMA 281:621–626, 1999.
12. Kempe CH, Silverman FN, Steele BF, et al: The battered-child syndrome. JAMA 181:105–112, 1962.
13. Ludwig S: Child abuse. In Fleisher GR, Ludwig S (eds): Textbook of Pediatric Emergency Medicine, 2nd ed. Baltimore, Williams & Wilkins, 1988, pp 1127–1163.
14. Hanigan WC, Peterson RA, Njus G: Tin ear syndrome: Rotational acceleration in pediatric head injuries. Pediatrics 80:618–622, 1987.
15. Harcourt B, Hopkins D: Ophthalmic manifestations of the battered-baby syndrome. BMJ 3:398–401, 1971.
16. Elner SG, Elner VM, Arnall M, et al: Ocular and associated systemic findings in suspected child abuse. Arch Ophthalmol 108:1094–1101, 1990.
17. Klein M, Stern L: Low birth weight and the battered child syndrome. Am J Dis Child 122:15–18, 1971.
18. Meservy CJ, Towbin R, McLaurin RL, et al: Radiographic characteristics of skull fractures resulting from child abuse. Am J Radiol 149:173–175, 1987.
19. Caffey J: On the theory and practice of shaking infants: Its potential residual effects of permanent brain damage and mental retardation. Am J Dis Child 124:161–169, 1972.
20. Ommaya AK, Yarnell P: Subdural hematoma after whiplash injury. Lancet 2:237–239, 1962.

21. Ommaya AK, Faas F, Yarnell P: Whiplash injury and brain damage: An experimental study. JAMA 204:285–289, 1968.
22. Ommaya AK, Gennarelli TA: Cerebral concussion and traumatic unconsciousness: Correlation of experimental and clinical observations on blunt head injuries. Brain 97:633–654, 1974.
23. Guthkelch AK: Infantile subdural hematoma and its relationship to whiplash injuries. BMJ 2:430–431, 1971.
24. Duhaime AC, Gennarelli TG, Thibault LE, et al: The shaken baby syndrome: A clinical, pathological, and biomechanical study. J Neurosurg 66:409–415, 1987.
25. Duhaime AC, Sutton LN, Schut L: The "shaken baby syndrome": A misnomer? J Pediatr Neurosci 4:77–86, 1988.
26. Hahn YS, Raimondi AJ, McLone DG, et al: Traumatic mechanisms of head injury in child abuse. Childs Brain 10:229–241, 1983.
27. Gennarelli TA, Thibault LE: Biomechanics of head injury. In Wilkins RH, Rengachary SS (eds): Neurosurgery, vol 2. New York, McGraw-Hill, 1985, pp 1531–1536.
28. Bruce DA, Zimmerman RA: Shaken impact syndrome. Pediatr Ann 18:482–489, 1989.
29. Duhaime AC, Christian CW, Rorke LB, et al: Nonaccidental head injury in infants—the "shaken baby syndrome." N Engl J Med 338:1822–1829, 1998.
30. Alexander R, Sato Y, Smith W, et al: Incidence of impact trauma with cranial injuries ascribed to shaking. Am J Dis Child 144:724–726, 1990.
31. Starling SP, Holden JR, Jenny C: Abusive head trauma: The relationship of perpetrators to their victims. Pediatrics 95:259–262, 1995.
32. Zimmerman RA, Bilaniuk LT, Bruce D, et al: Computed tomography of craniocerebral injury in the abused child. Radiology 130:687–690, 1979.
33. Sato Y, Yuh WTC, Smith WL, et al: Head injury in child abuse: Evaluation with MR imaging. Radiology 173:653–657, 1989.
34. Plunkett J: Sudden death in an infant caused by rupture of a basilar artery aneurysm. Am J Forensic Med Pathol 20:45–47, 1999.
35. Feldman KW, Brewer DK, Shaw DW: Evolution of the cranial computed tomography scan in child abuse. Child Abuse Negl 19:307–314, 1995.
36. Dias MS, Backstrom J, Falk M, et al: Serial radiography in the infant shaken impact syndrome. Pediatr Neurosurg 29:77–85, 1998.
37. Whyte KM, Pascoe M: Does "black" brain mean doom? Computed tomography in the prediction of outcome in children with severe head injuries: "Benign" vs "malignant" brain swelling. Australas Radiol 33:344–347, 1989.
38. Duhaime AC, Bilaniuk L, Zimmerman R: The "big black brain": Radiographic changes after severe inflicted head injury in infancy. J Neurotrauma 10(Suppl 1):S59, 1993.
39. Johnson DL, Boal D, Baule R: Role of apnea in nonaccidental head injury. J Pediatr Neurosurg 23:305–310, 1995.
40. Shaver E, Duhaime AC, Curtis M, et al: Experimental acute subdural hematoma in infant piglets. Pediatr Neurosurg 25:123–129, 1996.
41. Hadley MN, Sonntag VKH, Rekate HL, et al: The infant whiplash-shake syndrome: A clinical and pathological study. Neurosurgery 24:536–540, 1989.
42. Hymel KP, Abshire TC, Luckey DW, et al: Coagulopathy in pediatric abusive head trauma. Pediatrics 99:371–375, 1997.
43. American Academy of Pediatrics, Section on Radiology: Diagnostic imaging in child abuse. Pediatrics 87:262–264, 1991.
44. Ludwig S, Warman M: Shaken baby syndrome: A review of 20 cases. Ann Emerg Med 13:104–107, 1984.
45. Luerssen TG, Huang JC, McLone DG, et al: Retinal hemorrhages, seizures, and intracranial hemorrhages: Relationships and outcomes in children suffering traumatic brain injury. In Marlin AE (ed): Concepts in Pediatric Neurosurgery, vol 11. Basel, Karger, 1991, pp 87–94.
46. Johnson DL, Braun D, Friendly D: Accidental head trauma and retinal hemorrhage. Neurosurgery 33:234–235, 1993.
47. Christian C, Taylor AA, Hertle R, et al: Retinal hemorrhages due to accidental household trauma. J Pediatr 135:125–127, 1999.
48. Goetting MG, Sowa B: Retinal hemorrhage after cardiopulmonary resuscitation in children: An etiologic reevaluation. Pediatrics 85:585–588, 1990.
49. Green MA, Lieberman G, Milroy CM, et al: Ocular and cerebral trauma in non-accidental injury in infancy: Underlying mechanisms and implications for paediatric practice. Br J Ophthalmol 80:282–287, 1996.
50. Yoffe G, Buchanan GR: Intracranial hemorrhage in newborn and young infants with hemophilia. J Pediatr 113:333–335, 1988.
51. Ryan CA, Gayle M: Vitamin K deficiency, intracranial hemorrhage, and a subgaleal hematoma: A fatal combination. Pediatr Emerg Care 8:143, 1992.
52. Parsch CS, Krauss J, Hofmann D, et al: Arachnoid cysts associated with subdural hematomas and hygromas: Analysis of 16 cases, long-term follow-up, and review of the literature. Neurosurgery 40:483–490, 1997.
53. Tokoro K, Nakajima F, Yamataki A: Infantile chronic subdural hematoma with local protrusion of the skull in a case of osteogenesis imperfecta. Neurosurgery 22:595–598, 1988.
54. Haworth JC, Booth FA, Chudley AE, et al: Phenotypic variability in glutaric aciduria type I: Report of fourteen cases in five Canadian Indian kindreds. J Pediatr 118:52–58, 1991.
55. Duhaime AC, Christian C, Armonda R, et al: Disappearing subdural hematomas in children. Pediatr Neurosurg 25:116–122, 1996.
56. Willman KY, Bank DE, Senac M, et al: Restricting the time of injury in fatal inflicted head injuries. Child Abuse Negl 21:929–940, 1997.
57. Kelly JP, Nichols JS, Filley CM, et al: Concussion in sports: Guidelines for the prevention of catastrophic outcome. JAMA 266:2867–2869, 1991.
58. Cantu RC: Cerebral concussion in sport: Management and prevention. Sports Med 14:64–74, 1992.
59. Cho D, Wang Y, Chi C: Decompressive craniotomy for acute shaken/impact baby syndrome. Pediatr Neurosurg 23:192–198, 1996.
60. Gilles EE, Nelson MD Jr: Cerebral complications of nonaccidental head injury in childhood. Pediatr Neurol 19:119–128, 1998.
61. Bonnier C, Nassogne M, Evrard P: Outcome and prognosis of whiplash shaken infant syndrome: Late consequences after a symptom-free interval. Dev Med Child Neurol 37:943–956, 1995.
62. Duhaime AC, Christian C, Moss E, et al: Long-term outcome in children with the shaking-impact syndrome. Pediatr Neurosurg 24:292–298, 1996.
63. Haines DE, Harkey HL, Al-Mefty O: The "subdural" space: A new look at an outdated concept. Neurosurgery 32:111–120, 1993.
64. McLone DG, Gutierrez FA: Ultrastructure of subdural membranes of children. Concepts Pediatr Neurosurg 1:174–187, 1989.
65. Parent AD: Pediatric chronic subdural hematoma: A retrospective comparative analysis. Pediatr Neurosurg 18:266–269, 1992.
66. McLaurin RL, Isaacs E, Lewis HP: Results of nonoperative treatment in 15 cases of infantile subdural hematoma. J Neurosurg 34:753–759, 1971.
67. Kooh SW: Metabolic abnormalities of the skull and axial skeleton. In Hoffman H, Epstein F (eds): Disorders of the Developing Nervous System: Diagnosis and Treatment. Boston, Blackwell Scientific, 1986, pp 449–463.
68. Ingraham FD, Matson DD: Subdural hematoma in infancy. J Pediatr 24:1–37, 1944.
69. Gutierrez FA, McLone DG, Raimondi AJ: Pathophysiology and a new treatment of chronic subdural hematoma in children. Childs Brain 5:216–232, 1979.
70. Duhaime AC, Sutton LN: Delayed sequelae of pediatric head injury. In Barrow D (ed): Complications and Sequelae of Head Injury. Park Ridge, Ill, American Association of Neurological Surgeons, 1992, pp 169–186.
71. Aoki N, Masuzawa H: Unilateral subdural-peritoneal shunting for bilateral chronic subdural hematomas in infancy. J Neurosurg 63:134–137, 1985.
72. Aoki N: Chronic subdural hematoma in infancy: Clinical analysis of 30 cases in the CT era. J Neurosurg 73:201–205, 1990.
73. Gilles FH, Massoud B, Sotrel A: Infantile atlantooccipital instability. Am J Dis Child 133:30–37, 1979.
74. Bailey DK: The normal cervical spine in infants and children. Radiology 59:712–719, 1952.
75. Sullivan CR, Bruwer AJ, Harris LE: Hypermobility of the cervical spine in children: A pitfall in the diagnosis of cervical dislocation. Am J Surg 95:636–640, 1958.

76. Townsend EH, Rowe ML: Mobility of the upper cervical spine in health and disease. Pediatrics 10:567–573, 1952.

77. Pang D, Pollack IF: Spinal cord injury without radiographic abnormality in children—the SCIWORA syndrome. J Trauma 29:654–664, 1989.

78. McGrory BF, Fenichel GM: Hangman's fracture subsequent to shaking in an infant. Ann Neurol 2:82, 1977.

79. Kleinman PK: Spinal trauma. In Kleinman PK (ed): Diagnostic Imaging of Child Abuse. Baltimore, Williams & Wilkins, 1987, pp 91–102.

80. Levin HS, Aldrich EF, Saydjari C, et al: Severe head injury in children: Experience of the Traumatic Coma Data Bank. Neurosurgery 31:435–444, 1992.

81. Kriel RL, Krach LE, Panser LA: Closed head injury: Comparison of children younger and older than 6 years of age. Pediatr Neurol 5:296–300, 1989.

82. McClelland CQ, Rekate H, Kaufman B, et al: Cerebral injury in child abuse: A changing profile. Childs Brain 7:225–235, 1980.

83. Fischer H, Allasio D: Permanently damaged: Long-term followup of shaken babies. Pediatrics 33:696–698, 1994.

84. Han DP, Wilkinson WS: Late ophthalmic manifestations of the shaken baby syndrome. J Pediatr Ophthalmol Strabismus 27:299–303, 1990.

85. U.S. Department of Health, Education, and Welfare: The Abused Child: Principles and Suggested Language for Legislation on Reporting of the Physically Abused Child. Washington, DC, Children's Bureau, U.S. Government Printing Office, 1963.

86. Faller KC: Unanticipated problems in the United States child protection system. Child Abuse Negl 9:63–89, 1985.

87. Brent R: The irresponsible expert witness: A failure of biomedical education and professional accountability. Pediatrics 70:754–762, 1982.

88. Krugman RD: Advances and retreats in the protection of children. N Engl J Med 320:531–532, 1989.

89. Showers J, Apolo J: Criminal disposition of persons involved in 72 cases of fatal child abuse. Med Sci Law 26:243–247, 1986.

90. Marx S, Toth P, Dinsmore J: Investigation and Prosecution of Child Abuse, 2nd ed. Alexandria, Va, American Prosecutors Research Institute, 1993.

91. Widom CS: The cycle of violence. Science 244:160–166, 1989.

92. Martin JA, Elmer E: Battered children grown up: A follow-up study of individuals severely maltreated as children. Child Abuse Negl 16:75–87, 1992.

93. Sills JA, Thomas LJ, Rosenbloom L: Non-accidental injury: A two-year study in central Liverpool. Dev Med Child Neurol 19:26–33, 1977.

94. Olds DD, Henderson CR, Chamberlain R: Preventing child abuse and neglect: A randomized trial of nurse home visitation. Pediatrics 78:65–78, 1986.

95. Gray JD, Cutler CA, Dean JG, Kempe CH: Prediction and prevention of child abuse. Semin Perinatol 3(1):85–90, 1979.

96. McCauley K: Preventing child abuse through the schools. Children Today 21:8–10, 1992.

97. Showers J: "Don't shake the baby": The effectiveness of a prevention program. Child Abuse Negl 16:11–18, 1992.

Pediatric Vertebral Column and Spinal Cord Injuries

DACHLING PANG ■ PETER P. SUN

Injuries to the spinal cord and vertebral column are relatively uncommon in the pediatric age range from birth to 17 years. The incidence is 1% to 10% of all spinal injuries.[1–13] Data from major pediatric spinal trauma centers[11, 14–20] indicate that injury to the juvenile spine differs from its adult counterpart in anatomic and biomechanical features, mechanism of injury, response to deformation, injury pattern, and outcome. Several injury types are also unique to or prevalent in children, such as spinal cord injury without radiographic abnormality (SCIWORA), pure ligamentous injuries, atlanto-occipital dislocation (AOD), and atlantoaxial rotatory fixation (AARF). Finally, special problems are encountered in immobilizing the child's inherently mobile yet fragile spinal column. This chapter deals with all these issues.

CLASSIFICATION OF INJURY TYPE

Pediatric spinal injuries are classified according to findings on plain x-ray films and computed tomography (CT). Although magnetic resonance imaging (MRI) reveals abnormalities in the soft tissues, which can be helpful in assessing stability, it is less useful in the classification of injury types. Thus, based on skeletal information alone, four injury patterns are seen in children: (1) fracture of the vertebral body or posterior elements with subluxation; (2) fracture without subluxation; (3) subluxation without fracture, that is, pure ligamentous injury; and (4) spinal cord injury (SCI) without fracture or subluxation, or SCIWORA. A rough measure of the degree of instability of the injury is implicit in this classification. Similar to the adult counterpart, fracture-subluxations in the juvenile spine are unstable, whereas fractures without subluxation may or may not be unstable, depending on the amount of ligamentous disruption. Thus, a small compression fracture of the vertebral body is stable, but an undisplaced type II odontoid fracture and some spinous process fractures may not be stable. Pure ligamentous injuries (with displacement) are, by definition, unstable, even though in some cases the instability does not

manifest until months later as a progressive kyphotic deformity. SCIWORA is associated with a kind of "radiographically occult" instability that is not demonstrable by conventional radiographs but poses a serious risk of recurrent injury to the spinal cord if no immobilization measures are taken (see later).

BIOMECHANICAL CONSIDERATIONS

In contrast to the adult spine, the juvenile vertebral column is inherently more malleable to deforming forces. This physiologic hypermobility allows considerable movement between vertebral segments without damage, but at the expense of providing less protection to the underlying spinal cord, which suffers deformation poorly. Several unique features of the juvenile spine account for this physiologic hypermobility. First, the ligaments and joint capsules are elastic and can withstand considerable stretching without tearing.[21–25] This explains the phenomenon in young children of pseudosubluxation, or seemingly "excessive" angular displacement between C2 and C3 and, to a lesser extent, C3 and C4.[21–29] Second, owing to their high water content, the intervertebral disk and annulus in children are also exceedingly expansile in the longitudinal axis, allowing the vertebral column of neonates to lengthen by as much as 2 inches without rupture when forcefully distracted.[30] Third, the facet joints are shallow and oriented more horizontally than in adults,[21, 24–26] permitting translational as well as flexion and extension movements. Fourth, the immature vertebral bodies are wedged anteriorly,[21–26] so that forward slippage between adjacent segments is enhanced. Fifth, the uncinate processes of the mature vertebral body, which normally restrict lateral and rotational movements, are absent in children younger than 10 years.[31, 32] Sixth, the biologically active and hypervascular growth zone in the end plate represents another potential site of shifting; this structurally brittle zone splits readily from the primary centrum with even moderate shearing stresses.[33] Last, the proportionally large size of the infant's head, coupled with the relatively delicate nuchal musculature, predisposes the infant's neck to wide flip-flop swings when subjected to flexion and extension forces.[34]

Dynamic radiographs show that the upper cervical segments in infants and young children are especially hypermobile in flexion and thus most susceptible to flexion injuries. The fulcrum for maximal flexion is at C2-3 in infants and young children. The horizontal orientation of the facets and the anterior wedging of the vertebral bodies are more prominent in the upper four segments of the cervical spine in this age group.[21, 23]

The atlanto-occipital articulation in neonates also allows excessive sliding movements between the occipital condyle and the lateral mass of C1, due partly to the disparate matching between a large foramen magnum and a small C1 arch, the flimsy atlanto-occipital ligaments and condylar capsules,[1] and the convexity of the articulating surfaces.[2] Moreover, the protective groove on C1 for the vertebral artery, as it winds behind the C1 articular process to enter the cranium, is so shallow in neonates that during hyperextension the artery may be crushed between the condyle and the C1 arch, as was found on postmortem angiography in some victims of sudden infant death syndrome.[35]

Many of these features of the juvenile spine transform into "adult states" around age 8 or 9 years.[21, 22, 25, 26] In particular, the vertebral bodies become less wedged and more rectangular, the facet joints deepen and become more vertical, the uncinate processes enlarge, and the ligaments gain in tensile strength. With increasing age, the head also assumes a smaller proportion of the body and thus lessens its own lever effect. With this normal transition, pseudosubluxation is seen less often,[23, 36, 37] and the fulcrum for maximal flexion shifts from the upper cervical spine to C3-4 at around age 6 years, and then to C5-6 in adolescence and early adulthood.[24, 38, 39]

The age distribution of SCIWORA lesions[11, 14, 18, 27, 34, 40] suggests that this biomechanical maturation takes place much more abruptly and successfully in the upper cervical segments, so that the upper neck, although vulnerable to flexion forces before the age of 8 years, becomes much more resistant to injury shortly afterward. The lower cervical spine, in contrast, seems to mature more gradually; lower cervical injuries occur with relatively equal frequency from birth to 16 years, even though the serious lower cervical cord injuries tend to be more prevalent in younger age groups.

The preceding biomechanical data form the pathophysiologic basis of pediatric spinal cord and vertebral column injuries. Four basic premises can be deduced from these data: (1) a malleable vertebral column with elastic (stretchable) ligaments is less likely to sustain bony breakage and frank rupture of ligaments when subjected to deforming forces; (2) a malleable vertebral column permits more intervertebral displacement in the presence of external stresses and affords less protection to the underlying spinal cord, making it possible for the cord to be damaged without evidence of fracture or malalignment; (3) a more adult-like vertebral column with a sturdier osseoligamentous constitution provides better protection for the spinal cord; and (4) the adult constitution is much less yielding to deforming forces and is therefore more likely to suffer bony breakage and frank ligamentous rupture when subjected to high stresses.

Based on these premises, the following clinicopathologic predictions can be made: (1) in the younger age group (birth to 8 years), there should be fewer fractures and subluxations and more SCIWORA; (2) SCI in young children should be more severe than in older children (9 to 16 years); (3) because the upper cervical spine is inherently more unstable in the younger age group, there should be more upper cervical injuries, and most of these should be associated with severe cord damage but minimal bony injuries; (4) in the older age group, there should be more fractures and subluxations than SCIWORA; (5) SCI in the older age group from whatever mechanism should be less severe than in the younger age group; and (6) the distribution of spinal injuries among older children should more closely resemble the adult pattern, with a preponderance of lower cervical injuries. Data from large clinical series of pediatric spinal injuries bear out these predictions.

CLINICAL CHARACTERISTICS OF PEDIATRIC SPINAL INJURIES

Epidemiology

There is a seasonal peak for all categories of pediatric spinal injuries from June to September, owing to the increase in extracurricular activities during the summer break from school. The only other solitary peak in the otherwise smooth distribution curve is in the 2 weeks around the Christmas holiday.[17]

The cause of injury varies with age (Table 226–1). In the younger age group (0 to 9 years), the two predominant causes of injury are pedestrian-versus-vehicle accidents and falls, together accounting for more than 75% of the injuries.[14, 16, 37] In the intermediate age group (10 to 14 years), motor vehicle accidents, including motorcycle crashes, account for 40%, and falls and pedestrian accidents become less prevalent. This reflects the increasing role of older children as illegal drivers. In the late adolescent group (15 to 17 years), motor vehicle and motorcycle accidents become the leading cause of injury (>70%), and sports accidents also rise in number.[14, 16–18, 37] In keeping with these statistics, injuries in the 0- to 9-year age group tend to occur at or near home, such as the basement steps, upstairs window ledges, and local playgrounds. Older children and adolescents are more likely to sustain injuries at a greater distance from home.[17]

The male-female ratio in pediatric spinal injuries varies with age, which may indirectly reflect gender differences in injury-prone activities in the different age brackets. The boy-girl ratio is smallest in the 0- to 9-year group (1.1 to 1.3:1),[14, 16, 18] because pedestrian accidents affect both sexes equally, and boys are slightly more susceptible to falls. The ratio increases marginally in the 10- to 14-year group but markedly in

TABLE 226-1 ■ Cause of Spinal Injury Related to Age in 296 Children

CAUSE OF INJURY	NO. OF PATIENTS	NO. OF PATIENTS (%), BY AGE		
		0–9 yr	10–14 yr	15–17 yr
Motor vehicle accident	138	5 (14)	24 (32)	109 (59)
Fall	39	14 (38)	13 (18)	12 (7)
Pedestrian–motor vehicle accident	26	14 (38)	6 (8)	6 (3)
Sports activity	46	2 (5)	14 (19)	30 (16)
Motorbike accident	20	0	6 (8)	14 (8)
Miscellaneous (bicycle-, diving-related, etc.)	27	2 (5)	11 (15)	14 (8)
Total no. of patients	296	37	74	185

Data from Hadley MN, Zabramski JM, Browner CM, et al: Pediatric spinal trauma: Review of 122 cases of spinal cord and vertebral column injuries. J Neurosurg 68:18–24, 1988; and Hamilton MG, Myles ST: Pediatric spinal injury: Review of 174 hospital admissions. J Neurosurg 77:700–704, 1992.

the 15- to 17-year age group (2.3 to 2.5:1),[14, 16, 18] when aggressive sports and reckless driving are signatures of adolescent masculine behavior.

Age and Injury Pattern

In most series of pediatric spinal trauma,[14, 16–18, 37] the cases are split evenly between those with SCI and those who are neurologically intact. Among the SCI group (50% of the total), almost one third are complete cord injuries (Frankel grade A)[41] and two thirds are incomplete cord injuries of varying severity (Frankel grades B to D). Also, about 30% to 40% of the SCI patients have SCIWORA,[14, 16, 18] although the reported incidence of SCIWORA among children with traumatic myelopathy varies widely from 5% to 67%,[1–3, 7, 11, 12, 14, 18, 27, 42–46] depending on the availability of diagnostic tests and the awareness of this syndrome in the local medical community.

The patient's age profoundly affects the injury pattern. There is a significantly higher incidence of neurological injury in the 0- to 9-year group compared with the 10- to 17-year group. Among SCI patients, younger children are also much more likely to sustain complete (Frankel grade A) and severe (Frankel grades B and C) cord injuries than are older children.[14, 16] These trends reflect the inadequacy of the immature vertebral column as protector of the spinal cord. In addition, there are more SCIWORA and pure ligamentous injuries in the 0- to 9-year group than in the 15- to 17-year group and, conversely, more fracture-subluxations in the 10-

to 17-year group (Table 226–2).[14, 16, 18, 22] In several studies, the incidence of cervical spine fractures is 20% to 25% in the 0- to 8-year age range, versus 70% to 80% in children older than 13 years.[6, 16, 17] These statistics are also a reflection of the suppleness of the younger spine and its ability to yield without breakage against deforming forces, in contrast to the more "brittle" consistency of the adult-like spine in older children.

Besides the age factor, the degree of neurological compromise also correlates with the presence of subluxation. Children with only fractures tend to have fewer neurological injuries (20% to 25%) than do those with fracture-subluxations or subluxations without fracture (>50%).[14]

Age and Injury Site

The majority of spinal cord and vertebral column injuries in children occur in the cervical region. Osenbach and Menezes reported that all pure ligamentous injuries, 76% of SCIWORA, and 70% of fracture-subluxations are in the cervical spine.[18] Kewalramani and colleagues also found that 76% of pediatric SCIs are in the cervical spinal cord and only 24% are in the thoracic cord and conus.[7, 8]

The patient's age is a strong determinant of the injury site, as predicted by the developmental changes in biomechanics (Table 226–3). Upper cervical and craniovertebral junction injuries are two to three times as frequent in children younger than 3 years[14, 18, 47] because of the extreme hypermobility at these joints in

TABLE 226-2 ■ Type of Spinal Injury Related to Age in 296 Children

AGE (YR)	NO. OF PATIENTS	TYPE OF INJURY, NO. OF PATIENTS (%)			
		Fracture Only	Fracture Subluxation	Subluxation Only	SCIWORA
0–9	37	9 (24)	8 (21)	6 (16)	14 (39)
10–17	259	137 (53)	83 (32)	11 (4)	28 (11)
Total no. of patients	296	146	91	17	42

SCIWORA, spinal cord injury without radiographic abnormality.
Data from Hadley MN, Zabramski JM, Browner CM, et al: Pediatric spinal trauma: Review of 122 cases of spinal cord and vertebral column injuries. J Neurosurg 68:18–24, 1988; and Hamilton MG, Myles ST: Pediatric spinal injury: Review of 174 hospital admissions. J Neurosurg 77:700–704, 1992.

TABLE 226–3 ▪ **Level of Injury Related to Patient's Age in 301 Children**

LEVEL OF INJURY	AGE GROUP, NO. OF PATIENTS (%)	
	0–9 yr	10–16 yr
Upper cervical (to C3)	42 (53)	47 (21)
Lower cervical (C4-7)	20 (25)	76 (34)
Thoracic	8 (10)	26 (11)
Thoracolumbar	4 (5)	37 (18)
Lumbar	6 (7)	35 (16)
Total no. of patients	80	221

Data from Hadley MN, Zabramski JM, Browner CM, et al: Pediatric spinal trauma: Review of 122 cases of spinal cord and vertebral column injuries. J Neurosurg 68:18–24, 1988; and Osenbach RK, Menezes AH: Pediatric spinal cord and vertebral column injury. Neurosurgery 30:385–390, 1992.

this age group. Lower cervical and thoracic injuries occur with equal frequency in both the 0- to 9-year group and the 10- to 17-year group, because maturation at these joints occurs much more gradually than at the upper cervical articulations.[18, 27] Thoracolumbar and lumbar injuries are primarily lesions of adolescence.

Finally, multiple noncontiguous spinal injuries are found in 10% to 16% of cases,[14, 16] emphasizing the need to survey the entire vertebral column carefully in every injured child.

TREATMENT

The same general principles that apply to adults also apply to children regarding the assignment of instability, fracture reduction, spinal immobilization, and surgical fusion. Early surgical intervention is seldom mandated after the fracture has been reduced and the spine immobilized. The only undisputed indication for emergency surgery is progressive neurological deterioration due to either an irreducible subluxation, in which case open reduction and fixation are necessary, or cord compression by a hematoma, extruded disk, or bony fragments, for which decompression and simultaneous fusion are recommended. These circumstances are quite rare in children. In the majority of cases, nonoperative management is the rule for at least the first few days, during which the cord edema may resolve, serious extraneural injuries are dealt with, and the general prognosis is clarified. Thereafter, the indications for delayed surgery include irreducible fracture-subluxations, markedly unstable fractures, and pure ligamentous instability (see later).[14, 16, 29, 48–50] The specific treatment varies with the injury type. SCIWORA is, by definition, not associated with overt instability and requires only external immobilization.[27, 51]

Among upper cervical spine injuries, such as epiphysiolysis of the odontoid process, hangman's fracture, C2-3 subluxation, AOD, and AARF, all but the last probably require internal fixation. Among lower cervical injuries, most fracture-subluxations and tear-drop fractures are extremely unstable and require surgical fusion. Burst fractures with compromise of the spinal canal should have an anterior corpectomy and strut graft fusion reinforced with an anterior cervical plate. Most simple compression body fractures without significant loss of vertebral height, as well as uncomplicated spinous process fractures ("clay shuffler's" fractures), are stable and can be treated with an external orthosis. On the whole, about 25% to 30% of all pediatric spinal injuries require surgical treatment. About 60% of the fracture-subluxations are surgically fused, whereas only 10% to 15% of patients with fracture but no subluxation require fusion.[14, 16, 18] Most pure ligamentous injuries should probably be treated with internal fixation, because ligaments tend to heal poorly with just immobilization.[18] The management details and fusion techniques for specific injury types are discussed later in separate sections.

OUTCOME

In one large review, the mortality rate for pediatric spinal injury was 28%.[15] This is astounding when compared with an 11% mortality for adult spinal injury during the same study period. The majority of these pediatric deaths occurred at the accident scene and were invariably associated with unsalvageable multiorgan injuries. Only a small number of deaths were directly attributable to the SCI, all of which involved the upper cervical cord and had fatal cardiorespiratory complications. The study predicted that the mortality of pediatric spinal injury will not be influenced significantly by changes in treatment strategy, and injury prevention is still the most effective way to improve survival.[15, 52]

In spite of the high mortality, children who survive have a good prognosis for neurological improvement.[14, 16, 18, 50, 53, 54] The sole determinant of functional outcome is the initial neurological status. In the majority of patients with complete cord syndrome at admission, the injury remains complete; only 5% to 10% show some improvement, and virtually none make a full recovery.[5, 16–18, 27] Patients with severe cord injuries also tend to remain severely impaired. However, significant improvement is expected in those with mild to moderate cord injuries; 75% to 85% of these patients improve by one to two Frankel grades, and more than half of these patients enjoy a full recovery.[5, 16] The good outcome in pediatric SCI may be related to the enhanced plasticity of the young nervous system.

SPECIAL INJURY TYPES

SCIWORA

The acronym SCIWORA was first coined and described as a distinct syndrome by Pang and Wilberger[34] in 1982. Children with SCIWORA suffer a traumatic myelopathy without identifiable fracture or subluxation on plain spine films, tomography, and CT. Increasing recognition of this entity over the past decade has accrued a large pool of clinical data.[7, 14, 16–18, 27, 47]

BIOMECHANICS AND MECHANISMS OF SPINAL CORD INJURY

The pathogenetic concept of SCIWORA is based on the premise that the inherently elastic juvenile spine can accommodate considerable intersegmental displacement without fracture or ligamentous rupture, but at the sacrifice of the underlying spinal cord. Four mechanisms may be involved in the pathogenesis: hyperextension, flexion, distraction, and spinal cord ischemia.

Hyperextension of the cervical spine forces the interlaminar ligaments to bulge forward into the spinal canal and may cause up to 50% narrowing of the canal diameter.[55, 56] In addition, the cord thickens as it shortens during hyperextension.[57] Thus the space available for the cervical cord within the canal is reduced during moderate hyperextension. During violent hyperextension, Taylor and Blackwood[56] and Bourmer[58] demonstrated rupture of the anterior longitudinal ligament, shearing of the intervertebral disk from the end plates, and retrodisplacement of the upper vertebra. Dynamic radiography on fresh cadavers showed that elastic recoil of the displaced segment could bring about perfect spontaneous reduction to give a normal radiographic appearance.[59] With its elastic constituents, the juvenile spine is especially susceptible to this sequence of momentary dislocation and spontaneous reduction. Intersegmental movement in children is further facilitated by their horizontal facet joints,[21, 23–26, 32] and the immature vertebral body splits readily from its end plate within the brittle growth zone and leaves no radiographic trace.[33] The elastic elements,[21, 32, 60] horizontal facets,[21, 24–26] wedge-shaped bodies,[21, 23] and absence of uncinate processes likewise predispose the juvenile spine to hyperflexion myelopathy.[31, 32]

The spines of infants and young children are also uniquely vulnerable to distraction.[42, 61] Leventhal found that although the elastic spinal column of neonatal cadavers could be stretched up to 2 inches without structural damage, the inelastic spinal cord ruptures if stretched more than 0.25 inch.[62] The clinical counterpart of Leventhal's study is the finding of frank rupture of the cord and meninges within a completely intact vertebral column in infants who had undergone forceful breech extraction.[24, 63] In nonobstetric SCIWORA, the best evidence of distraction is found in cases when the thoracic spine is forcefully distracted in lap-belt injuries. Rupture of the dura and spinal cord in these patients is evidenced by the resultant cerebrospinal fluid–pleural fistula.[64] Finally, the precarious architecture of the neonatal atlanto-occipital articulations predisposes the upper cervical cord to ischemic necrosis from vertebral artery occlusion.

THE AGE FACTOR

As predicted by the biomechanics, age influences SCIWORA in three ways. First, many studies[14, 44, 46, 65] have shown that the incidence of SCIWORA is higher than that of other injury types among young children (0 to 9 years) with traumatic myelopathy, and vice versa in older children (Fig. 226–1). Second, young

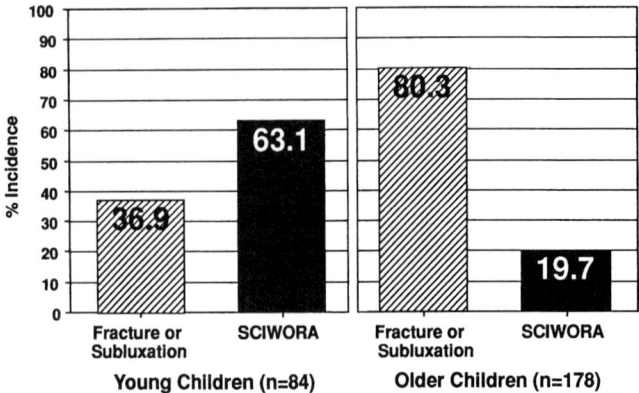

FIGURE 226–1. The incidence of spinal cord injury without radiographic abnormality (SCIWORA) versus overt spinal column injury in children with traumatic myelopathy as a function of age. "Young" children are those younger than 9 years or 10 years. (Data from references 14, 37, 40, 44, 188, 229.)

patients with SCIWORA typically have more severe neurological injuries than do their older counterparts (Fig. 226–2).[5, 46] In our own series, 21 of 30 children younger than 8 years suffered complete or severe injuries, compared with only 1 of 25 children older than 8 years ($P < .000001$).[27] Similarly, Osenbach and Menezes noted severe (Frankel grades B and C) injuries in 21 of 22 patients younger than 9 years, versus comparable injury severity in only 1 of 9 older children.[18] Severe SCI in older children is more typically associated with vertebral column disruption[14] rather than SCIWORA. Third, several studies have shown that young children are far more prone to upper cervical SCIWORA, whereas lower cervical lesions occur more often in older children. In our series, 9 of 10 upper cervical injuries occurred in children younger than 8 years, compared with 21 of 33 lower cervical injuries in older children (Fig. 226–3).[27] In the series of Osenbach and Menezes, all seven nonobstetric upper cervical injuries occurred in children younger than 9 years.[18] Unlike cervical lesions, SCIWORA involving the thoracic cord

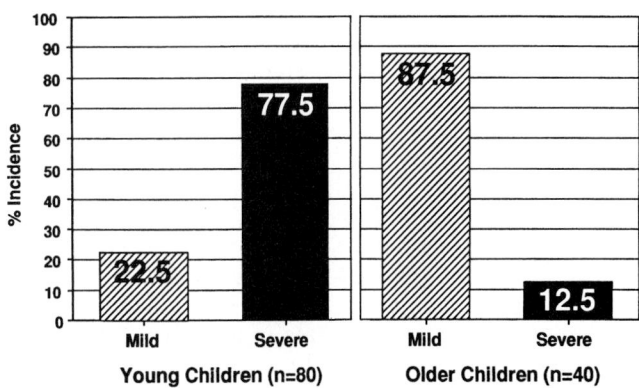

FIGURE 226–2. The severity of neurological injury in children with spinal cord injury without radiographic abnormality (SCIWORA) as a function of age. "Young" children are those younger than 9 years. (Data from references 3, 18, 31, 44, 46, 188.)

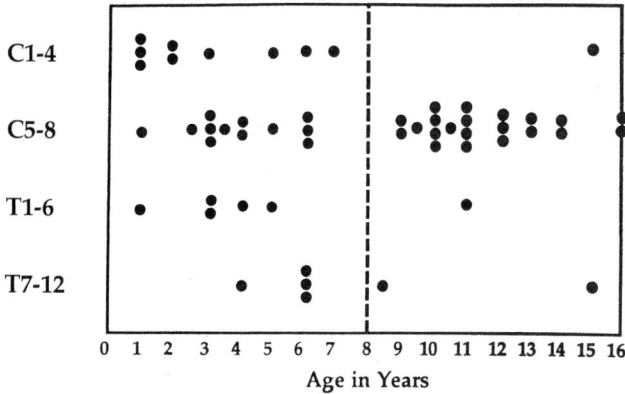

C1-4

C5-8

T1-6

T7-12

0 1 2 3 4 5 6 7 8 9 10 11 12 13 14 15 16

Age in Years

FIGURE 226–3. Correlation between patient's age and level of neurological injury in spinal cord injury without radiographic abnormality (SCIWORA). The *vertical dotted line* denotes the age (8 years) at which physiologic properties of the juvenile spine change. The upper cervical spine was most prone to injury in infants and young children, whereas the lower cervical spine was at risk in all ages up to 16 years.

is distributed evenly over the pediatric age range, with no age predilection.[18, 27, 46] Thus, because young children tend to have upper cord injuries, and most of these are complete or near complete, the rehabilitation potential of this age group is very limited, and the socioeconomic burden is accordingly prohibitive.

RADIOGRAPHICALLY OCCULT INSTABILITY

It is important to distinguish between radiographically occult instability in SCIWORA and overt instability seen in fracture-subluxation and subluxation without fracture (pure ligamentous injury). In SCIWORA, the spinal cord is injured without radiographic evidence of a fracture or subluxation that would indicate extensive ligamentous tear and gross instability. Yet there had to have been sufficient bony displacement at impact to inflict damage to the cord. This implies that the stabilizing ligaments and fibrocartilaginous structures, although sufficiently elastic to stretch and recoil without rupturing, may have been severely sprained or even partially torn to render the involved vertebral segments vulnerable to *repeated* stress. The resulting instability or biomechanically precarious state is therefore "occult" rather than overt.[20, 21, 24–27, 33] The fact that flexion-extension radiographs fail to disclose abnormal movements in SCIWORA does not argue against the existence of occult instability, because even gross instability can be masked by muscle spasm.[37] Later, when spasms have subsided, motion studies executed with deliberate caution cannot compare with the random and unguarded neck movements in real-life activities. It is therefore not surprising that post-SCIWORA dynamic films do not reveal the precarious state of the injured segments but do disclose overt instability.[27]

Until the advent of MRI, the existence of occult instability in SCIWORA was unproved although strongly suggested by two phenomena: delayed neurological deterioration and recurrent SCIWORA. In a number of children with SCIWORA, neurological deficits are not detectable immediately after trauma but develop and worsen after a latent period of 30 minutes to 4 days, apparently in the absence of further trauma.[27, 40, 43, 66–68] The mechanism of this delayed deterioration remains speculative. A few cases may result from post-traumatic occlusion of radicular arteries due to thrombosis or spasm, with subsequent delayed infarction of the cord,[43, 66] but this must be rare. The majority of cases probably result from repeated "punch-drunk" trauma to the cord during the latent period. This presumption is supported by two observations. First, many of these children recall transient neurological symptoms at the time of the initial trauma, such as subjective weakness, acroparesthesia, or Lhermitte's phenomenon, indicating that the cord had been distracted or hit by the supporting structures during the intersegmental displacement. This displacement may well have overstretched or partially torn crucial ligaments, rendering the segments susceptible to repeated shifts during otherwise innocuous neck movements. Second, the incidence of delayed deterioration at our institution has decreased dramatically (13 of 24 cases treated before 1982,[34] versus 2 of 33 since 1982[27]), owing to the rigorous implementation of prompt neck immobilization and neurosurgical referral for any child with neck pain and transient neurological symptoms. Many of these children have been found to have subtle neurological deficits that could easily have been missed on cursory examination, or they show evidence of myelopathy on somatosensory evoked potential testing. Such patients would presumably have been at risk for reinjury (i.e., delayed deterioration) if they had not been immobilized expeditiously.

The phenomenon of delayed neurological deterioration in SCIWORA suggests that the spinal column has been weakened temporarily by the impact, even if the initial neurological symptoms are mild. This concept of a postimpact period of vulnerability is supported by the phenomenon of recurrent SCIWORA, noted up to 10 weeks after initial SCIWORA in 8 of 42 children treated before 1986.[69] Before 1986, it had been our practice to immobilize children in hard collars for 2 months after SCIWORA. Four of the children with recurrent SCIWORA had removed their hard collars and were reinjured while engaging in forbidden sports such as wrestling, gymnastics, or basketball. The others were reinjured while wearing their collars. The neurological deficits resulting from the recurrent SCIWORA were much worse than those of the initial trauma, which in all cases were mild.[69] It is noteworthy that none of these children had overt instability on dynamic radiographs either at the first SCIWORA or at the time of reinjury. These normal studies belie the precarious state of the "once touched" spinal cord when the unprotected neck is subjected to the erratic motions of a child at play.

MAGNETIC RESONANCE IMAGING FINDINGS

The discovery of MRI abnormalities in the soft tissues of the spine represents the first direct evidence of occult ligamentous damage in SCIWORA.[70] These abnormalities are *extraneural,* involving mainly ligaments and intervertebral disks, and *neural,* involving the cord itself.

Extraneural Abnormalities

The extraneural soft tissue injury demonstrated on MRI is well correlated with the mechanism of injury.[70] For example, rupture of the anterior longitudinal ligament, seen as a loss of continuity of the low-signal prevertebral line, widening of the anterior intervertebral space, and anterior disk herniation (Fig. 226–4), is found in cases of hyperextension. Rupture of the posterior longitudinal ligament, seen as a loss of continuity of the retrovertebral line and small posterior disk herniation (Fig. 226–5), is correlated with hyperflexion. Intradiskal hemorrhages are seen when a translational interbody shearing mechanism is suspected. Tectorial membrane hemorrhage (tear) has been associated with the violent shaking of child abuse (Fig. 226–6), and hemorrhages in the interspinous and interlaminar ligaments are seen with distraction injury. Further, the level of these soft tissue injuries corresponds exactly to the level of the neurological lesion.[19]

These extraneural MRI findings strongly support the hypothesis that SCIWORA is associated with spraining or partial tearing of crucial stabilizing structures of the vertebral column.[19, 27] For years, these ligamentous and diskal injuries, which are responsible for the post-SCIWORA vulnerable period, had escaped detection

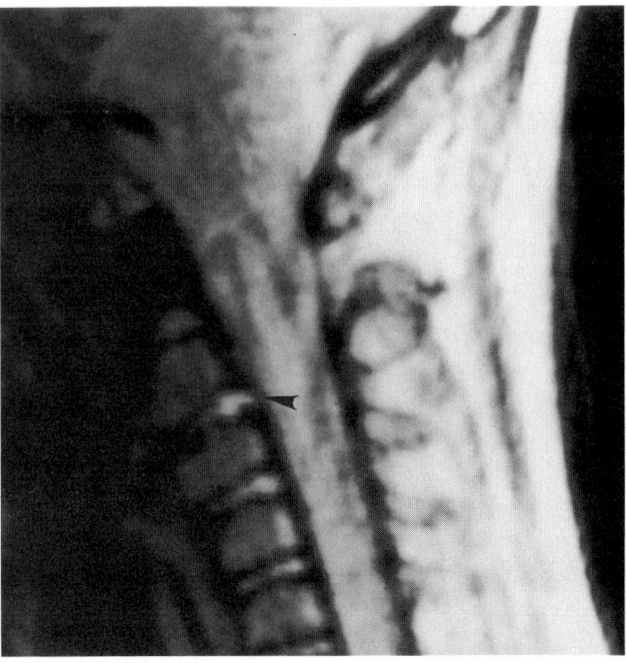

FIGURE 226–5. A 9-year-old boy sustained a lateral flexion injury and had complete Brown-Séquard syndrome at presentation. Sagittal long TR (TR, 4000; TE, 18) magnetic resonance imaging scan shows interruption of the retrovertebral line of signal void, suggesting a disrupted posterior longitudinal ligament and C2-3 disk herniation *(arrowhead).*

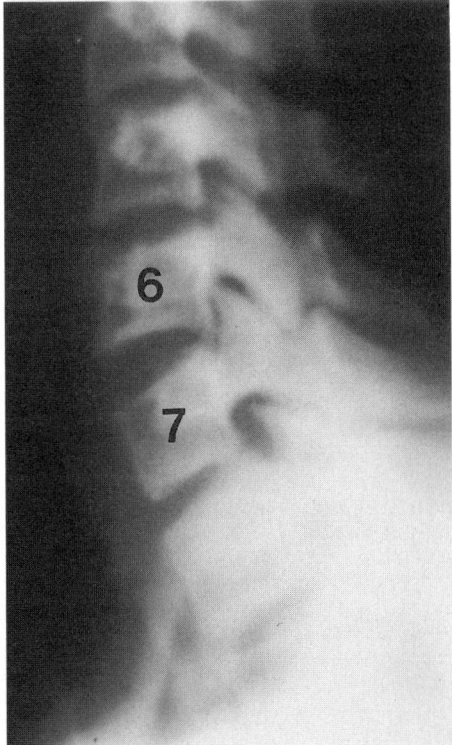

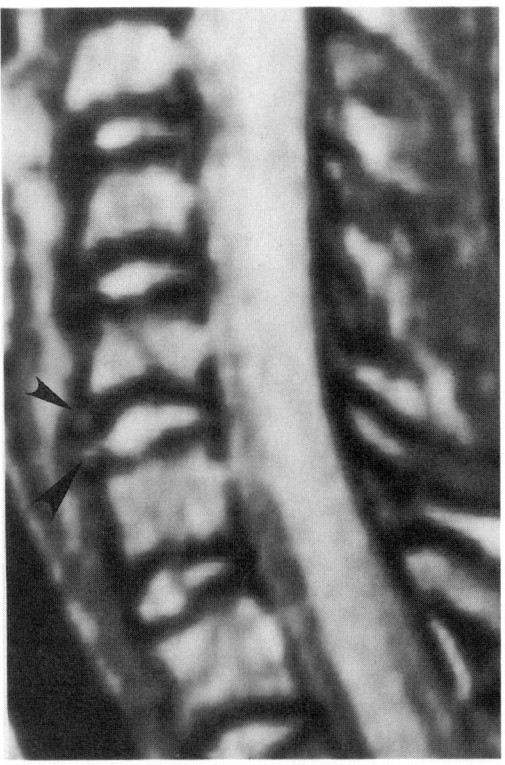

FIGURE 226–4. A 13-year-old girl who had mild partial C7 myelopathy after a hyperextension injury. *Left,* Plain film reveals sight separation of the disk space at C6-7. *Right,* Sagittal magnetic resonance imaging scan (TR, 2200; TE, 30) obtained 3 days after injury shows discontinuity of the prevertebral line of signal void, suggesting an anterior longitudinal ligament tear, anterior C6-7 disk herniation *(large arrowhead),* and possible end plate separation *(small arrowhead).*

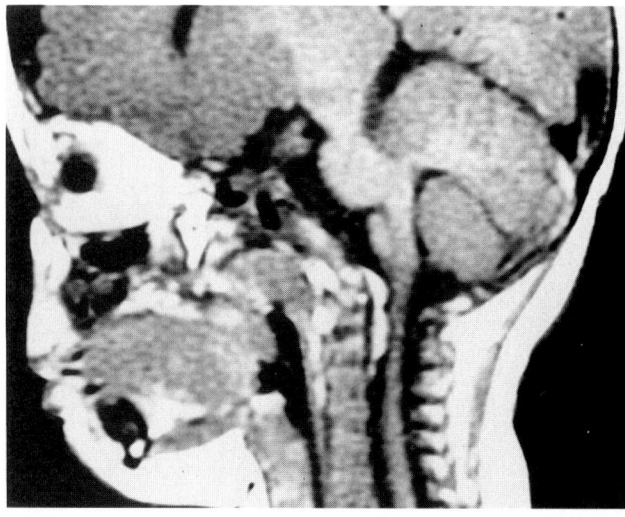

FIGURE 226–6. Sagittal magnetic resonance imaging scan in an infant with tectorial membrane tear resulting from whiplash-shake syndrome, seen as a subacute hemorrhage (hyperintense on short TR) within the soft tissue behind the odontoid process.

by conventional radiology but are now "exposed" by MRI. The continued use of MRI is expected to reveal more information about SCIWORA.

The signal characteristics of hemorrhage within non-neural tissues are detectable within hours of the injury on T1-weighted images as lines of hyperintensity, because extravasated blood is converted within hours into methemoglobin (MHb) in non-neural tissues, versus days to weeks in neural tissues (see later).[4, 30, 71, 72] Extraneural injuries in SCIWORA can thus be diagnosed by MRI within hours after the injury. The problem is that the adjacent fascial, muscular, and fat planes also produce high signals and can overwhelm small streaks of MHb. The use of fat-suppression sequences reduces the high signal of fat but not blood on short relaxation time (TR) (T1-weighted) images and is effective in highlighting the soft tissue hemorrhages in SCIWORA.

Neural Abnormalities

The MRI abnormalities seen within the traumatized spinal cord correspond to the signal characteristics of the various metabolized forms of extravasated hemoglobin (Table 226–4). Fresh blood from spinal cord hemorrhage contains intracellular oxyhemoglobin, which rapidly converts to deoxyhemoglobin (DHb) within 3 hours. DHb is a stable intracellular compound and appears hypointense on long TR (T2-weighted) images.[4, 10, 30, 71, 73] Gradient-echo techniques, which are particularly sensitive to paramagnetic substances such as DHb, detect acute hemorrhage even better than do standard long TR sequences.[12, 30, 71, 73, 74] Oxidation of intracellular DHb to MHb begins after approximately 3 days, although DHb may still be detectable up to 8 days after injury, especially in larger hematomas. Intracellular MHb is hyperintense on short TR images but hypointense on long TR images, whereas extracellular MHb appears hyperintense on both short and long TR images. Subsequent hemolysis around day 7 liberates MHb into extracellular tissues, where it may persist for months. Extracellular MHb is finally converted to hemosiderin following phagocytosis; this substance, which may persist for life, is markedly hypointense on long TR images and slightly hypointense on short TR images.[73] The larger the hemorrhage, the longer it takes for all the DHb to be converted to MHb and ultimately for MHb to become hemosiderin. Signal characteristics are thus dependent not only on the time elapsed since injury but also on hematoma size.

Five patterns of parenchymal (cord) findings are seen on the post-SCIWORA MRI scan.[70] (1) Complete disruption of the spinal cord is seen in severe distraction injuries in very young children (Fig. 226–7). This is usually accompanied by hypointensities on gradient-echo sequences (DHb) of the rostral cord stump. The common sites of cord disruption are the upper cervical and upper thoracic levels. Severe flexion injury occasionally produces a similar picture. (2) Major cord hemorrhage occurs when more than 50% of the cross-sectional area of the cord on axial MRI shows evidence of extravasated hemoglobin (Fig. 226–8). Depending on

T A B L E   2 2 6 – 4 ■ **Magnetic Resonance Imaging Signal Alterations in Spinal Cord Injury as a Function of the Chemical State of Blood**

CHEMICAL STATE OF BLOOD	AGE OF BLOOD AFTER INJURY (INTRAMEDULLARY)	AGE OF BLOOD AFTER INJURY (EXTRANEURAL)	MAGNETIC RESONANCE IMAGING APPEARANCE (GRADIENT ECHO)	MAGNETIC RESONANCE IMAGING APPEARANCE, SHORT REPETITION TIME (T1-WEIGHTED)	MAGNETIC RESONANCE IMAGING APPEARANCE, LONG REPETITION TIME (T2-WEIGHTED)
Oxyhemoglobin	0–3 hr	Minutes	?	Isointense	Isointense
Deoxyhemoglobin	2 hr–8 days	Minutes to 1 hr	Hypodense	Isointense to slightly hypointense	Hypointense
Intracellular methemoglobin	3–12 days	1–2 hr	?	Hyperintense	Hypointense
Extracellular methemoglobin	7 days–months	After 2 hr	?	Hyperintense	Hyperintense
Hemosiderin	Weeks to years	NA	?	Slightly hypointense	Very hypointense
Edema*	Hours to weeks	NA	Slightly hyperintense	Isointense	Very hyperintense

* Edema is not a chemical state of blood but often is a concomitant pathologic finding in cord injury.
?, no consensus as to the magnetic resonance imaging appearance with gradient echo; NA, not applicable.

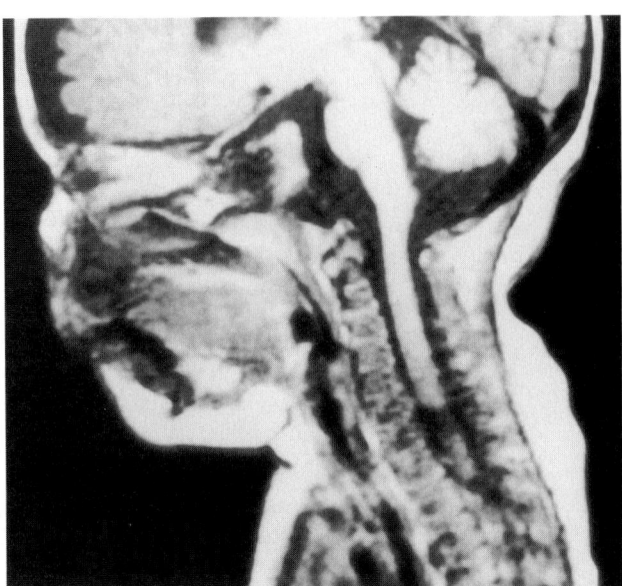

FIGURE 226–7. A 2-month-old with a complete C6 injury subsequent to a motor vehicle accident. Sagittal short TR (TR, 800; TE, 30) magnetic resonance imaging scan obtained 6 days after injury shows loss of cord continuity consistent with cord transection.

the timing of the MRI, the signal characteristics may be those of DHb, intracellular or extracellular MHb, or hemosiderin. This pattern is associated with severe neural deficits and a dismal prognosis. (3) Minor cord hemorrhage occurs when less than 50% of the cross-sectional area of the cord shows evidence of hemorrhage. It is associated with moderately severe initial deficits but a decent chance for recovery. (4) Edema only, without hemorrhage, is noted if the T1-weighted image shows iso- or slight hypointensity but the T2-weighted image is intensely bright. No stage of hemoglobin metabolism produces this pattern of signal characteristics. Edema is predictive of a good outcome. (5) Approximately 25% of patients with clinically proven SCIWORA do not have MRI abnormalities in their spinal cords. These patients have an excellent prognosis for complete recovery (authors' unpublished data).

It is our policy to repeat the MRI on days 6 to 9 after the injury, regardless of whether the acute MRI (on days 0 to 3) was abnormal. Edema takes 3 to 4 hours to develop, and small dots of DHb may not be easily detectable until it is converted to MHb, when the contrast between spinal cord and hemoglobin is greater. If the initial MRI is abnormal, a chronic study at 3 to 6 months is obtained to detect syrinx formation and marked atrophy of the cord.

THORACOLUMBAR SCIWORA

About 15% of SCIWORA involves the thoracic cord. SCIWORA of the thoracic spine typically involves violent trauma, such as high-speed automobile accidents or crushing injuries.[3, 18, 42, 44, 46, 61, 64, 67, 68, 75–78] Accordingly, these patients have a high incidence of associated tho-

racic, abdominal, and pelvic injuries. Two discrete subgroups of thoracic SCIWORA are encountered. One subgroup comprises children who sustain severe distraction injuries related to lap seat belts and high-speed vehicular collisions.[64] CT–myelography frequently shows spinal cord and dural rupture and free flow of contrast into the mediastinum.[25, 42, 75, 76] The splinting effect of the rib cage normally protects the thoracic spine against horizontal displacement due to flexion and extension forces. However, because the sternocostal joints normally permit a fair amount of "bucket-handle" movements, the rib cage provides little protection against longitudinal distraction. The mechanisms postulated for lap-belt injuries all involve a component of forceful distraction generated by the forward propulsion of the upper chest while the pelvis is harnessed by the lap belt. The elasticity of the juvenile spinal column far exceeds that of the spinal cord and dura[62]; the bony column recoils like a spring to restore normal configuration after having stretched enough to allow rupture of the cord and dura. As with upper cervical SCIWORA, thoracic SCIWORA from distraction occurs almost exclusively in children younger than 8 years. In older patients, fractures, dislocations, or both are more typical with such severe stresses.[64]

A second subgroup of thoracic SCIWORA comprises children who are crushed by slow-moving vehicles.[3, 27] Such thoracic crushing almost invariably leaves tire marks on the child's back, in addition to causing concomitant retroperitoneal injuries. In contrast, children with tire marks on the abdomen or anterior chest typically suffer intraperitoneal injuries but rarely SCI. It is postulated that in the group with ventral tire marks, the thoracic spinal column is buttressed by the ground at the time of the crush and is thus protected against excessive intersegmental displacement; the abdominal viscera bear the brunt of the injury. In the group with dorsal tire marks, the spinal column is hyperextended into the chest and abdominal cavities, thus causing hyperextension cord injury and rupture of retroperitoneal organs while sparing the well-protected intraperitoneal contents.

MANAGEMENT

The initial management of a child with a presumed SCI begins in the field (Fig. 226–9). Patients with symptoms or a mechanism of injury compatible with SCI should be immobilized supine in a hard collar and on a fracture board. If the child's head is large, the body from the shoulders down is propped up with folded blankets or foam sheets to prevent forced flexion of the neck.

When possible, a careful history is obtained from the patient or eyewitnesses to determine the cause and mechanism of injury. In addition, an interpretation of the associated non-neural injuries frequently gives clues to the mechanism of the spinal injury. All patients receive complete cervical spine films, and a full spine survey is obtained in patients with presumed thoracic cord lesions or severe multisystem trauma. Patients with SCI but without abnormalities on plain films un-

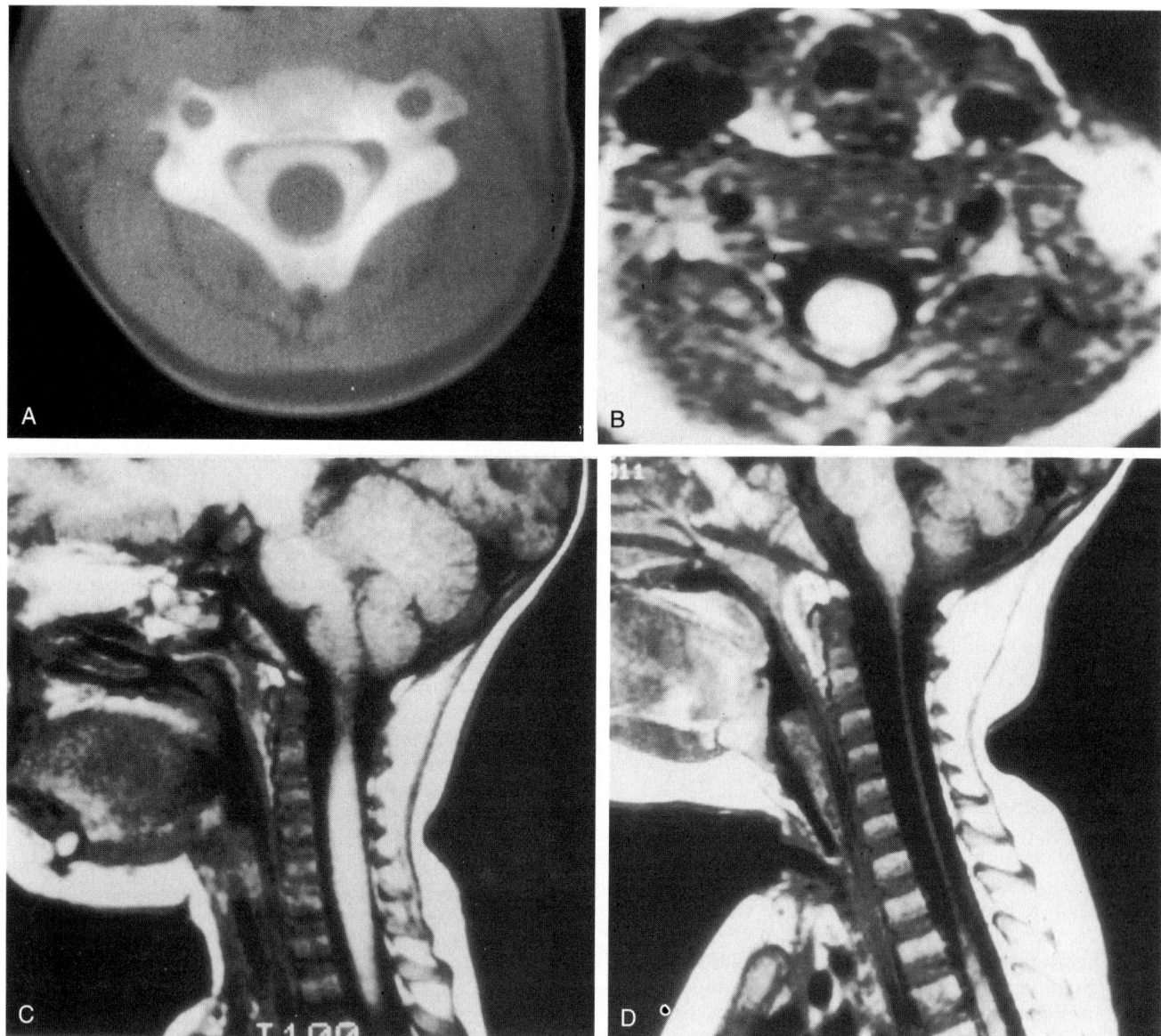

FIGURE 226–8. A 21-month-old boy who had a complete C3 injury after suffering physical abuse. *A*, Computed tomography–myelography scan obtained 15 days after injury shows marked enlargement of the cord; the cause (hemorrhage or edema) could not be discerned. *B*, Axial short TR (TR, 600; TE, 20) magnetic resonance imaging (MRI) scan obtained 16 days after injury shows intraparenchymal hyperintensity expanding and replacing the cord substance, consistent with methemoglobin. *C*, Sagittal short TR (TR, 600; TE, 20) MRI scan at day 16 shows the methemoglobin-suffused segment of the cord extending from C2 to T1. *D*, Sagittal short TR (TR, 600; TE, 20) MRI scan obtained 3 months after injury shows marked cervical cord atrophy.

dergo thin-section axial CT with bone algorithms to rule out an occult fracture at the level of the neurological lesion, followed by MRI. The radiographic evaluation is not complete until good-quality flexion and extension films of the affected area of the spine are obtained to rule out overt ligamentous instability. In many patients, severe spasm of the paraspinal muscles precludes adequate flexion for several days; in this case, the dynamic study must be repeated later.

Children with severe cord injuries diagnosed within 8 hours of the injury are begun on a 24-hour course of high-dose corticosteroids. This recommendation is based on the beneficial effects of high-dose methylprednisolone reported by the National Acute Spinal Cord Injury Study II.[79] Patients are maintained in a hard collar (for cervical SCIWORA) or on flat bed rest with log-rolling (for thoracic SCIWORA) until other serious systemic injuries have been treated. Those with cervical cord injuries are then immobilized in a Guilford brace (BA Guilford & Sons Orthotic Laboratory Ltd., Cleveland, OH) for 3 months. Thoracic lesions are treated with a thoracolumbar orthosis. Physical and occupational therapies are begun in the intensive care unit. Patients with severe residual deficits are dis-

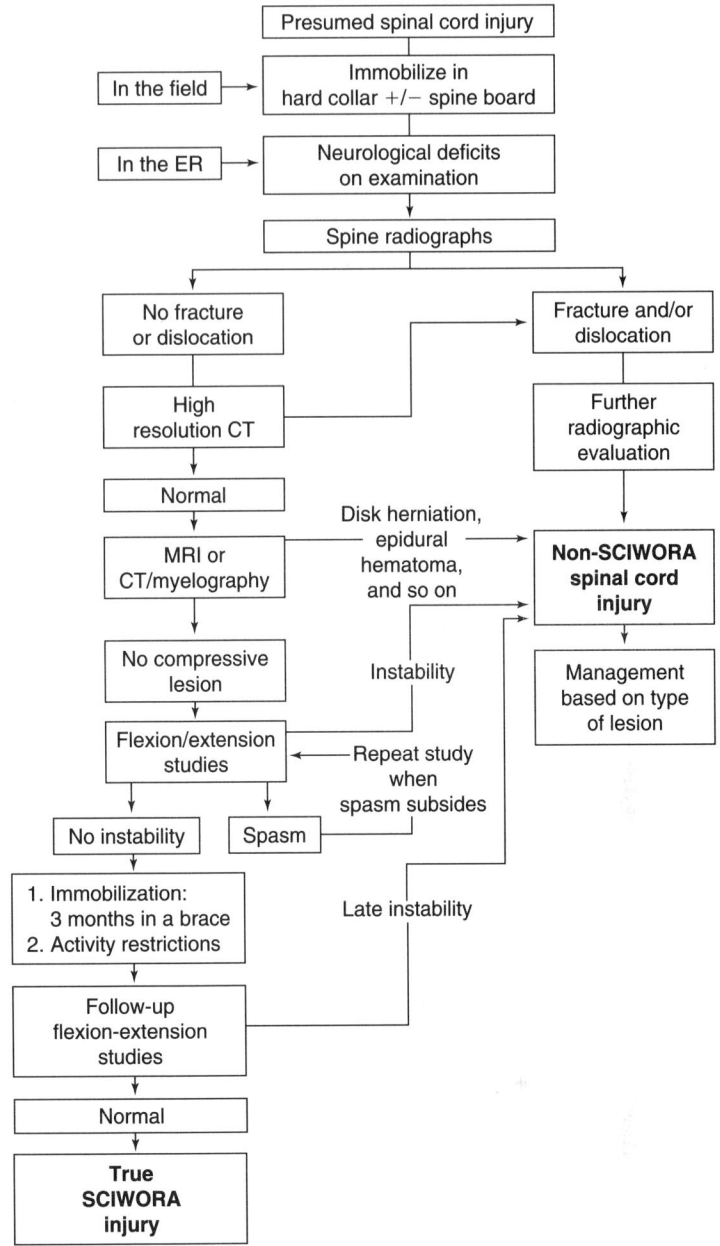

FIGURE 226–9. Management algorithm for the evaluation and treatment of children with spinal cord injuries. Emphasis is placed on our recommendations for patients with possible spinal cord injury without radiographic abnormality (SCIWORA). CT, computed tomography; ER, emergency room; MRI, magnetic resonance imaging. (Data from Pollack IF, Pang D: Spinal cord injury without radiographic abnormality [SCIWORA]. In Pang D [ed]: Disorders of the Pediatric Spine. New York, Raven Press, 1995, pp 575–604.)

charged to a rehabilitation facility when they are medically stable.

Children with mild SCIs are allowed to ambulate as soon as they are fitted with a Guilford brace or a thoracolumbar orthosis. Those with residual weakness are enrolled in an outpatient physical therapy program. Cervical bracing is maintained for 3 months, during which time both contact and noncontact sports are strictly prohibited. These stringent guidelines have essentially eliminated recurrent SCIWORA, an entity seen only under our old protocol of more lenient restrictions and the use of only a hard collar. The brace is favored for several reasons.[51] First, it can be tailored to fit children as young as 1 year old. Second, it imparts greater limitation of motion. Third, it produces less neck irritation and fewer skin complications than a collar. Fourth, and most important, a child cannot easily remove the brace, which also interferes with play activities, helping to maintain compliance. The compliance issue is further reinforced by frank discussions about the implications of inadequate healing with both the patient and the family. Our decision to continue immobilization for 3 months is based empirically on the fact that one patient treated with only 2 months of immobilization suffered reinjury 10 weeks after the initial SCIWORA. We have seen no recurrent injury since extending brace immobilization to 3 months. After the 3 months, flexion-extension radiographs are repeated without the brace to rule out late instability. In our experience, this is rarely a problem with SCIWORA, nor is late deformity such as scoliosis or kyphosis.

OUTCOME

Numerous studies have shown that the main or perhaps only predictor of long-term outcome in children with SCIWORA is the admission neurological status.[5, 18, 27] Children with complete lesions rarely improve. Those with severe but incomplete lesions often improve with time but seldom regain normal function. Only patients with mild to moderate initial deficits can hope for a full recovery (Fig. 226–10). Thus, the overall outcome for SCIWORA can best be improved by preventing serious neurological damage. Primary prevention programs within the community (e.g., Think First) have helped lower the overall incidence of SCI in children. In addition, it is desirable to minimize the extent of neuronal damage once SCI has occurred. This can be achieved through three avenues: (1) rule out other (non-SCIWORA) categories of SCI, (2) anticipate and prevent delayed neurological deterioration, and (3) prevent recurrent injury.

SCIWORA must be considered a diagnosis of exclusion. It is crucial that occult fractures, disk herniation, epidural hematoma, and overt ligamentous instability be excluded with dynamic radiographs, CT, and MRI before the diagnosis of SCIWORA is established, because each of these lesions merits specific intervention that is more urgent and vigorous than simple bracing. The results from our studies[27, 69] suggest that the incidence of delayed neurological deterioration and recurrent SCIWORA can be lowered by compulsive prehospital care and a low threshold for applying spinal immobilization to any injured child with symptoms or mechanisms suggestive of SCIWORA.

Pure Ligamentous Injuries (Subluxation without Fracture)

Unlike for SCIWORA, the diagnostic criteria and management guidelines for overt instability in children are not well defined. Certainly, if the radiograph shows extensive bony fractures or subluxation, the implication of gross instability is obvious. However, the biomechanics of many subtler kinds of ligamentous instability in children has not been studied as intensely as it has been in adults, and recommendations for children are often extrapolated from adult data. For example, cadaver studies by Fielding and coworkers regarding stability of the atlantoaxial joint showed that (1) the atlantodental interval (ADI) in normal adults seldom exceeds 3 mm, (2) an ADI of 3 to 5 mm implies rupture of the transverse ligament, (3) an ADI of 5 to 10 mm suggests additional incompetence of the alar ligaments, and (4) an ADI of greater than 10 mm exists only if all other accessory odontoid ligaments are also ruptured.[80, 81] Thus, an ADI greater than 3 mm in adults is considered unstable.[82] Equivalent scientific data are unavailable in children. From purely empirical observations, taking into account the elasticity of the juvenile ligaments, an ADI of 4 mm has been regarded as the upper limit of normal in children younger than 8 years.[80, 83] Other studies have also shown that 20% to 30% of children with trisomy 21 and an ADI greater than 6 mm deteriorate with time, suggesting that 6 mm should be used as the threshold for treatment in children with Down syndrome.[84–87]

Similar biomechanical studies of the subaxial spine by White and Panjabi and their associates showed that the angle between adjacent vertebrae in normal adults is always less than 11 degrees, and deformities greater than 11 degrees in adults are considered unstable.[82, 88–92] For children, however, the upper limit of normal should be less than 11 degrees. The reason is as follows: because the juvenile spine is so elastic and apt to recoil, the final resting position of the displaced segment may lie well short of its actual maximal excursion at the time of impact. The presenting angle of displacement on the lateral radiograph is thus deceptively small,

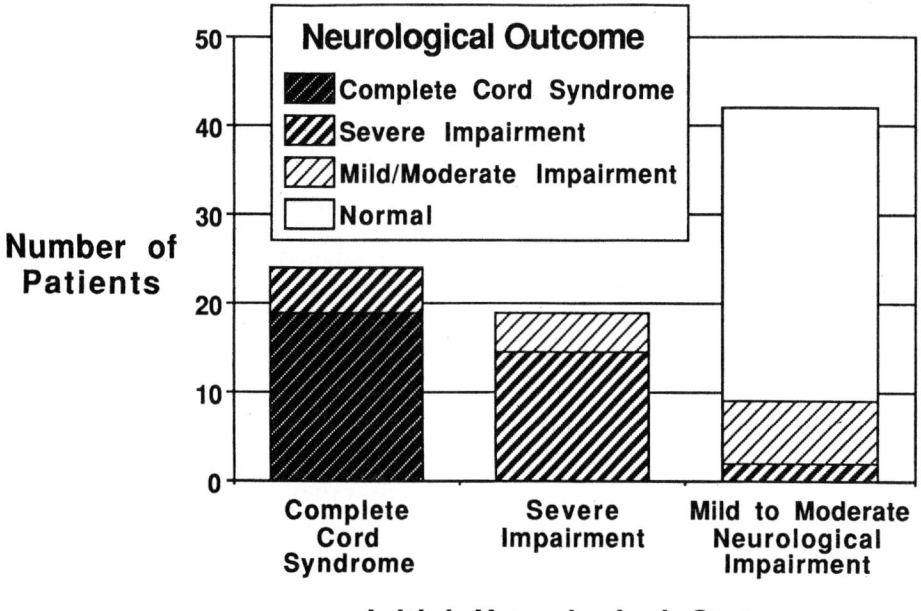

FIGURE 226–10. Long-term neurological outcome in children with spinal cord injury without radiographic abnormality (SCIWORA) as a function of initial neurological status. Both patients with severe long-term impairment and two of seven with mild to moderate impairment sustained recurrent SCIWORA. All four had initially regained normal neurological function after their first SCIWORA. (Data from references 18, 20, 31.)

and the actual ligamentous disruption may have been profound. This scenario is illustrated by the case of a 10-year-old boy who suffered a flexion injury and presented with an asymmetrical central cord syndrome and a radiograph showing a kyphotic deformity of 8 degrees and a horizontal displacement of 2 mm at C4-5. No dynamic radiographs were obtained for fear of aggravating the neurological deficits, but because the angulation did not satisfy the 11-degreee adult rule, he was initially treated with a halo vest and not surgical fusion. When the halo was removed 3 months later, he had rapid progression of his kyphosis and ultimately required a posterior fusion (Fig. 226–11).

This case illustrates the dilemma when the neutral radiograph does not meet the 11-degree instability rule yet the neural deficits suggest ligamentous damage but also preclude a flexion study. In retrospect, this boy's instability was obviously present in spite of the 8-degree angulation on the initial film. Such examples are common in pediatric neck injury. To avoid underdiagnosis, we recommend the following algorithm for children with angular deformities in the subaxial cervical spine (Fig. 226–12):

1. If the neutral radiograph shows greater than 11 degrees angulation, with or without neurological defi-cits, overt instability is assumed. No flexion-extension study is obtained, and surgical fusion is done.

2. If the neutral radiograph shows an angulation greater than 7 degrees but less than 11 degrees and there is neurological deficit, the injury is considered unstable, based on the assumption that the actual dis-placement must have been greater to cause myelopa-thy. No dynamic study is obtained.

3. If the neutral radiograph shows an angulation greater than 7 degrees but less than 11 degrees and the child is neurologically normal, flexion-extension studies are obtained. If the angulation increases to 11 degrees or greater, surgical fusion is done. If the angu-lation is unchanged, the dynamic study is repeated in 3 to 5 days to eliminate the effect of spasm. If the angle is again less than 11 degrees, the child is fitted with a cervicothoracic brace for 2 months, after which dy-namic radiographs are obtained to confirm solid liga-mentous healing.

4. If the initial angulation is less than 7 degrees but the patient has severe pain and spasm, a collar is worn until dynamic studies can be repeated in a few days to rule out instability.

Another case illustrates the importance of flexion studies (Fig. 226–13). A 12-year-old girl suffered a

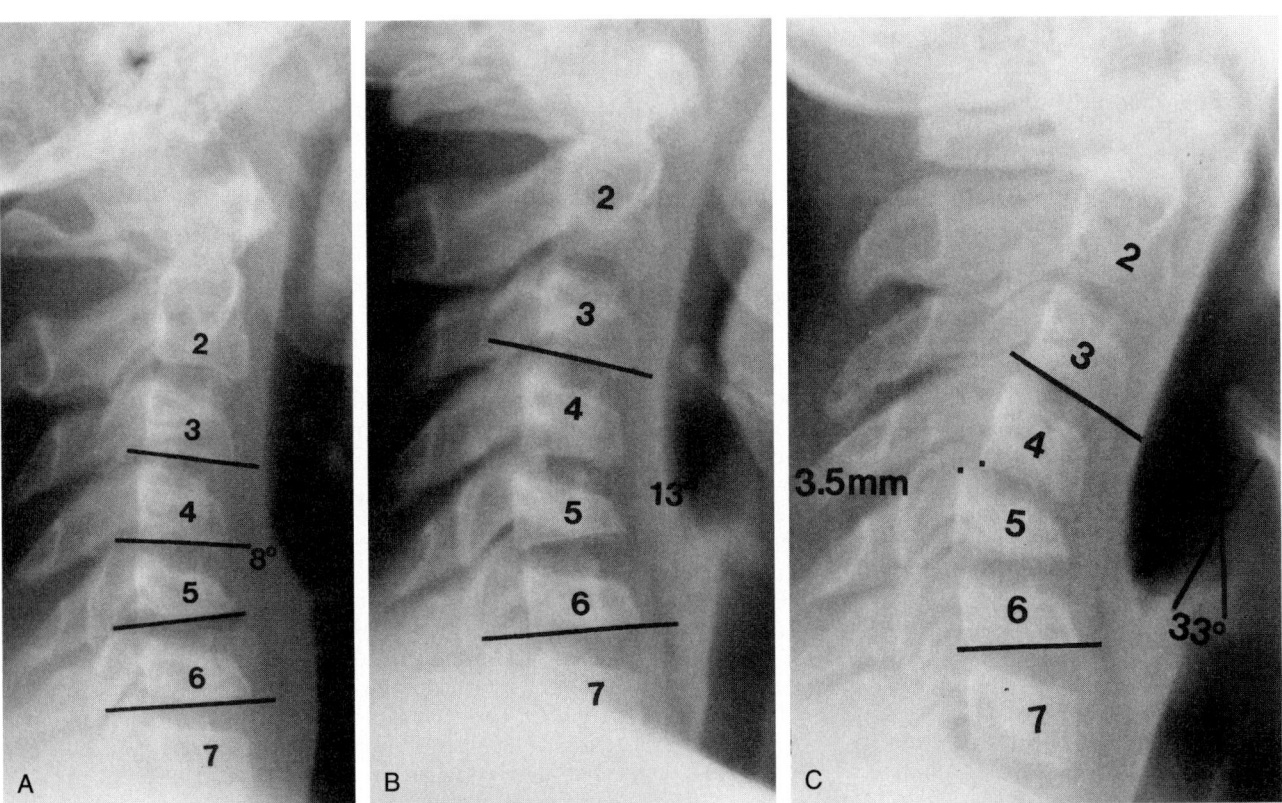

FIGURE 226–11. Flexion injury in a 10-year-old boy who presented with an asymmetrical central cord syndrome. *A,* Lateral radiograph shows a kyphotic deformity of 8 degrees at C4 and C5, horizontal displacement of less than 2 mm, slight widening of the C4-5 interspinous space, and compression fractures of the C5 and C6 vertebral bodies. He was treated with a halo for 3 months. *B,* Immediately after removal of the halo, a lateral radiograph shows an angulation of 13 degrees. *C,* One week after removal of the halo, angulation increased to 33 degrees. Horizontal displacement increased to 3.5 mm.

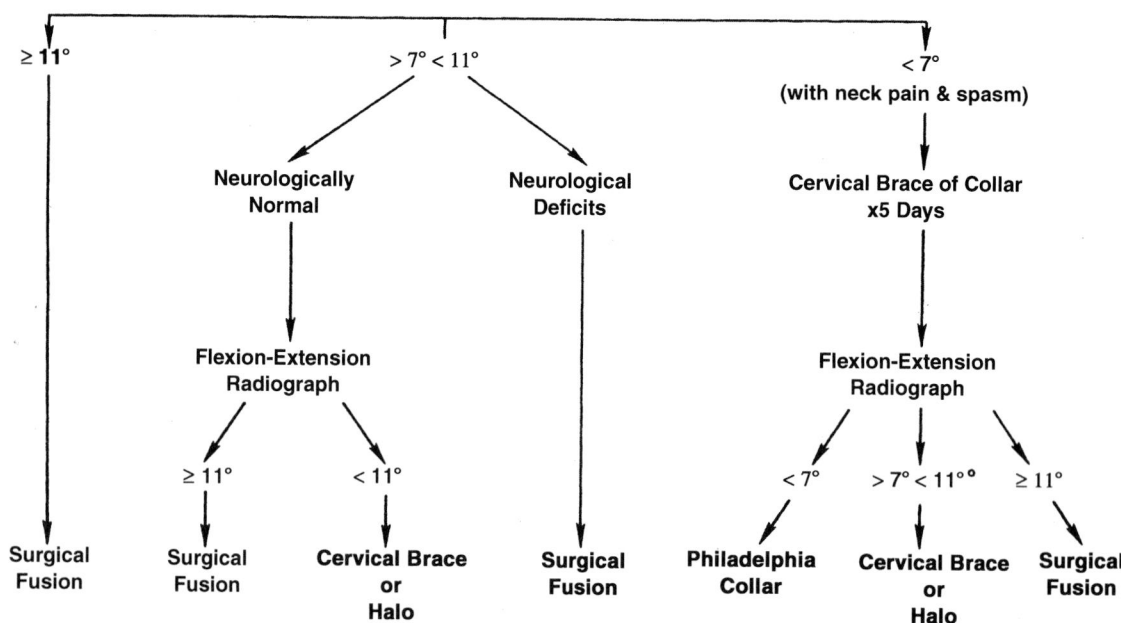

Lateral Cervical Spine Radiograph
Showing Angular Deformity

FIGURE 226–12. Management algorithm for ligamentous instability in children if the lateral radiograph shows a kyphotic deformity.

flexion injury and presented with a painful stiff neck, a normal neurological examination, and a neutral film that showed an angulation of 9 degrees at C4 and C5. A flexion study showed that the angle increased to 12 degrees. In spite of this, the child was only immobilized with a Philadelphia collar for 14 days, at which time a repeat radiograph showed that the kyphosis had increased to 17 degrees. Under present guidelines, this patient would have received a surgical fusion after the flexion study.

Besides the 11-degree rule, the White and Panjabi studies[82, 90–92] showed that a horizontal interbody displacement of greater than 3.5 mm in adults implies significant ligamentous rupture that will result in delayed instability. The juvenile spine, however, exhibits much greater physiologic horizontal movement than the adult spine, and a displacement greater than 3.5 mm may be considered normal. Sullivan and coworkers noted a forward glide of 3.5 to 4 mm between C2 and C3 in 13 of 100 normal children.[23] Cattell and Filtzer observed similar findings in 19% of normal children younger than 8 years.[26] In all probability, this "pseudosubluxation" between C2 and C3 and, to a lesser extent, between C3 and C4 is due to the elastic supporting soft tissues. The following recommendations are helpful in distinguishing clinical instability from physiologic hypermobility in the subaxial segments of children:

1. Children older than 8 years are similar to adults, and a horizontal displacement greater than 3.5 mm at any level should be considered unstable.

2. Children younger than 8 years have increased physiologic mobility at the C2-3 and C3-4 joints, but a horizontal displacement at these levels greater than 4.5 mm should be considered unstable.

3. In children younger than 8 years, if a horizontal displacement of 3.5 mm at the upper levels is accompanied by muscle spasm, pain, neurological findings, or additional abnormalities, such as an avulsed spinous process or widened interspinous space, clinical instability is assumed.

4. Even in children younger than 8 years, the physiologic mobility below C4 is not significantly different from that in adults; therefore, a horizontal displacement greater than 3.5 mm suggests instability.

Atlanto-occipital Dislocation

Traumatic AOD is one of the most common fatal cervical spine injuries. Autopsy and postmortem radiographic examinations of traffic fatalities revealed a 20% to 35% incidence of AOD.[93–95] Improvements in emergency resuscitation and prehospital care have increased survival in this previously almost invariably fatal injury. AOD is a particularly important entity in pediatric spine trauma, not only because it occurs more than twice as frequently in children as in adults,[96] but also because those children who survive the initial crisis often make good recoveries despite the severe presenting neurological deficits.

ANATOMY AND BIOMECHANICS

The occipitoatlantoaxial (O-C1-C2) articulations function as a single unit that procures movements of the

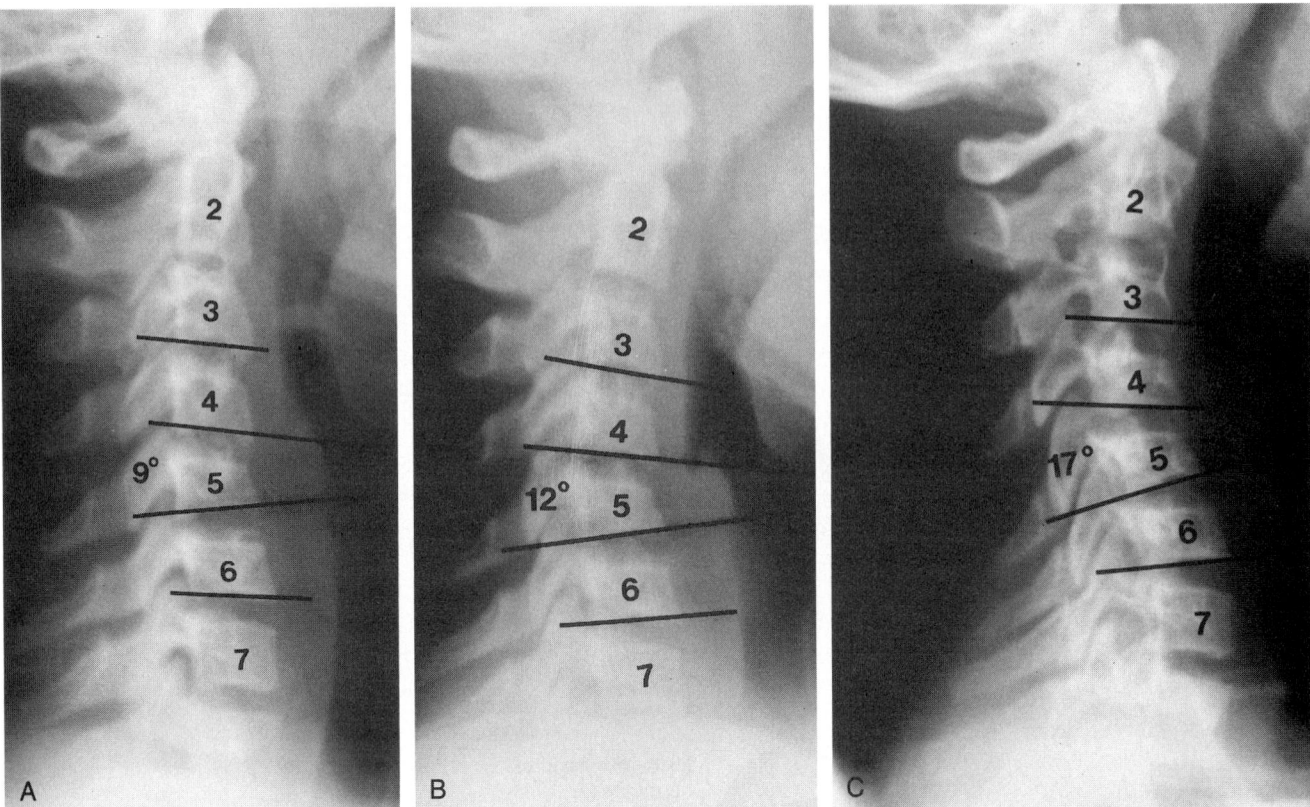

FIGURE 226–13. Flexion injury in a 12-year-old girl with a painful stiff neck and normal neurological status. *A,* Lateral radiograph shows an angulation of 9 degrees between C4 and C5. *B,* Flexion study shows an increase in angulation to 12 degrees. The child was immobilized in a Philadelphia collar. *C,* Fourteen days after injury, angulation between C4 and C5 increased to 17 degrees, indicating overt instability.

head about the spine. The atlas works as a biconcave washer between two spheres of motion. The upper articulation, between the occipital condyles and the atlas, is cup shaped in the sagittal plane and medially tilted in the coronal plane. This orientation allows flexion, extension, and some lateral bending, but minimal rotation. In contrast, the biconvex and laterally tilted facet articulation between the atlas and axis allows a large degree of rotation centered about the dens. Sagittal movement of the anterior arch of the atlas along the slightly pointed dens provides additional flexion and extension.

Movements within the O-C1-C2 unit are facilitated by the redundant articular capsules and thin occipitoatlantal and atlantoaxial membranes, which in turn impart minimal stability.[92] Rather, stability is provided by the strong internal ligaments between C2 and the occiput, chiefly the tectorial membrane, a well-developed continuation of the posterior longitudinal ligament that straps the body of C2 to the clivus; the paired alar ligaments that connect the dens to the occipital condyles; the cruciate ligament; and the apical dental ligament (Fig. 226–14). Flexion of the basion beyond the tip of the dens is limited by the tectorial membrane, whereas extension is checked by the tectorial membrane and by bony contact between the opisthion and

the arch of C1. Lateral bending and rotation are controlled by the alar ligaments.[97] The importance of the tectorial membrane and the alar ligaments was demonstrated by Werne,[98] who found that sectioning of the former results in excessive flexion and extension as well as vertical separation of the basion from the dens beyond the normal range of 1 cm, whereas sectioning of the latter results in increased lateral bending and rotation. When both the alar ligaments and tectorial membrane are cut, complete occipitoaxial dissociation occurs. The remainder of the internal ligaments—namely, the ascending band of the cruciate ligament and the apical ligament—are ineffectual in limiting motion. Finally, cadaver studies showed that paraspinal muscle action also contributes to the stability of the O-C1-C2 unit.[99, 100]

PATHOLOGY AND PATHOGENESIS

Traumatic AOD results from high-energy impacts that cause rupture of the tectorial membrane and alar ligaments.[65, 93, 95, 96, 101–103] Pedestrian-vehicle accidents are the most common cause. Three factors make children more vulnerable to AOD than adults. First, children are more frequently involved in pedestrian-vehicle accidents.[104] Second, the relatively larger head in children

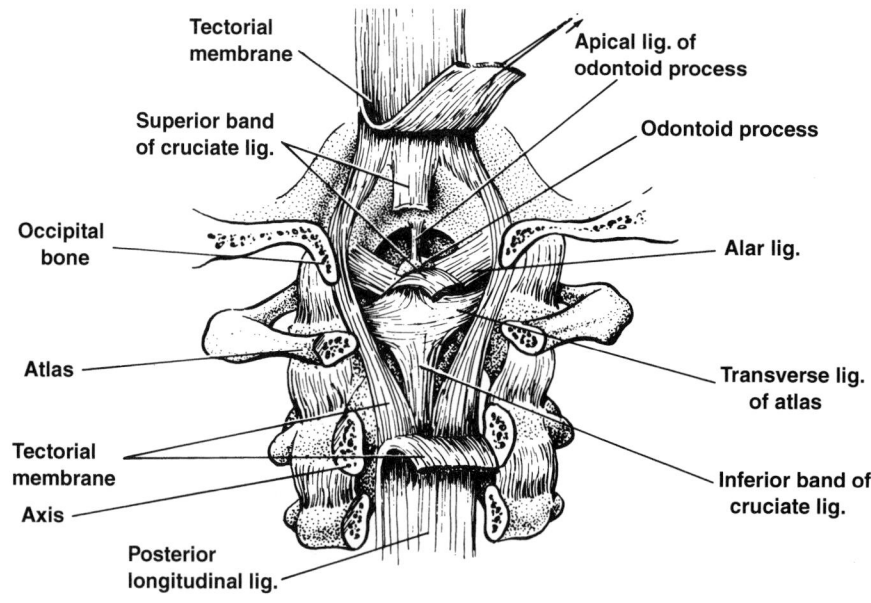

POSTERIOR VIEW

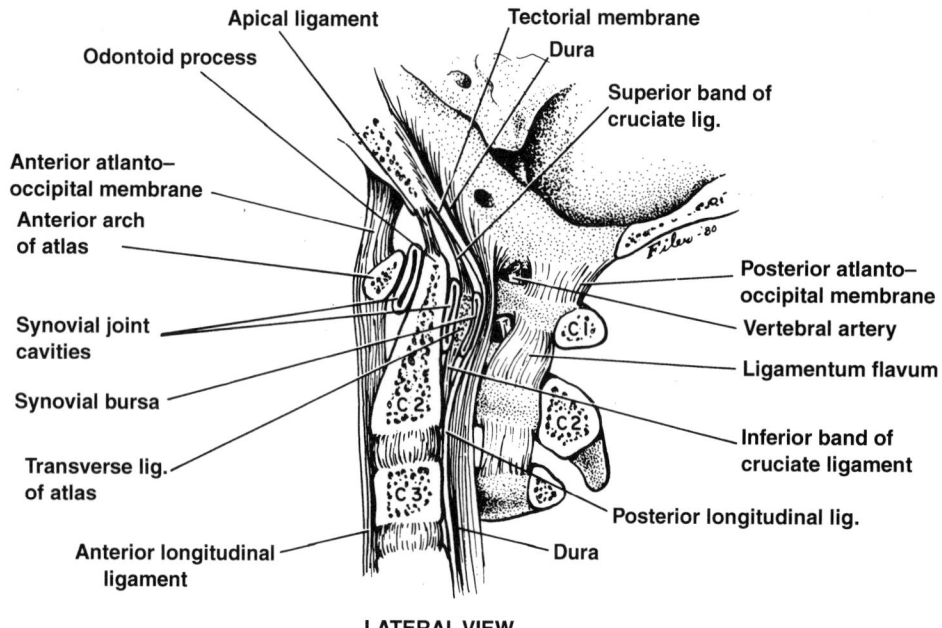

LATERAL VIEW

FIGURE 226–14. The joints and ligaments of the cranioverte- bral junction. *Top,* Posterior view. *Bottom,* Lateral view. Lig, Ligament. (From Wolf JW, Johnson RM: Cervical orthoses. In Bailey DW, Sherk HH [eds]: The Cervical Spine. Philadel- phia, JB Lippincott, 1983, pp 54–61.)

in comparison to the torso generates a greater shearing moment. Third, the occipitoatlantal joint is inherently more unstable in children.[105]

The force vectors involved in AOD may be recon- structed by circumstantial evidence. Adams' study re- vealed a high incidence of associated submental lacera- tions and mandibular fractures,[93] and others have reported posterior atlas fractures,[106] both of which point to a hyperextension mechanism. Further, 9 of Adams' 12 subjects had pontomedullary lacerations,[93] a le- sion that is characteristic of hyperextension and rota- tion.[107–109] However, approximately 25% of AOD cases have coexistent anterior atlantoaxial subluxation, and other cases are seen with spinomedullary transection

by a posteriorly pointing dens.[93, 102] These findings sug- gest a hyperflexion mechanism.[110] Because the alar ligaments—the check ligaments for rotation—are also ruptured in AOD, the forces must be directed obliquely to the head.[97, 111–113] Thus, AOD is most often caused by hyperextension-distraction forces obliquely directed to the chin, but hyperflexion-distraction forces to the occi- put are involved in some cases.

Recently, Sun and colleagues reported a series of 20 children with injury to the O-C1 region.[114] Using high- resolution MRI, they described a progressive pattern of disruption of structures responsible for the stability of the O-C2 joint. Thus, progressing from minor to severe injuries, the sequence of successive and additive involvement of structures is as follows: suboccipital musculature, atlanto-occipital and atlantoaxial membranes, apical and alar ligaments, tectorial membrane, and bilateral atlanto-occipital joint capsules. These authors postulated that involvement of the tectorial membrane is a critical threshold for instability at the O-C2 joint. Tectorial membrane damage can consist of frank rupture (Fig. 226–15) or, more commonly, stripping of the membrane from the clival or C2 attachments (Fig. 226–16). In both cases, the mechanical advantage of the membrane's stabilizing function is rendered ineffective. Weakening of this membrane appears to "expose" the O-C1 joint capsules to overt disruption, the denouement of the AOD scenario, leaving the cord vulnerable to all manner of traction and crushing injuries. In the four patients with SCI in Sun's series, the tectorial membrane was invariably damaged (in addition to all the other structures mentioned), but not in those patients in whom neither immediate nor subsequent instability of the O-C2 region could be demonstrated. These findings are consistent with the senior author's (DP) own data in a larger population of AOD patients.

Traynelis and coworkers classified AOD into three types.[110] Type I, the most common, is characterized by anterior displacement of the occiput on the atlas. Type II is a longitudinal separation of the two structures, and type III is posterior displacement of the occiput. The prevalence of anterior AOD seems contradictory

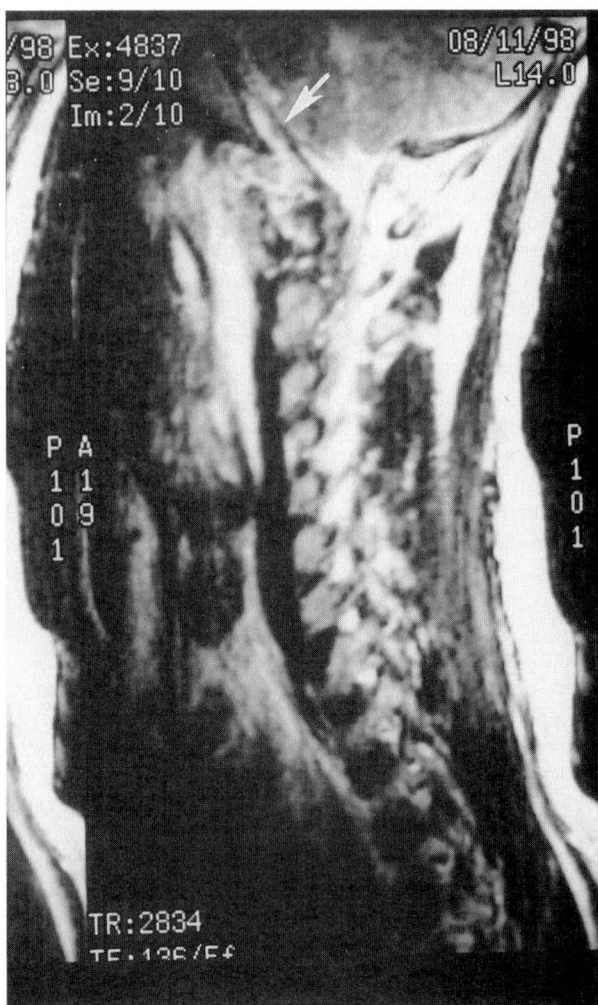

FIGURE 226–16. Sagittal T2-weighted magnetic resonance imaging scan in a 9-year-old child with atlanto-occipital dislocation. The tectorial membrane *(arrow)* is lifted off the clivus. The clival-dens space contains blood or edema fluid.

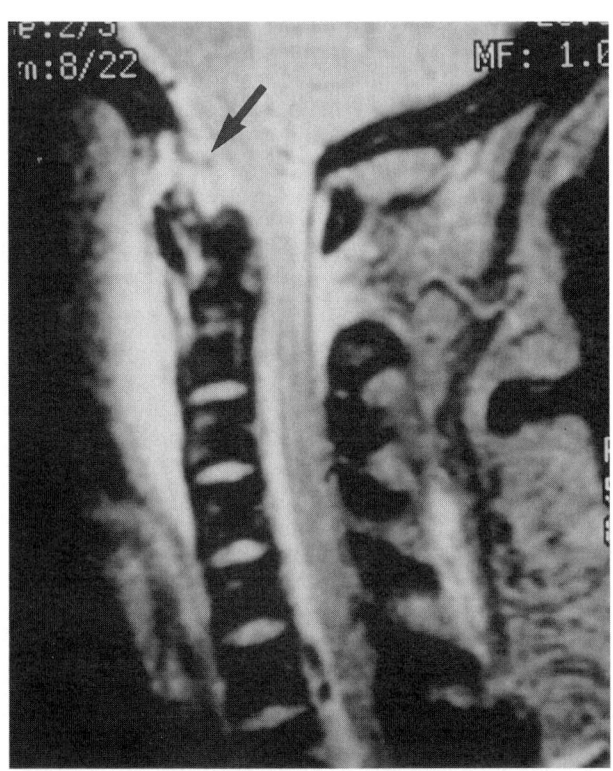

FIGURE 226–15. Sagittal T2-weighted magnetic resonance imaging scan in a 7-year-old child with atlanto-occipital dislocation. The tectorial membrane is completely disrupted. The upper stump *(arrow)* is still attached to the clivus. The alar ligaments are not visualized above the tip of the dens, suggesting that they have also ruptured.

to the postulated hyperextension vector, but given the highly unstable nature of this injury, the location of the head relative to C1 may be more a function of postimpact positioning than of the dynamics of impact. As the child lies on a flat board, the occipital prominence of the large head forces the neck into flexion, artificially creating an anterior displacement pattern. In addition to the three types of AOD, isolated examples of pure lateral dislocation,[115] as well as pure rotatory subluxation, have been reported in children, the latter in conjunction with AARF.[116, 117]

CLINICAL PRESENTATION

Children with traumatic AOD present with signs of brainstem, spinal cord, and cranial nerve injuries. Thirty percent of children who survive AOD are apneic or in full cardiorespiratory arrest at the scene of the accident.[47, 118–124] Other brainstem findings include pupillary abnormalities, rotatory nystagmus, ocular bobbing, decerebrate posturing, and variable alterations in consciousness. The motor deficits include quadriparesis, cruciate paralysis, crossed hemiplegia, or hemiparesis, depending on the level of the pyramidal tract lesions. Brainstem injury in AOD is due to a combination of actual disruption of tissues, spinal medullary compression by bony structures or epidural hematoma, and ischemia secondary to vertebral artery spasm or thrombosis.[125] Thrombosis of the anterior spinal artery produces the unique syndrome of ipsilateral hypoglossal palsy and crossed hemiplegia.[126] The caudal six pairs of cranial nerves may also be injured from downward traction of the medulla against the fixed points at their exit foramina.[127] However, the most common cranial neuropathy in AOD, sixth nerve palsy, is probably caused by the concomitant head injury. Post-traumatic hydrocephalus must be ruled out if the abducens palsy persists.

The true mortality rate of AOD is unknown. Of 35 nonfatal cases of pediatric AOD reported in the literature,[103, 113, 120–124, 127–137] only 5 presented with no initial deficits except for neck pain and torticollis. Of the 30 patients with deficits, 12 recovered fully; 3 remained quadriplegic and ventilator dependent, 2 of whom died 8 months after injury. The remaining 15 patients had various intermediate recoveries. Thus, children with AOD who have incomplete initial paralysis often make significant improvements, but in isolated cases, even initially flaccid paralysis does not preclude a good recovery.

RADIOGRAPHIC DIAGNOSIS

The diagnosis of AOD is contingent on a high level of suspicion in trauma victims, especially those with mandibular and facial fractures or with instantaneous cardiorespiratory instability. Casting of the brainstem with subarachnoid blood, seen in 25% of head computed tomographic scans in patients with AOD, should immediately suggest a distraction injury at the atlanto-occipital junction. The radiographic "chase" for the diagnosis should be relentless, because survival depends on recognition. Whereas gross separation of the occiput and atlas is obvious on plain x-ray films, horizontal luxations are much harder to diagnose. The literature is replete with diagnostic criteria, but no single criterion has reached fail-safe status. A critical review of these criteria allows the clinician to employ multiple methods to augment the positive yield.

One of the oldest criteria is the interval between the tip of the dens and the basion (DB interval) (Fig. 226–17). Wholey and associates examined 480 adult and 120 pediatric cervical spine radiographs and determined that the upper limit of the DB interval is 5 mm in adults and 10 mm in children, the age difference being attributed to incomplete summit ossification of the dens in children.[138] Earlier application of the DB interval revealed considerable overlap between normal subjects and patients with AOD, possibly because of the mixed age groups.[103] The most recent use of the DB interval exclusively in children showed that the value for normal children is less that 12.5 mm; the values in

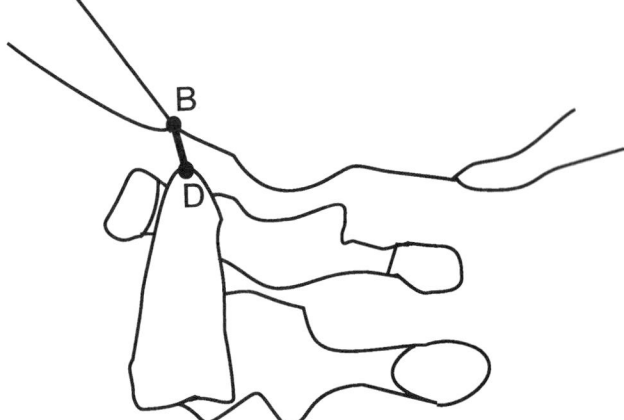

FIGURE 226–17. The dens-basion interval introduced by Wholey and colleagues.[138] An interval of 10 mm is abnormal, and 14 mm is indicative of atlanto-occipital dislocation in children. B, basion; D, dens.

11 children with proven AOD were all greater than 14 mm.[129] However, several problems are inherent in this method. First, as with any absolute radiographic measurement, the number depends on the target-film distance. Wholey's original measurements were done on an upright film at a target-film distance of 6 feet. When the DB intervals in 400 subjects were measured on supine films taken at 40 inches, Harris and colleagues found the upper limit to be 12 mm in adults.[139] Second, the variable ossification of the odontoid summit in children makes universal application of a maximal DB interval unreliable. Third, the measurement varies with flexion, extension, and axial traction in normal subjects. Nevertheless, a DB interval greater than 14 mm in a child is almost certainly indicative of AOD, but values between 10 and 14 mm still defy precise designation.

In 1980, Dublin measured the distances from the posterior cortex of the mandible to the anterior arch of C1 (A) and to the odontoid (B) (Fig. 226–18).[62] In anterior AOD, both A and B should be increased. However,

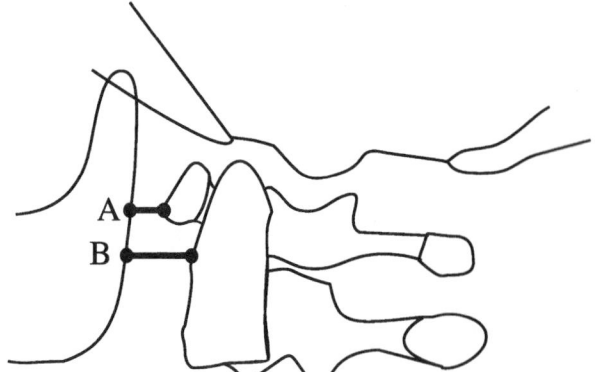

FIGURE 226–18. Dublin's method, using the distances between the posterior cortex of the mandible to the anterior arch of C1 (A) and to the odontoid (B). In anterior atlanto-occipital dislocation, both A and B should increase. Normal range of A is −10 to +9 mm; normal range of B is +2 to +17 mm.

because the mandible and the dens are not sagittally coplanar, these measurements vary greatly with the incident angle of the x-ray beam and are not consistently reproducible.[34] We do not recommend this method.

To circumvent the problems with noncoplanar landmarks, Kaufman and coworkers measured the width of the atlanto-occipital joint itself.[49] They found that the distance between any two opposing points along the joint surface should not exceed 5 mm in children on lateral or anteroposterior skull films. The problem with their original description is the use of plain films; superimposition of the mastoids and imperfect overlap of the two atlanto-occipital joints often make interpretation impossible.

Two methods using dimensionless numbers have been devised to eliminate the error due to radiographic magnification. The Powers ratio[103] is obtained by dividing the distance between the basion (B) and the posterior arch of C1 (C) by the distance between the opisthion (O) and the anterior arch of C1 (A) (Fig. 226–19A). Survey of a normal population gives a mean BC/AO ratio of 0.77 ± 0.09. In type I AOD (the most common), the BC/OA ratio is increased because BC widens while OA shortens. Powers found that ratios greater than 1 are always indicative of anterior dislocation. Although highly predictive for type I dislocation, the Powers ratio has two major shortcomings: it fails to diagnose type II and type III dislocations, and the opisthion is often difficult to pinpoint on the lateral spine films. In addition, anomalies of the posterior arch of C1 and the foramen magnum invalidate the ratio. The use of sagittally reconstructed CT has greatly simplified localization of the opisthion (see Fig. 226–19B).

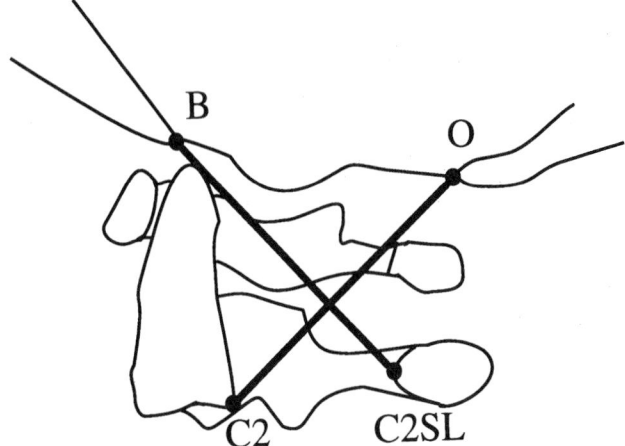

FIGURE 226–20. Lee's X line. A line drawn between the basion (B) and the midpoint of the spinolaminar line of C2 (C2SL) should tangentially intersect the posterosuperior aspect of the dens. A line drawn from the opisthion (O) to the posteroinferior corner of the C2 body (C2) should also tangentially intersect the C1 spinolaminar line. If both lines miss their respective intersections, atlanto-occipital dislocation is suspected.

The second dimensionless method uses the X lines proposed by Lee and colleagues,[125] formed by a line drawn between the basion and the base of the C2 lamina (BC2L) and one drawn between the opisthion and the inferior margin of the C2 body (C2O) (Fig. 226–20). Normally, the BC2L and C2O should tangentially intersect the posterior superior dens and the highest point on the C1 spinolaminar line, respectively. If both lines miss their respective tangential points,

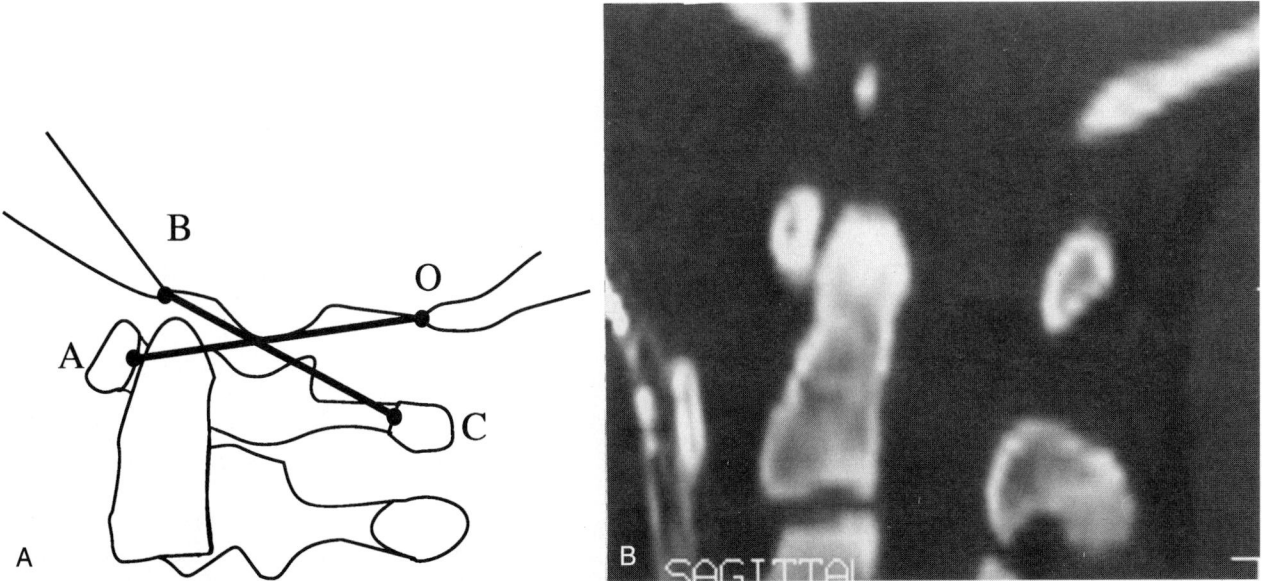

FIGURE 226–19. Powers ratio. *A*, The ratio is obtained when the distance between the basion (B) and the midpoint of the posterior arch of C1 (C) is divided by the distance between the opisthion (O) and the midpoint of the anterior arch of C1 (A). The mean BC/OA is 0.77. Any value greater than 1 is indicative of atlanto-occipital dislocation (AOD). *B*, Sagittal computed tomographic reconstruction in a patient with AOD. The BC/OA ratio is greater than 1.

AOD is suspected. This method is seldom applied in children because its validity depends on atlantoaxial integrity and a fully developed dens.

In 1993, Harris and coauthors began using the basion-axial interval (BAI), defined by a line drawn tangential to the posterior cortical surface of the axis (posterior axial line [PAL]) on the lateral cervical radiograph taken at 40 inches.[139, 140] The BAI is the distance between this line and a parallel line drawn through the basion (Fig. 226–21A). The normal BAI in adults ranges from +12 mm (basion anterior to the PAL) to −4 mm (basion behind the PAL). With anterior dislocation, the basion moves away from the dens, and the BAI exceeds 12 mm (see Fig. 226–21B), whereas with posterior dislocation, the basion moves far behind the dens and the BAI becomes less than −4 mm. In 50 children studied, the anterior limit of the BAI is still +12 mm, but the basion never moves behind the PAL. These authors showed that, used in conjunction with the DB interval, the BAI is more accurate in adults than either the Powers ratio or X lines. In very young children with a pointed dens, however, the PAL becomes excessively oblique forward. This artificially moves the posterior reference point of the measurement forward and, in effect, underestimates the true extent of the anterior basion displacement.

Recently, Sun and colleagues introduced the C1-2/C2-3 posterior interspinous ratio to assess the integrity of the atlanto-occipital joint.[114] This ratio is obtained from the lateral plain radiograph by dividing the shortest distance between the lower cortex of the posterior C1 ring and upper cortex of the C2 spinous process by the corresponding shortest distance between the spinous processes of C2 and C3 (Fig. 226–22). These authors found that normal children and those with neck injuries but intact tectorial membranes have an interspinous ratio of less than 2.5, whereas seven of eight children whose tectorial membranes had been damaged had a ratio greater than 2.5.

The hypothetical mechanism underlying an abnormal interspinous ratio in AOD, according to Sun and colleagues, was related to forward rocking and downward pressing of the occipital condyle on the anterior rim of the C1 facet secondary to a loose atlanto-occipital joint, thereby forcefully "jacking up" the posterior arch of C1 away from C2.[114] Like all the other radiographic criteria, this method has its share of inherent problems. The mode of postinjury immobilization can dramatically alter the contact relationship between the occipital condyle and the anterior rim of C1, thus unpredictably varying the interspinous distance between C1 and C2. A concomitant rupture of the transverse C1 ligament will cause C1-2 luxation and affect the ratio, as will congenital craniovertebral anomalies and other dysmorphic C1 and C2 arches. Muscle relaxants may also artificially widen the C1-2 interspinous distance. Last, there are no normative measurements of this ratio for adults and older children, and the reliability of the upper normal limit of 2.5 has not been vigorously tested on a large enough population of children with proven AOD. As did all its predecessors at one time, the interspinous ratio presently enjoys the status

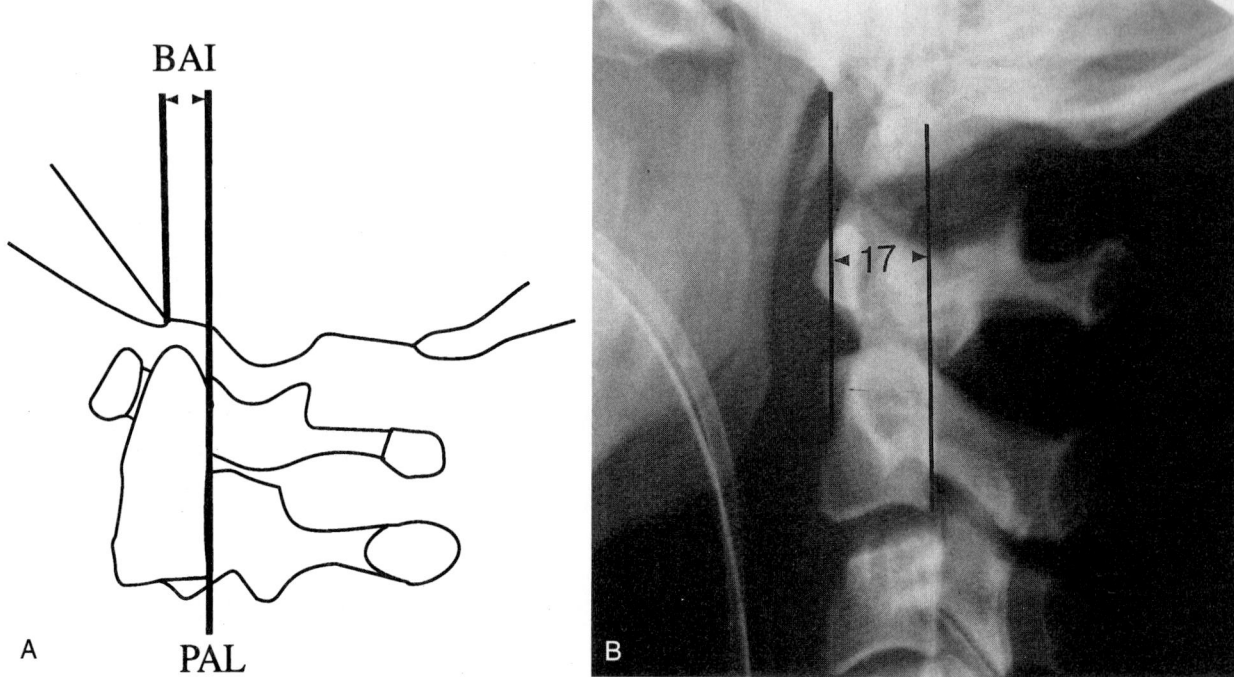

FIGURE 226–21. Harris' basion-axial interval (BAI). *A,* The BAI is the distance between the posterior axial cortical line (PAL) and a parallel line drawn through the basion. The normal BAI is between 0 and 12 mm in children. *B,* Lateral cervical radiograph of a patient with atlanto-occipital dislocation showing the BAI to be greater than +17 mm.

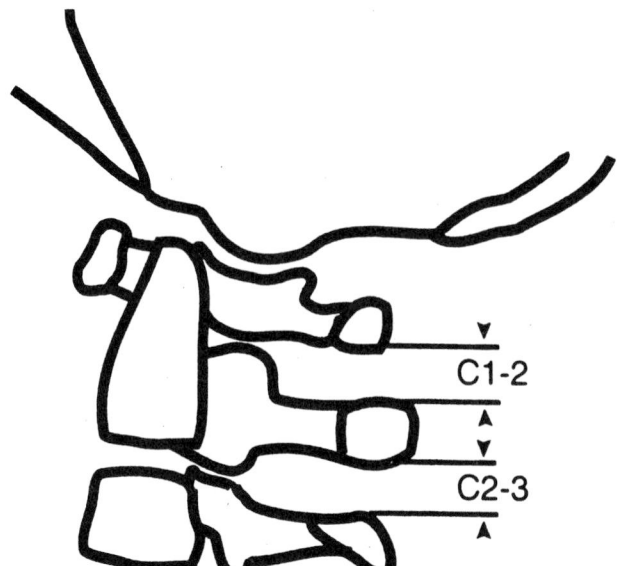

FIGURE 226–22. The C1-2/C2-3 ratio. Sun and colleagues[114] suggest that the ratio should be less than 2.5 with a stable atlanto-occipital relationship.

of a tantalizing promise, but it has yet to be tested by time and use.

Despite such a large array of available radiographic criteria, it is ironic that two of the senior author's recent cases of AOD fell into the diagnostic borderland between normal and abnormal. This was particularly distressing because the ambiguity involved the supposedly most reliable methods—the Powers ratio and Harris's BAI (Fig. 226–23). This led to the realization that, with the exception of Kaufman and associates flawed study,[49, 122] all the prior measurements use bony landmarks that do not actually participate in the atlanto-occipital articulation. It stands to reason that a direct measurement of the O-C1 joint interval should be a more precise indicator of O-C1 integrity (Fig. 226–24).

Such a study using both coronal and sagittal reconstructions of CT images through each of the condyle-C1 joints in children is in progress (authors' unpublished data). Our preliminary findings in more than 50 normal children reveal a mean occipital condyle–C1 interval of 1.8 mm, with a sagittal-coronal variation of less than 15% and a left-right variation of less than 8% (Fig. 226–25). Virtually no measurement in any projection exceeds 2.5 mm. Using 3 mm as the upper limit of normal, we found that at least one but usually both condyle-C1 joints were separated in all our patients with AOD, regardless of type (Fig. 226–26). The joint surfaces were very well delineated if thin axial CT cuts (1.5 or 2 mm thick) were acquired, and they often showed "water plane" horizontal displacement (Fig. 226–27) or even fractures in addition to separation, both of which are sure signs of ligamentous rupture and instability. Individual evaluation of each joint also disclosed cases with unilateral separation, usually accompanied by translational displacement of the joint, suggesting that the head was pried apart from the neck on one side and then pivoted on the opposite condyle-C1 joint.

So far, an abnormal occipital condyle–C1 interval has been found in every AOD patient who had two-dimensional reconstructed CT images. This is true even for those with equivocal readings from other radiographic criteria. The measurement is simple to obtain as long as good-quality reconstructed images are available. The occipital condyle–C1 interval as seen on CT reconstruction has proved to be the most reliable diagnostic criteria of AOD to date.

Thus, all patients with suspicious plain radiographs, basal subarachnoid blood, and a compatible mechanism of injury should undergo thin (1.5 to 2 mm) axial CT from the clivus to C3. All measurements can now be checked on the two-dimensional reconstructed CT images. Coronal reconstruction through the occipital condyles demonstrates the true extent of the atlanto-occipital separation. Asymmetry of the two joint surfaces on the coronal image suggests a rotatory component to the displacement (Fig. 226–28).

As mentioned, atlanto-occipital dissociation can be present without anteroposterior occipital displacement and thus can escape radiographic detection that depends on an abnormal relationship between bony landmarks other than the condyle-C1 joints themselves.[128, 141] In this situation, MRI performed in the neutral position may reveal rupture or lifting of the tectorial membrane off C2 or the clivus, as well as hemorrhages and edema around the alar ligaments, the retropharyngeal space, and the posterior nuchal soft tissues. AOD is presumed in the presence of such findings even if reconstructed CT is unavailable for determining the occipital con-

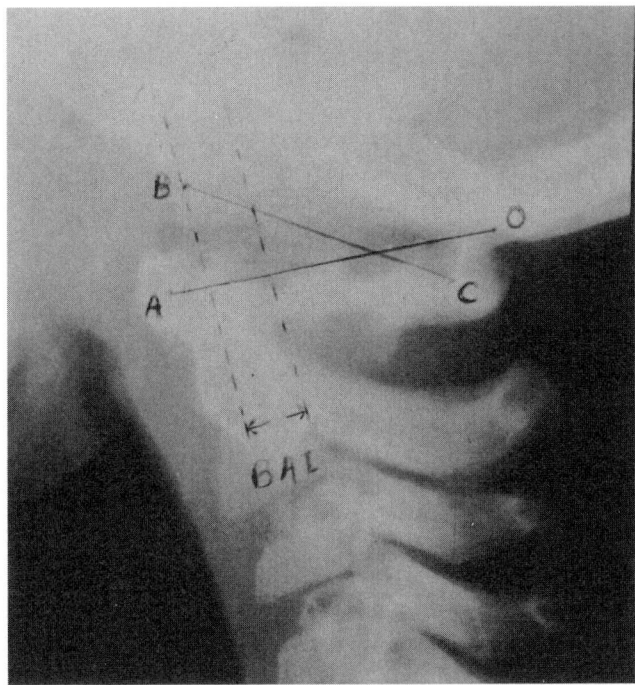

FIGURE 226–23. Lateral cervical spine radiograph of a child with atlanto-occipital dislocation proved by a widely separated occipital–C1 interval on reconstructed computed tomography (see Fig. 226–26). Harris' basion-axial interval is 10 mm, and the Powers ratio is 0.9. Both values put this case in the "normal" range according to these two criteria.

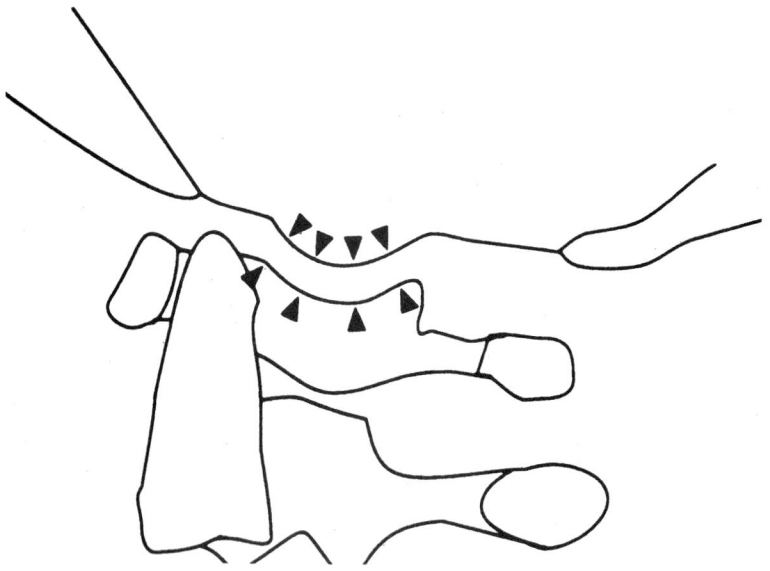

FIGURE 226–24. Occipital condyle–C1 interval (OCI). Four points *(arrowheads)* equidistant from each other are picked for measurement of the joint interval to compensate for the slight unevenness of the joint space.

dyle–C1 interval. It is worth re-emphasizing that in every suspicious situation, *all* of the previously mentioned methods should be employed, but a single positive result is enough to make the diagnosis of AOD.

TREATMENT

As soon as an airway is secured, immobilization is provided by a standard stiff collar with the head strapped down to the backboard. Elevation of the thorax with firm padding or blankets eliminates the flexion caused by the prominent occiput of a child. The highly unstable nature of AOD precludes the use of axial traction as a means of reduction.[133, 142] We recom-

mend reducing any horizontal displacement with simple repositioning of the head using suitable padding under fluoroscopy. The halo vest should be applied as soon as the alignment is satisfactory and the patient's vital functions are stabilized. Children who reportedly survived AOD were all 2 years or older in whom a low-torque multiple-pin–type halo ring could be safely used. Evolving brainstem findings after immobilization should raise the possibility of vertebral artery dissection, which requires angiographic confirmation and cautious anticoagulation.

Definitive stabilization of AOD requires surgical fusion across the entire occipitoatlantoaxial unit. Although fibrous union has been reported in children with immobilization alone,[111, 126, 142] persistent instability is the rule because pure ligamentous injuries of the cervical spine heal poorly.[103, 113, 121, 133] The fusion must incorporate the axis, because the stabilizing ligaments

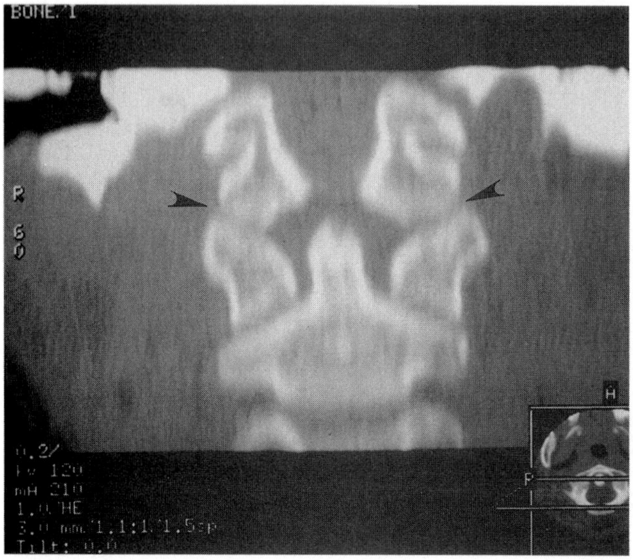

FIGURE 226–25. Coronal computed tomographic reconstruction through the midpoints of the occipital condyle–C1 joints in a normal child aged 3.5 years. The mean occcipital condyle–C1 interval (OCI) on each side, averaged from four points in each joint, measures less than 1.3 mm. The occipital–C1 joint relationship is perfectly symmetrical *(arrowheads)*.

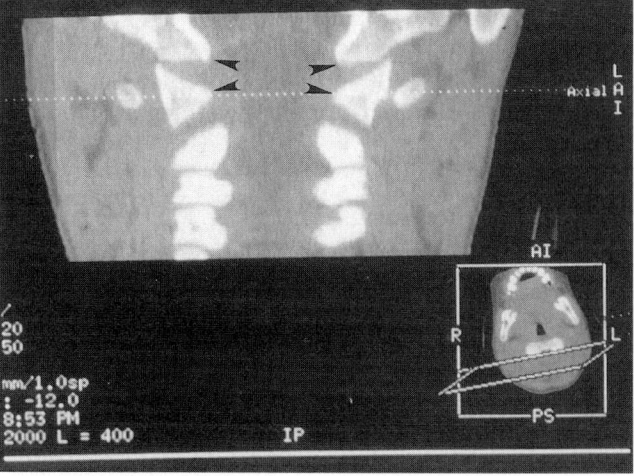

FIGURE 226–26. Coronal computed tomographic reconstruction in a child with atlanto-occipital disilocation. Both joints are widely dissociated *(arrowheads)*. The mean occipital condyle–C1 interval is greater than 7 mm on each side.

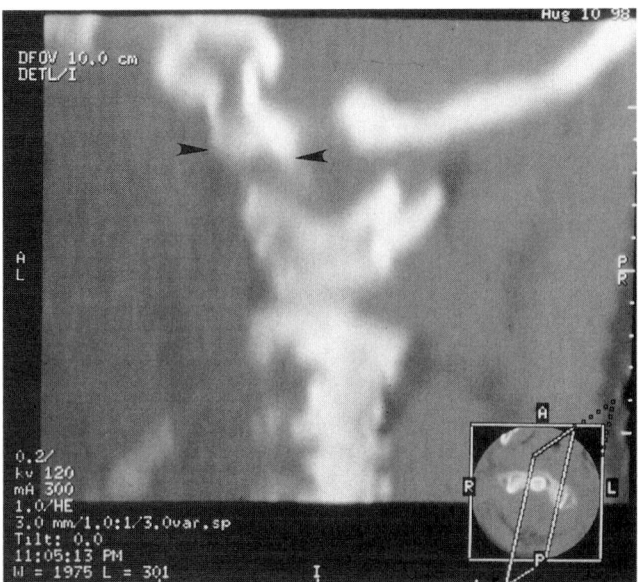

FIGURE 226–27. Sagittal computed tomographic reconstruction of the left occipital–C1 joint in a child with atlanto-occipital dislocation, showing wide separation (>9 mm) and anterior displacement of the occipital condyle *(between arrowheads)* in relation to the C1 joint surface.

of the entire O-C1-C2 unit all use the axis as the anchor. The operation is performed 5 to 7 days postinjury, after all other life-threatening injuries have been dealt with and brainstem swelling is on the wane. Once reduction is confirmed by a radiograph on the operating table, fusion is performed with the halo in situ, but it may occasionally be necessary to remove the posterior bars

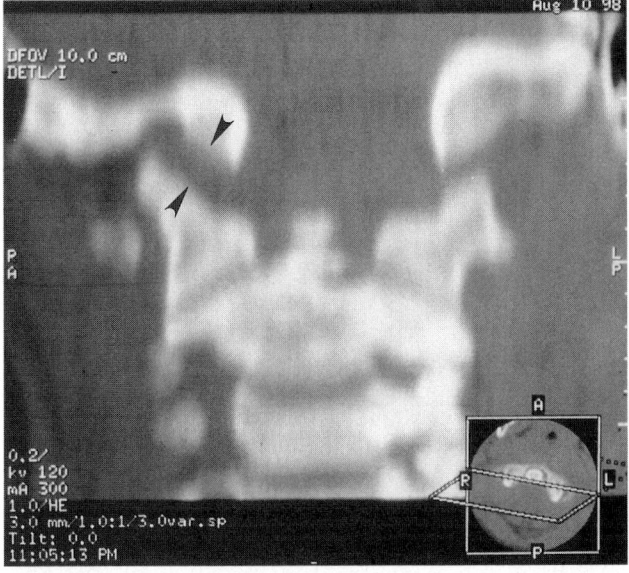

FIGURE 226–28. Coronal computed tomographic reconstruction of a child with atlanto-occipital dislocation, showing wide separation of the right occipital–C1 joint *(arrowheads)* and marked asymmetry in the left occipital condyle–C1 relationship. This results from complete anterior luxation of the left condyle so that section through the midpoint of the C1 joint surface "catches" only the posterior edge of the condyle.

and jacket. The cornerstone of long-term stability is bony arthrodesis across a wide area of the occipital squama and both the C1 and C2 arches. For immediate rigid fixation, in the past we used contoured Steinmann pins or appropriately sized Luque rectangles affixed to the occiput and neural arches with bur holes and sublaminar titanium cables.[141, 143–145] Cranial plates and screws are available for segmental fixation,[146] but most are unsuitable in children because of the thin skull. With either rectangular bars or plate and screw, postoperative halo immobilization is necessary for 12 to 16 weeks, or whenever adequate callus can be demonstrated across the fusion site on radiographs. We have now switched to the "inside-outside" occipital screwplate construct, which is particularly recommended for young children with thin skulls (see later).

Atlantoaxial Rotatory Fixation

AARF is most commonly encountered after otolaryngologic procedures, with cervical infections, or without an identifiable cause. Traumatic AARF accounts for only 30% of all cases. The inciting trauma is typically minor.[147, 148] The child presents with a painful neck that is laterally flexed and with the chin rotated to the contralateral side, aptly called the "cock robin" deformity. The pain worsens with attempted rotation to the corrective side. The neurological examination is usually negative; rarely, the patient may have signs of myelopathy or C2 radiculopathy.[149–152] Death directly attributable to AARF is extremely uncommon but has been reported.[153, 154]

The diagnosis of AARF has been the subject of intense debate for many years. In 1994, Li and Pang were the first to set down diagnostic criteria based on the normal and abnormal associated movements between the atlas and axis during head rotation, as seen on dynamic CT screening. A classification of AARF was also made based on the degree of abnormal "yoking" between C1 and C2.[155]

ANATOMY, BIOMECHANICS, AND PATHOPHYSIOLOGY

The most important ligament in maintaining a normal atlantoaxial relationship is the transverse atlantal ligament, which is actually the horizontal component of the cruciate ligament. This structure tightly straps the dens to the anterior arch of the atlas. Of secondary importance are the paired alar ligaments that connect the lateral masses of C1, the dens, and the occipital condyles and provide support against excessive rotation. The atlantoaxial joint provides most of the rotation in the cervical spine. The positions of C1 and C2 during rotation are readily depicted in a motion curve (Fig. 226–29). The C1 angle in relation to the vertical axis (0 degrees) is depicted on the x-axis. The angle between C1 and C2, the C1-2 angle (i.e., C1 minus C2), is depicted on the y-axis. As C1 rotates through the first 20 degrees, C2 remains stationary. The normal motion curve is linear in this range of C1 angles, because the C1 angle and C1-2 angle are the same. Be-

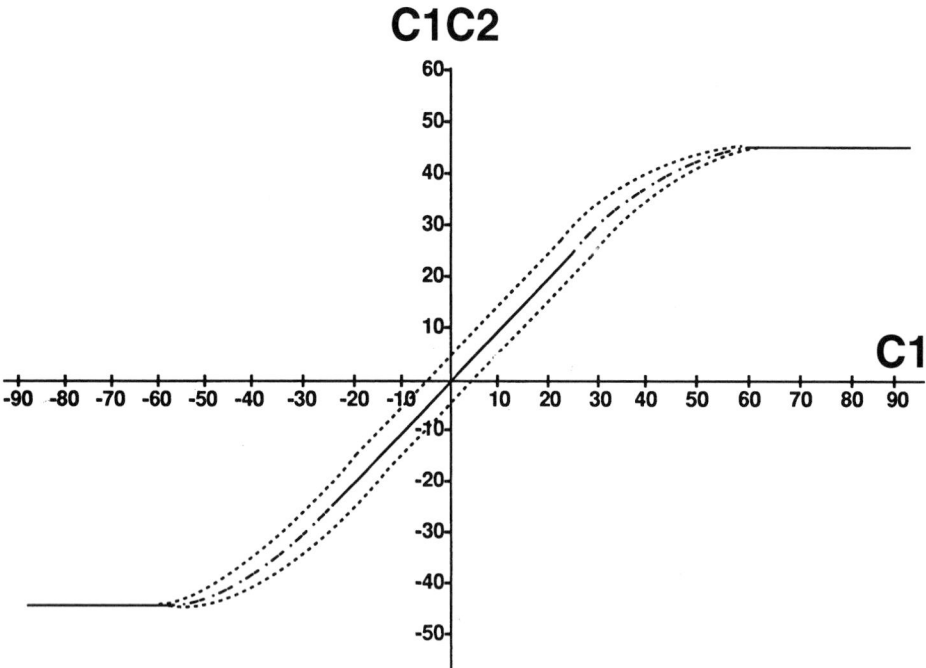

FIGURE 226–29. Normal motion curve of C1 and C2 rotation. The dotted lines denote the 5 degrees of normal variance of the C1 and C2 positions to either side of vertical zero and of each other. See text for details.

yond 20 degrees of C1 rotation, C2 begins rotating in the same direction because the alar ligaments become taut and pull on the dens, but C1 always rotates faster than C2, so the C1-2 angle continues to enlarge to a maximum of 47 degrees. Further rotation of C1 does not enlarge the C1-2 angle, and the motion curve plateaus. Rotation at the atlantoaxial joint is facilitated by the biconvex nature of the C1-2 articular surfaces and the relatively horizontal orientation of the joints.[82, 91] All the joints in this region are synovial, which makes them susceptible to a variety of arthropathies.

The physiologic hypermobility of the atlantoaxial articulation in children predisposes the joint to rotatory subluxation during sudden and vigorous turning of the head. This can result in true bony lock if the pathologic rotation is extreme, although this is rare. Also, the redundant synovial folds in children may be caught in the joint spaces at the extremity of rotation and jam any counterrotation. In addition, protrusion of parts of the articular surface through a tear in the joint capsule produces a "buttonhole" block. Finally, the muscle spasm that frequently accompanies neck trauma helps maintain the rotatory deformity.[23, 156]

RADIOGRAPHIC DIAGNOSIS AND CLASSIFICATION

Several hours after the onset of AARF, the child's conscious effort to realign the frontal visual axis causes involuntary counterrotation of the subaxial spine and deviation of the spinous process of the axis toward the side of the chin tilt. This so-called Sudeck's sign, shown on the anteroposterior radiograph, used to be considered pathognomonic of AARF.[60] However, plain and dynamic radiographs and even cineradiography have proved unreliable. The diagnostic method of choice

endorsed here is a CT protocol done with the patient's head in specified positions. Nonoverlapping 3-mm axial computed tomographic scans from the occiput to C3 are obtained on a mildly sedated child in three head positions with the body placed flat on the scanner table: (1) in the presenting position (P), in which the neck is most comfortable; (2), in the zero position (P_0), with the head turned perpendicular to the scanner table so that the sagittal axis of the skull and C1 are at anatomic zero; and (3) in the extreme corrected position (P−), with the head turned as far as possible without undue discomfort toward the side opposite the original rotatory deformity. The C1 angle is plotted against the C1-2 angle for the three head positions. A positive C1 angle signifies rotation toward the side of the chin tilt, whereas a negative C1 angle signifies rotation to the opposite side past the vertical zero. In type I AARF, the C1-2 angle is fixed as the head turns in the corrective direction so that the motion curve remains parallel to the y-axis at both the P_0 and P− positions (Fig. 226–30). This likely represents a true bony lock and is a rare form of AARF. In type II AARF, the C1-2 angle diminishes with corrective rotation. Because this could not happen with bony lock, type II cases likely result from soft tissue interposition within the joint. In type IIA AARF, C1 never crosses to the other side of C2, and the C1-2 angle never becomes 0 degrees (Fig. 226–31). This is the most common form of AARF. In type IIB, C1 does cross to the other side of C2, but only when C1 is at or less than −10 degrees—that is, way past the midline where they should normally overlap— suggesting a pathologically sticky C1-2 articulation (Fig. 226–32).

In practice, the three sets of C1 and C1-2 angles from one rotation sequence are plotted on a diagram of the motion curve on which five diagnostic domains

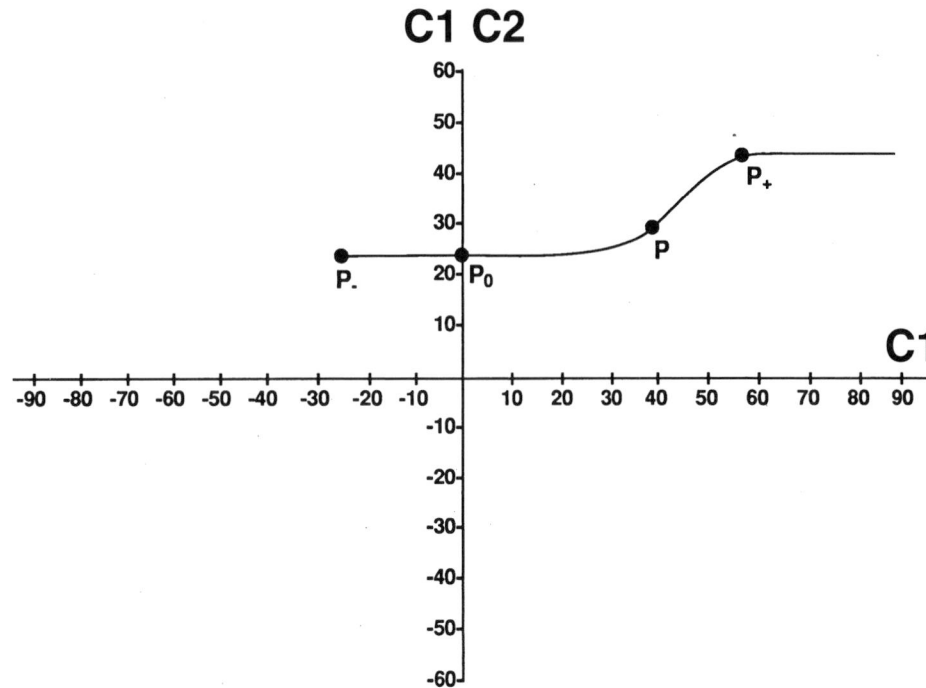

FIGURE 226–30. Type I atlantoaxial rotatory fixation. The C1 angle does not change as the head is rotated in the corrective (P−) position. This represents a true bony lock of C1 and C2.

have been superimposed (Fig. 226–33). If any of these points falls in any of the five domains, the diagnosis of AARF is made. Domain 1 (criterion 1) represents the area of the motion curve in which C1-2 is positive despite a C1 angle of less than −10 degrees; that is, the abnormal C1-2 angle is maintained despite forceful push of C1 past the midline. This criterion is met by all type I and IIA AARF patients as long as the head can be turned at least 10 degrees past midline on the

corrective side. Domain 2 represents criterion 2, which is met if the C1-2 angle is greater than 8 degrees when C1 is between −10 degrees and +3 degrees. This is most useful when C1 cannot be pushed back much beyond the P_0 position. This criterion can be met by all AARF types. Domain 3 represents criterion 3, which requires that the head of the patient be in the P_0 or P− position. In these positions, if C2 is less than −5 degrees (C1-2 > 8 degrees) when C1 is between 3 and 30

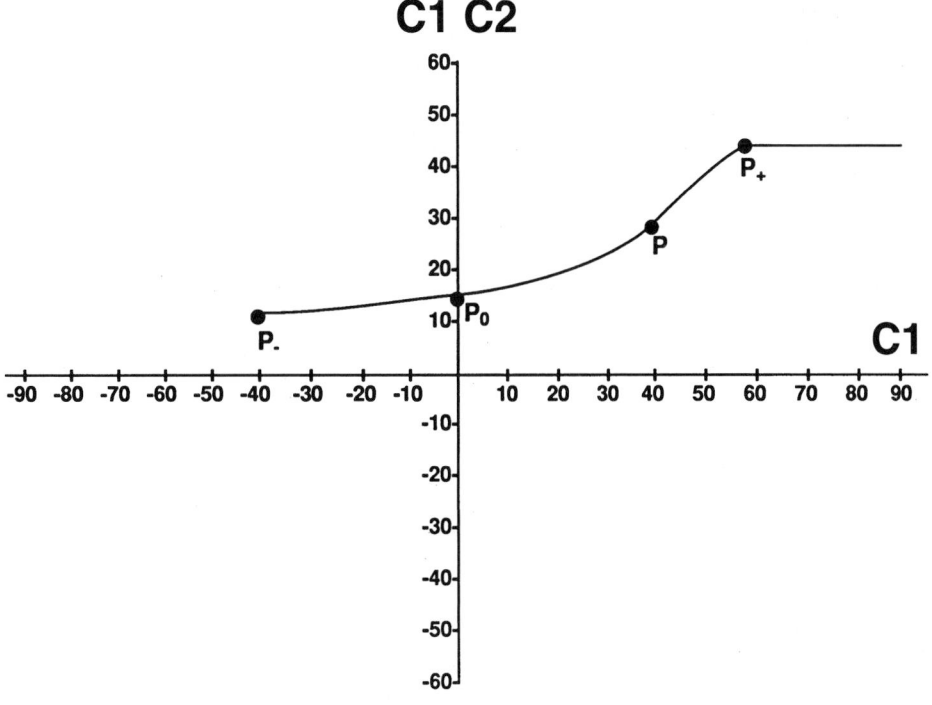

FIGURE 226–31. Type IIa atlantoaxial rotatory fixation. The C1-2 angle diminishes as the head is rotated in the corrective (P−) position; however, the curve never crosses the x-axis (C1 never crosses over C2). This represents a soft tissue interposition within the joint.

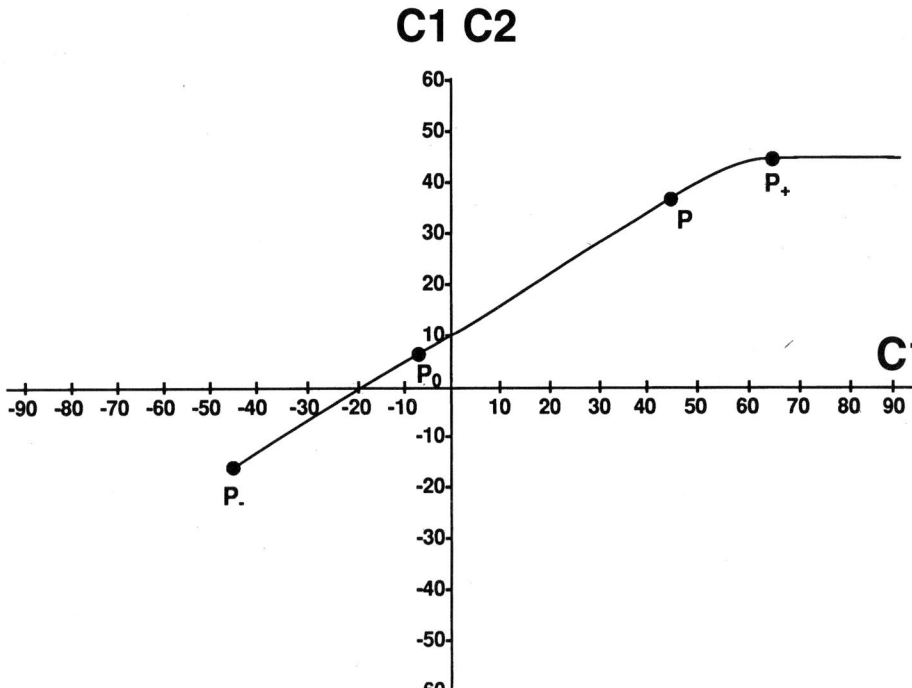

FIGURE 226–32. Type IIb atlantoaxial rotatory fixation. The C1-2 angle diminishes as the head is rotated in the corrective (P−) position. The curve crosses the x-axis, but at C1 less than −10 degrees. This represents abnormal "stickiness" within the joint.

degrees, any type of AARF may be present (Fig. 226–34). Criterion 4 in domain 4 requires that the head be in the P− position; if C1 is greater than 30 degrees despite maximal efforts to correct the deformity, severe limitation of head rotation is present, as in a bony lock (type I AARF). Finally, domain 5 is useful in detecting type IIB AARF. This criterion is met if the C1-2 crossover (i.e., when the C1-2 angle

is 0 degrees as the curve intersects the x-axis) takes place when C1 is less than −10 degrees. Diagnostic uncertainties occur when the study is suboptimal, as with neck spasm or poor cooperation, or if the angles are just outside the diagnostic domains but stray suspiciously far from the normal curve. In these cases, the study is repeated after several days of wearing a neck collar to soften the spasm.[155]

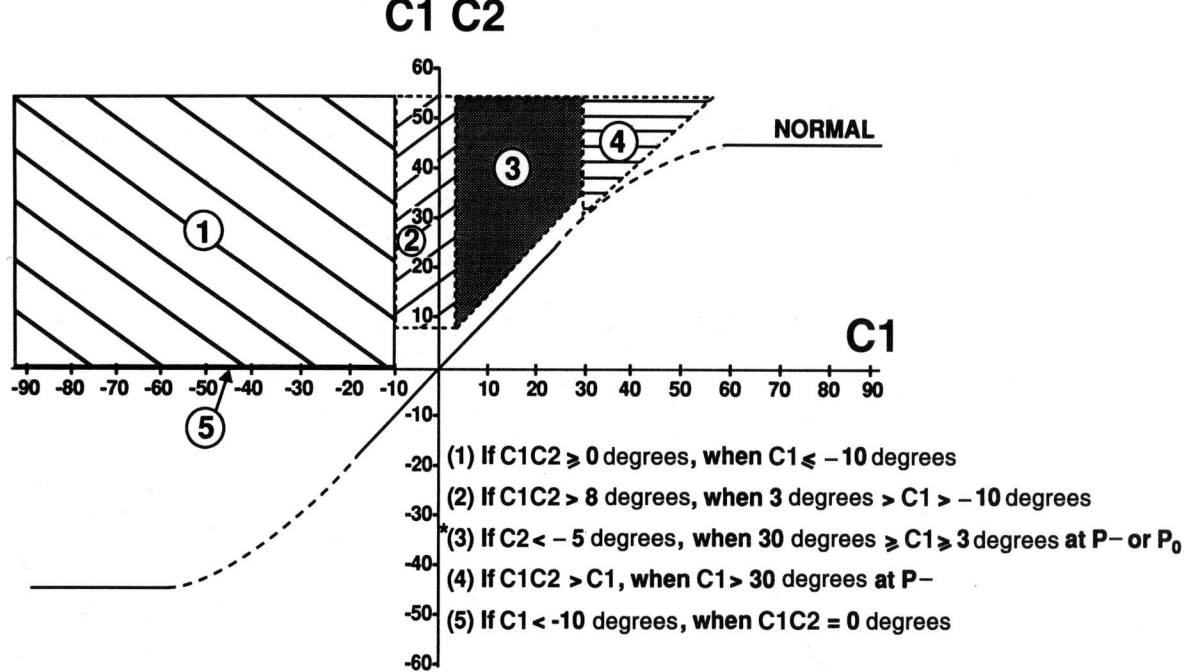

(1) If C1C2 ≥ 0 degrees, when C1 ≤ −10 degrees
(2) If C1C2 > 8 degrees, when 3 degrees > C1 > −10 degrees
*(3) If C2 < − 5 degrees, when 30 degrees ≥ C1 ≥ 3 degrees at P− or P_0
(4) If C1C2 > C1, when C1 > 30 degrees at P−
(5) If C1 < -10 degrees, when C1C2 = 0 degrees

FIGURE 226–33. Diagnostic domain diagram for atlantoaxial rotatory fixation. The head of the patient must be in the P_0 or P− position. See text for details.

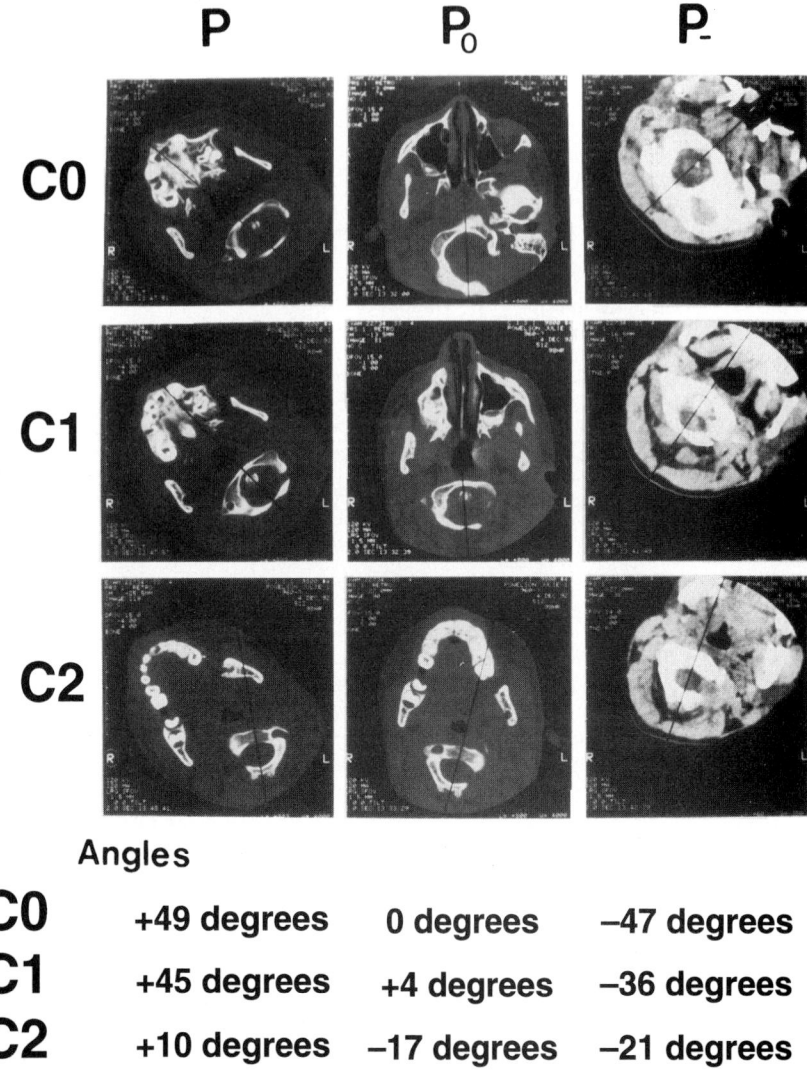

	P	P₀	P₋
C0			
C1			
C2			

Angles

	P	P₀	P₋
C0	+49 degrees	0 degrees	–47 degrees
C1	+45 degrees	+4 degrees	–36 degrees
C2	+10 degrees	–17 degrees	–21 degrees
C0C1	+4 degrees	–4 degrees	–11 degrees
C1C2	+35 degrees	+21 degrees	–15 degrees

FIGURE 226–34. Dynamic computed tomographic scan of a patient with type IIb atlantoaxial rotatory fixation (AARF). Scans in the P *(left column)*, P₀ *(middle column)*, and P– *(right column)* positions were obtained, and the angles were calculated: C0 = angle between occiput and vertical zero; C0C1 = angle between occiput and C1; C1C2 = angle between C1 and C2; C1 = angle between C1 and vertical zero; C2 = angle between C2 and vertical zero. C1 crosses C2 in the P– position. At P₀, however, the C1-2 angle is +21 degrees, which satisfies criterion 3 for AARF.

TREATMENT

In evaluating a child with possible traumatic AARF, it is important to rule out fractures and gross instability with complete cervical spine radiographs and flexion-extension studies. The "three-position" CT is then performed. An equivocal computed tomographic scan is repeated after 5 to 7 days of collar immobilization. If AARF is proved on CT, reduction in halter traction with incremental weights is begun (Fig. 226–35). Once the head resumes a midline position in traction, CT is done only in the P₀ position to confirm reduction, when C1 and C2 should be almost superimposable. The child is then immobilized for 2 to 3 months in a Guilford brace with a customized deep chin plate to restrict rotation. Final resolution is confirmed by CT in the P–, P₀, and P+ positions (P+ is when the head is fully turned to the side of the original chin rotation).

Recurrent subluxation occurs occasionally, so close follow-up is necessary. Recurrence is treated with re-reduction and halo immobilization. A second recurrence or failure of reduction is treated with open reduction and C1-2 fusion. At surgery, every effort should be made to reduce the deformity, because severe, permanent atlantoaxial rotation can result in compensatory atlanto-occipital laxity.[117, 157]

Translational Atlantoaxial Subluxation

In contrast to rotatory fixation, translational atlantoaxial subluxation occurs as a result of violent trauma. The true incidence of this injury is unknown, but it is probably extremely rare, at least among survivors.[158–160] Most affected children are in the 0- to 9-year age group, in which occipitoatlantoaxial injuries are more com-

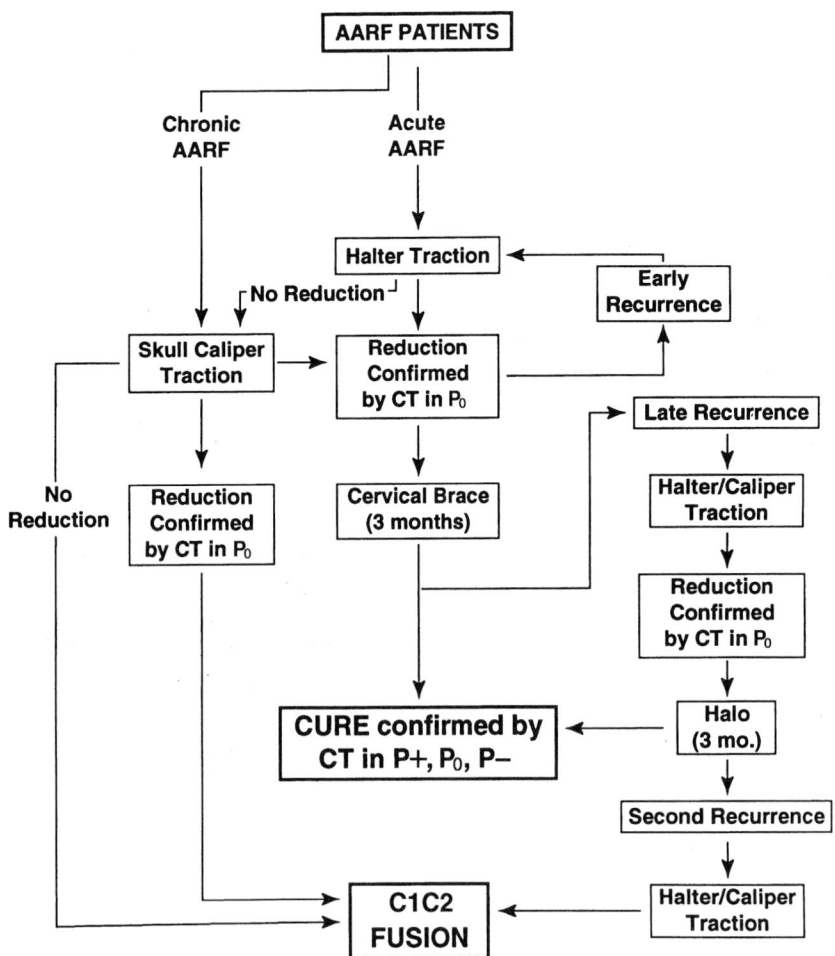

FIGURE 226–35. Treatment algorithm for acute, chronic, and recurrent atlantoaxial rotatory fixation.

mon.[11, 14, 17, 147] The majority of cases result from high-speed pedestrian-vehicular accidents.[14, 147, 161, 162] Children who survive the initial moments after injury tend to present at two extremes: either they have severe head injury, frequently aggravated by anoxic encephalopathy,[81] or they have only minor neck pain, subtle myelopathy, or C2 hypesthesia. Some cases are not initially diagnosed at all.[81, 147, 161, 163–165] Long-term survivors of this injury seldom have severe myelopathy, possibly because of selected survival at the injury scene.

Most cases of translational atlantoaxial subluxation are anterior and result from flexion injuries.[166] Exceptions are the very rare posterior C1-2 subluxation due to hyperextension[16, 167] and the even rarer C1-2 distraction. The transverse ligament is chiefly responsible for preventing excessive anterior translation of the atlantoaxial joint. Secondary support is provided by the alar ligaments. It is tempting to assume rupture of the transverse ligament as the likely cause of translational C1-2 subluxation, but Adams could find no such correlation in his autopsy study.[158] In fact, the most common abnormality in his patients was in the facet joints and their capsules. Braakman and Penning also noted that the dental synchondrosis has less strength than the transverse ligament in children, because most children younger than 8 years suffer epiphysiolysis of the odontoid rather than translational C1-2 subluxation.[168] If this is true, it would be unusual to encounter isolated rupture of the transverse ligament without dental epiphyseal separation. Therefore, "pure" traumatic translational C1-2 subluxation occurs only under very specific circumstances and likely in the presence of certain predisposing factors.

In most cases, the diagnosis is obvious on the lateral cervical radiograph. In the absence of other fractures, an atlantodental interval greater than 4 mm is abnormal in children.[81, 162, 169, 170] The retropharyngeal soft tissues are usually widened. Levine and Edwards reported an avulsed C1 tubercle (where the transverse ligament inserts on the C1 arch) on open-mouth views of the odontoid.[171] Occasionally, flexion-extension films are required to bring out an otherwise hidden instability.

Although immobilization alone has been tried on translational C1-2 subluxation,[147, 161, 163, 165] it is generally thought that extensive ligamentous injury requires C1-2 fusion.[81, 162, 171] As suggested by Levine and Edwards, halo immobilization after fusion is recommended.[171]

SPECIAL CONSIDERATIONS

A discussion of the atlantoaxial joint is not complete without mention of the various systemic disorders that can affect the strength of the synovial joints and ligamentous structures in this region. Approximately 20% of trisomy 21 (Down syndrome) patients have atlantoaxial instability.[172] Among these patients, there are reports of atlanto-occipital dislocation,[87, 173, 174] atlantoaxial instability,[85, 173, 175, 176] and AARF.[177] Because a child with Down syndrome has more lax ligaments and a higher incidence of vertebral anomalies that predispose the cord to injury,[86, 87, 175, 178–180] the index of suspicion for SCI after trauma should be raised in these children. Atlantoaxial instability has also been reported in patients with dens anomalies (e.g., os odontoideum and dental hypoplasia), juvenile rheumatoid arthritis, Morquio's syndrome, Scott's syndrome, pseudochondroplasia, spondyloepiphyseal dysplasia, spondylometaphyseal dysplasia, and cartilage-hair hypoplasia.[181–185] Special consideration should be given to investigating the spine and spinal cord in these patients, even after what would usually be considered trivial trauma.

SPINAL STABILIZATION IN CHILDREN: PROBLEMS AND PITFALLS

Problems Related to Immediate Stabilization

The application of skull caliper traction is still the simplest and most effective method of immediate stabilization, but it must be modified according to the age of the child.[51] Caliper traction is not recommended for children younger than 6 years because it is liable to cause ping-pong or other depressed skull fractures. Children in traction also tend to thrash about in bed and are at higher risk than if a one-piece orthosis is worn. Thus, for children between 1 and 6 years of age, the halo device is used for immediate stabilization. If the unstable segments in these young children are grossly malaligned, especially when the cord injury is incomplete, they should be reduced by fluoroscopically guided manual manipulation under general anesthesia, preferably with electrophysiologic monitoring. Afterward, fine-tuning and maintenance of the reduction can be achieved by adjusting the halo ring. If closed reduction is unsuccessful, the surgeon should proceed with open reduction and simultaneous fusion.

For children younger than 1 year, the problems are even greater, because halo rings are not designed for such fragile crania. If the fracture is unstable, there is no safe and effective means of emergency stabilization except open reduction and fusion. An appropriate external orthosis (see later) should then be applied in the operating room. Fortunately, unstable cervical fracture-dislocations are uncommon in this age group.

Skull caliper traction can be safely used on children from 7 to 12 years old, but with a modified protocol. First, strong sedatives are used to contain body motions and relax the nuchal muscles. Second, in young children, the forces required for reduction are much less than those required for adults, and the degree of ligamentous instability is often underestimated. The traction weight must therefore be reduced from the usual 5 pounds per level in adults to 2 or 3 pounds per level, with increments of 2 pounds, up to a maximum of 25% of the child's body weight. Each weight increment must be monitored by a lateral x-ray film to guard against overdistraction.[51] Finally, we recommend the pediatric Rotorest bed (Kinetic Concepts Inc., San Antonio, TX), in which the child's entire body can be fit snugly between adjustable side panels so that he or she feels more secure and is less disposed to thrash about. Upward sliding of the body is checked by well-padded shoulder stoppers.[51] The gentle rotation of the Rotorest bed is also helpful for reducing skin complications, which can develop rapidly in children.

Problems with External Orthoses

HALO FIXATION DEVICE

Among all the available cervical orthoses, the halo vest provides the most rigid immobilization of the cervical spine.[167, 186–188] It also permits the most precise positioning of the neck to obtain and maintain alignment. It is the only external orthosis that does not have a chin support, so it interferes the least with mandibular motion and eating.[189] Early mobilization enables the patient to participate in rehabilitation, which is an especially important advantage for children, who tend to sabotage the immobilization if they are not allowed some physical activity.

The halo vest is currently the orthosis of choice for most children with unstable cervical spines.[51, 88, 190, 191] However, the complications associated with the halo are also higher in children than in adults,[190] and most of them are related to the thinness of the child's calvaria. The anterior pins should be placed immediately above the eyebrows, to take advantage of the thick lateral supraorbital buttress,[190] and laterally to avoid injuring the supraorbital and supratrochlear nerves. The torque used for pin tightening should be between 2 and 4 inch-pounds, depending on the size of the child. For children 10 months to 3 years of age, "tiny tot" haloes are available with a small ring and up to 10 small pins that should only be finger-tightened.[192] However, one great disadvantage of the multipin system is that it leaves few unused holes on the ring for pin changes in case of pin site infection or loosening (see later).

The frequency of pin loosening is much higher in children than in adults.[190, 193] Some pins migrate cephalad because they were inserted above the skull equator, where the skull contour is sloping upward. Pins may also loosen because the correct degree of tightness was not rechecked. Owing to the viscoelastic properties of the skull, the pins frequently loosen up to 4 inch-pounds after the vest and uprights are attached to the ring, and they must be retightened to the correct torque 24 hours later. If a loose pin is discovered 2 to 3 weeks after insertion, the management depends on the age of the patient. Garfin and colleagues found that with 6 inch-pounds of torque, the halo pin only partially penetrates the outer table of the adult skull, and there is usually a solid margin of cortical bone to allow safe retightening.[193] Thus, it is usually safe to retighten loose pins in older children, provided definite resistance can be felt on tightening. The skull tables in young children are much thinner. Accelerated osteoclasis around the pin site softens the bone so much that retightening can cause full-thickness penetration and intracranial abscess.[194] Loose pins should be replaced and not tightened in these children.[51]

Pin site infections are also much more common in children than in adults. Baum and coworkers reported a 31% incidence of pin infection in children, versus 6% in adults.[190] The pin sites should be cleansed thoroughly with 10% hydrogen peroxide solution four times daily, and all scabs and crust around the pins must be removed to allow drainage. If the infection is mild and superficial, with only minimal surrounding scalp erythema and drainage, and the pin remains tight, oral antibiotics are prescribed. If the scalp is red and swollen, the drainage becomes copious and purulent, or the child complains of constant local pain or headaches, the pin should be removed and intravenous antibiotics given to prevent the dreaded cranial osteomyelitis. A computed tomographic scan should be done to rule out an intracranial abscess.[194–197]

Children in haloes also have a greater likelihood than adults to show alignment slippage, partly because of unrecognized pin loosening, and partly because children do not protect their haloes. Direct contact of the ring and posterior uprights with the bedding should be avoided to minimize transmitted flexion stresses. We use a large foam wedge to prop up the back of the vest so that the child can recline comfortably with the head and halo ring hanging free and still be able to watch television, read, play board games, and self-feed.[51] In addition, children sometimes undergo rapid and drastic changes in body weight and contour after SCI, so the original vest may become ill fitting and need to be recustomized.

Finally, children tend to be very unforgiving if the head position is not adjusted exactly to their liking. Because most unstable injuries are unstable in flexion, it is always tempting to set the neck in slight extension. However, children develop mechanical dysphagia when the neck is even slightly extended, due to restricted upward movement of the larynx during the pharyngeal phase of swallowing. Also, if the child's visual axis cannot command a full frontal view of the surroundings when the head is tilted too far back, the child will simply stop walking. Thus, the neck should be put in the "military salute" position, in which posterior translation is substituted for extension. For a young child, the top-heavy halo bars and vest in effect shift the center of gravity upward, and he or she must be patiently coached to relearn the basic skills of walking and navigating.

MINERVA CAST

On rare occasions, the Minerva cast has been used on young children who do not tolerate the halo pins. The thermoplastic jacket is constructed of polyfoam, a splinting material made from a polyester polycaprolac-tone, and polycushion, a closed-cell foam for padding.[198] This lightweight material solves the problems of hyperthermia and encumbered ambulation. Clinical trials also found that the thermoplastic Minerva jacket actually restricts intersegmental "snaking" movements in the cervical spine better than the halo vest. It deserves further evaluation for adaptation for use in children.

GUILFORD BRACE

The Guilford brace has been used extensively in our institution on children with SCIWORA.[19, 27, 69, 192] This brace has padded mandibular and occipital supports that interlock to form a rigid metal ring below the ears. The ring is connected by strong metal strips to anterior and posterior thoracic plates that are attached to each other by shoulder and axillary straps. The Guilford brace is comparable to other cervicothoracic braces in its ability to limit flexion, extension, and rotation, especially of the mid- to lower cervical segments.[167, 187] Like the other orthoses, the Guilford brace is not as effective in controlling lateral bending. Its main advantage over other braces is that it can be custom-made within 24 hours to fit any body size down to that of a 1-year-old. With deepening of the chin and occipital plates to restrict rotation, it is also suited for maintaining reduction in AARF.

MOLDED BODY SPLINT

There is no ideal orthosis for long-term immobilization of infants with grossly unstable necks. One example of this condition is diastrophic dwarfism, in which the affected infant has ligamentous laxity at multiple segments and usually presents in the first few months of life with apnea and quadriplegic spells due to multilevel subluxations and cervicomedullary injury. These neurological manifestations are completely reversible as long as the neck can be kept in a neutral or slightly extended position. Because no orthosis can reliably eliminate intersegmental motions in these infants, wiring and bone graft fusion often end in nonunion, and we usually do not attempt surgical fusion until these patients reach 3 years of age. In the interim, the infant is immobilized in a thermoplastic body and head splint molded to the contour of the thorax, head, and neck in the desired degree of extension.[51] The body section incorporates the pelvis and hip joints and has a crotch strap that interlocks with cross-shoulder straps over the chest and abdomen, based on the same principle as an infant car seat. The head section has a padded headband that is strapped across the forehead to secure the head. The back slab can be fenestrated if the infant develops hyperthermia, which happens not infrequently (Fig. 226–36). Diastrophic dwarfs are usually not ambulatory for many months after birth anyway, and with proper skin care, they can be kept safely in this molded body splint for up to 3 years (Fig. 226–37), at which time extensive surgical fusion has a better chance of success.

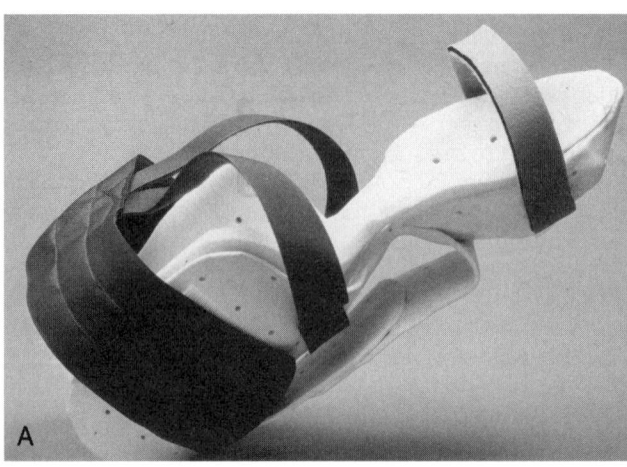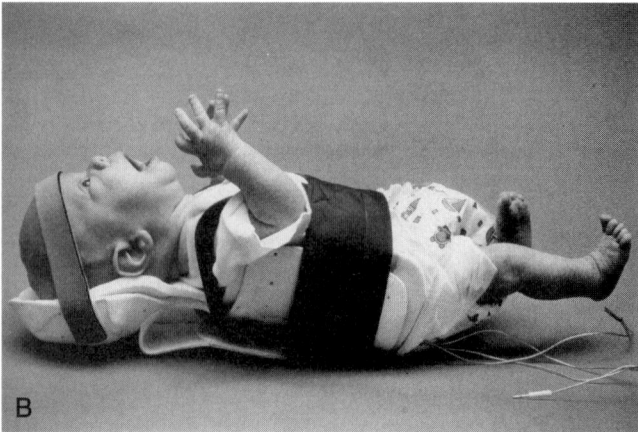

FIGURE 226–36. Thermoplastic body splint for long-term immobilization of the head and neck in young infants. *A*, Note the Velcro head and chest straps, fenestrations in the back slab for ventilation, and the flat shelf under the back section for more stable positioning on a bed or hard surface and to provide a secure hand grip for manual handling of the body splint. *B*, Body splint molded to the contour of the infant's neck, head, and thorax. The head position is adjustable, usually to slight extension.

Problems Related to Internal Surgical Fixation

GENERAL PRINCIPLES

As in adults with displaced fractures, it is always preferable to reduce any malalignment in children as soon as possible. Cord compression should be relieved promptly, and subsequent fusion can be rendered with minimal manipulation of the unstable segments. In older children, preoperative reduction can be accomplished with skull traction. In children younger than 7 years, reduction is best done in the operating room manually under fluoroscopy and general anesthesia.

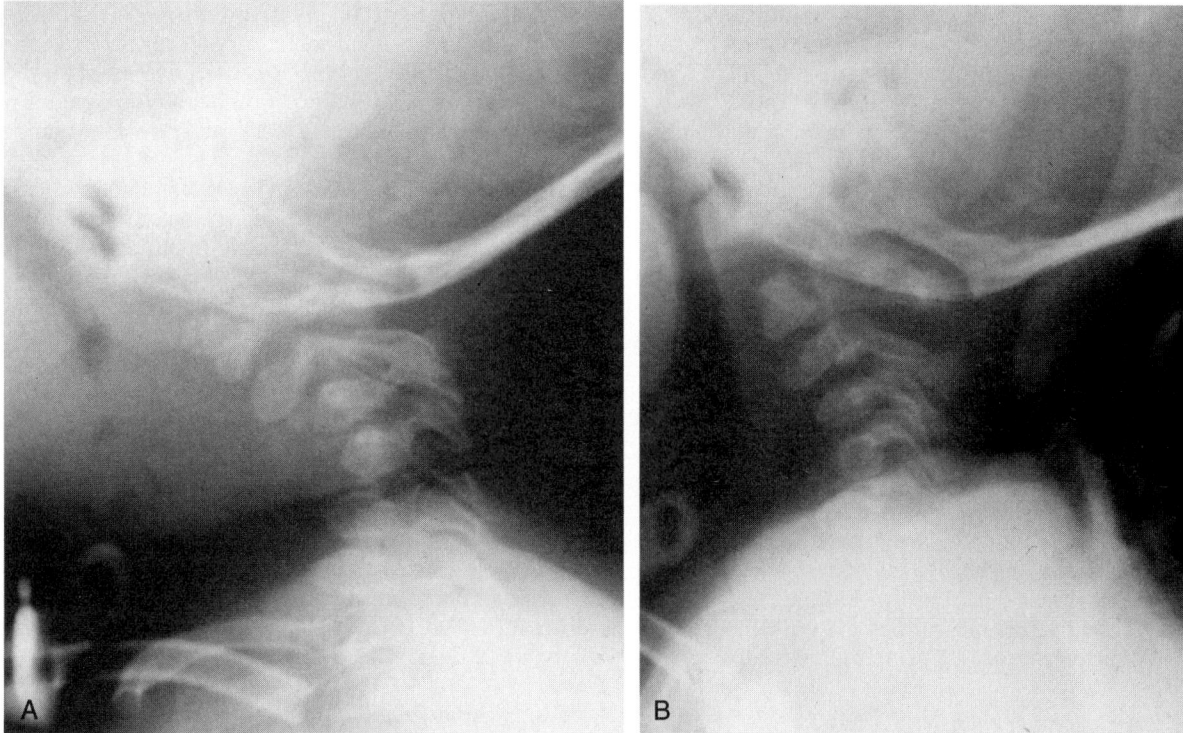

FIGURE 226–37. *A*, Lateral radiograph of an infant with diastrophic dwarfism showing multilevel severe anterior subluxation of the upper cervical spine. The infant had apnea in this position. *B*, Moderate reversal of the kyphotic curvature maintained by the molded body splint. The infant was asymptomatic in this position.

The halo should be applied to maintain the reduction before surgical fusion is begun.

It is common practice at many SCI centers to intubate adult patients with unstable injuries while they are awake so that any sudden changes in the patient's neurological status can be recognized. Awake intubation is seldom tolerated by children, even with potent local anesthetic spray and intravenous sedation. Young children, especially, tend to resist vigorously and may actually jeopardize the unstable injury further. We prefer to perform fiber-optic nasotracheal intubation on children *after* induction of general anesthesia with intravenous thiopental and vecuronium bromide. This way, the airway can be quickly and atraumatically secured with minimal head movement. Spinal cord function is monitored with real-time somatosensory evoked potentials throughout intubation, halo application, and the surgical fusion that follows.[51]

It is our and others' impression that bone bank bone has less chance of inducing successful fusion in children than autologous bone grafts do.[199] The amount of available bone is obviously limited by the size of the child, and both iliac crests should be prepared for use. Other bone sources include ribs, fibula, and split-thickness cranial bone from the occiput.[200]

Permanent stability at the fusion site ultimately depends on the amount of new bone that manages to form across the fusion surfaces. The larger the fusion surface available for new bone formation, the more exuberant the callus and the stronger the subsequent bony bridge. Although methyl methacrylate incorporated into a wiring construct enhances the immediate stability of the construct,[201] it also diminishes the available fusion surface for new bone formation and ultimately weakens the permanent strength of the fusion.[202] This is a particularly relevant issue in children, in whom the fusion surface is already limited. Also, acrylic does not bind to bone, weakens with time, and remains a permanent foreign body.[203, 204] Methyl methacrylate is therefore not used on children except when a malignancy is involved.

Continuous micromotions between fusion segments are strongly correlated with nonunion. As mentioned, halo immobilization in children is sometimes complicated by pin loosening and position slippage. Nonhalo orthoses provide even less satisfactory external stabilization.[167] Thus, for children with unstable injuries, the burden of immediate stabilization rests largely on the immediate strength of the fusion construct; this is in contrast to adult patients, in whom the halo can be depended on to provide more reliable external immobilization. Thus, one should always select the construct that gives maximal *immediate internal stability*, that is, the one that is most effective in eliminating intersegmental motion. Fusion techniques for children should be judged on this important principle.

INJURIES INVOLVING C2-7

In most unstable injuries in children involving the C2-7 levels, we favor the sublaminar wiring technique in the form of simple bilateral loops around the adjacent laminae.[51] The ligamenta flava are detached completely from the deep side of the laminae to facilitate visually locating the wire tip over the dura during the sublaminar passage. The 16- or 18-gauge Luque wire had been a popular choice because of its tensile strength and rounded tip, but recently, braided, MRI-compatible titanium Codman or Songer cables have been used instead of wires because of their malleability, sliding quality, and crimp-lock mechanism, enabling safe passage and strenuous tightening. Iliac crest bone grafts are then secondarily wired to the fusion surface or tightly pressed down against it by strapping sutures strung across the deep muscles.

The soft cables have substantially reduced the risk of cord injury due to the sublaminar passage. The construct is extremely strong and stable, ensuring a high rate of union in children. Regardless of the age of the child, the laminae are still the strongest bone buttress to support any wiring. Even in children 3 to 5 years old, 18-gauge cables can be used without producing laminar fracture. Tightening the cables usually makes the two adjacent laminae crunch against each other to produce a more stable friction block than either the interfacetal or interspinous wiring techniques.[201]

POSTERIOR MID- TO LOWER CERVICAL FUSION WITH INSTRUMENTATION

Posterior cervical fusion with instrumentation is not commonly used in young children, mainly because the delicate bone structures will not support internal bracing by large pieces of rigid metal. The latter also reduce the bony surface available for new bone formation. However, cervical instrumentation is occasionally indicated in children with postlaminectomy kyphosis when laminar wiring is not practicable or when a necessary multilevel fusion exceeds the holding capacity of a strut bone graft.

Kyphotic deformity involving more than two vertebral segments requires a corrective strut that can withstand rigorous stress. Particularly in children with connective tissue disease, such as Ehlers-Danlos syndrome and diastrophic dwarfism, the chronic curvature is not usually correctable by the halo device, and the internal fixation must bear most of the deforming strain. In such cases, a metal strut tailored to the length and contour of the deformed segments is fastened to the laminae with sublaminar cables. Choices of strut include a titanium Steinmann pin bent to an appropriate-sized rectangle or prefabricated Luque rectangles (Zimmer USA, Warsaw, IN) and Codman subaxial rectangles. Autologous cancellous bone grafts are laid over the exposed fusion surfaces. Because of the unstable nature of these conditions, a halo is used postoperatively for at least 4 to 5 months to reinforce the fusion construct.

The ultimate challenge is attempting to stabilize a child with kyphotic instability following extensive laminectomy. Not only are the fusion surfaces drastically reduced, but the best support for the wiring, the laminae, are gone. The use of interfacetal wiring or facetal strut grafts is limited by the fragility of the facets in young children. We have had excellent success using a contoured Luque rectangle with the top and bottom bars fastened to one or two intact laminae at each end of the laminectomy defect, but the fusion necessarily includes at least two extra levels beyond the laminectomy defect.

A sometimes feasible alternative that gives a more conservative fusion is lateral mass screws and plates.[205] Holes with measured depths are drilled through the precise center of the involved articular pillar by angling the drill bit slightly superiorly (10 degrees) and laterally (10 to 15 degrees). The titanium plates (Leotech, Jacksonville, FL) are curved slightly to aid in restoring the normal lordotic curvature. The plate length is chosen based on the number of unstable segments and whether fracture of a lateral mass requires skipping a level with the screws. After lining them up over the drill holes, the plates are secured with self-tapping cancellous bone screws. These posterior plates have not been used extensively in children because of the variable size of the articular pillars, the closeness of the vertebral artery to the screw path, and the dependency on the state of ossification of the pedicles. They should be used selectively, according to the size and age of the child. Usually the lower age limit for lateral mass screws and plates is 8 or 9 years.

INJURIES INVOLVING THE C1-2 JOINT

Different fusion techniques are used for the atlantoaxial articulation because of its unique anatomic and biomechanical characteristics. For example, the atlas does not have a spinous process for interspinous wiring. Because of the wide gap between the posterior arches of C1 and C2, simple sublaminar wiring does not impart extension stability unless the two arches are actually made to approximate. Moreover, the inclination of the atlantoaxial facet joints and the interfacet ligaments is teleologically "suited" to a 47-degree range of axial rotation[90, 197] and a high degree of translational freedom. Any fusion technique for this extremely mobile joint must therefore withstand all four planes of motion—flexion, extension, rotation, and translation.

The Gallie method, which uses a single midline wire loop around the arch of C1 and the spinous process of C2, does not meet the desired objectives because it eliminates neither extension nor rotation.[206] Extension is largely unchecked because the arches of C1 and C2 rarely approximate with the single wire loop, and axial rotation is only moderately restricted by the single fixation point provided by the midline loop. The Gallie fusion is particularly unsuitable for children because the midline synchondrosis between the two neural arches of C1 remains cartilaginous until age 5 or 6 years and brittle until 10 or 12 years, and it can easily be cut through by the midline wire.

In contrast to the Gallie method, the Brooks fusion offers much greater biomechanical advantage.[104] In this construct, bilateral wires are passed around the arch of C1 and the lamina of C2 and then tightened separately over a corticocancellous bone graft compressed against

the C1 and C2 rings. A modification of the Brooks technique by Griswold and associates uses an almost T-shaped bone graft wedged between the C1 and C2 bony rings; the flat part of the T prevents the graft from being displaced into the spinal canal.[207] With the modified Brooks construct, there is stability in both flexion and extension: flexion is eliminated by the circumferential wires, and extension is stopped by the bone graft, which serves as a buttressing block.[90] The bone graft also serves as a friction block between the two bony arches and offers stability against axial rotation and translation. The modified Brooks fusion is very effective in children with atlantoaxial instability, especially when the C1 arch is fixed in an upward tilt that leaves a wide gap between it and the C2 neural arch (Fig. 226–38). A newer modification of the Brooks method using two separate interposing bone grafts, one on each side of the midline, allows the Brooks principle to be used in cases in which the middle third of the C1 arch has to be removed for decompression, such as when C1-2 realignment is less than perfect.[51] Levy and McComb reported excellent results with this modification in 13 children.[208]

There is, however, a caveat when using the Brooks method in young children. It seems that the incidence of rapid graft absorption is higher in young children than in adults, possibly because halo fixation in young children does not provide the same degree of stability, and the continued micromotions at the fusion site promote graft resorption and retard bone formation, leading ultimately to graft shrinkage. Because the original wires are wound over the combined bulk of the lamina and the graft, graft shrinkage causes the wire loops to loosen and more intersegmental motion to occur, thereby completing the vicious circle and resulting in nonunion.[51]

Thus, in young children with atlantoaxial instability, we prefer to pass bilateral sublaminar wires around the arches of C1 and C2 and then tighten them until the two arches touch.[20, 51] This is quite easily and safely achieved in most young children without placing excessive strain on the arch of C1 (Fig. 226–39). The conjoined bony rings offer stability in both flexion and extension, and the two-point fixation provided by the double wires also increases friction between the twin rings and reduces axial rotation and translation. Onlaid bone grafts are then compressed tightly against the fusion surface by deep sutures. The inherent strength of this construct is undiminished by any interim changes in the grafts, and fusion is almost guaranteed as long as the bony rings and wires hold up against breakage.

ATLANTOAXIAL FUSION WITH INSTRUMENTATION

In older children, other options are available for instrumentation of the C1-2 joint. Magerl pioneered the use of transarticular screw fixation of C1-2 in 1979, and he and Seemann reported their experience in a large series of adults in 1986.[209] Modern adaptations of the original technique using newer drill assembly and precise tra-

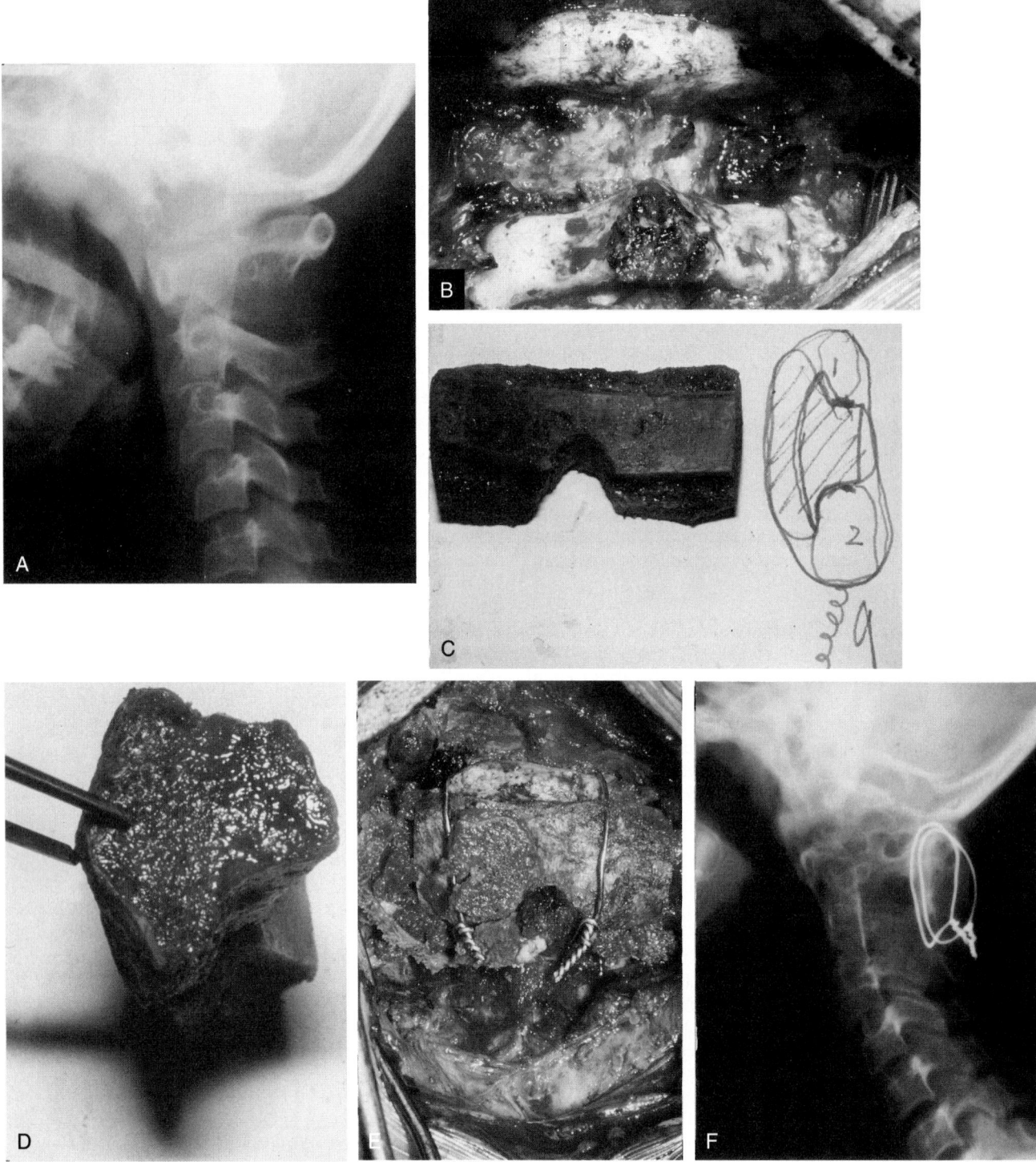

FIGURE 226–38. Modified Brooks fusion in an 8-year-old girl with untreated C1-2 rotatory fixation. The right lateral mass of C2 is rotated to the left and "stepped off" in front of the C2 facet, preventing reduction in spite of prolonged traction. Because of the unreduced C2 lateral mass, the posterior arch of C1 is "jacked up" in relation to the C2 laminae. *A,* Lateral radiograph demonstrates the persistently jacked-up position of the C1 arch. *B,* Intraoperative exposure shows the wide gap between the C1 arch and the C2 laminae. The C1 arch did not budge with earnest attempts to bring it down by instruments. *C,* Posterior view of the tricorticate T-shaped interposition graft from the iliac crest. Its natural curvature fits the transverse contour of the neural arches, and a notch was cut for the spinous process of C2. The inset drawing is an end-on sagittal section of the T-shaped graft interposed between C1 and C2 arches. *D,* Lateral view of the graft shows the T-shaped fitting for the adjacent neural arches. *E,* Bone graft wired into place by two wires looping around both neural arches and the graft. *F,* Postoperative radiograph showing the fusion construct.

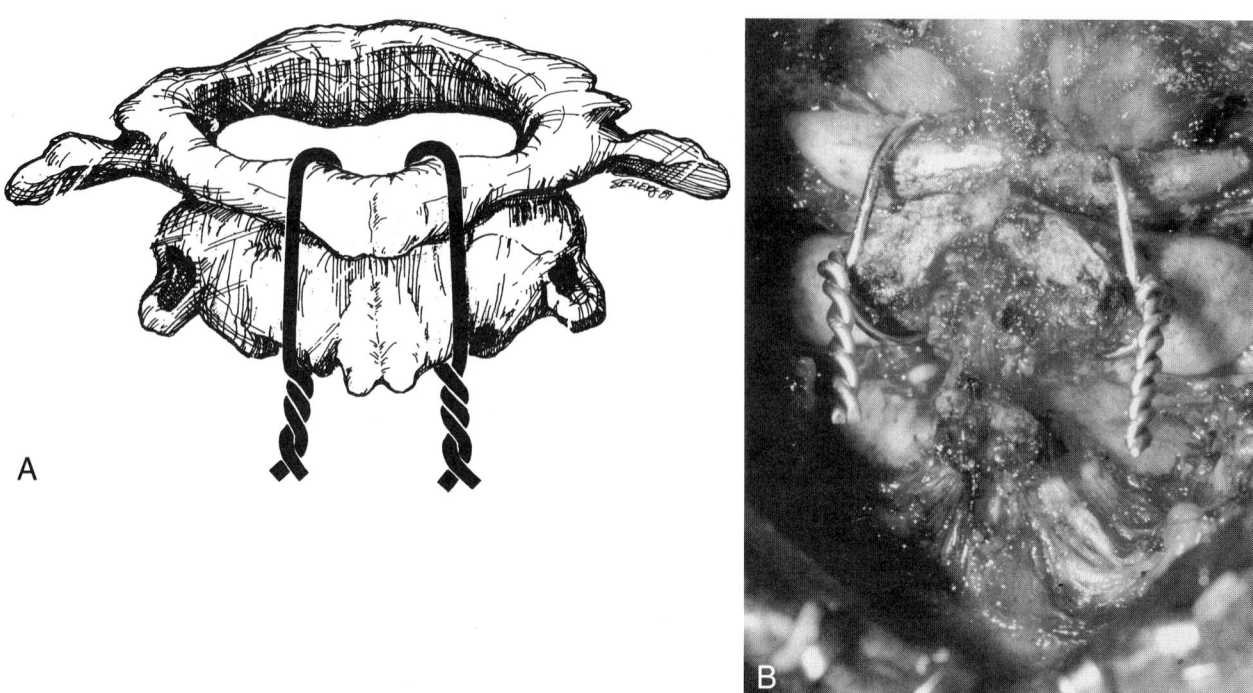

FIGURE 225–39. Posterior wire fusion of C1 and C2 in a 6-year-old child. Note approximation of the bony rings of C1 and C2 by the two sublaminar wire loops that are tightly twisted below the C2 ring. *A,* Drawing. *B,* Intraoperative appearance.

jectory planning and guidance with frameless stereotactic navigation have been described.[210] The chief advantages of this technique include excellent fixation against translation and rotation; when supplemented by an interposing bone graft between the arches of C1 and C2, which prevents flexion and extension, use of the postoperative halo can be avoided.[211] In addition, it is useful even when the arches of C1 or C2 have been removed for decompression. The reported successful fusion rates are 95% to 98%,[212, 213] compared with 80% to 86% when wire-graft techniques are used with the halo.[208, 212] The complication rates for vertebral artery injury, ischemic stroke, and neural injury are exceedingly low when proper precautions are taken.[210, 212–214] With the addition of bilateral vertical plates, the C1-2 transarticular screw construct can be extended to incorporate lateral mass screw fixation of the subaxial spine.

The bulk of the literature on C1-2 transarticular screw fixation concerns adults. In the last 5 years, this technique has been cautiously used on a small number of children, and emerging data suggest great promise (Fig. 226–40). Wang and colleagues reported a series of 13 children (the youngest 4 years old) with a 100% fusion rate, no complications, and no postoperative halo,[215] compared with an 84% fusion rate with a wire-graft method and halo reported by others.[216] With children, a number of special precautions must be heeded.

In some adults, the bony groove for the vertebral artery at C2 may be so large as to reduce the width of the pars interarticularis (isthmus) to below safety limits for passage of a 3.5-mm screw. Madawi and associates[217] and Paramore and coworkers[218] reported a 20%

exclusion rate for at least one isthmus on account of the vertebral artery anatomy, and in 4% to 5%, neither side was deemed safe. The isthmus in children is accordingly narrower than in adults (Fig. 226–41). Especially in younger children, the absolute dimension of the isthmus must be premeasured and the screw path preplanned on a virtual image before surgery. Triplane

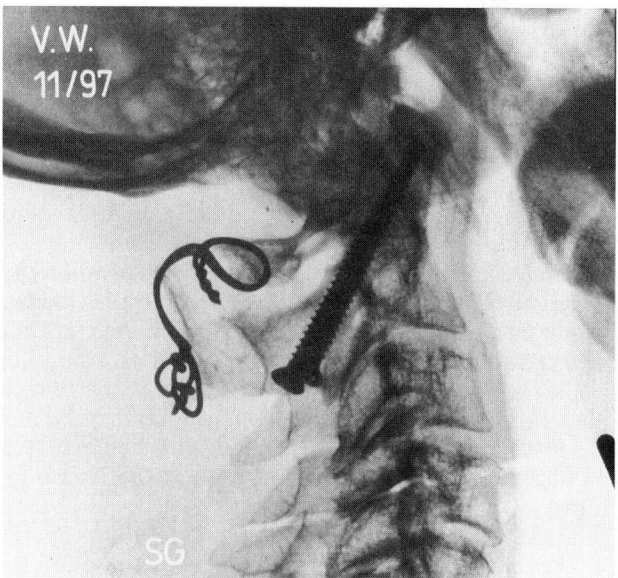

FIGURE 226–40. Lateral radiograph showing C1-2 transarticular screw fixation in a 12-year-old child with congenital C1-2 instability. Flexion and extension motions are eliminated by the simultaneous Sonntag-type posterior wiring.

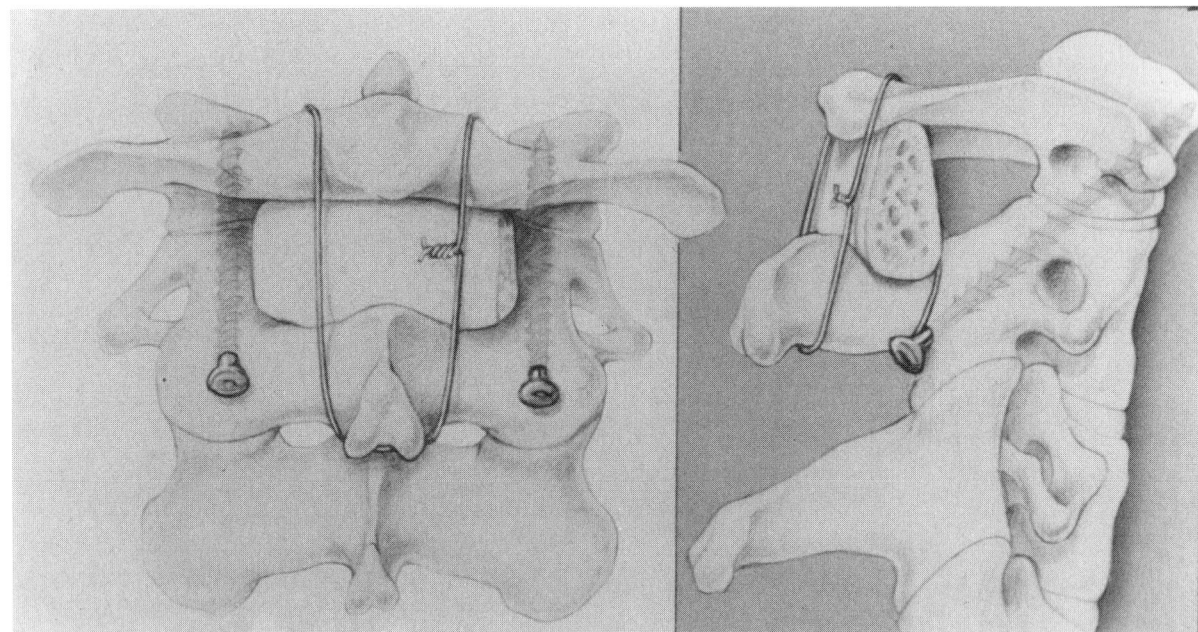

FIGURE 226–41. Drawings of C1-2 transarticular screw fixation. The desired screw trajectory is through the C2 isthmus and the C1-2 articulation. The medial side of the C2 pedicle serves as a direction guide. In children and in some adults with a wide vertebral artery groove, the isthmus may be too narrow for the screw path. (From Apfelbaum R: Posterior Transarticular C1-C2 Screw Fixation for Atlanto-Axial Instability. Aesculap Scientific Information No. 25. South San Francisco, CA, Aesculap, 1993.)

computer reconstruction with the cursor traversing the long axis of the isthmus (simulating the screw path) should be done on every child. If only unilateral screw placement is feasible, a postoperative halo should be used.

The lateral mass of C1 may be hypoplastic in some children (as in Down syndrome), and the distal purchase of the screw is therefore poorly sustained. The anterior tubercle of the atlas may be hypoplastic or absent, which makes fluoroscopic monitoring of the drill trajectory difficult, because the posterior cortex of the C1 tubercle is the target point on the lateral radiograph. Frameless stereotactic navigation can now bypass this problem. Madawi and associates also reported a higher incidence of screw malpositioning if the C1-2 subluxation is poorly reduced, with considerable offset in the facet contact surfaces.[217] Good alignment is therefore very important in pediatric patients.

Children usually have a wide space between the arches of C1 and C2, and in order to buttress against flexion and extension, a solid, well-fitting interposition bone graft must be affixed to the arches using the Brooks or Sonntag technique.[214, 219] Even if the middle third of the C1 and C2 arches has been removed, laterally placed bone grafts on each side can be fixed with separate titanium cables looped around the lateral extremes of both arches.[20, 208]

Finally, the fusion bed should be carefully prepared by decortication, avoidance of excessive use of the Bovie cautery, vigorous curettage of the facetal cartilage, and packing of cancellous bone chips into the C1-2 joint gaps.

One final word on C1-2 instrumentation: anterior odontoid screw fixation has been used on a few children with type II odontoid fractures that were perfectly reduced. The advantage of this technique over the transarticular screw is the preservation of C1-2 rotation, which is especially desirable in children. Further experience is needed before the use of this technique in children can be widely endorsed.

OCCIPITAL-CERVICAL FUSION WITH INSTRUMENTATION

Occasionally, an anteriorly dislocated C1 arch cannot be reduced by traction or manipulation. This happens in some cases of os odontoideum, chronic post-traumatic anterolisthesis, and several forms of mucolipidoses in which abnormal tissues interpose between the dens and the anterior arch of C1. Sublaminar wire fusion of the unreduced ring of C1-2 may add to the spinal cord compression. In such instances, it is safer to remove the arch of C1 to decompress the cord before attempting to fuse the occiput, C2, and C3 together. For this situation and for the progressive kyphosis sometimes seen after occipitocervical decompression for Chiari malformation, we use a Steinmann pin shaped in an inverted U with the bend contoured to conform to the occipital boss.[51] The two vertical bars are wired to the top two available laminae, and the curved U bend is wired to the occiput via bur holes on both sides of the midline (Fig. 226–42). A recent modification using the Luque rectangle adds a measure of inferior stability by fixing the lower rim of the rectangle to the lower intact lamina (Fig. 226–43).[20] Cancellous bone grafts are packed into the lateral gutters at

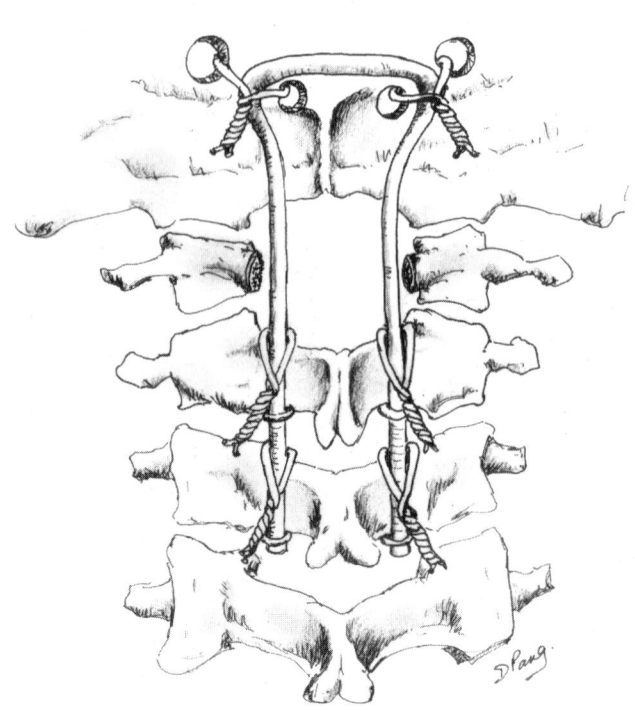

FIGURE 226–42. Steinmann pin fixation in occiput-C2-C3 fusion. The steel or titanium pin is first bent in an inverted U, and the bend is contoured to the occiput. The bend is wired to the occiput via bur holes, and the vertical arms are fixed to C2 and C3 with sublaminar wires.

C1, on the decorticated laminae, and on the occipital squama. A halo is necessary for this method of occipital-cervical fusion. This construct has excellent inherent strength and results in a very high union rate, even in young children.

The chief disadvantage of the rigid U-bar technique is that the sliding motion between the metal bar and the metallic cables cannot be totally eliminated. Completely rigid fixation is not obtained, and considering the great angular momentum of the child's heavy head working against the cable-bar contact, a halo vest is always recommended postoperatively to reinforce stability. Plates have been affixed more rigidly with screws to the occiput and the cervical spine,[144, 220–228] but with children, bone thickness of the occiput is of great concern, in terms of both providing adequate bony purchase for the traditional outside-to-inside screws and avoiding dural penetration. In fact, the unevenness of bone thickness in the occipital squama of a child is such that screw purchase is secure only into the midline keel and far laterally near the mastoid process.

Pait and colleagues described the "inside-outside" technique, which obviates most of the problems related to screw purchase in thin skulls and is eminently suitable for occipital-cervical fusion in children.[229] In this technique, a lateral mass plate is contoured to fit the shape of the occiput and the cervical spine, and the plate is affixed to the occiput by means of a flat-headed screw placed through a bur hole in the calvaria so that the head of the screw is in the epidural space and the threads face outward—hence the sobriquet "inside-outside." The bur hole marks the "entry site" of the inside-outside screw. After the dura is separated from the inner table of the skull, a "keyhole" is cut from the entry site some distance away to the premarked "exit site" for the screw using a craniotome footplated saw blade. The size of the exit site is cut to the size of the screw stem, always much smaller than the bur hole. The inside-outside screw is attached to the guide rod (Dyna-lok T bolt and nut; Sofamor Danek, Memphis, TN) and then carefully placed epidurally into the entry site and guided to the exit site (Fig. 226–44*A*). The reconstruction plate is placed "through" the out-pointing screw stem, and a nut is semitightened on the exposed screw threads with a socket wrench (see Fig. 226–44*B*). After the C1-2 transarticular screw (or C2 pedicle screw) and all the subaxial cervical lateral mass screws have been inserted and tightened on the plate, the occipital inside-outside screw is firmly tightened against the nut with the socket wrench while a screwdriver is inserted through the socket wrench into the hex in the hollow inside-outside screw to provide countertorque (see Fig. 226–44*C*).

Different plate systems can be linked to the inside-outside screw, depending on the size and age of the child. Children as young as 2 years old have been

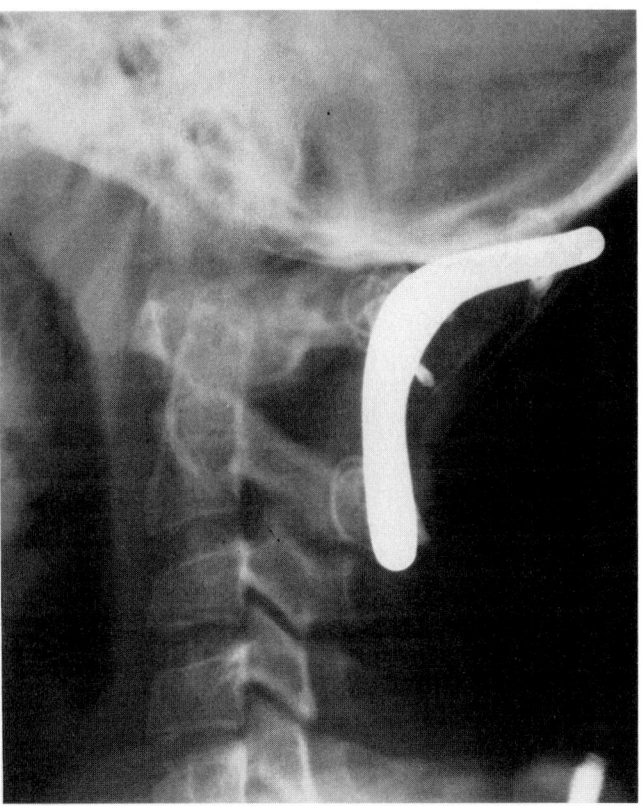

FIGURE 226–43. Occipitoatlantoaxial fusion with the Luque rectangle fixed to the occiput with titanium cables through bur holes, and to the C1 and C2 arches with sublaminar cables.

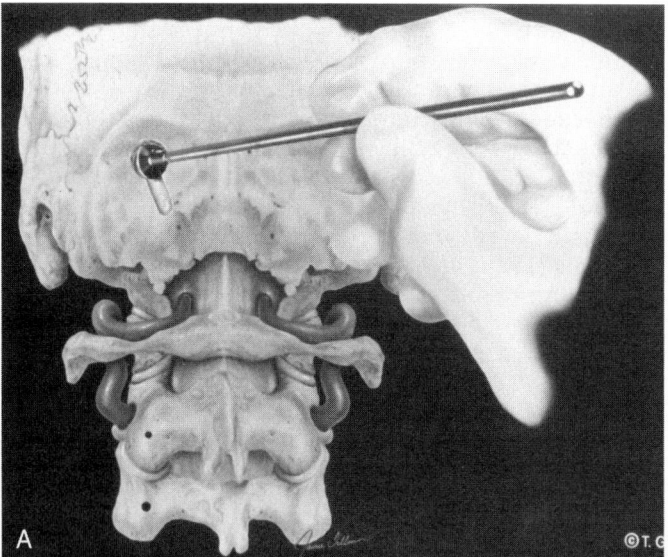

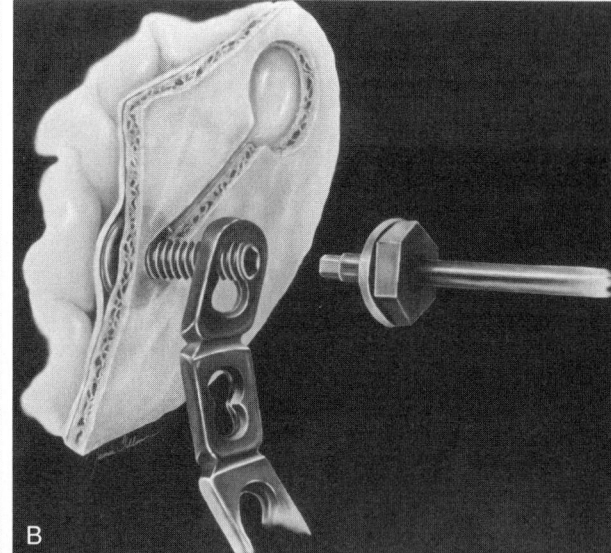

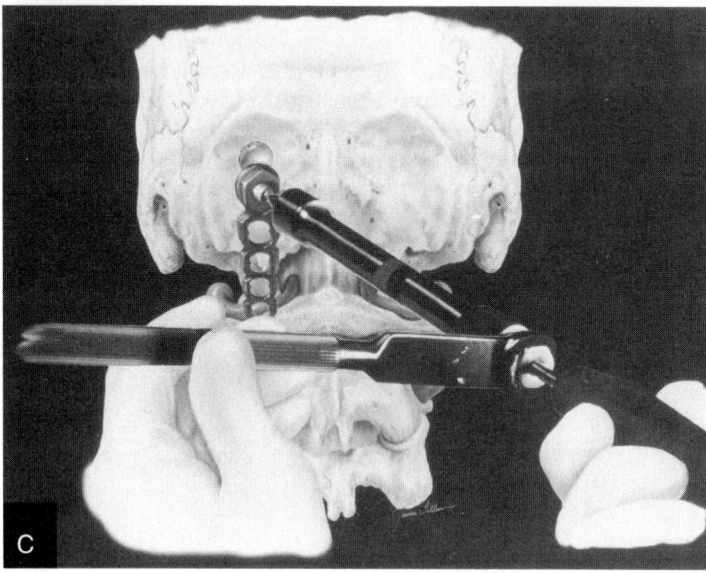

FIGURE 225–44. Pait's "inside-outside" screw technique. *A,* The inside-outside screw is attached to a guide rod and inserted into the entry bur hole. *B,* The reconstruction plate is placed over the inside-outside screw, and the nut is loosely attached to the screw. *C,* After adjustments for the suboccipital screws on the reconstructed plate, the nut is firmly tightened on the inside-outside screw by a socket wrench while a screwdriver is inserted through the wrench into the hex of the hollow screw head to provide countertorque. (From Pait TG, Al-Mefty O, Boop FA, et al: Inside-outside technique for posterior occipitocervical spine instrumentation and stabilization: Preliminary results. J Neurosurg [Spine 1] 90:1–7, 1999.)

treated with the AO/Synthes Posterior Cervical Plates (Synthes Spine, Paoli, PA), but with this plate system, the locations of the apertures for the cervical screws are restricted. The locations for the exit sites of the inside-outside screws can be marked on the occiput only *after* accurate designation of the trajectories of the C1-2 transarticular screw and the subaxial lateral mass screws on the plate. A malleable template is useful to compensate for the undulating bony surfaces. With the newer Star Lock Cervifix System, the screw heads on the cervical spine are attached to the vertical bars via sliding links. The inside-outside screws as well as all the cervical screws can be placed individually before application of the vertical elements and final adjustment of alignment, thereby eliminating a great deal of the "fidget factor" of the procedure (Fig. 226–45).

With this technique, children as young as 18 months can be instrumented safely for occipital C1-2 fusion, although sublaminar wires are used to affix the plate to the cervical spine in the very young. The thinness of the occipital bone in young children can be compensated for by choosing screw heads with larger diameters to distribute the crushing forces. Postoperative halo devices are usually not necessary. Preliminary fusion rates are very promising (authors' unpublished data).[229]

Problems with Fusion Extension

Unintentional inclusion of adjacent "bystander" vertebrae into the fusion mass sometimes occurs in children.[83] Bystander fusion can include the whole neck, even though the bone grafts were originally laid down over one or two levels.[51, 80, 83] The process appears to be related to a combination of overzealous subperiosteal dissection of the bystander laminae and spinous process and denudation of the cortical bone, migration of the bone grafts into adjacent sites, and rigid immobili-

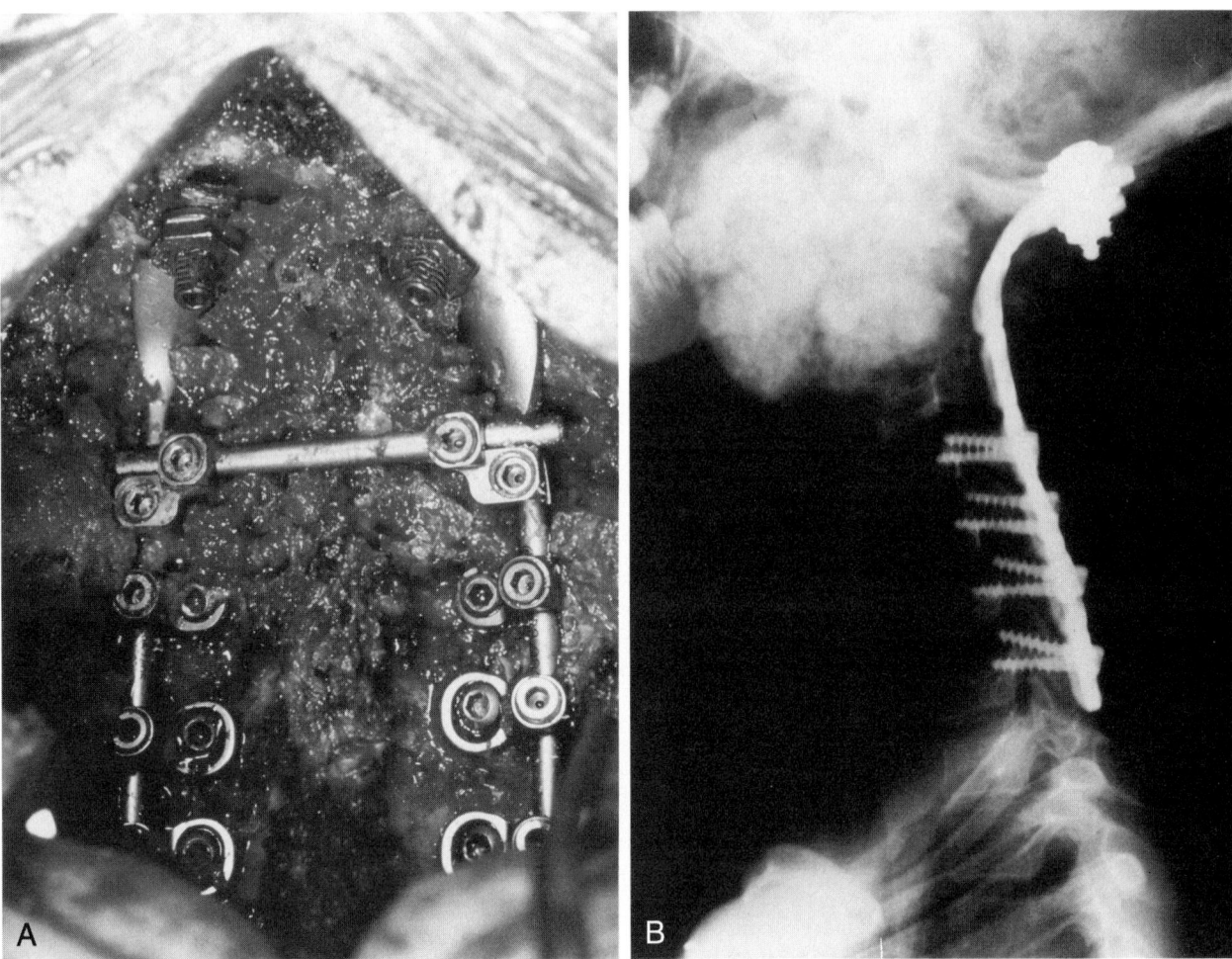

FIGURE 226–45. Inside-outside screw fixation construct in a 6-year-old child. *A*, Vertical bars and sliding screwhead links for the cervical screws. *B*, Lateral radiograph.

zation of the whole cervical spine. Children have a greater capacity than adults to form exuberant callus whenever the periosteum is breached and the neck is effectively immobilized. Migration of bone grafts seems to be less important, because as long as the periosteum is intact, stray grafts do not promote bystander fusion.

The obvious disadvantage of overfusion is unnecessary loss of mobility, but there is also a theoretical threat of accelerated spondylogenesis in the remaining mobile segments that are now burdened with excessive motions and stresses. The two factors are directly related: the greater the combined loss of mobility at the fusion, the greater the compensatory increase in stress at the remaining mobile segments. Fusion of a single level below C2 results in the loss of 8 to 17 degrees of flexion-extension and 8 to 12 degrees of axial rotation, depending on the level and the age of the patient.[90, 230] Inadvertent inclusion of the occiput into an atlantoaxial fusion means the loss of 13 degrees of flexion-extension at the occiput-C1 joint, in addition to the loss of 47 degrees of axial rotation at the C1-2 joint (>50% of total axial rotation).[90] Both situations represent a potential

handicap and should be avoided. The most effective preventive measure is meticulous preservation of the periosteum and other soft tissue overlying the bony surfaces adjacent to the intended fusion surface.

REFERENCES

1. Anderson M, Schutt A: Spinal injury in children: A review of 156 cases seen from 1950 through 1978. Mayo Clinic Proc 55: 499–504, 1980.
2. Andrews L, Jung S: Spinal cord injuries in children in British Columbia. Paraplegia 17:442–451, 1979.
3. Burke DC: Spinal cord trauma in children. Paraplegia 9:1–14, 1971.
4. Geisler FH, Dorsey FC, Coleman WP: Recovery of motor function after spinal cord injury—a randomized, placebo-controlled trial with GM-1 ganglioside. N Engl J Med 324:1829–1838, 1991.
5. Hadley MN, Sonntag VKH, Rekate HL: Pediatric vertebral column and spinal cord injuries. Contemp Neurosurg 10:1–6, 1988.
6. Henrys P, Lye ED, Lifton C, Salciccioli G: Clinical review of cervical spine injuries in children. Clin Orthop 129:172–176, 1977.
7. Kewalramani LS, Kraus JF, Sterling HM: Acute spinal cord lesions in a pediatric population: Epidemiological and clinical features. Paraplegia 18:206–219, 1980.
8. Kewalramani LS, Tori JA: Spinal cord trauma in children: Neu-

rologic patterns, radiologic features, and pathomechanics of injury. Spine 5:11–18, 1980.

9. Melzak J: Paraplegia among children. Lancet 2:45–48, 1969.
10. Mendelsohn DB, Zollars L, Weatherall, Girson M: MR of cord transection. J Comput Assist Tomogr 14:909–911, 1990.
11. Ruge JR, Sinson GP, McLone DG, Cerullo LJ: Pediatric spinal injury: The very young. J Neurosurg 68:25–30, 1988.
12. Schaeffer DM, Flanders AE, Osterholm JL, Northrup BE: Prognostic significance of magnetic resonance imaging in the acute phase of cervical spine injury. J Neurosurg 76:218–223, 1992.
13. Wilberger JE Jr: Spinal Cord Injuries in Children. Mount Kisco, NY, Futura, 1986.
14. Hadley MN, Zabramski JM, Browner CM, et al: Pediatric spinal trauma: Review of 122 cases of spinal cord and vertebral column injuries. J Neurosurg 68:18–24, 1988.
15. Hamilton MG, Myles ST: Pediatric spinal injury: Review of 61 deaths. J Neurosurg 77:705–708, 1992.
16. Hamilton MG, Myles ST: Pediatric spinal injury: Review of 174 hospital admissions. J Neurosurg 77:700–704, 1992.
17. Hill SA, Miller CA, Kosnik EJ, Hunt WE: Pediatric neck injuries: A clinical study. J Neurosurg 60:700–706, 1984.
18. Osenbach RK, Menezes AH: Spinal cord injury without radiographic abnormality in children. Pediatr Neurosci 15:168–175, 1989.
19. Pang D: Spinal cord injury without radiographic abnormality (SCIWORA) in children. In Betz R (ed): The Child with a Spinal Cord Injury. Rosemont, IL, AAOS and Shriners Hospital, 1996, pp 139–160.
20. Pang D: Pediatric spinal cord injuries. In McLone DG (ed): Paediatric Neurosurgery, 4th ed. Philadelphia, WB Saunders, 2001, pp 660–694.
21. Bailey D: The normal cervical spine in infants and children. Radiology 59:712–719, 1952.
22. Fesmire FM, Luten RC: The pediatric cervical spine: Developmental anatomy and clinical aspects. J Emerg Med 7:133–142, 1989.
23. Sullivan CR, Bruwer AJ, Harris E: Hypermobility of the cervical spine in children: A pitfall in the diagnosis of cervical dislocation. Am J Surg 95:636–640, 1958.
24. Townsend EH Jr, Rowe ML: Mobility of the upper cervical spine in health and disease. Pediatrics 10:567–573, 1952.
25. Von Torklus D, Gehle W: The Upper Cervical Spine. New York, Grune & Stratton, 1972.
26. Cattell HS, Filtzer DL: Pseudosubluxation and other normal variations in the cervical spine in children: A study of one hundred and sixty children. J Bone Joint Surg 47:1295–1309, 1965.
27. Pang D, Pollack IF: Spinal cord injury without radiographic abnormality in children—the SCIWORA syndrome. J Trauma 29:654–664, 1989.
28. Papvasiliou V: Traumatic subluxation of the cervical spine during childhood. Orthop Clin North Am 9:945–954, 1978.
29. Sherk HH, Schut L, Lane JM: Fractures and dislocations of the cervical spine in children. Orthop Clin North Am 7:593–604, 1976.
30. Kalfas I, Wilberger J, Goldberg A, Prostko ER: Magnetic resonance imaging in acute spinal cord trauma. Neurosurgery 23:295–299, 1988.
31. Braakman R, Penning L: Injuries of the Cervical Spine. Amsterdam, Excerpta Medica, 1971.
32. Todury G: The cervical spine: Its development and changes during life. Acta Orthop Belg 25:602–607, 1959.
33. Aufdermaur M: Spinal injuries in juveniles: Necropsy findings in twelve cases. J Bone Joint Surg 56:513–519, 1974.
34. Pang D, Wilberger JE: Spinal cord injury without radiographic abnormalities in children. J Neurosurg 57:114–129, 1982.
35. Gilles FH, Bina M, Sotrel A: Infantile atlantooccipital instability: The potential danger of extreme extension. Am J Dis Child 133:30–37, 1979.
36. Scher AT: Anterior cervical subluxation: An unstable position. AJR Am J Roentgenol 133:275–280, 1979.
37. Webb JK, Broughton RBK, McSweeney T, et al: Hidden flexion injury of the cervical spine. J Bone Joint Surg Br 58:322–327, 1976.
38. Baker D, Berdon W: Special trauma problems in children. Radiol Clin North Am 4:289–305, 1966.

39. Braakman R, Penning L: The hyperflexion sprain of the cervical spine. Radiol Clin North Am 37:309–320, 1968.
40. Osenbach RK, Menezes AH: Pediatric spinal cord and vertebral column injury. Neurosurgery 30:385–390, 1992.
41. Frankel HL, Hancock DO, Hyslop G, et al: The value of postural reduction in the initial management of closed injuries of the spine with paraplegia and tetraplegia. Paraplegia 7:179–192, 1969.
42. Burke DC: Traumatic spinal paralysis in children. Paraplegia 11:268–276, 1974.
43. Choi JU, Hoffman HJ, Hendrick EB, et al: Traumatic infarction of the spinal cord in children. J Neurosurg 65:608–610, 1986.
44. Hachen HJ: Spinal cord injury in children and adolescents. Paraplegia 16:55–64, 1977.
45. Hasue M, Hoshino R, Omata S, et al: Cervical spine injuries in children. Fukushima J Med Sci 20:115–123, 1974.
46. Yngve DA, Harris WP, Herndon WA, et al: Spinal cord injury without osseous spine fracture. J Pediatr Orthop 8:153–159, 1988.
47. Rockswald GL, Seljeskog EL: Traumatic atlantocranial dislocation with survival. Minn Med 62:151–154, 1979.
48. Fielding J: Injuries of the cervical spine in children. In Rockwood CA Jr, King RE (eds): Fracture in Children, vol 3. Philadelphia, JB Lippincott, 1984, pp 683–705.
49. Kaufman RA, Carrol CD, Buncher CR: Atlantooccipital junction: Standards for measurement in normal children. AJNR Am J Neuroradiol 8:995–999, 1987.
50. Zabramski JM, Hadley MN, Browner CM, et al: Pediatric spinal cord and vertebral column injuries. BNI Q 2:11–17, 1986.
51. Pang D: Principles and pitfalls of spinal stabilization in children. In Pang D (ed): Disorders of the Paediatric Spine. New York, Raven Press, 1995, pp 575–604.
52. Werthem SB, Bohlman HH: Occipitocervical fusion: Indications, techniques, and long-term results in thirteen patients. J Bone Joint Surg 69:833–836, 1897.
53. Beatson T: Fractures and dislocations of the cervical spine. J Bone Joint Surg 45:21–35, 1963.
54. Hubbard DD: Injuries of the spine in children and adolescents. Clin Orthop 100:56–65, 1974.
55. Alexander EJ, Davis C, Field C: Hyperextension injuries of the cervical spine. Arch Neurol Psychiatry 79:146–150, 1958.
56. Taylor AR, Blackwood W: Paraplegia in hyperextension cervical injuries with normal radiographic appearances. J Bone Joint Surg Br 30:245–248, 1948.
57. Breig A, El-Nadi AF: Biomechanics of the cervical spinal cord: Relief of contact pressure on and over-stretching of the spinal cord. Acta Radiol (Diag) 4:602–624, 1966.
58. Bourmer HR: Zur Frage der Halsmarkschadigung bei Hyperestensionsverletzungen der Wirbelsaule. Arch Klin Chir 268:409–416, 1951.
59. Marar BC: Hyperextension injuries of the cervical spine: The pathogenesis of damage to the spinal cord. J Bone Joint Surg 56:1655–1662, 1974.
60. Sudeck P: Uber Drchungsverrenkung des atlas. Dtsch Z Chir 183:289–303, 1923.
61. Glasauer F, Cares HL: Biomechanical features of traumatic paraplegia in infancy. J Trauma 13:166–170, 1973.
62. Leventhal HR: Birth injuries of the spinal cord. J Pediatr 56:447–453, 1960.
63. Abroms I, Brosnan, MJ, Zuckerman, JE, et al: Cervical cord injuries secondary to hyperextension of the head in breech presentations. Obstet Gynecol 41:369–378, 1973.
64. Pollack IF, Pang D, Hall WA: Subarachnoid pleural and subarachnoid-mediastinal fistulae. Neurosurgery 26:519–525, 1990.
65. Davis D, Bohlman H, Walker E, et al: The pathological finding in fatal craniospinal injuries. J Neurosurg 34:603–613, 1971.
66. Ahmann PA, Smith SA, Schwartz JF, et al: Spinal cord infarction due to minor trauma in children. Neurology 25:301–307, 1975.
67. Cheshire D: The pediatric syndrome of traumatic myelopathy without demonstrable vertebral injury. Paraplegia 15:74–85, 1977.
68. Walsh JW, Steven DB, Young AB: Traumatic paraplegia in children without contiguous spinal fracture of dislocation. Neurosurgery 12:439–445, 1983.
69. Pollack IF, Pang D, Sclabassi R: Recurrent spinal cord injury

without radiographic abnormalities in children. J Neurosurg 69: 177–182, 1988.

70. Grabb PA, Pang D: Magnetic resonance imaging in the evaluation of spinal cord injury without radiographic abnormality (SCIWORA) in children. Neurosurgery 35:406–414, 1994.

71. Flanders AE, Schaeffer DM, Doan HT, et al: Acute cervical spine trauma: Correlation of MR imaging findings with degree of neurologic deficit. Radiology 177:25–33, 1990.

72. Weirich SD, Cotler HB, Narayana PA, et al: Histopathologic correlation of magnetic resonance imaging signal patterns in a spinal cord injury model. Spine 15:630–638, 1990.

73. Yamashita Y, Takahashi M, Matsuno Y, et al: Acute spinal cord injury: Magnetic resonance imaging correlated with myelopathy. Br J Radiol 759:201–209, 1991.

74. Levitt MA, Flanders AE: Diagnostic capabilities of magnetic resonance imaging and computed tomography in acute cervical spinal column injury. Am J Emerg Med 9:131–135, 1991.

75. DePinto D, Payne T, Kittle CF: Traumatic subarachnoid-pleural fistula. Ann Thorac Surg 25:477–478, 1978.

76. LeBlanc HJ, Nadell J: Spinal cord injuries in children. Surg Neurol 2:441–444, 1974.

77. Rocha Campus BA, Silva LB, Ballalai N, Negrao MM: Traumatic subarachnoid-pleural fistula. J Neurol Neurosurg Psychiatry 37: 269–270, 1974.

78. Scher AT: Trauma of the spinal cord in children. S Afr Med J 50:2023–2025, 1976.

79. Bracken M, Shepard MJ, Collins WF, et al: A randomized, controlled trial of methylprednisolone or naloxone in the treatment of acute spinal-cord injury: Results of the second National Acute Spinal Cord Injury Study. N Engl J Med 322:1405–1411, 1990.

80. Fielding J: Selected observations on the cervical spine in the child. Curr Pract Orthop Surg 5:31–55, 1973.

81. Fielding JW, Cochran GVB, Lawsing JF, Hohl M: Tears of the transverse ligament of the atlas. J Bone Joint Surg 56:1683–1691, 1974.

82. White AA, Panjabi MM: The clinical biomechanics of the occipitoatlanto-axial complex. Orthop Clin North Am 9:867–878, 1978.

83. Fielding JW, Hawkins RJ: Roentgenographic diagnosis of the injured neck. Am Assoc Orthop Surgeons Int Course Lect 25: 149–170, 1976.

84. Martel E, Tishler J: Observations on the spine in mongoloidism. AJR Am J Roentgenol 97:630–638, 1966.

85. Pueschel S, Scola FH: Atlanto-axial instability in individuals with Down's syndrome: Epidemiologic, radiographic and clinical studies. Pediatrics 80:555–560, 1987.

86. Pueschel S, Scola FH, Perry CD, Pezzullo JC: Atlanto-axial instability in children with Down's syndrome. Pediatr Radiol 10: 129–132, 1981.

87. White KS, Ball WS, Prenger EC, et al: Evaluation of craniocervical junction in Down syndrome: Correlation of measurements obtained with radiography and MR imaging. Radiology 186: 377–382, 1993.

88. Kopits SE, Steingass MH: Experience with the "halo-cast" in small children. Surg Clin North Am 50:935–943, 1970.

89. Rogers W: Treatment of fracture dislocation of the cervical spine. J Bone Joint Surg 24:245–258, 1942.

90. White AA, Panjabi MM: The basic kinematics of the human spine. Spine 3:12–20, 1978.

91. White AA, Panjabi MM: Clinical Biomechanics of the Spine, 2nd ed. Philadelphia, JB Lippincott, 1990.

92. White AA, Panjabi MM: The problem of clinical stability in the human spine: A systemic approach. In White AA, Panjabi MM (eds): Clinical Biomechanics of the Spine. Philadelphia, JB Lippincott, 1978, p 196.

93. Adams VI: Neck injuries. I. Occipitoatlantal dislocation—a pathological study of twelve traffic fatalities. J Forensic Sci 37: 556–564, 1992.

94. Alker G, Oh Y, Leslie E: High cervical spine and craniofacial junction injuries in fatal traffic accidents: A radiographic study. Orthop Clin North Am 9:1003–1010, 1978.

95. Bucholz RW, Burkhead WZ: The pathological anatomy of fatal atlanto-occipital dislocations. J Bone Joint Surg 61:248–250, 1979.

96. Bohlman H: Acute fractures and dislocations of the cervical spine: An analysis of three hundred hospitalized patients and review of the literature. J Bone Joint Surg 61:1119–1142, 1979.

97. Dvorak J, Panjabi MM: Functional anatomy of the alar ligaments. Spine 12:183–189, 1987.

98. Werne S: Studies in spontaneous atlas dislocation. Acta Orthop Scand 23:1–150, 1957.

99. Goel VK, Clark CR, Callaes K, Liu YK: Moment-rotation relationships of the ligamentous occipito-atlanto-axial complex. J Biomech 21:673–680, 1988.

100. Menezes AH, Muhonen M: Management of occipital-cervical instability. In Cooper P (ed): Management of Post Traumatic Instability. Park Ridge, IL, American Association of Neurological Surgeons Publications Committee, 1990, pp 65–76.

101. Dublin AB, Marks WM, Wienstock D, Newton TH: Traumatic dislocation of the atlanto-occipital articulation (AOA) with short-term survival. J Neurosurg 52:541–546, 1980.

102. Grobovschek M, Scheibelbrandner W: Atlanto-occipital dislocation. Neuroradiology 25:173–174, 1983.

103. Powers B, Miller MD, Kramer RS, et al: Traumatic anterior atlanto-occipital dislocation. Neurosurgery 4:12–17, 1979.

104. Brooks A, Jenkins EB: Atlanto-axial arthrodesis by the wedge compression method. J Bone Joint Surg 60:279–284, 1978.

105. Englander O: Non-traumatic occipito-atlanto-axial dislocation: A contribution to the radiology of the atlas. Br J Radiol 15: 341–345, 1942.

106. Eismont FJ, Bohlman HH: Posterior atlanto-occipital dislocation with fractures of the atlas and odontoid process: Report of a case with survival. J Bone Joint Surg 60:397–399, 1978.

107. Britt R, Herrick MK, Mason RT, Dorfman LJ: Traumatic lesions of the pontomedullary junction. Neurosurgery 6:623–631, 1980.

108. Leetsma JE, Kalelkar MB, Teas S: Ponto-medullary avulsion associated with cervical hyperextension. Acta Neurochir (Wien) 32:69–73, 1983.

109. Lindenberg R, Freytag E: Brainstem lesions characteristic of traumatic hyperextension of the head. Arch Pathol 90:509–515, 1970.

110. Traynelis VC, Marano GD, Dunker RO, Kaufman HH: Traumatic atlanto-occipital dislocation: Case report. J Neurosurg 65: 863–870, 1986.

111. Georgopoulos G, Pizzutillo PD, Lee MS: Occipito-atlantal instability in children. J Bone Joint Surg 69:429–436, 1987.

112. Pang D, Wilberger JE: Traumatic atlantooccipital dislocation with survival: Case report and review. Neurosurgery 7:503–508, 1980.

113. Woodring JH, Selke AC, Duff DE: Traumatic atlantooccipital dislocation with survival. AJR Am J Roentgenol 137:21–24, 1981.

114. Sun PP, Poffenbarger J, Durhan S, Zimmerman RA: Spectrum of occipitoatlantoaxial injury in young children. J Neurosurg (Spine) 1:28–39, 2000.

115. Watridge CB, Orrison WW, Arnold H, Woods GA: Lateral atlantooccipital dislocation: Case report. Neurosurgery 17:345–347, 1985.

116. Altongy J, Fielding JW: Combined atlanto-axial and occipito-atlantal rotatory subluxation. J Bone Joint Surg Am 72:923–926, 1990.

117. Clark CR, Kathol MH, Walsh T, El-Khoury GY: Atlantoaxial rotatory fixation with compensatory counter occipitoatlantal subluxation. Spine 11:1048–1050, 1986.

118. Bools J, Rose B: Traumatic atlantooccipital dislocation: Two cases with survival. AJNR Am J Neuroradaiol 7:901–904, 1986.

119. Collato PM, Demuth WW, Schwentker EP, Boal DK: Traumatic atlanto-occipital dislocation: Case report. J Bone Joint Surg 68: 1106–1109, 1986.

120. Dibenedetto T, Lee CK: Traumatic atlanto-occipital instability: A case report with follow-up and a new diagnostic technique. Spine 15:595–597, 1990.

121. Farley FA, Graziano GP, Hensinger RN: Traumatic atlantoccipital dislocation in a child. Spine 17:1539–1541, 1992.

122. Kaufman RA, Dunbar JS, Botsfor JA, McLaurin RL: Traumatic longitudinal atlanto-occipital distraction injuries in children. AJNR Am J Neuroradiol 3:415–419, 1982.

123. Montane I, Eismont FJ, Green BA: Traumatic occipitoatlantal dislocation. Spine 16:112–116, 1991.

124. Putman WE, Straaton FT, Rohr RJ, et al: Traumatic atlanto-occipital dislocation: Value of the Powers ratio in diagnosis. J Am Osteopath Assoc, 86:798–804, 1986.

125. Lee C, Woodring JH, Goldstein SJ, et al: Evaluation of traumatic

atlantooccipital dislocations. AJNR Am J Neuroradiol 8:19–26, 1987.

126. Page CP, Story JL, Wissinger JP, Branch CL: Traumatic atlantoccipital dislocation: Case report. J Neurosurg 39:394–397, 1973.

127. Fruin AH, Pirotte TP: Traumatic atlantooccipital dislocation: Case report. J Neurosurg 46:663–666, 1977.

128. Ajuja A, Glasauer F, Alker G, et al: Radiology in survivors of traumatic atlantoccipital dislocation. J Neurol 41:112–118, 1994.

129. Bulas DI, Fitz CR, Johnson DL: Traumatic atlanto-occipital dislocation in children. Radiology 188:155–158, 1993.

130. Bundschuh CV, Alley JB, Ross M, et al: Magnetic resonance imaging of suspected atlantooccipital dislocation: Two case reports. Spine 17:245–248, 1992.

131. Cohen A, Hirsch M, Katz M, Sofer S: Traumatic atlanto-occipital dislocation in children: Review and report of five cases. Pediatr Emerg Care 7:24–27, 1991.

132. Evarts C: Traumatic occipito-atlantal dislocation: Report of a case with survival. J Bone Joint Surg 52:1653–1660, 1970.

133. Farthing J: Atlantocranial dislocation with survival: A case report. N C Med J 9:34–36, 1948.

134. Harmanli O, Koyfman Y: Traumatic atlanto-occipital dislocation with survival: A case report and review of the literature. Surg Neurol 39:324–330, 1993.

135. Hosono N, Yonenobu K, Kawagoe K, et al: Traumatic anterior atlanto-occipital dislocation: A case with survival. Spine 18:786–790, 1993.

136. Lee C, Woodring JH, Walsh JW: Carotid and vertebral artery injury in survivors of atlanto-occipital dislocation: Case reports and literature review. J Trauma 31:401–407, 1991.

137. Matava MJ, Whitesides TE, Davis PC: Traumatic atlanto-occipital dislocation with survival: Serial computerized tomography as an aid to diagnosis and reduction: A report of three cases. Spine 18:1897–1903, 1993.

138. Wholey MH, Bruwer AJ, Baker HL Jr: The lateral roentgenogram of the neck: With comments on the atlanto-odontoid relationship. Radiology 71:350–356, 1958.

139. Harris J Jr, Carson GC, Wagner LK: Radiologic diagnosis of traumatic occipitovertebral dislocation. 1. Normal occipitovertebral relationships on the lateral radiographs of supine subjects. AJNR Am J Neuroradiol 162:881–886, 1993.

140. Harris JH Jr, Carson GC, Wagner LK, Kerr N: Radiologic diagnosis of traumatic occipitovertebral dislocation. 2. Comparison of three methods of detecting occipitovertebral relationships on lateral radiographs of supine subjects. AJNR Am J Neuroradiol 162:887–892, 1993.

141. Ransford AO, Crockard HA, Pozo JL, et al: Craniocervical instability treated by contoured loop fixation. J Bone Joint Surg Br 68:173–177, 1986.

142. Gabrielsen TO, Maxwell JA: Traumatic atlantooccipital dislocation: With case report of patient who survived. AJNR Am J Neuroradiol 97:624–629, 1966.

143. Belzberg A, Tranmer B: Stabilization of traumatic atlanto-occipital dislocation: Case report. J Neurosurg 75:478–482, 1991.

144. Heywood AW, Learmonth ID, Thomas M: Internal fixation for occipito-cervical fusion. J Bone Joint Surg Br 70:708–711, 1988.

145. Mackenzie A, Uttley D, Marsh HT, Bell BA: Craniocervical stabilization using Luque/Hartshill rectangles. Neurosurgery 26:32–36, 1990.

146. Sasso RC, Jeanneret B, Fischer K, Magerl F: Occipitocervical fusion with posterior plate and screw instrumentation: A long term follow-up study. Spine 19:2364–2368, 1994.

147. Birney T, Hanley E: Traumatic cervical spine injuries in childhood and adolescence. Spine 14:1277–1282, 1989.

148. Fielding JW, Hawkins RJ, Hensinger RN, Francis WR: Atlantoaxial rotatory deformities. Orthop Clin North Am 9A:955–967, 1978.

149. Dugan MC, Locke S, Gallagher JR: Occipital neuralgia in adolescents and young adults. N Engl J Med 267:1166–1172, 1962.

150. Dyck P: Os odontoideum in children: Neurologic manifestations and surgical management. Neurosurgery 2:93–99, 1978.

151. Fielding JW, Hawkins RJ: Atlantoaxial rotatory fixation. J Bone Joint Surg 59:37–44, 1977.

152. Van Hosbeeck EMA, Mackay NNS: Diagnosis of acute atlantoaxial rotatory fixation. J Bone Joint Surg Br 71:90–91, 1989.

153. Corner E: Rotatory dislocations of the atlas. Ann Surg 45:9–26, 1907.

154. Coutts M: Atlanto-epistropheal subluxations. Arch Surg 29:297–311, 1934.

155. Li V, Pang D: Atlanto-axial rotatory fixation. In Pang D (ed): Disorders of the Pediatric Spine. New York, Raven Press, 1995, pp 531–553.

156. Kawabe N, Hirotani H, Tanaka O: Pathomechanism of atlanto-axial rotatory fixation in children. J Pediatr Orthop 9:569–574, 1989.

157. Phillips W, Hensinge RN: The management of rotatory atlanto-axial subluxation in children. J Bone Joint Surg 71:664–668, 1989.

158. Adams VI: Neck injuries. II. Atlantoaxial dislocation—a pathologic study of 14 traffic fatalities. J Forensic Sci 37:565–573, 1992.

159. Bohn D, Armstrong D, Becker L, et al: Cervical spine injuries in children. J Trauma 30:463–469, 1990.

160. McGory BJ, Klassen RA, Chao EYS, et al: Acute fractures and dislocations of the cervical spine in children and adolescents. J Bone Joint Surg 75:988–995, 1993.

161. DeBeer JDV, Thomas M, Walters J, Anderson P: Traumatic atlanto-axial subluxation. J Bone Joint Surg Br 70:652–655, 1988.

162. Floman Y, Kaplan L, Elidan J, Umansky F: Transverse ligament rupture and atlantoaxial subluxation in children. J Bone Joint Surg Br 73:640–643, 1991.

163. Hamilton AR: Injuries of the atlantoaxial joint. J Bone Joint Surg Br 33:434–435, 1951.

164. Spitzer R, Rabinowitch JY, Wybar KC: A study of the abnormalities of the skull, teeth and lenses in mongolism. Can Med Assoc J 84:567–572, 1961.

165. Wigren A, Amici F: Traumatic atlanto-axial dislocation without neurologic disorder. J Bone Joint Surg 55:642–644, 1973.

166. Maiman DJ, Cusick JF: Traumatic atlantoaxial dislocation. J Neurol 18:388–392, 1982.

167. Wolf JW, Johnson RM: Cervical orthoses. In Bailey DW, Sherk HH (eds): The Cervical Spine. Philadelphia, JB Lippincott, 1983, pp 54–61.

168. Braakman R, Penning L: Upper cervical spine. In Injuries of the Cervical Spine. Amsterdam, Excerpta Medica, 1971, pp 125–157.

169. Locke GR, Gardner JI, Van Epps EF: Atlas-dens interval (ADI) in children. Am J Radiol 97:135–140, 1966.

170. Steel HH: Anatomical and mechanical considerations of the atlanto-axial articulations. J Bone Joint Surg 50:1481–1482, 1968.

171. Levine AM, Edwards CC: Treatment of injuries in the C1-C2 complex. Orthop Clin North Am 17:31–44, 1986.

172. Hreidarsson S, Magram G, Singer H: Symptomatic atlantoaxial dislocation in Down's syndrome. Pediatrics 69:568–571, 1982.

173. Hungerford GD, Akkaraju V, Rawe SE, Young GF: Atlanto-occipital and atlanto-axial dislocations with spinal cord compression in Down's syndrome: A case report and review of the literature. Br J Radiol 54:758–761, 1981.

174. Stein SM, Kircner SG, Horev G, Hernanz-Schulman M: Atlanto-occipital subluxation in Down's syndrome. Pediatr Radiol 21:121–124, 1991.

175. Burke SW, French HG, Roberts JM, et al: Chronic atlantoaxial instability in Down's syndrome. J Bone Joint Surg 67:1356–1360, 1985.

176. Tishler J, Martel W: Dislocation of the atlas in mongolism. Radiology 84:904–906, 1965.

177. Sherk HH, Nicholson JT: Rotatory atlanto-axial dislocation with ossiculum terminale and mongolish. J Bone Joint Surg 51:957–964, 1969.

178. Aung M: Atlanto-axial dislocation in Down's syndrome. Bull Los Angeles Neurol Soc 38:197–201, 1973.

179. Levack B, Roper AB: Dislocation in Down's syndrome. Dev Med Child Neurol 26:122–125, 1984.

180. Semine AA, Ertel AN, Goldberg MJ, Bull MJ: Cervical-spine instability in children with Down's syndrome (trisomy 21). J Bone Joint Surg 60:649–652, 1978.

181. Beighton P, Craig J: Atlanto-axial subluxation in the Morquio syndrome. J Bone Joint Surg Br 55:478–481, 1973.

182. Dawson EG, Smith L: Atlanto-axial subluxation in children due to vertebral anomalies. J Bone Joint Surg 61:582–587, 1979.

183. Herring JA: Cervical instability in Down's syndrome and juvenile rheumatoid arthritis. J Pediatr Orthop 2:205–207, 1982.

184. Kopits SE, Perovic MN, McKusick V, et al: Congenital atlantoaxial dislocations in various forms of dwarfism. J Bone Joint Surg 54:1349–1350, 1972.

185. Stevens JC, Cartlidge NEF, Saunders M, et al: Atlanto-axial subluxation and cervical myelopathy in rheumatoid arthritis. Q J Med 159:391–408, 1971.

186. Callahan RA, Johnson RM, Margolis RN, et al: Cervical facet fusion for control of instability following laminectomy. J Bone Joint Surg 59:991–1002, 1977.

187. Johnson R, Owen JR, Hart BA, et al: Cervical orthoses. Clin Orthop 154:34–45, 1981.

188. Johnson R, Owen JR, Panjabi MM, et al: Immediate strength of certain cervical fusion techniques [abstract]. Orthop Trans 4: 42, 1980.

189. Prolo DJ, Runnels JB, Jameson RM: The injured cervical spine: Immediate and long-term immobilization with the halo. JAMA 224:591–594, 1973.

190. Baum J, Hanley E, Pullekines J: Comparison of halo complications in adults and children. Spine 14:251–252, 1989.

191. Chan RC, Schweigel JF, Thompson GB: Halo-thoracic brace immobilization in 188 patients with acute cervical spine injuries. J Neurosurg 58:508–515, 1983.

192. Mubarak SJ, Camp JF, Vuletich W, et al: Halo immobilization for cervical spine instability in the infant [abstract]. Paper presented at the Annual Meeting of the Pediatric Orthopedic Society of North America, 1988, Colorado Springs, CO.

193. Garfin SR, Bott MJ, Waters RL, et al: Complications in the use of the halo fixation device. J Bone Joint Surg 68:320–325, 1986.

194. Victor DI, Bresnan MJ, Keller RB: Brain abscess complicating the use of halo traction. J Bone Joint Surg 55:635–639, 1973.

195. Goodman ML, Nelson PB: Brain abscess complicating the use of a halo orthosis. Neurosurgery 20:27–30, 1987.

196. Hoffman GR, Merckx J, Vercauteren M: Abces cerebral consecutif a la "halo traction." Neurochirurgie 20:263–266, 1974.

197. Humbyrd DE, Latimer FR, Lonstein JE, et al: Brain abscess as a complication of halo traction. Spine 6:365–368, 1981.

198. Benzel E, Hadden A, Saulsbery C: A comparison of the Minerva and halo jackets for stabilization of the cervical spine. J Neurosurg 70:411–414, 1989.

199. Anderson L: Fractures of the Odontoid Process of the Axis. Philadelphia, JB Lippincott, 1983.

200. Walter BC: Cranial bone grafts for use in posterior fixation of the cervical spine. J Neurosurg 79:286–288, 1993.

201. Johnson RM, Wolf JW: Stability. In Bailey R, Sherk HH (eds): The Cervical Spine. Philadelphia, JB Lippincott, 1983, pp 35–53.

202. Johnson R, Southwick WO: Surgical approaches to the spine. In Rothman R, Simeone FA (eds): The Spine, 2nd ed. Philadelphia, WB Saunders, 1981, pp 67–147.

203. Eismont F, Bohlman HH: Posterior methylmethacrylate fixation for cervical trauma. Spine 6:347–353, 1981.

204. Whitehill R, Stowers SF, Fechner RE, et al: Posterior cervical fusions using cerclage wires, methylmethacrylate cement and autogenous bone graft: An experimental study of a canine model. Spine 12:12–22, 1987.

205. Cooper PR, Cohen A, Rosiello A, Koslow M: Posterior stabilization of cervical spine fractures and subluxations using plates and screws. Neurosurgery 23:300–306, 1988.

206. Gallie WE: Fractures and dislocations of the cervical spine. Am J Surg 10:495–499, 1939.

207. Griswold DM, Albright JA, Schiffman E, et al: Atlanto-axial fusion for instability. J Bone Joint Surg 60:285–292, 1978.

208. Levy ML, McComb JG: C1-C2 fusion in children with atlantoaxial instability and spinal cord compression: Technical note. Neurosurgery 38:221–217, 1996.

209. Magerl F, Seemann PS: Stable posterior fusion of the atlas and axis by transarticular screw fixation. In Kehr P, Weidner A (eds): Cervical Spine. Berlin, Springer-Verlag, 1986, pp 322–327.

210. Apfelbaum RI: Posterior C1-2 screw fixation for atlantoaxial instability. Neurosurg Operative Atlas 4:19–28, 1995.

211. Grob D, Crisco JJ III, Panjabi MM, et al: Biomechanical evaluation of four different posterior atlantoaxial fixation techniques. Spine 17:480–490, 1992.

212. Dickman CA, Sonntag VKH: Posterior C1-C2 transarticular screw fixation for atlantoaxial arthrodesis. Neurosurgery 43: 275–281, 1998.

213. Grob D, Jeanneret B, Aebi M, et al: Atlanto-axial fusion with transarticular screw fixation. J Bone Joint Surg Br 73:972–976, 1991.

214. Dickman CA, Sonntag VKH, Papadopoulos SM, Hadley MN: The interspinous method of posterior atlantoaxial arthrodesis. J Neurosurg 74:190–198, 1991.

215. Wang J, Vokshoor A, Kim S, et al: Pediatric atlantoaxial instability: Management with screw fixation. Pediatr Neurosurg 30: 70–78, 1999.

216. Lowry DW, Pollack IF, Clyde B, et al: Upper cervical spine fusion in the pediatric population. J Neurosurg 87:671–676, 1997.

217. Madawi AA, Casey ATH, Solanki GA, et al: Radiological and anatomical evaluation of the atlantoaxial transarticular screw fixation technique. J Neurosurg 86:961–968, 1997.

218. Paramore CG, Dickman CA, Sonntag VKH: The anatomical suitability of the C1-2 complex for transarticular screw fixation. J Neurosurg 85:221–224, 1996.

219. Dickman CA, Crawford NR, Paramore CG: Biomechanical characteristics of C1-C2 cable fixations. J Neurosurg 85:316–322, 1996.

220. Brattstrom H: Surgery in atlanto-axial dislocation in rheumatoid arthritis. Reconstr Surg Traumatol 18:16–29, 1981.

221. Cregan JC: Internal fixation of the unstable rheumatoid cervical spine. Ann Rheum Dis 25:242–252, 1966.

222. Dickman CA, Sonntag VK, Marcotte PJ: Techniques of screw fixation of the cervical spine. BNI Q 8:9–26, 1992.

223. Fehlings MG, Errico T, Cooper P, et al: Occipitocervical fusion with a five-millimeter malleable rod and segmental fixation. Neurosurgery 32:198–207, 1993.

224. Kerschbaumer F: Rheumatoid instability. In Bauer R, Kerschbaumer F, Poisel S (eds): Atlas of Spinal Operations. New York, Thieme, 1993, pp 347–376.

225. Roy-Camille R, Saillant G, Mazel C: Internal fixation of the unstable cervical spine by a posterior osteosynthesis with plates and screws. In Society CSR (ed): The Cervical Spine, 2nd ed. Philadelphia, JB Lippincott, 1989, pp 390–403.

226. Sonntag VK, Dickman CA: Craniocervical stabilization. Clin Neurosurg 40:243–272, 1993.

227. Sonntag VK, Dickman CA: Occipitocervical instrumentation. In Hitchon PW, Traynelis VC, Rengachary SS (eds): Techniques in Spinal Fusion and Stabilization. New York, Thieme, 1995, pp 107–121.

228. Sumi M, Kataoka O, Ikeda M, et al: Atlantoaxial dislocation: A follow-up study of surgical results. Spine 22:759–764, 1997.

229. Pait TG, Al-Mefty O, Boop FA, et al: Inside-outside technique for posterior occipitocervical spine instrumentation and stabilization: Preliminary results. J Neurosurg (Spine 1) 90:1–7, 1999.

230. Jofe MH, White AA, Panjabi MM: Kinematics. In Bailey RW, Sherk HH (eds): The Cervical Spine. Philadelphia, JB Lippincott, 1983, pp 23–35.

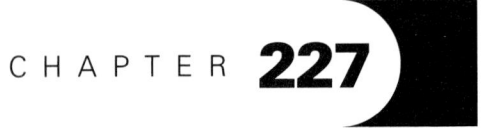

CHAPTER **227**

Intervertebral Disk Disease in Children

SHENANDOAH ROBINSON ■ ALAN R. COHEN

Although many aspects of intervertebral disk disease in children and adults are similar, there are distinct differences that warrant a separate discussion. Intervertebral disk herniation occurs in children and adolescents much less frequently than in adults. Because the clinical presentation of intervertebral disk disease in children can be difficult to distinguish from that of other disorders that affect the spine, the differential diagnosis of intervertebral disk disease in children is also reviewed. Characteristics of back pain associated with significant lesions in children are listed in Table 227–1.

HISTORY

Wahren reported the first lumbar diskectomy in a child in 1945.[1] He described a 12-year-old girl who developed a right S1 radiculopathy after gymnastics. She failed to improve after 1 month of nonoperative therapy but had complete resolution of her symptoms after surgical resection of the offending herniated disk. Several series of children treated surgically for symptomatic herniated lumbar disks were published in the 1960s.[2-4]

Other entities affecting the intervertebral disk in children were identified during the early part of the 20th century. Calcified cervical intervertebral disk (CCID), a presumed inflammatory process, can mimic cervical disk herniation in children. CCID was first described in 1924 by Baron.[5] In 1952 Weingartner first described disk protrusion associated with calcification of the disk.[6] Another entity that affects children, slipped epiphysis, was first described in an adolescent by Techakapuch in 1981.[7]

ANATOMY AND DEVELOPMENT

During embryologic development, the future intervertebral disk is located between two adjacent halves of the provertebrae. The notochord is extruded into the intervertebral space and eventually becomes the nucleus pulposus.[8] The intervertebral disks are the components of the spine located farthest from the growth plates and the intersegmental arteries. A vascular supply to the intervertebral disk is present for the first 8 years of life, after which the cells receive nutrition via diffusion. The nerve supply to intervertebral disks is from the nerve of Luschka via primary rami of the dorsal roots. In the fetus and neonate, this nerve innervates the anterior and posterior longitudinal ligaments, the peripheral annulus, the vertebral body, and the facet joints. By adulthood, the innervation decreases to just the fibers around the annulus; no fibers innervate the disk or the bone.[8]

The components of the intervertebral disk are the inner nucleus pulposus, the circular annulus fibrosus,

TABLE 227–1 ■ **Characteristics of Back Pain Associated with Significant Lesions in Children**

Back pain in a child 4 years old or younger
Symptoms persisting longer than 4 weeks
Pain that interferes with school or athletic activities
Pain associated with systemic symptoms and signs (fever, sweats, weight loss, poor appetite, malaise)
Pain with sleep
Progressive pain
History of sports-related or other trauma
Gait abnormality
Bladder or bowel dysfunction
Lower extremity deformity
Motor weakness
Positive Lasègue's sign
Pain below the knee
Painful scoliosis
Exaggerated kyphosis
Midline cutaneous lesion

From Hollingworth P: Back pain in children. Br J Rheumatol 35:1022–1028, 1996.

and adjacent hyaline cartilage end plates. The proteoglycan gel of the nucleus pulposus provides cushioning for radial and axial compression due to the fluid held in the gel. The gel water content decreases from 90% in the fetus to 80% in children and to 50% to 60% by adulthood. The nucleus is ultimately replaced by fibrous tissue. The annulus fibrosus is well developed by 6 months of age, and its development is complete by 10 years. The annulus fibrosus contains type I collagen fibrils attached to the vertebral body in layers and to the anterior and posterior longitudinal ligaments.

Ossification of the epiphyseal ring occurs during the first 2 decades of life. The epiphyseal ring lies outside the epiphyseal plates. Until adolescence, the epiphyseal ring fibers are attached only through the cartilage of the growth plate. The epiphyseal ring ossifies anteriorly first, laterally second, and posteriorly last. Calcification of the epiphyseal plate begins at age 6 years and is complete by age 13 years. Initial fusion of the epiphyseal ring to the vertebral body begins at age 13 to 15 years in girls and 15 to 17 years in boys; it is complete by age 20 years.

PATHOPHYSIOLOGY

In children, early degeneration of the disk may occur, or the mechanics of the disk space may be altered by other processes such as trauma, infection, or inflammation. Multiple disk herniations occur much less frequently in children than in adults.

CLINICAL PRESENTATION

Cervical and Thoracic Disk Disease

Cervical and thoracic disk herniation in children is rare. Cervical disk herniation in children is almost always associated with other pathology such as trauma or inflammatory lesions, including diskitis and CCID. The clinical presentation of cervical disk herniation in children, consisting of a new onset of radiculopathy or myelopathy, is similar to that in adults. Most entities that affect cervical disks in children cause pain in the neck or upper extremities.

Lumbar Disk Disease

EPIDEMIOLOGY

Ethnicity and Age

In several large series of patients of all ages with lumbar disk herniation, children constitute a small percentage of the total. In series with white patients, children account for 0.4% to 3.8% of the total,[9–13] whereas in series with Asian patients, children account for 3% to 15.4% of the total.[14, 15] Lumbar disk herniation occurs very infrequently during the first decade of life. Four 10-year-old children and a 27-month-old child who developed a symptomatic herniated disk have been reported in the literature.[16–19]

Most other lesions that affect the lumbar intervertebral disks in children are also rare. Slipped epiphysis is seen in only 0.07% of all patients with back pain and occurs most commonly in the second decade.[20] Other processes that mimic disk herniation, such as inflammatory disorders and tumors, occur more frequently in the first decade.

Gender Predominance

The gender predominance of lumbar disk herniation in children is controversial. Some authors have found a female predominance,[9, 10, 14, 16, 21–23] which was attributed to the earlier onset of puberty and growth in girls.[9] In other pediatric series, there was a slight predominance of males.[12, 15, 17, 24, 25] Some disorders that mimic lumbar disk herniation in children are found more commonly in males, including slipped epiphysis[20] and Scheuermann's kyphosis.[26] In contrast, there was a 2:1 female predominance found in children with diskitis.[27, 28]

Familial Predisposition

Several authors have found a familial predisposition to lumbar disk herniation. In two series, children who required lumbar disk surgery had an approximately fivefold increased likelihood of a family history of lumbar disk herniation compared with controls.[25, 29] Familial predisposition has also been described among patients with spondylolysis and spondylolisthesis, with 27% and 3%, respectively, having a first-order relative with the same abnormality.[30]

CLINICAL HISTORY

Precipitating Events

The presenting history and symptoms of lumbar disk disease in children differ from those in adults (Table 227–2). Thirty percent to 60% of children with symptomatic lumbar disk herniation have a history of trauma or sports-related injury before the onset of pain.[8, 10, 15, 17, 21, 23, 24] Children with lumbar disk herniation also tend to have grown more than their peers without disk herniation have.[12, 24]

Pain

Children with symptomatic lumbar disk herniation usually have pain in the back and a lower extremity. Less than 10% of children presenting with low back pain, however, have disk herniation as the cause, and less than half of those children require surgery.[8, 12, 31] Children usually provide a less specific description of pain than do adults. Half the patients have intermittent pain, and half have incapacitating pain. The average duration of symptoms before the diagnosis of lumbar disk herniation is 10.7 months.[10]

In addition to pain, scoliosis often prompts evaluation of the spine in children. In a large series of children with idiopathic scoliosis, about one quarter (23%) had back pain at presentation.[32] Among those who had back pain initially, only 9% had significant structural

TABLE 227-2 ■ **Symptoms of Herniated Lumbar Disks in Children and Adults**

	CHILDREN %	ADULTS %
Mean length of symptoms	9.7–11	4.7
History of trauma	16–73	57
Lifting	16	31
Fall	21	10
Sports	31	10
Family history	55–60	—
Back pain alone	2–15	1
Sciatica alone	17–34	7
Sciatica plus back pain	55–95	91–99
Bladder or bowel symptoms	1.4	0

Summary of Symptoms Found More Frequently in Children Than in Adults

Longer duration of symptoms before diagnosis
History of trauma, particularly sports related
Family history of lumbar disk disease
Back pain without sciatica

Data for children from references 9, 10, 12, 15, 16, 21–24, 31; data for adults from references 11, 49.

pathology—less than 2% of the entire series. There was no association between the direction of the curve (left or right) and the presence of significant pathology in this series.[32]

Other disorders that cause back and lower extremity pain can mimic lumbar disk herniation, including slipped epiphysis, symptomatic spondylolysis or spondylolisthesis, and Scheuermann's kyphosis (congenital kyphosis from anterior wedging of a vertebra). The pain from these disorders is worse with activity and often includes back pain referred to the legs in a nonradicular distribution. Patients with a tethered spinal cord due to occult spinal dysraphism may present with back and lower extremity pain.

In patients with diskitis, back pain usually predominates over radicular pain. Children younger than 3 years may refuse to walk. Children between 3 and 9 years old may complain of abdominal pain predominantly, and children older than 9 years often complain of back and radicular pain.[33] These children are more comfortable lying down and often appear hyperextended.[26]

Back pain is an unusual early feature of rheumatologic disorders in children.[34] The pain in juvenile-onset ankylosing spondylitis is worse with morning stiffness,[26] and in contrast to most other lesions of the spine, the pain improves with movement.[26] Back pain associated with juvenile rheumatoid arthritis becomes progressively worse through the day.[30]

Patients with a spinal mass typically have a shorter duration of symptoms before presentation. This pain is unremitting and bilateral, worse with recumbency, and typically worse at night.[13, 30] Aneurysmal bone cysts may not cause pain until after a minor episode of trauma.[30]

EXAMINATION

The prevalence of signs found on the general and neurological examinations in children with herniated lumbar disks is listed in Table 227–3. These signs are also frequently found with other spinal lesions that mimic disk herniation in children.

General Examination

Children with lumbar disk herniation tend to have more limitation of movement than do most adults. Most children with herniated lumbar disks have a positive straight leg raising (SLR) sign (Lasègue's sign), and about one third have a positive crossed SLR sign as well.[9, 10, 15, 17] Flattening of the lumbar lordosis, scoliosis, forward pelvic tilt, antalgic gait, and paraspinal muscle spasm with limitation of lumbar flexion are often observed. Scoliosis secondary to intervertebral disk herniation occurs more frequently in children than in adults. Patients usually complain of pain with sneezing, coughing, and straining.

Other entities may mimic lumbar disk herniation on examination. The majority of patients with slipped epiphysis have lumbar spasm and decreased lumbar lordosis.[20] Children with spondylolysis and spondylolisthesis often have paraspinal muscle spasm that limits lumbar flexion, and tight hamstrings are occasionally present.[26] These children may have tenderness to palpation, but a palpable step-off rarely is present. Children with Scheuermann's kyphosis often have an exaggerated thoracic kyphosis with attempted hyperextension, compensatory hyperlordosis, and mild scoliosis.[26] Children with occult spinal dysraphism often have a midline cutaneous signature on the back. It may be difficult to distinguish diskitis from disk herniation on examination. Children with diskitis often have a positive SLR sign, abnormal spinal posture, and difficulty standing and walking. These children also usually have irritability, decreased range of motion in the spine, and fever

TABLE 227-3 ■ **Signs of Herniated Lumbar Disk in Children and Adults**

	CHILDREN %	ADULTS %
General Examination		
Lasègue's sign (SLR)	86–100	76
Crossed Lasègue's sign (SLR)	14–68	19
Flattening of lumbar lordosis	66–90	85
Scoliosis	6–56	—
Lumbar spasm	87–96	—
Limited range of motion	100	85
Lumbar tenderness	39–50	—
Neurological Examination		
Sensory loss	9–58	38
Motor weakness	7–86	27–95
Diminished reflexes	9–68	72
Gait abnormality	13–48	—
Cauda equina syndrome	0–1.4	—

Summary of Differences in Signs Between Children and Adults

Crossed Lasègue's sign is more frequent in children
Scoliosis is more frequent in children
Neurological signs are less common in children

Data for children from references 9, 10, 12, 14–16, 21–24, 31; data for adults from references 11, 49.

(26%).[26, 35] Less than half the patients with spinal tumors have a positive SLR sign.[13] Tumors may cause painful scoliosis, spine tenderness, and disproportionate anemia.[26]

Neurological Examination

Children with lumbar disk herniation are less likely than adults to present with neurological findings in a radicular distribution (see Table 227–3). If present, neurological signs of disk herniation in children include unilateral or bilateral motor weakness, sensory loss, and diminished deep tendon reflexes. Bladder and bowel dysfunction occurs infrequently.

Other disorders that affect the lumbar spine in children may have neurological signs that are difficult to distinguish from lumbar disk herniation. About half the children with slipped epiphysis have neurological signs. With spondylolysis and spondylolisthesis, neurological symptoms and signs are less common.[26] Children with tethered cord due to occult spina bifida have neurological dysfunction, particularly bladder and bowel abnormalities, significantly more frequently than do patients with lumbar disk herniation. More than half the children with spinal mass lesions have abnormalities on neurological examination.

Lumbar Herniated Disk Location

The segmental distribution of lumbar disk herniation in children is similar to that in adults. About half of pediatric patients with surgically treated lesions have lumbar disk herniation at L4-5 or L5-S1.[9, 10, 22] Multilevel disk herniations are rare in children.

IMAGING STUDIES

Radiography

CERVICAL DISK DISEASE

Plain radiographs of a child with a cervical herniated disk may demonstrate a decrease in disk height. Osteophytes are rare in children. After trauma, spondylosis, spondylolisthesis, fracture, or malalignment due to ligamentous disruption may be present. In CCID, one or more disks may have a calcified nucleus pulposus that appears as a dense mass in the center of the disk space.

LUMBAR DISK DISEASE

Plain radiographs of the lumbar spine may be obtained to aid in the diagnosis of lumbar disk herniation and to exclude other structural abnormalities that cause chronic back pain. Radiographs are abnormal in 50% to 70% of children with herniated lumbar disks.[8] Other structural abnormalities, including loss of disk height at the level of herniation or loss of lumbar lordosis secondary to spasm, fracture, dislocation, stenosis, or a slipped epiphysis, are present in 5% of children with lumbar disk herniation requiring surgery (Table 227–4). Plain radiographs can be helpful in diagnosing other

TABLE 227–4 ■ Structural Abnormalities Associated with Lumbar Disk Herniation
Occult spina bifida
Extra lumbar vertebra
Sacralization of the fifth lumbar vertebra
Transitional vertebra
Spinal stenosis
Lateral recess stenosis
Spondylolisthesis

From Epstein J, Epstein N, Marc J, et al: Lumbar intervertebral disk herniation in teenage children: Recognition and management of associated anomalies. Spine 9:427–432, 1984.

disorders of the lumbar spine in children. Oblique films provide the best view of the pars interarticularis in the evaluation of spondylolysis. The prevalence of asymptomatic pars abnormalities on plain radiographs is 2% to 7% in children.[26]

In children with diskitis, paravertebral swelling and disk space narrowing may be observed on radiographs.[36] End plate erosion and bone destruction can lag 7 to 10 days behind the clinical course.[36] In diskitis, the degree of disk space narrowing and end plate destruction observed on plain radiographs is not predictive of the clinical course.[35] Other abnormalities that can be observed on plain radiographs include structural changes due to erosion or remodeling of bone by a tumor or intraspinal cyst, hemivertebrae, bifid lamina, or other abnormalities associated with occult spinal dysraphism.

Computed Tomography

In general, magnetic resonance imaging (MRI) has supplanted computed tomography as the initial study, except in the evaluation of acute traumatic spine fractures. Disk herniation can be accurately diagnosed by computed tomography in 67% to 100% of cases.[30]

Magnetic Resonance Imaging

Because MRI is noninvasive and provides excellent resolution of both neural elements and soft tissues, it is usually the preferred modality for imaging the spine in children, except for the evaluation of acute traumatic spine fractures. Interpretation of MRI signals in infants differs from that in older children. From birth to 1 month of age, the ossification centers are hypointense, and the cartilaginous end plates are hyperintense.[36] Between 1 and 6 months of age, increased intensity progresses from the ossification centers toward the end plates, and the prominent signal intensity in the cartilage decreases. From age 7 months to 2 years, there is increasing signal intensity in the more rectangular vertebral bodies. The signal in the cartilage continues to decrease.[36]

MRI may demonstrate disk herniation with compression of nerve roots or the thecal sac (Fig. 227–1). Decreased signal on T2-weighted images suggestive of disk degeneration is rarely found in children. No

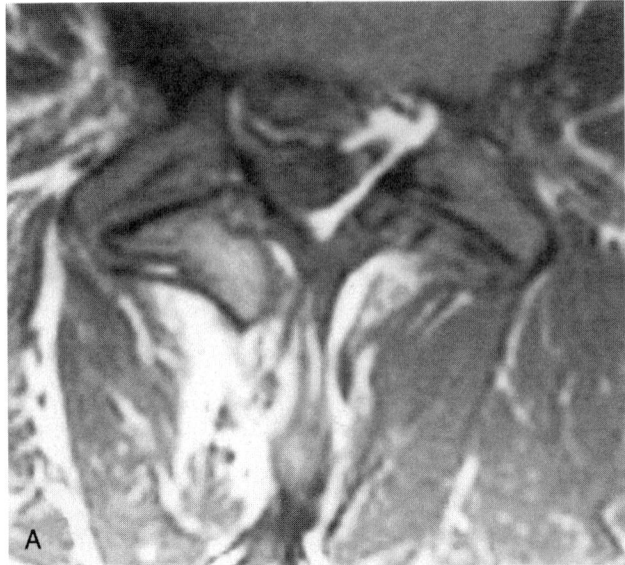

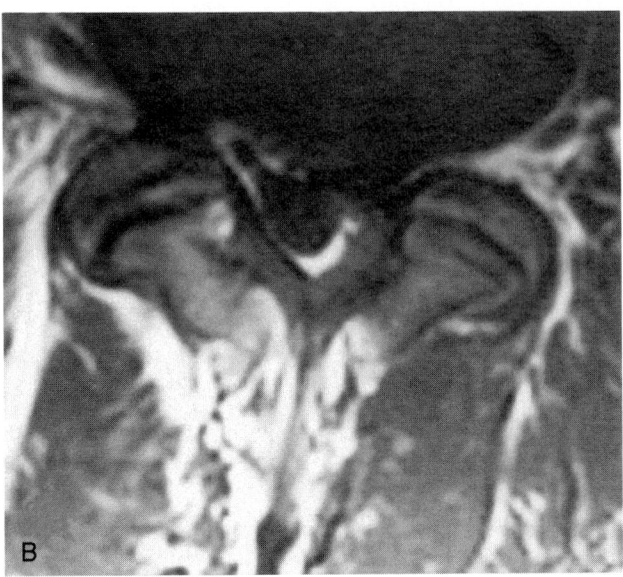

FIGURE 227–1. Lumbar disk herniation. A 13-year-old boy with a family history of lumbar disk herniation developed low back pain and left sciatica after playing football. Paresthesias resolved after several weeks. Magnetic resonance imaging (MRI) demonstrated a left posterolateral disk herniation at L4-5. He was treated with nonoperative therapy and experienced improvement. After 1 year he continued to have back pain and had thoracolumbar scoliosis, bilateral positive straight leg raising signs, and left extensor hallucis longus weakness. A year and a half after the initial onset of pain, he moved a heavy object and developed severe back pain with bilateral sciatica and numbness that failed to improve with 2 weeks of nonoperative therapy. Repeat MRI showed *(A)* a large right L3-4 disk herniation with a free fragment and *(B)* the old left L4-5 herniation on axial images. The patient underwent microsurgical diskectomies at the two levels, with resolution of his pain and neurological signs. He has remained asymptomatic for 4 years.

difference in the prevalence of disk degeneration between symptomatic children and age-matched controls was found on MRI.[37] A pars fracture in spondylolisthesis is hypointense on T1-weighted images.[26, 30] MRI may detect prespondylolisthesis changes, as well as healing fractures.[30] MRI is the preferred study for evaluating processes that involve neural elements, such as infections, tumors, and myelodysplasia. If MRI is nondiagnostic or contraindicated, myelography with a high-resolution computed tomographic scan is recommended.[36]

Myelography

In older series reported before the widespread use of MRI, myelograms were frequently obtained to better delineate the herniated disk. Myelograms were abnormal in 84% to 88% of children who underwent lumbar diskectomy.[9, 10] Because MRI is noninvasive and provides excellent visualization of the spinal and neural structures, it has replaced myelography except when MRI is contraindicated.

Radionuclide Scanning

Since the advent of MRI, with its superior diagnostic accuracy, the indications for bone scans have decreased. Radionuclide bone scans use technetium 99 to localize areas of increased blood flow in bone. A needle biopsy usually does not cause a false-positive bone scan. For the evaluation of diskitis in a child, if MRI is not an option, a bone scan is recommended. A gallium 67 citrate scan may be useful instead of a technetium 99 scan, because a gallium 67 scan can demonstrate the progression and resolution of inflammation and is less affected by other confounding factors such as previous surgery, pseudarthrosis, or neuropathologic changes.[36]

NONOPERATIVE TREATMENT

In general, the treatment of intervertebral disk herniation in children is similar to that in adults. If a motor deficit or sphincter dysfunction is present, urgent surgical treatment for decompression of neural structures may be indicated. If these deficits are not present, a trial of nonoperative therapy is recommended. Nonoperative treatment consists of bed rest and nonsteroidal analgesics for 1 to 2 weeks. Activity is gradually increased over several months, and physical therapy may be beneficial. The child is advised to avoid significant physical activity for 6 to 12 months. Muscle relaxants are rarely indicated in children. Trigger point injections and pelvic traction are not recommended.[8]

Although the majority of children with symptomatic disk herniation improve with nonoperative therapy, it is generally less effective for the treatment of lumbar disk herniation in children than in adults. Adults with symptomatic disk herniation require surgery in 10% to 20% of cases, compared with 20% to 30% of children.[8, 38] The more viscous disks found in children may contribute to the greater failure rate of nonoperative therapy.[23]

OPERATIVE TREATMENT

Cervical Disk Herniation

In children, the indications for surgical treatment of cervical disk herniation include progressive myelopathy or radiculopathy, incapacitating pain, and chronic debilitating pain. An anterior cervical diskectomy is performed using the same general techniques as in adults. Fusion with autograft or allograft bone is recommended.

Lumbar Disk Herniation

Because children with lumbar disk herniation generally have fewer neurological signs than do adults, even those with relatively few signs may benefit from lumbar diskectomy. In one pediatric series, 40% of children who underwent lumbar diskectomy had only a positive SLR sign and paraspinal muscle spasm on physical examination.[9] Indications for surgery include failure of nonoperative therapy, progressive neurological deficit, nerve root compression with a fixed neurological deficit, or intractable pain. The operative techniques for lumbar disk herniation in children are similar to those used in adults. If the disk is accessible, a unilateral microsurgical diskectomy through a hemilaminotomy is preferred. If there is a central disk herniation or a slipped epiphysis, laminectomy is often required. The viscous intervertebral disk in children is usually more difficult to remove than the desiccated disk commonly found in adults.[24]

If there is significant instability or severe spondylolisthesis, or if a bilateral procedure is performed, fusion is usually indicated.[12, 14, 31] Fusion after lumbar diskectomy in children has not been shown to improve outcome or decrease the recurrence rate.[12] Although fusion with instrumentation may rarely be needed after lumbar diskectomy, instrumentation has been used with minimal complications in children.[39] No experience with endoscopic diskectomy has been reported in children. Chemonucleolysis is not recommended for children.[8]

OUTCOME AND COMPLICATIONS

Children usually have excellent results after surgery, with more than 90% reporting an excellent or good outcome, defined as no or minimal pain 1 year after surgery (Table 227–5). A formal prospective study of outcome has not been performed in children undergoing lumbar diskectomy. In a retrospective study of children who underwent lumbar diskectomy, no significant predictors of poor outcome were identified, as has been found in adult studies.[21] Three percent to 12% experience recurrent pain.[8]

Disk herniation during childhood usually does not predispose a patient to disk herniation later in life.[8] With long-term follow-up, the percentage of children with recurrent symptoms remains low but slowly increases.[31] DeOrio and Bianco found that 76% of children had recurrence of low back pain or sciatica over a mean follow-up of 19 years.[31] The rate of reoperation varies from 0% to 24% with long-term follow-up.[14, 21]

Operative complications after diskectomy in children are similar to those in adults, with 4% suffering wound hematoma and 3% experiencing delayed

T A B L E   2 2 7 – 5 ■ **Outcome after Lumbar Diskectomy in Children and Adults**

	CHILDREN	ADULTS
At follow-up		
Minimal or no limitation (%)	72–88	80–89
Back Pain (%)	19–76	—
Radicular pain (%)	17	—
Leg numbness (%)	7–8	—
Leg weakness (%)	3–8	—
Reoperation (%)	0–24	6–11
Same level (%)	38–50	50
Different level (%)	50–62	25
For fusion (%)	24	—
Time to reoperation (yr)	3.1	4.3

Data for children from references 12, 14, 15, 21–24, 31; data for adults from references 11, 49.

wound healing.[15, 31] In children, diskitis secondary to infection at the time of surgery rarely occurs as a postoperative complication.

DIFFERENTIAL DIAGNOSIS

Because other entities that cause pain or symptoms referable to the spine are as common as intervertebral disk disease in children, the disorders in the differential diagnosis of a child with symptoms and signs referable to the spine are briefly reviewed (Table 227–6).

Structural Lesions

TRAUMATIC SPINE INJURY

Traumatic disk herniation may occur along with an acute spine injury. Acute myelopathy may be due to disk herniation, but spinal cord injury without persistent malalignment or disk herniation can occur in children after traumatic transient subluxation. Spinal cord injury without radiographic abnormalities was diagnosed more frequently before the advent of MRI.[40, 41]

SLIPPED EPIPHYSIS

Slipped epiphysis is a fracture of a triangular portion of the epiphyseal ring along with disk herniation, and it often mimics lumbar disk herniation in its presentation. The epiphyseal plate is more vulnerable to injury in children, as opposed to the desiccated disk in adults. In movements involving hyperextension or rapid flexion with axial loading, the greatest stress to the spine in children is transferred to the epiphyseal plate, particularly the posterior portion.[20] Slipped epiphysis occurs most commonly at the inferior portion of L4, causing a clinical picture similar to L4-5 disk herniation. In Epstein and colleagues' series of 30 children, only 18% improved with nonoperative therapy; with surgical therapy, 93% had excellent results.[22]

A limbus vertebra refers to an anterior slipped epiphysis with intrabody disk herniation, also called an anterior Schmorl's node. In a pediatric series of

TABLE 227-6 ■ **Differential Diagnosis for Lumbar Disk Herniation in Children**

Structural
Slipped epiphysis
Spondylolysis
Spondylolisthesis
Facet injury

Inflammatory
Vertebral osteomyelitis
Diskitis
Spinal epidural abscess
Juvenile-onset ankylosing spondylosis

Metabolic
Storage diseases

Mass Lesions
Benign tumors
  Osteoid osteoma
  Osteblastoma
  Neurofibromatosis
  Aneurysmal bone cyst
Malignant tumors
  Metastasis
  Lymphoma
  Leukemia
  Wilms' tumor
Ewing's sarcoma
Spinal chordoma
Teratoma
Rhabdomyosarcoma
Intraspinal cysts
  Extradural arachnoid cyst
  Tarlov's cyst
  Synovial cyst

Other Disorders
Conversion disorder
Dysmenorrhea
Fibromyalgia
Retroperitoneal mass
Chronic recurrent multicentric osteomyelitis
Idiopathic juvenile osteoporosis
Cystic fibrosis
Fibrodysplasia ossificans
Sickle-cell disease
Cushing's disease
Arachnoiditis

children with limbus vertebra, all the children had back pain, and 13% also had radicular pain. The majority of the patients were treated nonoperatively.[42]

SPONDYLOLYSIS AND SPONDYLOLISTHESIS

Spondylolysis is a unilateral or bilateral defect in the pars interarticularis without forward displacement of the adjacent vertebral body. Spondylolisthesis is subluxation of a vertebra due to a defect in the pars interarticularis. The types of spondylolisthesis observed in children include dysplastic, isthmic, traumatic, and pathologic, according to the Wiltse-Newman-MacNab classification.[43] Dysplastic spondylolisthesis is caused by a congenital deficiency in the pars interarticularis. In isthmic spondylolisthesis, the defect is due to (1) a lytic fatigue fracture of the pars, (2) an elongated pars without a true fracture, or (3) an

acute fracture. Traumatic spondylolisthesis results from disruption of a portion of the posterior arch except for the isthmus. Pathologic spondylolisthesis occurs in children with defects in bone formation such as osteogenesis imperfecta, Marfan's syndrome, Ehlers-Danlos syndrome, achondroplasia, osteopetrosis, and neurofibromatosis.[44, 45]

Children with spondylolisthesis may be asymptomatic, or they may become symptomatic once they reach a growth spurt.[30] Asymptomatic isthmic spondylolisthesis is found in 4.4% of 6-year-olds.[45] Sports that have a high risk of spondylolisthesis include gymnastics, ballet dancing, football, wrestling, hockey, the high jump, and weight lifting.[26, 46] If imaging confirms the diagnosis of isthmic spondylolisthesis, the fracture can usually be treated by having the child refrain from physical activity. A lumbar orthosis may be necessary.[46] If a fracture is evident on the plain radiographs but the bone scan is negative, a nonunion pseudarthrosis may have formed. If severe spondylolisthesis is present, or if there is persistent pain, fusion is recommended.[26]

SPINAL STENOSIS

Spinal stenosis has been described in children. In contrast to the 80% of adults that improve with a trial of nonoperative treatment, only 40% of children improve.[47]

SCHEUERMANN'S DISEASE

In Scheuermann's disease, there is a congenital kyphosis of the thoracic spine, with anterior wedging of a vertebral body. Asymptomatic kyphosis is present in 20% to 30% of plain radiographs from adults.[26] The typical adolescent patient with Scheuermann's disease presents with thoracic back pain or a painless thoracic kyphosis.[26] Radiographs show increased kyphosis with anterior wedging, irregularity of the end plates, and herniation of the disk into a vertebral body (Schmorl's node). Similar findings can occur with osteoporosis, hyperparathyroidism, tumor, or degenerated disk.[26] Other causes of slipped epiphysis anteriorly are osteonecrosis of the ring epiphysis and osteochondritis. Patients can be effectively treated with a brace.

TETHERED SPINAL CORD AND OCCULT SPINAL DYSRAPHISM

In children with tethered cord from occult spinal dysraphism, MRI is the imaging modality of choice to define the location of the conus and any abnormal components within the spinal canal, such as a dermoid cyst, dermal sinus, split cord malformation, or lipomyelomeningocele.

KYPHOS DEFORMITY

Children with congenital metabolic storage diseases can develop progressive kyphotic deformities of the spine. Localized gibbus of the upper lumbar spine develops, with preservation of the disk space. The hypotonia and poor muscle tone from the storage disease usually potentiate the kyphos.

Inflammatory Lesions

DISKITIS

Several authors have suggested that diskitis may be a milder, more indolent form of vertebral osteomyelitis.[27, 36] Diskitis also has been termed *infectious spondylitis*.[36] Diskitis occurs most frequently by hematogenous spread as metaphyseal osteomyelitis. *Staphylococcus* is the most common organism; other common organisms are *Streptococcus* and *Mycobacterium*. Disk herniation can occur in the setting of diskitis.

Diskitis can usually be treated successfully with an orthosis and empirical intravenous antibiotics.[27] Once the symptoms have abated, the child can be treated with oral antibiotics and physical therapy. Biopsy is usually not indicated unless the child fails to improve with empirical antibiotics or tuberculosis or tumor is suspected.[30, 36] Patients treated with intravenous antibiotics have a more rapid resolution of symptoms and a much lower incidence of recurrence than do patients treated with oral or no antibiotics.[35]

Tubercular spondylitis usually requires a more aggressive surgical approach than that needed for bacterial disease. In one series, 80 children with tubercular spondylitis were treated with either radical surgery or débridement.[36] Although the tuberculosis was successfully treated in all cases, 60% of the children treated with débridement had a residual kyphosis of 10 degrees or more.[36] Opportunistic infections, including vertebral osteomyelitis and diskitis, occur more frequently in children infected with human immunodeficiency virus. The opportunistic infections include cytomegalovirus, cryptococcal infections, toxoplasmosis, tuberculosis, and aspergillosis.

Infarcts from sickle cell disease may predispose children to spinal infections. Areas of necrotic bone provide a hospitable site for secondary infection by staphylococcus and salmonella organisms.[27] Radionuclide scans with both technetium 99 and gallium 67 may be necessary to differentiate the area of bone infarction from osteomyelitis. MRI is not good at differentiating between osteomyelitis and osteonecrosis.[27]

Spinal epidural abscess usually has a distinct presentation that can be distinguished from disk herniation. Children with spinal epidural abscess have tenderness, spasm, decreased range of motion in the spine, neurological signs, fever, leukocytosis, and an elevated sedimentation rate. MRI is the imaging modality of choice to distinguish diskitis from a spinal abscess. In most cases, laminectomy for drainage, combined with a long course of intravenous antibiotics, is the recommended treatment.

An entity termed *chronic recurrent multicentric osteomyelitis* has been described in children. Affected children are usually 5 to 15 years old, and there is a 2:1 female predominance.[27] The child typically has an indolent, sometimes recurrent course of inflammation, with single or multiple lesions in the spine. The child rarely has systemic symptoms. Laboratory values are usually normal, and no pathogen is identified. Plain radiographs may show lytic changes in the acute period, lytic or mixed changes in the subacute period, and sclerotic changes in the chronic stages. Supportive treatment, including nonsteroidal analgesic medications, is recommended.[27]

CALCIFIED CERVICAL INTERVERTEBRAL DISK

CCID can mimic cervical disk herniation in children. In adults, the annulus fibrosus calcifies 10-fold more than the nucleus does. In CCID in children, the nucleus pulposus calcifies prematurely, without calcification of the annulus fibrosus (Fig. 227–2). More than 100 cases of CCID in children have been reported. The typical age at presentation ranges from 5 to 10 years, but CCID has been reported in an infant.[5] There is a 1.5:1 male

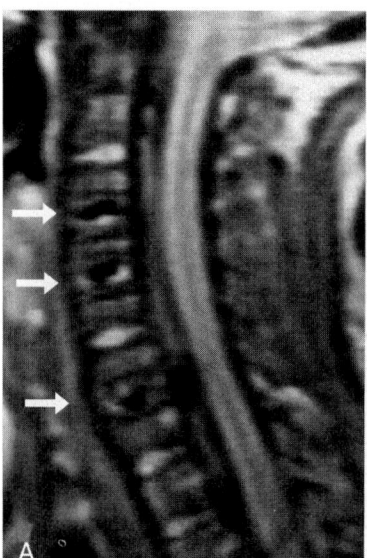
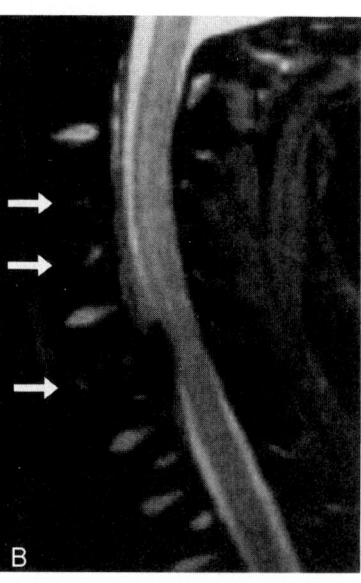

FIGURE 227–2. Calcified cervical intervertebral disk (CCID). A 5-year-old boy presented with a 1-week history of gait abnormality, meningismus, and fever. The cerebrospinal fluid was unremarkable. Examination showed left upper extremity weakness, diminished triceps reflex bilaterally, no signs of myelopathy, limited neck range of motion, and an abnormal gait with the neck in marked hyperextension. Plain radiographs and magnetic resonance imaging scans revealed CCID at C3-4, C4-5, and C6-7 *(arrows)* and disk herniation at C6-7, with mild impingement on the thecal sac and spinal cord, as illustrated here by sagittal T1-weighted *(A)* and T2-weighted *(B)* images. He underwent a C6-7 diskectomy with an iliac crest autograft. Postoperatively he recovered his strength and triceps reflexes and had no recurrence after 5 years.

predominance among symptomatic children, in contrast to a 2:1 female predominance among asymptomatic children.[26] Most symptomatic children have neck pain and tenderness, decreased range of motion, and torticollis of sudden onset.[5] Radiculopathy is rare. The most commonly affected level is C6-7. One third of children have multiple levels affected. There is frequently a history of fever, and laboratory studies show leukocytosis, an elevated erythrocyte sedimentation rate, and an elevated C-reactive protein level.[5, 36] Blood cultures are positive in 50% of children, and needle aspiration is positive in 60%.[36] Plain radiographs show the calcified nucleus pulposus as a mass. On MRI, at the level of the disk calcification, protrusion of the noncalcified portion of the disk is present in 38% of the disk levels,[5] although children rarely have neurological signs.[6] After the symptoms resolve, reimaging often shows resolution of the disk protrusion.[5]

If the child is symptomatic with neurological signs, particularly motor weakness, and fails to improve with a trial of nonoperative therapy, anterior cervical diskectomy is recommended. Five percent of children with CCID require surgery.[5] The cause of CCID is unknown.[5]

JUVENILE-ONSET ANKYLOSING SPONDYLITIS

Juvenile-onset ankylosing spondylitis is characterized by the gradual progression from peripheral arthritis to ankylosing spondylitis over 5 to 10 years. Two subsets of juvenile-onset ankylosing spondylitis exist, one of which is characterized by early axial involvement. Patients with axial involvement have decreased spinal mobility, morning stiffness, and tenderness of the spine to palpation. About 20% have no peripheral arthritis, and about 36% have fever and malaise. Juvenile rheumatoid arthritis may also cause spine pain. Pain that worsens throughout the day is typical of juvenile rheumatoid arthritis, whereas the pain of juvenile-onset ankylosing spondylitis improves through the day.[30]

Mass Lesions

NEOPLASMS

Children with malignancies can present with pain and neurological signs that mimic disk herniation. A study compared the clinical presentation of children with lumbar disk herniation with that of children with spine neoplasms.[13] The average age of children with lumbar disk herniation was 14.5 years, compared with 6.8 years for children with neoplasms. The children with neoplasms also had a shorter period of symptoms before diagnosis—15 weeks—compared with 46 weeks for the children with lumbar disk herniation. In addition, most children with neoplasms had bilateral lower extremity pain.

Osteoblastoma and Osteoid Osteoma

Osteoblastoma and osteoid osteoma are benign tumors of adolescence that occur in the posterior vertebral elements. Osteoid osteomas are usually less than 1 cm in diameter, and osteoblastomas are usually more

than 1 cm in diameter. Osteoblastomas typically cause tenderness and scoliosis.[26] On plain radiographs, osteoid osteomas have sclerosis, with a radiolucent center. Initial plain radiographs may be normal, and the lesion may be demonstrated on a bone scan.[26] Surgery is usually curative.

Spinal Chordoma

Chordomas are slow-growing tumors that arise from the notochord; half occur in the sacrum. Chordomas rarely occur in children. Imaging often shows a soft tissue sacral mass with bony destruction. The preferred treatment is gross total resection. External beam radiation is advised after subtotal resection.[8]

Eosinophilic Granuloma (Langerhans' Histiocytosis)

Histiocytosis lesions are more common in the thoracic spine than in the lumbar or cervical spine.[26] An eosinophilic granuloma usually presents as a well-marked lytic lesion on plain radiographs. If multiple vertebrae are involved, histiocytosis X may be present, and chemotherapy may be required.[26]

Malignant Vertebral Tumor

Malignant vertebral tumors can present with pain and physical findings that mimic a herniated disk. Malignant vertebral tumors include metastasis, rhabdomyosarcoma, Ewing's sarcoma, primary lymphoma, leukemia, teratoma, and neuroblastoma.[26, 30] Gangliogliomas may be benign or malignant. Often the preferred treatment for these tumors is resection of the intracanalicular portion, followed by adjuvant chemotherapy and radiation.

Intraspinal Tumor

Intraspinal tumors can present with back and lower extremity pain and physical signs that simulate the clinical presentation of disk herniation. Forty percent of patients with intraspinal tumors present with pain, and 60% have neurological signs.[26] Seventy percent of intraspinal lesions are benign.

Aneurysmal Bone Cyst

An aneurysmal bone cyst arises from pressurized venous blood that causes expansion of the underlying bone. Aneurysmal bone cysts constitute 1.4% of all bone tumors.[8] Most aneurysmal bone cysts occur in the spine, with lumbar cysts more frequent than thoracic cysts[26]; they rarely occur in the cervical spine. Typically, adolescent patients present with a history of pain for a few months, but the lesions may also cause painless scoliosis or limitation of spinal range of motion. The lesions are treated by surgical excision. Needle biopsy is not recommended.[26] Presurgical embolization may minimize intraoperative blood loss. Adjuvant therapy with 20 Gy of radiation is recommended if subtotal resection is achieved.

INTRASPINAL CYSTS

Intraspinal cysts can cause back pain and radiculopathy that mimic disk herniation. Intraspinal cysts include congenital extradural arachnoid cysts, Tarlov's perineurial cysts, spontaneous meningeal diverticula along nerve roots, and occult intrasacral meningoceles.[48]

Congenital extradural arachnoid cysts usually become symptomatic in the second decade, with a 4:3 female predominance. Most of the cysts occur in the thoracic spine. Extradural arachnoid cysts are usually attached by a narrow pedicle to the dura and are frequently located in the midline posteriorly or posterolaterally.[48] The cysts are usually solitary, are lined by arachnoid-like cells, and contain cerebrospinal fluid. Cysts in the cervical and thoracic spine often cause a fluctuating but progressive spastic quadriparesis or paraparesis with pain. In the lumbar spine, the cysts usually cause radicular pain.[48] Cysts are visualized well on MRI. The treatment is surgical resection with ligation of the pedicle and dural closure.

Tarlov's cysts arise in the potential space between the perineurium and endoneurium of spinal nerve roots.[48] These lesions are usually sacral and rarely occur in pediatric patients. Ganglion cysts have no synovial lining and are filled with a viscid gelatinous material. Synovial cysts are lined with synovium from the adjacent facet joint and are usually posterolateral and attached to the facet joint, particularly near L4-5. The cysts usually cause root compression and thus can mimic disk herniation. Synovial cysts may be bilateral.[48]

Conversion Hysteria

This syndrome is more common in adolescent girls. Typically, the primary complaint is back pain. Diffuse tenderness is often present on examination. Notably, the patient usually has a remarkably cheerful affect, and the parent tends to speak for the child.[26] Imaging, if performed, is unremarkable. A treatment program of physical therapy and gradual return to activities is often successful.

REFERENCES

1. Wahren H: Herniated nucleus pulposus in a child of twelve years. Acta Orthop Scand 16:40–42, 1945.
2. Bradford D, Garcia A: Herniations of the lumbar intervertebral disc in children and adolescents. JAMA 210:2045–2051, 1969.
3. Epstein J, Lavine L: Herniated lumbar intervertebral disc herniation in teen-age children. J Neurosurg 21:1070–1075, 1964.
4. Matson D: Neurosurgery of Infancy and Childhood. Springfield, Ill, Charles C Thomas, 1969, pp 376–380.
5. Heinrich S, Zembo M, King A, et al: Calcific cervical intervertebral disc herniation in children. Spine 16:228–231, 1991.
6. Oga M, Terada K, Kikuchi N, et al: Herniation of calcified cervical intervertebral disc causes dissociated motor loss in a child. Spine 18:2347–2350, 1993.
7. Techakapuch S: Rupture of the lumbar cartilage plate into the spinal canal in an adolescent: Case report. J Bone Joint Surg 63:481–482, 1981.
8. Hahn Y: Intervertebral disc diseases. In Albright L, Pollack I, Adelson D (eds): Principles and Practice of Pediatric Neurosurgery. New York, Thieme Medical, 1999, pp 433–445.
9. Borgesen S, Vang P: Herniation of the lumbar intervertebral disk in children and adolescents. Acta Orthop Scand 45:540–549, 1974.
10. Bradford D, Garcia A: Lumbar intervertebral disk herniations in children and adolescents. Orthop Clin N Am 2:583–592, 1971.
11. Davis R: A long-term outcome analysis of 984 surgically treated herniated lumbar discs. J Neurosurg 80:415–421, 1994.
12. Ebersold MJ, Quast LM, Bianco AJ Jr: Results of lumbar discectomy in the pediatric patient. J Neurosurg 67:643–647, 1987.
13. Martinez-Lage J, Martinez Robledo A, Lopez F, et al: Disc protrusion in the child. Childs Nerv Syst 13:201–207, 1997.
14. Ishihara H, Matsui H, Hirano N, et al: Lumbar intervertebral disc herniation in children less than 16 years of age. Spine 22:2044–2049, 1997.
15. Kurihara A, Kataoka O: Lumbar disc herniation in children and adolescents. Spine 5:443–451, 1980.
16. Garrido E, Humphreys R, Hendrick E, et al: Lumbar disc disease in children. Neurosurgery 2:22–26, 1978.
17. Giroux J-C, Leclercq T: Lumbar disc excision in the second decade. Spine 7:168–170, 1982.
18. Grass J, Dockendorff I, Soto V, et al: Progressive scoliosis with vertebral rotation after lumbar intervertebral disc herniation in a 10-year-old girl. Spine 18:336–338, 1993.
19. Revuelta R, DeJuambelz P, Fernandez B, et al: Lumbar disc herniation in a 27-month-old child. J Neurosurg Spine 92:98–100, 2000.
20. Martinez-Lage J, Poza M, Arcas P: Avulsed lumbar vertebral rim plate in an adolescent: Trauma or malformation? Childs Nerv Syst 14:131–134, 1998.
21. Durham S, Sun P, Sutton L: Surgically treated lumbar disc disease in the pediatric population: An outcome study. J Neurosurg Spine 92:1–6, 2000.
22. Epstein J, Epstein N, Marc J, et al: Lumbar intervertebral disk herniation in teenage children: Recognition and management of associated anomalies. Spine 9:427–432, 1984.
23. Gennuso R, Humphreys R, Hoffman H, et al: Lumbar intervertebral disc disease in the pediatric population. Pediatr Neurosurg 18:282–286, 1992.
24. Shillito JJ: Pediatric lumbar disc surgery: 20 Patients under 15 years of age. Pediatr Neurosurg 46:14–18, 1996.
25. Varlotta G, Brown M, Kelsey J, et al: Familial predisposition for herniation of a lumbar disc in patients who are less than twenty-one years old. J Bone Joint Surg Am 73:124–128, 1991.
26. Hollingworth P: Back pain in children. Br J Rheumatol 35:1022–1028, 1996.
27. Mandell G: Imaging in the diagnosis of musculoskeletal infections in children. Curr Probl Pediatr 26:218–237, 1996.
28. Ventura N, Gonzalez E, Terricabras L, et al: Intervertebral discitis in children: A review of 12 cases. Int Orthop 20:32–34, 1996.
29. Matsui H, Kanamori M, Ishihara H, et al: Familial predisposition for lumbar degenerative disc disease. Spine 23:1029–1034, 1998.
30. Payne WK III, Ogilvie JW: Back pain in children and adolescents. Pediatr Clin N Am 43:4899–4917, 1996.
31. DeOrio J, Bianco AJ Jr: Lumbar disc excision in children and adolescents. J Bone Joint Surg Am 64:991–996, 1982.
32. Ramirez N, Johnston C, Browne R: The prevalence of back pain in children who have idiopathic scoliosis. J Bone Joint Surg Am 79:364–368, 1997.
33. Wong-Chung J, Naseeb S, Kaneker S, et al: Anterior disc protrusion as a cause for abdominal symptoms in childhood discitis. Spine 24:918–920, 1999.
34. Cabral D, Tucker L: Malignancies in children who initially present with rheumatic complaints. J Pediatr 134:53–57, 1999.
35. Ring D, Wenger DR: Pyogenic infectious spondylitis in children. Am J Orthop 25:342–348, 1996.
36. Glazer P, Hu S: Pediatric spinal infections. Orthop Clin N Am 27:111–123, 1996.
37. Salo S, Paajanen H, Alanen A: Disc degeneration of pediatric patients in lumbar MRI. Pediatr Radiol 25:186–189, 1995.
38. Ghabrial Y, Tarrant M: Adolescent lumbar disc prolapse. Acta Orthop Scand 60:174–176, 1989.
39. Brown C, Lenke L, Bridwell K, et al: Complications of pediatric thoracolumbar and lumbar pedicle screws. Spine 23:1566–1571, 1998.
40. Felsberg G, Tien R, Osumi A, et al: Utility of MR imaging in pediatric spinal cord injury. Pediatr Radiol 25:131–135, 1995.

41. Grabb P, Pang D: Magnetic resonance imaging in the evaluation of spinal cord injury without radiographic abnormality in children. Neurosurgery 35:406–414, 1994.

42. Henales V, Hervas J, Lopez P, et al: Intervertebral disc herniations (limbus vertebrae) in pediatric patients: Report of 15 cases. Pediatr Radiol 23:608–610, 1993.

43. Wiltse L, Newman P, MacNab I: Classification of spondylolysis and spondylolithesis. Clin Orthop 117:23–29, 1976.

44. Martin R, Deanne R, Collett V: Spondylolysis in children who have osteopetrosis. J Bone Joint Surg Am 79:1685–1689, 1997.

45. Sampson J, Wilkins R: Lumbar spondylolisthesis. In Wilkins R, Rengachary S (eds): Neurosurgery. New York, McGraw-Hill, 1996, pp 3851–3858.

46. Cook P, Leit M: Issues in the pediatric athlete. Orthop Clin N Am 26:453–464, 1995.

47. Epstein N, Epstein J, Carras R: Spinal stenosis and disc herniation in a 14-year-old male. Spine 13:938–941, 1988.

48. Wilkins R: Intraspinal cysts. In Wilkins R, Rengachary S (eds): Neurosurgery. New York, McGraw-Hill, 1996, pp 3509–3519.

49. Pappas C, Harrington T, Sonntag V: Outcome analysis in 654 surgically treated lumbar disc herniations. Neurosurgery 30:862–866, 1992.

CHAPTER 228

Spondylolisthesis

DIANA BARRETT WISEMAN ■ DAVID LUNDIN ■ CHRISTOPHER I. SHAFFREY

In 1782, Herbiniaux, a Belgian obstetrician, first described spondylolisthesis.[1] The term is derived from Greek roots: *spondylos*, meaning "vertebra," and *listhesis*, meaning "movement" or "slippage." Kilian, in 1854, used the term to describe the forward displacement of L5 on S1 secondary to the overlying body weight.[2] Neugebauer, in 1888, examined anatomic museum specimens with the condition and concluded that it was caused primarily by injury.[3] Blake described the first case of spondylolisthesis in the United States in 1866.[4] His patient was a 26-year-old multiparous woman who had gained 100 pounds. Meyerding, writing in 1932, thought that trauma in patients with an underlying lumbosacral defect was the cause of spondylolisthesis.[4] By the 1960s, spondylolisthesis was attributed to one of five different mechanisms. Those categories, first described by Newman,[5] are still in use today.

EPIDEMIOLOGY

The incidence of spondylolisthesis differs with regard to gender and race, based on the underlying cause. More than one third of lumbar fusions are performed for spondylolisthesis, lumbar stenosis, or both.[6] The level most commonly affected differs, again depending on the underlying cause. For example, degenerative spondylolisthesis affects females more frequently than males, and the level most commonly involved is L4-5 (Fig. 228–1). In contrast, isthmic spondylolisthesis affects males more commonly than females, and the level most commonly involved is L5-S1 (Fig. 228–2). However, high-grade isthmic listhesis is four times more common in females than in males; the highest rate is found among female Eskimos from Alaska.

Hereditary factors appear to play a part in congenital as well as isthmic conditions. An increased incidence among first-degree relatives ranging from 19% to 69% has been cited in different series.[7–11] The dysplastic elongated pars, a type of isthmic spondylolisthesis, has a strong familial component.[12] Spondylolisthesis also has many strong environmental factors that play a role in its development.

CLASSIFICATION

Spondylolisthesis was classified into five groups by Newman in 1963[5] and presented by Wiltse and coworkers in *Clinical Orthopaedics* in 1976.[13]

1. Dysplastic (congenital)
   a. Articular processes with a transverse orientation
   b. Facet articulations with a sagittal orientation
   c. Anomalies of the lumbosacral junction
2. Isthmic
   a. Lytic lesion of the pars interarticularis
   b. Elongated pars
   c. Acute fracture of the pars

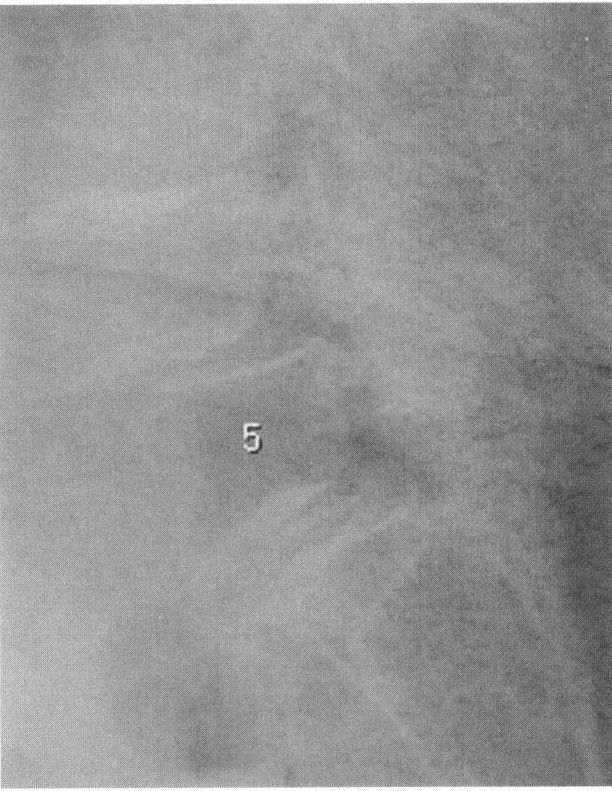

FIGURE 228–1. Plain lateral radiograph shows anterolisthesis of L4 on L5.

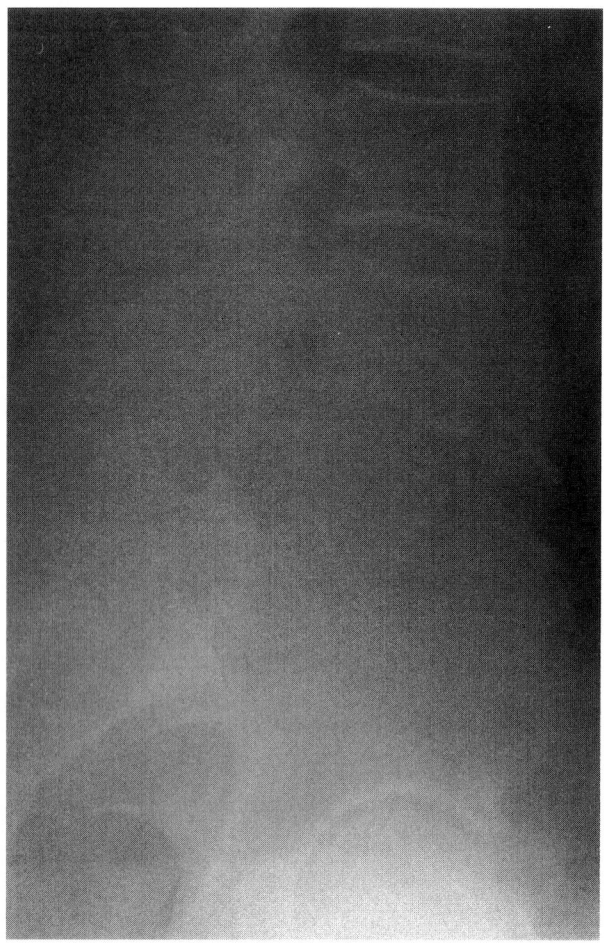

FIGURE 228–2. Lateral plain radiograph demonstrates anterolisthesis of L5 on S1.

3. Degenerative
4. Traumatic
5. Pathologic

A sixth group can be added secondary to iatrogenic causes: postsurgical.

MEASUREMENT

When spondylolisthesis is present, the Meyerding classification is used to grade it. On lateral plain radiographs, the anteroposterior diameter of the superior surface of the vertebra is divided into quarters. A grade of I to IV is assigned, based on slippage of one to four quarters of the anteroposterior diameter (Fig. 228–3). Slip angle, a measure of the kyphosis caused by the spondylolisthesis, is also measured and described. The angle is the intersection of a line drawn parallel to the L5 superior end plate and one drawn perpendicular to a line along the posterior cortex of the S1 and S2 bodies (Fig. 228–4).

PRESENTATION

Symptomatic patients most commonly present with low back pain. This is largely mechanical in nature;

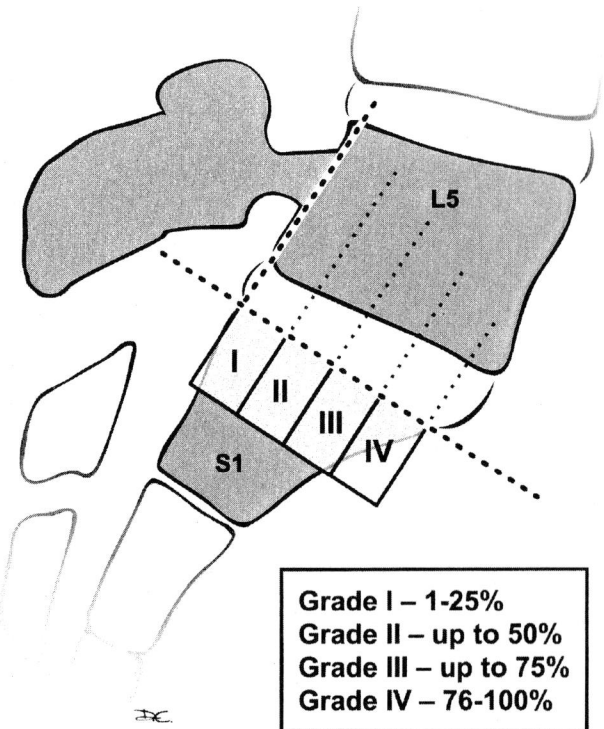

Grade I – 1-25%
Grade II – up to 50%
Grade III – up to 75%
Grade IV – 76-100%

FIGURE 228–3. Meyerding classification

therefore, it is worse with activity and improved with lying down. Physical examination findings in patients with isthmic spondylolisthesis include hyperlordotic posture with tight hamstrings. Hyperextension and ro-

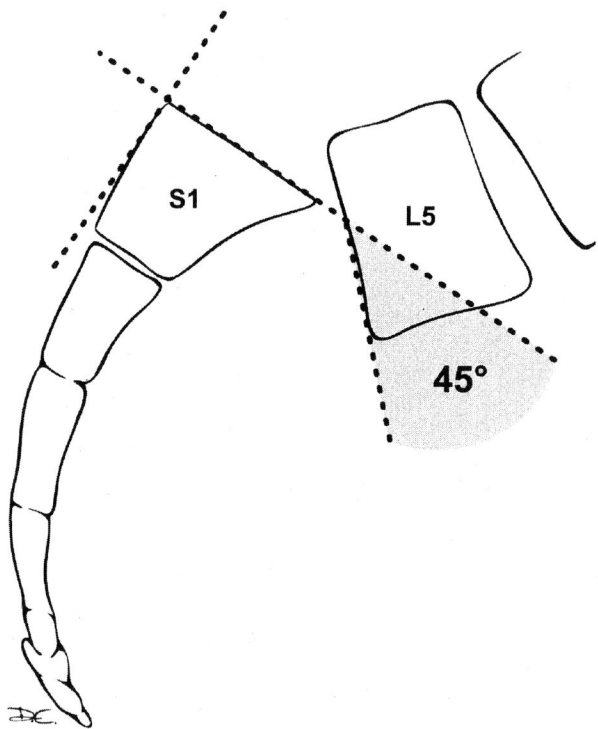

FIGURE 228–4. Slip angle measurement.

tation may aggravate symptoms, as may standing on one leg while leaning backward. Saraste found that listhesis greater than 25%, L4 spondylolisthesis, and disk degeneration at the level of slippage were associated with a higher incidence of back pain.[14] In cases of spondylolisthesis associated with stenosis (i.e., degenerative cases), patients may also complain of symptoms consistent with neurogenic claudication. Patients may relate that forward flexion, such as bending over a shopping cart or riding a bicycle, helps alleviate their symptoms, whereas extension aggravates them. One way that neurogenic claudication can be differentiated from vascular claudication is that neurogenic patients can bend forward and ride a bicycle with decreased symptoms, whereas this position does not affect vascular patients. In patients with significant spondylolisthesis, however, flexion may accentuate the listhesis, thereby increasing the degree of spinal stenosis. In these cases, extension may actually help relieve symptoms of spinal stenosis.

In general, patients have normal sensation and strength on lower extremity testing. Reflexes are often normal to decreased. Patients should not have pain with provocative hip motion. Osteoarthritis of the hip is present in 11% to 17% of patients with degenerative spondylolisthesis.[15] When hip arthritis is present, this may be responsible for some or all of the patient's symptoms.

Patients with isthmic spondylolisthesis may demonstrate the tight hamstring syndrome. A patient with this syndrome has a stooped posture, with flexion at the hips and knees, and walks with a waddling gait.[16] The flexed posture allows the patient to maintain his or her center of balance secondary to the exaggerated lumbar lordosis associated with high-grade dysplastic or isthmic spondylolisthesis. In addition, flexion can reduce tension on the involved nerve root.

DIFFERENTIAL DIAGNOSIS

The differential diagnosis of low back pain by itself or associated with radicular symptoms is large. Care must be taken to ensure that the back pain or lower extremity symptoms are originating from the spondylolisthesis itself. Because spondylolisthesis is often asymptomatic, other conditions such as osteoarthritis of the hip, sacroiliac joint arthritis, or diabetic neuropathy should be entertained. Other pathologic spinal conditions such as disk degeneration, disk herniation, or facet joint arthropathy can coexist with spondylolisthesis.

We will now discuss the different types of spondylolisthesis in the following order: dysplastic, traumatic, pathologic, and isthmic. Because of the importance and common occurrence of degenerative spondylolisthesis, this type will be covered last and in detail.

DYSPLASTIC SPONDYLOLISTHESIS

Dysplastic (congenital) spondylolisthesis is the result of a congenital defect at the L5-S1 facet joint. The pars

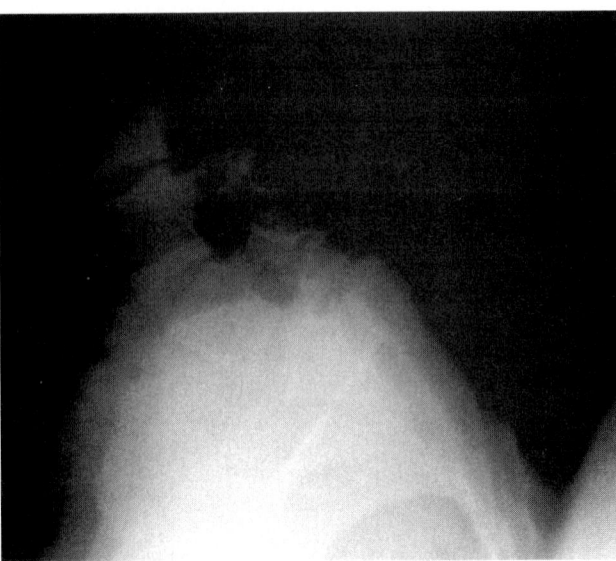

FIGURE 228-5. Severe dysplastic spondylolisthesis (spondyloptosis).

interarticularis may be poorly formed but is intact, and anterior translation results in stenosis of the segment. This condition occurs approximately twice as frequently in females as in males,[13, 17] and it accounted for 14% to 21% of treated cases in two series.[17, 18] Risk of progression of the listhesis is more common in patients with dysplastic spondylolisthesis than in those with isthmic spondylolisthesis.[19] This risk is secondary to the lack of a buttress effect of the dysplastic facets, which permits the superior vertebral body to slip out over the inferior one.

Dysplastic spondylolisthesis is subdivided into three categories:

1. In subtype A, the facet joints have a horizontal (transverse) orientation. Spina bifida is often associated with this dysplastic type, and a high-grade spondylolisthesis may result. This subtype often presents earlier than the others, with a more severe listhesis (Fig. 228-5).

2. In subtype B, the facet joints have a sagittal orientation. These patients often present with back and leg pain. The degree of listhesis is not as severe as that seen in subtype A.

3. In subtype C, there are congenital anomalies of the vertebral body. These anomalies range from failure of vertebral body formation to angular deformities of the sacrum.[20]

TRAUMATIC SPONDYLOLISTHESIS

Traumatic spondylolisthesis results from a fracture of the posterior elements, excluding the pars interarticularis. Listhesis of the involved segment is more likely to occur at L4-5 or L5-S1 than at the superior lumbar segments. This increased incidence at the lumbosacral junction is secondary to the presence of anterior-inferior force vectors at these levels that are absent at higher lumbar levels.[21]

Treatment of dorsal element fractures usually involves bracing alone. Progressive displacement of the involved level may require surgical stabilization.

PATHOLOGIC SPONDYLOLISTHESIS

In pathologic spondylolisthesis, a generalized or localized condition may be the cause of the listhesis; these conditions are categorized as subtype A and subtype B, respectively. Localized conditions cause listhesis by compromising the bone, ligaments, or both. Examples of localized conditions causing spondylolisthesis are infection, tumor, and iatrogenic causes (Fig. 228–6). Generalized conditions causing listhesis include osteoporosis, syphilitic disease, arthrogryposis, and Paget's disease.

ISTHMIC SPONDYLOLISTHESIS

As described by Wiltse and coworkers in 1976, spondylolysis and spondylolisthesis of the isthmus can be classified into one of three types: (1) lytic lesion—fatigue fracture of the pars, (2) elongated intact pars, and (3) acute fracture.[13] Type 2 lesions typically present clinically in adolescents and are the most common subtype in this age group (Fig. 228–7). The majority of spondylitic defects occur at the L5 level (85% to 95%); the next most common level is L4 (5% to 15%).[22]

The incidence of spondylolysis is reportedly between 3% and 7%.[19, 23, 24] Upon reviewing 4200 cadaver spines, Roche and Rowe found that the incidence varies with race and gender.[24] White males and females have rates of 6.4% and 2.3%, respectively; African-

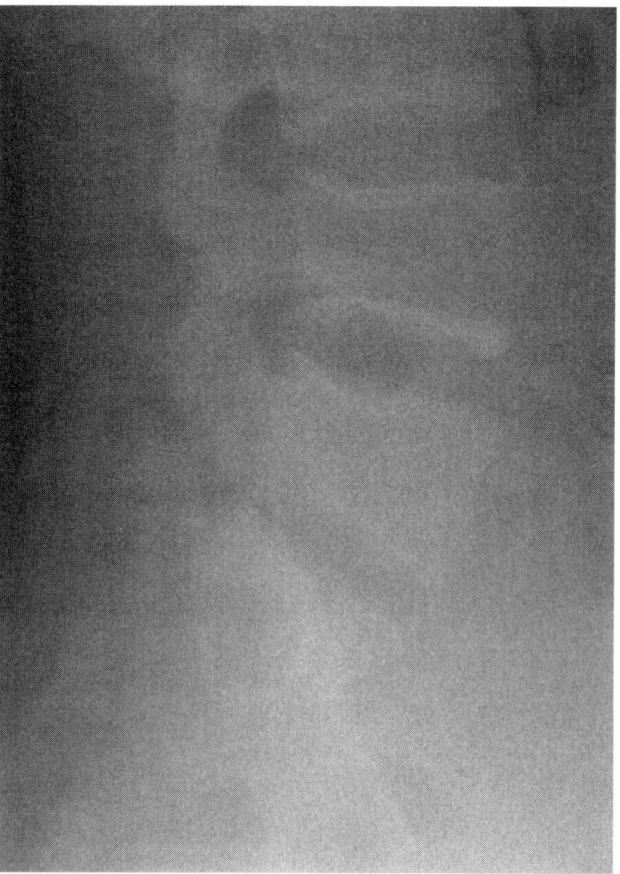

FIGURE 228–7. Fifteen-year-old boy with low back pain. Lateral radiograph reveals an L5 pars defect.

American males and females have rates of 2.8% and 1.1%, respectively. In general, males are affected two to three times more commonly than females. Age beyond childhood does not appear to change the rate of occurrence.[24] When spondylolysis is radiographically visible, there is an associated spondylolisthesis approximately 25% of the time. In one radiographic study of 500 newborns, no cases of spondylolysis were found.[19] Rosenberg and colleagues evaluated 143 adult patients who had been nonambulatory their entire lives and found no cases of pars defects.[25] Among 500 6-year-olds, an overall incidence of 4.4% was found, which increased to 6% by adulthood in the same population.[19] Most frequently, these defects are seen in correspondence with the adolescent growth spurt and are associated with activity. Participation in strenuous activities such as gymnastics, rowing, diving, swimming, weight lifting, and football is frequently implicated.

Jackson and associates studied 100 young female gymnasts and found an 11% rate of spondylolysis, which was significantly higher than expected according to previous population-based studies.[26] Rossi, in a review of 1430 adolescent athletes, noted a 15% incidence of spondylolysis, with wrestlers, gymnasts, divers, and weight lifters representing a majority within this affected group.[27] Soler and Calderon evaluated 3152 athletes and found an overall incidence of 8.02%. Among athletes participating in throwing sports (discus, shot

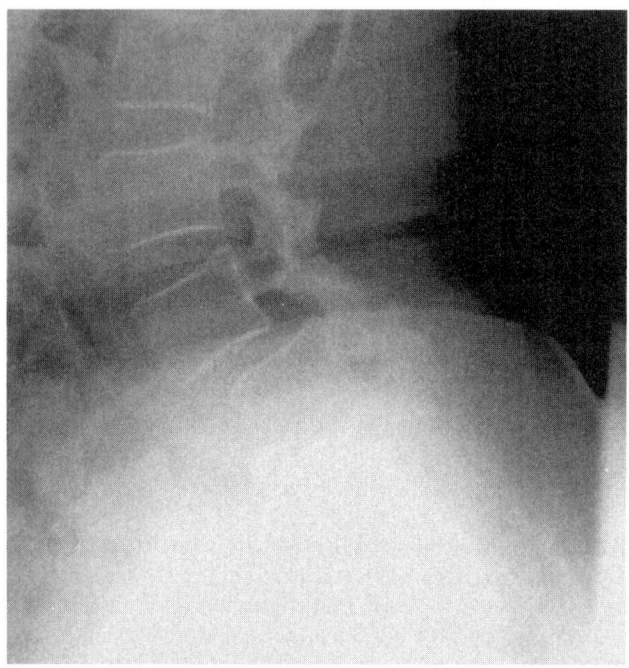

FIGURE 228–6. Postlaminectomy spondylolisthesis.

put), the incidence was 26.7%; in gymnastics, 16.9%; rowing, 16.9%; and swimming, 10.2%.[28] Jones and colleagues reviewed preparticipation radiographs of Division 1 college football players and compared them with controls.[29] They found comparable rates of spondylolysis among athletes and controls: 4.8% in athletes, and 6% in controls. The rate of spondylolisthesis was 3.8% in athletes and 3.6% in controls. Other studies reported 10.1% to 50% spondylolysis rates for downlinemen.

Diagnostic Studies

Radiographic evaluation begins with plain radiographs. Anteroposterior, lateral, and bilateral oblique radiographs make up the basic set of films. On plain oblique films, the defect in the pars interarticularis has been described as a collar on the "Scotty dog." Amato and coworkers found that a spot lateral view of the lumbosacral junction was the most sensitive view in their series of radiographs, disclosing the defect 84% of the time.[23] Bone scan is often positive in new lesions but negative in long-standing lesions. Bone scan may be helpful in identifying symptomatic pars lesions by showing increased activity at the defect. Computed tomographic scanning is more sensitive than plain films or nuclear medicine studies in identifying pars lesions, but it is not considered 100% sensitive or specific. Single photon emission computed tomography has advantages over bone scan and plain radiographs, but unfortunately, it has greater sensitivity than specificity for demonstrating a pars defect. Magnetic resonance imaging has a less defined role in imaging pars lesions, but it is useful for evaluating other possible pathology such as disk herniation, disk degeneration, annular disruption, or the presence of infection or tumor.

Risk of Progression

The risk of progression of spondylolisthesis depends on a number of factors. Younger age (decreased skeletal maturity), slip greater than 50%, slip angle greater than 40 to 50 degrees (0 to 10 degrees is normal), female gender, dome-shaped sacrum, and dysplastic lumbosacral junction are all associated with an increased risk of progressive listhesis. The risk of progression was noted by Frennered and associates to be 4%,[30] whereas Saraste noted a 5% risk.[14] There are conflicting opinions about contributing factors that lead to the progression of listhesis. Grobler and associates compared computed tomographic scans of normal lumbar spines with those of isthmic spondylolysis patients.[31] They found that the only significant morphologic difference was a smaller transverse articular dimension in the isthmic group. Fredrickson and colleagues found progression to be rare in adolescence,[19] whereas other authors attributed progression in adolescence to disk degeneration.[32, 33] Progression of listhesis has been associated with the adolescent growth spurt, lumbosacral kyphosis, and an initial listhesis greater than 50%.[19, 34] Kim and Suk evaluated the effect of transitional vertebrae on spondylolysis and isthmic spondylolisthesis in a retrospective study of 182 patients.[35] Thirty-three of the 182 patients had transitional vertebra—12 with lumbarization and 21 with sacralization. The remaining patients constituted the controls. The authors found that the subgroup of patients with sacralization and an isthmic defect at L4 had more slippage than similar patients without transitional vertebrae. Patients with sacralization and an isthmic defect at L5 showed less slippage than similar patients without transitional vertebrae. Blackburne and Velikas noted than no patient with a slip less than 30% progressed to beyond 30%.[36] Any progressive slippage that did occur was noted predominantly during puberty and had an association with spina bifida occulta. Saraste, in a study of 255 patients followed for a minimum of 20 years, noted a mean slip progression of 4 mm, with 11% of adolescents and 5% of adults progressing to more than 10 mm.[14] Muschik and coworkers reported on 86 young athletes, 6 to 20 years old, with spondylolysis.[37] Twelve percent of patients showed slip progression of more than 10% over a period of 4.8 years. Progression greater than 20% occurred in 1 of 86 patients. The mean initial degree of slip was 10.1%. Forty-seven percent of patients had no progression, 44% had slip progression, and 9% improved. An increased risk of progression was found during puberty and in those with an increased slip angle and sacral inclination. No increased risk was associated with spina bifida occulta or continued activity.

Treatment

Although the majority of cases of spondylolysis are asymptomatic and require no treatment, occasionally these lesions can be associated with significant low back pain. This is often the case with adolescents and young adults who ultimately present to spine surgeons with complaints of severe focal low back pain that can be debilitating and prevents participation in sports. The pain is often exacerbated by activities involving lumbar extension and rotation; occasionally, pain can extend into the buttock or proximal lower extremities, although true radiculopathy is less common.[38] True radicular symptoms require evaluation for disk herniation, foraminal stenosis, or significant instability; radiographic evaluation, including dynamic radiographs and magnetic resonance imaging, should be considered. The presence of decreased flexibility and tight hamstrings often leads to more frequent muscle strains.[22, 39] The combination of these findings often limits physical function and optimal performance in athletic programs. Therefore, all treatment options aim to relieve pain, optimize physical function, and promote bony healing of the underlying defect of the pars interarticularis.

Reviews of the literature on the standard treatment of spondylolysis can be confusing, because the natural history of symptoms is not clearly defined. The medical literature is also confounded by clinical reviews involving diverse groups of patients, often mixing groups containing children, adolescents, and adults, as well as the types and degrees of spondylolisthesis treated. Considerable debate exists over the indications for nonoperative treatment, including the indications for bracing, the type of brace that is best tolerated and best relieves symptoms, the value of physical therapy, and the time required to define a failure of nonoperative therapy. A number of treatment options have demonstrated effectiveness, and the clear superiority of one specific treatment regimen has not been shown.

Initial treatment options for isthmic spondylolisthesis focus on nonoperative management, including limitation of activity, bracing, and a rehabilitation program (as defined later). Surgical intervention is reserved for cases of definite failure of such treatment regimens.

Initial treatment plans encompass some degree of activity restriction. Activities resulting in repetitive flexion, extension, and rotation of the lumbar spine are specifically restricted in the early treatment phase. Thoracolumbosacral bracing and abdominal strengthening exercises often supplement these programs.

Steiner and Micheli reported on 67 patients with spondylolysis or low-grade spondylolisthesis treated in a modified Boston brace for 6 months, followed by a 6-month weaning period in which physical therapy was performed and a gradual return to athletics was allowed.[40] They noted an 18% rate of bony healing, although 78% of patients had good to excellent clinical results, including a full return to activity.

Blanda and colleagues reported their experience treating young patients with pars defects.[41] Initially, all patients were managed with activity restriction and bracing for 2 to 6 months, followed by a gradual exercise and stretching program. Radiographic union of these defects was noted in 37% of patients. However, only 15% of patients failed nonoperative management after more than 6 months without relief and therefore required surgical intervention. Notably, 96% of all patients had good or excellent results, defined as a return to normal activities and either no lumbago or minimal symptoms with strenuous activity.

In a study of 185 adolescent athletes with spondylolysis, Morita and associates classified pars defects with plain radiographs and computed tomography as early, progressive, or terminal stage.[42] Patients were then restricted from sporting activities and braced with a conventional lumbar corset for 3 to 6 months, followed by rehabilitation and bracing with an extension-limiting corset. They confirmed bony fusion with follow-up imaging in 37.9% of all patients. They noted, however, that 73% of early defects, 38.5% of progressive defects, and 0% of terminal defects healed. They concluded that pars defects diagnosed in the early stages can be effectively treated with conservative measures. The Boston brace is most commonly used for this condition.[39] It is molded to a 0-degree lordosis to help reduce the load on the posterior elements and is usually worn 23 hours a day for at least 4 months, although 6 to 9 months of bracing may be required in some cases.[40, 43]

In children who have significant or complete resolution of symptoms after conservative measures, a gradual reconditioning program is initiated before the return to routine sports activities. A physical therapy program focused on stretching the lumbodorsal fascia and strengthening the paraspinous and abdominal musculature without hyperextension of the spine is performed. Following reconditioning, the asymptomatic patient is allowed a gradual return to full activity. However, for those patients who fail such treatment or develop a recurrence of symptoms after resumption of full activity, further evaluation is warranted. Workup often starts with a bone scan and single photon emission computed tomography, which can detect early stress fractures of the pars interarticularis and determine whether the injury is acute or chronic in nature. An acute spondylolysis has greater potential for healing than does a chronic process. In our younger patients (younger than 21 years), a positive bone scan after failure of bracing and reconditioning is followed by a second course of activity restriction and bracing, in combination with electrical stimulation.

The addition of external electrical stimulation to promote the healing of pars defects has gained attention in recent years. The first indication that this technology might promote the healing of pars defects was its effect on healing after other types of spinal fusion. Mooney tested the effect of pulsed electromagnetic fields on interbody lumbar fusions in 195 patients operated on for various diagnoses, including spondylolisthesis.[44] In patients who had actively used the electromagnetic device in addition to standard bracing, he observed a 92.2% fusion rate, compared with a 67.9% fusion rate in the control group. Pettine and colleagues treated an adolescent with acute spondylolysis with intermittent bracing and daily external electric stimulation, noting progressive bony healing within 3 months of starting electrical treatments.[45] In a similar study, Fellander-Tsai and Micheli successfully treated two patients with bracing and electrical stimulation who had previously failed conservative treatment without such stimulation.[46] In young adults, however, the indications for electrical stimulation have not been clearly defined; therefore, only continual bracing and activity restriction are generally recommended.

The vast majority of patients with spondylolysis can be managed nonoperatively. The reported incidence of cases that ultimately require surgery varies from 9% to 53%.[22, 38, 40, 41, 47] Traditionally, intertransverse fusion procedures have been performed in children, adolescents, and adults who have failed nonoperative treatment. Indications for surgery include uncontrolled pain or major symptoms despite activity modification and bracing, slip greater than 50% on initial presentation or progressive slip from 25% to 50%, high slip angle greater than 30% with significant growth remaining, presence of significant nerve root irritation causing sciatic scoliosis, or progressive neurological deficit.[37]

In rare cases, less invasive surgical approaches, such as decompression alone or direct pars interarticularis repair, can be effective alternatives to traditional spinal fusion and can maintain the integrity of the motion segment. Some authors have advocated the use of decompression alone, especially if an isolated radiculopathy exists. Lapras and associates used simple decompression in 45 patients (44 adults) with grade I and II spondylolisthesis and obtained 68% good or excellent results.[48] However, this technique has a high risk of progressive slippage, especially in children. Decompression alone is therefore not generally advocated, except in adults with spondylolysis or minimal spondylolisthesis without motion on dynamic radiographs and with isolated unilateral radiculopathy.

Selected young patients (younger than 25 years) with spondylolysis or who fail nonoperative management may be considered for repair of the pars defects primarily. Several studies have demonstrated the efficacy of direct repair of pars defects in this patient population.[49-51] Buck originally described the repair of defects in the pars interarticularis in 1970.[52] The advantage of such a procedure is that it preserves the anatomic integrity and motion of the affected segment. In a recent study, Dai and associates examined the efficacy of direct pars repair in 46 patients with lumbar spondylolysis or mild (Meyerding grade I or II) isthmic spondylolisthesis.[49] They attained an excellent or good functional outcome in 93.4% of all patients. No significant improvement was found with the addition of facet fusion. They noted, however, that the success of such a procedure was highly dependent on the presence of normal adjacent disks, as assessed by magnetic resonance imaging. This is based on the notion that in the presence of significant disk degeneration, the segment with the spondylolysis or spondylolisthesis is predisposed to instability, and bony fusion is impaired. Szypryt and coworkers stated that, given the increased

degree of disk degeneration of the affected spinal segment with age, segmental fusion is recommended in patients older than 25 years with spondylolysis.[33] Kakiuchi described results in patients with spondylolysis and spondylolisthesis using a variable-angle screw in the pedicle and a laminar hook compressing across the pars defect[51] (Fig. 228–8). Direct repair of the pars interarticularis in cases of multilevel pars defects has also been reported.[53]

Early disk degeneration in patients with spondylolysis and spondylolisthesis is common. If there is any question whether the disk or the pars is the source of pain, direct pars injection with local anesthetic may help make the determination. Wu and colleagues showed that patients with a positive pars injection were highly likely to have a good or excellent outcome with operative repair.[47] In their evaluation of 100 patents who had positive pars injections, defined as reproduction of the patient's pain with needle insertion and at least 70% pain relief for more than 6 hours after anesthetic injection, 85 patients (91.3%) had good or excellent outcomes after an average of 30.4 months. In patients without relief of symptoms with a pars injection, other sources of pain such as intervertebral disk disruption or facet joint arthropathy must be considered. Further investigation, such as diskography, might be warranted. In cases of substantial disk degeneration or segmental instability, posterolateral fusion with or without instrumentation is the procedure of choice.

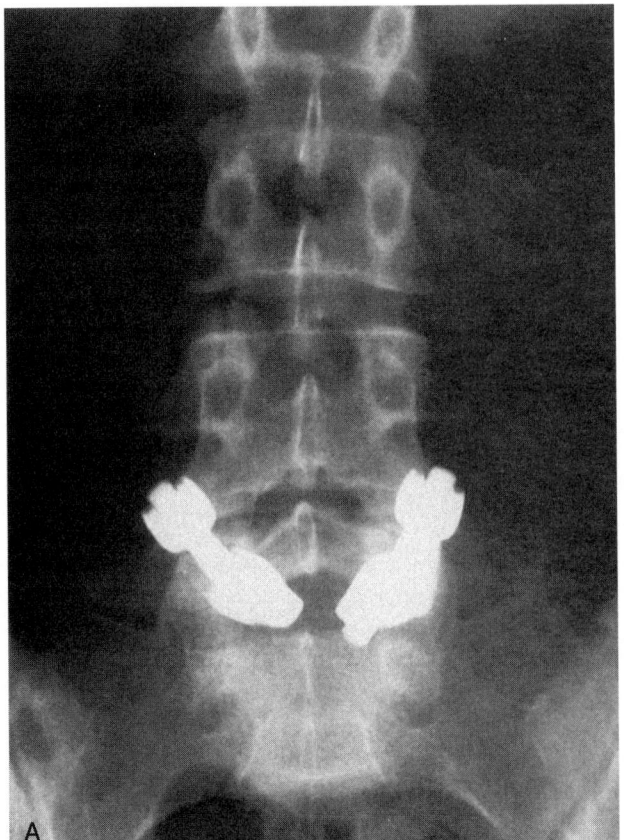
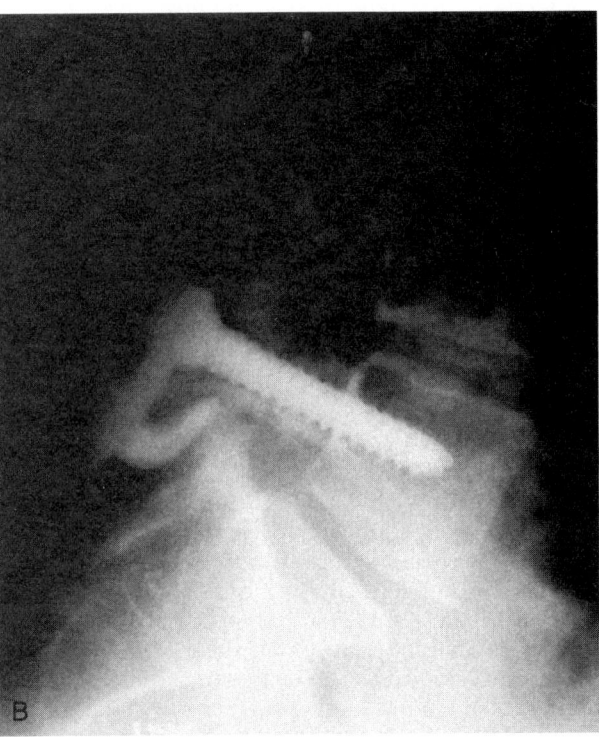

FIGURE 228–8. Anteroposterior *(A)* and lateral *(B)* radiographs of a pars defect repair.

Gill popularized decompression of symptomatic spondylolisthesis by removal of the lamina and the pars fibrocartilage.[54] This procedure without an associated fusion, however, has been associated with an increase in listhesis and back pain. Noninstrumented (in situ) posterolateral fusion is also an effective option is some cases of spondylolysis and spondylolisthesis, especially in younger patients (children and adolescents). This procedure has been shown to reduce symptoms in 70% to 100% of cases, although overall fusion rates are slightly lower and can range from 40% to 100%.[55-60] Fusion rates are lower in patients with higher-grade spondylolisthesis, especially those with an increased slip angle. Traditionally, patients undergoing noninstrumented procedures were managed with pantaloon spica casting until the fusion consolidated. There has been an increasing trend toward the use of a thoracolumbar or thoracolumbosacral orthosis with thigh extension in this patient population.

Lenke and colleagues evaluated 56 patients with isthmic spondylolisthesis who underwent posterolateral fusion without decompression.[61] Clinically, 80% of patients reported improvement; however, paradoxically, only 50% of patients were definitely fused, and 18% were likely fused. In contrast, adult isthmic spondylolisthesis often does not respond as well to the same procedure. Haraldsson and Willner compared the results of 22 adolescents and 23 adults who underwent posterolateral in situ fusion without decompression for isthmic spondylolisthesis.[62] Although fusion was noted in all patients, 95% of adolescents reported significant pain relief, but only 57% of adults did. The difference was thought to be due to a higher rate of degenerative disk disease and nerve root compression in adults.

Posterolateral fusion, although an effective treatment modality for most cases of spondylolisthesis, frequently does not improve the slip angle found in those with higher-grade spondylolisthesis. Although noninstrumented fusion can be accompanied by decompression, there is a higher risk of slip progression and nonunion. This is especially true for patients with a slip angle greater than 25 degrees, grade III and IV spondylolisthesis, trapezoidal L5 segment or dome-shaped sacrum, or hyperlordotic (>50%) lumbar spine.[57, 58, 60, 63-68] Complications ranging from mild sensory deficits to cauda equina syndrome can occur with in situ fusion. Schoenecker and colleagues noted a 6% rate of cauda equina syndrome in patients with grade III or IV spondylolisthesis.[69]

The advent and success of transpedicular instrumentation and fusion for other spinal disorders have led several authors to advocate various combinations of such procedures for spondylolisthesis. Posterior segmental instrumentation and fusion can be performed with or without reduction; the advantage over noninstrumented fusion is that it permits correction of the slip angle, which improves body posture and mechanics. Instrumentation increases the fusion rate in higher-grade spondylolisthesis while allowing full neural decompression. Molinari and coworkers noted that noninstrumented arthrodesis had a higher nonunion rate compared with posterior segmental instrumentation or

circumferential procedures in high-grade spondylolisthesis patients.[70] In adults with grade I or II isthmic spondylolisthesis, the advantages of instrumentation are less evident. In a recent prospective, randomized study, Moller and Hedlund compared the role of instrumented versus noninstrumented posterolateral fusion in 77 patients with isthmic spondylolisthesis and greater than 1 year of low back pain or sciatica.[71] They included patients 18 to 55 years old and those with grades I, II, and III spondylolisthesis. Counterintuitively, radiographic fusion was higher (78%) in the noninstrumented patients than in the instrumented group (65%). Although pain and disability indexes were significantly improved in both groups, there were no significant differences between the groups. Further, blood loss was greater and operating time was longer in instrumented patients, and two patients (5.4%) had pedicle screw–related nerve root injuries.

Treatment of high-grade spondylolisthesis may require the use of anterior or combined anterior-posterior procedures to relieve symptoms and obtain a solid arthrodesis.[70] The addition of an anterior procedure allows the fusion to heal under compression, and it is frequently used as a salvage procedure for failed posterior fusions. Theoretically, additional complications, such as retrograde ejaculation, can occur, although the overall incidence has not been quantified. Muschik retrospectively evaluated the use of anterior in situ fusion versus anterior spondylodesis with posterior transpedicular instrumentation and reduction and found significantly lower rates of pseudarthrosis, reduced degree of slip, reduced lumbosacral kyphosis, and decreased fusion time in patients undergoing transpedicular instrumentation. Although there was a trend toward improved clinical outcome with combined approaches—87% of patients symptom free at follow-up, versus 69% undergoing anterior approaches only—this difference was not statistically significant. Bohlman and Cook described a posterior decompression with anterior interbody fusion via a hole drilled through the posterior part of S1 into the L5 body. A piece of fibula or a cage filled with bone can be placed in the hole for fusion. A posterolateral fusion is performed concurrently (Fig. 228–9).[72]

Gaines and Nichols were the first to describe the anterior vertebral body resection followed by posterior decompression and instrumented fusion.[73] Although this procedure produces an excellent anatomic reduction of high-grade spondylolisthesis, complication rates can be high.[73, 74]

A posterior reduction of spondylolisthesis was developed by Schollner.[75] This involved a posterior decompression, diskectomy, and reduction of the listhesis, followed by a posterior lumbar interbody fusion. This procedure has also been associated with a high rate of neurological deficits, although the majority of these resolved.[65]

Summary

The majority of cases of spondylolysis or isthmic spondylolisthesis are asymptomatic and require no treat-

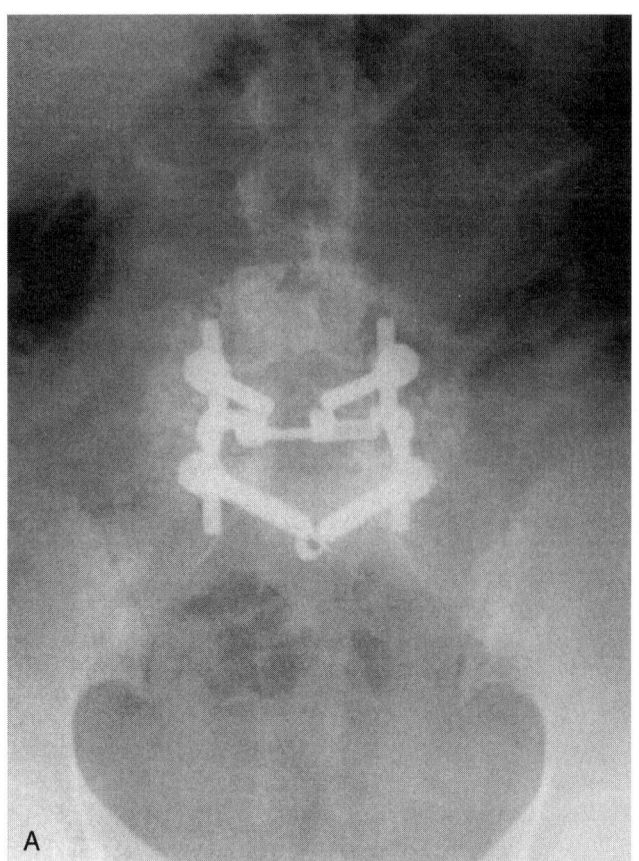

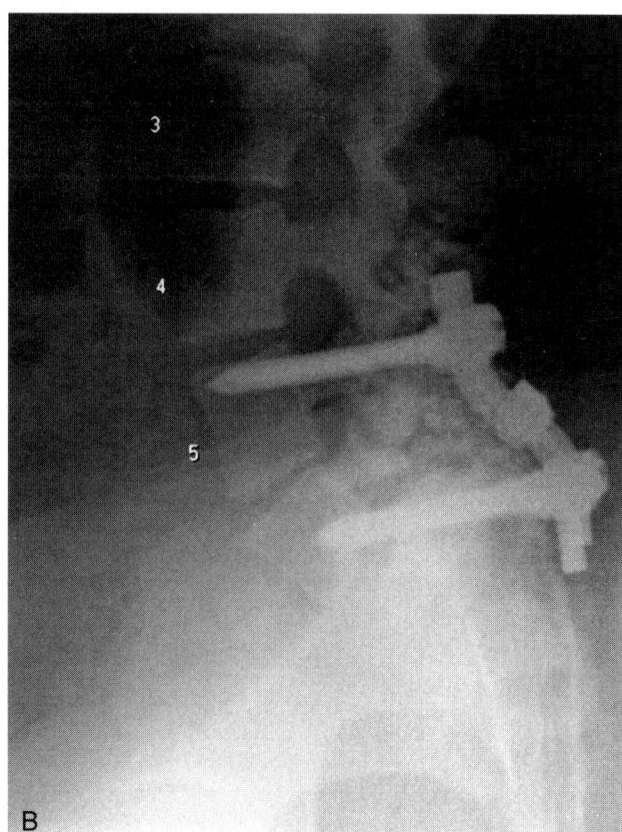

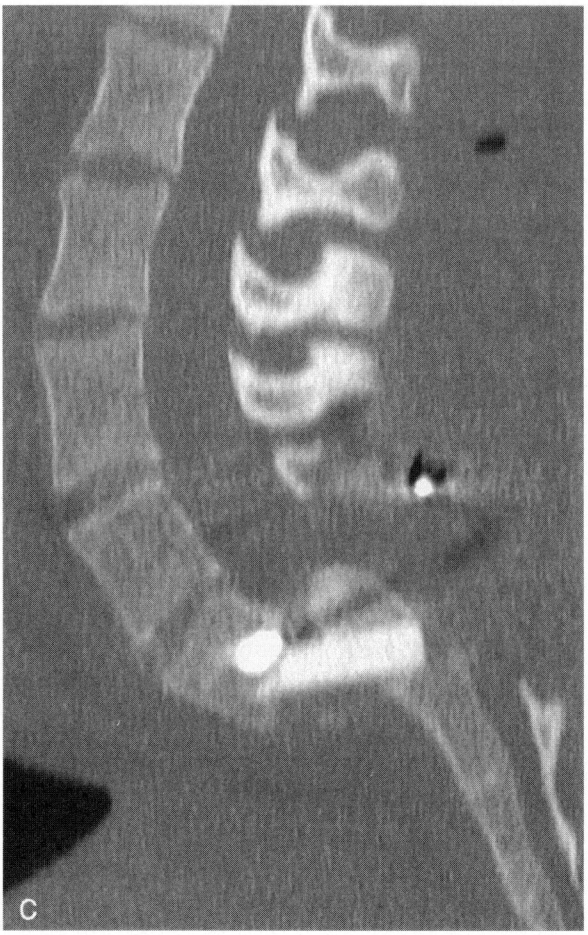

FIGURE 228–9. Anteroposterior *(A)* and lateral *(B)* radiographs of a Bohlman fusion performed for high-grade dysplastic spondylolisthesis. Sagittal reformatted computed tomographic scan *(C)* demonstrates the fibular allograft.

ment. In symptomatic cases, nonoperative measures that include activity restriction and bracing are usually sufficient to eliminate symptoms. It is unusual for younger patients to present with significant radicular pain or neurological deficits, and further investigation, including magnetic resonance imaging, should be considered in these cases. Surgical intervention is reserved for clear failures of nonoperative management. The range of such procedures is dependant on the age of the patient, the presence of neurological deficits, and the specific type of lesion present. If treated appropriately, most patients do well from a clinical perspective and should be able to return to a regular lifestyle.

DEGENERATIVE SPONDYLOLISTHESIS

In 1930, Junghanns first described lumbar spondylolisthesis without a pars defect as *pseudospondylolisthesis*.[76] Newman is credited with coining the term *degenerative spondylolisthesis*.[77] This condition affects primarily an older population and occurs most frequently at the L4-5 level. Rosenberg studied 20 skeletons and 200 patients with degenerative spondylolisthesis to determine predisposing factors.[78] He found that this condition occurs up to six times more frequently at the L4-5 level than at adjoining levels. Sacralization of L5 resulted in a fourfold greater rate of listhesis. Females are affected five times more frequently than males, and black females are affected three times more commonly than white females. On anatomic review, the superior facet of the affected level developed hypertrophic new bone anteriorly, causing lateral recess stenosis and spinal stenosis. Clinical review found that the maximal amount of slippage was 30%, and the mean amount was 14%. The percentage of slippage did not necessarily correlate with clinical symptoms; however, Rosenberg found that at the L3 level, even a small amount of listhesis often produced pronounced symptoms.[78] Patients with degenerative spondylolisthesis were noted to have less lordosis (a higher lumbosacral angle) than normal. The most common complaint was pain in the back, buttock, or thigh. Periods of remission of symptoms are not uncharacteristic. Symptoms are often improved by sitting. Rosenberg found that when objective physical findings were present, they were most often attributable to the L5 nerve root.[78]

Ligamentous laxity has been proposed as an underlying factor in the higher incidence of degenerative spondylolisthesis in females. Hormonal factors have been proposed as a possible cause.[67] Imada and colleagues demonstrated a three times higher incidence of degenerative spondylolisthesis in women who had been oophorectomized compared with matched controls who had not.[79] Nadaud and associates, however, found no immunohistochemical evidence of estrogen receptors on facet joint capsular ligaments from 14 patients undergoing spinal fusion.[80] Anatomic factors do play an important role. Grobler and associates studied the computed tomographic morphology of facet joints in degenerative spondylolisthesis and normal lumbar spines.[31] They found that the facet joint at L4-5 was more sagittally oriented in those with spondylolisthesis than in normal subjects. In addition, transverse articular dimension and joint surface depth were greater in the degenerative group than in the normal subjects. This finding may be related to osteophyte formation involving the joint.

The natural history of degenerative spondylolisthesis has been evaluated. In a prospective study, Matsunaga and colleagues followed 40 patients for a minimum of 5 years.[81] The demographics of their study revealed that women, mean age 55 years, were predominantly affected. L4 was most commonly involved (87.5% of patients), followed by L5 (10% of patients). Progression of slippage by 5% or more occurred in 30% of patients. The mean initial slippage rate was 12.4% in the progression group and 14.5% in the nonprogression group. A correlation between sex and progression of slippage was not found. A positive correlation between activity, particularly repetitive anterior flexion, and progression of slippage was found. Among the progression group, 75% were involved in activities that required repetitive flexion, compared with 10% who performed similar activities in the nonprogression group. No significant difference in lumbosacral angle, lamina angle, and facet inclination angle was found between the groups. Patients with spur formation of the involved vertebral body, sclerosis of the end plates, and ossification of the ligaments did not show progression of disk slippage. A greater percentage of patients with degenerative spondylolisthesis were noted to have joint laxity, defined by Carter's criteria, compared with normal individuals. Clinically, deterioration in symptoms was not correlated with progression of slippage. Low back pain and gluteal pain were present in 98% of patients, and lower extremity pain and numbness were present in 48%. Intermittent claudication was present in 13%, and one patient had bowel and bladder dysfunction. Matsunaga and colleagues, in a follow-up article, reviewed the 10-year results of nonsurgically treated patients.[82] Progressive spondylolisthesis was found in 34% of patients; however, this did not correlate with symptoms. Low back pain was noted to improve with a decrease in intervertebral space size. Patients who had presented with no neurological deficits at the primary examination remained deficit free at 10-year follow-up. Of the patients with neurological symptoms at presentation, 83% experienced further neurological deterioration.

Rosenberg found that of 200 patients with degenerative spondylolisthesis, 153 had lower extremity symptoms, 85 of whom had objective neurological findings.[78] Thirty-nine of his patients developed signs and symptoms that required hospitalization, and ultimately, 29 required operative treatment for symptoms failing conservative treatment.

Conservative Treatment

The course of symptoms in degenerative spondylolisthesis is often intermittent in nature. Rosenberg found that nonsteroidal anti-inflammatory drugs, bed rest, bracing, heat, exercise, and traction were unpredictable in their effects.[78] Epidural steroid injections may offer short-term relief but seldom have a long-term effect; in one series, less than 25% of patients had any long-term relief of symptoms.[83] Over time, patients with significant back pain may develop such significant disk space collapse, with end plate and facet joint osteophyte formation, that a functional "autofusion," resulting in diminution of symptoms, can occur. Matsunaga and associates evaluated the natural history of degenerative spondylolisthesis and found that patients with disk space collapse, end plate sclerosis, and spurring rarely slipped further with time.[81] The degree of spondylolisthesis does not necessarily correlate with symptoms. Patient series have shown that approximately 10% to 15% of patients fail conservative treatment and require surgery.[78, 84]

Surgical Treatment

Controversy exists about the optimal treatment of patients with degenerative spondylolisthesis. There are advocates of decompression of the involved segments alone, as well as advocates of decompression with fusion. Among those who advocate fusion, there is further debate whether to perform instrumentation or place interbody devices to optimize surgical outcome.

A wide range of outcomes has been reported for patients undergoing decompression without fusion.[85–92] A number of variables may ultimately affect the amount of decompression performed and whether that decompression leads to additional instability. Residual neural compression or progressive instability may degrade the clinical outcome, ultimately necessitating a second procedure to stabilize the spine. In 1985, Lombardi and colleagues reviewed their experience with 47 patients with degenerative spondylolisthesis who were treated by one of three posterior surgical approaches.[92] Patients who had midline decompression with preservation of the articular processes or preservation of the articular processes and an in situ intertransverse fusion had good to excellent results in 80% and 90% of cases, respectively. Among those patients undergoing midline decompression and removal of the articular processes without fusion, 33% had good to excellent outcomes. Herron and Trippi performed decompression without fusion and had an 83% good outcome in their series.[91] They preserved the pars as well as the integrity of the facet joints. Average preoperative slip was 7 mm, and no patient's listhesis increased by more than 4 mm postoperatively.

A strong case for combining decompression with intertransverse process fusion for the treatment of degenerative spondylolisthesis was made by Herkowitz and Kurz.[93] They performed a randomized, prospective clinical trial consisting of 50 patients, comparing decompression versus decompression and intertransverse process arthrodesis. Patients who had decompression and arthrodesis had significantly better outcomes than those who had decompression alone. Patients without arthrodesis had significantly more back and leg pain. Patients without arthrodesis also had a significant increase in listhesis and angular motion. Of note, within the arthrodesis group, nine patients had pseudarthroses; however, their outcomes were excellent in five patients and good in four.

Fischgrund and associates went on to evaluate the effect on clinical outcome when spinal instrumentation was added to arthrodesis for degenerative spondylolisthesis.[68] It had been shown previously that adding spinal instrumentation to an intertransverse process arthrodesis significantly improved fusion rates.[94] Fischgrund's group showed in a prospective, randomized clinical trial that although the addition of instrumentation to an intertransverse process arthrodesis improved fusion rates from 45% to 83%, it did not significantly affect clinical outcome.

Mardjetko and colleagues performed a meta-analysis of the literature in 1994, evaluating decompression of degenerative spondylolisthesis without arthrodesis, with arthrodesis, and with arthrodesis and instrumentation.[95] They found that decompression without arthrodesis left 69% of patients with satisfactory outcomes. The satisfactory outcome rate was improved to 90% when arthrodesis was added, and it was 86% when instrumentation was combined with arthrodesis. Fusion rates were 86% and 93%, respectively, for arthrodesis alone and with instrumentation. There are many articles supporting arthrodesis with decompression for the treatment of degenerative spondylolisthesis.[68, 93, 96–107]

Cost analysis of fusion with and without instrumentation for patients with degenerative stenosis found that lumbar decompression with a noninstrumented fusion raises hospital costs by 50%. Decompression with instrumented fusion raises costs by 100% compared with decompression alone.[96] Kuntz and colleagues evaluated the cost-effectiveness of fusion with and without instrumentation for patients with degenerative spondylolisthesis and stenosis.[108] They found that decompression and noninstrumented fusion costs $56,500 per quality-adjusted year of life, versus laminectomy without fusion. For decompression and instrumented fusion, the cost rises to $3,112,800 per quality-adjusted year of life.[108]

Surgical Approaches

The previous section cited several clinical studies that support arthrodesis and decompression of degenerative spondylolisthesis. Surgical decompression often involves a laminectomy of the involved levels or a hemilaminectomy of the superior and inferior lamina. Adequate decompression also involves a medial facetectomy; however, occasionally a more extensive facet removal, as well as removal of the pars interarticularis, may be required for decompression.

The arguments for intertransverse process arthrodesis were made earlier. Standard pedicle screw fixation is often added to that arthrodesis to improve fusion rates and better maintain reduction of the listhesis, even though some studies have found no positive effect on clinical outcome. There is support from several authors for a more aggressive surgical approach for younger, physically active patients with degenerative spondylolisthesis. Over time, some patients with a pseudarthrosis resulting from in situ fusion become symptomatic, with deterioration of clinical outcome. Kornblum and associates evaluated the long-term results of patients decompressed and fused with and without instrumentation.[109] Average follow-up was 7 years and 8 months. There was a statistically significant difference in outcome between those with a solid arthrodesis and those with a pseudarthrosis. This difference was apparent with regard to both back pain and lower extremity pain. The authors noted that previous studies had shown that spinal instrumentation improves fusion rates and therefore recommended its addition to posterolateral fusion for degenerative spondylolisthesis. Spinal realignment with improvement of sagittal balance may theoretically reduce back pain and adjacent segment degenerative changes while improving fusion rates.[110–112] Lee noted that reduction of unstable degenerative spondylolisthesis without decompression resulted in an 89% satisfactory outcome in back pain and a 93% improvement in radicular pain.[113] A solid posterolateral fusion was noted in 87% of patients. Improvement in alignment alone was therefore significant in contributing to better outcomes (Fig. 228–10).

As with any emerging technology, there are few studies evaluating the effectiveness of interbody fusion techniques for degenerative spondylolisthesis. A biomechanical analysis of degenerative lumbar spondylolisthesis focused on the immediate stability achieved by different instrument constructs in the degenerated and surgically decompressed spine. Cagli and associates evaluated in a cadaver study the effectiveness of stand-alone threaded cortical dowels or cages versus posterior instrumented fusion alone versus dowels or cages with supplemental posterior instrumentation in degenerative spondylolisthesis.[114] They found that stand-alone cages provided the least stable construct. Posterior instrumentation plus interbody threaded cages or dowels proved to be the most stable.

Kawakami and colleagues retrospectively reviewed how sagittal balance affected outcome in decompression and posterolateral arthrodesis with and without instrumentation for degenerative spondylolisthesis.[112] They found a positive correlation between recovery rates and lumbar lordosis of the fused segments. Further, patients with attempted reduction of slippage and pedicle screw fixation had better clinical results with regard to back pain than did similar patients with posterolateral arthrodesis alone (Fig. 228–11). The authors concluded that pedicle screw fixation improves outcome by reducing slippage in patients who had

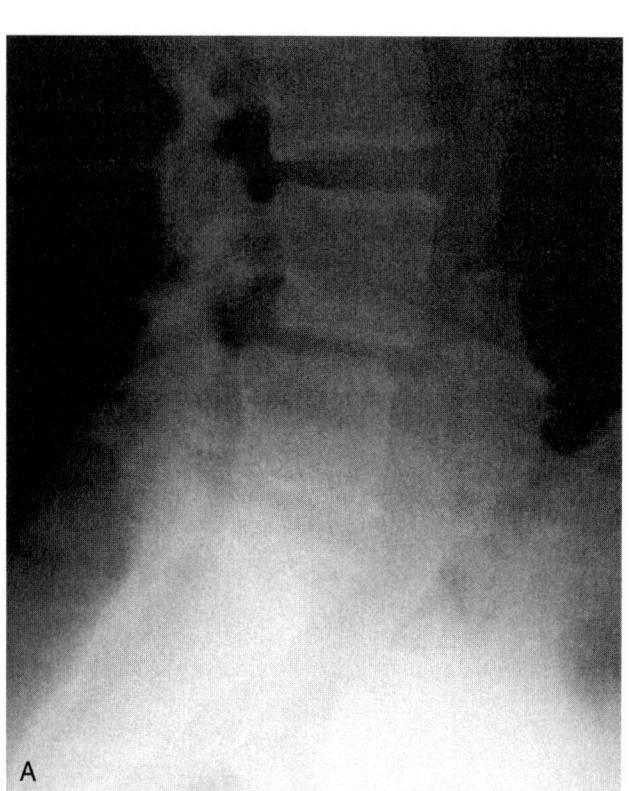
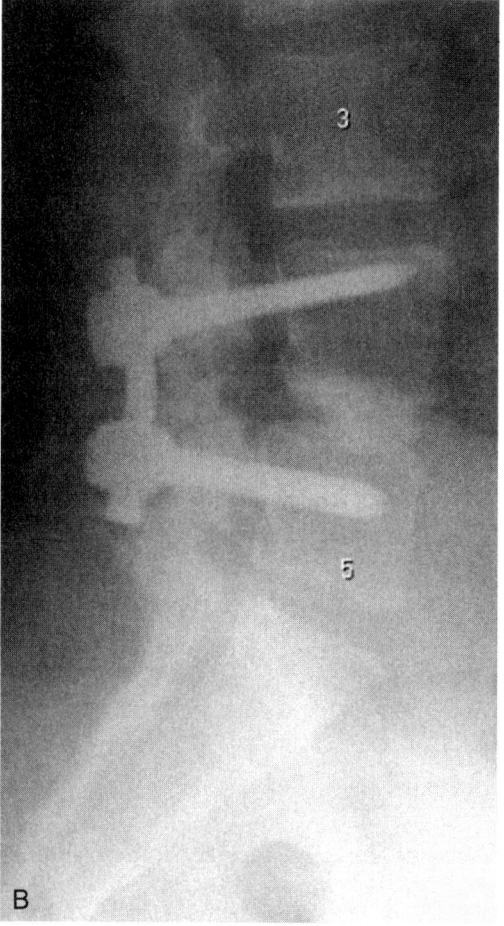

FIGURE 228–10. Preoperative *(A)* and postoperative *(B)* lateral radiographs demonstrate reduction of spondylolisthesis via a transforaminal interbody fusion and posterolateral fusion.

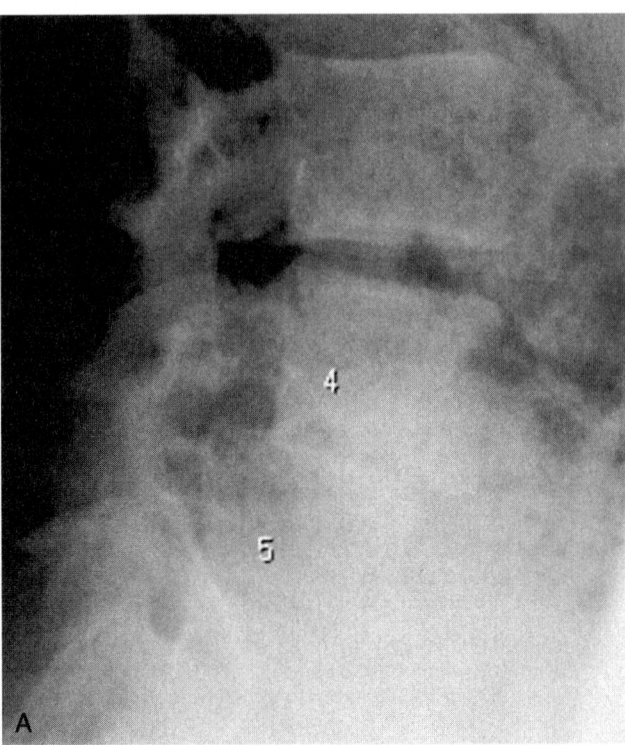

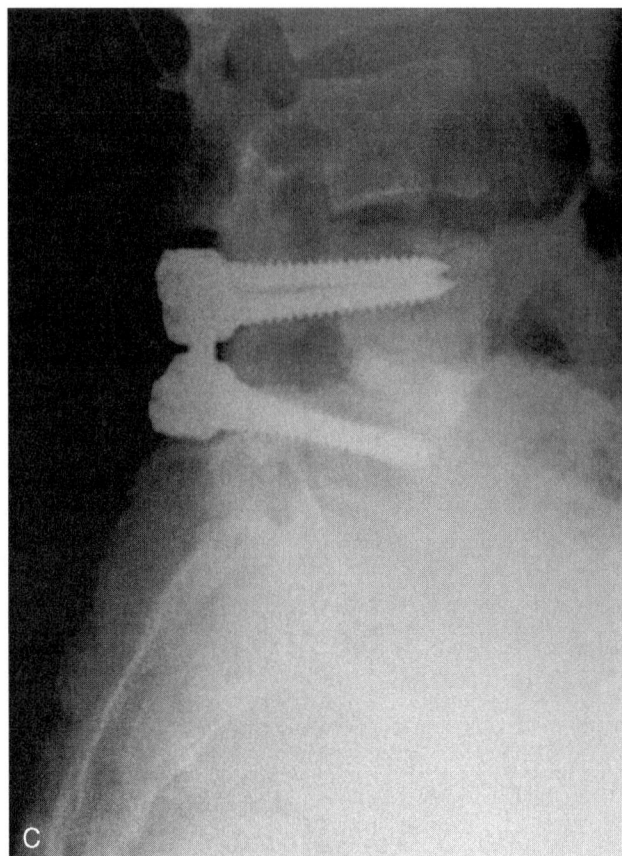

FIGURE 228–11. Preoperative *(A)* and postoperative *(B)* lateral radiographs of degenerative spondylolisthesis. After reduction, the patient had complete resolution of back pain and lower extremity radiculopathy.

sagittal imbalance preoperatively. Nonunion did not affect clinical outcomes in this study.

Suk and associates noted that in patients with spondylolytic spondylolisthesis, posterior lumbar interbody fusion combined with posterolateral instrumentation increased the rate of excellent outcomes for back pain from 45% to 75% when compared with posterolateral fusion with instrumentation.[110] They also compared posterolateral instrumentation and fusion with anterior lumbar interbody fusion and posterior instrumented fusion and found a 100% fusion rate with the latter. In addition, anterior lumbar interbody fusion was superior to posterolateral fusion in preventing loss of reduction.

Minimally invasive spine surgery is becoming more widely studied and practiced. Minimally invasive posterior instrumented fusion and posterior interbody fusion have been described. Khoo and associates published their results with this procedure in three patients.[115] Their average operative time was 3½ hours per level, with an estimated blood loss of 185 mL; the average inpatient stay was 2.8 days. With these promising early results, minimally invasive fusion may play an increasingly larger role in the treatment of spondylolisthesis. Studies are needed to compare the results of these procedures with those of open treatment.

CONCLUSION

Spondylolisthesis results from many factors, and treatment strategies are not standardized.

Isthmic Spondylolisthesis
- Most common at L5-S1.
- Most common in males.
- Most patients respond to conservative treatment.
- Children have better outcomes with posterolateral fusion without decompression than adults do.
- Improvement in sagittal balance and a 360-degree fusion improves fusion rates and outcomes in adults.
- Reduction of high-grade spondylolisthesis is associated with a greater risk of neurological injury.

Degenerative Spondylolisthesis
- More common at L4-5.
- More common in females.
- Most patients respond to conservative treatment.
- Surgical treatment outcomes are significantly improved if decompression is supplemented with arthrodesis.
- Long-term outcome studies find that solid fusions have better outcomes than pseudarthroses.
- Reduction of listhesis and improved sagittal bal-

ance can contribute to improved outcomes with regard to both fusion and symptoms.

The nonsurgical and surgical approaches to this complicated condition will benefit in the future from well-planned randomized, prospective studies and from the development of new technology.

REFERENCES

1. Herbiniaux G: Traite sur divers accouchements laborieux et sur les polypes de la matrice. Brussels, JL Boubers, 1782.
2. Kilian HF: Schilderungen neuer Beckenformen and ihres Verhaltens in Leben. Mannheim, Verlag von Bassermann & Mathey, 1854.
3. Neugebauer FL: A new contribution to the history and etiology of spondylolisthesis. New Sydenham Soc Select Monogr 121B: 1–64, 1888.
4. Meyerding HW: Spondylolisthesis. Surg Gynecol Obstet 54:371–377, 1932.
5. Newman PH: The etiology of spondylolisthesis. J Bone Joint Surg Br 45:39–59, 1963.
6. Davis H: Increasing rates of cervical and lumbar spine surgery in the United States, 1979–1990. Spine 19:1117–1123, discussion 1123–1124, 1994.
7. Friberg S: Studies on spondylolisthesis. Acta Chir Scand 82(Suppl):56, 1932.
8. Laurent L: Spondylolisthesis in children and adolescents. Acta Orthop Scand 31:45–64, 1961.
9. Turner RH, Bianco AJ Jr: Spondylolysis and spondylolisthesis in children and teen-agers. J Bone Joint Surg Am 53:1298–1306, 1971.
10. Wynne-Davies R, Scott JH: Inheritance and spondylolisthesis: A radiographic family survey. J Bone Joint Surg Br 61:301–305, 1979.
11. Albanese M, Pizzutillo PD: Family study of spondylolysis and spondylolisthesis. J Pediatr Orthop 2:496–499, 1982.
12. Lonstein JE: Spondylolisthesis in children: Cause, natural history, and management. Spine 24:2640–2648, 1999.
13. Wiltse LL, Newman PH, Macnab I: Classification of spondylolysis and spondylolisthesis. Clin Orthop 117:23–29, 1976.
14. Saraste H: Long-term clinical and radiological follow-up of spondylolysis and spondylolisthesis. J Pediatr Orthop 7:631–638, 1987.
15. Fitzgerald JA, Newman PH: Degenerative spondylolisthesis. J Bone Joint Surg Br 58:184–192, 1976.
16. Newman PH: A clinical syndrome associated with severe lumbo-sacral subluxation. J Bone Joint Surg Br 47:472–481, 1965.
17. Newman PH: Surgical treatment for spondylolisthesis in the adult. Clin Orthop 117:106–111, 1976.
18. Boxall D, Bradford DS, Winter RB, Moe JH: Management of severe spondylolisthesis in children and adolescents. J Bone Joint Surg Am 61:479–495, 1979.
19. Fredrickson BE, Baker D, McHolick WJ, et al: The natural history of spondylolysis and spondylolisthesis. J Bone Joint Surg Am 66:699–707, 1984.
20. Wiltse LL, et al: Spondylolisthesis: Classification, diagnosis, and natural history. Semin Spine Surg 1:78, 1989.
21. Nicoll E: Fractures of the dorso-lumbar spine. J Bone Joint Surg Br 31:376–394, 1949.
22. Standaert CJ, Herring SA: Spondylolysis: A critical review. Br J Sports Med 34:415–422, 2000.
23. Amato M, Totty WG, Gilula LA: Spondylolysis of the lumbar spine: Demonstration of defects and laminal fragmentation. Radiology 153:627–629, 1984.
24. Roche MA, Rowe RG: The incidence of separate neural arch and coincident bone variations: A survey of 4200 skeletons. Anat Rec 109:233–252, 1951.
25. Rosenberg NJ, Bargar WL, Friedman B: The incidence of spondylolysis and spondylolisthesis in nonambulatory patients. Spine 6:35–38, 1981.
26. Jackson DW, Wiltse LL, Cirincoine RJ: Spondylolysis in the female gymnast. Clin Orthop 117:68–73, 1976.
27. Rossi F: Spondylolysis, spondylolisthesis and sports. J Sports Med Phys Fitness 18:317–340, 1978.
28. Soler T, Calderon C: The prevalence of spondylolysis in the Spanish elite athlete. Am J Sports Med 28:57–62, 2000.
29. Jones DM, Tearse DS, el-Khoury GY, et al: Radiographic abnormalities of the lumbar spine in college football players: A comparative analysis. Am J Sports Med 27:335–338, 1999.
30. Frennered AK, Danielson BI, Nachemson AL: Natural history of symptomatic isthmic low-grade spondylolisthesis in children and adolescents: A seven-year follow-up study. J Pediatr Orthop 11:209–213, 1991.
31. Grobler LJ, Robertson PA, Novotny JE, Pope MH: Etiology of spondylolisthesis: Assessment of the role played by lumbar facet joint morphology. Spine 18:80–91, 1993.
32. Schlenzka D, Poussa M, Seitsalo S, Osterman K: Intervertebral disc changes in adolescents with isthmic spondylolisthesis. J Spinal Disord 4:344–352, 1991.
33. Szypryt EP, Twining P, Mulholland RC, Worthington BS: The prevalence of disc degeneration associated with neural arch defects of the lumbar spine assessed by magnetic resonance imaging. Spine 14:977–981, 1989.
34. Speck GR, McCall IW, O'Brien JP: Spondylolisthesis: The angle of kyphosis. Spine 9:659–660, 1984.
35. Kim NH, Suk KS: The role of transitional vertebrae in spondylolysis and spondylolytic spondylolisthesis. Bull Hosp Jt Dis 56: 161–166, 1997.
36. Blackburne JS, Velikas EP: Spondylolisthesis in children and adolescents. J Bone Joint Surg Br 59:490–494, 1977.
37. Muschik M, Hahnel H, Robinson PN, et al: Competitive sports and the progression of spondylolisthesis. J Pediatr Orthop 16: 364–369, 1996.
38. Standaert CJ, Herring SA, Halpern B, King O: Spondylolysis. Phys Med Rehabil Clin N Am 11:785–803, 2000.
39. Omey ML, Micheli LJ, Gerbino PG II: Idiopathic scoliosis and spondylolysis in the female athlete: Tips for treatment. Clin Orthop 372:74–84, 2000.
40. Steiner ME, Micheli LJ: Treatment of symptomatic spondylolysis and spondylolisthesis with the modified Boston brace. Spine 10: 937–943, 1985.
41. Blanda J, Bethem D, Moats W, Lew M: Defects of pars interarticularis in athletes: A protocol for nonoperative treatment. J Spinal Disord 6:406–411, 1993.
42. Morita T, Ikata T, Katoh S, Miyake R: Lumbar spondylolysis in children and adolescents. J Bone Joint Surg Br 77:620–625, 1995.
43. Micheli LJ, Wood R: Back pain in young athletes: Significant differences from adults in causes and patterns. Arch Pediatr Adolesc Med 149:15–18, 1995.
44. Mooney V: A randomized double-blind prospective study of the efficacy of pulsed electromagnetic fields for interbody lumbar fusions. Spine 15:708–712, 1990.
45. Pettine KA, Salib RM, Walker SG: External electrical stimulation and bracing for treatment of spondylolysis: A case report. Spine 18:436–439, 1993.
46. Fellander-Tsai L, Micheli LJ: Treatment of spondylolysis with external electrical stimulation and bracing in adolescent athletes: A report of two cases. Clin J Sports Med 8:232–234, 1998.
47. Wu SS, Lee CH, Chen PQ: Operative repair of symptomatic spondylolysis following a positive response to diagnostic pars injection. J Spinal Disord 12:10–16, 1999.
48. Lapras C, Pierluca P, Pernot P, Mottolese C: [Treatment of spondylolisthesis (stage I–II) by neurosurgical decompression without either osteosynthesis or reduction.] Neurochirurgie 30:147–152, 1984.
49. Dai LY, Jia LS, Yuan W, et al: Direct repair of defect in lumbar spondylolysis and mild isthmic spondylolisthesis by bone grafting, with or without facet joint fusion. Eur Spine J 10:78–83, 2001.
50. Gillet P, Petit M: Direct repair of spondylolysis without spondylolisthesis, using a rod-screw construct and bone grafting of the pars defect. Spine 24:1252–1256, 1999.
51. Kakiuchi M: Repair of the defect in spondylolysis: Durable fixation with pedicle screws and laminar hooks. J Bone Joint Surg Am 79:818–825, 1997.
52. Buck JE: Direct repair of the defect in spondylolisthesis: Preliminary report. J Bone Joint Surg Br 52:432–437, 1970.

53. Eingorn D, Pizzutillo PD: Pars interarticularis fusion of multiple levels of lumbar spondylolysis: A case report. Spine 10:250–252, 1985.

54. Gill GG, Manning JG, White HL: Surgical treatment of spondylolisthesis without spine fusion. J Bone Joint Surg 37:493–520, 1955.

55. Harris IE, Weinstein SL: Long-term follow-up of patients with grade III and IV spondylolisthesis: Treatment with and without posterior fusion. J Bone Joint Surg Am 69:960–969, 1987.

56. Freeman BL III, Donati NL: Spinal arthrodesis for severe spondylolisthesis in children and adolescents: A long-term follow-up study. J Bone Joint Surg Am 71:594–598, 1989.

57. Johnson JR, Kirwan EO: The long-term results of fusion in situ for severe spondylolisthesis. J Bone Joint Surg Br 65:43–46, 1983.

58. Laurent LE, Osterman K: Operative treatment of spondylolisthesis in young patients. Clin Orthop 117:85–91, 1976.

59. Hensinger RN, Langm JR, MacEwen GD: Surgical management of spondylolisthesis in children and adolescents. Spine 1:206–216, 1976.

60. Burkus JK, Lonstein JE, Winter RB, Denis F: Long-term evaluation of adolescents treated operatively for spondylolisthesis: A comparison of in situ arthrodesis only with in situ arthrodesis and reduction followed by immobilization in a cast. J Bone Joint Surg Am 74:693–704, 1992.

61. Lenke LG, Bridwell KH, Bullis D, et al: Results of in situ fusion for isthmic spondylolisthesis. J Spinal Disord 5:433–442, 1992.

62. Haraldsson S, Willner S: A comparative study of spondylolisthesis in operations on adolescents and adults. Arch Orthop Trauma Surg 101:101–105, 1983.

63. Dimar JR, Hoffman G: Grade 4 spondylolisthesis: Two-stage therapeutic approach of anterior vertebrectomy and anterior-posterior fusion. Orthop Rev 15:504–509, 1986.

64. Carragee EJ: Single-level posterolateral arthrodesis, with or without posterior decompression, for the treatment of isthmic spondylolisthesis in adults: A prospective, randomized study. J Bone Joint Surg Am 79:1175–1180, 1997.

65. Matthiass HH, Heine J: The surgical reduction of spondylolisthesis. Clin Orthop 203:34–44, 1986.

66. Schnee CL, Freese A, Ansell LV: Outcome analysis for adults with spondylolisthesis treated with posterolateral fusion and transpedicular screw fixation. J Neurosurg 86:56–63, 1997.

67. Bassewitz H, Herkowitz H: Lumbar stenosis with spondylolisthesis: Current concepts of surgical treatment. Clin Orthop 384:54–60, 2001.

68. Fischgrund JS, Mackay M, Herkowitz HN, et al: 1997 Volvo Award winner in clinical studies. Degenerative lumbar spondylolisthesis with spinal stenosis: A prospective, randomized study comparing decompressive laminectomy and arthrodesis with and without spinal instrumentation. Spine 22:2807–2812, 1997.

69. Schoenecker PL, Cole HO, Herring JA, et al: Cauda equina syndrome after in situ arthrodesis for severe spondylolisthesis at the lumbosacral junction. J Bone Joint Surg Am 72:369–377, 1990.

70. Molinari RW, Bridwell KH, Lenke LG, et al: Complications in the surgical treatment of pediatric high-grade, isthmic dysplastic spondylolisthesis: A comparison of three surgical approaches. Spine 24:1701–1711, 1999.

71. Moller H, Hedlund R: Instrumented and noninstrumented posterolateral fusion in adult spondylolisthesis—a prospective randomized study: Part 2. Spine 25:1716–1721, 2000.

72. Bohlman HH, Cook SS: One-stage decompression and posterolateral and interbody fusion for lumbosacral spondyloptosis through a posterior approach: Report of two cases. J Bone Joint Surg Am 64:415–418, 1982.

73. Gaines RW, Nichols WK: Treatment of spondyloptosis by two stage L5 vertebrectomy and reduction of L4 onto S1. Spine 10:680–686, 1985.

74. Lehmer SM, Steffee AD, Gaines RW Jr: Treatment of L5-S1 spondyloptosis by staged L5 resection with reduction and fusion of L4 onto S1 (Gaines procedure). Spine 19:1916–1925, 1994.

75. Schollner D: One stage reduction and fusion for spondylolisthesis. Int Orthop 14:145–150, 1990.

76. Junghanns H: Spondylolisthesen ohne Spalt in Zwischengelenkstuck. Arch Orthop Unfallchir 29:118–127, 1930.

77. Newman PH: Spondylolisthesis, its cause and effect. Ann Roy Coll Surg 16:305–323, 1955.

78. Rosenberg NJ: Degenerative spondylolisthesis: Predisposing factors. J Bone Joint Surg Am 57:467–474, 1975.

79. Imada K, Matsui H, Tsuji H: Oophorectomy predisposes to degenerative spondylolisthesis. J Bone Joint Surg Br 77:126–130, 1995.

80. Nadaud MC, McClure S, Weiner BK: Do facet joint capsular ligaments contain estrogen receptors? Application to pathogenesis of degenerative spondylolisthesis. Am J Orthop 30:753–754, 2001.

81. Matsunaga S, Sakou T, Morizono Y, et al: Natural history of degenerative spondylolisthesis: Pathogenesis and natural course of the slippage. Spine 15:1204–1210, 1990.

82. Matsunaga S, Ijiri K, Hayashi K: Nonsurgically managed patients with degenerative spondylolisthesis: A 10- to 18-year follow-up study. J Neurosurg 93(2 Suppl):194–198, 2000.

83. Rosen CD, Berstein R, et al: A retrospective analysis of the efficacy of epidural steroid injections. Clin Orthop 228:270–272, 1998.

84. Postacchini F, Cinotti G, Perugia D: Degenerative lumbar spondylolisthesis. II. Surgical treatment. Ital J Orthop Traumatol 17:467–477, 1991.

85. Epstein JA, Lavine LS: Nerve root compression associated with narrowing of the lumbar spinal canal. J Neurol Neurosurg Psychiatry 25:165–176, 1962.

86. Epstein NE, Epstein JA, Carras R, Lavine LS: Degenerative spondylolisthesis with an intact neural arch: A review of 60 cases with an analysis of clinical findings and the development of surgical management. Neurosurgery 13:555–561, 1983.

87. Epstein NE: Decompression in the surgical management of degenerative spondylolisthesis: Advantages of a conservative approach in 290 patients. J Spinal Disord 11:116–122, discussion 123, 1998.

88. Silvers HR, Lewis PJ, Asch HL: Decompressive lumbar laminectomy for spinal stenosis. J Neurosurg 78:695–701, 1993.

89. Kinoshita T, Ohki I, Roth KR, et al: Results of degenerative spondylolisthesis treated with posterior decompression alone via a new surgical approach. J Neurosurg 95(1 Suppl):11–16, 2001.

90. Kristof RA, Aliashkevich AF, Schuster M, et al: Degenerative lumbar spondylolisthesis-induced radicular compression: Non-fusion-related decompression in selected patients without hypermobility on flexion-extension radiographs. J Neurosurg 97(3 Suppl):281–286, 2002.

91. Herron LD, Trippi AC: L4-5 degenerative spondylolisthesis: The results of treatment by decompressive laminectomy without fusion. Spine 14:534–538, 1989.

92. Lombardi JS, Wiltse LL, Reynolds J, et al: Treatment of degenerative spondylolisthesis. Spine 10:821–827, 1985.

93. Herkowitz HN, Kurz LT: Degenerative lumbar spondylolisthesis with spinal stenosis: A prospective study comparing decompression with decompression and intertransverse process arthrodesis. J Bone Joint Surg Am 73:802–808, 1991.

94. Zdeblick TA: A prospective, randomized study of lumbar fusion: Preliminary results. Spine 18:983–991, 1993.

95. Mardjetko SM, Connolly PJ, Shott S: Degenerative lumbar spondylolisthesis: A meta-analysis of literature 1970–1993. Spine 19(20 Suppl):2256S–2265S, 1994.

96. Katz JN, et al: Lumbar laminectomy alone or with instrumented or noninstrumented arthrodesis in degenerative lumbar spinal stenosis: Patient selection, costs, and surgical outcomes. Spine 22:1123–1131, 1997.

97. Katz JN, Lipson SJ, Lew RA, et al: The role of fusion and instrumentation in the treatment of degenerative spondylolisthesis with spinal stenosis. J Spinal Disord 6:461–472, 1993.

98. Ido K, Urushidani H: Radiographic evaluation of posterolateral lumbar fusion for degenerative spondylolisthesis: Long-term follow-up of more than 10 years vs midterm follow-up of 2–5 years. Neurosurg Rev 24:195–199, 2001.

99. Hansraj KK, O'Leary PF, Cammisa FP Jr, et al: Decompression, fusion, and instrumentation surgery for complex lumbar spinal stenosis. Clin Orthop 384:18–25, 2001.

100. Fujiya M, Saita M, Kaneda K, Abumi K: Clinical study on stability of combined distraction and compression rod instru-

mentation with posterolateral fusion for unstable degenerative spondylolisthesis. Spine 15:1216–1222, 1990.

101. Kaneda K, Kazama H, Satoh S, Fujiya M: Follow-up study of medial facetectomies and posterolateral fusion with instrumentation in unstable degenerative spondylolisthesis. Clin Orthop 203:159–167, 1986.

102. McCulloch JA: Microdecompression and uninstrumented single-level fusion for spinal canal stenosis with degenerative spondylolisthesis. Spine 23:2243–2252, 1998.

103. Bednar DA: Surgical management of lumbar degenerative spinal stenosis with spondylolisthesis via posterior reduction with minimal laminectomy. J Spinal Disord Tech 15:105–109, 2002.

104. Booth KC, Bridwell KH, Eisenberg BA: Minimum 5-year results of degenerative spondylolisthesis treated with decompression and instrumented posterior fusion. Spine 24:1721–1727, 1999.

105. Nork SE, Hu SS, Workman KL, et al: Patient outcomes after decompression and instrumented posterior spinal fusion for degenerative spondylolisthesis. Spine 24:561–569, 1999.

106. Unnanantana A: Posterolateral lumbar fusion for degenerative spondylolisthesis: Experiences of a modified technique without instrumentation. J Med Assoc Thai 80:570–574, 1997.

107. Hanley EN Jr: Indications for fusion in the lumbar spine. Bull Hosp Jt Dis 55:154–157, 1996.

108. Kuntz KM, Snider RK, Weinstein JN, et al: Cost-effectiveness of fusion with and without instrumentation for patients with degenerative spondylolisthesis and spinal stenosis. Spine 25:1132–1139, 2000.

109. Kornblum M, Herkowitz H, Abraham D, et al: Degenerative lumbar spondylolisthesis with spinal stenosis: A prospective long-term study comparing fusion and pseudarthrosis. In AAOS. Orlando, FL, 2000.

110. Suk SI, Lee CK, Kim WJ, et al: Adding posterior lumbar interbody fusion to pedicle screw fixation and posterolateral fusion after decompression in spondylolytic spondylolisthesis. Spine 22:210–219, discussion 219–220, 1997.

111. Suk KS, Jeon CH, Park MS, et al: Comparison between posterolateral fusion with pedicle screw fixation and anterior interbody fusion with pedicle screw fixation in adult spondylolytic spondylolisthesis. Yonsei Med J 42:316–323, 2001.

112. Kawakami M, Tamaki T, Ando M, et al: Lumbar sagittal balance influences the clinical outcome after decompression and posterolateral spinal fusion for degenerative lumbar spondylolisthesis. Spine 27:59–64, 2002.

113. Lee TC: Reduction and stabilization without laminectomy for unstable degenerative spondylolisthesis: A preliminary report. Neurosurgery 35:1072–1076, 1994.

114. Cagli S, Crawford NR, Sonntag VK, Dickman CA: Biomechanics of grade I degenerative lumbar spondylolisthesis. Part 2. Treatment with threaded interbody cages/dowels and pedicle screws. J Neurosurg 94(1 Suppl):51–60, 2001.

115. Khoo LT, Palmer S, Laich DT, Fessler RG: Minimally invasive percutaneous posterior lumbar interbody fusion. Neurosurgery 51(5 Suppl):166–171, 2002.

CHAPTER 229

Benign Tumors of the Vertebral Column in Children

NALIN GUPTA ■ DAVID M. FRIM

Primary tumors of the spinal column are rare in children and, fortunately, the majority are benign.[1, 2] These tumors usually arise from the osseous elements and must be differentiated from more common conditions in children, such as congenital spinal anomalies, intramedullary spinal cord tumors, and paraspinal tumors such as neuroblastoma and Wilms' tumor. A number of non-neoplastic diseases such as fibrous dysplasia and eosinophilic granuloma can present similar to typical primary spinal tumors. The hallmark feature of most spinal tumors in children is persistent back pain, usually without neurologic deficit; this should alert the physician to the presence of a pathologic lesion. The management of each neoplasm is determined by the natural history of the actual tumor. Unfortunately, because of the rarity of these lesions, detailed information regarding incidence and prevalence is not available. Therefore, certain information has to be gleaned from data obtained from adult patients. We discuss seven entities that can be defined as benign tumors of the vertebral column in children: osteoid osteoma, osteoblastoma, giant cell tumor, aneurysmal bone cyst, vertebral hemangioma, fibrous dysplasia, and eosinophilic granuloma.

CLINICAL PRESENTATION

In general, the spinal level of the tumor, degree of bony or soft tissue involvement, and impingement on neural elements determine the clinical presentation. In most patients, pain is the most common presenting symptom.[3] This is often a difficult diagnosis in infants, in whom irritability or preference of a specific position may be the only clue. A variety of pain patterns is observed. The usual source is bony expansion or destruction, and inflammation of the overlying periosteum. This pain is usually localized to the involved level and is worsened by movement. If local nerve roots are compressed or irritated, a radicular component may also be present. Spinal instability may cause excessive motion at one segment, producing pain that is characteristically worsened by activity and relieved by rest. Finally, vertebral body collapse may result in a sudden worsening of pain, paraspinal muscle spasm, neurologic deficit, or visible spinal deformity. The classic example of loss of vertebral body height is the finding of vertebra plana described with eosinophilic granuloma of the spine (see Fig. 229–5).

Neurologic deficit is less commonly seen with benign spinal tumors; if it is present in the absence of other mechanical symptoms, other diagnoses should be entertained. In particular, intrinsic spinal cord tumors, myelodysplasia, syringomyelia, and transverse myelitis must be considered. Other important presenting signs include progressive scoliosis, torticollis, urinary incontinence, or a palpable mass.

DIAGNOSTIC IMAGING AND PROCEDURES

Conventional plain films of the spine may be useful as an initial screening tool. Suggestive abnormalities include lytic lesions, alignment deformities, scoliosis, and associated congenital abnormalities such as spinal dysraphism. Conventional radiography does not exclude bony lesions but may help direct further imaging studies. If an abnormality is found on initial imaging, magnetic resonance imaging (MRI) should be the next step in order to define the anatomy of the neural elements in relationship to the bony lesion. If a lesion cannot be localized on initial imaging, a nuclear medicine bone scan is useful as a localizing study. Once a lesion is identified or a bony origin is noted, the superior resolution of thin-cut computed tomography (CT) is needed to define the anatomy of the spinal elements. For primary spinal neoplasms, the tandem of CT and MRI is virtually always required to demonstrate the relationship between the primary neoplasm and the neural elements. Rarely, spinal angiography coupled with embolization may be required for highly vascular lesions. Extraspinal pathologic conditions such as neuroblastoma or sarcoma is best localized by MRI.

OSTEOID OSTEOMA

Osteoid osteomas are benign tumors of bone, 10% of which are found in the vertebral column. The nidus of the lesion consists of osteoid trabeculae containing a vascular fibrous stroma. The surrounding bone is histologically normal but is formed of dense cortical and trabecular bone and represents the reactive zone. This correlates with the imaging appearance of a lytic lesion surrounded by a sclerotic margin (Fig. 229–1). Localization of this tumor is facilitated by radionucleotide bone scanning, which invariably demonstrates increased activity. The classic presentation is night pain, although this is not the rule. Torticollis in association with pain is reported for cervical osteomas.[4] In one series, 63% of patients with osteoid osteoma or osteoblastoma had significant scoliosis.[5] Neurologic deficit is reported in up to 22% of patients at presentation.[6] There is a striking 6:1 male-to-female predominance for spinal osteomas.[7] Salicylate medications have been reported to relieve the pain of osteoid osteomas dramatically, but this is not the case in the majority of patients. The mechanism of this response is unknown, but prostaglandins are involved, and curiously, osteoid osteomas appear to have nerve endings distributed throughout the reactive zone.[8, 9] Inflammation involving these nerve endings may account for the common occurrence of pain as a presenting symptom.

On MRI scans, there is increased signal in the surrounding bone marrow on T2-weighted sequences. The zone of dense mineralization is seen as a ring of decreased signal on both T1- and T2-weighted sequences.[10] The nidus itself demonstrates homogeneous enhancement. Although some cases of osteoid osteoma demonstrate this typical appearance on CT and MRI scans, others overlap with osteoblastoma and giant cell tumor, sometimes prompting a surgical procedure for histologic diagnosis.[11, 12]

For patients with unremitting pain that does not respond to analgesics, intralesional surgical excision is the treatment of choice, with complete excision resulting in cure. Fusion, with or without instrumentation, is rarely required unless instability results from a large lesion or from surgical exposure and resection. Diagnosis and treatment with minimally invasive radiologically guided techniques have been reported.[13, 14] These offer the advantages of reduced operative risk and a smaller likelihood of compromising the structural integrity of the spine. The long-term efficacy of these techniques compared with surgical excision is not yet known.

OSTEOBLASTOMA

Osteoblastomas are also lytic lesions that contain immature bone and osteoid and are often highly vascular. In general, the pathologic features of osteoblastomas are the same as those of osteoid osteomas, with fibrous stroma surrounded by multinucleated giant cells and vascular channels. Grossly, osteoblastomas are defined as being larger than 2 cm. Approximately 30% to 50%

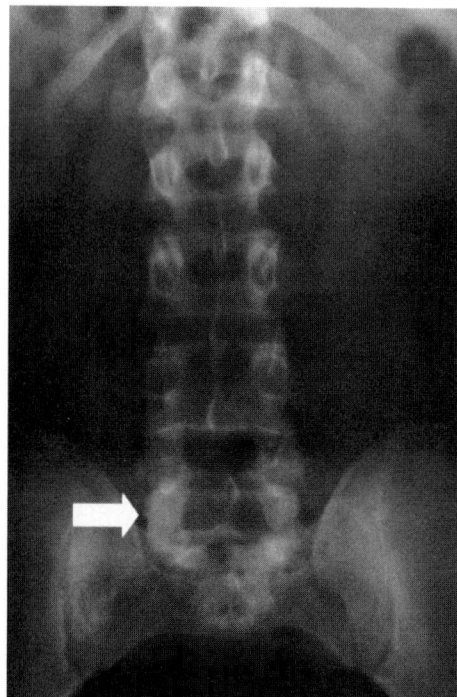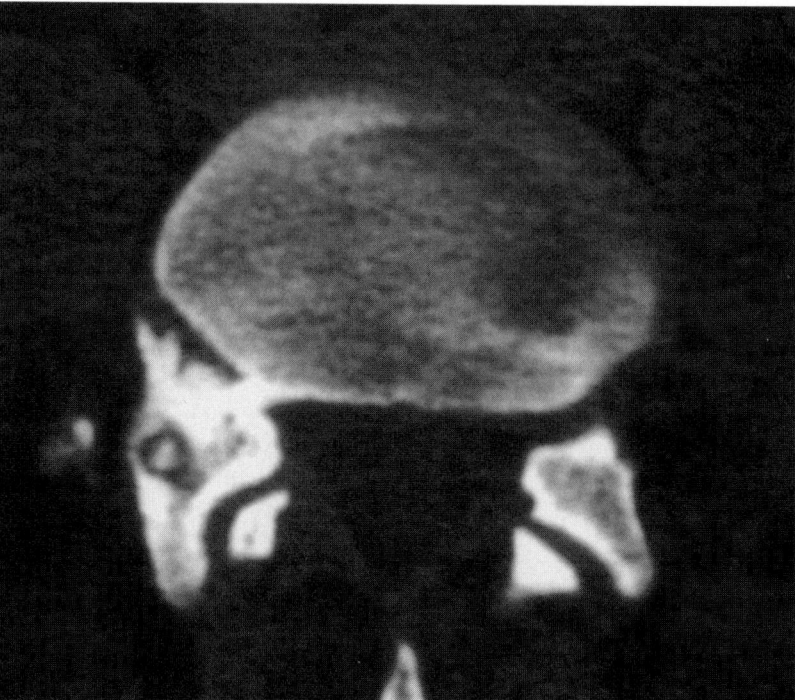

FIGURE 229–1. Osteoid osteoma of the lumbar spine. Imaging studies are of a teenage boy with a several-month history of low back pain. *Left,* Anteroposterior view of the lumbar spine demonstrates a sclerotic area in the vicinity of the right L5 pedicle *(arrow). Right,* Axial computed tomographic image shows a central nidus surrounded by a reactive margin, localized to the right superior facet of L5. (Courtesy of Dr. Daniel Mass, Section of Orthopedic Surgery, University of Chicago.)

of all osteoblastomas occur in the spine; the reason for this predilection is unknown.[15, 16] The majority of these lesions occur in adolescents and young adults. The most common presenting symptom is pain, but it tends to be less well localized than the pain of osteoid osteoma.[3, 17] Scoliosis is also commonly seen and seems to be secondary to the presence of asymmetrical muscle spasm.[18] Probably because of their proximity to the spinal canal and their larger size when compared with osteoid osteoma, osteoblastomas more commonly present with neurologic symptoms.[4, 6]

On imaging studies, as with osteoid osteoma, a lytic center is surrounded by a dense ring of reactive bone, but the overall appearance is less consistent.[19, 20] The central portion of the tumor invariably enhances after gadolinium administration. Reactive changes involving the bone marrow and surrounding soft tissues visible on MRI scans can overstate the extent of the tumor.[19] A curious geographic feature of osteoblastomas is their predilection for the posterior elements.[21]

Osteoblastoma can behave in an aggressive manner. In a report summarizing more than 300 cases from the records of the Mayo Clinic, approximately 20% of tumors recurred.[16] Histologic appearance, surprisingly, did not predict aggressive behavior.[22] Surgical excision with clean margins is the preferred treatment option, although radiation can be used for subtotally excised or recurrent lesions.[23, 24]

GIANT CELL TUMOR

Giant cell tumors are expansile, vascular lesions of bone. They produce lytic lesions in bone and display features consistent with repeat hemorrhage. The usual presentation is spinal pain. Although rare in children, giant cell tumors are usually found in the long bones but can occur in the spine.[25] They are characteristically located in the posterior elements and expand the bone without breaking through the periosteal layer. Although the histologic features are not typically malignant, giant cell tumors can be locally invasive and can recur and metastasize. Molecular studies suggest that expression of specific genes can affect biologic behavior. Expression of a matrix metalloproteinase-9 that is responsible for degrading various basement membrane proteins was found to correlate with the rate of lung metastasis.[26] Similarly, Gamberi and colleagues found that 38% of primary giant cell tumors overexpressed c-myc mRNA, compared with 69% of the lung metastases isolated from the original cohort of primary tumors.[27] Although these studies are suggestive, clear prognostic indicators are not available for predicting aggressive behavior.

Treatment of giant cell tumors is usually wide resection with bone grafting. Radiation has also been used with success to control tumor growth.[28, 29] Primary surgical treatment followed by radiation (35 Gy in 15 fractions) achieved excellent control in a mixed series of patients with a mean follow-up of 15 years.[30] Although not supported by some studies, there is reluctance to offer radiation for fear of sarcomatous transformation.[31]

ANEURYSMAL BONE CYST

Aneurysmal bone cysts (ABCs) are non-neoplastic vascular lesions of bone that consist of lytic areas filled with blood products, sometimes of various ages. There may be flimsy fibrous strands or septations traversing the blood-filled cavities. The cause of these lesions is unknown, and karyotypically they are normal.[32] It is possible that these lesions are primarily arteriovenous malformations located in mature bone. Curiously, one third of ABCs are associated with preexisting bony neoplasms such as osteoblastoma, angioma, or chondroblastoma.[33, 34] Treatment of these so-called secondary ABCs is directed toward the primary pathology. As a group, ABCs are clustered in children and adolescents, with 80% occurring in patients younger than 20 years.[33] In one large retrospective review of approximately 1000 cases, the median age of patients was 13 years.[35] Approximately 25% of all ABCs are found in the vertebral column. Pain is the most common presenting symptom, often lasting several months before diagnosis. The imaging appearance can be inconsistent, with varying degrees of cortical destruction, sclerosis, or fibrosis. The bony margins are often remodeled, giving the appearance of being ballooned outward (Figs. 229–2 and 229–3). Blood products of varying ages and fluid-fluid levels seen on MRI scans are highly suggestive of the diagnosis.

The conventional treatment of these lesions has been intralesional excision and bone grafting.[36] It appears that recurrence rates are high with this technique (19% in the Mayo Clinic series) unless an adjunctive therapy is added.[37–39] Intralesional excision followed by application of liquid nitrogen (cryotherapy) is reported to reduce recurrence rates greatly when compared with curettage alone.[40, 41] In addition, some reports describe excellent results with only selective arterial embolization.[42]

VERTEBRAL HEMANGIOMA

Vertebral hemangiomas are probably the most common spinal tumor by prevalence (~10%) and are often seen as solitary lesions on routine CT or MRI. Their prevalence in the pediatric population is rare, with only case reports available in the literature.[43, 44] Information regarding their management must be extrapolated from the experience in adults. The classic appearance on axial computed tomographic images is a polka-dot pattern produced by thickened vertical trabeculae in the absence of horizontal trabeculae. Vertebral hemangiomas consist of clusters of thin-walled vessels often located in the vertebral bodies, although they can extend into the posterior elements and span several levels. They are usually asymptomatic, but hemorrhage and extension into the spinal canal can result in pain with neurologic deficit.[45]

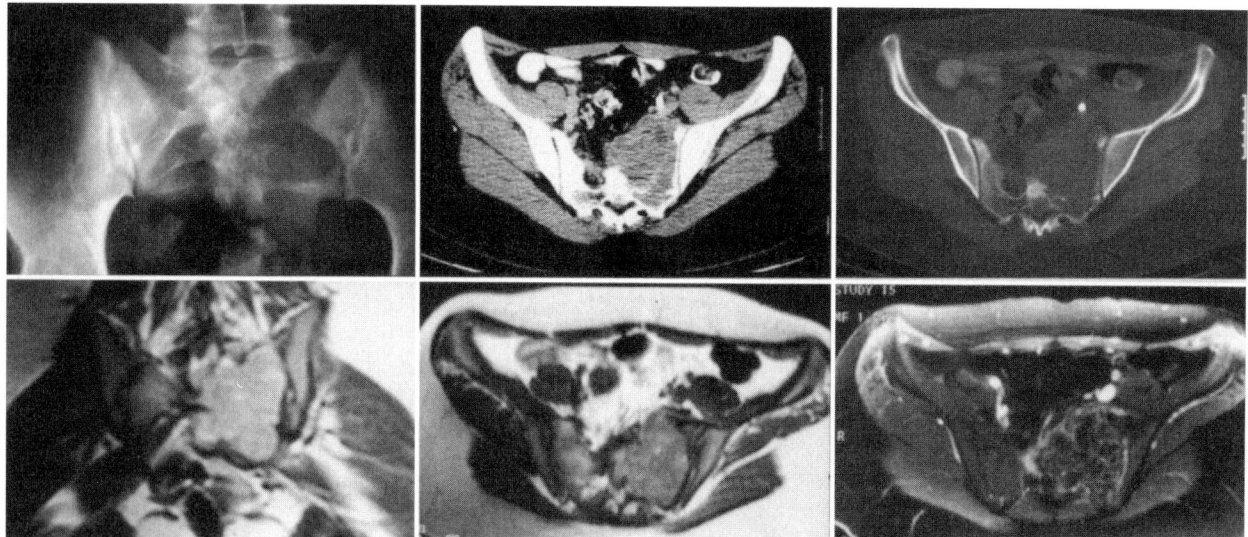

FIGURE 229–2. Aneurysmal bone cyst located in the sacrum of a 16-year-old girl. The mass is destructive *(top left)* and expands the bony margins of the sacrum (computed tomographic images, *top, middle* and *right*). Magnetic resonance images *(bottom)* demonstrate a soft tissue mass with heterogeneous signal characteristics and a delicate reticulated pattern (T2-weighted image, *bottom right*). (Courtesy of Dr. Daniel Mass, Section of Orthopedic Surgery, University of Chicago.)

Incidentally discovered lesions are not usually followed with sequential imaging. Although the natural history of these lesions is unclear, following numerous patients with incidental vertebral hemangiomas is not practical. Lesions that produce pain or neurologic deficits should be treated. Surgical management can present significant technical challenges. Preoperative embolization followed by surgical excision is recommended, because massive blood loss has been described during routine excision of these lesions.[46] Various strategies for embolization are available, and intralesional injection of pure ethanol was shown to be effective.[47–49] Radiation therapy alone is also effective in controlling symptoms.[50–52] In one report, the dose of radiation appeared to be important, with recurrences developing in only those patients receiving less than 26 Gy.[45] In children who have not reached skeletal maturity, radiation may alter spinal growth and should be avoided if possible. The role of conformal radiotherapy for these lesions has yet to be defined.

FIBROUS DYSPLASIA

Fibrous dysplasia is a benign disease in which normal bone is replaced by connective tissue that has a prominent fibrous component. Histologically, the tissue is composed of fibroblasts, collagen, and thin trabeculae of bone. Although most cases of fibrous dysplasia are sporadic, the triad of endocrinopathy, café au lait spots, and polyostotic fibrous dysplasia is known as *McCune-Albright syndrome.* The gene defect with this disease is known to be an activating mutation in the α chain of the signal transduction protein Gs.[53, 54] The overactivity of this protein is presumed to lead to increased activity of adenylate cyclase and cyclic adenosine monophosphate (a second messenger), and eventually to increased cell proliferation.[55] Sporadic forms of fibrous dysplasia also appear to carry mutations in the *Gs* gene, suggesting that a common biochemical pathway is responsible for the same histologic bone lesions.[56, 57]

Monostotic and polyostotic forms of fibrous dysplasia exist. Monostotic fibrous dysplasia restricted to the spine is rare, with few case reports in the literature.[58–62] The presenting symptoms can be diverse, including pain, progressive scoliosis, and paraparesis.[63–65] Neurologic compromise, spinal instability, and the possibility

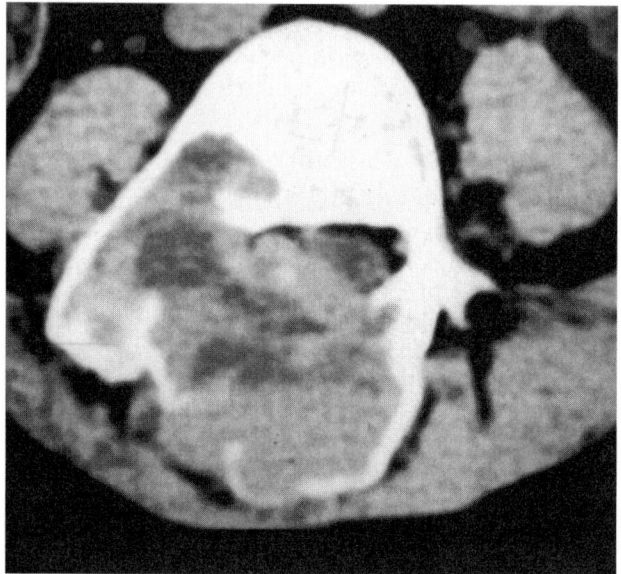

FIGURE 229–3. Expansile aneurysmal bone cyst located within the posterior elements of L5. Clinical presentation was scoliosis and radicular pain, likely related to compression of neural elements. (Courtesy of Dr. Daniel Mass, Section of Orthopedic Surgery, University of Chicago.)

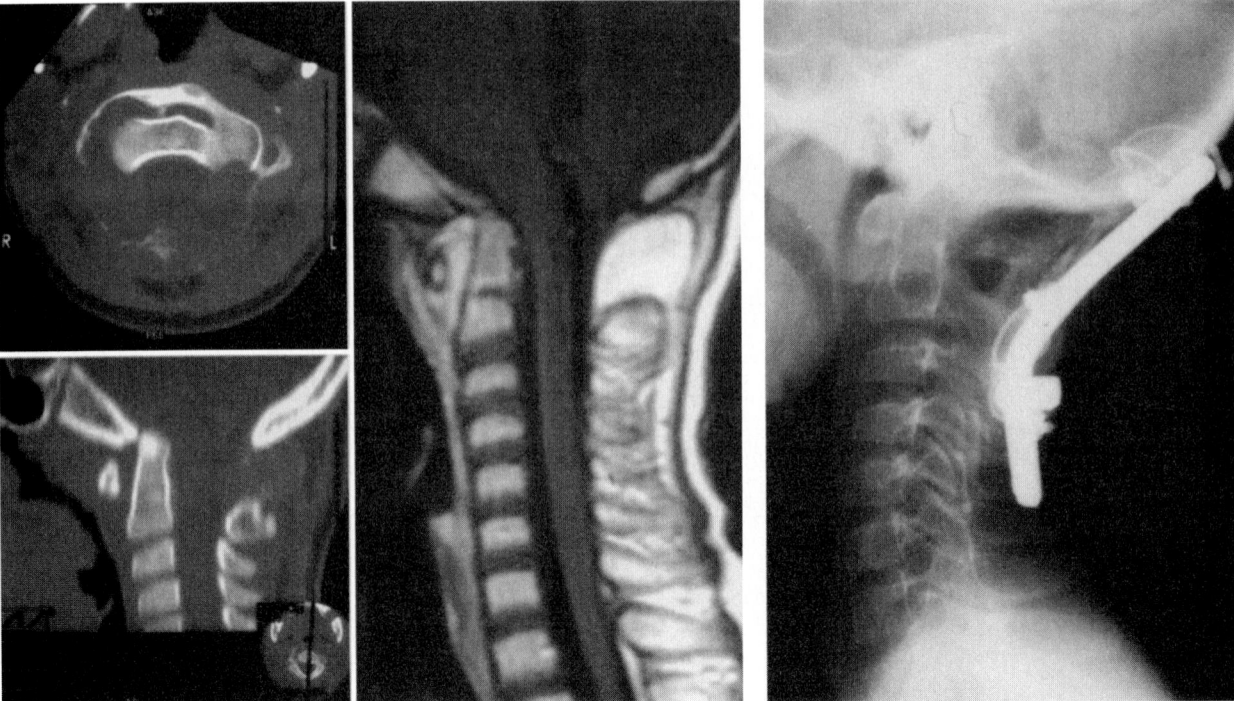

FIGURE 229–4. Fibrous dysplasia of C1. A 5-year-old boy presented with neck pain secondary to a soft tissue lesion that replaced the posterior arch and lateral masses of C1 (CT images, *far left*). C1–2 instability prompted a posterior fusion from the occiput to C3. Note also the upward migration of the odontoid into the foramen magnum (magnetic resonance imaging scan, *middle*). The 3-month postoperative lateral radiograph *(right)* demonstrates formation of a fusion mass at the operative site.

of sarcomatous transformation are absolute indications for surgical intervention (Fig. 229–4). Although the exact treatment is unclear, most reports describe an attempt at complete removal, followed by fusion with bone graft and instrumentation. Intracranial fibrous dysplasia is known to undergo remission, or "burnout," in adulthood. It is unknown whether spinal fibrous dysplasia has a similar natural history.

EOSINOPHILIC GRANULOMA

Eosinophilic granuloma of bone is the localized and most benign form of Langerhans' cell histiocytosis (also known as *histiocytosis X*). Although it is not formally a neoplastic process, its appearance and presentation overlap those of true spinal neoplasms, and it must be included in the differential diagnosis. Pathologically, there is a proliferation of histiocytes, producing lytic lesions of one or more bones. It is a disease of children and adolescents and rarely affects adults. Replacement of the normal vertebral bony structure leads to collapse of the vertebral body, thereby creating the classic radiologic appearance of vertebra plana (Fig. 229–5). This feature is probably seen in only half of patients with eosinophilic granuloma.[66, 67] The presenting symptom is usually pain, although neurologic deficit is also reported.[68–70] Imaging findings demonstrate a lytic lesion surrounded by a reactive sclerotic region of bone. The amount of edema surrounding the central soft tissue core is less than that observed with osteomyelitis or malignant lesions.[71] Diagnosis can usually be accomplished through CT-guided needle biopsy. The treatment of solitary eosinophilic granuloma of the spine without neurologic involvement is usually conservative, relying on rest, analgesics, and bracing. Remarkably, reconstitution of the vertebral body height can often be demonstrated over time.[72–74] Surgery is reserved for nondiagnostic biopsies and for patients with progressive spinal deformity or neurologic deficit, or both. Decompression of the neural elements, with reconstruction as needed, leads to resolution of symptoms.[68, 75]

CONCLUSIONS

Benign tumors of the pediatric spine are rare. They are usually self-limited, but confusion can occur with highly malignant tumors such as Wilms' tumor and osteosarcoma. The most common presenting symptom is back pain, at times accompanied by scoliosis or neurologic deficit. After imaging studies, the first goal of intervention must be diagnosis. Total excision is the preferred approach for osteoid osteoma, osteoblastoma, giant cell tumor, and ABCs. Total resection may not be required for fibrous dysplasia. Eosinophilic granuloma of the spine without deformity or neurologic compromise can be treated conservatively. Destabilizing surgery and spinal fusion in children should be carefully considered, because the potential for limiting spinal growth can have significant long-term effects.

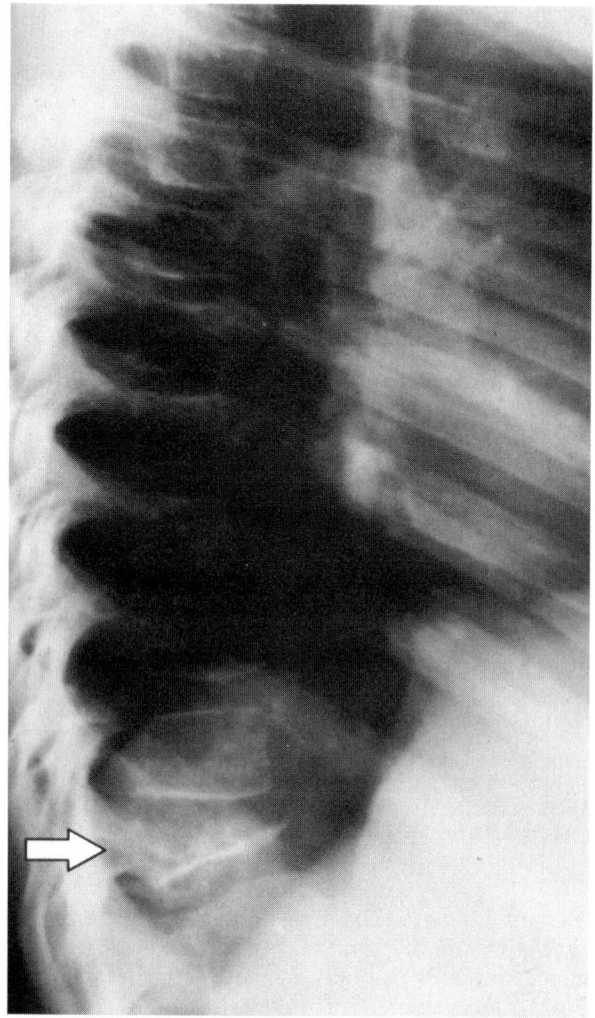

FIGURE 229–5. Lumbar eosinophilic granuloma. Lateral radiograph of the thoracic spine demonstrates a classic vertebra plana *(arrow)*. (Courtesy of Dr. Daniel Mass, Section of Orthopedic Surgery, University of Chicago.)

REFERENCES

1. Beer SJ, Menezes AH: Primary tumors of the spine in children: Natural history, management, and long-term follow-up. Spine 22:649–658, 1997.
2. Menezes AH, Sato Y: Primary tumors of the spine in children—natural history and management. Pediatr Neurosurg 23:101–113, 1995.
3. Payne WK, Ogilvie JW: Back pain in children and adolescents. Pediatr Clin North Am 43:899–917, 1996.
4. Raskas DS, Graziano GP, Herzenberg JE, et al: Osteoid osteoma and osteoblastoma of the spine. J Spinal Disord 5:204–211, 1992.
5. Pettine KA, Klassen RA: Osteoid-osteoma and osteoblastoma of the spine. J Bone Joint Surg Am 68:354–361, 1986.
6. Janin Y, Epstein JA, Carras R, et al: Osteoid osteomas and osteoblastomas of the spine. Neurosurgery 8:31–38, 1981.
7. MacLellan DI, Wilson FC: Osteoid osteoma of the spine: A review of the literature and report of six new cases. J Bone Joint Surg 49:111–121, 1967.
8. Hasegawa T, Hirose T, Sakamoto R, et al: Mechanism of pain in osteoid osteomas: An immunohistochemical study. Histopathology 22:487–491, 1993.
9. O'Connell JX, Nanthakumar SS, Nielsen GP, et al: Osteoid osteoma: The uniquely innervated bone tumor. Mod Pathol 11:175–180, 1998.
10. Greenspan A: Benign bone-forming lesions: Osteoma, osteoid osteoma, and osteoblastoma. Clinical, imaging, pathologic, and differential considerations. Skeletal Radiol 22:485–500, 1993.
11. Youssef BA, Haddad MC, Zahrani A, et al: Osteoid osteoma and osteoblastoma: MRI appearances and the significance of ring enhancement. Eur Radiol 6:291–296, 1996.
12. Radcliffe SN, Walsh HJ, Carty H: Osteoid osteoma: The difficult diagnosis. Eur J Radiol 28:67–79, 1998.
13. Simon MA: Percutaneous radiofrequency coagulation of osteoid osteoma compared with operative treatment. J Bone Joint Surg Am 81:437–438, 1999.
14. Baunin C, Puget C, Assoun J, et al: Percutaneous resection of osteoid osteoma under CT guidance in eight children. Pediatr Radiol 24:185–188, 1994.
15. Boriani S, Capanna R, Donati D, et al: Osteoblastoma of the spine. Clin Orthop 278:37–45, 1992.
16. Lucas DR, Unni KK, McLeod RA, et al: Osteoblastoma: Clinicopathologic study of 306 cases. Hum Pathol 25:117–134, 1994.
17. Frassica FJ, Waltrip RL, Sponseller PD, et al: Clinicopathologic features and treatment of osteoid osteoma and osteoblastoma in children and adolescents. Orthop Clin North Am 27:559–574, 1996.
18. Saifuddin A, White J, Sherazi Z, et al: Osteoid osteoma and osteoblastoma of the spine: Factors associated with the presence of scoliosis. Spine 23:47–53, 1998.
19. Shaikh MI, Saifuddin A, Pringle J, et al: Spinal osteoblastoma: CT and MR imaging with pathological correlation. Skeletal Radiol 28:33–40, 1999.
20. Cerase A, Priolo F: Skeletal benign bone-forming lesions. Eur J Radiol 27:S91–S97, 1998.
21. Nemoto O, Moser RP Jr, Van Dam BE, et al: Osteoblastoma of the spine: A review of 75 cases. Spine 15:1272–1280, 1990.
22. Della Rocca C, Huvos AG: Osteoblastoma: Varied histological presentations with a benign clinical course. An analysis of 55 cases. Am J Surg Pathol 20:841–850, 1996.
23. Di Lorenzo N, Delfini R, Ciappetta P, et al: Primary tumors of the cervical spine: Surgical experience with 38 cases. Surg Neurol 38:12–18, 1992.
24. Myles ST, MacRae ME: Benign osteoblastoma of the spine in childhood. J Neurosurg 68:884–888, 1988.
25. Schutte HE, Taconis WK: Giant cell tumor in children and adolescents. Skeletal Radiol 22:173–176, 1993.
26. Masui F, Ushigome S, Fujii K: Giant cell tumor of bone: An immunohistochemical comparative study. Pathol Int 48:355–361, 1998.
27. Gamberi G, Benassi MS, Bohling T, et al: Prognostic relevance of C-*myc* gene expression in giant-cell tumor of bone. J Orthop Res 16:1–7, 1998.
28. Chakravarti A, Spiro IJ, Hug EB, et al: Megavoltage radiation therapy for axial and inoperable giant-cell tumor of bone. J Bone Joint Surg Am 81:1566–1573, 1999.
29. Khan DC, Malhotra S, Stevens RE, et al: Radiotherapy for the treatment of giant cell tumor of the spine: A report of six cases and review of the literature. Cancer Invest 17:110–113, 1999.
30. Malone S, O'Sullivan B, Catton C, et al: Long-term follow-up of efficacy and safety of megavoltage radiotherapy in high-risk giant cell tumors of bone. Int J Radiat Oncol Biol Phys 33:689–694, 1995.
31. Sanjay BK, Sim FH, Unni KK, et al: Giant-cell tumours of the spine. J Bone Joint Surg Br 75:148–154, 1993.
32. Pfeifer FM, Bridge JA, Neff JR, et al: Cytogenetic findings in aneurysmal bone cysts. Genes Chromosomes Cancer 3:416–419, 1991.
33. Kransdorf MJ, Sweet DE: Aneurysmal bone cyst: Concept, controversy, clinical presentation, and imaging. AJR Am J Roentgenol 164:573–580, 1995.
34. Ruiter DJ, van Rijssel TG, van der Velde EA: Aneurysmal bone cysts: A clinicopathological study of 105 cases. Cancer 39:2231–2239, 1977.
35. Leithner A, Windhager R, Lang S, et al: Aneurysmal bone cyst: A population based epidemiologic study and literature review. Clin Orthop 363:176–179, 1999.
36. Capanna R, Albisinni U, Picci P, et al: Aneurysmal bone cyst of the spine. J Bone Joint Surg Am 67:527–531, 1985.
37. Ozaki T, Halm H, Hillmann A, et al: Aneurysmal bone cysts of the spine. Arch Orthop Trauma Surg 119:159–162, 1999.

38. Vergel De Dios AM, Bond JR, Shives TC, et al: Aneurysmal bone cyst: A clinicopathologic study of 238 cases. Cancer 69: 2921–2931, 1992.

39. de Kleuver M, van der Heul RO, Veraart BE: Aneurysmal bone cyst of the spine: 31 cases and the importance of the surgical approach. J Pediatr Orthop B 7:286–292, 1998.

40. Schreuder HW, Veth RP, Pruszczynski M, et al: Aneurysmal bone cysts treated by curettage, cryotherapy and bone grafting. J Bone Joint Surg Br 79:20–25, 1997.

41. Marcove RC, Sheth DS, Takemoto S, et al: The treatment of aneurysmal bone cyst. Clin Orthop 311:157–163, 1995.

42. De Cristofaro R, Biagini R, Boriani S, et al: Selective arterial embolization in the treatment of aneurysmal bone cyst and angioma of bone. Skeletal Radiol 21:523–527, 1992.

43. Duprez T, Lokietek W, Clapuyt P, et al: Multiple aggressive vertebral haemangiomas in an adolescent: A case report. Pediatr Radiol 28:51–53, 1998.

44. Paige ML, Hemmati M: Spinal cord compression by vertebral hemangioma. Pediatr Radiol 6:43–45, 1977.

45. Fox MW, Onofrio BM: The natural history and management of symptomatic and asymptomatic vertebral hemangiomas. J Neurosurg 78:36–45, 1993.

46. Raco A, Ciappetta P, Artico M, et al: Vertebral hemangiomas with cord compression: The role of embolization in five cases. Surg Neurol 34:164–168, 1990.

47. Goyal M, Mishra NK, Sharma A, et al: Alcohol ablation of symptomatic vertebral hemangiomas. AJNR Am J Neuroradiol 20:1091–1096, 1999.

48. Lonser RR, Heiss JD, Oldfield EH: Tumor devascularization by intratumoral ethanol injection during surgery: Technical note. J Neurosurg 88:923–924, 1998.

49. Heiss JD, Doppman JL, Oldfield EH: Treatment of vertebral hemangioma by intralesional injection of absolute ethanol. N Engl J Med 334:1340, 1996.

50. Faria SL, Schlupp WR, Chiminazzo H Jr: Radiotherapy in the treatment of vertebral hemangiomas. Int J Radiat Oncol Biol Phys 11:387–390, 1985.

51. Asthana AK, Tandon SC, Pant GC, et al: Radiation therapy for symptomatic vertebral haemangioma. Clin Oncol (R Coll Radiol) 2:159–162, 1990.

52. Sakata K, Hareyama M, Oouchi A, et al: Radiotherapy of vertebral hemangiomas. Acta Oncol 36:719–724, 1997.

53. Rao VV, Schnittger S, Hansmann I: G protein Gs alpha (GNAS 1), the probable candidate gene for Albright hereditary osteodystrophy, is assigned to human chromosome 20q12–q13.2. Genomics 10:257–261, 1991.

54. Schwindinger WF, Francomano CA, Levine MA: Identification of a mutation in the gene encoding the alpha subunit of the stimulatory G protein of adenylyl cyclase in McCune-Albright syndrome. Proc Natl Acad Sci U S A 89:5152–5156, 1992.

55. Marie PJ, de Pollak C, Chanson P, et al: Increased proliferation of osteoblastic cells expressing the activating Gs alpha mutation in monostotic and polyostotic fibrous dysplasia. Am J Pathol 150: 1059–1069, 1997.

56. Alman BA, Greel DA, Wolfe HJ: Activating mutations of Gs protein in monostotic fibrous lesions of bone. J Orthop Res 14: 311–315, 1996.

57. Shenker A, Chanson P, Weinstein LS, et al: Osteoblastic cells derived from isolated lesions of fibrous dysplasia contain activating somatic mutations of the Gs alpha gene. Hum Mol Genet 4: 1675–1676, 1995.

58. Resnik CS, Lininger JR: Monostotic fibrous dysplasia of the cervical spine: Case report. Radiology 151:49–50, 1984.

59. Troop JK, Herring JA: Monostotic fibrous dysplasia of the lumbar spine: Case report and review of the literature. J Pediatr Orthop 8:599–601, 1988.

60. Wright JF, Stoker DJ: Fibrous dysplasia of the spine. Clin Radiol 39:523–527, 1988.

61. Mezzadri JJ, Acotto CG, Mautalen C, et al: Surgical treatment of cervical spine fibrous dysplasia: Technical case report and review. Neurosurgery 44:1342–1346, 1999.

62. Nishiura I, Koyama T, Takayama S: Fibrous dysplasia of the cervical spine with atlanto-axial dislocation. Neurochirurgia (Stuttg) 35:123–126, 1992.

63. Przybylski GJ, Pollack IF, Ward WT: Monostotic fibrous dysplasia of the thoracic spine: A case report. Spine 21:860–865, 1996.

64. Oba M, Nakagami W, Maeda M, et al: Symptomatic monostotic fibrous dysplasia of the thoracic spine. Spine 23:741–743, 1998.

65. Guille JT, Bowen JR: Scoliosis and fibrous dysplasia of the spine. Spine 20:248–251, 1995.

66. Villas C, Martinez-Peric R, Barrios RH, et al: Eosinophilic granuloma of the spine with and without vertebra plana: Long-term follow-up of six cases. J Spinal Disord 6:260–268, 1993.

67. Floman Y, Bar-On E, Mosheiff R, et al: Eosinophilic granuloma of the spine. J Pediatr Orthop B 6:260–265, 1997.

68. Kumar A: Eosinophilic granuloma of the spine with neurological deficit. Orthopedics 13:1310–1312, 1990.

69. Scarpinati M, Artico M, Artizzu S: Spinal cord compression by eosinophilic granuloma of the cervical spine: Case report and review of the literature. Neurosurg Rev 18:209–212, 1995.

70. Boriani S, Biagini R, De Iure F, et al: Low back pain in tumors: Diagnosis and treatment. Chir Organi Mov 79:93–99, 1994.

71. Davies AM, Pikoulas C, Griffith J: MRI of eosinophilic granuloma. Eur J Radiol 18:205–209, 1994.

72. Seimon LP: Eosinophil granuloma of the spine. J Pediatr Orthop 1:371–376, 1981.

73. Mammano S, Candiotto S, Balsano M: Cast and brace treatment of eosinophilic granuloma of the spine: Long-term follow-up. J Pediatr Orthop 17:821–827, 1997.

74. Raab P, Hohmann F, Kuhl J, et al: Vertebral remodeling in eosinophilic granuloma of the spine: A long-term follow-up. Spine 23: 1351–1354, 1998.

75. Maggi G, de Sanctis N, Aliberti F, et al: Eosinophilic granuloma of C4 causing spinal cord compression. Childs Nerv Syst 12: 630–632, 1996.

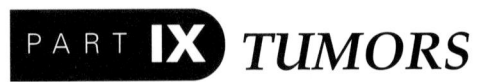

CHAPTER **230**

Optic Pathway and Hypothalamic Gliomas in Children

JEFFREY H. WISOFF

Optic pathway tumors constitute a spectrum of lesions ranging from tubular thickening of the optic nerves and chiasm to massive exophytic tumors of the hypothalamus. Optic pathway gliomas represent 3% to 6% of all pediatric brain tumors and occur with equal frequency in males and females.[1, 2] Approximately 10% to 30% are confined to a unilateral optic nerve, whereas the majority involve some combination of optic chiasm, optic tracts, hypothalamus, and third ventricle.[1-4] The association between these tumors, especially prechiasmatic optic nerve gliomas, and neurofibromatosis type 1 is well known: 20% to 50% of patients with optic pathway gliomas have neurofibromatosis, and 15% of patients with neurofibromatosis have a lesion in the visual pathway.[1-10]

The natural history of these neoplasms is variable. The benign histology of some of these tumors is often in marked contrast to their malignant clinical course in children. Some reports have suggested that optic gliomas behave similarly to hamartomas, remaining quiescent for years and requiring only expectant observation.[6, 11-13] The majority of tumors, particularly those involving the optic chiasm and hypothalamus, progress insidiously, leading to visual loss, vegetative compromise, and, if untreated, death.[1-4, 8, 9, 14, 15]

The anatomic location of these neoplasms and their intimate association with the visual pathways, hypothalamus, and limbic system predispose patients to severe visual, endocrine, and cognitive deficits, both at presentation and as a result of treatment. Although most children can compensate for neurological deficits and endocrine deficiencies, the cognitive and psychosocial sequelae may be functionally devastating, interfering with education, limiting independence, and adversely affecting the quality of life as these children approach adulthood.[16]

PATHOLOGY

Pilocytic astrocytoma is the most frequent histology in optic pathway gliomas and is almost universally present in optic nerve tumors. Low-grade fibrillary astrocytoma is the other common tumor type, whereas ganglioglioma, malignant astrocytoma, and glioblastoma are rare.[1] Mathematical models suggest that these tumors have a wide but continuous range of growth rates. Some grow rapidly enough to be explained by simple exponential doubling at a constant rate but may behave as though their growth decelerates.[3, 17]

Optic pathway gliomas tend to be more aggressive in children younger than 2 to 5 years, with an increased recurrence rate, a tendency to disseminate along the cerebrospinal fluid pathways, and a higher mortality rate.[1-4, 7, 9, 14, 15, 18-20] In my experience, the MIB-1 labeling index is significantly higher in tumors in children younger than 2 years. Recently, a variant of pilocytic astrocytoma with a distinctive monomorphous pilomyxoid histologic pattern was described.[21] Rosenthal fibers were not seen, and eosinophilic granular bodies were rare. The majority of these tumors occurred in infants and young children, involved the hypothalamic-chiasmatic region, and had a high rate of recurrence and dissemination.

Visual pathway gliomas in children with neurofibromatosis differ from those in children without neurofibromatosis. In general, lesions tend to be more extensive in patients with neurofibromatosis, infiltrating and following the optic radiations with a variable clinical course.[1, 7, 22]

CLINICAL PRESENTATION

The signs and symptoms of all suprasellar tumors are dependent on their direction of growth and compression of adjacent structures, not their histology. Optic pathway tumors have two basic patterns of clinical presentation: (1) neurological, ophthalmic, or neuropsychological deficits from mass effect or tumor infiltration, and (2) partial or complete hypopituitarism.

Often there is a combination of hormonal deficits and mass effect. Formal preoperative neuro-ophthalmologic, endocrinologic, and neuropsychological evaluations are mandatory.

A number of classification schemes have been suggested based on anatomic staging and visual function,[23] radiographic appearance,[5] and patient age.[20] I use a three-level classification based on preoperative magnetic resonance imaging (MRI) to guide surgical intervention[2, 15]: prechiasmatic optic nerve glioma, diffuse chiasmatic glioma, and exophytic chiasmatic-hypothalamic glioma.

Prechiasmatic Optic Nerve Glioma

Prechiasmatic optic nerve glioma presents over 6 to 9 months with progressive visual loss and proptosis.[4, 6, 9, 24, 25] The affected eye is displaced inferiorly and laterally. In infants, nystagmus and strabismus may be the first signs of visual deficits. Funduscopic examination usually demonstrates papilledema with venous engorgement, although optic atrophy may occasionally be seen with a longer prodrome. Asymptomatic tumors are often diagnosed in children with neurofibromatosis type 1, who are routinely screened with MRI.[7]

The differential diagnosis of proptosis in children includes primary and metastatic orbital tumors, fibrous dysplasia, paranasal mucocele, and agenesis of the sphenoid wing.

Diffuse Chiasmatic Glioma

Diffuse chiasmatic glioma manifests a combination of diminished visual acuity and bilateral, often incongruous, visual field deficits. Endocrinopathy and hydrocephalus are rare. Most children with this tumor have neurofibromatosis and may be diagnosed on surveillance MRI scans.

Exophytic Chiasmatic-Hypothalamic Glioma

These tumors have three distinct age-related patterns of clinical presentation. Infants (younger than 2 years) present with macrocephaly, failure to thrive–diencephalic syndrome, and visual failure. Severe hydrocephalus with signs of incipient herniation may mandate emergency cerebrospinal fluid shunting. The tumors are typically massive on imaging studies.

In children 2 to 5 years old, endocrine dysfunction, often with precocious puberty or short stature, is the most common presentation.[2, 9] Although visual deficits are demonstrated in most children, they are seldom the presenting complaint. Headache and vomiting may indicate extension into the third ventricle and consequent hydrocephalus. Rarely, seizure, hemiparesis, loss of developmental milestones, and deteriorating academic performance may initiate a neurological evaluation.

Older children and young adults most often present with visual complaints. Hypopituitarism is common,

and a complete endocrinologic evaluation is mandatory.

RADIOLOGY

Neuroimaging often establishes the histologic diagnosis as well as defining the location and extent of the cystic and solid portions of the tumor and its relationship to the distorted normal anatomy. The initial radiographic evaluation includes both noncontrast computed tomography and gadolinium-enhanced MRI. Vascular anatomy can be well demonstrated by MRI and magnetic resonance angiography, obviating the need for invasive cerebral angiography.[26]

When available, additional biologic and diagnostic information may be obtained through magnetic resonance spectroscopy.[26–28] Proton magnetic resonance spectroscopy demonstrates unique profiles that may assist in the differential diagnosis of suprasellar tumors.[27] Craniopharyngiomas show a dominant peak consistent with lactate or lipids and only trace amounts of other metabolites. Pituitary adenomas show either choline peaks or no metabolites at all. In contrast, gliomas demonstrate choline, *N*-acetylaspartate, and creatine, with an increased ratio of choline to *N*-acetylaspartate compared with normal brain. High normalized choline values may identify histologically low-grade gliomas with a propensity for more aggressive behavior.[29]

Computed tomography and MRI have complementary roles in the diagnosis of suprasellar tumors.[26, 28, 30, 31] Computed tomography better demonstrates the extent and nature of tumor calcification, as well as showing secondary changes in the skull base, such as enlargement of the sella turcica or erosion of the dorsum sellae. The presence of calcification in a newly diagnosed suprasellar tumor is strongly suggestive of craniopharyngioma.

MRI and magnetic resonance angiography provide valuable information about the tumor's relationships to surrounding structures, delineating the involvement or displacement of the visual pathways, hypothalamus, ventricles, and vessels of the circle of Willis. The surgeon's impression of the extent of tumor resection must be confirmed by neuroimaging. Postoperative imaging with enhanced MRI is best done within 48 hours to avoid the artifacts of surgical trauma.[26]

Prechiasmatic optic nerve gliomas demonstrate fusiform enlargement of the nerve within the orbit, within the optic canal, or intracranially, but without involvement of the optic chiasm. T2-weighted images do not demonstrate increased signal in the chiasm or optic tracts. Bilateral lesions may be seen in neurofibromatosis.

Diffuse chiasmatic gliomas demonstrate diffuse enlargement of the optic chiasm with variable extension into the optic tracts and nerves. Gadolinium-enhanced and T2-weighted MRI scans are particularly helpful in delineating these tumors and the involvement of contiguous structures. MRI findings are pathognomonic in the presence of neurofibromatosis. Germ cell tumors, sarcoidosis, and suprasellar dermoid should be considered in the absence of neurofibromatosis.

Exophytic chiasmatic-hypothalamic gliomas have large, bulky, exophytic extension into the suprasellar-parasellar spaces and third ventricle. It is often difficult to delineate whether the optic nerve is incorporated into the tumor or is being extrinsically compressed by the exophytic mass. These tumors usually enhance with gadolinium in a diffuse or patchy pattern. Intratumoral cysts may be present. In infants, associated nonneoplastic arachnoid cysts are often immediately adjacent to the tumor and extend into the sylvian fissure. Lack of calcification on computed tomography helps differentiate these tumors from craniopharyngiomas. Complete neuraxis imaging is essential, particularly in children younger than 5 years, because dissemination may be present at diagnosis.

TREATMENT

The management of visual pathway gliomas is controversial. Some of the confusion in interpreting outcomes is a result of inadequate organization of the spectrum of tumors and historically limited therapeutic options. The erratic natural history of these tumors confounds evaluation of the efficacy of the chosen regimen.[32] Categorization of the pattern and extent of growth assists in evaluating treatment options and potential surgical approaches and in predicting outcome.

Surgery

All intracranial surgery is performed with the operating microscope, usually under moderate to high magnification. Surgical adjuncts, including the ultrasonic aspirator, frameless stereotaxy, and rigid and flexible neuroendoscopes, should be available and used when appropriate.

PRECHIASMATIC OPTIC NERVE GLIOMA

Surgical excision is curative for lesions confined to a single optic nerve without extension to the chiasm.[3, 25] The goal of surgery is preservation of the globe and prevention of tumor extension into the chiasm. Total excision is indicated in children with increasing proptosis, progressive visual loss, radiographic evidence of an enlarging tumor, and a blind eye. Proptosis alone may be an indication for surgery when it produces pain, endangers the health of the cornea or globe, or causes significant cosmetic disfigurement.[4]

The entire lesion is removed en bloc through a unilateral pterional craniotomy. After an intradural inspection of the intracranial optic nerve and chiasm to ensure that there is no posterior extension of the tumor, the orbit and optic canal are unroofed with a high-speed microdrill and diamond bits. The nerve is identified within the orbit and divided just posterior to the globe. The globe is left in situ so that it may continue normal growth and prevent a future cosmetic deficit. Intracranially, the nerve is sectioned at the posterior limit of the tumor, which is variable distance from the chiasm. The low-grade histology of these tumors makes intraoperative biopsy and frozen section unreliable in delineating a clean margin. The surgical specimen should have the posterior aspect "tagged" by the surgeon so that a clean margin can be confirmed by pathologic examination. Residual tumor anterior to the chiasm is an indication for reoperation. Unfortunately, 25% of optic nerve tumors have invaded the chiasm at the time of diagnosis.[3]

In the absence of progressive symptoms or radiographic evidence of tumor growth, most authors support a more moderate approach.[2, 4, 11, 25, 33, 34] The frequent indolent course of these tumors, particularly in children with neurofibromatosis, supports expectant management. Serial visual acuity and visual field examinations, or visual evoked potentials in younger children, and periodic MRI scans permit therapy to be deferred until definitive clinical or radiographic progression is documented, with an extremely low risk of significant visual loss or posterior extension into the chiasm.

DIFFUSE CHIASMATIC GLIOMA

Surgical intervention is rarely indicated for diffuse chiasmatic tumors. The characteristic MRI appearance in the setting of neurofibromatosis is pathognomonic of a chiasmal tumor and obviates the need for histologic confirmation. Biopsy may be indicated when the radiographic or clinical presentation is atypical.

EXOPHYTIC CHIASMATIC-HYPOTHALAMIC GLIOMA

Large, exophytic tumors extending into the suprasellar and parasellar cisterns or superiorly into the third ventricle may be amenable to radical resection. Several reports noted that many of these patients had visual symptoms secondary to compression of the optic chiasm and tracts by the exophytic component of the tumor.[2, 9, 15, 35, 36] The operative approach depends on the direction of maximal tumor growth: suprasellar or perimesencephalic extension requires a pterional approach, whereas a predominantly third ventricular tumor indicates the need for a transcallosal route. Frameless stereotaxy, the operating microscope, and the ultrasonic aspirator are indispensable adjuncts. My experience with visual evoked potentials has been unsatisfactory; they are difficult to record and may not correlate with postoperative visual function.

The initial approach is identical to the pterional craniotomy for craniopharyngioma as advocated by Yasargil and colleagues.[37] This approach offers the shortest, most direct route to the suprasellar region and, with splitting of the sylvian fissure, minimizes or eliminates retraction of normal brain. Tumors extending from the pontomedullary junction to above the foramen of Monro can be removed through the pterional approach. This approach has been used for the other suprasellar tumors with certain modifications based on histology and potential intra-axial extension.

Dexamethasone (0.1 mg/kg), phenytoin (15 mg/kg), and cephalothin (25 mg/kg) are administered after induction and intubation. Mannitol (0.25 g/kg) is given at the time of skin incision to help maximize brain relaxation. The diuretic effect is maximal within the first hour of surgery, long before manipulation of the pituitary stalk and hypothalamus may produce diabetes insipidus, which complicates fluid and electrolyte management. A 7-cm frontotemporal craniotomy is performed, with removal of the sphenoid wing; when necessary, the orbital rim and zygomatic process of the frontal bone can be removed with the craniotomy flap to obtain a wider operative corridor and shorter distance to the tumor. Before opening the dura, frameless stereotaxy is used to determine the location and extent of the tumor and its relationship to the operative exposure.

Throughout the surgery, retraction of the brain is minimized. Mannitol, hyperventilation, and gradual drainage of cerebrospinal fluid through the opened sylvian fissure and basal cisterns usually provide excellent relaxation, even in the presence of moderate degrees of hydrocephalus. Ventricular drainage is reserved for cases refractory to these maneuvers. Preoperative shunting is reserved for patients with severe symptoms of increased intracranial pressure that is unresponsive to medical management.

Identification of the vascular anatomy, from distal to proximal, is crucial, because these tumors extend diffusely throughout the suprasellar cisterns, displacing and distorting normal anatomy. In my experience, approximately half these tumors involve one or both optic nerves, and the other half extrinsically compress the visual apparatus. Because these tumors often extended diffusely throughout the suprasellar cisterns, displacing and distorting normal structures, identification of the vascular anatomy provides essential landmarks. Starting laterally, the sylvian fissure is widely split, and the distal branches of the middle cerebral artery are identified. Bipolar cauterization is limited to avoid fusing arachnoid planes. The arachnoidal dissection proceeds medially to the main trunk of the middle cerebral artery, which is followed proximally to the ipsilateral carotid bifurcation, anterior cerebral artery, and internal carotid artery. As the carotid is followed proximally to the clinoid, the optic nerve, chiasm, or tracts are identified in relation to the tumor.

As the branches of the carotid artery and circle of Willis are identified, an arachnoidal plane can be established around the tumor. Working in the prechiasmatic, opticocarotid, and carotidotentorial triangles, one may develop and maintain an arachnoidal plane between the intact tumor and the branches of the ipsilateral carotid artery and vessels of the circle of Willis, preserving all vessels and their perforating branches. Because the tumor is originating from the chiasm and hypothalamus, perforating arteries may be directly involved with the tumor and must be preserved. When possible, this plane is developed posteriorly until the basilar artery is identified.

When both optic nerves can be identified, the initial resection is between the nerves, anterior to the enlarged chiasm. Resection of this portion of the tumor decompresses the nerves and may result in an improvement in visual acuity. If the nerves cannot be clearly delineated, dissection proceeds along the tuberculum sellae to both optic foramina. The tumor is incised midway between the foramina, and an internal decompression is performed with the ultrasonic aspirator. Often, as the tumor is resected, the markedly attenuated nerves become visible.

The remainder of the exophytic component can be resected by internally debulking the tumor with either bipolar and fine suction or the ultrasonic aspirator and then gradually dissecting the capsule free of the vessels and "rolling" the tumor in on itself. As the tumor is aspirated, additional glioma often spontaneously descends to "deliver" itself into the resection cavity. When appropriate, the lamina terminalis can be opened to aid internal decompression. Resection is complete when all suprasellar structures not contiguous with the tumor are cleanly dissected and no further tumor can be internally resected.

Tumors located primarily in the third ventricle are approached transcallosally. Frameless stereotaxy guides both the approach and the extent of lateral and deep tumor resection. The corpus callosum is incised for less than 2 cm. I previously used an interforniceal entry into the third ventricle[2]; however, a transforaminal approach through the foramen of Monro, and opening of the choroidal fissure when necessary, avoids potential injury to the fornices and provides excellent exposure. The posterior aspect of the tumor is usually free of the ependyma and can easily be identified. The tumor is gradually resected until the lateral ependymal walls or glial tumor interface is encountered. Stereotaxy helps confirm the relationship of the tumor to normal parenchyma. As the floor of the third ventricle is approached, fine suction and the bipolar forceps are used to resect the tumor in a piecemeal fashion. Overzealous resection may result in removal of normal, laterally displaced hypothalamus or unexpected penetration into the suprasellar cistern, with the potential for vascular injury.

Irradiation

Although there is no consensus about the optimal treatment of subtotally resected tumors, therapeutic irradiation has been the traditional adjuvant therapy for children with optic pathway gliomas and progressive disease.[3, 9, 38–40] Doses over 4500 cGy are required to obtain local control of tumor growth,[3] with most authors recommending 5000 to 5500 cGy.[3, 4, 9, 38–40] Even with conformal techniques, the typical large exophytic chiasmatic-hypothalamic tumor requires radiation fields that encompass the normal temporal lobe, frontal lobe, and pituitary.

Chemotherapy

Chemotherapy has been advocated as an alternative to irradiation for young children with chiasmatic-hypothalamic gliomas.[9, 32, 41–51] The decision to use chemotherapy is based on several factors: (1) patient age, (2) whether the child has neurofibromatosis type 1, (3) tumor size and location, (4) potential sequelae of radiotherapy, and (5) acute and long-term toxicity of the chemotherapeutic approach used.[32] Several different therapeutic protocols have been reported, including vincristine and actinomycin D,[49, 51] carboplatin,[45] vincristine and carboplatin,[48] oral etoposide,[41] and a five-drug nitrosourea-based regimen.[50]

OUTCOME

Surgery

In my experience, older children with newly diagnosed and recurrent exophytic chiasmatic-hypothalamic gliomas had an excellent response to radical surgery, with 70% achieving a 5-year event-free survival.[2, 15] These children tolerated surgical resection with acceptable morbidity and no operative mortality. Among older children, 75% are stable or improved after surgery. A recent multi-institutional study of the natural history of low-grade gliomas of childhood from the Children's Oncology Group showed a greater than 50% 5-year progression-free survival for subtotally resected chiasmatic-hypothalamic gliomas.[52] Further spontaneous involution of tumor after surgery has been reported[14, 53] and was seen in five of my patients. Deterioration in visual acuity or fields may be seen in approximately 15% of these children following operation, particularly among those with diffuse extension of the tumor into the optic nerves. Permanent new diabetes insipidus occurred predominantly with large third ventricular tumors that underwent radical subtotal or near-total resections using a transcallosal approach.

Infants and young children fared considerably worse than older children. Prognosis for survival and functional outcome was generally dismal, although symptomatic improvement was usually obtained, with relief of mass effect in all infants presenting with increased intracranial pressure. In those infants and young children presenting with diencephalic syndrome, radical resection resulted in resolution of the symptoms. In agreement with other reported series[20, 54, 55] and my own early experience,[2, 15] almost all the infants had a malignant course in spite of a benign histology. The early progression in infants is related to age and tumor biology rather than tumor size or location. The recent description of pilomyxoid astrocytomas[21] and their separation from other low-grade gliomas may explain this phenomenon. The high failure rate demonstrates the inadequacy of surgical resection as the sole therapy in infants and mandates the use of multimodality adjuvant treatments.

Irradiation

Stabilization of tumor size or diminished tumor volume following irradiation has been well documented,[10, 38, 56–58] yet clinical improvement in visual function and neurological deficits occurs in only a minority of children.[8] Approximately 50% of the tumors regress,[9, 59] with a median time to maximal radiographic response as long as 5 years.[4]

The recurrence rate appears to be significantly lower in irradiated children, but documentation of improved survival is lacking.[9, 60] Ten-year progression-free survival varies between 55% and 100%.[8, 10, 38, 56, 58] Long-term sequelae of irradiation include neuropsychological deficits, endocrinopathy, vasculopathy (Moyamoya syndrome), visual failure, and radiation-induced secondary neoplasms.[1, 8, 14, 22, 61, 62] Radiation may also induce anaplastic transformation of low-grade gliomas in childhood after a latency of several years.[63]

Chemotherapy

Chemotherapy is an increasingly important component in the management of chiasmatic-hypothalamic gliomas. The primary rationale for using chemotherapy has been to delay the need for irradiation in children younger than 5 years. Clinical trials have demonstrated that optic pathway gliomas may be successfully treated and stabilized with single-agent or multiagent regimens.[9, 32, 41–51] Initial disease control can be established in more than 90% of children; however, less than half of patients have a significant reduction in tumor volume.[44, 64]

The relative efficacy of one regimen compared with another has not been established. Progression-free survival is similar among the various regimens: 62% at 4 years for vincristine–actinomycin D,[49] 74% at 3 years for carboplatin-vincristine,[48, 64] 58% at 3 years for carboplatin alone,[45] and 132 weeks median time to progression for the five-drug nitrosourea-based regimen.[50] The Children's Oncology Group is currently conducting the first randomized trial between carboplatin-vincristine and a multiagent regimen (6-thioguanine, procarbazine, dibromodulcitol, CCNU, and vincristine).

Histology (juvenile pilocytic astrocytoma versus low-grade fibrillary astrocytoma) and presence of neurofibromatosis type 1 did not influence the response to chemotherapy.[64] Chemotherapy has permitted more than 70% of children to have irradiation treatment postponed until after age 5 years.[44]

CONCLUSION

In the post-MRI era, long-term survival and cure following excision of a unilateral optic nerve glioma approach 100%.[3, 25] Historically, with involvement of the chiasm and hypothalamus, 10-year progression-free survival has been poor; however, despite a high incidence of recurrent disease, actuarial survival is greater than 85%.[3, 10, 39, 51] Radical surgery in older children and the introduction of various chemotherapeutic regimens have improved the chance of prolonged progression-free survival. Age and the presence of neurofibromatosis also impact both recurrence and overall survival.

Because optic pathway gliomas are a chronic disease, sequential or combined use of different treatment modalities may be required to optimize both progression-free survival and the quality of life. Survivors may have visual, endocrine, and neuropsychological deficits.[44, 57, 65] Some may be present at diagnosis, and others are sequelae of treatment. The relative impact of different therapeutic strategies on the quality of life is unclear.[57]

REFERENCES

1. Hoffman HJ, Rutka JT: Optic pathway tumors in children. In Albright AL, Pollack IF, Adelson PD (eds): Principles and Practice of Pediatric Neurosurgery. New York, Thieme, 1999, pp 535–543.
2. Wisoff JH: Management of optic pathway tumors of childhood. Neurosurg Clin N Am 3:791–802, 1992.
3. Alvord EC Jr, Lofton S: Gliomas of the optic nerve or chiasm: Outcome by patients' age, tumor site, and treatment. J Neurosurg 68:85–98, 1988.
4. Tenny RT, Laws ER Jr, Younge BR, et al: The neurosurgical management of optic glioma: Results in 104 patients. J Neurosurg 57:452–458, 1982.
5. Fletcher WA, Imes RK, Hoyt WF: Chiasmal gliomas: Appearance and long-term changes demonstrated by computerized tomography. J Neurosurg 65:154–159, 1986.
6. Hoyt WF, Bagdassarian S: Optic glioma of childhood: Natural history and rationale for conservative management. Br J Ophthalmol 53:793–798, 1969.
7. Packer RJ, Bilaniuk LT, Cohen BH, et al: Intracranial visual pathway gliomas in children with neurofibromatosis. Neurofibromatosis 1:212–222, 1988.
8. Packer RJ, Savino PJ, Bilaniuk LT, et al: Chiasmatic gliomas of childhood: A reappraisal of natural history and effectiveness of cranial irradiation. Childs Brain 10:393–403, 1983.
9. Rodriguez LA, Edwards MS, Levin VA: Management of hypothalamic gliomas in children: An analysis of 33 cases. Neurosurgery 26:242–246, discussion 246–247, 1990.
10. Wong JY, Uhl V, Wara WM, et al: Optic gliomas: A reanalysis of the University of California, San Francisco, experience. Cancer 60:1847–1855, 1987.
11. Borit A, Richardson EP Jr: The biological and clinical behaviour of pilocytic astrocytomas of the optic pathways. Brain 105:161–187, 1982.
12. Imes RK, Hoyt WF: Childhood chiasmal gliomas: Update on the fate of patients in the 1969 San Francisco Study. Br J Ophthalmol 70:179–182, 1986.
13. Robertson AG, Brewin TB: Optic nerve glioma. Clin Radiol 31:471–474, 1980.
14. Hoffman HJ, Humphreys RP, Drake JM, et al: Optic pathway/hypothalamic gliomas: A dilemma in management. Pediatr Neurosurg 19:186–195, 1993.
15. Wisoff JH, Abbott IR, Epstein F: Surgical management of exophytic chiasmatic-hypothalamic tumors of childhood. J Neurosurg 73:661–667, 1990.
16. Fischer EG, Welch K, Shillito J Jr, et al: Craniopharyngiomas in children: Long-term effects of conservative surgical procedures combined with radiation therapy. J Neurosurg 73:534–540, 1990; see comments.
17. Lazareff J, Suwinski R, De Rosa R, et al: Tumor volume and growth kinetics in hypothalamic-chiasmatic pediatric low grade gliomas. Pediatr Neurosurg 30:312–319, 1999.
18. Bruggers CS, Friedman HS, Phillips PC, et al: Leptomeningeal dissemination of optic pathway gliomas in three children. Am J Ophthalmol 111:719–723, 1991.
19. Gajjar A, Bhargava R, Jenkins JJ, et al: Low-grade astrocytoma with neuroaxis dissemination at diagnosis. J Neurosurg 83:67–71, 1995.
20. Sugita K, Kageyama N: Treatment and follow up studies of the optic nerve gliomas: Infant and child types. Shoni No Noshikei 2:97–103, 1977.
21. Tihan T, Fisher PG, Kepner JL, et al: Pediatric astrocytomas with monomorphous pilomyxoid features and a less favorable outcome. J Neuropathol Exp Neurol 58:1061–1068, 1999.
22. Hoffman HJ, Soloniuk DS, Humphreys RP, et al: Management and outcome of low-grade astrocytomas of the midline in children: A retrospective review. Neurosurgery 33:964–971, 1993.
23. McCoullough D, Epstein F: Optic pathway tumors: A review with proposals for clinical staging. Cancer 56(Suppl):1789–1791, 1985.
24. Lloyd LA: Gliomas of the optic nerve and chiasm in childhood. Trans Am Ophthalmol Soc 71:488–535, 1973.
25. Wright JE, McNab AA, McDonald WI: Optic nerve glioma and the management of optic nerve tumours in the young. Br J Ophthalmol 73:967–974, 1989.
26. Harwood-Nash DC: Neuroimaging of childhood craniopharyngioma. Pediatr Neurosurg 21:2–10, 1994.
27. Sutton L, Wang Z, Wehrli S, et al: Proton spectroscopy of suprasellar tumors in pediatric patients. Neurosurgery 41:388–394, 1997.
28. Zimmerman R: Imaging of intrasellar, suprasellar, and parasellar tumors. Semin Roentgenol 25:174–197, 1990.
29. Lazareff J, Bockhorst K, Curran J, et al: Pediatric low-grade gliomas: Prognosis with proton magnetic resonance spectroscopic imaging. Neurosurgery 43:809–818, 1998.
30. Dattoli MJ, Newall J: Radiation therapy for intracranial germinoma: The case for limited volume treatment. Int J Radiat Oncol Biol Phys 19:429–433, 1990.
31. Tsuda M, Takahashi S, Higano S, et al: CT and MR imaging of craniopharyngioma. Eur Radiol 7:464–469, 1997.
32. Packer RJ: Chemotherapy: Low-grade gliomas of the hypothalamus and thalamus. Pediatr Neurosurg 32:259–263, 2000.
33. Hoyt WF, Fletcher WA, Imes RK: Chiasmal gliomas: Appearance and long-term changes demonstrated by computerized tomography. Prog Exp Tumor Res 30:113–121, 1987.
34. Laws ER, Taylor WF, Clifton MB, et al: Neurosurgical management of low-grade astrocytoma of the cerebral hemispheres. J Neurosurg 61:665–673, 1984.
35. Albright AL, Sclabassi RJ: Cavitron ultrasonic surgical aspirator and visual evoked potential monitoring for chiasmal gliomas in children: Report of two cases. J Neurosurg 63:138–140, 1985.
36. Gillett GR, Symon L: Hypothalamic glioma. Surg Neurol 28:291–300, 1987.
37. Yasargil MG, Curcic M, Kis M, et al: Total removal of craniopharyngiomas: Approaches and long-term results in 144 patients. J Neurosurg 73:3–11, 1990.
38. Flickinger JC, Torres C, Deutsch M: Management of low-grade gliomas of the optic nerve and chiasm. Cancer 61:635–642, 1988.
39. Kovalic JJ, Grigsby PW, Shepard MJ, et al: Radiation therapy for gliomas of the optic nerve and chiasm. Int J Radiat Oncol Biol Phys 18:927–932, 1990.
40. Pierce SM, Barnes PD, Loeffler JS, et al: Definitive radiation therapy in the management of symptomatic patients with optic glioma: Survival and long-term effects. Cancer 65:45–52, 1990.
41. Chamberlain MC: Recurrent chiasmatic-hypothalamic glioma treated with oral etoposide. Arch Neurol 52:509–513, 1995.
42. Chamberlain MC, Levin VA: Chemotherapeutic treatment of the diencephalic syndrome: A case report. Cancer 63:1681–1684, 1989.
43. Charrow J, Listernick R, Greenwald MJ, et al: Carboplatin-induced regression of an optic pathway tumor in a child with neurofibromatosis. Med Pediatr Oncol 21:680–684, 1993.
44. Janss AJ, Grundy R, Cnaan A, et al: Optic pathway and hypothalamic/chiasmatic gliomas in children younger than age 5 years with a 6-year follow-up. Cancer 75:1051–1059, 1995.
45. Mahoney D, Cohen ME, Friedman HS, et al: Carboplatin is effective therapy for young children with progressive optic pathway tumors: A Pediatric Oncology Group phase II study. Neurooncology 2:213–220, 2000.
46. Moghrabi A, Friedman HS, Burger PC, et al: Carboplatin treatment of progressive optic pathway gliomas to delay radiotherapy. J Neurosurg 79:223–227, 1993.
47. Nishio S, Morioka T, Takeshita I, et al: Chemotherapy for progressive pilocytic astrocytomas in the chiasmal-hypothalamic regions. Clin Neurol Neurosurg 97:300–306, 1995.
48. Packer RJ, Lange B, Ater J, et al: Carboplatin and vincristine for recurrent and newly diagnosed low-grade gliomas of childhood. J Clin Oncol 11:850–856, 1993.
49. Packer RJ, Sutton LN, Bilaniuk LT, et al: Treatment of chiasmatic/

hypothalamic gliomas of childhood with chemotherapy: An update. Ann Neurol 23:79–85, 1988.

50. Petronio J, Edwards MS, Prados M, et al: Management of chiasmal and hypothalamic gliomas of infancy and childhood with chemotherapy. J Neurosurg 74:701–708, 1991.

51. Rosenstock JG, Packer RJ, Bilaniuk L, et al: Chiasmatic optic glioma treated with chemotherapy: A preliminary report. J Neurosurg 63:862–866, 1985.

52. Wisoff JH, Sanford RA, Sposto R, et al: Low grade gliomas of childhood: Impact of surgical resection. A report from the Children's Oncology Group protocol CCG-9891/POG-9130: Treatment of newly diagnosed low-grade astrocytomas. Presented at the annual meeting of the American Association of Neurological Surgeons, 2002, Chicago.

53. Venes JL, Latack J, Kandt RS: Postoperative regression of optico-chiasmatic astrocytoma: A case for expectant therapy. Neurosurgery 15:421–423, 1984.

54. Davis PC, Hoffman JC Jr, Weidenheim KM: Large hypothalamic and optic chiasm gliomas in infants: Difficulties in distinction. AJNR Am J Neuroradiol 5:579–585, 1984.

55. Nishio S, Takeshita I, Fujiwara S, et al: Optico-hypothalamic glioma: An analysis of 16 cases. Childs Nerv Syst 9:334–338, 1993.

56. Erkal HS, Serin M, Cakmak A: Management of optic pathway and chiasmatic-hypothalamic gliomas in children with radiation therapy. Radiother Oncol 45:11–15, 1997.

57. Sutton LN, Molloy PT, Sernyak H, et al: Long-term outcome of hypothalamic/chiasmatic astrocytomas in children treated with conservative surgery. J Neurosurg 83:583–589, 1995.

58. Tao ML, Barnes PD, Billett AL, et al: Childhood optic chiasm gliomas: Radiographic response following radiotherapy and long-term clinical outcome. Int J Radiat Oncol Biol Phys 39:579–587, 1997.

59. Fisher B, Bauman G, Leighton C, et al: Low-grade gliomas in children: Tumor volume response to radiation. J Neurosurg 88:969–974, 1998.

60. Imes RK, Hoyt WF: Childhood chiasmal gliomas: Update on the fate of patients in the 1969 San Francisco Study. Prog Exp Tumor Res 30:108–112, 1987.

61. Duffner PK, Cohen ME, Thompson P, et al: The long term effects of cranial irradiation on the central nervous system. Cancer 56:1841–1847, 1985.

62. Sinsawaiwong S, Phanthumchinda K: Progressive cerebral occlusive disease after hypothalamic astrocytoma radiation therapy. J Med Assoc Thai 80:338–342, 1997.

63. Dirks PB, Jay V, Becker LE, et al: Development of anaplastic changes in low-grade astrocytomas of childhood. Neurosurgery 34:68–78, 1994.

64. Packer RJ, Ater J, Allen J, et al: Carboplatin and vincristine chemotherapy for children with newly diagnosed progressive low-grade gliomas. J Neurosurg 86:747–754, 1997.

65. Collet-Solberg PF, Sernyak H, Satin-Smith M, et al: Endocrine outcome in long-term survivors of low-grade hypothalamic/chiasmatic glioma. Clin Endocrinol (Oxf) 47:79–85, 1997.

CHAPTER 231

Intracranial Germ Cell Tumors

ALYSSA T. REDDY ■ TIMOTHY B. MAPSTONE

Intracranial germ cell tumors are a relatively rare central nervous system (CNS) malignancy, accounting for 5% or less of brain tumors in published series.[1, 2] As a group, however, they present many unique and complex challenges, from clinical and pathologic diagnosis to formulation of the most beneficial treatment plan.

Germ cell tumors of the CNS are a histologically diverse group, much like their gonadal counterparts, with six subtypes recognized by the World Health Organization (Table 231–1). The classification of germ cell tumors was first outlined by Teilum in 1976, who proposed that all germ cell tumors arise from a primordial germ cell (Fig. 231–1). This cell can either differentiate into a germinoma or be the origin of totipotential cells that give rise to the other types of germ cell tumors, often collectively referred to as *nongerminoma germ cell tumors* (NG-GCTs). According to this theory, the totipotential cell gives rise to embryonal carcinoma, which in turn may give rise to other germ cell tumors. Primitive embryonal carcinoma may differentiate into benign tumors such as teratomas, dermoids, or epidermoids. If neoplastic transition occurs with differentiated embryonal tissue, a malignant teratoma will develop. Embryonal carcinoma can also differentiate into tumor derived from extraembryonic tissue, such as trophoblastic tissue (choriocarcinoma), or yolk sac elements (endodermal sinus tumor).

Despite the acceptance of this theory by the World Health Organization, some authors have disputed it and formulated other hypotheses. It has been pointed out that according to the germ cell theory, choriocarcinoma and yolk sac tumor should be the most differentiated among germ cell tumors, yet they are considered to be the most malignant.[3] Germinoma, which is the most undifferentiated, has the most favorable outcome.

This contradicts the general principle of oncology that the more differentiated a tumor is, the more benign it is. Sano has suggested that each of the so-called germ cell tumors may represent the neoplastic equivalent of an embryonic stage of development (Fig. 231–2).[3] In this theory, tumors composed of cells resembling the cells that appear in the early stages of embryogenesis are more malignant than those composed of cells resembling the cells that appear in later stages.

Despite the unclear pathogenesis of these tumors, they are, in varying degrees, amenable to multimodal therapy. For treatment purposes, these tumors are broadly divided into the two groups mentioned earlier: pure germinoma and NG-GCT, including mixed germ cell tumors. Treatment is further tailored depending on the presence or absence of spinal dissemination and multicentric disease. Surgery has become much safer and plays a definite role in the management of germ cell tumors. Tissue diagnosis is vital to both prognosis and treatment. However, the appropriate degree of surgical resection is an evolving issue. These tumors often invade eloquent structures, precluding safe, complete resection in many cases. Germ cell tumors have also been shown to be both radiation- and chemotherapy-sensitive. As in

TABLE 231–1 ■ **World Health Organization Classification of Germ Cell Tumors**

Germinoma
Embryonal carcinoma
Yolk sac tumor (endodermal sinus tumor)
Choriocarcinoma
Teratoma
Mixed germ cell tumor

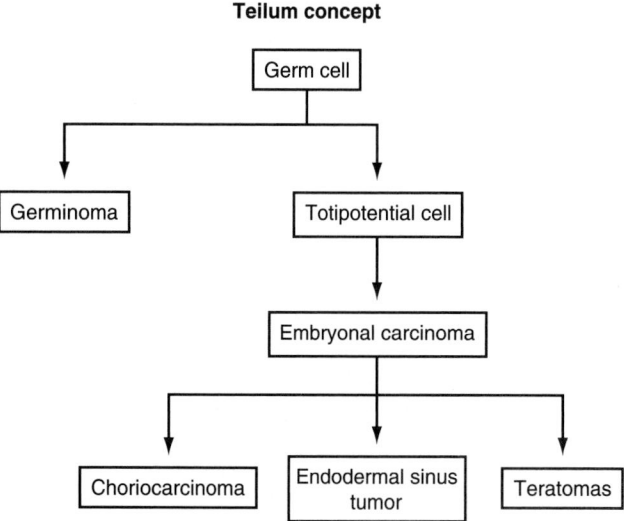

FIGURE 231–1. Teilum's concept of germ cell tumorigenesis.

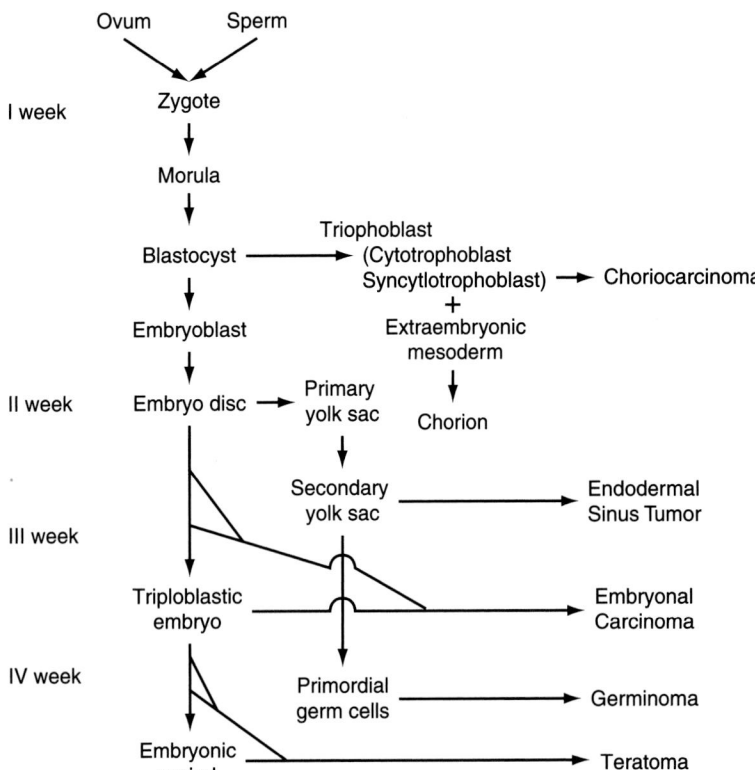

FIGURE 231–2. Sano's proposed hypothesis for germ cell tumorigenesis. (From Sano K: So-called intracranial germ cell tumors: Are they really of germ cell origin? Br J Neurosurg 9:391–401, 1995.)

other areas of neuro-oncology, our ability to control disease must be balanced against treatment sequelae. For germ cell tumors, the most successful treatment plan has not yet been determined. This chapter examines the epidemiology and classification of germ cell tumors, how patients typically present, what diagnostic studies are appropriate, and the role of surgery and adjuvant therapy in the management of patients with these tumors.

EPIDEMIOLOGY

Germ cell tumors have been reported to occur at all ages but are most frequent around puberty, between 11 and 15 years.[4] Seventy percent are diagnosed between 10 and 21 years.[1] Males develop germ cell tumors more frequently than do females, in a ratio of 2:1.[1, 5] This finding seems limited to pineal region tumors and not germ cell tumors that arise in other locations.[3]

Like other extragonadal germ cell tumors, most CNS tumors originate in the midline structures, particularly the pineal and suprasellar regions. The pineal region is the most common site, and 5% to 10% of patients have multicentric disease in both sites at presentation.[1, 3, 6] This latter finding seems to be restricted to patients with pure germinoma. Germ cell tumors may also occur in the basal ganglia, thalamus, infundibulum, fourth ventricle, cerebral cortex, and spine (Fig. 231–3). It is not clear how cells of germ cell origin are "misplaced" within the CNS. Sano hypothesized that the embryonic cells of various stages of embryogenesis may be misplaced in the bilaminar embryonic disk at the time of primitive streak formation, where they be-

come involved in the stream of lateral mesoderm and are carried to the neural plate and incorrectly enfolded into the brain at the time of neural tube formation.[3]

The most common germ cell tumor is the pure germinoma, which accounts for about 40% of all germ cell tumors.[7] NG-GCTs include embryonal cell carcinoma and endodermal sinus tumor (5% to 9%), teratoma (12% to 18%), choriocarcinoma (3% to 5%), and mixed germ cell tumor (8% to 20%).[1, 3, 8, 9]

PRESENTATION

Germ cell tumors are uncommon tumors arising predominantly in children. The clinical signs and symptoms leading to the diagnosis of germ cell tumors are generally a manifestation of the tumor location and rarely the cell of origin. These tumors typically arise in the pineal or suprasellar regions, although they have been reported in the basal ganglia, thalamus, fourth ventricle, cerebellopontine angle, and spinal cord. Age at diagnosis, duration of symptoms, sex, and tumor location can be useful in narrowing the differential diagnosis. Furthermore, 10% to 15% of germ cell tumors have CNS metastases at presentation.

Congenital tumors are by far most likely to be teratomas, to arise in the pineal region, and to be seen in female patients.[3, 9, 10] In the 0- to 3-year age group, NG-GCTs predominate; in the later years and into the second decade, germinomas predominate.[1, 3, 9, 10]

Pure germinomas arise far more often in males than in females, and there is a strong male trend for pineal region germinomas (>90%). Germinomas arising in the

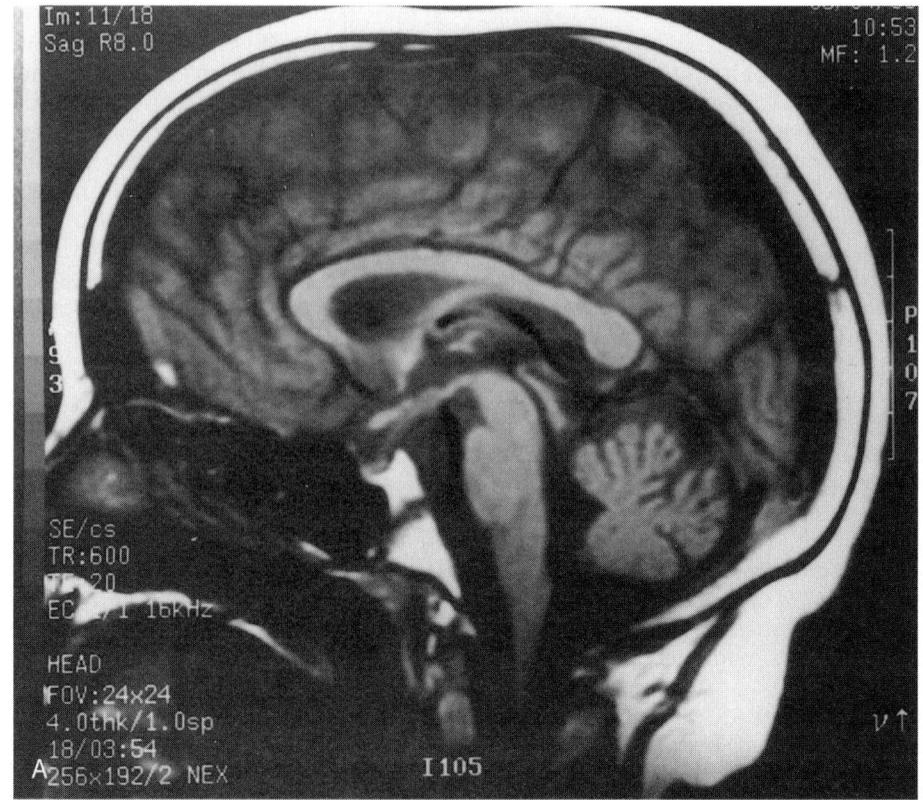

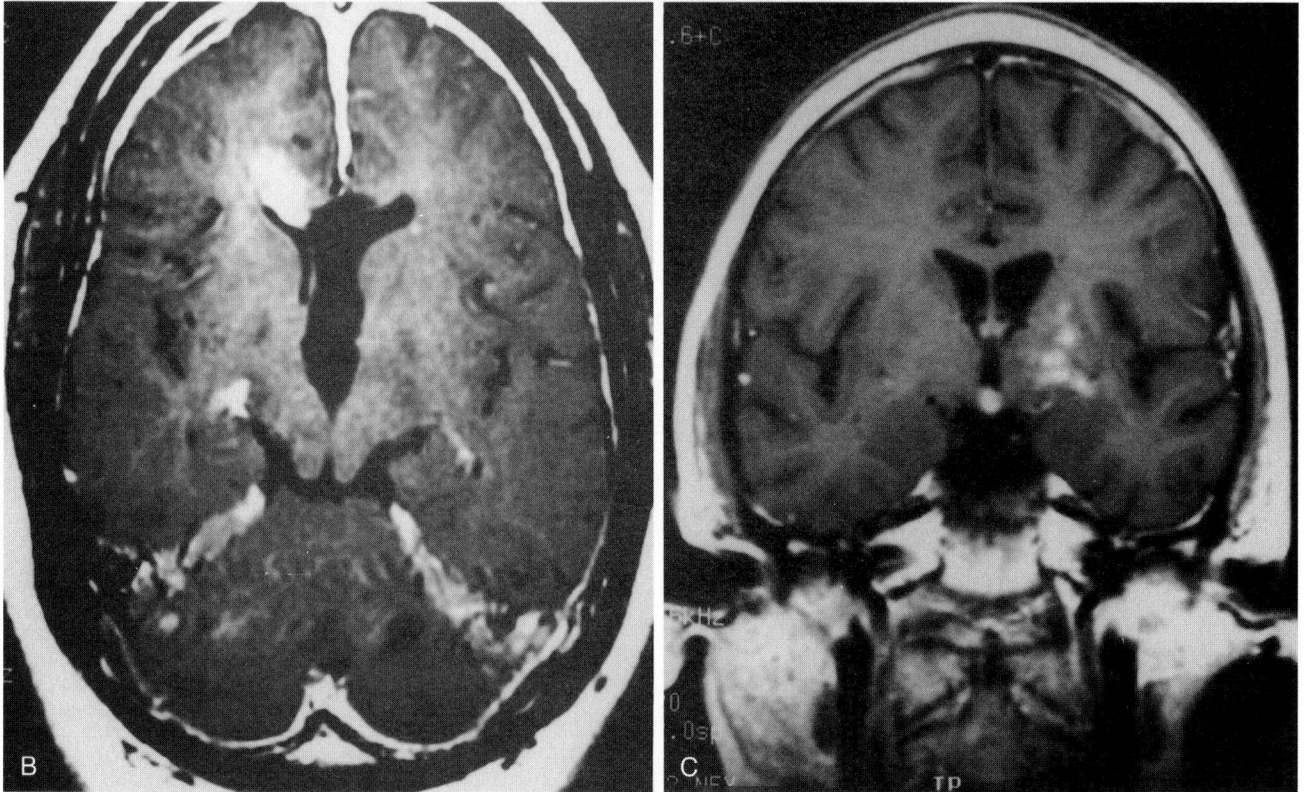

FIGURE 231–3. *A,* Sagittal magnetic resonance imaging (MRI) scan of germinoma showing thickened infundibulum. *B,* Axial enhanced MRI scan of germinoma showing atypical location of tumor. *C,* Coronal enhanced MRI scan of germinoma showing a lesion in the basal ganglia and area of the hypothalamus-infundibulum recess.

suprasellar region are about equally divided between males and females. Rarely, germinomas arise in other locations (e.g., basal ganglia); there is also a male predominance for these sites. Depending on the reporting country of origin, there is a tendency for germinomas to arise mainly in the pineal region, although some series report a roughly equal split between pineal and suprasellar locations.[1, 3, 5, 9]

Those tumors arising in the pineal region are commonly associated with hydrocephalus and consequently present with headache, Parinaud's syndrome, diplopia, and papilledema. They can also cause symptoms of hypothalamic-pituitary axis dysfunction, which can be a result of hydrocephalus or possibly spread of the tumor to the hypothalamus.[1, 10] Germinomas that arise in the suprasellar area most commonly present with diabetes insipidus and disturbances of visual acuity and visual fields. Headache is also seen, but not as commonly as interruption of the function of the hypothalamic-pituitary axis, manifesting as growth delay, menstrual irregularities, and precocious puberty.[8, 11]

Of particular note is that the duration of symptoms can be extended in patients with germinomas, with 30% to 40% having symptoms for more than 6 months. One series reported that 9 of 10 patients with germ cell tumors and symptoms in excess of 5 years had germinomas.[1] Germinomas arising in the basal ganglia or thalamus have been reported to present with seizures, hemiparesis, and dementia.

NG-GCTs are far more likely to occur in the pineal region than in the suprasellar region and to be present at other sites than are germinomas. There is a clear male predominance, especially for tumors presenting

in the second decade of life. The male-female discrepancy is not seen in the first decade of life.[1, 10, 11]

Consequently, NG-GCTs are more likely to present with signs or symptoms of intracranial hypertension and tectal plate compression. In addition, because they are more likely to be located outside the pineal–third ventricle–hypothalamus axis, their presentation can be more protean than that of germinomas. The prodrome for these tumors is also much shorter than that for germinomas, with the overwhelming majority of patients diagnosed within 6 months of the onset of symptoms; only 10% have symptoms for more than 24 months. Choriocarcinomas have a propensity to hemorrhage, so rapid symptom onset or worsening can occur.[1, 3, 9, 10]

DIAGNOSTIC EVALUATION

Germ cell tumors are relatively unusual brain tumors in that their evaluation includes not only neuroimaging but also assessment of protein markers in both blood and cerebrospinal fluid (CSF). These markers can be useful in suggesting specific tumor cell presence and may raise the suspicion that there are multiple cell types within a tumor when the biopsy result is consistent with only germinoma. These tests are used as a guide and do not replace neuropathologic examination of the tumor specimen.

Germinomas are generally well demarcated and iso- or hyperdense to brain on computed tomographic scans. There may be a cystic component. This is in contrast to astrocytomas, which are usually hypodense. Germinomas have uniform enhancement. Magnetic

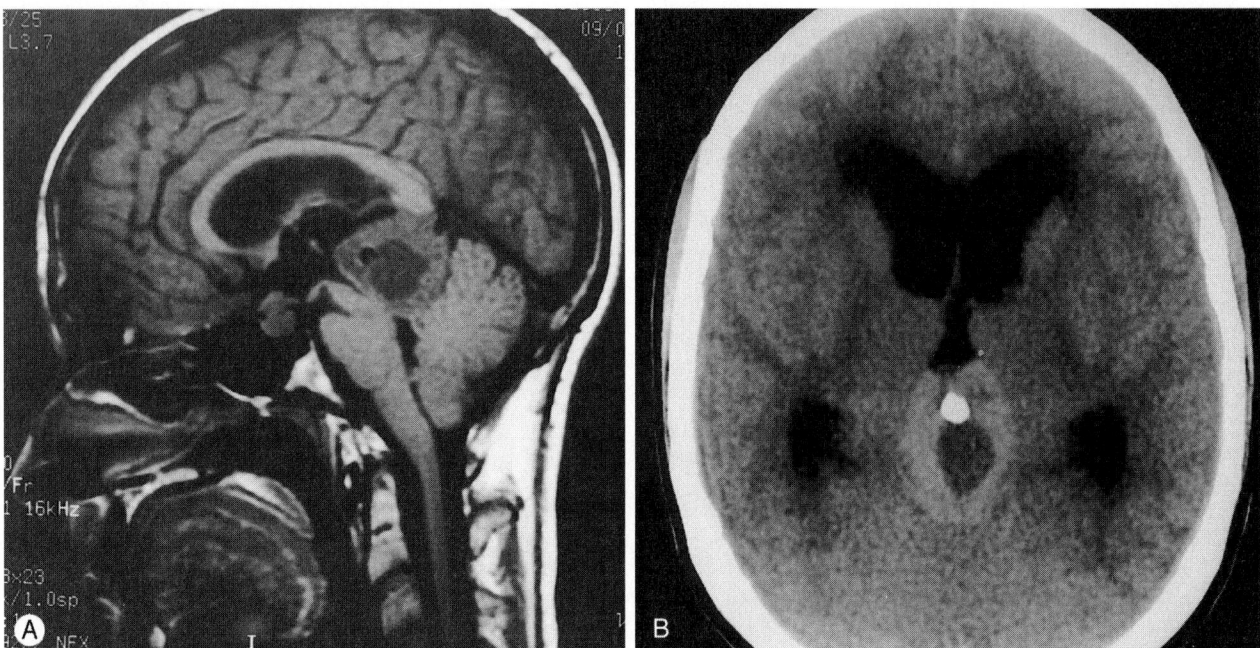

FIGURE 231–4. *A*, Sagittal unenhanced MRI scan of germinoma showing typical pineal location and calcium in the gland. This cystic area is uncommon. *B*, Axial unenhanced computed tomographic scan of germinoma showing the lesion as hyperdense to brain, a cystic component, and calcium.

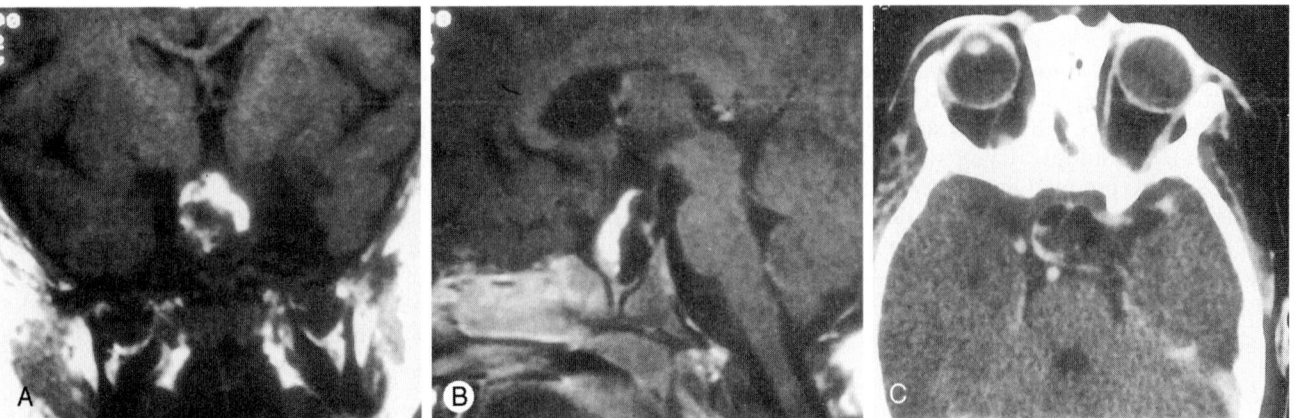

FIGURE 231–5. *A,* Coronal unenhanced MRI scan of mature teratoma. *B,* Sagittal unenhanced MRI scan of mature teratoma. *C,* Axial computed tomographic scan showing calcium and hypodensity, which are often seen in teratomas.

resonance imaging scans show prolonged T1 and T2 relaxation times, again with uniform enhancement. Germinomas can involve the infundibulum, which helps differentiate them from astrocytomas. These tumors generally do not calcify (Fig. 231–4).[12]

Germinomas are generally negative with respect to alpha fetoprotein (AFP) and human chorionic gonadotropin (hCG), although there are reports of elevated levels of hCG in germinomas with syncytiotrophoblastic giant cells. Germinomas can express placental alkaline phosphatase.[1, 9, 10]

Teratomas present a distinct neuroradiologic image of significant heterogeneity, as one would predict from

their pathologic characteristics. As a rule, enhancement is not seen except in areas of malignant degeneration. Teratomas that have a more homogeneous appearance are more likely to be malignant (Fig. 231–5).[12]

Mature teratomas are generally negative for tumor markers, but immature or malignant teratomas can be positive for hCG and placental alkaline phosphatase.

The other NG-GCTs do not have neuroradiologic features that make them reliably diagnosable, except for choriocarcinoma, which has a higher likelihood of hemorrhage (Fig. 231–6). Because most tumors arising in the pineal or suprasellar region are not hemorrhagic, the presence of blood suggests a choriocarcinoma. Cho-

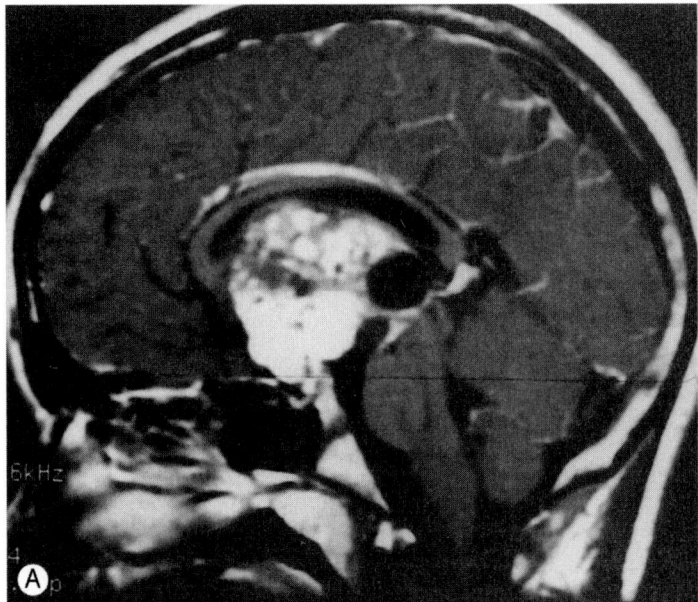
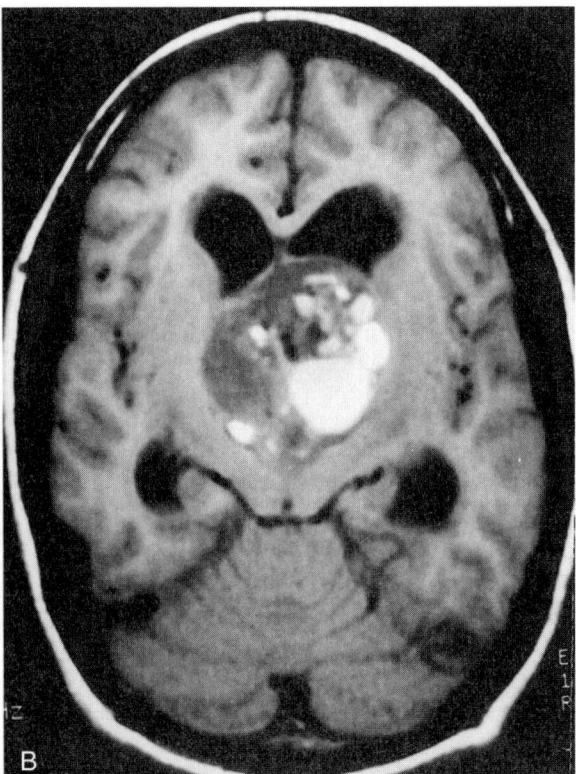

FIGURE 231–6. *A,* Sagittal enhanced MRI scan of endodermal sinus tumor showing heterogeneous enhancement and cyst. *B,* Same patient, axial view.

riocarcinoma is the tumor most associated with hCG expression. AFP expression is most likely to be seen with endodermal sinus tumor, and both hCG and AFP are reported to be elevated with embryonal cell carcinoma. Elevation of tumor markers in blood or CSF can support the pathologic diagnosis and, when only small tissue samples are available, may suggest the presence of mixed tumors. Although radiologic imaging and tumor marker assessment provide a reasonable approximation of tumor type, they are used as an adjuvant to tissue sampling.[1, 3, 10]

SURGICAL MANAGEMENT

The role of the neurosurgeon in the management of germ cell tumors is both to provide tissue for diagnosis and to alleviate the patient's symptoms. Because many of these tumors occur in the pineal region and the vast majority arise in the midline, hydrocephalus is common.

Options for the management of hydrocephalus are ventriculoperitoneal (or other terminus) shunt, endoscopic third ventriculostomy, temporary external ventricular drain, and tumor removal. The disadvantages of shunting are the possibility of spreading the tumor via the system, occlusion of the system as a result of tumor debris, and the fact that up to 80% of patients may not need a shunt once the tumor burden is diminished.[5, 10, 13] However, shunting does permit CSF sampling and provides safe CSF diversion until the tumor burden resolves.

Endoscopic third ventriculostomy seems ideal in that it allows CSF sampling and may permit biopsy if the tumor is visible. It carries a higher risk than ventriculoperitoneal shunt for complications and in our hands has not been as successful in alleviating hydrocephalus in patients with germ cell tumors as in patients with aqueductal stenosis or tectal gliomas.

External ventricular drainage relieves CSF pressure without an increased risk of extra-CNS spread and allows CSF sampling. There is a slightly increased risk of infection as one waits for treatment to shrink the tumor and open CSF pathways. If open craniotomy is planned, this approach may be preferred. There are reports of subgaleal shunts being used in other circumstances to relieve increased CSF pressure temporarily; we have no experience with them in this environment, although we have kept them functional an average of 3 to 4 weeks in premature infants with posthemorrhagic hydrocephalus and persistent CSF debris.

The role of craniotomy for anything other than extensive biopsy remains controversial for a multitude of reasons. Primarily, neurosurgeons have been reluctant to operate on these lesions because of their location in areas with a high surgical risk of injury, because of the lack of data indicating that aggressive surgery for tumors other than teratomas is efficacious, and because effective nonsurgical therapy is available.[1, 10, 14] Nonetheless, neurosurgeons have an important role in the management of this tumor.

If the tumor appears on imaging to be a teratoma,

an attempt at surgical excision is warranted unless it is clear that there are malignant elements that have metastasized. In all other situations, obtaining tissue for neuropathologic examination is warranted. Should biopsy prove the tumor to be a germinoma (especially if AFP and hCG levels are normal), adjunctive therapy (discussed later) is efficacious and should be the initial treatment, forgoing tumor resection. If the biopsy shows NG-GCT or germinoma with other elements, the decision becomes more complex. In the presence of germinoma plus other cell types, one must consider adjunctive therapy with a second-look surgery for residual disease after the germinoma elements have been treated, along with whatever response the other cell types may have. There is no evidence that this necessarily prolongs survival, but there are anecdotal reports that it makes surgical management less complex. Should the biopsy specimen show no germinoma elements, a safe, aggressive resection should be undertaken. There are as yet no data to suggest that complete resection of NG-GCTs provides survival advantage. Thus, surgery should be carried out with as little risk to the patient as possible. Consideration of a second-look surgery after adjunctive therapy may be contemplated, and there are reports of planned chemotherapy-surgery-chemotherapy successes (Fig. 231–7).[15, 16]

An uncommon surgical dilemma faced by neurosurgeons in this disease is the presentation of a child with diabetes insipidus and a small enhancing mass in the infundibulum. The differential diagnosis includes germinoma, Langerhans' cell histiocytosis, sarcoid, and infundibulitis. Before our improved understanding of germ cell tumors and other lesions arising in the infundibulum, a trial of radiation therapy was often considered.[17] However, careful observation, with detailed neuroimaging and biopsy if there are any changes, is now preferred.

RADIATION THERAPY

Germinomas are highly radiosensitive, and treatment with whole-brain radiation alone produces excellent long-term survival rates approaching 90%.[10, 18] In fact, radiation treatment has been the standard of care for germ cell tumors for more than 50 years, although optimal management in terms of volume and dose remains undecided.[18] In many of the older series, patients were treated without biopsy, making interpretation of the data difficult. In one review, data from approximately 800 patients were available, and 46% of the patients had not undergone biopsy.[8] This reflected the older practice of giving a test dose of radiation and then continuing with further treatment if the patient showed a response. However, in view of improved neuroimaging and surgical techniques, a therapeutic trial of radiation therapy is never warranted.

Modern series have evaluated lowering the dose of radiation. One series compared high-dose radiation therapy with low-dose radiation therapy, which was defined as less than or equal to 25.5 Gy to the whole brain, less than 50 Gy to the tumor site, and less than

Treatment Algorithm for Central Nervous System Germ Cells Tumors

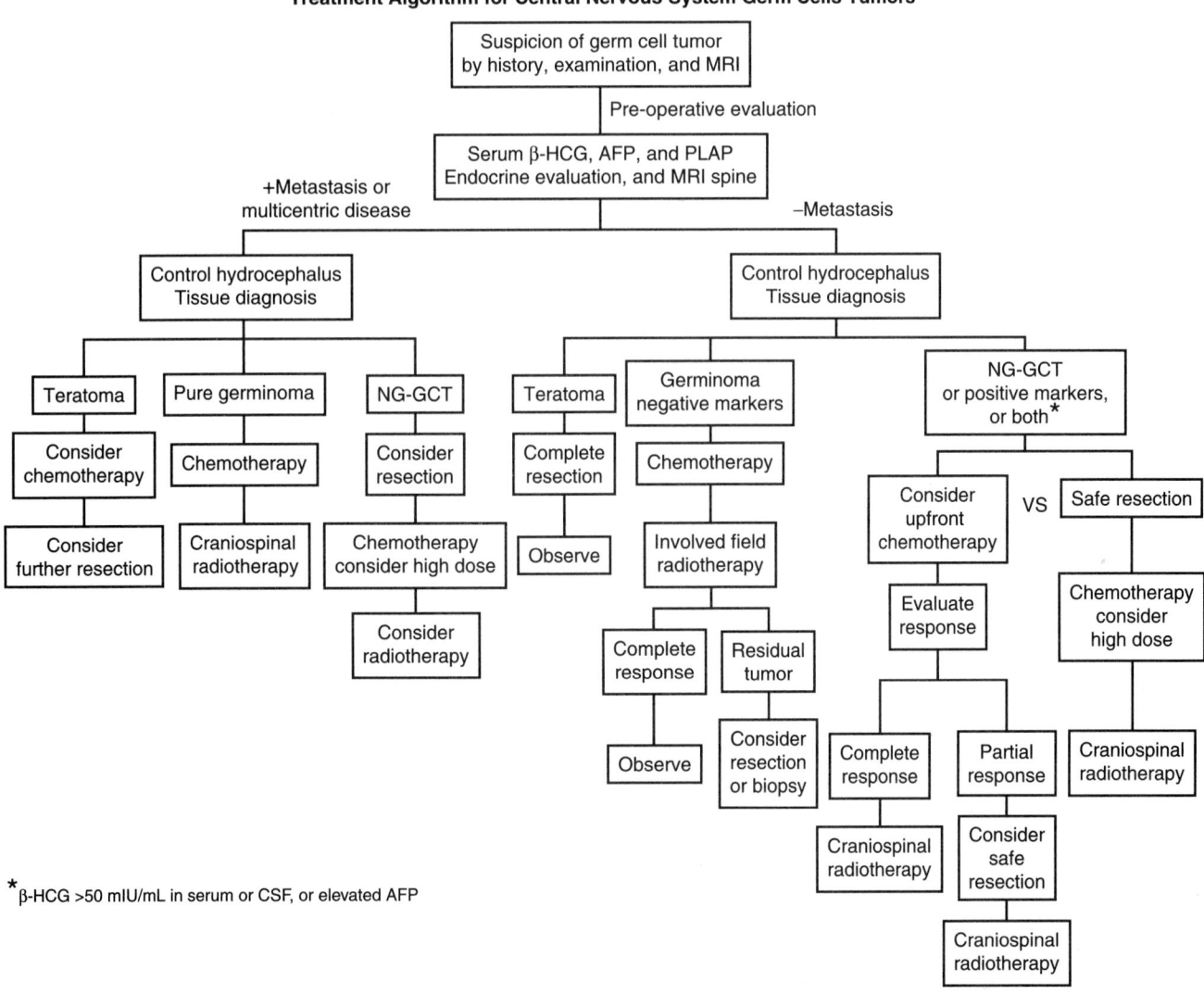

FIGURE 231–7. Treatment algorithm for patients with central nervous system germ cell tumors at the Children's Hospital of Alabama. AFP, alpha fetoprotein; β-HCG, beta-human chorionic gonadotropin; MRI, magnetic resonance imaging; NG-GCT, nongerminoma germ cell tumor; PLAP, placental alkaline phosphatase.

22 Gy to the spine.[18] This study included 40 patients, 13 with biopsy-proven germinoma and 23 who had clinical histories, imaging studies, and tumor markers consistent with the diagnosis. The 5-year disease-free survival and overall survival for these patients were 97%. Outcome was not affected by the dose of radiation. Interestingly, outcome was unchanged regardless of CSF dissemination or elevation of hCG. This group recommends reducing the dose of whole brain radiation to 25 Gy, tumor volume to 45 Gy, and spinal radiation to 22 Gy if disseminated. Others have advocated local treatment alone if there is no clinical evidence of seeding and the lesion is proved to be pure germinoma.[19–21] The rationale for reducing the dose of radiation and eliminating craniospinal radiation if possible is the same as it is for medulloblastoma and other diseases—to reduce or avoid the known deleterious side effects of whole-brain radiation on intellectual, psychological, and hormonal development.

There has never been a cooperative group trial in the United States directed at the study of CNS germinoma. The Pediatric Oncology Group is currently evaluating the treatment of patients with histologically proven germinoma with a reduced dose of radiation. Craniospinal radiation is given only to patients with disseminated or multicentric disease. This trial involves chemotherapy before radiation and is discussed later in the chemotherapy section.

As mentioned earlier, patients with NG-GCT have a much poorer outcome than patients with pure germinoma treated with similar therapy. A review of the literature found a 5- and 10-year survival of 36% for patients with biopsy-proven NG-GCT treated with radiation therapy alone.[22] Another study found a long-term disease-free survival rate of less than 25%, with virtually no chance of survival with some of the histologic subtypes.[1] There seems to be little justification for reducing the dose of radiation in these patients, with the outcome being so poor. Current treatment strategies include the combination of chemotherapy and radiation. The current Pediatric Oncology Group protocol treats patients with high-risk disease—those with NG-GCT histologic features or elevated tumor markers—with high-dose craniospinal radiation and high-dose chemotherapy.

CHEMOTHERAPY

There is a unique precedent for treating CNS germ cell tumors with chemotherapy because of the histologic similarities of germ cell tumors throughout the body. Cisplatin-based chemotherapy regimens have been successful in the treatment of germ cell tumors outside the CNS.[8] Cure rates for testicular cancer, the most common cancer in young men, are reported at 60% to 90% with regimens that include cisplatin or carboplatin and etoposide.[23, 24]

The activity of these agents in CNS germinoma has been reported in several small series.[25, 26] More recent clinical trials have given chemotherapy followed by radiation treatment. One study treated newly diagnosed patients with histologically confirmed germinoma with carboplatin, followed by varying dosing of irradiation and 21 to 30 Gy if disseminated.[6] Of 10 assessable patients, 7 had a complete response and 3 a partial response, with 91% of patients remaining in continuous remission for a median of 25 months. Another study treated six patients with solitary pure germinoma with cisplatin and etoposide, followed by 24 Gy to the involved field.[14] In the same study, 11 patients were treated with ifosfamide, cisplatin, and etoposide, followed by 24 Gy to the involved field. The patients in the latter group were considered high risk because they had elevated hCG (four patients), multifocal disease (four patients), or dissemination (three patients). The patients with dissemination were also treated with 24 Gy craniospinal irradiation. A complete response to chemotherapy was achieved in all patients, and 16 of 17 patients (94%) were free from recurrence at the median follow-up of 24 months (range 6 to 60 months). The one failure in this study had a recurrence outside the radiation port. He was retreated with ifosfamide, carboplatin, and etoposide chemotherapy and craniospinal radiation and remained disease free at 22 months.

With such excellent results, the possibility of treating germinoma with chemotherapy alone has been explored. An international cooperative group trial treated 45 patients with germinoma and 26 patients with NG-GCT using four cycles of carboplatin, etoposide, and bleomycin.[27] Those with a complete response received two further cycles; others received two more cycles intensified by cyclophosphamide. There were 71 patients in this study, and 55 (78%) achieved a complete response with six cycles of chemotherapy and no irradiation. Despite these initial promising results, 28 of 71 patients had recurrence. Of these, 26 of 28 underwent successful salvage therapy. Pathologic features were the only variable that was predictive of survival. The probability of surviving 2 years was 84% for germinoma patients and 62% for NG-GCT patients. Seven patients (10%) died of treatment-related toxicity. Although these investigators successfully treated 50% of their patients with chemotherapy alone, the overall results were not as good as those obtained with radiation alone or with a combination of chemotherapy and radiation.

These studies demonstrate the activity of chemotherapy in the treatment of germ cell tumors and justify the role of preirradiation chemotherapy in an attempt to improve survival for patients with NG-GCT and reduce the dose of radiation for patients with germ cell tumors who respond to chemotherapy. The Pediatric Oncology Group study treats all patients with CNS germ cell tumors with chemotherapy that includes cisplatin, VP-16, vincristine, and cyclophosphamide, followed by irradiation. For patients with pure germinoma, chemotherapy is given every 3 weeks for four cycles, after which a radiographic assessment of response is performed. For patients with a complete response to chemotherapy, a reduced dose of 30.6 Gy irradiation is given to the tumor bed. For those with less than a complete response, 50.4 Gy is given. If patients have dissemination or multicentric disease at diagnosis, craniospinal radiation is also given. For patients with high-risk disease (NG-GCT or elevated markers), more intensive chemotherapy, with higher doses of cisplatin and cyclophosphamide, is given. Radiation doses remain standard, and all patients receive craniospinal treatment. Only a modest dose reduction is made for those who respond to treatment.

CONCLUSIONS

Advances in the treatment of CNS germ cell tumors are exciting. Improved surgical techniques have made it possible to diagnose these tumors more safely and accurately. Several surgical questions remain: What degree of resection is appropriate? What is the role of second-look surgery? What is the safest way to manage hydrocephalus?

Radiation therapy continues to play a vital role in the management of these patients, regardless of pathologic subtype. For patients with pure germinoma, the addition of preirradiation chemotherapy may allow for lower doses of radiation in an attempt to reduce the long-term sequelae of treatment in patients who have good long-term survival rates. In the future, identifying subsets of patients who may be cured by chemotherapy alone may be possible.

Much work remains in improving the outcome for patients with high-risk disease—those with NG-GCT histologic features or elevated hCG or AFP. It is likely that patients with elevated tumors markers have mixed pathologic characteristics. Current investigational protocols treat these patients aggressively, with intensified chemotherapy and fairly high doses of craniospinal radiation. Again, identifying subsets of patients and how they respond to treatment may help tailor regimens in the future. It is likely that not all NG-GCTs are created equal, and a better understanding of the biologic underpinnings of these diseases may lead to refinements in treatment.

REFERENCES

1. Jennings MT, Gelman R, Hochberg F: Intracranial germ-cell tumors: Natural history and pathogenesis. J Neurosurg 63:155–167, 1985.
2. Jellinger K: Primary intracranial germ cell tumours. Acta Neuropathol 25:291–306, 1973.
3. Sano K: Pathogenesis of intracranial germ cell tumors reconsidered. J Neurosurg 90:258–264, 1999.
4. Ho DM, Liu HC: Primary intracranial germ cell tumor: Pathologic study of 51 patients. Cancer 70:1577–1584, 1992.
5. Hoffman HJ, Yoshida M, Becker LE, et al: Pineal region tumors in childhood: Experience at the Hospital for Sick Children, 1983. Pediatr Neurosurg 21:91–103, 1994; discussion 104.
6. Allen JC, DaRosso RC, Donahue B, Nirenberg A: A phase II trial of preirradiation carboplatin in newly diagnosed germinoma of the central nervous system. Cancer 74:940–944, 1994.
7. Horowitz MB, Hall WA: Central nervous system germinomas: A review. Arch Neurol 48:652–657, 1991.
8. Kretschmar CS: Germ cell tumors of the brain in children: A review of current literature and new advances in therapy. Cancer Invest 15:187–198, 1997.
9. Bigner D, McLendon RE, Bruner J: Russell and Rubinstein's Pathology of Tumors of the Nervous System. New York, Oxford University Press, 1998.
10. Matsutani M, Sano K, Takakura K, et al: Primary intracranial germ cell tumors: A clinical analysis of 153 histologically verified cases. J Neurosurg 86:446–455, 1997.
11. Bigner SH, McLendon RE, Fuchs H, et al: Chromosomal characteristics of childhood brain tumors. Cancer Genet Cytogenet 97:125–134, 1997.
12. Barkovich J: Pediatric Neuroimaging. New York, Raven Press, 1995.
13. Rickert CH: Abdominal metastases of pediatric brain tumors via ventriculo-peritoneal shunts. Childs Nerv Syst 14:10–14, 1998.
14. Sawamura Y, Shirato H, Ikeda J, et al: Induction chemotherapy followed by reduced-volume radiation therapy for newly diagnosed central nervous system germinoma. J Neurosurg 88:66–72, 1998.
15. Knappe UJ, Bentele K, Horstmann M, Herrmann HD: Treatment and long-term outcome of pineal nongerminomatous germ cell tumors. Pediatr Neurosurg 28:241–245, 1998.
16. Herrmann HD, Westphal M, Winkler K, et al: Treatment of nongerminomatous germ-cell tumors of the pineal region. Neurosurgery 34:524–529, 1994; discussion 529.
17. Atkins D, Sanford R, Thomas B, Joyner R: Infundibuloneurohypophysitis in children. Pediatr Neurosurg 30:267–271, 1999.
18. Hardenbergh PH, Golden J, Billet A, et al: Intracranial germinoma: The case for lower dose radiation therapy. Int J Radiat Oncol Biol Phys 39:419–426, 1997.
19. Shibamoto Y, Abe M, Yamashita J, et al: Treatment results of intracranial germinoma as a function of the irradiated volume. Int J Radiat Oncol Biol Phys 15:285–290, 1988.
20. Linstadt D, Wara WM, Edwards MS, et al: Radiotherapy of primary intracranial germinomas: The case against routine craniospinal irradiation. Int J Radiat Oncol Biol Phys 15:291–297, 1988.
21. Chao CK, Lee ST, Lin FJ, et al: A multivariate analysis of prognostic factors in management of pineal tumor. Int J Radiat Oncol Biol Phys 27:1185–1191, 1993.
22. Fuller BG, Kapp DS, Cox R: Radiation therapy of pineal region tumors: 25 new cases and a review of 208 previously reported cases. Int J Radiat Oncol Biol Phys 28:229–245, 1994.
23. Peckham MJ, Horwich A, Hendry WF: Advanced seminoma: Treatment with cis-platinum-based combination chemotherapy or carboplatin (JM8). Br J Cancer 52:7–13, 1985.
24. Bajorin DF, Sarosdy MF, Pfister DG, et al: Randomized trial of etoposide and cisplatin versus etoposide and carboplatin in patients with good-risk germ cell tumors: A multiinstitutional study [see comments]. J Clin Oncol 11:598–606, 1993.
25. Edwards MS, Hudgins RJ, Wilson CB, et al: Pineal region tumors in children. J Neurosurg 68:689–697, 1988.
26. Allen JC, Bosl G, Walker R: Chemotherapy trials in recurrent primary intracranial germ cell tumors. J Neurooncol 3:147–152, 1985.
27. Balmaceda C, Heller G, Rosenblum M, et al: Chemotherapy without irradiation—a novel approach for newly diagnosed CNS germ cell tumors: Results of an international cooperative trial. The First International Central Nervous System Germ Cell Tumor Study. J Clin Oncol 14:2908–2915, 1996.

Choroid Plexus Tumors

RICHARD G. ELLENBOGEN ▪ R. MICHAEL SCOTT

HISTORY AND CLINICAL SIGNIFICANCE

Tumors of the choroid plexus are rare tumors. They often present a formidable surgical challenge, even to the most experienced neurosurgeons. Choroid plexus tumors account for only 0.4% to 1% of all intracranial tumors.[1] They arise from the neuroepithelial lining of the choroid plexuses.[2, 3] Choroid plexus tumors demonstrate a wide spectrum of histologic and biologic properties, from the well-demarcated benign papilloma to the highly anaplastic, infiltrative carcinoma. Benign choroid plexus papilloma is resectable and thus potentially curable.[4, 5] Malignant choroid plexus carcinoma has a poor prognosis, but it is slightly less ominous than that associated with most malignant brain tumors, with reports of selected survivors living more than 5 years.[4–8]

Papilloma of the choroid plexus was described in only 0.6% of Cushing's 2023 verified intracranial tumors in 1932 and in only 0.5% of Zulch's review of 6000 intracranial tumors reported in 1956.[9, 10] Among children, however, they are more common, representing 1% to 5% of pediatric brain tumors in various published series, and 4% to 12% among patients younger than 1 year.[11–14]

The first description of a primary choroid plexus tumor was by Guerard in the early 19th century, in an autopsy specimen of a 3-year-old girl.[15] Between 1833 and 1925, publications on neoplasms of the choroid plexus emphasized the rarity of the lesion or its association with hydrocephalus.[16–25] Bielschowsky and Unger reported the first surgical resection of a choroid plexus tumor in an adult, in 1906.[26] However, the patient later died. In 1919, Perthes reported the first long-term survival of an adult with a choroid plexus tumor.[20] Van Wagenen in 1930 reported excision of a tumor from the lateral ventricle of a 3-month-old child.[25] Dandy in 1934 described the removal of a choroid plexus tumor from a 14-year-old girl.[27] Dandy also pioneered the transcallosal route to the third ventricle and was the first to describe it for excision of a choroid plexus tumor in 1922. The first successful removal of a third ventricle papilloma was through a transfrontal approach and was reported by Masson in 1934.[28]

A wide variety of surgical approaches has been described to remove these surgically imposing neoplasms, and the choice must be based on the individual characteristics and location of each tumor. Choroid plexus tumors should be included in the differential diagnosis of any intraventricular mass, especially in a young child. When resectable, choroid plexus tumor is often a welcome diagnosis, compared with other tumors in this location.

CLINICAL FEATURES

Primary choroid plexus neoplasms can be found in patients of any age, from birth to the eighth decade of life. More than 70% of reported choroid plexus neoplasms occur in children, and at least 50% are found in children younger than 2 years.[4, 14, 29–32] Reports of choroid plexus tumors discovered in utero by prenatal ultrasonography indicate a congenital origin for some of these tumors.[33, 34] However, they are also discovered in adults after a short course of presenting symptoms. A preponderance of male patients has been described in a several series.[4, 35–39] However, other series show a fairly even distribution between males and females.[1, 40] There seems to be no difference in age at diagnosis, sex, symptoms, or location of tumor for patients with papillomas versus those with carcinomas in the pediatric age group.[4]

An interesting feature of choroid plexus tumors is their anatomic distribution. They are most commonly found in the lateral ventricles in children and less commonly in the posterior fossa. In contrast, in adults, the majority of these tumors are found in the fourth ventricle and its lateral recesses.[2, 31, 32, 37, 41–44] No anatomic or developmental feature adequately explains this unique distribution. Approximately 75% of the tumors in children are found in the lateral ventricles. Most tumors in the lateral ventricles are found in the atrium or trigone, but they can also be seen in the temporal horn or near the foramen of Monro. There appear to be a relatively equal number in the right and left lateral ventricles.[4, 25]

Location in the third ventricle is much less common but has been described in both children and adults.[37, 40, 45–47] Third ventricular choroid plexus neoplasms are uncommon in pediatric series, averaging approximately 10% and ranging from 0% to 29%.[4, 14, 39, 45, 48, 49]

Primary extraventricular locations are the rarest sites, but tumors have been described in the cerebellopontine angle, cerebellomedullary cistern, suprasellar cistern, foramen magnum, and the spinal subarachnoid space.[2] Extension of the tumor from one ventricle into another, through a ventricular foramen, or into a subarachnoid cistern is occasionally noted.[32, 47] Tumor in multiple locations is extremely rare but has been reported.[50] All choroid plexus neoplasms likely arise in a ventricle or cistern, but particularly large or invasive ones may interdigitate with the parenchyma over such a large area that they appear to arise from within the parenchyma and not the ventricle.

The patient's initial clinical features can be grouped into four overlapping sets of signs: increased intracranial pressure, seizures, hemorrhage, and focal neurologic abnormalities. Adults can present with headache, cranial nerve palsy, or signs of increased intracranial pressure. Most children are brought to the hospital for investigation of signs of increased intracranial pressure, such as a tense fontanelle, macrocephaly, vomiting, lethargy, or irritability.[4, 14, 39] Choroid plexus tumors in children, like other intraventricular tumors in adults, are often large by the time of diagnosis; in one series, they averaged 4 cm in diameter at diagnosis.[4] The symptoms of choroid plexus tumors in children are caused predominantly by the hydrocephalus that occurs in the majority of pediatric patients. The duration of symptoms ranges from several weeks to 6 months. Although most infants present with intracranial hypertension, the presentation in young children may be more nonspecific. Less common but well-documented presentations include head tilt, titubation, weakness, failure to thrive, developmental delay, and shunt-resistant hydrocephalus.[47, 51-54] Shunt-resistant hydrocephalus is secondary to a choroid plexus tumor (papilloma) that produces several times the normal amount of cerebrospinal fluid (CSF).[55] This overproduction of CSF can be significant enough to cause abdominal ascites if a ventriculoperitoneal shunt is placed before surgical removal of the tumor.[47]

Adult and pediatric patients with posterior fossa lesions may exhibit signs of brainstem compression, cranial nerve paresis, and cerebellar signs. Adult patients may present with symptoms and magnetic resonance imaging (MRI) findings similar to those of a patient with a meningioma in that location.[56] Hydrocephalus is also a prominent finding with tumors in the posterior fossa, especially if the CSF pathways of the fourth ventricle are blocked.[49, 57, 58] In a series of 12 adult patients with cerebellopontine angle choroid plexus tumors, 8 had hydrocephalus.[56] Patients with tumors of the third ventricle present with hydrocephalus but may also exhibit endocrine disturbances such as menstrual irregularities, obesity, precocious puberty, diabetes insipidus, bobble-head phenomenon, psychosis, or diencephalic disorders.[24, 46, 48, 59]

HYDROCEPHALUS

Hydrocephalus, which is a cardinal manifestation of choroid plexus neoplasms, can be the result of obstruction of CSF pathways or overproduction of CSF. The subject of overproduction of CSF by choroid plexus neoplasms has attracted a great deal of interest.[22, 32, 55, 60-66] Initially, the resolution of hydrocephalus after the complete resection of choroid plexus tumors was the basis for postulating that oversecretion of CSF was responsible for the hydrocephalus.[1] However, only in a limited number of patients has an increased rate of CSF production been unequivocally demonstrated.[31, 55, 60, 65-67] Although overproduction of CSF can cause hydrocephalus, a complex combination of overproduction and limited absorption of CSF may be the cause of hydrocephalus in many patients.[68]

Tumor mass, blood products, tumor products, cellular debris, and metastases can mechanically obstruct the normal absorption of CSF, causing hydrocephalus. Necrosis, tumor hemorrhage, operative hemorrhage, and ependymitis have all been implicated as causes of hydrocephalus in patients with these choroid tumors.[38, 49, 53, 69-72] Elevation of CSF protein is found in the majority of patients, and xanthochromia in the CSF is common; frank hemorrhage is less common.[1] The obstruction of CSF absorptive pathways may also explain why hydrocephalus sometimes persists despite gross total excision of the tumor. Approximately one third to one half of patients with choroid plexus neoplasms require permanent CSF diversion postoperatively, even when the tumor is completely removed.[4, 5, 39, 49, 70, 71]

Another interesting entity reported is *diffuse villous hypertrophy* of the choroid plexus, a term originally coined by Davis in 1924 to describe a bilateral choroid plexus lesion.[17] Because there is only a minor histopathologic difference between papillomas and normal choroid plexus tissue, it is difficult to determine whether this entity represents a true neoplasm or simple hypertrophy. Bilateral papilloma is a rare condition, demonstrated by its absence from series of choroid plexus papillomas.[1, 29, 32, 42-44] The observation that overproduction of CSF can result from villous hypertrophy of the choroid plexus or from papilloma has been reported by several investigators.[17, 31, 53, 66, 67, 73] Performing a ventriculostomy and measuring CSF formation may help document the overproduction of CSF. Laurence described six cases of his own but was cautious about recommending the removal of these lesions.[31] However, several surgeons have shown that resection of these rare bilateral choroid plexus lesions results in resolution of the CSF overproduction and alleviation of the concomitant hydrocephalus.[66, 67, 73] Coagulation of this lesion through a minimally invasive endoscopic approach, and the subsequent resolution of CSF overproduction, has also been reported.[74]

DIAGNOSTIC EVALUATION

In the current era of imaging, patients are initially diagnosed by computed tomography or MRI. Previously, skull radiography, pneumoencephalography, ventriculography, and angiography were used to show these tumors to be intraventricular masses with associated hydrocephalus.[1] Plain radiographs showed marked calcification and nonspecific signs of increased pressure.[1, 29, 75]

The introduction of computed tomography followed by MRI improved the safety and accuracy of diagnosis, and ultimately the outcome, in all patients harboring these tumors.[32] Both papillomas and carcinomas appear isodense to hyperdense on computed tomographic scans, with frequent calcification and usually marked enhancement. Tumors are spherical or multilobular and sometimes cystic. They infrequently extend into another ventricle or CSF cistern, a finding that is not specific for choroid plexus tumors.

MRI scans most often show a mass that is isointense or slightly hypointense to gray matter on T1-weighted images and hyperintense on T2-weighted images. The tumor is often a lobulated, homogeneous, intraventricular mass on both short T1-weighted sequences.[76] Enhancement with paramagnetic substances such as gadolinium-DTPA is markedly intense and usually homogeneous, although various patterns can be seen, including nodular, peripheral enhancement and cyst wall enhancement (Fig. 232–1). A frequent finding is the presence of serpentine signal voids, indicating the presence of an enlarged blood vessel supplying the tumor.[77, 78] MRI is the diagnostic imaging study of choice because of its detailed anatomic delineation and triplanar imaging ability. Magnetic resonance angiography may provide additional information regarding the vascular supply of the tumor. Magnetic resonance angiography is replacing transfemoral cerebral angiography in the management of these tumors in some patients. In select children and adults, angiography still has a great deal of utility, especially if preoperative embolization of the feeding vessels is desired. Furthermore, angiography provides the most definitive anatomic configuration of the feeding vessels. The angiogram can provide the surgeon with the most efficacious route to occlude the tumor vessels for a safe resection.

Both papilloma and carcinoma can compress the surrounding brain, although brain invasion is a characteristic of carcinoma.[79] Some authors have commented on the peritumor vasogenic edema in the surrounding white matter in carcinoma.[77, 79] Carcinoma has a greater tendency to invade the brain, but it can also be found in an entirely intraventricular location (Fig. 232–2).

The radiologic differential diagnosis of choroid plexus tumors includes ependymoma, meningioma, primitive neuroectodermal tumor, astrocytoma, germinoma, teratoma, and metastases to the choroid plexus. Despite the significant difference in histologic appearance, on MRI scans, these tumors can appear homogeneous and similar in appearance to choroid plexus tumors. Other unusual tumor-like masses that can appear similar include inflammatory pseudotumor, choroid plexus cysts, and xanthogranulomas.

PATHOLOGY AND DIFFERENTIAL DIAGNOSIS

On visual inspection, choroid plexus papillomas have cauliflower-like surfaces and are generally well-circum-scribed masses arising from a ventricle. The papillomas can extend into the brain parenchyma, compressing it along a broad margin. Heavily calcified tumors may be difficult to section without first decalcifying them.[2] Microscopically, choroid plexus tumors typically appear as a single layer of cuboid epithelial cells surrounding a delicate fibrovascular stalk, arranged in a papillary configuration with finger-like projections of tissue (Fig. 232–3). A well-formed continuous basement membrane is a prominent feature noted in all cases. Choroid plexus tumors span the histologic spectrum from extremely well-differentiated tumors to anaplastic tumors with minimal epithelial differentiation. Both well-differentiated and poorly differentiated components may be seen in a single tumor.[2] However, the majority of choroid plexus neoplasms are well differentiated. It is occasionally difficult to differentiate normal choroid plexus from a papilloma, but the latter contains cells that are more crowded, columnar in shape, and pleomorphic and that demonstrate more variation in nuclear size. The nuclear-to-cytoplasmic ratio is often increased.[2]

Ultrastructural observations include apical microvilli, scattered cilia, and interdigitating lateral cell borders sitting atop a basement membrane seated on a delicate fibrovascular stalk. Stromal calcification or xanthomatous changes may be evident. Atypical microscopic features may be observed in papilloma and include increased cellularity (two or three cell layers thick, as opposed to one), mitoses, nuclear pleomorphism, and poorly formed papillary structures. These intermediate tumors may possess one or two of these features and are called *atypical papillomas*, but they do not necessarily have a more aggressive natural history and are not classified as carcinomas. However, anaplastic transformation of well-differentiated tumors has been reported to occur over time. Although uncommon, a lesion that is initially well differentiated or atypical can become anaplastic, as documented during a subsequent resection.[80, 81] This "gray area" adds to the confusion in planning treatment for neoplasms that are classified as papilloma but have one or two features that are found in carcinoma.

The histologic features of papilloma versus carcinoma have been subject to both close scrutiny and controversy. The focus in diagnosis often centers on this important question: Which particular characteristics differentiate papilloma from carcinoma? Review of the literature reveals that, from a historical perspective, the criteria for differentiation of papilloma from carcinoma have not been uniform. The definition of choroid plexus carcinoma has varied slightly in several studies based on histologic criteria.[4, 11, 38, 82, 83] Dohrmann and Collias,[11] using Russell and Rubinstein's[38] and Lewis's[84] criteria for carcinoma, reviewed 22 cases of primary choroid plexus carcinoma in the literature from 1844 to 1975 and found that only 11 satisfied the criteria of carcinoma. Similarly, Lewis's review of the literature resulted in the dismissal of many other cases of carcinoma.[84]

In our experience, the consistent histologic features of choroid plexus tumors that unequivocally differenti-

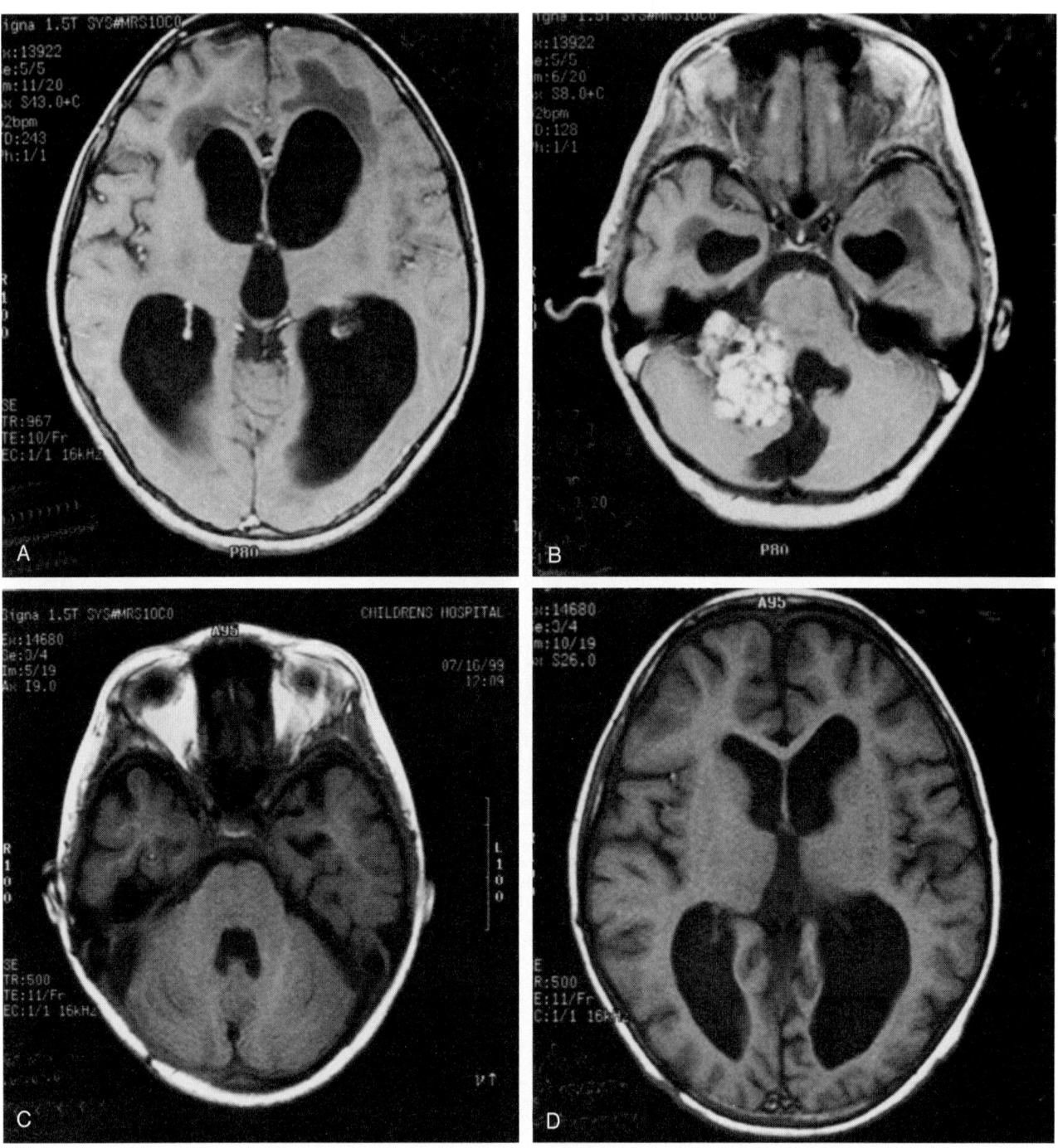

FIGURE 232–1. This axial magnetic resonance imaging (MRI) scan with gadolinium is of a 10-year-old child who presented with blindness as a result of previously untreated hydrocephalus secondary to a posterior fossa choroid plexus papilloma. *A,* An emergently performed ventriculostomy yielded approximately 40 mL/hour of cerebrospinal fluid (CSF) drainage with the ventriculostomy level 15 cm above the tragus. This CSF-producing tumor was a rare choroid plexus papilloma of the right foramen of Luschka and the fourth ventricle. *B,* Note how the tumor demonstrates nodular enhancement as it fills the foramen and creeps into the cerebellopontine angle. The patient underwent a corticectomy through the right lateral cerebellar hemisphere with a gross total excision of this vascular papilloma, which was adherent to cranial nerves VII through X. Despite intraoperative cranial nerve monitoring, the patient suffered paresis of cranial nerves IX and X, which improved. She did not recover her sight. She remains tumor free, and the CSF oversecretion halted after the excision of this tumor *(C* and *D).*

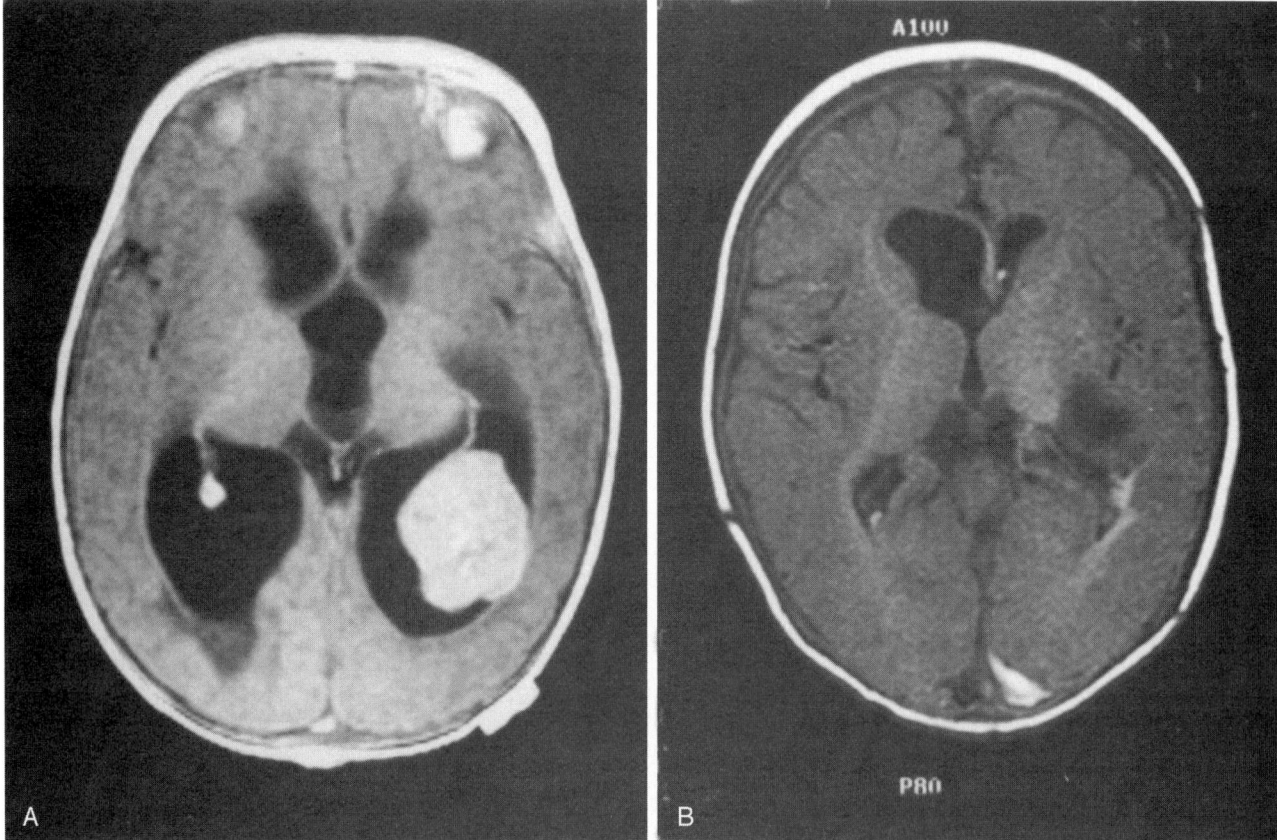

FIGURE 232–2. Preoperative T1-weighted axial MRI scan *(A)* and postoperative axial MRI scan *(B)* with gadolinium administration in an 8-month-old child with a choroid plexus carcinoma of the left lateral ventricle. At this time, there are no specific MRI characteristics that can reliably differentiate this carcinoma from a papilloma. This patient underwent a magnetic resonance angiogram, which showed a hypertrophied posterior medial and lateral choroidal feeding vessel. Intraoperative color flow Doppler ultrasonography was used to plan the trajectory to the vascular pedicle. The tumor was exceptionally vascular and invaded the wall of the lateral ventricle. As a result, it was difficult to mobilize the tumor before ligating the vascular pedicle. A parietal approach was chosen, and the tumor was successfully excised with minimal morbidity consisting of a transient visual field cut. A staged approach was undertaken to limit morbidity from blood loss. The patient underwent postoperative adjuvant chemotherapy and remains tumor free after 1 year.

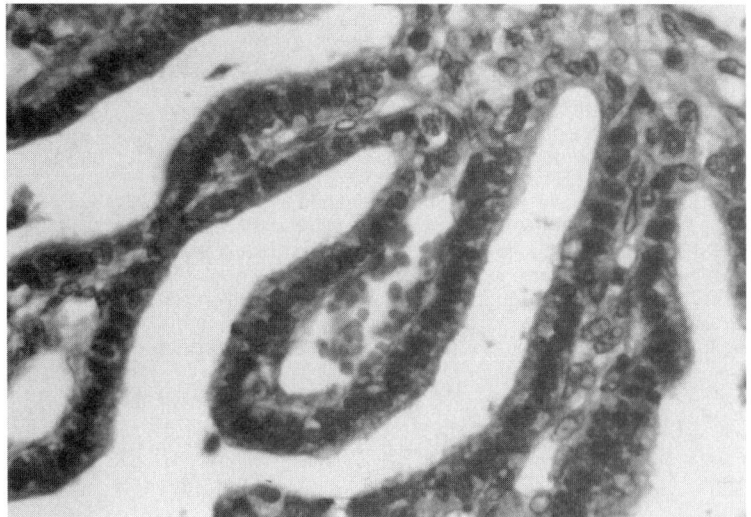

FIGURE 232–3. This pathology slide represents the typical papillary appearance of a choroid plexus papilloma excised from the lateral ventricle. Note the single layer of columnar cells with organized papillary architecture based on a delicate fibrovascular stroma. The cells are more columnar and pleomorphic than normal choroid plexus cells. (Hematoxylin and eosin, ×80.)

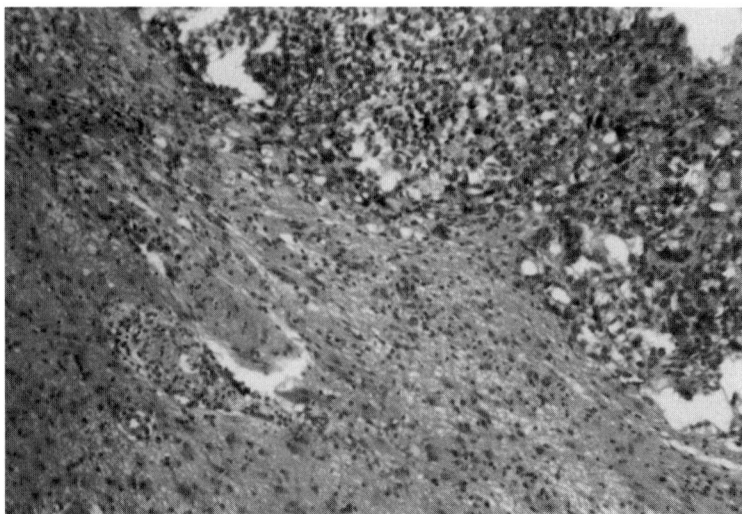

FIGURE 232–4. This sample is taken from a large choroid plexus carcinoma that invaded the wall of the lateral ventricle. Note the sheet of cells with loss of differentiated papillary architecture (compared with Fig. 232–3) and nuclear pleomorphism. This tumor clearly invades and infiltrates the brain, seen on the lower aspect of the field. (Hematoxylin and eosin, ×10.)

ate carcinoma from papilloma include cellular anaplasia, loss of differentiated papillary choroid architecture, nuclear pleomorphism, mitosis, necrosis, and giant cell formation. At the extreme end of the spectrum are sheets of anaplastic cells without appreciable papillae. These tumors are very cellular, with complex cribriform structures and a high mitotic index (Fig. 232–4). One issue of contention is whether brain invasion is required for the diagnosis of carcinoma or whether invasion by itself confirms the diagnosis. Some authors insist that invasion be demonstrated histologically; others do not.[83] It is noteworthy that not all surgical specimens have brain tissue insinuated within the tumor projections, especially when the surgeon uses ultrasonic aspiration or microsurgical suction to remove the specimen at the brain-tumor interface and brain is not included in the surgical specimen. Thus, the absence of finger-like projections invaginating into the brain parenchyma does not necessarily eliminate the diagnosis of carcinoma. Some tumors may invade the stroma but, on careful histopathologic analysis, not invade the brain. In addition, some choroid tumors with relatively benign histologic features are invasive, whereas some anaplastic tumors seem to have circumscribed borders.[4, 85] Often, the diagnosis of invasion can be inferred by MRI scans and not by histologic evidence. Thus, although invasion of the brain makes the diagnosis of carcinoma highly likely, it is not invariably secured unless there are associated malignant cellular features.

Some have reported choroid plexus papilloma macro- and microscopic implants found in the leptomeninges, the subarachnoid space of the spinal cord, and the ventricular system.[86–88] A rare case of pulmonary metastases from a choroid plexus papilloma in an 11-year-old girl was reported.[89] Another case of a 19-year-old woman with extensive craniospinal metastases from a fourth ventricular papilloma was also reported.[86]

The diagnostic utility of immunohistochemistry is unclear. Immunohistochemistry of choroid plexus tumors reveals both epithelial and glial characteristics. Choroid neoplasms can be positive for cytokeratin (epithelial), S-100 protein (diffuse staining), vimentin, and synaptophysin.[90–92] Positivity for carcinoembryonic antigen is more common in carcinoma, whereas S-100 protein positivity is more common in papilloma.[93]

The differential diagnosis in children often focuses on how to differentiate choroid plexus tumors from ependymoma and embryonal tumors. Ependymoma is characterized by nonepithelial glial elements as well as epithelial components. Ependymomas lack the prominent basement membrane possessed by choroid plexus tumors seen on periodic acid–Schiff preparations, electron microscopy, or immunohistochemical stains for laminin.[94] The presence of a basal lamina viewed by electron microscope is a feature of choroid plexus tumor but not ependymoma.[95] Choroid plexus neoplasms are positive for cytokeratin, but ependymomas are not. Ependymomas are often positive for glial fibrillary acidic protein, whereas choroid plexus tumors are diffusely but not uniformly positive for the same protein. In an adult with an intraventricular mass, S-100 protein positivity favors a primary choroid plexus tumor rather than a metastatic tumor.[2]

DNA sequences similar to those found in simian virus 40 have been found in choroid plexus tumors. This provocative finding is supported by the observation that some transgenic mice (SV11) infected with simian virus 40 have developed choroid plexus neoplasms, which is indicative of the oncogenic properties of polyomaviruses.[96, 97] However, in summary, no clearcut immunochemical or molecular criteria have emerged with any consistency to separate papilloma from carcinoma or to establish prognostic significance.

SURGICAL TREATMENT AND CONSIDERATIONS

Many different surgical approaches have been described to remove choroid plexus tumors. The location of these lesions in the ventricle makes passing through neural structures mandatory in all surgical approaches, with the possible exception of small tumors in the cerebellopontine angle or fourth ventricle.[98] These tumors are technically challenging not only because of their location but also because of their exuberant, friable blood supply, which is often deep to the tumor bulk and not accessible until much of the tumor has been excised. It is for this reason that we attempt preoperative tumor embolization when possible. In small children, this may not always be technically feasible, but the assistance of a skilled interventional neuroradiologist or neurosurgeon can make the tumor resection immeasurably easier. We have embolized large, highly vascular tumors in children as young as 3 years and large hemispheric lesions in adults. Such embolization, when successful, can markedly lessen the blood loss in these difficult cases. A similar experience has been reported by other surgeons.[5] Other investigators have commented on the successful use of preoperative chemotherapy to shrink these tumors rather than risk a large intraoperative blood loss.[83, 99–101]

The successful excision of a choroid plexus neoplasm takes the concerted effort of a team that includes members from neuroradiology, neuroanesthesiology, neuro–intensive care, and nursing. Because blood loss and hemodynamic instability account for much of the operative morbidity, judicious and early use of the appropriate blood products is essential. Ventricular drainage lessens intracranial pressure, and careful monitoring of intravascular volume and mean arterial blood pressure ensures an adequate cerebral perfusion pressure, even during periods of continuous blood loss.

The basic principles of tumor removal are an appropriately placed cortical incision, early isolation of the vascular supply (both arterial and venous), mobilization of the tumor, and microdissection or resection to reduce blood loss. It is sometimes difficult to mobilize choroid plexus neoplasms, especially large ones. Vigorous manipulation of an extremely large tumor is unwise, as the arterial supply may be disrupted before its visualization. Piecemeal resection must often be performed. Debulking of the tumor's papillary regions with bipolar electrocautery or ultrasonic suction can make a large tumor more manageable. However, if the blood supply to these tumors remains intact, piecemeal excision can be like encountering a friable vascular malformation. Once the vascular supply is identified, it can be occluded so that the more vascular tumor mass can be excised en bloc or piecemeal.

An appreciation of the relevant anatomy is helpful in surgical approaches to the ventricles. The primary arteries to the choroid plexus are the anterior and posterior choroidal arteries. The arterial supply of these tumors usually arises from hypertrophied branches of these choroidal arteries. The anterior choroidal artery rises from the internal carotid artery, distal to the posterior communicating artery, and courses posteriorly through the choroidal fissure to lie near the posterior choroidal artery. The anterior choroidal artery often supplies tumors in the atrium and temporal horn. Because the choroidal arteries pass through the choroidal fissure, opening this fissure permits proximal control of the feeding vessels.

The posterior choroidal arteries have lateral and medial divisions. The lateral posterior choroidal artery arises from the posterior cerebral artery, pierces the ventricle, and traverses the choroidal fissure at the level of the crus of the fornix. This vessel supplies the temporal horn, atrium, and body of the lateral ventricle, as well as tumors contained within those cavities.[98] The medial posterior choroidal artery, which also originates from the posterior cerebral artery, travels through the velum interpositum, sending inconstant branches to the lateral ventricles through the choroidal fissure and foramen of Monro. The medial posterior choroidal artery can supply tumors in the third ventricle and the lateral ventricle, as well as the choroid plexus in the roof of the third ventricle. Tumors may be supplied by one enlarged artery or by multiple feeders from the anterior and posterior choroidal arteries simultaneously.[98]

Fourth ventricle tumors are often fed by choroidal branches of the posterior inferior cerebellar artery or superior cerebellar arteries. Venous drainage is often deep, through the subependymal veins, internal cerebral veins, vein of Rosenthal, vein of Galen, and quadrigeminal or precentral cerebellar veins. There are many important veins composing the deep lateral and medial groups, but perhaps the best known for surgical and angiographic orientation during tumor removal in the lateral ventricle is the thalamostriate vein, which runs along the floor of the lateral ventricle in a lateral to medial direction toward the foramen of Monro.

The appropriate approach is determined by the tumor location, vascular supply, and experience and preference of the surgeon. Extremely large tumors may require a combination of more than one approach so that the cortical excision and retraction are minimal. The different approaches can be grouped according to location in the lateral, third, and fourth ventricles.

The transcortical approaches are useful because they permit access to all five regions of the lateral ventricle through one or a combination of approaches. Conversely, the low risk of neuropsychological sequelae and seizure after a well-performed callosal section make this route attractive and appropriate in selected patients. Tumors in the frontal horn, although uncommon, can become large and cause obstruction of the foramen of Monro, with subsequent ventricular dilatation. The transcortical middle frontal gyrus approach is an excellent approach for tumors in the ipsilateral anterior horn. Tumors that extend inferiorly from the lateral ventricle into the third ventricle and require a subchoroidal exposure for removal are better visualized through a transcortical approach than a transcallosal approach. In patients who have small ventricles, tumor in both lateral ventricles, or tumor in the body of the lateral ventricle, a transcallosal route may be preferable.

The superior parietal approach is a natural approach for neurosurgeons because it uses a path to the lateral ventricle that is taken when placing a parietal occipital catheter for CSF diversion. Placing a catheter into the ventricle and performing a corticectomy down its pathway is a helpful maneuver. It is a reasonable approach for reaching choroid plexus neoplasms in the collateral trigone, posterior part of the body, atrium, and glomus regions of the ventricle. The lateral posterior choroidal artery, which may be obscured by the tumor mass, should be uncovered in the choroidal fissure between the pulvinar and the crus of the fornix and be isolated and secured to devascularize the tumor. This approach is more risky in the dominant than in the nondominant hemisphere.

No single middle fossa approach permits early control of both the anterior and posterior choroidal arteries initially.[102] The middle temporal gyrus approach provides a direct route to middle fossa choroid plexus neoplasms with minimal morbidity and early control of the anterior choroidal artery feeding vessels. The lateral temporoparietal junction approach is used in rare cases when a large tumor is harbored in the nondominant atrium. The risk of a field deficit and damage to the angular gyrus is high, but this may be the shortest and most direct route to the tumor below.

Posterior fossa tumors can be removed by a standard posterior fossa craniectomy using retrosigmoid or extreme lateral approaches. Tumors confined to the fourth ventricle can be reached through a vermian split or corticectomy through the cerebellar hemisphere. Tumors that exit through the foramen of Luschka or those that creep anterior to the cerebellopontine angle may require a more laterally placed skull base approach. Cerebellopontine angle tumors are challenging to excise because of their location, a complex vascular supply that can include both branches of the posterior and anterior inferior cerebellar artery, and the tumor's intimate relationship with the cranial nerves. It sometimes requires hours of meticulous microsurgery to peel the well-vascularized tumor off each of the lower cranial nerves (VII to XII) before the tumor exits the foramen of Luschka. Care must be taken not to sacrifice the anterior inferior cerebellar branch adjacent to the cranial nerve VII to cranial nerve III complex or cause vasospasm in any of the small arterial vessels near the brainstem. Papaverine on pledgets placed over these essential vessels may ameliorate the effects of manipulation in this region. Intraoperative cranial nerve monitoring for cerebellopontine angle tumors can be used, but it may have limited utility. Often, tumor bulk must be dissected from each cranial nerve, causing the intraoperative spontaneous electromyogram to fire incessantly. Ultimately, the surgeon must make the decision whether to peel the tumor off the nerve or to leave residual tumor.

PROGNOSIS AND COMPLICATIONS

Before 1958, the morbidity and mortality from excision of these tumors were as high as 50%.[1] Fortuna and colleagues in 1979 reported a 48% surgical mortality in their review of 25 cases of choroid plexus neoplasms removed from the third ventricle.[103] The intraventricular location, associated hydrocephalus, and abundant vascular supply are the principal features of all these tumors and are responsible for their associated morbidity and mortality. Since the 1970s, surgical mortality in series has been reported as high as 24% and as low as 0%.[29, 43, 49]

Improved outcomes were achieved by progressive developments in CSF shunting techniques, imaging technology, microsurgical technique, anesthesiology, and perioperative care. Several series report a 100% perioperative survival in patients with papilloma undergoing surgery after 1961.[4, 39, 49]

The complications of transcortical and transcallosal surgery are specific to the approach, preoperative condition of the patient, location of the tumor, and difficulty encountered in removing it. The risks and potential complications are well described and include hematoma, hemiparesis, seizure disorders, developmental delay, neuropsychological deficits, visual field deficits, and cranial nerve deficits.[40, 47]

The series on choroid plexus neoplasms are too small to make general statements concerning neurologic outcome. Histopathologic features do not always correlate with outcome, but not surprisingly, both children and adults with papilloma tend to have significantly more favorable outcomes than do those with carcinoma. In a series of 40 pediatric choroid plexus neoplasms studied over a 45-year period, only 50% with carcinoma survived, compared with 84% with papilloma. The major morbidity in the survivors was hemiparesis (23%) and seizures (25%). Twenty-three percent of the patients with papilloma enjoyed an excellent outcome without neurologic deficit, whereas only 14% of those with carcinoma had a good long-term outcome with reasonable function.

There is controversy over the prognosis of choroid plexus carcinoma and considerable disagreement over the ability of surgical excision to extend survival in those with malignant lesions. Some groups maintain a pessimistic posture despite survivors in their own series, arguing that these tumors possess a uniformly grave outcome.[12, 83] Carpenter and coworkers, in 1982, reviewed 25 patients in the literature with choroid plexus carcinoma and concluded that only 4 of them enjoyed "relatively good results."[104] The groups with survivors have been impressed that aggressive surgical intervention (multiple times, if necessary), followed or preceded by adjuvant therapy, has been rewarded by a few long-term survivors, an observation previously thought to be impossible.[4, 7, 8] In 1998, Berger and associates from France reported a 5-year survival rate of 26% after aggressive surgical intervention for choroid plexus carcinoma.[6] Patients with a documented gross total excision had an 86% survival rate. Nearly all patients with an incomplete resection had recurrence and a poor outcome. The sole significant prognostic parameter was the extent of surgical excision.[6]

The complete removal of a neoplasm of the choroid plexus does not obviate the need for placement of a shunt in all patients.[49, 70, 71] One of the more problematic complications of intraventricular surgery for choroid neoplasms is the development of symptomatic subdural fluid collections, which has been discussed in detail by several authors.[14, 40, 105] Although this complication is not unique to the removal of choroid plexus tumors, it has occurred with both transcortical and transcallosal approaches.[45] In Boyd and Steinbok's surgical series of 11 choroid plexus neoplasms, 2 patients developed postoperative collections requiring a subdural peritoneal shunt after transcortical surgery.[40] The authors argued that this complication may be avoided by making a smaller corticectomy, filling the ventricles with physiologic saline before dural closure, and placing a fine pial suture or using tissue glue to close the fistula.[40]

The extent of surgical resection of choroid plexus tumors is the single most important determinant in achieving long-term disease-free survival.[4, 6, 8, 30, 37, 106, 107] Adjuvant therapy may be required for tumors that are incompletely resected or malignant or those that have shown neuraxis or leptomeningeal spread. External beam irradiation is a reasonable form of adjuvant therapy in older children and adults, especially craniospinal irradiation for those patients with drop metastases, leptomeningeal spread, and tumors invading the parenchyma.[108] However, the efficacy of radiation therapy, both conventional and focused beam, remains undefined in the treatment of this disease. Case reports of successful treatment of choroid plexus tumors with stereotactic radiation therapy are just beginning to appear in the literature.

The documented neuropsychological sequelae of radiation therapy on the developing brain[109] have led to alternative approaches in young children. Patients younger than 3 years have received chemotherapy instead of radiation to spare them the cognitive dysfunction and short stature associated with this form of treatment. Gianella-Borradori and colleagues successfully treated two children with subtotal resected malignant carcinomas with eight-drug-a-day chemotherapy without radiation therapy. They concluded that chemotherapy may provide long-term survival, but more trials are needed.[110]

There are other reports of aggressive multimodality therapy consisting of combined pre- or postresection chemotherapy and radiotherapy. This approach is also used for subsequent attempts at radical resection of choroid plexus carcinomas that could not be removed initially. The conclusion is that pretreatment with chemotherapy shrinks the tumor, making the subsequent surgery easier and the disease-free survival period longer.[83, 99–101] A report from the Pediatric Oncology Group in 1995 described eight infants with choroid plexus carcinoma who underwent surgery and successful prolonged postoperative chemotherapy and delayed radiation. The conclusion was that this aggressive multimodality approach prolongs survival even in children with subtotally resected choroid plexus neoplasms. However, the danger of delayed disease recurrence from meningeal carcinomatosis in carcinoma still exists, despite this aggressive multimodality therapy.[111]

CONCLUSIONS

Choroid plexus tumors represent a spectrum of neoplasia from hypertrophy of normal choroid plexus to aggressive and highly mitotic carcinoma. Regardless of the histologic characteristics, they are challenging lesions to excise, even for experienced surgeons. They possess an impressive vascular supply, often buried deep to the tumor mass. The anatomy of the ventricles and their relationship to the tumor permit a variety of surgical approaches. The location and size of the lesion, preoperative deficits, associated hydrocephalus, vascularity of the lesion, and experience of the surgeon contribute to the ultimate selection of a surgical approach. A combination of approaches and a staged approach are occasionally required to excise these lesions adequately with minimal morbidity.

The treatment of choroid plexus papilloma has yielded excellent results with exceptionally high survival rates in the microsurgical era. It is a curable tumor with surgical extirpation alone in the majority of cases. The management of postoperative subdural effusions and hydrocephalus is often the most confounding perioperative challenge in the treatment of these lesions. Significant neurologic deficits can and do occur but are less common in the microsurgical era.

Prolonged survival after surgical excision of choroid plexus carcinoma was originally thought to be uniformly unlikely. However, since 1989, there have been small series and scattered case reports of survival after removal of this malignant form of choroid plexus neoplasm.[4-8] Some groups are encouraged based on an aggressive surgical posture, appropriate adjuvant therapy, and vigilant follow-up and maintain that there is some hope for survival, albeit limited and guarded. The series of choroid plexus carcinoma are too small to derive any conclusive prognostic data on long-term survival. Advances in microsurgical techniques and the use of multiple surgical resections, chemotherapy, and radiation therapy have been partly responsible for the measured improvement over the previously dismal survival statistics. Currently, as long as the lesion remains localized and the patient's condition permits, an attempt at an aggressive therapeutic approach is justified.

REFERENCES

1. Matson D: Tumors of the choroid plexus. In Matson DD (ed): Neurosurgery of Infancy and Childhood, 2nd ed. Springfield, Ill, Charles C Thomas, 1969, pp 581–595.
2. Burger PC, Scheithauer BW: Tumors of neuroglia and choroid plexus epithelium. In Burger PC, Scheithauer BW (eds): Tumors of the Central Nervous System, vol 3. Washington, DC, Armed Forces Institute of Pathology, 1994, pp 136–161.
3. Rubinstein L: Tumors of the choroid plexus and related structures. In Firminger HI (ed): Tumors of the Central Nervous System, vol 2. Washington, DC, Armed Forces Institute of Pathology, 1972.
4. Ellenbogen RG, Winston KR, Kupsky WJ: Tumors of the choroid plexus in children. Neurosurgery 25:327–335, 1989.
5. Pencalet P, Sainte-Rose C, Lellouch-Tubiana A, et al: Papillomas and carcinomas of the choroid plexus in children. J Neurosurg 88:521–528, 1998.
6. Berger C, Thiesse P, Lellouch-Tubiana A, et al: Choroid plexus carcinomas in childhood: Clinical features and prognostic factors. Neurosurgery 42:470–475, 1998.
7. Lena G, Genitori L, Molina J, et al: Choroid plexus tumors in children: Review of 24 cases. Acta Neurochir 106:68–72, 1990.
8. Packer R, Perilongo G, Johnson D, et al: Choroid plexus carcinoma of childhood. Cancer 69:580–585, 1992.

9. Cushing H: Intracranial Tumors. Springfield, Ill, Charles C Thomas, 1932.

10. Zulch K: Biologie und pathologie der hirngeschwulste. In Olvecrona H, Tonnis W (eds): Handbuch der Neruochirurgie, vol 3. Berlin, Springer-Verlag, 1956.

11. Dohrmann G, Collias J: Choroid plexus carcinoma. J Neurosurg 43:225–232, 1975.

12. Humphreys R, Nemoto S, Hendrick EB, Hoffman HJ: Childhood choroid plexus tumors. Concepts Pediatr Neurosurg 7:1–18, 1987.

13. Koos W, Miller M: Intracranial Tumors of Infants and Children. St. Louis, Mosby, 1971, pp 239–244.

14. Matson D, Crofton F: Papilloma of the choroid plexus in childhood. J Neurosurg 17:1002–1027, 1960.

15. Guerard M: Tumeur Fongeuse dans le ventricle droit du cerveau chez une petite fille de trois ans. Anat Paris 8:211–214, 1832.

16. Boudet G, Clunet J: Contribution a l'etude des tumeurs epitheliales primitives de l'encephale. Arch Med Exp Anat Pathol 22:379–411, 1910.

17. Davis L: A physiopathological study of the choroid plexus with the report of a case of villous hypertrophy. Med Res 44:521–534, 1924.

18. Davis L, Cushing H: Papillomas of the choroid plexus: A report of six cases. Arch Neurol Psychiatry 13:681–710, 1925.

19. Garrod: Papillomatous tumor in the fourth ventricle of the brain. Lancet 1:303, 1873.

20. Perthes G: Entfernung eines Tumors des Plexus Choriodeus an dem Seitenventrikel des Cerebrums. Munch Med Wschr 66:677–678, 1919.

21. Rand C, Reeves D: Choroid plexus tumors in infancy and childhood: Report of four cases. Bull Los Angeles Neurol Soc 5:405–410, 1940.

22. Sachs E: Papillomas of the fourth ventricle. Arch Neurol Psychiatry 8:379–382, 1922.

23. Slaymaker S, Elias F: Papilloma of the choroid plexus with hydrocephalus: Report of a case. Arch Intern Med 3:289–294, 1909.

24. Turner O, Simon M: Malignant papillomas of the choroid plexus: Report of two cases with review of the literature. Am J Cancer 30:289–297, 1937.

25. Van Wagenen W: Papillomas of the choroid plexus: Report of two cases, one with removal of tumor and one with "seeding" of the tumor in the ventricular system. Arch Surg 20:199–231, 1930.

26. Bielschowsky M, Unger E: Kenntnis der primaren Epithelgeschwulste der Adergeflechte des Gehirns. Arch Klin Chir 81:61–82, 1906.

27. Dandy W: Benign Encapsulated Tumors of the Lateral Ventricle. Baltimore, Williams & Wilkins, 1934.

28. Masson C: Complete removal of two tumors of the third ventricle with recovery. Arch Surg 28:527–537, 1934.

29. Hawkins JCI: Treatment of choroid plexus papillomas in children: A brief analysis of twenty years' experience. Neurosurgery 6:380–384, 1980.

30. Johnson DL: Management of choroid plexus tumors in children. Pediatr Neurosci 15:195–206, 1989.

31. Laurence K: The biology of choroid plexus papilloma and carcinoma of the lateral ventricle. In Vinken P, Bruyn G (eds): Tumors of the Brain and Skull. Part 2. Handbook of Clinical Neurology, vol 17. New York, Elsevier, 1974, pp 555–595.

32. Pascual-Castroviejo I, Villarejo F, Perez-Higueras A, et al: Childhood choroid plexus neoplasms: A study of 14 cases less than 2 years old. Eur Pediatr 140:51–56, 1983.

33. Body G, Darnis E, Pourcelot D, et al: Choroid plexus tumors: Antenatal diagnosis and follow-up. J Clin Ultrasound 18:575–578, 1990.

34. Tomita T, Naidich TP: Successful resection of choroid plexus papillomas diagnosed at birth: Report of two cases. Neurosurgery 20:774–779, 1987.

35. Kahn E, Luros J: Hydrocephalus from overproduction of cerebrospinal fluid (and experiences with other papilloma of the choroid plexus). J Neurosurg 9:59–67, 1952.

36. Knierim DS: Choroid plexus tumors in infants. Pediatr Neurosurg 16:276–280, 1990.

37. McGirr SJ, Ebersold MJ, Scheithauer BW, et al: Choroid plexus papillomas: Long-term follow-up results in a surgically treated series. J Neurosurg 69:843–849, 1988.

38. Russell D, Rubinstein L: Pathology of Tumors of the Nervous System, 2nd ed. London, Edward Arnold, 1971.

39. Tomita T, McLone DG, Flannery AM: Choroid plexus papillomas of neonates, infants and children. Pediatr Neurosci 14:23–30, 1988.

40. Boyd M, Steinbok M: Choroid plexus tumors: Problems in diagnosis and management. J Neurosurg 66:800–805, 1987.

41. Aicardi JGJ, Lepintre J, Cherrie JJ, Thieffry S: Les papillomes des plexus choroides chez l'enfant. Arch Fr Pediatr 25:673–686, 1968.

42. Bohm J, Strange R: Choroid plexus papillomas. J Neurosurg 18:493–500, 1961.

43. Guidetti B, Spallone A: The surgical treatment of choroid plexus papillomas: The results of 27 years' experience. Neurosurgery 6:380–384, 1981.

44. Zhang W: Clinical significance of anterior inferior cerebellar artery in angiographic diagnosis of choroid plexus papilloma at the cerebellopontine angle. Chin Med J (Engl) 96:275–280, 1983.

45. Jooma R, Grant D: Third ventricle choroid plexus papillomas. Childs Brain 10:242–250, 1983.

46. Pollack IF, Schor NF, Martinez JA, Towbin R: Bobble-head doll syndrome and drop attacks in a child with a cystic choroid plexus papilloma of the third ventricle. J Neurosurg 83:729–732, 1995.

47. Schijman E, Monges J, Raimondi A, Tomita T: Choroid plexus papillomas of the III ventricle in childhood. Childs Nerv Syst 6:331–334, 1990.

48. Pecker J, Ferrand B, Javalet A: Tumeurs du troisieme ventricule. Neurochirurgie 12:1–136, 1966.

49. Raimondi A, Gutierrez F: Diagnosis and surgical treatment of choroid plexus papillomas. Childs Brain 1:81–115, 1975.

50. Rovit R, Schechter M, Chodroff P: Choroid plexus papillomas—observation on radiologic diagnosis. AJR Am J Roentgenol 110:608–617, 1970.

51. Abbott K, Rollas Z, Meagher J: Choroid plexus papilloma causing spontaneous subarachnoid hemorrhage. J Neurosurg 14:566–570, 1957.

52. Ernsting J: Choroid plexus papilloma causing spontaneous subarachnoid hemorrhage. J Neurol Neurosurg Psychiatry 18:134–136, 1955.

53. Ray B, Peck F Jr: Papilloma of the choroid plexus of the lateral ventricles causing hydrocephalus in an infant. J Neurosurg 13:405–410, 1956.

54. Shaw J: Papilloma of the choroid plexus. In Amador L (ed): Brain Tumors in the Young. Springfield, Ill, Charles C Thomas, 1983, pp 655–670.

55. Milhorat T, Hammock M, Davis D, Fenstermacher J: Choroid plexus papilloma: Proof of cerebrospinal overproduction. Childs Brain 2:273–289, 1976.

56. Talacchi A, DeMicheli E, Lombardo C, et al: Choroid plexus papilloma of the cerebellopontine angle: A twelve patient series. Surg Neurol 51:621–629, 1999.

57. Hammock M, Milhorat T, Breckbill D: Primary choroid plexus papilloma of the cerebellopontine angle, presenting as brain stem tumor in a child. Childs Brain 2:132–142, 1976.

58. Wilkins R, Rutledge B: Papillomas of the choroid plexus. J Neurosurg 18:14–18, 1961.

59. Cassinari V: Tumori della parte anteriore del terzo ventricolo. Acta Neurochir 11:236–271, 1963.

60. Eisenberg H, McComb G, Lorenzo A: Cerebrospinal fluid overproduction and hydrocephalus associated with choroid plexus papilloma. J Neurosurg 40:380–385, 1974.

61. Fairburn B: Choroid plexus papilloma and its relationship to hydrocephalus. J Neurosurg 17:166–171, 1958.

62. Johnson R: Clinicopathological aspects of the cerebrospinal fluid circulation. In Wilstenholme G, O'Conner M (eds): Ciba Foundation Symposium on Cerebrospinal Fluid Production, Circulation and Absorption. Boston, Little, Brown, 1957, pp 265–281.

63. Portnoy H, Croissant P: A practical method of measuring hydrodynamics of cerebrospinal fluid. Surg Neurol 5:173–177, 1976.

64. Sahar A, Feinsod M, Beller A: Choroid plexus papilloma: Hydrocephalus and cerebrospinal fluid dynamics. Surg Neurol 13:476–478, 1980.

65. Vigouroux A: Ecoulement de liquide cephalorachidien. Hydrocephalie papillome des plexus chorides du IV ventricule. Rev Neurol 16:281–285, 1970.

66. Welch K, Strand R, Bresnan M, Cavazzuti V: Congenital hydrocephalus due to villous hypertrophy of the telencephalic choroid plexuses: Case report. J Neurosurg 59:172–175, 1983.

67. Gudeman S, Sullivan H, Rosner M, Becker D: Surgical removal of bilateral papillomas of the choroid plexus of the lateral ventricles with resolution of hydrocephalus. J Neurosurg 50:677–681, 1979.

68. Rekate HL, Erwood S, Brodkey JA, et al: Etiology of ventriculomegaly in choroid plexus papilloma. Pediatr Neurosci 12:196–201, 1985–1986.

69. Husag L, Costabile G, Probst C: Persistent hydrocephalus following removal of choroid plexus papilloma of the lateral ventricle. Neurochirurgia (Stuttg) 27:82–85, 1984.

70. Jellinger K, Grunert V, Sunder-Plassmann M: Choroid plexus papilloma associated with hydrocephalus in infancy. Neuropaediatrics 1:344–348, 1970.

71. McDonald J: Persistent hydrocephalus following the removal of papillomas of the choroid plexus of the lateral ventricles. J Neurosurg 30:736–740, 1969.

72. Smith J: Hydrocephalus associated with choroid plexus papillomas. Neuropathol Exp Neurol 14:442–449, 1933.

73. Hirano H, Hirahara K, Tetsuhiko A, et al: Hydrocephalus due to villous hypertrophy of the choroid plexus in the lateral ventricles. J Neurosurg 80:321–323, 1994.

74. Philips M, Shanno G, Duhaime A: Treatment of villous hypertrophy of the choroid plexus by endoscopic contact coagulation. Pediatr Neurosurg 28:252–256, 1998.

75. Crofton F, Matson D: Roentgenologic study of choroid plexus papillomas in children. Am J Roentgenol Radium Ther Nucl Med 84:273–311, 1950.

76. Vazquez E, Ball WS, Prenger EC, et al: Magnetic resonance imaging of fourth ventricular choroid plexus neoplasms in childhood. Pediatr Neurosurg 17:48–52, 1991.

77. Coates TL, Hinshaw DB Jr, Peckman N, et al: Pediatric choroid plexus neoplasms: MR, CT, and pathologic correlation. Radiology 173:81–88, 1989.

78. Schellhas KP, Siebert RC, Heithoff KB, Franciosi RA: Congenital choroid plexus papilloma of the third ventricle: Diagnosis with real-time sonography and MR imaging. AJNR Am J Neuroradiol 9:797–798, 1988.

79. Morrison G, Sobel D, Kelly W, Norman D: Intraventricular mass lesions. Radiology 153:435–442, 1984.

80. Gullotta F, de Melo A: Plexus chorioideus. Klinishe, lightmikroskopische und elektronenoptische untersuchungen. Neurochirurgia (Stuttg) 22:1–9, 1979.

81. Paulus W, Janisch W: Clincopathologic correlations in epithelial choroid plexus neoplasms: A study of 52 cases. Acta Neuropathol (Berl) 80:635–641, 1990.

82. Matsuda M, Uzura S, Nakasu S, Handa J: Primary carcinoma of the choroid plexus in the lateral ventricle. Surg Neurol 36:294–299, 1991.

83. St. Clair SK, Humphreys RP, Pillay PK, et al: Current management of choroid plexus carcinoma in children. Pediatr Neurosurg 92:225–233, 1991.

84. Lewis P: Carcinoma of the choroid plexus. Brain 90:177–186, 1967.

85. Ausman J, Shrontz C, Chason J, et al: Aggressive choroid plexus papilloma. Surg Neurol 22:472–476, 1984.

86. Leblanc R, Bekhor S, Melanson D, Carpenter S: Diffuse craniospinal seeding from a benign fourth ventricle choroid plexus papilloma: Case report. J Neurosurg 88:757–760, 1998.

87. Ringertz N, Reymond A: Ependymomas and choroid plexus papillomas. J Neuropathol Exp Neurol 8:355, 1949.

88. Russell D, Rubinstein L: Pathology of Tumors of the Nervous System, 2nd ed. Baltimore, Williams & Wilkins, 1963, pp 141–142.

89. Vraa-Jensen G: Papilloma of the choroid plexus with pulmonary metastases. Acta Psychtr (Koln) 25:299–306, 1950.

90. Ang L, Taylor A, Bergin D, Kaufmann J: An immunohistochemical study of papillary tumors of the central nervous system. Cancer 65:2712–2719, 1990.

91. Cruz-Sanchez F, Rossi M, Hughes J, et al: Choroid plexus papillomas: An immunohistological study of 16 cases. Histopathology 15:61–69, 1989.

92. Kepes J, Collins J: Choroid plexus epithelium (normal and neoplastic) expresses synaptophysin: A potentially useful aid in differentiating carcinoma of the choroid plexus from metastatic papillary carcinomas. J Neuropathol Exp Neurol 58:1111–1112, 1999.

93. Coffin C, Wick M, Braun J, Dehner L: Choroid plexus neoplasms: Clinicopathological and immunohistochemical studies. Am Surg Pathol 10:394–404, 1986.

94. Furness P, Lowe J, Tarrant G: Subepithelial basement deposition and intermediate filament expression in choroid plexus neoplasms and ependymomas. Histopathology 16:251–255, 1990.

95. Hirano A: Some contributions of electron microscopy to the diagnosis of brain tumors. Acta Neuropathol (Berl) 43:119–128, 1978.

96. Bergsagel D, Finegold M, Butel J, et al: DNA sequences similar to those of simian virus 40 in ependymomas and choroid plexus tumors of childhood. N Engl J Med 326:988–993, 1992.

97. Patrick T, Kranz D, van Dyke T, Roy E: Folate receptors as potential therapeutic targets in choroid plexus tumors of SV40 transgenic mice. J Neurooncol 32:111–123, 1997.

98. Timurkaynak E, Rhoton A, Barry M: Microsurgical anatomy and approaches to the lateral ventricles. Neurosurgery 19:685–723, 1986.

99. Araki K, Aori T, Takahashi J, et al: A case report of choroid plexus carcinoma. No Shinkei Geka 25:853–857, 1997.

100. Kumabe T, Tominaga T, Kondo T, et al: Intraoperative radiation therapy and chemotherapy for huge choroid plexus carcinoma in an infant: Case report. Neurol Med Chir (Tokyo) 36:179–184, 1996.

101. Souweidane M, Johnson JJ, Lis E: Volumetric reduction of a choroid plexus carcinoma using preoperative chemotherapy. J Neurooncol 43:167–171, 1999.

102. Jun C, Nutic S: Surgical approaches to intraventricular meningiomas of the trigone. Neurosurgery 16:416–420, 1985.

103. Fortuna A, Celli P, Ferrante L, Turano C: A review of papillomas of the third ventricle. J Neurosurg 23:61–72, 1979.

104. Carpenter D, Michelsen W, Hays A: Carcinoma of the choroid plexus. J Neurosurg 56:722–777, 1982.

105. Shillito J, Matson D: An Atlas of Pediatric Neurosurgical Operations. Philadelphia, WB Saunders, 1982.

106. Pierga J, Kalifa C, Terrier-Lacombe MJ, et al: Carcinoma of the choroid plexus: A pediatric experience. Med Pediatr Oncol 21:480–487, 1993.

107. Sharma R, Rout D, Gupta A, Radhakrishnan V: Choroid plexus papillomas. Br J Neurosurg 8:169–177, 1994.

108. Geerts Y, Gabreels F, Lippens R, et al: Choroid plexus carcinoma: A report of two cases and review of the literature. Neuropediatrics 27:143–148, 1996.

109. Duffner P, Cohen M, Thomas P, et al: The long term effects of cranial irradiation in the central nervous system. Cancer 56:1841–1847, 1985.

110. Gianella-Borradori A, Zeltzer PM, Bodey B, et al: Choroid plexus tumors in childhood. Cancer 69:809–816, 1992.

111. Peschgens T, Stollbrink-Peschgens C, Mertens R, et al: Zur Therapie des Plexus-chorioideus-Karzinomas im Kindesalter. Fallbeispiel und Literaturubersicht. Klin Padiatr 207:52–58, 1995.

Intracranial Ependymomas

LESLIE N. SUTTON ■ JOEL GOLDWEIN

Cerebral ependymomas are uncommon tumors with a peak incidence in early childhood. They were first classified as a distinct entity in 1926 by Bailey and Cushing,[1] and in the past, they were considered favorable tumors. If one excludes subependymomas (which are believed to be related to hamartomas and astrocytomas) and ependymoblastomas (which are currently classified with primitive neuroectodermal tumors), they are usually histologically benign and slow growing. Despite their relatively benign histologic appearance, they recur relentlessly and are among the most difficult neoplasms to cure. Surgical excision is the mainstay of treatment, but the location of ependymomas often makes complete surgical resection a morbid procedure. When there is brainstem involvement, the surgeon faces a dilemma: attempt a radical resection and risk serious neurological complications, or leave tumor behind and await the inevitable recurrence.

EPIDEMIOLOGY

Intracerebral ependymomas occur with an incidence of 0.3 per 100,000 patient-years (adults and children)[2] and account for 1.2% to 7.8% of brain tumors overall.[3–5] They present more commonly in children, representing 10% of brain tumors in children younger than 14 years but only 1.9% of brain tumors in adults.[6] They are the third most common histologic type of brain tumor in children, after primitive neuroectodermal tumors and astrocytomas. Peak incidence is between birth and 4 years of age, with little variation after that age.[7–9] Males are 1.4 times more likely to develop ependymomas than females are.[2]

More than 90% of childhood ependymomas arise within the cranium; two thirds occur below the tentorium, and one third above it. In contrast, in adults, more than 75% occur within the spinal canal, and the majority of intracranial ependymomas arise within the supratentorial compartment.[10]

The cause of ependymomas is unknown. No environmental factor has been implicated, and recent work has concentrated on cytogenetic abnormalities. Because ependymomas are found in 2% to 5% of patients with neurofibromatosis type 2,[11] particular attention has been paid to chromosome 22, the site of the recently cloned neurofibromatosis gene. There have been several reports of loss of material from chromosome 22 in ependymoma tissue.[12–16] The consistent loss of a specific chromosomal region in a tumor often indicates the presence of a tumor suppressor gene, and the early age at which ependymomas typically present is consistent with the hypothesis that there is a germline mutation that predisposes these children to develop cancer at an early age. Recent work, however, has not shown mutations of the neurofibromatosis gene in patients with ependymomas.[12] At least one family without neurofibromatosis has been reported to have a predisposition for both ependymomas and meningiomas,[17] and it is possible that lack of a functional tumor suppressor gene at a locus distinct from the neurofibromatosis gene on chromosome 22 is responsible for both familial and sporadic ependymomas. One patient developed a malignant ependymoma at age 5 and was found to have a de novo constitutional translocation with a breakpoint in the region between ARVCF and D22S264, but this does not appear to be a consistent breakpoint in sporadic ependymomas.[18]

PATHOLOGY AND PATHOBIOLOGY

Ependymomas presumably arise from ependymal cells or rests, so they should occur only in relation to the ventricular surface. In fact, although most do arise adjacent to a ventricle, they may occur in the supratentorial parenchyma, in the filum terminale, or within the substance of the spinal cord. Ependymomas of the spinal cord and filum terminale represent special cases and are discussed elsewhere. Ependymomas have been reported in the posterior mediastinum in adults, without a connection to the central nervous system.[19]

Grossly, most ependymomas are grayish or red, lobulated, gritty, and firm. They are relatively well circumscribed and, although frequently vascular, are typically less so than medulloblastomas or rhabdoid-teratoid tumors. Some have a papillary appearance, which may suggest a choroid plexus tumor. Supratentorial tumors are often periventricular and may have a large lobulated portion within the ventricle with a subcortical extension.

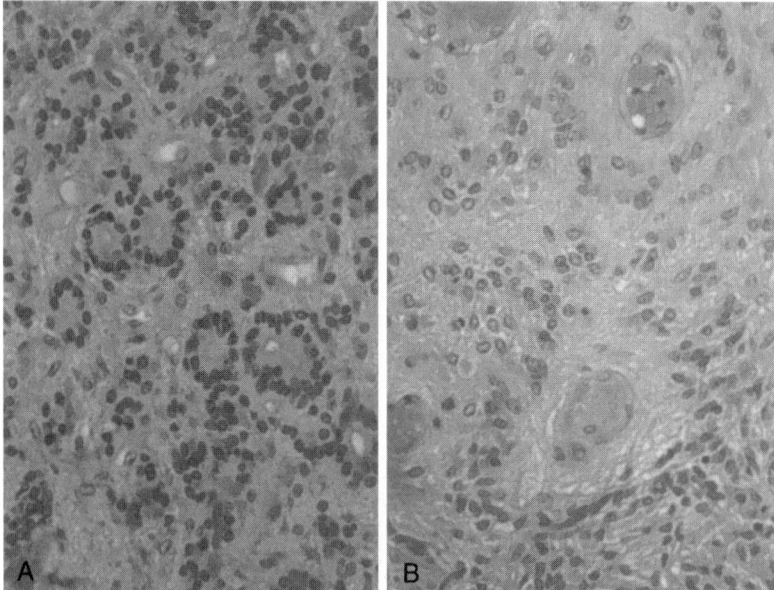

FIGURE 233–1. Histopathologic appearance of a typical ependymoma (hematoxylin-eosin, ×400). The background is composed of round or polygonal cells of roughly the same size. *A,* The round structures are true rosettes, which recapitulate the central canal. There is no blood vessel within. *B,* The round structures are pseudorosettes, with a central blood vessel. Both are characteristic of ependymomas. (From Sutton L, Goldwein J, Schwartz D: Ependymomas. In Albright A, Pollack I, Adelson P [eds]: Principles and Practice of Pediatric Neurosurgery. New York, Thieme, 1999.)

Microscopically, the degree of cellularity is variable, even within a single tumor.[20] The cells are typically polygonal and form a uniform background. A diagnostic feature is the presence of rosettes, representing the tumor's attempt to recapitulate an ependyma-lined central canal. Most also contain perivascular pseudorosettes, in which a blood vessel is surrounded by an eosinophilic halo composed of radiating processes of the cells, which are oriented toward it (Fig. 233–1). Blepharoplasts may occasionally be seen using light microscopy but are better seen using electron microscopy. Common to ependymomas are vascular hyalinization and microcalcifications, and some may even suggest metaplastic bone or cartilage.[21] Histopathologic curios include melanin-producing variants[22] and tumors containing so-called signet-ring cells.[23] Specific immunohistochemical stains for intermediate filament proteins are typically positive for glial fibrillary acidic protein and vimentin and may be positive for neuron-specific enolase and S-100. Ependymomas are typically negative for alpha-fetoprotein, carcinoembryonic antigen, and desmin.[24]

There is considerable variation in the way ependymomas are graded. Several systems have been used in the past, but the current system is that of the World Health Organization,[25] which includes the designations "ependymoma" and "anaplastic ependymoma." This may partly explain the lack of consensus regarding histology as a prognostic factor. Whereas some series have reported a worse prognosis for malignant or "high-grade" lesions,[26–31] others have not.[32–35] Other explanations for this lack of agreement include disease and treatment variability and the fact that multivariate analysis has not been used in all these series. Further, ependymoblastomas, which are now regarded as a type of primitive neuroectodermal tumor, were often classified with ependymomas in the past. Recently, attempts have been made to correlate various growth factors[36] and proliferative indices with outcome. MIB-1 and p53 immunolabeling might be objective indicators of high grade in ependymomas that do not otherwise meet routine histologic criteria for a high-grade designation,[37] but some studies have found little predictive value for MIB-1.[38] In addition to histologic criteria of dense cellularity and conspicuous mitotic activity, prominent expression of these indices might justify the diagnosis of anaplastic ependymoma.[39] Regardless of the histologic grading system used, however, the majority of lesions are histologically benign.

SIGNS AND SYMPTOMS

Presentation is determined by the location of the tumor within the central nervous system. In children, most originate within the posterior fossa and typically present with the "midline posterior fossa syndrome" of headache, vomiting, and lethargy. These symptoms are nonspecific manifestations of raised intracranial pressure, and a similar picture is seen with medulloblastomas and astrocytomas. Because all these tumors may arise within the fourth ventricle, obstructive hydrocephalus occurs early and is usually the cause of early symptoms. The midline syndrome typically begins insidiously, with occasional morning headache and vomiting that improve throughout the day and may initially be attributed to a viral illness. Later in the course of the disease, symptoms become more persistent, and if the diagnosis is not made at this stage, signs of truncal ataxia, nystagmus, and sixth nerve palsy due to hydrocephalus may develop. Some patients are noted to have a head tilt from impaction of the cerebellar tonsils into the cervical spinal canal. If tumor progression is permitted to continue, pressure waves, opisthotonos, bradycardia, apnea, and death ensue. In adults, in whom these tumors most often arise in the cerebral hemispheres or in relation to the third ventri-

TABLE 233-1 ■ **Signs and Symptoms of 51 Children with Intracranial Ependymomas**

SYMPTOM	PERCENTAGE OF PATIENTS
Vomiting	61
Headache	57
Ataxia	38
Cranial nerve dysfunction	20
Head tilt	5
Hemiparesis	5
Other	23

Data from Goldwein J, Laehy J, Packer R, et al: Intracranial ependymomas in children. Int J Radiat Oncol Biol Phys 19:1497–1502, 1990.

cle, symptoms are headaches, diplopia, hemiparesis, and seizures.[10]

Atypical presentations are not unusual. The propensity of ependymomas to arise in the region of the area postrema and obex explains the predominance of vomiting even in the absence of hydrocephalus, which may initially lead to referral to a gastroenterologist (Table 233–1). Ependymomas often extend through the foramen of Luschka into the cerebellopontine angle, and cranial nerve dysfunction, especially facial weakness, hearing loss, and swallowing dysfunction, may be noted. Rarely, an ependymoma presents as an acute spontaneous hemorrhage.[40] This appears to be more likely in young children with more malignant tumors. Supratentorial ependymomas may present with signs and symptoms of generalized intracranial hypertension, seizures, or neurological symptoms referable to the area of brain involvement.

DIAGNOSTIC STUDIES

On computed tomographic scans, ependymomas are typically isointense to cerebellar cortex and heterogeneous. Hemorrhage is present in up to 13% of cases, and calcifications are frequent, occurring in 25% to 50% of cases. Cysts and necrotic areas are of low density. Fourth ventricular ependymomas are sometimes surrounded by a "peritumoral halo" of edema or cerebrospinal fluid (CSF), but this is not specific and may also be seen with other tumor types. At least partial contrast enhancement is present in virtually all ependymomas, but it is usually heterogeneous and irregular.[41] Hydrocephalus is present in virtually all posterior fossa lesions.

Supratentorial lesions are frequently extremely large at diagnosis. They may have a site of origin within the ventricle or may be entirely intraparenchymal. They typically enhance irregularly and may have low-density necrotic centers, mimicking malignant gliomas (Fig. 233–2).

Magnetic resonance imaging (MRI) is extremely valuable in defining the anatomy of posterior fossa tumors as they relate to the brainstem, spinal cord, and cerebellopontine angle.[41, 42] The most characteristic appearance is that of a mass arising from the lower brainstem

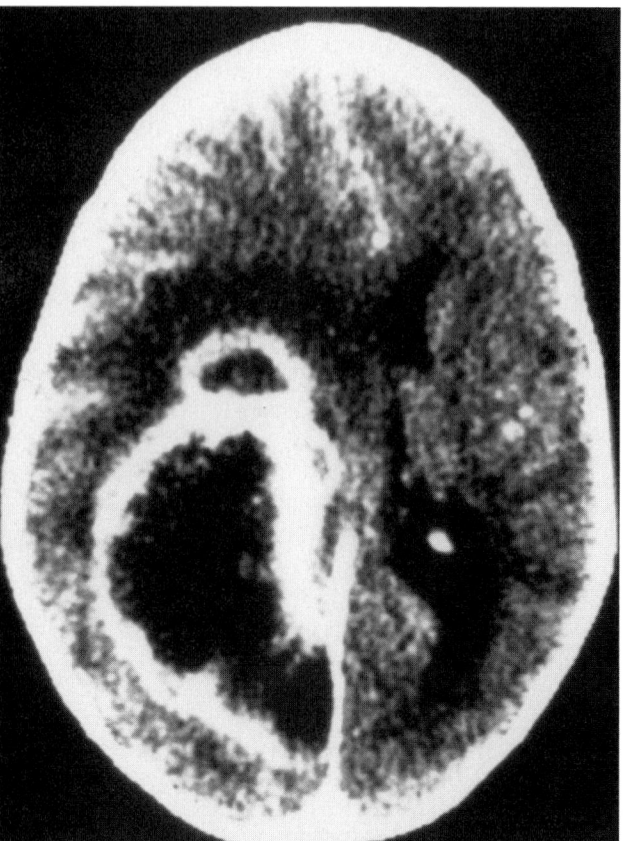

FIGURE 233–2. Contrast-enhanced computed tomographic scan of a supratentorial ependymoma in a child. The large, ring-enhancing appearance with central necrosis is typical and may be impossible to distinguish from a malignant glioma.

and projecting into the fourth ventricle. Ependymomas have a particular tendency to project through the foramen of Luschka into the cerebellopontine angle and to have tonguelike portions of tumor dorsal and lateral to the upper cervical cord. The vertebral arteries and posterior inferior cerebellar arteries may be displaced or encased (Table 233–2). As with computed tomography, the MRI appearance of ependymomas is characterized by inhomogeneity. The tumors are typically isointense or of low density on T1-weighted images, and isointense or of increased signal on T2-weighted and proton-density images. There is usually inhomogeneous enhancement with intravenous contrast material (Fig. 233–3).

Because of the lack of specificity of standard imaging modalities, newer techniques such as proton magnetic resonance spectroscopy have been used to increase diagnostic accuracy. The three major histologic groups of pediatric posterior fossa tumors show different metabolic patterns. Cerebellar astrocytomas show a somewhat decreased ratio of *N*-acetyl aspartate to choline compared with control brain, ependymomas on average have an even lower ratio, and medulloblastomas have the lowest ratio of all.[43] Neural network–based computer algorithms are capable of using both quantitative spectroscopy data and standard imaging data to predict histology in pediatric posterior fossa

TABLE 233-2 ■ **Radiographic Findings in Nine Patients with Posterior Fossa Ependymomas**

FINDING	PERCENTAGE OF PATIENTS
Encasement of vessels	33
Hydrocephalus	100
Structural heterogeneity	65
Calcification	57
Hemorrhage	22
Isodense on computed tomography	86
T1-weighted images	
Isointense	56
Low intensity	33
High intensity	11
Proton density	
High intensity	75
Isointense	25
T2-weighted images	
Isointense	67
High intensity	33

Data from Tortori-Donati P, Fondelli M, Cama A, et al: Ependymomas of the posterior cranial fossa: CT and MRI findings. Neuroradiology 37:238–243, 1995.

tumors with remarkable accuracy, which is helpful when discussing the likely risks of surgery with patients and their families.[44]

It is unusual for ependymomas to have disseminated at the time of diagnosis, with an incidence of only 11% to 17%.[30, 32] Nonetheless, it is important to demonstrate its presence or absence, because disseminated disease is a strong adverse prognostic factor. It is preferable to perform a staging spinal MRI scan preoperatively, because after posterior fossa surgery, the associated blood may give a false-positive result. In addition, the presence of disseminated disease should restrain the surgeon from risking neurological morbidity associated with removal of small portions of tumor in the primary area, because the child will be left with residual disease in any event. Unfortunately, infants and small children with ependymomas are often extremely ill at presentation, and sedation to obtain an extended spinal study may be unwise. In these cases, it is best to defer the staging study until after surgery.

If the results are confusing or equivocal, a second spinal MRI is repeated in 2 to 3 weeks when the blood has cleared.

TREATMENT

The optimal treatment of ependymomas is not fully defined, but careful analysis of prognostic factors provides insight and guidance. It is clear that an aggressive surgical resection offers the best hope of cure.[30, 32, 45–47]

Management of Hydrocephalus

Children with ependymomas are often acutely ill at the time of presentation. Occasionally, hemorrhage within a tumor may precipitate acute deterioration resulting in coma and posturing, particularly in infants. These symptoms are usually the result of acute obstructive hydrocephalus rather than the mass itself, and considerable controversy has centered on the management of this hydrocephalus. Options include preoperative steroids followed by tumor excision,[48, 49] external ventricular drainage,[50] and placement of a CSF shunt before tumor removal.[51–57] Those who favor the use of preoperative shunting point out that this option allows time to prepare the patient and the family for surgery, perform diagnostic tests, and schedule major surgery electively; in addition, surgery in the posterior fossa may be safer after the intracranial pressure is decreased. In one series, the operative mortality rate was decreased with preoperative shunting.[52] Others point out that there are disadvantages with this strategy. First, not all patients require shunts after the tumor has been excised, and preoperative shunting condemns the patient to the possibility of long-term shunt complications. Second, a preoperative shunt delays definitive treatment of the tumor. Third, shunts serve as a source of dissemination of tumor, which may spread by CSF pathways.[50, 58] The use of millipore filters has been described to prevent this problem,[59] but these filters frequently obstruct, resulting in shunt failure. And fourth, upward herniation[60] and tumor hemorrhage[61, 62] have been reported after acute decompression of the

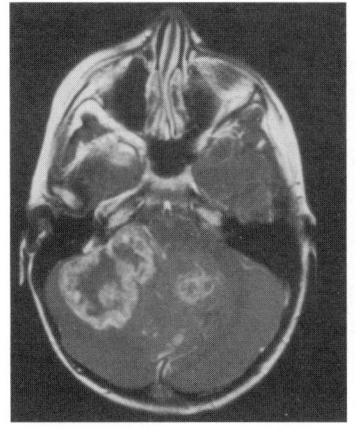
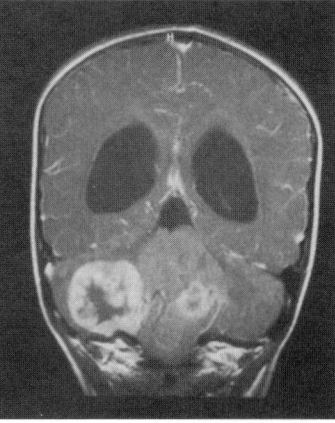

FIGURE 233–3. Contrast-enhanced magnetic resonance imaging scan of a very large ependymoma with a component in the cerebellopontine angle and a component filling the region of the fourth ventricle. (From Sutton L, Goldwein J, Schwartz D: Ependymomas. In Albright A, Pollack I, Adelson P [eds]: Principles and Practice of Pediatric Neurosurgery. New York, Thieme, 1999.)

supratentorial compartment when the posterior fossa mass is not removed. McLaurin[60] concluded that these risks and benefits probably balance each other and that either approach is acceptable.

The use of preoperative endoscopic third ventriculostomy a few days before definitive surgery has been described.[63] Following tumor resection, however, in most patients the obstructive component of the hydrocephalus is relieved; patients with persistent hydrocephalus have primarily a communicating type that would not be relieved by third ventriculostomy. It is the policy of the authors to begin dexamethasone (1 mg/kg per day) on admission, avoid preoperative shunting in most cases, and perform intraoperative ventriculostomy and definitive surgery on the next elective operative day. If the child deteriorates suddenly, the tumor is removed on an emergent basis.

Management of the Tumor

Although ependymomas can be quite vascular, arteriography and embolization are rarely indicated. The blood supply to the tumor is from small branches of the posterior inferior cerebellar artery, and the risks of embolization are significant.

For surgery on posterior fossa ependymomas, the patient is placed in the prone position. The risk of air embolism, frontal pneumocephalus, and systemic hypotension associated with the sitting position is minimized, and the surgeon's arms become less fatigued. Children 3 years of age or older and adults are flexed and held in position with three-point pin fixation. It is recommended that short "pediatric" pins be used in prepubertal children, at a pressure of 40 pounds. In children younger than 3 years old, in whom pins might perforate the skull, the head is supported with a padded horseshoe-shaped rest. By standing at the side of the patient facing the head, the operating surgeon obtains an excellent view, and exposure is excellent as far upward as the upper vermis and tentorial notch. Occasionally, the flexion of the neck occludes the endotracheal tube, which results in high inflating airway pressures and venous bleeding in the operative field. This requires immediate readjustment of the head holder. The risk of this problem may be lessened by using an armored tube or nasotracheal intubation, resulting in a gentler curve of the tube.

Surgery is begun by placing an occipital bur hole to provide access to the ventricle. In patients with hydrocephalus, a catheter is inserted into the ventricle and tunneled subcutaneously to an exit site. CSF can then be vented as the dura is opened and during the postoperative period, if necessary.

In most cases, a midline vertical incision is made from the inion to the midcervical region, and a wide craniectomy is performed from the transverse sinuses to the foramen magnum. Even tumors that are laterally placed can be well exposed through a midline approach, because the skin is quite elastic in children, and retraction is readily achieved to the sigmoid sinus. If the tumor arises entirely within the cerebellopontine angle, a retrosigmoid approach may be considered.

Free craniotomy flaps for posterior fossa procedures have been described[64] and can be created by placing bur holes on either side of the midline in the upper posterior fossa, drilling down the keel between them, and using a high-speed drill to cut the flap, which is replaced at the end of the procedure. The arch of C1 is removed when the tumor extends into the cisterna magna and upper cervical area.

The dura is opened with a Y-shaped incision extending to the level of C1. Large dural venous sinuses are frequent at the level of the foramen magnum in children; they are occluded with MRI-compatible dural clips or oversewn. CSF is vented through the ventriculostomy at this point to reduce the tension in the posterior fossa; if the ventricles are small, mannitol is used for this purpose. The cisterna magna is opened, and the cerebellar tonsils are separated with self-retaining retractors. The tumor may be visible as a gray-tan, usually well-circumscribed mass presenting in the vallecula. The vermis is then opened in the midline to expose the superior pole of the tumor using bipolar cautery and gentle suction until the dorsal surface of the tumor is totally exposed. With some smaller tumors, it is possible to gain access to the fourth ventricle by sharply incising the tela choroidea laterally to the foramen of Luschka to open the lateral recess on each side and avoid opening the vermis.[65]

Ependymomas are not truly encapsulated, but a clear interface can often be developed between the tumor and surrounding brain. A gross total excision can be accomplished if an effort is made to define this plane circumferentially around the tumor as the inside of the tumor is gutted using suction or the ultrasonic surgical aspirator. The dissection is accomplished using bipolar cautery, suction, and cottonoid sponges as the retraction is gradually deepened. Retraction must be done gently, under direct vision. The tumor is usually not removed as a single specimen but is internally decompressed as the margins are defined. A midsagittal MRI scan is useful to delineate where CSF of the fourth ventricle separates tumor from brainstem, and these portions of the tumor are removed first. The position of the brainstem must be inferred from the MRI scan and continuously kept in mind as tumor resection proceeds. Ependymomas often arise in the subependymal region of the lateral wall of the fourth ventricle, and the ventricle itself is displaced laterally by the tumor mass. Removal of areas where the brainstem may be attached is deferred until there is less tumor bulk to obscure the anatomy. Similarly, tumor removal from the foramen of Luschka and the cerebellopontine angle is deferred until the major midline bulk of tumor has been resected. At the superior depth of the tumor, a tongue of tumor often occludes or fills the aqueduct, and this is removed with suction.

If the tumor is attached to the brainstem or peduncles, it is carefully shaved down. In patients with known disseminated disease, removal of an additional small amount of tumor from the primary site would not be expected to improve outcome. In the absence of dissemination, however, there is no easy answer to how aggressive one should be in removing tumor from

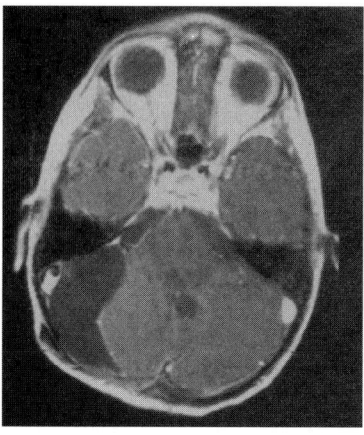 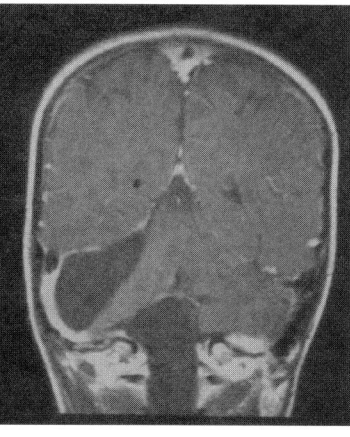

FIGURE 233–4. Postoperative magnetic resonance imaging scan of the same patient as in Figure 233–3. This lesion was totally resected in two stages, with acceptable morbidity. (From Sutton L, Goldwein J, Schwartz D: Ependymomas. In Albright A, Pollack I, Adelson P [eds]: Principles and Practice of Pediatric Neurosurgery. New York, Thieme, 1999.)

the brainstem. Because ependymomas have a predilection to attach at the obex, the major risks are sleep apnea, swallowing dysfunction, and chronic aspiration. Unless a complete removal of bulky disease can be accomplished, however, the tumor almost always progresses if it is followed long enough. The surgeon must base the decision on the nature of the brainstem attachment, and it is essential to prepare the patient and family for possible problems in the postoperative period. A similar situation arises with tumor in the cerebellopontine angle. It may be possible to use the operating microscope to dissect the tumor from multiple cranial nerves, and loss of facial movement or hearing may be acceptable if a gross total resection can be achieved (Fig. 233–4). Unfortunately, the tumor often encases the lower cranial nerves and branches of the posterior inferior cerebellar artery, and even if these structures are anatomically intact at the end of the procedure, a tracheostomy and feeding gastrostomy are often necessary, at least for a while.[66] These deficits may resolve over several months.[67] Electrophysiologic monitoring may be of some help (see later), but its value remains unproved.[68] Brainstem infarct is a major complication, and in the authors' view, no attempt should be made to resect any portion of a tumor that encases brainstem perforators.

During the first 24 to 48 hours, the ventriculostomy is drained at 100 mm H_2O by elevating the drainage bag or by attaching the system to a pressure transducer and intermittently opening the system to drainage when needed. During the next 24 to 48 hours, the drain is clamped, and if this is well tolerated, the ventriculostomy is removed. Some surgeons believe that intermittent spinal taps are useful for a few days to promote CSF drainage and to clear blood. This requires that the CSF pathways be open and may be hazardous if there is tumor or blood clot within the aqueduct or fourth ventricle. If a large subcutaneous CSF collection (pseudomeningocele) develops at the operative site, or if symptoms of hydrocephalus occur with cessation of CSF drainage, a shunt is required.

Dissection of the paraspinal muscles results in considerable discomfort in the immediate postoperative period. Although the compassionate physician's instinct is to alleviate pain, analgesia must be carefully monitored so as not to interfere with neurological assessment. Oral acetaminophen with codeine is usually sufficient, but patients may have persistent vomiting, precluding the oral route. Morphine may be given cautiously in this setting under close nursing supervision. A decrease in alertness must not be ascribed to sedative medication and ignored. Any narcotic must be reversed if there is concern, and other causes for the change should be investigated. Newer nonsteroidal anti-inflammatory medications such as ketorolac have considerable analgesic effects but have been associated with perioperative bleeding complications.[69] Their safety following neurosurgical procedures is yet to be established.

Supratentorial ependymomas are approached using standard techniques, depending on location. The tumors are typically large, and localization is not difficult. Adjuncts such as functional MRI localization of eloquent areas of cortex and image-assisted volumetric resection for deep tumors[70] are used at some centers.

COMPLICATIONS

Clinical or subclinical air embolism can occur even in the prone position.[71] Air embolism usually occurs during the craniectomy but may become apparent at any point in the procedure, including insertion of the pin fixation head holder. The significance of venous air embolism is that the entrance of a large quantity of air can produce an air lock that prevents adequate filling of the heart, leading to cardiac arrest. Nitrous oxide tends to expand the bubble, making the situation worse. If there is a patent foramen ovale, air may enter the left side of the heart and be deposited in the coronary sinuses or the cerebral vessels, leading to myocardial ischemia or stroke. The most sensitive sign of venous air embolism is Doppler monitoring, followed by a drop in end-tidal carbon dioxide, as measured by mass spectrometer or capnograph. With greater amounts of air, there is an increase in central venous pressure and a drop in cardiac output. Eventually, clinical signs are evident, such as systemic hypotension, cardiac arrhythmias, and the "mill wheel" murmur heard with the esophageal stethoscope. The incidence of venous air embolism in children is probably similar to that in adults, with at least subclinical air being detected in 33% of sitting cases,[72] 26% of "lounging" cases,[73] and 10% of prone cases.[74] The relatively low incidence with the prone position probably does not justify the routine use of atrial catheters in most cases.

Treatment of a suspected venous air embolism requires cooperation between the surgeon and the anesthesiologist. As the anesthesiologist ventilates the patient with 100% oxygen and aspirates from the atrial catheter, if one is in place, the surgeon applies bone wax to the edges of the craniectomy and floods the wound with irrigation to prevent additional air entry. The head is lowered, if possible, and unilateral or bilateral jugular vein compression is applied, with care being taken not to occlude the carotid arteries as well. Cardiac medications are administered to support the circulation. Increased airway pressure as a means of elevating central venous pressure is avoided, because it also reduces venous return to the heart. If cardiac instability requires resuscitation, a few large sutures or towel clips are used to approximate the skin, and the patient is turned to the supine position.

The prone position requires some form of support for the head, which can present problems, particularly in infants or small children. If a padded horseshoe-shaped support is used, careful attention to positioning is necessary to avoid retinal ischemia and blindness due to orbital compression, possibly combined with low arterial blood pressure and poor cerebral venous drainage. Pressure necrosis of the forehead is also encountered after long procedures. Other points of potential pressure necrosis include the axilla, iliac crests, knees, breasts, and penis.[75] The use of pin fixation devices is not without risk either. Complications may include scalp laceration from pin slippage, venous air embolism through the pin sites, depressed skull fracture, supratentorial arterial or venous epidural hematoma, or delayed brain abscess. The liberal use of a topical iodine paste at pin sites is useful in providing a seal against air leaks.

Following tumor removal and wound closure, the patient should awaken promptly from anesthesia. Failure to do so should provoke a search for the cause. If residual anesthetics or relaxants cannot explain the persistent lack of responsiveness, an emergency computed tomographic scan is obtained. Treatable possibilities include acute hydrocephalus with a blocked ventriculostomy, supratentorial epidural or subdural hematoma from a pin perforation or rapid decompression of hydrocephalus, or a clot in the operative site. Pneumocephalus is commonly seen on immediate postoperative scans but is rarely the cause of failure to awaken following surgery. If none of these problems is found, the patient is kept intubated and observed in the intensive care unit. The concern in this situation is brainstem dysfunction due to vascular occlusion or manipulation associated with retraction or tumor removal. Patients with compromise of lower cranial nerve function are at risk for aspiration and respiratory failure, which may further impair brainstem function-

ing by ischemic damage.[76] These patients should be kept intubated and may require tracheostomy. The ventriculostomy is kept open at a level of 50 to 100 mm H_2O, because development of acute hydrocephalus may not be immediately recognized in the setting of altered level of consciousness.

Removal of tumor from the brainstem carries risk, even when the surgeon is aided by adjuncts such as evoked potential monitoring, surgical laser, and the ultrasonic aspirator. Patients may have carbon dioxide retention, inability to swallow, ataxia, vocal cord paralysis, recurrent aspiration pneumonia, or quadriparesis. Such patients may require feeding gastrostomy, tracheostomy, or prolonged ventilatory support. Some of these problems have been attributed to respiratory insufficiency in the immediate postoperative period, but it seems likely that they are due, at least in part, to direct trauma to the medulla or to vascular compromise of the tumor bed.

Delayed development of altered consciousness or focal neurological signs in the postoperative period should prompt imaging studies. In addition to the problems of hydrocephalus and hematoma, a peculiar syndrome of pseudobulbar palsy has been described in which stupor, irritability, emotional lability, dysarthria, mutism, nystagmus, and facial diplegia may occur about 72 hours after surgery for midline extrinsic posterior fossa tumors.[77] This syndrome tends to resolve over several weeks to months and has been attributed to retraction-induced edema of the cerebellar peduncles, upper pons, and midbrain. It may be extremely difficult to distinguish this syndrome clinically from decompensated hydrocephalus, especially in a young child. If a repeat scan shows ventricular enlargement that is unchanged or greater compared with the preoperative scan, it may be wisest to place a shunt.

Mutism is seen in 5% to 30% of patients undergoing surgery for large vermian tumors.[78-80] Typically, the patient speaks for a day or so following the procedure, then becomes abruptly mute, retaining receptive language function. The deficit recovers with time, usually over a few weeks to 6 months. Recovery is heralded by the immediate return of full words and sentences, rather than just sounds, suggesting an inhibition of speech rather than aphasia, apraxia, or dysarthria. Patients are often left with a "scanning" cerebellar speech. The substrate for this phenomenon remains controversial. Most authorities place the lesion in the dentate nuclei or the superior cerebellar peduncles.

Aseptic meningitis is another well-recognized postoperative syndrome. This was reported by Cushing,[81] who described fever, photophobia, nuchal rigidity, and CSF pleocytosis occurring in association with blood-stained spinal fluid; he recommended serial spinal taps to clear the CSF. The syndrome typically appears 5 to 14 days after surgery, often as steroids are being weaned. If there is concern about infection, CSF is obtained by lumbar puncture or from the shunt or ventriculostomy to rule out bacterial meningitis, and antibiotics are begun pending cultures. If these prove to be negative, the corticosteroid dose is increased, or nonsteroidal anti-inflammatory medications are given.

It is difficult to achieve a truly watertight closure after posterior fossa tumor surgery in children, and a postoperative pseudomeningocele is common. Wound revision is rarely necessary. Occipital pseudomeningoceles can be treated initially with intermittent lumbar puncture and removal of 10 to 20 mL of CSF daily and wrapping of the head with an elastic bandage. If a follow-up imaging study shows persistent ventricular enlargement, if the wound is threatening to leak spinal fluid, or if the child develops persistent headache, lethargy, or ataxia, a ventriculoperitoneal shunting procedure is required. Otherwise, the meningocele can simply be left alone. In most cases it eventually disappears as the suboccipital bone reforms. Approximately 30% of posterior fossa tumors in children require shunts.

Postoperative melena, abdominal pain and distention, and hematemesis in a child with a posterior fossa tumor should raise the suspicion of a stress-induced "Cushing ulcer." The period of maximal risk appears to be 7 to 10 days postoperatively.[82] The first suggestion of a relationship between conditions affecting the central nervous system and gastrointestinal disease was made by Hunter in 1772, who described two patients with gastromalacia and head injuries.[83] Cushing presented 11 cases of ulcers in association with central nervous system disease, 3 of which were children with posterior fossa tumors.[84] He speculated that there might be a center extending from the hypothalamus to the vagal nucleus in the brainstem that was irritated in certain brain conditions, resulting in excess parasympathetic activity and gastric erosions. Recent work has implicated a spiral enteric pathogen, *Campylobacter pylori,* in gastritis and ulcer disease, but the relationship between this entity and stress ulcer is unclear.[85] Factors associated with stress ulcers include coma, inappropriate secretion of antidiuretic hormone, pyogenic infections of the central nervous system, and other postoperative complications.[86] Peptic ulcer disease is uncommon in children, so it is striking that there appears to be such a predilection for gastrointestinal hemorrhage in association with posterior fossa tumors in this group, especially in the setting of tumor involvement of the lower brainstem.[82] Steroids are not a risk factor.

The value of prophylactic antacids and H$_2$ blockers is controversial, despite their frequent use by neurosurgeons. Studies have indicated that the prophylactic use of cimetidine, ranitidine, or antacid to keep the gastric pH greater than 4 is helpful in protecting patients with severe head injuries or other critically ill patients.[87] Others, however, have questioned the wisdom of neutralizing gastric acidity, which may be an important component of the antibacterial defense of the gastrointestinal tract and may actually increase the incidence of nosocomial pneumonia.[88] In the absence of a randomized clinical trial demonstrating the benefit of giving prophylactic medications to prevent ulcers in children with posterior fossa tumors, there is no strong reason to recommend it.

Treatment of a stress ulcer once it has developed is clearer. Suspicion of the problem should prompt consultation with a gastroenterologist and endoscopy.

If the symptoms are not life threatening, medical management is appropriate, using H$_2$ blockers and antacids. Major upper gastrointestinal hemorrhage requires emergent surgery, with oversewing of the ulcer and vagotomy-pyloroplasty or even gastrectomy.[82]

Late-onset cervical spine instability, swan-neck deformity, or C1-2 rotatory fixation is unusual, occurring in 4 of 72 patients in one series.[89] It is typically seen within a year of surgery. Factors associated with this problem include laminectomy of C2 or lower and local infection. The use of laminaplasty techniques has not prevented this unusual complication. Cervical fusion may be required.

Cognitive deficits are usually not attributed to surgery for posterior fossa ependymomas, because the cerebellum and brainstem are not usually associated with intellectual function. Nonetheless, some perioperative factors, such as shunt or ventriculostomy infection, postoperative bacterial meningitis, CSF leak, subdural hematoma and hygroma, and the need for repeat craniotomy, do appear to be associated with neurocognitive deficits, particular in younger children. In one series, 81% of children with one or more of these factors experienced a 20-point decline in fullscale intelligence quotient, compared with no drop greater than 13 points among patients with none of these problems. The need for a postoperative shunt did not correlate with cognitive deficits.[90]

Because ependymomas often involve the brainstem and cerebellopontine angle, many centers use intraoperative neurophysiologic monitoring in an attempt to decrease morbidity and allow more aggressive surgical resection. The underlying rationale is that stimulation of structures in the surgical site aids the surgeon in identifying structures to be preserved, and early changes in electrical signals warn of impending permanent neurological injury. Monitoring of the facial nerve during surgery for vestibular schwannoma has gained wide acceptance.[91] Monitoring of other cranial nerves and brainstem auditory evoked responses are routinely employed for selected posterior fossa tumors by many pediatric neurosurgeons, but their value has never been demonstrated in a randomized, controlled manner. Although the value of these techniques has been questioned,[68] they may be helpful in some instances.[92] Electromyographic recording of muscles innervated by the cranial nerves may be performed as the surgeon stimulates portions of tumor in the cerebellopontine angle. This requires an anesthetic technique that does not rely on muscle relaxants. Mapping of the brainstem in the floor of the fourth ventricle can also be done, but it is not clear that this decreases complications when an ependymoma infiltrates the brainstem. The respiratory drive center cannot be localized using current techniques. General brainstem function can be assessed continuously by recording brainstem auditory evoked responses and median nerve cortical somatosensory evoked potentials simultaneously. Distortion of brainstem pathways from retraction, direct trauma, or vascular compromise is manifested by a greater than 50% amplitude reduction and loss of waveform definition of one or both modalities. When this occurs, further tumor manipulation is discontinued, retractors are released, and blood pressure is allowed to rise. Damage to either the vestibulocochlear nerve or the cochlear artery can result in alteration or loss of the ipsilateral brainstem auditory evoked response. Deterioration of both brainstem auditory evoked responses and somatosensory evoked potentials and loss of bilateral recordings suggest a global insult.

ADJUNCTIVE TREATMENT

Radiation Therapy

Radiation therapy has been used as a postoperative adjunct for decades. Although there have been no randomized, prospective trials to demonstrate its efficacy, the value of radiotherapy has been established in retrospective series in which patients treated with postoperative radiotherapy fared significantly better than those treated with surgery alone (Table 233–3).[4, 45] In some centers, clinical trials are under way in which routine postoperative radiotherapy is withheld in selected supratentorial ependymomas with complete radiographic surgical resection and no evidence of dissemination.[93–95]

In the past, there has been controversy over the optimal extent of irradiation (local field versus whole brain versus craniospinal axis) needed for the treatment of ependymomas. The debate arose from data from the 1970s and early 1980s that demonstrated improved survival with craniospinal axis radiation,[29] as well as autopsy reports demonstrating a high incidence of leptomeningeal dissemination.[26, 29] More recent studies, in which patients have been staged with myelography, computed tomography, and MRI, however, have demonstrated a low incidence (11%) of dissemination at the time of diagnosis.[30] Furthermore, even at relapse, dissemination is usually preceded by failure at the local site.[30, 32–34, 96, 97] Finally, the adverse cognitive effects of whole-brain and craniospinal axis radiation on young children are now well recognized,[98, 99] and craniospinal axis radiation is reserved for patients with disseminated disease at the time of diagnosis.[100] Few would argue against craniospinal axis radiation in these patients, although the toxicity is significant. Anaplastic histology does not appear to be an indication for craniospinal axis radiation in the absence of disseminated disease,

and there is evidence that it may actually worsen survival.[101] Adult patients are treated in a similar fashion to children.[102]

The dose of radiation for the treatment of ependymoma has traditionally been in the range of 4500 to 5600 cGy. In series in which dose response was studied, doses below this range were associated with higher relapse rates.[26, 27, 29, 33, 103, 104] Perhaps owing to statistical limitations of small numbers, selection biases, and the presence of other confounding factors, this dose effect has not been found in all reports.[31, 45, 46]

Conventional fractionation of 180 to 200 cGy daily has generally been used. The use of hyperfractionated radiotherapy to increase efficacy without an increase in toxicity has been studied.[105] A recent pilot study[106] using fractions of 100 cGy twice a day, up to a total dose of 7200 cGy, followed by chemotherapy, reported an 80% progression-free survival in totally resected patients, but follow-up was not long enough to ascertain late toxicity and the ultimate control rate.

Because the primary problem with ependymomas is local tumor control, brachytherapy with [125]iodine has been used at recurrence.[107] The number of such cases is small, and many centers have abandoned brachytherapy in favor of radiosurgical techniques for all but the largest tumors. Radiosurgical techniques are currently being used to treat local recurrence, using either the linear accelerator[108] or the gamma knife.[109] Fraction sizes between 1000 and 2000 cGy have been administered as a single dose. Results of this form of treatment are preliminary, but the technique appears to be well tolerated. Some have used a radiosurgery boost for localized ependymomas at diagnosis, but these results are preliminary as well.[110] Fractionated stereotactic radiotherapy, in which dose fractions of 1.8 to 2 Gy/day are administered using 25 to 30 fractions and a relocatable head frame, is now available at many centers.[108] This technique is not likely to significantly improve tumor control, but its more focused localization may decrease the late effects of radiation.

Chemotherapy

Because the prognosis of ependymomas is so poor, considerable effort has gone into evaluating chemotherapy as a postsurgical adjunct (for a review, see reference 111). Ependymomas are relatively uncommon tumors, and studies have of necessity been small and nonrandomized. Several studies have noted tumor responses and improved survival with *cis*-platinum–based regimens for recurrent ependymomas.[112–118] Unfortunately, there is no convincing evidence that adjuvant chemotherapy improves survival when added to standard surgery and radiation therapy for newly diagnosed ependymomas (Fig. 233–5). Most retrospective studies in which children received chemotherapy as an adjuvant failed to demonstrate benefit,[32, 119] although a 74% 5-year progression-free survival was reported in a small group of children treated with carboplatin, vincristine, ifosfamide, and etoposide.[106] There have been a limited number of studies randomizing chemotherapy plus radiation therapy versus radiation alone. Lefkowitz and colleagues,[120]

TABLE 233–3 ■ **Long-term Survival for Ependymomas Treated with Surgery Alone versus Surgery and Radiation Therapy**

AUTHOR	YEAR	SURGERY ALONE (%)	SURGERY + RADIATION (%)
Davidoff[146]	1940	20	
Ringertz and Reymond[134]	1949	26	
Fokes and Earle[148]	1969	21	
Grant[149]	1956	7	
Mork and Loken[4]	1977	17	40
Rousseau et al[45]	1994	0	45

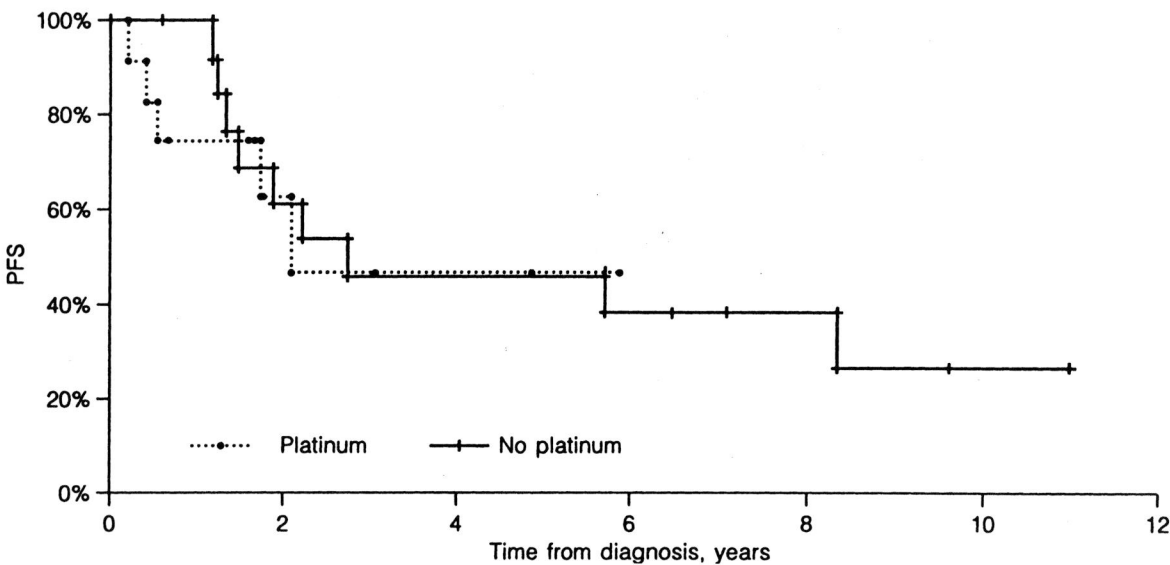

FIGURE 233–5. Effect of adjuvant chemotherapy with cisplatin on 5-year progression-free survival in intracranial ependymoma. There was no difference in outcome between patients receiving cisplatin and those receiving chemotherapy without cisplatin or those receiving no chemotherapy at all. (From Sutton L, Goldwein J, Perilongo G, et al: Prognostic factors in childhood ependymomas. Pediatr Neurosurg 16:57–65, 1990–1991.)

using a combination of CCNU, vincristine, and prednisone, found no difference in outcome for the 33 patients in the study, though the small number prevents assigning strong significance to the results. In Children's Cancer Group study CCG-942, children were randomized to be treated following surgery with craniospinal axis radiotherapy alone or in conjunction with chemotherapy (vincristine, CCNU, and prednisone). The overall difference in 10-year survival did not reach statistical significance, being 40% and 35%, respectively.[121]

Other reports have focused on infants, in whom chemotherapy has been used to substitute for, or delay, radiation therapy in order to avoid its deleterious effects on the immature nervous system.[122–125] In a study by the Pediatric Oncology Group, 48 children younger than 3 years at diagnosis were treated with postoperative vincristine, cyclophosphamide, *cis*-platinum, and etoposide.[126] Radiation was given after the children reached 3 years of age. The overall 2-year progression-free survival rate was 43%, which compares favorably with that of older children receiving radiation therapy at diagnosis, suggesting that this is a worthwhile strategy.

High-dose chemotherapy followed by autologous bone marrow transplantation has been tried on a limited basis, usually at the time of progression.[127–129] The results have generally been disappointing, and this form of therapy should be considered experimental. Chemotherapy has also been used following subtotal resection in an attempt to render the residual tumor more amenable to second-look surgery. Preliminary experience shows that although some tumors were "totally resected" at reoperation, histology of the surgical specimens revealed viable tumor with little evidence of chemotherapeutic effect.[130]

In comparison with medulloblastomas and even astrocytomas, ependymomas are quite chemoresistant.

The reasons for this are unclear but may involve expression of the multiple drug resistance gene, *MDR-1*. The product of this gene, P-glycoprotein, is expressed on the cell membrane and enhances drug efflux from tumor cells. A high expression of the *MDR-1* gene in ependymomas has been reported.[131, 132] Overexpression of the DNA repair protein O6-methyl-guanine DNA methyltransferase in ependymomas has also been reported.[133]

SURVIVAL AND PROGNOSTIC FACTORS

Intracranial ependymomas present one of the most difficult therapeutic challenges in pediatric neuro-oncology. In Olivecrona's surgically treated series reported in 1949,[134] the 5-year survival rate was only 15% for supratentorial tumors, and 33% for those of the posterior fossa. The advent of radiation therapy and improved surgical techniques resulted in improved survival, and contemporary series consistently show 5-year progression-free survival rates of about 40% (Table 233–4). Relapse-free survival is the best indicator of long-term success in the treatment of ependymomas, because patients who develop recurrent disease after conventional therapy (surgery and radiotherapy) are rarely cured.[115] The advent of modern imaging techniques for staging and postoperative surveillance has permitted a more objective assessment of postoperative disease and time of recurrence[32, 46] and has permitted detailed and valid assessment of prognostic factors.

Among the patient variables that have been correlated with outcome are age, tumor location, histology, and presence of dissemination at diagnosis, which may be interrelated. Some studies have suggested that younger children fare somewhat worse than older

TABLE 233-4 ▪ **Survival in Contemporary Series of Ependymomas**

AUTHOR	YEAR	NO. OF PATIENTS	MEDIAN FOLLOW-UP (YR)	5-YR RELAPSE-FREE SURVIVAL (%)	10-YR RELAPSE-FREE SURVIVAL (%)
Schwartz et al[10]*	1999	23		42	27
Needle et al[106]	1997	19		74	
McLaughlin et al[150]	1998	41			46
Horn et al[135]	1999	83		42	
Carrie et al[100]	1995	37	6	40	
Sutton et al[32]	1991	45	6	36	
Healey et al[46]	1991	29	6.8	40	
Rousseau et al[45]	1994	80	4.5	38	
Robertson et al[137]	1998	32	6.5	50	
Vanuytsel et al[31]	1992	93	8	41	

* Adult series of supratentorial ependymomas.

ones,[35, 135, 136] but others have noted little or no difference.[28, 137] Although children as a group appear to enjoy better survival rates than adults with intracranial ependymomas, age does not appear to be a major independent determinant of outcome within the pediatric age group.[28, 29, 32] Similarly, tumor location (supratentorial versus infratentorial) does not appear to be a strong determinant of outcome. Although some studies have suggested a more favorable outcome for supratentorial tumors,[4, 138] others have reported a more favorable outlook for tumors in the posterior fossa[103] or no significant difference at all.[26, 28, 29, 32, 35, 139] Tumor location may be associated with more robust predictive factors such as resectability and likelihood of seeding, and it is likely that location as a prognostic factor is overshadowed by other variables. The impact of histology is difficult to evaluate because of the myriad schemes used to classify ependymomas. Malignant ependymomas are unusual in any event, accounting for only 7%

of ependymomas.[26, 28, 29, 32, 35, 46, 139] One study found a high proliferative index to be an adverse prognostic factor,[30] but others have found no predictive value.[38] Disease dissemination at diagnosis is unusual, occurring in only 10% of cases,[30] and is most likely in younger patients, those with subtotal resections, and those with more aggressive tumors. When present, however, it carries a poor prognosis.

Most modern series in which postoperative scans were used to evaluate the extent of resection have reported a strong association between postoperative residual tumor and tumor progression or recurrence. In fact, this may be the single most important prognostic factor (Fig. 233–6).[31, 32, 34, 45, 46, 97] The effects of the other treatment variables—radiation therapy and chemotherapy—have already been discussed.

Based on these factors, the current management of childhood ependymoma begins with an attempt at maximal surgical resection, followed by staging MRI

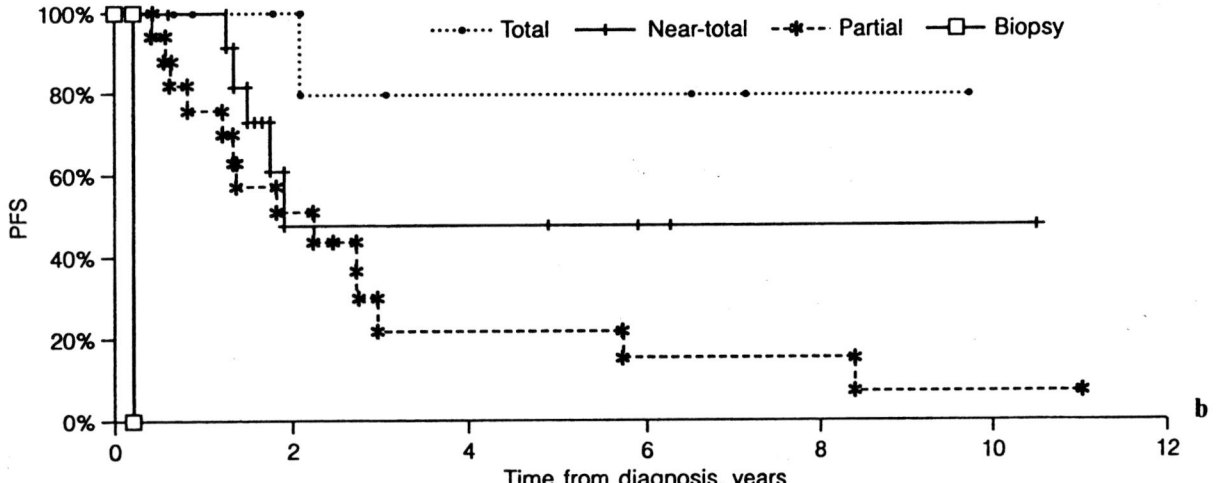

FIGURE 233–6. Effect of surgical resection on progression-free survival in childhood cerebral ependymoma. Stratification based on degree of resection, as determined by the surgeon's impression and postoperative imaging, shows a 5-year progression-free survival of 80% for total resection, 48% for near-total resection, 22% for partial resection, and 0% for biopsy. (From Sutton L, Goldwein J, Perilongo G, et al: Prognostic factors in childhood ependymomas. Pediatr Neurosurg 16:57–65, 1990–1991.)

to assess residual tumor. Involved field radiation is offered in most instances, except in the case of infants, who receive postoperative chemotherapy. Chemotherapy is considered if there is residual disease.

Infants pose a particular treatment challenge because of the potential for morbidity from conventional doses of radiotherapy. In many centers, children younger than 3 years are treated with chemotherapy alone, and radiation is deferred or withheld. Two reports have described the results of this strategy. In one, 48 young children and infants were treated initially with vincristine and cyclophosphamide, alternating with cisplatin and etoposide. In this series, 7 of 25 patients evaluated for chemotherapy response had complete tumor disappearance after two cycles of chemotherapy, and the 2-year actuarial progression-free survival was 42%.[126] In another series, 15 infants were treated with chemotherapy alone, and the 3-year progression-free survival was 26%.[123] In both studies, the protocol design called for radiation therapy to be given when the infant got older, but in many instances, the parents declined this therapy. Although it is not possible to draw firm conclusions from these small series, together they suggest that some infants can be "cured" with surgical resection and chemotherapy alone.

RECURRENT DISEASE

It is the practice at many centers to perform routine surveillance head MRI scans at regular intervals to detect asymptomatic recurrences. Whereas this practice is controversial with medulloblastomas and primitive neuroectodermal tumors,[140] it seems rational in the case of ependymomas, because recurrences are often local and amenable to surgery, which is presumably safer and more effective when the tumor is small. Furthermore, the yield appears to be relatively high. In the one study that addressed this issue, 7 of 11 recurrences of fourth ventricular ependymomas were detected by surveillance scans in asymptomatic patients.[141] The ideal frequency and duration of surveillance scanning for ependymomas have not been established, although the methodology to do so exists.[142] It is currently the practice at many centers to perform scans every 6 months for 2 years, every year for an additional 3 years, and then every 2 years for a prolonged period thereafter.

Most recurrences develop with a local component, either alone or in association with disseminated disease. It is desirable to restage the patient with complete contrast-enhanced MRI scans of the brain and spine before undertaking surgery, because tumor dissemination carries a poor prognosis.[115] Patients with only local recurrences should be considered for resection and may experience prolonged remissions, even after several repeat resections. The time until the next recurrence usually accelerates after each resection, however. Treatment with radiosurgery, implants, or chemotherapy may also be considered.

Patients with unresectable tumors, multiple recurrences, or disseminated disease are candidates for phase I or phase II clinical trials. Most phase II studies in recurrent disease have included only a small number of ependymomas, reflecting their rarity and the generally pessimistic attitude toward their treatment with chemotherapy.[143] The results have been poor. In a Pediatric Oncology Group report, a group of 153 patients with recurrent ependymoma were treated with single-agent or multiagent chemotherapy. Partial or complete responses were seen in only 14.5%, and moderate responses and stabilization of disease was seen in another 30%.[144] The 2-year progression-free survival was 25%. Probably the most effective agents are the platinum compounds. Cisplatin is the best studied, but its toxicity is significant, particularly ototoxicity and renal toxicity. Carboplatin has a more favorable toxicity profile, and its use is limited primarily by hematologic problems. The low response rate to conventional chemotherapy has led to trials of high-dose chemotherapy with autologous stem cell support. Overall, the results have been disappointing.[129]

QUALITY OF LIFE

Until recently, most reports of childhood brain tumors emphasized survival, with little attention to quality of life issues. Those who follow children with brain tumors and their families for long periods appreciate that there is a significant impact on both psychosocial adjustment and academic achievement. Patients who receive extensive cranial radiation at a young age will almost certainly experience loss of IQ, and many experience depression, adjustment problems at school, and impairment of academic function.[145] The impact of severe neurological handicaps on the patient and family is difficult to quantitate, but it must be kept in mind by the neuro-oncology teams considering treatment options for children with ependymomas. In particular, loss of airway protective reflexes, necessitating a tracheostomy and feeding tube, is devastating. In some cases, however, it is worth the risk of permanent lower cranial nerve dysfunction if recovery will take place over time and the tumor will be cured.

REFERENCES

1. Bailey P, Cushing H: Classification of the Tumors of the Glioma Group on a Histogenic Basis with a Correlated Study of Prognosis. Philadelphia, JB Lippincott, 1926.
2. Central Brain Tumor Registry of the United States: First Annual Report. 1995.
3. Svien H, Mabon R, Kernohan J, Craig W: Ependymoma of the brain: Pathologic aspects. Neurology 3:1–15, 1952.
4. Mork S, Loken A: Ependymomas—a follow-up study of 101 cases. Cancer 40:907–915, 1977.
5. Barone B, Elvidge A: Ependymomas: A clinical survey. J Neurosurg 33:428–38, 1970.
6. Jellinger K: Pathology of human intracranial neoplasia. In Jellinger K (ed): Therapy of Malignant Brain Tumors. Vienna, Springer-Verlag, 1987, pp 1–90.
7. Polednak A, Flannery J: Histology of cancer incidence and prognosis: SEER population-based data, 1973–1987. Brain, other central nervous system, and eye cancer. Cancer 75:330–337, 1994.
8. Pollack I: Brain tumors in children. N Engl J Med 331:1500–1507, 1994.

9. Miller R, Young J, Novakovic B: Histology of cancer incidence and prognosis: SEER population-based data, 1973–1987. Childhood cancer. Cancer 75:395–405, 1994.
10. Schwartz T, Kim S, Glick R, et al: Supratentorial ependymomas in adult patients. Neurosurgery 44:721–731, 1999.
11. Russell D, Rubinstein LJ: Pathology of Tumors of the Nervous System. Baltimore, Williams & Wilkins, 1994.
12. Slavc I, MacCollin MM, Dunn M, et al: Exon scanning for mutations of the NF2 gene in pediatric ependymomas, rhabdoid tumors and meningiomas. Int J Cancer 64:243–247, 1995.
13. Rubio M, Correa K, Ramesh V, et al: Analysis of the neurofibromatosis 2 gene in human ependymomas and astrocytomas. Cancer Res 54:45–47, 1994.
14. Sawyer J, Sammertino G, Husain M, et al: Chromosome aberrations in four ependymomas. Cancer Genet Cytogenet 74:132–138, 1994.
15. Vagner-Capodano A, Gentet G, Gambarelli D, et al: Cytogenetic studies in 45 pediatric brain tumors. Pediatr Hematol Oncol 9:223–235, 1992.
16. Weremowicz S, Kupsky W, Morton C, Letcher J: Cytogenetic evidence for a chromosome 22 tumor suppressor gene in ependymoma. Cancer Genet Cytogenet 61:193–196, 1992.
17. Sieb J, Pulst S, Buch A: Familial CNS tumors. J Neurol 239:343–344, 1992.
18. Rhodes C, Call K, Budarf M, et al: Molecular studies of an ependymoma-associated constitutional t(1;22)(p22;q11.2). Cytogenet Cell Genet 78:247–252, 1997.
19. Wilson R, Moran C: Primary ependymoma of the mediastinum: A clinicopathologic study of three cases. Ann Diagn Pathol 2:293–300, 1998.
20. Russell D, Rubenstein L: Pathology of Tumors of the Nervous System, 5th ed. Baltimore, Williams & Wilkins, 1989, pp 251–279.
21. Matthews T, Moossy J: Gliomas containing bone and cartilage. J Neuropathol Exp Neurol 33:456–471, 1974.
22. Rosenblum M, Erlandson R, Aleksic S, Budzilovich G: Melanotic ependymoma and subependymoma. Am J Surg Pathol 14:729–736, 1990.
23. Zuppan C, Mierau G, Weeks D: Ependymoma with signet-ring cells. Ultrastruct Pathol 18:43–46, 1994.
24. Birgisson S, Blondal H, Bjornsson J, Olafsdottir K: Tumours in Iceland. 15. Ependymoma: A clinicopathological and immunohistological study. APMIS 100:294–300, 1992.
25. Rorke L, Gilles F, Davis R, Becker L: Revision of the World Health Organization classification of brain tumors for childhood brain tumors. Cancer 56:1869–1886, 1985.
26. Kim Y, Fayos J: Intracranial ependymomas. Radiology 124:805–808, 1977.
27. Garett P, Simpson W: Ependymomas: Results of radiation treatments. Int J Radiat Oncol Biol Phys 9:1121–1124, 1983.
28. Shaw E, Evans R, Scheithauer B, et al: Post-operative radiotherapy of intracranial ependymoma in pediatric and adult patients. Int J Radiat Oncol Biol Phys 13:1457–1462, 1987.
29. Salazar O, Castro-Vita H, Van Houtte P, et al: Improved survival in cases of intracranial ependymoma after radiation therapy: Late report and recommendations. J Neurosurg 59:652–659, 1983.
30. Rezai A, Woo H, Lee M, et al: Disseminated ependymomas of the central nervous system. J Neurosurg 85:618–624, 1996.
31. Vanuytsel L, Bessell E, Ashley S, et al: Intracranial ependymoma: Long-term results of a policy of surgery and radiotherapy. Int J Radiat Oncol Biol Phys 23:313–319, 1992.
32. Sutton L, Goldwein J, Perilongo G, et al: Prognostic factors in childhood ependymomas. Pediatr Neurosurg 16:57–65, 1990–1991.
33. Goldwein J, Laehy J, Packer R, et al: Intracranial ependymomas in children. Int J Radiat Oncol Biol Phys 19:1497–1502, 1990.
34. Chiu J, Woo S, Ater J, et al: Intracranial ependymoma in children: Analysis of prognostic factors. J Neurooncol 13:283–290, 1992.
35. Pierre-Kahn A, Hirsch J, Roux F, et al: Intracranial ependymomas in childhood: Survival and functional results of 47 cases. Childs Brain 10:145–156, 1983.
36. Chan A, Leung S, Wong M, et al: Expression of vascular endothelial growth factor and its receptors in the anaplastic progression of astrocytoma, oligodendroglioma, and ependymoma. Am J Surg Pathol 22:816–826, 1998.
37. Rushing E, Brown D, Hladik C, et al: Correlation of bcl-2, p53, and MIB-1 expression with ependymoma grade and subtype. Mod Pathol 11:464–470, 1998.
38. Prayson R: Clinicopathologic study of 61 patients with ependymoma including MIB-1 immunohistochemistry. Ann Diagn Pathol 3:11–18, 1999.
39. Rosenblum M: Ependymal tumors: A review of their diagnostic surgical pathology. Pediatr Neurosurg 28:160–165, 1998.
40. Ernestus R, Schroder R, Klug N: Spontaneous intracerebral hemorrhage from an unsuspected ependymoma in early infancy. Childs Nerv Syst 10:357–360, 1992.
41. Atlas S, Lavi E: Intra-axial brain tumors. In Atlas S (ed): Magnetic Resonance Imaging of the Brain and Spine, 2nd ed. Philadelphia, Lippincott-Raven, 1996, pp 378–383.
42. Tortori-Donati P, Fondelli M, Cama A, et al: Ependymomas of the posterior cranial fossa: CT and MRI findings. Neuroradiology 37:238–243, 1995.
43. Wang A, Sutton L, Cnann A, et al: Proton MR spectroscopy of pediatric cerebellar tumors. AJNR Am J Neuroradiol 16:1821–1833, 1995.
44. Arle J, Morris C, Wang Z, et al: Posterior fossa tumor prediction in children using MR image properties, spectroscopy, and neural networks. J Neurosurg 86:755–761, 1997.
45. Rousseau P, Habrand JL, Sarrazin D, et al: Treatment of intracranial ependymomas of children: Review of a 15-year experience. Int J Radiat Oncol Biol Phys 28:381–386, 1994.
46. Healey E, Barnes P, Kupsky W, et al: The prognostic significance of postoperative residual tumor in ependymoma. Neurosurgery 28:666–671, 1991.
47. Kovalic JJ, Flaris N, Grigsby PW, et al: Intracranial ependymoma: Long term outcome, patterns of failure. J Neurooncol 15:125–131, 1993.
48. Lapras C, Palet J, Lapras C, et al: Cerebellar astrocytomas in childhood. Childs Nerv Syst 2:55–59, 1986.
49. Wilson C: Diagnosis and surgical treatment of childhood brain tumors. Cancer 35:950–956, 1975.
50. Kessler L, Dugan P, Concannon J: Systemic metastases of medulloblastoma promoted by shunting. Surg Neurol 3:147–152, 1975.
51. Abraham J, Chandy J: Ventriculo-atrial shunt in the management of posterior fossa tumor—preliminary report. J Neurosurg 20:252–253, 1963.
52. Albright L, Reigel D: Management of hydrocephalus secondary to posterior fossa tumors. J Neurosurg 46:52–55, 1977.
53. Albright A: Posterior fossa tumors. Neurosurg Clin N Am 3:881–891, 1992.
54. Elkins C, Fonesca J: Ventriculo-venous anastomosis in obstructive and acquired hydrocephalus. J Neurosurg 18:139–144, 1961.
55. Hekmatpanah J, Mullan S: Ventriculo-caval shunt in the management of posterior fossa tumors. J Neurosurg 26:609–613, 1967.
56. Jane J, Kaufman B, Nulsen F, et al: The role of angiography and ventriculovenous shunting in the treatment of posterior fossa tumors. Acta Neurochir (Wien) 28:13–27, 1973.
57. Raimondi A, Yashon D, Matsumoto S, Reyes C: Increased intracranial pressure without lateralizing signs: The midline syndrome. Neurochirurgia 10:197–209, 1967.
58. Hoffman H, Hendrick E, Humphreys R: Metastasis via ventriculoperitoneal shunt in patients with medulloblastoma. J Neurosurg 44:562–566, 1976.
59. Park T, Hoffman H, Hendrick E, et al: Medulloblastoma, clinical presentation and management: Experience at the Hospital for Sick Children, Toronto, 1950–1980. J Neurosurg 58:543–552, 1983.
60. McLaurin R: On the use of precraniotomy shunting in the management of posterior fossa tumors in children: A cooperative study. In Chapman P (ed): Concepts in Pediatric Neurosurgery. Basel, Karger, 1985, pp 1–5.
61. Vaquero J, Cabezudo J, DeSola R: Intratumoral hemorrhage in posterior fossa tumors after ventricular drainage. J Neurosurg 54:406–408, 1981.
62. Waga S, Shimizu T, Shimosaka S, Tochio H: Intratumoral hemorrhage after a ventriculo-peritoneal shunting procedure. Neurosurgery 9:249–252, 1981.

63. Cobbs C, McDonald J, Edwards M: Ependymomas. In Youmans J (ed): Neurological Surgery, 4th ed. Philadelphia, WB Saunders, 1996, pp 2552–2569.

64. Tomita T, McLone D: Medulloblastoma in childhood: Results of radical resection and low-dose neuroaxis radiation therapy. J Neurosurg 64:238–242, 1986.

65. Kellogg J, Piatt JJ: Resection of fourth ventricle tumors without splitting the vermis: The cerebellomedullary fissure approach. Pediatr Neurosurg 27:28–33, 1997.

66. Nagib M, O'Fallon M: Posterior fossa lateral ependymoma in childhood. Pediatr Neurosurg 24:299–305, 1996.

67. Sanford R, Kun L, Heideman R, Gajjar A: Cerebellar pontine angle ependymoma in infants. Pediatr Neurosurg 27:84–91, 1997.

68. Grabb P, Albright A, Sclabassi R, Pollack I: Continuous intraoperative electromyographic monitoring of cranial nerves during resection of fourth ventricular tumors in children. J Neurosurg 86:1–4, 1997.

69. Rusy L, Houck C, Sullivan L, et al: A double-blind evaluation of ketorolac tromethamine versus acetaminophen in pediatric tonsillectomy: Analgesia and bleeding. Anesth Analg 80:226–229, 1995.

70. Morita A, Kelly P: Resection of intraventricular tumors via a computer-assisted volumetric stereotactic approach. Neurosurgery 32:920–927, 1993.

71. Shenkin H, Goldfedder P: Air embolism from exposure of posterior cranial fossa in prone position. JAMA 210:726, 1969.

72. Cucchiara R, Bowers B: Air embolism in children undergoing suboccipital craniotomy. Anesthesiology 57:338–339, 1982.

73. von Gosseln H-H, Samii M, Suhr D, Bini W: The lounging position for posterior fossa surgery: Anesthesiological considerations regarding air embolism. Childs Nerv Syst 7:368–374, 1991.

74. Albin M, Carroll R, Maroon J: Clinical considerations concerning detection of venous air embolism. Neurosurgery 3:380–384, 1978.

75. Shapiro H: Neurosurgical anesthesia and intracranial hypertension. In Miller R (ed): Anesthesia, 2nd ed. New York, Churchill Livingstone, 1986, pp 1563–1589.

76. Abbott R, Shiminski-Maher T, Wisoff J, Epstein F: Intrinsic tumors of the medulla: Surgical complications. Pediatr Neurosurg 17:239–244, 1991–1992.

77. Wisoff J, Epstein F: Pseudobulbar palsey after posterior fossa operation in children. Neurosurgery 15:707–709, 1984.

78. Crutchfield J, Sawaya R, Meyers C, Moore B: Postoperative mutism in neurosurgery: Report of two cases. J Neurosurg 81:115–121, 1994.

79. Ferrante L, Mastronardi L, Acqui M, Fortuna A: Mutism after posterior fossa surgery in children: Report of three cases. J Neurosurg 72:959–963, 1990.

80. Humphreys R: Mutism after posterior fossa tumor surgery. Concepts Pediatr Neurosurg 9:57–64, 1988.

81. Cushing H: Experiences with the cerebellar astrocytomas: A critical review of seventy-six cases. Surg Gynecol Obstet 52:129–204, 1931.

82. Ross A, Siegel K, Bell W, et al: Massive gastrointestinal hemorrhage in children with posterior fossa tumors. J Pediatr Surg 22:633–636, 1987.

83. Hunter J: On the digestion of the stomach after death. Philos Trans (Lond) 62:447–454, 1772.

84. Cushing H: Peptic ulcers and the interbrain. Surg Gynecol Obstet 55:1–34, 1932.

85. Bartlett J: *Campylobacter pylori*: Fact or fantasy? Gastroenterology 94:229–232, 1988.

86. Chan K-H, Mann K, Lai E, et al: Factors influencing the development of gastrointestinal complications after neurosurgery: Results of multivariate analysis. Neurosurgery 25:378–382, 1989.

87. Levine B, Sirinek K, Mcleod C, et al: The role of cimetidine in the prevention of stress induced gastric mucosal injury. Surg Gynecol Obstet 148:399–402, 1979.

88. MacLean L: Prophylactic treatment of stress ulcers: First do no harm. Can J Surg 31:76–77, 1988.

89. Steinbok P, Boyd M, Cochrane D: Cervical spine deformity following craniotomy and upper cervical laminectomy for posterior fossa tumors in children. Childs Nerv Syst 5:25–28, 1989.

90. Kao G, Goldwein J, Schultz D, et al: The impact of perioperative factors on subsequent intelligence quotient deficits in children treated for medulloblastoma/posterior fossa primitive neuroectodermal tumors. Cancer 74:965–971, 1994.

91. Harner S, Daube J, Ebersold M, Beatty C: Improved preservation of facial nerve function with use of electrical monitoring during removal of acoustic neuroma. Laryngoscope 62:92–107, 1987.

92. Sutton L, Goldwein J, Schwartz D: Ependymomas. In Albright A, Pollack I, Adelson P (eds): Principles and Practice of Pediatric Neurosurgery. New York, Thieme, 1999, pp 609–628.

93. Awaad Y, Allen J, Miller D, et al: Deferring adjuvant therapy for totally resected intracranial ependymoma. Pediatr Neurol 14:216–219, 1996.

94. Hukin J, Epstein F, Lefton D, Allen J: Treatment of intracranial ependymoma by surgery alone. Pediatr Neurosurg 29:40–45, 1998.

95. Palma L, Celli P, Cantore G: Supratentorial ependymomas of the first two decades of life: Long-term follow-up of 20 cases (including two subependymomas). Neurosurgery 32:169–175, 1993.

96. Kovnar E, Kun L, Burger P, et al: Patterns of dissemination and recurrence in childhood ependymoma: Preliminary results of the Pediatric Oncology Group #8532. Ann Neurol 30:457, 1991.

97. Nazar G, Hoffman H, Becker L, et al: Infratentorial ependymomas in childhood: Prognostic factors and treatment. J Neurosurg 72:408–417, 1990.

98. Radcliffe J, Packer R, Atkins T, et al: Three- and 4-year cognitive outcome in children with non-cortical brain tumors treated with whole-brain radiotherapy. Ann Neurol 32:551–554, 1992.

99. Packer R, Sutton L, Atkins T, et al: A prospective study of cognitive function in children receiving whole-brain radiotherapy and chemotherapy: 2-year results. J Neurosurg 70:707–713, 1989.

100. Carrie C, Mottolese C, Bouffet E, et al: Non-metastatic childhood ependymomas. Radiother Oncol 36:101–106, 1995.

101. Merchant T, Haida T, Wang M, et al: Anaplastic ependymoma: Treatment of pediatric patients with or without craniospinal therapy. J Neurosurg 86:943–949, 1997.

102. Donahue B, Steinfeld A: Intracranial ependymoma in the adult patient: Successful treatment with surgery and radiotherapy. J Neurooncol 37:131–133, 1998.

103. Marks J, Adler S: Comparative study of ependymomas by site of origin. Int J Radiat Oncol Biol Phys 13:37–43, 1982.

104. Phillips T, Sheline G, Boldrey E: Therapeutic considerations in tumors affecting the central nervous system: Ependymomas. Radiology 83:98–105, 1964.

105. Bernstein M, Rutka J: Brain tumor protocols in North America. J Neurooncol 17:231–251, 1993.

106. Needle M, Goldwein J, Grass J, et al: Adjuvant chemotherapy for the treatment of intracranial ependymoma of childhood. Cancer 80:341–347, 1997.

107. Sneed P, Russo C, Scharfen C, et al: Long-term follow-up after high-activity ^{125}I brachytherapy for pediatric brain tumors. Pediatr Neurosurg 24:314–322, 1996.

108. Dunbar S, Tarbell N, Kooy H, et al: Stereotactic radiotherapy for pediatric and adult brain tumors: Preliminary report. Int J Radiat Oncol Biol Phys 30:531–539, 1994.

109. Hirato M, Nakamura M, Inoue H, et al: Gamma knife radiosurgery for the treatment of brainstem tumors. Stereotact Funct Neurosurg 64(Suppl):32–41, 1995.

110. Aggarwal R, Yeung D, Kumar P, et al: Efficacy and feasibility of stereotactic radiosurgery in the primary management of unfavorable pediatric ependymoma. Radiother Oncol 43:269–273, 1997.

111. Souweidane M, Bouffet E, Finlay J: The role of chemotherapy in newly diagnosed ependymoma of childhood. Pediatr Neurosurg 28:273–278, 1998.

112. Allen J, Walker R, Luks E, et al: Carboplatin and recurrent brain tumors. Clin Oncol 5:459–463, 1987.

113. Bertolone S, Baum E, Krivit W, Hammond D: Phase II trial of cisplatinum diamino-dichloride (CPDD) in recurrent childhood brain tumors: A CCSG trial. J Neurooncol 7:5–11, 1989.

114. Gaynon P, Ettinger L, Moel D: Pediatric phase I trial of carboplatin: A Children's Cancer Study Group report. Cancer Treat Rep 71:1039–1042, 1987.

115. Goldwein J, Glauser T, Packer R, et al: Recurrent intracranial ependymomas in children: Survival, patterns of failure, and prognostic factors. Cancer 66:557–563, 1990.

116. Sexauer C, Khan A, Burger P, et al: Cisplatin in recurrent pediatric brain tumors: A POG phase II study. Cancer 56:1497–1501, 1985.

117. Tamura M, Ono N, Kurihara H: Adjunctive treatment for recurrent childhood ependymoma of the IV ventricle: Chemotherapy with CDDP and MCNU. Childs Nerv Syst 6:186–189, 1990.

118. Walker RW, Allen JC: Cisplatin in the treatment of recurrent childhood primary brain tumors. J Clin Oncol 6:62–66, 1988.

119. Bloom H: Intracranial tumors: Response and resistance to therapeutic endeavors, 1970–1980. Int J Radiat Oncol Biol Phys 8:1083–1132, 1982.

120. Lefkowitz I, Evans A, Sposto R, et al: Adjuvant chemotherapy of childhood posterior fossa (PF) ependymoma: Craniospinal irradiation with or without CCNU, vincristine (VCR) and prednisone (P). Proc Am Soc Clin Oncol 8:87, 1989.

121. Evans AE, Anderson JR, Lefkowitz-Boudreaux IB, Finlay JL: Adjuvant chemotherapy of childhood posterior fossa ependymoma: Cranio-spinal irradiation with or without adjuvant CCNU, vincristine, and prednisone: A Children's Cancer Group study. Med Pediatr Oncol 27:8–14, 1996.

122. Duffner P, Cohen M, Meyers M: Survival of children with brain tumors: SEER program, 1973–1980. Neurology 36:597–601, 1986.

123. Geyer J, Zeltzer P, Boyett J, et al: Survival of infants with primitive neuroectodermal tumors and malignant ependymomas of the CNS treated with eight drugs in 1 day: A report from the Children's Cancer Group. J Clin Oncol 12:1607–1615, 1994.

124. Strauss L, Killmond T, Carson B: Efficacy of postoperative chemotherapy using cisplatin plus etoposide in young children with brain tumors. Med Pediatr Oncol 19:16–21, 1991.

125. White L, Johnson H, Jones R, et al: Postoperative chemotherapy without radiation in young children with malignant non-astrocytic brain tumours: A report from the Australia and New Zealand Childhood Cancer Study Group (ANZCCSG). Cancer Chemother Pharmacol 32:403–406, 1993.

126. Duffner P, Horowitz M, Kirscher J: Postoperative chemotherapy and delayed radiation in children less than three years of age with malignant brain tumors. N Engl J Med 328:1725–1731, 1993.

127. Mahoney D, Strother D, Camitta B, et al: High-dose melphalan and cyclophosphamide with autologous bone marrow rescue for recurrent/progressive malignant brain tumors in children: A pilot Pediatric Oncology Group study. J Clin Oncol 14:382–388, 1996.

128. Mason WP, Goldman S, Yates AJ, et al: Survival following intensive chemotherapy with bone marrow reconstitution for children with recurrent intracranial ependymoma—a report of the Children's Cancer Group. J Neurooncol 37:135–143, 1998.

129. Grill J, Kalifa C, Doz F: A high-dose busulfan-thiotepa combination followed by autologous bone marrow transplantation in childhood recurrent ependymoma: A phase II study. Pediatr Neurosurg 25:7–12, 1996.

130. Foreman N, Love S, Gill S, Coakham H: Second-look surgery for incompletely resected fourth ventricle ependymomas: Technical case report. Neurosurgery 40:856–860, 1997.

131. Geddes J, Vowles G, Ashmore S, et al: Detection of multidrug resistance gene product (P-glycoprotein) expression in ependymomas. Neuropathol Appl Neurobiol 20:118–121, 1994.

132. Chou P, Barquin N, Gonzalez-Crussi F, et al: Ependymomas in children express the multidrug resistance gene: Immunohistochemical and molecular biologic study. Pediatr Pathol Lab Med 16:551–561, 1996.

133. Silber J, Mueller B, Ewers T, Berger M: Comparison of O6-methylguanine-DNA-methyltransferase activity in brain tumors and adjacent normal brain. Cancer Res 53:3416–3420, 1993.

134. Ringertz N, Reymond A: Ependymomas and choroid plexus papillomas. J Neuropathol Exp Neurol 8:355–380, 1949.

135. Horn B, Heideman R, Geyer R, et al: A multi-institutional retrospective study of intracranial ependymoma in children: Identification of risk factors. J Pediatr Hematol Oncol 21:203–211, 1999.

136. Papadopoulos D, Giri S, Evans R: Prognostic factors and management of intracranial ependymomas. Anticancer Res 10:689–692, 1990.

137. Robertson P, Zeltzer P, Boyett J, et al: Survival and prognostic factors following irradiation and chemotherapy for ependymomas in children: A report of the Children's Cancer Group. J Neurosurg 88:695–703, 1998.

138. Dohrmann G, Farwell J, Flannery J: Ependymomas and ependymoblastomas in children. J Neurosurg 45:273–283, 1976.

139. Undijian S, Marinov M: Intracranial ependymomas in children. Childs Nerv Syst 6:31–34, 1990.

140. Torres C, Rebsamen S, Silber J, et al: Surveillance scanning of children with medulloblastoma. N Engl J Med 330:892–895, 1994.

141. Steinbok P, Hentschel S, Cochrane D, Kestle J: Value of postoperative surveillance imaging in the management of children with some common brain tumors. J Neurosurg 84:726–732, 1996.

142. Sutton L, Cnaan A, Klatt L, et al: Postoperative surveillance imaging in children with cerebellar astrocytomas. J Neurosurg 84:721–725, 1996.

143. Siffert J, Allen J: Chemotherapy in recurrent ependymoma. Pediatr Neurosurg 28:314–319, 1998.

144. Weitman S, Ochoa S, Sullivan J, et al: Pediatric phase II cancer chemotherapy trials: A Pediatric Oncology Group study. J Pediatr Hematol Oncol 19:187–191, 1997.

145. Seaver E, Geyer R, Xulzbacher S, et al: Psychosocial adjustment in long-term survivors of childhood medulloblastoma and ependymoma treated with craniospinal irradiation. Pediatr Neurosurg 20:248–253, 1994.

146. Davidoff L: Thirteen year follow-up of a series of cases of verified tumors of brain. Arch Neurol Psychiatry 44:1246–1261, 1940.

147. Cushing H: Intracranial Tumors: Notes upon a Series of Two Thousand Verified Cases with Surgical Mortality Percentages Pertaining Thereto. Springfield, Ill, Charles C Thomas, 1932.

148. Fokes E, Earle K: Ependymomas: Clinical and pathological aspects. J Neurosurg 30:588–594, 1969.

149. Grant F: A study of the results of surgical treatment in 2326 consecutive patients with brain tumors. J Neurosurg 13:479–488, 1956.

150. McLaughlin M, Marcus R, Buatti J, et al: Ependymoma: Results, prognostic factors and treatment recommendations. Int J Radiat Oncol Biol Phys 40:845–850, 1998.

Medulloblastoma

BRUCE A. KAUFMAN

Medulloblastomas were first described as a cohesive group of tumors by Bailey and Cushing in 1924, using the term *spongioblastoma cerebelli*.[1] The word *medulloblastoma* was subsequently chosen based on their assumption that the tumor derived from a presumed primitive pluripotential cell, the medulloblast. In 1983, Rorke proposed including medulloblastomas in the group of tumors called *primitive neuroectodermal tumors* (PNETs), derived from the transformation of primitive neuroepithelial cells.[2] This grouping with PNETs has been widely debated, but it has been adopted by the World Health Organization. Most neurosurgeons, however, continue to refer to such tumors as medulloblastomas.

Since Cushing's first large series of patients, the surgical treatment of this tumor has evolved. Initial attempts at surgical resection had a high operative mortality rate, which decreased to less than 10% by the late 1970s.[3, 4] More recent reports describe a nearly absent surgical mortality.[5, 6]

The adjunctive therapy of medulloblastoma also evolved. Bailey and Cushing recognized that this tumor was radiosensitive, but it was not until the 1950s that craniospinal radiotherapy became the standard treatment.[1, 7] Throughout the 1960s and 1970s, radiotherapy techniques were modified to provide a dose that controlled the tumor with tolerable side effects.

Chemotherapy as an adjunctive therapy for medulloblastoma began with the treatment of tumor recurrences. It has now become a third component of primary treatment, particularly for patients younger than 3 years old, in whom the morbidity of craniospinal radiotherapy is prohibitive.[8] There is ongoing investigation into the use of adjunctive chemotherapy as a means of reducing the effective radiotherapy dose and its associated sequelae.

EPIDEMIOLOGY

Medulloblastoma is one of the most common tumors of the posterior fossa, constituting 20% to 25% of all pediatric brain tumors.[9–12] The median age at diagnosis is between 5 and 7 years, with up to 80% of cases diagnosed before age 16 years.[13, 14] There are two presentation peaks in childhood—an early one at 2 to 4 years, and a later one at 6 to 8 years.[9, 12, 14, 15] Medulloblastoma can occur through adulthood, with another peak in incidence from 20 to 24 years of age, when it is usually located more laterally in the posterior fossa (30% to 49% lateral tumors in adults versus 7% in children).[16–21]

A nearly 2:1 male predominance has been consistently reported.[6, 9, 14–16, 22–26] The overall incidence is approximately five cases per million children per year.[12, 27, 28] There is a debate whether this incidence has been dropping in the past few decades.[9, 27] There is no obvious reason for this drop in incidence, but it does not appear to be due to the reclassification of medulloblastoma as a PNET.

An increased frequency of medulloblastoma has been reported in two genetic syndromes: nevoid basal cell carcinoma (or Gorlin's syndrome), and multiple colonic polyposis (Turcot's syndrome). Approximately 3% to 5% of children with nevoid basal cell carcinoma develop medulloblastoma, frequently before age 5 years.[29, 30] The frequency with which Turcot's syndrome patients develop medulloblastoma is not known. Medulloblastoma does not appear to have an increased incidence in the phakomatoses—neurofibromatosis and tuberous sclerosis.

PATHOLOGY AND GENETICS

The "medulloblast" hypothesized by Bailey and Cushing has never been found. Earlier theories of medulloblastoma development were based on the "static" concept of the tumor arising from remnants of cells in a particular location, such as the fetal external granule cell layer.[31–33] In experimental tumor induction studies, JC virus was found to infect cells of the external granule cell layer, which could be tracked migrating and forming medulloblastoma-like tumors.[34]

A more "dynamic" concept of tumorigenesis suggests that these tumors derive from the transformation of normal neural progenitor cells. The persistent undifferentiated cells of the subependymal fourth ventricular and pineal regions can migrate outward and laterally to form the granule cell layer, and this is compatible with the observed locations of medulloblastomas.[35] Subpopulations of medulloblastoma cells have shown differentiation that partially recapitulates stages of normal neuronal cell differentiation.[31, 36, 37] Medulloblastomas harbor at least some of the molecular markers that are normally expressed in a temporal fashion during neuronal differentiation.[38–40] Less frequently, medulloblastomas demonstrate glial differentiation, further supporting their derivation from a pluripotential cell.

On light microscopic examination, the "classic" diffuse medulloblastomas are extremely cellular, composed of small cells with scant cytoplasm and poorly defined cell margins. The nuclei are round to oval and variable in size, but they stain densely with hematoxylin. Mitotic activity can be quite brisk. The tumor cells typically form irregular masses, with a thin stroma of blood vessels and only occasional endothelial proliferation. Light microscopic evidence of neuronal or glial differentiation may be seen in up to 50% of cases.[41] More obvious neuroblastic differentiation with well-formed Homer Wright rosettes may occur in 35% to 40% of cases. Rarely, such differentiation is extensive, and the term *cerebellar neuroblastoma* may be applied. Perivascular pseudorosettes can be encountered, though they are typically not as prominent as those seen in ependymomas.

The desmoplastic variant of medulloblastoma accounts for 20% of cases.[13, 16, 42] These tumors are often lateral and superficial, with pial invasion and a prominent reticulin-rich stromal reaction. A common subset, often referred to as *nodular medulloblastoma*, consists of reticulin-poor islands of pale staining cells with reticulin-rich internodular zones. The centers of these islands typically demonstrate the greatest degree of neuronal differentiation and maturation.

Several rare variants associated with different degrees of neuronal maturation have been described. These variants generally have a better prognosis.[43–45] There can also be extensive neurocyte-predominant maturation after chemotherapy.[46] These findings suggest that the development of a treatment capable of inducing neuronal maturation in medulloblastomas could improve patient management, possibly delaying or replacing radiotherapy.

The recently recognized large cell or anaplastic medulloblastomas are associated with a particularly dismal prognosis; patients often present with cerebrospinal fluid (CSF) dissemination and survive less than a year.[47, 48] This subtype constitutes 4% to 14% of all medulloblastomas, depending on the stringency of inclusion criteria.[49] These tumors have a high frequency of *c-MYC* amplification and isochromosome 17q (see later).[48–50] The morphologic, clinical, and genetic data suggest that this variant is the result of anaplastic progression of classic medulloblastoma.

The differential diagnosis of a tumor suspected of being a medulloblastoma must include the atypical teratoid-rhabdoid tumor of childhood and the cellular ependymoma. On frozen section, the cellular ependymoma can appear just like a medulloblastoma. However, this ependymoma has better defined perivascular pseudorosettes. On immunohistochemistry, there are no neuronal markers present, as it is a purely glial tumor. The atypical teratoid-rhabdoid tumor is often misdiagnosed as a PNET or medulloblastoma.[51, 52] However, the atypical teratoid-rhabdoid tumor occurs in a younger age group and is found less frequently in the cerebellum. In 70% of these tumors, the microscopic appearance is indistinguishable from medulloblastoma. The correct diagnosis can be made by obtaining an adequate sample and using careful immunohistochemical analysis for markers. Epithelial membrane antigen is almost never positive in medulloblastoma. Unfortunately, atypical teratoid-rhabdoid tumor has a grim prognosis, with most patients dying of progressive disease within 1 year, despite surgery and radiotherapy.

The immunohistochemistry of medulloblastomas is variable. The great majority demonstrate at least focal primitive neuronal differentiation with immunoreactivity for synaptophysin and neuron-specific enolase. The majority of medulloblastomas also show reactivity to antibodies against class III tubulin, a presumptive neuron-specific form of tubulin.[53, 54] There is variable reactivity to the different neurofilament protein antibodies, and chromogranin is typically negative. In reported series, the number of tumors that express glial fibrillary acidic protein (GFAP) varies widely from 11% to 85%.[10, 54–59] This likely reflects the difficulty in some cases of distinguishing tumoral GFAP expression from expression within entrapped reactive astrocytes.

In medulloblastoma, the proliferative index has not been correlated with any biologic behavior or prognosis.[60–62] DNA histograms describing ploidy show that medulloblastomas have a wide variation; many are diploid, but a large number are aneuploid.[42, 61, 63] The significance of ploidy is unclear.[60, 61, 64] Of the gross histologic types of medulloblastoma, only the desmoplastic variant seems to have a consistent histogram, typically diploid.[65, 66] CSF dissemination has not been associated with a particular ploidy, but extraneural metastasis has been described as occurring more frequently among diploid tumors.[61, 63]

The most common genetic abnormalities found in medulloblastoma are alterations of chromosome 1, including extra copies of 1q; gain of chromosome 7; loss of chromosome 22; and loss of chromosome 17p.[67, 68] The loss of chromosome 17p occurs in up to half of cases and manifests cytogenetically as an isochromosome 17q, with p-arm deletion and q-arm duplication.[50, 68–70] The minimal region of common loss includes 17p12 through 17p13.1.[71–73] The location of common loss on 17p seems to exclude the p53 locus.[50, 68, 69, 74]

Based on the presumption that medulloblastoma derives from a differentiating cell, attention has focused on the effects of growth factors in these tumors. The *MYC* family of genes may have a roll in cell differentiation and cell proliferation signal transduction. Amplification of the *c-MYC* gene has been frequently seen in medulloblastoma cell lines but infrequently seen in the tumor tissue, and it is not clear that *c-MYC* is actually involved in medulloblastoma tumorigenesis.[75] It is frequently amplified in the aggressive large cell or anaplastic variant. Data suggest that *c-MYC* amplification likely has more to do with tumor progression than with tumorigenesis. The *c-ERB2* oncogene encodes a transmembrane growth factor receptor. The expression of this oncogene has been associated with a poorer prognosis in medulloblastoma.[76] One class of neurotrophin growth factor receptor (TrkC) has been associated with a better outcome in medulloblastoma.[77] In a larger study, medulloblastomas with high TrkC expression were associated with an 89% 5-year survival rate, whereas patients whose tumors demonstrated low TrkC expression had a 46% 5-year survival rate.[78] These studies suggest that molecular characterization may play a more significant role in the future diagnostic workup of patients with medulloblastoma.

If medulloblastomas are derived from tissues that are migrating and differentiating, genes associated with organizing the development of the cerebellum may be involved. These include the homeobox genes, such as the *PAX* genes. There have been reports of deregulated or overexpressed *PAX5* gene function in medulloblastoma, but others have not identified overt genetic changes compared with wild-type *PAX* genes.[79–81]

Unlike with other pediatric tumors, no large prospective studies using genetic markers have verified the utility of such tests to subcategorize medulloblastomas and thus guide treatment decisions. Initial reports correlated specific regions of 17p loss with worse outcomes, but larger studies failed to confirm this association.[69, 70]

IMAGING

Imaging has greatly aided the preoperative diagnosis of and surgical planning for medulloblastoma, the detection of metastatic disease, and the evaluation of treatment. However, the pathologic diagnosis of a tumor cannot be discerned by imaging alone. Medulloblastomas can look like oligodendrogliomas, astrocytomas, or ependymomas.

Computed tomography (CT) is widely available, and high-quality images can be obtained in just a few seconds, precluding the need for sedation. CT remains the easiest method of detecting calcification and hemorrhage and evaluating for hydrocephalus. On nonenhanced CT, medulloblastomas typically show a homogeneous mass that is isodense to hyperdense relative to cerebellar tissue (Fig. 234–1). As a group, medulloblastomas are more homogeneous than ependymomas.[82] Calcification is seen in nearly 30% of tumors, and hydrocephalus is present in nearly 90% of medulloblastoma patients presenting with moderate to large tumors.[5, 83, 84]

Magnetic resonance imaging (MRI) yields exquisite anatomic detail. Axial images define the relationship of the tumor to the cerebellar peduncles and floor of the fourth ventricle. Sagittal images show the superior and inferior extent of the tumor and the relationship to the brainstem anteriorly. Although the various images can show apposition of tumor to the fourth ventricular floor, actual invasion of the floor cannot be accurately predicted from imaging alone. Limitations

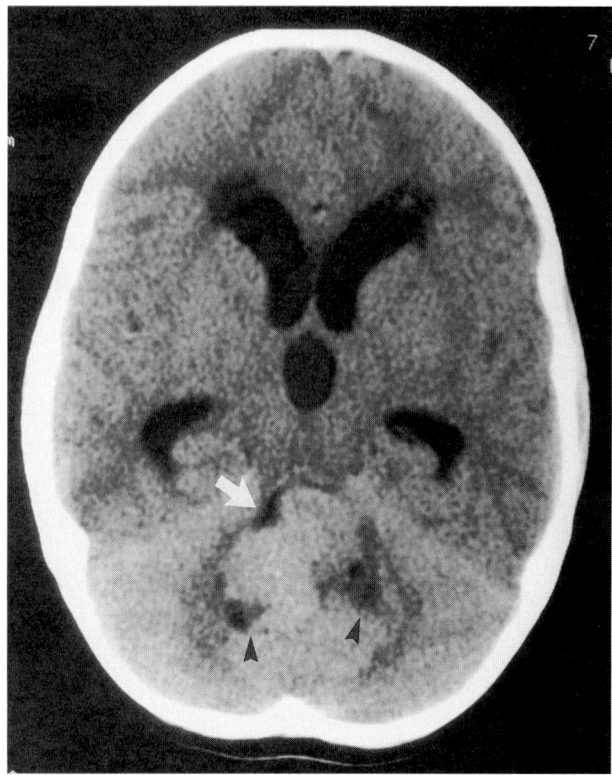

FIGURE 234–1. Nonenhanced axial computed tomographic scan. The midline posterior fossa tumor is isodense to hyperdense. It has displaced the fourth ventricle *(arrow)* and has caused obstructive hydrocephalus. Several small areas of hypodensity on the posterior aspect of the mass *(arrowheads)* are probably cysts.

of MRI include lack of availability and the frequent need for sedation. Sedation must be carefully monitored in patients with severely increased intracranial pressure.

Medulloblastoma has a variable appearance on MRI. On T1-weighted sequences, the tumor is typically of low to intermediate signal[85, 86] (Fig. 234–2). T2-weighted sequences show a variably low to hyperintense signal relative to the white matter.[85, 86] Some of the signal heterogeneity is due to vessels, cysts, and calcification within the tumor. Enhancement can be quite variable, with some areas of nonenhancement[85–87] (Fig. 234–3). Significant amounts of tumor or metastases may be nonenhancing and thus poorly visualized.

Overall, medulloblastomas are relatively well differentiated from the surrounding brain. Cysts may be present in up to 40% to 75% of cases, typically within the tumor.[84, 86, 87] The cysts are usually isointense to hyperintense to CSF on both T1- and T2-weighted sequences. Medulloblastomas are less likely than ependymomas to extend through the outlets of the fourth ventricle (occurring in only 15% of cases).[87, 88]

In older children and adults, the appearance is less "classic," with up to 50% to 66% presenting in the cerebellar hemisphere[20, 21, 82, 89, 90] (Fig. 234–4). These tumors can be contiguous with the tentorium in the cerebellopontine angle and can be mistaken for meningiomas. There is only slight to moderate enhancement, with 82% having cystic or necrotic foci.[89]

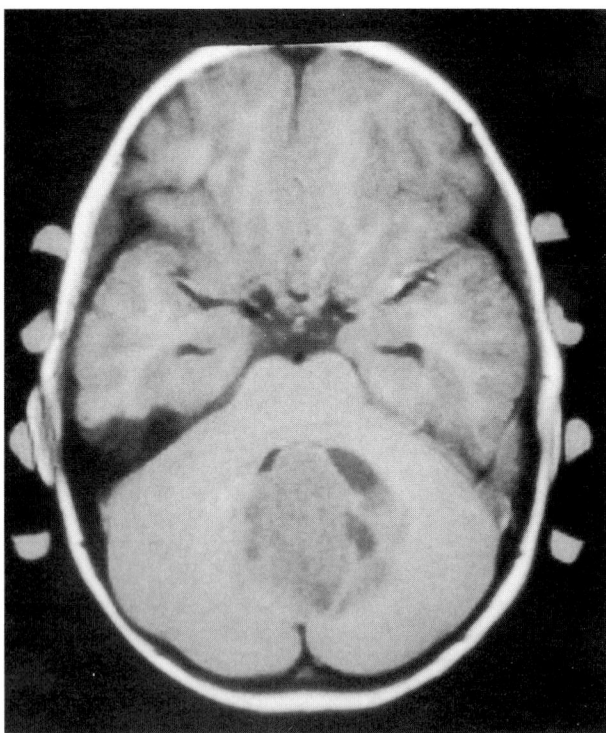

FIGURE 234–2. Nonenhanced, T1-weighted, axial magnetic resonance imaging scan. The mass shows a large amount of signal variation, with the suggestion of cysts along the periphery. The fourth ventricle is seen, but invasion of the fourth ventricle floor cannot be fully evaluated.

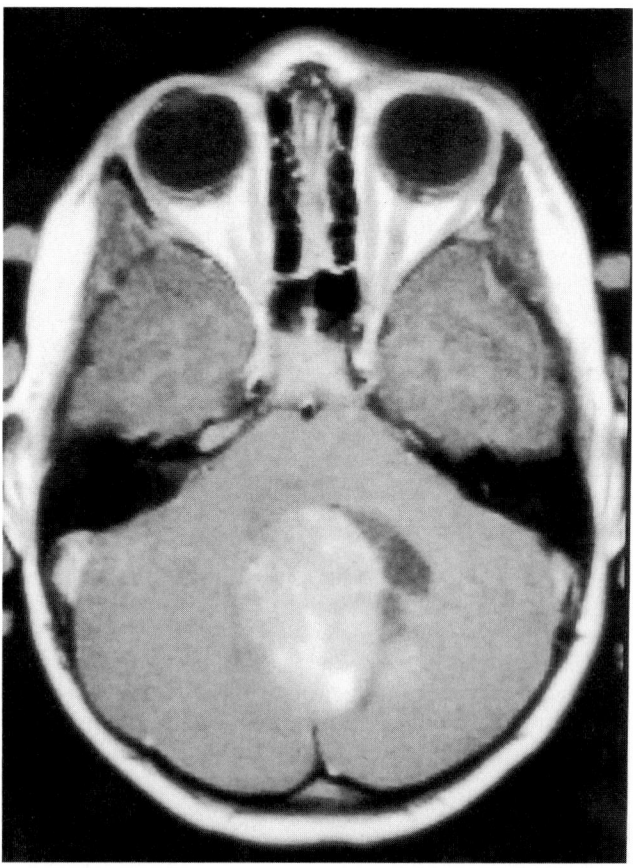

FIGURE 234–3. Gadolinium-enhanced, T1-weighted, axial magnetic resonance imaging scan. A variable pattern of enhancement is seen in this medulloblastoma. In addition, the margins with the cerebellum are not distinct, somewhat different from most low-grade astrocytomas.

Angiography of these tumors is needed infrequently. When undertaken for posterior fossa tumors, it shows the pattern typical of a vermian mass, with posterior stretching and lateral displacement of the vermian arteries and veins. The choroidal point and the retrobasilar and posterior medullary portions of the posterior inferior cerebellar artery are displaced forward and inferiorly. However, a tumor that envelops these vessels may show paradoxical displacement.

Immediate postoperative MRI should be performed to assess for the presence of residual disease, because this can affect the adjunctive therapy. MRI should be obtained both without and with the use of a contrast agent, to better define any residual disease from artifacts of the surgery. The scan should be obtained within 48 hours of surgery, and preferably within 24 hours. Beyond 72 hours, there is extensive enhancement of the surgically traumatized brain, precluding the definition of residual disease. Even when scanning within 24 hours, edge enhancement unrelated to tumor is seen.[91] The possibility of residual tumor must be correlated with the preoperative images and the pattern of tissue enhancement. Hemostatic materials (Gelfoam, Surgicel, Oxycel) left in the surgical bed trap blood and can effectively obscure the area on MRI.[91]

Spinal imaging is required in all cases of medulloblastoma, because the most common form of metastasis is subarachnoid seeding.[92] Medulloblastoma is disseminated at the time of diagnosis in 11% to 71% of patients.[10, 93–101] Dissemination at diagnosis is more frequent in patients younger than 5 years of age.[97, 98] MRI with contrast enhancement has effectively replaced CT–myelography as the procedure of choice for evaluating spinal disease.[93, 102] Spinal imaging should include sagittal and axial images, without and with contrast, of the entire CSF spinal space.[82]

When to perform the initial spinal canal evaluation is controversial. Some authors recommend obtaining the spinal images at the time of the initial cranial imaging.[82] This can lead to unnecessary imaging studies or result in suboptimal studies in patients who are uncomfortable and cannot remain still. However, blood, air, and artifactual dural enhancement can obscure the spinal canal for up to 14 days postoperatively. In some cases, these artifacts look just like neoplastic tissue, leading to an incorrect diagnosis of dissemination.[88, 91, 93, 103] A 2-week delay in the staging study is not clinically significant, because adjunctive therapy is rarely required so soon after surgery.

Long-term follow-up imaging, so-called surveillance imaging, has also become standard in the treatment of medulloblastoma.[104] Obtained at 3- to 6-month intervals postoperatively, this imaging is meant to detect recurrent tumor before symptoms or signs appear, allowing additional treatment to begin promptly. The effectiveness of this strategy has been challenged; crit-

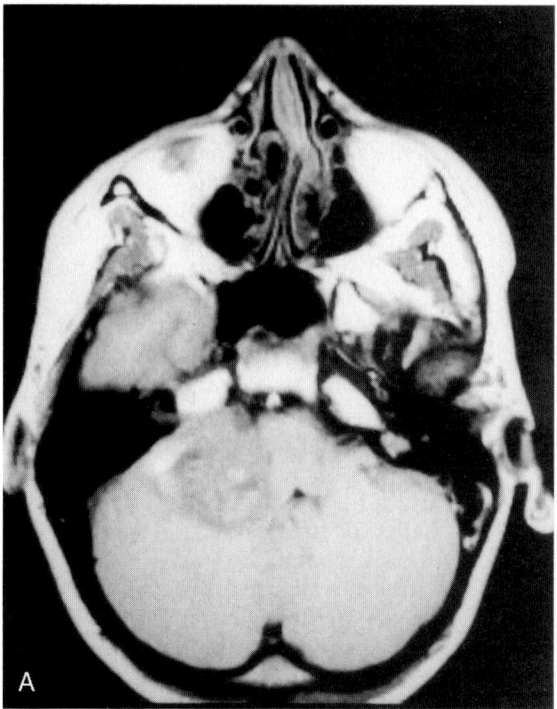

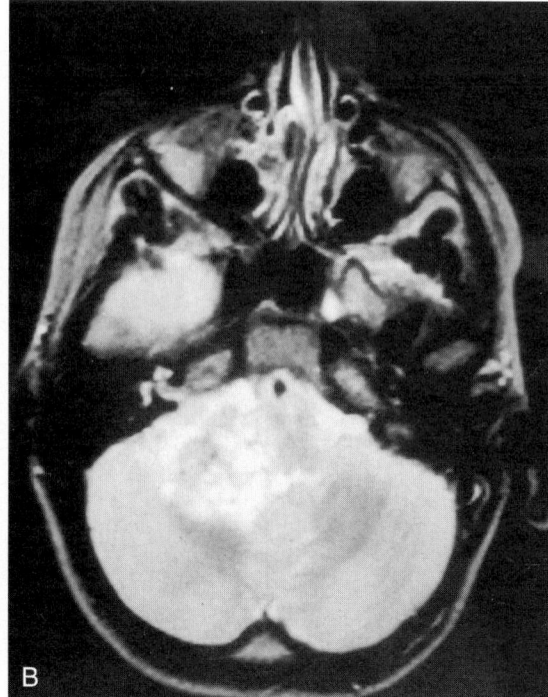

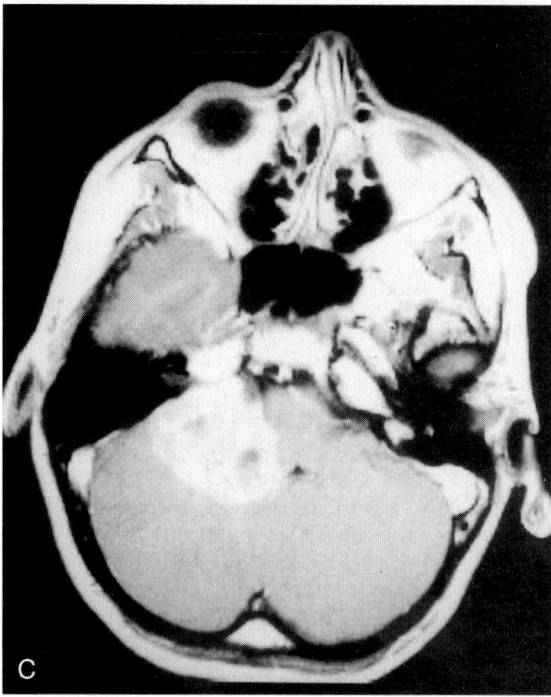

FIGURE 234–4. Seven-year-old boy with headaches. *A,* Nonenhanced, T1-weighted, axial magnetic resonance imaging (MRI) scan. The tumor is seen in the left cerebellopontine angle. There is signal inhomogeneity, and at other levels (not shown) there are cysts. The tumor extends through the lateral foramen of the fourth ventricle, which has been displaced. *B,* T2-weighted, axial MRI scan. The signal is quite variable and suggests cyst formation within the tumor. However, at operation, some of the bright signal areas were found to be neoplasm rather than cyst. *C,* Gadolinium-enhanced, T1-weighted, axial MRI scan. The tumor is quite densely enhancing and appears dural based. Its location and signal changes could lead to the misdiagnosis of meningioma or ependymoma. The lateral angle location is unusual in this age group and highlights the inability of imaging to make a pathologic diagnosis.

ics note that there are other aspects to consider, such as resource utilization (imaging costs, sedation needs), and that the advantage of early detection has not been proved.[105, 106] Surveillance imaging does have a role in defining the effects of treatment and the complications related to treatment.

SURGERY

The goals of surgical therapy include establishing a diagnosis, resecting as much of the tumor as safely possible, and treating any concurrent hydrocephalus. Hydrocephalus is usually responsible for any sudden preoperative deterioration in the patient. It appears that treatment of significant hydrocephalus before an operation improves the patient's condition and subsequent clinical course.[4]

Although preoperative shunt placement successfully controls hydrocephalus, it commits every patient to a shunt when only 10% to 40% of medulloblastoma patients may ultimately need shunting.[4, 107, 108] There has also been concern that preoperative shunting in medulloblastoma increases the risk of extraneural metastasis. However, studies suggest that only a small portion of patients with extraneural metastases have shunts, and the shunt rarely contributes to the metastasis.[108, 109] Currently, the use of millipore filtering is also discouraged. There is no evidence that it prevents extraneural dissemination of tumor, but the filter does lead to shunt occlusion unrelated to tumor spread.

External ventricular drainage can be placed before or at the start of surgery and has assumed the dominant role in the perioperative treatment of hydrocephalus. External drainage that is continued postoperatively carries away bloody fluid and debris, possibly reducing the need for subsequent shunting or the risk of aseptic meningitis. Any drainage procedure before surgery carries some risk, perhaps as much as 3% to 6%, of creating upward herniation or hemorrhage into the tumor.[4, 5, 83, 110, 111]

Preoperative steroid use can reduce cerebral edema and intracranial pressure. Although steroid treatment usually improves a patient who is ill from hydrocephalus, it should not be used to the exclusion of ventricular drainage. Steroids are continued for several days postoperatively.[5] Prophylactic antacids or H_2 antagonists have been given in conjunction with steroids to prevent gastrointestinal complications. Perioperative antibiotics are used as in other operations.

Appropriate operative monitoring is used, with adequate arterial and venous access. Electromyographic monitoring of the facial muscles and lateral rectus eye muscles has been investigated as an adjunct to resection of a tumor on or in the fourth ventricle. There is no clear indication that this type of monitoring helps the surgeon prevent brainstem injury during the resection of these mostly extra-axial tumors.[112]

The sitting position was once the classic choice for posterior fossa surgery, but it has been supplanted by the prone position. The sitting position carries a significant risk of intraoperative air embolism, requiring the placement of a central venous catheter ending at the atrium. There can be extensive and uncontrollable ventricular CSF drainage during the operation, with severe postoperative pneumocephaly. The sitting position is also difficult to attain in a young infant who cannot be placed in a pin-type head holder. In addition, the surgeon is forced into an uncomfortable and difficult position to gain access to the posterior fossa. Infants and children younger than 3 years old are easily positioned in a horseshoe head holder in a straight prone position. Nasotracheal intubation can allow more neck flexion and ultimately better exposure of the superior aspect of the posterior fossa.

The operative field can be prepared to include an occipital bur hole for external ventriculostomy placement, with the catheter tunneled to a separate externalization site to minimize the risk of infection. The posterior fossa is exposed by a midline incision from just above the inion to approximately the midcervical region. The incision is deepened in the avascular midline between the strap muscles of the neck. These muscles are elevated from the cranium and upper cervical laminae. In infants and children, it is not necessary to incise

across the muscle insertion (a so-called T-cut). The strap muscles can be retracted far enough laterally so that all tumors, except those in the cerebellopontine angle, can be approached from the midline. With tumors that extend into the cervical canal, the laminae of C1 and C2 are removed as needed.

A posterior fossa craniotomy is just as easy to perform as a craniectomy and allows for some bone replacement just below the inion, which limits the cosmetic deformity. A line of small bur holes is placed just inferior to the level of the transverse sinus, along the lateral aspects of the exposure, and toward the foramen magnum inferiorly. No bur hole is needed in the superior midline, where the bone can be quite thick and may have venous channels. The dura is separated between the holes, and the craniotome creates the bone flap. Rongeurs are used to widen the exposure as needed, and intraoperative ultrasonography is used to define an adequate exposure.

The dura is opened in a Y-like fashion, starting from the superior lateral aspects of the exposure and directed to the midline just above the foramen magnum. The surgeon must be prepared to occlude and ligate an occipital dural sinus that is variably present in the midline of the posterior fossa. The dura at the foramen magnum is often quite thick and may contain a circular sinus that requires ligation. Suture ligatures are preferable to metal clips; they are more secure and do not produce any artifact on subsequent MRI.

The cerebellar tonsils can be separated, exposing the vallecula, entrance to the fourth ventricle, and dorsum of the cervical cord. In some cases, tumor is extruding from the fourth ventricle and extending into the cervical canal. A cottonoid can be placed along the fourth ventricular floor where it is clear of tumor. This protects the floor and begins to orient the surgeon to the direction of the superior brainstem. Cottonoids should not be inserted into the fourth ventricle except under direct vision to avoid injury to the floor, particularly where tumor may have invaded it.

Tumor resection begins with exposure of the dorsal tumor surface and dissection along the usually distinct tumor-cerebellum interface. In most cases, the dorsal exposure is performed by splitting the vermis. The posterior inferior cerebellar arteries are usually displaced laterally against the medial aspect of the cerebellar tonsils. After the margins are defined, the tumor is internally debulked, using bipolar coagulation and suction or a Cavitron ultrasonic surgical aspirator. The internal decompression allows room for further dissection along the tumor margin. During this debulking, specimens are obtained for pathologic evaluation and for investigational studies or tumor banking.

Wherever the fourth ventricle is entered, the normal tissue should be protected with patties. It is usually easiest to enter the fourth ventricle from an inferior direction and extend the resection along the lateral walls of the ventricle and cerebellar peduncles. If necessary, the velum interpositum can be divided to give access to the lateral recesses of the fourth ventricle. The fourth ventricle is often free at the superior pole of the tumor near the aqueduct. The exposed aqueduct can be occluded to prevent the dependent drainage of blood into the third ventricle.

Some surgeons use a "horizontal" approach to achieve appropriate exposure and limit injury to the vermis or deeper cerebellar structures.[113] The cerebellar tonsils can be gently displaced laterally, exposing the tela choroidea and the inferior medullary velum. Access to the floor and main body of the fourth ventricle can be obtained by sectioning the tela. Access to the lateral recesses and superior portions of the fourth ventricle can be achieved with more extensive incision of the tela, combined with incision of the inferior medullary velum.

Tumor attachment at the cerebellar peduncles and along the fourth ventricular floor, which occurs in 15% to 40% of cases, must be carefully isolated.[5, 10, 114] It can be quite easy to injure the brainstem or peduncles while following the margins of the tumor. Magnified vision is very helpful while resecting the tumor with aspiration until it is nearly flush with the floor or peduncle at the point of attachment. When tumor invades the brainstem, it is not necessary or advisable to attempt its complete removal.

In one multi-institutional report, a resection of greater than 90% could be obtained in 80% of patients, and a resection of 51% to 90% could be obtained in 14% of patients. Pediatric neurosurgeons were able to achieve radical resections more frequently than and with the same morbidity as general neurosurgeons.[115] This likely represents a greater familiarity with the regional anatomy and more experience in dealing with these particular tumors.

Hemostasis is obtained with bipolar coagulation along the cerebellar surfaces. On the brainstem and cerebellar peduncles, bleeding is controlled only with gentle pressure or small bits of thrombin-soaked gelatin sponge, because bipolar cauterization would transfer an unacceptable amount of energy through the tissue and might injure delicate adjacent structures. Valsalva's maneuver is performed to confirm hemostasis. The cavity is copiously irrigated, and the aqueduct is flushed free of any debris or blood. The dura is closed primarily as much as possible. Very small dural defects can be closed with a piece of muscle; larger defects require the use of a patch. Closure of the dura may reduce the incidence of chemical meningitis by limiting the seepage of blood into the posterior fossa from the overlying tissues.

I place a layer of compressed Gelfoam over the dura. The bone flap is replaced and secured along its superior aspect with nonabsorbable suture or with plates and screws. Metal plates and screws are used only in older children and adults; absorbable plating systems can be used in younger children. The muscles are closed in the midline in multiple layers. It is most important to close the fascial layer tightly, and care must be taken to get a good closure near the inion to avoid problems with CSF leakage. There is often a small amount of fluid collecting beneath the flap postoperatively, and this may persist for several weeks. However, development of a tense pseudomeningocele is usually due to the development of hydrocephalus.

If an external ventricular drain has been placed, drainage is maintained at normal pressure levels for 1 to 3 days. This allows removal of blood and debris from the ventricular system and keeps CSF from trying to exit through the posterior fossa wound. Over the next 1 to 2 days, the pressure level of the drain is gradually increased, observing for an appropriate decrease in drainage and no indication of leakage around the drain. If the drainage persists or the pressure increases, several additional days of drainage are warranted before trying to wean the patient from the ventriculostomy again. The incidence of shunting has been correlated with younger patient age, larger ventricles on presentation, and larger tumors.[107]

COMPLICATIONS OF SURGERY

The morbidity and mortality of posterior fossa surgery for medulloblastoma have been greatly reduced to approximately 1%.[116] However, immediate postoperative morbidity is quite common, from 26% to 46%.[5, 117] Most commonly this involves an increase in nystagmus and cerebellar ataxia, particularly truncal ataxia and gait changes. Cranial nerve dysfunction is also frequently seen and is related to tumor invasion into the brainstem or the operative manipulations required to remove tumor from the vicinity of the fourth ventricle.

Air embolism remains a risk of any posterior fossa surgery. Air embolism can be detected with Doppler monitoring over the heart or by monitoring for a drop in end-tidal carbon dioxide. Clinical signs, including hypotension or arrhythmia, occur quite late, after severe air embolism has occurred. Treatment of a significant air embolism requires aspiration of the air from the right side of the heart, with concurrent maneuvers to prevent additional air from entering the system. The central venous pressure is increased with fluid volume, the operative field should be flooded, and all exposed bone edges should be carefully waxed. In patients positioned prone, air embolism may occur in up to 10%, but it is usually asymptomatic.[116]

Aseptic meningitis can manifest as headache, photophobia, fever, and neck stiffness within a few days of the operation. Because no clinical evaluation can accurately distinguish aseptic meningitis from an acute bacterial infection, the patient should undergo CSF sampling for Gram staining and culture and should be given broad-spectrum antibiotics until the cultures are proved negative. In the absence of infection, an increased steroid dose can be used for symptomatic relief.

Cerebellar mutism, or postoperative pseudobulbar palsy, has an estimated incidence of 10% to 25%.[114, 118, 119] The patient has cessation of speech 24 to 72 hours postoperatively, increased emotional lability, pseudobulbar palsies, and possibly hemiparesis. The emotional lability and weakness subside over several weeks, but the mutism may persist for months. There is often some residual dysarthria. The cause of this syndrome is not known, but it has been associated with larger midline tumors. Resection of the vermis may play a role, but in one prospective study, even extensive resection of the vermis caused very little neurological deficit.[120] Injury to the dentate nucleus or the cerebellar peduncles has also been theorized as a causative factor. The treatment of cerebellar mutism is supportive; steroids are not helpful.

PROGNOSIS AND STAGING

Adjunctive therapies are typically limited or expanded based on a determination of the patient's risk of disease progression or recurrence. In lower-risk patients, adjunctive therapy and craniospinal radiation might be reduced or limited, whereas in higher-risk patients, additional or more intensive therapies might be used sooner.

Age at diagnosis is the most consistently identified patient-related prognostic factor. A patient younger than 3 years old at diagnosis generally has a worse prognosis,[24, 115, 121–125] but this may result from the reduction, delay, or avoidance of radiotherapy in these young children. In some reports, patients treated with the same regimen had similar survival regardless of age.[11, 25, 124] The difference in outcome may also be related to the fact that younger children more often have disseminated disease at diagnosis.[24, 126]

Standard histology, genetic attributes, and immunohistochemical markers have been assessed for prognostic significance. The apparent cytologic differentiation of medulloblastomas has not been clearly associated with differing outcomes.[41, 54, 58, 127, 128] The classification of medulloblastomas as either classic or desmoplastic has been of inconsistent prognostic value.[10, 16, 17] There have also been discordant prognostic results when classification was based on the cellular differentiation of the tumor.[41, 127]

Evaluation of tumor immunohistochemical and DNA markers has also shown divergent results. Ploidy (aneuploid versus diploid tumors) has not been shown to clearly affect outcome.[61–64] GFAP expression correlated with poor prognosis, and tumors that were negative for both GFAP and neuronal intermediate filament were nearly six times less likely to relapse than were tumors expressing GFAP.[116]

Extent of disease may be one of the most easily identified and important tumor-related prognostic factors. One component of the extent of disease is the presence of tumor dissemination at the time of diagnosis, which is found in 13% to 43% of cases.[97, 98, 126, 129] The extent of disease can also be defined by the amount of tumor remaining after surgical therapy. Assessing the extent of disease is called *staging*. The most commonly used staging system has been that of Chang and coworkers, describing the extent of tumor at presentation (T stage) and the absence or presence of metastatic lesions (M stage).[130] The T1 and T2 stages refer to smaller tumors limited to the cerebellum. T3- and T4-stage tumors have invaded adjacent structures or extended out of the fourth ventricle. The M stages are as follows: M0, no subarachnoid or gross metastasis; M1, tumor cells in the CSF; M2, gross disease in the cranial

CSF spaces, including the lateral or third ventricle; M3, gross spread into the spinal subarachnoid spaces; and M4, extraneural metastasis.

The Chang staging system has been used in a number of multi-institutional studies. However, the prognostic significance of preoperative tumor size has not been confirmed.[11, 23, 115, 126] As surgeons have achieved greater tumor resection, defining the extent of disease with postoperative imaging and staging has been replacing the Chang system, and this may be a more appropriate measure.[115, 126, 131]

Current methods of staging include imaging the primary site of tumor within 48 hours of surgery, imaging the spine (either preoperatively or several weeks postoperatively), and obtaining CSF for cytology (at the time of surgery or postoperatively).[93, 132] Most treatment protocols include bone marrow biopsy and bone scans as part of the initial staging, although extraneural metastasis at presentation is rare.

Patient age and tumor dissemination at diagnosis are unalterable, but the extent of resection may be under the surgeon's control, and it seems that a greater extent of tumor resection is associated with a better prognosis.[9, 17, 23, 26, 62, 124, 126, 133, 134] In single-institution studies, the 5-year survival of patients with gross total resection was 82% to 100%, but it was less than 40% for those with residual disease.[17, 58, 61, 62, 124, 134] Multi-institutional studies do not show a convincing difference in survival between patients with total versus subtotal resections, but they confirm the significantly improved outcome of these groups compared with patients receiving partial resections.[24, 115, 126, 127, 135–138]

There seems to be no difference in outcome between total resection (with or without any small amount left on the brainstem) and near-total resection (>90% resection, but postoperative imaging showing <1.5 cm² of tumor).[114, 116] Recent cooperative studies suggest that patients with a small amount of tumor attached to or invading the brainstem, but not visible on postoperative imaging, do as well as the "average-risk" group and should be included in that category.[134, 139, 140] Patients with no evidence of metastasis but brainstem residual disease less than 1.5 cm² had a 5-year progression-free survival of 78%, compared with a survival of 54% if they had more than 1.5 cm² disease remaining.

Currently, an "average-risk" group is defined as patients who are at least 3 years of age, have had a gross total resection (<1.5 cm² of residual tumor on postoperative imaging), and have no metastatic disease. A "high-risk" group includes those at least 3 years old with a subtotal resection, metastatic disease, or gross brainstem invasion. Patients younger than 3 years may be placed in a separate category or included in the high-risk group, regardless of the extent of postoperative disease.

ADJUNCTIVE TREATMENT

Radiotherapy

It has long been recognized that surgical excision of a medulloblastoma is not curative, and there is a need for adjunctive therapy.[114, 141] Cushing was the first to recognize that medulloblastoma was radiosensitive, and Patterson and Farr clearly demonstrated the utility of neuraxis radiotherapy in doubling the 3-year survival to more than 50%.[7]

Modern radiotherapy typically involves using 5400 to 5800 cGy to the primary site and any metastases and 3500 cGy to the neuraxis.[141, 142] This has resulted in a 50% to 70% survival rate at 5 years for standard-risk patients. It had been thought that using less than 5000 cGy to the posterior fossa would result in an increase in local recurrence or a decrease in survival.[13, 143] However, the least amount of radiotherapy needed to control disease outside the primary site has not been defined.

The morbidity of radiotherapy at these doses has prompted attempts to decrease the side effects without affecting the survival rate (see "Complications of Adjunctive Therapy"). In theory, delivering hyperfractionated treatment has the potential for a greater "kill" effect on the tumor, allowing either dose reduction or improved survival at the same dose. In practice, hyperfractionated treatment of medulloblastoma has shown no improvement over standard therapy, and the treatment schedule is difficult for young children who require sedation for treatment.[144, 145]

Treatments involving radiation dose reduction have been tried alone and in conjunction with adjunctive chemotherapy.[124, 138, 146–148] Reduction of the radiation dose was evaluated by the combined Pediatric Oncology Group–Children's Cancer Group study from 1986 to 1990. In this randomized trial, patients with "low-stage" medulloblastoma received either 3600 or 2340 cGy craniospinal irradiation. This study was terminated when there were early relapses in the reduced-dose group (the 3-year disease-free survival rate was 78% for the standard-treatment group and 52% for the reduced-radiation group).[149] Outcomes at 5 and 8 years continue to show a difference in event-free survival, although the difference is not statistically significant.[149, 150]

A number of studies have used chemotherapy before and during radiotherapy, with and without standard and reduced craniospinal radiation doses.[144, 147, 148, 151] Use of procarbazine before radiation and hydroxyurea during radiation yielded no difference in disease progress between those receiving standard radiation and those receiving reduced radiation.[147] There was a marked difference in survival rates between the good- and poor-risk groups, with 5-year survivals of 83% and 58%, respectively. The poor-risk group failed mostly at the primary site, suggesting a need to intensify therapy there. The International Society of Pediatric Oncology (SIOP) study did not show a benefit with the use of preradiation chemotherapy. There was a worse outcome in the chemotherapy–decreased radiation group, possibly due to a delay in starting radiotherapy as a result of chemotherapy complications.[151]

Stereotactic radiosurgery can be used to treat focal areas of residual tumor, attempting to improve initial tumor control.[152] It can also be used for recurrent tumor sites. However, this modality has not been tested in clinical trials.[135]

Chemotherapy

Beneficial effects of adjuvant chemotherapy for medulloblastoma were seen in the Children's Cancer Group study (CCG-942) that compared conventional radiotherapy to radiotherapy followed by chemotherapy with vincristine, CCNU, and prednisone.[24] Although the overall survival for the two groups did not significantly differ, there was an improvement in survival among patients with large residual tumors or metastatic disease at diagnosis (57% survival for the chemotherapy group versus 19% for the conventional radiotherapy group; progression-free survivals of 46% and 0%, respectively).

A European trial (SIOP I) using a chemotherapy regimen similar to that of CCG-942 had similar results, with no overall difference but improved outcomes in patients with incompletely resected tumors, brainstem invasion, or metastatic disease.[136] A Pediatric Oncology Group phase III trial used nitrogen mustard, vincristine, procarbazine, and prednisone after radiotherapy and demonstrated a better 5-year survival in the chemotherapy group (74% versus 56%).[153] This effect was not seen in patients younger than 5 years old.

Packer and coworkers used adjuvant chemotherapy in the treatment of a relatively small number of high-stage patients and reported a significant improvement (73%) in the 5-year disease-free survival.[123] The results remained good (85% 5-year progression-free survival) when the regimen was applied to a larger group of patients, and a similar improvement was even seen in patients younger than 5 years old who received reduced craniospinal radiotherapy (2400 cGy).[123]

Neoadjuvant chemotherapy (before radiotherapy) has a theoretical advantage, in that drug delivery is not impaired by any radiation-induced tissue changes. Pilot studies suggested a role for neoadjuvant therapy.[154–157] One study of "8-in-1" neoadjuvant chemotherapy (eight drugs given in one day) showed 5-year disease-free survival rates of 57% for high-stage disease and 62% for low-stage disease.[158] However, a phase III trial of neoadjuvant chemotherapy (CCG-921) in the treatment of high-risk patients showed that the 5-year event-free survival rate was better for the control arm (63%) than for the experimental group (45%).[134] Preliminary reports from Pediatric Oncology Group study 9031, comparing chemotherapy before and after radiation with chemotherapy after radiation, suggest no difference in the two treatment groups, with 7-year survival rates of approximately 68% to 75%.

From these and other studies, it appears that upfront chemotherapy is certainly feasible. But with no significant change in the disease-free progression or overall survival, there does not appear to be an obvious advantage to this treatment.[134, 142, 154, 158, 159] In one study, the risk of disease progression increased with a longer duration of preradiation chemotherapy.[160] It seems that radiotherapy should not be deferred by more than 6 to 8 weeks when using neoadjuvant chemotherapy.[154, 161]

Another strategy involves the use of high-dose chemotherapy and subsequent bone marrow rescue.[162, 163] This strategy is predicated on medulloblastoma's sensitivity to chemotherapeutic agents with primarily hematopoietic dose-limiting toxicity. Such treatment also requires the isolation of bone marrow regenerative cells that are free of tumor and can engraft and regenerate. Fortunately, medulloblastoma rarely metastasizes to the marrow, and newer techniques of isolating stem cells from the peripheral circulation have made the technique easier. This treatment has been used for patients with recurrence, as consolidation therapy in infants with no postoperative residual disease, and in conjunction with other standard chemotherapy regimens.[164] Unfortunately, this treatment has a high monetary cost, is quite labor-intensive, and has a serious toxic mortality ranging from 5% to 22%.[162, 163, 165, 166]

Infants younger than 3 years old with medulloblastoma have been described as having a worse prognosis, with reported 5-year survival rates of 20% to 40%.[123, 136, 167–169] As mentioned, this may be because these patients do not receive adequate radiotherapy.[170] However, infants treated with radiotherapy that differs significantly from standard treatment have not been shown to have disease-free survival rates that equal those achieved with standard radiotherapy delivered immediately after surgery.[122, 161, 168, 169, 171]

The Pediatric Oncology Group attempted to delay the start of radiotherapy in infants by using continuing chemotherapy.[122] For medulloblastoma patients, there was a 34% 2-year progression-free survival rate. Other groups have used chemotherapy and reduced radiotherapy,[161, 168, 172] reporting 5-year progression-free survival rates of 54% but also significant morbidity associated with the chemotherapy and radiotherapy. However, there are reports of long-term infant survivors treated with only surgery and chemotherapy.[121, 170]

COMPLICATIONS OF ADJUNCTIVE TREATMENT

Radiotherapy has clearly defined, significant physical and neuropsychological side effects that are often insidious in onset and mostly dose related. There are acute effects, such as cutaneous inflammation or leukopenia.[141] Radiation effects on the developing brain can be quite severe, with delayed or destroyed myelination resulting in leukoencephalopathy.[173] There may be microvascular injury, with subsequent ischemic damage and dystrophic calcification. Unusual complications of radiotherapy have been reported, including cardiac and pulmonary dysfunction resulting from spinal irradiation.[174, 175]

As many as 41% of long-term survivors of medulloblastoma have moderate to severe handicaps.[151, 176] Cognitive impairment, which can be subtle attention or learning deficits rather than frank retardation, has been seen in as many as 90% of survivors.[6, 177–182] These radiation effects are worse in patients who are younger at treatment or receive a greater dose.[6, 25, 161, 179, 182–190] Reflecting the multifactorial nature of treatment-induced cognitive decline, one study found that age at treatment, radiation, and the use of chemotherapy were all contributing factors. The patients receiving chemotherapy and radiation did worse than those receiving radiation alone.[191]

The functional decline may not be noticeable during the first year after treatment, but longitudinal studies have shown a progressive decline in intelligence.[178, 183, 184, 192, 193] In one study, 60% of patients had an intelligence quotient (IQ) greater than 90 at 1 year after therapy, but after 5 years, only 20% were above 90, and only 10% by 10 years.[194] The intellectual decline is thought to be due to bilateral hemispheric radiation exposure, because it is not seen in patients with posterior fossa ependymomas undergoing focal radiotherapy or in patients with cerebellar astrocytomas not treated with radiation.[176, 194] Also, dose reduction has resulted in a measurable sparing of IQ.[150, 151] Although patients still have declining IQs, this reflects the increasing gap between their abilities and those of their peers, rather than a loss of previously acquired skills.

Radiation can also cause endocrinologic side effects, including growth retardation, hypothyroidism, hypocortisolism, and hypogonadism.[10, 176, 195] Some of the effect is due to direct dose-related end-organ radiation exposure.[187, 196] There also appears to be a correlation with increasing dose delivered to the hypothalamus.[195] Patients receiving less than 1800 cGy had no growth hormone deficiency, whereas 56% of the group receiving 2400 cGy and 75% of the cohort receiving doses up to 4500 cGy developed growth hormone deficiency.[197]

Growth failure is the most common endocrinologic sequela.[6, 10, 172, 176, 179, 186, 198] However, craniospinal irradiation further impairs overall growth by interfering with vertebral growth.[199] The rapidity of onset is dose dependent.[195] The radiation effects on growth may be accentuated by the concurrent use of chemotherapy.[199, 200] Cranial irradiation greater than 2400 cGy may cause unusually early puberty, which limits the number of years available to catch up on growth.[201]

Careful monitoring of the growth rate and appropriate endocrinologic testing allow early treatment of short stature with recombinant growth hormone replacement. There is currently no evidence that the use of exogenous growth hormone puts these patients at greater risk of tumor recurrence, although this is a regular concern of patients and their families.[202] Long-term endocrinologic surveillance is necessary in medulloblastoma survivors, because these complications have an insidious onset, often occurring years after the completion of therapy.

The complications of chemotherapy are usually more acute than those of radiotherapy. Bone marrow depression is frequent and usually requires supportive care. With the platinum-based medications, a well-recognized sensorineural hearing loss is associated with the cumulative dose. Each of the chemotherapy agents has its own known systemic side effects, such as cardiomyopathy (doxorubicin), urinary bladder fibrosis (cyclophosphamide), and pulmonary fibrosis (carmustine).[172, 175, 203]

As the duration of survival after medulloblastoma

treatment increases, there is an increased likelihood of identifying second malignancies caused by the radiation and chemotherapy. In one series, after 20 years there was a 10% cumulative rate of second malignancy.[143] Another series reported a 16% incidence of second malignancy (thyroid adenoma, meningioma) occurring more than 5 years after treatment.[6] In a population study based on the United States and Sweden, a 5.4-fold increase in second malignancies (salivary gland, uterine cervix, brain, thyroid, acute lymphoblastic leukemia) was identified.[204] Most of the tumors seemed to be related to radiation fields. It is well recognized that high-grade gliomas and meningiomas are inducible by radiotherapy. Chemotherapy with alkylating agents is associated with later development of acute myelogenous leukemia.[205] Patients with Gorlin's syndrome—up to 5% of those with medulloblastoma—are at increased risk for additional malignancies.[172, 204]

RECURRENCE

Medulloblastoma most frequently recurs within 2 to 4 years of diagnosis.[25, 124] Although uncommon, recurrences more than 8 years after diagnosis do occur. Collin's rule—that a disease-free survival lasting longer than the patient's age at diagnosis plus 9 months is equivalent to a cure—does not hold true in 20% of medulloblastoma patients.[13, 25, 206, 207]

The primary site is also the most common site of recurrence, accounting for 56% to 80% of recurrences.[13, 137] That pattern may be changing with recent therapies, however. One study found that only 18% of recurrences were at the primary site in patients who had received at least 5300 cGy, and another study did not correlate relapse site with radiation dose to the primary site or neuraxis.[144, 208] In older radiotherapy reports, recurrence in the ethmoid or cribriform plate region was frequently identified and was thought to be due to improper radiation shielding of the eyes.

Imaging for late recurrences of medulloblastoma must take into consideration that not all recurrent tumors enhance.[209] Dural enhancement is frequently seen on postoperative imaging and by itself is not diagnostic of recurrence.[92] Nodular enhancement is seen in 26% of recurrent medulloblastomas, and pia-arachnoid enhancement in 63%.[92]

Extra-axial metastasis of medulloblastoma is typically a late event, occurring in approximately 5% to 20% of patients and found an average of 2 years after diagnosis.[210, 211] Bone lesions are the most common (80% to 90%), presenting with regional pain and a mass. They can be blastic or mixed lytic-blastic.[82, 109, 210, 212] Patients who have not had adjuvant chemotherapy may be at greater risk for bone metastasis.[208, 211] Lymph nodes are the next most common site of extraneural metastasis (30% to 65%), with liver, lung, and pleura being less frequent (15%).

Treatment for recurrent medulloblastoma is extremely limited by the prior radiation or chemotherapy and is usually only palliative. Repeat radiation treatment has a very high toxicity and adds only a limited time to survival.[213] Reoperation is of little value unless it is followed by chemotherapy or radiotherapy. Radiosurgery for focal recurrences has been tried with some limited success.[135]

High-dose chemotherapy with rescue of the bone marrow has been tried in some cases of recurrence.[162–164, 214, 215] Kaplan-Meier estimates of 34% event-free survival and 46% overall survival at 36 months have been reported.[215] There is a significant acute mortality associated with the treatment of recurrences (10% to 22%).[162, 163, 165, 166, 214, 215]

CONCLUSION

Through the evolution of surgical technique, diagnostic imaging, and adjunctive therapy, patients treated for medulloblastoma have achieved a progressively increasing rate of survival. The explosion of genetic information gives further hope that we can adjust and tailor treatments based on biologic expectations and perhaps find some unique treatments. Concurrent with the increased survival has been an awareness of the morbidity associated with successful treatment. Attention is being focused on the quality of that survival and on treatment techniques to enhance the quality of life without sacrificing better survival.

REFERENCES

1. Bailey P, Cushing H: Medulloblastoma cerebelli, a common type of midcerebellar glioma of childhood. Arch Neurol Psych 14: 192–224, 1925.
2. Rorke LB: The cerebellar medulloblastoma and its relationship to primitive neuroectodermal tumors. J Neuropathol Exp 42: 1–15, 1983.
3. Ingraham FD, Bailey OT, Barker WF: Medulloblastoma cerebelli: Diagnosis, treatment and survival, with a special report of fifty-six cases. N Engl J Med 238:171–174, 1948.
4. Raimondi AJ, Tomita T: Hydrocephalus and infratentorial tumors: Incidence, clinical picture, and treatment. J Neurosurg 55: 174–182, 1981.
5. Albright AL, Wisoff JH, Zelzer PM, et al: Current neurosurgical treatment of medulloblastoma in children: A report from the Children's Cancer Study Group. Pediatr Neurosci 15:276–282, 1989.
6. Helseth E, Due-Tonnessen B, Wesenberg F, et al: Posterior fossa medulloblastoma in children and young adults (0–19 years): Survival and performance. Childs Nerv Syst 15:451–456, 1999.
7. Paterson E, Farr RF: Cerebellar medulloblastomas: Treatment by irradiation of the whole central nervous system. Acta Radiol 39:323–336, 1953.
8. Gerosa MA, di Stefano E, Olivi A, et al: Multidisciplinary treatment of medulloblastoma: A 5-year experience with the SIOP trial. Childs Brain 8:107–118, 1981.
9. Agerlin N, Gjerris F, Brincker H, et al: Childhood medulloblastoma in Denmark 1960–1984: A population-based study. Childs Nerv Syst 15:29–37, 1999.
10. Park TS, Hoffman HJ, Hendrick EB, et al: Medulloblastoma: Clinical presentation and management. Experience at the Hospital for Sick Children, Toronto 1950–1980. J Neurosurg 58:543–552, 1983.
11. David KM, Casey ATH, Hayward RD, et al: Medulloblastoma: Is the 5-year survival rate improving? A review of 80 cases from a single institution. J Neurosurg 86:13–21, 1997.
12. Schoenberg BS, Schoenberg DG, Christine BW, et al: The epidemiology of primary intracranial neoplasms of childhood: A population study. Mayo Clin Proc 51:51–56, 1976.

13. Belza MG, Donaldson SS, Steinberg GK, et al: Medulloblastoma: Freedom from relapse longer than 8 years—a therapeutic cure? J Neurosurg 75:575–582, 1991.

14. Roberts RO, Lynch CF, Jones MP, et al: Medulloblastoma: A population-based study of 532 cases. J Neuropathol Exp Neurol 50:134–144, 1991.

15. Farwell JR, Dohrmann GJ, Flannery JT: Medulloblastoma in childhood: An epidemiological study. J Neurosurg 61:657–664, 1984.

16. Chatty EM, Earler KM: Medulloblastoma: A report of 201 cases with emphasis on relationship of histological variants to survival. Cancer 28:977, 1971.

17. Maleci A, Cervoni L, Delfini R: Medulloblastoma in children and adults: A comparative study. Acta Neurochir (Wien) 119: 62–67, 1992.

18. Sheikh BY, Kanaan IN: Medulloblastoma in adults. J Neurosurg Sci 38:229–234, 1994.

19. Haie-Meder C, Song PY: Medulloblastoma: Differences in adults and children. Int J Radiat Oncol Biol Phys 32:1255–1257, 1995.

20. Prados MD, Warnick RE, Wara WM, et al: Medulloblastoma in adults. Int J Radiat Oncol Biol Phys 32:1145–1152, 1995.

21. Carrie C, Lasset C, Alapetite C, et al: Multivariate analysis of prognostic factors in adult patients with medulloblastoma. Cancer 74:2352–2360, 1994.

22. Ringertz N, Tola JH: Medulloblastoma. J Neuropathol Exp Neurol 9:354–372, 1950.

23. Berry MP, Jenkin RD, Keen CW, et al: Radiation therapy for medulloblastoma: A 21-year review. J Neurosurg 55:43–51, 1981.

24. Evans AE, Jenkin RDT, Sposto R, et al: The treatment of medulloblastoma: Results of a prospective randomized trial of radiation therapy with and without CCNU, vincristine, and prednisone. J Neurosurg 72:572–582, 1990.

25. Hoppe-Hirsch E, Renier D, Lelouch-Tubiana A, et al: Medulloblastoma in childhood: Progressive intellectual deterioration. Childs Nerv Syst 6:60–65, 1990.

26. Raimondi AJ, Tomita T: Medulloblastoma in childhood: Comparative results of partial and total resection. Childs Brain 5: 310–328, 1979.

27. Thorne RN, Pearson ADJ, Nicoll JAR, et al: Decline in incidence of medulloblastoma in children. Cancer 74:3240–3244, 1999.

28. Clausen N, Garwics S, Glomstein A, et al: Medulloblastoma in Nordic children. I. Acta Paediatr Scand Suppl 371:5–11, 1990.

29. Evans DG, Farndon PA, Burnell LD, et al: The incidence of Gorlin syndrome in 173 consecutive cases of medulloblastoma. Br J Cancer 64:959–961, 1991.

30. Lacombe D, Chateil JF, Fontan D, et al: Medulloblastoma in the nevoid basal-cell carcinoma syndrome: Case reports and review of the literature. Genet Couns 1:273–277, 1990.

31. Smits A, van Grieken D, Hartman M, et al: Coexpression of platelet-derived growth factor α and β receptors on medulloblastomas and other primitive neuroectodermal tumors is consistent with an immature stem cell and neuronal derivation. Lab Invest 74:188–198, 1996.

32. Kershman J: The medulloblast and the medulloblastoma: A study of human embryos. Arch Neurol Psych 40:937–967, 1938.

33. Stevenson L, Echlin F: Nature and origin of some tumors of the cerebellum: Medulloblastoma. Arch Neurol 31:93–109, 1934.

34. Nagashima K, Yasui K, Kimura J, et al: Induction of brain tumors by a newly isolated JC virus (Tokyo-1 strain). Am J Pathol 116:455–463, 1984.

35. Rorke LB, Gilles FH, Davis RL, et al: Revision of the World Health Organization classification of brain tumors for childhood brain tumors. Cancer 56:1869–1886, 1985.

36. Trojanowski JQ, Fung KM, Rorke LB, et al: In vivo and in vitro models of medulloblastoma and other primitive neuroectodermal brain tumors in childhood. Mol Chem Neuropathol 21: 219–239, 1994.

37. Rubinstein LJ: Embryonal central neuroepithelial tumors and their differentiating potential: A cytogenetic view of a complex neurooncological problem. J Neurosurg 62:795–805, 1985.

38. Rostomily RC, Bermingham-McDonogh O, Berger MS, et al: Expression of neurogenic basic helix-loop-helix genes in primitive neuroectodermal tumors. Cancer Res 57:3526–3531, 1997.

39. Tohyama T, Lee VM, Rorke LB, et al: Monoclonal antibodies to a rat nestin fusion protein recognize a 220-kDa polypeptide in subsets of fetal and adult central nervous system neurons and in primitive neuroectodermal tumor cells. Am J Pathol 143: 258–268, 1993.

40. Fruhwald MC, O'Dorisio MS, Pietsch T, et al: High expression of somatostatin receptor subtype 2 (sst2) in medulloblastoma: Implications for diagnosis and therapy. Pediatr Res 45:697–708, 1999.

41. Packer RJ, Sutton LN, Rorke LB, et al: Prognostic importance of cellular differentiation in medulloblastoma of childhood. J Neurosurg 61:296–301, 1984.

42. Schoefield DE, Yonis ES, Geyer JR, et al: DNA content and other prognostic features in childhood medulloblastoma: Proposal of a scoring system. Cancer 69:1307–1314, 1992.

43. Giangaspero F, Perilongo G, Fondelli MP, et al: Medulloblastoma with extensive nodularity: A variant with favorable prognosis. J Neurosurg 91:971–977, 1999.

44. Soylemezoglu F, Soffer D, Onol B, et al: Lipomatous medulloblastoma in adults: A distinct clinicopathological entity. Am J Surg Pathol 20:413–418, 1996.

45. Giangaspero F, Cenacchi G, Roncaroli F, et al: Medullocytoma (lipidized medulloblastoma). Am J Surg Pathol 20:656–664, 1996.

46. Cai DX, Mafra M, Schmidt RE, et al: Medulloblastoma with extensive posttherapy neuronal maturation: Report of two cases. J Neurosurg 93:330–334, 2000.

47. Giangaspero F, Rigobello L, Badiali M, et al: Large-cell medulloblastoma: A distinct variant with highly aggressive behavior. Am J Surg Pathol 16:687–693, 1992.

48. Brown HG, Kepner JL, Perlman EJ, et al: "Large cell/anaplastic" medulloblastomas—a Pediatric Oncology Group study. J Neuropathol Exp Neurol 59:857–865, 2000.

49. Leonard J, Cai DX, Rivet D, et al: Large cell/anaplastic medulloblastomas and medullomyoblastomas: Clinicopathological and genetic features. J Neurosurg 95:82–88, 2001.

50. Bayani J, Zielenska M, Marrano P, et al: Molecular cytogenetic analysis of medulloblastomas and supratentorial primitive neuroectodermal tumors by using conventional banding, comparative genomic hybridization, and spectral karyotyping. J Neurosurg 93:437–448, 2000.

51. Rorke LB, Packer RJ, Biegel JA: Central nervous system atypical teratoid/rhabdoid tumors of infancy and childhood: Definition of an entity. J Neurosurg 85:56–65, 1996.

52. Burger PC, Yu IT, Tihan T, et al: Atypical teratoid/rhabdoid tumor of the central nervous system: A highly malignant tumor of infancy and childhood frequently mistaken for medulloblastoma: A Pediatric Oncology Group study. Am J Surg Pathol 22: 1083–1092, 1998.

53. Katsetos CD, Burger PC: Medulloblastoma. Semin Diagn Pathol 11:85–97, 1994.

54. Maraziotis T, Perentes E, Karamitopoulou E, et al: Neuron-associated class III beta-tubulin isotope, retinal S-antigen, synaptophysin, and glial fibrillary acidic protein in human medulloblastomas: A clinicopathological analysis. Acta Neuropathol (Berl) 84:355–363, 1992.

55. Mannoji H, Takeshita I, Fukui M, et al: Glial fibrillary acidic protein in medulloblastoma. Acta Neuropathol (Berl) 55:63–69, 1981.

56. Palmer JO, Kasselberg AG, Netsky MG: Differentiation of medulloblastoma: Studies including immunohistochemical localization of glial fibrillary acidic protein. J Neurosurg 55:161–169, 1981.

57. Roessmann U, Valesco ME, Gambetti P, et al: Neuronal and astrocytic differentiation in human neuroepithelial neoplasms. J Neuropathol Exp Neurol 42:113–121, 1983.

58. Taomoto K, Tomita T, Raimondi AJ, et al: Medulloblastomas in childhood: Histological factors influencing patients' outcome. Childs Nerv Syst 3:354–360, 1987.

59. Molenaar WM, Trojanowski JQ: Primitive neuroectodermal tumors of the central nervous system in childhood: Tumor biological aspects. Crit Rev Oncol Hematol 17:1–25, 1994.

60. Tait DM, Eeles RA, Carter R, et al: Ploidy and proliferative index in medulloblastoma: Useful prognostic factors? Eur J Cancer 29A:1383–1387, 1993.

61. Yasue M, Tomita T, Engelhard H, et al: Prognostic importance of DNA ploidy in medulloblastoma of childhood. J Neurosurg 70:385–391, 1989.

62. Schofield DE, Yunis EJ, Geyer JR, et al: DNA content and other prognostic features in childhood medulloblastoma. Cancer 69: 1307–1314, 1992.

63. Zerbini C, Gelber RD, Weinberg D, et al: Prognostic factors in medulloblastoma, including DNA ploidy. J Clin Oncol 11: 616–622, 1993.

64. Chou PM, Reyes-Mugica M, Barquin N, et al: Multidrug resistance gene expression in childhood medulloblastoma: Correlation with clinical outcome and DNA ploidy in 29 patients. Pediatr Neurosurg 23:283–292, 1995.

65. Bigner SH, Mark J, Friedman HS, et al: Structural chromosomal abnormalities in human medulloblastoma. Cancer Genet Cytogenet 30:91–101, 1988.

66. Giangaspero F, Chieco P, Ceccarelli C, et al: "Desmoplastic" versus "classic" medulloblastoma: Comparison of DNA content, histopathology and differentiation. Virchows Arch Pathol Anat 418:207–214, 1991.

67. Rasheed BKA, Bigner SH: Genetic alterations in glioma and medulloblastoma. Cancer Metastasis Rev 10:289–299, 1991.

68. Bigner SH, McLendon RE, Fuchs H, et al: Chromosomal characteristics of childhood brain tumors. Cancer Genet Cytogenet 97: 125–134, 1997.

69. Gogen PH, McDonald JD: Tumor suppressor genes and medulloblastoma. J Neurooncol 29:103–112, 1996.

70. Biegel JA, Janss AJ, Raffel C, et al: Prognostic significance of chromosome 17p deletions in childhood primitive neuroectodermal tumors (medulloblastomas) of the central nervous system. Clin Cancer Res 3:473–478, 1997.

71. Thomas GA, Raffel C: Loss of heterozygosity on 6q, 16q, and 17p in human central nervous system primitive neuroectodermal tumors. Cancer Res 51:639–643, 1991.

72. Cogen PH, Daneshvar L, Metzger AK, et al: Deletion mapping of the medulloblastoma locus on chromosome 17p. Genomics 8:279–285, 1990.

73. Cogen PH, Daneshvar L, Metzger AK, et al: Involvement of multiple chromosome 17p loci in medulloblastoma tumorigenesis. Am J Hum Genet 50:584–589, 1992.

74. Steichen-Gersdorf E, Baumgartner M, Kreczy A, et al: Deletion mapping on chromosome 17p in medulloblastoma. Br J Cancer 76:1284–1287, 1997.

75. Bruggers CS, Tai K-F, Murdock T, et al: Expression of the c-myc protein in childhood medulloblastoma. J Pediatr Hematol Oncol 20:18–25, 1998.

76. Gilbertson RJ, Pearson ADJ, Perry RH, et al: Prognostic significance of the c-erbB-2 oncogene product in childhood medulloblastoma. Br J Cancer 71:473–477, 1995.

77. Goumnerova LC: Growth factor receptors and medulloblastoma. J Neurooncol 29:85–89, 1996.

78. Grotzer MA, Janss AJ, Fung KM, et al: TrkC expression predicts good clinical outcome in primitive neuroectodermal brain tumors. J Clin Oncol 18:1027–1035, 2000.

79. Kozmik Z, Sure U, Rüedi D, et al: Deregulated expression of Pax5 in medulloblastoma. Proc Natl Acad Sci U S A 92: 5709–5713, 1995.

80. VandenBerg SR, May EE, Rubinstein LJ, et al: Desmoplastic supratentorial neuroepithelial tumors of infancy with divergent differentiation potential ("desmoplastic infantile gangliogliomas"). J Neurosurg 66:58–71, 1987.

81. Wang W, Kumar P, Whalley J, et al: The mutation status of Pax3 and p53 genes in medulloblastoma. Anticancer Res 18: 849–854, 1998.

82. Blaser SI, Harwood-Nash DCF: Neuroradiology of pediatric posterior fossa medulloblastoma. J Neurooncol 29:23–34, 1996.

83. Goel A: Whither preoperative shunts for posterior fossa tumours? Br J Neurosurg 7:395–399, 1993.

84. Chang T, Teng MMH, Lirng JF: Posterior cranial fossa tumors in childhood. Neuroradiology 35:274–278, 1993.

85. Meyers SP, Kemp SS, Tarr RW: MR imaging features of medulloblastomas. AJR Am J Roentgenol 158:859–865, 1992.

86. Vezina LG, Packer RJ: Infratentorial tumors of childhood. Neuroimaging Clin N Am 4:423–436, 1994.

87. Mueller DP, Moore SA, Sato Y, et al: MRI spectrum of medulloblastoma. Clin Imaging 16:250–255, 1992.

88. Barkovich AJ: Brain tumors of childhood. In Barkovich AJ (ed): Pediatric Neuroimaging, 2nd ed. Philadelphia, Lippincott-Raven, pp 321–438.

89. Bourgouin PM, Tampieri D, Grahovac SZ, et al: CT and MR imaging findings in adults with cerebellar medulloblastoma: Comparison with findings in children. AJR Am J Roentgenol 159:609–612, 1992.

90. Koci TM, Chiang F, Mehringer CM, et al: Adult cerebellar medulloblastoma: Imaging features with emphasis on MR findings. AJNR Am J Neuroradiol 14:929–939, 1993.

91. Oser AB, Moran CJ, Kaufman BA, Park TS: Intracranial tumor in children: MR imaging findings within 24 hours of craniotomy. Radiology 215:807–812, 1997.

92. Meyers SP, Wildenhain S, Chess MA, et al: Postoperative evaluation for intracranial recurrence of medulloblastoma: MR findings with gadopentetate dimeglumine. AJNR Am J Neuroradiol 15:1425–1434, 1994.

93. Meyers SP, Wildenhain SL, Chang JK, et al: Postoperataive evaluation for disseminated medulloblastoma involving the spine: Contrast-enhanced MR findings, CSF cytologic analysis, timing of disease occurrence, and patient outcomes. AJNR Am J Neuroradiol 21:1757–1765, 2000.

94. George RE, Laurent JP, McCluggage CW, et al: Spinal metastasis in primitive neuroectodermal tumors (medulloblastoma) of the posterior fossa: Evaluation with CT myelography and correlation with patient age and tumor differentiation. Pediatr Neurosci 12:157–160, 1985.

95. North C, Segall HD, Stanley P, et al: Early CT detection of intracranial seeding from medulloblastoma. AJNR Am J Neuroradiol 6:11–13, 1985.

96. Lee YY, Tien RD, Bruner JM, et al: Loculated intracranial leptomeningeal metastases: CT and MR characteristics. AJNR Am J Neuroradiol 10:1171–1179, 1989.

97. Deutsch M, Laurent JP, Cohen ME: Myelography for staging medulloblastoma. Cancer 56:1763–1766, 1985.

98. Deutsch M, Reigel DH: The value of myelography in the management of childhood medulloblastoma. Cancer 45:2194–2197, 1980.

99. Dorwart RH, Wara WN, Norman D, et al: Complete myelographic evaluation of spinal metastasis from medulloblastoma. Radiology 139:403–408, 1981.

100. Flannery AM, Tomita T, Radkowski MA, et al: Medulloblastoma in childhood: Post-surgical evaluation with myelography and cerebrospinal fluid cytology. J Neurooncol 8:149–151, 1990.

101. O'Reilly G, Hayward RD, Harkness WF: Myelography in the assessment of children with medulloblastoma. Br J Neurosurg 7:183–188, 1993.

102. Kramer ED, Vezina LG, Packer RJ, et al: Staging and surveillance of children with central nervous system neoplasms: Recommendations of the Neurology and Tumor Imaging Committees of the Children's Cancer Group. Pediatr Neurosurg 20: 254–263, 1994.

103. Wiener MD, Boyko OB, Friedman HS, et al: False-positive spinal MR findings for subarachnoid spread of primary CNS tumor in postoperative pediatric patients. AJNR Am J Neuroradiol 11: 1100–1103, 1990.

104. Friedman HS, Kun LE: More on surveillance of children with medulloblastoma. N Engl J Med 332:191, 1995.

105. Torres CF, Rebsamen S, Silber JH, et al: Surveillance scanning of children with medulloblastoma. N Engl J Med 330:892–895, 1994.

106. Shaw DWW, Geyer JR, Berger MS, et al: Asymptomatic recurrence detection with surveillance scanning in children with medulloblastoma. J Clin Oncol 15:1811–1813, 1997.

107. Lee M, Wisoff JH, Abbott R, et al: Management of hydrocephalus in children with medulloblastoma: Prognostic factors for shunting. Pediatr Neurosurg 20:240–247, 1994.

108. Berger MS, Baumeister B, Geyer JR, et al: The risks of metastases from shunting in children with primary central nervous system tumors. J Neurosurg 74:872–877, 1991.

109. Jamjoom ZAB, Jamjoom AB, Sulaiman A-H, et al: Systemic metastasis of medulloblastoma through ventriculoperitoneal shunt: Report of a case and critical analysis of the literature. Surg Neurol 40:403–410, 1993.

110. Hoffman HJ, Hendrick EB, Humphreys RP: Metastasis via ventriculoperitoneal shunt in patients with medulloblastoma. J Neurosurg 44:562–566, 1976.

111. Waga S, Shimizu T, Shimosaka S, et al: Intratumoral hemorrhage

after a ventriculoperitoneal shunting procedure. Neurosurgery 9:249–252, 1981.

112. Grabb PA, Albright AL, Sclabassi RJ, et al: Continuous intraoperative electromyographic monitoring of cranial nerves during resection of fourth ventricular tumors in children. J Neurosurg 86:1–4, 1997.

113. Mussi ACM, Rhoton AL Jr: Telovelar approach to the fourth ventricle: Microsurgical anatomy. J Neurosurg 92:812–823, 2000.

114. Gajjar A, Sanford RA, Bhargava R, et al: Medulloblastoma with brain stem involvement: The impact of gross total resection on outcome. Pediatr Neurosurg 25:182–187, 1996.

115. Albright AL, Wisoff JH, Zeltzer PM, et al: Effects of medulloblastoma resection on outcome in children: A report from Children's Cancer Group. Neurosurgery 38:934–939, 1996.

116. Sutton LN, Phillips PC, Molloy PT: Surgical management of medulloblastoma. J Neurooncol 29:9–21, 1996.

117. Cochrane DD, Gustavsson B, Poskitt KP, et al: The surgical and natural morbidity of aggressive resection for posterior fossa tumors in childhood. Pediatr Neurosurg 20:19–29, 1994.

118. Pollack IF, Polinko P, Albright AL, et al: Mutism and pseudobulbar symptoms after resection of posterior fossa tumors in children: Incidence and pathophysiology. Neurosurgery 37:885–893, 1995.

119. Wisoff JH, Epstein FJ: Pseudobulbar palsy after posterior fossa operation in children. Neurosurgery 15:707–709, 1984.

120. Bastian AJ, Mink JW, Kaufman BA, et al: Posterior vermal split syndrome. Ann Neurol 44:601–610, 1998.

121. Baram TZ, van Eys J, Dowell RE, et al: Survival and neurological outcome of infants with medulloblastoma treated with surgery and MOPP chemotherapy: A preliminary report. Cancer 60:173–177, 1987.

122. Duffner PK, Horowitz ME, Krischer JP, et al: Postoperative chemotherapy and delayed radiation in children less than three years of age with malignant brain tumors. N Engl J Med 328:1725–1731, 1993.

123. Packer RJ, Sutton LN, Goldwein JW, et al: Improved survival with the use of adjuvant chemotherapy in the treatment of medulloblastoma. J Neurosurg 74:433–440, 1991.

124. Tomita T, McLone DG: Medulloblastoma in childhood: Results of radical resection and low dose radiation therapy. J Neurosurg 64:238–242, 1986.

125. White L, Johnston H, Jones R, et al: Postoperative chemotherapy without radiation in young children with malignant non-astrocytic brain tumours: A report from the Australia and New Zealand Childhood Cancer Study Group (ANZCCSG). Cancer Chemother Pharmacol 32:403–406, 1993.

126. Jenkin D, Goddard K, Armstrong D, et al: Posterior fossa medulloblastoma in childhood: Treatment results and a proposal for a new staging system. Int J Radiat Oncol Biol Phys 19:265–274, 1990.

127. Caputy AJ, McCullough DC, Manz HJ, et al: A review of the factors influencing the prognosis of medulloblastoma: The importance of cell differentiation. J Neurosurg 66:80–87, 1987.

128. Coffin CM, Braun JT, Wick MR, et al: A clinicopathologic and immunohistochemical analysis of 53 cases of medulloblastoma with emphasis on synaptophysin expression. Mod Pathol 164–170, 1993.

129. Allen J, Epstein F: Medulloblastoma and other primary malignant neuroectodermal tumors of the CNS: The effect of patient's age and extent of disease on prognosis. J Neurosurg 57:446, 1982.

130. Chang CH, Houspian EM, Herbert C Jr: An operative staging system and megavoltage radiotherapeutic technique for cerebellar medulloblastoma. Radiology 93:1351–1359, 1969.

131. Laurent JP, Chang CH, Cohen ME: A classification system for primitive neuroectodermal tumors (medulloblastoma) of the posterior fossa. Cancer 56:1807–1809, 1985.

132. Harrison SK, Ditchfield MR, Waters K: Correlation of MRI and CSF cytology in the diagnosis of medulloblastoma spinal metastasis. Pediatr Radiol 28:571–574, 1998.

133. Massimino M, Gandola L, Cefalo G, et al: Management of medulloblastoma and ependymoma in infants: A single-institution long-term retrospective report. Childs Nerv Syst 16:15–20, 2000.

134. Zeltzer PM, Boyett JM, Finlay JL, et al: Metastasis stage, adjuvant treatment, and residual tumor are prognostic factors for medulloblastoma in children: Conclusions from the Children's Cancer Group 921 randomized phase III study. J Clin Oncol 17:832–845, 1999.

135. Woo C, Stea B, Lulu B, et al: The use of stereotactic radiosurgical boost in the treatment of medulloblastoma. Int J Radiat Oncol Biol Phys 37:761–764, 1997.

136. Tait DM, Thornton-Jones H, Bloom HJG, et al: Adjuvant chemotherapy for medulloblastomas: The first multi-centre control trial of the International Society of Pediatric Oncology (SIOP). Eur J Cancer 26:464–469, 1990.

137. Garton GR, Schomberg PJ, Scheithauer BW, et al: Medulloblastoma—prognostic factors and outcome of treatment: Review of the Mayo Clinic experience. Mayo Clin Proc 65:1077–1086, 1990.

138. Sutton LN, Packer RJ, Schut L: Medulloblastomas. Neurosurg Clin N Am 1-1:97–109, 1990.

139. Gajjar A, Kuhl J, Epelman S, et al: Chemotherapy of medulloblastoma. Childs Nerv Syst 15:554–562, 1999.

140. Zeltzer P, Boyett J, Finlay JL, et al: Tumor staging at diagnosis and therapy type for primitive neuroectodermal tumors (PNET) determine survival: Report from the Children's Cancer Group, CCG-921. p 238.

141. Hornback NB: Radiation therapy in treatment of medulloblastoma in childhood. In Zeltzer PM, Pochedly C (eds): Medulloblastoma in Children: New Concepts in Tumor Biology, Diagnosis, and Treatment. New York, Praeger, pp 164–181.

142. Prados MD, Wara W, Edwards MSB, et al: Treatment of high-risk medulloblastoma and other primitive neuroectodermal tumors with reduced dose craniospinal radiation therapy and multi-agent nitrosourea-based chemotherapy. Pediatr Neurosurg 25:174–181, 1996.

143. Jenkin D: The radiation treatment of medulloblastoma. J Neurooncol 29:45–54, 1996.

144. Wara WM, Le QT, Sneed PK, et al: Pattern of recurrence of medulloblastoma after low-dose craniospinal radiotherapy. Int J Radiat Oncol Biol Phys 30:551–556, 1994.

145. Prados MD, Edwards MSB, Chang SM, et al: Hyperfractionated craniospinal radiation therapy for primitive neuroectodermal tumors: Results of a phase II study. Int J Radiat Oncol Biol Phys 43:279–285, 1999.

146. Brand WN, Schneider PA, Tokars RP: Long-term results of a pilot study of low dose craniospinal irradiation for cerebellar medulloblastoma. Int J Radiat Oncol Biol Phys 13:1641–1645, 1987.

147. Halberg FE, Wara WM, Fippin LF, et al: Low dose craniospinal radiation therapy for medulloblastoma. Int J Radiat Oncol Biol Phys 20:651–654, 1991.

148. Levin VA, Rodriguez LA, Edwards MSB, et al: Treatment of medulloblastoma with procarbazine, hydroxyurea, and reduced radiation doses to whole brain and spine. J Neurosurg 68:383–387, 1988.

149. Deutsch M, Thomas PRM, Krischer J, et al: Results of a prospective randomized trial comparing standard dose neuraxis irradiation (3600 cGy/20) with reduced neuraxis irradiation (2340 cGy/13) in patients with low-stage medulloblastoma. Pediatr Neurosurg 24:167–177, 1996.

150. Thomas PM, Deutsch M, Kepner JL, et al: Low-stage medulloblastoma: Final analysis of trial comparing standard-dose with reduced-dose neuraxis irradiation. J Clin Oncol 18:3004–3011, 2001.

151. Bailey CC, Grekow A, Welleck S, et al: Prospective randomized trial of chemotherapy given before radiotherapy in childhood medulloblastoma. International Society of Paediatric Oncology (SIOP) and the (German) Society of Paediatric Oncology (GPO): SIOP II. Med Pediatr Oncol 25:166–178, 1995.

152. Patrice SJ, Tarbell NJ, Goumnerova LC, et al: Results of radiosurgery in the management of recurrent and residual medulloblastoma. Pediatr Neurosurg 22:197–203, 1995.

153. Krischer JP, Ragab AH, Kun L, et al: Nitrogen mustard, vincristine, procarbazine, and prednisone as adjuvant chemotherapy in the treatment of medulloblastoma: A Pediatric Oncology Group Study. J Neurosurg 74:905–909, 1991.

154. Kühl J, Müller HL, Berthold F, et al: Preradiation chemotherapy of children and young adults with malignant brain tumors:

Results of the German pilot trial HIT '88/'89. Klin Padiatr 210: 227–233, 1998.

155. Heideman RL, Kovnar EH, Kellie SJ, et al: Preirradiation chemotherapy with carboplatin and etoposide in newly diagnosed embryonal pediatric CNS tumors. J Clin Oncol 13:2247–2254, 1995.

156. Kovnar EH, Kellie SJ, Horowitz ME, et al: Preirradiation cisplatin and etoposide in the treatment of high-risk medulloblastoma and other malignant embryonal tumors of the central nervous system: A phase II study. J Clin Oncol 8:330–336, 1990.

157. Schell MJ, McHaney VA, Green AA, et al: Hearing loss in children and young adults receiving cisplatin with or without prior cranial irradiation. J Clin Oncol 7:754–760, 1989.

158. Gentet JC, Bouffet E, Doz E, et al: Preirradiation chemotherapy including "eight drugs in 1 day" regimen and high-dose methotrexate in childhood medulloblastoma: Results of the M7 French Cooperative Study. J Neurosurg 82:608–614, 1995.

159. Lopez-Aguilar E, Sepulveda-Vildosola AC, Rivera-Marquez H, et al: Survival of patients with medulloblastoma treated with carboplatin and etoposide before and after radiotherapy. Arch Med Res 29:313–317, 1998.

160. Hartsell WF, Gajjar A, Heideman RL, et al: Patterns of failure in children with medulloblastoma: Effects of preirradiation chemotherapy. Int J Radiat Oncol Biol Phys 39:15–24, 1997.

161. Gajjar A, Mulhern RK, Heideman RL, et al: Medulloblastoma in very young children: Outcome of definitive craniospinal irradiation following incomplete response to chemotherapy. J Clin Oncol 12:1212–1216, 1994.

162. Finlay JL, Goldman S, Wong MC, et al: Pilot study of high-dose thiotepa and etoposide with autologous bone marrow rescue in children and young adults with recurrent CNS tumors. J Clin Oncol 14:2495–2503, 1996.

163. Gururangan S, Dunkel IJ, Goldman S, et al: Myeloablative chemotherapy with autologous bone marrow rescue in young children with recurrent malignant brain tumors. J Clin Oncol 16: 2486–2493, 1998.

164. Graham ML, Herndon JE II, Casey JR, et al: High-dose chemotherapy with autologous stem cell rescue in patients with recurrent and high-risk pediatric brain tumors. J Clin Oncol 15: 1814–1823, 1997.

165. Kalifa C, Valteau D, Pizer B, et al: High-dose chemotherapy in childhood brain tumors. Childs Nerv Syst 15:498–505, 1999.

166. Dunkel IJ, Finlay JL: High dose chemotherapy with autologous stem cell rescue for patients with medulloblastoma. J Neurooncol 29:69–74, 1996.

167. Cohen BH, Packer RJ, Siegel KR, et al: Brain tumors in children under 2 years: Treatment, survival and long-term prognosis. Pediatr Neurosurg 19:171–179, 1993.

168. Saran FH, Driever PH, Thilmann C, et al: Survival of very young children with medulloblastoma (primitive neuroectodermal tumor of the posterior fossa) treated with craniospinal irradiation. Int J Radiat Oncol Biol Phys 42:959–967, 1998.

169. Geyer JR, Zeltzer PM, Boyett JM, et al: Survival of infants with primitive neuroepithelial tumors or malignant ependymomas of the CNS treated with eight drugs in 1 day: A report from the Children's Cancer Group. J Clin Oncol 12:1607–1615, 1994.

170. Di Rocco C, Ianelli A, Papacci F, et al: Prognosis of medulloblastoma in infants. Childs Nerv Syst 13:388–396, 1997.

171. Bouffet E, Bernard JL, Frappay D, et al: M4 protocol for cerebellar medulloblastoma: Supratentorial radiotherapy may not be avoided. Int J Radiat Oncol Biol Phys 24:79–85, 1992.

172. Kiltie AE, Lashford LS, Gattamaneni HR: Survival and late effects in medulloblastoma patients treated with craniospinal irradiation under three years old. Med Pediatr Oncol 28:348–354, 1997.

173. Schultheiss TE, Kun LE, Ang KK, et al: Radiation response of the central nervous system. Int J Radiat Oncol Biol Phys 31: 1093–1112, 1995.

174. Jackacki RI, Goldwein JW, Larsen RL, et al: Cardiac dysfunction following spinal irradiation during childhood. J Clin Oncol 11: 1033–1038, 1993.

175. Jackacki RI, Schramm CM, Donahue BR, et al: Restrictive lung disease following treatment for malignant brain tumors: A potential late effect of cranial irradiation. J Clin Oncol 13:1478–1485, 1995.

176. Hirsch JF, Renier D, Czernickow P, et al: Medulloblastoma in childhood: Survival and functional results. Acta Neurochir (Wien) 48:1–15, 1978.

177. Glauser TT, Packer RJ: Cognitive deficits in long-term survivors of childhood brain tumors. Childs Nerv Syst 7:2–12, 1991.

178. Duffner PK, Cohen ME, Thomas P: Late effects of treatment on the intelligence of children with posterior fossa tumors. Cancer 51:233–237, 1983.

179. Johnson DL, McCabe MA, Nicholson HS, et al: Quality of long-term survival in young children with medulloblastoma. J Neurosurg 80:1004–1010, 1994.

180. Kimmings E, Kleinlugtebeld AT, Casey A, et al: Medulloblastoma: Factors influencing the educational potential of surviving children. Br J Neurosurg 9:611–617, 1995.

181. Jenkin D, Danjoux C, Greenberg M: Subsequent quality of life for children irradiated for a brain tumor before age four years. Med Pediatr Oncol 31:506–511, 1998.

182. Mulhern RK, Kepner JL, Thomas PR, et al: Neuropsychologic functioning of survivors of childhood medulloblastoma randomized to receive conventional or reduced-dose craniospinal irradiation: A Pediatric Oncology Group study. J Clin Oncol 16: 1723–1728, 1998.

183. Packer RJ, Sutton LN, Atkins TE, et al: A prospective study of cognitive function in children receiving whole brain radiotherapy and chemotherapy: 2-year results. J Neurosurg 70:707–713, 1989.

184. Radcliffe J, Atkins TE, Packer RJ, et al: A prospective study of cognitive function in children with medulloblastoma receiving whole-brain radiotherapy and chemotherapy: 3- and 4-year results. 15. p 146.

185. Radcliffe J, Bunin GR, Sutton LN, et al: Cognitive deficits in long-term survivors of childhood medulloblastoma and other noncortical tumors: Age-dependent effects of whole brain radiation. Int J Dev Neurosci 12:327–334, 1994.

186. Suc E, Kalifa C, Brauner R, et al: Brain tumors under the age of three: The price of survival. Acta Neurochir (Wien) 106: 93–98, 1990.

187. Chin HW, Maruyama Y: Age at treatment and long-term performance results in medulloblastoma. Cancer 53:1952–1958, 1984.

188. Yang TF, Wong TT, Cheng LY, et al: Neuropsychological sequelae after treatment for medulloblastoma in childhood—the Taiwan experience. Childs Nerv Syst 13:77–81, 1997.

189. Dennis M, Spiegler BJ, Hetherington CR, et al: Neuropsychological sequelae of the treatment of children with medulloblastoma. J Neurooncol 29:91–101, 1996.

190. Packer RJ, Sutton LN, Elterman R, et al: Outcome for children with medulloblastoma treated with radiation and cisplatin, CCNU, and vincristine chemotherapy. J Neurosurg 81:690–698, 1994.

191. Carlson-Green B, Morris RD, Krawiecki N: Family and illness predictors of outcome in pediatric brain tumors. J Pediatr Psychol 20:769–784, 1995.

192. Bordeaux JD, Dowell RE, Copeland DR, et al: A prospective study of neuropsychological sequelae in children with brain tumors. J Child Neurol 3:63–68, 1988.

193. Seaver E, Geyer R, Sulzbacher S, et al: Psychosocial adjustment in long-term survivors of childhood medulloblastoma and ependymoma treated with craniospinal irradiation. Pediatr Neurosurg 20:248–253, 1994.

194. Hoppe-Hirsch E, Brunet L, Laroussinie F, et al: Intellectual outcome in children with malignant tumors of the posterior fossa: Influence of the field of radiation and quality of surgery. Childs Nerv Syst 11:340–345, 1995.

195. Clayton PE, Shalet SM: Dose dependency of time of onset of radiation-induced growth hormone deficiency. J Pediatr 118: 226–228, 1991.

196. Shalet SM, Gibson B, Swindell R, et al: Effect of spinal irradiation on growth. Arch Dis Child 62:461–464, 1987.

197. Rappaport R, Brauner R: Growth and endocrine disorders secondary to cranial irradiation. Pediatr Res 25:561–567, 1989.

198. Heikens J, Michiels EMC, Behrendt H, et al: Long-term neuroendocrine sequelae after treatment for childhood medulloblastoma. Eur J Cancer 34:1592–1597, 1998.

199. Ogilvy-Stuart AL, Shalet SM: Growth and puberty after growth hormone treatment after irradiation for brain tumors. Arch Dis Child 73:141–146, 1995.

200. Olsham JS, Gubernick J, Packer RJ, et al: The effects of adjuvant chemotherapy on growth in children with medulloblastoma. Cancer 70:2013–2017, 1992.

201. Ogilvy-Stuart AL, Clayton PE, Shalet SM: Cranial irradiation and early puberty. J Clin Endocrinol Metab 78:1286–1296, 1994.

202. Clayton PE, Shalet SM, Gattamaneni HR, et al: Does growth hormone cause relapse of brain tumours? Lancet 1:711–713, 1987.

203. O'Driscoll BR, Hasleton PS, Taylor PM, et al: Active lung fibrosis up to 17 years after chemotherapy with carmustine (BCNU) in childhood. N Engl J Med 322:378–382, 1990.

204. Goldstein AM, Yuen J, Tucker MA: Second cancers after medulloblastoma: Population-based results from the United States and Sweden. Cancer Causes Control 8:865–871, 1997.

205. Blatt J, Penchansky L, Phebus C, et al: Leukemia in a child with a history of medulloblastoma. Pediatr Hematol Oncol 8:77–82, 1991.

206. Bloom HJG, Wallace ENK, Henk JM: The treatment and prognosis of medulloblastoma in children: A study of 82 verified cases. AJR Am J Roentgenol 105:43–62, 1969.

207. Latchaw JP, Hahn J, Moylan DJ, et al: Medulloblastoma: Period of risk reviewed. Cancer 55:186–189, 1985.

208. Tarbell NJ, Loeffler JS, Silver B, et al: The change in patterns of relapse in medulloblastoma. Cancer 68:1600–1604, 1991.

209. Rollins N, Mendelsohn D, Mulne A, et al: Recurrent medulloblastoma: Frequency of tumor enhancement on Gd-DTPA MR imaging. AJNR Am J Neuroradiol 11:583–587, 1990.

210. Kleinman GM, Hochberg FH, Richardson EP Jr: Systemic metastases from medulloblastoma: Report of two cases and review of the literature. Cancer 48:2296–2309, 1981.

211. Tomita T, Das L, Radkowski MA: Bone metastases of medulloblastoma in childhood: Correlation with flow cytometric DNA analysis. J Neurooncol 8:113–120, 1990.

212. Algra PR, Postma T, Van Groeningen CJ, et al: MR imaging of skeletal metastases from medulloblastoma. Skeletal Radiol 21:425–430, 1992.

213. Wara WM, Wallner KE, Levin VA, et al: Retreatment of pediatric brain tumors with radiation and misonidazole: Results of CCSG/RTOG phase I/II study. Cancer 58:1636–1640, 1986.

214. Mahoney DH, Strother D, Camitta B, et al: High-dose melphalan and cyclophosphamide with autologous bone marrow rescue for recurrent/progressive malignant brain tumors in children: A pilot Pediatric Oncology Group study. Clin Oncol 14:382–388, 1996.

215. Dunkel IJ, Boyett JM, Yates A, et al: High dose carboplatin, thiotepa, and etoposide with autologous stem-cell rescue for patients with recurrent medulloblastoma. J Clin Oncol 16:222–228, 1998.

Cerebellar Astrocytomas in Children

JEFFREY W. CAMPBELL ■ R. MICHAEL SCOTT

Cerebellar astrocytomas are one of the most common pediatric brain tumors, constituting roughly 10% to 20% of intracranial tumors in children.[1] These tumors are notable not only for their prevalence but also for their unusually favorable prognosis in most patients.[2-7] Because of the relatively high incidence of these tumors, a tremendous body of literature exists regarding treatment, outcome, and prognostic factors, starting with Cushing's first report in 1931.[8] In four articles from 1986 and 1987, Ilgren and Stiller[7, 9-11] summarized the results of 40 major series published between 1926 and 1984, encompassing 2916 cases. Since that time, at least 23 major series have been published, describing an additional 1686 cases.[3-6, 12-30] Although certain aspects of management are clear, such as the benefit of complete surgical resection, there remains some disagreement regarding other aspects of these tumors, such as the prognostic role of histology and the benefits of postoperative radiotherapy. This chapter outlines the patient demographics, symptoms, imaging, histology, and treatment options for patients with cerebellar astrocytomas, with particular emphasis on prognostic factors.

PATIENT DEMOGRAPHICS

Age

Roughly 70% of cerebellar astrocytomas are diagnosed in children,[11] although a bimodal distribution has been described, with the second peak around the seventh decade of life.[23] The mean age of presentation in series that include patients of all ages is approximately 14 years,[6, 11, 13, 31] whereas in series that include only children, the mean age is 7 years.[3, 11-13, 15, 18, 25, 27] Children have a more favorable prognosis than their adult counterparts,[3, 6, 11, 13, 21] although patients younger than 5 years may do worse than older children.[18] This variation in prognosis likely results from differences in tumor biology,[6] with a greater incidence of malignant histology reported in adult patients.[10, 23]

Gender

The incidence of cerebellar astrocytomas is equal by gender.[3, 11, 13, 15, 30] Although a drop in tumor incidence for females around puberty has been reported,[11] most series have not confirmed this association. No series has found an association between prognosis and gender.[32]

PRESENTATION

Clinical Findings

The average duration of symptoms before diagnosis has fallen from 18.7 months reported by Ilgren and Stiller[11] to a mean of 5 months.[12, 23, 26, 32] Presenting symptoms and signs (Table 235–1), including headache, vomiting, and papilledema, are usually consistent with increased intracranial pressure from fourth ventricular compression and subsequent hydrocephalus. Gait disturbance and diplopia are also common, whether from increased intracranial pressure or direct compression of the cerebellum and brainstem, which can also lead to a variety of cranial neuropathies and motor system dysfunction. Some patients present with more subtle symptoms such as neck pain (perhaps due to cerebellar tonsillar herniation through the foramen magnum) or behavioral changes from hydrocephalus; others may present dramatically with coma or major brainstem dysfunction with respiratory failure and circulatory collapse. Hydrocephalus is evident at presentation in 60% to 93% of children.[23, 25, 28] Prognosis is not significantly affected by duration of symptoms, although patients with direct invasion of the brainstem, who are more likely to present cranial neuropathies or hemiparesis, appear to do worse.[11, 17, 26, 33, 34]

Imaging Findings

Computed tomographic scans typically reveal a tumor that is iso- or hypodense to the surrounding brain, with most solid portions of the tumor enhancing after intravenous contrast is given.[23, 35, 36] Foci of calcification are seen in 10% to 20% of cases, and cysts are present in approximately 70% to 85% of tumors. The cysts can be quite large, complex, or multiloculated, leading to considerable compression of adjacent cerebellum, brainstem, and fourth ventricle. The cyst walls rarely enhance, and many authorities consider them a reac-

T A B L E 2 3 5 – 1 ■ **Presenting Symptoms and Signs of Cerebellar Astrocytomas**

AUTHOR	NO. CASES	SYMPTOMS (%)			SIGNS (%)		
		Headache	Vomiting	Gait Disturbance	Papilledema	Ataxia	Cranial Nerve Palsy
Pencalet et al (1999)[25]	168	77	74	69	69	46	29
Sgouros et al (1995)[26]	97	85	84	79	88	89	39
Abdollahzadeh et al (1994)[12]	66	82	65	63	77	74	
Garcia et al (1989)[3]	84	82	81	—	86	82	37
Ilgren & Stiller (1987)[11]	112	76	—	—	—	86	—

tive, non-neoplastic component of the tumor[26]; some believe that enhancement of the cyst wall suggests neoplasia and the need for resection. The cyst volume may dwarf the solid portion of the tumor on or within the cyst wall—the so-called mural nodule.[35, 36]

Magnetic resonance imaging (MRI) likewise reveals a tumor that is hypo- or isointense to the surrounding brain on T1-weighted images and hyperintense to brain on T2-weighted images. Once again, the majority of these tumors enhance with intravenous gadolinium, in a pattern similar to that seen on computed tomography (Fig. 235–1). Magnetic resonance spectroscopy reveals characteristics typical for other brain tumors, with a decrease in both the ratio between *N*-acetyl-aspartate and choline and the ratio between creatine and choline; compared with more malignant tumors, however, the *N*-acetyl-aspartate–choline ratio is relatively closer to normal.[37]

TUMOR CHARACTERISTICS

Location

Although most studies report that the primary site of tumor is equally distributed between the vermis and the cerebellar hemispheres,[5, 11, 23, 26] some authors note a prevalence of vermian lesions.[25] Solid tumors are more frequently located in the vermis, and cystic tumors have a slight predilection for the hemispheres.[9, 26] Most tumors that invade the brainstem are solid[25, 26] and usually arise from the cerebellar hemispheres or cerebellar peduncles, although vermian lesions can invade the stem along the anterior medullary velum and then into the dorsal midbrain. Up to 40% of tumors invade the brainstem,[26] resulting in a worse prognosis in terms of survival and functional status[25]; however, this may be due to the difficulty of achieving complete excision of these lesions.[6, 11, 32]

Histology

The histologic classification of these tumors and the prognostic significance of histology remain somewhat controversial. Several classification systems for cerebellar astrocytomas have been reported in the literature, and the most widely cited systems divide astrocytomas into pilocytic and fibrillary cell types. Pilocytic tumors are described as biphasic, with compact bipolar cells

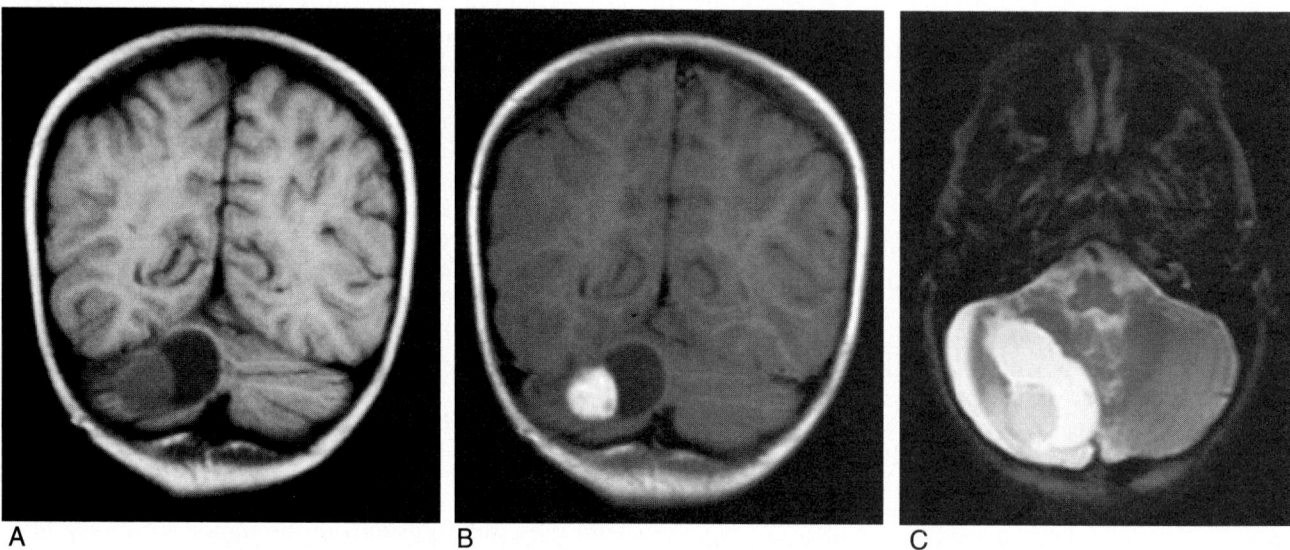

FIGURE 235–1. Magnetic resonance imaging scans of juvenile pilocytic astrocytoma. *A* and *B*, These T1-weighted coronal images reveal a contrast-enhancing mural nodule associated with a large cyst. The fluid within the cyst has imaging characteristics similar to those of cerebrospinal fluid, and the solid tumor is hypointense to brain before the infusion of gadolinium *(A)*. The mural nodule displays significant homogeneous enhancement after contrast *(B)*. *C*, This T2-weighted axial image of the same tumor demonstrates that the imaging characteristics of the fluid within the cyst are similar to those of cerebrospinal fluid. The solid portion of the tumor is hyperintense to normal brain.

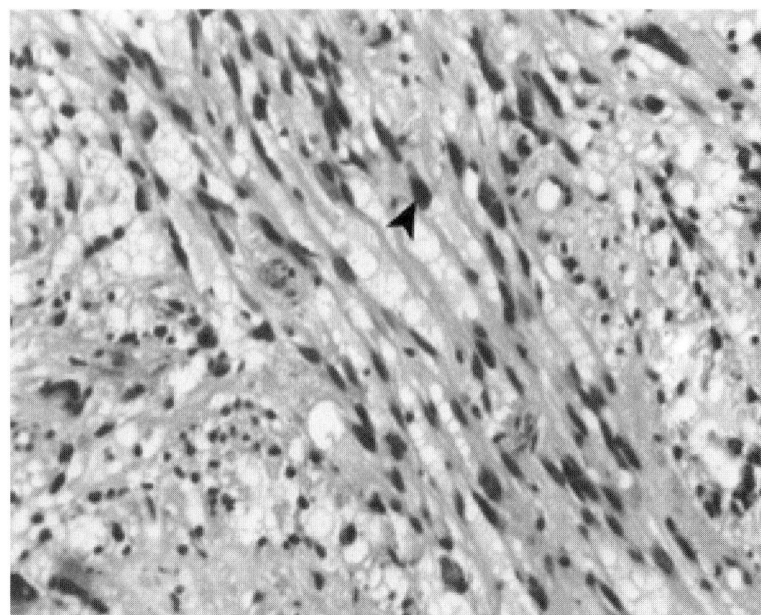

FIGURE 235–2. Juvenile pilocytic astrocytoma. This lesion demonstrates the characteristic biphasic pattern, consisting of regions of compact bipolar cells associated with Rosenthal fibers *(arrowhead)* interposed in areas of loose astrocytes and granular bodies (hematoxylin-eosin, ×200).

associated with Rosenthal fibers interposed in areas of loose astrocytes associated with granular bodies (Fig. 235–2). These tumors constitute roughly 80% to 85% of cerebellar astrocytomas[6, 24, 38] and are generally well circumscribed, although as many as 14% may invade into surrounding tissues.[6] Diffuse or fibrillary-type astrocytomas are histologically identical to astrocytomas found elsewhere within the central nervous system and often display invasion into surrounding parenchyma (Fig. 235–3).[6, 24] These constitute the remaining 15% to 20% of cerebellar astrocytomas.[6, 24] A small number of diffuse cerebellar astrocytomas closely resemble high-grade lesions (anaplastic astrocytoma or glioblastoma multiforme) seen supratentorially. In most reports, these constitute less than 2% of all cere-

bellar astrocytomas, and only 5% of high-grade astrocytomas are found in the cerebellum.[8, 10, 24] Their biologic behavior is similar to that of high-grade astrocytomas found elsewhere in the brain, with a very poor prognosis for long-term survival.[39] The World Health Organization classification system recognizes four types of astrocytomas: juvenile pilocytic, low grade, anaplastic, and glioblastoma multiforme.

It is controversial whether the distinction between a juvenile pilocytic astrocytoma and a low-grade astrocytoma is of clinical significance. Tumors often display characteristics of both variants, leading to difficulty in classification.[9, 24] The relative paucity of fibrillary astrocytomas, along with the overwhelming confounding effect of the degree of resection, has led to consider-

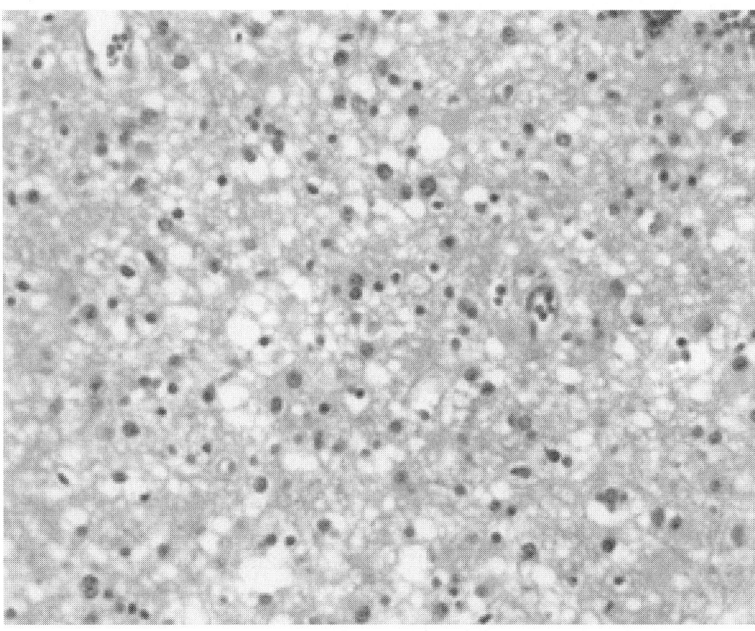

FIGURE 235–3. Astrocytoma. Low-grade astrocytomas display hypercellularity with moderate nuclear pleomorphism. Rarely do cerebellar astrocytomas in children have histologic indications of malignancy, such as significant mitoses, endothelial cell hyperplasia, or areas of necrosis (hematoxylin-eosin, ×200).

able disagreement in the literature. Some studies showed that both pilocytic and fibrillary astrocytomas have similar prognoses,[9, 18, 33, 40, 41] and others found that fibrillary tumors are more likely to progress.[6, 23, 26, 32] In a series of 72 patients from the Children's Hospital of Pittsburgh, histology was an independent predictor of progression-free survival (PFS) and total survival in children with incomplete resection of their tumors, although children with complete resection did uniformly well, regardless of histology (unpublished data).

In fibrillary astrocytomas, anaplasia consisting of hypercellularity, necrosis, calcifications, mitotic figures, and nuclear pleomorphism strongly correlates with poorer survival.[10, 24, 42] A similar association is not seen with pilocytic astrocytomas; in patients with these tumors, long-term PFS is often seen despite an atypical or malignant histology.[43] Some studies report improved prognosis with microcystic changes and endothelial hyperplasia when found in conjunction with perivascular pseudorosettes and vascular hyperplasia.[9, 42] There is little agreement as to the significance of hypercellularity, calcification, Rosenthal fibers, hemosiderin, endothelial cell proliferation, perivascular pseudorosettes, and areas of oligodendroglial differentiation when each is found in isolation.[9, 10, 14] Investigators have looked at molecular markers of growth potential, such as silver-binding nucleolar organizer regions, which seems to correlate with progression of residual tumors.[41]

TREATMENT

Surgical Resection

TECHNIQUE

The primary treatment of cerebellar astrocytomas is surgical excision, with significant improvement in prognosis when a gross total resection is achieved.[23, 26, 28, 32] This goal is possible with nearly all tumors that do not overtly invade the parenchyma of the brainstem or cerebellar peduncle. An additional consideration during resection is minimizing trauma to normal cerebellum, which should decrease the incidence of postoperative complications. Mutism, which occurs in as many as 30% of cerebellar tumor resections,[44] is thought to be secondary to edema into the deep cerebellar nuclei and may be related to the degree of manipulation of the vermis.[31, 45]

During surgery, the patient should be positioned prone, with consideration of nasotracheal intubation to minimize the chance of intraoperative extubation and to maximize neck flexion, particularly if exposure high beneath the tentorium will be required. All patients must have adequate intravenous access, and many centers place central venous lines in case an intraoperative air embolus is detected. In addition, patients should have a Foley catheter, which aids in the detection of hypovolemia, and a precordial Doppler, which allows for early detection of air embolism. In patients with hydrocephalus, either a ventriculostomy should be placed preoperatively or the operative field should be wide enough to provide access for intraoperative placement of a ventriculostomy if required. If the patient has a ventriculostomy, care must be taken to avoid overdrainage of cerebrospinal fluid and subsequent upward herniation before tumor resection.

We advocate a standard midline approach to all these lesions, even when the tumor is located entirely within one hemisphere of the cerebellum. Identification and protection of the brainstem are paramount, and this approach allows clear identification of midline structures, including the floor of the fourth ventricle. The patient is placed prone on rolls, with adequate padding of all pressure points. The head is held securely in rigid skeletal fixation, if possible, and positioned with no rotation in a military "sniffing" position, consisting of flexion at the craniospinal junction and a relatively straight midcervical spine. The degree of neck flexion should allow easy access to the upper cervical spine without compromising venous outflow through the jugular veins. The head of the operating table is elevated until the patient's head is parallel to or just above the heart, which decreases venous pressure within the sinuses and provides a flat operative site.

A midline incision is made from the spinous process of C2 to above the inion. The fascia is likewise opened in the midline, although the occipital musculature can be "T'd" below its nuchal attachment to facilitate a watertight and physiologic muscle closure. The muscle is opened in the midline avascular plane and dissected off the occipital bone with either electrocautery or periosteal instruments; because the periosteum and underlying skull in the pediatric population are often quite vascular, we prefer to use electrocautery here. The caudal dissection should expose the posterior ring of C1 to ensure adequate visualization of the inferior cerebellum when the retractors are placed. The craniotomy should extend from the foramen magnum to the transverse sinus, with the lateral extent on each side of midline dependent on the location of the tumor. The dura of the posterior fossa is opened in a Y fashion by first opening over each hemisphere and then carefully connecting across the occipital sinus. The dura can be extremely vascular in children because of large midline and paramedian venous sinuses within its leaves, and opening the dura over the hemispheres of the cerebellum first facilitates the control of these venous sinuses. It is important to anticipate their presence and to be ready to clip or suture-ligate these structures when they are encountered to avoid rapid loss of blood.

If there is considerable normal tissue displacement from tumor mass, the cyst can be tapped with a ventricular catheter or needle either before or after opening the dura. The tumor should be removed by establishing a plane of dissection between the tumor and the cerebellum, a maneuver often facilitated by entering the cyst cavity, identifying the tumor nodule, and dissecting it away from surrounding normal brain. Cerebellar astrocytomas are easy to differentiate from the surrounding brain because of their reddish brown or gray color, which contrasts with the pure white of the surrounding cerebellar white matter. Areas of gliosis around tumors can create some difficulty in identifying dissection planes. It is usually in these areas or in corners of the tumor that are difficult to visualize, such as the high vermis or anterolateral cerebellum, that tumor is inadvertently left behind. If the tumor lies beneath the vermis, care should be taken to minimize dissection of normal parenchyma superior and deep in the midline, in order to avoid damage to the dentate and other midline cerebellar nuclear groups, which could result in prolonged postoperative truncal ataxia or, occasionally, cerebellar mutism. If the tumor projects into the fourth ventricle, the vermis can be extensively elevated by dividing the tela choroidea that connects the choroid plexus in the roof of the fourth ventricle to its blood supply from the posterior inferior cerebellar artery, providing wide exposure of the fourth ventricle. The floor of the fourth ventricle is an important landmark to establish early in the procedure, and it should be protected with a cottonoid patty to prevent efflux of blood into the aqueduct and to protect the brainstem from inadvertent manipulation or entrance during tumor removal.

Some controversy exists with regard to the handling of cyst walls. Various authors advocate resection of cyst walls that enhance with contrast,[14] resection based on frozen sections of the cyst wall,[14] resection of macroscopically abnormal tissue,[25] or leaving the cyst wall alone.[26] In the vast majority of cases, it is safe to consider nonenhancing cyst walls as nonneoplastic.

Tumors that are mainly solid can be dissected in a variety of ways, depending on their consistency. Because many of these tumors are gelatinous and difficult to grasp without disrupting them, we frequently use a technique involving some degree of internal decompression to reduce tumor bulk. We then use broad dissectors to develop the plane of dissection around the outside of the tumor while displacing it inward away from normal tissue, using bipolar coagulation to deal with vessels supplying the tumor. Most of these operations are carried out with the microscope positioned so that the surgeon and the assistant are positioned opposite each other, with each having a binocular view of the dissection. The surgeon can develop the plane around the tumor using dissectors and the repositioning of self-retaining retractors, and the assistant can maintain hemostasis. Occasionally, nodules of tumor embed themselves into the lateral brainstem or deep into a cerebellar peduncle, and a technique of circumferential dissection could injure structures on the ventricular floor or brainstem. In this circumstance, an ultrasonic aspirator can remove tumor residua. We have also found that an yttrium-aluminum-garnet contact laser dissector can be used to great advantage to dissect and vaporize tumor in eloquent locations.

At the completion of the procedure, we close the dura watertight, with the aid of a dural graft if needed. When closure takes place, we often remove any clips previously placed on sinuses that were clip-ligated, oversewing the sinuses with 4–0 sutures as the clips are removed; this maneuver aids in obtaining watertight suture margins. It is our practice, as it is in other pediatric centers, to replace the bone flap before skin closure, using 2–0 or 3–0 absorbable suture in very small children and miniplates in children with bone thick enough to accept the instrumentation. The more solid fixation afforded by the miniplates accelerates bone healing and also probably reduces the incidence of cerebrospinal fluid accumulations in the subcutaneous space, because the dural closure is buttressed by the repositioned bone flap.

COMPLICATIONS

The rate of significant morbidity varies from 5% to 20% in several reports (Table 235–2), with few cases of surgical mortality.[1, 16, 25, 26] The likelihood of new postoperative neurological deficits is small but strongly depends on the location of the tumor and its adherence to the brainstem and cranial nerves. One of the more common postoperative complications is a pseudomeningocele at the site of closure, sometimes associated with a transcutaneous cerebrospinal fluid fistula. Preoperative ventricular dilatation significantly increases the risk of a postoperative pseudomeningocele, which can often be avoided with several days of postoperative drainage through a ventriculostomy. Intermittent measurement of intracranial pressure is often helpful in determining the need for a permanent shunt. Another particularly disturbing complication, previously mentioned, is mutism, which can develop anytime in the first several postoperative days and tends to resolve within several months.[25] As with any craniotomy for tumor resection, postoperative bleeding can occur within the resection bed, and subdural bleeding or cerebrospinal fluid hygromas can develop if ventricular decompression occurs rapidly during or after the procedure. Aseptic meningitis, a syndrome that results in fever, headache, and stiff neck following posterior fossa surgery in the pediatric age group, can also be seen; it frequently responds to high-dose steroid administration.

OUTCOME

As mentioned previously, prognosis is strongly influenced by the extent of resection. In reports before 1985, 10-year survival rates for patients with gross total re-

T A B L E 2 3 5 – 2 ■ **Operative Complications (%)**

AUTHOR	MORTALITY	HEMIPARESIS	CRANIAL NERVE PALSY	PSEUDO-MENINGOCELE	HEMATOMA	INFECTION	ASEPTIC MENINGITIS	MUTISM
Abdollahzadeh et al (1994)[12]	0	1.5	4.5	24	7.5	6	4.5	1.5
Dirven et al (1997)[16]	1.4	5.5	5.5	—	1.4	—	—	—
Pencalet et al (1999)[25]	1.2	—	—	—	—	—	—	6
Sgouros et al (1995)[26]	7.2	—	5	7	—	8	—	—

section of tumor ranged from 52% to 100%.[7] More recent reports indicate survival of more than 88% at 10 years after gross total resection,[4, 13, 16, 19, 20, 26, 30, 42, 46] and several series in the microsurgical era demonstrate 100% PFS after gross total resection, with up to 20 years of follow-up.[12, 19, 30] Extent of resection should be based on postoperative MRI when possible, because surgeons are notoriously inaccurate in judging the degree of resection, with up to a 30% error rate when compared to postoperative imaging.[16] We recommend postoperative imaging within 48 to 72 hours to detect the presence of any residual tumor. To simplify the MRI interpretation, we limit the use of Gelfoam and other hemostatic agents in the resection bed, which reduces the number of postoperative artifacts on the study. Suspected residual tumor can be managed by an early return to the operating room, if the area of concern was suspicious to the surgeon during the operation, or by sequential observation with MRI. With tumors that are small, solid, and poorly differentiated from surrounding cerebellum, we occasionally use intraoperative MRI to remove tumor residua from areas where visual guidance or other image-guided techniques do not provide enough information to effect tumor removal at a second procedure.

When gross total resection would result in unacceptable morbidity, such as in cases of diffuse infiltration of the brainstem or leptomeningeal spread,[47, 48] subtotal resection should be considered if the mass effect of the tumor can be safely reduced. In one series, the volume of residual tumor correlated with PFS, highlighting the need for appropriate surgical debulking.[32] The 5- and 10-year PFS reported before 1985 in patients with subtotal resection is between 29% and 46% and 17% and 32%, respectively.[7] Most recurrences are amenable to re-exploration and resection, so overall survival is as high as 60% at 10 years in these reports. More recent series report similar results, with 10-year PFS of 0% to 79% and overall survival of 59% to 86%.[4, 12, 13, 15, 19, 30]

Radiation Therapy

Given the results achieved with surgery, radiation therapy is not indicated after gross total resection of benign tumors,[12, 14] although high-grade lesions progress similarly to supratentorial tumors[10] and require postoperative irradiation, chemotherapy, or both, regardless of the extent of resection. The efficacy of postoperative irradiation after subtotal resection remains controversial. Most published series treat all patients alike with regard to irradiation, making it impossible to determine its effect on PFS or total survival in the absence of an appropriate control group. Several series that reported on patients both with and without postoperative irradiation did not demonstrate an improvement in survival,[3, 4, 7, 20, 32, 34, 42, 46] although one report suggested a slight improvement in PFS.[4] In addition, malignant degeneration of benign tumors, including juvenile pilocytic astrocytomas, has been reported in at least 13 patients, 11 of whom received postoperative irradiation.[25, 43, 49–51] Given the questionable efficacy of radiation therapy after subtotal resection and its possible deleterious effects on the developing nervous system, most centers do not routinely recommend traditional radiation therapy. Some centers have described the use of radiosurgery for both residual and recurrent astrocytomas, although the data are still sparse. As with all treatments of an inherently benign process, decades of follow-up will be required to fully assess the efficacy of radiosurgery in these lesions and to evaluate the incidence of secondary radiation-induced tumors in this population.

FOLLOW-UP

These tumors do not strictly follow Collins' law, which states that recurrences should occur within a period equal to the patient's age at diagnosis plus 9 months.[14] Recurrences appear to occur steadily during follow-up, as highlighted by one series that reported progression of disease in 26% of patients during the first 10 years of follow-up, and progression in an additional 33% during the next 10 years of follow-up.[30] Cerebellar astrocytomas are reported to recur as long as 39 years after initial resection,[14, 51, 52] making it difficult to declare a patient free from risk of recurrence at any particular time following treatment. Benign tumors may recur with malignant degeneration, and juvenile pilocytic astrocytomas can recur with leptomeningeal dissemination, despite benign histology.[53]

Long-term survival with residual tumor is surprisingly common,[5, 40] and some authors report that up to 25% of residual tumors undergo spontaneous involution.[32] Geissinger and Bucy[54] reported that 60% of patients who underwent subtotal resection had no progression of tumor, and five of these patients were followed more than 25 years after initial resection. It is unclear why these tumors remain quiescent for extended periods, but it may result from alterations in blood supply during partial resection.[7] Many of these reports also come from periods when sophisticated imaging technologies were not available.

CONCLUSION

Benign cerebellar astrocytomas have a better prognosis than do most other central nervous system tumors, although high-grade cerebellar astrocytomas are aggressive lesions that result in poor survival despite aggressive surgical resection and full adjuvant therapy. Gross total resection of benign lesions provides a high likelihood of long-term PFS. When postoperative imaging studies reveal residual tumor, the surgeon should consider immediate re-exploration if the entire residual is surgically accessible. If residual tumor remains, some authors suggest the use of conventional radiation therapy or radiosurgery, although to date, neither has demonstrated a significant effect on prognosis. In addition, radiation may increase the risk of malignant transformation of a previously benign process and lead to the development of secondary tumors elsewhere in the calvarium. We believe that these tumors should never be radiated unless unresectable growth makes treatment mandatory. Long-term PFS is common after subtotal resection alone, and some centers have noted spontaneous involution of residual tumor. We currently reserve radiation for patients with recurrent tumors that are not amenable to surgical resection or tumors that recur despite multiple gross total resections. Because of the risk of late recurrences, patients should be followed for many years; however, recurrences of tumors that have been totally resected as demonstrated by MRI after 10 years' follow-up are extremely rare.

REFERENCES

1. Larson D, Wara W, Edwards M, et al: Management of childhood cerebellar astrocytoma. Int J Radiat Oncol Biol Phys 18:971–973, 1990.
2. Fulchiero A, Winston K, Leviton A, et al: Secular trends of cerebellar gliomas in children. J Natl Cancer Inst 58:839–843, 1977.
3. Garcia D, Latifi H, Simpson J, et al: Astrocytomas of the cerebellum in children. J Neurosurg 71:661–664, 1989.
4. Garcia D, Marks J, Latifi H, et al: Childhood cerebellar astrocytomas: Is there a role for postoperative irradiation? Int J Radiat Oncol Biol Phys 18:815–818, 1990.
5. Gjerris F, Klinken L: Long-term prognosis in children with benign cerebellar astrocytoma. J Neurosurg 49:179–184, 1978.
6. Hayostek C, Shaw E, Scheithauer B, et al: Astrocytomas of the cerebellum: A comparative clinicopathologic study of pilocytic and diffuse astrocytomas. Cancer 72:856–869, 1993.
7. Ilgren E, Stiller C: Cerebellar astrocytomas: Therapeutic management. Acta Neurochir (Wien) 81:11–26, 1986.
8. Cushing H: Experiences with the cerebellar astrocytomas. Surg Gynecol Obstet 52:129–205, 1931.
9. Ilgren E, Stiller C: Cerebellar astrocytomas. Part I. Macroscopic and microscopic features. Clin Neuropathol 6:185–200, 1987.
10. Ilgren E, Stiller C: Cerebellar astrocytomas. Part II. Pathologic features indicative of malignancy. Clin Neuropathol 6:201–214, 1987.
11. Ilgren E, Stiller C: Cerebellar astrocytomas. J Neurooncol 4:293–308, 1987.
12. Abdollahzadeh M, Hoffman H, Blazer S, et al: Benign cerebellar astrocytoma in childhood: Experience at the Hospital for Sick Children 1980–1992. Childs Nerv Syst 10:380–383, 1994.
13. Akyol F, Atahan I, Zorlu F, et al: Results of post-operative or exclusive radiotherapy in grade I and grade II cerebellar astrocytoma patients. Radiother Oncol 23:245–248, 1992.
14. Austin E, Alvord E: Recurrences of cerebellar astrocytomas: A violation of Collins' law. J Neurosurg 68:41–47, 1988.
15. Conway P, Oechler H, Kun L, et al: Importance of histologic condition and treatment of pediatric cerebellar astrocytoma. Cancer 67:2772–2775, 1991.
16. Dirven C, Mooij J, Molenaar W, et al: Cerebellar pilocytic astrocytoma: A treatment protocol based upon analysis of 73 cases and a review of the literature. Childs Nerv Syst 13:17–23, 1997.
17. Ferbert A, Gullotta F: Remarks on the follow-up of cerebellar astrocytomas. J Neurol 232:134–136, 1985.
18. Gajjar A, Sanford R, Heideman R, et al: Low-grade astrocytoma: A decade of experience at St. Jude Children's Research Hospital. J Clin Oncol 15:2792–2799, 1997.
19. Heiskanen O, Lehtosalo J: Surgery of cerebellar astrocytomas, ependymomas and medulloblastomas in children. Acta Neurochir (Wien) 78:1–3, 1985.
20. Kehler U, Arnold H, Muller H, et al: Long-term follow-up of infratentorial pilocytic astrocytomas. Neurosurg Rev 13:315–320, 1990.
21. Laws E, Bergstrath E, Taylor W, et al: Cerebellar astrocytomas in children. Prog Exp Tumor Res 30:122–127, 1987.
22. Mandigers C, Lippens R, Hoogenhout J, et al: Astrocytoma in childhood: Survival and performance. Pediatr Hematol Oncol 7:121–128, 1990.
23. Morreale V, Ebersold M, Quast L, et al: Cerebellar astrocytoma: Experience with 54 cases surgically treated at the Mayo Clinic, Rochester, Minnesota, from 1978 to 1990. J Neurosurg 87:257–261, 1997.
24. Palma L, Russo A, Celli P, et al: Prognosis of the so-called diffuse cerebellar astrocytoma. Neurosurgery 15:315–317, 1984.
25. Pencalet P, Maixner W, Sainte-Rose C, et al: Benign cerebellar astrocytomas in children. J Neurosurg 90:265–273, 1999.
26. Sgouros S, Fineron P, Hockley A, et al: Cerebellar astrocytoma of childhood: Long-term follow-up. Childs Nerv Syst 11:89–86, 1995.
27. Slavef I, Salchegger C, Hauer C, et al: Follow-up and quality of survival of 67 consecutive children with CNS tumors. Childs Nerv Syst 10:433–443, 1994.
28. Tomita T, Chou P, Reyes M, et al: IV ventricle astrocytomas in childhood: Clinicopathological features in 21 cases. Childs Nerv Syst 14:537–546, 1998.
29. Undjian S, Marinov M, Georgiev K, et al: Long-term follow-up after surgical treatment of cerebellar astrocytomas in 100 children. Childs Nerv Syst 5:99–101, 1989.
30. Wallner K, Gonzales M, Edwards M, et al: Treatment results of juvenile pilocytic astrocytoma. J. Neurosurg 69:171–176, 1988.
31. Riva D, Giorgi C: The cerebellum contributes to higher functions during development: Evidence from a series of children surgically treated for posterior fossa tumours. Brain 123:1051–1061, 2000.
32. Smoots D, Geyer J, Lieberman D, et al: Predicting disease progression in childhood cerebellar astrocytoma. Childs Nerv Syst 14:636–648, 1998.
33. Pagni C, Giordana, M, Canavero S, et al: Benign recurrence of a pilocytic cerebellar astrocytoma 36 years after radical removal: Case report. Neurosurgery 28:606–609, 1991.
34. Schneider J Jr, Raffel C, McComb J, et al: Benign cerebellar astrocytomas of childhood. Neurosurgery 30:58–63, 1992.
35. Chang T, Teng M, Lirng J, et al: Posterior cranial fossa tumours in childhood. Neuroradiology 35:274–278, 1993.
36. Lee Y, van Tassel P, Bruner J, et al: Juvenile pilocytic astrocytomas: CT and MR characteristics. AJR Am J Roentgenol 152:1263–1270, 1989.
37. Wang Z, Sutton L, Cnaan A, et al: Proton MR spectroscopy of pediatric cerebellar tumors. AJNR Am J Neuroradiol 16:1821–1833, 1995.
38. Kleihaus P, Burger P, Scheithauer B: Histological Typing of Tumours of the Central Nervous System. New York, Springer-Verlag, 1993, pp 11–15.
39. Bristo R, Raco A, Vangelista T, et al: Malignant cerebellar astrocytomas in childhood. Childs Nerv Syst 14:532–536, 1998.
40. Austin E: Prognosis of cerebellar astrocytoma. J Neuropathol Exp Neurol 49:339, 1990.
41. Dirven C, Koudstaal J, Mooij J, et al: AgNOR staining may reflect the growth potential of pilocytic astrocytomas. Childs Nerv Syst 15:384–388, 1999.
42. Shapiro K, Shulman K: Spinal cord seeding from cerebellar astrocytoma. Childs Brain 2:177–186, 1976.
43. Tomlinson F, Scheithauer B, Hayostek C, et al: The significance of atypia and histologic malignancy in pilocytic astrocytoma of the cerebellum: A clinocopathologic and flow cytometric study. J Child Neurol 9:301–310, 1994.
44. Catsman C, Van Dongen H, Mulder P, et al: Tumour type and size are high risk factors for the syndrome of "cerebellar" mutism and subsequent dysarthria. J Neurol Neurosurg Psychiatry 67:755–757, 1999.
45. Pollack I, Polinko P, Pang D, et al: Mutism and pseudobulbar symptoms after resection of posterior fossa tumors in children. Neurosurgery 37:885–893, 1995.
46. Laws E: Cerebellar astrocytomas in children. Neurosurgery 19:322, 1986.
47. Auer R, Rice G, Hinton G, et al: Cerebellar astrocytoma with benign histology and malignant clinical course. J Neurosurg 54:128–132, 1981.
48. Pollack I, Hurtt M, Pang D, et al: Dissemination of low-grade intracranial astrocytomas in children. Cancer 73:2869–2878, 1994.

49. Casadei G, Arrigoni G, D'Angelo V, et al: Late malignant recurrence of childhood cerebellar astrocytoma. Clin Neuropathol 9: 295–298, 1990.
50. Schwartz A, Ghatak N: Malignant transformation of benign cerebellar astrocytoma. Cancer 65:333–336, 1990.
51. Scott R, Ballantine H Jr: Cerebellar astrocytoma: Malignant recurrence after prolonged postoperative survival. J Neurosurg 39: 777–779, 1973.
52. Mishima K, Nakamura M, Nakamura H, et al: Leptomeningeal dissemination of cerebellar pilocytic astrocytoma. J Neurosurg 77:788–791, 1992.
53. Tamura M, Zama A, Kurihara H, et al: Management of recurrent pilocytic astrocytoma with leptomeningeal dissemination in childhood. Childs Nerv Syst 14:617–622, 1998.
54. Geissinger J, Bucy P: Astrocytomas of the cerebellum in children. Arch Neurol 24:125–135, 1971.

CHAPTER 236

Brainstem Gliomas

A. LELAND ALBRIGHT ■ IAN F. POLLACK

HISTORY AND CLINICAL SIGNIFICANCE

Brainstem gliomas (BSGs) occur in the midbrain, pons, and medulla. Approximately 75% of BSGs occur in children, and 25% occur in adults. The median age at presentation in childhood is 6.5 years, with no sex predilection.[1] BSGs account for approximately 1% of all primary brain tumors, 10% of pediatric brain tumors, and 25% of pediatric posterior fossa tumors. They are unusual brain tumors in several regards: they have a relatively bimodal prognosis as either very malignant or very benign, they usually do not need to be treated surgically, and their prognosis often corresponds poorly with the histologic appearance seen on biopsy.

Historically, BSGs were considered a uniform type of tumor. However, computed tomography and magnetic resonance imaging (MRI) have shown them to be otherwise. BSGs, like supratentorial gliomas, are not homogeneous tumors in their location, histologic appearance, or prognosis. Several classifications have been proposed (Table 236–1). The importance of classification is to recognize the different biologic and therapeutic variants of BSGs. Approximately 75% of BSGs are diffuse and 25% are focal. Of the focal tumors, most are in the midbrain, with the remainder in the pons and medulla.

Dorsally exophytic pontine tumors were first described by Hoffman and colleagues in 1980 and are the only extramedullary BSGs. They originate from the pontine floor of the fourth ventricle and grow posteri-

orly, filling the fourth ventricle.[2] They present more like a typical posterior fossa tumor than an intramedullary one. In the past, thalamic tumors were sometimes considered to be brainstem tumors, but they should not be; the thalamus is not part of the brainstem, and thalamic tumors differ considerably from BSGs in their clinical presentation, surgical treatment, and prognosis. Some authors consider cervicomedullary tumors to be BSGs. However, cervicomedullary tumors behave more like cervical spinal cord tumors and are probably the most cephalic variant of such tumors. Their symptoms, signs, treatment (with open exposure, myelotomy, and tumor resection), and prognosis are virtually identical to those of intramedullary cervical cord tumors. We therefore do not include them as BSGs, and they are not discussed in this chapter.

SIGNS AND SYMPTOMS

Diffuse Brainstem Gliomas

These tumors cause cerebellar dysfunction (87%), cranial nerve palsies (77%), and paresis (53%) because of tumor infiltration into nuclei and tracts.[1] Less common symptoms include personality changes, anorexia, sensory abnormalities, sleep apnea, hypernasality of speech, and choking. The symptoms are often less severe than might be expected from the extent of tumor seen on MRI scans. Symptoms are present for less than 1 month before diagnosis in 55% of cases, 3 months or less in 80%, and 6 months or less in 94%.[1] The duration of symptoms before diagnosis correlates with prognosis, which is significantly worse for tumors with symptoms of less than 1 month's duration and significantly better for those with symptoms lasting 6 months or more.[1]

The cranial nerves affected most often are VI, VII, and IX and X. It is unclear whether the presence of cranial nerve palsies at diagnosis correlates with prognosis. Ataxia is both appendicular and axial. Paresis is more often unilateral than bilateral. The epicenter of diffuse BSG is the pons, which enlarges into the shape of an egg. Because there is no significant amount of tumor within the fourth ventricle, hydrocephalus is

TABLE 236–1 ■ Classifications of Brainstem Gliomas

ALBRIGHT ET AL.[28]	EPSTEIN AND CONSTANTINI[15]	RUBIN ET AL.[29]
Diffuse	Midbrain	Cervicomedullary
Focal	Pontine	Dorsally exophytic
Midbrain	Dorsally exophytic	Cystic
Pons—intrinsic	Cervicomedullary	Focal
Dorsally exophytic	Diffuse	Diffuse
Medulla		

uncommon, occurring in less than 20% of patients at the time of diagnosis.

Focal Tumors

Midbrain tumors almost always present with symptoms and signs of slowly worsening hydrocephalus. Other signs, such as Parinaud's syndrome, paresis of cranial nerve III or IV, and hemiparesis, are uncommon. Focal pontine tumors may present with diplopia, facial weakness, and hemiparesis, either singly or in combination. Dorsally exophytic pontomedullary tumors present with hydrocephalus, ataxia, and diplopia, but without paresis. Focal medullary tumors present with swallowing difficulty, vomiting, ataxia, and hemiparesis.

PATHOGENESIS

Molecular Biology

Diffuse BSGs resemble adult malignant glial tumors in their molecular biology, with mutation of p53, a tumor suppressor gene, and amplification of a mutated epidermal growth factor receptor gene; this may explain their similarly aggressive behavior.[3] In a cytogenetic analysis of six BSG cases, three had abnormal chromosomes (trisomy 1q, deletion of chromosome 19, and multiple abnormalities); tumors with chromosomal abnormalities progressed rapidly.[4]

Neurofibromatosis

Individuals with neurofibromatosis type I develop intramedullary lesions that may resemble, or may be, gliomas. Diffuse BSGs in individuals with neurofibromatosis may have a more benign course than in patients without this syndrome. Focal tumors may also have a more indolent course.[5, 6] Pollack and coworkers reported 21 patients with neurofibromatosis type I and brainstem masses.[7] During a median follow-up of 3.75 years, nine patients had radiographic evidence of disease progression, and only three had clinical evidence of progression. The authors also observed spontaneous involution of some lesions and recommended that intervention be limited to lesions that exhibit rapid or unrelenting clinical or radiographic changes.

DIFFERENTIAL DIAGNOSIS

The differential diagnosis of brainstem masses of children and adults differs considerably. In children, diffuse lesions are gliomas. In a Children's Cancer Group study of 41 predominantly diffuse BSGs, 15 cases were low-grade astrocytomas, 23 were anaplastic, and 2 were glioblastomas.[1] Although there was no significant correlation between histologic tumor grade and outcome, the true proportion of low-grade to high-grade tumors is probably unknown, because a minority of BSGs are biopsied; in those that are biopsied, the neces-

sarily limited specimen may not reveal the most malignant component of the tumor. Accordingly, many children have been reported to have low-grade astrocytomas from biopsy results, but glioblastomas at autopsy less than a year later. Biopsy sampling error seems to be a more likely explanation for these differences than tumor differentiation in such a short time. Focal enhancing masses are often benign gliomas, such as juvenile pilocytic astrocytomas.

In adults with brainstem masses, the differential diagnosis is considerably broader and includes lymphomas, metastases, demyelinating diseases, and vascular lesions, in addition to gliomas.

DIAGNOSTIC EVALUATION

Computed Tomography

On computed tomographic scans without contrast enhancement, diffuse BSGs are hypodense lesions that enlarge the pons and displace the fourth ventricle posteriorly. After contrast agents are given, the tumors enhance nonhomogeneously, sometimes with a ring of enhancement around a central nonenhancing region. Focal midbrain tumors may not be seen on computed tomographic scans, either with or without contrast administration, leading to a false diagnosis of idiopathic late-onset aqueductal stenosis. Computed tomographic scans are superior for demonstrating calcification, which is often present in occult vascular malformations but rarely occurs in BSG. Zimmerman reported only three BSG cases with calcification in 10 years: one in an oligodendroglioma of the brainstem, one in the cephalic component of a cervicomedullary astrocytoma, and one after irradiation.[8]

Magnetic Resonance Imaging

If MRI scans are available, there is no reason to obtain computed tomographic scans to diagnose BSG. Good-quality MRI scans can virtually make the diagnosis of diffuse BSG because of the pathognomonic features (Fig. 236-1). T1-weighted images demonstrate hypointensity of the pons, but the extent of tumor is usually better seen on T2-weighted images, with hyperintensity extending into the adjacent midbrain or medulla, or both, and throughout the transverse extent of the pons. Contrast enhancement patterns are similar to computed tomographic patterns: nonhomogeneous enhancement within or around the tumor. Enhancement is present at the time of diagnosis in one third of cases,[8] although there is no significant difference in the prognosis of contrast-enhancing and nonenhancing tumors.

Prognosis of BSG correlates well with two radiographic features: tumor site (midbrain, pons, or medulla) and whether the tumor is focal or diffuse. In Fishbein and colleagues' study, 5-year survival was 75% for those with midbrain tumors, 65% for those with tumors in the medulla, and 18% for those with tumors in the pons (Fig. 236-2).[9] Five-year survival for

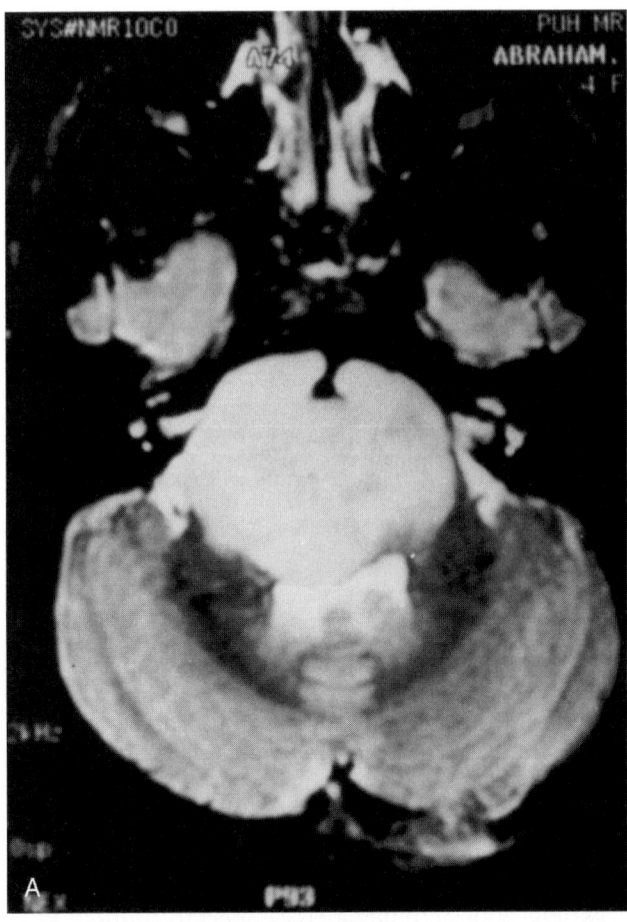

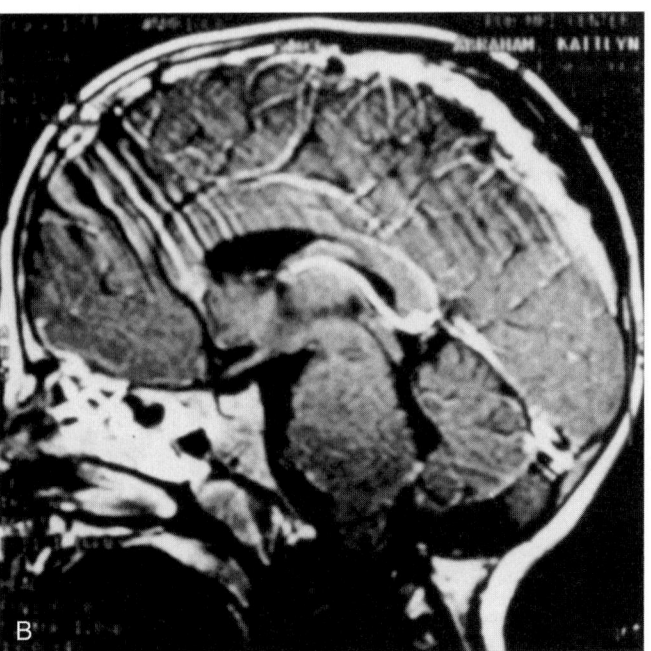

FIGURE 236–1. Magnetic resonance imaging (MRI) scans demonstrating a typical diffuse brainstem glioma. *A*, T2-weighted axial image. *B*, T1-weighted sagittal image.

those with focal tumors was 70%; for those with diffuse tumors, 22%. Other studies have reported lower survival rates for diffuse tumors. In Kaplan and associates' report of children treated with hyperfractionated radiation, 3-year survival was approximately 10%.[1]

There is probably no other intrinsic brainstem tumor with the same MRI appearance as diffuse BSG, with the possible exception of hamartoma, which is exceedingly rare and generally presents when the patient is younger than 2 months old.[8] The appearance of focal juvenile pilocytic tumors is also characteristic, although

other tumors (e.g., primitive neuroectodermal tumors, medulloepitheliomas, hemangioblastomas, and rhabdoid tumors) may rarely mimic focal, nonpilocytic astrocytomas. In the United States, it is unlikely that an intramedullary brainstem lesion is a tuberculoma, abscess, or focal inflammatory or demyelinating lesion. These rare cases usually have a clinical history dissimilar to that of BSG.

Focal tumors are of limited size, well circumscribed, and without associated edema or infiltration; they may be partially cystic. They are more common in the mid-

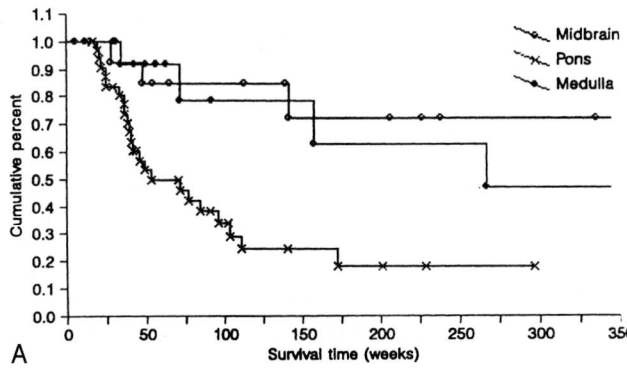

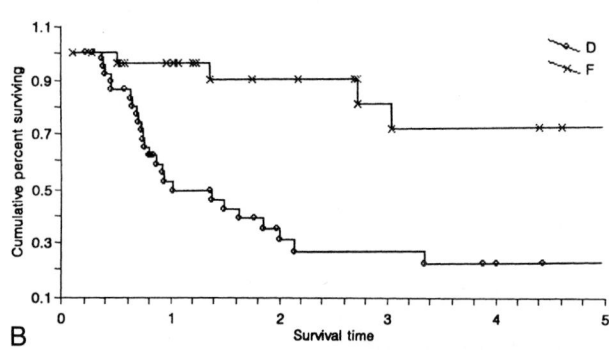

FIGURE 236–2. Survival for brainstem tumors by location *(A)* and by pattern of growth *(B)*. From Fishbein NJ, Prados MD, Wara W, et al: Radiologic classification of brain stem tumors: Correlation of magnetic resonance imaging appearance with clinical outcomes. Pediatr Neurosurg 24:9–23, 1996.)

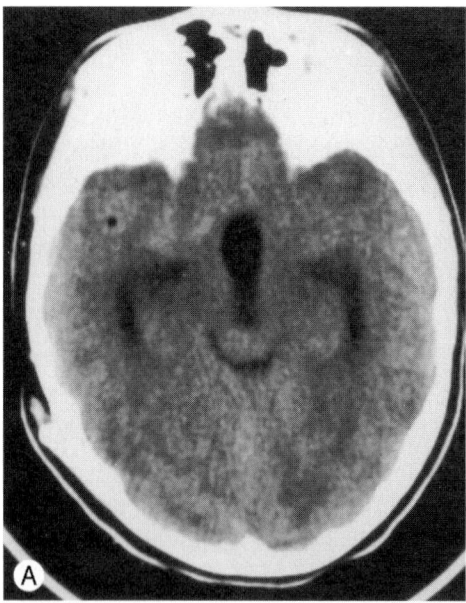
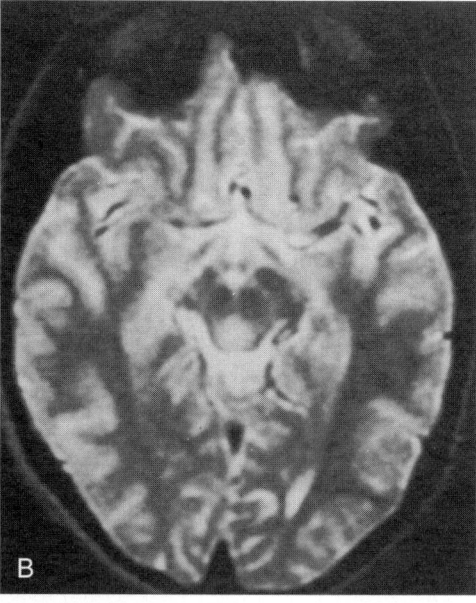

FIGURE 236–3. Axial computed tomographic *(A)* and MRI *(B)* scans without contrast enhancement of a child with a midbrain glioma. The tumor is not evident on the computed tomographic scan but is apparent on the MRI scan.

brain than in the medulla and are least common in the pons. Focal, intensely enhancing tumors with no associated edema, at any site, are usually juvenile pilocytic tumors. Focal midbrain tumors are isointense or mildly hypointense on T1-weighted images but hyperintense on T2-weighted images and may have a nidus of focal enhancement. Figure 236–3 demonstrates a focal midbrain tumor that was not evident on computed tomographic scans but was evident on MRI scans. Focal pontine and medullary tumors can have either MRI features similar to those of a diffuse BSG, but localized into one area, albeit with somewhat ill-defined margins, or, rarely, features of a juvenile astrocytoma.

Dorsally exophytic tumors appear as intra–fourth ventricle tumors, and their derivation from the brainstem often cannot be appreciated on scans. Their appearance resembles that of a vermian astrocytoma, which may also involve the floor of the fourth ventricle.

BSGs have been evaluated with single photon emission computed tomographic imaging using thallium-201; they accumulate thallium, although the specificity of that uptake is about 90%.[10] Thallium uptake is not correlated with tumor grade, gadolinium enhancement, or necrosis. Magnetic resonance spectroscopy has been used to evaluate brainstem enlargement in patients with gliomas and in those with neurofibromatosis type I.[11] Levels of *N*-acetyl aspartate and the sum of the metabolites choline and creatine-phosphocreatine are significantly lower in patients with diffuse BSGs than in those with neurofibromatosis or in normal controls.

TREATMENT

Surgical Treatment

In children with clinical signs and symptoms of BSG who have diffuse brainstem masses evident on good-

quality MRI scans, the diagnosis is so likely to be BSG that a biopsy is not indicated; the risks of the biopsy outweigh the remote possibility of diagnosing something other than a glioma. There is no evidence that partial tumor removal improves survival, and current treatment protocols are not altered by the pathologic diagnosis. Surgery is indicated only for some of the 20% of brainstem tumors that are focal, enhancing, and accessible with acceptable risks; the rare tumors with significant cystic components; or the few cases in which the diagnosis is in doubt. With high-quality MRI scans, the number of children in whom the diagnosis is questionable is certainly less than 5%.

When the diagnosis is in doubt, stereotactic biopsies usually provide diagnostic material and have relatively low risks.[12, 13] In the series of Rajshekhar and Chandy, a diagnosis was made in 68 of 69 cases.[12] In Steck and Friedman's series of 24 stereotactic biopsies of brainstem lesions in children and adults, a pathologic diagnosis was made in 23 (16 astrocytomas, 3 metastases, 1 lymphoma, 1 germinoma, 1 chordoma, 1 leukodystrophy); 6 of 6 children had astrocytomas, whereas 7 of 18 adults had lesions other than astrocytomas.[13]

In children with focal midbrain nonenhancing tumors associated with hydrocephalus, the hydrocephalus is treated—ideally by an endoscopic third ventriculostomy rather than a shunt—and the tumor is subsequently evaluated by serial MRI scans. If there is a small area of contrast enhancement in the tumor, suggestive of a pilocytic astrocytoma, the lesion is observed. If the area of contrast enhancement is suggestive of a different lesion or is of sufficient size that treatment is indicated, a biopsy is warranted. We prefer a stereotactic biopsy via a coronal trajectory for such lesions, rather than an open biopsy. If the biopsy reveals a pilocytic astrocytoma, it can generally be treated with external irradiation (stereotactic radiosurgery or conformal fields) as effectively as with either open resection or interstitial irradiation, and with

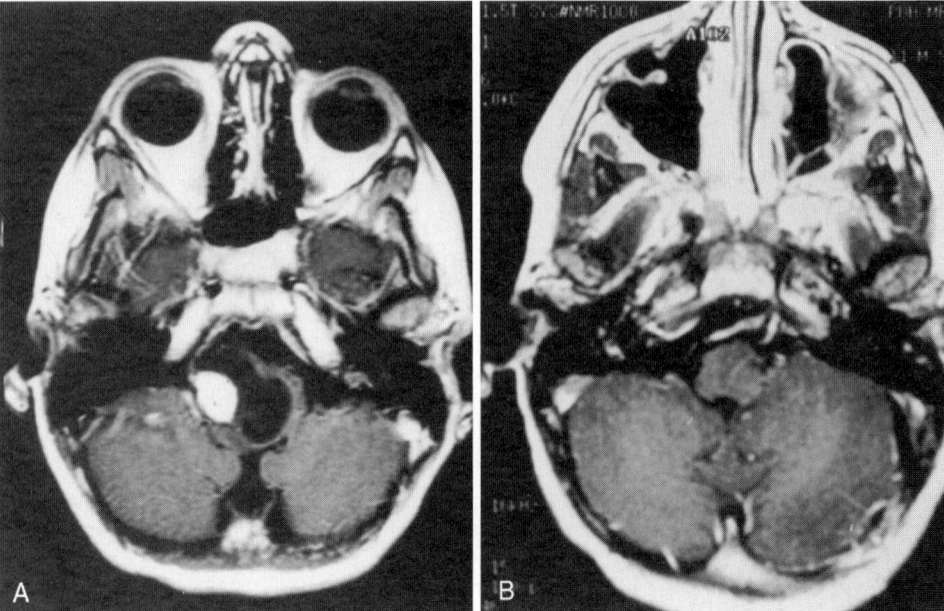

FIGURE 236–4. Axial enhanced MRI scan of a lateral medullary pilocytic astrocytoma that could be resected with acceptable risks. Preoperative *(A)* and postoperative *(B)* images.

lower risks. Resections of tumors in this area are associated with relatively high risks, even with current techniques.[14] We do, however, favor resecting large lesions with significant mass effect and well-defined tumor borders.

Focal tumors of the pons are rare and can be biopsied stereotactically via a coronal transpeduncular approach. The rare tumors that are located superficially can be surgically excised. Surgical techniques for brainstem lesions have been summarized by Epstein and Constantini, who demonstrated the inadvisability of operations on diffuse BSGs and the feasibility of operations for focal lesions.[15]

Dorsally exophytic pontine gliomas present as mass lesions within the fourth ventricle. These tumors require resection and are often not suspected until surgery is under way. There is a reasonable plane for dissection between the dorsum of the tumor and the adjacent cerebellum, but anteriorly, the tumor blends into the floor of the fourth ventricle. Tumor removal is performed with the ultrasonic surgical aspirator down to the level of the floor of the ventricle, but tumor below the floor is not removed because of the attendant risks.[2]

The treatment of focal tumors in the medulla varies, depending on the location of the tumor. If it is located laterally and appears to be approachable with acceptable risks (Fig. 236–4), resection is appropriate. If the tumor location is more central, it can probably be treated better by stereotactic biopsy and irradiation (Fig. 236–5), although the optimal approach for these difficult lesions is controversial.

SURGICAL COMPLICATIONS

The complication rate of open BSG resections is substantial, and it is uncommon to achieve complete tumor resection with no increase in morbidity. In a compila-

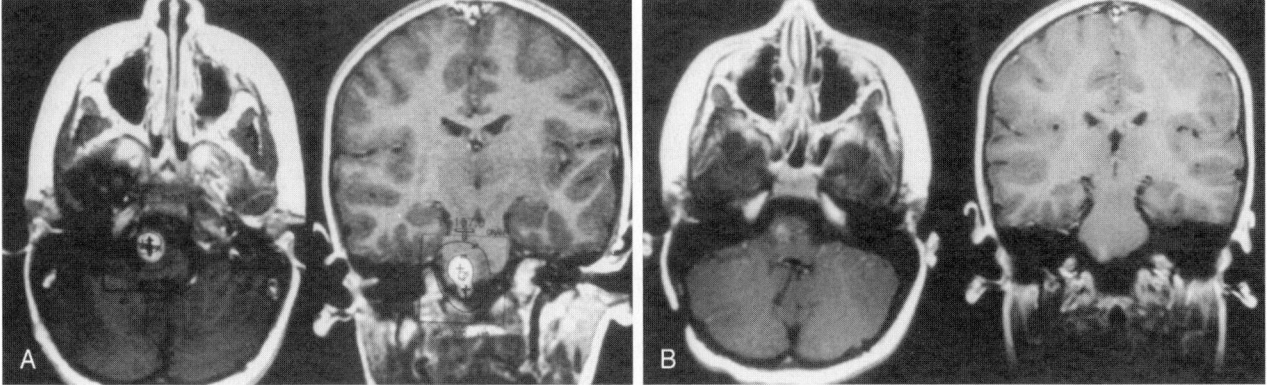

FIGURE 236–5. Axial enhanced MRI scan of a central medullary pilocytic astrocytoma that was treated with stereotactic irradiation rather than resection. Before radiosurgery *(A)* and 13 months after radiosurgery *(B)*.

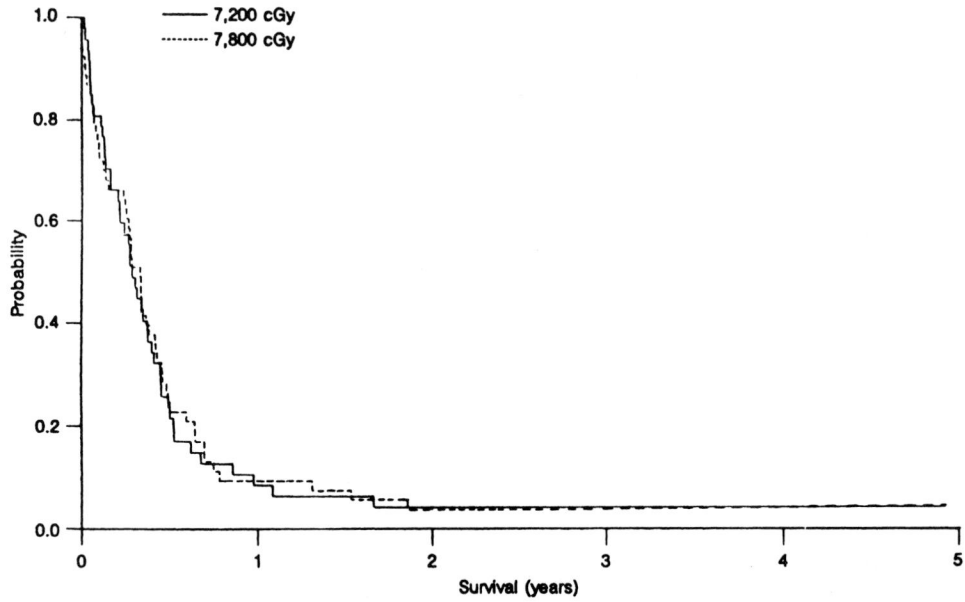

FIGURE 236–6. Survival for patients treated with hyperfractionated irradiation, 72 to 78 Gy. (From Packer RJ: Brain stem gliomas: Therapeutic options at time of recurrence. Pediatr Neurosurg 24:211, 1996.)

tion of BSG biopsy series involving predominantly stereotactic biopsies, morbidity was reported in 6% to 11% of cases.[16] In a series of 69 computed tomography–guided stereotactic biopsies of brainstem masses, transient morbidity occurred in 5.6% of cases and permanent morbidity in 1.4%.[12]

The value of intraoperative monitoring during BSG surgery is unclear. Some authors monitor electromyograms of muscles innervated by cranial nerves, whereas others monitor brainstem evoked potentials or somatosensory evoked potentials, or both. In our experience with such monitoring, electromyographic activity is often observed during tumor resections around cranial nerve nuclei, but determining whether the changes represent manipulation rather than damage is challenging, even for a skilled neurophysiology team. Brainstem evoked potential and somatosensory evoked potential monitoring may be used but has not been proved to increase the safety of tumor removal.

Nonsurgical Treatment

IRRADIATION

When children present with signs and symptoms characteristic of BSGs and have good-quality MRI scans demonstrating diffuse brainstem masses, they are commonly given corticosteroids, which improve symptoms, as they do for supratentorial gliomas. Irradiation is the standard treatment for diffuse BSGs and is given by external fractions. In the early 1980s, such irradiation consisted of 54 Gy given in once-daily fractions of 180 cGy. Since 1985, the Children's Cancer Group and the Pediatric Oncology Group have evaluated hyperfractionation—the administration of 100 cGy fractions twice daily—to treat BSGs, in the hope of increasing efficacy without increasing morbidity. Total doses began at 64 Gy and escalated to 78 Gy, with no evidence of dose-dependent improvement in 2-year survival (Fig. 236–6, Table 236–2).

Approximately 70% of patients undergoing irradiation have transient clinical stabilization or improvement. Prados and colleagues reported that tumor size decreased in 30% of patients receiving 78 Gy, was stable in 40%, and progressed in 30%.[17] Morbidity increases with increasing dosage, and at 78 Gy, patients develop steroid dependency, hearing loss, ischemic events, hormone deficits, and late seizures.[18] An important Pediatric Oncology Group study compared hyperfractionated irradition using 78 Gy with conventional irradiation of 54 Gy given in once-daily fractions, plus cisplatin.[19] The authors found no difference in

TABLE 236–2 ■ Hyperfractionated Irradiation for Brainstem Gliomas

STUDY	NUMBER OF PATIENTS	DOSE (GY)	MST (MO)	SURVIVAL (%)		
				One Year	Two Years	Three Years
Freeman et al.[30] (POG #8495)	38	66	11	48	6	3
Freeman et al.[30] (POG #8495)	57	70.2	10	40	23	21
Packer et al.[32] (CCG #9882)	53	72	9	38	14	8
Packer et al.[33] (CCG #9882)	—	78	9.5	35	22	6
Prados et al.[17] (UCSF)	78	78	13	—	—	—

CCG, Children's Cancer Group; MST, Median Survival Time; POG, Pediatric Oncology Group; UCSF, University of California at San Francisco.

survival between the groups and concluded that there is no role for hyperfractionated irradiation in the treatment of children with newly diagnosed diffuse BSG. Hyperfractionation has also been combined with beta-interferon, with acceptable toxicity but no change in survival.[20] Conventional external radiation has also been supplemented with interstitial iodine-125 implants safely, but without apparent improvement in survival rates.[21]

If focal BSGs are followed and then progress, they are treated with radiation. The optimal forms of irradiation are either stereotactic radiosurgery or conformal irradiation—the daily administration of external fractionated irradiation using stereotactic delivery techniques. Both methods result in excellent tumor control and probably have lower morbidity than conventional external radiation therapy.

CHEMOTHERAPY

Chemotherapy has been used since the 1970s to treat diffuse BSGs, mostly in phase II clinical trials using agents singly (cyclophosphamide, carboplatin, cisplatin, etoposide, and thiotepa) and in combination. Responses of 15% to 20% have been observed, but survival has not been prolonged. Some of the more recent chemotherapy series are listed in Table 236–3. Ongoing studies are evaluating the efficacy of agents that may potentiate the effects of radiation therapy, such as gadolinium texaphyrin, topotecan, and carboplatin combined with the blood-brain barrier disruption agent RMP-7.

OUTCOMES

In the past, several authors reported 5-year survivals of 20% to 30% among patients with BSGs. Most of those series were from the pre–computed tomography era, so they included lesions that may not have been BSGs, and they included patients with both focal and diffuse gliomas.

Within 6 to 24 months after diagnosis and irradiation, diffuse BSGs commonly progress at the original site and then lead almost inexorably to death, usually within 3 to 6 months after relapse is diagnosed.[22] In the 1996 series of Kaplan and associates, 37% of patients survived 1 year, 20% survived 2 years, and 13% survived 3 years.[1] The median time to death was 10 months. A single case report exists of spontaneous regression of a diffuse pontine glioma in a 2-year-old.[23] That tumor, confirmed as a fibrillary astrocytoma, regressed spontaneously and was not visible on scans when the child was 6.6 years old.

Spinal leptomeningeal metastases occur soon after local tumor relapse in approximately 30% of cases.[24] Systemic metastases have been reported but are rare. Treatment options at the time of recurrence are generally limited to the use of investigational chemotherapeutic agents. In a review of responses to chemotherapy given at the time of BSG relapse, 17 of 116 patients responded to single agents, and 8 of 96 responded to multiple agents.[22]

After irradiation, focal tumors gradually involute and become quiescent for a long time, perhaps permanently. As the tumor undergoes radionecrosis, symptoms may transiently worsen and are treated with corticosteroids. Months later, cysts may form and cause mass effect, requiring either stereotactic or open drainage. The instillation of radioactive colloids such as P32 may decrease the likelihood of cyst reaccumulation.

Dorsally exophytic gliomas have an excellent prognosis, even with subtotal resection. In Pollack and coworkers' review of 18 patients treated by subtotal excision and 2 others who also received irradiation, 17 patients were alive at a median follow-up of 9 years.[25] Tumor growth had occurred in 4 cases and was treated mainly with reoperation. The outcome of focal pontine tumors varies with histologic type and is excellent for the rare juvenile astrocytoma but dismal for more aggressive tumors. Excision of focal medullary tumors has substantial morbidity to lower cranial nerves but may provide long-term tumor control.[26]

Adults with BSGs appear to have considerably better prognoses than do children, probably because of their lower percentage of diffuse tumors. In a review of 19 adults with a median age of 40 years and a mixed pattern of BSG, the median survival was 54 months, and the 5-year survival rate was 45%.[27] Survival did not correlate with clinical or imaging features such as age at diagnosis, duration of symptoms, cranial nerve involvement, MRI enhancement, or treatment, which included irradiation in 12 patients and observation in 7. Adults with tectal and cervicomedullary tumors may have better prognoses than those with tumors in other brainstem sites, as is true in children.

CONCLUSIONS

The treatment of BSG has evolved since the 1980s, primarily because of better neuroimaging. Fewer pa-

---

T A B L E 2 3 6 – 3 ■ **Series Treating Brainstem Gliomas with Chemotherapy**

YEAR	RESPONSES/SUBJECTS	CHEMOTHERAPY AGENTS	REFERENCE
1987		Chloroethyl-cyclohexylnitrosourea, vincristine, prednisone	Jenkin et al.[36]
1993		Cisplatin, cyclophosphamide	Kretchmar et al.[34]
1994		Myeloablative + rescue	Dunkel et al.[35]
1995	0/10	Ifosfamide	Heideman et al.[37]
1996	0/14	Topotecan	Blaney et al.[38]
1998	1/10	Temozolomide	Estlin et al.[39]

tients are now operated on, but the outcomes of patients with BSG are essentially unchanged. Diffuse BSG remains the pediatric brain tumor type with the worst prognosis. For these tumors, operation, irradiation, and chemotherapy appear to have no long-lasting therapeutic benefits. Future advances will probably come from new chemotherapy agents or from altogether novel treatment approaches. The minor proportion of BSGs that are focal have good prognoses and can be effectively treated, when necessary, with resection and irradiation.

REFERENCES

1. Kaplan AM, Albright AL, Zimmerman RA, et al: Brainstem gliomas in children: A Children's Cancer Group review of 119 cases. Pediatr Neurosurg 24:185–192, 1996.
2. Hoffman HJ, Becker LE, Craven MA: A clinically and pathologically distinct group of benign brain stem gliomas. Neurosurgery 7:243–248, 1980.
3. Raffel C: Molecular biology of pediatric gliomas. J Neurooncol 28:121–128, 1996.
4. Chadduck WM, Boop RA, Sawyer JR: Cytogenic studies of pediatric brain and spinal cord tumors. Pediatr Neurosurg 17:57–65, 1991.
5. Pollack IF, Pang D, Albright L: The long term outcome in children with late-onset aqueductal stenosis resulting from benign intrinsic tectal tumors. J Neurosurg 80:681–688, 1994.
6. Raffel C, McComb JG, Bodner S, Gilles FE: Benign brain stem lesions in pediatric patients with neurofibromatosis: Case reports. Neurosurgery 25:959–964, 1989.
7. Pollack IF, Shultz B, Mulvihill JJ: The management of brainstem gliomas in patients with neurofibromatosis. Neurology 46:1652–1660, 1999.
8. Zimmerman RA: Neuroimaging of primary brainstem gliomas: Diagnosis and course. Pediatr Neurosurg 25:45–53, 1996.
9. Fishbein NJ, Prados MD, Wara W, et al: Radiologic classification of brain stem tumors: Correlation of magnetic resonance imaging appearance with clinical outcome. Pediatr Neurosurg 24:9–23, 1996.
10. Nadvi SS, Ebrahim FS, Corr P: The value of 201 thallium-SPECT imaging in childhood brainstem gliomas. Pediatr Radiol 28:575–579, 1998.
11. Broniscer A, Gajjar A, Bhargava R, et al: Brain stem involvement in children with neurofibromatosis type 1: Role of magnetic resonance imaging and spectroscopy in the distinction from diffuse pontine glioma. Neurosurgery 40:331–337, 1997.
12. Rajshekhar V, Chandy MJ: Computerized tomography–guided stereotactic surgery for brainstem masses: A risk-benefit analysis in 71 patients. J Neurosurg 82:976–981, 1995.
13. Steck J, Friedman WA: Stereotactic biopsy of brainstem mass lesions. Surg Neurol 43:563–567, 1995.
14. Lapras C, Bognar L, Turjman F, et al: Tectal plate gliomas. Part I. Microsurgery of the tectal plate gliomas. Acta Neurochir 126:76–83, 1994.
15. Epstein F, Constantini S: Practical decisions in the treatment of pediatric brain stem tumors. Pediatr Neurosurg 24:24–34, 1996.
16. Albright AL: Diffuse brainstem gliomas: When is a biopsy necessary? Pediatr Neurosurg 24:252–255, 1996.
17. Prados MD, Wara WM, Edwards MS, et al: The treatment of brain stem and thalamic gliomas with 78 Gy of hyperfractionated radiation therapy. Int J Radiat Oncol Biol Phys 32:85–92, 1995.
18. Freeman CR, Farmer JP: Pediatric brain stem gliomas: A review. Int J Radiat Oncol Biol Phys 40:265–271, 1998.
19. Mandell LR, Kadota R, Freeman C, et al: There is no role for hyperfractionated radiotherapy in the management of children with newly diagnosed diffuse intrinsic brainstem tumors: Results of a Pediatric Oncology Group phase III trial comparing conventional vs. hyperfractionated radiotherapy. Int J Radiat Oncol Biol Phys 43:959–964, 1999.
20. Packer RJ, Prados M, Phillips P, et al: Treatment of children with newly diagnosed brain stem gliomas with intravenous recombinant beta-interferon and hyperfractionated radiation therapy: A Children's Cancer Group phase I/II study. Cancer 77:2150–2156, 1996.
21. Chuba PJ, Zamarano L, Hamre M, et al: Permanent I-125 brain stem implants in children. Childs Nerv Syst 14:570–577, 1998.
22. Packer RJ: Brain stem gliomas: Therapeutic options at time of recurrence. Pediatr Neurosurg 24:211–216, 1996.
23. Lenard HG, Engelbrecht V, Janssen G, et al: Complete remission of a diffuse pontine glioma. Neuropediatrics 29:328–330, 1998.
24. Donahue B, Allen J, Siffert J, et al: Patterns of recurrence in brain stem gliomas: Evidence for craniospinal dissemination. Int J Radiat Oncol Biol Phys 40:677–680, 1998.
25. Pollack IF, Humphreys RP, Becker L: The long term outcome after surgical treatment of dorsally exophytic brain-stem gliomas. J Neurosurg 78:859–863, 1993.
26. Abbott R, Shimanski-Maher T, Wisoff JH, et al: Intrinsic tumors of the medulla: Surgical complications. Pediatr Neurosurg 17:239–244, 1991.
27. Landolfi JC, Thaler HT, DeAngelis LM: Adult brainstem gliomas. Neurology 51:1136–1139, 1998.
28. Albright AL, Packer RJ, Zimmerman R, et al: Magnetic resonance scans should replace biopsies for the diagnosis of diffuse brain stem gliomas: A report from the Children's Cancer Group. Neurosurgery 33:1026–1030, 1993.
29. Rubin G, Michowitz S, Horev G, et al: Pediatric brain stem gliomas: An update. Childs Nerv Syst 14:167–173, 1988.
30. Freeman CR, Krischer J, Sanford RA, et al: Hyperfractionated radiotherapy in brainstem tumors: Results of a Pediatric Oncology Group study. Int J Radiat Oncol Biol Phys 15:311–318, 1988.
31. Freeman CR, Krischer J, Sanford RA, et al: Hyperfractionated radiotherapy for brain-stem tumors: Results at the 7020 cGy dose level of Pediatric Oncology Group Study #8495. Cancer 68:474–481, 1991.
32. Packer RJ, Boyett JM, Zimmerman RA, et al: Hyperfractionated radiotherapy (72 Gy) for children with brain stem gliomas: A Children's Cancer Group phase I/II trial. Cancer 72:1414–1421, 1993.
33. Packer RJ, Boyett JM, Zimmerman RA, et al: Outcome of children with brain stem gliomas after treatment with 7800 cGy of hyperfractionated radiotherapy. Cancer 74:1827–1834, 1994.
34. Kretchmar CS, Tarbell NJ, Barnes PD, et al: Pre-irradiation chemotherapy and hyperfractionated radiation therapy 66 Gy for children with brainstem tumors: A phase II study of the Pediatric Oncology Group. Protocol 8833. Cancer 72:1404–1413, 1993.
35. Dunkel I, Garvin J, Goldman S, et al: High-dose chemotherapy with autologous bone marrow rescue does not cure children with brain stem tumors. Pediatr Neurosurg 21:219, 1994.
36. Jenkin RD, Boesel C, Ertel I, et al: Brain-stem tumors in childhood: A prospective randomized trial of irradiation with and without adjuvant CCNU, VCR and prednisone: A report from the Children's Cancer Study Group. J Neurosurg 66:227–233, 1987.
37. Heideman RL, Douglas EC, Langston JA, et al: A phase II study of every other day high-dose ifosfamide in pediatric brain tumors: A pediatric oncology study. J Neurooncol 25:77–84, 1995.
38. Blaney SM, Phillips PC, Packer RJ, et al: Phase II evaluation of topotecan for pediatric central nervous system tumors. Cancer 78:527–531, 1996.
39. Estlin EJ, Lashford L, Ablett S, et al: Phase I study of temozolomide in paediatric patients with advanced cancer: United Kingdom Children's Cancer Study Group. Br J Cancer 78:652–661, 1998.

CHAPTER 237

Craniopharyngiomas

PETER CARMEL

Tumors of disordered embryogenesis are a heterogeneous group that may have either neoplastic or nonneoplastic characteristics. They frequently have little growth potential and are often considered hamartomatous. This chapter reviews craniopharyngiomas, the most common type of tumor of disordered embryogenesis. Chapter 238 discusses colloid tumors, inclusion cysts, epidermoids, dermoids, teratomas, and lipomas.

Craniopharyngiomas have been recognized as a distinct tumor type for more than 100 years.[1] Their histologic and clinical features and natural history are well known. They are benign histologically but difficult to remove because of their location and their adhesion to vital vascular and neural structures. Surgical treatment remains controversial, and the surgeon's attitude will markedly affect his or her ability to deal with craniopharyngiomas. Neurosurgeons who do not believe that surgical excision is usually possible will rarely, if ever, achieve total removal. The author's bias is that surgical removal can potentially cure the patient and is the operative goal, recognizing that not all craniopharyngiomas can be removed.

HISTORY

An unusual group of epithelial tumors encountered in the sella and parasellar regions intrigued pathologists at the end of the 19th century. In 1899, Mott and Barrett[1] were the first to postulate that these tumors might arise from the hypophysial duct or Rathke's pouch. Rathke's pouch is an upward invagination of the primary oral cavity, the stomodeum, and is lined by epithelial cells of ectodermal origin. The pouch detaches from the stomodeum and becomes a rounded vesicle. When the infundibulum extends downward from the diencephalon, the vesicle surrounds its anterior surface and becomes the anterior lobe of the hypophysis, and its hollow center is reduced to a cleft between the anterior and posterior pituitary lobes.[2] This embryogenesis of the pituitary was described by Rathke[3] in 1838. In 1904, Erdheim[4] carefully characterized the histologic features of these tumors and postulated that they arose from embryonic squamous cell rests of an incompletely involuted hypophysial-pharyngeal duct.

This theory has been borne out by the subsequent discovery of craniopharyngiomas along the path of development of Rathke's pouch from the pharynx to the floor of the sella, as well as above and within the sella.[5]

In 1892, Onanoff[6] noted the resemblance of certain tumors of the infundibulum to adamantinomas of the jaw and applied the term *pituitary adamantinoma* to these neoplasms. More recently, a histologic similarity to the keratinizing and calcifying odontogenic cyst has been noted, which may more precisely mimic craniopharyngioma.[7, 8] Although craniopharyngiomas resemble these two tumors of odontogenic origin, the histologic pictures of craniopharyngioma and Rathke's cleft cyst differ greatly, despite their common origin.[9] Rathke's cleft cysts are lined with epithelium, which secretes a mucoid material. These cysts lack the true neoplastic transformation found in craniopharyngiomas.[9–11]

Several authors have noted differences in the histologic patterns of adult and pediatric craniopharyngiomas.[12, 13] These authors postulate that an embryonic origin for adult tumors is not required and that craniopharyngiomas appearing later in life may arise from metaplasia of pituitary cells. This theory gained some support from the fact that squamous epithelial cell rests in the hypophysis have long been known to exist.[14] Cell rests of this type are found in only 3% of neonates.[15] However, they are found with increasing frequency in each succeeding decade of life.[16] Although metaplasia probably accounts for these data, proof of neoplastic transformation of these rests is lacking.

PATHOLOGY

The microscopic appearance of most craniopharyngiomas consists of an external layer of high columnar epithelium, a variable amount of polygonal cells, and a central network of epithelial cells (Fig. 237–1). These epithelial bands are supported by a mesodermal connective tissue stroma. It has been postulated that regressive changes in the epithelial cells cause cellular liquefaction and deposition of keratin-like material.[4, 17, 18] The central stroma also may degenerate, leading to

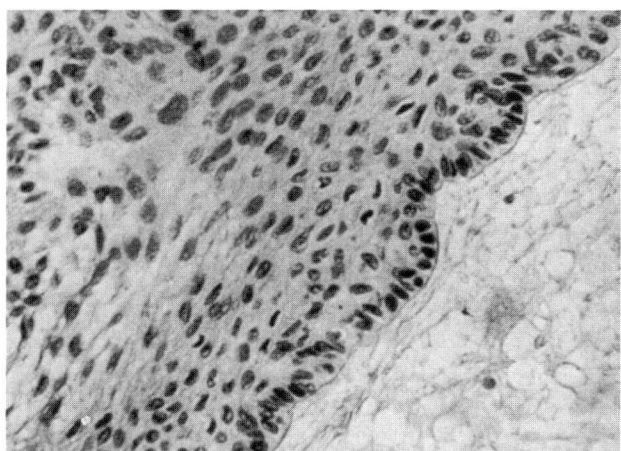

FIGURE 237–1. Microscopic appearance of a craniopharyngioma. A well-defined basement membrane is seen between the tumor and surrounding astroglial tissue. A band of high columnar cells forms the external tumor layer. Next, a layer of polygonal cells is seen, and then a central network of epithelial cells.

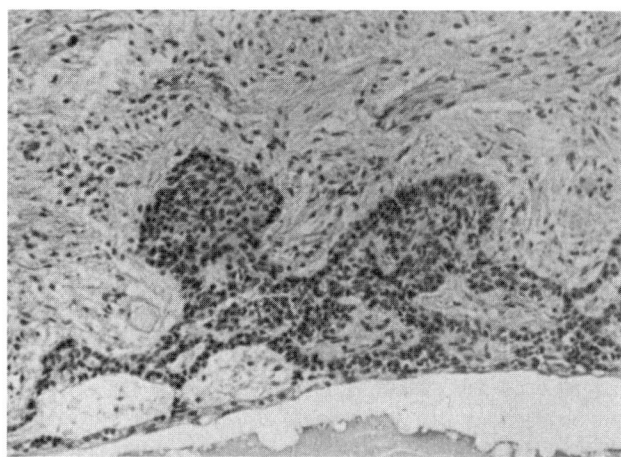

FIGURE 237–2. Pseudopod formation in a cystic craniopharyngioma. Inner cystic material is seen at the bottom. The tumor processes appear to project into the surrounding brain tissue. However, close inspection shows that this layer is almost entirely glial reactive tissue, with few neurons. Some authors maintain that this glial layer is a plane of cleavage that allows safe separation of tumor from brain. (From Sweet WH: Recurrent craniopharyngiomas: Therapeutic alternatives. Clin Neurosurg 27:206–229, 1980.)

cyst formation.[4] A collagenous basement membrane often forms the boundary between the tumor and the surrounding meninges or brain.[18] Cyst walls may vary from thin, diaphanous membranes to thick, tough structures that may also be hard and rigid because of calcium salt deposition. Calcification is found on microscopic examination in approximately half of adult craniopharyngiomas and in almost all pediatric cases.[19, 20]

Cases of craniopharyngiomas with rapid growth and aggressive recurrence are occasionally reported; however, these are generally not believed to represent malignant degeneration. Matson and Crigler[21] specifically denied that craniopharyngiomas invade brain. Some signs of anaplastic change have been reported in electron microscopic studies of particularly aggressive craniopharyngiomas.[22] Tissue culture studies of these tumors show little mitotic activity and a pronounced tendency to produce cysts.[23] A recent case purporting to demonstrate the transition of typical craniopharyngioma to squamous cell carcinoma must be questioned because of the three courses of radiotherapy used to treat the tumor.[24]

Craniopharyngiomas often cause an intense glial reaction in surrounding brain tissue.[25] This is particularly marked around small papillary tumor projections into the undersurface of the hypothalamus (Fig. 237–2). Because of this dense glial layer, some authors believed that traction on craniopharyngiomas always led to hypothalamic damage and precluded safe total removal.[26] Sweet,[27] however, pointed out that this "glial envelope" may provide a plane in which to dissect the craniopharyngioma safely from surrounding brain. Moreover, autopsy findings in several cases have shown only minimal attachment of the tumor at the level of the tuber cinereum.[19, 28]

Craniopharyngiomas are frequently densely adherent to major arteries at the base of the brain.[29] Attachment of tumor to the internal carotid artery was cited as preventing the total removal of 6 of 23 lesions in children.[28, 30] Review of incompletely removed craniopharyngiomas in children revealed that attachment to a major artery at the circle of Willis was a far more likely site of residual tumor than was adherence to the hypothalamus or chiasm (Fig. 237–3).[31, 32] It may be that the mesenchymal reaction of the vessel wall with the tumor produces a tougher and more tenacious attachment than does glial proliferation.[33]

The blood supply for suprasellar craniopharyngiomas is derived principally from small arterial feeders of the anterior circulation.[19] Direct branches from the internal carotid and posterior communicating arteries are also noted. However, craniopharyngiomas do not receive blood from the posterior cerebral arteries or from the basilar artery bifurcation unless the blood supply of the floor of the third ventricle is parasitized.[19] Within the sella, the tumor may be supplied by small perforating arteries from the cavernous sinuses.

INCIDENCE

Craniopharyngiomas constitute between 2.5% and 4% of all brain tumors.[34, 35] There is a preponderance of tumors in children between 5 and 15 years of age; however, childhood tumors constitute less than half of all craniopharyngiomas.[20] These tumors may become symptomatic at any age; the oldest patient in a large series was 71 years at the time of surgery.[20] The age distribution in a series of 109 patients is shown in Figure 237–4. Occasional series have reported a male preponderance; however, an equal sex incidence has been noted in groups of children.[20, 28, 32, 36] In Matson's[37] large series of tumors in children, craniopharyngiomas were the most common nonglial tumor and constituted 9% of his series. Although craniopharyngiomas ac-

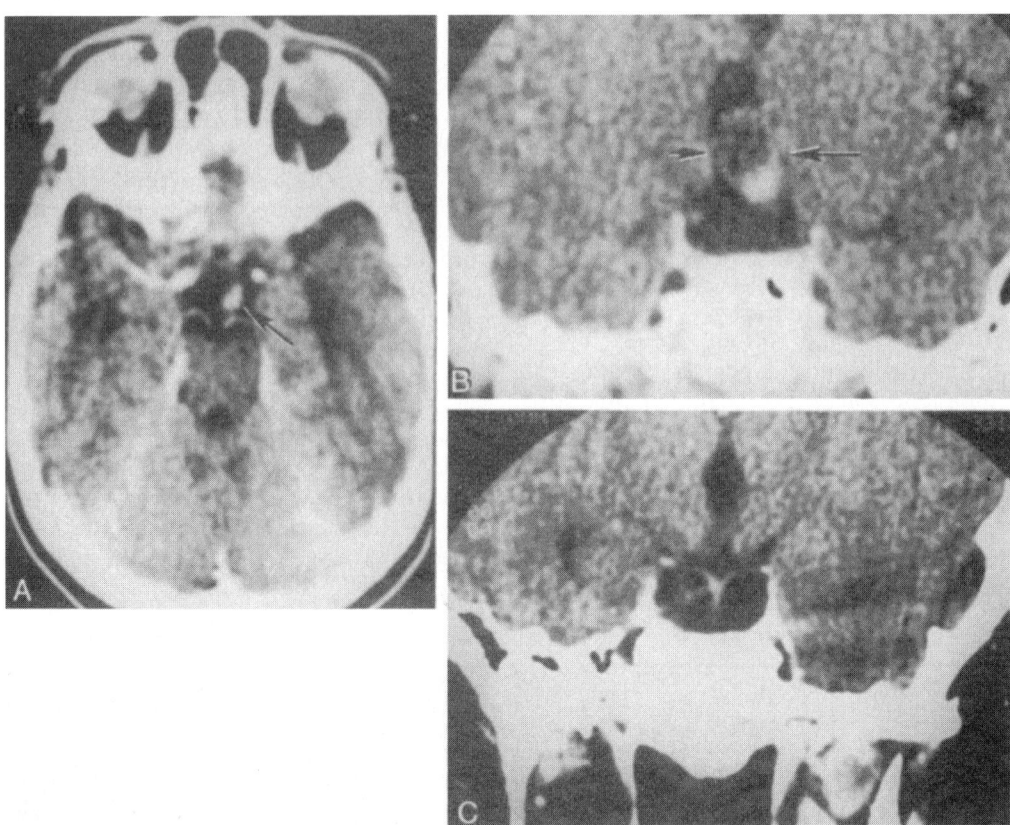

FIGURE 237–3. *A,* Axial contrast-enhanced computed tomographic scan taken a year after removal of a large craniopharyngioma in an 8-year-old girl. A small calcified fragment of tumor is seen adherent to basal arteries at the junction of the posterior communicating and posterior cerebral arteries *(arrow). B,* Coronal computed tomographic scan taken 7 months after the scan in *A.* A cyst has formed *(arrows),* which is expanding within the third ventricle and arising from the calcified remnant of tumor. At this point, the decision to reoperate was made. *C,* Coronal contrast-enhanced computed tomographic scan taken after the second operation. The tumor was removed by a subfrontal trans–lamina terminalis approach, and the lesion was sharply dissected from the arteries.

count for a high percentage of childhood brain tumors, 60% of these tumors are found in patients older than 16 years.[20, 38] The relative rarity of these tumors is shown in data from population-based tumor registries, which indicate an incidence of 0.13 per 100,000 person-years. Approximately 338 cases are expected to occur

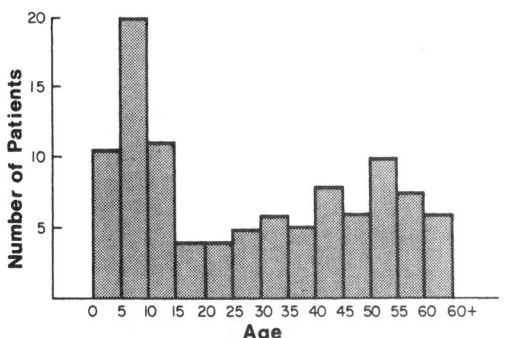

FIGURE 237–4. Age distribution in a series of 109 patients with craniopharyngioma. (Data from Sung DI, Chang CH, Harisiadis L, Carmel PW: Treatment results of craniopharyngioma. Cancer 47: 847–852, 1981.)

annually in the United States, with 96 cases in patients aged 14 years or younger.[39]

SIGNS AND SYMPTOMS

Endocrine dysfunction caused by craniopharyngioma is responsible for most signs and symptoms, even though these problems may not be the reason for the initial medical evaluation. Almost 93% of children have signs of growth failure, whereas most adults develop sexual or menstrual dysfunction (decreased sexual drive in 88% of men and primary or secondary amenorrhea in 82% of women).[40, 41]

Because craniopharyngiomas are slow-growing extra-axial tumors, they may become quite large before causing symptoms, especially in children. Children often tolerate a high degree of visual loss without complaint, continuing their schoolwork and watching television without arousing the suspicion of parents and teachers.[32] Adults generally are more sensitive to visual impairment, and about 90% of adult patients complain of vision loss.[33, 41]

Almost half of patients present with headache,

which is often related to associated hydrocephalus. Many tumors in children obstruct cerebrospinal fluid pathways and cause signs and symptoms of increased intracranial pressure. Large tumors in adults may cause psychiatric symptoms or memory loss and may or may not result in associated hydrocephalus.[42] In these patients, apathy, incontinence, depression, and hypersomnia may be noted. Long-standing mentation deficits and profound memory loss are associated with a poor prognosis.[10] Mental changes characteristic of Korsakoff's syndrome were found in 3 of 12 adult patients in the series by Kahn and coauthors.[12] Large cystic tumors may extend into the posterior fossa, and three cases of patients presenting with hearing loss have been reported.[43]

DIAGNOSTIC IMAGING

Almost all craniopharyngiomas have their origin from cells in the pituitary stalk, either above or below the level of the diaphragma sellae. Despite this common origin, the configuration, geometry, and growth pattern of these tumors vary greatly. Fahlbusch and coworkers[41] emphasized several important anatomic distinctions that must be made: whether the tumor (1) is below the diaphragma sellae, (2) above the diaphragma sellae and simply elevates the hypothalamus and third ventricle, or (3) actually penetrates and is within the third ventricle.

Both computed tomography (CT) and magnetic resonance imaging (MRI) are useful in showing the tumor mass, its general configuration, and its relationship to the ventricular system and major cranial arteries (Fig. 237–5). Enhancement with contrast agent, generally more sensitive on MRI, often brings out poorly defined cyst walls and allows visualization of the solid portions of the tumor. The cystic portion of craniopharyngiomas may be lucent or hyperintense on CT or MRI, depending on the protein content or suspension of calcium salts within the tumor cyst fluid.[43]

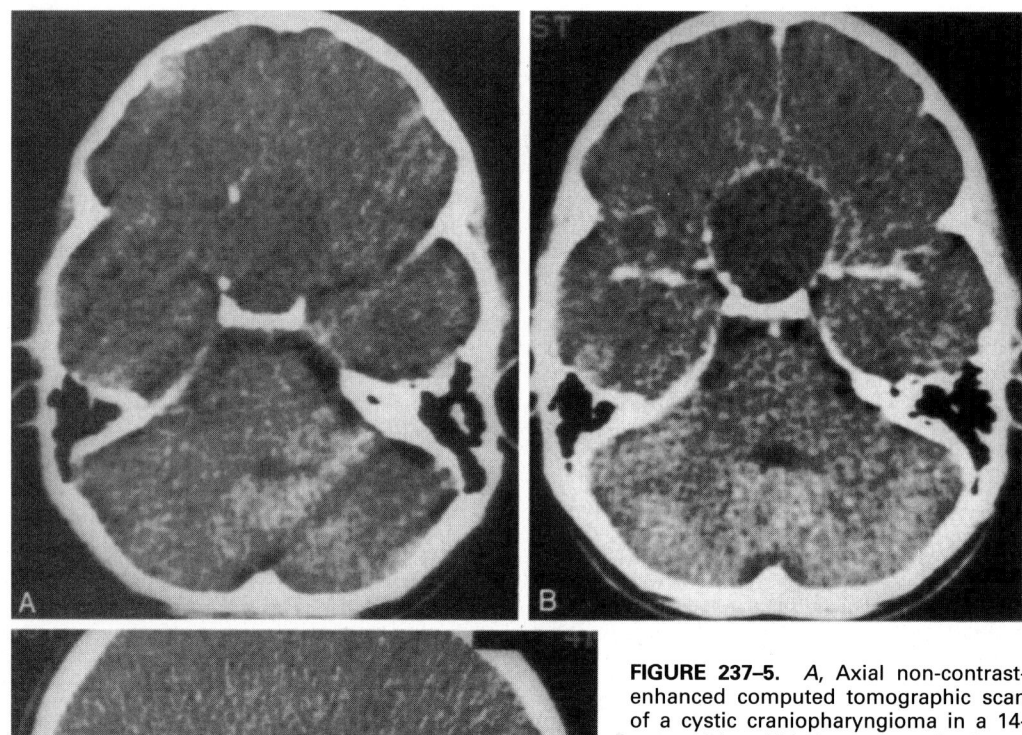

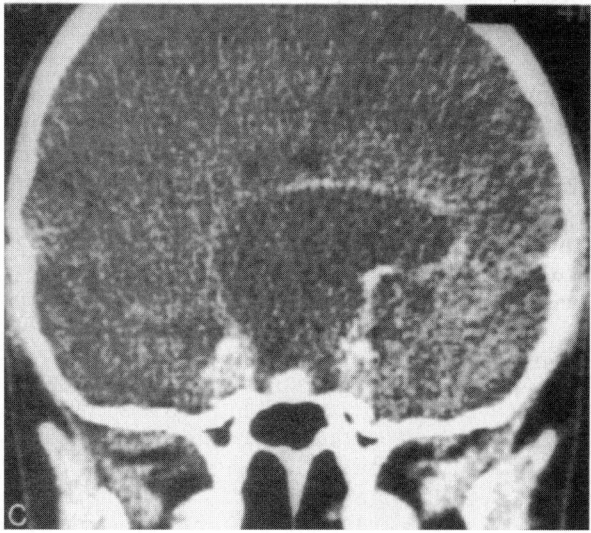

FIGURE 237–5. *A,* Axial non-contrast-enhanced computed tomographic scan of a cystic craniopharyngioma in a 14-year-old boy. This large tumor is almost isodense with the surrounding brain tissue and is poorly defined. Two calcified areas on the left side of the cyst wall are seen, suggesting the diagnosis. *B,* Axial computed tomographic scan of the same patient after contrast enhancement. The tumor is well defined, and the cyst wall and calcifications are seen. *C,* Coronal contrast-enhanced computed tomographic scan of the same child. The marked asymmetry of the tumor, which will modify the operative approach, is readily appreciated. This child was studied because of his small size and delayed maturation, but he was neurologically intact and had normal visual fields and acuity.

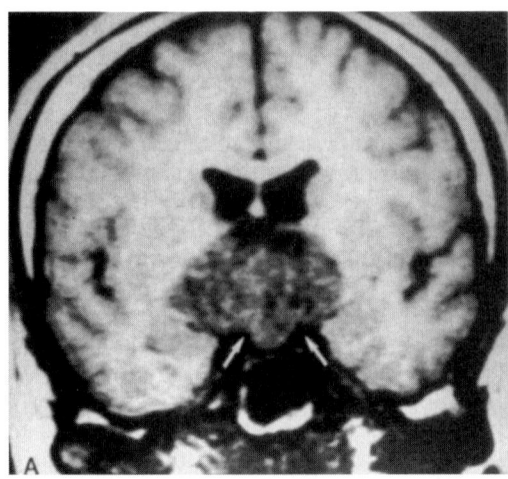
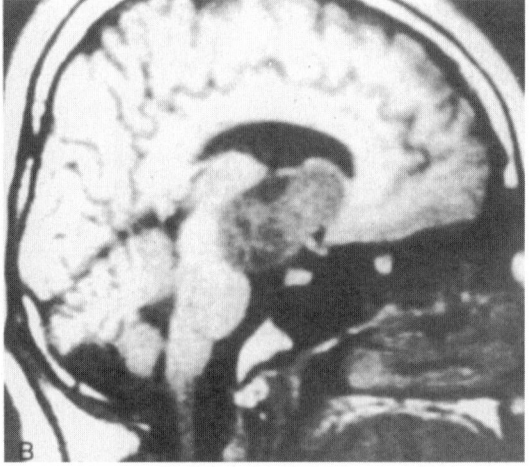

FIGURE 237–6. *A,* Coronal magnetic resonance imaging (MRI) scan of a 22-year-old woman who presented with marked mentation and personality changes, obesity, and amenorrhea. The tumor is not entirely contained within the third ventricle and is accessible through basal subarachnoid pathways *(arrows).* Small, dark regions within the lower part of the tumor are calcific areas, whereas the larger dark areas at the top of the tumor are cysts. *B,* Sagittal MRI scan of the same patient. The relationship of the tumor to the optic chiasm and the brainstem is delineated. The subfrontal and transcallosal routes, as a two-stage procedure, were used to approach the tumor. A portion of the tumor that remained after the second operation was treated by stereotactic radiotherapy.

The sagittal view on MRI is very useful, permitting definition of the relationship between the tumor and the optic nerves and chiasm. Heavily T2-weighted MRI scans help define the relationship of the anterior optic pathways in patients with suprasellar tumors.[44] On sagittal and coronal views, it is important to discern whether the tumor abuts the cerebrospinal fluid pathways in the suprasellar region. Tumors that appear to be entirely within the third ventricle on axial CT may actually be visible in the suprasellar cisterns. These tumors can be removed by a totally extra-axial approach once the basal portion of the tumor is identified and exposed in the basal cisterns (Fig. 237–6).

CT often reveals fine calcification within the tumor. It also shows the details of remolding of the basal skull anatomy by the tumor. Kucharczyk and Montanera,[45] however, pointed out that the solid, calcified portions of craniopharyngiomas may be completely overlooked on MRI alone. Visualization of the major arteries around the surface of the tumor may be easily revealed on either CT or magnetic resonance angiography. Direct angiography is no longer a requirement for this surgery.

EVALUATION OF ENDOCRINE FUNCTION

Evaluation of pituitary function is generally obtained preoperatively. Both hypoadrenalism and hypothyroidism may contribute to poor intra- or postoperative results.[32] Hypoadrenalism can be adequately treated by the high doses of steroids used to prevent edema resulting from brain retraction. Hypothyroidism is more difficult to correct and may take longer to normalize. Although the preoperative endocrine evalua-

tion may be interesting diagnostically, the more significant determination of endocrine status is made postoperatively, after all endocrine supplements have been stopped. The need for continuing endocrine, neuro-ophthalmologic, and neuropsychological follow-up must be emphasized.[31]

OPERATIVE MANAGEMENT

Hydrocephalus and Large-Volume Cysts

Many patients with craniopharyngioma present with symptoms of hydrocephalus, which is the most common presenting pattern in children with this tumor.[32] In many patients, the cystic portions of the tumor are of considerable volume. Managing the volume displacement caused by the amount of cyst fluid or tumor size is of primary importance.[46] When the presenting symptoms are related solely to hydrocephalus, a shunting procedure is indicted. If the tumor has obstructed both foramina of Monro, bilateral ventricular catheters, united to a single shunting system, may be required (Fig. 237–7). In tumors with a single large-volume cyst, it may be useful to drain the cyst to achieve volume reduction before surgery.

Decompression over a period of time is preferable to a single aspiration of fluid for the relief of hydrocephalus and drainage of cysts. For patients with hydrocephalus, overnight drainage may be useful to reduce intracranial pressure and reduce volume in a controlled manner. Similarly, overnight drainage of cyst fluid by way of an external catheter prevents sudden intracranial decompression.

Tumor Removal

Many operative approaches to craniopharyngiomas exist, and the choice is determined by the size and loca-

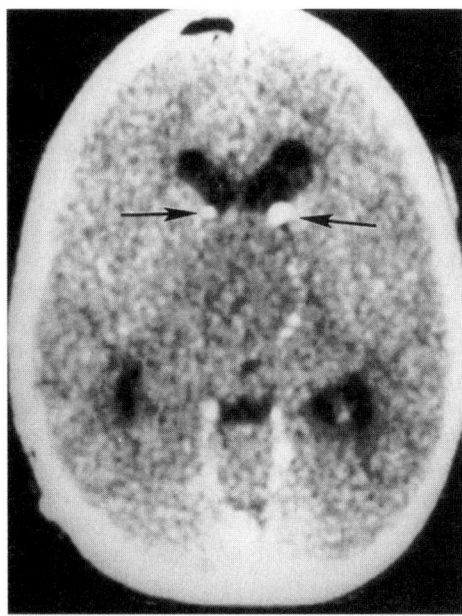

FIGURE 237–7. Axial computed tomographic scan of a 7-year-old boy with a large, partially cystic craniopharyngioma after bilateral ventricular shunting. The tumor fills the third ventricle, obstructing both foramina of Monro. The hydrocephalus had been largely relieved 4 days after shunting, at the time of this scan. The arrows point to the ventricular catheters.

tion of the tumor, degree of calcification, location of cystic portions, and accessibility to cerebrospinal fluid pathways. Within the range of choices, which are presented in Table 237–1, certain principles can be discerned. In general, extra-axial approaches are preferred

to transaxial routes, unilateral approaches are preferable to the elevation of both frontal lobes, and resection of functional neural tissue is rarely indicated to reach these tumors. The right subfrontal approach has the advantage of limiting retraction to the nondominant hemisphere and is easier for most right-handed surgeons. A left frontal or bifrontal approach, however, may be indicated when there is major tumor extension into the left frontal region or into the left middle fossa.[47, 48]

A bicoronal skin incision is preferred in most cases. The bone flap should be placed as low as possible along the base of the frontal fossa, usually avoiding the frontal sinus. When greater retrosellar exposure is desired, the lateral portion of the sphenoid wing is extensively removed, and a more generous craniotomy is performed, including the anterior temporal region. This approach allows opening of the sylvian fissure and exposure of the interpeduncular region. The subfrontal approach may be subdivided into several different routes (Fig. 237–8). Access between the optic nerves is achieved by either the subchiasmatic route or by removal of portions of the tuberculum sellae. Opening the lamina terminalis exposes portions of tumor that extend into the third ventricle. The tumor may be approached lateral to the optic nerve and optic tract on either side of the carotid artery. The surgeon should evaluate each of these possible routes and choose the one that allows the greatest exposure of tumor surface. A tumor filling the third ventricle pushes the chiasm forward and the optic tracts laterally. Displacement of the optic apparatus decreases the space available for dissection and creates the appearance of a prefixed chiasm.[33, 46]

T A B L E   2 3 7 – 1 ■ **Operative Approaches for Craniopharyngiomas**

APPROACH	ADVANTAGES	DISADVANTAGES
Extra-axial Approaches		
Subfrontal	Good visualization of optic nerve and chiasm Good visualization of ipsilateral carotid artery Below circle of Willis	Poor visualization of mass within third ventricle Poor visualization of undersurface of ipsilateral tract, chiasm
Pterional	Shortest distance to parasellar region Below circle of Willis	Essentially unilateral Poor visualization of contralateral optic nerve
Lamina terminalis	Good visualization of retrosellar region Good visualization of anterior third ventricle Allows separation of mass from choroid plexus, internal cerebral veins	Difficulty in locating lateral landmarks Highest risk of hypothalamic damage
Transaxial Approaches		
Transsphenoidal	Avoids craniotomy; direct visualization of tumor within sella Good decomposition of undersurface of chiasm	Poor visualization of anterior, lateral, or interpeduncular extension of tumor Difficult if both sella and pituitary gland are normal
Transcallosal	Largely extra-axial on medial hemispheric surface Good visualization of both walls of third ventricle Allows approach to both sides of anterior third ventricular tumor	Divides anterior corpus callosum Risk of bilateral fornix damage Difficulty in identifying landmarks
Transcortical	Ease of landmark identification Good visualization of ipsilateral foramen of Monro Good visualization of anterior and contralateral third ventricle walls	Requires hydrocephalus Poor visualization of third ventricle walls Divides frontal region cortex; possible postoperative seizure disorder

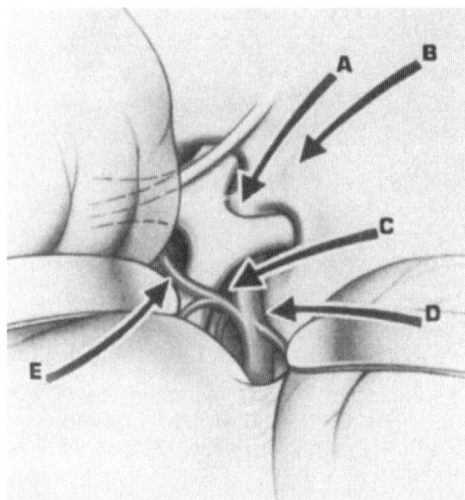

FIGURE 237–8. The subfrontal approach can be subdivided into several different routes: A, subchiasmatic; B, drilling into the sphenoid sinus to enlarge the subchiasmatic exposure; C, lateral to the optic chiasm and optic tract; D, lateral to the carotid artery; and E, opening of the lamina terminalis.

The tumor is exposed by opening the cisternal arachnoid along the edge of the sphenoid ridge, over the optic nerves, and across the tumor. It is important to identify the double (or more) layers of arachnoid and to distinguish the cisternal from the tumor arachnoidal plane (Fig. 237–9). Care is taken not to anneal arachnoid to the tumor capsule by the use of cautery, because preservation of the subarachnoid plane is a major aid in safe and total tumor removal. The optimal plane of dissection is between the tumor arachnoid and the tumor capsule, not in the cisternal plane.

All tumors should be aspirated, including those that appear to be quite solid on scans. Many tumors that appear dense or solid on scans have cystic portions, and aspiration of even a few milliliters of cyst fluid provides more room for dissection. In tumors with large cystic components, only a portion of the fluid is

removed initially, as the turgor of the cyst provides a ballotable surface that aids in separation of the tumor capsule and arachnoid. If too much cyst fluid is removed initially, the capsule may become redundant and make dissection of the planes more difficult.

When a sufficiently large portion of the tumor surface has been dissected, the tumor is entered and its mass reduced by internal debulking. As the tumor mass decreases, arterial feeders to the tumor may be coagulated and divided. Care must be taken to preserve the arterial anastomosis that surrounds the median eminence. This anastomotic ring also supplies the undersurface of the chiasm and optic tracts, and loss of vision may occur if this supply is not spared. The posterior portions of the tumor and those that extend upward into the third ventricle rarely have a major arterial supply and usually are not densely adherent. In reoperations, great caution must be used in removing portions of the tumor that directly underlie the basilar and posterior cerebral artery system, where adhesions are often very dense.

Portions of the capsule that are brought into view may be resected, with care being taken not to "lose the handle." Particularly with a shunt in place, those portions of the tumor within the third ventricle rapidly recede out of sight if released and are extremely difficult to retrieve. In children, the calcific portions of the tumor tend to be located at the base, often lying beneath the chiasm and optic nerves. These pieces of calcium must be crushed before delivering them past the optic apparatus, which is often difficult. Occasionally, it may be necessary to use the high-speed diamond drill to break up calcified fragments before removal.

The remaining fragments of the tumor are sharply dissected from the undersurface of the optic apparatus and hypothalamus. Small, angled dental mirrors are then used to inspect the undersurface of the chiasm and the median eminence for tumor remnants. Use of an endoscope to view areas not directly viewed through the microscope has proved useful.

Other Operative Approaches

Small craniopharyngiomas located entirely within the sella have been reported.[33, 49] On CT, these tumors appear as lucent areas within the sella turcica; in women, they may be mistakenly diagnosed as prolactinomas. Their removal by the transsphenoidal route is easily accomplished, and the tumor capsule is usually readily identified. Even tumors that have a considerable suprasellar component may be readily removed transsphenoidally if they have elevated the diaphragma sellae on their upper surface, with the tumor remaining subdiaphragmatic.[49]

Large tumors that have penetrated through the diaphragma sellae, especially those that are densely calcified, are difficult to remove transsphenoidally, even when the sella is widely eroded. Laws and coauthors[50] reported a case in which manipulation of a very large, calcified intrasellar tumor resulted in damage to both carotid arteries. Very large cystic tumors, however (even those with considerable suprasellar extension),

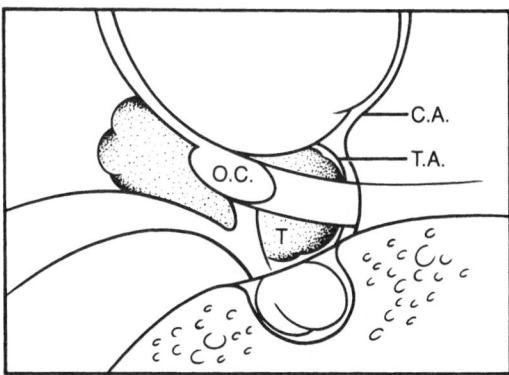

FIGURE 237–9. Schematic sagittal view of tumor (T) arising in the suprasellar region, appearing beneath the optic chiasm (O.C.). The tumor is invested by a layer of arachnoid (T.A.) and is covered by the cisternal arachnoid (C.A.). As the tumor grows, the layers may become fused over some or even most of the tumor surface.

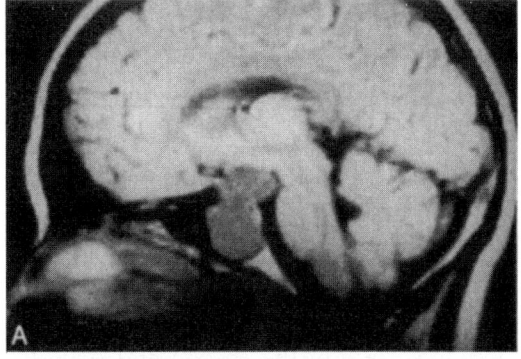
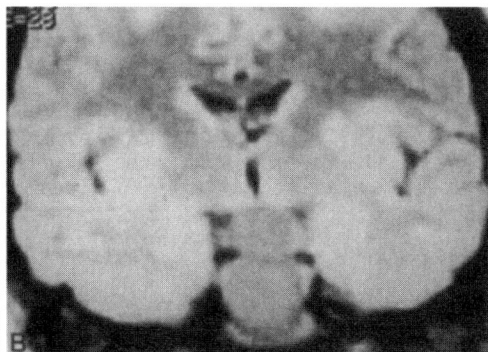
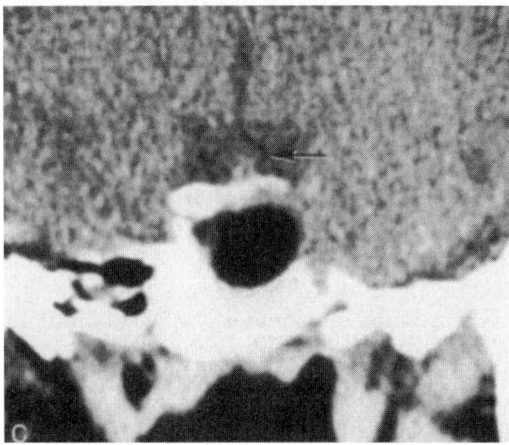

FIGURE 237–10. *A,* Sagittal magnetic resonance imaging (MRI) scan of a 20-year-old woman with a large cystic craniopharyngioma. She had experienced recent secondary amenorrhea and bifrontal headaches but no visual disturbance. *B,* Coronal MRI scan of the same patient. The tumor is constricted across the midportion by the diaphragma sellae. The diaphragm is occasionally difficult to enlarge, especially when the circular dural sinuses of this structure remain patent. A small diaphragmatic aperture may limit access to the suprasellar portion of the tumor. *C,* Coronal computed tomographic scan taken after tumor removal. The pituitary stalk *(arrow)* is preserved and is seen in the suprasellar cistern. The sella turcica has been packed with fat to prevent the syndrome of chiasmatic prolapse.

may be removed by this route (Figs. 237–10*A* and *B*). It may be useful to inject air intrathecally to outline the dome of the tumor on image intensification as the capsule is being removed, thus visualizing adherent structures on the superior surface of the tumor. When the tumor has caused extensive erosion of the sella, it may be necessary to pack the sella with fat to prevent the syndrome of chiasmatic prolapse (see Fig. 237–10*C*).

Use of the bifrontal approach for craniopharyngioma has been advocated and beautifully illustrated by Samii and Bini.[48] This approach requires very careful dissection of the olfactory tracts back to the olfactory trigone bilaterally, and it allows excellent visualization of the tumor on both sides. The lamina terminalis is then seen *en face,* which allows for excellent orientation to the midline. Samii persuaded me to use this approach, which was carried out in six consecutive cases. Having to operate around both olfactory tracts and both optic nerves was somewhat annoying, and in two cases, an olfactory tract was lost due to overretraction.

Opening of the lamina terminalis is an important step in adequately removing tumors that have invaded the third ventricle, as well as for many tumors that have only invaginated the ventricle. Gentle pressure on the floor of the third ventricle often allows one to see the small tumor remnant at the base of the ventricle, which is apparent in the suprasellar cistern. The bifrontal approach allows one to precisely locate the midline, and any approach that is laterally displaced correspondingly impairs one's perspective of the midline. The unilateral subfrontal approach distorts this perspective only minimally, whereas the pterional approach makes orientation and visualization within the third ventricle more difficult.

Approaches through and under the temporal lobe have been described. One series reported 20 patients who were operated on using resection of a portion of the anterior temporal lobe and attempting radical removal of the tumor.[29] Although this series had only one operative death, two additional patients died shortly after surgery as a result of an altered level of consciousness that led to pneumonia.

Transaxial approaches, either through the corpus callosum or transfrontally-transventricularly, can be used for craniopharyngiomas within the third ventricle. Yasargil and coauthors[51] described combining them with the subfrontal approach. For such tumors, it may be necessary to expose more of the third ventricle than can be visualized through the intact foramen of Monro. Several methods of opening the third ventricle are available: (1) dividing a single fornix, (2) dividing a vein near the foramen, (3) entering under the choroid plexus, and (4) separating the internal cerebral veins.[46, 52, 53]

Occasionally, it is necessary to stage operative procedures to achieve total tumor removal. Most often, this involves intracranial removal of the suprasellar portion of the tumor, followed later by transsphenoidal resection of intrasellar portions.[33, 36, 47] Portions of the tumor may extend into the middle or posterior fossa, making removal by a subfrontal route impossible. In these cases, a subsequent transtemporal or infratemporal approach, or even a posterior fossa approach, may be required.

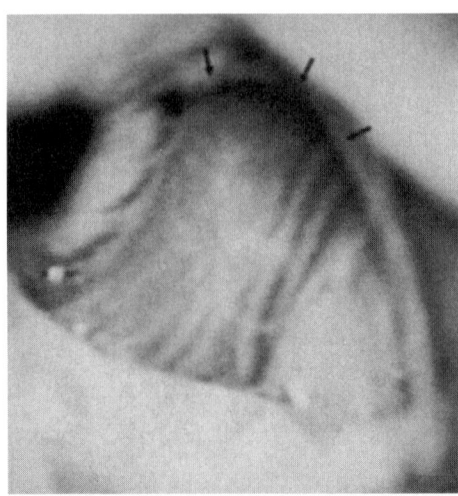

FIGURE 237–11. Operative view of the pituitary stalk after removal of the large craniopharyngioma seen in Figure 237–7. The stalk is identified by the constant location of penetration through the diaphragma sellae *(arrows)* and by its striate appearance. These striations are the long portal veins that run along the stalk surface. The striations remain parallel, even when the stalk is distorted by the tumor. (Reproduced from videotape.)

Preserving the Pituitary Stalk

Preservation of the pituitary stalk is now technically possible using contemporary microscopic visualization during radical removal of craniopharyngiomas.[33, 47, 48] Even when the stalk is damaged, a remnant of it reaching from the median eminence to the pituitary may serve as a matrix on which the pituitary portal system may re-form.[54, 55]

Identification of the stalk is basic to its preservation. Although the stalk may be displaced to any part of the tumor surface, it can be located as it penetrates the diaphragma sellae to reach the pituitary. A further identifying feature is the striate appearance caused by the long portal veins on the stalk surface. Even when the stalk is severely displaced, these vessels maintain their parallel arrangement (Fig. 237–11). These striations are unique among suprasellar structures.[31, 33]

Cyst Aspiration

Aspiration of cystic craniopharyngiomas, either before radiotherapy or for the treatment of cyst recurrence by isotope instillation, has been recommended by several authors.[56–58] Drainage has been used for cyst recurrence of childhood tumors until the child's growth is completed and radiotherapy can be given. An excellent course was reported in a patient with a cystic tumor that drained spontaneously through the nasopharynx for 3 decades.[59]

Insertion of a catheter connected to an Ommaya reservoir into the cystic portion of the tumor has been recommended to facilitate aspiration of fluid contents.[46, 60] This operative procedure is probably more widely used than most series indicate. It is rarely effective if the cyst wall has been resected before insertion of the catheter, because the catheter is excluded from the cystic portion of the tumor as the wall re-forms (Fig. 237–12). Even when the catheter is inserted directly into the cyst through a needle puncture, it may quickly become walled off by growth of a fibrous sheath around it.

Postoperative Care

Patients undergoing craniotomy usually receive large doses of high-potency synthetic corticosteroids to control cerebral swelling. These synthetic steroids have little of the mineralocorticoid effect of cortisone acetate. As the synthetic steroids are progressively tapered, cortisone replacement is given in physiologic doses. Patients who have undergone operations for craniopharyngiomas must be regarded as having hypoadrenalism and therefore need supplemental corticosteroids when fighting infection, under stress, or febrile. The death of a patient during a metyrapone test after removal of a craniopharyngioma was reported.[61]

Diabetes insipidus is an almost invariable consequence of total or radical subtotal removal of craniopharyngiomas. Fluid replacement is the best initial management. If excessive thirst or frequent urination poses difficulty for the patient, or if severe hypernatremia develops, short-acting preparations of vasopressin may be given. It must be remembered that the natural sequence of antidiuretic hormone (ADH) release after pituitary stalk section is triphasic.[62] After the initial cessation of ADH secretion owing to disruption of the pituitary stalk, axon terminals within the posterior pituitary degenerate and release their hormone (ADH) in supraphysiologic amounts. This release is usually seen between 48 and 96 hours after stalk damage. If patients have been given a long-acting antidiuretic preparation, they may be at risk for renal shutdown after the release of endogenous ADH. After total depletion of ADH from the degenerating terminals, diabetes insipidus returns. Desmopressin acetate by intravenous injection, pill, or nasal spray may be used. Careful and frequent observation of urine specific gravity, fluid intake and output, and serum electrolyte values is required for the successful management of postoperative diabetes insipidus.

Those patients who have diabetes insipidus combined with loss of thirst sensation pose a difficult management problem. This syndrome usually results from damage to osmoreceptors in the anterior hypothalamus, as well as division of the pituitary stalk.[54] Patients without thirst sensation are unable to help in the regulation of their serum electrolyte levels, and complications related to hypernatremia frequently result. Other hypothalamic deficit syndromes that occur after removal of craniopharyngiomas include disturbances of caloric balance, changes in wakefulness, changes in affective behavior, and memory disturbances.[47, 54]

Operative deaths after removal of craniopharyngiomas usually are attributed to hypothalamic injury, which causes a clinical syndrome characterized by hyperpyrexia and somnolence. In one case, a patient survived with fluctuating levels of consciousness for 15 months postoperatively before dying of pneumonia.[29]

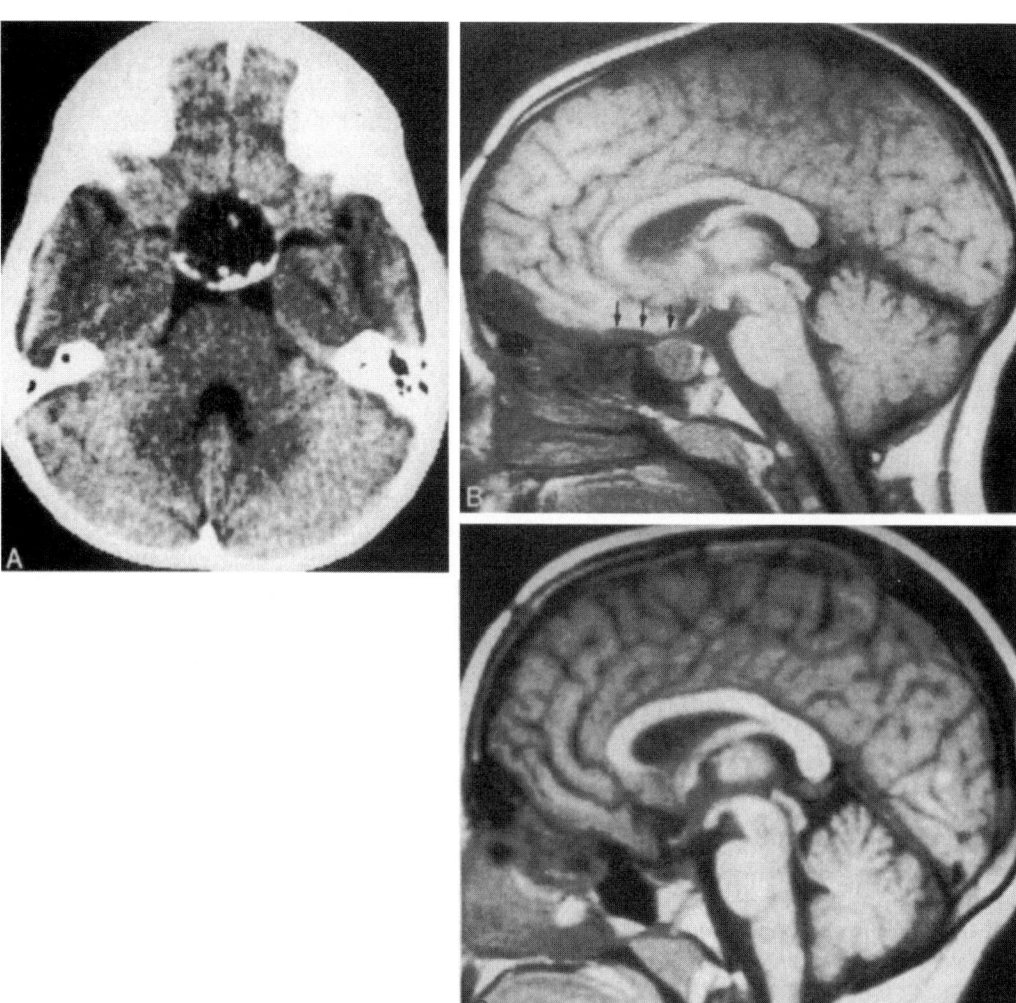

FIGURE 237-12. *A,* Axial computed tomographic scan of a 12-year-old girl with vision loss. This large cystic tumor was subtotally resected at another institution. The tumor recurred, and 10 months later a second craniotomy was performed. At that time, a calcified fragment was left under the left optic nerve, because the child had vision only in the left nasal field. A catheter was placed in the tumor bed and connected to an Ommaya reservoir. One course of radiotherapy was given. *B,* Sagittal magnetic resonance imaging (MRI) scan taken almost 2 years after the second craniotomy shows cystic tumor recurrence. Vision in the left nasal field was decreasing. The catheter *(dark line, arrows)* was excluded from the cyst as the tumor recurred. Aspiration from the reservoir did not yield cystic fluid, and the catheter was thought to be obstructed. *C,* Sagittal MRI scan taken after a third craniotomy performed 34 months after the first operation. At surgery, the catheter was found to be indenting the left chiasm and was being forced upward by the growing cyst. The tumor was thought to be totally removed, and vision returned in the left eye to the degree present after the second craniotomy.

Results

Most neurosurgeons would agree that total removal of craniopharyngiomas is the most desirable operative outcome and that it offers the best chance of cure.[32, 47, 48, 51, 63] The surgeon's judgment determines whether an attempt at total removal is worth the risk of possible operative mortality and functional impairment of the patient. Excellent results have been reported with attempted radical removal, including some series with zero mortality or very low risk.[47, 48, 51, 64, 65] Mortality rates after attempts at radical removal of craniopharyngiomas vary widely; however, most large series report rates from 1% to 10%. Mortality rates of 35%, even for

very large tumors treated contemporarily, would be regarded by most neurosurgeons as unacceptable.[66] Others regard craniopharyngiomas as malignant lesions with a dangerous location and growth pattern and believe that no forceful attempt at total extirpation should be made.[67]

Some craniopharyngiomas cannot be removed completely. The tumor may be so densely adherent to important neural or vascular structures that safe excision is precluded, and further treatment for the residual tumor is likely to be needed. There are also cases in which either immediate or long-term postoperative scans show a tumor fragment, even though the surgeon believed that total excision was achieved. These so-called inadvertent residuals may be treated by radiotherapy, watched for subsequent growth and then treated (as in Fig. 237–3), or immediately reoperated on. This last approach has been highly successful, leading to a number of surgical cures.

Data indicate that subtotal or partial resection alone is rarely satisfactory treatment for these tumors, which are likely to recur over time.[32, 68] Recurrence has an adverse effect on survival.[69] Sung and coauthors[20] reported that less than 10% of patients treated with subtotal removal alone are recurrence free 10 years postoperatively. Certain craniopharyngiomas may be quiescent for years after partial resection, and some patients may lead virtually symptom-free lives despite only partial tumor removal.[19, 40] These anecdotal cases may have been overemphasized in the treatment of craniopharyngiomas. In fact, the great majority of tumors that are removed subtotally will recur within 3 years. Tumors that are radically removed take longer to recur than do those that are only partially removed.[32, 68] Patients with subtotal tumor removal will likely require further therapy— either irradiation or reoperation.

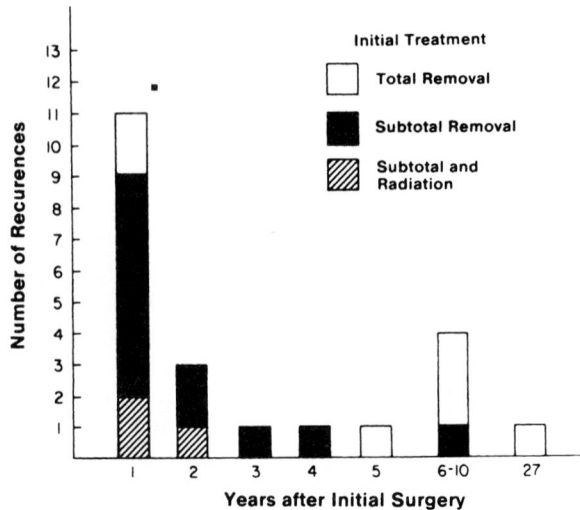

FIGURE 237–13. Time of recurrence of craniopharyngioma. Most tumors that recur do so within the first 3 years after surgery. (Data from Sung DI, Chang CH, Harisiadis L, Carmel PW: Treatment results of craniopharyngioma. Cancer 47:847–852, 1981.)

RADIOTHERAPY

More than 70 years ago, Carpenter and coauthors[57] reported on a small group of patients in whom radiotherapy for craniopharyngiomas produced marked improvement. These authors concluded that although the tumor was not destroyed by x-rays, the cells that produced secretions and formed cysts were killed.[70] After this preliminary report, doubt persisted that radiotherapy could destroy craniopharyngioma epithelium.[28] In the 1960s, Kramer and coauthors[71, 72] reported excellent results with subtotal tumor removal and supravoltage irradiation. After this report, many studies indicated that radiotherapy both increases survival and lengthens the interval before tumor recurrence.[20, 65, 70, 73] Survival rates for patients treated with operation and radiotherapy are better than for those treated with operation alone; the recurrence-free survival rates are improved to an even greater extent.[20] Excellent results have been reported with the use of radical subtotal removal followed by radiotherapy. Baskin and Wilson[40] reported that 91% of 74 patients treated by this method were in remission and that the operative mortality was 3%. Shapiro and coauthors[60] described better recurrence-free rates for patients undergoing radical subtotal removal before radiotherapy than for those undergoing simple biopsy and cyst drainage before irradiation. Merchant and coauthors[74] recently recommended conservative debulking of these tumors, followed by irradiation.

The hazards of radiotherapy must not be overlooked. Radiation necrosis, endocrine deficiency, optic neuritis, and dementia have all been reported as complications.[32] Radiation may actually induce tumors, including meningiomas, sarcomas, and gliomas (Figs. 237–13 and 237–14) . Particularly in children, radiotherapy may seriously damage the capacity for intellectual

performance.[75] Thus, there is an increasing tendency at my institution to defer radiotherapy in pediatric patients. It is not clear at what age the deleterious effects of radiation on maturation of the brain cease to be a major factor. Adverse effects of radical operative procedures on intellectual performance also have been reported.[75]

Data for late neuropsychological and cognitive function remain sparse and contradictory for both surgery and radiotherapy for craniopharyngioma. A group of 12 children treated by radical surgery alone showed no cognitive or short-term memory deficits, although three children were found to have mild attention deficits.[76] A prospective study in 13 adults showed that neuropsychological performance was not impaired and that quality-of-life measurements were improved after surgical removal of these tumors.[25]

A recent report of 30 patients, treated between 1984 and 1997, came to a different conclusion. The first 15 patients were treated by surgical attempts at removal, followed by radiotherapy (8 patients). The second group had "limited" surgery, followed by radiotherapy. The limited group had a lower decrease in intelligence quotient (IQ) and fewer endocrine and neurological complications than did the operative group.[74] These same authors, however, reported a later group of patients, treated since 1997 with conformal radiation, in whom neuropsychometric quantification of radiation-related central nervous system effects was determined. The authors concluded that although children with hemispheric or posterior fossa tumors showed no decline in full-scale IQ, those with central tumors showed a significant decline. In particular, the patients with craniopharyngiomas declined from an average IQ of 91 before radiotherapy to an average IQ of 78 in the first 30 months after therapy.[77]

Reoperation after either tumor recurrence or radiotherapy is widely regarded as being more difficult than

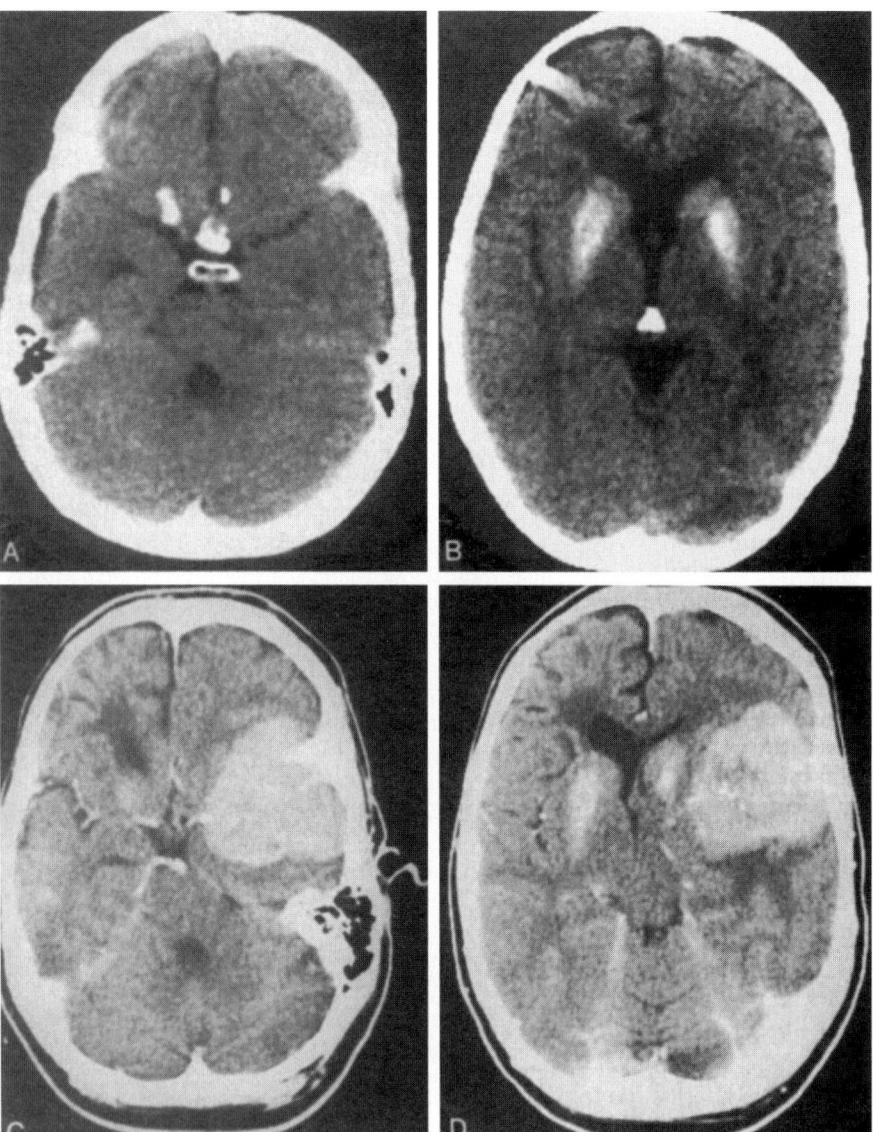

FIGURE 237-14. *A* and *B*, Axial computed tomographic scans of a 20-year-old man who had been treated 13 years earlier for craniopharyngioma. At age 7 years, the tumor was subtotally removed, and a course of radiotherapy (5000 rads) was given. At the time of this scan, the patient was suffering from the recent onset of generalized seizures but was neurologically intact. He was of short stature, somewhat obese, and mildly retarded. The scan shows typical postradiation changes: calcified tumor remnants, calcification in the basal ganglia, and mild atrophy. *C* and *D*, Contrast-enhanced computed tomographic scans taken 2 years after the scans in *A* and *B* (15 years after the initial treatment). This large sphenoid wing tumor was a benign meningioma, despite its apparent rapid growth. The tumor arose in the region of the radiation port on the left side and was believed to be totally removed at reoperation. Seizure frequency markedly decreased postoperatively.

primary surgery, and even surgeons who advocate radical tumor resection at the initial operation consider reoperation for recurrence unduly hazardous. Undoubtedly, it is true that locating arachnoidal planes and dealing with scarring are more difficult in tumors that have recurred or been irradiated; however, in my experience, this does not preclude successful removal of these tumors (Fig. 237–15).

Those who routinely attempt total removal of craniopharyngiomas are not always successful.[30, 31, 68] Even after apparent total removal by experienced neurosurgeons using micro-operative technique, there is a noticeable rate of tumor recurrence. Amacher[63] reviewed several series and documented 17 recurrences after 92 total excisions. Routine use of advance scanning reveals many, if not all, of these residual tumor fragments, and the "false cure rate" can be expected to decrease. Because of this propensity to recur, instead of referring to these tumors as being removed, many authors say that they have been *radically resected*. This

term should not be used for cases in which a major fragment of the tumor is known to be left.

Stereotactic Radiosurgery

A number of small studies using either gamma knife or linear accelerator stereotactic radiosurgery for craniopharyngioma have been published.[78–80] Stereotactic radiosurgery and intracavitary irradiation or chemotherapy, however, must still be regarded as investigational.[81] More than a decade ago, Lunsford[82] recognized that sudden impairment of the visual field was a complication of the earliest treated patients and recommended a target distance of 3 to 5 mm from optic pathways.

Chung and colleagues[79] have treated tumors with volumes up to 9 cm³. Of 31 patients, 10% had cystic enlargement and 13% had tumor progression over 3 years; one patient has some loss of visual field. Chiou and associates[78] treated 10 patients with a median mar-

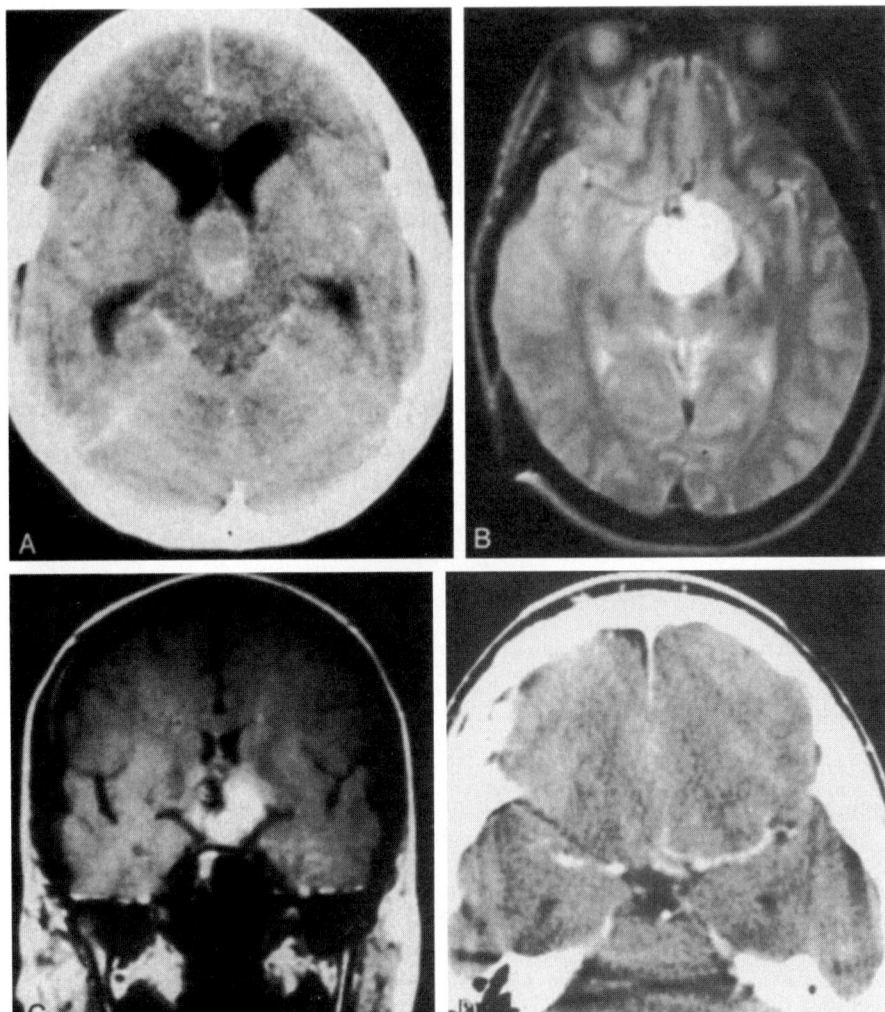

FIGURE 237–15. *A,* Axial contrast-enhanced computed tomographic scan of a 31-year-old woman with headache and some menstrual irregularity. This cystic craniopharyngioma has calcified basal portions. Headache was relieved by shunting. A course of proton beam irradiation was then given. *B* and *C,* Axial and coronal magnetic resonance imaging scans taken 16 months after proton beam irradiation. The patient has amenorrhea, headache, and some vision loss. These T2-weighted scans appear to show cystic areas; however, at surgery, most of the mass was found to be tumor. *D,* Postoperative computed tomographic scan in the same patient. At surgery, a small fragment of solid tumor was believed to have been left adhering to the anterior (A_1) artery on the right.

ginal dose of 16.4 Gy and a dose to optic apparatus limited to less than 8 Gy. Two patients required further radiosurgery. Prior visual defects improved in six patients; however, one patient had continued visual deterioration and lost vision 9 months after treatment.

INTRACYSTIC IRRADIATION OR CHEMOTHERAPY

Increasing experience has been gained in the instillation of radioisotopes into cystic portions of craniopharyngiomas.[56, 58, 83, 84] In most of these protocols, knowledge of cyst volume is necessary for calculating the amount of radioactive substance to be injected, and it is an important factor in determining the minimal effective dose to be delivered to the cyst wall.[85] Leksell[86] suggested that 100 Gy delivered to the cyst surface would collapse the cyst. In a very thin-walled cyst, however, this dosage would have significant penetration into surrounding brain.[28] Several workers have suggested that 200 Gy delivered to the cyst wall would be required.[56, 58] The isotopes most commonly used are phosphorous 32, colloidal gold 198, and colloidal yttrium 91.

Intracystic isotope treatment is limited to those craniopharyngiomas that have a large-volume cystic component. It is not applicable to solid tumors or tumors with very thick or calcified walls. Usually, the cyst volume does not noticeably change initially, but it progressively shrinks over the ensuing weeks and months.[58] There is disagreement whether this method should be employed stereotactically or by direct placement of a catheter into the cyst, with the catheter leading to an external reservoir. Some centers use intracystic isotope therapy primarily, whereas others reserve it for recurrent cystic tumors.[56, 58] A potential problem is radiation of adjacent visual pathways, and serious deterioration of visual function has been described.[87] Difficulty in evaluating this therapy is exemplified by a recent series of six patients treated with intracavitary yttrium 90. Most of the cysts required no further aspiration after isotope instillation (average follow-up was 3.5 years); however, two patients died—at least one of tumor progression.[88]

Bleomycin is a chemotherapeutic agent used to treat epithelial tumors. This led to studies of its use in tissue cultures of craniopharyngiomas (Kubo and coworkers, as cited in Fahlbusch and coauthors[47]). Broggi and colleagues[89] reported shrinkage of 13 of 18 cysts after stereotactic instillation of bleomycin. Current protocols recommend an initial course of 2 to 5 mg of bleomycin per dose, three times a week, for 3 to 5 weeks.[90] In a series of 24 patients, Mottolese and associates[91] found that 70% could be stabilized with intracavitary treatment alone.

Bleomycin can be toxic, and its injection should be preceded by a watertightness test. Despite this precaution, perhaps one third of patients experience transient fever, nausea, or vomiting. Other adverse reactions reported include blindness,[91] hypersomnia,[92] and fatal diencephalic damage.[93]

REFERENCES

1. Mott FV, Barrett JOW: Three cases of tumor of the third ventricle. Arch Neurol (Lond) 1:417–440, 1899.
2. Barrow DL, Spector HH, Takei Y, Tindall CT: Symptomatic Rathke's cleft cysts located entirely in the suprasellar region: Review of diagnosis, management and pathogenesis. Neurosurgery 16:766–772, 1985.
3. Rathke H: Ueber die Entsehung der Glandula pituitaria. Arch Anat Physiol Wissensch M:482, 1838.
4. Erdheim J: Ueher Hypophysengangsgeshwulste und Hirncholesteotome. Sitzungsber Akad Wiss (Wien) 118:537–726, 1904.
5. Podoshin L, Rolan L, Altman M, Peyser E: "Pharyngeal" craniopharyngioma. J Laryngol Otol 84:93–99, 1970.
6. Onanoff J: Sur un cas d'epithelioma (etude histologique). Paris, 1892. Cited in Seemayer TA: Pituitary craniopharyngioma with tooth formation. Cancer 29:423–430, 1972.
7. Bernstein HL, Buchino JJ: The histological similarity between craniopharyngioma and odontogenic lesions: A reappraisal. Oral Surg 56:502–511, 1983.
8. Gorlin RJ, Pindborg JJ, Redman BS, et al: The calcifying odontogenic cyst: A new entity and possible analogue of the cutaneous calcifying epithelioma of Malherbe. Cancer 17:723–729, 1964.
9. Shuangshoti S, Netsky MG, Nashold BS: Epithelial cysts related to sella turcica: Proposed origin from neuroepithelium. Arch Pathol Lab Med 90:444–450, 1970.
10. Bartlett JR: Craniopharyngiomas: An analysis of some aspects of symptomatology, radiology and histology. Brain 94:725–732, 1971.
11. McGrath P: Cysts of the sellar and pharyngeal hypophysis. Pathology 3:123–131, 1971.
12. Kahn EA, Cosch HH, Seeger JF, Hicks SP: Forty-five years experience with the craniopharyngioma. Surg Neurol 1:5–12, 1973.
13. Petito CK, DeGirolami U, Earle KM: Craniopharyngiomas: A clinical and pathological review. Cancer 37:1944–1952, 1976.
14. Carmichael HT: Squamous epithelial rests in the hypophysis cerebri. Arch Neurol Psychiatry 26:966–975, 1931.
15. Goldberg CM, Eshbaugh DE: Squamous cell rests of the pituitary gland as related to the origin of craniopharyngiomas: A study of their presence in the newborn and infants up to age four. Arch Pathol Lab Med 70:293–299, 1960.
16. MacCarty CS, Leavens ME, Love JG: Dermoid and epidermoid tumors in the central nervous system of adults. Surg Gynecol Obstet 108:191–198, 1959.
17. Critchley M, Ironside RN: The pituitary adamantinomata. Brain 49:437–481, 1926.
18. Russell DS, Rubinstein LJ: Pathology of Tumors of the Nervous System, 4th ed. Baltimore, Williams & Wilkins, 1977.
19. Pertuiset B: Craniopharyngiomas. In Vinken PJ, Bryun CW (eds): Handbook of Clinical Neurology, vol 18, pt 3. Amsterdam, North Holland, 1975, pp 531–572.
20. Sung DI, Chang CH, Harisiadis L, Carmel PW: Treatment results of craniopharyngiomas. Cancer 47:847–852, 1981.
21. Matson DD, Crigler JF Jr: Management of craniopharyngioma in childhood. J Neurosurg 30:377–390, 1969.
22. Liszczak T, Richardson EP, Phillips JP, et al: Morphological, biochemical, ultrastructural, tissue culture and clinical observations of typical and aggressive craniopharyngiomas. Acta Neuropathol (Berl) 43:191–203, 1978.
23. Cobb JP, Wright JC: Studies on a craniopharyngioma in tissue culture. I. Growth characteristics and alterations produced following exposure to two radiomimetic agents. J Neuropathol Exp Neurol 18:563–568, 1959.
24. Kristopaitis T, Thomas C, Petruzzelli GJ, Lee JM: Malignant craniopharyngiomas. Arch Pathol Lab Med 124:1356–1360, 2000.
25. Honegger J, Barockas A, Sadri B, Fuhlbusch R: Neuropsychological results of craniopharyngioma surgery in adults: A prospective study. Surg Neurol 50:19–28, 1998.
26. Kempe LC: Operative Neurosurgery, vol 1. New York, Springer-Verlag, 1968, pp 90–93.
27. Sweet WH: A review of dermoid, teratoid and teratomatous intracranial tumors. Dis Nerve Syst 1:228–238, 1940.
28. Hoffman HJ, Hendrick BB, Humphreys RP, et al: Management of craniopharyngioma in children. J Neurosurg 47:218–227, 1977.
29. Symon L, Sprich W: Radical excision of craniopharyngioma: Results in 20 patients. J Neurosurg 62:174–181, 1985.
30. Hoffman HJ, DaSilva M, Humphreys RP, et al: Aggressive surgical management of craniopharyngiomas in children. J Neurosurg 76:47–52, 1992.
31. Carmel PW: Management of brain tumors of developmental and congenital origin. In Tindall GT, Cooper PR, Barrow DL (eds): The Practice of Neurosurgery. Baltimore, Williams & Wilkins, 1996, pp 833–846.
32. Carmel PW, Antunes JL, Chang CH: Craniopharyngiomas in children. Neurosurgery 11:382–389, 1982.
33. Carmel PW: Craniopharyngiomas. In Wilkins RB, Rengachary SA (eds): Neurosurgery, vol 1. New York, McGraw-Hill, 1985, pp 905–916.
34. Kernohan JW: Tumors of congenital origin. In Minckler J (ed): Pathology of the Nervous System. New York, McGraw-Hill, 1971, pp 1927–1937.
35. Zulch KJ: Brain Tumors: Their Biology and Pathology, 2nd ed. New York, Springer-Verlag, 1965.
36. Koos WT, Miller MH: Intracranial Tumors of Infants and Children. Stuttgart, Georg Thieme, 1991.
37. Matson DD: Neurosurgery of Infancy and Childhood, 2nd ed. Springfield, IL, Charles C Thomas, 1969, pp 544–574.
38. Choux M, Lena G, Genitori L: Le craniopharyngiome de l'enfant. Neurochirurgie 37(Suppl 1):12–165, 1991.
39. Bunin GR, Surawicz TS, Witman PA, et al: The descriptive epidemiology of craniopharyngioma. J Neurosurg 89:547–551, 1998.
40. Baskin DS, Wilson CB: Surgical management of craniopharyngiomas. A review of 74 cases. J Neurosurg 65:22–27, 1986.
41. Fahlbusch R, Honegger J, Buchfelder M: Clinical features and management of craniopharyngiomas in adults. In Tindall GT, Cooper PR, Barrow DL (eds): The Practice of Neurosurgery, vol 1. Baltimore, Williams & Wilkins, 1996, pp 1159–1174.
42. Garcia-Uria J: Surgical experience with craniopharyngioma in adults. Surg Neurol 9:11–14, 1978.
43. Connally ES, Winfree CJ, Carmel PW: Giant posterior fossa cystic craniopharyngiomas presenting with hearing loss. Report of three cases and review of the literature. Surg Neurol 47:291–299, 1997.
44. Saeki N, Murai H, Kubota M, et al: Heavily T2 weighted MR images of anterior optic pathways in patients with sellar and parasellar tumors: Prediction of surgical anatomy. Acta Neurochir (Wien) 14:25–35, 2002.
45. Kucharczyk W, Montanera WJ: The sellar-parasellar region. In Atlas SW (ed): Magnetic Resonance Imaging of the Brain and Spine. New York, Raven Press, 1991, p 625.
46. Carmel PW: Tumours of the third ventricle. Acta Neurochir (Wien) 75:136–146, 1985.
47. Fahlbusch R, Honegger J, Paulus W, et al: Surgical treatment of craniopharyngiomas: Experiences with 168 patients. J Neurosurg 90:237–250, 1999.
48. Samii M, Bini W: Surgical treatment of craniopharyngiomas. Zentralbl Neurochir 52:17–23, 1991.
49. Honegger J, Buchfelder M, Fahlbusch R, et al: Transsphenoidal microsurgery for craniopharyngioma. Surg Neurol 37:189–196, 1992.
50. Laws ER Jr, Randall RV, Kern EB, Abboud CF: Management of Pituitary Adenomas and Related Lesions. New York, Appleton-Century Crofts, 1982.
51. Yasargil MG, Curic M, Kis M, et al: Total removal of craniopha-

ryngiomas: Approaches and long-term results in 144 patients. J Neurosurg 73:3–11, 1990.

52. Antunes JL, Muraszko K, Quest DO, Carmel PW: Surgical strategies in the management of tumours of the anterior third ventricle. In Brock M (ed): Modern Neurosurgery. Berlin, Springer-Verlag, 1982, pp 215–244.
53. Apuzzo MLJ, Chikovani OK, Gott PS, et al: Transcallosal interfornicial approaches for lesions affecting the third ventricle: Surgical considerations and consequences. Neurosurgery 10:547–554, 1982.
54. Carmel PW: Surgical syndromes of the hypothalamus. Clin Neurosurg 27:133–159, 1979.
55. Carmel PW, Antunes JL, Ferin H: Collection of blood from the pituitary stalk and portal veins in monkeys, and from the pituitary sinusoidal system of monkey and man. J Neurosurg 50:75–80, 1979.
56. Backlund EO: Studies on craniopharyngiomas. III. Stereotaxic treatment with intracystic yttrium-90. Acta Chir Scand 139:237–247, 1973.
57. Carpenter BC, Chamberlin GW, Frazier CH: The treatment of hypophyseal stalk tumors by evacuation and irradiation. Am J Radiol 38:162–177, 1937.
58. Julow J, Lauyi F, Hajda H, et al: The radiotherapy of cystic craniopharyngioma with intracystic instillation of ⁹⁰Y silicate colloid. Acta Neurochir (Wien) 74:94–99, 1985.
59. Maier HC: Craniopharyngioma with erosion and drainage into the nasopharynx: An autobiographical case report. J Neurosurg 62:132–134, 1985.
60. Shapiro K, Till K, Grant ON: Craniopharyngiomas in childhood: A rational approach to treatment. J Neurosurg 50:617–623, 1979.
61. Hoffman HJ: Comment on paper by Patterson RH Jr, Danvlevitch A. Neurosurgery 7:116–117, 1980.
62. Ranson SW, Fisher C, Ingram WR: Hypothalamico-hypophyseal mechanism in diabetes insipidus. Assoc Res Nerv Ment Dis 17:410–432, 1938.
63. Amacher AL: Craniopharyngioma: The controversy regarding radiotherapy. Childs Brain 5:57–64, 1980.
64. Caldarelli M, Colosimo C, DiRocco C: Intra-axial dermoid/epidermoid tumors of the brainstem in children. Surg Neurol 56:97–105, 2001.
65. Hoff JT, Patterson RH Jr: Craniopharyngiomas in children and adults. J Neurosurg 36:2922–2932, 1972.
66. Al-Mefty O, Hassounah M, Weaver P, et al: Microsurgery for giant craniopharyngiomas in children. Neurosurgery 17:585–595, 1985.
67. Mori K, Handa H, Murata T, et al: Results of treatment for craniopharyngioma. Childs Brain 6:303–312, 1980.
68. Sweet WH: Recurrent craniopharyngiomas: Therapeutic alternatives. Clin Neurosurg 27:206–229, 1980.
69. Banna MI: Craniopharyngioma in adults. Surg Neurol 1:202–204, 1973.
70. Kramer S: Craniopharyngioma: The best treatment is conservative surgery and postoperative radiation therapy. In Morley TP (ed): Current Controversies in Neurosurgery. Philadelphia, WB Saunders, 1976, pp 336–343.
71. Kramer S, McKissock W, Concannon JP: Craniopharyngiomas: Treatment by combined surgery and radiation therapy. J Neurosurg 18:217–226, 1961.
72. Kramer S, Southard M, Mansfield CM: Radiotherapy in the management of craniopharyngiomas: Further experiences and late results AJR Am J Roentgenol 103:44–52, 1968.
73. Richmond IL, Wara WM, Wilson CG: Role of radiation therapy in management of craniopharyngiomas in children. Neurosurgery 6:513–517, 1980.
74. Merchant TE, Kiehna EN, Sanford RA, et al: Craniopharyngiomas: The St. Jude Children's Research Hospital experience 1984–2001. Int J Radiat Oncol Biol Phys 53:533–542, 2002.
75. Fischer FC, Welch K, Beth J, et al: Treatment of craniopharyngiomas in children: 1972–1981. J Neurosurg 62:496–501, 1985.
76. Riva D, Pantalesi C, Devote M, et al: Late neuropsychological and behavioral outcome of children, surgically treated for craniopharyngioma. Childs Nerv Syst 14:179–184, 1998.
77. Honeycutt JH, Sanford RA, Kin LE, Merchant TE: Neuropsychometric testing in pediatric patients with localized primary brain tumors [abstract 819]. Paper presented at the annual meeting of the American Association of Neurological Surgeons, Apr 2002, Chicago.
78. Chiou SM, Lunsford LD, Niranjan A, et al: Stereotactic radiosurgery for residual or recurrent craniopharyngioma, after surgery, with or without radiation therapy. Neurooncology 3:159–166, 2001.
79. Chung WY, Pan DH, Shiau CY, et al: Gamma knife radiosurgery for craniopharyngiomas. J Neurosurg 93(Suppl 3):47–56, 2000.
80. Tekeuchi J, Mori K, Moritakes K, et al: Teratomas in the suprasellar region: Report of five cases. Surg Neurol 2:247–255, 1975.
81. Eisenstat DD: Craniopharyngioma. Curr Treatment Options Neurol 3:77–78, 2001.
82. Lunsford LD: Opinions. In Choux M, Lena G, Genetouri L (eds): Le craniopharyngioma de l'enfant. Neurochirurgie 37(Suppl 1):170–171, 1991.
83. Kobayashi T, Kageyama N, O'Hara K: Internal irradiation for cystic craniopharyngioma. J Neurosurg 55:896–903, 1981.
84. Kodama T, Matsukado Y, Uemura S: Intra-capsular irradiation therapy of craniopharyngiomas with radioactive gold: Indication and followup results. Neurol Med Chir (Tokyo) 21:49–58, 1981.
85. Loevinger R, Japha EM, Brownell CL: In Hine, Brownell CL (eds): Radiation Dosimetry. New York, Academic Press, 1956.
86. Leksell L: Stereotaxis and Radiosurgery: An Operative System. Springfield, IL, Charles C Thomas, 1971.
87. Van den Berge JH, Blaauw G, Bruman WAP, et al: Intracavitary brachytherapy of cystic craniopharyngiomas. J Neurosurg 77:545–550, 1992.
88. Blackburn TP, Doughty D, Plowman PN: Stereotactic intracavitary therapy of recurrent cystic craniopharyngioma by installation of 90 yttrium. Br J Neurosurg 13:359–365, 1999.
89. Broggi C, Giorgi C, Franzini A, et al: Preliminary results of intracavitary treatment of craniopharyngioma with bleomycin. J Neurosurg Sci 33:145–148, 1989.
90. Hader WJ, Steinbok P, Hukin J, Fryer C. Intratumoral therapy with bleomycin for cystic craniopharyngiomas in children. Pediatr Neurosurg 33:211–218, 2000.
91. Mottolese C, Stan H, Hermier M, et al: Intracystic chemotherapy with bleomycin in the treatment of craniopharyngiomas. Childs Nerv Syst 17:724–730, 2001.
92. Haisa T, Ueki K, Yoshida S: Toxic effects of bleomycin on the hypothalamus following its administration into a cystic craniopharyngioma. Br J Neurosurg 8:747–750, 1994.
93. Savas A, Erdem A, Tun K, Karplot Y: Fatal toxic effect of bleomycin on brain tissue after intracystic chemotherapy for a craniopharyngioma: Case report. Neurosurgery 46:213–217, 2000.

CHAPTER 238

Brain Tumors of Disordered Embryogenesis

PETER CARMEL

The tumors of disordered embryogenesis include craniopharyngiomas, colloid cysts, inclusion cysts, epidermoids, dermoids, teratomas, and lipomas. These tumors are a heterogeneous group of neoplasms that have in common their congenital origin and slow growth rate. Indeed, many of these tumors have so little growth potential that they are often considered hamartomatous. Because of their slow growth, it is not unusual for these congenital lesions to first appear clinically during adulthood. Despite their generally benign histologic character and extra-axial location, these tumors are not easily removed, and optimal therapy remains mired in controversy. Rarely, these neoplasms do have malignant potential.

Craniopharyngiomas are discussed separately in Chapter 237; the other tumors of disordered embryogenesis are covered in this chapter.

COLLOID CYST

Colloid cyst is a term applied to a group of cystic tumors filled with gelatinous, viscous material and generally found in the region of the foramen of Monro. It is a relatively rare tumor, constituting less than 1% of all intracranial tumors.[1, 2] Its importance in neurosurgical thinking is a result of its legendary ability to cause sudden death, the difficulty of diagnosing this tumor before computed tomography and magnetic resonance imaging, and the unresolved debate concerning its pathologic origin.

Wallman[3] first described this tumor in 1858 when he reported an autopsy of a 50-year-old man with gait abnormality and involuntary micturition and defecation. Premorbid diagnosis of colloid cysts was not possible until the introduction of ventriculography and pneumoencephalography by Dandy.[4, 5] Dandy later reported on five patients with colloid cysts who had been operated on, with successful removal in four patients.[5]

These tumors have been reported in patients of all ages, from young infants to the elderly. Colloid cysts are not infrequently found incidentally at autopsy, including that of Harvey Cushing.[6] The highest incidence is in patients from 20 to 40 years of age, and there is no gender preponderance.

Pathology

The walls of a colloid cyst usually consist of a single layer of ciliated and nonciliated columnar epithelium. This lining may be variable, and stratified epithelium of columnar, cuboidal, or squamosal cells has been described. This cellular layer abuts a collagenous connective tissue stroma. The material within the cyst is gelatinous and homogeneous and is positive on periodic acid–Schiff staining. The ratio of ciliated and nonciliated cells in the cyst is variable from area to area in the same patient and may also vary greatly from one patient to another.

On electron microscopy, the epithelial cells lining the cyst consist of two types. The first group is ciliated and has microvilli. The second type is more electron dense, has well-developed endoplasmic reticulum, and can contain prominent vacuolar spaces. This arrangement strongly suggests a secretory function for these cells.[7]

The pathologic picture just described and the usual location of these cysts at the foramen of Monro have led to at least four theories of pathogenesis. Derivation from choroidal epithelium, from ependymal cells, and from the paraphysis has been described.[8–12] In addition, Hirano and Ghatak[7] suggested that colloid cysts arise from an endodermal source rather than from the neuroepithelial sources just listed. These authors found that the secretory cells of a colloid cyst are covered by an electron-dense surface coat not found in neuroepithelium at any stage of development. Moreover, in colloid cysts, the epithelium rests on a prominent basement lamina not found with ependyma.

At the beginning of the 20th century, Sjovall[11] suggested that these peculiar cysts might arise from the paraphysis, which is an invagination in the roof of the third ventricle that occurs during embryogenesis. Although this structure has a secretory function in amphibians, it has lost all functional significance in humans and generally degenerates by the 100-mm embryonic stage. Because the paraphysis is located where most colloid cysts develop, this derivation is widely accepted.[13] However, this derivation cannot explain the colloid cysts found in the septum pellucidum, posterior portions of the third ventricle, and fourth ventricle.

Cystic structures are commonly found in the choroid plexus, and this finding raises the possibility that the choroid gives rise to colloid cysts. Choroidal cysts rarely contain cilia, however, and do not produce the same sort of colloid material found in colloid cysts.[14] Electron microscopic studies have shown a close morphologic relationship between colloid cysts and ependyma.[8] More than half a century ago, Fulton and Bailey[6] suggested the term *neuroepithelial cyst* for these tumors because their origin was and continues to be obscure; this term does not specify the exact embryologic derivation of the colloid cyst.

Signs and Symptoms

Headache is the most common symptom in patients with colloid cysts. It is the initial symptom in more than 75% of patients, and almost all patients with colloid cysts have headache as one of their complaints.[1] Headaches may be so severe initially that the patient is hospitalized, or they may be intermittent and occur at irregular intervals over a period of years. In some patients, the headaches are clearly positional, and these patients learn to lie down or change their head position to lessen the pain. In the past, the intermittent nature of these headaches and the lack of clinical symptoms between episodes made the colloid cyst one of the most difficult intracranial tumors to diagnose. In the years before scanning was available, the need for ventriculography or angiography with magnification for accurate diagnosis contributed to the problem. Most of these lesions are now easily diagnosed by scanning, usually during the initial episode.

Sudden attacks of leg weakness are also described in many patients, presumably owing to acute hydrocephalus that rapidly stretches the corticospinal nerve fibers to the legs. "Drop attack" episodes of leg weakness may be years apart, or they may occur almost daily. This peculiar symptom complex is rarely found in patients with intracranial tumors other than colloid cysts.[15]

Dementia may be a prominent finding in patients with colloid cysts. It may be progressive, as hydrocephalus increases, or it may be fluctuating or episodic in nature. Riddoch[16] first emphasized that these tumors can cause progressive ventricular enlargement and dementia without obvious signs of increased intracranial pressure. Seizures have been reported in about 20% of patients with colloid cysts[17]; however, most series report a somewhat lower percentage. Abnormalities of temperature regulation and endocrine dysfunction have also been described.

Sudden death of patients with colloid cysts is a widely reported complication. A review found 55 cases of sudden deterioration and death in these patients.[18] The authors concluded that most of these patients had prior symptoms and an adequate interval for diagnosis. Tumor size, degree of hydrocephalus, and duration of symptoms were not reliable prognostic indicators for the possibility of sudden death. A recent study of the risk of acute deterioration in patients who are already symptomatic from colloid cysts estimated that at least one third are at risk for precipitate decline or death.[19]

Diagnosis

The introduction of both CT and MRI greatly facilitated the diagnosis of tumors in the region of the anterior third ventricle. On CT, colloid cysts usually appear as radiodense lesions before injection of contrast agent (Fig. 238–1A). Occasionally, tumors may be radiolucent and show enhancement after the use of a contrast agent. On MRI, the relationship of the tumor to the structures of the anterior third ventricle is well seen on sagittal views.[19, 20] The differential diagnosis of tumors in this region includes the large-celled astrocytomas associated with tuberous sclerosis (epiloia), astrocytomas arising from the walls of the anterior third ventricle, subependymal glomerate astrocytomas (subependymomas), papillary ependymomas, and craniopharyngiomas. Colloid cysts may calcify; however, a calcified tumor in the foraminal region is more likely to be a craniopharyngioma or tuberous sclerosis.

Cysts that are radiodense on CT have higher viscosity than do those that are isodense or hypodense.[20] MRI does not predict the viscosity of cyst contents.

Operative Management

The initial operative approach for colloid cyst, described by Dandy[4] in 1922, involved traversing the right frontal lobe and the anterior horn of a dilated right lateral ventricle. In the first 2 decades after the introduction of this procedure, operative mortality ranged from 10% to 20%, and severe complications included subdural hematomas, seizures, stupor or coma, confusion, and Korsakoff's syndrome.[6] In response to the high mortality and morbidity, Torkildsen[21] proposed the use of a "palliative" method of shunting the lateral ventricles without directly attacking these slow-growing tumors. Results of this conservative method were generally good. Shunt dependency developed, however, and patients were left at risk for the progressive effects of local tumor pressure. For these reasons, a direct operative approach is generally preferred.

The transfrontal route is preferable when hydrocephalus is present, and it avoids manipulation of the contralateral fornix. However, a postoperative seizure rate of about 5% results.[22] The transcallosal approach is preferred in the absence of hydrocephalus, and it avoids postoperative seizures and behavioral disorders.[9, 22] However, damage to or division of the fornices may result in short-term memory deficits, which may be temporary or permanent.[21–24] With contemporary microscopic techniques, the transventricular, transcallosal, transventricular-subchoroidal, and transcallosal-interfornicial approaches have all been associated with

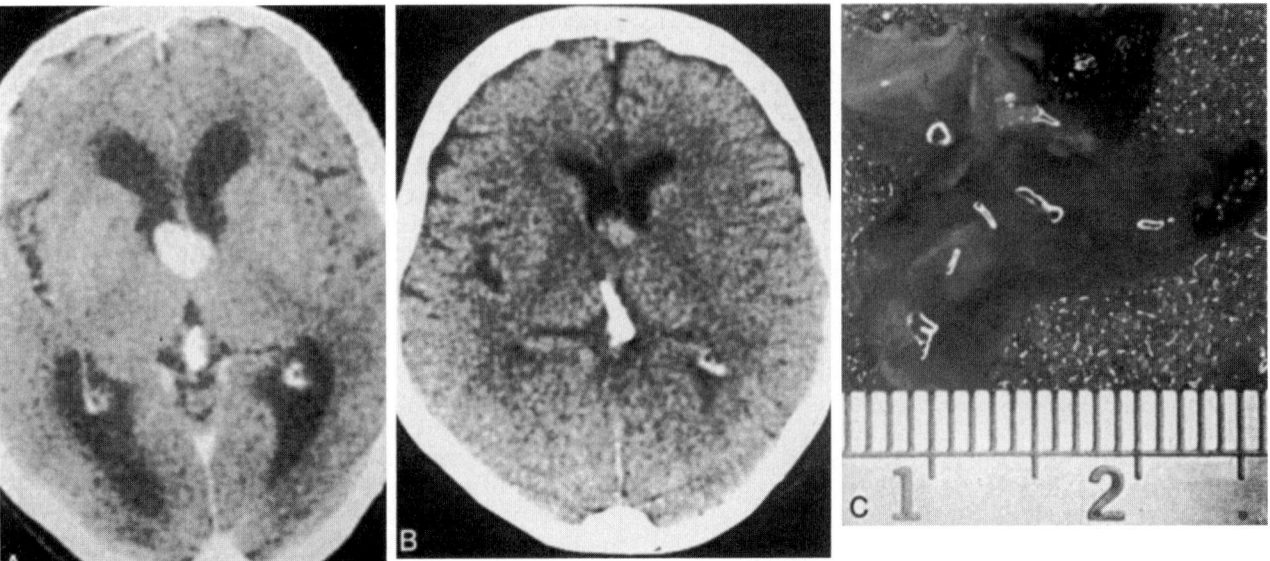

FIGURE 238–1. *A,* Axial computed tomographic scan in a 48-year-old woman complaining of headache with changes in mentation. Hydrocephalus had been relieved by shunting at another institution. The electron-dense lesion has blocked both foramina of Monro. *B,* Axial computed tomographic scan taken after stereotactic aspiration of the lesion. Although most of the tumor mass has been removed, it is not certain that the ventricular system has been unblocked. *C,* Viscid "colloid" material removed by stereotactic aspiration in the same patient. The specimen contains both cystic contents and portions of the cyst wall. (Courtesy of Dr. Robert Solomon.)

successful results.[24, 25] Operative mortality rates in these series approach zero. The cyst may be attached to the roof of the third ventricle, posterior to access through the dilated foramen of Monro. A number of methods for enlarging the foramen or opening the tela choroidea of the roof of the third ventricle have been described.[23, 25, 26]

Stereotactic aspiration of colloid cysts guided by CT was first reported in 1978 by Bosch and coauthors.[27] A series of seven patients initially treated by the stereotactic approach was reported by Hall and Lunsford[18] in 1987. Because of difficulties in aspirating the viscous cyst contents, there was one aspiration failure and three partial aspirations, and three patients had subsequent craniotomies. In a subsequent report on 22 patients treated with stereotactic aspiration, there were 11 satisfactory results; 50% of patients required further operative procedures.[20] One patient with a successful aspiration had a recurrence after only 5 weeks.[28]

Endoscopic approaches to colloid cysts allow puncture, aspiration, and partial wall removal under direct vision. The wall removal is carried out with cauterization or laser and is rarely total. Despite subtotal wall removal, long-term results have been quite good.[29, 30] An ingenious method of biportal neuroendoscopy, allowing complete removal of cysts, has been reported.[31]

INCLUSION TUMOR

Inclusion tumors arise from tissue displaced during the period of neural closure at 3 to 5 weeks' gestation. The nomenclature of these tumors is poorly standardized,

and the classification in Table 238–1 is presented as a guide. These tumors represent a spectrum of abnormalities reflecting the beginning of fetal development, with teratomas occurring at the early stages and single-tissue tumors arising later. In 1897, Bostroem[32] suggested that these tumors might arise from embryonic epithelial inclusions and called them *pial dermoid* and *pial epidermoid tumors.* Patten[33] stated that teratomas may arise from "unorganized growth of totipotential cells from the primitive streak region of the embryo." That this relationship is not entirely linear is shown by the finding of cartilage and muscle fiber rests in mature lipomas.[34]

Tumors resembling dermoid and epidermoid cysts may be created by implanting epithelial tissue into the central nervous system either experimentally or accidentally by lumbar puncture.[35] The latter cause is rare, and most inclusion tumors are congenital in origin. This is in marked contrast to cholesteatomas of the

TABLE 238–1 ■ **Simplified Classification of Inclusion Tumor**

Single-tissue type
 Epidermoid cysts (epidermal elements only)
 Lipomas
 Dermoid cysts (epidermis plus hair and dermal glands)
Teratoids—two germinal layers
 Usually epidermal or dermal tissue plus muscle, cartilage, fat
Teratomas
 All germinal layers
Embryomas
 All germinal layers plus formed organs (so-called inclusion twin)

middle ear, which are generally thought to arise after multiple bouts of otitis media. Unfortunately, in the past, cranial epidermoid lesions were also termed *cholesteatomas*, because the desquamated epithelial cells filling the cyst are rich in cholesterol crystals. This term should be avoided in describing intracranial epidermoid tumors.

EPIDERMOID TUMOR (EPIDERMOID CYST)

Intracranial epidermoid cysts constitute 0.5% to 1.8% of all brain tumors.[36] The incidence is higher in Japan, reaching 2.2%.[36] (A similar higher incidence is reported for teratomas in Japan.) There is no gender preponderance. The onset of symptoms is usually in the third to fifth decades.[36, 37]

Typically, epidermoid cysts spread along the cisterns at the base of the brain, often becoming adherent to adjacent structures, particularly blood vessels. The parasellar and cerebellopontine angle regions are the most common sites; however, epidermoid cysts have been found in the fourth and lateral ventricles, cerebrum, cerebellum, and brainstem.[38–41] About 25% of epidermoid tumors are found intradiploically in the skull or spine.[17]

Pathologically, these cysts consist of desquamated epidermal cellular debris, often in concentric layers, that arises from a capsule of stratified squamous epithelium. The capsule has a smooth, nodular, glistening white appearance[38] (Fig. 238–2). Although most neoplasms have an exponential growth rate, epidermoids increase in size by means of gradual accumulation of normally growing cells. Growth is linear, resembling that of human epidermis.[42] The slow growth rate and the ability of these tumors to travel along extra-axial planes cause a gradual onset of symptoms and a prolonged duration of "soft" signs.[36] Before the advent of computed scans, the duration of symptoms was often reported as decades long; however, in a contemporary report, the average duration had decreased to 4.3 years.[39]

Cysts in the cerebellopontine angle cause ataxia, nystagmus, partial or complete seventh and eighth cranial nerve dysfunction, and trigeminal neuralgia. Intradiploic epidermoids at the petrous apex also may cause fifth and seventh cranial nerve pain and dysfunction.[43] Epidermoid cysts in the sellar region are manifested by visual or endocrine losses or even hydrocephalus. Hydrocephalus is also the usual presenting feature in patients with repeated bouts of aseptic meningitis[44] or in those with fourth ventricle tumors.[45] The most common single symptom is seizures, and almost 50% of patients with intracranial epidermoid cysts have a seizure disorder.[35, 45]

Patients with epidermoid cysts may have repeated attacks of aseptic meningitis as a result of leakage of cyst contents into the cerebrospinal fluid (CSF) pathways.[36, 39] The cystic contents, rich in cholesterol and fatty acids, are highly irritating to the meninges. These patients have CSF findings of pleocytosis, decreased glucose concentration, and elevated protein levels.[44] CSF cultures are negative, and the meningismus usually clears in several days to a week.

Epidermoid cysts are best diagnosed by high-resolution scanning.[39] Axial, coronal, and sagittal sections are helpful in delineating the extent of the tumor (Fig. 238–3). On CT, these low-density tumors do not enhance with intravenous injection of contrast agents and may be mistaken for fluid-filled cavities. The use of nonionic iodine contrast cisternography combined with CT is often helpful in defining the lesion.[46] Rare epidermoid tumors enhance after intravenous injection of contrast agent, and this finding raises the possibility of a malignant epithelial component.[17, 39] Intradiploic epidermoids may be shown by the use of bone windows on axial CT.

Treatment of epidermoid tumors is operative.[37, 39] Some of these tumors are only slightly adherent to surrounding structures and can be removed entirely, especially those within the fourth ventricle.[38] Because of the dense attachment to vessels, however, many authors believe that complete removal is unwise and should be avoided.[39] The capsule is the living portion of the tumor, and after careful removal of the cyst contents, nonadherent portions of the capsule are excised as widely as possible. Viable portions of the capsule that remain will likely regrow, but often at rates so slow that the patient may not become symptomatic during the normal life span.

Intradiploic epidermoid cysts of the skull may remain small for long periods and are often discovered incidentally on skull films. Others may slowly expand, either as bony masses or as areas of the skull that are tender to palpation. Those that are growing or tender

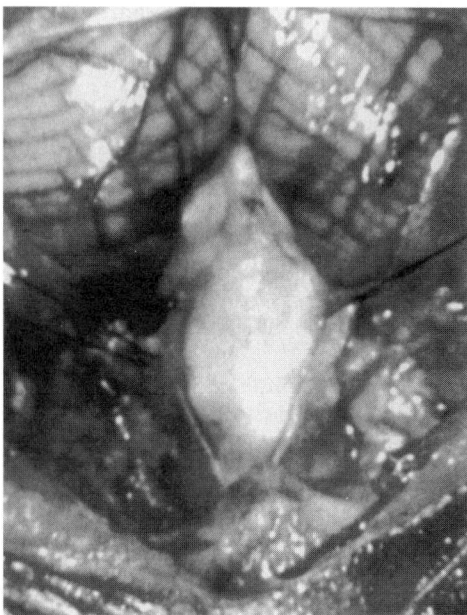

FIGURE 238–2. Epidermoid tumor in the fourth ventricle in a young woman with signs and symptoms of hydrocephalus. The tumor has the typical smooth, glistening, "mother-of-pearl" appearance. No clear point of attachment was seen, and the lesion was totally removed.

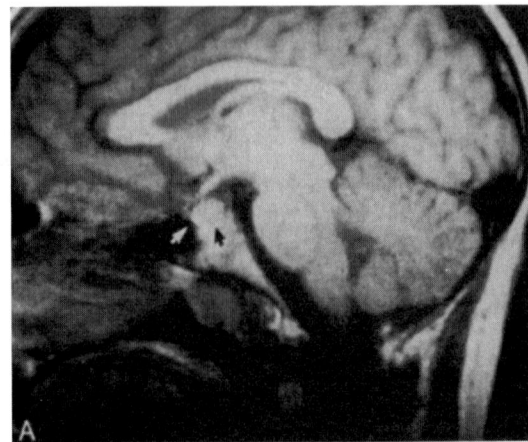

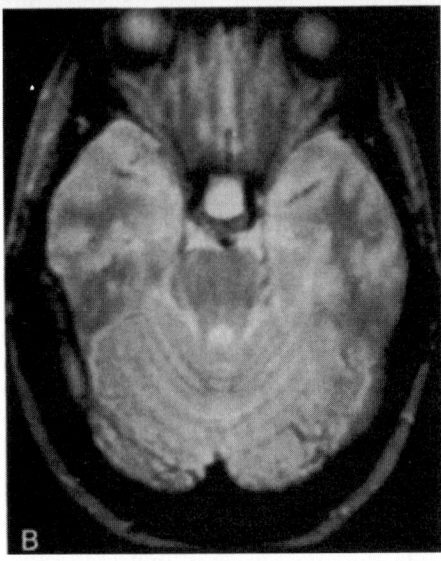

FIGURE 238–3. *A,* Sagittal magnetic resonance imaging (MRI) scan in a 12-year-old girl who had suffered three episodes of aseptic meningitis over a 14-month period. Neurological examination, growth and development, and pituitary function were all normal. On this T1-weighted MRI scan, the enlarged sella contains a rounded mass *(arrows)* with a density greater than that of cerebrospinal fluid. *B,* Axial MRI scan of the same patient. On this T2-weighted scan, the fluidlike content of the cyst is more apparent. At surgery, an epidermoid tumor with cystic fluid content was removed.

should be excised, and their removal is usually easily accomplished. Although these cysts have a low rate of malignant change, more than 12 cases of malignancy have been reported.[17]

Operative mortality for intracranial epidermoid tumors was very high during the first half of the 20th century, approaching 70%.[37, 38, 40] Recent technologic advances and, perhaps, a greater willingness to settle for subtotal removal have virtually eliminated operative death.[47]

Removal of posterior fossa epidermoids, in particular, has been complicated by multiple cranial nerve deficits, severe neurological impairment, and high mortality. Recent series have high survival rates, with large recurrence-free intervals.[41] Cautious, "conservative" resection of two intramedullary brainstem cysts produced good results.[48]

Postoperative aseptic meningitis, caused by spillage of cyst contents, is a common problem. This syndrome is often masked by the high-potency steroids given perioperatively, only to flare up again during tapering of these agents. Use of hydrocortisone in the operative irrigating solutions and a gradual tapering of steroids over 3 weeks after the patient is discharged from the hospital have been advocated.[39] The appearance of hydrocephalus in the postoperative period is not uncommon, presumably because of the meningeal reaction. Follow-up scans reveal those patients in whom hydrocephalus may be progressive.

DERMOID TUMOR (DERMOID CYST)

Dermoid cysts are less common than epidermoid cysts and constitute about 0.3% of all intracranial tumors.[37, 39, 45, 49] They generally grow more quickly than epidermoids do, and patients become symptomatic at a much earlier age. More than half of these tumors are diagnosed in childhood or early adolescence.[40, 45]

Whereas epidermoid cysts are often found laterally within the brain, dermoid cysts tend to be located in the midline.[45] About one third are in the fourth ventricular region.[37, 40] Almost 50% of patients with these tumors have associated congenital anomalies.[50] Dermal elements such as hair, hair follicles, or sebaceous glands may be found in only a small part of the capsule, and the rest of the cyst wall may closely resemble an epidermoid tumor. A greater proportion of dermal elements causes the cyst to be darker and to contain more watery contents. A dermal sinus tract may connect the cyst to the skin surface, especially when the tumor is located in the posterior fossa or quadrigeminal plate region.[39] This tract may allow bacteria to enter the CSF, and bacterial meningitis may be the initial presentation in patients with these tumors. Repeated bouts of bacterial meningitis associated with dermoid tumors are not rare and should raise suspicion of this lesion.[39] Because of the tendency for dermoid tumors to occur in the midline, obstruction of CSF pathways is frequently the cause of initial signs and symptoms. Both progression of symptoms and development of neurological impairment are more rapid with dermoid than epidermoid tumors.

Diagnosis is best achieved by high-resolution CT or MRI. Although calcification is rare with epidermoid tumors, about 20% of dermoid tumors have evidence of calcium deposition.[51] Scans may show a sinus tract not seen on physical examination, helping to establish the diagnosis.

Operative removal of dermoid tumors involves many of the same problems and hazards encountered with epidermoid cysts. Tumors adjacent to blood vessels often form dense, tenacious adhesions. Cysts in the ventricles appear to be more easily removed. The young age of most of these patients and the more rapid growth of these tumors impose greater operative demands on the surgeon.

As with epidermoid tumors, radiotherapy has little effect on dermoids. Postoperative irradiation does not shrink these tumors, nor does it prevent their recurrence.[51]

TERATOMA

Teratomas are more common than dermoid tumors but less common than epidermoid tumors. Although they constitute about 0.5% of all intracranial tumors, their incidence increases dramatically in younger age groups.[40] Teratomas account for 2% of all intracranial tumors in children.[52] This incidence increases to 9% for intracranial tumors in children younger than 2 years and to 50% for cerebral neoplasms in infants younger than 2 months.[53] In Japanese series, the incidence is two to three times higher, even when germinomas are excluded from the teratoma group. Teratomas are generally reported to be more common in males, even after the exclusion of germinomas.[54]

Almost half of all teratomas arise in the pineal region.[54, 55] The suprasellar region is probably the next most common site.[56] Those in the pineal region frequently have a germ cell tumor component, complicating their nomenclature. Classification of pineal tumors as *atypical teratomas* adds to the confusion.[54] If the term *teratoma* is restricted to those tumors in which tissue of all three germinal layers is found, three types can be defined: mature, immature (embryonic), and malignant. Malignant changes may affect either mature or immature teratomas, and some pathologists simply classify both malignant forms as teratocarcinomas.

Growth of teratomas may be extremely rapid, especially in neonates. Cases of fetuses with enlarged heads in whom the tumor has totally replaced supratentorial brain tissue have been reported.[53] With slower-growing mature teratomas, hydrocephalus may be the presenting feature, or local compression in the pineal region may be the first sign.

Diagnosis is usually accomplished by high-resolution CT and MRI.[57] Teratomas have a variegated, often polycystic appearance (Fig. 238–4). Half of mature teratomas have calcification, and mature bone or teeth may be identified. Calcification is rarely pronounced in immature teratomas and is unusual in lesions with anaplastic changes. In neonates and fetuses, an ultrasonic scan may be diagnostic; one series reported on three cases recognized in utero, and another case was diagnosed at 21 weeks' gestation.[53, 58] Teratoma in a fetus is usually first suspected because it is large for its gestational age. Sonographic examination may show cranial enlargement, a hyperechoic multicystic mass, and polyhydramnios.[53]

Teratomas are the most difficult of the inclusion tumors to treat because of their rapid growth, large size at discovery, tendency to recur, and young age of many patients. The outlook in neonates treated with surgery alone is particularly dismal.[53] Ventureyra and Herder[57] reported successful excision of an immature teratoma from a 6-day-old boy, with no evidence of recurrence at 4 months of age. Very few of these children survive beyond 2 years of age, however.[53] Better results with excision of mature teratomas have been reported.[40]

All teratomas have a variegated appearance at surgery, and well-encapsulated tumors that appear to be mature and benign may prove to be either immature or anaplastic on histologic examination. Almost all these tumors require adjunctive therapy. For germinomas, radiation alone generally controls the disease, and newer protocols reduce the cranial dose to 30 Gy. Both germinomas and mature teratomas have a high 5-year survival rate (96% and 100%, respectively); however, for immature teratomas, it is only 67%.[59] Patients with germinomas that secrete β-human chorionic gonadotropin have a 5-year survival rate of only 38%; patients with choriocarcinoma, embryonal carcinoma, and yolk sac tumors have lower survival rates. Immature teratomas have responded to various chemotherapeutic regi-

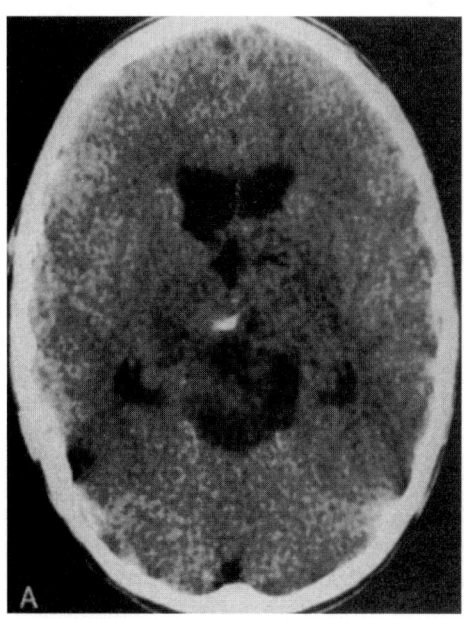 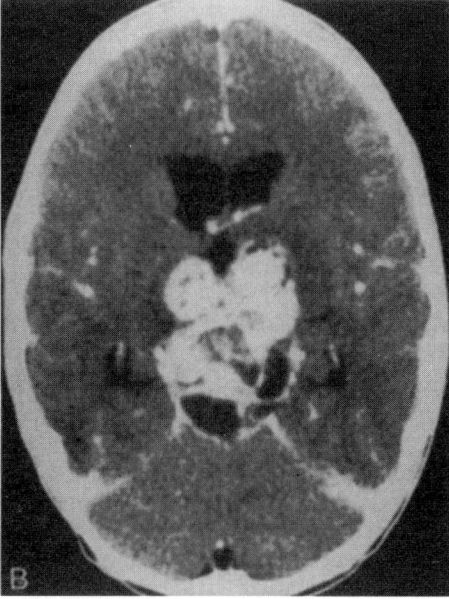

FIGURE 238–4. *A,* Axial non–contrast-enhanced computed tomographic scan in a 5-year-old boy with a malignant (immature) teratoma. Symptoms of headache and somnolence and signs of mesencephalic compression began 8 days before this scan. Shunting relieved the headache but did not improve the remaining deficits. The tumor has a fatty portion (right posterior), cystic areas, and a small calcification. *B,* Axial contrast-enhanced computed tomographic scan in the same patient. Operative debulking of this vascular tumor did not improve his condition, and a course of chemotherapy was given. He died approximately 7 weeks after this scan.

mens, with most including cisplatin and etoposide.[60] Further consolidation with radiotherapy is often recommended.[60]

LIPOMA

Intracranial lipomas are rare fatty tumors that often cause no symptoms during life and are discovered only at autopsy. Gerber and Plotkin[61] were able to find only 85 tumors that were diagnosed in living patients up to 1982. Most of these tumors are found in the region of the corpus callosum, followed by the cerebellopontine angles, with small numbers reported in the brainstem, cerebellum, basal cerebrum, quadrigeminal plate region, and lateral ventricles.[61–65]

Many lipomas are associated with other congenital anomalies, including agenesis of the corpus callosum, spina bifida, and myelomeningocele.[63] A patient with a corpus callosum lipoma and dysraphism was found to have trisomy 13.[66] Congenital anomalies of cranial nerves in association with lipoma also have been reported.[62] The tendency for lipomas to occur in the midline and their frequent association with dysraphic anomalies have led some authors to believe that they are caused by an imperfection of neural tube closure, relating them to inclusion tumors.[61–63] However, Zettner and Netsky[67] believe that their pathogenesis lies in faulty differentiation of primitive meninx tissue in the intrahemispheric fissure, which may later interfere with the development of midline structures.

Pathologically, lipomas consist of mature adipose tissue, with varying amounts of collagen at points of contact with nerve tissue and blood vessels. Use of the term *angiolipoma* to designate lipomas of greater vascularity adds little to the understanding of these tumors.[64] Growth patterns of lipomas are generally more like those of hamartomas than of neoplasms.[61, 67] These adipose cells respond to steroids, as do most fat cells, and patients with undiscovered lipomas have become symptomatic with steroid therapy.[68]

More than 50% of patients with intracranial lipomas present with seizures. This finding is not readily explained by tumor location, growth rate, or any associated anomalies. Whether it can be related to the collagenous reaction at the tumor-brain interface is debatable. Almost 20% of patients have mentation defects.[69] The presentation is related to tumor growth in only a small number of patients, and in this group, the symptoms are usually due to obstructive hydrocephalus.

Diagnosis is easily achieved by either high-resolution CT or MRI (Fig. 238–5). On CT, the attenuation values for lipomas are quite negative (−50 to −100 Hounsfield units) and are lower than those for epidermoid tumors. On MRI, T1-weighted scans show high intensity, which changes to low intensity on late-echo T2-weighted scans.[70] These MRI parameters are characteristic of fat. On both types of scans, the homogeneity of the lesion suggests that neither desquamated epithelium nor other tissue elements are present, helping to rule out both dermoid cysts and teratomas. Peritumoral calcification may be seen.[61, 63, 71]

Management of an intracranial lipoma should generally be conservative. Epilepsy, the most common symptom produced by the tumor, is unlikely to be relieved by surgery.[61] Hydrocephalus may be relieved by a shunting procedure. Only in unusual cases does the tumor require debulking or removal. The tenacious attachments to surrounding structures may account for the poor results seen after apparently satisfactory operative procedures.[61, 64] In a recent review of cerebellopontine angle lipomas, Tankere and coauthors[65] found that almost three fourths of patients were worse after surgery, and almost two thirds sustained a hearing loss. Clarici and Heppner[69] reported on a case of radical removal of a callosal lipoma with a carbon dioxide laser. The anterior cerebral arteries, however, are likely to be encased by tumor and are subject to injury even when the laser is used. Kudoh and coauthors[63] suggested that the Cavitron ultrasonic surgical aspirator (CUSA) might be effective in these tumors. I have used the CUSA on several intracranial lipomas. This instrument has the advantage of leaving major vascular structures intact. The dense septa within the lipoma, however, are quite resistant to the aspirator. In addition, if the vibration rate is high and the septum is thick, considerable heat may be generated.

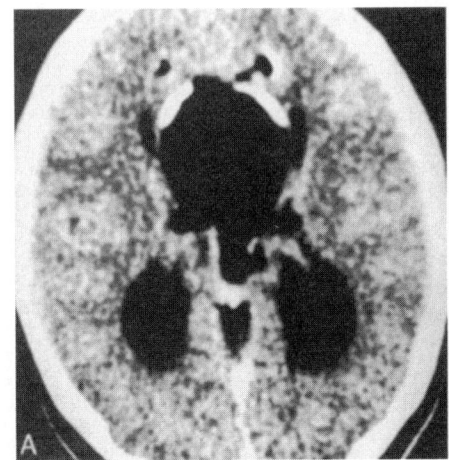
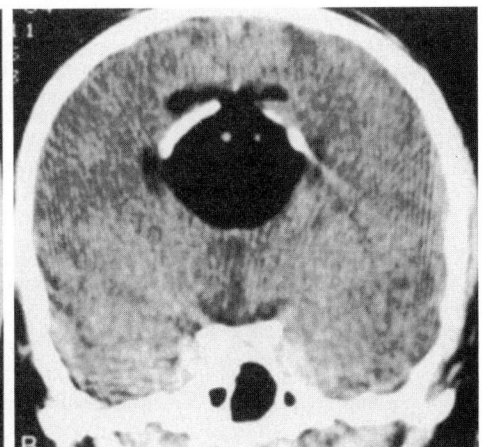

FIGURE 238–5. *A* and *B*, Corpus callosum lipoma in an 18-year-old girl with headaches and the recent onset of a focal seizure disorder. The fatty tumor has calcification on its border, which is not an unusual finding. The patient also had a fatty scalp tumor at the skull vertex, which was entirely extracranial.

REFERENCES

1. Yenermen NIH, Bowerman CI, Haymaker NV: Colloid cyst of the third ventricle: A clinical study of 54 cases in light of previous publications. Acta Neurosurg 17:211–277, 1958.
2. Zulch KJ: Brain Tumors: Their Biology and Pathology, 2nd ed. New York, Springer-Verlag, 1965.
3. Wallman H: Eine colloidcyste im dritten Hirnventrikel und eine lipom im Plexus choroides. Virchows Arch (Pathol Anat) 11:385–388, 1858.
4. Dandy WE: Diagnosis, localization, and removal of tumors of the third ventricle. Bull Johns Hopkins Hosp 33:188–189, 1922.
5. Dandy WE: Benign Tumors in the Third Ventricle of the Brain: Diagnosis and Treatment. Springfield, IL, Charles C Thomas, 1933.
6. Fulton JF, Bailey P: Contribution to the study of tumors in the region of the third ventricle: Their diagnosis and relationship to pathological sleep. J Nerv Ment Dis 69:1–25, 1929.
7. Hirano A, Ghatak NB: The fine structure of colloid cysts of the third ventricle. J Neuropathol Exp Neurol 33:333–341, 1974.
8. Coxe WS, Luse SA: Colloid cyst of the third ventricle: An electron microscopic study. J Neuropathol Exp Neurol 23:431–445, 1964.
9. Greenwood J: Paraphysial cysts of the third ventricle: With report of eight cases. J Neurosurg 6:153–159, 1949.
10. Katz FL: Late results of radical excision of craniopharyngiomas in children. J Neurosurg 42:86–90, 1975.
11. Sjovall E: Uber eine Epengymcyste embryonalen Charakters (Paraphyse?) im dritten Hirnventrikel mit todlichem Ausgang. Beitr Pathol Anat 47:248–269, 1910.
12. Fahlbusch R, Honegger J, Paulus W, et al: Surgical treatment of craniopharyngiomas: Experiences with 168 patients. J Neurosurg 90:237–250, 1999.
13. Kappers JA: The development of the paraphysis cerebri in man with comments on its relationship to the intercolumnar tubercle and its significance for the origin of cystic tumors in the third ventricle. J Comp Neurol 102:425–510, 1955.
14. Shuangshoti S, Roberts MD, Netsky MC: Neuroepithelial (colloid) cysts: Pathogenesis and relation to choroid plexus and ependyma. Arch Pathol 80:214–224, 1965.
15. Kelly R: Colloid cysts of the third ventricle: Analysis of twenty-nine cases. Brain 74:23–65, 1951.
16. Riddoch G: Progressive dementia, without headache or changes in the optic discs, due to tumors of the third ventricle. Brain 59:225–233, 1936.
17. Yanai Y, Tsuji R, Obmori S, et al: Malignant change in an intradiploic epidermoid: Report of a case and review of the literature. Neurosurgery 16:252–256, 1985.
18. Hall NA, Lunsford LD: Changing concepts in the treatment of colloid cysts. J Neurosurg 66:186–191, 1987.
19. deWitt Hamer PC, Verstegen MJ, De Haan RJ, et al: High risk of acute deterioration in patients harboring symptomatic colloid cysts of the third ventricle. J Neurosurg 96:1041–1045, 2002.
20. Kondziolka D, Lunsford LD: Stereotactic management of colloid cysts: Factors predicting success. J Neurosurg 75:45–57, 1991.
21. Torkildsen A: Should extirpation be attempted in cases of neoplasm in or near the third ventricle of the brain? Experiences with a palliative method. J Neurosurg 5:249–275, 1948.
22. Antunes JL, Louis KM, Ganti SB: Colloid cyst of the third ventricle. Neurosurgery 7:450–455, 1980.
23. Antunes JL, Muraszko K, Quest DO, Carmel PW: Surgical strategies in the management of tumours of the anterior third ventricle. In Brock M (ed): Modern Neurosurgery. Berlin, Springer-Verlag, 1982, pp 215–244.
24. Apuzzo MLJ, Chikovani OK, Gott PS, et al: Transcallosal interfornicial approaches for lesions affecting the third ventricle: Surgical considerations and consequences. Neurosurgery 10:547–554, 1982.
25. Lavyne MH, Patterson RH Jr: Subchoroidal transvelum interpositum approach to mid–third ventricular tumors. Neurosurgery 12:86–94, 1983.
26. Carmel PW: Tumours of the third ventricle. Acta Neurochir (Wien) 75:136–146, 1985.
27. Bosch DA, Hahn T, Backlund EO: Treatment of colloid cysts of the third ventricle by stereotactic aspiration. Surg Neurol 9:15–18, 1978.
28. Skirving DJ, Pell MF: Early recurrence from stereotactic aspiration of a colloid cyst of the third ventricle. J Clin Neurosci 8:570–571, 2001.
29. Kehler U, Brunori A, Glienroth J, et al: Twenty colloid cysts: Comparison of endoscopic and microsurgical management. Minim Invasive Neurosurg 44:12–17, 2001.
30. Longatti P, Martinuzzi A, Moro M, et al: Endoscopic treatment of colloid cysts of the third ventricle: 9 conservative cases. Minim Invasive Neurosurg 43:118–123, 2000.
31. Horvath Z, Veto F, Balas I, Doczi T: Complete removal of colloid cyst via CT-guided stereotactic biportal neuroendoscopy. Acta Neurochir (Wien) 142:539–546, 2000.
32. Bostroem E: Ueber die pialen Epidermoide, Dermoide und lipoma und duralen Dermoide. Zentralbl Allg Path Anat 8:1–98, 1897.
33. Patten BM: Patten's Human Embryology. New York, McGraw-Hill, 1976.
34. Schmid AH: A lipoma of the cerebellum. Acta Neuropathol (Berl) 26:75–80, 1973.
35. Choremis C, Economos D, Papadatos C, Cargonlas A: Intraspinal epidermoid tumours (cholesteatomas) in patients treated for tuberculous meningitis. Lancet 271:437–439, 1956.
36. Ulrich J: Intracranial epidermoids: A study of their distribution and spread. J Neurosurg 21:1051–1058, 1964.
37. Guidetti V, Gagliardi FM: Epidermoid and dermoid cysts: Clinical evaluation and late surgical results. J Neurosurg 47:12–18, 1977.
38. Bailey P: Cruveilhier's "tumeurs perlees." Surg Gynecol Obstet 31:390–401, 1920.
39. Berger MB, Wilson CB: Epidermoid cysts of the posterior fossa. J Neurosurg 21:1051–1058, 1984.
40. Sweet WH: A review of dermoid, teratoid and teratomatous intracranial tumors. Dis Nerve Syst 1:228–238, 1940.
41. Talacchi A, Sala F, Allessandrini F, et al: Assessment and management of posterior fossa epidermoid tumors: Report of 28 cases. Neurosurgery 42:242–252, 1998.
42. Alvord FC Jr: Growth rates of epidermoid tumors. Ann Neurol 2:361–370, 1977.
43. Jefferson C, Smalley AA: Progressive facial palsy produced by intratemporal epidermoids. J Laryngol 53:417–443, 1938.
44. Ellner JJ, Bennett JE: Chronic meningitis. Medicine 55:341–369, 1976.
45. Fleming JFB, Botterell EH: Cranial dermoid and epidermoid tumors. Surg Gynecol Obstet 109:403–411, 1959.
46. Critchley M, Ironside RN: The pituitary adamantinomata. Brain 49:437–481, 1926.
47. Bernstein HL, Buchino JJ: The histological similarity between craniopharyngioma and odontogenic lesions: A reappraisal. Oral Surg 56:502–511, 1983.
48. Caldarelli M, Colosimo C, DiRocco C: Intra-axial dermoid/epidermoid tumors of the brainstem in children. Surg Neurol 56:97–105, 2001.
49. Cobb CA, Youmans JB: Brain tumors of disordered embryogenesis in adults. In Youmans JB (ed): Neurological Surgery, 2nd ed. Philadelphia, WB Saunders, 1982, pp 2899–2935.
50. MacCarty CS, Leavens ME, Love JG: Dermoid and epidermoid tumors in the central nervous system of adults. Surg Gynecol Obstet 108:191–198, 1959.
51. Keville FJ, Wise BL: Intracranial epidermoid and dermoid tumors. J Neurosurg 16:564–569, 1959.
52. Ingraham FD, Bailey OT: Cystic teratomas and teratoid tumors of the central nervous system in infancy and childhood. J Neurosurg 3:511–532, 1946.
53. Lipman SP, Pretorius DH, Rumack CM, Manco-Johnson ML: Fetal intracranial teratoma: Ultrasound diagnosis of three cases and a review of the literature. Radiology 157:491–494, 1985.
54. Russell DS: The pinealoma: Its relationship to teratoma. J Pathol Bacteriol 56:145–150, 1944.
55. Russell DS, Rubinstein LJ: Pathology of Tumors of the Nervous System, 4th ed. Baltimore, Williams & Wilkins, 1977.
56. Tekeuchi J, Mori K, Moritakes K, et al: Teratomas in the suprasellar region: Report of five cases. Surg Neurol 2:247–255, 1975.
57. Ventureyra ECC, Herder S: Neonatal intracranial teratoma. J Neurosurg 59:879–883, 1983.
58. Horton D, Pilling DW: Early antenatal ultrasound diagnosis of fetal intracranial teratoma. Br J Radiol 70:1299–1301, 1997.

59. Brandes AA, Pasetto LM, Monfardini S: Treatment of cranial germ cell tumours. Cancer Treat Rev 26:233–242, 2000.
60. Youshida J, Sugita K, Kobayashi T, et al: Prognosis of intracranial germ cell tumours: Effectiveness of chemotherapy with cisplatin and etoposide (CDDP and VP-16). Acta Neurochir (Wien) 120: 111–117, 1993.
61. Gerber SS, Plotkin B: Lipoma of the corpus callosum. J Neurosurg 57:281–285, 1982.
62. Hori A: Lipoma of the quadrigeminal plate region with evidence of congenital origin. Arch Pathol Lab Med 110:850–851, 1986.
63. Kudoh H, Sakamoto K, Kobayashi N: Lipomas in the corpus callosum and the forehead associated with a frontal bone defect. Surg Neurol 22:503–508, 1984.
64. Pensak L VI, Glasscook ME, Gulya AJ, et al: Cerebellopontine angle lipomas. Arch Otolaryngol Head Neck Surg 112:99–101, 1986.
65. Tankere F, Vitte E, Martin-Duerneuil N, Soudant J: Cerebellopontine angle lipomas: Report of four cases and review of the literature. Neurosurgery 50:626–631, 2002.
66. Wainright H, Bowen R, Radcliffe M: Lipoma of corpus callosum associated with dysraphic lesions and trisomy 13. Am J Med Genet 57:10–13, 1995.
67. Zettner A, Netsky MC: Lipoma of the corpus callosum. J Neuropathol Exp Neurol 19:305–319, 1960.
68. Haga HJ, Thomassen E, Johannesen A, Krakenes J: Neural compressive symptoms appearing during steroid treatment in a patient with intracranial lipoma. Scand J Rheumatol 28:184–186, 1999.
69. Clarici C, Heppner F: The operative approach to lipomas of the corpus callosum. Neurochirurgia 22:77–81, 1979.
70. Fulton JF, Bailey P: Contribution of the study of tumors in the region of the third ventricle. J Nerv Ment Dis 60:1–25, 1925.
71. Friedman BB, Segal B, Latchaw BB: Computerized tomographic and magnetic resonance imaging of intra-cranial lipoma. J Neurosurg 65:407–410, 1986.

CHAPTER 239

Pediatric Cerebral Hemispheric Tumors

LOI K. PHUONG ■ COREY RAFFEL

Cerebral hemispheric tumors are one of the most common pediatric tumors. This chapter discusses the epidemiology, clinical presentation, diagnostic studies, histology, treatment, and prognosis of pediatric cerebral hemispheric tumors.

EPIDEMIOLOGY

Central nervous system tumors in children younger than 18 years of age have an incidence of 3.6 per 100,000 and cause 0.04% to 0.18% of deaths in children younger than 1 year of age. The Connecticut, Massachusetts, Missouri, and Utah registries report a prevalence of 37.8 cases per million among children.[1] There are reports that the incidence of pediatric central nervous system tumors has recently increased, particularly among males.[2, 3]

Intracranial brain tumors account for 90.7% to 93.6% of all childhood central nervous system neoplasms, with the remainder in the spine.[3, 4] Although infratentorial tumors predominate in children overall, supratentorial tumors are more common in the first 2 to 3 years of life. Sixty percent of hemispheric tumors in children are World Health Organization grade 1 or 2 astrocytomas, in contrast to the predominantly grade 3 or 4 tumors that occur in adults. Astrocytoma accounts for more than half of these low-grade neoplasms in children.[5–7] However, in children with brain tumors diagnosed in the first year of life, 77% to 85% of them are high grade.[8] In a review of 107 brain tumors in children younger than 4 years, the most common tumor was astrocytoma, accounting for 33.6%.[4] Ependymoma is the most common nonastrocytic supratentorial neoplasm in children, constituting 10% to 15% of such tumors. Supratentorial ependymomas account for 30% of intracranial ependymomas.[9] Primitive neuroectodermal tumor and ganglioglioma each account for 5% to 10% of pediatric hemispheric tumors. Eighty percent of supratentorial primitive neuroectodermal tumors occur in the first decade.[10] Oligodendroglioma accounts for 4% to 8% of supratentorial tumors in children. Other less common tumors include teratoma, dysembryoplastic neuroepithelial tumor, subependymal giant cell astrocytoma, meningioma, germinoma, sarcoma, chondroma, metastases, and lymphoma.

SIGNS AND SYMPTOMS

Children with supratentorial tumors tend to have a longer delay in diagnosis after presentation compared with those with infratentorial tumors.[11] Infratentorial tumors of childhood more commonly present with symptoms of increased intracranial pressure due to obstruction of cerebrospinal fluid outflow from the fourth ventricle. In contrast, supratentorial cerebral hemispheric tumors frequently cause seizures due to irritation of the cortical gray matter. Overall, 30% of patients present with seizures only.[12–15] The incidence of seizure is higher with tumors that invade the cortical surface (59% versus 15%). Because dysembryoplastic neuroepithelial tumor, oligodendroglioma, and ganglioglioma have a propensity to involve the temporal cortex, 80% of these patients have a history of seizures often refractory to anticonvulsant medications. The first seizure in these patients usually occurs before they reach age 20.[16] Patients with pleomorphic xanthoastrocytoma usually present with a history of seizures as well. The interictal neurological examination is normal in almost all cases. The seizure is primarily simple or complex partial, accounting for 28% and 55% of cases, respectively. Children with anaplastic astrocytoma and primitive neuroectodermal tumor have a lower incidence of seizures.

In addition to seizures, patients can present with nonspecific complaints. Approximately 80% have a personality change or failure to thrive. Among children who present with seizures, 90% have cognitive change. Other common presenting symptoms include headache, nausea, emesis, visual disturbance, and gait difficulty.

Focal neurological deficits such as hemiparesis, aphasia, and hemianesthesia can occur, depending on the location of the tumor. In more rapidly growing tumors, signs of increased intracranial pressure such as papilledema may occur. Bulging fontanelle and macrocephaly may be evident in infants.

DIAGNOSTIC STUDIES

Computed tomography (CT) with intravenous contrast administration is usually the first radiologic study for children suspected of having an intracranial mass lesion. The presence of calcification, hemorrhage, and contrast enhancement within the tumor, as well as surrounding vasogenic edema, can be demonstrated on CT. The ventricular size can also be assessed for hydrocephalus.

Magnetic resonance imaging (MRI) is the preferred imaging modality for evaluating brain tumors. The signal characteristics of the tumor on MRI are usually nonspecific, with the solid portion of the tumor hypo-

intense to isointense on T1-weighted images and isointense to hyperintense on T2-weighted images. The presence of intense gadolinium enhancement, surrounding edema, and mass effect suggests a malignant or higher-grade tumor. The pattern of contrast enhancement (homogeneous, heterogeneous, or peripheral), the presence of a cyst, and hemorrhage within the mass are important characteristics detected on MRI that help differentiate tumor types. Because patient movement during the MRI scan can greatly deteriorate

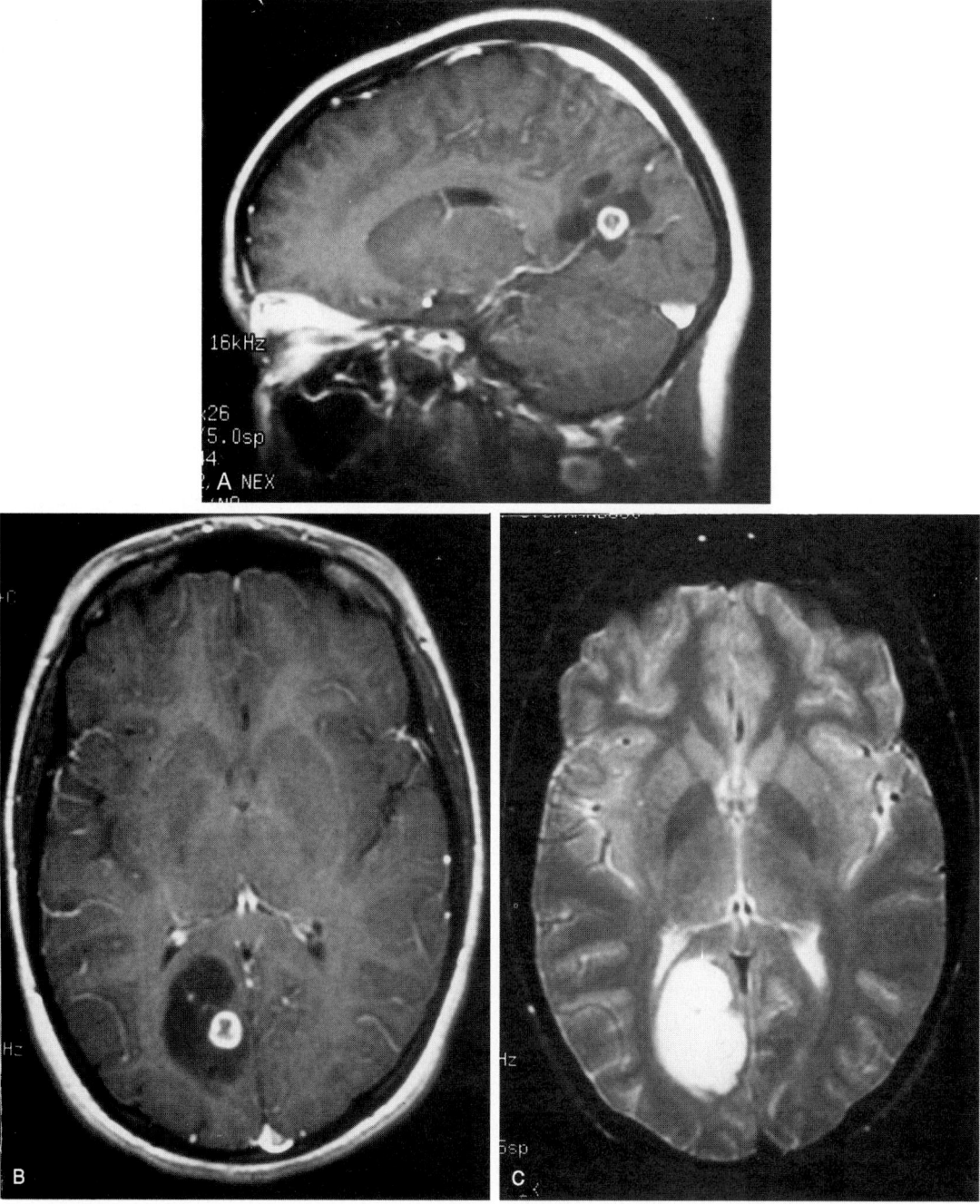

FIGURE 239–1. A 15-year-old girl presented with simple partial seizures that consisted of flashing lights and numbness of the left tongue and fingers. *A*, T1-weighted gadolinium-enhanced sagittal magnetic resonance imaging (MRI) scan. *B*, T1-weighted gadolinium-enhanced axial MRI scan. *C*, T2-weighted axial MRI scan. Note the cystic tumor with an enhancing nodule in the right parasagittal parieto-occipital lobe. Pathologic examination revealed a low-grade oligodendroglioma.

the quality and diagnostic value of the study, general anesthesia may be required in infants and young children.

Low-grade fibrillary astrocytoma is a diffusely infiltrating, poorly delineated tumor. On CT, it is hypo- to isointense, and calcification is seen in 15% to 20% of cases. Bone windows may show remodeling of the inner table adjacent to the tumor. On MRI, the tumor appears homogeneous and shows decreased or similar signal relative to gray matter on T1-weighted images and increased signal on T2-weighted images. There may be a cystic component. Enhancement and surrounding edema on CT and MRI are minimal or absent.

Oligodendroglioma is found predominantly in the cortex. Calcification occurs in 70% to 90% of these tumors and is best appreciated on CT.[17] The inner table of the skull may be remodeled by the growth of the tumor. MRI shows a poorly delineated tumor that may have heterogeneous enhancement with mild surrounding vasogenic edema. Cystic degeneration may also be seen (Fig. 239–1).[18]

Most ependymomas are located within 2 cm of the ventricular system but may extend to the cortex. Solely intraventricular ependymoma is less common. They appear isodense to slightly hyperdense on CT, and calcification may be seen within the tumor.[19] On MRI, they show a decreased to similar signal relative to gray matter on T1-weighted images and an increased signal on T2-weighted images with heterogeneous enhancement. A cystic component can sometimes be seen. Imaging of the neuraxis should be performed, as the tumor may disseminate.

Dysembryoplastic neuroepithelial tumor appears on CT scans as a low-attenuation mass involving the temporal and frontal cortical surfaces in 62% and 31% of cases, respectively.[17] A pseudocystic appearance is seen in 50%, calcification in 23%, and focal contrast enhancement in 18%. On MRI, it has a decreased signal relative to gray matter on T1-weighted images and an increased signal on T2-weighted images. The surrounding edema is minimal. Minimal focal or punctate contrast enhancement is seen in 30% of cases (Fig. 239–2). The tumor is well circumscribed at the margins. The adjacent calvaria is remodeled in 60% to 67% of cases. This tumor may resemble low-grade astrocytoma or ganglioglioma on MRI.[20, 21]

Supratentorial primitive neuroectodermal tumor occurs most frequently in the frontal or parietal lobe adjacent to the lateral ventricles. On CT, this tumor appears iso- or hyperintense and usually has heterogeneous enhancement. Half the cases have a cystic component.[22] MRI shows a heterogeneously enhancing tumor with necrosis, hemorrhage, and calcification (Fig. 239–3). The boundary between tumor and brain is relatively well delineated on CT and MRI, which differentiates primitive neuroectodermal tumor from high-grade astrocytoma. As in the case of ependymoma, spinal MRI should be done to evaluate for the presence of dissemination.

Ganglioglioma is most commonly found in the temporal lobe. Bone windows on CT may show remodeling of the inner calvarial table. A cystic appearance with an iso- or hypodense mural nodule that is partially calcified is characteristic. The enhancement pattern is variable. On MRI, hypointensity on T1-weighted images and hyperintensity on T2-weighted images

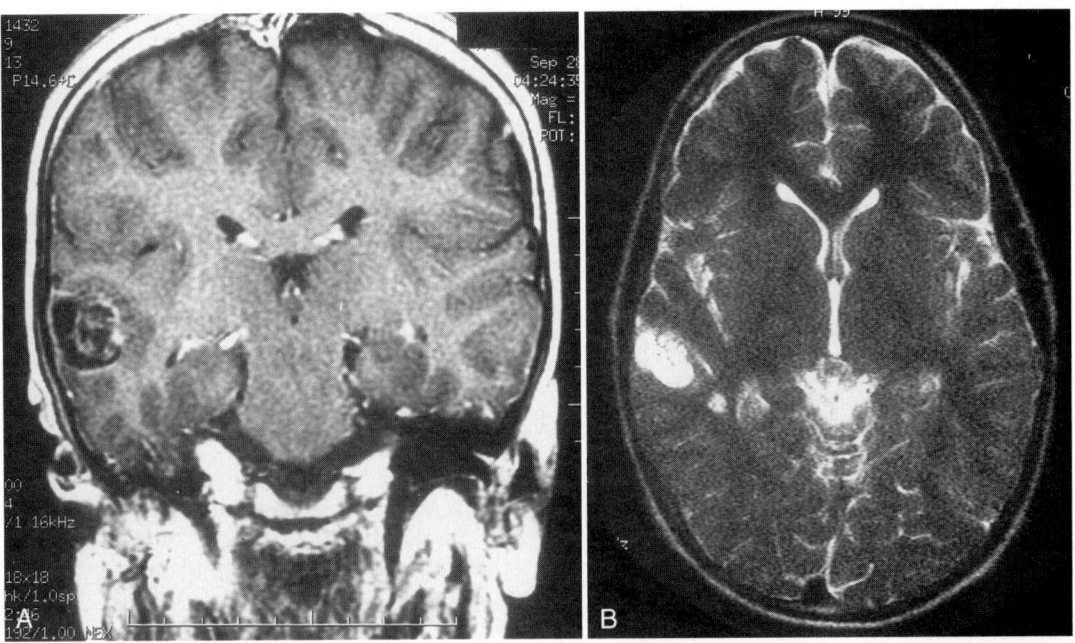

FIGURE 239–2. This 9-year-old boy experienced partial complex seizures consisting of staring spells and palpitations 5 months before admission. *A*, T1-weighted gadolinium-enhanced coronal magnetic resonance imaging (MRI) scan. *B*, T2-weighted axial MRI scan. Note the partially cystic tumor with punctate enhancement at the lateral right temporal lobe. Pathologic examination revealed a dysembryoplastic neuroepithelial tumor.

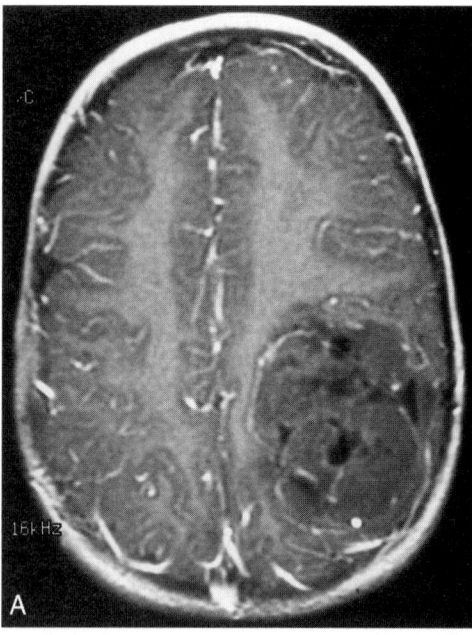

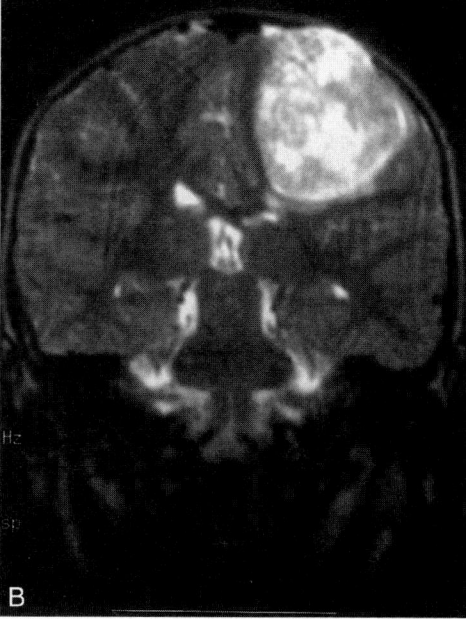

FIGURE 239–3. This 2-year-old girl had been experiencing simple partial seizures consisting of right hand jerking for several months before consultation. *A,* T1-weighted gadolinium-enhanced axial magnetic resonance imaging (MRI) scan. *B,* T2-weighted coronal MRI scan. Note the heterogeneous mass in the left posterior frontal lobe with mild contrast enhancement. Pathologic examination revealed a ganglioneuroblastoma.

with a well-delineated border are typical (Figs. 239–4 and 239–5).[23–26]

Pleomorphic xanthoastrocytoma is a well-delineated tumor that involves the cortical surface, most commonly at the temporal or parietal lobe, and may be contiguous with the leptomeninges.[17] It consists of cystic and nodular components. The mural nodule strongly enhances with contrast on CT or MRI and usually does not calcify (Fig. 239–6). It has a decreased to similar signal relative to gray matter on T1-weighted images and an increased signal on T2-weighted images.[27]

PATHOLOGIC FEATURES

The term *primitive neuroectodermal tumor* was initially coined by neuropathologists Hart and Earle in 1973.[28] They described a predominantly undifferentiated, malignant tumor found in the cerebral hemispheres of young patients. This tumor contains small, undifferentiated cells with dark, oval to irregular nuclei and malignant features such as high cellularity, pleomorphism, endothelial hyperplasia, mitotic figures, and necrotic areas. A prominent mesenchymal component is present in some cases, and there are a few focal areas of neuronal or glial differentiation. The primitive component usually accounts for 90% of the tumor.[10] Cerebral neuroblastoma, pineoblastoma, retinoblastoma, and ependymoblastoma are included in the classification of primitive neuroectodermal tumor.

Oligodendroglioma tends to infiltrate the cortex and is frequently calcified. Perinuclear cytoplasmic clearing with a "fried egg" appearance is an artifact that results from delayed fixation.[29] A "chicken wire" pattern of vascularization is sometimes seen. If the tumor contains a significant component of neoplastic astrocytes, it is classified as oligoastrocytoma.

Astrocytoma is diffuse and poorly marginated. The subtypes of astrocytoma include protoplasmic, fibrillary, gemistocytic, and giant cell forms.[29] Mitoses, necrosis, hypercellularity, nuclear atypia, and vascular proliferation within the tumor suggest a higher grade. Astrocytoma initially diagnosed as low grade may present years later with histologic features indicating a higher grade.

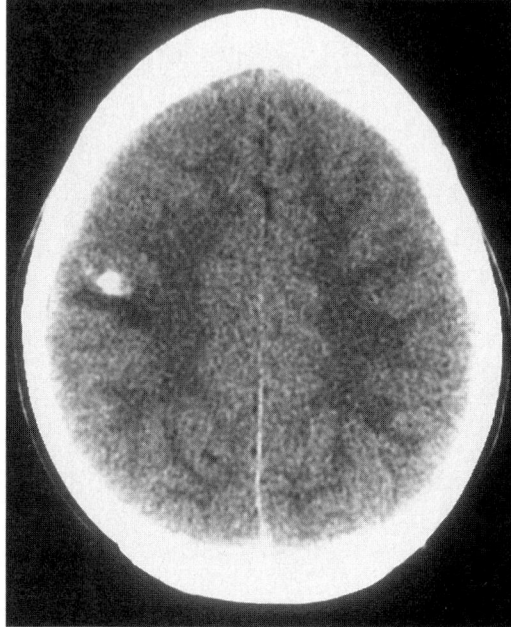

FIGURE 239–4. This 13-year-old boy had several episodes of left facial jerking. Axial head computed tomographic scan without contrast shows a calcified lesion in the right posterior frontal lobe. Pathologic examination revealed a ganglioglioma.

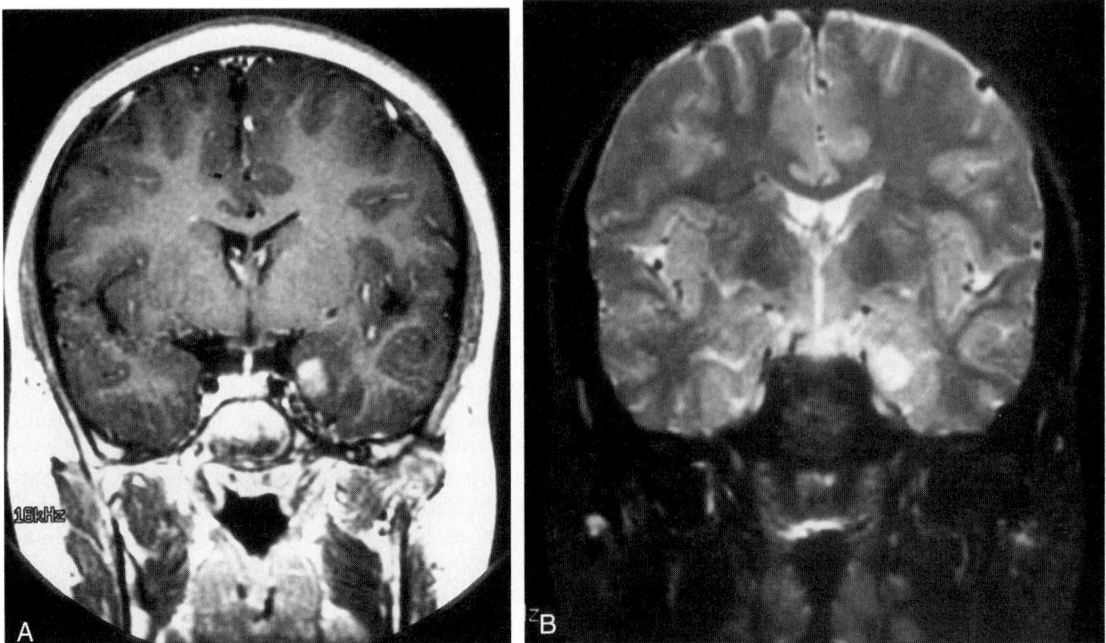

FIGURE 239-5. An 8-year-old girl presented with complex partial seizures consisting of staring spells and facial grimacing. *A,* T1-weighted gadolinium-enhanced coronal magnetic resonance imaging (MRI) scan. *B,* T2-weighted coronal MRI scan. Note the well-delineated, enhancing tumor in the left mesial temporal lobe with minimal mass effect. Pathologic examination revealed a ganglioglioma.

Ganglioglioma contains clusters of abnormal, mature, binucleate ganglion cells surrounded by collagen-rich stroma and lymphoid infiltrate.[29] Neoplastic astrocytes with cytoplasmic granular bodies are sometimes seen. The cyst wall is non-neoplastic.

The origin of dysembryoplastic neuroepithelial tumor is unknown. The presence of cortical dysplasia and the heterogeneity of cellular composition have led to the hypothesis that it is derived from the secondary germinal layers during embryogenesis. Histologically, the tumor is characterized by cellular pleomorphism with the presence of neurons, astrocytes, and oligoden-

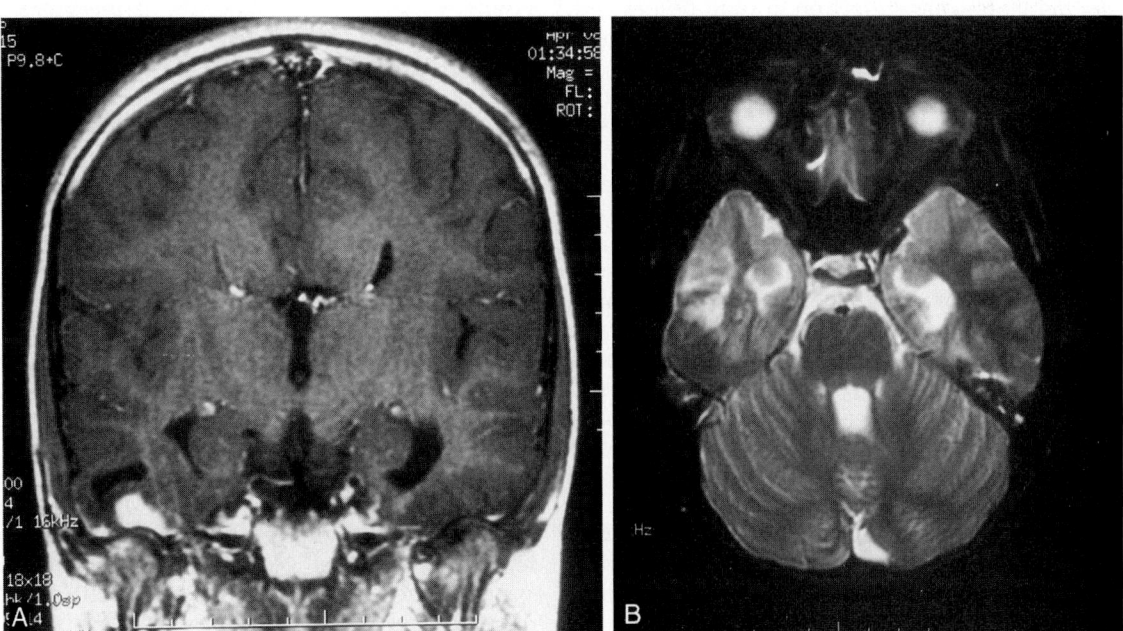

FIGURE 239-6. This 12-year-old boy had medically intractable seizures since age 5. *A,* T1-weighted gadolinium-enhanced coronal magnetic resonance imaging (MRI) scan. *B,* T2-weighted axial MRI scan. Note the cystic right temporal tumor with an enhancing mural nodule. Pathologic examination revealed a pleomorphic xanthoastrocytoma.

droglia that have variable morphology. It may have a specific glioneuronal element, a nodular component, or an association with cortical dysplasia.[16]

Pleomorphic xanthoastrocytoma contains lipid-rich cells and abundant reticulin reactivity. Mitotic activity is rarely seen. The cells exhibit nuclear atypia and are pleomorphic and multinucleated.[30] Malignant transformation occurs in 20%.

PERIOPERATIVE MANAGEMENT

A high-resolution MRI scan is necessary for surgical planning. If the tumor is small or located near eloquent cortex, imaging with fiducials for registration in a frameless stereotactic system may be useful for intraoperative tumor localization. If the imaging study shows significant edema surrounding the tumor and the patient is symptomatic, a loading dose of corticosteroid should be given at the time of admission, followed by a maintenance dose perioperatively. Antiulcer prophylaxis is given concurrently to minimize the risk of steroid-induced gastrointestinal hemorrhage. Unless the patient presents with a history of seizure, the use of anticonvulsant medication prophylactically has generally been found to be unnecessary. If there is a history of seizure, however, anticonvulsant medication is continued perioperatively and gradually tapered over 3 months to 1 year.

SURGICAL THERAPY

Gross total resection is the primary treatment for most cerebral hemispheric tumors. Removal of the tumor provides tissue for histologic diagnosis, achieves cytoreduction, alleviates mass effect on normal tissue, and, when it is the epileptogenic focus, offers definitive seizure control. Stereotactic biopsy is indicated if the tumor is deemed unresectable by virtue of its location or the extent of cerebral involvement.

A powerful tool to aid in the resection of small or deep-seated tumors is frameless stereotaxy. The craniotomy size and cortical resection can be minimized with this system. Although the accuracy of frameless stereotaxy can be up to 2 mm, the shifting of tissues after drainage of cerebrospinal fluid following dural opening and during tumor resection limits its accuracy.

Intraoperative ultrasonography is another valuable tool in tumor resection. It provides real-time images of the tumor, the lack of which is a significant drawback of frameless stereotaxy. The preparation time and cost of using intraoperative ultrasonography are also less than for frameless stereotaxy.

The risk of resecting hemispheric tumors located within or adjacent to functional cortex is lower with the advent of intraoperative stimulation mapping. Functional motor, sensory, or language areas were found within the tumor in 28 of 413 patients in one series.[31]

The resection can be guided with intraoperative electrocorticography, which is used to identify the seizure focus that extends beyond the tumor. In 60% of patients with medically refractory seizures, persistent seizure foci adjacent to the tumor were identified after tumor resection.[15] The use of electrocorticography must be considered when planning the operative approach.

The main treatment for low-grade astrocytoma is gross total resection whenever possible.[32, 33] Residual tumor should be followed by MRI, and if growth occurs, it should be resected again. Some lesions may be deep seated or may not be resectable without unacceptable neurological deficit. In those situations, CT- or MRI-guided stereotactic biopsy can be performed to obtain histologic diagnosis. Chemotherapy or radiation therapy is reserved for progressive or recurrent tumors.

The primary treatment for ganglioglioma is gross total resection. Long-term survival is the rule, even with incompletely resected lesions. Leptomeningeal and subarachnoid dissemination is very rare.[34]

Gross total resection is the primary treatment for dysembryoplastic neuroepithelial tumor.[16] The tumor is macroscopically visible on the cortical surface, with a variable degree of demarcation and firmness. Seizures either resolve completely or are significantly reduced after resection. No further adjuvant therapy is necessary. There is no radiographic or clinical recurrence, even following subtotal resection.

ADJUVANT THERAPY

Chemotherapy and radiation have been used extensively to treat pediatric tumors following resection. Radiation therapy is rarely used in children younger than 2 years, but chemotherapy can be used if residual tumor is left or if the tumor recurs. Chemotherapy allows radiation therapy to be delayed in children younger than 2 years, who are at the greatest risk of serious developmental delay from radiation injury. In older children, who are at less risk for significant psychomotor retardation, radiation therapy may be useful.

Chemotherapy is usually given in a multidrug regimen to reduce the possibility of developing resistance. A short course is usually used to minimize hematopoietic toxicity. The effectiveness of chemotherapy depends on four factors: (1) blood-brain barrier, (2) uptake into cells, (3) retention of chemotherapy agents, and (4) ability to inflict DNA damage on tumor cells. Resistance develops if drugs are exported from cells or if tumor cells are able to repair the drug-induced injury. Penetration of chemotherapeutic agents into the central nervous system is aided by agents that disrupt the blood-brain barrier.[35–37]

The efficacy of chemotherapy for supratentorial primitive neuroectodermal tumor has not been established.[38] Chemotherapy and radiation therapy are offered after resection to improve the dismal outcome. In a review of 27 patients with supratentorial primitive neuroectodermal tumor, Albright and colleagues found the overall 5-year survival to be 34% and the progression-free survival to be 31%.[39] These rates are worse than those of posterior fossa medulloblastoma. Patients younger than 3 years or with intracranial or intraspinal tumor dissemination or positive cerebrospinal fluid cytologic findings at the time of diagnosis have a significantly worse progression-free survival. There is no statistically significant difference in progression-free survival between subtotal and gross total resection, although there was a trend toward improved progression-free survival with gross total resection.

Children with newly diagnosed high-grade glioma obtain a modest benefit from chemotherapy. In a randomized study by the Children's Cancer Study Group in 1989, postsurgical radiation therapy and chemotherapy with chloroethyl-cyclohexyl-nitrosourea (CCNU) and vincristine improved the percentage of children who were free of disease 5 years after treatment to 46%, compared with 18% for children treated with postsurgical radiation therapy alone.[40] There was no difference in survival using the eight-drugs-in-one-day regimen in place of CCNU and vincristine.[41] The Pediatric Oncology Group trial, which looked at children younger than 36 months of age with biopsy-proven malignant brain tumors, demonstrated that cyclophosphamide, vincristine, and cisplatin are effective primary postoperative treatments that allow radiation therapy to be delayed.[42]

The use of chemotherapy for children with recurrent malignant glioma has not been encouraging. The median time to progression is usually less than 6 months following treatment.[43–47] Trials on the use of high-dose chemotherapy followed by autologous bone marrow rescue or peripheral stem cell rescue are under way.

The main prognostic factor in ependymoma is the extent of resection at the time of surgery. Chemotherapy offers no survival benefit in newly diagnosed cases. Recurrent tumor is treated with repeat resection, followed by a course of etoposide or cisplatin.[48]

Chemotherapy for the treatment of oligodendroglioma is of unknown benefit. There are no randomized, prospective studies of children with newly diagnosed or recurrent oligodendroglioma.

Biologic response modifiers have not proved useful in the treatment of gliomas. Adaptive immunotherapy with interleukin-2; passive immunotherapy with monoclonal antibodies injected intrathecally; and nonspecific immunotherapy with interferon beta, interferon gamma, and *Serratia marcescens* extract (Imuvert) are being studied.[49–54]

PROGNOSIS

Factors associated with a good prognosis include seizure at presentation, symptoms for more than 6 months, and a benign histology.[14] Children diagnosed with brain tumors between the ages of 10 and 14 years have a 5-year survival rate of 57%. The worst survival rate is in infants younger than 2 years, who have a 36% 5-year survival rate.[55] Reasons for this difference may be the smaller dose of radiation infants receive postoperatively and the higher proportion of malignant tumors in infants.[56] Combined loss of chromosome arms 1p and 19q is a statistically significant predictor of prolonged survival in patients with pure oligoden-

droglioma, independent of tumor grade.[57] The 5-year survival rate of children with low-grade supratentorial astrocytoma is 71%. Children with high-grade (grade 3 or 4) supratentorial astrocytoma have a survival rate between 16% and 35%. The survival rate at 5 years following gross total resection of an ependymoma is 75% to 80%, compared with a survival rate of 22% to 41% among patients with evidence of residual disease.[58, 59]

The probability of seizure control is highest after gross total resection of a low-grade glioma or ganglioglioma in children who present with a history of seizure for less than 1 year.[13, 60] Approximately 78% to 86% of these patients become seizure free following gross total resection. In addition, patients who present at a younger age and have no epileptiform discharge on postoperative electroencephalograms have a higher probability of seizure control.

A predictor of prognosis in children with grade 3 or 4 astrocytoma is the MIB-1 labeling index.[61] The MIB-1 antibody binds onto the Ki-67 nuclear antigen, which is expressed in actively cycling cells. The median progression-free survival and the overall survival in the group with low MIB-1 levels are both greater than 48 months, which is statistically different from the progression-free survival of 6 months and the overall survival of 16 months in the group with high MIB-1 levels. The MIB-1 labeling index reflects the proliferative activity of the tumor and can be used to improve the accuracy of predicting the tumor's biologic behavior.

CONCLUSION

Pediatric cerebral hemispheric tumors encompass a wide variety of histologies, and unlike those that occur in adults, a higher proportion of them are low grade. They present primarily with seizures and failure to thrive. Improvements in imaging techniques have led to earlier detection of cerebral tumors. Gross total resection is the treatment of choice. However, for recurrent or high-grade tumors, adjuvant radiation or chemotherapy is indicated. Advances in immunotherapy have the potential to improve our ability to control tumor growth following cytoreduction.[62–65]

REFERENCES

1. Davis F, Malinski N, Haenszel W: Primary brain tumor incidence rates in four United States regions, 1985–1989: A pilot study. Neuroepidemiology 15:103–112, 1996.
2. Desmeules M, Mikkelsen T, Mao Y: Increasing incidence of primary malignant brain tumors: Influence of diagnostic methods. J Natl Cancer Inst 84:442–445, 1992.
3. Staneczek W, Janisch W: Epidemiology of primary tumors of the central nervous system in children and adolescents: A population-based study. Pathologe 15:207–215, 1994.
4. Rickert C, Probst-Cousin S, Gullota F: Primary intracranial neoplasms of infancy and early childhood. Childs Nerv Syst 13:507–513, 1997.
5. Pollack I: Brain tumors in children. N Engl J Med 331:1500–1507, 1994.
6. Farwell J, Dohrmann G, Flannery J: Central nervous system tumors in children. Cancer 40:3123–3132, 1977.

7. Berger M, Keles G, Geyer J: Cerebral hemispheric tumors of childhood. Neurosurg Clin N Am 3:839–852, 1992.

8. Kumar R, Tekkok I, Jones R: Intracranial tumours in the first 18 months of life. Childs Nerv Syst 6:371–374, 1990.

9. Coulon R, Till K: Intracranial ependymomas in children: A review of 43 cases. Childs Brain 3:154–168, 1977.

10. Gaffney C, Sloane J, Bradley N, Bloom H: Primitive neuroectodermal tumours of the cerebrum: Pathology and treatment. J Neurooncol 3:23–33, 1985.

11. Flores L, Williams D, Bell B, et al: Delay in the diagnosis of pediatric brain tumors. Am J Dis Child 140:684–686, 1986.

12. Pollack I, Claassen D, al-Shboul Q, et al: Low grade gliomas of the cerebral hemispheres in children: An analysis of 71 cases. J Neurosurg 82:536–547, 1995.

13. Packer R, Sutton L, Patel K, et al: Seizure control following tumor surgery for childhood cortical low grade gliomas. J Neurosurg 80:998–1003, 1994.

14. Shady J, Black P, Kupsky W, et al: Seizures in children with supratentorial astroglial neoplasms. Pediatr Neurosurg 21:23–30, 1994.

15. Berger M, Ghatan S, Haglund M, et al: Low grade gliomas associated with intractable epilepsy: Seizure outcome utilizing electrocorticography during tumor resection. J Neurosurg 79:62–69, 1993.

16. Daumas-Duport C, Scheithauer B, Chodkiewicz J, et al: Dysembryoplastic neuroepithelial tumor: A surgically curable tumor of young patients with intractable partial seizures. Report of thirty-nine cases. Neurosurgery 23:545–556, 1988.

17. Osborn A: Diagnostic Neuroradiology. St Louis, Mosby, 1994.

18. Lee Y, Van Tassel P: Intracranial oligodendrogliomas: Imaging findings in 35 untreated cases. AJR Am J Roentgenol 152:361–369, 1989.

19. Furie D, Provenzale J: Supratentorial ependymomas and subependymomas: CT and MR appearance. J Comput Assist Tomogr 19:518–526, 1995.

20. Kuroiwa T, Bergey G, Rothman M, et al: Radiologic appearance of the dysembryoplastic neuroepithelial tumor. Radiology 197:233–238, 1995.

21. Koeller K, Dillion W: Dysembryoplastic neuroepithelial tumors: MR appearance. AJNR Am J Neuroradiol 13:1319–1325, 1992.

22. Davis P, Wichman R, Takei Y, Hoffman JJ: Primary cerebral neuroblastoma: CT and MR findings in 12 cases. AJR Am J Roentgenol 154:831–836, 1990.

23. Haddad S, Moore S, Menezes A, VanGilder J: Ganglioglioma: 13 years of experience. Neurosurgery 31:171–178, 1992.

24. Otsubo H, Hoffman J, Humphreys R, et al: Detection and management of gangliogliomas in children. Surg Neurol 38:371–378, 1992.

25. Hashimoto M, Fujimoto K, Shinoda S, Masuzawa T: Magnetic resonance imaging of ganglion cell tumours. Neuroradiology 35:181–184, 1993.

26. Benitez W, Glasier C, Husain M, et al: MR findings in childhood gangliogliomas. J Comput Assist Tomogr 14:712–716, 1990.

27. Yoshino M, Lucio R: Pleomorphic xanthoastrocytoma. AJNR Am J Neuroradiol 13:1330–1332, 1992.

28. Hart M, Earle K: Primitive neuroectodermal tumors of the brain in children. Cancer 32:890–897, 1973.

29. Okazaki H, Scheithauer B: Atlas of Neuropathology. New York, Gower Medical, 1988.

30. Kepes J, Rubinstein L, Eng L: Pleomorphic xanthoastrocytoma: A dinstinctive meningocerebral glioma of young subjects with relatively favorable prognosis. A study of 12 cases. Cancer 44:1839–1852, 1979.

31. Skirboll S, Ojemann G, Berger M, et al: Functional cortex and subcortical white matter located within gliomas. Neurosurgery 38:678–685, 1996.

32. Berger M: The impact of technical adjuncts in the surgical management of cerebral hemispheric low grade gliomas. J Neurooncol 28:129–155, 1996.

33. Hirsch J, Sainte Rose C, Pierre-Kahn A, et al: Benign astrocytic and oligodendrocytic tumors of the cerebral hemispheres in children. J Neurosurg 70:568–572, 1989.

34. Diepholder H, Schwechheimer K, Mohadjer M, et al: A clinicopathologic and immunomorphologic study of 13 cases of ganglioglioma. Cancer 68:2192–2201, 1991.

35. Kroll R, Pagel M, Muldoon L, et al: Improving drug delivery to intracerebral tumor and surrounding brain in a rodent model: A comparison of osmotic versus bradykinin modification of the blood-brain and/or blood-tumor barriers. Neurosurgery 43:879–886, 1998.

36. Zlokovic B, Apuzzo M: Strategies to circumvent vascular barriers of the central nervous system. Neurosurgery 43:877–878, 1998.

37. Elliot P, Hayward N, Huff M, et al: Unlocking the blood brain barrier: A role for RMP-7 in brain tumor therapy. Exp Neurol 141:214–224, 1996.

38. Cohen B, Zeltzer P, Boyett J, et al: Prognostic factors and treatment results for supratentorial primitive neuroectodermal tumors in children using radiation and chemotherapy: A Children's Cancer Group randomized trial. J Clin Oncol 13:1687–1696, 1995.

39. Albright A, Wisoff J, Zeltzer P, et al: Prognostic factors in children with supratentorial primitive neuroectodermal tumors. Pediatr Neurosurg 22:1–7, 1995.

40. Sposto R, Ertel I, Jenkin R, et al: The effectiveness of chemotherapy for treatment of high grade astrocytoma in children: Results of a randomized trial. A report from the Children's Cancer Study Group. J Neurooncol 7:165–177, 1989.

41. Finlay J, Boyett J, Yates A, et al: Randomized phase III trial in childhood high-grade astrocytoma comparing vincristine, lomustine, and prednisone with the eight-drugs-in-1-day regimen. J Clin Oncol 13:112–123, 1995.

42. Duffner P, Horowitz M, Krischer J: Post-operative chemotherapy and delayed radiation in children less than three years of age with malignant brain tumors. N Engl J Med 328:1725–1731, 1993.

43. Walker R, Allen J: Cisplatin in the treatment of recurrent childhood primary brain tumors. J Clin Oncol 6:62–66, 1988.

44. Allen J, Walker R, Luks E, et al: Carboplatin and recurrent childhood brain tumors. J Clin Oncol 5:459–463, 1987.

45. Bertolone S, Baum E, Krivit W, Hammond G: A phase II study of cisplatin therapy in recurrent childhood brain tumors: A report from the Children's Cancer Study Group. J Neurooncol 7:5–11, 1989.

46. Twelves C, Ash C, Miles D, et al: Activity and toxicity of carboplatin and iproplatin in relapsed high-grade glioma. Cancer Chemother Pharmacol 27:481–483, 1991.

47. van den Bent M, Schellens J, Vecht C, et al: Phase II study on cisplatin and ifosfamide in recurrent high grade gliomas. Eur J Cancer 34:1570–1574, 1998.

48. Goldwein J, Glauser T, Packer R, et al: Recurrent intracranial ependymomas in children: Survival, patterns of failure, and prognostic factors. Cancer 66:557–563, 1990.

49. Moseley R, Benjamin J, Ashpole R, et al: Carcinomatous meningitis: Antibody-guided therapy with I-131 HMFG1. J Neurol Neurosurg Psychiatry 54:260–265, 1991.

50. Farkkila M, Jaaskelainen J, Kallio M, et al: Randomised, controlled study of intratumoral recombinant gamma-interferon treatment in newly diagnosed glioblastoma. Br J Cancer 70:138–141, 1994.

51. Packer R, Kramer E, Ryan J: Biological and immune modulating agents in the treatment of childhood brain tumors. Neurol Clin 9:405–422, 1991.

52. Kemshead J, Jones D, Lashford L, et al: 131-I coupled to monoclonal antibodies as therapeutic agents for neuroectodermally derived tumors: Fact or fiction? Cancer Drug Delivery 3:25–43, 1986.

53. Allen J, Packer R, Bleyer A, et al: Recombinant interferon beta: A phase I–II trial in children with recurrent brain tumors. J Clin Oncol 9:783–788, 1991.

54. Jaeckle K, Mittleman A, Hill F: Phase II trial of *Serratia marcescens* extract in recurrent malignant astrocytoma. J Clin Oncol 8:1408–1418, 1990.

55. Duffner P, Cohen M, Myers M, Heise H: Survival of children with brain tumors: SEER Program, 1973–1980. Neurology 36:597–601, 1986.

56. Geyer J, Finlay J, Boyett J, et al: Survival of infants with malignant astrocytomas: A report from the Children's Cancer Group. Cancer 75:1045–1050, 1995.

57. Smith J, Perry A, Borell T, et al: Alterations of chromosome arms 1p and 19q as predictors of survival in oligodendrogliomas, astrocytomas, and mixed oligoastrocytomas. J Clin Oncol 18:636–645, 2000.

58. Pollack I, Gerszten P, Martinez A, et al: Intracranial ependymomas of childhood: Long-term outcome and prognostic factors. Neurosurgery 37:655–666, 1995.

59. Rousseau P, Habrand J, Sarrazin D, et al: Treatment of intracranial ependymomas of children: Review of a 15 year experience. Int J Radiat Oncol Biol Phys 28:381–386, 1993.

60. Morris H, Matkovic Z, Estes E, et al: Ganglioglioma and intractable epilepsy: Clinical and neurophysiologic features and predictors of outcome after surgery. Epilepsia 39:307–313, 1998.

61. Pollack I, Campbell J, Hamilton R, et al: Proliferation index as a predictor of prognosis in malignant gliomas of childhood. Cancer 79:849–856, 1997.

62. Zeltzer P, Moilanen B, Yu J, Black K: Immunotherapy of malignant brain tumors in children and adults: From theoretical principles to clinical application. Childs Nerv Syst 15:514–528, 1999.

63. Visse E, Siesjo P, Widegren B, Sjogren H: Regression of intracerebral rat glioma isografts by therapeutic subcutaneous immunization with interferon-gamma, interleukin-7, or B7-1-transfected tumor cells. Cancer Gene Ther 6:37–44, 1999.

64. Jean W, Spellman S, Wallenfriedman M, et al: Interleukin-12–based immunotherapy against rat 9L glioma. Neurosurgery 42:850–856, 1998.

65. Fakhrai H, Dorigo O, Shawler D, et al: Eradication of established intracranial rat gliomas by transforming growth factor beta antisense gene therapy. Proc Natl Acad Sci U S A 93:2909–2914, 1996.

CHAPTER 240

Intraspinal Tumors in Infants and Children

GEORGE I. JALLO ■ KARL F. KOTHBAUER ■ FRED J. EPSTEIN

The first successful resection of an intramedullary spinal cord tumor was performed in 1907 in Vienna by von Eiselsberg.[1] However, the first published report of such an operation appeared in 1911 by Elsberg and Beer in New York.[2] They developed a strategy of a two-stage operation. A myelotomy was performed at the first surgery, and by the second surgery (about a week later), the tumor had already partly extruded itself from the cord substance, facilitating further resection. The first intradural extramedullary tumor resection is credited to Macewen in 1883.[3]

After the early work of these pioneer neurosurgeons, the neurologic risk of surgery for intramedullary neoplasms was considered unacceptably high. This led to the development of a conservative treatment plan with biopsy, dural decompression, and subsequent radiation therapy, regardless of the histologic diagnosis.[4]

The advent of the operating microscope and the development of microsurgical techniques revolutionized all neurosurgery and opened new avenues in the treatment of spinal cord tumors. Computed tomography and particularly magnetic resonance imaging (MRI) have dramatically improved preoperative planning and significantly contributed to the development of modern treatment strategies for both intra- and extramedullary spinal cord tumors. In particular, the treatment strategy for intramedullary tumors changed from a conservative to an aggressive approach. Most of these tumors are histologically benign. Complete or nearly complete resection results in long-term progression-free survival with acceptable neurologic morbidity.[5–12]

This chapter describes the treatment approach to pediatric patients with intramedullary and intradural extramedullary spinal cord tumors.

EPIDEMIOLOGY

Intramedullary spinal cord tumors are relatively rare, accounting for only 5% to 10% of all central nervous system tumors.[9] About 55% of all intradural neoplasms in children have an intramedullary location.[13]

In a large series of more than 200 children with intramedullary spinal cord tumors operated on by the senior author, the median age at presentation was about 10 years, and the male-to-female ratio was 1: 1.1 (Table 240–1). Astrocytomas and gangliogliomas accounted for more than two thirds of the histologic diagnoses. The remainder were ependymomas, mixed gliomas, and miscellaneous tumors (Table 240–2). Astrocytomas and gangliogliomas were more prevalent in the younger age groups, whereas ependymomas were more frequent in older children.

Intradural extramedullary neoplasms are less common than intramedullary tumors.[14] They represent about 45% of intradural tumors in children. Dermoid and epidermoid tumors account for about one third of these lesions, and nerve sheath tumors account for another third. These lesions are often associated with neurofibromatosis type I.[15, 16] Meningiomas, unlike in the adult population, account for less than 5%.[13]

The rarest intradural lesions in children are diffuse leptomeningeal tumors. Either these are primary low-grade astrocytomas, which may present with diffuse leptomeningeal dissemination, or they arise as dissemination from posterior fossa tumors, mostly primitive neuroectodermal tumors or ependymomas. These disseminated tumors cannot be treated surgically. Surgery is performed only to obtain a histologic diagnosis.

TABLE 240–1 ■ **Characteristics of 164 Children with Intramedullary Spinal Cord Tumors**

Age	10.4 yr
Sex	
Male	79
Female	85
Location	
Cevicomedullary	14
Cervical	26
Cervicothoracic	44
Thoracic	64
Conus	16
Number of vertebra levels	5.4

TABLE 240–2 ■ **Tumor Histology in 164 Children with Intramedullary Spinal Cord Tumors**

HISTOLOGY	NUMBER (%)
Astrocytoma, low grade	58 (35)
Astrocytoma, high grade	18 (11)
Ganglioglioma	44 (27)
Mixed glioma	10 (6)
Ependymoma	19 (12)
Other	15 (9)

CLINICAL PRESENTATION

Intramedullary spinal cord tumors may remain asymptomatic for a long time and reach a considerable size before they are detected.[9] The onset of symptoms is often insidious, and symptoms may be present for months or even years before a diagnosis is established. Symptoms may also appear at the time of a trivial injury. Not infrequently, parents describe exacerbations and remissions. A common early symptom is back or neck pain, occurring in up to two thirds of all pediatric patients.[9] The pain may be diffuse, in which case an intramedullary tumor is the more likely cause, or the pain may have a radicular distribution, which is more common in intradural extramedullary lesions.[14] Young children may present with abdominal pain as a nonspecific symptom, which makes diagnosis particularly difficult. It is not uncommon for these children to have an extensive gastrointestinal evaluation before diagnosis of the intraspinal neoplasm[4] (Table 240–3).

Motor function appears to be affected early.[7, 9, 12] This may manifest as motor regression (e.g., refusal to stand or crawl after having learned to walk) or as gait abnormality. Children present with lower extremity weakness, clumsiness, or frequent falls. On examination, the majority of these patients have mild to moderate motor deficits, as well as upper motor neuron findings, such as spasticity, hyperreflexia, and clonus.

About one third of patients have some degree of kyphoscoliosis,[9] most of them with tumors in the thoracic region.[17] Paraspinal pain is common in this group and is attributed to the scoliosis. Torticollis is seen in about one fifth of children, being more common in cervical tumors.[8, 18]

TABLE 240–3 ■ **Reasons for Parental Concern in Children with Intramedullary Neoplasms**

PARENTAL CONCERN	PERCENTAGE
Motor regression	65
Pain	45
Gait abnormality	37
Kyphoscoliosis	32
Torticollis	18
Delayed milestones	3
Abdominal complaints	1

Sensory symptoms, mostly dysesthesias described as unpleasant hot or cold sensations, are also found in about 20% of patients. In glial tumors, as opposed to ependymomas, the sensory symptoms are frequently asymmetrical.

Sphincter dysfunction is present late in the clinical course, except for tumors located in the conus medullaris. However, changes in bladder function are difficult to detect in young children, especially before they are toilet trained.

Malignant intramedullary gliomas are rare.[6, 8, 12] The symptoms are similar, but the clinical history is significantly shorter. Children with malignant intramedullary tumors have a median prodrome of about 4.5 months, compared with 9.2 months in children with benign tumors.

Another associated finding in children with intramedullary neoplasms is hydrocephalus, which has been reported to occur in as many as 15%.[19, 20] The mechanisms for hydrocephalus include an increased concentration of protein in the cerebrospinal fluid, arachnoidal fibrosis, and subarachnoid dissemination. The incidence of hydrocephalus is substantially higher in children with malignant tumors (~35%) than in those with low-grade tumors (~15%). Children with cervical tumors are likely to develop hydrocephalus, most likely secondary to obstruction of the fourth ventricle outlets. The presence of hydrocephalus associated with an astrocytoma caudal to the cervicothoracic junction is suggestive of a malignant tumor with leptomeningeal dissemination and obstruction of the spinal fluid pathways.[20]

DIAGNOSTIC STUDIES

Magnetic Resonance Imaging

MRI is the study of choice to identify both intra- and extramedullary spinal cord neoplasms.[11, 21] Extramedullary lesions are readily identified as such, and their relation to the cord, attachment to dura, and displacement of the cord are visualized.

MRI scans should be performed both before and after intravenous administration of contrast agents (gadolinium diethylenetriaminepentaacetic acid), with T1-weighted images obtained in multiple planes.[22] These images demonstrate the solid tumor component. T2-weighted images optimally show the cerebrospinal fluid and tumor-associated cysts. Although MRI scans do not allow for a definite histologic diagnosis preoperatively, some typical imaging patterns have been identified for the most commonly encountered types of tumors. Ependymomas tend to enhance brightly and homogeneously. They often are associated with rostral and caudal cysts and are located primarily in the center of the cord (Fig. 240–1). Astrocytomas and gangliogliomas enhance less frequently, and if enhancement is seen, it is often weak and heterogeneous.[23, 24] In addition, these neoplasms are more often eccentric in the spinal cord and produce an asymmetrical enlargement of the cord (Figs. 240–2 and 240–3).

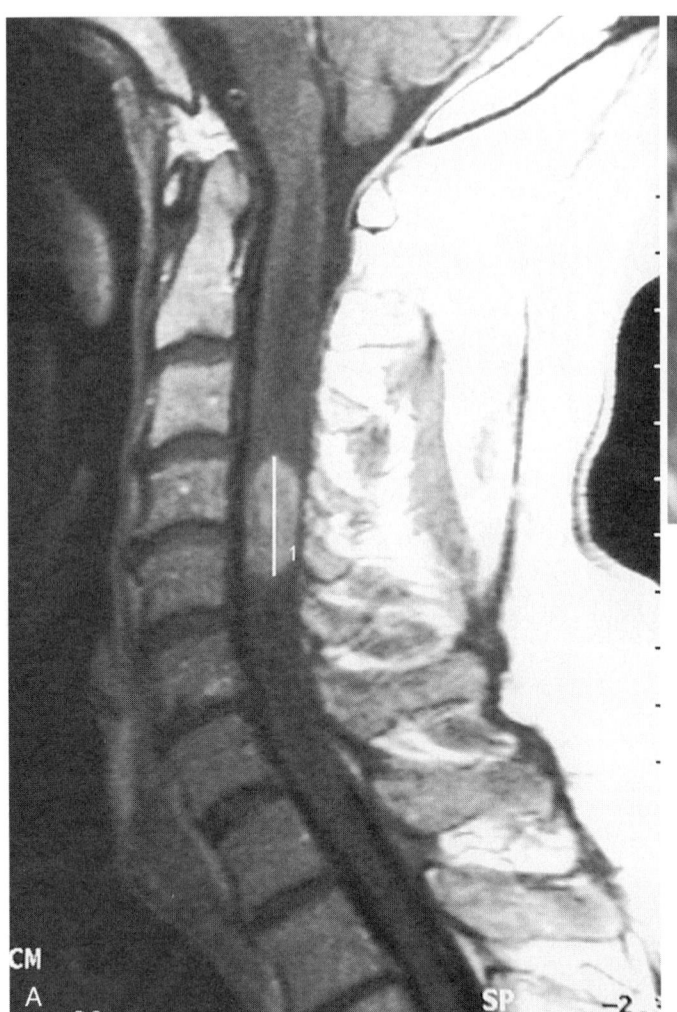

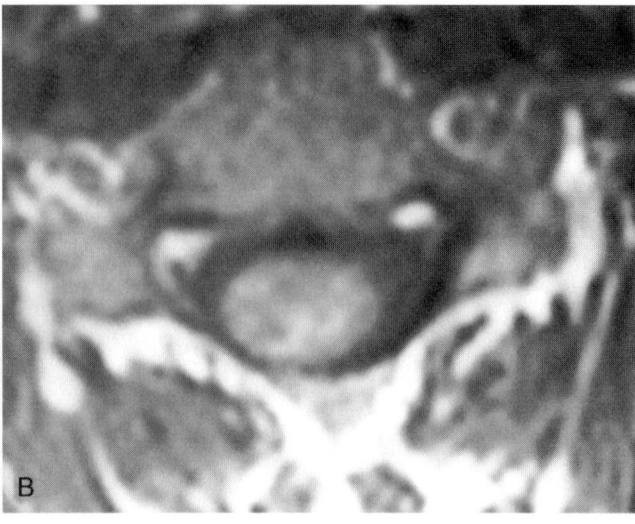

FIGURE 240–1. *A*, Sagittal T1-weighted magnetic resonance imaging (MRI) scan that shows a focal cervical intramedullary neoplasm. *B*, Axial T1-weighted MRI scan with gadolinium demonstrates the central location of the neoplasm, which proved to be an ependymoma.

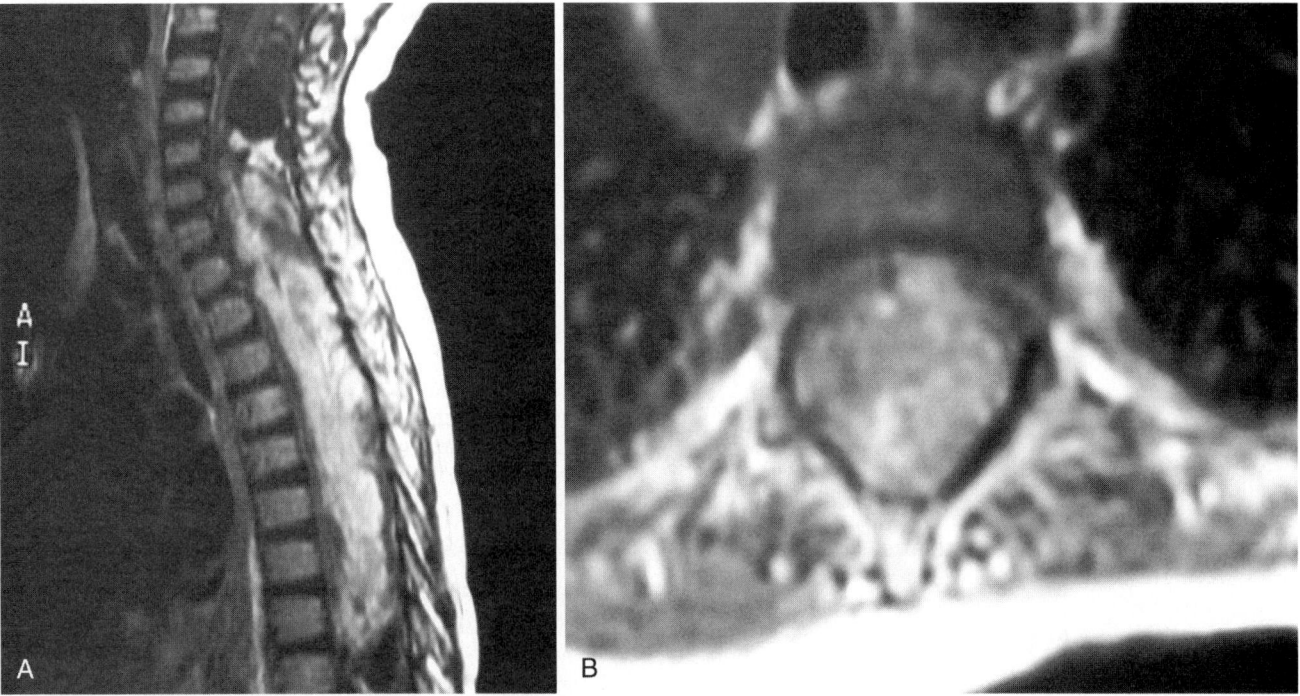

FIGURE 240–2. *A*, Sagittal T1-weighted MRI scan with contrast discloses a large cervicothoracic intramedullary ganglioglioma with the presence of rostral and caudal cysts in a 2-year-old boy. *B*, Axial T1-weighted MRI scan of the same patient shows the heterogeneous enhancement of the tumor and widened spinal cord.

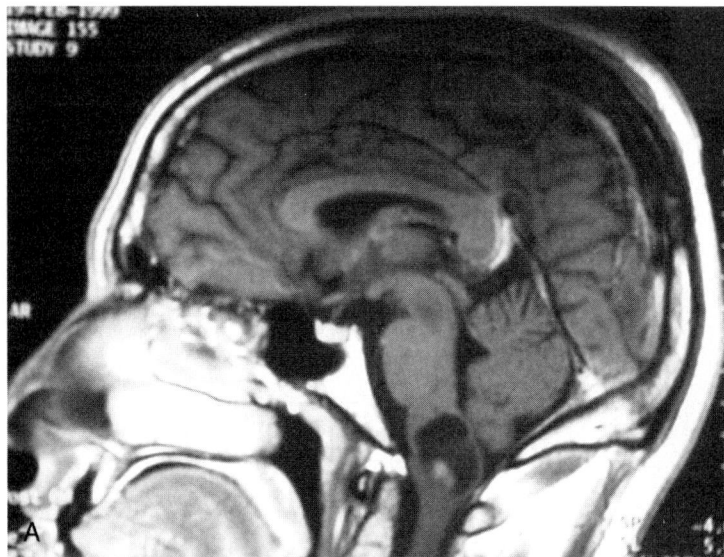
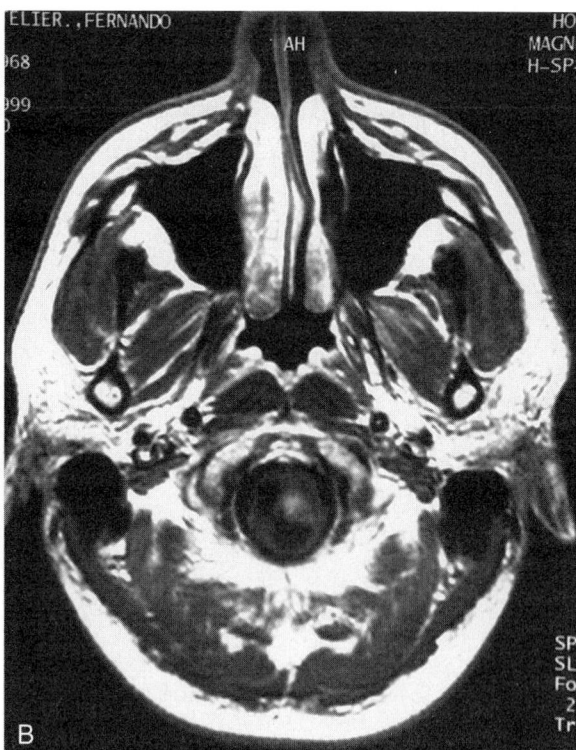

FIGURE 240–3. *A,* Sagittal T1-weighted MRI scan with contrast of a cervicomedullary juvenile pilocytic astrocytoma in a 21-year-old man. *B,* Axial postcontrast T1-weighted image shows the presence of the dorsal tumor–associated cyst.

Plain Radiographs

Plain radiographs are mandatory for children who present with scoliosis. These initial films serve as a baseline for the future management of the spinal deformity. Intradural extramedullary tumors can thin or cause sclerosis of the pedicles. A tumor that extends through a neural foramen enlarges that foramen and can be visualized on oblique films. Intramedullary neoplasms may show a diffusely widened spinal canal, with associated erosion of the pedicles and scalloping of the vertebrae.

Myelography and Computed Tomography

Myelography with water-soluble contrast agent combined with computed tomography was once used extensively in the evaluation of suspected intraspinal lesions.[6, 25] Today, computed tomography–myelography is reserved for the rare case in which MRI may be impossible to perform (e.g., owing to metallic implants) or impossible to interpret because of image distortion from metallic artifacts.

Computed tomographic scans delineate the bony anatomy better than MRI scans do. This technique may be used in conjunction with MRI scans for the rare malignant intradural neoplasms that have bone involvement.

SURGICAL MANAGEMENT OF INTRADURAL TUMORS

Surgical Instruments

Traditional suction and bipolar cautery for the removal of central nervous system neoplasms are now supple-
mented by a set of specialized instruments that aid in minimizing surgical trauma to normal neural tissue. Some of these specialized instruments have become essential for the microsurgical resection of spinal cord tumors.

ULTRASONIC ASPIRATOR

The Cavitron ultrasonic aspirator system was a significant advancement in the removal of spinal cord tumors.[26, 27] It uses high-frequency sound waves to fragment the tumor tissue, which is then aspirated by the suction apparatus at the tip of the device. This allows tumor removal with only minimal manipulation of the adjacent neural tissue compared with conventional suction-cautery.

LASER

The laser is an excellent surgical adjunct for spinal cord surgery. We prefer the Nd:YAG Contact Laser System (SLT, Montgomeryville, Pennsylvania) to other available laser technologies. This system has a touch-control handpiece and contact probes of various sizes. The contact probes are particularly useful as a scalpel to perform the myelotomy, demarcate the glial-tumor interface, and remove residual tumor fragments. This laser has minimal associated char, as seen with previous laser systems. This contact laser, at low intensity, is effective in preventing small arteriole or capillary bleeding. Firm lesions, such as meningiomas, neurofibromas, or rare types of intramedullary tumors, can be removed with reasonable safety only when the laser is available. These lesions cannot be manipulated with the bipolar cautery and scissors because of inevitable manipulation of the adjacent spinal cord tissue, and these lesions are too firm for the Cavitron ultrasonic aspirator to be internally decompressed. For lipomas, dermoids, and extramedullary tumors, the larger laser contact probes provide great precision for vaporization of fat and internal debulking.

Surgical Technique

Surgery is performed with the child in the prone position. A rigid head holder, such as the Sugita or Mayfield, is used for cervical and cervicothoracic tumors to secure the head in a neutral and unrotated position. In children younger than 6 years, we prefer the six-pin Sugita head holder. The horseshoe-shaped headrest should be avoided because it does not secure a neutral neck position.

A laminectomy or osteoplastic laminotomy[28] (for previously unoperated tumors) is performed with the Midas drill. The bone removal should expose the solid tumor component but does not need to expose the rostral or caudal cysts. The cyst fluid disappears after the neoplasm is removed, because the cyst walls are composed of non-neoplastic glial tissue.

Intraoperative ultrasonography visualizes the full extent of the tumor and its relation to the bone removal.[29] The spinal cord can be viewed in two dimensions, both sagittal and axial sections. Intramedullary astrocytomas and gangliogliomas have about the same echogenicity as the spinal cord. In these tumors, the spinal cord is diffusely enlarged, and the intratumoral cysts can be easily visualized.[30, 31] In contrast, ependymomas are usually hyperechogenic and can be differentiated from the spinal cord. Most often they are visible in the center of the cord. If the bone removal is not sufficient, the laminectomy is extended to expose the entire solid tumor before opening the dura.

The dura is then opened in the midline. The spinal cord is frequently expanded, and it may even be rotated and distorted. The asymmetrical expansion and rotation of the spinal cord may make identification of the midline raphe difficult. However, it is important to localize this raphe because this is the most frequent approach into the spinal cord. An alternative approach for extremely asymmetrical tumors is to enter the spinal cord through the dorsal root entry zone.

The neoplasm is usually located several millimeters underneath the dorsal surface of the spinal cord. The contact laser is used to perform the myelotomy with minimal neural injury. Each type of intramedullary tumor has a different macroscopic appearance. They can be differentiated by color and texture.

Ependymomas are red or dark gray and have a clear margin from the spinal cord. This interface can be separated with the plated bayonet[32] or the scalpel probe on the contact laser. The caudal pole of the tumor is identified, and the cleavage plane is separated in a rostral direction. The ventral aspect of ependymomas is adherent to the anterior median raphe because the feeding vessels originate from the anterior spinal artery. It is essential to preserve this vessel. The majority of these tumors can be removed en bloc.[5, 6, 33, 34]

Solid astrocytomas or gangliogliomas have a gray-yellow, glassy appearance. They must be removed from the inside out until the glial-tumor interface is recognized by the change in color and consistency of the tissue. Rarely, a true plane between tumor and normal spinal cord exists, and futile efforts to define this interface result in hazardous manipulation of normal spinal cord tissue.[7, 19]

The resection of astrocytomas is initiated at the midportion rather than at the poles of the tumor. The rostral and caudal poles are the least voluminous, and manipulation there may be the most dangerous to normal surrounding tissue. Intraoperative ultrasonography can be used to assess the extent of tumor resection. Residual fragments of tumor can be removed with the contact laser.

The excision of cystic neoplasms begins at the cyst-tumor junction. The neoplastic tissue is usually within cyst walls that encompass both the solid and the cystic components. It is unusual to have tumor tissue anterior to the cyst wall. Once the cyst-tumor junction is identified, the surgeon opens the cyst wall and localizes the solid tumor component.

Intramedullary lipomas require a different strategy from glial neoplasms. Although lipomas may appear well demarcated from the adjacent spinal cord, these lesions are densely adherent to the normal tissue. Therefore, total removal is impossible without incurring neurologic deficits. The contact laser is an excellent instrument for debulking the lipoma. The laser vaporizes the fatty tissue without surgical trauma to the spinal cord. The debulking of the lipoma may result in improvement of pain but rarely in improvement of neurologic function.[35] Further growth of the lipoma is unlikely.

After tumor removal, hemostasis is obtained with warm saline irrigation and oxidized microfibrillar collagen (Aviteno). The dura is then closed primarily in a watertight fashion. If an osteoplastic laminotomy was performed, the segments of bone are replaced and secured with a nonabsorbable suture.[28] The dural layer must be closed in a cerebrospinal fluid–tight fashion. The muscle and fascial closure must not be under tension. A subcutaneous drain is placed only for reoperations. The skin is then closed in several layers: a deep subcutaneous layer, a superficial layer, and running locked skin sutures. About 2 days of bed rest is recommended for reoperated cases. Children who have had previous surgery and received radiation therapy are at higher risk for wound dehiscence and cerebrospinal fluid leak.

NEUROPHYSIOLOGIC MONITORING

The use of intraoperative motor evoked potentials (MEPs) is a direct motor tract monitoring technique that is now the most important monitoring tool for spinal cord surgery.[36–40] Motor potentials are evoked with transcranial electrical stimulation of the motor cortex in two ways: a single-stimulus technique and a train-stimulus technique. With the single-stimulus technique, a volley of signals in fast-conducting corticospinal axons is generated, which is then recorded with an electrode placed on the spinal cord, usually in the epidural space. This signal is called a *D wave*,[41] because it results from direct activation of these fast-conducting axons. The D-wave amplitude is a relative measure of the number of functioning fast-conducting corticospinal fibers. The train-stimulus technique evokes a muscle response in target muscles (thenar, anterior tibialis).[42] These muscle MEPs are interpreted in an all-or-none fashion. Their presence indicates intact functional integrity of the voluntary motor system in the spinal cord. Their absence indicates jeopardized functional integrity of the motor pathways, which is highly associated with at least a temporary disruption of voluntary motor control. The stimulation and recording of D waves and muscle MEPs can be repeated every second; thus, it is fast and does not require averaging and therefore the information provided is real time. Figure 240–4 summarizes the technique of stimulation and recording.

D waves and muscle MEPs must be interpreted together. Loss of muscle MEPs during a spinal cord tumor resection indicates at least a temporary disruption of motor function of the spinal cord. The more incremental change in D-wave amplitude allows further interpretation of the motor outcome. A loss of muscle MEPs is highly associated with a temporary motor deficit in the lower extremities, even if the D-wave amplitude is unchanged. In the majority of cases, this is side-specific. As long as the D-wave amplitude remains above a cutoff value of about 50% of its baseline value,

this motor deficit is temporary, with the patient recovering to preoperative strength within hours to days, or sometimes weeks. A further decline in D-wave amplitude or its loss is associated with a long-term, severe motor deficit.[43]

The short-term neurologic morbidity of intramedullary tumor surgery is about 30%. The combined use of epidural and muscle MEP recording has been shown to detect all postoperative motor deficits intraoperatively.[40] Most importantly, the combination of epidural and muscle MEPs allows for the neurophysiologic identification of a reversible motor deficit. Thus, MEPs provide information about injury to the motor system before this injury results in permanent, irreversible neurologic deficit.

Somatosensory evoked potential recording is useful to assess the functional integrity of the sensory system. The correlation of somatosensory evoked potentials with postoperative motor function is poor, however. Particularly in intramedullary surgery, somatosensory evoked potentials tend to disappear when the midline myelotomy is performed and are of no further use in the critical assessment of the motor system.

Electromyographic mapping of nerve roots—that is, direct electrical stimulation of exposed nerves with a handheld probe and recording from lower extremity and sphincter ani muscles—is useful during resection of tumors in the conus and cauda equina region.[44]

Continuous monitoring of the bulbocavernosus reflex provides information about the functional integrity of oligosynaptic reflex arches involved in sphincter control. This has been shown to be feasible during general anesthesia,[45] and information is emerging about good correlation between bulbocavernosus reflex data and postoperative sphincter control.[46]

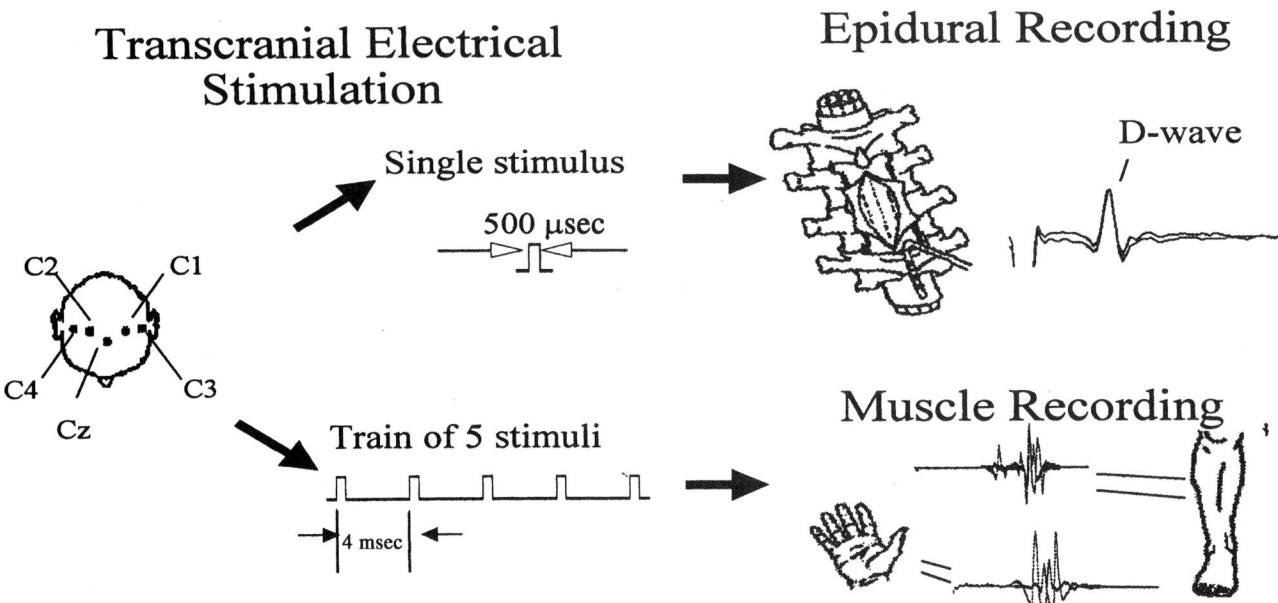

FIGURE 240–4. Schematic overview of the single- and multiple-stimulus techniques to elicit motor evoked potentials.

SURGICAL COMPLICATIONS

Functional Outcome

The major complication after intraspinal, and in particular intramedullary, tumor surgery is paralysis. Its incidence is related to preoperative functional status. Children who have no or minimal preoperative motor deficits have a less than 1% incidence of this complication. Children who have a significant motor deficit are more likely to deteriorate postoperatively.[43]

In the senior author's series of pediatric intramedullary tumors, a gross total resection was feasible in 77% of patients and subtotal (80% to 97%) resection in 20%. There was no surgical mortality. The short-term deterioration of motor function was significant. One third of patients experienced a transient motor deficit that resolved within hours to days.[40] The long-term functional outcome was much better and was directly related to preoperative neurologic function. Two thirds of the children were functioning at McCormick grade I or II at long-term follow-up.[47] In the children whose clinical status deteriorated, this was usually by one grade. Therefore, it is essential that children with known intramedullary tumors be operated on before the development of significant neurologic deficits.

Impaired joint position sense is a serious functional disability and should be included in preoperative discussions with the family. Children who have impaired proprioception may require extensive physical therapy to learn to compensate for this deficit, which is more common after intramedullary surgery for ependymomas than for astrocytomas. Astrocytomas (which are more common in children) tend to displace the posterior columns laterally, making the risk of injury from the surgical approach less likely than that for centrally located ependymomas.

Postoperative Spinal Deformity

Another potential complication is spinal deformity.[48] Scoliosis and kyphosis may evolve after surgery.[49, 50] Some deformity developed in approximately 70% of the children in our series. However, only one third of these children required an orthopedic procedure for correction or stabilization. Osteoplastic laminotomy appears to reduce the incidence of significant spinal deformities. Several surgeons recommend osteoplastic laminotomy for all children to reduce the incidence of spinal deformity.[28, 52] In a study of 58 patients younger than 25 years who underwent multilevel laminectomy for various conditions, deformity occurred in 46% of patients younger than 15 years and in 6% of patients older than 15 years. In this series, 100% of children (nine of nine) who had cervical laminectomy developed postoperative deformity, compared with 36% (4 of 11) undergoing thoracic laminectomy and none of six children after lumbar laminectomy.[50] It is essential that all children be followed closely with plain radiographs and receive routine orthopedic evaluation. Surgical indications for spinal fusion should be regarded as more urgent in these children than in those with idiopathic deformity. Children who develop progressive deformity should also have MRI scans to rule out tumor recurrence.

Spinal deformity is also a complication of radiation therapy to treat epidural tumors.[53, 54] Mayfield and colleagues reported that 32 of 57 children with neuroblastoma treated with radiation therapy and chemotherapy developed significant spinal deformities. A higher rate of deformity was associated with younger age at time of radiation, doses greater than 20 Gy, and asymmetrical radiation fields.[55]

Cerebrospinal Fluid Leak

Cerebrospinal fluid leak is rare in children who have not previously been operated on or received radiation therapy. However, children who have been irradiated are at risk for wound dehiscence and cerebrospinal fluid fistula. Early in our surgical experience, several children had problems with wound healing that resulted in either meningitis or local wound infection. Since then, we have used plastic surgery techniques for these complicated wounds.[56] We routinely close the fascia in a watertight fashion without tension. Occasionally, relaxing incisions are performed to provide a tension-free closure. A drain must be placed in the subcutaneous space for several days to allow healing of the tissues. In certain cases, muscle transposition from areas outside the radiated fields is performed by plastic surgeons.

ONCOLOGIC OUTCOME

It must be emphasized that despite gross total resection, residual microscopic fragments are left in the resection bed. This residual tissue (in particular for glial neoplasms) may remain dormant or may involute over time. The clinical significance of these minute fragments remains to be determined.

Long-term survival was significantly better for children with low-grade neoplasms than for those with high-grade and intermediate tumors. The 5- and 10-year survival was 88% and 82%, respectively, for patients with low-grade neoplasms in the senior author's series. The cause of death in these children was progression of disease and systemic complications after chemotherapy. The children with high-grade neoplasms fared poorly, with an 18% 5-year survival despite surgery and adjuvant therapy.

ADJUVANT THERAPY

There is abundant evidence that radiation has deleterious effects on the immature nervous and osseous systems,[57–59] and no study has convincingly demonstrated that radiation therapy has a beneficial effect on survival or neurologic function for low-grade tumors. Although some authors recommend radiation therapy for intramedullary spinal cord tumors,[60, 61] no prospective study has been performed on the effects of radiation therapy

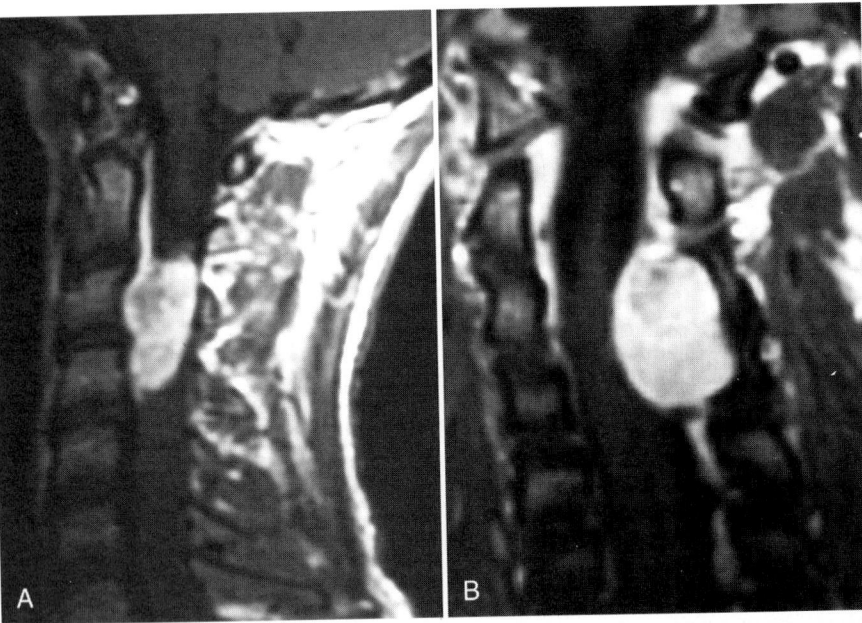
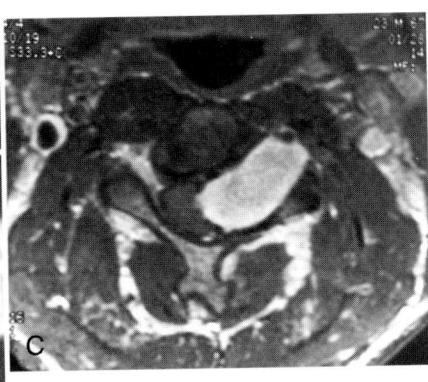

FIGURE 240–5. Nerve sheath tumor, schwannoma. *A,* Sagittal T1-weighted image with contrast. *B,* Coronal T1-weighted image with contrast reveals the homogeneously enhancing tumor. *C,* Axial T1-weighted image with contrast demonstrates the extension into left neural foramen.

for intramedullary neoplasms. There is no clear evidence that radiation therapy improves the outcome of patients with low-grade astrocytomas of the central nervous system.[62, 63] Children with low-grade intramedullary neoplasms who are treated with radical surgery have long-term, progression-free survival without the need for adjuvant therapy. Thus, these tumors should be recognized as a disease to be treated by surgery, both at presentation and at the time of recurrence.

Stein did not recommend radiotherapy for adult patients with low-grade intramedullary neoplasms, regardless of the extent of removal, and emphasized the deleterious effects of radiation on the spinal cord tissue adjacent to the tumor site.[10] Others have reported myelopathy in children who received doses of 30 Gy.[64] In addition, alterations of motor and somatosensory evoked potentials have been reported in patients who received radiation therapy to the spinal cord.[43, 65] Thus, we do not recommend radiation therapy for low-grade intramedullary neoplasms. Radiation therapy is reserved only for children with malignant tumors, children with documented postoperative rapid tumor regrowth, or those with substantial residual tumor who are not candidates for further surgery.

We use total neuraxis radiation for these highly malignant tumors. Unfortunately, it has been shown that glioblastomas invariably progress. Despite aggressive radiation therapy and chemotherapy, children with these neoplasms have a median survival of 12 months.[66] There is progressive tumor infiltration in the spinal cord and leptomeninges, resulting in paraplegia and death.

INTRADURAL EXTRAMEDULLARY AND EXTRADURAL TUMORS

The treatment of choice for intradural extramedullary tumors is surgery. The majority—nerve sheath tumors

and meningiomas—are benign, and gross total removal is possible in most cases. Frequently there is significant spinal cord compression, and it is mandatory to avoid excessive manipulation of the cord during resection. Here again, the contact laser is the safest and least traumatic way to deal with these tumors, particularly when they are firm and fibrous. Usually the prognosis of these tumors is good when they are completely resected, and adjuvant therapy is reserved for malignant variants. Some nerve sheath tumors extend into the extradural space through the neural foramen and into the paravertebral soft tissue (Fig. 240–5). In these cases, the surgeon may need to carry out a second extraspinal resection to remove the remaining tumor.

In children, most epidural tumors are extensions of malignant paravertebral neoplasms that infiltrate the spinal canal. The treatment options for these tumors are surgical decompression, radiation therapy, and chemotherapy. The most important factor in successful therapy is the tumor type. Ewing's sarcoma, neuroblastoma, and lymphoma can be successfully treated without surgery.[14]

REFERENCES

1. Koos WT, Day JD: Neurological surgery at the University of Vienna. Neurosurgery 39:583, 1996.
2. Elsberg CA, Beer E: The operability of intramedullary tumors of the spinal cord: A report of two operations with remarks upon the extrusion of intraspinal tumors. Am J Med Sci 142:636–647, 1911.
3. Sonntag VKH: History of degenerative and traumatic diseases of the spine. In Greenblatt SH (ed): A History of Neurosurgery. Park Ridge, Ill, American Association of Neurological Surgeons, 1997, pp 355–371.
4. Wood EH, Berne AS, Taveras JM: The value of radiation therapy in the management of intrinsic tumors of the spinal cord. Radiology 63:11–24, 1954.
5. Greenwood J: Surgical removal of intramedullary tumors. J Neurosurg 26:276–282, 1967.
6. Guidetti B, Mercuri S, Vagnozzi R: Long-term results of the surgical treatment of 129 intramedullary spinal gliomas. J Neurosurg 54:323–330, 1981.

7. Epstein FJ, Epstein N: Surgical treatment of spinal cord astrocytomas of childhood. J Neurosurg 57:685–689, 1982.

8. Epstein F: Spinal cord astrocytomas in childhood. In Homburger F (ed): Progress in Experimental Tumor Research. Basel, S Karger, 1987, pp 135–153.

9. Epstein FJ, Farmer J-P: Pediatric spinal cord tumor surgery. Neurosurg Clin N Am 1:569–590, 1990.

10. Stein BM: Intramedullary spinal cord tumors. Clin Neurosurg 30:717–741, 1983.

11. Brotchi J, Dewitte O, Levivier M, et al: A survey of 65 tumors within the spinal cord: Surgical results and the importance of preoperative magnetic resonance imaging. Neurosurgery 29:651–656, 1991.

12. Constantini S, Houten J, Miller DC, et al: Intramedullary spinal cord tumors in children under the age of 3 years. J Neurosurg 85:1036–1043, 1996.

13. Yamamoto Y, Raffel C: Spinal extradural neoplasms and intradural extramedullary neoplasms. In Albright AL, Pollack IF, Adelson PD (eds): Principles and Practice of Pediatric Neurosurgery. New York, Thieme Medical Publishers, 1999, pp 685–696.

14. Murovic J, Sundaresan N: Pediatric spinal axis tumors. Neurosurg Clin N Am 4:947–958, 1992.

15. Seppälä M, Haltia MJJ, Sankila RJ, et al: Long-term outcome after removal of spinal schwannoma: A clinicopathological study of 187 cases. J Neurosurg 83:621–626, 1995.

16. Seppälä M, Haltia MJJ, Sankila RJ, et al: Long-term outcome after removal of spinal neurofibroma. J Neurosurg 82:572–577, 1995.

17. Allen SS, Kahn EA: A case of scoliosis produced by spinal cord tumor. J Nerv Ment Dis 77:52–55, 1933.

18. Kiwak KJ, Deray MJ, Shields WD: Torticollis in three children with syringomyelia and spinal cord tumor. Neurology 33:946–948, 1983.

19. Cohen AR, Wisoff JH, Allen JC, et al: Malignant astrocytomas of the spinal cord. J Neurosurg 70:50–54, 1989.

20. Rifkinson-Mann S, Wisoff JH, Epstein FJ: The association of hydrocephalus with intramedullary spinal cord tumors: A series of 25 patients. Neurosurgery 27:749–754, 1990.

21. Sze G: Magnetic resonance imaging in the evaluation of spinal tumors. Cancer 67:1229–1241, 1991.

22. Goy AMC, Pinto RS, Raghavendra BN, et al: Intramedullary spinal cord tumors: MR imaging, with emphasis of associated cysts. Radiology 161:381–386, 1986.

23. Dillon WP, Norman D, Newton TH, et al: Intradural spinal cord lesions: Gd-DTPA-enhanced MR imaging. Radiology 170:229–237, 1989.

24. Patel U, Pinto RS, Miller DC, et al: MR of spinal cord ganglioglioma. AJNR Am J Neuroradiol 19:879–887, 1998.

25. DeSousa AL, Kalsbeck JE, Mealey J, et al: Intraspinal tumors in children: A review of 81 cases. J Neurosurg 51:437–445, 1979.

26. Flamm ES, Ransohoff JP, Wuchinich D, et al: Preliminary experience with ultrasonic aspiration in neurosurgery. Neurosurgery 2:240–245, 1978.

27. Constantini S, Epstein FJ: Ultrasonic dissection in neurosurgery. In Wilkins RH, Rengachary SS (eds): Neurosurgery. New York, McGraw-Hill, 1996, pp 607–608.

28. Abbott R, Feldstein N, Wisoff JH, et al: Osteoplastic laminotomy in children. Pediatr Neurosurg 18:153–156, 1992.

29. Epstein FJ, Farmer J-P, Schneider SJ: Intraoperative ultrasonography: An important surgical adjunct for intramedullary tumors. J Neurosurg 74:729–733, 1991.

30. Dohrmann GJ, Rubin JM: Intraoperative ultrasound imaging of the spinal cord: Syringomyelia, cysts, and tumors—a preliminary report. Surg Neurol 18:395–399, 1982.

31. Kawakami N, Mimatsu K, Kato F: Intraoperative sonography of intramedullary spinal cord tumors. Neuroradiology 34:436–439, 1992.

32. Epstein FJ, Ozek F: The plated bayonet: A new instrument to facilitate surgery for intra-axial neoplasms of the spinal cord and brain stem. Technical note. J Neurosurg 78:505–507, 1993.

33. Fischer G, Mansuy L: Total removal of intramedullary ependymomas: Follow-up study of 16 cases. Surg Neurol 14:243–249, 1980.

34. Epstein FJ, Farmer J-P, Freed D: Adult intramedullary spinal cord ependymoma: The result of surgery in 38 patients. J Neurosurg 79:204–209, 1993.

35. Lee M, Rezai AR, Abbott R, et al: Intramedullary spinal cord lipomas. J Neurosurg 82:394–400, 1995.

36. Boyd SG, Rothwell JC, Cowan JMA, et al: A method of monitoring function in corticospinal pathways during scoliosis surgery with a note on motor conduction velocities. J Neurol Neurosurg Psychiatry 49:251–257, 1986.

37. Burke D, Hicks RG, Stephen JPH: Corticospinal volleys evoked by anodal and cathodal stimulation of the human motor cortex. J Physiol (Lond) 425:283–299, 1990.

38. Deletis V: Intraoperative monitoring of the functional integrity of the motor pathways. In Devinsky O, Beric A, Dogali M (eds): Electrical and Magnetic Stimulation of the Brain and Spinal Cord. New York, Raven Press, 1993, pp 201–214.

39. Jones SJ, Harrison R, Koh KF, et al: Motor evoked potential monitoring during spinal surgery: Responses of distal limb muscles to transcranial cortical stimulation with pulse trains. Electroencephalogr Clin Neurophysiol 100:375–383, 1996.

40. Kothbauer KF, Deletis V, Epstein FJ: Motor evoked potential monitoring for intramedullary spinal cord tumor surgery: Correlation of clinical and neurophysiological data in a series of 100 consecutive procedures. Neurosurg Focus 4:1, 1998. Available at http://www.aans.org/journals/online_j/may98/4-5-1.

41. Patton HD, Amassian VE: Single- and multiple unit analysis of cortical stage of pyramidal tract activation. J Neurophysiol 17:345–363, 1954.

42. Taniguchi M, Cedzich C, Schramm J: Modification of cortical stimulation for motor evoked potentials under general anesthesia: Technical description. Neurosurgery 32:219–226, 1993.

43. Morota N, Deletis V, Constantini S, et al: The role of motor evoked potentials during surgery for intramedullary spinal cord tumors. Neurosurgery 41:1327–1336, 1997.

44. Kothbauer K, Schmid UD, Seiler RW, et al: Intraoperative motor and sensory monitoring of the cauda equina. Neurosurgery 34:702–707, 1994.

45. Deletis V, Vodusek DB: Intraoperative recording of the bulbocavernosus reflex. Neurosurgery 40:88–93, 1997.

46. Sala F, Krzan MJ, Epstein FJ, et al: Specificity of neurophysiological monitoring of the lumbosacral nervous system during tethered cord release: A preliminary report [abstract]. Paper presented at the 27th Annual Congress of the International Society for Pediatric Neurosurgery, Salt Lake City, Utah, 1999.

47. McCormick PC, Torres R, Post KD, et al: Intramedullary ependymoma of the spinal cord. J Neurosurg 72:523–532, 1990.

48. Winter RB, Hall JE: Kyphosis in childhood and adolescence. Spine 3:285–308, 1978.

49. Reimer R, Onofrio BM: Astrocytomas of the spinal cord in children and adolescents. J Neurosurg 63:669–675, 1985.

50. Tachdjian MO, Matson DD: Orthopedic aspects of intraspinal tumors in infants and children. J Bone Joint Surg Am 49:713–720, 1965.

51. Yasuoka S, Peterson H, MacCarty CS: Incidence of spinal column deformity after multilevel laminectomy in children and adults. J Neurosurg 57:441–445, 1982.

52. Raimondi AJ, Gutierrez FA, Di Rocco C: Laminotomy and total reconstruction of the posterior spinal arch for spinal canal surgery in childhood. J Neurosurg 45:555–560, 1976.

53. Katzman H, Waugh T, Berdon W: Skeletal changes following irradiation of childhood tumors. J Bone Joint Surg Am 51:825–842, 1969.

54. Riseborough EJ, Grabias SL, Burton RI, et al: Skeletal alterations following irradiation for Wilm's tumor. J Bone Joint Surg Am 58:526–536, 1976.

55. Mayfield JK, Riseborough EJ, Jaffe N, et al: Spinal deformity in children treated for neuroblastoma. J Bone Joint Surg Am 63:183–193, 1981.

56. Zide BM, Epstein FJ, Wisoff J: Optimal wound closure after tethered cord correction: Technical note. J Neurosurg 74:673–676, 1991.

57. Clayton PE, Shalet SM: The evolution of spinal growth after irradiation. Clin Oncol 3:220–222, 1991.

58. Duffner PK, Horowitz ME, Krischer JP, et al: Postoperative chemotherapy and delayed radiation in children less than three years of age with malignant brain tumors. N Engl J Med 328:1725–1731, 1993.

59. Marcus RBJ, Million RR: The incidence of myelitis after irradia-

tion of the cervical spinal cord. Int J Radiat Oncol Biol Phys 19: 3–8, 1990.

60. O'Sullivan C, Jenkin RD, Doherty MA, et al: Spinal cord tumors in children: Long-term results of combined surgical and radiation treatment. J Neurosurg 81:507–512, 1994.

61. Minehan KJ, Shaw EG, Scheithauer BW, et al: Spinal cord astrocytoma: Pathological and treatment considerations. J Neurosurg 83: 590–595, 1995.

62. Hardison HH, Packer RJ, Rorke LB, et al: Outcome of children with primary intramedullary spinal cord tumors. Childs Nerv Syst 3:89–92, 1987.

63. Rossitch E Jr, Zeidman SM, Burger PC, et al: Clinical and pathological analysis of spinal cord astrocytomas in children. Neurosurgery 27:193–196, 1990.

64. Sundaresan N, Gutierrez FA, Larsen MB: Radiation myelopathy in children. Ann Neurol 4:47–50, 1978.

65. De Scisciolo G, Bartelli M, Magrini S, et al: Long-term nervous system damage from radiation of the spinal cord: An electrophysiological study. J Neurol 238:9–15, 1991.

66. Kopelson G, Linggood RM: Intramedullary spinal cord astrocytoma versus glioblastoma: The prognostic importance of histologic grade. Cancer 50:732–735, 1982.

CHAPTER 241

Benign Tumors of the Skull, Including Fibrous Dysplasia

HERBERT E. FUCHS

Most pediatric skull tumors manifest as a lump, first noticed by a parent or pediatrician. The spectrum of skull tumors occurring in pediatric patients is distinctly different from that seen in adults. Most tumors are benign, but several have significant intracranial extensions or systemic manifestations.

EPIDEMIOLOGY

Many skull masses are first discovered after incidental trauma. The two most common traumatic skull masses are directly related to an obvious trauma. A calcified cephalohematoma may occur in the neonate after birth trauma. This diagnosis accounted for 9% of "nontraumatic" skull lesions in one series.[1] The growing skull fracture or leptomeningeal cyst occurs primarily in children younger than 3 years of age, occurring in approximately 1% of cases of infant skull fractures.[2]

Between 75% and 90% of the truly nontraumatic skull lesions in children are benign.[1, 3] The most common lesions are epidermoid and dermoid cysts, accounting for 30% to 60% of cases, with epidermoids occurring much more frequently. Histiocytosis X is next most common, accounting for 7% to 16% of cases. Dysraphic conditions (e.g., meningocele, encephalocele), fibrous dysplasia, hemangiomas, and hamartomas each account for approximately 3% of cases. True benign bony skull tumors, such as osteoma, are rare.

DIAGNOSTIC STUDIES

By the time a child is referred to a neurosurgeon, most patients have already undergone imaging with skull radiographs, computed tomography (CT), or magnetic resonance imaging (MRI). Skull radiographs and CT can provide the most information about bony involvement. The margins of the lesion should be carefully studied for evidence of sclerosis. Slowly growing lesions, such as dermoid or epidermoid cysts, allow surrounding bone reformation, but faster growing lesions, such as eosinophilic granuloma, do not.

Differential destruction of the outer and inner tables of the skull provides further diagnostic clues. Dermoid cyst and eosinophilic granuloma commonly arise extracranially and cause greater scalloping of the outer table. An arachnoid cyst or an enlarged pacchionian granulation causes greater scalloping of the inner table.

CT yields excellent definition of bony involvement and demonstrates intracranial extension. CT with three-dimensional reconstruction may be very useful in defining the anatomy of and planning the surgical approach to skull base or orbital tumors. MRI is critical in evaluating midline lesions for involvement of dural sinuses and in vertex lesions that are not depicted well on axial CT.

TRAUMATIC SKULL LESIONS

Calcified Cephalohematoma

The most common site of subperiosteal hematoma in the neonate is the parietal region. The hematoma is limited by suture lines and generally resolves over the next several weeks as the skull grows and remodels. Occasionally, however, the elevated periosteum triggers new diploic bone formation, resulting in a markedly thickened calvarium (Fig. 241–1). Treatment is reserved for unacceptable cosmetic appearance, and most cases consist of recontouring of the lesion to conform to the inner table, which has a normal contour.[4]

Growing Skull Fractures

Growing skull fractures (i.e., leptomeningeal cysts) result from pulsatile pressure of the brain and cerebrospinal fluid (CSF) at the site of a skull fracture with dural laceration. The fracture line is gradually enlarged, and cerebral tissue may herniate through the defect.[5] The term *leptomeningeal cyst* is a misnomer, because many growing skull fractures do not have an associated cyst, and on pathologic examination of those with a cyst, leptomeningeal elements may not be present.[6, 7]

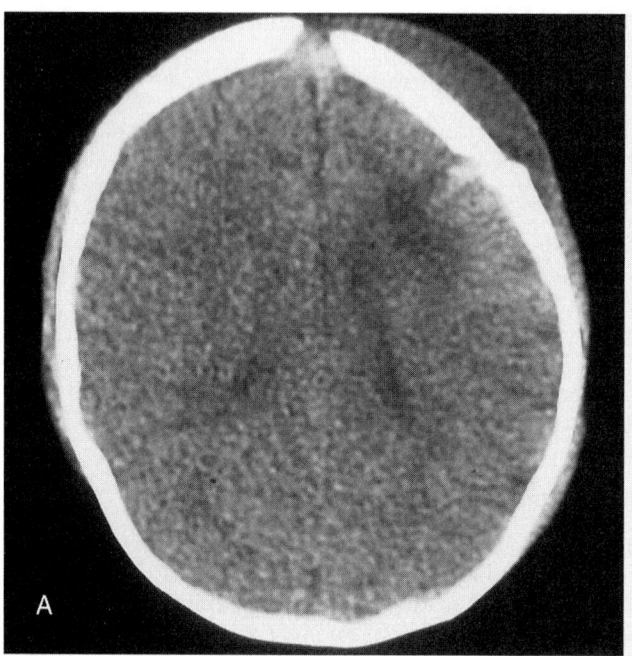

FIGURE 241–1. Axial computed tomographic scan of a patient with a large, right parietal, calcified cephalohematoma. Notice the expanded diploic space, with normal contour of the inner table.

Skull radiographs demonstrate an elliptical defect that is obviously enlarged compared with radiographs taken at the initial injury. The bony margins are often sclerotic, with greater erosion of the inner table. CT

demonstrates the expanded fracture line and herniated cerebral tissue (Fig. 241–2).[7]

Treatment of a growing skull fracture is surgical, with complete exposure and repair of the dural defect, which is often larger than the bony defect.[8] The calvarial defect should be repaired with autologous bone, such as with split-thickness cranioplasty. Recurrent cyst formation may require ventriculoperitoneal shunting.[9, 10]

CONGENITAL SKULL LESIONS

Dermoid and Epidermoid Tumors of the Skull

Dermoid and epidermoid tumors of the skull are the most common skull lesions encountered by the neurosurgeon. Dermoid cysts and dermal sinus tracts most commonly are encountered in younger children, with epidermoid cysts occurring intracranially in older children and adults. Dermoid cysts most commonly occur at the anterior fontanelle, around the orbit, or along cranial sutures, especially at the pterion.[1] The epidermoid cysts are composed of keratinizing, stratified squamous epithelium, with additional dermal appendages such as hair follicles and sebaceous glands included in dermoid cysts. These cysts are thought to arise because of failure of dysjunction of neuroectoderm from cutaneous ectoderm during neural tube closure.

Skull radiographs typically show a lytic lesion with sclerotic borders, with greater scalloping of the outer table. CT or MRI fully delineates the cyst, including

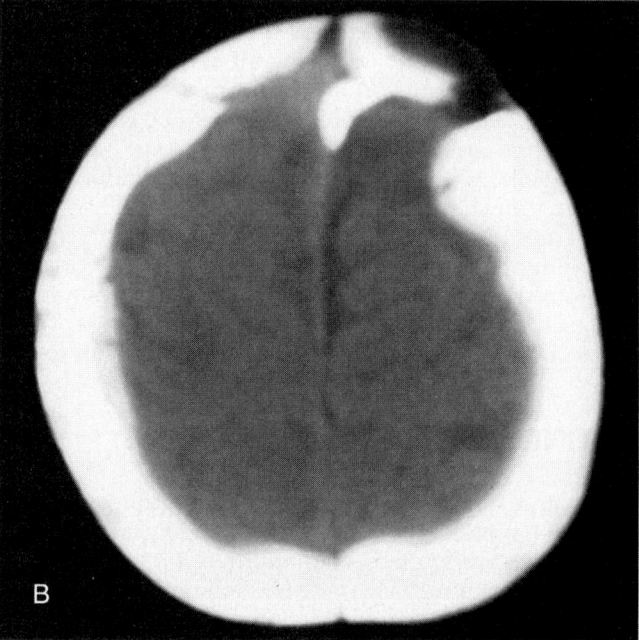

FIGURE 241–2. *A*, Axial computed tomographic scan of an infant with a left frontal linear skull fracture and underlying contusion after a motor vehicle accident. *B*, An axial computed tomographic scan of the same patient 3 months later, when the patient presented with a soft and fluctuant mass at the site of the previous fracture, demonstrated widening of the fracture line with a leptomeningeal cyst.

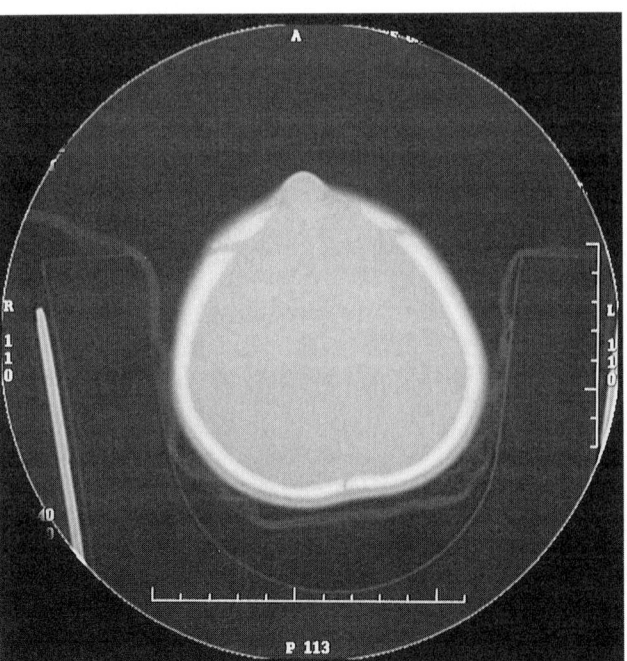

FIGURE 241-3. Axial computed tomographic scan of an infant with a midline dermoid cyst at the anterior aspect of the anterior fontanelle.

any intracranial extension (Fig. 241–3). For midline lesions with overlying cutaneous abnormalities, MRI may best demonstrate intracranial extension of a sinus tract and dural venous sinus involvement.

Fibrous Dysplasia

In fibrous dysplasia, normal bone marrow is replaced by a highly cellular, fibrous tissue, with collagen interspersed with immature woven bone. The process begins in the marrow space and expands, thinning the overlying cortical bone.[11] Involvement may be confined to a single bone (i.e., monostotic) or include multiple, usually contiguous bones (i.e., polyostotic). As an area of dysplasia expands, it may cross suture lines to involve adjacent bones.[12] This type of involvement is most common in the craniofacial bones and often is identified by the neurosurgeon and craniofacial surgeon.

When polyostotic fibrous dysplasia occurs in conjunction with precocious puberty or other hypersecretory endocrinopathies and hyperpigmented skin lesions (i.e., café au lait spots), the disorder is known as the McCune-Albright syndrome. Experimental studies using cell transplantation techniques have demonstrated that the fibrous dysplasia seen in this syndrome is associated with a mutation in a subtype of the common regulatory protein called *G protein*.[13] The mutation results in increased cyclic adenosine monophosphate levels and hyperactivity of affected cells. It appears that a mixture of mutant and normal stromal cells is required to produce the characteristic lesions of fibrous dysplasia, implying that the lesions seen clinically are a result of genetic mosaicism.[11]

Involvement of the skull occurs in up to 27% of patients with the monostotic form and in up to 50% of patients with the polyostotic form of fibrous dysplasia.[14, 15] Disease activity is greatest before skeletal maturation, often manifesting around the time of puberty, but it may persist into adulthood. The initial manifestation is often a painless, progressive deformity of the skull, with proptosis in cases of orbital involvement.[12] With skull base involvement, there is narrowing of cranial nerve exit foramina, with ensuing cranial neuropathies. Loss of visual acuity is usually gradual, but acute visual loss has been reported.[15, 16] Temporal bone involvement may cause tinnitus, hearing loss, or facial weakness.[17]

Imaging for patients with fibrous dysplasia is best accomplished with thin-section CT in the axial and coronal planes. The characteristic ground-glass appearance is readily apparent, and with biplanar imaging, skull base involvement of cranial nerve exit foramina can be thoroughly evaluated (Fig. 241–4). A grading system has been devised, dividing the skull into four zones to assist in preoperative planning.[18]

The goals of surgery include improvement or stabilization of neurological function, correction of cosmetic deformity, and total resection of involved bone, if feasible.[18] With extensive cranial base involvement, subtotal resection with maximal decompression and immediate reconstruction using an autologous bone graft provides good results, often with disease stabilization.[18] Improvement of visual or hearing loss has been reported with prompt decompression.[17, 19] The incidence of malignant degeneration (most commonly to osteosarcoma) is approximately 0.5%, usually occurring in the polyostotic form.[20] The role of irradiation for residual or recurrent disease is unclear, but such therapy may predispose the patient to malignancy.[21]

Histiocytosis X

Langerhans cell histiocytosis takes its name from the characteristic proliferation of Langerhans histiocytes seen in a spectrum of diseases. This group of diseases most likely represents a disorder of immune function, with an unidentified inciting stimulus, rather than a true neoplasm.[22] At one end of the spectrum is the patient with a single, isolated eosinophilic granuloma. Patients with Hand-Schüller-Christian disease have cranial involvement, exophthalmos, and diabetes insipidus. Most severely affected are patients with Letterer-Siwe disease, which has diffuse systemic involvement that often manifests in younger patients and that is often fatal.

Histiocytosis usually manifests before puberty, with the skull the most frequent site of involvement (80%).[22, 23] The most common presentation is a painful, immobile scalp mass that may have enlarged recently.[24–26] Skull radiographs show the characteristic "punched-out" lesion without sclerotic margins (Fig. 241–5). CT may demonstrate intracranial extension. In patients with diabetes insipidus, hypothalamic involvement is best demonstrated on MRI.[27, 28] Although unifocal skull involvement is common, multifocal involve-

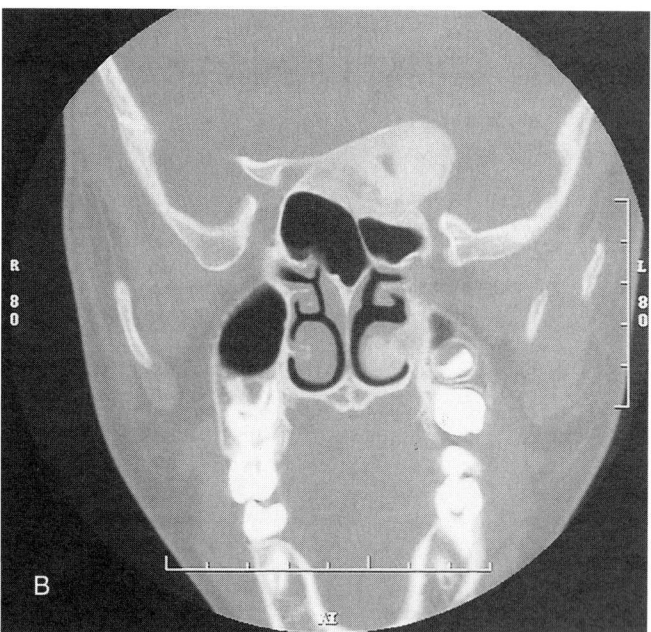

FIGURE 241–4. *A,* Axial computed tomographic scan of a patient with polyostotic fibrous dysplasia shows marked narrowing of the optic canal on the left. *B,* Coronal computed tomographic scan of the same patient shows marked narrowing of the optic canal and massive enlargement of the anterior clinoid process on the left.

ment occurs in more than 20% of patients and should be sought with further imaging studies.[22] Skeletal survey radiography appears most accurate for assessing the skull and long bones, but nuclear medicine bone scanning is best for rib and vertebral lesions. Both studies should be performed for complete radiographic evaluation.[29]

Treatment of unifocal histiocytosis of the skull should consist of complete resection of the lesion to clean bone margins, with split-thickness autologous cranioplasty performed at the time of resection. This treatment is associated with a very low recurrence rate,

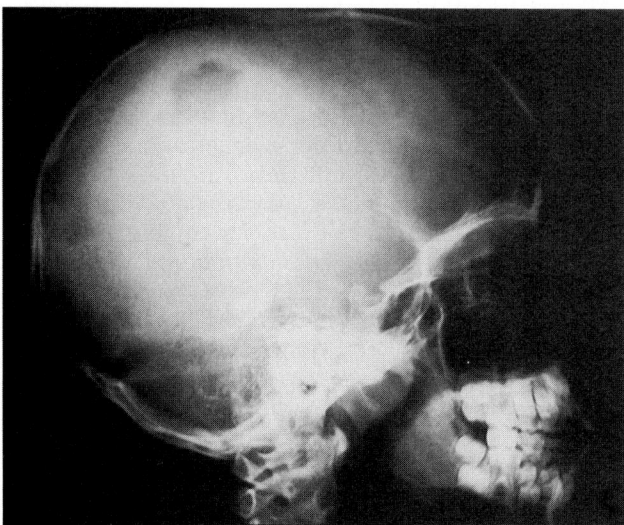

FIGURE 241–5. A characteristic punched-out lesion without sclerotic margins or histiocytosis is seen on skull radiography.

and adjuvant therapy is not indicated.[30] Patients with multiple organ system involvement who are younger than 2 years old at diagnosis, with hepatosplenomegaly, or with thrombocytopenia are considered to be at high risk for disease recurrence.[22] Patients with multifocal, recurrent, or progressive disease may be treated with low-dose radiation or chemotherapy. Optimal chemotherapeutic regimens have not been determined. Intralesional injection of corticosteroids has also been reported to be successful in the treatment of solitary bone lesions.[31]

The natural history of histiocytosis is poorly understood. Lesions have been reported to undergo spontaneous regression, and the relative benefits of surgery, irradiation, and chemotherapy have not been conclusively demonstrated.[22] A local recurrence rate of 6% is reported for all treatment modalities.[22] New lesions are seen in 22% of patients.[22] Because most recurrences are seen within 2 years of diagnosis, the minimum follow-up period, using skeletal survey radiographs and bone scans, for patients with histiocytosis should be 5 years.[22]

BONE NEOPLASMS OF THE SKULL

Hemangioma

Hemangiomas account for 3% to 5% of calvarial masses and are usually found in older children and adults.[1] They represent cavernous angiomas in the diploic bone and are most commonly located in the parietal bone. The appearance of a hemangioma on a skull radiograph is a lytic lesion with a characteristic "sunburst" pattern due to radiating bony spicules within the lesion. Treatment is excision and autologous split-thickness cranioplasty.

Aneurysmal Bone Cyst

Aneurysmal bone cysts are expansions of the diploic space that distort the overlying cortical bone. These lesions occur most commonly in older children and adults and only 2% occur in the bones of the skull.[32, 33] Patients usually present with a painful, expanding skull mass.[34]

Aneurysmal bone cysts have often been considered to result from other, adjacent bone lesions, such as osteoblastoma or giant cell tumor, and such lesions should be carefully sought when evaluating a patient with aneurysmal bone cyst.[32, 35] Aneurysmal bone cysts are highly vascular lesions and, particularly in young children, surgery for resection may be associated with significant blood loss. Preoperative angiography and embolization may significantly reduce surgical risk. Total resection should be the goal. Postoperative imaging to assess for residual disease or recurrence is also helpful in seeking other associated bone lesions.

Osteoblastoma

Osteoblastoma accounts for approximately 1% of benign bone tumors in children, with approximately 20% of all osteoblastomas occurring in the skull.[36] With variable calcification patterns, radiographic diagnosis is imprecise.[37] Histologically, these tumors are composed of osteoblasts in an immature osteoid matrix. Complete resection with split-thickness calvarial reconstruction is recommended.[37]

Osteoma

In contrast to osteoblastoma, osteoma is rarely seen in children.[1] The typical computed tomographic appearance is a hyperdense, sharply demarcated lesion. There is considerable controversy about treatment—whether drilling to a normal skull contour is sufficient or complete excision with reconstruction is required in all cases.

CONCLUSIONS

Pediatric skull lesions are relatively uncommon lesions, and true tumors of the skull are rare. Radiographic techniques, including plain radiography, CT, and MRI, may facilitate the differential diagnosis; however, surgery for biopsy or total resection with reconstruction is usually the preferred treatment. For lesions such as fibrous dysplasia or eosinophilic granuloma, complete skeletal and systemic evaluations are also necessary.

REFERENCES

1. Ruge JR, Tomita T, Naidich TP, et al: Scalp and calvarial masses of infants and children. Neurosurgery 22:1037–1042, 1988.
2. Locatelli D, Messina AL, Bonfanti N, et al: Growing fractures: An unusual complication of head injuries in pediatric patients. Neurochirurgia 32:101–104, 1989.
3. Choux M, Gomez A, Choux A, et al: Diagnostic and therapeutic problems concerning tumors of the vault. Childs Brain 1:207–216, 1975.
4. Kaufman HH, Hochberg J, Anderson RP, et al: Treatment of calcified cephalohematoma. Neurosurgery 32:1037–1039, 1993.
5. Scarfo GB, Mariottini A, Tomaccini D, et al: Growing skull fractures: Progressive evolution of brain damage and effectiveness of surgical treatment. Childs Nerv Syst 5:163–167, 1989.
6. Lende RA, Erickson TC: Growing skull fractures of childhood. J Neurosurg 18:479–489, 1961.
7. Tandon PN, Banerji AK, Bhatia R, et al: Cranio-cerebral erosion (growing fracture of the skull in children). Part II. Clinical and radiological observations. Acta Neurochir 88:1–9, 1987.
8. Pezzotta S, Silvani V, Gaetani P, et al: Growing skull fractures of childhood. Case report and review of 132 cases. J Neurosurg Sci 29:129–135, 1985.
9. Kashiwagi S, Abiko S, Aoki H: Growing skull fracture in childhood. A recurrent case treated by shunt operation. Surg Neurol 26:63–66, 1986.
10. Gupta SK, Reddy NM, Khosla VK, et al: Growing skull fractures: A clinical study of 41 patients. Acta Neurochir 139:928–932, 1997.
11. Bianco P, Kuznetsov SA, Riminucci M, et al: Reproduction of human fibrous dysplasia of bone in immunocompromised mice by transplanted mosaics of normal and Gsα-mutated skeletal progenitor cells. J Clin Invest 101:1737–1744, 1998.
12. DiRocco C, Marchese E, Velardi F: Fibrous dysplasia of the skull in children. Pediatr Neurosurg 18:117–126, 1992.
13. Weinstein LS, Shenker A, Gejman PV, et al: Activating mutations of the stimulatory G protein in the McCune-Albright syndrome. N Engl J Med 325:1688–1695, 1991.
14. Sassin JF, Rosenberg RN: Neurological complications of fibrous dysplasia of the skull. Arch Neurol 18:363–369, 1968.
15. Harris WH, Dudley HR, Barry RJ: The natural history of fibrous dysplasia: An orthopedic, pathological and roentgenographic study. J Bone Joint Surg 44:207, 1962.
16. Posnick JC, Wells MD, Drake JM, et al: Childhood fibrous dysplasia presenting as blindness: A skull base approach for resection and immediate reconstruction. Pediatr Neurosurg 19:260–266, 1993.
17. Morrissey DD, Talbot JM, Schleuning AJ: Fibrous dysplasia of the temporal bone: Reversal of sensorineural hearing loss after decompression of the internal auditory canal. Laryngoscope 107:1336–1340, 1997.
18. Chen YR, Noordhoof MS: Treatment of craniomaxillofacial fibrous dysplasia: How early and how extensive? Plast Reconstr Surg 86:835–842, 1990.
19. Chen YR, Breidahl A, Chang CN: Optic nerve decompression in fibrous dysplasia: Indications, efficacy and safety. Plast Reconstr Surg 99:22–30, 1997.
20. Taconis WK: Osteosarcoma in fibrous dysplasia. Skeletal Radiol 17:163–170, 1988.
21. Ruggieri P, Sim FH, Bond JR, et al: Malignancies in fibrous dysplasia. Cancer 73:1411–1424, 1994.
22. Kilpatrick SE, Wenger DE, Gilchrist GS, et al: Langerhans' cell histiocytosis (histiocytosis X) of bone. A clinicopathologic analysis of 263 pediatric and adult cases. Cancer 76:2471–2484, 1995.
23. Angeli SI, Alcalde J, Hoffman HT, et al: Langerhans cell histiocytosis of the head and neck in children. Ann Otol Rhinol Laryngol 104:173–180, 1995.
24. Rawlings CE, Wilkins RH: Solitary eosinophilic granuloma of the skull. Neurosurgery 15:155–161, 1984.
25. Puzzilli F, Mastronardi L, Farah JO, et al: Solitary eosinophilic granuloma of the calvaria. Tumori 84:712–716, 1998.
26. Yiannias JA, Brodland DB: Transcranial eosinophilic granuloma manifested by a subcutaneous scalp mass: Differential diagnosis in children. J Dermatol Surg Oncol 19:631–634, 1993.
27. Moore JB, Kulkarni R, Crutcher DC: MRI in multifocal eosinophilic granuloma: Staging disease and monitoring response to therapy. Am J Pediatr Hematol Oncol 11:174–177, 1989.
28. Grois N, Flucher-Wolfram B, Heitger A, et al: Diabetes insipidus in Langerhans' cell histiocytosis: Results from the DAL-HX 83 study. Med Pediatr Oncol 24:248–256, 1995.
29. Dogan AS, Conway JJ, Miller JH, et al: Detection of bone lesions

in Langerhans cell histiocytosis: Complementary roles of scintigraphy and conventional radiography. J Pediatr Hematol Oncol 18:51–58, 1996.

30. Martinez-Lage JF, Poza M, Cartagena J, et al: Solitary eosinophilic granuloma of the pediatric skull and spine: The role of surgery. Childs Nerv Syst 7:448–451, 1991.

31. Egeler RM, Thompson RC Jr, Voute PA, et al: Intralesional infiltration of corticosteroids in localized Langerhans' cell histiocytosis. J Pediatr Orthop 12:811–814, 1992.

32. Szendroi M, Cser I, Konya A, et al: Aneurysmal bone cyst: A review of 52 primary and 16 secondary cases. Arch Orthop Trauma Surg 111:318–322, 1992.

33. Kozlowski K, Campbell J, McAlister W, et al: Rare primary cranial vault and base of the skull tumors in children. Radiol Med 81:213–224, 1991.

34. O'Brien DP, Rashad EM, Toland JA, et al: Aneurysmal cyst of the frontal bone: Case report and review of the literature. Br J Neurosurg 8:105–108, 1994.

35. Wojno KJ, McCarthy EF: Fibro-osseous lesions of the face and skull with aneurysmal bone cyst formation. Skeletal Radiol 23: 15–18, 1994.

36. McLeod RA, Dahlin RC, Beabout JW: The spectrum of osteoblastoma. AJR Am J Radiol 126:321–325, 1976.

37. Choudhury AR, al Amin MC, Chaudhri KA, et al: Benign osteoblastoma of the parietal bone. Childs Nerv Syst 11:115–117, 1995.

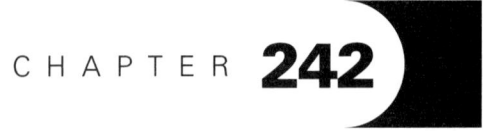

Cerebral Palsy: An Overview

CATHERINE J. DOTY

DEFINITION

Cerebral palsy is a diagnosis that represents a diverse collection of clinical syndromes. These disorders are nonprogressive and are characterized by alterations in movement and posture, which occur as a result of injury to the immature brain. Immaturity is generally defined as 3 years old and younger, although some sources include children up to the age of 7 years. The nonprogressive nature of cerebral palsy denotes that the neurological injury is not an ongoing process; however, the process of growth and development can cause tone and range of motion changes that alter gait patterns and the ability to accomplish tasks of daily living, resulting in functional losses or a failure to progress. This does not mean that affected children cannot improve in areas of motor control and language skills.

EPIDEMIOLOGY

Cerebral palsy is one of the leading causes of childhood neurological impairment and disability. There are more than 100,000 children younger than 18 years[1] and 300,000 to 400,000 individuals of all ages[2] with cerebral palsy in the United States. The overall incidence of cerebral palsy ranges from 1.5 to 3 per 1000 live births.[1, 3] The occurrence rate of cerebral palsy in low-birth-weight infants has increased since the 1980s—in concert with an improvement in their survival rate—to 13 to 14 per 1000 for infants weighing from 1501 to 2500 g and up to 90 to 91 per 1000 for infants weighing 1500 g or less.[4] However, the incidence of cerebral palsy in the full-term population has not changed significantly, despite falling rates of neonatal mortality, indicating that delivery-related hypoxia is an infrequent cause of cerebral palsy in these cases.[1, 5, 6] Predictive factors for the occurrence of cerebral palsy include maternal preeclampsia, infection, late gestational bleeding, multiple gestation, intrauterine growth retardation, nonvertex presentation, abruptio placentae, and fetal distress.

CAUSE

Cerebral palsy cannot be attributed to a single causative factor or event; rather, it is caused by a variety of conditions that result in injury to the developing brain and can be categorized by time frame as well as by pathology. These include problems such as migrational defects, infarction, intracranial hemorrhage, infection, chemical injury, and hypoxia (Table 242–1). The causative mechanisms can occur during gestation, in the case of insults such as stroke and TORCH (toxoplasmosis, other, rubella, cytomegalovirus, herpes) infections; during the perinatal period, in the case of hypoxia; and neonatally, in the case of group B streptococcal meningitis and intraventricular hemorrhage.[7] Early childhood events can result in cerebral palsy as well. These include traumatic brain injury secondary to abuse or accident, infections such as meningitis and encephalitis, and hypoxic-ischemic injury from near drownings, house fires, and even status epilepticus. However, despite improvements in diagnostic techniques and the quantity of information obtained during gestation, up to 20% of cases have no identifiable cause.[8]

CLASSIFICATION

The six primary clinical syndromes that constitute the diagnosis of cerebral palsy include the four forms of pyramidal cerebral palsy, one type of extrapyramidal cerebral palsy, and cerebellar or ataxic cerebral palsy.

TABLE 242–1 ■ **Time Line for Causes of Cerebral Palsy**

GESTATIONAL	PERINATAL	NEONATAL	EARLY CHILDHOOD
Chronic hypoxia	Hypotension	Prematurity	Traumatic brain injury
Placental insufficiency	Diminished cerebral	Germinal matrix	Child maltreatment
Umbilical vascular	perfusion	Ischemia	(shaken baby syndrome)
malformation	Bradycardia	Hemorrhage	Motor vehicle crash
Ischemic infraction	Hemorrhage	Intraventicular hemorrhage	Blunt trauma crash
Vascular instability	Abruptio placentae	Infection	Infection
Maternal cocaine use	Bleeding disorder	Herpes simplex virus	Meningitis
Infection	Hypoxia	Meningitis	Encephalitis
Cytomegalovirus	Respiratory depression	Group B streptococcus	
Toxoplasmosis	Nuchal cord	*Escherichia coli*	
Malformations/migrational	Meconium aspiration	Pneumococcus	
abnormalities			
Multiple gestation			

Data adapted from Kliegman RM, Behrman RE: Diseases of the newborn infant: Premature and full-term. In Behrman R, Vaughan V, Nelson W (eds) : Nelson Textbook of Pediatrics. Philadelphia, WB Saunders, 1987, pp 385–391; Molnar G: Cerebral palsy. In Molnar G (ed): Pediatric Rehabilitation. Baltimore, Williams & Wilkins, 1985, pp 420–467.

Pyramidal cerebral palsy accounts for three quarters of diagnosed cases and is distinguished by spasticity appearing as hyperactive deep tendon reflexes with hypertonia of a velocity-dependent, clasp-knife quality. This spastic type commonly takes the form of quadriplegia (27%), diplegia (21%), or hemiplegia (21%).[5] Hypertonia results in a diminished ability to dissociate limb and trunk movements. The lower limbs are more involved than the upper limbs in both spastic quadriplegia and spastic diplegia. Weakness and proximal hypotonia marked by poor head and trunk control are also prevalent features of both quadriplegia and diplegia; the two can be distinguished by the more generalized upper body and limb involvement in quadriplegia. The opposite pattern of involvement is commonly seen in spastic hemiplegia, with more upper limb than lower limb impairment on the involved side of the body.

Cerebral palsy with spastic quadriplegia generally implies a more diffuse insult to the cerebral cortex and is the second most common presentation in full-term infants. It is also frequently seen in premature, low-birth-weight infants and secondary to later injuries from meningitis, trauma, and child abuse. Diffuse brain injury can occur early as a result of chronic placental insufficiency; a catastrophic event during the perinatal period, such as hypoxia, stroke, or intraventricular hemorrhage; and infectious disease during gestation, such as cytomegalovirus and toxoplasmosis (part of the TORCH constellation).

Spastic diplegia is the pattern most closely associated with prematurity and is frequently linked with the finding of periventricular leukomalacia, which is thought to be attributable to hypoperfusion with watershed ischemia and to periventricular hemorrhage.[8, 9]

Hemiplegia is the most common clinical manifestation of cerebral palsy in term infants and is the second most common presentation in preterm infants.[9] Male infants are more frequently affected than are female infants, and right hemiplegia is the predominant form. Hemiplegia results from a relatively localized injury to the brain and is often the result of infarction, hemorrhage, or malformation, although the cause cannot always be determined.

Cerebral palsy with rigidity is seen in approximately 4% to 5% of the population and should be differentiated from severe spasticity.[8] Rigidity is characterized by a constant, high level of tone that does not change with the velocity of joint movement; rather, there is constant resistance.

Extrapyramidal or dyskinetic cerebral palsy types affect both trunk and limbs and manifest with abnormal movement and fluctuating tone. This form is attributable to injury of the basal ganglia and represents 25% of all cases.[10] Frequently diagnosed movement disorders in this type of cerebral palsy are athetosis, with slow, writhing movements of the face and distal (more so than proximal) extremity musculature, and dystonia, characterized by slow, rhythmic changes of posture and tone that affect the trunk and proximal limbs. The movements of both athetosis and dystonia are involuntary and can interfere with purposeful movement as well as resting posture. Other rarely occurring movement disorders associated with extrapyramidal cerebral palsy include tremor and choreiform or ballistic movements. Dyskinetic cerebral palsy can result from both ischemic and chemical injury to the basal ganglia and is found more often in full-term infants. Historically, hypoxic-ischemic injury, secondary to birth-related anoxia, and kernicterus were the most common causes of dyskinetic cerebral palsy, but new findings clearly indicate that birth asphyxia is a rare causative factor.[10, 11] The most probable mechanism of antepartum hypoxic injury is unstable cerebral perfusion, which has been associated with notable findings of basal ganglia injury, including patchy, symmetrical demyelination in the putamen, globus pallidus, caudate nucleus, and thalamus and hypermyelination of the glial fibers in the putamen. Both patchy demyelination and glial hypermyelination are linked with the arterial watershed and are associated with heterotopia in the white matter, which is thought to be a result of placental insufficiency early in gestation. Bilirubin-related encephalopathy is now a much less frequent phenomenon, owing to improved treatment options for hyperbilirubinemia.

Ataxic cerebral palsy is rare and presents with classic cerebellar signs. The pyramidal and extrapyramidal forms may present with early hypotonia, followed by the evolution of spasticity or a movement disorder, but a small number of patients remain hypotonic and are classified as having atonic cerebral palsy.

The last group in the classification of cerebral palsy represents mixed clinical types, with spastic-athetoid, spastic-dystonic, and spastic-rigid being the most common presentations.

DIAGNOSIS AND CLINICAL PRESENTATION

Early diagnosis has traditionally been difficult for a variety of reasons, including the wide variability in presentation and the lack of a single definitive diagnostic test. Cerebral palsy is a diagnosis of exclusion based on clinical signs. A key point to remember when working through the differential diagnosis is that cerebral palsy is nonprogressive, whereas other disorders follow a deteriorating course. The differential diagnosis must include diseases that affect tone, movement, strength, and developmental milestones. For example, a child with low tone may have cerebral palsy or benign hereditary infantile hypotonia, but the possibility of mitochondrial and metabolic myopathies must be investigated. In addition to laboratory testing, serial examination is vital. In the case of familial hypotonia, there is no accompanying weakness, and these children eventually become normotonic and catch up on their motor milestones, whereas myopathic diseases may progress. Weakness can be the presenting symptom in neonatal spinal cord injury, particularly if there is a history of a difficult delivery with a large infant or shoulder dystocia, and in lower motor neuron disorders such as infantile spinal muscular atrophy. Progressive loss of milestones is the hallmark of neurodegenerative diseases such as Lesch-Nyhan syndrome and the leukodystrophies and can be the presenting feature of intracranial neoplasms. These diseases must be ruled out because of the significant repercussions for treatment and prognosis and the need for genetic counseling.

The diagnosis of cerebral palsy may be suspected during the first 4 to 6 months of life, particularly in infants that are later determined to have spastic quadriplegia or hemiplegia. However, it is not until after 4 months of age—when the primitive reflexes are being integrated, gross motor milestone acquisition is under way, and clearly isolated volitional movement is expected—that a clear clinical picture emerges.[3, 8, 12] A definitive diagnosis of cerebral palsy can be made during the second half of the first year by thoroughly assessing the six major motor categories as defined by Levine[13]: posture and movement patterns, primitive reflexes, muscle tone and reflex patterns (deep tendon and plantar reflexes), evolution of postural reactions and milestones, oral motor patterns, and presence of strabismus.

Observation of movement patterns and posture is particularly important for the identification of dystonia, dyskinesia, and ataxia, but it also plays a role in discerning synergistic movement patterns that are typical of spasticity. Identification of primitive reflex patterns is a vital tool, because hyperactivity or persistence of these responses is well correlated with the diagnosis of cerebral palsy.[7, 10–12] The reflexes are under brainstem control and are elicited through the stimulation of the sensory end-organs in the vestibular system, as well as those providing proprioceptive feedback from the joints. Primitive reflexes are expected to be integrated or extinguished between the third and sixth months of life. The reflexes with the greatest predictive value are the Moro, asymmetrical tonic neck, crossed extension/stepping, and tonic labyrinthine reflexes; somewhat less significant are the palmar grasp, Landau reflex, and positive supporting response (Table 242–2). Primitive reflexes can be quantified with a 5-point grading scale ranging from 0 (absent reflex) to 4+ (obligate reflex), with a 2 indicating a normally present reflex.[10–12] The obligatory presence of the primitive reflexes is considered to be abnormal at any age. Each of the primitive reflexes plays a role in the development of necessary motor skills and should be evaluated for quality and symmetry of response. Tone can be evaluated by examining the deep tendon reflexes for hyperactivity and the plantar reflexes for an extensor response, as well as by using the modified Ashworth scale,[14] a reliable quantification tool (Table 242–3). This appraisal is necessary to differentiate spastic, rigid, and dyskinetic forms, as well as to determine prognosis and treatment. Acquisition of postural or protective responses and achievement of motor and language milestones are crucial developmental steps during the first year of life. Abnormal oral motor patterns—including tongue thrusting or retraction, reflexive bite during feeding, and oral defensiveness—and strabismus with esotropia or exotropia, combined with the presence of other motor deficits, can assist in making the diagnosis of cerebral palsy. Understanding the general pattern of skill refinement, from rolling over to walking, provides a basis for judging whether a delay is significant and pertinent to the diagnosis.

Once the diagnosis has been made, the next step is to provide the child's family with prognostic information. Determining the prognosis can be accomplished by understanding the different clinical types of cerebral palsy and performing serial examinations to determine the pace of motor development and the evolution of protective responses. Families generally want the answers to two questions: (1) Will my child walk? and (2) How will my child do in school? The youngest age at which motor prognosis can be reliably determined is 2 years old. Gross motor milestones that have assessment value are rolling, sitting, crawling, cruising, and walking.

In the pyramidal spastic types of cerebral palsy, children with hemiplegia have a 4- to 6-month delay in milestone achievement, but the majority walk within the first 2 years of life, and all are eventually ambula-

T A B L E   2 4 2 – 2   ■ **Primitive Reflexes Used in the Evaluation of Cerebral Palsy**

PRIMITIVE REFLEXES	ELICITING STIMULUS	DESCRIPTION	AGE OF APPEARANCE AND INTEGRATION
Moro	Semiseated position with head in midline—head drops back a few centimeters	Abduction with upward movement of the arms at the shoulders, with extension of the arms and hands open, followed by adduction and flexion toward midline	Birth 4–6 mo
Asymmetrical tonic neck	Head rotated 90 degrees to the right or left and position held for 5 sec	The fencing position is assumed, with the face-side limbs in extension and the occiput-side limbs in flexion	Birth 4–6 mo
Tonic labyrinthine	Supine position with extension of head 45 degrees from midline	Upper limb extension with shoulder retraction, followed by upper limb flexion Lower limbs extended Posture frequently accompanied by involuntary tongue thrusting	Birth 4–6 mo
Crossed extension stepping	Horizontal: crossed extension reflex elicited by unpleasant stimulus to sole of foot Vertical: stepping reflex—support in vertical with sole of foot contacting a surface	Phase I: flexion on side of stimulation and extension on contralateral side Phase II: adduction Phase III: extension on stimulated side In vertical, the same response occurs, but as weight is lifted, a stepping pattern emerges	Birth 2–3 mo
Palmar grasp	Pressure in palm of hand	Strong finger flexion	Birth 4 mo
Landau	Held suspended in prone with trunk support between shoulders and pelvis	Extension of head, trunk, and limbs	2–3 mo 12–24 mo
Positive supporting	Held suspended in vertical and forefeet placed against a supporting surface	Infantile response results in momentary extension of lower limbs with support of body weight Mature response results in extension of lower limbs with support of body weight	Birth and disappears at 3–4 mo Appears at 6 mo and integrates with voluntary standing and ambulation

Data adapted from Capute A: Early neuromotor reflexes in infancy. Pediatr Ann 15:217–226, 1986; Capute A, Palmer R, Shapiro B, et al: Primitive reflex profile: A quantitation of primitive reflexes in infancy. Dev Med Child Neurol 26:375–383, 1984; Capute A, Shapiro B, Accardo P, et al: Motor functions: Associated primitive reflex profiles. Dev Med Child Neurol 24:662–669, 1982.

T A B L E   2 4 2 – 3   ■ **Modified Ashworth Scale**

SCORE	DESCRIPTION	EXAMINATION
0	No increase	Moves freely at any velocity
1	Slight increase	Catch and release or minimal resistance at end range
1+	Slight increase	Catch and release with minimal resistance through remainder of range of motion
2	More marked increase	Moderate resistance throughout range, but joint is easily moved
3	Considerable increase	High tone is present—joint is difficult to move
4	Severe increase	Affected joints are rigid—cannot be moved from flexed or extended position

Data adapted from Bohannon R, Smith M: Interrater reliability of modified Ashworth scale of muscle spasticity. Phys Ther 67:206–207, 1986.

tory unless profound intellectual deficits exist.[15] Typically, 50% of children with spastic diplegia progress to independent, community-level ambulation, another 20% require assistive devices, and only 15% are totally dependent on a wheelchair as the primary means of mobility because of spasticity, increased energy demand, or intellectual deficits.[16] Motor deficits are more profound in spastic quadriplegia, and ambulation is often delayed past the age of 3 years. A wide range of abilities is found among those with quadriplegia; one third of patients require total assistance for mobility, self-care, and other activities of daily living, and approximately two thirds either need orthotics and assistive devices for ambulation and activities of daily living or are basically independent. Seventy-five percent of children diagnosed with athetoid-type cerebral palsy walk independently, and 50% ambulate before the age of 3 years; however, the population with mixed-type spastic-athetoid cerebral palsy has only a 50% rate of independent ambulation. The majority of children affected with the ataxic type do walk, but often not until school age. The rigid and atonic forms of cerebral palsy carry the worst prognosis, and these children are generally nonambulatory.[8, 16, 17]

The guidelines for determining ambulation potential are based on attainment of independent sitting. Ninety-six percent of ambulators sit by the age of 4 years, and 100% of children with cerebral palsy who sit by the age of 2 years will eventually ambulate community distances independently, without assistive devices.[17] Children who sit after age 3 years generally require assistive devices and ambulate limited distances.

The second question, related to cognitive prognosis, is far more difficult. Approximately 50% of children with cerebral palsy have intelligence quotients (IQs) within normal limits, another 25% to 30% have mild to moderate retardation, and the same number have severe to profound retardation.[18] The same statistics indicate that children with the most severe motor involvement are more likely to have severe intellectual deficits. However, there is wide variability in cognitive skills, and the discrepancy between the degree of motor involvement and IQ can be significant. Therefore, a child with severe spastic or athetoid quadriplegia can have a high level of intelligence, and a child with hemiplegia can be profoundly retarded. Many children with normal or near-normal IQs have been considered intellectually deficient because of motor deficits that interfere with oral motor and fine motor skills and therefore make traditional means of communication impossible. Children with cerebral palsy also have a high incidence of dyspraxia, visual motor–visual perceptual deficits, and sensory integration deficits that may interfere with their ability to progress and complete self-care tasks. It is important that all children, even those with profound motor deficits, be followed closely to determine their potential.

COMPLICATIONS

The disorders of movement, posture, and tone that exemplify cerebral palsy can result in complications that involve multiple systems. Feeding problems and growth failure are frequently an issue. The children most often affected by weight and linear growth retardation are those with severe motor involvement and dystonia. A study by Stevenson and coworkers found that in this group of severely affected children, 38% had heights below the 2.5th percentile, 42% had weights below the 2.5th percentile, and 30% had triceps skinfold measurements below the 3rd percentile for gender and age.[19] Although feeding issues are more common in children with severe motor involvement, significant problems can be present in any of the subtypes. The cause of feeding and growth problems is multifactorial. Neuromotor issues include oral motor dyspraxia, dyskinesia, and pseudobulbar palsy. Altered sensation and oral motor coordination are seen, with clinical evidence of oral hypersensitivity, hyperactive bite reflex, inadequate lip and cheek closure, drooling, abnormal tongue thrusting, hyperactive or hypoactive gag reflex, and defects in coordinating the timing of the swallow reflex and airway protection. These factors lead to delayed and often inadequate bolus formation, distal propulsion, and initiation of the swallow reflex.[8, 20] Incoordination of respiratory timing and swallowing is associated with prolonged ventilatory recovery time[20] and diminished airway protective mechanisms, which lead to increased energy consumption, fatigue, and ultimately aspiration associated with feeding. Mealtime thus becomes an exhausting and unpleasant experience that may be nutritionally ineffective and can heighten symptoms of oral aversion, thus perpetuating the cycle and leading to malnutrition. Oral motor impairment not only affects the ability to eat but also plays a significant role in other complications. Drooling causes problems with oral hygiene and skin management, in addition to having social repercussions for the children.

Diminished selective muscle control and coordination of breath support can severely alter a child's ability to communicate. The most common impediments to independent verbal communication are dyspraxia and dysarthria secondary to spasticity and dystonia.

Gastrointestinal disturbances are common. Constipation and its associated encopresis are multifactorial and have medical, hygienic, and psychosocial implications. Diminished activity levels and immobility can exacerbate the problem, but the primary issue is the upper motor neuron lesion that alters bowel motility. Failure to implement an effective bowel program can result in problems ranging from uncontrolled soiling, leading to skin breakdown due to insufficient cleanup, to impaction with symptoms of bowel obstruction and megacolon. Gastroesophageal reflux is also associated with neurological impairment and can place children with compromised oropharyngeal motor skills and mechanisms for airway protection at high risk for aspiration pneumonia.

Respiratory complications are a significant source of morbidity and mortality. Neonatal respiratory distress syndrome is a complication of premature birth, mechanical ventilation, and chemical injury (e.g., meconium aspiration) and can lead to restrictive lung disease. Risk for pneumonia is also increased by less effective clearance of secretions, incoordination of cough, and a higher risk of aspiration during reflux episodes and swallowing.

Infants and children with cerebral palsy have a greater risk of developing epilepsy. Seizures occur in 30% to 50% of the population but are most common in those with spastic hemiplegia; the incidence is between 50% and 70%, based on whether the hemiplegia occurred pre- or postnatally.[4, 8] Fifty percent of children with spastic quadriplegia have epilepsy, but in those with diplegia, ataxia, and athetosis, the incidence of epilepsy is less than 30%.[8] A wide range of seizure types is noted and can significantly affect prognosis, particularly in the case of infantile spasms. Visual and auditory deficits associated with cerebral palsy can have a significant impact on self-care, mobility, communication, education, and instrumental activities of daily living, including access to computers, augmentative communication devices, environmental control systems, and powered mobility aids and the independent use of a motor vehicle or public transportation. More than 50% of children with cerebral palsy have strabismus,[21] most commonly esotropia; in addition, visual field defects are not uncommon in children with hemiplegia, and refractive errors are found among all the subtypes. The sequelae of retinopathy of prematurity range from myopia that is correctable with refractive lenses to blindness. Cortical visual loss is also a complication, most commonly affecting children with more severe impairments. TORCH syndrome, particularly cytomegalovirus and toxoplasmosis, can result in vision loss from chorioretinitis and optic atrophy. Hearing loss is found in approximately 10% of children with cerebral palsy and is most commonly sensorineuronal in origin.[22] Potential causes of deafness include kernicterus, hypoxia, neonatal meningitis, and the ototoxic antibiotics used in the treatment of meningitis, sepsis, and the TORCH infections.[8]

Urinary incontinence is multifactorial. It can be the result of altered sensation, cognition, communication, and mobility skills. Some individuals may not sense bladder fullness, some may not be capable of understanding the concept of continence, and others may be fully aware of the need to urinate but are unable to communicate it to caregivers. Impaired mobility may present an obstacle to reaching the toilet and removing clothing in time. Another cause of urinary incontinence in children with cerebral palsy is a neurogenic bladder. The most common presenting symptoms are frequency and urgency, which are most often attributable to detrusor hyperreflexia and diminished bladder capacity. Stress incontinence can also be observed and may be the result of a lower motor neuron lesion of the distal urethra secondary to a hypoxic injury or poor coordination of voluntary sphincter control.[23]

Bone density is a major concern for individuals who are not ambulatory or regularly weight bearing, because bone mass is maintained through forces placed on the bones by gravity and muscle contraction. In unimpaired individuals, this occurs as normal activities of daily living and mobility are carried out. A program of weight-bearing activity, consisting of upper body strengthening and supported standing, for a minimum of 2 hours a day is necessary to prevent osteopenia, which occurs as bone mass rapidly diminishes. This places the child at high risk for fractures during bed mobility, transfers, stretching activities, and participation in therapy programs.

Myofascial pain syndrome is three to four times more prevalent in children with cerebral palsy than in age-matched controls.[24] The identifiable trigger points and tender, taut bands follow the classic patterns of presentation outlined by Travell and colleagues,[25] with more than 50% occurring in the shoulder girdle. The increased incidence of myofascial pain appears to be the result of muscle overload and altered biomechanics due to abnormal muscle control, weakness, spasticity, and diminished range of motion.

Joint contractures, dislocations, and scoliosis are frequently encountered musculoskeletal complaints in children with cerebral palsy. Contractures occur for a variety of reasons, including joint imbalance secondary to spasticity in one group of muscles and concomitant weakness of the antagonistic group. Muscles are stimulated to grow longitudinally by stretching them. In children who do not have hypertonia and motor deficits, stretch is applied daily through antigravity weight bearing. Children with selective motor control deficits, spasticity, and weakness are susceptible to a relative shortening of affected muscle groups across joints because bone growth continues even though muscle growth is impeded. Growth spurts are the periods of greatest risk for developing joint contractures, especially during adolescence, when it is common for therapies to be discontinued. Joint contractures and deformities can be avoided by instituting a therapeutic home program that includes a daily stretching regimen and using appropriate nighttime bracing to administer prolonged stretch across selected joints. The muscle groups most likely to be involved are those that cross two joints, such as the biceps, hamstrings, and triceps surae. The thumb adductors and wrist and finger flexors are often involved as well, creating an unbalanced and functionally limited hand.[26–28] If fixed contractures occur, orthopedic intervention will be necessary.

Joint subluxation and dislocation can occur as a result of muscle imbalance, with an incidence between 22% and 45%.[29] Severe spasticity, early onset of hip position changes, lack of ambulation and weight bearing, and migration index greater than 50% significantly increase the risk of hip dislocation.[30] Hip radiographs should be obtained routinely to monitor for coxa valga, subluxation, and progression to dislocation, which occurs in as many as 12% to 15% of cases.[29] Progressive changes in the hip joint appear to be secondary to imbalance of the hip flexors and adductors, causing the center of rotation to shift from the femoral head to the lesser trochanter, effectively levering the femoral head from the acetabulum.[30] Hip pain, loss of range of motion, diminished ambulation, impaired sitting ability, and degenerative joint disease can all occur as a result of dislocation.

Scoliosis is a significant problem, occurring in approximately 15% of all children with cerebral palsy and in 25% to 40% of those with quadriplegia.[31] The curve is neuromuscular in nature, arising from weakness or hypotonia of the trunk musculature.[32] A number of conservative methods for controlling scoliotic curves are used, including trunk strengthening through physical therapy, electrical stimulation modalities, and orthotics; however, these are often ineffective in children or teenagers with progressive curvature. Once scoliosis has been identified, monitoring should be carried out regularly, and the possibility of surgical intervention should be discussed with the patient and family. As with scoliosis of any cause, there are fewer growth complications when spinal fusion and instrumentation are done as close to skeletal maturity as possible.[31, 32] If severe scoliosis is not addressed, there may be major ramifications related to pulmonary function, seating and positioning, skin management, and mobility. A teenager or adult with a high-degree curvature is at risk for respiratory insufficiency, sleep disturbance, and pressure breakdown over bony prominences. This results in the need for complicated and costly pressure-relief mattresses and wheelchair seating systems. Mobility and weight bearing can also be profoundly affected, with loss of ambulation and even transfer and standing skills; this can result in less independence, as well as an increased risk of osteopenia with fractures. Surgical correction is also associated with functional complications, most notably loss of trunk flexibility and neck extension. Independent dressing activities are adversely affected, and prone positioning, an effective means of prolonged hip flexor stretch, becomes painful and difficult.

GAIT AND ORTHOTICS

The disorders of movement, posture, and tone that characterize cerebral palsy have a major impact on ambulation through changes in the gait cycle and static and dynamic balance and their effect on energy expenditure and oxygen consumption. The alterations in motor control occur secondary to an upper motor neuron injury and result in a diminished ability to dissociate movement of the limbs and trunk and to maintain balance while standing and moving. The loss of selective muscle control—including muscle agonist-antagonist co-contractions and muscle group imbalances across joints—the use of compensatory primitive reflex patterns, and the presence of abnormal tone are all major contributors to pathologic gait.[33] To understand how these changes affect gait in children, one needs a basic knowledge of what makes normal gait work.

Gait is a complex, symmetrical pattern of movement that occurs in a coordinated fashion not only to propel the body forward in space but also to do so in a manner that is energy efficient against the force of gravity. This is accomplished by means of fine-tuned motor control, packaged as the movements that make up the six determinants and the three rockers of the gait cycle. The six determinants of gait were first outlined by Saunders in 1953 and revised by Inman in 1981 and Rose and Gamble in 1994.[34] They function to

smooth the path of the center of gravity, which lies just anterior to the S1 or S2 segment, by minimizing vertical and horizontal excursions of the trunk during the gait cycle. The first determinant is pelvic rotation around the vertical axis. The second determinant is pelvic obliquity or Trendelenburg positioning, which involves tipping the pelvis on the anterior-posterior axis. The third, fourth, and fifth determinants are interdependent and involve knee flexion in stance, ankle flexion and extension mechanisms, and knee and ankle rotation. These mechanisms also result in the three rockers, which are events that occur during the gait cycle and represent shifts in momentum and the ground reaction force. The sixth determinant of gait, lateral displacement, limits the horizontal movements of the trunk.[33–36] The integrity of the six determinants and the three rockers is vital to the energy-efficient execution of walking, reducing vertical excursion by 50% and horizontal excursion by 30%; this limits displacement of the center of gravity to 4 to 5 cm in both planes.[34, 35, 37]

The gait abnormalities associated with the various forms of cerebral palsy are the result of disturbances in symmetry and in the rockers and determinants. In pyramidal cerebral palsy, spasticity and motor planning and motor control problems make dissociated movements of the pelvis and lower limbs difficult or impossible. This results in derangement or loss of the first and second determinants, with severely compromised stride length and excessive upward motion of the trunk. Weakness and spasticity make a notable contribution to the disruption of the third, fourth, and fifth determinants and the three rockers. Dynamic control of agonist and antagonist muscle groups is diminished, with muscle group cocontraction and relative weakness of the hip, knee, and ankle extensors when compared with the spasticity of the flexors. This is particularly evident in the severely compromised ability to eccentrically contract the lower limb musculature to control knee flexion during loading response, plantarflexion at the first rocker, and dorsiflexion at the second rocker. As a result, the most typical pattern observed is plantarflexion at first contact, with adducted, internally rotated hips and excessive hip and knee flexion. This creates a crouched gait pattern prohibitive of the flexion-extension movements at the knee and ankle that limit vertical displacement of the center of gravity and allow for the efficient transfer of energy.[34] The sixth determinant of gait is severely compromised by the loss of a stable base of support, secondary to scissoring and equinovarus or excessively pronated foot positioning, which prevents successful weight shifting to the stance-phase limb.[33, 34] In other forms of cerebral palsy, many of the same issues are present, owing to diminished motor control and significant losses in static and dynamic balance secondary to proprioceptive abnormalities, dyskinesias, and ataxia. These disturbances not only alter the way the child perceives limb and joint position but also remove the child's ability to control extraneous movement and maintain equilibrium. In general, muscle weakness, poor limb positioning, and changes in tone can significantly affect a child's ability to support body weight against gravity and can negatively influence step length and generation of power. The end result in most forms of cerebral palsy in which the abnormalities do not preclude ambulation is excessive displacement of the center of gravity, poor use of momentum, and inefficient transfer of energy from one segment to another. This drives the energy cost of walking three to four times higher than in a more normal gait pattern.[37]

Orthotics and assistive devices can be used to compensate for losses in motor control. The purpose of orthotics or bracing is to prevent and correct deformity, provide a stable base of support, facilitate skill acquisition, and improve gait efficiency. When choosing orthotics for children with cerebral palsy, it is important to assess their tone carefully. Unless the child has the hypotonic-atonic form of cerebral palsy, it is necessary to remember that tone is dynamic in nature and that strength and motor control issues are of equal importance. A balance must be achieved between supporting the involved joint and minimizing the loss of strength in the muscles acting across the joint—in other words, one must avoid "overbracing." The natural inclination of many practitioners is to attempt to completely control each joint and to correct problems at every segment where they occur. This frequently leads to the application of extensive, heavy bracing, which dramatically increases energy expenditure, as measured by oxygen consumption, and results in loss of functional strength and flexibility. Orthotics must be matched to the particular patient. For example, bracing that works well for someone with muscular dystrophy or myelodysplasia is often inappropriate for an individual with cerebral palsy. When prescribing orthotics, it is paramount that the practitioner understand the materials making up the brace and the style being used. For example, children and young adults with cerebral palsy are fully capable of strengthening weak musculature and should be given every opportunity to do so, rather than perpetuating dependence on a brace made of heavy, rigid materials. The design is also important. A hinge is often added at the ankle of pediatric ankle-foot orthotics, but this style should be used only when there is active dorsiflexion present or in the rare case when a child needs the ability to crawl while wearing the brace and needs plantarflexion but not dorsiflexion resistance while in stance. If plantarflexion resistance is not needed, a supramalleolar trim-line brace will suffice. The best rule to follow is that less is more: The least restrictive bracing that serves the need should be used. Once the relationship between normal gait and the causes of pathologic gait in cerebral palsy has been examined, the problems related to functional ambulation and the means to treat them become much clearer.

TREATMENT

The treatment of cerebral palsy is aimed not at a cure but at optimization of functional gains. When setting treatment priorities, quality of life is the primary concern; therefore, a means of functional communication and independence in daily living skills should come first, followed by mobility and ambulation.[33] No matter what treatment course is implemented, the plan must attend to the needs of the whole child, not just an isolated issue such as disturbance in body mechanics. Therefore, problems in nutritional, psychosocial, and school-related areas should be identified, as well as those related to language and communication, self-care, and mobility skills. The projected effects of growth and development must be analyzed, and a variety of treatment alternatives should be considered, including no treatment. Finally, a set of functional short-term, long-term, and end-range goals should be defined.[37] Once the planning process has been set in motion, the myriad options, including physical therapy, medication, and surgical intervention, can be considered.

A speech and language evaluation is recommended for most children with cerebral palsy. A large number of individuals have dysarthria as well as oral motor dyspraxia, which can affect spontaneous speech patterns. For children with significant language delays, an augmentative communication evaluation must be done in conjunction with speech and language pathology and occupational therapy. The ability to communicate basic wants and needs is intrinsic to even the youngest infants and becomes increasingly clear and sophisticated as children develop language skills. A wide array of devices is available to make functional community-level communication possible. Many children who are severely impaired are fully capable of understanding the use of such a device and activating it to express their feelings and desires.

Occupational therapy is a vital component of the treatment regimen, but the term *occupational* is deceptive. Occupational therapists work with children to help them gain the ability to perform self-care activities, including feeding, grooming, dressing, and toileting as independently as possible at age-appropriate levels. This requires evaluation and execution of a therapy program for fine motor coordination, upper limb gross motor planning, visual motor and visual perceptual skills, problem solving, and processing skills. In addition, occupational therapists can assess the quality of sensory integration and provide therapeutic intervention to assist children with significant problems such as oral and tactile defensiveness, which is common in those with cerebral palsy. Abnormalities in these areas can lead to failure to thrive, mother-child detachment, and the inability to explore the environment effectively. In the 1970s, Ayers developed a therapy program based on the theory that defective sensory integration abilities prevent children from integrating the primitive reflexes and gaining the righting and equilibrium reactions.[38] Providing tactile, proprioceptive, and vestibular input in a controlled manner is thought to allow children to learn to process information in a more organized fashion and then respond to their environment with improved motor planning and adaptive capabilities. This form of therapy does not appear to rectify children's developmental delays and tone abnormalities,[39] but it has been successful in improving their response to the sensory stimuli encountered when interacting with caregivers and the community.[38]

Physical therapy is the standard treatment for the impairments of cerebral palsy. There are numerous treatment techniques; some are methodologic, and others are less structured but based on a unified set of concepts. Some of the most notable are neurodevelopmental treatment, the Vojta technique, conductive education, and the Rood technique. Neurodevelopmental treatment was developed by Karel and Berta Bobath and is based on the theory that the disturbances of movement and tone in cerebral palsy are the result of the failure to extinguish primitive reflex patterns, which interferes with the development of normal postural control.[40, 41] The goal of neurodevelopmental treatment is to inhibit abnormal patterns and facilitate normal ones through handling of the child and using "key points of control." Vojta also based his method on controlling or modifying primitive reflex patterns and developing more mature postural reflex patterns. Conductive education involves immersion of the child and family in a structured program that emphasizes patterning of movement.[39] Rood based her treatment on the concept of tactile stimulation, via brushing, to alter tone and patterns of movement through facilitation.[42] Therapeutic modalities also play an important role in treatment. The use of ice, moist heat, and ultrasonography can facilitate stretching for range of motion and is helpful in the treatment of musculoskeletal pain.

Therapeutic electrical stimulation is used in several forms. Functional electrical stimulation uses enough intensity to elicit muscle contraction and has been shown to increase strength and alter fiber type. Threshold electrical stimulation as described by Pape and associates involves the overnight application of low-intensity stimulation below the level that produces muscle contraction. Improvements in gross motor function have been reported, but more in-depth inquiries are needed to determine efficacy.[43, 44]

Studies examining the outcome of therapeutic interventions show that the method used is not the key factor; rather, intensive family and patient involvement in therapy and life adjustment is critical.[39, 45, 46] The majority of therapies today consist of an eclectic mix of techniques with the goal of improving functional performance and adaptation, as well as training to correct problems with movement and posture.

Pharmacologic treatment plays a significant role in the management of spasticity and dyskinesias. The mainstays of treatment are antispasticity medications such as baclofen (Lioresal), dantrolene (Dantrium), and diazepam (Valium). Baclofen is a centrally acting gamma aminobutyric acid (GABA) analog, which is thought to act by suppressing the release of excitatory neurotransmitters at the presynaptic level in the spinal cord. The most common side effects are drowsiness, fatigue, dizziness, and a risk of seizures and hallucinations with abrupt withdrawal.[47, 48] Dantrolene acts at the level of the muscles and elicits its effect by suppressing the release of calcium from the sarcoplasmic reticulum. Weakness, drowsiness, lethargy, and hepatic injury can occur, and routine liver function studies

should be performed while dantrolene is being administered. Diazepam acts in the central nervous system to enhance the effects of GABA. It can be sedating and cause memory disturbance, and tolerance to diazepam can develop, requiring escalating doses to maintain effectiveness. When the side effects of these medications are understood and the functional needs of children with cerebral palsy are carefully considered, it is clear that dantrolene and diazepam are less suitable alternatives for the long-term management of this population, which has significant issues with weakness and the resultant loss of independence. In addition, there is evidence that dantrolene, although physiologically active, does not have a significant effect on the functional status of children with cerebral palsy relative to changes in upper limb dexterity, range of motion, and mobility skills.[49]

Other oral medications that are useful in the management of spasticity are the centrally acting α_2-agonists, including clonidine, which acts at the level of the brainstem and spinal cord, and tizanidine (Zanaflex), which appears to increase presynaptic inhibition at the level of the spinal cord. Additionally, gabapentin (Neurontin) has been found to be effective in pediatric patients.[50] The treatment of movement abnormalities is a more complicated issue, but some success has been achieved in treating athetosis with carbidopa-levodopa (Sinemet) and dystonia with clonazepam (Klonopin).

Options for the treatment of spasticity and dystonia also include injection of neurolytic agents and surgical intervention. Neurolytics have been used for many years, primarily in the form of absolute alcohol washes and phenol (carbolic acid) motor point injections, but during the past 20 years, the use of type A botulinum toxin has also become an accepted procedure. Absolute alcohol has been shown to reduce spasticity temporarily when diluted to a 50% solution with normal saline and injected intramuscularly. This method is reported to have few side effects, and no muscle fiber fibrosis is evident on biopsy.[51] The application of 5% to 7% phenol, via electromyographic guidance into the motor point, produces more lasting effects by nonselectively destroying axons, but the procedure is painful and can result in fibrosis and dysesthesias. Phenol can also result in cardiorespiratory depression and seizures if intravascular injection should occur.[35, 47, 52] Type A botulinum toxin acts by permanently binding to the presynaptic terminal at the neuromuscular junction and inhibiting the release of acetylcholine vesicles, thus functionally denervating that portion of muscle. The amount of weakness obtained is dose dependent and reverses over time as terminal sprouting occurs and new end plates are formed.[53] Botox is the preparation used in the United States and is approximately three times more potent than Dysport, the preparation used in the United Kingdom.[52, 54] Pediatric administration is calculated in units per kilogram of body weight; the maximum recommended dose is the lesser of 12 units/kg or 400 units.[55] An effect is expected within 3 to 7 days, with maximal response occurring at approximately 2 weeks and lasting for an additional 6 to 16 weeks in the majority of patients, although more prolonged responses have been documented. The frequency of injections should be minimized to avoid anti–botulinum A antigen formation, a major reason for diminished efficacy with repeated use. In addition, Botox appears to be far more effective when combined with therapeutic interventions for stretching, including serial casting, muscle re-education and strengthening, and proper fitting with resting and functional orthotics. The use of Botox in the management of spasticity has shown preliminary promise, with improvements in tone, positioning, and range of motion and diminished cocontraction of antagonist and agonist muscle groups. Additional controlled studies are still required to define the most successful way of using this treatment modality.

Spasticity management is a priority for individuals with cerebral palsy, but treatment of other complications that affect health and independence is equally important. Bowel and bladder incontinence is a major issue for all patients with cerebral palsy because it not only can result in skin and hygienic problems but also can affect community-level independence. In some cases, these problems are secondary to cognitive deficits, but they are frequently a result of neurogenic bowel and bladder. Stool incontinence or constipation should be managed with a routine bowel program using stool softeners, bulking agents, and, when necessary, suppositories to train the gut to empty at a chosen time. Urinary incontinence as a result of either upper or lower motor neuron injury can be improved with medication. Anticholinergic agents such as oxybutynin (Ditropan), hyoscyamine (Levsin), and propantheline can be very effective in the treatment of the low-volume, hyperreflexive bladder in upper motor neuron lesions. Adrenergic agonists such as ephedrine can be helpful in the case of lower motor neuron injury with sphincter dysfunction.

Drooling is another common complication and is often the result of diminished oral motor planning and control and decreased swallowing frequency. Speech and language therapy techniques, particularly those that include biofeedback, can be effective, but medications such as glycopyrrolate, benzhexol, and transdermal scopolamine can greatly reduce the quantity of secretions, allowing improved management.[56–58]

Surgical intervention also plays a role in the management of tone, positioning, and range of motion. Orthopedic intervention for joint deformity, dislocation, and scoliosis can be a vital component of treatment. Care must be taken to choose the appropriate time and situation for procedures such as tenodesis and tendon transfers. Lengthening of tendons diminishes tone, but the effect can be transient, because growth and "resetting" of the muscle length-tension relationship can occur. In addition, each time a tendon or muscle is lengthened it is weakened, which can result in a different set of joint imbalances than those treated initially. Therefore, the most appropriate use of tendon or muscle lengthening procedures is to relieve fixed contractures. Tendon transfers are performed to create balance across a joint and improve function. When these procedures are timed correctly, performed

on muscle groups for which there is adequate control and motor planning ability, and followed by therapeutic intervention, the end result can be very good.[24–26] However, rotational changes secondary to growth, hypertonia, and movement disorders can significantly alter the anatomy postoperatively, resulting in the recurrence of contractures and the emergence of new joint imbalances. Motor dyspraxia and neurological neglect can also have a negative effect on the ability to benefit from surgical alterations intended to balance joints and produce functional movement. The patient must be willing and able to work as a team with his or her therapists after surgery, and most young children are not cognitively able to do so. It is therefore imperative for every surgical candidate to undergo a screening examination and for the procedure to be delayed until the patient is able to derive substantial functional benefits, with less risk of recurrence of the deformity.

Implantation of an intrathecal baclofen pump can allow fine-tuned control of severe spasticity that cannot be achieved with oral medications. Finally, selective dorsal rhizotomy, in a carefully chosen population of patients, can produce excellent results.

EQUIPMENT

The use of assistive devices for communication, weight bearing, positioning, ambulation, and mobility, as well as to facilitate activities of daily living, is an important part of treating children with cerebral palsy. Language and communication skills are often affected by the motor impairments resulting from the original injury. Providing children with the ability to communicate with family, peers, and the outside world is a vital component of their cognitive and psychosocial development. An absolute priority when treating children with significantly delayed language development is to obtain a thorough augmentative communication evaluation by a trained team consisting of an occupational therapist, a speech and language therapist, and, if possible, a rehabilitation engineer, with follow-up at regular intervals. Techniques and devices that can be used range from learning American Sign Language to using computer-assisted technology that allows children with severe motor impairments to clearly communicate their wants and needs.

All children who are chronologically old enough to be standing but are not yet ambulatory for community distances need to be placed in a position of weight bearing for a minimum of 2 hours every 24 hours. This is most easily accomplished with a stander, which can provide a variable amount of trunk support and can be positioned in supine, vertical, or prone, based on the child's trunk and head control. With a passive-style stander, the child must be placed in it. Other standers can be operated independently; these types come both in a manual style and as a feature on a power wheelchair and should be strongly considered for adolescent and adult patients for whom greater independence and control are appropriate. Other devices such as feeder seats, corner chairs, and car seats assist with safety and support and provide alternative seating for positioning.

Assistive devices for mobility include crutches, most commonly Lofstrand forearm crutches; walkers, both reverse and standard; gait trainers; and wheelchairs. The choice of ambulatory aid should be based on the individual's need for balance and support. Individuals with anterior balance issues can do well with crutches, but children with balance disturbances in more than one plane may require walkers. Gait trainers provide more support than walkers and have straps that can be used to help control scissoring and foot placement problems. An intermediate type of walker is a reverse walker with a seat, which is helpful for children with low endurance who choose to ambulate in the community.

Independent mobility is intrinsic to one's exploration of the outside world and is necessary if children are to develop a sense of self and avoid the feeling of helplessness that often affects individuals with disabilities.[37] This factor is often overlooked in children with moderate and severe motor deficits. Too often, children with moderate motor impairments are not given wheeled mobility because they will eventually walk, or because if they have wheelchairs they will not have an incentive to walk. Yet these children have significant motor delays that deprive them of the opportunity to move under their own control. Conversely, children with moderate to severe involvement may be placed in stroller-style devices that cannot be self-propelled, making them entirely dependent on others for mobility. This deprives them of the experience of independently exploring the outside world, creates a sense of frustration, and fosters a dependent self-image. A key factor in this issue is communication. Children who have spastic quadriplegia, dystonia, and athetosis may appear to have cognitive deficits that, in the view of the average practitioner, preclude the use of powered mobility. However, appearances can be deceptive, and some of these children will eventually be found to have normal to only mildly affected cognition, despite significant communication problems. Therefore, until a trial with a powered chair and appropriately modified controls has been completed, no child should be denied the opportunity to be independently mobile. Age is not necessarily a controlling factor either, because children as young as 18 months are capable of operating powered mobility.[37]

Assistive devices for activities of daily living are often overlooked in older children and adolescents with cerebral palsy because of the long-standing nature of their disabilities. The original insult occurred early in life, when children are expected to be dependent on their parents for care. But as these children grow older, they should begin to perform as many self-care tasks as possible. By providing simple tools, greater independence can be facilitated. Items such as button and zipper hooks for dressing, an electric toothbrush, a long-handled brush or a brush with a universal strap for grooming, a rocker knife for cutting food, and a reacher (which can be used with a wrist-hand orthotic) for retrieving items on the floor or otherwise out of reach should be included. Access to equipment that enhances independence in all facets of life should be a priority in the treatment of children with cerebral palsy.

ADJUNCTIVE ACTIVITIES

Traditional therapies are extremely important in the management of the tone, movement, and postural problems associated with cerebral palsy, but a number of recreational activities also have strong therapeutic value. These include resistance strength training with isometric or isokinetic techniques, aquatic therapy or therapeutic swimming, therapeutic horsemanship, and participation in organized sports.

Resistance exercise training has clearly been shown to increase strength, improve muscle balance across joints and biomechanics in gait, reduce contractures, and improve gross motor function.[59, 60] Aquatic therapy has tremendous value in improving aerobic conditioning, strength, and balance and in treating sensory integration problems. Equestrian therapy provides the opportunity for sustained adductor stretch and use of the lower paraspinal, abdominal, hip abductor and extensor, and knee extensor musculature. Horse riding has been shown to increase grip strength and supply proprioceptive stimulation through weight shifting, which not only stimulates the vestibular system but also encourages the appropriate use of equilibrium responses and the development of head and trunk control.[61] Organized sports are a vital component of the therapeutic program for children and young adults with cerebral palsy. This can include participation in such activities as martial arts or self-defense training, basketball, soccer, and even dance and gymnastics. All these activities encourage stretching and help increase aerobic conditioning, strength, balance, and motor coordination.[62, 63] The most critical benefits of such adjunctive therapies are not physical but mental and include increased self-confidence, improved self-esteem, and revision of the dependent self-image. This may make the difference between success and failure in adult life.

SUMMARY

Cerebral palsy is the result of a nonprogressive lesion of the immature brain. The survival rate after the first year of life, even for the most severely affected, is 60%; for those with milder involvement, it is 90%.[64] The transition to adulthood must be considered when planning childhood treatment. Optimizing independence in communication, self-care, and mobility, and thereby reducing dependence on caregivers, is the primary goal of patient management. This requires a multidisciplinary effort with participation from primary care, neurosurgery, pediatric physiatry, neurology, and orthopedic surgery and from a competent and knowledgeable team of therapists. To achieve these goals, it is imperative that the patient be evaluated and treated as a whole person, rather than as a collection of individual impairments. In addition, the family must be empowered with the knowledge that improvement is possible. The medical team has the opportunity to affect outcome by improving family adaptation and compliance, as well as patient self-perception and motivation. Individuals who have family support and have experienced success as youngsters are far more likely to become productive adults. Such individuals can exceed expectations, based on their disabilities, related to independent self-care and employment.[64] In addition, by providing young people affected by cerebral palsy with the knowledge and confidence to be self-advocates, the treatment team can help prevent the adult complications that can result from inadequate intervention and medical care.[2, 16]

REFERENCES

1. Kuban K, Leviton A: Cerebral palsy review article. N Engl J Med 330:188–195, 1994.
2. Murphy K, Molnar G, Lankasky K: Medical and functional status of adults with cerebral palsy. Dev Med Child Neurol 37:1075–1084, 1995.
3. Goodlin R: Do concepts of causes and prevention of cerebral palsy require revision? Am J Obstet Gynecol 172:1830–1836, 1995.
4. Eicher P, Batshaw M: Cerebral palsy, the child with developmental disabilities. Pediatr Clin North Am 40:537–551, 1993.
5. Freeman J, Nelson K: Intrapartum asphyxia and cerebral palsy. Pediatrics 82:240–249, 1988.
6. Catto-Smith A, Yu V, Bajuk B, et al: Effect of neonatal periventricular haemorrhage on neuro-developmental outcome. Arch Dis Child 60:8–11, 1985.
7. Pinto-Martin J, Riolo S, Cnaan A, et al: Cranial ultrasound prediction of disabling and nondisabling cerebral palsy at age two in a low birth weight population. Pediatrics 95:249–254, 1995.
8. Molnar G: Cerebral palsy. In Molnar G (ed): Pediatric Rehabilitation. Baltimore, Williams & Wilkins, 1985, pp 420–467.
9. Khaw C, Tidemann A, Stern L: Study of hemiplegic cerebral palsy with a review of the literature. J Paediatr Child Health 30:224–229, 1994.
10. Foley J: Dyskinetic and dystonic cerebral palsy at birth. Acta Paediatr 81:57–60, 1992.
11. Menkes J, Curran J: Clinical and MR correlates in children with extrapyramidal cerebral palsy. AJNR Am J Neuroradiol 15:451–457, 1994.
12. Capute A: Identifying cerebral palsy in infancy through study of primitive reflex profiles. Pediatr Ann 8:34–42, 1979.
13. Levine M: Cerebral palsy diagnosis in children over age 1 year: Standard criteria. Arch Phys Med Rehabil 61:385–389, 1980.
14. Bohannon R, Smith M: Interrater reliability of a modified Ashworth scale of muscle spasticity. Phys Ther 67:206–207, 1986.
15. Bleck E: Locomotor prognosis in cerebral palsy. Dev Med Child Neurol 17:18–25, 1975.
16. Molnar G, Gordon S: Cerebral palsy: Predictive value of selected clinical signs for early prognostication of motor function. Arch Phys Med Rehabil 57:153–158, 1976.
17. Molnar G: Cerebral palsy: Prognosis and how to judge it. Pediatr Ann 8:43–56, 1979.
18. Kudrjavcev T, Schoenberg B, Kurland L, Groover R: Cerebral palsy: Survival rates, associated handicaps, and distribution by clinical subtype. Neurology 35:900–903, 1985.
19. Stevenson R, Hayes R, Carter L, Blackman J: Clinical correlates of linear growth in children with cerebral palsy. Dev Med Child Neurol 36:135–142, 1994.
20. Casas M, Kenny D, McPherson K: Swallowing/ventilation interactions during oral swallow in normal children and children with cerebral palsy. Dysphagia 9:40–46, 1994.
21. Schenk-Rootlieb A, van Nieuwenhuizen O, van der Graaf Y, et al: The prevalence of cerebral visual disturbance in children with cerebral palsy. Dev Med Child Neurol 34:473–480, 1992.
22. Cunningham C, Holt K: Problems in the diagnosis and management of children with cerebral palsy and deafness. Dev Med Child Neurol 19:479, 1997.
23. Reid C, Borzyskowski M: Lower urinary tract dysfunction in cerebral palsy. Arch Dis Child 68:739–742, 1993.
24. McKenzie M, Taylor L, Cummings G, Andrew P: Prevalence of muscle trigger points in children with cerebral palsy. Phys Occup Ther Pediatr 17:47–59, 1997.
25. Travell J, Simons D, Simons L: Travell and Simons' Myofascial Pain and Dysfunction: The Trigger Point Manual. Baltimore, Williams & Wilkins, 1998.
26. Dahlin L, Komoto-Tufvesson Y, Salgeback S: Surgery of the spastic hand in cerebral palsy: Improvement in stereognosis and hand function after surgery. J Hand Surg [Br] 23:334–339, 1998.
27. Wolf T, Clinkscales C, Hamlin C: Flexor carpi ulnaris tendon transfers in cerebral palsy. J Hand Surg [Br] 23:340–343, 1998.
28. Harilaos T, Kirvin F: Management of the unbalanced wrist in cerebral palsy by tendon transfer. Ann Plast Surg 35:90–94, 1995.
29. Root L, LaPlaza F, Brourman S, Angel D: The severely unstable hip in cerebral palsy. J Bone Joint Surg Am 77:703–712, 1995.
30. Bragg M, Farlier J, Miller F: Long term follow-up of hip subluxation in cerebral palsy patients. J Pediatr Orthop 13:32–36, 1993.
31. Allen B, Ferguson R: L-rod instrumentation for scoliosis in cerebral palsy. J Pediatr Orthop 2:87–96, 1982.
32. Cassidy C, Clifford C, Perry A, et al: A reassessment of spinal stabilization in severe cerebral palsy. J Pediatr Orthop 14:731–739, 1994.
33. Gage J: Gait analysis in cerebral palsy. Clin Dev Med 121:37–131, 1991.
34. Whittle M: Gait Analysis: An Introduction. Oxford, Reed Educational and Professional Publishing, 1996, pp 53–154.
35. Stempien L, Gaehler-Spira D: Rehabilitation of children and adults with cerebral palsy. In Braddom R (ed): Physical Medicine and Rehabilitation. Philadelphia, WB Saunders, 1996, pp 1113–1128.
36. Hoffinger S: Gait analysis in pediatric rehabilitation. Clin Phys Med Rehabil 2:817–845, 1991.
37. Butler C: Effects of powered mobility on self-initiated behaviors of very young children with locomotor disability. Dev Med Child Neurol 28:325–332, 1986.
38. White R: Sensory integrative therapy for the cerebral-palsied child. In Scrutton D (ed): Management of the Motor Disorders of Children with Cerebral Palsy. Oxford, Blackwell Scientific, 1984, pp 86–95.
39. Graves P: Therapy methods for cerebral palsy. J Paediatr Child Health 31:24–28, 1995.
40. Bobath B: Motor development, its effect on general development, and application to the treatment of cerebral palsy. Physiotherapy 57:526–532, 1971.
41. Bobath K, Bobath B: The neuro-developmental treatment. In Scrutton D (ed): Management of the Motor Disorders of Children with Cerebral Palsy. Oxford, Blackwell Scientific, 1984, pp 6–18.
42. Rood M: Neurophysiological mechanisms utilized in the treatment of neuromuscular dysfunction. Am J Occup Ther 10:220–224, 1956.
43. Hazelwood M, Brown J, Rowe P, Salter P: The use of therapeutic electrical stimulation in the treatment of hemiplegic cerebral palsy. Dev Med Child Neurol 36:661–673, 1994.
44. Gowland C, Boyce W, Wright V, et al: Reliability of the gross motor performance measure. Phys Ther 75:597–613, 1995.
45. Mayo N: The effect of physical therapy for children with motor delay and cerebral palsy. Am J Phys Med Rehabil 70:258–267, 1991.
46. Bower E, McLellan D: Effect of increased exposure to physiotherapy on skill acquisition of children with cerebral palsy. Dev Med Child Neurol 34:25–39, 1992.
47. Massagli T: Spasticity and its management in children. Clin Phys Med Rehabil 2:867–884, 1991.
48. Graziani V: Spasticity management: Oral antispasticity drugs. In Managing Severe Spasticity: A Multidisciplinary Approach. Minneapolis, Minn, Medtronic, 1998.
49. Joynt R, Leonard J: Dantrolene sodium suspension in treatment of spastic cerebral palsy. Dev Med Child Neurol 22:755–767, 1980.

50. Gruenthal M, Mueller M, Olson W, et al: Gabapentin for the treatment of spasticity in patients with spinal cord injury. Spinal Cord 35:686–689, 1997.

51. Carpenter E, Seitz D: Intramuscular alcohol as an aid in management of spastic cerebral palsy. Dev Med Child Neurol 122:497–501, 1980.

52. Francisco G: Spasticity management: Injection therapy, nerve blocks, Botox. In Managing Severe Spasticity: A Multidisciplinary Approach. Minneapolis, Minn, Medtronic, 1998.

53. Cosgrove A, Corry I, Graham H: Botulinum toxin in the management of the lower limb in cerebral palsy. Dev Med Child Neurol 39:635–640, 1997.

54. Forssberg H, Tedroff K: Botulinum toxin treatment in cerebral palsy: Intervention with poor evaluation? Dev Med Child Neurol 39:635–640, 1997.

55. Gracies J, Elovic E, McGuire J, et al: Traditional pharmacologic treatments for spasticity. Part I. Local treatments. Muscle Nerve 20(Suppl 6):S61–S91, 1997.

56. Koheil R, Sochaniwskyj A, Bablich K, et al: Biofeedback techniques and behavior modification in the conservative remediation of drooling by children with cerebral palsy. Dev Med Child Neurol 29:19–26, 1987.

57. Reddihough D, Johnson H, Staples M, et al: Use of benzhexol hydrochloride to control drooling of children with cerebral palsy. Dev Med Child Neurol 32:985–989, 1990.

58. Siegel L, Klingbeil M: Control of drooling with transdermal scopolamine in a child with cerebral palsy. Dev Med Child Neurol 33:1010–1014, 1991.

59. Diamo D, Vaughn C, Abel M: Muscle response to heavy resistance exercise in children with spastic cerebral palsy. Dev Med Child Neurol 37:731–739, 1995.

60. McPhail H, Kramer J: Effect of isokinetic strength-training on functional ability and walking efficiency in adolescents with cerebral palsy. Dev Med Child Neurol 37:736–775, 1995.

61. MacKinnon J, Noh S, Lariviere J, et al: A study of therapeutic effects of horseback riding for children with cerebral palsy. Dev Med Child Neurol 37:731–739, 1995.

62. Rowland R, Boyajian A: Aerobic response to endurance exercise training in children. Pediatrics 96:654–658, 1995.

63. van der Berg-Emons H, Saris W, Barbanson D: Daily physical activity of school children with spastic diplegia and of healthy control subjects. J Pediatr 127:578–584, 1995.

64. O'Grady R, Crain L, Kohn J: The prediction of long-term functional outcomes of children with cerebral palsy. Dev Med Child Neurol 37:997–1005, 1995.

Selective Dorsal Rhizotomy for Spastic Cerebral Palsy

T. S. PARK

Cerebral palsy (CP) is an important neurological problem, inflicting lifelong disabilities on more than 500,000 children and adults in the United States alone.[1–3] The prevalence of CP has not declined in recent years, despite remarkable advances in neonatal care.[4] In the United States, approximately 8600 new patients are diagnosed each year with the disorder.[5] The past decade has seen a remarkable increase in the role of neurosurgeons in caring for patients with CP, largely due to the reintroduction of dorsal rhizotomy. A large volume of information is available on selective dorsal rhizotomy (SDR) as a therapeutic modality for CP. This chapter synthesizes that information, as well as the author's own experience with the procedure.

PATHOGENESIS OF SPASTIC CEREBRAL PALSY

Spastic CP is the most common subtype of CP. Spastic diplegia and spastic quadriplegia affect approximately 60% of patients. Additionally, spasticity coexists with dyskinesia and ataxia in mixed subtypes of CP. Thus, as a whole, spasticity afflicts 80% to 90% of all patients with CP.[5, 6] A distinct epidemiologic feature of CP is the close association between spastic CP and premature birth and low birth weight.[7] In particular, the prevalence of spastic diplegia increases sharply with decreasing gestational age and birth weight.[8, 9] This relationship does not exist in other subtypes of the disease, such as athetoid and dyskinetic CP.

A neuropathologic substrate for the high prevalence of spastic CP among prematurely born children is periventricular leukomalacia[10] (Fig. 243–1). In fact, periventricular leukomalacia is the most common magnetic resonance imaging finding among children who develop spastic CP—particularly spastic diplegia—following premature birth.[11, 12] The periventricular leukomalacia is a result of ischemic necrosis, and the white matter injury is related to the fact that in the immature brain, the periventricular and subcortical white matter is more predisposed to selective depriva-

tion of adequate blood flow than is the cerebral cortex during hypotension.[13]

The high incidence of spastic diplegia in infants with periventricular leukomalacia is explained in part by topographic arrangements in the white matter of projection fibers descending from the motor homunculus. As seen in Figure 243–2, the leg fibers traverse the white matter closer to the ventricle than do the arm fibers. Thus, periventricular leukomalacia is more likely to injure the leg fibers while sparing the arm fibers. Extensive leukomalacia injures other projection fibers as well, resulting in spastic quadriplegic CP.

The cellular mechanisms by which injury of the immature brain causes CP spasticity are not known, and direct experimental evidence is lacking. One can only infer from previous experimental studies of spinal cord spasticity that CP spasticity may result from hyperactive alpha motor neurons in the spinal cord and consequent stretch reflex activities.[14] There is evidence, however, that the nature of CP spasticity may be substantially different from that of adult-onset spasticity. It has been shown that patients with CP spasticity are incapable of normal reciprocal relaxation of the

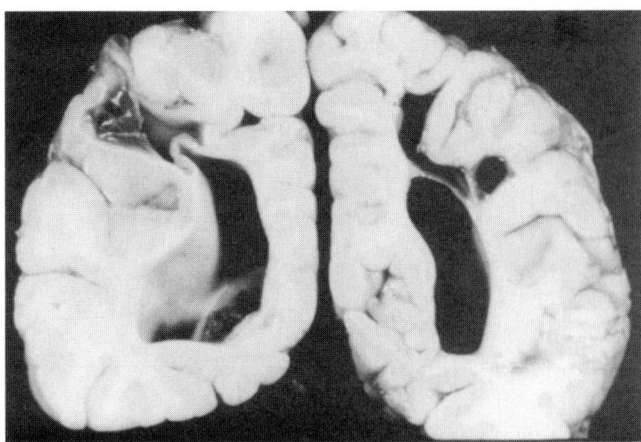

FIGURE 243–1. Coronal section of the brain showing periventricular leukomalacia with markedly reduced white matter adjacent to the posterior lateral ventricle and subcortical infarct.

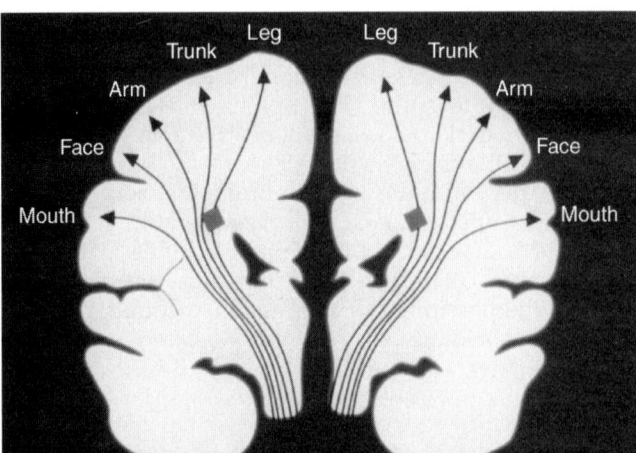

FIGURE 243–2. Schematic drawing of projection fibers from the motor cortex in relation to the lateral ventricle.

antagonist muscle during voluntary leg movements and thus exhibit cocontraction of agonist and antagonist muscles. Such abnormal cocontraction of muscles is not seen in patients with spasticity due to stroke in adulthood.[15]

DELETERIOUS EFFECTS OF CEREBRAL PALSY SPASTICITY

CP spasticity is particularly harmful to growing children (Table 243–1) ; thus, it requires optimal treatment at an early age. The most significant deleterious effect of CP spasticity is that it inhibits motor activities, as attested to by the improvement in motor function as spasticity is reduced in patients who undergo SDR.[16] Spasticity-induced inhibition of motor activities does not abate if spasticity is left untreated.

Another important deleterious effect of CP spasticity is that it decreases muscle and bone development and causes deformities of the affected extremities. Normally, longitudinal muscle growth proceeds as new myofilaments and sarcomeres are added to the ends of the muscle fibers.[17] The greatest increase in sarcomere numbers takes place at an early age, occurring much more actively during development than after maturation. In parallel with the addition of sarcomeres, longitudinal muscle growth occurs rapidly during develop-

ment.[17] The increase in sarcomere number is not under neural control but is induced mainly by the amount of tension the muscle is subjected to (i.e., repeated muscle stretch).[18, 19] Thus, when muscles are immobilized, there is a rapid decrease in the number of already existing sarcomeres, as well as in the number of new sarcomeres that should form with normal development.[18, 20] Because CP spasticity in developing children limits muscle stretch in daily activities, it causes a loss of sarcomeres and inhibition of longitudinal muscle growth.[18, 20] The effect of spasticity on muscle growth was clearly shown in a study in which longitudinal muscle growth was reduced by 45% in spastic mice as compared with control animals.[21] The loss of sarcomeres accompanies a significant decrease in muscle elasticity[22] and makes muscles resistant to passive stretch.[23] Additionally, muscles of children with spastic CP undergo atrophy of type I and II muscle fibers, concurrent with type II hypertrophy in some cases.[24] The pathologic events in the muscle cells cause abnormally shortened muscles, long tendons,[23] and "muscle contracture" (i.e., increased resistance of the muscle to passive stretch in the absence of muscle contraction). The muscle contractures typically worsen as a child grows,[25] producing various bone and joint deformities in the extremities.[26]

INDICATIONS FOR SELECTIVE DORSAL RHIZOTOMY

Indications for SDR vary among medical centers; current indications used in the author's practice are given in Table 243–2. Primary beneficiaries of SDR are children with spastic diplegia secondary to premature birth. Children with spastic quadriplegic CP can also benefit from SDR (Table 243–3). In spastic hemiplegic CP, spasticity is not a predominant cause of motor impairment, and reduction of spasticity does not greatly improve motor function. The optimal age for SDR is 2 to 6 years. Because of the significant deleterious effects of spasticity, early treatment is recommended to reduce the chance of severe orthopedic deformities of the lower extremities. SDR is not considered for children younger than 2 years, because 30% of children who are diagnosed with CP at 1 year old subsequently become symptom free.[6] Adolescents and adults younger than 40 years can also make good functional gains after SDR.[27] The risk of dorsal rhizotomy in adolescents and adults is no greater than that in

TABLE 243–1 ■ Harmful Effects of Spasticity in Children with Spastic Cerebral Palsy

Reduction of protein synthesis in myocytes
Loss of sarcomeres
Reduction of muscle extensibility
Inhibition of longitudinal muscle growth
Shortening of muscles
Inhibition of voluntary movements
Development of muscle contractures
Development of bone and joint deformities

TABLE 243–2 ■ Indications for Selective Dorsal Rhizotomy in Spastic Cerebral Palsy

Diagnosis—spastic diplegia or quadriplegia
Age—2 to 40 yr
History of premature birth or neonatal asphyxia
Bilateral schizencephaly underlying spastic diplegia
Emerging locomotive functions
Potential for significant postoperative functional gains

TABLE 243-3 ■ **Subtypes of Spastic Cerebral Palsy Treated with Selective Dorsal Rhizotomy (St. Louis Children's Hospital, 1987–2000)**

SUBTYPES	NO. OF PATIENTS	PERCENTAGE
Diplegia	584	77
Quadriplegia	166	22
Triplegia	9	1
Hemiplegia	2	<1
Total	761	100

young children, when it is performed through a single-level laminectomy. It is possible that reduction of spasticity lessens the impact of aging on the physical stresses caused by CP (e.g., abnormal stress on bones and muscles, wear and tear on joints, increasing joint and muscle pain).

Patients should have sufficient motor function underlying the spasticity to potentially become ambulators, either assisted or independent (Table 243–4). In some patients with spastic quadriplegia, SDR is recommended to improve sitting posture and upper extremity movement. Patients are not candidates when their motor impairment is so severe that support is required even for sitting. In such patients, SDR often fails to reduce muscle tone owing to coexistent rigidity and dystonia, and long-term benefits are generally negligible.

When selecting patients older than 18 years for SDR, additional factors should be taken into consideration: (1) independent ambulation, (2) fixed orthopedic deformities, (3) back pain, (4) level of motivation, and (5) other medical problems. Because the main goal of SDR is to improve function and quality of life, the author limits SDR to those who can walk alone or with a cane. At this time, it is unclear whether SDR benefits adults who walk with walkers or who cannot walk at all. Severe orthopedic deformities render improvement or functional gains unlikely, making such patients unsuitable for SDR. Spinal deformities in independently walking adults with CP include lumbar hyperlordosis, spondylolysis, spondylolisthesis, and scoliosis. These

TABLE 243-4 ■ **Preoperative Ambulatory Function in Patients Undergoing Selective Dorsal Rhizotomy for Spastic Cerebral Palsy (St. Louis Children's Hospital, 1987–2000)**

WALKING ABILITY	NO. OF PATIENTS	PERCENTAGE
Walking with walker	283	37
Walking with crutches or cane	40	5
Independent walking	224	29
Some locomotion	111	15
Crawling	84	11
No independent mobility	19	3
Total	761	100

deformities do not preclude the performance of SDR through a single-level lumbar laminectomy. Back pain in older adult patients may be due to degenerative diseases of the spine. The spinal abnormalities and severity of back pain should be taken into consideration. In patients older than 10 years, the patient's level of motivation and desire to improve his or her quality of life are important factors in postoperative rehabilitation and achievement of maximal benefits from SDR. With regard to other medical problems, one should be alert to the possibility of depression, a common condition in disabled adults.

CONTRAINDICATIONS FOR SELECTIVE DORSAL RHIZOTOMY

Table 243–5 lists contraindications for SDR. Patients who are not candidates for SDR are those with severe congenital hydrocephalus, severe neonatal bacterial meningits, intrauterine encephalitis such as toxoplasmosis and cytomegalovirus infection, severe head trauma, or brain injury following drowning. The presence of extensive neuronal migration disorders is another contraindication. However, schizencephaly involving the sensory motor area is a rare cause of spastic diplegia, and these patients can show reduced spasticity and functional improvements after SDR. The main reason for precluding SDR in all patients is basal ganglia damage and associated rigidity and dystonia, which can coexist with spasticity. Likewise, severe basal ganglia damage following perinatal difficulties is a contraindication in children younger than 5 years, because dystonia generally manifests during the first 5 years of life.[28] After the age of 5 years, however, SDR can be considered even in the presence of demonstrable basal ganglia damage if spasticity is an overwhelming problem.

Predominant athetosis, ataxia, and dystonia are also contraindications. However, if spasticity is predominant in patients with concomitant athetosis and dystonia, SDR can be helpful. In such patients, SDR can

TABLE 243-5 ■ **Contraindications for Selective Dorsal Rhizotomy for Spastic Cerebral Palsy (CP)**

CP associated with intrauterine encephalitis
Mixed CP with predominant dystonia, rigidity, athetosis, or ataxia
Spastic hemiplegia
CP due to widespread neuronal migration disorder
Severe head injury and hypoxic encephalopathy (e.g., after drowning) as a cause of CP
Familial spastic paraplegia and other progressive neurological disorders
Severe basal ganglia damage in children younger than 5 yr
Severe thoracolumbar scoliosis
Severe lumbar lordosis
Multiple prior muscle and tendon releases
Profound motor impairment with no head control
Psychiatric disorder in adults
Lack of commitment to carry out postoperative therapy

reduce spasticity, but the athetosis and dystonia remain unchanged postoperatively.

Severe scoliosis precludes a rhizotomy, necessitating a multilevel lumbosacral laminectomy. However, patients with an early stage of scoliosis can undergo SDR if it is performed via a single-level laminectomy. When no functional gain is anticipated in a child, parents should be dissuaded from SDR. In adults, the presence of severe depression or other psychiatric disorders is considered a contraindication.

PREOPERATIVE EVALUATION

Patient evaluation starts with a careful review of the perinatal history, including hypoxic-ischemic events, gestational age, birth weight, twin birth, intraventricular hemorrhage, neonatal infection, and seizures. A history of premature birth is among the most important factors in evaluating patients for SDR. Next, one should ascertain that the patient's motor impairment dates back to infancy and has steadily improved rather than progressively deteriorated during the preschool years. If a child had a period of normal motor development and subsequently showed signs of motor impairment, one should consider a neurological disorder rather than CP. The author has seen children who were erroneously diagnosed with CP and later found to have spinal cord tumors or craniovertebral junction anomalies.

Prior treatments for spasticity and orthopedic surgeries should also be reviewed. If a child received intramuscular injection of botulinum toxin type A (Botox) and intrathecal baclofen infusion, the extent of improvement following these treatments can help assess the effect of spasticity on the child's motor function. A history of orthopedic surgery should be reviewed in detail and taken into account during the physical examination.

A neurological examination determines signs of spasticity, including increased muscle tone, hyperactive deep tendon reflexes, and ankle clonus. Ankle clonus is an unequivocal sign of spasticity. Spasticity increases as the child repeats movements rapidly. Thus, an easy way to elicit spasticity in a young child is to instruct the child to walk, stand, crawl, and sit. The attempted movements increase not only muscle tone but also abnormal postures. For example, equinus postures of the ankles, tiptoe walking, and scissoring of the lower extremities become prominent during the attempted movements. This also helps determine whether spasticity significantly inhibits motor activities. The presence of concomitant ataxia, athetosis, and dystonia is also ascertained. It is, however, nearly impossible to detect ataxia in a child with CP spasticity, unlike athetosis and dystonia.

Motor strength can be determined by testing individual muscles. In young children, past motor milestones, speed of movement, and ability to isolate joint movements are reliable indices of motor strength. If the motor milestone is close to normal and, for instance, the child can sit alone by the age of 2 years, he or she most likely has adequate motor strength and will walk in the future. Crawling or walking in a walker and making rapid transitions between positions are also signs of relatively good motor function. As a rule, the greater the motor impairment, the slower the movement. One neurological sign that can be an excellent predictor of gait outcome in children younger than 3 to 4 years is isolated joint movements in the lower extremities[29] (see the discussion of gait under "Outcome").

In addition, the severity of orthopedic deformities and their effect on a patient's motor performance are assessed in detail. Neurosurgeons performing SDR should be knowledgeable about the ramifications of orthopedic deformities and the standard orthopedic management for those deformities. Also, it is particularly important to determine muscle weakness caused by prior muscle releases and the effects on walking and posture. Common problems include excessive foot dorsiflexion and consequent crouch gait following heel cord release, genu recurvatum following hamstring release, and excessive hip abduction and valgus deformities of the foot following adductor release. These problems are generally refractory to treatment.

Physical therapy evaluation is essential and includes a review of previous physical therapy provided to the child, gross motor function measurements, determination of orthopedic deformities, assessment of braces, and videotaping of patients. Videotaping is useful not only for gross motor function measurements but also to record changes in the child's condition over time.

Radiologic studies include magnetic resonance imaging scans of the head and radiographs of the lumbosacral spine and hip. Magnetic resonance imaging detects disorders that make SDR inappropriate and helps predict the long-term outcome of SDR, but routine head or spine magnetic resonance imaging scans are unnecessary. Spine radiographs demonstrate the presence of lumbar hyperlordosis, scoliosis, spondylolysis, spondylolisthesis, and congenital anomalies. Hip radiographs reveal hip subluxation and dislocation—deformities that influence the timing of surgical interventions. Gait analysis with a dynamic electromyogram (EMG) helps confirm the presence of spasticity before SDR and assess postoperative changes in motor performance.

SURGICAL TREATMENT

Between 1987 and 1991, the author performed dorsal rhizotomies on 173 patients through a laminectomy at the L2-S2 levels, as described by Peacock and coworkers.[30] In 1991, however, the potential risk of late spinal deformities following the procedure led to the development of a dorsal rhizotomy procedure through an L1-2 or L1 laminectomy.[31] This surgical technique, described here, was performed on 588 children and adults between 1991 and 2000, with no postoperative complications.

Anesthesia and Preparation. The patient is premedicated with oral midazolam, if necessary, then intubated under deep halothane anesthesia; intubation may be facilitated by short-lasting muscle relaxants (e.g., atracurium, vecuronium). Anesthesia is induced with thiopental, halothane, and nitrous oxide and is maintained by fentanyl (2 μg/kg/hr), 1% halothane, and 70% nitrous oxide. Propofol is avoided because it greatly alters EMG activity. The patient receives a dose of antibiotic before the skin incision is made. A bladder catheter is placed.

The patient is placed prone in a Trendelenburg position on the operating table to minimize cerebrospinal fluid loss from the intracranial compartment. Needle electrodes are placed bilaterally in the adductor longus, vastus lateralis, anterior tibialis, peroneus, medial hamstring, and medial gastrocnemius muscles in preparation for intraoperative EMG examinations.

Laminectomy. In children, the spinous process of the L1 vertebra is estimated by counting the lumbar spinous processes. In adolescents and adults, the L1 is precisely localized by lateral lumbosacral radiography. The lower thoracic and entire lumbar regions of the back are exposed in the operating field. The paraspinal muscles at the presumed L1-2 segments are injected bilaterally with saline solution containing 1:400,000 epinephrine.

Normally, the conus medullaris terminates between the T12 and L3 spinal levels.[32] It is thus necessary to use intraoperative ultrasonography to localize the conus in a laminectomy. The L1-2 interlaminar space is exposed, or, in adults, a keyhole laminotomy is done on the lower margin of the L1 lamina. Through the interlaminar space, intradural structures are examined by ultrasonography. On the ultrasound examinations, the conus is easily distinguished from the cauda equina. A sagittal examination reveals the conus as a hypodense triangle tapering caudally, whereas the cauda equina appears hyperdense. Axial views localize the conus more reliably than do sagittal views. On axial views, the conus is typically a hypodense circular structure centered in the dural sac; also, one can notice a narrow gap between the dorsal and ventral spinal roots, lateral to the conus. If the caudal end of the conus is visualized, the lamina overlying the conus is removed. After the single-level laminectomy is completed, location of the conus is confirmed again by ultrasonography.

The laminectomy should cover 5 to 10 mm of the caudal conus so that the dorsal roots are safely separated from the ventral roots at a later stage of the operation. In children 2 years of age, it is necessary to extend the laminectomy to a part of the lamina above or below the total laminectomy. In older children, a single-level laminectomy is performed. The laminectomy is extended to the medial margin of the facet using a Midas Rex craniotome with a B5 attachment (Midas Rex Pneumatic Tools, Inc., Fort Worth, Tex).

Separation of Dorsal Roots. Saline irrigation is not used after the dura is opened because it alters EMG responses. An operating microscope is brought into the field and used during EMG testing and sectioning of

dorsal root fascicles. The operating table is rotated slightly away from the surgeon as the contralateral spinal roots are dissected. The arachnoid is removed, and the filum terminale is identified. Next, the L1-2 spinal roots are identified at the neural foramen, and the dorsal root is separated from the ventral root (Fig. 243–3). The L2 ventral and dorsal roots are traced back to the conus until the cleft between the ventral and dorsal roots is identified. Then the L2 and adjacent dorsal roots are gently retracted medially, and a cotton patty is placed over the ventral roots. The L1 root is left untouched at this point. Next, the conus and the filum terminale are examined, and the S2-5 sacral roots exiting the conus are identified. The S2 dorsal root can be bulky, especially in patients with postfixed lumbosacral plexus, but there is always an abrupt and marked decrease in its size. The individual S3-5 spinal roots appear as thin threads. The dorsal and ventral roots at this level are close together without intervening space, so all the S3-5 spinal roots are left intact. The lower sacral roots can best be identified by gently lifting the dorsal roots from the entry zone on the dorsal aspect of the conus. Whenever the surgeon is unsure of the exact identification of S3-5, it is prudent to spare the S2 dorsal root. It should be emphasized that direct electrical stimulation of the dorsal roots does not help identify the sacral nerve roots.[33]

Once the L2-S2 dorsal roots are identified, a 5-mm-wide blue Silastic sheet is placed around all the dorsal roots and distant from the conus (see Fig. 243–3); the Silastic keeps the L2-S2 dorsal roots safely separate from the ventral and lower sacral roots during the rest of operation. Before starting EMG testing, to ensure that no ventral root or lower sacral root is over the Silastic material, the surgeon again examines three structures: the L2 foraminal exit, the cleft lateral to the conus between the ventral and dorsal roots, and the S3-5 roots.

Identification of Individual Dorsal Roots. A shortcoming of this particular dorsal rhizotomy procedure is the difficulty in identifying individual dorsal roots with certainty. However, precise identification of the dorsal roots is not critical for SDR for the following reasons: (1) the dorsal roots project to multiple segments in the spinal cord[34]; (2) all major muscles of the lower extremity in children with spastic CP receive motor innervation from several segments[35]; and (3) somatotopic reorganization occurs in the spinal cord and brain following deafferentation.[36]

The L2 dorsal root is readily identified at the neural foramen. The L3-S2 dorsal roots below the conus are close together without a natural demarcation, so unequivocal identification of the individual dorsal root is difficult. Nevertheless, dorsal root fibers of individual segments are roughly identified as follows. First, the dorsal roots are spread on top of the Silastic sheet. The L3 and L4 dorsal roots, which are located medial to the L2 root, are identified; each of the roots consists of two to three naturally separated rootlets. The L5 and S1 roots are medial to the L4 root and are the largest of the lumbosacral roots. The L5 and S1 dorsal roots

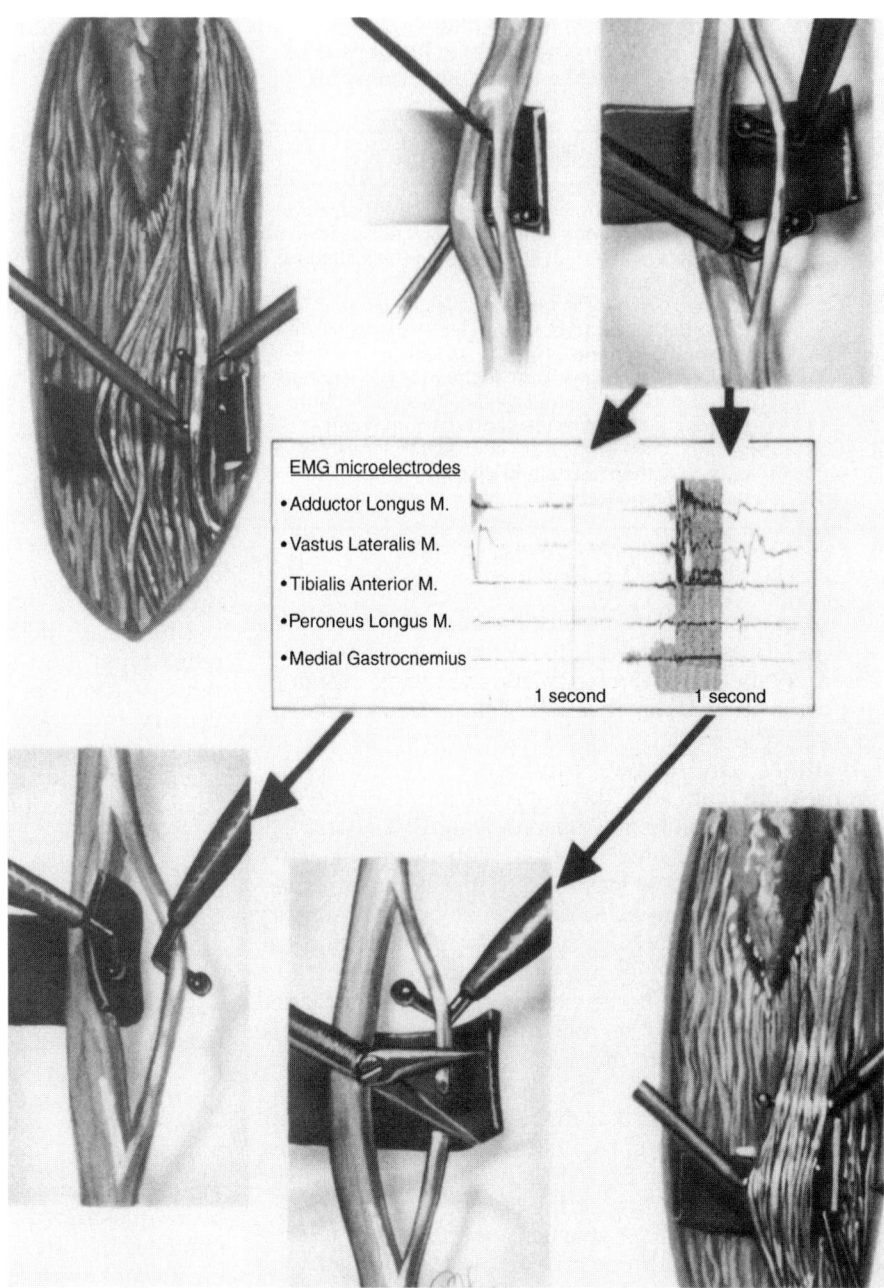

FIGURE 243–3. Schematic drawing showing the steps of selective dorsal rhizotomy: identification and separation of the L1-S2 dorsal spinal roots from the ventral spinal roots, division of the spinal root into rootlet fascicles, intraoperative electromyographic testing, and sectioning of dorsal rootlets.

consist of three or four rootlets with natural demarcation. The S2 root has a single fascicle. Second, the innervation pattern of each root is examined by EMG testing. An individual dorsal root is placed over two hooks of the rhizotomy probes (Aesculap Instrument Co., Burlingame, Calif), and responses to electrical stimulation with a threshold voltage are recorded from the lower extremity muscles. The entire dorsal root is tested at each level immediately before subdividing the dorsal root into rootlets.

Electromyogram Examination and Sectioning of Dorsal Roots. Whether intraoperative EMG tests help determine the dorsal root fibers to be cut is a topic of controversy. The author continues to use intraoperative EMG testing, because there is no conclusive evidence

invalidating it, and the test helps identify spinal root levels during the operation. After the innervation of a dorsal root is determined by EMG responses to electrical stimulation of the whole spinal root, the root is sharply subdivided with a Scheer needle (Storz, St. Louis, Mo) into four to seven smaller rootlet fascicles of equal size (see Fig. 243–3). The rootlet fascicles are suspended over two hooks of the rhizotomy probes. Single, constant, square wave pulses of 0.1-msec duration are applied to the rootlet at a rate of 0.5 Hz. The stimulus intensity is increased stepwise until a reflex response appears from the ipsilateral muscles. After the reflex threshold is determined, a 50-Hz train of tetanic stimulation is applied to the rootlet for 1 second. The reflex response is then graded according to the criteria in Table 243–6. In the author's experience,

TABLE 243–6 ■ **Criteria for Grading Electromyographic Responses to Selective Dorsal Rhizotomy for Spastic Cerebral Palsy**

GRADE	ELECTROMYOGRAPHIC RESPONSE
0	Unsustained or single discharge to a train of stimuli
1+	Sustained discharges from muscles innervated through the segment stimulated in the ipsilateral lower extremity
2+	Sustained discharges from muscles innervated through the segment stimulated and immediately adjacent segments
3+	Sustained discharges from segmentally innervated muscles as well as muscles innervated through segments distant to the segment stimulated
4+	Sustained discharges from contralateral muscles with or without sustained discharges from the ipsilateral muscles

the great majority of rootlets produce 1+ to 4+ responses. Thus the decision to section a given rootlet is based on the number of rootlets producing sustained responses at that level and the intensity of the responses. The rootlets that produce a response of 0 are left intact. The rootlets producing 3+ and 4+ responses are cut, and those producing 1+ and 2+ responses are sometimes spared. If only 1+ and 2+ responses are detected, rootlets with the most active responses are cut. At least one rootlet is left, irrespective of EMG responses, to avoid postoperative sensory loss. The dorsal rootlets spared from sectioning are placed behind the Silastic sheet and kept separated from rootlets yet to be tested. The procedure is carried out in sequence on the remaining L3-S2 dorsal roots. Using the criteria in Table 243–6, the author sections 50% to 75% of the rootlets examined. Last, the L1 dorsal root is identified at the neural foramen, and half of the dorsal root is cut without EMG testing, because in the author's experience, EMG testing of the L1 root is unreliable. Sectioning of the L1 dorsal root is necessary to further reduce spasticity in hip flexors, especially in patients with a large L1 root associated with prefixed lumbosacral plexus. The rhizotomy is repeated on the contralateral side.

The intradural space is irrigated with saline solution. Bipolar cautery is seldom required to control bleeding from the cut ends of fascicles. The dura is closed in a running fashion with 4–0 monofilament nylon. Fentanyl at a dose of 0.5 μg/kg body weight is injected intradurally, after which the Trendelenburg position is reversed. The wound is closed in layers.

Postoperative Care. Patients stay overnight in the intensive care unit, where they receive fentanyl at a dose of 1 to 3 μg/kg per hour. Benzodiazepam is also administered intravenously to augment pain management. Patients are transferred to the ward the next day, and the fentanyl drip is continued for another 24 hours. On the third postoperative day, patients are allowed to sit, and physical therapy is started. Patients are discharged home on the sixth postoperative day and receive outpatient physical therapy from local therapists. Postoperative inpatient rehabilitation is not recommended.

Postoperative Course and Complications. Reduction of spasticity is apparent immediately after SDR. Patients typically complain of numbness, tingling, and a feeling of heaviness in the lower extremities for 5 to 10 days. Voluntary urination is regained within 72 hours. Most patients who were independent walkers preoperatively walk with assistance by the 5th postoperative day and resume full independent walking by the 14th day. Patients who walked with aids preoperatively have a slower postoperative course; it often takes more than 6 weeks for their motor performance to reach preoperative levels. The recovery of motor performance is faster after this variation of dorsal rhizotomy than after the operation introduced by Peacock. The rapid recovery is attributed to the lack of traction on the ventral spinal roots and to the consequent neurapraxic injury during the latter operation.

Immediate postoperative complications include cerebrospinal fluid leak, meningitis, neurogenic bladder, sensory loss, ileus, bronchospasm, pneumonia,[37] and urinary tract infection. None of the author's patients has developed neurological complications, but a small number developed bronchospasm, pneumonia, or urinary tract infection.

Potential delayed complications include sensory loss, dysesthesia, muscle hypotonia, impotence, and spinal deformities related to extensive laminectomy. Sensory loss of clinical significance did not occur in the author's patients. Some patients reported numbness in a small area of the upper lumbar dermatomes, and hypesthesia could be detected on examination. Dysesthesia following SDR involves hypersensitivity in the foot. It may be severe enough to hinder walking for the first few months but improves or resolves in several months. There is no report of the occurrence of sexual dysfunction in the absence of neurogenic bladder following the rhizotomy. The author's male patients have been questioned about penile function at follow-up clinic visits, and none has reported impairments of erection or ejaculation.

Spinal deformities such as spondylosis, spondylolisthesis,[38] lumbar spinal stenosis,[39] and lumbar hyperlordosis[40] have been reported in patients who underwent SDR through a multilevel lumbosacral laminectomy or laminotomy. Peter and colleagues found that 20% of 99 patients developed isthmic spondylolysis or grade I spondylolisthesis following five-level lumbosacral laminectomies for SDR.[38] In 19 of their patients, the isthmic defects involved L3-4, L4-5, or L5-S1 levels, and six patients had spondylolisthesis. The majority of patients were ambulatory and active.

Spinal stenosis occurred in 2 of 130 patients who underwent SDR for spastic diplegia 4 years after L1-S2 laminectomy and 2 years after L2-S2 laminotomy.[39] Both children required decompressive procedures to relieve the symptoms. Lumbar hyperlordosis occurred in two nonambulatory children with spastic quadriplegia who had significant trunk weakness.[40] The reported spinal deformities following SDR through an extensive laminectomy highlights the importance of limited laminectomy. Although some claim that osteoplastic laminotomy may reduce the risk of spinal deformities, convincing evidence remains to be demonstrated.

OUTCOME

Of all the neurosurgical and orthopedic procedures currently used in the management of CP, SDR has undergone the most rigorous scientific scrutiny. Over the past 14 years, neurosurgeons, orthopedic surgeons, pediatricians, therapists, and biomedical engineers have examined the safety and efficacy of the operation. Evidence amassed to date indicates that SDR is an excellent option in the management of spastic CP. Outcome studies of SDR have addressed multiple facets of CP, and extensive information is available concerning the efficacy of the operation.

Spasticity. Reduction of spasticity is a principal goal of SDR. This can be achieved in nearly all patients with spastic diplegia[16, 41–44] and in most patients with spastic quadriplegia. The marked reduction of spasticity is apparent shortly after the operation. Muscle tone may increase later but remains reduced from the preoperative level, and SDR is never followed by total flaccidity of the lower extremities. The reduction of spasticity can be assessed clinically by decreased muscle tone, decreased knee and ankle jerks, and absence of ankle clonus. Additionally, the change in spasticity can be quantified.[43]

An important observation is that spasticity can be reduced permanently in patients with spastic diplegia. In support of this claim, none of the author's patients with spastic diplegia who underwent SDR 5 to 12 years ago has developed recurrent spasticity equal to the preoperative level, and it seems unlikely that these patients will develop recurrent spasticity after so many years of reduced spasticity. Because spasticity in CP adversely affects the muscles and does not undergo spontaneous resolution, benefits from the early reduction of spasticity extend into adult life.

In contrast, in patients with spastic quadriplegia, SDR carries a substantial risk of failure to reduce spasticity. The precise reason for this is unclear, but the severity of the patient's motor impairment is a factor. The highest failure rate is seen among nonambulatory and severely involved quadriplegics in whom SDR is performed to improve hygiene and sitting. In such patients, spasticity increases progressively over 6 weeks, reaching preoperative levels of severity by 2 years after the operation. Quadriplegic patients who can walk with aid are less likely to have persistent spasticity after SDR. In this group, spasticity can recur, but it is usually much less severe than before the operation.

Strength. Motor weakness of varying degrees is invariably present in CP. When spasticity is reduced or eliminated, motor weakness underlying the spasticity surfaces, giving the impression that SDR produces mo-

tor weakness. Although it is true that SDR produces transient motor weakness immediately after the operation, especially when performed through a multilevel laminectomy, it is untrue that SDR produces lasting motor weakness. Based on quantitative strength measurements, strength in CP patients was less than that in able-bodied children, but 6 months after SDR, strength had increased over preoperative levels.[43] An additional observation indicating the lack of persistent motor weakness after SDR is that SDR does not lower the level of walking in ambulatory children.

Motor Function. The effects of SDR on changes in gross motor function have been examined in three controlled studies.[16, 41, 42] All the studies used gross motor function measures to assess changes in motor function. These measures evaluate several gross motor functions: lie/roll, sit, crawl/kneel, stand, walk/run/jump.[45] The three studies included a group receiving physical therapy alone and another group receiving SDR combined with physical therapy. Two studies found the SDR group to have significantly higher gross motor function scores at 9 months and 12 months than the group receiving physical therapy alone.[16, 41] In contrast, one study found no beneficial effect of SDR on gross motor function assessed at 12 and 24 months postoperatively.[42] All three studies were limited in scope because quality of gait and other motor performance, efficiency of gait, quality of life, and deformities of the lower extremities were not examined. Moreover, the followup was too short to determine the long-term effects of reduced spasticity, such as increasing deformities and higher rates of orthopedic surgery in later life.

Gait. Walking is a part of gross motor function, but gait outcome deserves a separate discussion because it is a primary concern to many parents of children with CP. A frequently asked question is, what will a child's level of walking be after SDR? To answer the question, one should take into consideration the diagnosis of CP, the level of motor development, and the ability to dorsiflex the foot. All hemiplegics walk independently, and 87% of diplegics walk with or without assistive devices.[46] No quadriplegics can walk independently; they are either nonambulatory or walk with assistive devices.[47] Regarding motor development for the prediction of gait outcome, the child should sit and stand before taking steps. Thus, children who can sit alone at 2 years of age will most likely walk independently or with aids.[46] Sitting ability is a predictor of independent or assisted walking, but it does not specifically predict independent walking. One can use the child's ability to dorsiflex as a predictor of independent walking after SDR[29]; in the author's experience, virtually all children who can dorsiflex the foot bilaterally without associated simultaneous movements of other joints, either before or after SDR, become independent walkers. If the dorsiflexion is unilateral and without associated movements of other joints, there is a good chance that the child will become an independent walker; the gait, however, will be significantly abnormal because of the more involved extremity. If the dorsiflexion is bilateral but associated with other joint movements, household independent walking can be achieved. If dorsiflexion of the foot is lacking bilaterally, independent walking after SDR is impossible, and a walker or crutches will be needed. The predictive value of foot dorsiflexion stems from the fact that active foot movements are most vulnerable to cerebral lesions[48]; thus, the ability to dorsiflex the foot indicates a relatively mild injury to the motor area.

Several investigators have used computerized gait analysis to assess changes of gait following SDR.[49–52] Gait analysis quantitatively assesses gait parameters in children with CP, including cadence (steps/minute), velocity (meters/second), stride length, pelvic tilt, hip extension and abduction, knee range, and ankle range. Early studies demonstrated significant improvement of many gait parameters, with improvement maintained for as long as 10 years postoperatively.[52]

Orthopedic Surgery. Because spasticity is a cause of muscle contractures and deformities, one can expect a decreased rate of orthopedic surgery after SDR in patients with spastic CP. An earlier study suggests that SDR performed between 2 and 4 years of age reduces the need for orthopedic surgery for heel cord, hamstring, and adductor releases.[53] It is rare to encounter the need for late orthopedic surgery in diplegic children who walk unaided after undergoing SDR at 2 to 4 years old. In contrast, children who walk with assistive devices or cannot walk at all often need orthopedic surgery. The rate of orthopedic surgery is highest among children with more severe involvement. The limited muscle stretching in daily activities produces increasing deformities, even in the absence of spasticity. Delayed SDR in independent ambulators and limited muscle stretching in assisted ambulators or nonambulators could necessitate later orthopedic surgery.[54–56] These assisted or nonambulatory patients in particular should have orthopedic follow-up after SDR.

Hip Deformities. Hip subluxation and dislocation are common problems in children with spastic CP, occurring in 3% to 59% of patients.[57, 58] The cause of hip deformities is multifactorial, but spasticity in the hip adductor and iliopsoas muscles, combined with lack of normal weight bearing, plays an important role in their development. Because it decreases spasticity, SDR might decrease the incidence of hip subluxation in children with CP. The author and colleagues examined changes in lateral hip migration in spastic diplegic and quadriplegic children undergoing SDR. First, 67 diplegics between 2 and 11 years of age at the time of surgery were followed for 6 to 46 months postoperatively. Of all the hips examined radiographically, 75% remained unchanged, 17% improved, and 7% worsened.[59] Next, 45 quadriplegics were examined in a similar manner. In these more involved children, 80% of hips remained unchanged, 9% improved, and 11% worsened.[60] These results contradict a suggestion in a previous report[61] and indicate that SDR prevents progressive hip subluxation in the majority of children with spastic diplegia and quadriplegia who undergo the operation.

Because of the high incidence of hip abnormalities in CP, it is essential to obtain hip radiographs at the initial evaluation. The severity of hip abnormalities influences decisions about the timing and performance of the operation. It is also important to follow up after SDR to avoid delayed orthopedic intervention in the case of progressive hip subluxation due to dysplastic acetabulum. Postrhizotomy follow-up of hips is especially important in children younger than 5 years, whose hips are not completely mature.[62, 63]

Cognitive Performance, Speech, Upper Extremity Movement, and Bladder Function. Some children who appear mentally retarded before SDR show marked improvements in their attention, language, temperament, mood, and interactions with people after SDR. These improvements may result in part from the alleviation of spasticity-associated physical discomfort or from intensified therapy following SDR. Also, the improvements may be related to "suprasegmental effects" of SDR on neural circuits beyond the lumbosacral segments. Although the idea of suprasegmental effects of SDR remains to be substantiated, positive changes in cognitive performance following SDR were shown by a neuropsychological study.[64] Groups of children with spastic diplegia and able-bodied children were tested for visual-attention tasks and Woodcock-Johnson psychoeducational battery measures (vocabulary, spatial relations, quantitative concepts, phonemic blending, memory for sentences, and visual-auditory associated learning). The children with spastic diplegia received either SDR plus therapy or therapy only. In a 6-month interval, those who underwent SDR made more improvements in visual-attention tasks and visual-auditory associated learning than those receiving therapy only. Those cognitive performances are believed to be part of frontal lobe functioning.

Regarding speech improvement, parents frequently report that children speak more clearly and in longer sentences shortly after SDR. The speech improvements often parallel improvements in sitting, pointing to the role of peripheral effects of SDR on speech. Other undefined factors must also underlie speech improvements following SDR.

The positive effects of SDR on upper extremity function have been documented,[65, 66] and, as a rule, these improvements manifest as increased range of motion. Spastic quadriplegic children who have some upper extremity movement are likely to show improvement after SDR. In contrast, children who have either severe spastic quadriplegia with little upper extremity movement or mild spastic quadriplegia with full range of motion do not show upper extremity improvement following SDR. Fine motor skills are generally not affected by SDR.

Bladder dysfunction is not uncommon in CP; more than one third of children with CP show dysfunctional voiding symptoms such as dribbling, stress incontinence, enuresis, urgency, and frequency.[67] The urinary symptoms are caused mainly by upper motor neuron lesions. Thus, urodynamic studies of incontinent children reveal uninhibited contractions of the bladder, detrusor-sphincter dyssynergia, small bladder capacity, or hypertonic bladder.[68] Sweetser and coworkers reported improvements in incontinence and urgency in patients with spastic diplegia following SDR but found no beneficial effects on voiding symptoms in those with spastic quadriplegia.[69] Likewise, the author has seen young children with spastic diplegia who could complete potty training within a few months after SDR.

Long-Term Outcome. The long-term outcome of SDR was studied by a group in Cape Town, South Africa.[52, 56] Fifty-one children with spastic CP were studied 3 to 7 years after undergoing SDR. Ages at the time of surgery ranged from 20 months to 14 years. The group reported that spasticity remained reduced in all patients, motor function continued to improve in 80%, sensory disturbances were insignificant, and 47% required orthopedic surgeries to further improve their functioning.[56] Repeat gait analysis 10 years after SDR in children with spastic diplegia demonstrated sustained improvement in hip and knee ranges of motion, step length, and velocity of gait.[52] Similar long-term outcome studies remain to be reported from centers in the United States.

CONCLUSIONS

SDR is an excellent treatment option for many patients with spastic CP, with reported data on surgical outcome overwhelmingly in favor of SDR. At this time, it is evident that SDR can produce a sustained reduction of spasticity, long-term morbidity of the procedure is minimal, and SDR is the only treatment available that can permanently reduce CP spasticity. Thus, physicians caring for patients with CP must inform them of SDR when discussing treatment options. Neurosurgeons who perform SDR on patients with CP should be knowledgeable about all aspects of CP and should be able to counsel parents regarding orthopedic surgery and various physical therapy regimens. Future efforts should be directed toward refinement of criteria for patient selection for SDR, investigation of long-term benefits of SDR, and studies of SDR in adult patients.

REFERENCES

1. Newacheck PW, Taylor WR: Childhood chronic illness: Prevalence, severity, and impact. Am J Public Health 82:364–371, 1992.
2. Murphy KP, Molnar GE, Lankasky K: Medical and functional status of adults with cerebral palsy. Dev Med Child Neurol 37:1075–1084, 1995.
3. Kuban KC, Leviton A: Cerebral palsy. N Engl J Med 330:188–195, 1994.
4. Rosen MG, Dickinson JC: The incidence of cerebral palsy. Am J Obstet Gynecol 167:417–423, 1992.
5. Grether JK, Cummins SK, Nelson KB: The California Cerebral Palsy Project. Paediatr Perinatal Epidemiol 6:339–351, 1992.
6. Nelson KB, Ellenberg JH: Children who "outgrew" cerebral palsy. Pediatrics 69:529–536, 1982.
7. Ellenberg JH, Nelson KB: Cluster of perinatal events identifying infants at high risk for death and disability. J Pediatr 113:546–552, 1988.
8. Stanley F, Alberman E: Birthweight, gestational age and the cerebral palsies. Clin Dev Med 87:57–68, 1987.
9. Hagberg B, Hagberg G, Olow I, Von Wendt L: The changing panorama of cerebral palsy in Sweden: The birth year period 1979–82. Acta Paediatr Scand 78:283–290, 1989.
10. Banker BQ: The neuropathological effects of anoxia and hypoglycemia in the newborn. Dev Med Child Neurol 9:544–550, 1967.
11. Okumura A, Hayakawa F, Kato T, et al: MRI findings in patients with spastic cerebral palsy. I. Correlation with gestational age at birth. Dev Med Child Neurol 39:363–368, 1997.
12. Park TS, Phillips LH, Torner JC: Magnetic resonance imaging in selective dorsal rhizotomy for spastic cerebral palsy. In Park TS, Phillips LH, Peacock WJ (eds): Neurosurgery: State of the Art Reviews: Management of Spasticity in Cerebral Palsy and Spinal Cord Injury. Philadelphia, Hanley & Belfus, 1989, pp 485–495.
13. Young RSK, Hernandez MJ, Yagel SK: Selective reduction of blood flow to white matter during hypotension in newborn dogs: A possible mechanism of periventricular leukomalacia. Ann Neurol 12:445–448, 1982.
14. Bishop B: Spasticity: Its physiology and management. Phys Ther 57:371–401, 1977.
15. Myklebust BM, Gottlieb GL, Penn RD, Agarwal GC: Reciprocal excitation of antagonistic muscles as a differentiating feature in spasticity. Ann Neurol 12:367–374, 1982.
16. Steinbok P, Reiner AM, Beauchamp R, et al: A randomized clinical trial to compare selective posterior rhizotomy plus physiotherapy with physiotherapy alone in children with spastic diplegic cerebral palsy. Dev Med Child Neurol 39:178–184, 1997.
17. Williams PE, Goldspink G: Longitudinal growth of striated muscle fibres. J Cell Sci 9:751–767, 1971.
18. Goldspink G, Tabary C, Tabary JC, et al: Effect of denervation on the adaptation of sarcomere number and muscle extensibility to the functional length of the muscle. J Physiol 236:733–742, 1974.
19. Huet de la Tour E, Tabary JC, Tabary C, Tardieu C: The respective roles of muscle length and muscle tension in sarcomere number adaptation of guinea-pig soleus muscle. J Physiol 75:589–592, 1979.
20. Hayat A, Tardieu C, Tabary JC, Tabary C: Effects of denervation on the reduction of sarcomere number in cat soleus muscle immobilized in shortened position during seven days. J Physiol 74:563–567, 1978.
21. Ziv I, Blackburn N, Rang M, Koreska J: Muscle growth in normal and spastic mice. Dev Med Child Neurol 26:94–99, 1984.
22. Tabary JC, Tardieu C: Experimental rapid sarcomere loss with concomitant hypoextensibility. Muscle Nerve 4:198–203, 1981.
23. Tardieu C, Huet de la Tour E, Bret MD, Tardieu G: Muscle hypoextensibility in children with cerebral palsy. I. Clinical and experimental observations. Arch Phys Med Rehabil 63:97–102, 1982.
24. Castle ME, Reyman TA, Schneider M: Pathology of spastic muscle in cerebral palsy. Clin Orthop 142:223–233, 1979.
25. Hoffer MM, Knoebel RT, Roberts R: Contractures in cerebral palsy. Clin Orthop 219:70–77, 1987.
26. Bleck EE: Orthopaedic Management in Cerebral Palsy. London, Mac Keith Press, 1987, pp 1–497.
27. Peter JC, Arens LJ: Selective posterior lumbosacral rhizotomy in teenagers and young adults with spastic cerebral palsy. Br J Neurosurg 8:135–139, 1994.
28. Burke RE, Fahn S, Gold AP: Delayed-onset dystonia in patients with "static" encephalopathy. J Neurol Neurosurg Psychiatry 43:789–797, 1980.
29. Chicoine MR, Park TS, Vogler GP, Kaufman BA: Predictors of ability to walk after selective dorsal rhizotomy in children with cerebral palsy. Neurosurgery 38:711–714, 1996.
30. Peacock WJ, Arens LJ, Berman B: Cerebral palsy spasticity: Selective posterior rhizotomy. Pediatr Neurosci 13:61–66, 1987.
31. Park TS: Selective dorsal rhizotomy for the spasticity of cerebral palsy. In Neurosurgical Operative Atlas, vol 4. Rolling Meadows, IL, American Association of Neurological Surgeons Publications Committee, 1995, pp 183–190.
32. Wilson DA, Prince JR: MR imaging determination of the location of the normal conus medullaris throughout childhood. AJNR Am J Neuroradiol 10:258–262, 1989.
33. Ojemann JG, Park TS, Komanetsky R, et al: Lack of specificity in electrophysiological identification of lower sacral roots during selective dorsal rhizotomy. J Neurosurg 86:28–33, 1997.
34. Imai Y, Kusama T: Distribution of the dorsal root fibers in the

cat: An experimental study with the Nauta method. Brain Res 13:338–359, 1969.

35. Phillips LH, Park TS: Electrophysiologic mapping of the segmental anatomy of the muscles of the lower extremity. Muscle Nerve 14:1213–1218, 1991.

36. Basbaum AI, Wall PD: Research reports: Chronic changes in the response of cells in adult cat dorsal horn following partial deafferentation: The appearance of responding cells in a previously non-responsive region. Brain Res 116:181–204, 1976.

37. Abbott R: Complications with selective posterior rhizotomy. Pediatr Neurosurg 18:43–47, 1992.

38. Peter JC, Hoffman EB, Arens LJ: Spondylolysis and spondylolisthesis after five-level lumbosacral laminectomy for selective posterior rhizotomy in cerebral palsy. Childs Nerv Syst 9:285–288, 1993.

39. Gooch JL, Walker ML: Spinal stenosis after total lumbar laminectomy for selective dorsal rhizotomy. Pediatr Neurosurg 25:28–30, 1996.

40. Crawford K, Karol LA, Herring JA: Severe lumbar lordosis after dorsal rhizotomy. J Pediatr Orthop 16:336–339, 1996.

41. Wright FV, Sheil EM, Drake JM, et al: Evaluation of selective dorsal rhizotomy for the reduction of spasticity in cerebral palsy: A randomized controlled trial. Dev Med Child Neurol 40:239–247, 1998; see comments.

42. McLaughlin JF, Bjornson KF, Astley SJ, et al: Selective dorsal rhizotomy: Efficacy and safety in an investigator-masked randomized clinical trial. Dev Med Child Neurol 40:220–232, 1998.

43. Engsberg JR, Olree KS, Ross SA, Park TS: Spasticity and strength changes as a function of selective dorsal rhizotomy. J Neurosurg 88:1020–1026, 1998.

44. Peacock W, Staudt L: Functional outcomes following selective posterior rhizotomy in children with cerebral palsy. J Neurosurg 74:380–385, 1991.

45. Russell DJ, Rosenbaum PL, Cadman DT, et al: The gross motor function measure: A means to evaluate the effects of physical therapy. Dev Med Child Neurol 31:341–352, 1989.

46. Molnar GE, Gordon SU: Cerebral palsy: Predictive value of selected clinical signs for early prognostication of motor function. Arch Phys Med Rehabil 57:153–158, 1976.

47. Watt JM, Robertson CM, Grace MG: Early prognosis for ambulation of neonatal intensive care survivors with cerebral palsy. Dev Med Child Neurol 31:766–773, 1989.

48. Foerster O: The motor cortex in man in the light of Hughlings Jackson's doctrines. Brain 59:135–159, 1936.

49. Boscarino LF, Ounpuu S, Davis RB, et al: Effects of selective dorsal rhizotomy on gait in children with cerebral palsy. J Pediatr Orthop 13:174–179, 1993.

50. Cahan L, Adams J, Perry J, Beeler L: Instrumented gait analysis after selective dorsal rhizotomy. Dev Med Child Neurol 32:1037–1043, 1990.

51. Thomas SS, Aiona MD, Pierce R, Piatt JH: Gait changes in children with spastic diplegia after selective dorsal rhizotomy. J Pediatr Orthop 16:747–752, 1996.

52. Subramanian N, Vaughan CL, Peter JC, Arens LJ: Gait before and 10 years after rhizotomy in children with cerebral palsy spasticity. J Neurosurg 88:1014–1019, 1998.

53. Chicoine MR, Park TS, Kaufman BA: Selective dorsal rhizotomy and rates of orthopedic surgery in children with spastic cerebral palsy. J Neurosurg 86:34–39, 1997.

54. Carroll KL, Moore KR, Stevens PM: Orthopedic procedures after rhizotomy. J Pediatr Orthop 18:69–74, 1998.

55. Marty GR, Dias LS, Gaebler-Spira D: Selective posterior rhizotomy and soft-tissue procedures for the treatment of cerebral diplegia. J Bone Joint Surg 77:713–718, 1995.

56. Arens LJ, Peacock WJ, Peter J: Selective posterior rhizotomy: A long-term follow-up study. Childs Nerv Syst 5:148–152, 1989.

57. Lonstein JE, Beck K: Hip dislocation and subluxation in cerebral palsy. J Pediatr Orthop 6:521–526, 1986.

58. Samilson RL, Tsou P, Aamoth G, Green WM: Dislocation and subluxation of the hip in cerebral palsy. J Bone Joint Surg Am 54:863–873, 1972.

59. Park TS, Vogler GP, Phillips LH II, et al: Effects of selective dorsal rhizotomy for spastic diplegia on hip migration in cerebral palsy. Pediatr Neurosurg 20:43–49, 1994.

60. Heim RC, Park TS, Vogler GP, et al: Changes in hip migration after selective dorsal rhizotomy for spastic quadriplegia in cerebral palsy. J Neurosurg 82:567–571, 1995.

61. Greene WB, Dietz FR, Goldberg MJ, et al: Rapid progression of hip subluxation in cerebral palsy after selective posterior rhizotomy. J Pediatr Orthop 11:494–497, 1991.

62. Vidal J, Deguillaume P, Vidal M: The anatomy of the dysplastic hip in cerebral palsy related to prognosis and treatment. Int Orthop 9:105–110, 1985.

63. Harris NH, Lloyd-Roberts GC, Gallien R: Acetabular development in congenital dislocation of the hip. J Bone Joint Surg Br 57:46–52, 1975.

64. Craft S, Park TS, White DA, et al: Changes in cognitive performance in children with spastic diplegic cerebral palsy following selective dorsal rhizotomy. Pediatr Neurosurg 23:68–74, 1995.

65. Kinghorn J: Upper extremity functional changes following selective posterior rhizotomy in children with cerebral palsy. Am J Occup Ther 46:502–507, 1992.

66. Beck AJ, Gaskill SJ, Marlin AE: Improvement in upper extremity function and trunk control after selective posterior rhizotomy. Am J Occup Ther 47:704–707, 1993.

67. McNeal DM, Hawtrey CE, Wolraich ML, Mapel JR: Symptomatic neurogenic bladder in a cerebral-palsied population. Dev Med Child Neurol 25:612–616, 1983.

68. Decter RM, Bauer SB, Khoshbin S, et al: Urodynamic assessment of children with cerebral palsy. J Urol 138:1110–1112, 1987.

69. Sweetser PM, Badell A, Schneider S, Badlani GH: Effects of sacral dorsal rhizotomy on bladder function in patients with spastic cerebral palsy. Neurourol Urodyn 14:57–64, 1995.

Intrathecal Baclofen Infusion

PAUL STEINBOK ■ MAUREEN O'DONNELL

Intrathecal baclofen, which was first introduced by Penn and Kroin in 1984,[1] is well established as an effective treatment of spasticity of both spinal and cerebral origin. In the adult population, the treatment is used predominantly for spasticity of spinal origin; this aspect is covered in another section of this book. This chapter focuses on the use of intrathecal baclofen for the treatment of spasticity in children. In the pediatric population, spasticity is almost always of cerebral origin and most commonly occurs in the context of cerebral palsy. Spasticity is often associated with other motor disorders such as dystonia, and the use of intrathecal baclofen to treat dystonia is also discussed.

CEREBRAL PALSY

Cerebral palsy refers to a persistent abnormality of control of movement and posture, resulting from non-progressive pathology in the immature brain. The incidence of cerebral palsy ranges from 1.5 to 2.5 per 1000 live births,[2–4] with approximately 90% resulting from insults occurring antenatally, at the time of birth, or in the first postnatal month (congenital cerebral palsy). In up to 16% of children, cerebral palsy is caused by cerebral damage after the first month of life, usually from infection, trauma, or ischemia (acquired cerebral palsy).[5] In order to cause cerebral palsy, the cerebral insult must generally occur before 2 years of age, but some have raised the upper limit to 5 years.[6, 7]

Although the insult to the brain causing spastic cerebral palsy typically occurs before 1 month of age, the presence of a disorder of motor function is rarely recognized before 6 months, reflecting the immaturity of the motor pathways in infants. The synaptic projections from the corticospinal pathways to motor neurons develop in the first postnatal year concurrent with the emergence of independent finger movements, and myelination of the corticospinal pathways is not complete until 2 years of age.[8] The more severe the cerebral palsy, the earlier the problem is apparent, with moderately severe cases diagnosed by 1 year and the mildest cases not diagnosed until close to 2 years. In children with moderate or severe spastic cerebral palsy, the disturbance of motor function typically becomes more obvious and disabling as the child grows. This may also be the case for some children with mild involvement, but it is important to recognize that a significant number of children diagnosed with mild cerebral palsy at 1 year of age are free of motor impairment by 7 years without any specific intervention.

The most common pattern of spastic cerebral palsy is involvement of both lower limbs, termed *spastic diplegia*, even though there is not complete paralysis of the lower limbs. Spastic diplegia is particularly associated with a preterm delivery and periventricular leukomalacia, and there is often some involvement of the upper limbs. In children born at term, the most common pattern is involvement of all limbs (*spastic quadriplegia*), with the lower limbs usually more affected than the upper. These children often have associated intellectual delay and cortical visual impairment, which contribute to their overall functional disabilities. The motor disorder is often fairly symmetrical, but significant asymmetry may be present, often with involvement of both lower limbs and the upper limb on the more affected side. Such a triplegic pattern is commonly associated with a grade 4 intraventricular hemorrhage in a premature neonate, with the area of cerebral infarction contralateral to the more affected side of the body. There is no clear-cut definition of how bad the upper limb involvement in a spastic diplegic child has to be to call the disorder spastic quadriplegia, so the same child may be labeled differently by different observers.

Nature of the Motor Disorder

The motor disorder in children with spastic cerebral palsy is complex and results from a combination of spasticity, weakness, incoordination, excessive reflex irradiation, muscle and joint contractures, and impaired sensory perception. The spasticity is only one element of an upper motor neuron syndrome. Invariably there is associated weakness and usually some incoordination of the affected limbs. Increased tone usually is not due to spasticity alone, and there is typically some dystonia or athetosis in addition to the spasticity. In children with spastic quadriplegia, the hypertonia may be caused more by rigidity than by spasticity, and because of the therapeutic implications, it is important to determine how much of the hypertonia is due to spasticity. Spasticity implies a velocity-dependent increase in muscle tone, typically demonstrated as a clasp-knife response, and is associated with exaggerated deep tendon reflexes. In addition to the spasticity and weakness, children with spastic cerebral palsy demonstrate reflex irradiation to other muscle groups, which results in difficulty isolating movements in the affected limbs. Agonist and antagonist muscles contract together, rather than the normal pattern in which antagonists of contracting muscles relax. They also demonstrate mirror movements, such that when they try to extend the knee on one side, the other knee extends at the same time. As the child gets older, contractures and deformities of the spine and extremities often develop, with hip dislocations, knee flexion contractures, rocker-bottom feet, and scoliosis commonly adding to the motor disability.

Pathophysiology of the Motor Disorder

The pathophysiology of the motor disorder in cerebral palsy is not well understood. The spasticity results from increased output from the spinal alpha motor neuron pool and not, as was once proposed, by increased gain in the muscle spindle or increased excitation of Ia afferents.[9] The hyperexcitability of the alpha motor neurons is secondary to partial loss of the predominantly inhibitory modulating influences carried in descending pathways, such as the corticospinal, vestibulospinal, and reticulospinal tracts.[10] At the level of the spinal interneuron pool, potential pathophysiologic mechanisms with some experimental support include (1) decreased reciprocal inhibition of antagonist motor neuron pools by Ia afferents, (2) reduced presynaptic inhibition of Ia afferents, and (3) decreased nonreciprocal inhibition by Ib fibers.[10] In addition, there are a number of changes that occur in response to cerebral injury, particularly in the immature nervous system. Developing corticospinal pathways become redirected to innervate both agonist and antagonist muscles, which could explain the observed simultaneous contraction of antagonists and agonists and the mirror movements observed in children with spastic cerebral palsy.[8] Unaffected spinal interneurons, more of which are excitatory than in the normal situation, may sprout and make synapses at sites vacated by the dying axons. Thus, there may be less inhibitory activity as well as more excitatory activity, with axons having larger fields than normal. It has also been hypothesized, but not proved, that the membrane properties of alpha motor neurons may change in response to the cerebral injury, resulting in primary hyperexcitability of these neurons.[11]

In addition to these changes in the spinal cord, it is known that the intrinsic mechanical properties of muscle change in the presence of long-standing spasticity, and this may be responsible for part of the motor impairment in a child with cerebral palsy.[12, 13] A major stimulus for muscle growth is stretch of the muscle. In a spastic child, the tonically spastic muscle resists stretch and attempts to maintain its shortest length, whereas the antagonist to that muscle is stretched excessively. This leads to inadequate growth and a decreased number of sarcomeres of the agonist, and excessive growth and lengthening of the antagonist, resulting in growth contractures.

BACLOFEN

Baclofen (β-[4-chlorophenyl]-GABA) is a synthetic γ-aminobutyric acid (GABA) agonist that acts selectively on both pre- and postsynaptic GABA$_B$ receptors to reduce excitatory synaptic transmission. Activation of presynaptic GABA$_B$ receptors by baclofen results in decreased release of excitatory neurotransmitters, such as glutamate and aspartate, but the mechanism for this effect is not clear.[14] Most studies have suggested that the presynaptic effect of baclofen is related to a restriction of calcium influx into the presynaptic terminals. Activation of postsynaptic GABA$_B$ receptors by baclofen causes increased potassium conductance at postsynaptic terminals, which results in prolonged hyperpolarization of the neuronal membrane and decreased neuronal activity.[14, 15] Baclofen also acts at nociceptive afferent nerve endings, where it reduces the release of excitatory neurotransmitters, including substance P, which can cause flexor spasms.[16] In human studies, the antispastic effect of intrathecal baclofen seems to be primarily related to postsynaptic inhibition.[17]

Commercially available baclofen is a racemic mixture of the L- and D-isomers. A number of in vivo behavioral and electrophysiologic studies and in vitro electrophysiologic studies have indicated that the L-isomer is the effective moiety in reducing spasticity, with up to 100-fold more potency than the D-isomer.[15] There have been conflicting reports that D-baclofen may antagonize the effects of L-baclofen.[15, 18]

GABA$_B$ receptors are located throughout the central nervous system but are particularly concentrated in the thalamus and in layers II and III of the dorsal gray matter of the spinal cord.[19] Baclofen relieves spasticity by its action on the spinal cord receptors; the major side effects of sedation and respiratory depression reflect the supraspinal effects of the drug.

Oral Baclofen

Baclofen has been used orally since the early 1970s as an antispastic agent. The drug is absorbed well after oral administration but has low lipid solubility and does not cross the blood-brain barrier readily.[20, 21] The usual starting dose in children is 5 to 10 mg daily in three divided doses, working up to doses as high as 160 mg daily, with the usual therapeutic doses in the range of 40 to 60 mg/day.[21] Oral baclofen has been shown in a number of randomized, controlled studies involving children and adults to improve spasticity associated with spinal cord lesions.[22, 23] Oral baclofen has not been as effective in reducing spasticity of cerebral origin, specifically in children with cerebral palsy.[23–25] The value of oral baclofen is limited by the common occurrence of sedation at the dose levels needed to relieve spasticity. Other less frequent side effects include behavioral changes, confusion, ataxia, urinary frequency, and insomnia.[21, 23] These adverse effects are thought to be related to the effects of baclofen on intracranial GABA_B receptors.

Intrathecal Baclofen

Because the target site for relief of spasticity is the GABA_B receptors in the superficial layers of the spinal cord, and because baclofen does not cross the blood-brain barrier readily, it was rationalized that direct instillation of the drug into the spinal subarachnoid fluid might relieve spasticity while minimizing the centrally mediated side effects. With oral doses of baclofen up to 100 mg/day, lumbar cerebrospinal fluid (CSF) levels of the drug were never more than 12 ng/mL.[20, 26] With continuous intrathecal infusions of 50 to 1200 μg/day, lumbar CSF levels of baclofen ranged from 130 to 950 ng/mL.[26] Intraspinal subarachnoid baclofen diffuses cephalad in the CSF by bulk flow, as does any hydrophilic compound. With a continuous infusion into the subarachnoid space at the L1 level, the concentration in the cisterna magna is one quarter that in the lumbar subarachnoid space,[27] which explains why the effect is more marked in the lower limbs than in the upper limbs. Because the concentrations of baclofen typically achieved with continuous intrathecal infusions are 10 to 80 times those present after oral administration, and because the CSF levels of baclofen at the cisterna magna are only one quarter those in the lumbar CSF, other factors must explain why sedation is seen relatively infrequently with intrathecal baclofen. It may be that the intracranial GABA_B receptors are not as close to the surface as the spinal GABA_B receptors, and because baclofen diffuses poorly into neural tissue, the baclofen tissue concentration at the intracranial receptor sites is relatively less than that at the spinal receptor sites.[28]

A bolus injection of intrathecal baclofen typically reduces lower limb spasticity at about 60 minutes, affects upper extremities by about 2 hours, and has its maximal effect at about 4 hours; the effect wears off by 8 to 10 hours.[29, 30] There is wide individual variation in the pharmacokinetics of intrathecal baclofen, with the elimination half-life ranging from 0.9 to 5 hours.[31, 32] In order to achieve a clinically useful prolonged effect, intrathecal baclofen must be given by continuous infusion via an implanted pump.

PUMP TECHNOLOGY

Two basic types of implantable pumps are available: programmable and nonprogrammable. In children with spasticity of cerebral origin, the severity of spasticity tends to fluctuate, and the ability to program the rate of infusion of intrathecal baclofen is often helpful. The only programmable pump available, the Synchromed pump (Medtronic, Inc., Minneapolis, Minnesota; Fig. 244–1), is battery powered. It is adjusted

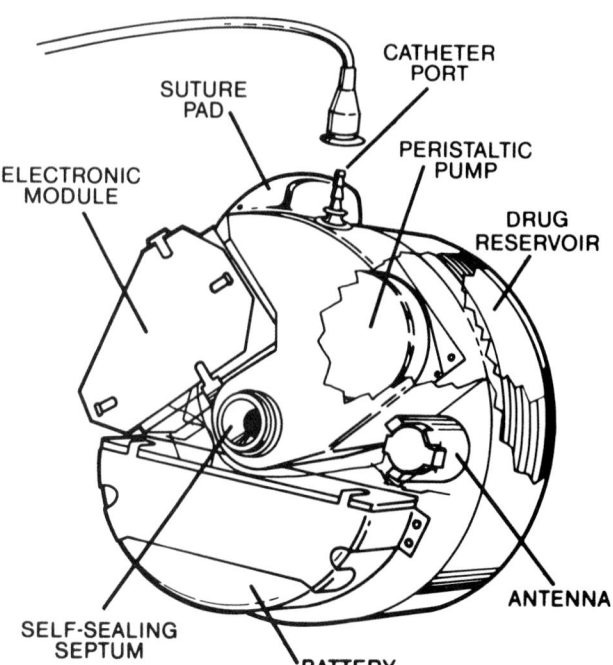

FIGURE 244–1. Line drawing showing the essential features of the Synchromed programmable pump. (Courtesy of Medtronic, Inc., Minneapolis, MN.)

using a radiofrequency-controlled external wand and a programming computer (Fig. 244–2) to deliver variable flow rates or continuous or bolus infusions, or both, or to set a total dose. The pump is powered by a lithium thionyl-chloride battery that lasts for 5 to 7 years, at which time the pump must be replaced. The pump contains a drug reservoir and is covered by a titanium casing with a central aperture, which can be punctured

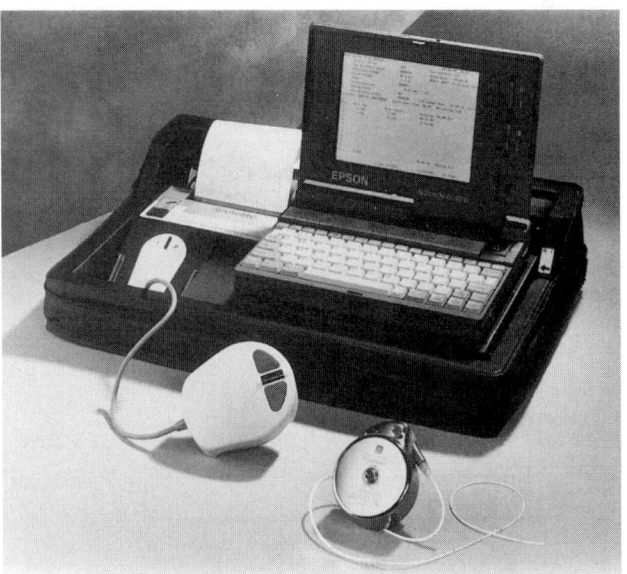

FIGURE 244–2. The programming device and computer for the Synchromed pump, with a Synchromed pump and attached catheter in the foreground. (Courtesy of Medtronic, Inc., Minneapolis, MN.)

for filling of the chamber. The standard pump, with an 18-mL reservoir, has a diameter of 7.5 cm and a thickness of 2.8 cm, approximately the size of an ice hockey puck. The pediatric version has the same diameter but is 2.3 cm thick, and the reservoir has a capacity of 10 mL.

The nonprogrammable implantable pumps, such as the Arrow (Arrow International, Inc., Reading, Pennsylvania), Isomed (Medtronic, Inc., Minneapolis, MN), and Anschutz (Tricumed GmbH, Kiel, Germany), deliver a fixed flow rate and express fluid by the expansion of a propellant gas, which is compressed by refilling the pump (Fig. 244–3). In the nonprogrammable pumps, the rate of infusion is set by the manufacturer, and the inability to change the rate is a major disadvantage. The advantage of these pumps is that, in theory, they have an indefinite life span, but in practice, the pumps usually have to be replaced within 10 years because of some malfunction. The nonprogrammable pumps are more tapered than the Synchromed pump and may be easier to implant in a small child.

These delivery systems cost between $5000 and $10,000 in the United States, with the programmable Synchromed pump costing slightly more than the nonprogrammable pumps.

In most centers, a trial of baclofen injections into the spinal subarachnoid space is performed to determine which patients are likely to benefit from continuous intrathecal baclofen. Responders to this preliminary trial have pumps implanted for long-term continuous infusion. In children with spasticity, the screening trial involves boluses of intrathecal baclofen, which may be given by repeated lumbar punctures to inject the drug or by repeated injections into the external portion of a lumbar subarachnoid catheter or into an implanted reservoir attached to a lumbar subarachnoid catheter. The tone in the limbs is assessed by a physiotherapist before and multiple times during the first 8 hours after each bolus injection, using a quantitative scale such as the Ashworth scale (Table 244–1).[33] During this trial, it is important to avoid being misled by a placebo effect, and placebo and baclofen are often injected in a

TABLE 244–1 ■ **Ashworth Scale for Grading Spasticity**

SCORE	DEFINITION
0	Hypotonic: less than normal muscle tone; floppy
1	Normal: no increase in muscle tone
2	Mild: slight increase in tone; "catch" in limb movement or minimal resistance to movement through less than half the range of motion
3	Moderate: more marked increase in tone through most of the range of motion, but affected part is easily moved
4	Severe: considerable increase in tone; passive movement difficult
5	Extreme: affected part rigid in flexion or extension

blinded fashion. This is particularly important in patients whose tone fluctuates from time to time. In most cases in which there is a response to the intrathecal bolus of baclofen, however, the spasticity is so dramatically reduced that a placebo trial may appear superfluous.[34]

The initial dose of baclofen is usually 25 μg, and this can be doubled each day to a maximum of 100 μg until a response is achieved or it is determined that the patient is a nonresponder. In children with cerebral palsy, muscle tone in the lower extremities was decreased by 1 point or more on the Ashworth scale (considered clinically significant) in 68% of patients after a 25-μg dose and in an additional 17% of patients after a 50- or 100-μg dose of baclofen.[21] The response to intrathecal boluses of baclofen is useful in determining whether the patient is likely to respond to a continuous intrathecal infusion but does not predict the functional outcome with continuous intrathecal baclofen.[34]

Intrathecal baclofen has also been used for the treatment of generalized dystonia in cerebral palsy.[35, 36] In this situation, bolus doses of intrathecal baclofen are usually ineffective in reducing the dystonia, whereas a continuous infusion may be effective. Hence, the screening trial is carried out via a lumbar subarachnoid catheter connected to an external microinfusion pump.[36] The baclofen is infused at an initial rate of 100 μg/day, increasing the dose every 8 to 12 hours by 50 μg until the dystonia improves, side effects occur, or the daily infusion rate reaches 900 μg/day with no response. The degree of dystonia is graded on a dystonia scale (Table 244–2), and a 30% decrease in the dystonia score indicates clinically significant improvement and justifies implantation of a pump.[36]

The risks associated with these screening trials are small. Meningitis is a possibility, especially if a lumbar subarachnoid catheter or implanted reservoir is used for multiple injections.[37] Sedation is the most common adverse neurologic effect of bolus doses of baclofen and has been noted with doses as low as 10 μg.[34, 37]

PUMP IMPLANTATION AND FOLLOW-UP

In patients with a successful response to screening doses of intrathecal baclofen, a pump is implanted in

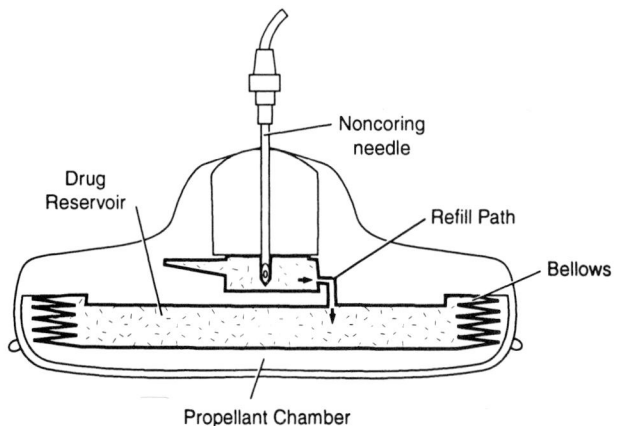

FIGURE 244–3. Line drawing showing the essential features of the Arrow nonprogrammable pump. Other nonprogrammable pumps use a similar mechanism.

TABLE 244-2 ■ **Dystonia Scale**

EYES	TRUNK
0 No dystonia present	0 No dystonia present
1 Slight dystonia; occasional blinking or eye movements noted <10% of the time	1 Slight dystonia; clinically insignificant, noted <10% of the time
2 Mild; frequent blinking without prolonged spasms of eye closure, *or* eye movements <50% of the time	2 Mild; definite lateral flexion or resistance to forward flexion, *or* dystonia that does not interfere with sitting, standing, or walking
3 Moderate; prolonged spasms of eyelid closure, but eyes open most of the time, *or* eye movements >50% of the time that interfere with tracking	3 Moderate lateral flexion or extension of the trunk >50% of the time, *or* dystonia that interferes with sitting, standing, or walking
4 Severe; prolonged spasms of eyelid closure, with eyes closed at least 30% of the time, *or* eye movements >50% of the time that prevent tracking	4 Severe lateral flexion or extensor thrust of the trunk >50% of the time, *or* dystonia that prevents positioning in a standard wheelchair, standing, or walking

MOUTH	UPPER EXTREMITIES
0 No dystonia present	0 No dystonia present
1 Slight dystonia; occasional grimacing or other mouth movements noted <10% of the time (e.g., jaw open or clenched, tongue movement)	1 Slight dystonia; clinically insignificant, noted <10% of the time
2 Mild; movement present <50% of the time	2 Mild; dystonic movements or contractions noted <50% of the time, *or* dystonia that does not interfere with upper limb function
3 Moderate dystonic movements or contractions present >50% of the time, *or* dystonia that interferes with speech or normal feeding	3 Moderate dystonic movements or contractions >50% of the time, *or* dystonia that interferes with upper limb function
4 Severe dystonic movements or contractions present >50% of the time, *or* dystonia that prevents speech or normal feeding	4 Severe dystonic movements or contractions >50% of the time, *or* dystonia that prevents upper limb function (e.g., arms restrained in wheelchair to prevent injury)

NECK	LOWER EXTREMITIES
0 No dystonia present	0 No dystonia present
1 Slight dystonia; clinically insignificant, noted <10% of the time	1 Slight dystonia; clinically insignificant, noted <10% of the time
2 Mild; definite pulling noted <50% of the time, *or* dystonia that does not interfere with sitting, standing, or walking	2 Mild; dystonic movements or contractions noted <50% of the time, *or* dystonia that does not interfere significantly with function
3 Moderate pulling >50% of the time, *or* dystonia that interferes with sitting, standing, or walking	3 Moderate dystonic movements or contractions >50% of the time, *or* dystonia that interferes with functional movement or weight bearing
4 Severe pulling >50% of the time, *or* dystonia that interferes with sitting in standard wheelchair, standing, or walking (e.g., requires more than standard headrest on wheelchair)	4 Severe dystonic movements or contractions >50% of the time, *or* dystonia that prevents functional movement or weight bearing

From Albright A: Intrathecal baclofen in cerebral palsy movement disorders. J Child Neurol 11:S29–S35, 1996.

a subcutaneous pocket in the anterior abdominal wall. A catheter is inserted into the lumbar subarachnoid space at the L3-4 or L4-5 level and is threaded superiorly so that the tip is at the T11-12 level in patients with disabling lower limb spasticity. If the intent is to reduce upper limb spasticity as well, the catheter may be threaded higher into the midthoracic region. This can be performed most precisely under fluoroscopic control, but it can also be achieved by measuring the length of catheter to be inserted and directing it superiorly. The catheter is inserted via a Tuohy needle. The technique that we use, in an attempt to avoid displacement of the catheter or CSF leak, is to insert a Tuohy needle into the subarachnoid space. With the needle still in position, a small incision is made incorporating the needle, and a figure-of-eight suture is placed into the lumbar fascia around the needle. The catheter is threaded into the subarachnoid space, the needle is removed, and the figure-of-eight suture is tied snugly

around the catheter. The catheter is then pulled through a subcutaneous tunnel into the anterior abdominal wall, where it is connected to the pump. The pump is filled with intrathecal baclofen, and if it is programmable, the pump is programmed in the operating room. Our practice is to perform the procedure as day surgery in an acute care hospital, but the children return to a rehabilitation facility for observation for at least 24 hours after surgery.

Thereafter, the pump is refilled every 2 to 3 months and reprogrammed as necessary. The refilling is often delegated to the family physician or a clinic nurse, but the reprogramming is performed under the direction of the team involved in the intrathecal baclofen program. The daily dose of baclofen varies from 25 to 1000 μg/day, and each patient has to be titrated initially to determine the best dose and schedule. The daily dose of intrathecal baclofen usually has to be increased over the first year to control spasticity; it then tends to stabilize.[38] In some adults, most of whom had multiple sclerosis, lasting reduction of spasticity was noted when continuous intrathecal baclofen, which had been used for many years, was discontinued.[39] The mechanism of this phenomenon is unclear, and whether it would apply to children with cerebral palsy is not known.

OUTCOMES

The efficacy of intrathecal baclofen in children with cerebral palsy is reviewed here with consideration of the quality of the evidence supporting the treatment's use and the "dimensions," or "domains," in which that treatment has been demonstrated to have an effect. The National Center for Medical Rehabilitation Research has proposed that outcomes be considered in one of five dimensions: pathophysiology, impairment, functional limitations, disability, and societal limitations (Table 244–3).

The majority of work studying the efficacy of intrathecal baclofen has involved adults with spinal cord injury. The evidence regarding this population is presented elsewhere in this book, but it should be said that there is strong evidence of the efficacy of intrathecal baclofen in adults with spinal cord injury. This evidence comes from both double-blind placebo-controlled trials and a number of open trials.[40–43] These studies demonstrate statistically significant effects on outcomes in impairment, including decreases in lower extremity tone (using the Ashworth scale) and fewer spasms. The improved spasticity and spasms are said to be associated with less discomfort and easier care. However, in this group, there is little scientifically documented evidence of positive outcomes in functional limitations, disability, or societal limitations, such as activities of daily living, motor performance, self-care, or participation in school or work.

Much less is known about the efficacy of intrathecal baclofen in the treatment of spasticity of cerebral origin, particularly in children. A number of studies have been published, but most are case reports or case series.[37, 44–52] Although these case series can be helpful and provide direction for further systematic study, their results must be approached with caution. Armstrong and Almeida and their colleagues reported on N-of-1 randomized clinical trials that provide stronger evidence of the treatment's efficacy.[37, 53] In Armstrong's study, the randomized trial involved only bolus doses of intrathecal baclofen, and this part of the study was performed to determine whether the patients improved enough to justify implantation of the continuous infusion pump. The strongest study design (and therefore the strongest evidence) is presented by Albright and coworkers in the only double-blind, placebo-controlled study reported to date.[30] This study involved 19 children and 4 adults with spasticity due to cerebral palsy or of cerebral origin who participated in a randomized, multiple-crossover study of bolus doses (not continuous infusion) of intrathecal baclofen.

These studies have provided evidence of the efficacy of intrathecal baclofen at the impairment level (e.g., tone, clonus, spasms, strength, and range of motion). In Albright's randomized study, lower extremity muscle tone, as measured by the Ashworth scale, was significantly reduced, but a significant change in upper extremity muscle tone could not be demonstrated.[30] In a later retrospective case series, there was a mild reduction in spasticity in the upper limbs, which was similar to that noted in patients treated by selective dorsal rhizotomy.[54] Latash and Penn and Almeida and colleagues reported significant improvements in ankle clonus, exaggerated reflexes, and spasms.[50, 53] In their case series of children receiving continuous infusion of intrathecal baclofen, Armstrong and colleagues found a significant decrease in hip adductor tone, as measured on the Ashworth scale, with less improvement in elbow flexor spasticity.[37] Almeida's study also demonstrated a desirable short-term improvement of range of movement, but this did not persist over time.[53] Although a number of the case series have examined the effect of intrathecal baclofen on range of motion and the need for subsequent orthopedic procedures, at this time there is only weak evidence of efficacy in this regard.[47] An effect on motor control, particularly relating to the upper limb, has been sought but is not yet strongly supported.[30, 44, 50, 53, 54]

Outcomes within the dimension of functional limitations, such as activities of daily living, have been examined less frequently. In the N-of-1 study of Almeida and colleagues, self-reported improvement in dressing, transferring, and toileting was documented in the one

TABLE 244–3 ■ **National Center for Medical Rehabilitation Research Model of Dimensions of the Disabling Process**

DIMENSION	DESCRIPTION
Pathophysiology	Cellular and molecular processes of injury or disease pertinent to a particular condition
Impairment	Dysfunction at the organ system level resulting from a disease process or injury (e.g., tone, spasms, strength)
Functional limitations	Limitation in the set of skills required to perform specific activities, either of the whole body or of body segments (e.g., limitations in gait, sitting, manipulating objects)
Disability	Difficulties in carrying out the role or function expected of an individual (e.g., attending school, returning to work, partaking in age-appropriate recreation, performing activities of daily living)
Societal limitations	Barriers placed by society that limit full participation by people with disabilities; these barriers may be physical, economic, or attitudinal (e.g., wheelchair-unfriendly architecture, inability to afford a power wheelchair)

patient studied, but there was no improvement in gross and fine motor function during the randomized trial.[53] Albright and associates also found that children previously able to perform self-care rated their own self-care as improved.[44] With both these studies, however, one must be cautious about the self-reported outcome measure used. In the case series reported by Gerszten and coworkers, the effect of intrathecal baclofen on ambulation was assessed in 24 children who were ambulatory to some extent with or without assistive devices before the intervention.[46] Gait was thought to be improved in 20 of the 24 children, as reported by the patients or their families. The level of ambulation, as graded retrospectively using a four-level functional scale, improved in 9 patients, remained the same in 12, and was worse in 3. Thus, there is only weak evidence of improved motor function after intrathecal baclofen in children with spastic cerebral palsy.

For the disability and societal limitation dimensions, no significant evidence of the efficacy of intrathecal baclofen has been demonstrated. At this time, there is no evidence that intrathecal baclofen increases a child's ability to attend school, participate in developmentally appropriate activities, or have an improved quality of life. Thus, although there is demonstrated effectiveness of intrathecal baclofen for the treatment of spasticity, spasms, and exaggerated reflex responses for children with spasticity of cerebral origin, further study is required to delineate its effect on gross and fine motor function, activities of daily living, and quality of life.

Although relatively little is known about the effects of intrathecal baclofen on spasticity of cerebral origin, even less is known about its effects on dystonia and athetosis. Narayan and colleagues were the first to report improvement in axial dystonia in an 18-year-old patient receiving continuous intrathecal baclofen.[35] Other studies have had mixed results for both segmental and generalized dystonia.[36, 51, 55, 56] The strongest study of the effects of intrathecal baclofen on dystonia in cerebral palsy is that of Albright and colleagues.[56] In this case series, the impairment-level outcome of dystonia was examined, using a dystonia measurement scale (see Table 244–2). The effects of intrathecal baclofen in a screening test infusion were examined, and then a smaller subset of patients was followed. Of the 12 patients with cerebral palsy studied, 10 had improvement with the test infusions, and 8 of these 10 underwent pump implantation for continuous infusion. As the patients were followed over the longer term, the positive effects were maintained in six of the eight patients receiving continuous intrathecal baclofen. To date, there are insufficient data to comment on the effects of baclofen on other dimensions of the disabling process, such as functional limitations and disability. The data support the need for additional investigation of the utility of intrathecal baclofen for this population of patients.

COMPLICATIONS

Complications associated with intrathecal baclofen are common and may be related to the drug or to local problems with the surgical procedure or the hardware. The most common drug-related problem from intrathecal baclofen is mild sedation, which requires a decrease in the dose of the drug. Less commonly there may be dizziness, blurred vision, and slurred speech.[21, 57] An increased frequency or precipitation of seizures has also been reported.[40, 58, 59]

Life-threatening overdoses, characterized by severe respiratory depression, coma, hypotension, and bradycardia, also occur. In most cases, the overdose has been associated with the use of bolus doses of intrathecal baclofen, especially if the bolus is given on top of a continuous infusion or if intrathecal baclofen is used concurrently with oral baclofen, but programming errors and pump malfunction have also been responsible.[28, 37, 60] In patients with suspected drug overdose, the diagnosis is supported by the findings of weakness, flaccidity, and areflexia in both lower and upper limbs. These patients should be admitted to an intensive care unit, where ventilatory support can be provided if needed. The intrathecal infusion should be discontinued or the pump reservoir emptied of baclofen. Intravenous physostigmine has been used with variable success in the treatment of overdoses,[61–63] but because of the potential side effects, it is not recommended. Removal of baclofen from the lumbar subarachnoid space via lumbar puncture may be helpful.[21, 63] With appropriate supportive care, the outcome after overdose has been uniformly good, with no lasting sequelae.

A complication that is related to the expected reduction in lower limb tone with intrathecal baclofen is deep venous thrombosis in the lower limbs and pulmonary embolus. This has been noted in the adult population but not in children.[64, 65]

Sudden withdrawal of intrathecal baclofen after long-term use, as might occur with a blockage in the system or pump failure, may result in hallucinations, seizures, confusion, psychotic behavior, rebound severe spasticity, and hyperthermia.[66–69] If the diagnosis is made, reinfusion of baclofen into the subarachnoid space via the pump as a bolus or by lumbar puncture may reverse the symptoms, and in patients with hyperthermia, dantrolene has been useful.[68, 70] If it is decided to discontinue continuous intrathecal baclofen, this should be carried out gradually, and the patient should be placed on oral baclofen.

Failure of the pump occurs in 5% to 10% of cases, necessitating replacement.[40, 57] Other local problems related to the infusion system are common and include seromas around the pump, erosion of the skin over the pump, disconnection at a connector site, breakage of the catheter, kinking of the catheter, displacement of the intrathecal catheter, and leak of CSF at the catheter insertion site.[21, 37, 71] Some of these complications have been reduced as surgeons have gained experience inserting the pumps and with improved catheter systems, particularly the development of thicker walled catheters.[72] However, even in series carried out in the 1990s, reoperations for catheter-related problems are performed in more than 20% of patients.[21, 28] In children, the local problems tend to be aggravated. The pumps are large and protrude markedly in the anterior abdominal wall, especially in young or thin children (Fig. 244–4). In spastic quadriplegic children, who are often restrained in wheelchairs and who tend to be thin, the protruding pump may be irritated repeatedly by the restraints, leading to a higher incidence of local complications.

Another potential complication of the administration of intrathecal baclofen is spinal arachnoiditis, associated with the drug or the catheter, but there is no definite case report of such a complication.[73]

As in any surgery involving implants, infection is a major concern. Local infection of the wound or subcutaneous pump pocket has been reported in up to 20% of patients.[71, 74] Pump erosion through the skin with subsequent contamination of the pump is not unusual, especially in children. Local infections can sometimes be eradicated with the use of systemic antibiotics, but more often the pump has to be removed. Meningitis has been documented, both during the trial of repeated intrathecal injections before insertion of the pump and after pump implantation. Treatment of meningitis using systemic antibiotics in addition to intrathecal antibiotics administered through the pump reservoir or side port may be successful and avoids removal of the pump.[74]

A further consideration is that continuous intrathecal baclofen requires chronic medical attention to refill the pump, adjust the dose to obtain the desired effect, replace the pump when the battery fails, and address the various complications previously mentioned. Should spasticity recur in a patient receiving continuous intrathecal baclofen, one needs to determine whether tolerance to the drug has occurred or whether there is a problem with the intrathecal drug delivery system. Hence, pump failure or some other mechanical problem has to be ruled out. Plain anteroposterior and lateral radiographs of the infusion system may demonstrate an obvious break or disconnection or may show that the catheter has migrated out of the subarachnoid space. If the system appears to be intact and positioned appropriately, a number of techniques may be helpful in determining the cause of the problem.[21] If the pump is programmable, it can be programmed to deliver a bolus of baclofen to see if this relieves spasticity.

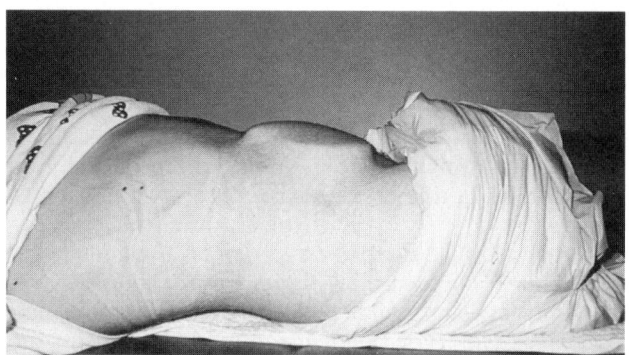

FIGURE 244–4. Photograph of a 9-year-old child with an implanted Synchromed pump demonstrates the marked protrusion of the pump in the anterior abdominal wall.

Alternatively, radioactive isotope or water-soluble contrast material can be injected into the reservoir. After waiting a few hours to allow the material to reach the end of the catheter, a scan or radiograph is then performed. The infusion rate can be increased or a bolus given to speed up the investigation, but if this is carried out, the baclofen should be removed from the reservoir first. Even then, there is a risk of overdose as the baclofen in the catheter is infused rapidly into the subarachnoid space. If there is a side port associated with the pump, the contrast material or radionuclide can be injected into this side port, outlining the catheter system immediately. Assay of CSF obtained by lumbar puncture to determine the concentration of baclofen may also be helpful.

MANAGEMENT

The goals of management of a child with spasticity of cerebral origin are improved motor function, increased mobility, increased independence, decreased painful spasms and, for severely affected quadriplegics, increased ease of care. It is critical for all parties involved, including the caregivers, to appreciate that the goals of treatment are not simply relief of spasticity or improved range of movement.

SELECTION OF PATIENTS FOR NEUROSURGICAL TREATMENT

In order to make the most appropriate recommendations, the treating physicians must be familiar with and must be prepared to discuss the pros and cons of the various options available. These include physiotherapy; occupational therapy; oral spasmolytics; orthopedic procedures, such as tendon lengthening; botulinum toxin injections; therapeutic electrical stimulation; and selective dorsal rhizotomies.

The first issue in the assessment of a hypertonic child is to determine the nature of the increased tone. Is the hypertonia due to spasticity, rigidity, dystonia, or some combination? This determination is crucial, because interventions designed to relieve spasticity may be of little or no benefit for other types of hypertonia. In children with cerebral palsy, there is often a combination of spasticity and dystonia. If spasticity is significant, there is always a clasp-knife reaction to flexing of the knees and often a similar response to abducting of the hips. This type of response may be difficult to demonstrate at the ankles, which may be held fairly rigidly in plantar flexion. Hyperreflexia of the deep tendon jerks and upgoing plantar responses are usually present.

The next question is whether it is the spasticity or some other problem, such as contractures, dystonia, or weakness, that is inhibiting the child's function or the caregivers' ability to look after the child. It is often instructive to ask the parents or other caregivers how they think the child would benefit if spasticity in the lower or upper limbs were reduced. If it is thought that reducing spasticity would not improve function, the child is not a candidate for a spasticity-relieving procedure. In children in whom the functionally important spasticity is in predominantly one muscle group—for example, the ankle plantar flexors or hamstrings—consideration is given to a simpler orthopedic tendon-lengthening procedure or administration of botulinum toxin. We recognize that even when the functionally important spasticity affects one muscle group, there is usually spasticity throughout the lower limbs, and one can make a case for performing a dorsal rhizotomy or using intrathecal baclofen to decrease the lower limb spasticity more diffusely in this patient population. However, we opt for a simpler procedure if the functional results might reasonably be expected to be similar.

If the child might benefit functionally from relief of spasticity diffusely in the lower limbs, options such as intrathecal baclofen or dorsal rhizotomy are considered. The ambulatory potential must be assessed, and an attempt is made to determine whether reduction in lower limb spasticity might be detrimental to the child's ambulatory function, because the child may be using the spasticity to support weight in the upright position. This is one of the most difficult issues. In our experience, children who are walking independently without a walker or crutches, and younger children who crawl on knees and arms, have enough underlying strength in the lower limbs and are not a concern. For other patients, the child's ability to rise in a slow, graded fashion from the squatting position is assessed. If the child is able to do this with the examiner supporting the arms or upper body minimally, the probability is high that there is adequate underlying quadriceps strength to support the child's weight if the spasticity is reduced. One clearly needs to be concerned about this issue in children with ambulatory potential, but this must be considered even in spastic quadriplegics, in whom ambulation is not a realistic goal. Many of these children, who get around in wheelchairs, use their spasticity to assist in standing transfers. They may be worse functionally if that spasticity is reduced and they are no longer able to support their weight. This may not be a major issue for a young child who is easily lifted, but it attains increasing importance as the child gets older, heavier, and more difficult to lift.

At the completion of the assessment, it is critical that one ascertain the expectations and hopes of the parents or other primary caregivers and ensure that these expectations are realistic. This should be documented, because almost all parents are seeking a cure for their child's motor problems or at least have the hope that their child will walk, and many have unrealistic expectations of proposed treatments. These parents may not be happy even if the child improves functionally, because the child does not achieve their expectations. In most cases, many months can pass before treatment of the spasticity becomes crucial, and the parents are usually counseled to take some time to think about the recommendations, especially if an operation is advised. Occasionally, when the hips of the child are dislocating because of excessive hip abductor spasticity, a more urgent intervention is recommended.

If it is determined that treatment of the spasticity is indicated, one needs to decide what intervention is most appropriate. Intrathecal baclofen is the intervention of choice in spastic, dystonic, quadriplegic children after near drowning.[37] In patients in whom dystonia, rather than spasticity, is inhibiting function, preliminary studies suggest that intrathecal baclofen may be indicated.[56] Children with spastic, quadriplegic cerebral palsy affecting the upper limbs more than the lower limbs or with severe opisthotonic posturing may be considered for intrathecal baclofen, because it may be possible to increase the dose of baclofen or direct the subarachnoid catheter higher in the spinal canal so that upper limb spasticity is reduced.[75]

Intrathecal baclofen is often preferred over rhizotomy in children with spastic diplegic cerebral palsy when there is concern that spasticity is needed for standing or walking support.[34] The argument is that the dose of baclofen can be titrated, and if the result is unsatisfactory, the treatment is reversible. This concern about the possible loss of the ability to stand or walk may be more theoretical than real. Our experience is that these patients do well after selective dorsal rhizotomy, with no child losing the ability to walk or stand after that procedure. Hence, we recommend a selective dorsal rhizotomy in this situation as opposed to intrathecal baclofen.

Other indications for intrathecal baclofen include older patients with diplegia, particularly those older than 16 years, and children with spastic quadriplegia in whom the lower limb spasticity is disabling or making care difficult.[34] These children may also meet the criteria for selective dorsal rhizotomy, but there are no studies that compare these two treatment modalities in these populations. When intrathecal baclofen and selective dorsal rhizotomy are considered to be equally effective and indicated options, our practice is to recommend rhizotomy. Our rationale is that compared with intrathecal baclofen, selective dorsal rhizotomy requires little long-term management, does not require reoperation, has fewer complications, has a better-documented effectiveness in improving function, and is less costly overall to the health care system.[52]

CONCLUSIONS

Management of the motor impairment in a child with spastic cerebral palsy should be multidisciplinary and usually involves a physiotherapist, occupational therapist, developmental pediatrician, orthopedic surgeon, and orthotist, in addition to the neurosurgeon. The neurosurgeon is usually asked for an opinion about the management of the spasticity. It is important that he or she appreciates the various neurosurgical and non-neurosurgical interventions available for the relief of spasticity and also recognizes that the goal of treatment is not the relief of spasticity per se but the improvement of motor function. The neurosurgeon should work as part of a team to identify the best management option to optimize the functional outcome. Furthermore, if a neurosurgical intervention directed at the relief of spasticity is indicated, the best outcome is achieved with input from physiotherapists, occupational therapists, orthotists, and orthopedic surgeons in the postoperative period.

REFERENCES

1. Penn RD, Kroin JS: Intrathecal baclofen alleviates spinal cord spasticity. Lancet 1:1078, 1984.
2. Paneth N, Kiely J: The frequency of cerebral palsy: A review of population studies in industrialized nations since 1950. In Stanley F, Alberman E (eds): The Epidemiology of the Cerebral Palsies. London, Spastics International Medical Publications, 1984, pp 46–56.
3. Stanley FJ, Blair E: Why have we failed to reduce the incidence of cerebral palsy? Med J Aust 154:623–626, 1991.
4. Newacheck PW, Taylor WR: Childhood chronic illness: Prevalence, severity and impact. Am J Public Health 82:364–371, 1992.
5. Murphy CC, Yeargin-Allsopp M, Decoufle P, et al: Prevalence of cerbral palsy among ten-year-old children in metropolitan Atlanta. J Pediatr 123:S13–S20, 1993.
6. Albright AL: Spasticity and movement disorders in cerebral palsy [editorial]. J Child Neurol 11:S1–S4, 1996.
7. Dabney KW, Lipton GE, Miller F: Cerebral palsy. Curr Opin Pediatr 9:81–88, 1997.
8. Brouwer B, Ashby P: Do injuries to the developing human brain alter corticospinal projections? Neurosci Lett 108:225–230, 1990.
9. Harrison A: Spastic cerebral palsy: Possible spinal interneurone contributions. Dev Med Child Neurol 30:769–780, 1989.
10. Filloux FM: Neuropathophysiology of movement disorders in cerebral palsy. J Child Neurol 11:S5–S12, 1996.
11. Young RR: Spasticity: A review. Neurology 44:S12–S20, 1994.
12. Dietz V, Quintern J, Berger W: Electrophysiological studies of gait in spasticity and rigidity: Evidence that altered mechanical properties of muscle contribute to hypertonia. Brain 104:431–449, 1981.
13. Hufschmidt A, Mauritz KH: Chronic transformation of muscle in spasticity: A peripheral contribution to increased tone. J Neurol Neurosurg Psychiatry 48:676–685, 1985.
14. Kerr DIB, Ong J: GABA$_B$ receptors. Pharmacol Ther 67:187–246, 1995.
15. Zieglgansberger W, Howe JR, Sutor B: The neuropharmacology of baclofen. In Muller H, Zierski J, Penn RD (eds): Local Spinal Therapy of Spasticity. Berlin, Springer-Verlag, 1988, pp 37–49.
16. Young RR, Delwaide PJ: Drug therapy: Spasticity. N Engl J Med 304:96–99, 1981.
17. Azouvi P, Roby-Brami A, Biraben A, et al: Effect of intrathecal baclofen on the monosynaptic reflex in humans: Evidence for a postsynaptic action. J Neurol Neurosurg Psychiatry 56:515–519, 1993.
18. Fromm GH, Shibuya T, Nakata M, et al: Effects of D-baclofen and L-baclofen on the trigeminal nucleus. Neuropharmacology 29:249–254, 1990.
19. Price GW, Wilkin GP, Turnbull MJ, et al: Are baclofen-sensitive GABA$_b$ receptors present on primary afferent terminals of the spinal cord? Nature 307:71–74, 1984.
20. Knutsson E, Lindblom U, Beissinger RL, et al: Plasma and cerebrospinal fluid levels of baclofen (Lioresal) at optimal therapeutic responses in spastic paraparesis. J Neurol Sci 23:473–484, 1974.
21. Albright AL: Baclofen in the treatment of cerebral palsy. J Child Neurol 11:77–83, 1996.
22. Hattab JR: Review of European clinical trials with baclofen. In Feldman RG, Young RR, Koella WP (eds): Spasticity: Disordered Motor Control. Chicago, Year Book Medical Publishers, 1980, pp 71–85.
23. O'Donnell M, Armstrong R: Pharmacologic interventions for management of spasticity in cerebral palsy. Ment Retard Dev Disabil Res Rev 3:204–211, 1997.
24. Van Hemert JCJ: A double blind comparison of baclofen and placebo in patients with spasticity of cerebral origin. In Feldman RG, Young RR, Koella WP (eds): Spasticity: Disordered Motor Control. Chicago, Year Book Medical Publishers, 1980.
25. Milla PJ, Jackson ADM: A controlled trial of baclofen in children with cerebral palsy. J Int Med Res 5:398–404, 1977.

26. Muller H, Zierski J, Dralle D, et al: Pharmacokinetics of intrathecal baclofen. In Muller H, Zierski J, Penn RD (eds): Local Spinal Therapy of Spasticity. Berlin, Springer-Verlag, 1988, pp 223–226.
27. Kroin JS, Ali A, York M, et al: The distribution of medication along the spinal canal after chronic intrathecal administration. Neurosurgery 33:226–230, 1993.
28. Ochs GA: Intrathecal baclofen. Baillieres Clin Neurol 2:73–86, 1993.
29. Muller H, Zierski J, Dralle D, et al: Intrathecal baclofen in spasticity. In Muller H, Zierski J, Penn RD (eds): Local Spinal Therapy of Spasticity. Berlin, Springer-Verlag, 1988, pp 155–214.
30. Albright AL, Cervi A, Singletary J: Intrathecal baclofen for spasticity in cerebral palsy. JAMA 265:1418–1422, 1991.
31. Sallerin-Caute B, Lazorthes Y, Monsarrat B, et al: CSF baclofen levels after intrathecal administration in severe spasticity. Eur J Clin Pharmacol 40:363–365, 1991.
32. Penn RD, Kroin JS: Long-term intrathecal baclofen infusion for treatment of spasticity. J Neurosurg 66:181–185, 1987.
33. Bohannon RW, Smith MB: Interrater reliability of a modified Ashworth scale. Phys Ther 67:206–207, 1987.
34. Albright AL: Intrathecal baclofen in cerebral palsy movement disorders. J Child Neurol 11:S29–S35, 1996.
35. Narayan RK, Loubser PG, Jankovic J, et al: Intrathecal baclofen for intractable axial dystonia. Neurology 41:1141–1142, 1991.
36. Albright AL, Barry MJ, Fasick P, et al: Continuous intrathecal baclofen infusion for symptomatic generalized dystonia. Neurosurgery 38:934–938, 1996; discussion 938–939.
37. Armstrong RW, Steinbok P, Cochrane DD, et al: Intrathecally administered baclofen for treatment of children with spasticity of cerebral origin. J Neurosurg 87:409–414, 1997.
38. Akman MN, Loubser PG, Donovan WH, et al: Intrathecal baclofen: Does tolerance occur? Paraplegia 31:516–520, 1993.
39. Dressnandt J, Conrad B: Lasting reduction of severe spasticity after ending chronic treatment with intrathecal baclofen. J Neurol Neurosurg Psychiatry 60:168–173, 1996.
40. Coffey RJ, Cahill D, Steers W, et al: Intrathecal baclofen for intractable spasticity of spinal origin: Results of a long-term multicenter study. J Neurosurg 78:226–232, 1993.
41. Hugenholtz H, Nelson RF, Dehoux E, et al: Intrathecal baclofen for intractable spinal spasticity—a double-blind cross-over comparison with placebo in 6 patients. Can J Neurol Sci 19:188–195, 1992.
42. Loubser PG, Narayan RK, Sandin KJ, et al: Continuous infusion of intrathecal baclofen: Long-term effects on spasticity in spinal cord injury. Paraplegia 29:48–64, 1991.
43. Meythaler JM, Steers WD, Tuel SM, et al: Continuous intrathecal baclofen in spinal cord spasticity: A prospective study. Am J Phys Med Rehabil 71:321–327, 1992.
44. Albright AL, Barron WB, Fasick MP, et al: Continuous intrathecal baclofen infusion for spasticity of cerebral origin. JAMA 270:2475–2477, 1993.
45. Albright AL, Barry MJ, Hoffmann P: Intrathecal L-baclofen for cerebral spasticity: Case report. Neurology 45:2110–2111, 1995.
46. Gers17ten PC, Albright AL, Barry MJ: Effect on ambulation of continuous intrathecal baclofen infusion. Pediatr Neurosurg 27:40–44, 1997.
47. Gerszten PC, Albright AL, Johnstone GF: Intrathecal baclofen infusion and subsequent orthopedic surgery in patients with spastic cerebral palsy. J Neurosurg 88:1009–1013, 1998.
48. Gilmartin R, Rawlins P: Seizures in epileptic cerebral palsy patients receiving intrathecal baclofen infusion. Epilepsia 36:12, 1995.
49. Krach L, Gilmartin R, Bruce D, et al: Functional changes noted following treatment of individuals with cerebral palsy with intrathecal baclofen. Dev Med Child Neurol Suppl 75:D1, 1997.
50. Latash ML, Penn RD: Changes in voluntary motor control induced by intrathecal baclofen in patients with spasticity of different etiology. Physiother Res Int 1:229–246, 1996.
51. Penn RD, Gianino JM, York MM: Intrathecal baclofen for motor disorders. Mov Disord 10:675–677, 1995.
52. Steinbok P, Daneshvar H, Evans D, et al: Cost analysis of continuous intrathecal baclofen versus selective functional posterior rhizotomy in the treatment of spastic quadriplegia associated with cerebral palsy. Pediatr Neurosurg 22:255–264, 1995; discussion 265.

53. Almeida GL, Campbell SK, Girolami GL, et al: Multidimensional assessment of motor function in a child with cerebral palsy following intrathecal administration of baclofen. Phys Ther 77: 751–764, 1997.
54. Albright AL, Barry MJ, Fasick MP, et al: Effects of continuous intrathecal baclofen infusion and selective posterior rhizotomy on upper extremity spasticity. Pediatr Neurosurg 23:82–85, 1995.
55. Ford B, Greene P, Louis ED, et al: Use of intrathecal baclofen in the treatment of patients with dystonia. Arch Neurol 53: 1241–1246, 1996.
56. Albright AL, Barry MJ, Painter MJ, et al: Infusion of intrathecal baclofen for generalized dystonia in cerebral palsy. J Neurosurg 88:73–76, 1998.
57. Penn RD: Intrathecal baclofen for spasticity of spinal origin: Seven years of experience. J Neurosurg 77:236–240, 1992.
58. Kofler M, Kronenberg MF, Rifici C, et al: Epileptic seizures associated with intrathecal baclofen application. Neurology 44:25–27, 1994.
59. Rifici C, Kofler M, Kronenberg M, et al: Intrathecal baclofen application in patients with supraspinal spasticity secondary to severe traumatic brain injury. Funct Neurol 9:29–34, 1994.
60. Lazorthes Y, Sallerin-Caute B, Verdie JC, et al: Chronic intrathecal baclofen administration for control of severe spasticity. J Neurosurg 72:393–402, 1990.
61. Muller-Schwefe G, Penn RD: Physostigmine in the treatment of intrathecal baclofen overdose: Report of three cases. J Neurosurg 71:273–275, 1989.
62. Saltuari L, Baumgartner H, Kofler M, et al: Failure of physostigmine in treatment of acute severe intrathecal baclofen intoxication. N Engl J Med 322:1533–1534, 1990.
63. Delhaas EM, Brouwers JR: Intrathecal baclofen overdose: Report of 7 events in 5 patients and review of the literature. Int J Clin Pharmacol Ther Toxicol 29:274–280, 1991.
64. Broseta J, Morales F, Garcia-March G, et al: Use of intrathecal baclofen administered by programmable infusion pumps in resistant spasticity. Acta Neurochir Suppl 46:39–45, 1989.
65. Armstrong RW: Intrathecal baclofen and spasticity: What do we know and what do we need to know? Dev Med Child Neurol 34:739–745, 1992.
66. Kofler M, Arturo LA: Prolonged seizure activity after baclofen withdrawal. Neurology 42:697–698, 1992.
67. Mandac BR, Hurvitz EA, Nelson VS: Hyperthermia associated with baclofen withdrawal and increased spasticity. Arch Phys Med Rehabil 74:96–97, 1993.
68. Reeves RK, Stolp-Smith KA, Christopherson MW: Hyperthermia, rhabdomyolysis, and disseminated intravascular coagulation associated with baclofen pump catheter failure. Arch Phys Med Rehabil 79:353–356, 1998.
69. Siegfried RN, Jacobson L, Chabal C: Development of an acute withdrawal syndrome following the cessation of intrathecal baclofen in a patient with spasticity. Anesthesiology 77:1048–1050, 1992.
70. Khorasani A, Peruzzi WT: Dantrolene treatment for abrupt intrathecal baclofen withdrawal. Anesth Analg 80:1054–1056, 1995.
71. Gardner B, Jamous A, Teddy P, et al: Intrathecal baclofen—a multicentre clinical comparison of the Medtronics Programmable, Cordis Secor and Constant Infusion Infusaid drug delivery systems. Paraplegia 33:551–554, 1995.
72. Penn RD, York MM, Paice JA: Catheter systems for intrathecal drug delivery. J Neurosurg 83:215–217, 1995.
73. Armstrong RW, Steinbok P, Farrell K, et al: Continuous intrathecal baclofen treatment of severe spasms in two children with spinal-cord injury. Dev Med Child Neurol 34:731–738, 1992.
74. Müller H: Treatment of severe spasticity: Results of a multicenter trial conducted in Germany involving the intrathecal infusion of baclofen by an implantable drug delivery system. In Lakke JPWF, Delhaas EM, Rutgers AWF (eds): Parenteral Drug Therapy in Spasticity and Parkinson's Disease. Lancaster, UK, Parthenon, 1992, pp 103–113.
75. Hugenholtz H, Nelson RF, Dehoux E: Intrathecal baclofen—the importance of catheter position. Can J Neurol Sci 20:165–167, 1993.

CHAPTER **245**

Recognition of Surgical Candidates and the Presurgical Evaluation

NANCY FOLDVARY ■ ELAINE WYLLIE

GENERAL CONCEPTS

The goal of the presurgical evaluation in patients of all ages is to define the epileptogenic zone, the region of cortex capable of generating seizures. The complete removal or disconnection of this zone is required to produce a seizure-free state.[1] The evaluation includes clinical history, ictal and interictal electroencephalograms (EEGs), seizure symptoms, neuroimaging, and neuropsychological assessment. A recommendation for surgery is made when the evaluation successfully delineates the epileptogenic zone and the proposed resection is believed to carry a low risk of neurologic morbidity. In this respect, epilepsy surgery in infants and children is similar to that in older patients. However, the causes of epilepsy, types of resection, and goals and risks of epilepsy surgery in pediatric patients differ considerably from those in adults. An understanding of the unique aspects of epilepsy surgery in children is paramount to the selection of appropriate surgical candidates.

Causes of Medically Refractory Epilepsy in Children. The most common causes of refractory epilepsy in pediatric surgical series are malformations of cortical development and low-grade tumors.[2-4] Hippocampal sclerosis, the most common pathologic substrate in adults with refractory epilepsy, is uncommon in children.[5] In a pediatric series from the Cleveland Clinic Foundation, only 12% of 62 children and 15% of 74 adolescents had hippocampal sclerosis.[2] Focal cerebral dysgenesis and low-grade tumors were the cause of epilepsy in 90% of infants younger than 3 years, 70% of children, and 57% of adolescents.[2] In the series of Duchowny and colleagues, cortical dysplasia ac-

counted for 68%, developmental tumors for 23%, and peri- or postnatal lesions for 10% of cases of medically refractory partial epilepsy in infants younger than 3 years.[6] Five patients had hippocampal sclerosis, which was associated with cortical dysplasia or tumor in all five patients.[6] Other less common causes of epilepsy in children include head injury, central nervous system infection, vascular malformation, and arachnoid cyst.[2] Causes affecting an entire hemisphere, such as Sturge-Weber syndrome, hemimegacephaly, and perinatal cerebral infarction, are much more common in infants and children than in adults.

Types of Surgery. The types of surgical procedures performed in children for medically refractory partial epilepsy vary considerably from those in adult series. The most common surgical procedure performed in adults with refractory partial epilepsy is temporal lobe resection.[7] In the series of Duchowny and colleagues, 45% of patients younger than 3 years underwent functional hemispherectomy, 10% had multilobar resections, and the remainder had lobar resections.[6] Temporal lobectomies constituted only 36% of lobar resections. Extratemporal or multilobar resections or hemispherectomies constituted 44% of surgeries in adolescents, 50% in children, and 90% in infants in the Cleveland Clinic series.[2]

Surgical Complications. Despite the tendency for more widespread pathology and the need for larger resections, the rate of surgical complications, neurologic morbidity, and mortality remain relatively low in young patients after epilepsy surgery. Among the nearly 150 pediatric patients who underwent epilepsy surgery in the Cleveland Clinic series, 2 (1.3%) died in the immediate postoperative period.[2] Wound infections occurred in four patients (2.9%), three of whom underwent subdural electrode investigation. Superficial infections were treated with antibiotics alone in three cases, and removal and subsequent repair of the bone flap was required in one case. Transient language disturbance and ipsilateral superior oblique paresis occurred in one patient. Three patients had hemiparesis postoperatively, which was expected in two cases of perirolandic resection. After functional hemispherectomy, one patient developed deep venous thrombosis, one developed contralateral subdural hematoma, and one had an entrapped temporal horn relieved by marsupialization. Some patients had transient worsening of hemiparesis, with recovery to baseline within weeks. In another series, 2 of 31 infants (6%) died postoperatively—one as a result of sepsis, syndrome of inappropriate antidiuretic hormone, and dehydration, and another with unrecognized hydrocephalus.[6] No deaths or permanent disabling complications were incurred in 47 children who underwent epilepsy surgery consisting mostly of temporal lobe resections.[8] However, permanent, nondisabling complications occurred in 4.2% and transient neurologic deficits in 6.4% of patients. Four perioperative deaths occurred out of 58 patients after hemispherectomy for Rasmussen's syndrome, malformations of cortical development, and Sturge-Weber syndrome or other vascular lesions, highlighting the risk of larger resections in the very young.[9]

Plasticity. Plasticity of the developing brain allows for some young children to undergo epilepsy surgery involving language and sensorimotor cortices with minimal risk of loss of function. In 1977, Rasmussen reported that some children transfer language dominance to the right hemisphere after an injury to the left hemisphere before the age of 6 years.[10] More recent studies support and extended this early observation.[11, 12] Duchowny and colleagues reported the results of six children with perinatal or postnatal cerebral insults and refractory epilepsy who underwent left hemisphere language mapping.[11] No language areas were identified in three children who were 5 years or younger at the time of insult, but language cortex was identified in the other three patients, all of whom suffered left hemisphere insults after the age of 5 years. In children with epilepsy caused by developmental pathology and tumors near left hemisphere language areas, language function is not displaced even when the epileptogenic cortex and language areas overlap.[12] Similarly, motor function may be displaced in patients with lesions involving the perirolandic area and unaffected after resection of the lesion.[13]

Seizure Outcome. Despite different causes and different surgery types, seizure outcome after epilepsy surgery in children is comparable to that in adults. In the series of Duchowny and colleagues, 61% of infants were free of seizures, and 15% achieved greater than 90% seizure reduction.[6] A better seizure outcome was achieved in patients with single structural lesions seen on magnetic resonance imaging (MRI) scans in whom complete resection of the epileptogenic zone was performed. In the Cleveland Clinic series, patients were more likely to be rendered free of seizures after temporal resection (78%) than after hemispherectomy (68%) or multilobar resection (54%), when cause was not considered.[2] However, independent of type of surgery and age, a seizure-free outcome was more likely in patients with low-grade tumor (82%) than in those with focal cerebral dysgenesis (52%). Sixty-seven percent of children with hippocampal sclerosis were rendered free of seizures after temporal lobectomy, a figure that compares favorably with adult series.[2] In the single largest hemispherectomy series, 54% of patients were rendered free of seizures, 24% had nondisabling seizures, and 23% had persistent disabling seizures.[9]

Developmental Outcome. The goals of epilepsy surgery in infants and children differ greatly from those in adolescents and adults. The primary goals among adolescents and adults with medically refractory epilepsy center on driving, employment, independence, and the establishment of interpersonal relationships. For infants and young children with catastrophic epilepsy, improvement of seizures and behavior and resumption of developmental progress are the expectations of parents and caregivers. Few data are available on the effects of epilepsy surgery on development in infants and young children. Duchowny and colleagues found no significant changes in development postoperatively, despite reports of accelerated motor and cognitive development by parents of seizure-free children.[6] However, in another series, developmental gains were observed in 24 children with infantile spasms who underwent epilepsy surgery at a mean of 20.8 months of age.[14] Earlier age at surgery and higher presurgical developmental status were associated with better developmental outcomes postoperatively. In their series of 100 pediatric patients who underwent resection for intractable focal epilepsy, Vasconcellos and colleagues found that younger age at seizure onset was associated with lower Full-Scale Intelligence Quotient (FSIQ) scores.[15] The frequency of mental retardation was significantly greater for patients with onset of epilepsy before 24 months of age (46%) than for older patients (12%), independent of the cause of the epilepsy. This was particularly true for the subgroup of patients with daily seizures, highlighting the importance of the timing of surgery in young patients with catastrophic focal epilepsy.

RECOGNITION OF SURGICAL CANDIDATES

Medical Intractability. Advances in neuroimaging have revolutionized the identification and evaluation of surgical candidates. Patients are now being considered for surgery who would have been rejected even in the early 1990s. Identification of surgical candidacy begins with the determination of medical intractability. Unfortunately, the concept of medical intractability is not strictly defined. Adults are generally considered to have medically intractable epilepsy once they have failed adequate trials of two or more conventional antiepileptic drugs (AEDs) over a period of approximately 2 years.[16] For most epileptologists, these drugs include phenytoin and carbamazepine. However, the application of stringent criteria of intractability to infants and young children with catastrophic epilepsy not only may delay referral to a comprehensive epilepsy center but also may have devastating consequences for the developing brain. Neuropsychological performance appears to be worse in children who develop generalized motor seizures before 5 years of age compared with those who are older at seizure onset.[17]

Gilman and colleagues studied records of 72 pediatric epilepsy surgery candidates to determine patterns of AED therapy before consideration of surgery.[18] Medical intractability was defined as seizures persisting despite treatment with trials of first-line AEDs (carbamazepine, phenytoin, sodium valproate); first-line agents as both monotherapy and in at least one combination; first-line agents using maximally tolerated serum AED concentrations or documentation of adverse drug effects limiting therapy; and one adjunctive or second-line therapy (if a child is stable), including benzodiazepines and methsuximide. Using this definition, 21 of the 72 children (29%) did not meet medical intractability criteria. The most common deficiency was failure to attain maximally tolerated serum concentrations with agents administered as monotherapy, which was documented in 15 cases. Correction of the criterion omission failed to produce a significant reduction in seizures in 19 children (90%), although two patients responded to high concentrations of carbamazepine monotherapy.

In infants and children with catastrophic epilepsy, the risk of frequent seizures often outweighs the risks and cost of surgical intervention. In a 12-year study of prognosis of childhood epilepsy in Sweden, 11 of 194 children died during the course of the study; all had active epilepsy.[19] Abnormal neurologic examination, mental retardation, and frequent seizures predicted a worse seizure outcome; only 20% of children having all three factors were free of seizures at study termination, compared with 37% with two factors, 63% with one factor, and 89% with none of the factors present. The risk of mortality was found to be 1 in 295 in a cohort of children and adolescents with severe epilepsy and learning disabilities.[20] These data highlight the importance of aggressive treatment and caution against the application of strict intractability criteria to infants and children with poorly controlled epilepsy.

Infants and children should be referred for surgical consideration when seizures continue despite adequate trials of the major AEDs (documentation of serum concentrations or intolerable adverse effects, or both) and seizures interfere with behavior or development. Patients with clearly defined lesions on MRI that can be completely removed with minimal risk should be considered for surgery even before multiple drug trials, because complete excision of the lesion has a high likelihood of eliminating seizures.[21] Furthermore, the impact of long-term AED therapy on cognition and behavior is unknown. Infants with devastating seizures due to hemispheric lesions, such as large perinatal infarction, Sturge-Weber syndrome, and hemimegacephaly, should be considered for early surgery to optimize cognitive and motor development. Rarely, patients with multiple lesions, such as tuberous sclerosis, are surgical candidates if it can be demonstrated that a single lesion is responsible for most or all of the seizures. Children with poorly controlled benign focal epilepsy must be excluded and differentiated from those with symptomatic focal epilepsy. This distinction is crucial, because seizures tend to remit spontaneously during the second decade of life in patients with benign focal epilepsy of childhood.

Establishing the Focus. Aside from determining medical intractability, establishing the focal nature of epilepsy is the earliest step in the consideration of surgical candidacy. In older children and adults, it is rarely difficult to demonstrate a focus when using the clinical history, seizure symptoms, video electroencephalogram (VEEG) evaluation, and neuroimaging. However, this proves to be a challenging task in some infants and young children. Seizures may be difficult to classify, and lateralizing features are often absent in very young patients.[22, 23] Similarly, the EEG may show generalized or multifocal epileptiform abnormalities, even in patients with focal epileptogenic lesions.[24–26] The studies of Chugani and colleagues demonstrating regional or lateralized hypometabolic defects on fluorodeoxyglucose F 18 (^{18}F) positron emission tomography (PET) or focal MRI lesions in children with infantile spasms with hypsarrhythmia highlight the importance of neuroimaging in infants and young children with seemingly generalized epilepsy based on seizure symptoms and EEGs alone.[24–26]

THE PRESURGICAL EVALUATION

As mentioned earlier, the goal of the presurgical evaluation is to demonstrate the focal nature of epilepsy by localizing the epileptogenic zone using the clinical history, ictal symptoms, ictal and interictal EEGs, neuroimaging, and neuropsychological assessment. A recommendation for surgery is made only when the epileptogenic zone is delineated and its complete removal is believed to have a high likelihood of alleviating seizures with minimal risk of neurologic compromise.

Video Electroencephalogram Monitoring

VEEG monitoring is the simultaneous recording of an EEG and clinical behavior, usually performed over several days in patients with paroxysmal disturbances of cerebral function.[27] The technique is useful in the differentiation of epilepsy and nonepileptic paroxysmal disorders, including syncope, cardiac arrhythmias, transient ischemic attacks, narcolepsy, and psychiatric disorders; for the quantification of seizures and interictal epileptiform activity in patients with epilepsy; and in the documentation of a response to therapeutic interventions. With few exceptions, the technology of VEEG in the pediatric population is the same as in adults.

The technical aspects of pediatric VEEG monitoring are reviewed elsewhere.[28]

In children with refractory epilepsy, VEEG allows the identification and localization of interictal epileptiform and nonepileptiform abnormalities and the correlation of clinical behavior with EEGs. VEEG monitoring is usually performed once seizures have continued despite appropriate trials of AEDs if a focal abnormality is suspected. Information obtained from the clinical history, including descriptions of auras and seizure symptoms; neuroimaging; and routine EEGs help guide electrode placement during the monitoring evaluation. Modified electrode placement over the suspected epileptogenic region and placement of sphenoidal electrodes increase the likelihood of detecting epileptiform abnormalities and enhance the precision of localization (Figs. 245–1 and 245–2). Special recording techniques are particularly helpful in the localization of focal epilepsy arising from deep or midline regions and in patients in which the epileptogenic zone is confined to a small area of cortex. Anterior temporal discharges are better defined using additionally placed electrodes designed to record from the basal or mesial temporal regions. Surface electrodes placed 1 cm above a point one third the distance between the external auditory meatus and the external canthus (T_1, T_2)—FT_9 and FT_{10} in the 10–10 system—or sphenoidal electrodes are most commonly used.[29] Sphenoidal electrodes are placed beneath the zygomatic arch approximately 2.5 cm anterior to the incisura intertragica, roughly 10 degrees superior to the horizontal plane and posterior to the coronal plane.[30] Sphenoidal electrodes are well tolerated, are relatively free of artifacts, and have a low complication rate. Closely spaced scalp and semi-invasive electrodes improve the yield of spike detection over the standard 10–20 system.[31] At least 16 channels of EEG are required during VEEGs, although most surgical centers record 32 or more channels.

During VEEG monitoring, withdrawal from anticonvulsant medication allows the expedient recording of habitual seizures without affecting their clinical and electrographic manifestations.[32] However, this may not be required in infants and children with frequent seizures. During behavioral events, trained hospital personnel interact with patients to assess level of consciousness, language, memory, and presence of focal neurologic sensory or motor deficits, if possible. These features may help establish the epileptic nature of an event, as well as assist in the localization and lateralization of seizures.

An understanding of the value of VEEG monitoring requires some knowledge of the localizing value of epileptiform abnormalities. The distribution of scalp-recorded epileptiform activity provides a reasonable estimate of the epileptogenic zone. However, spikes and sharp waves do not necessarily originate from cortical tissue directly beneath or even in the vicinity of the recording electrodes. Their distribution on the scalp is dependent on the recording technique, the spatial characteristics of the generator, the conductive properties of the surrounding tissue, and the duration and synchronization of an epileptic discharge.[33] Consequently, the distribution of interictal epileptic discharges and ictal patterns may fail to localize or even mislocalize the region or hemisphere of seizure origin. Epileptiform activity recorded from subdural or depth electrodes is frequently not seen on surface EEGs.[34] As a result, epileptiform activity, particularly when arising

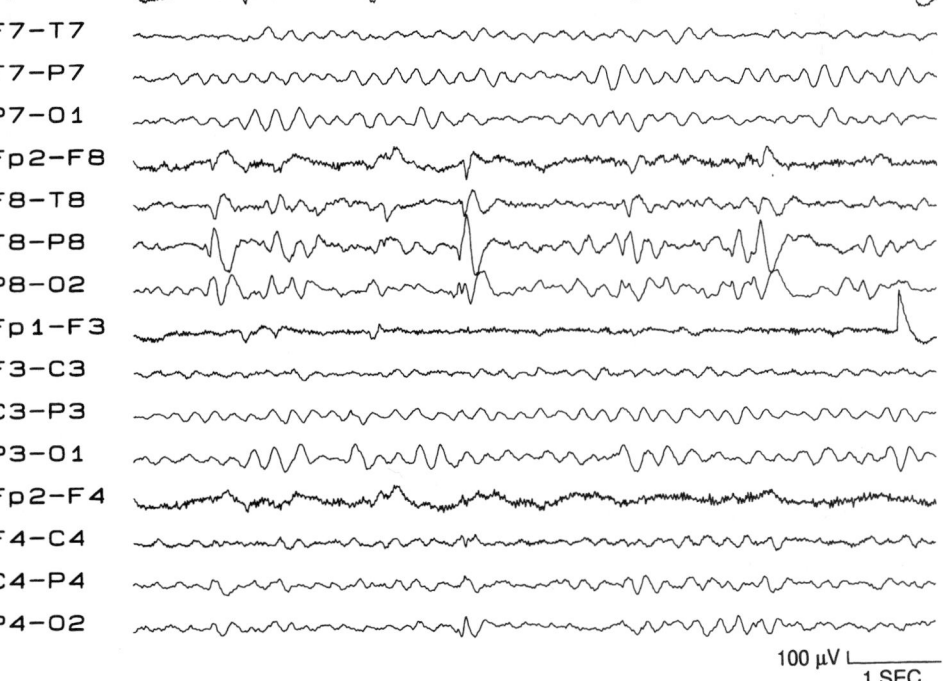

FIGURE 245–1. Interictal electroencephalogram (EEG) from an 8-month-old boy with seizures since birth. Seizures were characterized by bilateral eyelid blinking and clonic arm activity occurring 10 to 40 times per day and asymmetrical spasms. Focal slowing, decreased background activity, and frequent sharp waves in the right posterior temporal region maximal at the T_8 and P_8 electrodes are seen. (From Wyllie E [ed]): The Treatment of Epilepsy: Principles and Practice, 3rd ed. Philadelphia, Lippincott Williams & Wilkins, 2001.)

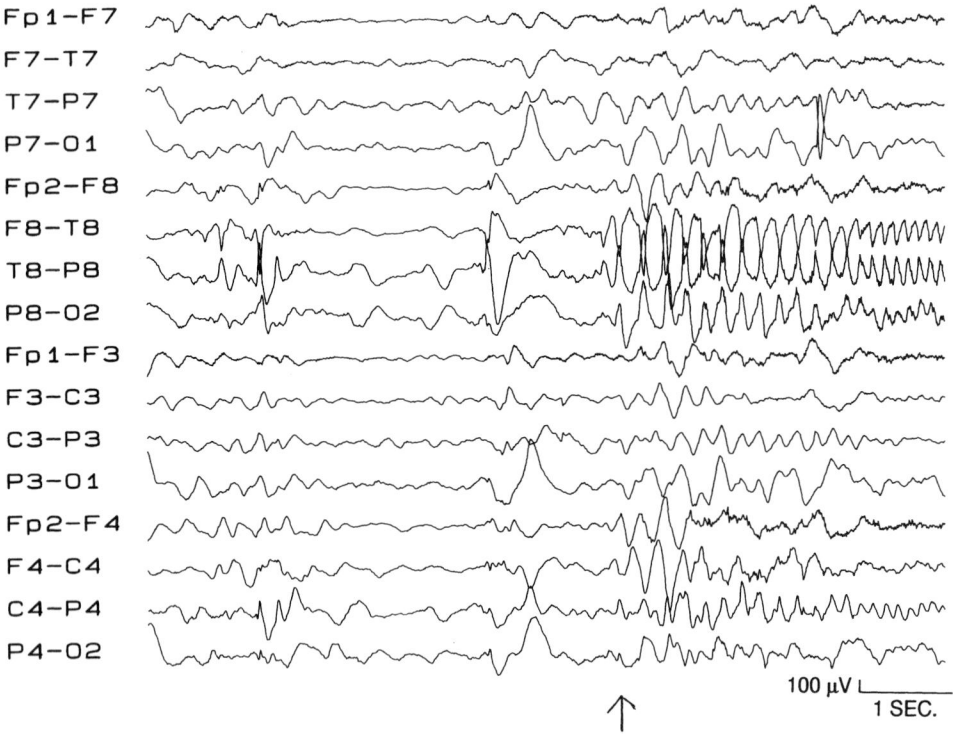

FIGURE 245–2. Ictal EEG of the same patient as in Figure 245–1. Bilateral eyelid blinking and clonic arm seizures were characterized by rhythmic theta activity in the right posterior temporal (T_8) region *(arrow).* (Adapted from Wyllie E [ed]: The Treatment of Epilepsy: Principles and Practice, 3rd ed. Philadelphia, Lippincott Williams & Wilkins, 2001.)

from deep regions, is apt to escape detection or appear widespread and of limited localizing value. The extent of interictal epileptiform abnormalities tends to be larger than the area of cortex from which a clinical seizure originates.[1] Nevertheless, interictal epileptiform activity generally provides more reliable localizing information than do ictal EEGs. This is because a seizure has usually spread outside the zone of ictal onset to contiguous or even remote areas by the time an ictal pattern is detected by scalp electrodes. Furthermore, seizures originating in functionally silent cortex produce symptoms only when the ictal discharge spreads to symptomatic areas that may be at some distance from the generator. The state of the patient, seizure type, and seizure frequency also affect the yield of the VEEG evaluation. Non–rapid eye movement sleep and sleep deprivation are potent activators of interictal epileptiform activity and seizures.[35, 36] Spike rate is increased during non–rapid eye movement sleep and reduced during rapid eye movement sleep relative to wakefulness.[37, 38] Spike rate increases markedly during the first 24 to 48 hours after a clinical seizure.[39, 40] Unlike sleep and sleep deprivation, hyperventilation and photic stimulation rarely activate epileptiform activity in patients with focal epilepsy. Epileptiform activity is more commonly observed in patients with complex partial seizures of temporal lobe origin, compared with epilepsy arising from deep or midline regions. This is particularly true when sphenoidal or additional scalp electrodes are used.

In addition to the EEG, seizure symptoms provide valuable clues to the localization of partial seizures. The International League Against Epilepsy defines partial (focal, location-related) seizures as those in which the first clinical or electroencephalographic manifestations suggest initial activation of a population of neurons limited to part of one cerebral hemisphere.[41] Partial seizures are further subdivided based on the presence or absence of alteration of consciousness. Simple partial seizures are those in which consciousness is preserved, whereas complex partial seizures are focal seizures with alteration of awareness. Focal clonic activity, unilateral dystonic posturing, postictal language disturbances, ictal speech, and automatisms with preserved awareness are helpful clues in the lateralization of focal seizures. Clonic activity of a limb or face and version (forced, unnatural turning of the head or eyes) occurring in the early part of a clinical seizure reliably predict seizure origin from the contralateral hemisphere in older children and adults, although version may be misleading in infants.[22] Unilateral dystonic posturing of a limb contralateral to the epileptogenic focus is observed in approximately 25% of patients with temporal lobe epilepsy.[42] Postictal language disturbances are predictive of epilepsy arising from the dominant temporal lobe, whereas ictal speech strongly suggests nondominant temporal lobe origin.[43] Ictal vomiting and automatisms with preserved responsiveness are less common manifestations of temporal lobe epilepsy, but both are believed to suggest nondominant temporal lobe origin.[44, 45] However, the localizing value of these behaviors is based almost exclusively on studies of adolescents and adults.

Seizure symptoms in infants and young children may differ from those in adults and adolescents. The current classification of epileptic seizures does not take into account the difficulty of classifying seizures in infants and children. It is often impossible to assess level of consciousness and amnesia in young patients, and infants and young children are unable to describe auras. To address these limitations, seizure classifications designed specifically for infants and young children have been proposed.[23, 42] Acharya and colleagues from the Cleveland Clinic studied seizure symptoms in 23 infants with focal epilepsy.[23] In their series, seven patients had seizures characterized by either an arrest or marked reduction of behavioral motor activity, with minimal or no automatisms and an indeterminate level of consciousness (hypomotor seizures), arising from the temporal or temporoparietal region. In 13 cases, localized or bilateral clonic, tonic, versive, or atonic seizures arose from the frontal, frontocentral, or frontoparietal region. Two infants with infantile spasms had epileptogenic zones in the frontal and temporoparietal regions. The absence of features of partial seizures that are typical in older children and adults, including automatisms and unilateral dystonic posturing, and the inability to assess level of consciousness in infants with partial epilepsy have also been reported by others.[22, 46] The presence of focal features, including asymmetrical spasms, partial seizures, hemiparesis, focal radiologic findings, and lateralized hypsarrhythmia, was strongly predictive of focal pathology in 66% of 66 infants with West's syndrome.[47] Of nine infants with West's syndrome who underwent epilepsy surgery, six became free of seizures, several of whom had diffuse hemispheric pathology due to malformations of cortical development. This finding highlights the importance of subtle, focal clinical and electroencephalographic manifestations during VEEG evaluation (Fig. 245–3).

When noninvasive VEEGs and neuroimaging fail to delineate the epileptogenic zone adequately, invasive electroencephalography may be indicated. The decision to proceed with invasive monitoring is made only when the noninvasive evaluation provides enough information to ensure that electrodes can be placed in or over the suspected ictal generator, that successful localization of the epileptogenic zone will lead to surgical resection that has minimal or no risk of significant neurologic sequelae, and that patient cooperation and maturity are sufficient to ensure safety and the attainment of the necessary data for surgical decision making. Consequently, very young patients and children with developmental delay are not ideal candidates for invasive evaluation. The morbidity of depth and subdural electrode placement in children and adolescents appears to be comparable to that in adults.[48]

Neuroimaging

Advancements in neuroimaging have had a major impact on pediatric epilepsy surgery. This is perhaps best exemplified by the growing numbers of infants and children undergoing surgery in whom seizure symptoms and EEGs failed to identify the focal nature of a seizure disorder but neuroimaging studies revealed a well-delineated epileptogenic lesion. Newer imaging techniques have also increased the appreciation of the varying types of pathologic substrates operative in infants and children with refractory epilepsy and how they differ from those seen in adolescents and adults. The reader is referred elsewhere for detailed reviews of the most widely used neuroimaging techniques in

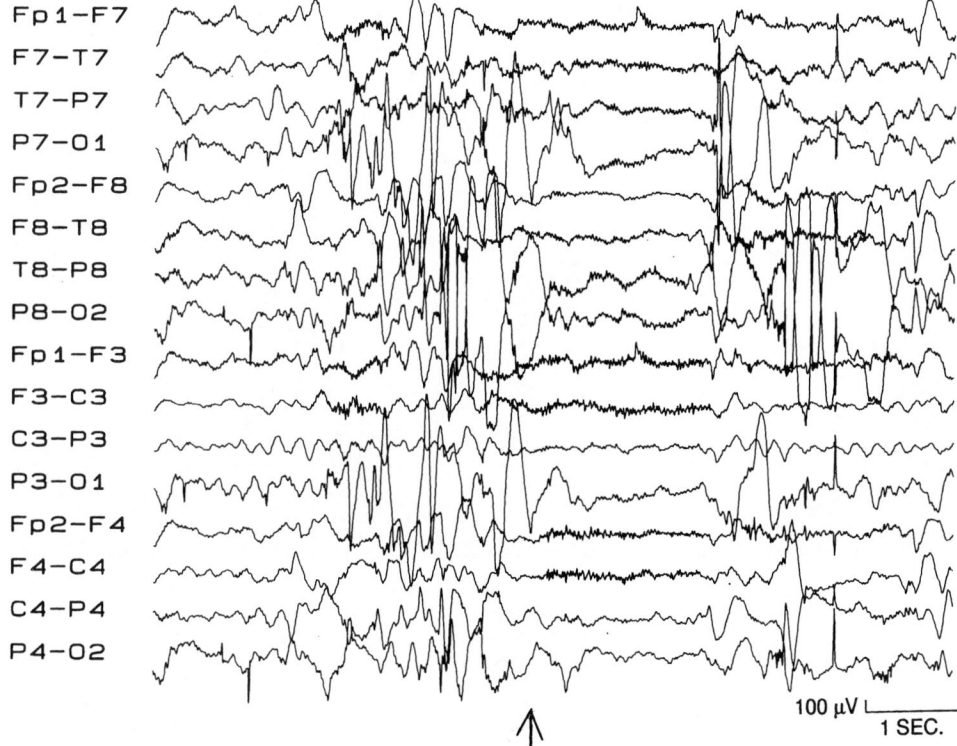

FIGURE 245–3. During asymmetrical spasms, the EEG of the same patient as in Figures 245–1 and 245–2 shows a diffuse electrodecremental response *(arrow)* preceded by myogenic artifact. (Adapted from Wyllie E [ed]: The Treatment of Epilepsy: Principles and Practice, 3rd ed. Philadelphia, Lippincott Williams & Wilkins, 2001.)

100 μV

1 SEC.

the evaluation of pediatric epilepsy surgery candidates.[49, 50]

Magnetic Resonance Imaging. MRI has essentially replaced computed tomography in the evaluation of patients with epilepsy. The greater resolution of brain parenchyma, the ability to image the brain in multiple planes without bony artifact, and the absence of exposure to ionizing radiation are major advantages of MRI over computed tomography.[49] Volumetric analysis of the hippocampus and fluid-attenuated inversion recovery sequences are now incorporated into the MRI protocol of virtually all epilepsy surgery centers. Fluid-attenuated inversion recovery enhances the appearance of small lesions in both temporal and extratemporal regions and improves the detection of malformations of cortical development and tumors that are common substrates of focal epilepsy (Fig. 245–4).

Positron Emission Tomography. [18]F PET measures cerebral glucose metabolism, which is reduced in the epileptogenic region in some patients with focal epilepsy. Temporal lobe hypometabolism is seen in more than 70% of patients with intractable temporal lobe epilepsy.[51] The extent of abnormality is usually larger than the epileptogenic zone, frequently extending into the ipsilateral basal ganglia, thalamus, and frontoparietal cortices. The yield of PET in nonlesional extratemporal epilepsy is significantly lower. However, PET may be especially useful in infants to identify regional malformations of cortical development that are difficult to appreciate on MRI[24–26] (Fig. 245–5). Owing to the short half-life of the isotope, ictal studies using ^{18}F PET are not feasible.

Single-Photon Emission Computed Tomography. Single-photon emission computed tomography (SPECT) is more readily available than PET because the technique uses commercially available isotopes and does not require an on-site cyclotron. The ligands that are now used include technetium 99m (^{99m}Tc)-hexamethylpropyleneamine oxime (HMPAO, Ceretec) and ^{99m}Tc-ethyl cysteinate dimer (ECD, Neurolite). Interictal SPECT reveals hypoperfusion in the epileptogenic temporal lobe in more than 50% of patients with temporal lobe epilepsy, although false lateralization has been reported in 10% to 20% of cases.[52] The resolution of SPECT is inferior to that of PET, and quantitative analysis is not available. The long half-lives of the isotopes

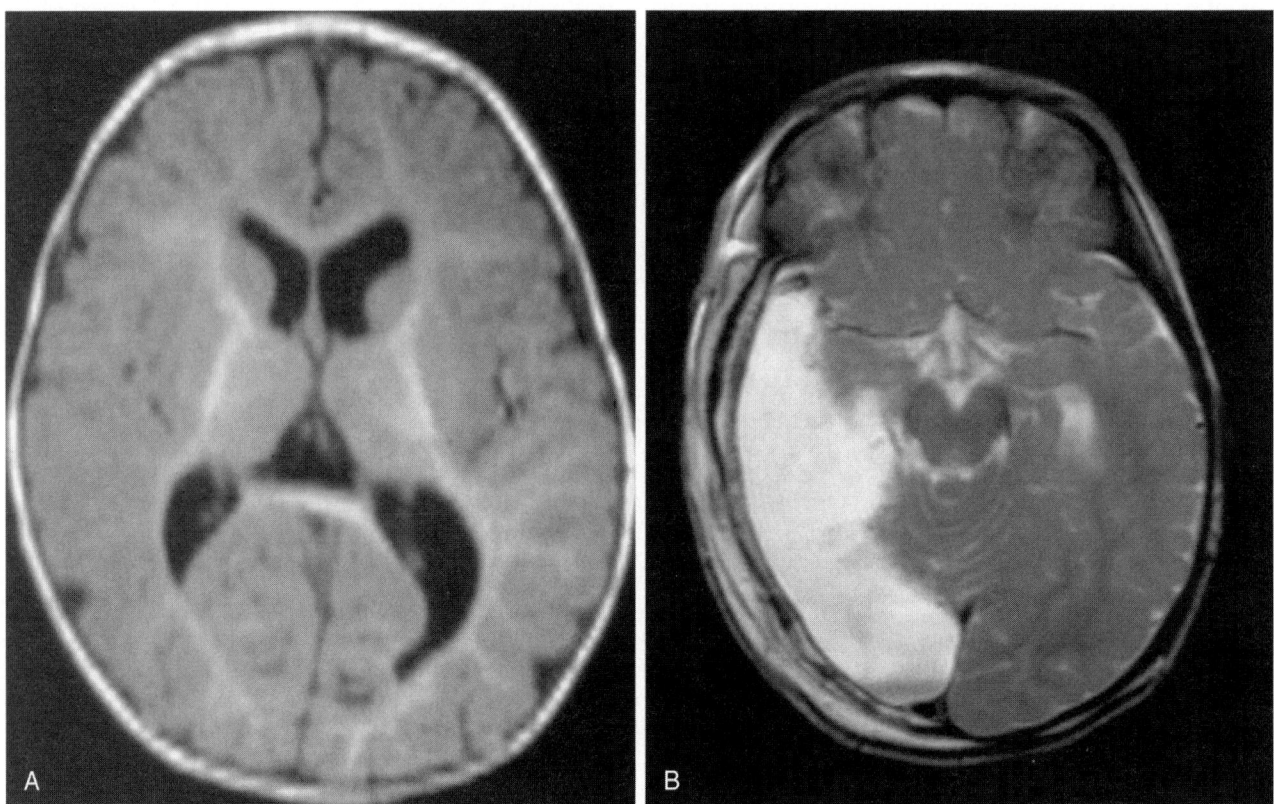

FIGURE 245–4. *A,* Preoperative axial magnetic resonance imaging (MRI) scan of an 8-month-old boy (same subject as in previous figures) showing a malformation of cortical development in the right temporo-occipital region. Decreased arborization of the white matter and thickened, poorly sulcated cortex were observed. *B,* Postoperative MRI shows evidence of a right temporo-occipital resection performed at 22 months of age. Fourteen months later, the child is still developmentally delayed but remains free of seizures and is no longer taking antiepileptic medications. (From Wyllie E [ed]: The Treatment of Epilepsy: Principles and Practice, 3rd ed. Philadelphia, Lippincott Williams & Wilkins, 2001.)

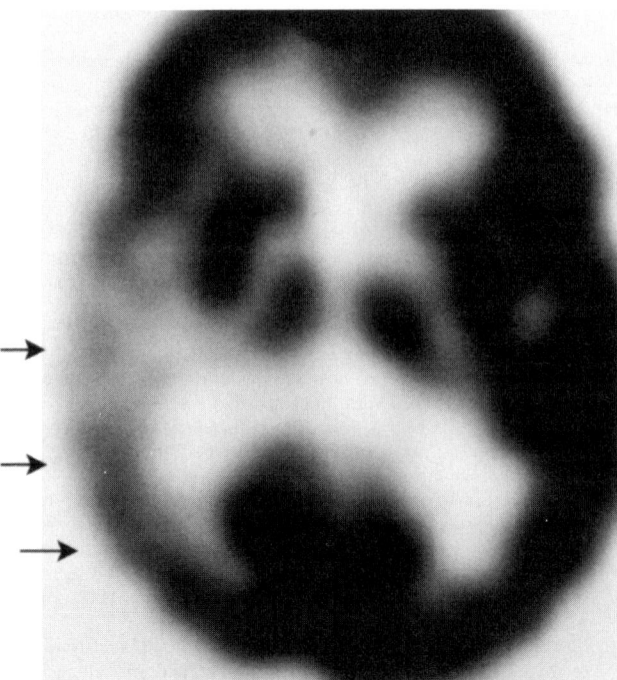

FIGURE 245–5. Fluorodeoxyglucose-18 positron emission tomography scan of the same patient as in previous figures, showing glucose hypometabolism in the right temporo-occipital region *(arrows)*. (From Wyllie E [ed]: The Treatment of Epilepsy: Principles and Practice, 3rd ed. Philadelphia, Lippincott Williams & Wilkins, 2001.)

make ictal and immediate postictal SPECT a useful noninvasive localizing tool. The results of ictal SPECT depend on the time of injection of the isotope from seizure onset. Under optimal circumstances, 65% to 95% of studies demonstrate hyperperfusion ipsilateral to seizure origin.[52] Delayed injections produce widespread hyperperfusion and a higher incidence of false lateralization. Abnormalities on ictal or interictal SPECT concordant with clinical or electroencephalographic localization were found in 73% to 93% of children with medically refractory epilepsy.[53, 54]

Magnetic Resonance Spectroscopy. Magnetic resonance spectroscopy is the newest technique being applied to patients with epilepsy. The technique measures a variety of metabolic markers, including *N*-acetyl-aspartate, which is present in neurons and is a marker of neuronal loss, and creatine, which is present in glial cells. Localized reductions in the *N*-acetyl-aspartate–creatine ratio are observed in and around the epileptogenic zone in patients with focal epilepsy, providing an additional noninvasive tool for seizure localization.

Other Methods. Additional techniques that are currently being investigated for their localizing value in epilepsy surgery candidates include functional MRI, diffusion-weighted MRI, and magnetoencephalography. These techniques have the potential to improve the noninvasive localization of epileptogenic cortex and reduce the need for invasive EEG recordings while increasing our understanding of plasticity in patients with epileptogenic lesions involving eloquent areas. It

remains unknown whether these modalities will assume an integral role in the presurgical evaluation of patients with intractable epilepsy.

Neuropsychological Assessment

In adolescents and adults, the presurgical neuropsychological assessment includes formal neuropsychological testing, the intracarotid amobarbital test for lateralization of language and memory, and a psychosocial evaluation. Formal neuropsychological testing consists of a battery of standardized tests that measure global intelligence, language, memory, and other cognitive faculties. Preoperative cognitive and language functioning is used to predict the risk of loss of function after a given type of surgery. Material specific memory deficits after temporal lobectomy have been reported extensively in adults and are more common after dominant hemisphere temporal resection.[55] Higher preoperative memory scores and absence of a lesion on MRI are predictive of postoperative memory deficits in adults.[56] The value of neuropsychological testing in predicting the outcome of epilepsy surgery in the pediatric population is unknown. However, a psychosocial evaluation, including an assessment of the goals of the patient or parents and any developmental and behavioral issues that may adversely affect outcome, should be performed in all pediatric epilepsy surgery candidates.

The intracarotid amobarbital test is performed routinely in adolescents and adults with temporal lobe epilepsy to identify the hemisphere of language dominance and establish whether the contralateral temporal lobe can support memory. Because the study is performed in an angiography suite and requires patient cooperation, this test is not performed routinely during the presurgical evaluation of infants and young children. However, in cases in which lateralization of memory or language is necessary to proceed with a recommendation for surgery, the modified intracarotid amobarbital test using pictures or pictures with simple words can be performed safely and effectively even in young children.[57]

CONCLUSIONS

Epilepsy surgery has become a treatment option for an increasing number of infants and children with intractable focal epilepsy. Epilepsy in young patients differs from that in adolescents and adults in a variety of ways, including causes, types of surgical procedures, goals and risks of surgery, and seizure symptoms. In appropriately chosen patients, epilepsy surgery can produce rewarding results, including dramatic improvements in seizure frequency, seizure severity, and neural development.

REFERENCES

1. Luders HO, Awad I: Conceptual considerations. In Luders H (ed): Epilepsy Surgery. New York, Raven Press, 1991, pp 1063–1070.

2. Wyllie E, Comair YG, Kotagal P, et al: Seizure outcome after epilepsy surgery in children and adults. Ann Neurol 44:740–748, 1998.

3. Adelson PD, Peacock WJ, Chugani HT, et al: Temporal and extended temporal resections for the treatment of intractable seizures in early childhood. Pediatr Neurosurg 18:169–178, 1992.

4. Duchowny M, Levin B, Jayakar P, et al: Temporal lobectomy in early childhood. Epilepsia 33:298–303, 1992.

5. Weiser HG, Engel J Jr, Williamson PD, et al: Surgically remedial temporal lobe syndromes. In Engel J Jr (ed): Surgical Treatment of the Epilepsies, 2nd ed. New York, Raven Press, 1993, pp 49–63.

6. Duchowny M, Jayakar P, Resnick T, et al: Epilepsy surgery in the first three years of life. Epilepsia 39:737–743, 1998.

7. Engel J Jr, Van Ness PC, Rasmussen TB, Ojemann LM: Outcome with respect to epileptic seizures. In Engel J Jr (ed): Surgical Treatment of the Epilepsies, 2nd ed. New York, Raven Press, 1993, pp 609–621.

8. Ventureyra ECG, Higgins MJ: Complications of epilepsy surgery in children and adolescents. Pediatr Neurosurg 19:40–56, 1993.

9. Vining EPG, Freeman JM, Pillas DJ, et al: Why would you remove half a brain? The outcome of 58 children after hemispherectomy—the Johns Hopkins experience: 1968–1996. Pediatrics 100:163–171, 1997.

10. Rasmussen TB: Surgical aspects. In Wise G (ed): Topics in Child Neurology. Englewood Cliffs, NJ, Spectrum Publications, 1997, pp 143–153.

11. Duchowny M, Jayakar P, Harvey SA, et al: Language cortex representation: Effects of developmental versus acquired pathology. Ann Neurol 40:31–38, 1996.

12. DeVos KJ, Wyllie E, Geckler C, et al: Language dominance in patients with early childhood tumors near left hemisphere language areas. Neurology 45:349–356, 1995.

13. Wyllie E, Bingaman W: Epilepsy surgery in infants and children. In Wyllie E (ed): The Treatment of Epilepsy: Principles and Practice, 3rd ed. Philapdelphia, Lippincott Williams & Wilkins, in press.

14. Asarnow RF, LoPresti C, Guthrie D, et al: Developmental outcomes in children receiving resection surgery for medically intractable infantile spasms. Dev Med Child Neurol 39:430–440, 1997.

15. Vasconcellos E, Wyllie E, Sullivan S, et al: Mental retardation in pediatric candidates for epilepsy surgery: The role of early seizure onset (submitted for publication).

16. Wilensky A: History of focal epilepsy and criteria for medical intractability. Neurosurg Clin N Am 4:193–198, 1993.

17. Dikman S, Matthews CG, Harley JP: Effect of early versus late onset of major motor epilepsy on cognitive-intellectual performance: Further considerations. Epilepsia 18:31–36, 1977.

18. Gilman JT, Duchowny M, Jayakar P, et al: Medical intractability in children evaluated for epilepsy surgery. Neurology 44:1341–1343, 1994.

19. Brorson LO, Wranne L: Long-term prognosis in childhood epilepsy: Survival and seizure prognosis. Epilepsia 28:324–330, 1987.

20. Nashef L, Fish DR, Garner S, et al: Sudden death in epilepsy: A study of incidence in a young cohort with epilepsy and learning difficulties. Epilepsia 36:1187–1193, 1993.

21. Awad IA, Katz A, Hahn JF, et al: Extent of resection in temporal lobectomy for epilepsy. I. Interobserver analysis and correlation with seizure outcome. Epilepsia 30:756–762, 1989.

22. Nordli DR, Bazil CW, Scheuer ML, et al: Recognition and classification of seizures in infants. Epilepsia 38:553–560, 1997.

23. Acharya JN, Wyllie E, Luders HO, et al: Seizure symptomatology in infants with localization-related epilepsy. Neurology 48:189–196, 1997.

24. Chugani HT, Shewmon DA, Peacock WJ, et al: Surgical treatment of intractable neonatal-onset seizures: The role of positron emission tomography. Neurology 38:1178–1188, 1988.

25. Chugani HT, Shields WD, Shewmon DA, et al: Infantile spasms. I. PET identifies focal cortical dysgenesis in cryptogenic cases for surgical treatment. Ann Neurol 27:406–413, 1990.

26. Chugani HT, Shewmon DA, Shields WD, et al: Surgery for intractable infantile spasms: Neuroimaging perspectives. Epilepsia 34:764–771, 1993.

27. AEEGS guidelines for long-term monitoring for epilepsy. J Clin Neurophysiol 11:88–110, 1994.

28. Mizrahi EM: Pediatric electroencephalography video monitoring. J Clin Neurophysiol 16:100–110, 1999.

29. Silverman D: The anterior temporal electrode and the ten-twenty system. Electroencephalogr Clin Neurophysiol 12:735–737, 1960.

30. King DW, So EL, Marcus R, et al: Techniques and applications of sphenoidal recording. J Clin Neurophysiol 3:51–65, 1986.

31. Morris HH III, Luders H, Lesser RP, et al: The value of closely spaced scalp electrodes in the localization of epileptiform foci: A study of 26 patients with complex partial seizures. Electroencephalogr Clin Neurophysiol 63:107–111, 1986.

32. Marciani MG, Gotman J: Effects of drug withdrawal on location of seizure onset. Epilepsia 27:423–431, 1986.

33. Jayakar P, Duchowny M, Resnick TJ: Localization of seizure foci: Pitfalls and caveats. J Clin Neurophysiol 8:414–431, 1991.

34. Abraham K, Ajmone Marsan C: Patterns of cortical discharges and their relation to routine scalp electroencephalography. Electroencephalogr Clin Neurophysiol 10:447–461, 1958.

35. Rossi GF, Colicchio G, Pola P: Interictal epileptic activity during sleep: A stereo-EEG study in patients with partial epilepsy. Electroencephalogr Clin Neurophysiol 58:97–106, 1984.

36. Ajmone Marsan C, Ziven LS: Factors related to the occurrence of typical paroxysmal abnormalities in the EEG records of epileptic patients. Epilepsia 11:361–381, 1970.

37. Montplaisir J, Laverdiere M, Saint-Hilaire J, et al: Nocturnal sleep recording in partial epilepsy: A study with depth electrodes. J Clin Neurophysiol 4:383–388, 1987.

38. Sammaritano M, Gigli GM, Gotman J: Interictal spiking during wakefulness and sleep and the localization of foci in temporal lobe epilepsy. Neurology 41:290–297, 1991.

39. Gotman J, Koffler DJ: Interictal spiking increases after seizures but does not after decrease in medication. Electroencephalogr Clin Neurophysiol 72:7–15, 1989.

40. Sundarum M, Hogan T, Hiscock M, et al: Factors affecting interictal spike discharges in adults with epilepsy. Electroencephalogr Clin Neurophysiol 75:358–360, 1990.

41. Commission on Classification and Terminology of the International League against Epilepsy: Proposal for revised classification of epilepsies and epileptic syndromes. Epilepsia 30:389–399, 1989.

42. Kotagal P, Luders H, Morris HH, et al: Dystonic posturing in complex partial seizures of temporal lobe onest: A new lateralizing sign. Neurology 39:196–201, 1989.

43. Gabr M, Luders H, Dinner D: Speech manifestations in lateralization of temporal lobe seizures. Ann Neurol 25:82–87, 1989.

44. Ebner A, Dinner DS, Noachtar S: Automatisms with preserved responsiveness: A lateralizing sign in psychomotor seizures. Neurology 45:61–64, 1995.

45. Kramer RE, Luders H, Goldstick LP, et al: Ictus emeticus: An electroclinical analysis. Neurology 38:1048–1052, 1988.

46. Duchowny MS: Complex partial seizures of infancy. Arch Neurol 44:911–914, 1987.

47. Kramer U, Sue WC, Mikati MA: Focal features of West syndrome indicating candidacy for surgery. Pediatr Neurol 16:213–217, 1997.

48. Kramer U, Riviello JJ, Carmant L, et al: Morbidity of depth and subdural electrodes: Children and adolescents versus young adults. J Epilepsy 7:7–10, 1994.

49. Zupanc ML: Neuroimaging in the evaluation of children and adolescents with intractable epilepsy. I. Magnetic resonance imaging and the substrates of epilepsy. Pediatr Neurol 17:19–26, 1997.

50. Zupanc ML: Neuroimaging in the evaluation of children and adolescents with intractable epilepsy. II. Neuroimaging and pediatric epilepsy surgery. Pediatr Neurol 17:111–121, 1997.

51. Henry TR, Chugani HT: Positron emission tomography. In Engel J Jr, Pedley TA (eds): Epilepsy: A Comprehensive Textbook. Philadelphia, Lippincott-Raven, 1997, pp 947–968.

52. Berkovic SF, Newton MR: Single photon emission computed tomography. In Engel J Jr, Pedley TA (eds): Epilepsy: A Comprehensive Textbook. Philadelphia, Lippincott-Raven, 1997, pp 969–975.

53. Cross JH, Gordon I, Jackson GD, et al: Children with intractable focal epilepsy: Ictal and interictal ^{99m}Tc HMPAO single photon emission computed tomography. Dev Med Child Neurol 37:673–681, 1995.

54. Lynch BJ, O'Tuama LA, Treves ST, et al: Correlation of ^{99m}Tc-HMPAO SPECT with EEG monitoring: Prognostic value for outcome of epilepsy surgery in children. Brain Dev 17:409–417, 1995.

55. Chelune GJ: Hippocampal adequacy versus functional reserve: Predicting memory functions following temporal lobectomy. Arch Clin Neuropsychol 10:413–432, 1995.

56. Chelune GJ, Najm I: Risk factors associated with postsurgical decrements in memory. In Lüders HO, Comair Y (eds): Epilepsy Surgery, 2nd ed. Philadelphia, Lippincott-Raven, 1999.

57. Szabo CA, Wyllie E: Intracarotid amobarbital testing for language and memory dominance in children. Epilepsy Res 15:230–246, 1993.

CHAPTER 246

Temporal and Extratemporal Lobe Resections for Childhood Intractable Epilepsy

GLENN MORRISON

Epilepsy has been recognized as a clinical entity for centuries, perhaps as early as 2080 BC.[1] The treatment of epilepsy has always included surgery, although the early attempts would be considered barbaric and futile by modern standards. Hippocrates spoke of epilepsy as a disease of the brain in about 400 BC.[2] In the ensuing thousands of years, much has changed, and it can now be emphatically stated that intractable epilepsy in childhood is a progressive and debilitating condition that should be treated aggressively.

Intractable epilepsy is defined as persistent seizure activity of such frequency or severity that it prevents the individual from normal function or development. This designation is made only after a satisfactory trial of multiple anticonvulsant medications, singly and in combination, for an adequate time, with documented therapeutic drug levels. Whereas patients with medically resistant epilepsy are a minority of seizure patients, they are significant users of medical resources. Attempts to control their seizures typically involve innovative medical or dietary regimens, but most remain medically resistant, and early seizure remission is rare.[3] Because the majority of patients with medically intractable epilepsy are identified in childhood, this is when an appropriate assessment using a comprehensive children's epilepsy program should occur.

In recent decades, there has been increasing interest in the surgical treatment of patients with intractable seizures.[4–6] The number of procedures performed at major epilepsy surgery centers between 1986 and 1990[7] was more than twice that reported before 1985.[8] This increase has been the result of technologic advances in neuroimaging and electroencephalography, new appreciation of the devastating personal and socioeconomic effects of recurrent seizures, delineation of surgically remediable epilepsy syndromes, and recognition of the long-term benefits of early surgical intervention. The use of surgical options increased exponentially in the 1990s,[9–12] and the trend will probably continue in the 21st century.

EPIDEMIOLOGY

The estimated lifetime cumulative incidence and prevalence of epilepsy are 3% and 0.5%, respectively, with approximately 60% of patients manifesting partial seizures.[13, 14] The prevalence of epilepsy in the United States was previously noted to be from 5 to 10 per 1000 population (0.5% to 2%).[15] In childhood, the incidence and prevalence of epilepsy are higher, and 90% of all new cases of epilepsy occur before age 20 years.[16, 17] Although most patients with new-onset epilepsy have few seizures or are well controlled, an estimated 5% to 10% of patients become sufficiently medically intractable to consider surgical therapy.[14, 18] Data from a Danish registry of unselected patients with partial epilepsy suggest that the cumulative incidence of intractable epilepsy is 135 per 100,000.[19] Intractable epilepsy is a major risk factor for personal injury, poor quality of life, and, in some instances, mortality. Further, recurrent seizures have a significant socioeconomic cost to the individual and society. The majority of children with chronic medically intractable epilepsy also have behavioral and cognitive disorders.[20–25] Considerable emotional stress and upheaval are present in the families of children with chronic seizures.[26–28]

Based on the previously mentioned data, there are at least 1.5 million people in the United States with epilepsy.[29] It has been estimated that as many as 5000 new patients annually in the United States might benefit from epilepsy surgery,[18] yet less than one third receive treatment at the major centers.[8] Underuse of epilepsy surgery is also apparent in other countries.[19, 30] Educating primary care physicians to refer patients with medically intractable epilepsy, instructing health insurers and government health agencies regarding reimbursement for epilepsy surgery, and refining epilepsy surgical protocols should increase the appropriate referral of patients with intractable epilepsy who may benefit from surgical intervention.

DIFFERENCES BETWEEN CHILDREN AND ADULTS

It is important to recognize that the treatment of children with intractable epilepsy is not the same as the treatment of adults with intractable epilepsy. Children are *not* "little adults." This is particularly apparent with regard to epilepsy and the surgical implications thereof. The common locations of the seizure loci are different in children; there are more extratemporal foci in children, and multilobar foci are more common.[31–33] The pathology is different as well; children have less mesial temporal sclerosis and many more developmental tumors (dysembryoplastic neuroepithelial tumors or gangliogliomas) and cortical dysplasias. In addition, the presentation, the underlying neuropsychological situation, and the previous, and thus subsequent, functional situations may be quite different. While age is an obvious difference, some of the social and familial issues may not be so readily apparent. Children have a "plasticity" that adults do not have; children can recover function that adults cannot.

SYMPTOMS AND SIGNS

Temporal Lobe

Epilepsy of temporal lobe origin, and especially mesial temporal lobe epilepsy, has been the sine qua non of the candidate for epilepsy surgery. Temporal lobe resections make up approximately two thirds of all procedures currently performed at epilepsy surgery centers, reflecting the predominance of adult patients with intractable temporal lobe epilepsy. As alluded to earlier, in pediatric epilepsy surgery centers, a greater proportion of patients undergo extratemporal, multilobar, and hemispheric resections.[31–33]

Some of the typical semiology of temporal lobe seizures may actually arise from extratemporal locations, especially in children. Typically, seizures of temporal lobe origin have auras and vegetative or visceral symptoms and a form of behavioral arrest with a motionless stare. These are simple partial seizures if there is no alteration of consciousness, and complex partial seizures if there is such an alteration. Associated automatisms and sometimes head turning and posturing are common accompaniments. Although temporal lobe epilepsy is often relatively easy to define electrically, extratemporal foci (which may cause identical symptoms) may be difficult to detect or localize with surface electroencephalograms (EEGs). This is particularly true if the extratemporal seizures spread rapidly to limbic structures, in which case the ictal manifestations mimic, and may be clinically indistinguishable from, temporal lobe epilepsy.[34, 35] Rasmussen[96, 102–105] recognized that extratemporal epileptogenic foci are considerably more variable in extent and topographic configuration than temporal lobe epileptogenic foci.

Frontal Lobe

There are several fairly distinct types of frontal lobe epilepsy.[27, 37–41] However, there can be considerable overlap, thus making it difficult to identify the seizure's exact origin. Typical complex partial seizures can originate from the frontal lobe,[37, 42, 43] but they are usually brief, occur in clusters, and are often nocturnal. They usually have motor signs that include motor automatisms,[44] dystonic posturing, head and eye deviation, and tonic, clonic, or atonic activity. There may be bipedal, bimanual automatisms and vocalization. Typically, there is minimal postictal confusion. When the seizure spreads to the temporal lobe, there is a mixed seizure pattern with characteristics of both lobes involved.

Seizures arising from the *cingulate gyrus* present with complex partial seizures, absences, and autonomic signs. However, they may also be manifested by generalized tonic-clonic activity[45] and even complex limbic automatisms, vocalization, and urinary incontinence.

Orbitofrontal seizures[46–49] may be complex partial seizures, along with motor automatisms, visceral sensory symptoms, and autonomic signs. If olfactory manifestations or hallucinations are present, they are helpful in localization. The episodes may begin with dystonic athetoid posturing of the arms associated with thrashing, kicking, and bicycling movements.[41] They may begin abruptly with arousal, may be nocturnal, and may involve trunk rotation, head deviation, vocalization, fear, and even screaming.

Lateral frontal (dorsolateral) seizure foci[50] involve tonic contralateral head and eye deviation, and there may be speech arrest. The seizures may begin with focal motor signs such as aversive head and eye deviation or tonic hand and face posturing. They have a propensity to spread and generalize.[51, 52]

Supplementary motor area seizures may also have speech arrest or hoarse vocalizations, but there is usually complex tonic posturing without loss of consciousness.[53] The tonic posturing of the contralateral limbs includes elevation of the shoulder, flexion of the elbow, and abduction of the arm. This has been likened to the fencing position. There may be associated aversive head and eye deviation.[54–57]

Seizures arising from the *motor* or *prerolandic area* are usually simple partial seizures with focal clonic activity, as recognized by Jackson.[58] *Opercular region* seizures are also often simple partial with clonic movements (face), and they may involve autonomic signs and speech arrest. Events such as olfactory auras, déjà vu or jamais vu phenomena, and auditory or visual phenomena preclude a frontal origin.[59]

Parietal Lobe

There have been reports of somatosensory auras and sensations,[60, 61] but other data suggest that seizures of parietal lobe origin are frequently silent until they spread to the frontal and central area (high parietal) or to the posterior temporal region (low parietal).[62]

Occipital Lobe

Simple or complex visual phenomena are usually indicative of occipital lobe seizures.[63, 64] Ictal amaurosis has been reported as the second most common symptom of occipital lobe epilepsy.[63] This has not been reported with temporal lobe epilepsy, but elementary visual symptoms have been described in patients with temporal lobe epilepsy,[65] especially if the focus involves the posterior temporal lobe.

Multilobar Symptoms and Signs

It is not uncommon for more than one lobe to be involved in children with intractable epilepsy. Frontal and temporal lobe involvement is fairly common, as is inferior temporal lobe involvement going posteriorly into the occipital lobe. It is important to remember that some clinical phenomena are not localizing; for example, gustatory hallucinations may involve the parietal operculum, the uncinate region, or the insula.[66]

DIAGNOSTIC STUDIES

Clinical

It is important that a comprehensive team of health care professionals be brought together to assess every child who may be a surgical candidate. This obviously includes a pediatric neurologist and pediatric neurological surgeon, each of whom takes a careful history and performs a physical examination. Additionally, a clinical neuropharmacologist is valuable to report on the pharmacokinetics of the various antiepileptogenic medications to be certain that the child is truly intractable. A clinical neuropsychologist is needed to evaluate the child and the family dynamics, to help establish realistic goals, and, on occasion, to provide clinical help that allows the child and family to work through the whole process. The other members of the comprehensive team include an electroencephalographer, neurophysiologist, neuroradiologist, and neuropathologist.

Electrical

Electroencephalograpy and electrocorticography are the basis for electrical diagnosis. Most centers now use hard-wired, closed-circuit, split-screen, 24-hour video EEG monitoring. Aside from standard montages (64 channel), closely spaced surface electrodes often prove helpful in localizing an epileptogenic focus. More invasive sphenoidal or nasopharyngeal electrodes are used much less commonly than in the past. Although interictal data are of value, there is controversy about whether the epileptogenic area in lesional cases can be sufficiently defined by interictal data alone.[67] Most centers rely on ictal information to devise a specific treatment plan for each child and to maximize the benefit derived from treatment.[11, 31] Several of the child's typical seizures are captured and studied carefully for reproducibility as well as localization.

Neuroimaging

The most valuable neuroimaging study, which is essential in every evaluation, is magnetic resonance imaging (MRI). Thin cuts with and without gadolinium are obtained through areas that are thought to be involved as a result of previous imaging studies or clinical semiology. The MRI scan has a focal abnormality in about two thirds of children with intractable epilepsy. Other abnormalities may be seen that are nonlocalizing, such as atrophy or multiple areas of cortical dysplasia. In cases with a focal abnormality (cortical dysplasia or developmental tumor), this can be very helpful, particularly if there is convergent information about the epileptogenic focus (electrical and semiology). Computed tomography has been relegated to specific roles, such as to judge the amount of calcification present or the presence of bony involvement.

Functional imaging is also important, but it is relied on to varying degrees, depending on the center's experience, availability of the testing mode, and so forth. Some centers have found positron emission tomography (PET) to be very helpful.[68–71] PET is a measure of metabolic activity and may lateralize an abnormality. This may help in evaluating a child with intractable epilepsy, but the studies are usually interictal and may lack the specificity required for precise cortical resective planning. PET correlates with video EEG and extraoperative monitoring with subdural electrodes, but because of its lack of specificity, PET is not necessary in the majority of cases. Snead and coworkers concluded that a child should not be excluded from surgical consideration if PET is normal and that most children require extraoperative monitoring regardless of the PET.[72] Ictal single photon emission computed tomography has been helpful on occasion.[73, 74] This is a measure of blood flow and, when obtained during a seizure, identifies the area of increased flow, correlating with an epileptogenic focus. It is thought that further refinements of these functional, metabolically active studies hold great promise for the future.[75] Additionally, noninvasive methods of identifying eloquent cortex (such as functional MRI studies) will become increasingly important. Some centers (mostly dealing with adults) have found magnetoencephalography helpful in evaluating patients for epilepsy surgery.[76, 77] Magnetoencephalography is based on the principle that a magnetic field generated by intraneuronal electrical current can be detected outside the head with highly sensitive biomagnetometers with superconducting quantum interference device technology.[78]

Decision Making

After everyone on the comprehensive epilepsy team has evaluated the child and the child has had sufficient ictal events recorded, the group meets to formally present the data and make a treatment decision. The decision may be that further testing or medication trials should be conducted, but any specific decisions should be agreed on. For the child to be a candidate for surgical intervention, he or she needs to be certifiably intractable, and the seizures must be coming from an area that can be surgically treated, with or without some preconceived (and agreed on) functional loss.

Next, the choice of operation is discussed. There

are certain clear indications for hemispherectomy and corpus callostomy, and these are dealt with elsewhere. There has been increasing interest in the use of vagal nerve stimulators for intractable epilepsy, but the follow-up data are still too limited to draw any worthwhile conclusions. Sometimes the data are so clear and convergent that a single surgical procedure is recommended. This is especially true for temporal lobe epilepsy when there is an abnormality shown by MRI and the clinical and surface EEG data all point to the nondominant temporal lobe. This may also be true for the dominant temporal lobe if the abnormality is thought to be medial and thus very unlikely to involve language. However, when language is a consideration in temporal lobe epilepsy, functional cortical mapping with precise epileptogenic focus identification may be required. This is best done via a planned two-stage operation with implantation of subdural electrodes[79, 80]—strips, grids, or both—and extraoperative electrocorticography monitoring and mapping.

Extraoperative monitoring or mapping is more likely to be necessary with extratemporal epilepsy than with temporal lobe epilepsy.[76] If a child has a well-defined lesion by MRI and the clinical and electrical data agree that this is the source of the epilepsy, the child can safely be operated on in one stage. However, if the evaluation reveals nonconvergent data or that functional cortical mapping is required, a two-stage operative plan is in the child's best interest. This reflects the difficulty in defining the epileptogenic zone in extratemporal epilepsy, wherein the focus is more often diffuse or ill defined and frequently involves eloquent areas.[34, 81–84] Although good results have been obtained with intraoperative electrocorticography[85] and functional cortical mapping in awake patients,[86] these are largely adult series, and the principles have much less applicability to children.[5]

SURGICAL INTERVENTION

History

Hippocrates suggested trephination on the side opposite a clinical seizure in 400 BC.[87] Although this was the first mention of the surgical treatment of epilepsy, Horsley is credited with performing the first operation designed specifically for seizure control. This was an extratemporal resection performed on May 25, 1886, at the National Hospital for the Paralyzed and Epileptic in London.[88, 89] Horsley correctly noted that in some focal epilepsies, part of the central cortex could be resected with good clinical results.[90] Clinical electroencephalography became available 43 years later,[91] and in 1935 human electrocorticographic studies were reported by Foerster and Altenburger.[92] Penfield, after spending time with Foerster in 1928, established his program at the Montreal Neurological Institute in 1929[34] and began reporting his experience operating on patients with intractable epilepsy.[93] A wealth of experience was gained thereafter by Penfield and others.[34, 94–98] Most of this experience was with temporal lobe epilepsy in an adult population.[34, 99–101] Whereas 32% of Penfield's 2177 operations were for extratemporal epilepsy (and 11% multilobar), Olivier and Awad's more recent series of 560 patients included only 14% extratemporal, with 2.5% being multilobar.[34] Most of these patients were adults. Sachs reported subpially resecting the central cortex,[36] and Rasmussen published several reports on extratemporal lobe resections,[102–105] but again, mostly in an adult population. Rasmussen also reported operations for intractable epilepsy arising outside the temporal or frontal lobe.[106, 107] Thereafter, a few reports involved operating on children.[108–110] The procedures were mostly temporal lobe resections,[17, 111–113] and the patients were mostly adolescents; very few children younger than 10 years of age received surgical treatment.[55] Falconer was an early champion of operating on young patients with intractable epilepsy.[109, 111, 112] He recognized that once the diagnosis of intractability was made, there was nothing to be gained from waiting, and in actuality, harm was being done. The concept of the plasticity of the young brain was being developed, such that if one operates early, there is a greater potential for functional recovery or attainment of functionality.[114–117]

By the 1980s the concept of operating on children with intractable epilepsy was fairly well advanced,[118–127] but it was not until the 1990s that very young children were recognized as surgical candidates.[128, 129] Indeed, there is no lower age limit at which a child should not be considered a surgical candidate[130, 131] if he or she has the clinical stigmata of intractability and the clinical constellation that predicts a reasonably good outcome.[132] The last decade saw an explosion of interest in the surgical treatment of epilepsy,[7, 9, 10, 12, 58] and the age at surgery has continued to fall.[128] In addition to the seizures per se, epileptic children and their families face a constellation of difficulties.[133] Therefore, as soon as a child has been diagnosed as having intractable epilepsy, he or she should be considered for a surgical procedure. The earlier surgery is done, the greater the likelihood that the child's functional and developmental potential will be maximized.[134] Thus, all children with intractable epilepsy should be evaluated by video EEG. If they have clear bilateral or multifocal epileptogenic discharges, they are not candidates for a resective procedure; perhaps a corpus callosotomy could be offered for drop attacks. Recently, use of a vagal nerve stimulator has been introduced,[135–137] and although there have been some promising results, only a few studies have been done on children.[138–140] Only long-term follow-up will determine the true place for the procedure.

If the child has a focal abnormality by MRI, there is convergent data by surface video EEG that this area is the epileptogenic zone, and functional mapping is not required, one can proceed with a one-stage resection with intraoperative electrocorticography. If, however, there is no lesion, it is not clear where the epileptogenic zone resides, or if functional mapping is required, a two-stage procedure should be considered. Children with intractable epilepsy that is nonlocalized by surface EEG but who have a reasonable chance of having a resectable area (perhaps intrahemispheric, cingulate, or orbital-frontal) should be considered for invasive monitoring.

One Stage

When the clinical, EEG, and neuroradiologic data are all convergent, the child may safely, and reasonably securely, undergo a planned one-stage procedure. The physiologic and anatomic limits of the seizure focus have been identified from clinical, scalp EEG, and neuroimaging information.[141] There remain, however, special considerations when operating on a child with intractable epilepsy.[134, 142] Anticonvulsants are usually continued until surgery.

The child is placed under general anesthesia. When electrocorticography or motor cortical stimulation is to be performed, propofol (Diprivan), less than 0.5% isoflurane, or both are recommended as the anesthesia. The skin incision is outlined. If the child has reasonably long hair, only the hair along the planned incision is shaved. Usually the outlined incision is considerably larger than that needed for the planned resection. This is done so that adequate electrocorticography or some form of mapping can be performed. Once the scalp flap is turned, the bone is elevated via standard neurosurgical technique. An osteoplastic bone flap is theoretically preferred to a free flap because of concerns about healing and infection. Therefore, the bone may be hinged on the temporalis muscle. Mannitol may or may not be given before opening the dura, depending on the circumstances. If a lesion has been identified by MRI, it may be helpful to use ultrasonography before dural opening to transdurally outline the lesion. This can be repeated after the dura is opened and may be used throughout the resection to assess its thoroughness. A frameless stereotactic system, if available, is also of value. Once the cortex has been exposed and viewed, any planned mapping or electrocorticography is performed. Various sized grids, strips, or both may be placed on the surface. Additionally, ground and reference electrodes are placed subgaleally. Rarely, a depth electrode is of some use or interest. This surface recording is not always necessary but may be helpful in confirming the information obtained preoperatively from scalp recordings. The electrical information obtained is, of course, usually interictal and thus not as helpful as ictal data.

If the partial epilepsy is associated with a discrete neocortical lesion (abnormal MRI showing tumor, vascular malformation, focal cortical dysplasia), the potential to cure the child's epilepsy is quite good with a minimum of electrophysiologic investigation and a localized resection. However, on occasion, the surrounding cortex may harbor occult pathology and be epileptogenic, necessitating a more thorough electrophysiologic investigation and a wider resection.[74, 143, 144] Foerster and Penfield reported reproducing the typical seizure via electrical stimulation of the cortex.[93] This is not recommended. Stimulation is used to functionally map the cortex and not to produce seizure activity, because even if the produced seizures are typical, which is rare, removing this cortex does not guarantee that the epilepsy will be cured. The central sulcus can usually be identified via phase reversal, as seen with peripheral stimulation (somatosensory evoked responses), or motor responses may be obtained by direct cortical stimulation. The motor responses may be motor movement or electromyographic activity. There is a direct relationship between the age of the patient and the probability of obtaining a motor response from direct cortical stimulation. It is very unlikely that a child younger than 1 year will give any response; thereafter, the response is fairly linear with respect to age.

The resection is then carried out. Magnification is usually employed, because it allows for a more careful pial incision and subpial resection. Interestingly, Horsley first described the technique of subpial dissection in 1906,[36] and it has continued to be the preferred technique of cortical excision. The ultrasonic aspirator is useful on occasion, but the carbon dioxide laser is no better than bipolar coagulation and suction. Of course, every attempt is made not to manipulate cortex that will not be resected. Often a corticectomy is the procedure of choice. Here the subpial resection is of the gray matter alone. The resection is carried down to the white matter, and the gyral folds are carefully followed into the sulci so that no epileptogenic cortex is left behind. Postresection electrocorticography is of some interest but rarely leads to further resection, so it is not routinely done. The usual careful closure is then performed.

Postoperative anticonvulsants are used. They may be the same drugs the child was taking preoperatively, or fosphenytoin may be given if oral intake is a problem. Within a few days, most children can be managed with a single anticonvulsant at a tailored therapeutic dose. Antibiotics are used intraoperatively and for 1 day postoperatively. Dexamethasone is used intraoperatively and weaned over 5 to 7 days postoperatively.

Two Stages

Two operative procedures are planned when it is necessary to obtain precise ictal data from the cortical surface or when functional cortical mapping is required.[145] This is especially true if language may be affected, because although some children can be operated on while awake, the electrical data obtained are interictal, and language mapping, while possible, is not as satisfactory as it is in an extraoperative setting. Moreover, the only way to accurately assess the interhemispheric cortex, cingulate gyrus, and orbital-frontal cortex (not to mention the mesial temporal structures) is with implanted subdural electrodes. Although epidural electrodes have been used and have been very helpful in seizure focus localization,[146] they cannot be used for functional cortical mapping; therefore, subdural electrodes are preferred.[147] Further, the use of subdural electrodes and extraoperative monitoring obviates the need for other forms of preoperative anatomic planning (e.g., angiography, callosal reference).[34] In cases in which there is a clearly demonstrable lesion (defined as a focal abnormality by MRI) and there are convergent clinical, electrical, and neuroimaging data, a single operation is often very successful. However, there is general agreement that nonlesional epilepsy requires intracranial electrodes to record ictal events.[11, 148]

The initial craniotomy is done as described earlier for a one-stage procedure. Operative details have been outlined by Uematsu.[149] The various strips and grids are placed on, under, or around the cortex as required. The electrodes may be made of either platinum-indium or stainless steel. The former are preferred because they are less prone to ionic deposition during current passage and are MRI compatible.

The placement of interhemispheric strips is sometimes aided by knowing the venous anatomy. This may be obtained preoperatively by the use of magnetic resonance venous angiography.

On occasion, depth electrodes are also used.[150] The position of these depth electrodes may be verified via intraoperative ultrasonography.[151, 152] The electrodes are brought out through separate stab wounds using a large-bore needle with a trocar. A record is made of the electrodes' placement. Some make a detailed drawing, while others use a photograph (digital or Polaroid). The strips and grids are sewn to the dura, if possible, to minimize the risk of postoperative movement. The electrode wires are sutured to the scalp, again to minimize movement. The subdural space may need to be enlarged to accommodate the electrodes. A piece of freeze-dried dura or other dural substitute is used for the duraplasty. This may not be necessary in all cases and is clearly related to the number of electrodes, the amount of dural shrinkage, and the fullness of the brain; however, it is done as a precautionary measure in most cases (see "Complications"). The bone flap is not fixed tightly to the skull but is loosely replaced. However, the temporalis fascia and periosteum are approximated to minimize tissue retraction. Postoperative radiographs show the electrode positions and are referred to if there is any concern about electrode movement during the monitoring process. Children with subdural electrodes are usually placed on an antibiotic and a low dose of dexamethasone and kept on these medications until after the electrodes are removed.

The child is monitored until several typical seizures are recorded. Modifications are made pertaining to long-term monitoring in the pediatric population.[153] Reduction of anticonvulsant medication may be necessary. This reduction is usually done slowly so as not to precipitate status epilepticus. Once an adequate number of seizures have been recorded, functional mapping can be carried out. Cortical mapping should not be performed before the typical seizures have been completely and adequately recorded, because the cortical stimulation may cause a nontypical seizure. The advantage of extraoperative cortical stimulation is that the child can be fully awake, in the presence of reassuring family members, and in a more relaxed atmosphere. The mapping can be repeated if the child tires or reproducibility is desired.

The response to stimulation may be motor, sensory, or language arrest clinically (a functional response) or electrically, as seen by an afterdischarge at a maximum of 15 mA. Pulse durations are increased in a stepwise fashion starting at 0.3 msec to a maximum of 1 msec. There is wide variation in the afterdischarge threshold among patients and among adjacent electrodes, so the stimulation protocol needs to individualized.[154–156] There is a linear age-related response threshold; the younger the child, the higher the threshold. Mapping of children younger than 4 years is difficult and at times ineffective.[157, 158] This does not preclude young children from surgical consideration, however. Immature cortex and nonmyelinated nerve fibers typically have longer chronaxies that shift the strength-duration curve to the right and therefore require longer pulse durations to be successful. Stimulation paradigms based on stepwise increments of both stimulus intensity and pulse duration converge to the tissue chronaxie and are usually effective for mapping children.[155] Sensorimotor response, in general, has a lower threshold than afterdischarges in nonfunctional areas. Additionally, epileptogenic areas have a lower threshold for afterdischarges and seizure production than do other regions of the brain.

Infants and children do not complain of pain or cry in response to stimulation. Thus, functional areas may be missed because of the absence of response to stimulation intensities at or below 15 mA. In older children, it is less likely that these areas could be missed because even though nonfunctional and nonepileptogenic regions have very high thresholds, the sensorimotor areas usually have a response threshold below 15 mA. The utility of subdural stimulation is limited in infants and children who are unable to cooperate. Here, a sensory response may be missed, as well as a negative motor response, and language cannot be assessed. However, with careful repetitive sessions, a reliable anatomic homunculus can usually be established.[159]

All dressings are done under a nursing protocol requiring sterile technique.[160] There is almost always some leakage of fluid around the electrodes, but it is rarely a problem. Further radiographs or scans can be done to confirm electrode placement and correlation with the electrical recordings and stimulations. On rare occasions, subdural strip electrodes move during the extraoperative monitoring time frame. The position of the electrodes is documented initially postoperatively and again before the second operation with radiographs. If there has been electrode movement, appropriate adjustments are made during the resective surgery. The previously obtained operative photographs or anatomic drawings are used as a template during the second surgical procedure. Some electrodes allow for thick-slice MRI wherein the electrodes can be well viewed on the cortical surface. This allows electrical data to be directly correlated with anatomy and helps in planning the resection.

After all the pertinent data are obtained, the child is re-evaluated by the comprehensive epilepsy team, and a decision is made regarding a planned resection. The extent of the planned resection is defined according to the electrical, structural, and functional data.[161] Ideally, all the ictal, secondary ictal activation, and prominent interictal cortex should be removed. This is especially important if a focal lesion was not seen on preoperative MRI. If this can be accomplished, the results are predictably quite good; conversely, if this is not possible due to the presence of eloquent cortex, the results are adversely affected.

After a surgical plan has been formulated, the child is returned to the operating room, and the craniotomy is reopened. Care is taken not to dislodge the electrodes. The area of the planned resection is cut out from the grid, and the resection is carried out as outlined for a single-stage resection. As noted before, postresective electrocorticography is not helpful in deciding about further resection and is rarely done. The resection is tailored, depending on the location and presumed pathology. Sometimes a corticectomy is performed with preservation of the white matter, and sometimes a more generous resection that includes white matter is carried out.

Rarely, the subdural electrodes are removed and no resective surgery is performed. This occurs if no epileptogenic focus can be found or if the epileptogenic focus involves an area in which resection would result in an unacceptable neurological deficit. What is unacceptable to one family may not be unacceptable to another family; thus, the term is relative and not absolute. A field cut is usually more acceptable than a language or motor deficit. But even these may be acceptable (especially in a child younger than 5 years) if the seizures represent a significant disability. The electrodes are also removed when the extraoperative monitoring reveals a more global or generalized discharge than anticipated (or bilateral independent discharges).

Additionally, a technique of *multifocal subpial transection* (MST) may be carried out. This technique, as put forth by Morrell and colleagues,[162] allows for the preservation of vertical axons in a given gyrus while disconnecting the horizontally projecting axons. Thus, an epileptogenic focus may still fire but not propagate and therefore have no clinical manifestation. This procedure is helpful when eloquent cortex is involved. Pial openings are made at 5-mm intervals on the side of a given gyrus, and a blunt instrument is passed across the gyrus to the other side and then brought up to the subpial surface. The instrument is then pulled back across the gyrus to the original opening and removed. An immediate ecchymosis identifies the transection. The instrument used consists of a heavy steel wire, the end of which is flattened and turned up at a right angle to the shaft for a distance of 4 mm. Various angulations allow for entrance into differently arranged gyri. When dealing with abnormally configured gyri, transections may be done at lesser intervals (e.g., 3 mm). This isolates an epileptogenic zone into segments that are not discharging but are functioning.[34] A deafferentation mechanism involving different fiber systems may contribute to the antiseizure effects of MST.[163]

Reoperation

Although it is not common, some children require reoperation sometime after the first procedure or procedures. If the child had a single-stage operation, the reoperation is not too difficult. If the child had electrodes implanted in the subdural space, the procedure can be quite tedious, because the pial surface densely adheres to the dura and often requires microsurgical dissection. This adherence is in contrast to other clinical settings, such as reoperation for a brain tumor, where the exposure can usually be done fairly easily.

PATHOLOGY

There are diverse pathologic substrates for childhood epilepsies (Table 246–1). In virtually every case examined, there is some abnormality.[164] Many of these abnormalities, especially in nonlesional cases, are of the migrational type, wherein neurons have not migrated to where they should have, or there are other developmental abnormalities such as cortical dysplasia. There may be degeneration or absence of neurons, neuronal ectopias or heterotopias, or gliosis. In lesional cases (a *lesion* is defined as a focal abnormality seen on MRI), all these abnormalities may be seen, and a number of developmental tumors must be considered as well. Dysembryoplastic neuroepithelial tumors have been recognized as being very epileptogenic, as have gangliogliomas and gangliocytomas. Cortical dysplasia in and of itself can be epileptogenic. Regardless of the scans, there is usually a pathologic substrate for the epileptogenic foci, and, commonly, more than one pathologic abnormality will be found.[11, 165–168] Hippocampal sclerosis, which is common in adults, is much less common in children but has been reported in a child as young as 12 months.[169] As more experience is gained with epilepsy surgery in childhood, the even-

TABLE 246–1 ■ Pathology of Childhood Epilepsy

Cortical dysplasia
Developmental
  Neuronal
    Heterotopia
    Ectopia
    Degeneration or loss
  Schizencephaly
  Hemimegalencephaly
  Pachygyria
  Polymicrogyria
  Dyslamination
Atrophic/sclerotic
Gliosis
Neurocutaneous disorder
  Sturge-Weber syndrome
  Tuberous sclerosis
Tumors
  Dysembryoblastic neuroepithelial tumor
  Gangliocytoma
  Ganglioglioma
  Hamartoma
Vascular
  Infarct (encephalomalacia)
  Malformation
Inflammation
  Encephalitis

tual pathologic substrate may be correlated preoperatively with the diagnostic MRI.[168]

RESULTS AND OUTCOME

Results are generally reported in terms of the percentage of seizure relief and the length of time since surgery.[170] Engel and coworkers proposed a classification of I to IV.[171] Class I is seizure free, but whereas some authors require 100% absence of seizures,[129] Engel allows "nondisabling simple partial seizures" and "generalized convulsion with antiepileptic drug withdrawal." Class II is a "rare disabling seizure." This class equates with a 90% reduction of seizures, with most occurring nocturnally. Class III is "worthwhile improvement," equivalent to a 50% reduction in seizure frequency. Class IV is "no worthwhile improvement," which equates with a less than 50% reduction in seizure frequency.

An additional feature is the functionality of the child. This is especially applicable when the resection of eloquent cortex would result in loss of function. Behavioral improvement further strengthens the argument for early operation in children with intractable epilepsy, whether the seizure focus is inside or outside the temporal lobe.[172, 173] It is unusual for a patient to achieve a normal lifestyle after surgery without being seizure free.[174] Quality-of-life issues are difficult to assess but are related to the degree of improvement after epilepsy surgery.[165] Frequently, behavior, socialization, and higher cognitive functions improve after a cortical resection with elimination of seizure activity and reduction of anticonvulsant medication. Whether these favorable changes are due to the absence of seizures or the reduction in medication (or both) is difficult to assess. Paradoxically, curative epilepsy surgery may create unanticipated psychosocial problems due to newly acquired independence or upward vocational mobility.[175] The psychosocial benefits of epilepsy surgery[176–178] have been better defined for temporal lobe surgery than for extratemporal surgery, but the principles are similar.[173, 179]

The majority of children who are surgically treated for intractable epilepsy undergo a focal cortical resection (as differentiated from a lobar or hemispheric resection). Although the temporal lobe is the single most involved lobe, the frontal lobe (in contrast to an adult series) is involved almost as frequently. Extratemporal resections as a group represent the majority of resections.

The results of cortical resection for intractable epilepsy are that about 50% to 67% of the children are seizure free, and about 75% to 85% receive some benefit from the operative procedure with a mean follow-up of 3 years. Although temporal lobe resections provide better results than extratemporal resections, the differences are marginal in most series. However, there are significant differences among reported resective series. In a series of 200 children undergoing resective surgery, 71% were seizure free, and 90% had some benefit from surgery.[180] Virtually all children in a small series were helped by temporal lobectomy without invasive EEG.[181] Interestingly, children (*n* = 46) with temporal lobectomies may do much better (76% Engel class I and 96% improved) than adults (*n* = 193; 53% Engel class I and 84% improved).[182] Temporal lobectomies may be done in early childhood with good results (69% seizure free and 90% improved).[153] It appears that temporal lobe surgery is cost-effective in the adult population,[183, 184] and this is probably more true for children so treated.

Goldring reported significant improvement in 63% of children undergoing extratemporal resections.[123] Zentner and colleagues reported that 86% of extratemporal resection patients received some benefit from the surgery.[11] This number compares favorably with Engel and coworkers' survey of 1098 extratemporal resections.[171] The best determinant of seizure relief is the completeness of the excision of the epileptogenic focus.[11] If a lesion is present and it can be totally removed, the reported results are excellent. Some authors report that only the lesion needs to be resected,[146, 185] while others emphasize the need to resect associated epileptogenic cortex.[145, 186–189] On occasion, it is necessary to remove some adjacent epileptogenic cortex as well as the lesion itself.[143, 144]

In children with lesions, three quarters become seizure free following surgery, and in those without lesions, only slightly more than half become seizure free.[190] In nonlesional temporal and extratemporal cases, it is even more imperative to remove the entire epileptogenic focus (the ictal focus, any secondary ictal activation, and any prominent interictal focal abnormality).[190] Awad and colleagues reported excellent results (mostly in adults): 94% seizure free with total excision of a lesion, 83% seizure free with incomplete lesion excision but complete seizure focus excision, and 52% seizure free with incomplete lesion excision and incomplete seizure focus excision.[191] If the entire epileptogenic focus can be removed, more than 95% will receive some benefit, and 75% will be seizure free; if eloquent cortex precludes a complete epileptogenic resection, less than 15% will be seizure free, and less than 50% will receive some benefit.[190] Therefore, although patients may benefit from incomplete seizure focus resection or incomplete lesion resection, the goal of surgery should be to remove both as completely as possible. This tenet is independent of the lobe of seizure origin or the underlying pathology.

The use of MST may increase the percentage of seizure freedom in cases in which eloquent cortex is involved and a permanent deficit is not acceptable. Initially, most MST procedures were done in conjunction with a cortical resection, so it was difficult to know whether to ascribe the results to the resection or the MST. Now, however, more patients are being treated with MST alone, and over time, the true contribution of MST will be better known. Complete seizure control is rare when MST is done without resection.[192] Further, MST commonly results in functional deficits; these deficits are usually transient, but they need to be anticipated. The results appear to be independent of the pathology or the lobe of origin.[74]

TABLE 246-2 ■ **Complications of Childhood Epilepsy Surgery**

Neurological
  Cognitive, level of consciousness
  Weakness
  Sensory deficit
  Visual field deficit
  Language dysfunction
Bleeding
  Intraoperative
  Postoperative
    Parenchymal
    Extraparenchymal
Inflammatory
  Wound
  Bone
  Brain
Seizures

COMPLICATIONS

As with any surgical procedure, there are a number of complications of epilepsy surgery in childhood.[143, 193–196] The reported mortality is less than 0.5%,[196] and the morbidity is between 5% and 10%.[74, 118, 123, 196] Surgical complications include cerebral infarction, intracranial hemorrhage or infection, cranial nerve or cortical injury, subdural or subgaleal fluid collections, and a spectrum of new neurological deficits (Table 246–2). The deficits may be temporary or permanent. Children implanted with electrodes may begin to deteriorate neurologically and require a return to the operating room sooner than anticipated. This risk may be reduced by using a duraplasty and treating the children with steroids. Infectious complications are usually reduced as experience increases. Early reports included mortality rates of 12%,[146] and only 37% of the patients operated on where helped by the surgical procedure. Rasmussen's series of frontal resections included an operative mortality of 2%.[29] Even current series report complication rates as high as 10%.[11] Therefore, it is imperative that families be fully informed before surgery is undertaken.

CONCLUSIONS

Children with intractable epilepsy should be evaluated by a comprehensive epilepsy center as soon as the diagnosis is made. An aggressive approach is justified in light of the strong evidence that, if untreated, the child will not do well functionally or socially. Although temporal resections are important in children, extratemporal cortical resections play a much larger role in the treatment of children with intractable epilepsy than they do in the adult population. Children frequently require two operative procedures to maximize the clinical results. They may need the placement of subdural electrodes so that the epileptogenic focus can be precisely identified with ictal recordings in an extraoperative setting, and so that functional cortical mapping

can be carried out. As more experience is gained with the surgical treatment of childhood epilepsy and new modalities are introduced, the results will continue to improve. This will be further aided by the development of better neuroimaging that includes more precise functional and metabolic scanning. There are significant complications associated with epilepsy surgery, but considering the alternative, they are acceptable. Finally, as the medical and lay public better understands the consequences of intractable epilepsy in childhood, children will be referred to comprehensive epilepsy centers at younger and younger ages.

REFERENCES

1. Wilder BJ, Bruni J: Seizure Disorders. New York, Raven Press, 1981, pp 1–3.
2. Chadwick J, Manon W (trans): The Sacred Disease in the Medical Works of Hippocrates. Oxford, Blackwell Scientific, 1950.
3. Huttenlocher PR, Hapke RJ: A follow-up study of intractable seizures in childhood. Ann Neurol 28:699–705, 1990.
4. Duchowny M: Surgery for intractable epilepsy: Issues and outcome. Pediatrics 84:886–894, 1989.
5. Resnick T: Evaluation of children for epilepsy surgery. Int Pediatr 3:136–142, 1988.
6. Zupanc ML: Update on epilepsy in pediatric patients. Mayo Clin Proc 71:899–916, 1996.
7. Second Palm Desert Conference on Surgical Treatment of the Epilepsies, American Epilepsy Society, Palm Desert, Calif, February 18–24, 1992.
8. Engel J Jr, Shevmon DA: Who should be considered a surgical candidate? In Engel J Jr (ed): Surgical Treatment of the Epilepsies. New York, Raven Press, 1993, pp 23–24.
9. Engel J Jr (ed): Surgical Treatment of the Epilepsies. New York, Raven Press, 1993.
10. Ludders HO (ed): Epilepsy Surgery. New York, Raven Press, 1992.
11. Zentner J, Hufnagel A, Ostertun B, et al: Surgical treatment of extratemporal epilepsy: Clinical, radiologic, and histopathologic findings in 60 patients. Epilepsia 37:1072–1080, 1996.
12. Adelson PD, Black PM: Surgical treatment of epilepsy in children. Neurosurg Clin N Am 6, 1995.
13. Hauser WA, Annegers JF, Kurland LT: Prevalance of epilepsy in Rochester, Minnesota: 1940–1980. Epilepsia 32:429–445, 1991.
14. Hauser WA: The natural history of seizures. In Wyllie E (ed): The Treatment of Epilepsy: Principles and Practice. Philadelphia, Lea & Febiger, 1993, pp 165–170.
15. Hauser WA, Kurlan LT: The epidemiology of epilepsy in Rochester, Minnesota, 1935–1967. Epilepsia 16:1–66, 1975.
16. O'Donohoe NV: Epilepsies of Childhood. Boston, Butterworth, 1985, p 4.
17. Davidson S, Falconer MA: Outcome of surgery in children with temporal lobe epilepsy. Lancet 1:1260–1263, 1975.
18. NIH Consensus Conference: Surgery for epilepsy. JAMA 264:729–733, 1990.
19. Mackenzie RA, Matheson JM, Smith JS, Dwyer M: Surgery for refractory epilepsy. Med J Aust 153:69–76, 1990.
20. Lindsay J, Ounsted C, Richards P: Long-term outcome in children with temporal lobe seizures. V. Indications and contraindications for neurosurgery. Dev Med Child Neurol 26:25–32, 1984.
21. Ounsted C, Lindsay J, Norman R: Biological Factors in Temporal Lobe Epilepsy, No. 22. London, The Spastics Society Medical Education and Information Unit in association with William Heinemann Medical Books, Ltd. 1966.
22. Flor-Henry P: Ictal and interictal psychiatric manifestations in epilepsy: Specific or non-specific? A critical review of some of the evidence. Epilepsia 13:767–772, 1972.
23. Kaminer Y, Apter A, Aviv A, et al: Psychopathology and temporal lobe epilepsy in adolescents. Acta Psychiatr Scand 77:640–644, 1988.
24. Bourgeois BF, Prensky AL, Palkes HS, et al: Intelligence in

epilepsy: A prospective study in children. Ann Neurol 14:438–444, 1983.

25. Rodin EA, Schmaltz S, Twitty G: Intellectual functions of patients with childhood-onset epilepsy. Dev Med Child Neurol 28: 25–33, 1986.

26. Hoare P: Psychiatric disturbances in the families of epileptic children. Dev Med Child Neurol 26:14–19, 1984.

27. Williamson PD, Wieser HG, Delgado-Escueta A: Clinical characteristics of partial seizure. In Engel J Jr (ed): Surgical Treatment of the Epilepsies. New York, Raven Press, 1987, pp 101–121.

28. Mims J: Self-esteem, behavior, and concerns surrounding epilepsy in siblings of children with epilepsy. J Child Neurol 12: 187–192, 1997.

29. Hauser WA, Hesdorffer DC: Epilepsy: Frequency, Causes and Consequences. New York, Demos, 1990, pp 21–28.

30. Polkey CE: Surgical treatment of epilepsy. Lancet 336:553–555, 1990.

31. Morrison G, Duchowny M, Resnick T, et al: Epilepsy surgery in childhood. Pediatr Neurosurg 18:291–297, 1990.

32. Wyllie E: Cortical resection for children with epilepsy. Perspectives in pediatrics. Am J Dis Child 145:314–320, 1991.

33. Holmes GL: Surgery for intractable seizures in infancy and early childhood. Neurology 43(Suppl 5):s28–s37, 1993.

34. Olivier A, Awad I: Extratemporal resection. In Engel J Jr (ed): Surgical Treatment of the Epilepsies, 2nd ed. New York, Raven Press, 1993, pp 489–500.

35. Schneider RC, Crosby EC, Farhat SM: Extratemporal lesions triggering the temporal-lobe syndrome. J Neurosurg 22:246–263, 1964.

36. Sachs E: The subpial resection of the cortex in the treatment of jacksonian epilepsy (Horsley operation) with observations on areas 4 and 6. Brain 58:492–523, 1935.

37. Delgado-Escueta AV, Swartz B, Maldonado H, et al: Complex partial seizures of frontal lobe origin. In Wieser HD, Elger CE (eds): Presurgical Evaluation of Epileptics: Basics, Techniques, Implications. New York, Springer-Verlag, 1987, pp 268–299.

38. Penfield WG, Jasper H: Epilepsy and the Functional Anatomy of the Human Brain. Boston, Little, Brown, 1954.

39. Penfield WG, Kristiansen K: Epileptic Seizure Patterns. Springfield, Ill, Charles C Thomas, 1951.

40. Geier S, Bancaud J, Talairach J, et al: The seizures of frontal lobe epilepsy: A study of clinical manifestations. Neurology 27: 951–958, 1977.

41. Resnick T: Seizures of frontal lobe origin: Clinical semiology. Int Pediatr 9(Suppl 1):78–84, 1944.

42. Williamson PD, Spencer DD, Spencer SS, et al: Complex partial seizures of frontal lobe origin. Ann Neurol 18:497–504, 1985.

43. Waterman K, Purves SJ, Kosaka B, et al: An epileptic syndrome caused by mesial frontal lobe foci. Neurology 37:577–582, 1987.

44. Geier S, Bancaud J, Talairach J, et al: Automatisms during frontal lobe epileptic seizures. Brain 99:447–458, 1976.

45. Mazars G: Cingulate gyrus epileptogenic foci as an origin for generalized seizures. In Gastaut H, Bancaud J, Waltregny A (eds): The Physiopathogenesis of the Epilepsies. Springfield, Ill, Charles C Thomas, 1969, pp 186–189.

46. Ludwig B, Ajmone-Marsan C, Van Buren J: Cerebral seizures of probable orbitofrontal origin. Epilepsia 16:141–158, 1975.

47. Tharp BR: Orbital frontal seizures: A unique electroencephalographic and clinical syndrome. Epilepsia 13:627–642, 1972.

48. Pinard JM, Duchowny M, Resnick T, et al: Clinical features of orbitofrontal seizures in young children. Epilepsia 32(Suppl 3): 32–71, 1991.

49. Tharp BR: Orbital frontal seizures: A unique electroencephalographic and clinical syndrome. Epilepsia 13:627–642, 1972.

50. Quesney LF, Constain M, Rasmussen T: Seizures from the dorsolateral frontal lobe. In Chauvel P, Delgado-Escueta AV, Halgren E, et al (eds): Frontal Lobe Seizures and Epilepsies: Advances in Neurology. New York, Raven Press, 1992, pp 233–244.

51. Bancaud J, Talairach J: Clinical semiology of frontal lobe seizures. In Chauvel P, Delgado-Escueta AV, Halgren E, et al (eds): Frontal Lobe Seizures and Epilepsies: Advances in Neurology. New York, Raven Press, 1992, p 57.

52. Sutherling WW, Risinger MW, Crandall PH, et al: Focal functional anatomy of dorsolateral seizures. Neurology 40:87–98, 1990.

53. Morris HH, Dinner DS, Luders H, et al: Supplementary motor seizures: Clinical and electroencephalographic findings. Neurology 38:1075–1082, 1988.

54. Ajmone-Marsan C, Ralson BL: The Epileptic Seizure: Its Functional Morphology and Diagnostic Significance. Springfield, Ill, Charles C Thomas, 1957.

55. Penfield W, Welch K: The supplementary motor area of the cerebral cortex: A clinical and experimental study. Arch Neurol Psychiatry 66:289–317, 1951.

56. Wieser HG: Stereo electroencephalographic correlates of focal motor seizures. In Speckman EJ, Elger CE (eds): Epilepsy and the Motor System. Baltimore, Urban & Schwarzenberg, 1983, pp 287–309.

57. VanBuren JM, Fedio P: Functional representation on the medial aspect of the frontal lobes in man. J Neurosurg 44:275–289, 1976.

58. Jackson JH: Selected Writings of John Hughlings Jackson. London, Staples Press, 1931.

59. Morris HH: Frontal lobe epilepsies. In Luders HO (ed): Epilepsy Surgery. New York, Raven Press, 1992, pp 157–165.

60. Williamson PD, Boon PA, Thadani VM, et al: Parietal lobe epilepsy: Diagnostic considerations and results of surgery. Ann Neurol 31:193–201, 1992.

61. Palmini A, Gloor P: The localizing value of auras in partial seizures: A prospective and retrospective study. Neurology 42: 801–808, 1992.

62. Resnick T, Duchowny M, Jayakar P, et al: Clinical semiology of parietal epilepsy. Epilepsia 34(Suppl 6):29, 1993.

63. Williamson PD, Thadani VM, Darcey TM, et al: Occipital lobe epilepsy: Clinical characteristics, seizure spread patterns and results of surgery. Ann Neurol 31:3–13, 1992.

64. Sveinbjornsdottir S, Duncan JS: Parietal and occipital lobe epilepsy: A review. Epilepsia 34:493–521, 1993.

65. King DW, Ajmone-Marsan C: Clinical features and ictal patterns in epileptic patients with EEG temporal lobe foci. Ann Neurol 2:138–147, 1977.

66. Hausser-Hauw C, Bancaud J: Gustatory hallucinations in epileptic seizures: Electrophysiological, clinical and anatomical correlates. Brain 110:339–359, 1987.

67. Engel J: Approaches to localization of the epileptogenic lesion. In Engel J (ed): Surgical Treatment of the Epilepsies. New York, Raven Press, 1987, pp 75–79.

68. Chugani HT, Shields WD, Shewmon DA, et al: Infantile spasms. I. PET identifies focal cortical dysgenesis in cryptogenic cases for surgical treatment. Ann Neurol 27:406–413, 1990.

69. Chugani H, Shewmon DA, Khanna S, Phelps ME: Interictal and postictal focal hypermetabolism on positron emission tomography. Pediatr Neurol 9:10–15, 1993.

70. Chugani HT: PET in preoperative evaluation of intractable epilepsy. Pediatr Neurol 9:411–443, 1993.

71. Chugani HT, Rintahaka PJ, Shewmon DA: Ictal patterns of cerebral glucose utilization in children with epilepsy. Epilepsia 35:813–822, 1994.

72. Snead OC, Chen LS, Mitchell WG, et al: Usefulness of 18F fluorodeoxyglucose positron emission tomography in pediatric epilepsy surgery. Pediatr Neurol 14:98–107, 1996.

73. Harvey AS, Hopkins IJ, Bowe JM: Frontal lobe epilepsy: Clinical seizure characteristics and localization with ictal 99mTc-HMPAO SPECT. Neurology 43:1966–1980, 1993.

74. Duchowny M, Harvey AS: Pediatric epilepsy syndromes: An update and critical review. Epilepsia 37:S26–S40, 1996.

75. Fois A, Farnetani MA, Balestri P, et al: EEG, PET, SPECT and MRI in intractable childhood epilepsies: Possible surgical correlations. Childs Nerv Syst 11: 672–678, 1995.

76. Ebersole JS: Magnetoencephalography/magnetic source imaging in the assessment of patients with epilepsy. Epilepsia 38(Suppl 4): S1-S5, 1997.

77. Ko DY, Kufta C, Scaffidi D, Sato S: Source localization determined by magnetoencephalography and electroencephalography in temporal lobe epilepsy: Comparison with electrocorticography: Technical case report. Neurosurgery 42:414–421, 1998.

78. Cohen D: Magnetoencephalography: Detection of the brain's electrical activity with a superconducting magnetometer. Science 175:664–666, 1972.

79. Wyler AR, Ojemann GA, Lettich E, Ward AA Jr: Subdural strip electrodes for localizing epileptogenic foci. J Neurosurg 60:1195–1200, 1984.

80. Wyllie E, Luders H, Morris HH, et al: Clinical outcome after complete or partial cortical resection for intractable epilepsy. Neurology 37:1634–1641, 1987.

81. Haglund MM, Ojemann GA: Extratemporal resective surgery for epilepsy. Neurosurg Clin N Am 4:283–292, 1993.

82. Quesney LF: Extratemporal epilepsy: Clinical presentation, preoperative EEG localization and outcome. Acta Neurol Scand Suppl 140:81–94, 1992.

83. Williamson PD, Spencer SS: Clinical and EEG features of complex partial seizures of extratemporal origin. Epilepsia 27(Suppl 2):S46–S63, 1986.

84. Talairach J, Bancaud J, Boris A, et al: Surgical therapy for frontal epilepsies. In Chavel P, Delgado-Escueta AV, Halgren E (eds): Advances in Neurology. New York, Raven Press, 1992, pp 707–732.

85. Ojemann GA: Surgical therapy for medically intractable epilepsy. J Neurosurg 66:489–499, 1987.

86. Ojemann GA, Ojemann J, Lettich E, Berger M: Cortical language localization in left, dominant hemisphere. J Neurosurg 71:316–326, 1989.

87. Chadwick J, Manon W (trans): The Sacred Disease in the Medical Works of Hippocrates. Oxford, Blackwell Scientific, 1950.

88. Horsley V: Brain surgery. BMJ 2:670–675, 1886.

89. Horsley V: Discussion of the treatment of epilepsy: Medical Society of London. BMJ 3:371–372, 1903.

90. Horsley V: The origin and seat of epileptic disturbance. BMJ 1:693–696, 1892.

91. Gloor P: Hans Berger—psychophysiology and the discovery of the human electroencephalogram in epilepsy. In Harris P, Mawdsley C (eds): Proceedings of the Hans Berger Centenary Symposium. New York, Churchill Livingstone, 1974, pp 353–373.

92. Foerster O, Altenburger H: Electrobiologische Vorgange und der Menschlichen Hirnrinde. Dtsch Z Nervenheilk 135:277–288, 1935.

93. Foerster O, Penfield W: The structural basis of traumatic epilepsy and the results of radical operations. Brain 53:99–119, 1930.

94. Bailey P, Gibbs FA: The surgical treatment of psychomotor epilepsy. JAMA 145:365–370, 1951.

95. Penfield W, Paine K: Results of the surgical therapy for focal epileptic seizures. Can Med Assoc J 73:515–531, 1955.

96. Rasmussen T: Surgical treatment of patients with complex partial seizures. In Purpura DP, Penry JK, Walter RD (eds): Advances in Neurology vol 8. New York, Raven Press, 1975, pp 415–449.

97. Falconer MA, Hin D, Meyer A: Treatment of temporal lobe epilepsy by temporal lobectomy: A survey of findings and results. Lancet 1:827–835, 1955.

98. Falconer MA, Serafetinides EA: A follow-up study of surgery in temporal lobe epilepsy. J Neurol Neurosurg Psychiatry 26:154–165, 1963.

99. Penfield W, Flanigan H: Surgical therapy of temporal lobe seizures. Arch Neurol Psychiatry 64:491–500, 1950.

100. Penfield W, Baldwin M: Temporal lobe seizures and the technic of subtotal temporal lobectomy. Ann Surg 136:625–634, 1952.

101. Walker AE: Temporal lobectomy. J Neurosurg 26:642–649, 1967.

102. Rasmussen T: Surgical therapy of frontal lobe epilepsy. Epilepsia 4:181–198, 1963.

103. Rasmussen T: Surgery of frontal lobe epilepsy. In Purpura DP, Penry JK, Walter RD (eds): Advances in Neurology, vol 8. New York, Raven Press, 1975, pp 139–144.

104. Rasmussen T: Commentary: Extratemporal cortical excisions and hemispherectomy. In Engel J Jr (ed): Surgical Treatment of the Epilepsies. New York, Raven Press, 1987, pp 417–424.

105. Rasmussen T: Surgery of frontal lobe epilepsy. In Purpura DP, Penry JK, Walter RD (eds): Neurosurgical Management of the Epilepsies. New York, Raven Press, 1975, pp 197–205.

106. Rasmussen T: Focal epilepsies of non-temporal and non-frontal origin. In Wieser HD, Elger CE (eds): Presurgical Evaluation of Epileptics: Basics, Techniques and Implications. Berlin, Springer-Verlag, 1987, pp 344–351.

107. Rasmussen T: Surgery for epilepsy arising in regions other than the temporal and frontal lobes. In Purpura DP, Penry JK, Walter RD (eds): Advances in Neurology. New York, Raven Press, 1975, pp 207–226.

108. Green JR: Surgical treatment for epilepsy in childhood and adolescence. Surg Neurol 8:72–80, 1977.

109. Falconer MA: Significance of surgery for temporal lobe epilepsy in childhood and adolescence. J Neurosurg 33:233–252, 1970.

110. Walker AE: Surgical treatment of epilepsy. In Levingston S (ed): Comprehensive Management of Epilepsy in Infancy, Childhood, and Adolescence. Springfield, Ill, Charles C Thomas, 1972, pp 406–436.

111. Falconer MA: Place of surgery for temporal lobe epilepsy during childhood. BMJ 2:631–635, 1971.

112. Falconer MA: Reversibility by temporal lobe resection of the behavioral abnormalities of temporal lobe epilepsy. N Engl J Med 289:451–455, 1973.

113. Falconer M: Temporal lobe epilepsy in children and its surgical treatment. Med J Aust 1:1117–1121, 1972.

114. Hoffman HJ, Hendrick EB, Dennis M, et al: Hemispherectomy for Sturge-Weber syndrome. Childs Brain 5:233–238, 1979.

115. Duchowny M: Surgical outcome in children. In Luders HO (ed): Epilepsy Surgery. New York, Raven Press, 1992, pp 669–676.

116. Kennard MA: Reorganization of motor function in the cerebral cortex of monkeys deprived of motor and premotor areas in infancy. J Neurophysiol 1:477–496, 1938.

117. Wyllie E: Candidacy for epilepsy surgery: Special considerations in children. In Luders HO (ed): Epilepsy Surgery. New York, Raven Press, 1992, pp 127–130.

118. Meyer FB, Mersh WR, Laws ER, Sharbrough FW: Temporal lobectomy in children with epilepsy. J Neurosurg 64:371–376, 1986.

119. Green JR, Sidell AD, Walker ML: Neurosurgery of epilepsy in childhood and adolescence with comments about 50 patients. In Thompson RA, Green JR (eds): Pediatric Neurology and Neurosurgery. New York, Med Sci Book, 1978.

120. Goldring S: A method for surgical management of focal epilepsy, especially as it relates to children. J Neurosurg 49:344–356, 1978.

121. Vaernet K: Temporal lobotomy in children and young adults. In Parsonage M (ed): Advances in Epileptology: Fourteenth Epilepsy International Symposium. New York, Raven Press, 1983, pp 255–261.

122. Goldring S: Pediatric epilepsy surgery. Epilepsia 28(Suppl 1): S82–S102, 1987.

123. Goldring S: Surgical management of epilepsy in children. In Engel J Jr (ed): Surgical Treatment of the Epilepsies. New York, Raven Press, 1987, pp 445–464.

124. Wheless J: Evaluation of children for epilepsy surgery. Pediatr Ann 20:41–49, 1991.

125. Mizrah EM, Kellaway P, Grossman R, et al: Anterior temporal lobectomy and medically refractory temporal lobe epilepsy of childhood. Epilepsia 31:303–312, 1990.

126. Larkins MV, Hehn JF: Epilepsy surgery in children and young adults. Cleve Clin J Med 56(Suppl Pt 2):S262–S268, 1989.

127. Morrison G: Surgical management of epilepsy in children. Int Pediatr 3:143–147, 1988.

128. Duchowny M, Resnick T, Alvarez L, Morrison G: Focal resection for malignant partial seizures in infancy. Neurology 40:980–984, 1990.

129. Morrison G, Duchowny M, Resnick T, et al: Epilepsy surgery in childhood. Pediatr Neurosurg 18:291–297, 1992.

130. Duchowny M, Alvarez L, Resnick T, Morrison G: Surgery in infancy for partial seizures. Cleve Clin J Med 56:275, 1989.

131. Jayakar P, Resnick T, Duchowny M, et al: Outcome of very early frontal lobectomy. Epilepsia 31:680, 1990.

132. Duchowny M, Jayakar P, Resnick T, et al: Epilepsy surgery in patients under age 3 years. Ann Neurol 40:286, 1996.

133. Ziegler RG: Impairments of control and competence in epileptic children and their families. Epilepsia 22:339–346, 1981.

134. Wheless J: Evaluation of children for epilepsy surgery. Pediatr Ann 20:41–49, 1991.

135. Amar AP, Heck CN, Levy ML, et al: An institutional experience with cervical vagus nerve trunk stimulation for medically refractory epilepsy: Rationale, technique, outcome. Neurosurgery 43:1265–1280, 1998.

136. Ben-Menachem E, Manon-Espaillat R, Ristanovic R, et al: Vagus nerve stimulation for the treatment of partial seizures. 1. A controlled study of effect on seizures. First International Vagus Nerve Stimulation Study Group. Epilepsia 35:616–626, 1994.

137. Handforth A, DeGiorgio CM, Schachter SC, et al: Vagus nerve stimulation therapy for partial-onset seizures: A randomized active-control trial. Neurology 51:48–55, 1998.

138. Hornig GW, Murphy JV, Schallert G, Tilton C: Left vagus nerve stimulation in children with refractory epilepsy: An update. South Med J 90:484–488, 1997.

139. Murphy JV: Pediatric VNS study group: Left vagal nerve stimulation in children with medically refractory epilepsy. J Pediatr 134:563–566, 1999.

140. Parker APJ, Polkey CE, Binnie CD, et al: Vagal nerve stimulation in epileptic encephalopathies. Pediatrics 103:778–782, 1999.

141. Blume WT, Kaibara M: Localization of epileptic foci in children. Can J Neurol Sci 18:570–572, 1991.

142. Peacock WJ, Comair Y, Hoffman HJ, Morrison G: Special considerations for epilepsy surgery in childhood. In Engel J Jr (ed): Surgical Treatment of the Epilepsies, 2nd ed. New York, Raven Press, 1993, pp 541–547.

143. Berger MS, Ghatan S, Geyer JR, et al: Seizure outcome in children with hemispheric tumors and associated intractable epilepsy: The role of tumor removal combined with seizure foci resection. Pediatr Neurosurg 17:185–191, 1991.

144. Berger MS, Ghatan S, Haglund MM, et al: Low-grade gliomas associated with intractable epilepsy: Seizure outcome utilizing electrocorticography during tumor resection. J Neurosurg 79: 62–69, 1993.

145. Wyllie E, Luders H, Morris HH, et al: Clinical outcome after complete or partial cortical resection for intractable epilepsy. Neurology 37:1634–1641, 1987.

146. Goldring S, Gregorie M: Surgical management of epilepsy using epidural recording to localize the seizure focus. J Neurosurg 60: 457–466, 1984.

147. Luders H, Lesser RP, Dinner D, et al: Commentary: Chronic intracranial recording and stimulation with subdural electrodes. In Engel J Jr (ed): Surgical Treatment of the Epilepsies. New York, Raven Press, 1987, pp 297–321.

148. Bladin PF, Woodward J: Epilepsy and the frontal lobe. Proc Aust Assoc Neurol 11:229–237, 1974.

149. Uematsu S: Detection of an epileptic focus and cortical mapping using a subdural grid. In Rengachary SS, Wilkins RD (eds): Neurosurgical Operative Atlas, vol 2. Chicago, American Association of Neurological Surgeons, 1992.

150. Ludwig BL, Ajmone-Marsan C, Van Buren J: Depth and direct cortical recording in seizure disorders of extratemporal origin. Neurology 26:1085–1099, 1976.

151. Altman N, Duchowny M, Jayakar P, et al: Placement of intracerebral depth electrodes during excisional surgery for epilepsy: Value of intraoperative ultrasound. AJNR Am J Neuroradiol 13: 254–256, 1992.

152. Duchowny M, Altman N, Morrison G, et al: Ultrasound localization of intraoperative subdural and depth electrode placement. Epilepsia 30:717–718, 1989.

153. Duchowny M, Levin B, Jayakar P, et al: Temporal lobectomy in early childhood. Epilepsia 33:298–303, 1992.

154. Duchowny M, Jayakar P: Functional mapping in children. Adv Neurol 63:149–154, 1993.

155. Jayakar P, Alvarez L, Duchowny M, Resnick T: A safe and effective paradigm to functionally map the cortex in childhood. J Clin Neurophysiol 9:288–293, 1992.

156. Lesser R, Luders H, Klem G, et al: Cortical afterdischarge and functional response thresholds: Results of extraoperative testing. Epilepsia 25:615–621, 1984.

157. Alvarez LA, Jayakar P: Cortical stimulation with subdural electrodes: Special considerations in infancy and childhood. J Epilepsy 3:125–130, 1990.

158. Nespeca M, Wyllie E, Luders H, et al: EEG recording and functional localization studies with subdural infants and young children. J Epilepsy 3(Suppl 1):107–124, 1990.

159. Duchowny M, Jayakar P: Functional cortical mapping in children. In Beric A, Dogali M, Devinski O (eds): Electrical and Magnetic Stimulation of the Brain and Spinal Cord. New York, Raven Press, 1993, pp 149–154.

160. Dean P: Grids for kids: The pediatric patient undergoing invasive extraoperative EEG monitoring. J Neurosci Nurs 26:352–356, 1994.

161. Davies KG, Weeks RD: Cortical resections for intractable epilepsy of extratemporal origin: Experience with seventeen cases over eleven years. Br J Neurosurg 7:343–353, 1993.

162. Morrell F, Whisler WW, Bleck TP: Multiple subpial transection: A new approach to the surgical treatment of focal epilepsy. J Neurosurg 70:231–239, 1989.

163. Kaufmann WE, Krauss GL, Uematsu S, Lesser RP: Treatment of epilepsy with multiple transections: An acute histologic analysis in human subjects. Epilepsia 37:342–351, 1996.

164. Wolf HK, Zentner J, Hufnagel A, et al: Surgical pathology of chronic epileptic seizure disorders: Experience with 63 specimens from extratemporal corticectomies, lobectomies and functional hemispherectomies. Acta Neuropathol (Berl) 86:466–472, 1993.

165. Robitaille Y, Rasmussen T, Dubeau F, et al: Histopathology of non-neoplastic lesions in frontal lobe epilepsy: Review of 180 cases with recent MRI and PET correlation. In Chavel P, Delgado-Escueta AV, Halgren E, Bancaud J (eds): Frontal Lobe Seizures and Epilepsies. New York, Raven Press, 1992, pp 499–513.

166. Babb TL, Brown WJ: Pathological findings in epilepsy. In Engel J Jr (ed): Surgical Treatment of the Epilepsies. New York, Raven Press, 1987, pp 511–540.

167. Farrell MA, DeRosa MJ, Curran JG, et al: Neuropathologic findings in cortical resections (including hemispherectomies) performed for the treatment of intractable childhood epilepsy. Acta Neuropathol (Berl) 83:246–259, 1992.

168. Altman N, Birchansky S, Goldstein T, et al: Preliminary report of neuroimaging and pathologic correlations in children operated on for intractable focal epilepsy. Int Pediatr 9:85–93, 1994.

169. Duchowny M, Jayakar P, Harvey AS, et al: Epilepsy surgery in the first three years of life. Epilepsia 39:737–743, 1998.

170. Van Ness PC: Surgical outcome for neocortical (extrahippocampal) focal epilepsy. In Luders J (ed): Epilepsy Surgery. New York, Raven Press, 1991, pp 613–624.

171. Engel J, Van Ness PC, Rasmussen TB, Ojemann LM: Outcome with respect to epileptic seizures. In Engel J Jr (ed): Surgical Treatment of the Epilepsies, 2nd ed. New York, Raven Press, 1993, pp 609–621.

172. Adler J, Erba G, Winston KR, et al: Results of surgery for extratemporal partial epilepsy that began in childhood. Arch Neurol 48:133–140, 1991.

173. Fraser RT: Improving function rehabilitation outcome following epilepsy surgery. Acta Neurol Scand 117(Suppl):122–128, 1988.

174. Malmgren K, Sullivan M, Ekstedt G, et al: Health-related quality of life after epilepsy surgery: A Swedish multicenter study. Epilepsia 38:830–838, 1997.

175. Bladin PF: Psychosocial difficulties and outcome after temporal lobectomy. Epilepsia 33:898–907, 1992.

176. Taylor DC, Falconer MA: Clinical, socio-economic, and psychological changes after temporal lobectomy. Br J Psychiatry 114: 1247–1261, 1968.

177. Jensen I: Temporal lobe epilepsy: Social conditions and rehabilitation after surgery. Acta Neurol Scand 54:22–44, 1976.

178. Lindsay J, Ounsted C, Richards P: Long-term outcome in children with temporal lobe seizures. Dev Med Child Neurol 21: 285–298, 433–440, 630–636, 1979.

179. Augustine EA, Novelly RA, Mattson RH, et al: Occupational adjustment following neurosurgical treatment of epilepsy. Ann Neurol 15:68–72, 1984.

180. Bourgeois M, Sainte-Rose C, Lellouch-Tubiana A, et al: Surgery of epilepsy associated with focal lesions in childhood. J Neurosurg 90:833–842, 1999.

181. Blume WT, Girvin JP, McLachlan RS, Gilmore BE: Effective temporal lobectomy in childhood without invasive EEF. Epilepsia 38:164–167, 1997.

182. Polkey CE: Temporal lobe resections. In Oxbury JM, Polkey CE, Duchowny M (eds): Intractable Focal Epilepsy. London, WB Saunders, 2000, pp 667–696.

183. Langfitt JT: Cost-effectiveness of anterotemporal lobectomy in medically intractable complex partial epilepsy. Epilepsia 38:154–163, 1997.

184. King JT, Sperling MR, Justice AC, O'Connor MJ: A cost-effectiveness analysis of anterior temporal lobectomy for intractable temporal lobe epilepsy. J Neurosurg 87:20–28, 1997.

185. Petrovici AC: Epilepsy in temporal lobe tumors. Eur Neurol 5: 201–214, 1971.

186. Spencer DD, Spencer SS, Mattson RH, Williamson PD: Intracerebral masses in patients with intractable partial epilepsy. Neurology 34:432–436, 1984.
187. Drake J, Hoffman HJ, Kobayashi J, et al: Surgical management of children with temporal lobe epilepsy and mass lesions. Neurosurgery 21:792–797, 1987.
188. Boon PA, Williamson PD, Fried I, et al: Intracranial, intraaxial, space-occupying lesions in patients with intractable partial seizures: An anatomoclinical, neuropsychological and surgical correlation. Epilepsia 32:467–476, 1991.
189. Zentner J, Hufnagel A, Wolf HK, et al: Surgical treatment of neoplasms associated with medically intractable epilepsy. Neurosurgery 41:378–387, 1997.
190. Morrison G, Jayakar P, Duchowny M, et al: Resective epilepsy surgery in childhood—with and without a lesion. J Neurosurg 86:351A, 1997.
191. Awad IA, Rosenfeld J, Ahl J, et al: Intractable epilepsy and structural lesions of the brain: Mapping, resection strategies, and seizure outcome. Epilepsia 32:179–186, 1991.
192. Hufnagel A, Zentner J, Fernandez G, et al: Multiple subpial transection for control of epileptic seizures: Effectiveness and safety. Epilepsia 38:678–688, 1997.
193. Van Buren JM: Complications of surgical procedures in the diagnosis and treatment of epilepsy. In Engel J Jr (ed): Surgical Treatment of the Epilepsies. New York, Raven Press, 1987, pp 465–475.
194. Ventureyra ECG, Higgins MJ: Complications of epilepsy surgery in children and adolescents. Pediatr Neurosurg 19:40–56, 1993.
195. Kramer U, Riviello JJ, Carmant L, et al: Morbidity of depth and subdural electrodes: Children and adolescents versus young adults. J Epilepsy 7:7–10, 1994.
196. Behrens E, Schramm J, Zentner J, Konig R: Surgical and neurological complications in a series of 708 epilepsy surgery procedures. Neurosurgery 41:1–10, 1997.

CHAPTER 247

Acute Pediatric Neurorehabilitation

MICHAEL J. NOETZEL

Rehabilitation, in its most literal sense, is the process of restoration following disease, illness, or injury in the hope of recovering the ability to function in a normal or near-normal manner.[1] In its broadest sense, rehabilitation extends far beyond the bounds of traditional medicine, because one of its chief aims is to protect or restore personal and social identity.[2] Within this context, neurorehabilitation can be defined as two separate but overlapping concepts. First, neurorehabilitation is the subspecialty of medicine that treats patients with disabling (and therefore often chronic) diseases of the central and peripheral nervous systems.[3] Under this definition, rehabilitation should be perceived as an active process that seeks to reduce the effects of a primary neurological disease on a person's daily life. Second, neurorehabilitation comprises the specific therapeutic modalities required to overcome or improve any neurological impairment that has been demonstrated to interfere with daily life.[2] Both aspects of this definition clearly have practical implications for the use of neurorehabilitation in the pediatric population.[4]

To better understand the principles and goals of neurorehabilitation, it is helpful to start by defining those terms that have gained wide acceptance as the nomenclature of rehabilitation, based on the international classification of impairments, disabilities, and handicaps (ICIDH).[5] One caution is that these terms are currently undergoing revision as a result of updating and field-testing. As originally defined by the World Health Organization (WHO) in 1980, *impairment* is the loss or abnormality of physiologic, psychological, or anatomic structure or function. *Disability* is the lack of or restricted ability to perform a functional task, within the range or in the manner considered normal at specific ages, due to an impairment. A disability therefore describes the interaction between a child and his or her environment and is dependent on that individual's environment. This concept has significant implications for one of the ways that the neurorehabilitation can be carried out, namely, to modify or adapt the environment. The concept of disability is also a normative one. Thus, a clear understanding of normal development, as well as the ramifications of abnormal development, is key to the appropriate neurorehabilitation of an infant, child, or adolescent. When a disability limits or prevents a person from fulfilling a normal role in life, the original ICIDH referred to that condition as a *handicap*. A handicap was viewed as the subjective impact of a disease, that is, the disadvantage it confers on a person's ability to function normally. Unfortunately, disadvantage is particularly difficult to quantify, and in children, it often cannot be directly inferred from disability.[2] Although physicians' training is directed toward an understanding of the pathologic processes resulting in the impairment of organ function, such an understanding does not readily lend itself to predicting the disability that will stem from such impairment, much less to defining the disadvantage it will confer on a particular individual.[6, 7] To correct these (and other) deficiencies in the classification system, the most recent version of the ICIDH views disablement as a three-dimensional construct consisting of impairment, activity limitations, and participation restrictions.[8] Each dimension is conceptualized as being the result of interaction between the biologic features intrinsic to the individual's medical condition and the person's physical and social environment.[6] Thus, in this manner, the WHO hopes to broaden the range of disablement and to negate the assumption that disability stems solely and directly from the type and degree of impairment.

Concomitant with these new definitions, the concept of dependency has arisen as a fundamental aspect of medical rehabilitation.[2] Unlike some of the components of disablement, dependency is more readily quantifiable. In addition, degree of dependency has been shown to have a critical influence on quality of life, as well as on the cost of ongoing medical and neurorehabilitative care. A variety of scales have been developed to measure a patient's potential autonomy or, conversely, the burden imposed on a caregiver.[2] Unfortunately, such scales are particularly difficult to use in the pediatric population because of the interrelated issues of anticipated development and maturation.

Nonetheless, the disablement-disadvantage paradigm is important in pediatric neurorehabilitation. The paradigm emphasizes movement toward appropriate functional outcomes, as well as diagnosis. Thus, it is much more informative than traditional neurodiagnostic categories.[4] There are three other distinct advantages to conceptualizing neurorehabilitation using this paradigm. First, neurorehabilitation is a process that requires the participation of a multidisciplinary team comprising physicians, nurses, therapists, and other health care professionals who work in collaboration with the patient and the patient's family. Second, the paradigm emphasizes that therapeutic considerations and treatment modalities should be based primarily on the disablement and resultant activity limitations, as opposed to the underlying pathologic process producing the impairment. In practical terms, this means that treatment techniques can often be successfully transferred from one patient to another regardless of their primary neurological diagnosis.[2] Finally, the paradigm provides a framework for patient care that can easily be expanded to encompass the multifaceted aspects of neurorehabilitation inherent in the practice of child neurology. For example, the paradigm works equally well for an adolescent with seizures (impairment) who is prohibited from driving an automobile (disablement) as for a child with a lower thoracic spinal cord injury causing paralysis of the legs and thus a limited capacity to ambulate. In both cases there are resultant activity limitations that affect social life and future employment opportunities.

MECHANISMS UNDERLYING FUNCTIONAL RECOVERY IN THE NERVOUS SYSTEM

Implicit in any consideration of the neurorehabilitation process is the recognition that the potential for recovery of function exists. Without this potential of restoring a normal condition, the field of neurorehabilitation would be severely limited. Although recovery is rarely complete following injury to the nervous system, the development of an appropriate neurorehabilitation program begins with a better understanding of the cellular and molecular bases of neuronal dysfunction, as well as the potential mechanisms by which recovery of function occurs. In this latter regard, it is especially important to recognize that each proposed mechanism of recovery follows a different time course, the implications of which are important in defining an appropriate therapy program.

Although much about the recovery of neurological function is, at best, poorly understood, several general conclusions can be made based on a variety of scientific evidence. First, the nervous system has a rather significant capability to undergo biologic modifications

in response to injury and developmental aberrations. Second, the mechanisms by which the nervous system can respond to injury are more varied and dynamic than previously realized.[9] Third, meaningful recovery of function continues for a much greater period than was previously recognized.[10] These findings stand in contrast to the former belief that recovery was, in essence, a biphasic process. Any recovery that occurred within the first few months following an injury was thought to be due to the reversibility of factors affecting dysfunctional, as opposed to dead, tissue. Any later increase in functional capabilities was attributed to nonphysiologic factors such as learning and behavior modification. As will be described later, it is clear that in many instances, changes in neuronal circuitry, rather than psychological factors, may be mediating the recovery of function.[10] At present, however, the basis of scientific information does not allow us to separate one set of factors from another. Thus, at least in terms of acquired injury to the nervous system, it is perhaps best to simply acknowledge that there is ongoing debate concerning the relative contributions of biologic healing and learned adaptations to the process of functional recovery.

Resolution of Temporary Dysfunction

Various theories have been proposed to explain the recovery of neurological function that occurs within hours to days following injury to the nervous system. The mechanisms underlying recovery of function in these circumstances most likely relate to resolution of temporary dysfunction in areas of the brain that have not been damaged irreversibly. Potential factors causing impairment of function include (1) raised intracranial pressure, (2) hypoxia, (3) small contusions or focal hematomas, (4) edema (both cytotoxic and vasogenic), and (5) transient depression of metabolic and enzymatic activity in areas of the nervous system remote to the primary injury.

Both clinical and experimental evidence supports each of the first four factors.[11] In addition, other studies have demonstrated that focal brain injury can result in depression of metabolic activity in noncontiguous brain areas secondary to transient reduction in levels of transmitter synthesizing enzymes in the damaged brain regions.[12] In a similar fashion, the concept of diaschisis has arisen. This is a form of neural shock in which uninvolved areas of the brain are rendered temporarily nonfunctional following damage to a remote area of the brain. It is postulated that the intact areas of the brain cease to function in a normal fashion when deprived of appropriate input from the injured brain tissue. Recovery of function presumably transpires as a result of increased neurotransmitter synthesis or, more likely, elevated production of neurotransmitter receptors. Thus, it has been suggested that some portion of early recovery in humans following brain injury may relate to resolution of a similar metabolic derangement.[13] Such recovery would necessarily take place relatively early, starting perhaps 12 to 24 hours after injury and lasting for about 7 to 10 days.

Reorganization of Neuronal Connections

Modification of active neural connections is another potential mechanism of recovery following nervous system injury. Recent research in neurobiology now provides some insight into how reorganization might be mediated at both the physiologic and anatomic levels.

Over the last 2 decades, three specific modifications of neural connections have been touted as the most promising examples of reorganizational mechanisms in the nervous system. These are axonal regeneration, axon retraction, and collateral sprouting, also termed *reactive synaptogenesis*. Axonal regeneration, the process by which damaged axons regrow to their normal target, clearly plays a role in recovery in the peripheral nervous system. At times, this regeneration may establish connections with incorrect synaptic contacts if the normal locus of termination is damaged. Regeneration in the mammalian central nervous system has rarely been documented, however, and only under highly artificial conditions.[14] Thus, it is unlikely that it plays any significant role in the recovery of function in humans. With regard to axon retraction, it is well documented that in early development, certain axons project branches that ultimately are destined to be retracted later on. The time course of programmed retraction of axon collaterals has not been clearly established, but typically it seems to be confined to early development.[15] Research now suggests that this normal retraction process may not occur if nervous system injury is sustained early on, thus providing a mechanism for retention of function.[16] Collateral sprouting involves the outgrowth of axons from undamaged neurons in the establishment of synaptic contact at sites vacated by degenerating or dying neurons. Collateral sprouting is typically confined to regions normally innervated by that particular grouping of nerve cells under normal circumstances. This collateral growth does not cross certain anatomic boundaries, so it does not affect novel nervous system domains. Collateral sprouting appears to be greatly influenced by growth and apoptotic factors.[17] In this regard, it is not surprising that experimental data indicate that the magnitude and rate of sprouting following an acute injury to the nervous system appear to be much greater in the immature brain.

There is also a fourth anatomic mechanism involving the reestablishment of neuronal connections in response to brain injury. Based on recent research, it now appears that there is a resting population of neural progenitor cells in the brain that retains the capacity to proliferate, divide, and differentiate when activated by the correct signals.[18] Whether these cells can respond to central nervous system injury and, through neurogenesis, promote restoration of function has not been established.

Plasticity of the Nervous System

Another explanation for the gradual recovery of neurological function following neuronal injury is that the nervous system has developed characteristics that allow a certain degree of malleability both during development and in reaction to injury. Researchers have suggested that this "plasticity" may relate to both the redundancy of the nervous system and a process of vicarious functioning. *Redundancy* is a term implying that there are latent neural connections and silent synapses that can subserve a particular function if the primary control pathway is damaged.[19] It is a form of compensation in which a damaged neural system comes to rely on new cues or different receptors. This type of acute adaptation is commonly seen in experimental conditions. In human recovery, its role is gradually gaining acceptance. The best evidence to date supporting its existence comes from positron emission tomography studies,[20] as well as clinical and research observations about the recovery of function in young patients undergoing surgical hemispherectomy.[21] Both these lines of evidence indicate that various neurological functions, especially motor performance, can shift from an injured side of the brain to the corresponding area in the opposite hemisphere. Based on positron emission tomography studies, the time course for this mechanism of recovery is somewhat variable but is most likely in the range of weeks.

Vicarious functioning is a process by which neural tissues not normally involved in the performance of a particular task alter their properties to assume control of the task.[10] Vicarious functioning is typically described as occurring in an area of the brain adjacent to the injured site or systemically related to the damaged tissue. Evidence supporting this construct comes from two-stage lesion studies and research on the immature visual cortex.[22] Most investigators recognize, however, that the concept implies a high level of central nervous system reorganizational ability, which typically is not attributed to the mature nervous system. Thus, although a role for vicarious functioning in the pediatric population has been suggested, its role in the recovery of adults is obscure.

Mechanisms of Late Recovery

Probably the most important mechanism for late recovery in humans is functional substitution. This concept implies that there is an overt or covert adaptation of an altered strategy to achieve a desired goal. By definition, it is a recovery of the "ends" and not a recovery of the "means" to that end. In essence, the task is modified to fit the capabilities of the uninjured neural tissue. The tissue subserving this recovery does not alter its intrinsic properties; rather, by using novel strategies, a performance goal is achieved. Neurorehabilitation has its greatest impact on this form of recovery, because functional substitution depends on new learning and repetitive problem solving. This form of recovery is clearly related to specific eliciting experiences that typically take place during rehabilitation therapy.[23] Thus, the process requires an awake patient capable of at least some degree of learning and consolidating memory.

Summary

Recovery following damage to the nervous system is a highly complex and often remarkable process. All the postulated mechanisms seem to favor the immature or developing brain, thus accounting for the relatively better outcomes typically reported in the pediatric literature. This is not surprising. All the proposed events of neural reorganization that emerge in response to injury are better recognized as normal developmental processes of maturation that are reactivated or potentiated in response to neuronal cell loss.[24] It is anticipated that with a better understanding of these mechanisms of recovery, neurorehabilitative therapy will eventually be custom-made to fit the particular circumstances of nervous system injury and recovery.

PRINCIPLES OF PEDIATRIC NEUROREHABILITATION

Neurological disorders represent a large proportion of all severe and complex disabilities, especially those secondary to trauma and other acquired injury. This is especially true in the pediatric population, where injury to the brain and spinal cord account for the vast majority of children referred for rehabilitation. Thus, pediatric neurologists are in an excellent position to contribute meaningfully to pediatric rehabilitation services.[4]

The process of pediatric neurorehabilitation has several guiding principles based on both the nature of the discipline and the age of the patients involved. One distinguishing principle of neurorehabilitation is that the process requires a coordinated multidisciplinary team working together to provide integrated evaluations and therapeutic interventions. Of necessity, the team must include individuals who can address a variety of nonmedical issues such as home and school accessibility, psychosocial adaptation to disability, and so on. A second guiding principle is that the team should concentrate on issues of true functional significance rather than treatments that merely decrease symptoms without improving a patient's functional capabilities. In pediatrics, this means focusing on practical management decisions that are endorsed by both the patient and the family. To do this, the team must have a clear understanding of the physical, emotional, cognitive, and social consequences of a child's injury.[25] Differences in degree, extent, and rate of recovery among children, as well as the variability of functioning from setting to setting and task to task in a single child, mandate continual reassessment. As previously described, the immature brain responds to injury in a varied but dynamic manner. The resultant biologic recovery, in combination with substitute or alternative movement patterns and thought processes, requires an ongoing program of assessment and reassessment. In addition, it is hoped that there will be changes in the baseline condition based on a positive response to treatment. Thus, neurorehabilitation has been described as a spiral management process in which evaluation initiates a therapy program that is then constantly revised and updated in view of successive reassessments that take into consideration changes secondary to treatment.[2]

Another essential principle of pediatric neurorehabilitation is that these frequent reassessments of cognitive, psychosocial, and motor deficits, especially when resulting from acquired brain injury, must be guided by an understanding of normal development. Knowledge of age-appropriate patterns of cognitive development is especially important in the neurorehabilitation of infants and children for several reasons. First, normative milestones of cognitive development can serve as sequential goals in an individual's rehabilitation program.[25] Second, the developmental age of the patient as a result of the injury necessarily limits the direction of therapy and the patient's ability to respond. This is especially true early in the neurorehabilitative process, when individuals lack the developmental skills necessary to learn the complex strategies on which functional substitution is predicated. Finally, an understanding of cognitive development allows one to predict more accurately the long-term effects of neuronal injury in young children. This is particularly significant in areas of the brain subserving functions that normally blossom later in childhood or in early adolescence, such as executive functioning of the frontal lobes.

The final guiding principle of pediatric neurorehabilitation is that interventions must begin as early as possible. For most pediatric patients with acquired injuries, this means while the child is still in the intensive care unit but medically stable.[25, 26] Coma is not a contraindication to the initiation of neurorehabilitation management strategies. This phase of early intervention is designed to limit maladaptive movement patterns and prevent complications that can take months to resolve if they are not properly addressed during the acute phase of injury. Specific goals include maintenance of skin integrity; prevention of physical deformities, such as contractures due to abnormal spasticity and prolonged immobilization; and limitation of those aspects of systemic autonomic instability related to fluctuation in muscle tone and bladder distention.

Nutritional support is also a key element of the acute management process.[27] In particular, pediatric patients with acquired nervous system injuries are at high risk for compromised nutrition secondary to a variety of causes, including a hypermetabolic state associated with systemic trauma or infection[28]; intestinal stasis and delayed gastric emptying; oral pharyngeal dysfunction, which, if unrecognized, can result in aspiration pneumonia; and underestimation of caloric requirements for growth.[29] Early on, nasogastric feedings are usually indicated. In cases of major intra-abdominal injury, hyperalimentation may be warranted. As neurological recovery proceeds, gradual introduction of oral feeding begins with a commensurate decrease in supplemental alimentation. Swallowing difficulties are an almost universal complication of acquired brain injury in the pediatric population due to bihemispheric injury or lower cranial nerve involvement.[30] Thus, careful evaluation by a rehabilitation feeding team is necessary.[31]

Other medical issues often have an impact on acute neurorehabilitation management or impair the accuracy of the neurorehabilitation team's assessment. Infection and associated fever are near-universal complications seen in pediatric patients in need of acute neurorehabilitation.[32] In those with intracranial trauma, the possibility of central nervous system infection must be considered.[33] The risk of brain abscess and bacterial meningitis is increased in patients with penetrating brain injuries and basilar or compound skull fractures. Other more obvious sources of infection include intravascular lines and indwelling urinary catheters. Sinusitis is a relatively common infection in view of the frequent need for nasotracheal intubation or long-term nasogastric tubes. In children with acquired brain injuries, fever of central origin secondary to hypothalamic injury can occur. Typically, other clinical features of autonomic dysregulation are observed, most notably, hypertension and tachycardia.[34] The diagnosis of fever of central origin cannot be made until other sources of infection have been carefully evaluated and excluded, including drug-induced fever. Disturbances in endocrine function, although much less common than infection, can complicate severe acquired brain injury.[32, 35] Hypothalamic and pituitary damage can result in the syndrome of inappropriate antidiuretic hormone secretion or, conversely, central diabetes insipidus, in which antidiuretic hormone secretion is insufficient. Although generally transient, both these conditions mandate judicious fluid and electrolyte management, as well as pharmacologic treatment with desmopressin acetate in cases of diabetes insipidus.

Gastrointestinal disorders are also common in the pediatric population with acquired nervous system injuries, including hemorrhage secondary to gastric hyperacidity, stress ulceration, and reflux esophagitis.[36] In addition, any child with a feeding tube is at risk for damage to the gastric mucosa and should be treated prophylactically with H_2-receptor blockers. Finally, in children with traumatic injuries to the nervous system, the incidence of skeletal fractures, typically of the long bones, is high.[37] Such fractures may not be apparent in a comatose patient but reveal themselves during the early course of neurorehabilitation treatment.[38] Close coordination between the orthopedic surgeon and the therapy team with regard to range-of-motion exercises and weight-bearing status is essential to optimize the response to therapy.

MANAGEMENT OF SPASTICITY

Almost every patient requiring acute neurorehabilitation services manifests an alteration in tone as a result of injury or illness. In the early phase following trauma, absent or reduced tone is common; with time, spasticity is typically encountered as one part of the upper motoneuron syndrome.[39] Spasticity is defined as an exaggerated response to passive movement of a limb, inducing a velocity-dependent involuntary resistance of the stretched muscle. Spasticity is characterized by excessive and inappropriately timed activation of skeletal muscles. The clinical manifestations of spasticity are varied, reflecting the different locations within the central nervous system that, when damaged, give rise to the upper motoneuron syndrome. Extent of injury, as well as intrinsic characteristics of recovery, also influences the presentation of spasticity. In almost all cases, however, spasticity affects passive movement and static postural alignment.[39] Spasticity is often accompanied by impaired activation of voluntary movement, resulting in weakness and clumsiness.[40] Spasticity must be differentiated from other manifestations of impaired movement such as dystonia and rigidity, both of which typically occur within the context of associated or secondary injury due to ischemia and hypoxia.

As indicated previously, treatment of spasticity is predicated on establishing goals that improve a child's functional capabilities.[41] Thus, the main reason for attempting to decrease spasticity in the pediatric population is to improve functional movement, most typically ambulation or upper extremity use in activities of daily living. In some instances, improvement of head, neck, and trunk posture by lessening spasticity may have the additional benefits of increasing oral feeding and providing better breath support for speech. Early in neurorehabilitation, however, the main focus of relieving spasticity is to minimize the complication of joint and muscle contractures, with a secondary goal of eliminating painful spasms.[26] In comatose or obtunded patients, spasticity management begins with proper positioning, range-of-motion exercises, and splinting, typically used in combination.[39] In addition, it is important to eliminate any potential exacerbating causes of spasticity, such as inappropriate external sensory stimuli (e.g., a catheter leg bag), bladder or bowel distention, occult fractures, and skin irritation or sores.[40]

Range-of-motion exercises should be carried out daily in all joints, regardless of alteration of tone.[25] As recovery progresses, range-of-motion exercises are tailored to specific affected muscle groups and often combined with physical treatment modalities. Temperature variation (hot and cold) and use of water and electrical stimulation are effective adjuncts in the treatment of spasticity, with few side effects. The mechanism of action of these measures is to facilitate the antagonists of a spastic muscle, which in turn causes relaxation by reciprocal inhibition.[42] Alternatively, physical modalities may induce relaxation of spastic muscles directly through inhibition and fatigue. In either case, the duration of benefit is rather short and is dependent on treatment duration.

Proper positioning is designed to improve postural alignment and symmetry and to correct weight-bearing distribution throughout the body to reverse flexible postural imbalances. In addition, position can promote relaxation of tone by using gravity to stretch spastic muscles. In the latter stages of recovery, proper position can facilitate active contraction of functionally weak muscle groups. Proper therapeutic alignment of the body is based on the abnormal position assumed by the body at rest or when moved. In addition, specific positions or exercises should be avoided if they promote the disinhibited reflexes that underlie abnormal trunk and neck postures.

Casting and splinting are also mainstays in the treatment of spasticity. It is clear that these measures can increase range of motion and prevent the formation or worsening of contractures in a spastic extremity.[40] Inhibitive casting may also result in a lowering of tone, although clear scientific documentation is not available. Proponents of this technique assert that the reduction of spasticity may result from several mechanisms, including the effects of neutral warmth and constant pressure on the spastic muscle, reduction in sensory input from cutaneous receptors resulting in habituation, and inhibition of the excitability of gamma motoneurons or the sensitivity of muscle spindles to stretch.[43] In patients who have progressed further in their recovery, splints or orthotics are often used to produce functional benefit without necessarily altering spasticity. For example, a properly fitted extension splint may improve function in hand activities such as keyboarding without altering the underlying tone.

Pharmacologic agents are the final treatment modality for the management of spasticity in pediatric patients undergoing acute neurorehabilitation. Although a number of antispasticity medications have been available for many years, the available data are insufficient to conclude that any of these agents is truly effective in reducing spasticity in acutely brain-injured pediatric patients. The problem is largely a lack of the multicenter protocols that are typically necessary to resolve these issues adequately. In addition, the side effects of antispasticity medications in the pediatric population are a concern. Thus, antispasticity medication should be used only when severe spasticity cannot be adequately managed by other therapeutic modalities. Unfortunately, at St. Louis Children's Hospital, this represents roughly 40% to 50% of the patients with acquired brain injuries. Finally, the use of antispasticity medication should be limited to those situations in which meaningful functional goals, such as greater independence in activities of daily living or improved ambulation, can be achieved as opposed to mere clinical goals, such as decreased resistance to stretch or a reduction in clonus.

Baclofen, diazepam, and dantrolene sodium are the three most common antispasticity medications prescribed.[25, 41] The use of diazepam, especially in acute brain-injured patients, is severely limited by its sedative side effects, which often produce underarousal and impaired attention even at relatively low doses. Baclofen is much better tolerated because its mode of action appears to be via polysynaptic inhibitory pathways within the spinal cord.[44] In my experience, baclofen has been moderately effective in reducing spasticity secondary to acquired brain injury, although the doses required to achieve this result are quite variable. Dantrolene sodium is the least sedating of the antispasticity medications because its site of action is in the muscle. This agent suppresses the release of

calcium ions from the sarcoplasmic reticulum, thus uncoupling electrical excitation from muscle contraction.[45] The efficacy of dantrolene sodium is limited by the need for careful titration to minimize the potential for severe generalized weakness. In addition, liver function tests must be carefully monitored, and treatment is limited to 3 to 6 months because of the risk of chemical hepatitis.[41] Clonidine has also been reported to reduce tone.[46] Tizanidine, another of the α-adrenergic agonists, is a promising new agent, but its use in children with spasticity of cerebral origin has not been studied sufficiently.[47]

In addition to oral antispasticity medications, botulinum toxin may be helpful in managing severe spasticity that involves only a few muscles or muscle groups.[48, 49] The total dose of botulinum toxin that can be administered at one time is limited. Thus, only a few select muscles or muscle groups can be injected. In addition, there must be appropriate spacing between injections (even to different muscles) to minimize the development of antibodies to the toxin. Nonetheless, judicious use of this agent, often in patients who are intolerant of splinting or with severe postural deformities, can be a beneficial adjunct to maintain range of motion. The vast majority of children with spasticity secondary to acquired nervous system injury demonstrate significant motor recovery and lessening of spasticity within 6 to 12 months.[39] Thus, the reversible denervation caused by botulinum toxin on the neuromuscle junction must be viewed as a positive attribute.

ACQUIRED BRAIN INJURY

Acquired brain injury is one of the major causes of pediatric disability and medical expense in the United States. It is also the most common condition necessitating treatment in an acute neurorehabilitation setting. At St. Louis Children's Hospital, traumatic brain injury represents 40% of all admissions to our acute neurorehabilitation service. Cerebrovascular accident, hypoxic-ischemic brain injury, and brain tumor each contribute 10%. With the addition of central nervous system infection, acquired brain injury accounts for nearly 75% of our pediatric patients.

Neurorehabilitation of a pediatric patient with acquired brain injury is complicated, in part, by the nature of the injury. In the majority of cases, the damage to the central nervous system occurs at multiple locations, even though the primary injury may be a focal one. In addition, secondary injury from hypoxia or ischemia or raised intracranial pressure from cerebral edema may inflict diffuse damage. Unfortunately, this latter scenario is particularly common in infants and children, especially those with nonaccidental traumatic brain injury secondary to abuse.[39] Although the neuropathology of acquired brain injury is extremely varied, there are a number of neurorehabilitation issues, such as the previously discussed problem of spasticity, that must be addressed in almost every child recovering from this form of injury.

Behavioral Disturbances

One nearly universal consideration is the issue of behavior.[50, 51] Aberrations in behavior can be observed at all stages of recovery once coma resolves. Early on, the disturbances in behavior are typically characterized by agitation, such as random, nonpurposeful motor and verbal activity, as well as emotional regression and impaired information processing. These behaviors are unlikely to respond to sedative medication, and in fact, the symptoms may be aggravated by further clouding the sensorium. At this stage, the goal should be to prevent these behaviors from becoming learned patterns that will slow the pace of recovery. Typically, these early behavioral aberrations persist for days or weeks.

In the middle stages of recovery, the typical manifestation is intolerance of sensory stimulation associated with exceedingly poor understanding of deficits.[25] In children younger than 8 years, this is manifested by hyperactivity and impulsive or even destructive behavior. In older children or adolescents, lethargy combined with decreased motivation and poor initiation of action are typically observed. Management of these behaviors requires careful, ongoing assessment of the child's attention and arousal patterns. Medications that are likely to produce cognitive or behavioral side effects should be withdrawn. Unfortunately, this is easier said than done, because many medications have unpredictable central nervous system side effects in individuals with acquired brain injury.[52] Nonetheless, it is important to reassess on an ongoing basis the need for any medication in such a patient. In addition, it is important to carefully modulate a child's environment to prevent prolonged sensory deprivation or overstimulation.[25] In some cases, it may be necessary to eliminate background noise or activity; in other cases, constancy of background noise (so-called white noise) may be helpful. Alerting a child and preparing him or her for any activity or treatment are also appropriate. In many cases, consistency in approaching the child or modulating the environment is key. It is also essential to monitor the child's response to determine whether environmental adaptations are actually beneficial.[50]

When aberrant behavior persists despite careful changes in the environment, pharmacologic management is typically needed. Unfortunately, the use of pharmacologic therapy for behavioral management in children with acquired brain injury has not been scientifically investigated to any significant degree.[53] The proposed benefit of most agents is based on a relatively limited number of case studies, often carried out on adult patients in a nonblinded fashion and without appropriate controls. For other medications, efficacy is extrapolated from the benefits reported in patients with mental retardation or psychiatric disorders. The most pressing behavioral issues involve patients with aggression and severe agitation. Reasonable medications to try in these situations include clonidine, amantadine, buspirone, carbamazepine, and valproate.[53–55]

Communication and Cognitive Deficits

Communication and cognitive deficits secondary to an acquired brain injury are exceedingly common in all stages of recovery and represent the largest cause of long-term disability in these patients. Various cognitive impairments are observed in children and adolescents with acquired brain injury, the most common of which affect arousal and attentional skills, memory and learning of new information, and higher executive functioning. Some intellectual deficits may not become apparent until years after the injury, when these skills fail to emerge at the expected developmental age. Early on, however, maintenance of an appropriate level of arousal and sustained attention is key to any successful program of pediatric neurorehabilitation. This has led to the consideration of pharmacologic management of underarousal or reduced attention, with major emphasis on agents that act on the cholinergic, adrenergic, dopaminergic, and serotonergic neurotransmitter systems. Stimulant medications, in particular methylphenidate, have been shown to improve neurobehavioral tasks of attention and concentration in at least one double-blind placebo-controlled crossover study.[56] Dopaminergic agents, such as amantadine, and tricyclics have also been used in clinical situations.[52, 57] The results are equivocal but suggest an overall beneficial impact on arousal and attention. With regard to memory and learning of new information, no credible published reports exist on the efficacy of pharmacologic intervention in children or adolescents.

Neurorehabilitation of communication and cognitive impairment is based on several guiding principles. First, like the treatment of spasticity, therapy must begin in the acute setting, with a main focus on providing appropriate sensory modulation. Second, cognitive retraining should pervade all aspects of the neurorehabilitation process, including time spent with nursing and child-life specialists. For example, informal memory training can occur during any therapeutic activity to which the patient is exposed. Finally, therapy should be based on the dual approach of enhancing preserved function and remediating deficits.[25] Neurorehabilitation of communication and intellectual deficits mandates ongoing assessment of cognitive and linguistic capabilities using standardized tests, from which a systematic structured program of therapeutic intervention can be framed.[50] Sensory deficits, especially auditory and visual difficulties, may have an impact on the neurological assessment as well as the response to therapy. Clinical suspicion of these problems should be high in any child with an acquired brain injury, and appropriate evaluations (audiogram, brain evoked auditory potentials, visual evoked responses, ophthalmologic consultation, and so on) should be carried out.

Post-traumatic Seizures

Seizures secondary to acquired brain injury typically have their onset in the first 7 to 10 days following injury.[58] These early seizures are much more common in children than in adults, with a 5% to 10% incidence in children with traumatic brain injuries.[59, 60] The risk is highest in those younger than 3 years, in those with nonaccidental brain injury, and in children of any age with severe injuries; in the last group, the incidence may be as high as 30%.[59-61] However, it should be emphasized that in children, most early seizures follow relatively minor head injury, often within minutes of the trauma. In contrast, the risk of late post-traumatic epilepsy is much lower in childhood than in adulthood. In fact, the incidence of post-traumatic epilepsy in pediatric patients with mild to moderate traumatic brain injury is less than 1%.[60] Even in children with severe traumatic brain injury, the incidence of post-traumatic epilepsy is roughly half that observed in adults (7.4% versus 13.3%). In the pediatric population, severity of traumatic brain injury seems to be the single most important predictive factor. Other risk factors include intracranial hemorrhage, focal neurological signs, and nonaccidental traumatic brain injury.[58, 62]

Early seizures, especially those that occur within days of the acute injury, do not require treatment. In patients with recurrent early seizures, short-term anticonvulsant therapy, typically with phenytoin, may be indicated in some circumstances. The goal of treatment is to suppress additional seizures that may cause increased cerebral edema secondary to seizure-induced acidosis and increased blood flow.[58] This consideration is most appropriate in patients with raised intracranial pressure, because additional seizures may raise the pressure even further, resulting in impaired cerebral blood flow and extension of injury. Some investigators have suggested that initiation of anticonvulsant therapy is also indicated in patients with early seizures and additional risk factors for late seizures, such as intracranial hemorrhage, focal neurological signs, and penetrating cerebral injury.[58] A similar situation is the prophylactic administration of anticonvulsants in patients without seizures but with raised intracranial pressure or intracranial hemorrhage. It must be recognized, however, that there is no convincing evidence that prophylactic therapy is effective in preventing the development of post-traumatic epilepsy in children.[63] This fact, combined with the potential deleterious effects of antiepileptic drugs on cognition and behavior, has led most authors to conclude that there is little justification for prophylactic anticonvulsant administration in the pediatric population. In patients started on anticonvulsant therapy to suppress early seizures, the treatment duration should be limited. At St. Louis Children's Hospital, it is our policy to taper and then discontinue antiepileptic drugs before discharge, unless multiple focal seizures have occurred. In the latter case, we obtain a follow-up electroencephalogram; if that study is without epileptiform activity, tapering of the medication is initiated. In patients with persistent epileptiform discharges, we recommend longer-term treatment (typically 6 to 12 months) but switch the medication from phenytoin (or, less commonly, phenobarbital) to carbamazepine to minimize cognitive side effects.

FUTURE DIRECTIONS

Neurorehabilitation of acutely injured pediatric patients has improved dramatically over the last quarter century. Advances in surgical and medical management and technology have produced a dramatic impact on the mortality, morbidity, and quality of life of these children and adolescents. Our understanding of the biologic mechanisms of recovery has accelerated, leading to the hope that this knowledge can be translated into neurospecific therapies that can serve as the basis for restorative neurorehabilitation. The more immediate concern for the future, however, is to upgrade the provision of neurorehabilitation treatment to our patients. Few of the pharmacologic agents, physical modalities, and therapeutic approaches used to treat children and adolescents with acquired brain injuries have been subjected to rigorous scientific research with appropriate controlled subjects. Most of the published investigations involved limited populations, with little regard for the impact of normal development and recovery, and many failed to assess the achievement of functional goals as clinically appropriate end points. Even the use of such agents as heat and cold, which have been around for centuries and have a theoretic basis for efficacy, still prompts discussion. Objective research investigations with quantifiable, clinically relevant end points using double-blind protocols are essential for the future growth of neurorehabilitation and the improved care of neurologically injured children.

REFERENCES

1. Stedman's Medical Dictionary, 25th ed. Baltimore, Williams & Wilkins, 1990, p 1341.
2. Ward C, McIntosh S: The rehabilitation process: A neurological perspective. In Greenwood R, Barnes MP, McMillan TM, et al (eds): Neurological Rehabilitation. Edinburgh, Churchill Livingston, 1993, pp 13–28.
3. Selzer ME: Neurological rehabilitation. Ann Neurol 32:695–699, 1992.
4. Taylor DA: Neurorehabilitation in child neurology. J Child Neurol 6:97–100, 1991.
5. World Health Organization: The international classification of impairments, disabilities and handicaps (ICIDH). WHO, 1980.
6. Bickenbach JE, Chatterji S, Bradley EM, et al: Models of disablement, universalism and the international classification of impairments, disabilities and handicaps. Soc Sci Med 48:1173–1187, 1999.
7. Halbertsma J, Heerkens YF, Hirs WM, et al: Towards a new ICIDH: International classification of impairments, disabilities and handicaps. Disabil Rehabil 22:144–156, 2000.
8. World Health Organization: The international classification of impairments, activities and participation (ICIDH-2). WHO, 1997.
9. Taub E, Uswatte G, Elbert T: New treatments in neurorehabilitation founded on basic research. Nat Rev Neurosci 3:228–236, 2002.
10. Whyte J: Mechanisms of recovery of function following CNS damage. In Rosenthal M, Griffith ER, Bond MR, et al (eds): Rehabilitation of the Adult and Child with Traumatic Brain Injury, 2nd ed. Philadelphia, FA Davis, 1990, pp 79–88.
11. Waxman SG: Functional recovery in diseases of the nervous system. Adv Neurol 47:1–7, 1988.
12. Dail WG: Responses to cortical injury II. Widespread depression of the activity of an enzyme in cortex remote from a focal injury. Brain Res 211:79–89, 1981.
13. Hovda DA, Lee SM, Smith ML, et al: The neurochemical and metabolic cascade following brain injury: Moving from animal models to man. J Neurotrauma 12:903–906, 1995.
14. Fawcett JW, Rosser AE, Dunnett SB: Anatomical plasticity. In Fawcett JW, Rosser AE, Dunnett SB (eds): Brain Damage, Brain Repair. Oxford, Oxford University Press, 2001, pp 171–195.
15. Cowan WM, Fawcett JW, O'Leary DDM, et al: Regressive events in neurogenesis. Science 225:1258–1265, 1984.

16. Eyre JA, Taylor JP, Villagra F, et al: Evidence of activity-dependent withdrawal of corticospinal projections during human development. Neurology 57:1543–1554, 2001.

17. Conner JM, Fass-Holmes B, Varon S: Changes in nerve growth factor immunoreactivity following entorhinal cortex lesions: Possible molecular mechanism regulating cholinergic sprouting. J Comp Neurol 345:409–418, 1994.

18. Craig CG, Tropepe V, Morshead CM, et al: In vivo growth factor expansion of endogenous subependymal neural precursor cell populations in the adult mouse brain. J Neurosci 16:2649–2658, 1996.

19. Jenkins WM, Merzenich MM: Reorganization of neocortical representations after brain injury: A neurophysiological model of the bases of recovery from stroke. Prog Brain Res 71:249–266, 1987.

20. Chollet F, DiPiero V, Wise RJ, et al: The functional anatomy of motor recovery after stroke in humans: A study with positron emission tomography. Ann Neurol 29:63–71, 1991.

21. Villablanca JR, Hovda DA: Developmental neuroplasticity in a model of cerebral hemispherectomy and stroke. Neuroscience 95:625–637, 2000.

22. Elli KR, Danilov YP, Ahmad A, et al: Functional plasticity in extrastriate visual cortex following neonatal visual cortex damage and monocular enucleation. Brain Res 882:241–250, 2000.

23. Caplan B: Neuropsychology in rehabilitation: Its role in evaluation and intervention. Arch Phys Med Rehabil 63:362–366, 1982.

24. Finger S, Almli CR: Brain damage and neuroplasticity: Mechanisms of recovery or development. Brain Res Rev 10:177–186, 1985.

25. Gans BM, Mann NR, Ylisaker M: Rehabilitation management approaches. In Rosenthal M, Griffith ER, Bond MR, et al (eds): Rehabilitation of the Adult and Child with Traumatic Brain Injury, 2nd ed. Philadelphia, FA Davis, 1990, pp 593–615.

26. Michaud LJ, Duhaime AC, Batshaw ML: Traumatic brain injury in children. Pediatr Clin North Am 40:553–565, 1993.

27. McLean DE, Kaitz ES, Keenan CJ, et al: Medical and surgical complications of pediatric brain injury. J Head Trauma Rehabil 10:1–12, 1995.

28. Feldman Z, Contant CV, Pahwa R, et al: The relationship between hormonal mediators and systemic hypermetabolism after severe head injury. J Trauma 34:806–816, 1993.

29. Phillips R, Ott L, Young B, Walsh J: Nutritional support and measured energy expenditure of the child and adolescent with head injury. J Neurosurg 6:846–851, 1987.

30. Bruce DA: Head injuries in the pediatric population. Curr Probl Pediatr 20:61–107, 1990.

31. Logemann JA, Ylvisaker M: Therapy for feeding and swallowing disorders after traumatic brain injury. In Ylvisaker M (ed): Traumatic Brain Injury Rehabilitation: Children and Adolescents. Boston, Butterworth-Heinemann, 1998, pp 85–99.

32. Jaffe KM, Hays RM: Pediatric head injury rehabilitative medical management. J Head Trauma Rehabil 1:30–40, 1986.

33. Bell LM, Baker MD, Beatty D: Infections in severely traumatized children. J Pediatr Surg 11:1394–1398, 1992.

34. Krach LE, Kriel RL, Morris WF, et al: Central autonomic dysfunction following acquired brain injury in children. J Neurol Rehabil 11:41–45, 1997.

35. Barzilay Z, Somekh E: Diabetes insipidus in severely brain damaged children. J Med Clin Exp Ther 19:47–64, 1988.

36. Cochran EB, Phelps SJ, Tolley EA, Stidham GL: Prevalence of, and risk factors for, upper gastrointestinal tract bleeding in critically ill pediatric patients. Crit Care Med 1:1519–1523, 1992.

37. Blasier D, Letts M: The orthopaedic manifestations of head injury in children. Orthop Rev 18:350–358, 1989.

38. Sobus KM, Alexander MA, Harcke HT: Undetected musculoskeletal trauma in children with traumatic brain injury or spinal cord injury. Arch Phys Med Rehabil 74:902–904, 1993.

39. Noetzel MJ, Miller G: Traumatic brain injury as a cause of cerebral palsy. In Clark G, Miller G (eds): The Cerebral Palsies: Causes, Consequences and Management. Newton, MA, Butterworth-Heinemann, 1998, pp 185–207.

40. Barnes M, McLellan L, Sutton R: Spasticity. In Greenwood R, Barnes MP, McMillan TM, et al (eds): Neurological Rehabilitation. Edinburgh, Churchill Livingston, 1993, pp 161–172.

41. Whyte J, Robinson KM: Pharmacologic management. In Glenn MB, Whyte J (eds): The Practical Management of Spasticity in Children and Adults. Philadelphia, Lea & Febiger, 1990, pp 201–226.

42. Giebler KB: Physical modalities. In Glenn MB, Whyte J (eds): The Practical Management of Spasticity in Children and Adults. Philadelphia, Lea & Febiger, 1990, pp 118–148.

43. Feldman PA: Upper extremity casting and splinting. In Glenn MB, Whyte J (eds): The Practical Management of Spasticity in Children and Adults. Philadelphia, Lea & Febiger, 1990, pp 149–166.

44. Price GW, Wilkin GP, Turnbull MJ, Bowery NG: Are baclofen-sensitive GABA$_B$ receptors present on primary afferent terminals of the spinal cord? Nature 307:71–74, 1984.

45. Pinder RM, Brogden RN, Speight TM, et al: Dantrolene sodium: A review of its pharmacological properties and therapeutic efficacy in spasticity. Drugs 13:3–23, 1977.

46. Dall JT, Harmon RL, Quinn CM: Use of clonidine for treatment of spasticity arising from various forms of brain injury: A case series. Brain Inj 10:453–458, 1996.

47. Milanov I, Georgiev D: Mechanisms of tizanidine action on spasticity. Acta Neurol Scand 89:274–279, 1994.

48. Yablon SA, Agana BT, Ivanhoe CB, et el: Botulinum toxin in severe upper extremity spasticity among patients with traumatic brain injury: An open-labeled trial. Neurology 47:939–944, 1996.

49. Wilson DJ, Childers MK, Cooke DL, et al: Kinematic changes following botulinum toxin injection after traumatic brain injury. Brain Inj 11:157–167, 1997.

50. Ylivsaker M, Chorazy AJL, Feeney TJ, et al: Traumatic brain injury in children and adolescents: Assessment and rehabilitation. In Rosenthal M, Griffith ER, Kreutzer JS, et al (eds): Rehabilitation of the Adult and Child with Traumatic Brain Injury, 3rd ed. Philadelphia, FA Davis, 1999, pp 356–392.

51. Chorazy AJL, Crumrine PK, Hanchett JM, et al: Rehabilitation medical management. In Ylvisaker M (ed): Traumatic Brain Injury Rehabilitation: Children and Adolescents. Boston, Butterworth-Heinemann, 1998, pp 27–39.

52. O'Shanick GJ: Pharmacologic intervention. In Ylvisaker M (ed): Traumatic Brain Injury Rehabilitation: Children and Adolescents. Boston, Butterworth-Heinemann, 1998, pp 53–59.

53. Parmelee DX, O'Shanick GJ: Neuropsychiatric interventions with head injured children and adolescents. Brain Inj 1:41–47, 1987.

54. Connor DF, Steingard RJ: A clinical approach to the pharmacotherapy of aggression in children and adolescents. Ann N Y Acad Sci 794:290–307, 1996.

55. Krach LE, Kriel RL: Traumatic brain injury. In Molnar GE, Alexander MA (eds): Pediatric Rehabilitation, 3rd ed. Philadelphia, Hanley & Belfus, 1999, pp 245–268.

56. Mahalick DM, Carmel PW, Greenberg JP, et al: Psychopharmacologic treatment of acquired attention disorders in children with brain injury. Pediatr Neurosurg 29:121–126, 1998.

57. Kraus MF, Maki PM: Effect of amantadine hydrochloride on symptoms of frontal lobe dysfunction in brain injury: Case studies and review. J Neuropsychiatry Clin Neurosci 9:222–230, 1997.

58. Kennedy CR, Freeman JM: Post-traumatic seizures and post-traumatic epilepsy in children. J Head Trauma Rehabil 1:66–73, 1986.

59. Hendrick EB, Harris L: Post-traumatic epilepsy in children. J Trauma 8:547–555, 1968.

60. Annegers JF, Grabow JD, Groover RV, et al: Seizures after head trauma: A population study. Neurology 30:683–689, 1980.

61. Gilles EE, Nelson MD Jr: Cerebral complications of non-accidental head injury in childhood. Pediatr Neurol 19:119–128, 1998.

62. Barlow KM, Sowart JJ, Minns RA: Early post-traumatic seizures in non-accidental head injury: Relation to outcome. Dev Med Child Neurol 42:591–594, 2000.

63. Young B, Rapp RP, Norton JA: Failure of prophylactically administered phenytoin to prevent post-traumatic seizures in children. Childs Brain 10:185–192, 1983.

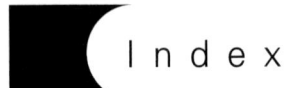

I n d e x

Note: Page numbers followed by f indicate illustrations; those by a b, boxes; those by a t, tables.

ABC system, of cervical spine anterior
    screw-plate fixation, 4630t, 4635–4636,
    4636f
ABCDEs, 5087–5088
Abdomen, trauma assessment of, 5089
Abducens nerve, 29, 316, 316f, 1899, 1974
  examination of, 266
    pediatric, 3173–3174
  injury to, in atlanto-occipital dislocation,
    4929
  paresis of, 317, 318t, 320, 320f
Abortion, CNS transplantation tissue from,
    2833, 2835
Abscess
  epidural. See Epidural abscess; Pyogenic
    infection, spinal.
  tuberculous, 1443
Absolute alcohol wash, for cerebral palsy,
    3731
ABT-627, as angiogenesis antagonist, 779t
Abulia, 285
  in frontal lobe tumors, 830
Abuse, reporting obligations in, 411
Academic practice, legal issues regarding,
    409–410
Accessory nerve, 1973–1974
Acetaminophen, for pain, 2959
Acetazolamide
  for brain edema, 802
  for elevated intracranial pressure, 1429
  for infantile posthemorrhagic
    hydrocephalus, 3411
Acetyl coenzyme A, synthesis of, 1483t
Acetylcholine, in action potential, 3814
Achilles tendonitis, vs. distal tibial nerve
    entrapment, 3936
Achondroplasia, 3362–3371
  apnea in, 3363–3364
  cervicomedullary compression in,
    3364–3365
    decompression of, 3367–3368
      outcome of, 3369
      ventriculostomy for, 3367
  craniovertebral region, 3343, 3344f
  epidemiology of, 3362–3363
  genetics of, 3362–3363
  hydrocephalus in, 3365–3366, 3398
  intracranial pressure in, 3365–3366
  jugular bulb dehiscence in, 3364
  medical complications of, 3363–3364,
    3363t
  neurologic complications of, 3363t
  neurologic vs. orthopedic aspects of,
    3366
  psychosocial problems in, 3363
  reproduction in, 3363
  spinal stenosis in, 3365, 3366–3367
    decompression of, 3368–3369
      outcome of, 3369–3370
    recurrence of, 3370–3371, 3370f, 3371f
Acid-base metabolism, 123–126, 125f
Acidosis, cerebral, in head injury, 5050
Acoustic meatus, internal, 36f, 40f
Acoustic neuroma, 1147–1164. See also
    Brainstem, glioma of.

Acoustic neuroma (Continued)
  arterial involvement in, 1159, 1159t
  cerebellopontine angle
    anatomic distortions in, 1158–1159,
      1158t
    auditory tests in, 335f–336f
    treatment of, 1163–1164, 1163f
  diagnosis of, 1149–1150, 1149f, 1152,
    1153f
  facial nerve distortions in, 1158–1159,
    1158t, 1159t
  features of, 1147, 1147f
  historical review of, 1147–1150, 1148f,
    1149f
  in pregnancy, 872
  intracanalicular, 1162–1163, 1163f
  magnetic resonance imaging of, 1149,
    1149f
  pathology of, 1152–1153, 1154f
  posterior fossa anatomic variations in,
    1158–1159, 1158t
  radiosurgery for, 1154–1155, 4055–4056,
    4059f
    complications in, 574
    linac, 4112
    vs. microsurgery, 1164, 4056, 4057t,
      4058f
  surgery for, 1154–1158, 1158t
    complications of, 1161–1162
      avoidance of, 570–571
    cranial nerve preservation in,
      1160–1161
    evolution of, 1150–1152
    facial nerve monitoring during,
      1159–1160
    facial nerve paralysis after, 1161
    headache after, 1162
    middle fossa approach to, 1155
    morbidity in, 1161–1162
    mortality in, 1161
    neurophysiologic monitoring during,
      1160
    outcome in, 1164
    posterior fossa intradural approach to,
      925–926
    suboccipital approach to, 1156–1158,
      1156f–1158f
    translabyrinthine approach to,
      1148–1149, 1155–1156
  treatment of, 1147, 1150
    tumor size and, 1162–1164, 1163f
  venous involvement in, 1159, 1159t
  vs. facial nerve schwannoma, 1147,
    1147f, 1148f
  vs. meningioma, 1153
  vs. peripheral schwannoma, 1153, 1154f
Acoustic radiation, 9
Acoustic reflex, hearing assessment with,
    334, 335f–336f
Acquired immunodeficiency syndrome
    (AIDS)
  neuropathy in, 3841
  primary central nervous system
    lymphoma in, 1069–1070, 1071f

Acquired immunodeficiency syndrome
    (AIDS) (Continued)
  pyogenic spinal infections in, 4363–4364
    differential diagnosis of, 4371
    medical management of, 4379
  reporting obligations in, 411–412
  systemic lymphoma in, 1070, 1072
Acromegaly
  carpal tunnel syndrome in, 3890
  diagnosis of, in pregnancy, 868
  dopamine agonists for, 1193
  growth hormone excess and, 1189, 1190
  neuropathy in, 3843
  radiation therapy for, 1193, 4035–4036
  radiosurgery for, 4062
  recurrence of, 1193–1194
  somatostatin analogs for, 1192–1193
  surgery for, 1176
Actin, in axonal regeneration, 197
Actinomyces israelii, spinal infection with,
    4295
Actinomycin, for Ewing's sarcoma, 4850
Actinomycosis, spinal, 4385
Action potential, 73
  calcium, 219, 220, 222–224
  conductance changes during, 220–221,
    221f
  electrodiagnostic testing of, 3851–3852,
    3851f
  generation of, 220–221, 221f
  glial, 221
  ion currents in, 219
  maintenance of, 224–225
  motor unit, polyphasic nature and,
    3856–3857, 3856f
  muscle fiber, spontaneous, peripheral
    nervous system abnormalities with,
    3856, 3856t
  neuronal, 3813, 3813f, 3814b
  repolarization of, 220, 224–225
  sodium, 220–222
Adamantinoma, pituitary, 1207
Adaptive development, 3170, 3170t
Adductor reflex testing, pediatric, 3180
Adenoassociated viruses
  as central nervous system gene therapy
    vector, 4166–4167
  as vectors, 818
Adenocarcinoma, paranasal sinus, 1312
Adenohypophysis, morphology of,
    1171–1172
Adenoid cystic carcinoma, paranasal sinus,
    1312, 1313f
Adenoma, pituitary. See Pituitary
    adenoma.
Adenosine
  for pain, 2966
  in cerebral autoregulation, 1475
  in cerebral blood flow–metabolism
    coupling, 1489
Adenosine triphosphate, 119–120
  after brain injury, 2455–2456
  generation of, 118–119, 119f
  in cerebral metabolism, 1479, 1482
  in focal cerebral ischemia, 134, 134f
  in neurons, 1486

Baclofen *(Continued)*
  intrathecal
    cerebrospinal fluid concentration of, 2883–2884, 2884f, 3749
    complications of, 3753–3754
    delivery systems for, 2886
    distribution of, 2883–2884, 2884f
    dosage of, 3750, 3751–3752
    duration of action of, 3749
    efficacy of, 2884–2885, 2885f, 2885t, 3752–3753, 3752t
    for cerebral palsy, 3732, 3749–3756
    for dystonia, 2748, 2748f, 2749t
    for spasticity, 2750–2751, 2751t, 2866t, 2867, 2882–2887, 3788
    GABA receptors and, 3748, 3749
    kinetics of, 2883–2884, 2884f
    mechanism of action of, 3748
    patient selection for, 2886–2887, 2886t, 3750, 3751t, 3754–3755
    pharmacokinetics of, 3749
    physiologic effects of, 2883, 2883f
    pump for, 3749–3754, 3749f, 3750f
    response to, 3750
    side effects of, 2885–2886, 3748–3749
    tolerance to, 2885–2886
    vs. dorsal rhizotomy, 3752–3753, 3752t
Bacteremia, pyogenic spinal infections in, 4364
Bacterial infection. *See also* specific infection.
  myelitis from, 4312t, 4313
  pyogenic. *See* Pyogenic infection.
Bacteriology, neoplastic disease treatment and, 711–712
Bacteroides, spinal infection from, 4365
Bad, 719
Bak, 719
Baker's cyst, 3934
Balance disturbance, after temporal bone fracture, 5281
Baldness, headrests and, 610
Ballism, 2720
Ballismus, 2676
Balloon angioplasty
  for carotid restenosis, 1666
  for cerebral vasospasm, 1856–1857, 1857f, 1858f
Balloon cells, proliferation of, 2492
Balloon compression, for trigeminal neuralgia, 3000–3002, 3001f
Balloon occlusion, of aneurysms, 2057–2060, 2058f
Baló's concentric sclerosis, 1452
Band of Giacomini, 27
Bands of Büngner, 3961, 3962f
Barbiturate coma
  in bullet wounds, 5231
  intracranial hypertension treatment by, 5133–5134
Barbiturates, 1508
  after head injury, 5097
  brain protection with, 5059
  cerebral metabolic rate of oxygen and, 1532
  in carotid endarterectomy, 1626–1627
  in craniotomy, 5150
  in hypothermic circulatory arrest, 1511
  in ischemia protection, 1521
  intracranial pressure and, 188–189
Barthel Index, 243t, 5288
Basal arteries, craniopharyngioma attached to, 3672, 3673f
Basal cell carcinoma
  scalp, 1409–1410

Basal cell carcinoma *(Continued)*
  skull, 1398, 1399f
  staging of, 1410
Basal ganglia, 11
  anatomy of, 2671, 2672f, 2683–2695, 2699, 2700f, 2730–2731
  "anterior," 19
  in dystonia, 2795–2796, 2796f
  in micturition, 359
  in movement disorders, 2699–2701, 2700f–2701f, 2702t, 2703, 2824–2825
  in obsessive-compulsive disorders, 2854–2855
  in psychiatric disorders, 2855
  in urologic dysfunction, 373
  input to, 2671–2672
  intrinsic connections of, 2672–2673
  motor thalamic nuclei inputs from, 2691, 2692f
  organization of, 2683, 2684f
  output projections of, 2673
  synaptic connectivity of, 2683–2695, 2730–2731. *See also* specific structure, e.g., Striatum.
  thalamic nuclei inputs to, 2693, 2694f
  thalamocortical circuit and, 2699–2701, 2700f, 2702t, 2703
    in Huntington's disease, 2718
  venous drainage of, 1238
Basal vein, 10f, 15f, 35f, 36f
  segments of, 23–24, 24f
Basement membrane, 3814
  glioma spread through, 760
Basic fibroblast growth factor, 51
  in angiogenesis, 719, 771, 773
  in brain injury recovery, 5031–5032
  in recurrent carotid artery stenosis, 1663
Basic helix-loop-helix structure, 51
Basigin gene, 158
Basilar apex
  anatomy of, 1974–1975, 1975f
  aneurysms of, 1975, 2025, 2041–2052
    arteriovenous malformations with, 1976
    coil embolization for, 2051–2052
    complications in, 2051
    endovascular treatment of, 2051–2052
    extended orbitozygomatic approach to, 1982, 1985, 1985f
    medial petrosectomy for, 1986–1987
    orbitozygomatic-pterional approach to, 1982, 1983f–1984f
    pterional approach to, 2049–2050
    pterional-transsylvian approach to, 1978, 1978f–1981f, 1982
    pure transsylvian approach to, 2042–2047, 2043f
      clipping in, 2047
      craniotomy in, 2043–2044, 2045f, 2046f
      positioning in, 2043, 2044f
      scalp incision in, 2043, 2045f
      subarachnoid exposure in, 2044, 2046–2047
    skull base approach to, 1985–1987, 1986f
    subtemporal approach to, 1977–1978, 1977f, 2042, 2047–2049, 2047f, 2048f
    surgery for, 2042–2051
      anatomy in, 2041–2042
      approaches to, 1977–1987, 2025
      temporary occlusion for, 2050–2051
    transclinoidal approach to, 1985
    transclinoidal-extracavernous approach to, 1986, 1986f

Basilar apex *(Continued)*
    transclinoidal-transcavernous approach to, 1985
    treatment timing for, 2050
  giant aneurysm of, deep hypothermic circulatory arrest for, 1529, 1530f
  perforating arteries of, 1974–1975, 1975f
Basilar artery, 22f, 36f, 37, 38f
  anatomy of, 1974, 2026
  aneurysms of, 2025–2038
    clinical presentation of, 2025–2026
    combined petrosal approach to, 2030–2032, 2031f–2033f
    combined supra-/infratentorial approach to, 1990–1991, 1990f
    complications of, 2036–2038
    embolization of, 2067–2068
    extended retrolabyrinthine approach to, 1987f–1988f, 1988–1989
    extradural temporopolar approach to, 2029–2030, 2030f, 2031f
    extreme lateral inferior transtubercular approach to, 2034–2036, 2035f–2037f
    middle fossa approach to, 1991, 1992f, 1993
    results of, 2038
    retrolabyrinthine transsigmoid approach to, 2032–2034, 2033f–2035f
    subtemporal transtentorial approach to, 2026–2027, 2026f, 2027f
    surgical approaches to, 1985, 1987–1993, 2026–2036
      hypothermic circulatory arrest in, 2037
      rupture during, 2037
    transcochlear approach to, 1987f–1988f, 1989–1990
    translabyrinthine approach to, 1987f–1988f, 1989
    transoral approach to, 1993, 1993f
    transpetrosal approach to, 1987–1990, 1987f–1988f, 1988t
    transsylvian approach to, 2027–2029, 2028f, 2029f
  blunt trauma to, 5212
  fusiform aneurysms of, 1593, 1594f
  intermittent insufficiency of, 1692
  occlusion of, 5212
  paramedian perforating branches of, rupture of, 1739
Basilar impression, 3340
  congenital developmental, 3341–3343, 3343f
Basilar invagination, 3340–3341, 3341f
Ballismus, 2729
Bathrocephaly, 428–429
Batimastat (BB-94), for glioma invasion, 766
Battered child syndrome, evaluation of, 3499–3500, 3500f
Bax, 719
Bayliss effect, 1475
BB-94 (batimastat), for glioma invasion, 766
Bcl-2, 718, 743
  cell protection by, 1519
  in carotid body tumors, 1678
Bcl-x, 718
Bcl-xl, 718–719
Becquerel, 4007
Behavior management, in traumatic brain injury, 5294–5295
Behavioral disturbances, pediatric, neurorehabilitation of, 3789

Behavioral therapy, pain treatment with, 2966
  regression of benefit in, 2940–2941
Bell's cruciate paralysis, 4871, 4871f
Bence Jones protein, in multiple myeloma, 4854
BendMeister rod bender, 4659f, 4660
Benedikt's syndrome, 273
Benton Controlled Oral Word Association Test (COWAT), 5186
Benzel-Kesterson interspinous wiring modification, 4645, 4647f
Benzodiazepines, 1508
  for dystonia, 2796
  for pain, 2966
  in intracranial pressure management, 5127, 5127t
  in pregnancy, 2422
Beriberi, neuropathy in, 3844
Bernard-Horner syndrome, in nerve plexus injury, 3970
Bethanechol, for multiple sclerosis, 1455t
Biceps reflex testing, pediatric, 3180
Biglycan, 4230
Bilharziosis, spinal, 4390
Bing's sign, 268
Bioartificial materials, for central nervous system repair, 4163
Biochemical markers, for neoplastic meningitis, 1232
Biomechanics
  of atlantoaxial joint, 4187, 4188
  of axis, 4939
  of cervical spine, 4187–4190, 4193–4194, 4432
  of craniovertebral junction, 3333–3334
  of facet joints, 4185
  of internal spinal fixation, 4592–4596, 4593f, 4594f
  of intervertebral disk, 4185–4186
  of lumbar spine, 4191, 4714–4715
  of pediatric atlantoaxial joint, 3537–3538, 3538f
  of pediatric atlanto-occipital joint, 3528–3529
  of pediatric spinal injury, 3515–3516
  of spinal cord injury without radiographic abnormality, 3516
  of spine, 4181–4199, 4586, 4587f, 4588–4589
  of spondylolisthesis, 4543–4547
  of thoracic spine, 4190–4191, 4953–4954, 4953f–4955f
  of thoracic spine fixation, 4195–4198
  of thoracic spine fractures, 4192, 4195–4198
  of thoracic spine posterior procedures, 4694–4695
  of vertebrae, 4184–4185
Biopsy
  complications in, 573, 573t
  endoscopic, 3430
  in frameless stereotactic surgery, 945–946
  in pyogenic spinal infection, 4369, 4370f
  muscle, 3963–3964
  of pineal region tumors, 1014–1016, 1014f, 1014t
  of third ventricle tumors, 1248–1249
  peripheral nerve, 3837, 3838f, 3962–3963
  surgical navigation in, 945–946
Birbeck granules, in eosinophilic granuloma, 4843
Birth history, 3169–3170
Birth trauma, 3481–3486

Birth trauma (*Continued*)
  brachial plexus injury in, 3488–3495, Brachial plexus, obstetric injury to
  epidural hematoma in, 3483–3484, 3483f
  incidence of, 3481
  intracranial hemorrhage in, 3483–3485, 3483f–3486f
  posterior fossa subdural hematoma in, 3484–3485, 3485f, 3486f
  risk factors for, 3481
  scalp injury in, 3481–3482
  subdural hematoma in, 3484, 3484f
Bisphosphonates, in bone metabolism, 4233
Bisulfan, for ependymoma, 1048t
Bithermal caloric test, 344–345, 344f
Biventral lobule, 30f, 33f
Bladder
  anatomy of, 357–358, 357f, 358f
  autonomic receptors in, 358, 358f
  distention of, 364
  dysfunction of, in cerebral palsy, 3728, 3732, 3744–3745
  filling dysfunction of, 364–365, 365f
  neuromuscular function of, 363
  reflex contraction of, 377
  storage dysfunction of, 364–365, 365f
    treatment of, 378–379
  storage function of, 363
  voiding dysfunction of, 365
Bladder outlet resistance, 359
Bladder outlet retention, treatment of, 379–380
Blastocyst, development of, 4239, 4240f
Blastomycosis
  cranial destruction in, 430, 430f
  spinal, 4388f, 4389
Bleomycin, for craniopharyngioma, 1219, 3683–3684
Blepharospasm, 2729
Blindness
  in trigeminal schwannoma, 1345, 1345f
  monocular, 2541, 2542f
    optic nerve lesions, 2542, 2542f
  patient positioning and, 612–614
  prone positioning and, 603–604
Blink response, pediatric, 3173
Blood pressure. *See also* Arterial pressure.
  in cervical spine trauma, 4888, 4889
  in intracerebral hemorrhage, 1740
  in pregnancy, 2421
  in stroke, 1500–1501
  in trauma, 5090
Blood transfusion, 2829
Blood vessels, lumbar spine and, surgical anatomy of, 4706
Blood viscosity
  hypothermia effects on, 1532
  in head injury, 5058–5059
Blood-brain barrier, 153–170
  adherens junctions in, 157
  amino acid transport across, 160–161, 160t, 161f
  anatomic, 159
  capillaries of, 154
  cell biology of, 154–159, 155f
  contrast media penetration of, 164
  diseases affecting, 163–167
  disruption of, in chemotherapy, 879
  drug delivery across, 15–18, 16f
  endothelial cells forming, 153–154
  functional, 159
  gap junctions in, 157
  glucose transport across, 154, 159–160, 159f

Blood-brain barrier (*Continued*)
  GLUT-1 in, 158–159
  glutamate transport across, 161–162
  γ-glutamyltranspeptidase in, 158, 161
  immune cell passage through, 890
  in aging, 166–167
  in brain injury, 166
  in brain tumors, 164–165, 165t
  in cerebral edema, 165–166
  in cerebral ischemia, 166
  in cerebral metabolism, 1487
  in chemotherapy, 878
  in epilepsy, 166
  in experimental allergic encephalomyelitis, 164
  in hypertension, 166
  in immune response, 673
  in multidrug resistance, 162–163
  in multiple sclerosis, 164
  in radiation injury, 166
  in stress, 166
  inflammation effects on, 163–164
  ion transport across, 162
  ketone body transfer across, 1485
  lipoprotein transport across, 162
  macromolecular passage through, 154–155
  markers of, 157–159
  maturation of, 158
  microenvironmental influences on, 157–159
  morphology of, 154–155, 155f
  neurotransmitter transport in, 154, 161–162
  opening of
    chemotherapy delivery via, 153
    for brain edema, 802–803
  pediatric, 3462
  pericytes in, 153
  perivascular glia in, 153
  permeability of, 154, 155f
    cellular mechanisms of, 163
    disease effects on, 11–15
    lipophilicity and, 15, 16f
    to nucleosides, 158
    to nucleotides, 157–158
  physiology of, 791–792, 792f
  protective metabolic function of, 161
  receptor-mediated transport across, 163
  regulation of, astrocytes in, 109–110
  tight junctions in, 156–157, 159f
  transcellular endocytosis in, 159f
  transcellular lipophilic pathway in, 159f
  transcytosis through, 163
  transendothelial pathways of, drug delivery via, 159, 159f
  transport across, 156, 159–163, 159f
Blood–cerebrospinal fluid barrier, 791–792, 792f
Blood-tumor barrier, 17
Bmp4, 53t
Bobble-head doll syndrome, in suprasellar cysts, 3294
Bohlman triple-wire technique, 4645–4646, 4647f–4648f
Bone
  abnormalities of, head shape and, 3300
  anatomy of, 4227–4229, 4228f, 4613–4614
  biochemistry of, 4614–4615
  calcium in, 4231
  cancellous, 4227–4229, 4228f, 4613–4614
  cellular elements of, 4229, 4230f, 4614
  cortical, 4227, 4228f, 4613
  formation of, 4231–4233, 4231f, 4232t, 4613
  in spondyloarthropathies, 4460

Catheters (*Continued*)
  ventricular
    in cerebrospinal fluid shunt,
      3379–3380, 3380f
    obstruction of, 3382–3383
Cauda equina, 4989f
  compression of
    decompression for, 4998
    in pyogenic spinal infection, 4364
    in spinal stenosis, 4521
    treatment of, 4374
  recovery of, 4989–4990
  sensory loss in, 272, 272f
Cauda equina syndrome, 4872
  in lumbosacral spine tumors, 4041
  lumbar diskectomy and, 580
Caudal agenesis, 4269–4270, 4269f
Caudal point, 38
Caudal regression syndrome, 4317
Caudate
  arteriovenous malformation of, 2246
  hematoma of, 1737
Caudate nucleus. *See* Nucleus caudalis.
Caudomedial artery, 39
Causalgia, 3831
  definition of, 3094
  pain in, 3820–3821
  sympathectomy for, 3094
  vicious cycle hypothesis of, 3094
Cavernoma. *See* Cavernous malformations.
Cavernous angioma. *See* Cavernous
  malformations.
Cavernous angiomatosis, familial multiple,
  2394
Cavernous carotid fistula, 1771, 2341–2350,
  5211
  carotid-jugular compression for, 2345
  classification of, 2343–2344
  clinical presentation of, 5212, 5214
  embolic agents for, 2346
  embolization of
    balloon, 2345–2346
    coil, 2346
  endovascular treatment of, 2342–2343,
    2345
  historical aspects of, 2341, 2342f
  in pregnancy, 2429
  in type IV Ehlers-Danlos syndrome,
    1771
  intracaverous internal carotid artery
    aneurysm and, 1882, 1884–1885
  microsurgery for, 2341–2342, 2346, 2347f
  radiosurgery for, 2349–2350
  surgery for, 2346, 2348–2349, 2348f
  symptoms of, 2344
  treatment of, 2344–2350
Cavernous hemangioma. *See* Cavernous
  malformations.
Cavernous malformations, 1373,
  2142–2147, 2167–2171, 2292–2298,
  4315t
  anesthesia in, 1512
  arteriovenous malformations and, 2154
  asymptomatic, 2169
  behavior of, 2171
  brainstem, 2294–2295, 2295f, 2321–2338.
    See also Brainstem, cavernous
    malformations of.
  capillary telangiectasia and, 2153
  capsular, 2314–2316
  central skull base, 1268
  cerebral
    familial, 2299
      CCM1 in, 2300–2301
      genetic markers in, 2300

Cavernous malformations (*Continued*)
    genetics of, 2299–2303
    historical background for, 2299
    Krev-1/rap1a pathway in, 2303
    KRIT1 mutations in, 2301–2302, 2303
    linkage analysis of, 2299–2300
    magnetic resonance imaging of,
      2300
    sporadic, 2299
  classification of, 2167–2168, 2167t
  clinical presentation of, 2138t, 2144,
    2169–2170, 2293–2295, 2293f–2297f
  cryptic, 2167
  definition of, 2167–2168
  developmental venous anomalies and,
    2153
  dural-based, 2317
  epidemiology of, 2142, 2168–2169,
    2292–2293
  extradural, 4821
  familial, 2293, 2293f, 2295
  focal deficit in, 2170
  genetics of, 2168
  hemorrhage in, 2169–2170, 2170t,
    2293–2294, 2293f–2296f, 2295, 2296
    morbidity and mortality of, 2170–2171
  imaging of, 2138t, 2144–2145, 2145f,
    2146f, 2167–2168
  in extratemporal lobe epilepsy, 2598
  incidence of, 2292, 2293t
  infratentorial, 2321–2338. *See also*
    Brainstem, cavernous malformations
    of.
  intradural, 4826, 4830f
  magnetic resonance imaging of, 471,
    471f, 2167–2168, 2167t, 2292,
    2293f–2297f
  natural history of, 2138t, 2144,
    2295–2296, 2297f
  neurological deficit in, 2294, 2295f
  occult, 2167
  optic pathway, 2316
  outcome in, 2170–2171
  pathology of, 2138t, 2142–2144, 2143f
  pineal, 2316, 2316f
  scalp, 1413–1414
  seizure in, 2169, 2171, 2294, 2294f
  spinal cord, 2353–2354, 2355f, 2356. *See
    also* Spinal cord, cavernous
    malformations of.
  sporadic, 2293, 2295
  supratentorial, 2305–2317
    clinical scenarios associated with,
      2305, 2305t
    epilepsy in, 2310
    expectant management of, 2305–2306
    hemorrhage in, 2305, 2307–2308, 2308f,
      2309f
    incidental, 2306–2307, 2307f
    intractable epilepsy with, 2314
    lesions mimicking, 2310–2311, 2310f,
      2312f
    long-standing seizure in, 2310
    mass effect in, 2309
    medical management of, 2306
    multiple, 2316–2317, 2317f
    neurological deficits in, 2309
    new-onset seizure in, 2309
    radiotherapy for, 2306
    stereotactic radiosurgery for, 2306
    surgery for, 2306, 2311–2318
      imaging before, 2311
    venous malformations associated
      with, 2311, 2313f, 2314
    vs. arteriovenous malformation, 2311,
      2312f

Cavernous malformations (*Continued*)
  synonyms for, 2167
  thalamic, 2314–2316, 2314f, 2315f
  third ventricular, 1247
  treatment of, 2138t, 2146–2147
  vascular anatomy of, 2386
Cavernous sinus, 1895
  anatomy of, 918–919, 919f, 920f
  frontotemporal surgical approach to,
    2346, 2348–2349, 2348f
  inferior, artery of, 1896
  injury to, transsphenoidal surgery and,
    1182
  internal carotid artery and, fistula
    between. *See* Cavernous carotid
    fistula.
  lateral triangle of, 2341–2342
  meningioma of, 1118, 1118f, 1278
  septic thrombosis of, 1421
  triangles of, 2346, 2348–2349, 2348f
  tumors of, 1265
Cavernous sinus syndrome, intracavernous
  internal carotid artery aneurysm and,
  1881–1882
Cavitation
  post-traumatic, 206
  spinal cord, 4317
CCM1, 2142, 2168
  KRIT1 mutations and, 2301–2302, 2301t
  localization of, 2300–2301
CCM2, 2142, 2168
  localization of, 2300–2301
CCM3, 2142, 2168
  localization of, 2300–2301
CD4
  in antigen recognition, 678
  in multiple sclerosis, 1450
CD8, in antigen recognition, 678
CD40–CD40 ligand system, in antigen-
  presenting cell activation, 893
CDK4, 1411
CDKN2, 1411
CDKN2/p16/INK4a, 741
Celecoxib, for pain, 2959
Celiac plexus block, 2983–2984
  fluoroscopy in, 2973, 2973f, 2974f
Cell(s)
  calcium metabolism in, 122f
  electrical measurements in, 216, 217f
  electrical properties of, 215–216, 216f,
    218–219, 219f
  major histocompatibility complex
    expression in, 678
  migration of, 681–683
  proliferation of, in malignant phenotype,
    771, 772f
Cell adhesion molecules
  in central nervous system repair,
    4156–4157, 4162
  in malignant glioma, 760–761, 763
Cell cycle, 716–718, 717f
  regulation of, tumor suppressor genes
    in, 741
Cell cycle analysis, cytometric, tumor
  proliferation marking by, 694–695
Cell cycle arrest pathways, in glioma,
  717–718, 717f
Cell cycle modulators, in gene therapy,
  820–821
Cell death, 82–83. *See also* Apoptosis.
  apoptotic vs. necrotic, 130–132, 131f
  calcium hypothesis of, 126
  calcium-related, 126–128
  excitotoxic hypothesis of, 126
  genetic program for, 133

Cell death *(Continued)*
glutamate-related, 126–128
in global ischemia, 132–133
mitochondrial failure and, 132–133
pathways for, 133
programmed, 718–719
protein synthesis and, 132
Cell membrane, ion selectivity of, 219
Cell Saver system, 4968
Cell swelling, 228
Cell-cell signaling, 774t
Cellular signaling proteins, as tumor
suppressor genes, 741–743
Central deafferentation syndromes, 3018t
Central herniation, 826, 826t, 5055t, 5056
rostral-caudal progression of, 292, 292f
Central lobule, 30f, 31f
Central nervous system
abnormal sensory feedback to, in
parkinsonian tremor, 2774
antigen presentation in, 887, 889–890
B cells in, 683
congenital tumors of, 811
disorders of, blood-brain barrier in, 153
drug penetration of, 17–18
electrophysiology of, 215–232
hemangioblastoma of, 1053–1060. *See
also* Hemangioblastoma.
immune-inflammatory network in,
673–685. *See also* Immune response;
Inflammation.
in urinary tract function, 359–360, 359f,
360f
inflammation of, 135–136
neuroimmunology and, 4155
injury to, 202–206
apoptosis after, 4155–4156
astrocytes in, 86, 204–205
chronic responses to, 4156
gene expression after, 4154–4155
inflammation in, 205–206
neurons in, 202–203
oligodendrocytes in, 203–204
pediatric, 3463
recovery from, 5025–5033
response to, 202
retrograde neuronal changes after,
4156
secondary effects of, 206
sequelae to, 4154–4156
transneuronal degeneration after, 4156
vs. peripheral nervous system injury,
3968–3969
wallerian degeneration after, 4156
lymphocytes in, 890
malformations of, gene mutations and,
46t
metastases to
chemotherapy for, 17
classification of, 671–672
magnetic resonance imaging of, 457,
457f, 458f
peripheral nervous system and, 3809
physiology of, 216, 217f
primary lymphoma of. *See* Lymphoma,
primary central nervous system.
regulation of, astrocytes in, 86
repair of, 4153–4169
after incomplete injury, 4157
bioartificial regeneration environments
in, 4163
biologic methods in, 4158
developmental rationale for,
4156–4157
dorsal root entry zone in, 4161–4162

Central nervous system *(Continued)*
embryonic tissue transplantation in,
4158
ensheathing glia in, 4162–4163
evaluation of, 4158
evidence supporting, 4156–4157
extracellular matrix in, 4168
gene therapy in, 4166–4167
glial cellular transplantation in,
4161–4163
glial scarring in, 4167–4168
in chronic injury, 4169
in immature mammals, 4156
in nonmammalian species, 4156
inflammatory cell transplantation in,
4164
inhibition reduction in, 4168, 4169
intraspinal embryonic tissue
transplantation in, 4159
intrinsic regenerative capacity in,
4164–4169
mammalian lower extremity function
and, 4157
mechanisms of, 4153–4154
models for, 4157–4158
myelin inhibition of, 4168–4169
myelin repair in, 4164
peripheral nerve grafts in, 4161, 4162
physical methods in, 4164
Schwann cells in, 4162
strategies for, 4158–4169
trophic molecules in, 4164–4166
undifferentiated, renewable cells in,
4159–4161
vs. plasticity, 4154
replacement in, 4154
secondary lymphoma of, 1074
stimulation of, 3119
transplantation in, 2829–2847. *See also*
Transplantation.
tuberculosis of, 1439–1443
tumors of
chemotherapy for, 877–878
classification of, 4023
cyst with, 671t
extra-axial
radiologic features of, 835, 836–839
vs. intra-axial, 835
functional magnetic resonance
imaging of, 852–853, 853f
intra-axial
radiologic features of, 835, 842–852
vs. extra-axial, 835
intraparenchymal, radiologic features
of, 835, 840–841
radiologic features of, 835–854
xanthogranuloma of, 1443–1444
Central spinal cord syndrome, 4397, 4890,
4890f
Central sulcus, 3, 4f, 24f
in craniometrics, 630–631
localization of, 2532, 2532f
magnetic resonance imaging of, 2532
of insula, 5, 6f
topography of, 2533
Centromedian-parafascicular nuclear
complex, subthalamic nucleus
projections from, 2690
Centrum semiovale, venous drainage of,
1238
Cephalocele, 3198
Cephalohematoma
calcified, pediatric, 3717, 3718f
linear skull fracture and, 3482
scalp injury and, 3482
skull, 1404

Cephalothin, in pediatric glioma surgery,
3598
Ceramic bone graft, 4618
c-ERB2, in medulloblastoma, 3641
Cerebellar artery
anterior inferior, 36f, 37–39, 40f, 1974,
2026
embolization of, 2258
in arteriovenous malformations,
2256–2257, 2257f
occlusion of, ischemia risk with, 2107
origin of, aneurysms arising at, 2025
saccular aneurysm of, 1975
basilar superior, 2026
inferior, aneurysms of, 2025
rupture of, 1787
posterior inferior, 36f, 37–39, 40f,
1973–1974
anastomosis of, 2115
aneurysms of, 1975
clinical significance of, 2007–2008
diagnosis of, 2013–2014
endovascular occlusion of, 2019,
2021
far lateral suboccipital approach to,
2015, 2017f
lateral/medial suboccipital
approach to, 2018
midline suboccipital approach to,
2018–2019
outcome in, 2020–2021
preoperative evaluation for, 2014
presentation of, 2009, 2010t–2012t,
2013, 2013f
rupture of, 2009
subarachnoid hemorrhage in, 2013,
2013f
surgical complications of, 2019–2020
treatment indications for, 2007–2008,
2008f
embolization of, 2258
in arteriovenous malformations,
2256–2257, 2256f, 2257f
occlusion of, ischemia risk with, 2107
superficial temporal artery bypass to,
2115
superior, 36f, 38f, 39–40, 1974, 1975
aneurysms of, 1975
embolization of, 2258
in arteriovenous malformations,
2256–2257, 2256f, 2257f
trigeminal nerve compression by, 3013
trigeminal nerve and, 1344
Cerebellar astrocytoma
pediatric, 3655–3660
age in, 3655
clinical presentation of, 3655, 3656t
complications of, 3659, 3659t
fibrillary, 3657, 3657f, 3658
follow-up for, 3660
histology of, 3656–3658, 3657f
imaging of, 3655–3656, 3656f
location of, 3656
outcome in, 3659–3660
radiation therapy for, 3660
sex in, 3655
surgery for, 3658–3659
pilocytic, juvenile, 3656–3657, 3657f
Cerebellar ataxia
after medulloblastoma surgery, 1037
urologic disorders in, 373–374
Cerebellar fissure, precentral, 32
Cerebellar hemisphere
arteriovenous malformations of, 2251
arterial supply/venous outflow in,
2256–2257, 2257f, 2258f

Compound nerve action potential
(*Continued*)
nerve assessment by, 3866
within surgical field, 3864
Compression, peripheral nerve injury in, 3827–3828
Compression fracture. *See* Fracture(s), compression.
Compression sleeves, 4968
Compression therapy, for transverse-sigmoid dural arteriovenous malformation, 2288
Compton effect, in radiation therapy, 4006, 4006f
Computed tomography, 5019
before epilepsy surgery, 2483–2485, 2484f, 2485f
in surgical navigation, 946
skull, 419, 432–433
spinal, 501–503, 502f, 4145
xenon. *See* Xenon computed tomography.
Computer, in image-guided spinal navigation, 4743–4756
Concentration
after hyperextension-hyperflexion injury, 4919
after traumatic brain injury, 5186–5187
Concentrative nucleoside transporters, 158
Concorde position, 597t, 604, 604f
Concussion, 5045
labyrinthine, 5281
pediatric, 3463
temporal bone fracture and, 5281
vestibular, 5281
Conditioning lesions, in central nervous system repair, 4164
Conduction, during action potential, 220–221, 221f
Conduction block, nerve conduction studies of, 3860
Conductor, 215
Confusion, in pregnancy, 295, 295t
Congenital anomalies
cranial destruction in, 429–430
spinal, imaging of, 533–536
vertigo in, 2902
Congenital deformities, of axial skeleton, 4317–4318
Congenital lumbosacral lipoma. *See* Lipoma, congenital lumbosacral.
Congenital malformations. *See also* specific malformations.
neural, 4256–4271, 4256t
spinal, 4148, 4276–4281, 4276f–4281f, 4315t, 4316–4319, 4317f, 4318f
Congenital spondylolisthesis, 4541, 4542f
pathogenesis of, 4543–4544
treatment of, 4550–4551
Coning, 1504–1505
Connective tissue, in spasticity, 2879–2880
Connective tissue disorders, heritable, aneurysms with, 1769–1773, 1770t
Connexins, in astrocytes, 101
Conotoxin, peripheral nerve effects of, 3816
Conradi's syndrome, 3334
Consciousness
after surgery, 906–907
altered states (loss) of, 275, 283–286, 285t
brainstem auditory evoked potentials in, 297
causes of, 282, 282t
diagnosis of, 294t
differential diagnosis of, 277–298

Consciousness (*Continued*)
electroencephalography in, 296–297, 296f
in injury severity estimation, 5195–5196
in mild head injury, 5073
intracranial pressure monitoring in, 295–296
mechanisms of, 277–278, 278f
respiratory failure in, 282–283, 283f
somatosensory evoked potentials in, 297
treatment of, 292–295
assessment of, 281–292, 281t
Glasgow Coma Scale in, 286–287, 286t
in herniation syndromes, 290–292, 291t, 292f
in intracranial catastrophe, 289–292, 291t, 292f
ocular movement abnormalities in, 288–289
oculovestibular response testing in, 289, 290f, 290t
Pediatric Coma Scale in, 287–289, 288f
physical examination in, 282–283, 283f
pupillary response in, 287–288
clouding of, 283
definition of, 277, 393
level of, in bullet wounds, 5227–5228, 5228f
neuroanatomy of, 278–280, 279f
neurophysiology of, 280–281, 280f
self-awareness in, 283
Constipation, in cerebral palsy, 3727, 3732
Contact guidance, in peripheral nerve regeneration, 3804–3805
Contractures, in cerebral palsy, 3728, 3732
Contrast media, blood-brain barrier effects of, 164
Contusion(s)
brain, 5041–5042
cerebral, 5159, 5159f
evacuation of, 5159, 5160f–5161f, 5162
hemorrhagic, in traumatic brain injury, 5107f, 5108
in mild head injury, 5070, 5071t
magnetic resonance imaging of, 469
pediatric, 3463
peripheral nerve injury from, 3827
shaking-impact syndrome and, 3501, 3504f
Conus medullaris, 4989f
arteriovenous malformations of, 2371–2372, 2371f
ascent of, 4245, 4247f
dysraphic anomalies of, 3247–3248
lesions of, sensory loss in, 272, 272f
lipoma of, 3229
tethering of, by tight filum terminale, 3247
Conus medullaris syndrome, 4872
Conversion hysteria, pediatric, back pain in, 3568
Coordination, examination of, 267–268
pediatric, 3179
Copper chelators, as angiogenesis antagonists, 778t, 781–782, 782f
Copper depletion, in angiogenesis, 775, 776f
Coprolalia, 2730
Copropraxia, 2730
Copula pyramidis, 31f
Copular point, 31f, 32, 37
Cordectomy, for spasticity, 2870
Cordotomy

Cordotomy (*Continued*)
anatomy for, 3059–3061, 3060f
complications of, 3068–3070
for pain, 3059–3070
historical aspects of, 2913–2914, 3059
lateral spinothalamic tract in, 3060, 3060f
open, 3067–3068
anterior, 3068, 3068f
posterior, 3067–3068, 3067f
patient selection for, 3061
percutaneous technique of, 3061–3067
anatomic localization in, 3062–3063, 3063f–3066f
anesthesia for, 3062
anterior, 3063, 3066f
bilateral, 3066–3067
care after, 3067
computed tomography–guided, 3063, 3064f, 3065f
dentate ligament in, 3063, 3066f
electrode system calibration in, 3061, 3062f
instrumentation in, 3061, 3062f
lesions in, 3065–3066
physiologic localization in, 3063, 3065
positioning for, 3062
preparation before, 3061–3062
x-ray–guided, 3063, 3066f
results of, 3068–3070
Cornea, assessment of, 302, 304, 304f
Cornu ammonis, 2486, 2487f
Corona radiata, 7f
Coronal suture, 423f
Corpectomy
cervical, anterior, 4439–4440, 4441f
complications of, 577
for pyogenic spinal infection, 4372f, 4374–4376, 4377f–4379f
in cervical spine fixation, 4625–4626, 4628f
thoracic, 4767, 4768f
anterior, 4974–4978, 4976f–4977f
vertebral reconstruction after, 4767, 4768f, 4769
Corpus callosotomy
complications of, 1243–1244
for extratemporal lobe epilepsy, 2596
for third ventricle tumors, 1253–1254
seizure outcome after, 2578–2579
Corpus callosum, 4f, 7f, 8f, 9, 24f, 1237, 1238f
agenesis of, in Dandy-Walker syndrome, 3286
anterior
arteriovenous malformation of, 2242, 2242f
damage to, 265
genu of, 14f
glioma spread through, 757, 759–760
hematoma of, in distal anterior cerebral artery aneurysms, 1948
lipoma of, 3693
median artery of. *see* Cerebral artery, anterior.
posterior
arteriovenous malformation of, 2242–2243, 2243f
damage to, 265
rostrum of, 15f
splenium of, 13
surgical complications of, 1258–1259
venous drainage of, 1238
Cortex
abnormal organization of, 2493
anterior cingulate, 2932–2933

Death *(Continued)*
  determination of, 415
  diagnosis of, 393–394
Débridement
  for postoperative spinal infection, 4384
  for pyogenic spinal infection, 4375–4376,
    4376f, 4378
  for spinal tuberculosis, 4387
  of bullet wounds, 5236–5237, 5237t
Decompression
  for cervical degenerative disease,
    4409–4428
  for cubital tunnel syndrome, 3909–3910
  for degenerative spondylolisthesis,
    3581–3583
  for failed back syndrome, 4337–4339
  for lumbar fracture, 5004–5005
  for pyogenic spinal infection, 4374–4375,
    4379
  for spinal cord injury, 4878–4880
  for spinal metastases, 4858–4862,
    4860f–4863f
  for spinal stenosis, 3368–3369
  for spinal tuberculosis, 4387
  for thoracic disk herniation, 4981
  for thoracic spine fracture, 4972–4978,
    4974f–4977f, 4980
  for thoracolumbar scoliosis, 4562
  for thoracolumbar spine fracture,
    5000–5002, 5000t, 5001f, 5001t
  microvascular, of trigeminal nerve,
    3005–3014
  neurovascular, for vertigo, 2909
  of cauda equina compression, 4998
  of cervicomedullary compression,
    3367–3368
  of spinal cord compression, 4998
  of ulnar nerve entrapment, 3909–3910
  of vertebral arteries, 1700, 1702, 1703,
    1705f, 1709
  stereotactic, for craniopharyngioma,
    1216
  thoracic spine
    anterior, 4973–4978, 4974f–4977f
    posterolateral, 4972–4973
  transoral, for upper cervical spine,
    4751–4752, 4752f
  transthoracic, 4974, 4975–4978, 4975f
Decorin, 4230–4231
Deep brain stimulation, 3026–3027
  chronic pain treatment with, 3119–3129,
    3123
    complications of, 3128–3129
    electrode implantation in, 3125–3126
    functional magnetic resonance
      imaging in, 3122
    generator implantation in, 3126
    head frame for, 3123
    hemorrhage in, 3128, 3128t
    historical aspects of, 3119–3120
    mechanisms of, 3121–3122
    microelectrode recording in, 3124
    outcomes in, 3126–3128, 3127t, 3128t
    paresthesia-producing targets in,
      3121–3122, 3122t
    patient selection in, 3120–3121, 3121t
    periaqueductal gray targets in, 3121,
      3121t, 3122, 3125, 3125f
    periventricular gray targets in, 3121,
      3121t, 3122, 3125
    procedure in, 3126–3127
    site selection in, 3121, 3121t, 3122t
    stimulation trial in, 3126
    target selection in, 3123, 3124
    technique of, 3122–3126

Deep brain stimulation *(Continued)*
  for Parkinson's disease, 2662, 2662f
  movement disorder treatment with,
    2803–2825. *See also* specific target,
    e.g., Globus pallidus, internal.
    atlases in, 2808–2809
    basal ganglia targeting in, 2804
    clinical validation in, 2809
    complications of, 2822–2824
    computed tomography in, 2808
    coordinates in, 2809, 2809f
    costs of, 2825
    electrode implantation in, 2810, 2811f,
      2812–2813, 2812f
    electrophysiologic studies in, 2813,
      2814f–2816f, 2815–2817
    generators in, 2817–2819, 2818f, 2824
    indications for, 2819–2820
    lesion targeting in, 2805–2810
    magnetic resonance imaging in,
      2804–2805, 2806f–2808f, 2807–2808
    microadjustments in, 2815–2817
    microrecording in, 2813, 2815, 2815f
    parallel processing model and, 2819
    patient selection in, 2819–2820
    radiography in, 2804
    results of, 2820–2822
    side-effects of, 2824
    software for, 2810
    target localization in, 2819, 2824
    ventriculography in, 2804, 2805–2807,
      2805f
    vs. ablation, 2824
    vs. neural grafts, 2824
  seizure outcome with, 2579
  vs. thalamotomy, 2780
Deep hypothermic circulatory arrest,
    1528–1537, 2108
  cannulation sites in, 1534
  cerebral ischemia pathophysiology and,
    1532
  complications in, 1536
  for posterior circulation aneurysms,
    2000, 2002
  history of, 1528
  in aneurysm treatment, 1511, 1528–1529,
    1529f–1531f, 1531, 1807
  indications for
    anatomic factors in, 1528–1529,
      1529f–1531f, 1531
    patient-related factors in, 1531–1532,
      1531t
  medical evaluation before, 1533–1534
  neuroanesthetic management in,
    1534–1535
  patient preparation for, 1534
  results of, 1536–1537
  surgical management in, 1535–1536
  technical preparations before, 1533
  techniques for, 1533–1536
Deep tendon reflexes
  in peripheral neuropathy, 3833
  testing of, 3824–3825
Deep venous thrombosis, 563–564
Degenerative disease
  neuronal, 4315t–4316t, 4319–4321, 4320f
  spinal, 4147–4148
    cervical. *See* Cervical disk disease.
    lumbar. *See* Lumbar disk disease.
    thoracic. *See* Thoracic disk herniation.
    vs. pyogenic infection, 4371
Degenerative spondylolisthesis
  pathogenesis of, 4545–4546, 4545f, 4546f
  treatment of, 4551–4553, 4552f
Dehydration, intracranial hypertension
    treatment by, 5133

Dejerine-Sottas disease, 536, 537f
Delirium, 286
  after traumatic brain injury, 5296
Delivery
  brachial plexus injury in, 3488–3495. *See
    also* Brachial plexus, obstetric injury
    to.
  epidural hematoma in, 3483–3484, 3483f
  in neoplastic disease, 873
  intracranial hemorrhage in, 3483–3485,
    3483f–3486f
  intraparenchymal hemorrhage in, 3485
  posterior fossa subdural hematoma in,
    3484–3485, 3485f, 3486f
  scalp injury in, 3481–3482
  skull fracture in, 3482–3483, 3482f
  subdural hematoma in, 3484, 3484f
  traumatic. *See also* Birth trauma; Brachial
    plexus, obstetric injury to.
  vertex, brachial plexus injury in, 3488,
    3489f
Delta, 53t
Dementia, 285–286
  colloid cyst and, 3688
  Lewy body
    apoptosis in, 2710
    clinical features of, 2712
    forms of, 2708–2709
    neuritic Alzheimer's disease changes
      in, 2712
    pathology of, 2712–2713
    substantia nigra pars compacta in,
      2706f
  positron emission tomography of,
    484–485
  thalamic, strategic infarcts and, 1609
Demyelination, 3961, 3961f
  imaging of, 541, 543f
  in multiple sclerosis, 1450–1451
  in sensory nerve action potential, 3853,
    3853f
  primary, 3962
  radiation-induced, 854
  secondary, 3962
  segmental, 3962
  urologic disorders in, 375
  vertigo in, 2902
Dendrite(s), 72f, 73
  antigen presentation by, 893
  structure of, 77
Denervation
  prolonged, 201
  urologic disorders in, 375
Denervation hypersensitivity, in cerebral
  vasospasm, 1849
Dens
  aplasia-hypoplasia of, 3341
  fracture of. *See also* Odontoid fracture.
    imaging of, 519, 519f
Dentate gyrus, 26f, 27, 2486, 2487f
Dentate ligament, 3060, 3060f
  in cordotomy, 3063, 3066f
  triangular processes of, 36f
Dentate tubercle, 31f
Dentatorubropallidoluysian atrophy,
  2718–2719, 2740
Dentition, in craniofacial trauma,
  5248–5249
2-Deoxyglucose, in positron emission
  tomography, 480, 481t, 482
Dependency
  definition of, 3783–3784
  in traumatic brain injury response, 5193t
Depolarization, 3813, 3813f
Depolarizing potentials, 228

Dystonia *(Continued)*
  definition of, 2729
  dopa-responsive, 2737, 2765
  dorsal column stimulation for, 2797
  focal, 2738
  heredodegenerative, 2721
  idiopathic torsion, positron emission
    tomography of, 2764–2765
  in cerebral palsy, 3724, 3725, 3731–3732,
    3747–3748, 3751t
  intrathecal baclofen for, 2748, 2748f,
    2749t
  medical therapy for, 2796
  nonkinesigenic, 2737
  pallidotomy for, 2797–2798
  parkinsonism and, 2678, 2721, 2737
    vs. dopa-responsive dystonia, 2765
    x-linked (Lubac), 2721
  paroxysmal, 2737
  paroxysmal kinesigenic, 2737
  pediatric, assessment of, 3179–3180
  peripheral denervation for, 2797
  plus, 2737
  primary, 2737, 2795
  primary inherited, 2721
  primary torsion, 2721
  reciprocal innervation in, 2891
  secondary, 2721, 2737, 2795
  severity of, 3751t
  spasmodic torticollis in, 2891
  surgery for, 2748, 2796–2799
    microelectrode recording in,
      2798–2799
    patient selection in, 2796–2797
  thalamic stimulation for, 2821
  thalamotomy for, 2797–2798
  treatment of, 2737–2738
  with myoclonus, 2721
Dystopia, orbital, 5257, 5262
  in roof fracture, 5261f, 5262f
Dysuria, 365
DYT1, in primary dystonia, 2721
DYT5, 2737
DYT11, 2737

EAAC1, 103
EAAT4, 103
EAAT5, 103
Ear(s)
  hair cell of, 74, 74f
  in craniofacial trauma, 5251
Ebselen, for cerebral vasospasm, 1854
E-cadherin, in meningioma, 1103
Echinococcal infection, spinal, 4390
Eclampsia, 2425
Edema
  brain. *See* Cerebral edema.
  dependent, prone positioning and, 563
  in arteriovenous malformation, 2188
  in astrocytoma, 836
  ischemic, 5055
  neurotoxic, 5055
  postoperative, 566
  tumor-associated, 13
Edward's sleeves, in thoracic spine
  fixation, 4969f
EGFR
  in glioblastoma, 950
  in glioblastoma multiforme, 726
  in glioma, 716
EGR2, 53t
Ehlers-Danlos syndrome type IV,
  1770–1771, 1771t
  intracranial aneurysms in, 1771

Eicosanoids
  in blood-brain barrier function, 12
  in cerebral blood flow regulation,
    1472–1473, 1472f
  in cerebral vasospasm, 1848–1849
Ejaculation
  in neurogenic disorders, 366
  retrograde, anterior lumbar approach
    and, 580
Elbow
  brachial plexus obstetric palsy and,
    3980t
  ulnar nerve entrapment at, 3897–3917.
    See also Ulnar nerve, entrapment of,
    elbow-level.
  ulnar nerve surgery and, 652
Electrical auditory brainstem response,
  with cochlear implants, 337
Electrical injury, peripheral nerve, 3828
Electrical stimulation, 3107–3116
  deep brain. *See* Deep brain stimulation.
  electrode computer adjustment in,
    3115–3116, 3115f
  electromyographic recording and,
    4223–4224
  for cerebral palsy, 3731
  for chronic pain, 3107–3116
  for failed back surgery syndrome,
    3112–3113
  for urinary retention, 378
  implanted pulse generators for,
    3110–3111, 3111f
  mechanisms of, 3107–3108
  peripheral nerve, 3112–3114
    electrodes for, 3109–3110, 3110f
  screening protocols for, 3111–3112
  spinal cord, 3112–3114
    complications of, 3115t
    contraindications to, 3115t
    electrodes for, 3108–3109, 3108f–3110f
    for angina pectoris, 3113
    for ischemic pain, 3113
    for low back pain, 3113
    for peripheral nerve injury, 3113
    for reflex sympathetic dystrophy,
      3113–3114
    indications for, 3112–3114
    outcomes of, 3114–3115, 3114f
    vs. reoperation, 3112–3113
Electrocardiogram, subarachnoid
  hemorrhage effects on, 553–554
Electrocorticogram, in ischemia
  prevention, 1523f
Electrodes
  computer adjustment for, in electrical
    stimulation, 3115–3116, 3115f
  depth, 2555, 2555f, 2558–2559, 2558f,
    2559f
  epidural peg, 2556–2557
    insertion of, 2561
  for electrophysiologic studies,
    2554–2557, 2555f, 2556f
  foramen ovale, 2557, 2561
  implantable
    deep brain stimulation with, 2810,
      2811f, 2812–2813, 2812f, 3125–3126
    spinal cord stimulation with,
      3108–3109, 3108f–3110f
  in cordotomy, 3061, 3062f
  in epilepsy, 2486, 2486f, 2529, 2530, 2535,
    2599
  in peripheral nerve surgery monitoring,
    3863
  in trigeminal neuralgia, 2997, 2998f

Electrodes *(Continued)*
  intracranial monitoring with, 2554–2557,
    2555f, 2556f
    insertion of, 2558–2561, 2558f–2560f
  percutaneous, peripheral nerve
    stimulation with, 3109–3110, 3110f
  sphenoidal, 2557
  subdural, 2555, 2556f, 2559–2560, 2560f
Electrodiagnostic studies. *See*
  Electromyography; Electrophysiologic
  studies; Nerve conduction studies.
Electroencephalography, 230–231
  desynchronization of, 280
  in altered consciousness, 296–297, 296f
  in anesthesia, 1506–1507, 1506f
  scalp, 2551
Electrolytes
  in altered consciousness, 295
  in anterior communicating artery
    aneurysms, 1937
  in subarachnoid hemorrhage, 554,
    1829–1830, 1830t
  management of, in traumatic brain
    injury, 5130–5131, 5130f
Electromagnetic stimulation, in bone
  healing, 4619
Electromyography, 3851
  fundamentals of, 3851–3852, 3851f
  in selective dorsal rhizotomy, 3741–3742,
    3741f, 3742t
  indications for, 3851
  intraoperative, 4219–4222, 4220t, 4221f,
    4222f
  needle, 3856–3857, 3856f, 3856t
    interference pattern in, 3857
    motor unit action potential size and,
      3856–3857, 3856f
    of carpal tunnel syndrome, 3858
    of peripheral nerve trauma, 3860–3861
    of radiculopathy, 3859
    of ulnar neuropathy, 3858–3859
    positive sharp waves in, 3856, 3856f
    recruitment in, 3857
    spontaneous muscle fiber action
      potentials in, 3856, 3856t
  spontaneous free-running
    in peripheral nerve surgery
      monitoring, 3863, 3865
    of thenar muscles, 3866, 3867f
  triggered
    in median nerve tumor surgery, 3866,
      3867f
    in peripheral nerve surgery
      monitoring, 3862, 3864
Electronystagmography, 343–346, 344f,
  346f
Electrophysiologic studies
  electrodes for, 2554–2557, 2555f, 2556f
  in neurosurgery, 230–232, 232t
  in thoracic spine fracture, 4967–4968
  intraoperative
    historical review of, 4203–4204
    medicolegal aspects of, 4224–4225
    methodological overview of, 4204
    nerve root involvement and,
      4216–4222
    of spinal cord and nerve roots,
      4203–4225
    space-occupying lesions and,
      4222–4224
    spinal cord function and, 4204–4215
    tethered cords and, 4222–4224
  of central nervous system, 215–232
  physical principles of, 216, 217f
  recording equipment for, 2557
  terminology in, 216t

Failed back syndrome *(Continued)*
  pathology of, 4328–4329
  physical examination of, 4332–4333
  physiologic testing of, 4334
  physiology of, 4327–4328
  psychological, social, economic testing
    of, 4334, 4336
  psychosocioeconomic, 4332
  treatment of, 4336–4343
    decompressive surgery in, 4337–4339
    epidural fibrosis after, 4337
    ganglionectomy in, 3042
    neuropathic pain surgery in, 4343
    pharmacologic, 4336–4337
    psychosocioeconomic, 4338
    rehabilitation in, 4336
    stabilization-arthrodesis surgery in,
      4339–4343, 4341f, 4342f
    surgical, 4338–4343
  types of, 4329–4332
False negative, 497
False positive, 4⌗
Falx cerebri
  in Chiari malformation type II, 3351,
    3351f
  meningioma of, 1112–1113
Familial cancer syndrome, 969
Familial polyposis, brain tumors in, 812t,
  813
Family, in life-sustaining treatment refusal,
  415
Family history, 263–264
Farnesyl transferase inhibitors,
  angiosuppressive therapy with, 780
Fas ligand, in astrocytoma development,
  891
Fas/Apo1/CD95, 743
Fasciculations, 268
Fastigium, 31f
Fat, in Cushing's disease, 1195
Fatigue, in neuromuscular junction
  disorders, 270
Fatty acids, free, after traumatic brain
  injury, 5026
Fazio-Londe syndrome, 4319, 4320
FCMD, in lissencephaly, 61
Fecal incontinence, in cerebral palsy, 3727,
  3732
Feeding problems, in cerebral palsy, 3727
Felbamate, pharmacology of, 2470t,
  2471–2472
Femoral cutaneous nerve, lateral,
  entrapment of, 3933
Fertility, prolactinoma and, 1188–1189
Fetal tissue, in neurogenesis, 5033
Fetal tissue transplantation, 2830–2843,
  4158
  abortion in, 2833, 2833t
  assessment before, 2832–2833, 2832t
  chromaffin cells in, 2831
  donation protocols in, 2833
  donor age determination in, 2833, 2834f,
    2834t, 2835
  mesencephalic tissue in, 2831–2832
    grafting procedures for, 2836–2837
    preparation techniques for, 2835–2836,
      2835f
  patient selection in, 2832
  postoperative care in, 2837–2838
  results of, 2838–2839, 2840t, 2841, 2842t,
    2843t
Fetus
  central nervous system development in,
    2833, 2834f
  Parkinson's disease effects on, positron
    emission tomography of, 2757–2758,
    2758f

Fever
  in pediatric neurorehabilitation, 3787
  in traumatic brain injury, 5124, 5124f,
    5128, 5136
  pain associated with, 4290–4295, 4291t
  treatment of, 5136
FGFR3, in achondroplasia, 3362, 3363
Fibrillation potentials, 3856, 3856t
Fibrillin-1, 1772
Fibrinolysis, for intracerebral hemorrhage,
  1753–1754
Fibrinolytic agents, spontaneous
  intracerebral hemorrhage with, 1735
Fibroblast growth factor
  in axonal regeneration, 200
  in brain tumors, 727–728
  in central nervous system repair, 4160,
    4162
  in glioma, 716
Fibroblast growth factor receptor
  in brain tumors, 728
  in craniofacial syndromes, 3315–3316
Fibrolysis, subarachnoid blood clot, 1852
Fibroma, ossifying, 1367
Fibromuscular cushions, 2148
Fibromuscular dysplasia, carotid artery,
  1681–1682, 1682f
Fibromyalgia, 4331
Fibromyositis, 4331
Fibromyxochondroma, 1365
Fibronectin, in malignant glioma, 761
Fibrosarcoma, 1142–1143, 1143f
  skull, 1389–1390, 1390f
Fibrosis, cerebral arterial, in vasospasm,
  1847–1848
Fibrous dysplasia, 1365–1367
  monostotic, 3590–3591
  orbital, 1374–1375
  osteogenic sarcoma with, 1389, 1389f
  radiologic aspects of, 1365–1366, 1365f
  signs/symptoms of, 1366
  skull, 1401–1402, 1402f, 1403f
    pediatric, 3719, 3720f
  spinal, pediatric, 3590–3591, 3591f
  treatment of
    indications for, 1366
    surgical, 1366–1367, 1367f
Fibrovascular stroma, in bone graft
  incorporation, 4619
Fick equation, 5048
Field potentials, 230–231
Filum terminale
  dysgenesis of, 3264–3266, 3265f, 3266f
  dysraphic anomalies of, 3247–3248
  ependymoma of, 4296t, 4300–4301, 4819
    treatment of, 4824
  hypertrophic, 3264, 3265f
  lipoma of, 3229
    split spinal cord from, 3248, 3248f
  paraganglioma of, classification of,
    666–667
  thickened, 4266–4267
  tight, 4316
    development of, 3247
Fimbria, 9, 2486, 2487f
Finger-to-nose test, 3179
Fishes, spinal cord regeneration in, 4156
Fistula
  arteriovenous. *See* Arteriovenous fistula.
  cavernous carotid. *See* Cavernous
    carotid fistula.
  cerebrospinal fluid. *See* Cerebrospinal
    fluid fistula.
  perilymph
    temporal bone fracture and, 5281–5282

Fistula *(Continued)*
  tympanotomy for, 2907
  vertigo in, 2903–2904
  traumatic, 2132
Fixation, internal. *See* Internal fixation.
Flap(s), galea-frontalis, in craniofacial
  trauma, 5258f–5259f
Flexion injury
  to cervical spine, 4890, 4896, 4909, 4909f
  to thoracic spine, 4958–4959, 4959f, 4962,
    4962t
Flexion-rotation injury, to thoracic spine,
  4959–4960, 4960f, 4980–4981
Flexor carpi ulnaris, in ulnar nerve
  compression, 3903
Flexor superficialis muscle, median nerve
  entrapment at, 3924
Flexor synovialis, in carpal tunnel
  syndrome, 3890
Flexor-pronator aponeurosis, in ulnar
  nerve compression, 3903
FLNA, 53t
Flocculus, 30, 30f, 31, 31f, 34, 36f, 40f
  peduncle of, 32, 33f
Floor plate, notochord and, in primary
  neurulation, 4254–4255
Flow cytometry, in tumor proliferation
  marking, 694–695
Fluid management
  in traumatic brain injury, 5130–5131,
    5130f
  intracranial pressure and, 188
Fluid pressure injury
  hippocampus effects of, 2449, 2450
  synaptic modification from, 2452, 2453f
Fluid shifts, in deep hypothermic
  circulatory arrest, 1536
^{11}C-Flumazenil, neuronal marking by, 1609
2-[^{18}F]Fluoro-2-deoxy-D-glucose (FDG),
  positron emission tomography with,
  480, 481t, 482
  in brain tumors, 487, 487f–489f
  in Huntington's disease, 483, 484f
  of regional hypermetabolism, 490, 491f
[^{18}F]6-Fluoro-L-dopa, in positron emission
  tomography, 482, 483f
^{18}F-Fluoromisonidazole, hypoxia marking
  by, 1609
Fluoroscopy, image-guided spinal
  navigation and, 4754–4755, 4755f
5-Fluorouracil, for paranasal sinus tumors,
  1327
Foam cells, in xanthogranuloma formation,
  1444
Folate
  deficiency of, neural tube defects from,
    3217–3218
  supplemental, 3218, 3218t
Foley catheter, complications of, patient
  positioning and, 614
Folic acid
  deficiency of, in occult spinal
    dysraphism, 3257–3258
  recommended daily allowances for, 3218
  supplemental, in pregnancy, 871
Folium, 34
Folstein Mini-Mental Status Testing, 242t
Fontan's space, 4674
Foot
  abnormalities of, nerve damage and,
    3833, 3833f
  digital nerve entrapment in, 3936
Foot drop, nerve injury and, 3823

Glial cell(s)
  abnormal proliferation of, 2492
  in central nervous system repair,
    4162–4163
  in potassium spatial buffering, 2455
  potassium ion distribution by, 102, 104f
  radical, 79f, 80, 84, 97, 98f
Glial cell line–derived growth factor
  delivery of, positron emission
    tomography in, 492–493, 493f
  in axonal regeneration, 199–200
Glial cell line–derived neurotrophic factor
  in axonal regeneration, 200
  in central nervous system
    transplantation, 2843–2844
Glial fibrillary acidic protein, 97
  after central nervous system injury, 4168
  in Alexander's disease, 111
  in diffuse fibrillary astrocytoma, 661
  in medulloblastoma, 3640, 3646
Glial membrane potential, in potassium
    redistribution, 2455
Glial scar, in axonal regeneration, 205
Glial tumors, 4296t
  in pregnancy, 870–871, 870f
  mixed, classification of, 665–667, 666t
  oligodendrocyte progenitor cells and,
    92–93
  radiosurgery for, 4063–4065, 4064t
  spinal cord, 4825
  third ventricular, 1246
Glioblastoma
  brachytherapy for, 4097
  classification of, 662
  contiguous spread of, 757
  deep vein thrombosis risk in, 939
  EGFR amplification in, 950
  fibroblast growth factor receptor in, 728
  gene alterations in, 751t
  low copper diet in, 781
  multifocal spread of, 758, 758f
  mutations in, 715
  platelet-derived growth factor receptor
    in, 730
  vascular endothelial growth factor
    receptor in, 733
Glioblastoma multiforme
  anaplastic, 969
  bromodeoxyuridine marking of, 693
  cytometric cell-cycle analysis of, 695
  diagnosis of, 972, 973f
  DNA polymerase marking of, 694
  genetics of, 726, 969–970
  histopathology of, 970–971, 971f
  incidence of, 4018
  interstitial brachytherapy for, 4097
  Ki-67/MIB-1 marking of, 696
  necrosis in, 843f–844f, 844
  prognosis for, 977–978
  proliferating cell nuclear antigen
    marking of, 694
  radiation therapy for, 975
  radiologic features of, 842, 842f
  radiosurgery for, 4063–4065, 4064t
  recurrent, treatment of, 976–977, 977f
  seizures in, 828
  third ventricular, 1246
  ³H-thymidine marking of, 692
  vascular endothelial growth factor in,
    733
Glioblastosis cerebri, classification of,
    662–663
Gliofibroma, 990
Gliogenesis, 97, 98f

Glioma, 981–994. *See also* specific type, e.g.,
    Astrocytoma.
  angionecrotic, 772
  brain edema in, 795
  brainstem. *See* Brainstem, glioma of.
  bromodeoxyuridine marking of, 692–693
  "butterfly," 970f
  cell cycle arrest pathways in, 717–718
  cellular biology of, 714–720
  chordoid, third ventricle, 664
  cystic, intracavitary brachytherapy for,
    4106–4107
  diffuse chiasmatic, pediatric, 3596, 3597
  DNA polymerase marking of, 694
  electrophysiologic abnormalities in, 230
  endothelial proliferation in, 771–772
  exophytic chiasmatic-hypothalamic,
    pediatric, 3596, 3597, 3598
  gene therapy for, 711–721
  incidence of, 808–809, 809t, 950
  insulin-like growth factors in, 728–729
  intramedullary, pediatric, 3708
  low-grade, 950–966
    chemotherapy for, 964
    computer-assisted stereotactic
      resections of, 956
    histopathology of, 951–953, 951f, 952f
    magnetic resonance imaging of, 953,
      954f
    magnetic resonance spectroscopy of,
      954, 955f
    malignant transformation of, 954–956
    misdiagnosis of, 955
    outcome in, 965–966
    preoperative characteristics of,
      953–954, 954f, 955f
    prognostic factors in, 964–965
    radiation therapy for, 962–964, 963t
    stereotactic biopsy of, 955–956
    surgery for, 955–962
      frameless navigation systems in,
        956, 958f
      imaging during, 956–957
      magnetic source imaging in, 956,
        957f
      prognosis of, 957, 959, 959t–962t
      sonographic navigation in, 956, 958f
      stimulation mapping techniques in,
        956, 956f
      timing of, 955–956
      type of, 956–957
  magnetic resonance imaging of, 449–450,
    450f–454f, 452–453
  malignant, 757–766, 969–978, 4018
    adhesion molecules in, 760–763
    brachytherapy for, 757
    cadherins in, 763
    cell surface adhesion molecules in, 763
    chemotherapy for, 975–976
    collagen in, 761
    computed tomography of, 758–759
    contiguous spread of, 757
    diagnosis of, 972, 973f
    distant recurrence of, 757–758
    epidemiology of, 969
    extracellular matrix molecules in,
      761–763
    familial, 969–970
    fibronectin in, 761
    genetics of, 969–970
    glycoproteins in, 762
    glycosaminoglycan in, 762
    grading of, 970–972, 970f–972f
    histopathology of, 970–972, 970f–972f
    hyaluronate receptors in, 763

Glioma (*Continued*)
  immunoglobulin superfamily in, 763
  integrins in, 763
  interstitial brachytherapy for,
    4101–4104, 4102t, 4103t
  intraoperative mapping techniques
    for, 974, 974f
  invasion in, 757–766
  laminin in, 761
  magnetic resonance imaging of,
    758–759
  multifocal, 758, 758f
  neutron therapy for, 4020–4021
  pediatric, chemotherapy for, 3703
  prognosis for, 977–978
  proteoglycans in, 762–763
  radiation therapy for, 974–975
    high-dose, 4019, 4019t
    particle beam radiation in,
      4020–4021
    prognostic factors in, 4021, 4021t
  radiosensitization of, 4019–4020
  radiosurgery for, 758, 4063–4065, 4064t
  recurrent, 4103–4104, 4103t
  seizures in, 828
  spread of
    along basement membrane, 760,
      760f
    animal models of, 764–765
    anti-invasion therapy for, 765–766
    by cerebrospinal fluid, 760
    clinical patterns of, 757–758
    cytostatics for, 765–766
    experimental models for, 763–765
    mechanism of, 759–760, 760f
    molecular basis of, 760
    through white matter, 759–760
  surgery for, 972–974, 974f
  tenascin in, 761–762
  thrombospondin in, 762
  treatment of, 972–977
molecular biology of, 714–720
mutations in, 714–715
optic nerve, 309, 1373
  focal manifestations of, 831
  prechiasmatic, pediatric, 3596
optic pathway, pediatric, 3595–3599. *See
    also* Optic pathway glioma,
    pediatric.
proliferating cell nuclear antigen
    marking of, 693
proliferation markers for, 689–705, 690f,
    690t
  mitotic activity as, 689–692
  molecular, 692–696
signal transduction in, 715–716, 716f
surgery for
  complication avoidance in, 566–567,
    566t, 567t
  tumor removal in, 905
³H-thymidine marking of, 692
treatment of
  angiogenesis in, 720
  cell cycle arrest pathways in, 717f, 718
  invasion and, 720
  molecular targets for, 720, 721f
  programmed cell death in, 719
  signal transduction in, 716, 716f
usual types of, 981–994
vascular endothelial growth factor in,
    733
vascular endothelial growth factor
    receptors in, 733
ventricular, endoscopic treatment of,
    3429, 3429f

Hemosiderosis
  seizures from, 2314
  superficial cerebral, 2580
Hemostasis
  in cervical laminoforaminotomy, 4416
  in cervical laminoplasty, 4419
  in supratentorial arteriovenous
    malformation surgery, 2237
Hensen's node, 47, 4239, 4240f, 4241
Heparan sulfate proteoglycans, in
  malignant glioma, 762
Heparin
  in carotid endarterectomy, 1633–1634
  in cerebral venous thrombosis,
    1726–1727
  in deep venous thrombosis prevention,
    564
  in pregnancy, 2423
  in recurrent carotid artery stenosis,
    1662–1663
  spontaneous intracerebral hemorrhage
    with, 1735
Hepatitis
  neuropathy from, 3842
  transmission of, by allograft bone, 4617
Hepatocyte growth factor–scatter factor,
  773
Hepatolenticular degeneration, 2735
Hereditary motor and sensory neuropathy,
  imaging of, 536, 537f
Hereditary neuropathy, 3845–3846
  with liability to pressure palsy,
    3845–3846
Herniation syndromes, 290–292
  central, 826, 826t, 5055t, 5056
    rostral-caudal progression of, 292, 292f
  definition of, 291
  effects of, 293
  in brain tumors, 826–827, 826f, 826t
  intracranial pressure in, 183
  posterior (tectal), 5055t, 5056
  sites for, 5055, 5055t
  subfalcine (cingulate), 5055, 5055t
  tonsillar, 826t, 827, 5055t, 5056, 5091,
    5092f
    bullet wounds and, 5224
    in Chiari malformation type I, 3349,
      3350f
  transtentorial, 826
  treatment of, 827
  types of, 291t
  uncal, 826, 826t, 5055–5056, 5055t, 5091,
    5091f
    Duret's hemorrhage in, 5091, 5092f
Heroin
  blood-brain barrier transport of, 15
  spontaneous intracerebral hemorrhage
    from, 1735
Herpes simplex virus
  as central nervous system gene therapy
    vector, 4166–4167
  multiple sclerosis from, 1449
  mutant, cytopathic-oncolytic capability
    of, 822
Herpes simplex virus thymidine kinase
  gene, vector transfer of, 818–820, 819f,
    820f
Herpes zoster infection
  myelitis in, 4312–4313
  neuropathy from, 3841–3842
Herpesvirus B, myelitis from, 4311, 4312t
Herpesviruses
  as vectors, 818
  myelitis from, 4311, 4312t
Heschl's gyrus, 5, 6f, 14, 15f

HESX1, 53t
Heterotopia
  magnetic resonance imaging of, 2493,
    2493f
  periventricular, 61
  subcortical laminar, 61, 62f
Heterotopic nodules, 63, 63f
Heterotopic ossification, in brain injury
  rehabilitation, 5295
Heubner's artery, 22f
Hieron osteon, 5011
Hindbrain herniation
  in Chiari malformation, 3353–3354
  posterior fossa volume reduction and,
    3340
Hip dislocation/subluxation, in cerebral
  palsy, 3728
  after dorsal rhizotomy, 3744
Hippel-Lindau syndrome, 4302
Hippocampal sulcus, remnant of, magnetic
  resonance imaging of, 2495, 2495f
Hippocampal vein, 17
  longitudinal, 24f
  transverse, 1239
Hippocampectomy, 2607
Hippocampus, 7f, 8f, 9, 10f, 11, 12f, 15f,
  18f, 26f
  atrophy of, 2487, 2489
    as developmental abnormality, 2490
  gray matter structures of, 2486, 2487f
  long-term potentiation in, after
    traumatic brain injury, 2452, 2453f
  magnetic resonance imaging of,
    2486–2487, 2488f
  neuronal loss in, in post-traumatic
    epilepsy, 2449–2450, 2450f
  regions of, 2486, 2487f
  resection of, memory loss and, 2618
  sclerosis of
    magnetic resonance imaging of,
      2486–2487, 2487f–2490f, 2489–2491
    surgical algorithm for, 2490–2491,
      2490f
Hippus, 288
Histamine, release of, 2953, 2954f
Histiocytoma, fibrous, 1143
  orbital, 1375
Histiocytosis, Langerhans cell
  pediatric, 3591
  skull, 1400–1401, 1401f
    pediatric, 3719–3720, 3720f
  spinal, 4355, 4837, 4843, 4845f
    pediatric, 3567
Histiocytosis X, pediatric, 3591
  skull, 3719–3720, 3720f
History, 263–264
Histrionic personality, in traumatic brain
  injury response, 5193, 5193t
H-neu, 744
Hoarseness, 267
Hoffman reflex, 4410
Holoprosencephaly, 52, 56–57, 56f, 57f, 81
  alobar, 56
  middle interhemispheric variant of, 57
  semilobar, 56–57
Homeoboxes, 51
Homeodomain, 48, 51
Homeostasis, extracellular, maintenance of,
  228, 229f, 230
Homocystine, stroke risk in, 1617
Hook-rod construct
  lumbar, 4733, 4733f
    complication avoidance in, 582
    multiple hooks in, 4734, 4734f
  thoracic, 4969–4972, 4970f–4972f

Hooks
  sublaminar, 4971–4972, 4972f
  transverse, 4972, 4972f
Hormonal therapy, for meningioma,
  1110–1111
Hormones, in pregnancy, 2422
Horner's syndrome, 322, 323f, 5212
  avoidance of, in thoracic
    sympathectomy, 3099f, 3100f
  stellate ganglion block and, 2982
  thoracic endoscopic sympathectomy
    and, 3101
  vagus nerve stimulator implantation
    and, 2643
  vs. thoracic disk herniation, 4492
House/Brackman Scale for Facial Nerve,
  242t
Hox, 52, 53t, 3332
H-reflex, 3855, 3855f
HT7 antigen, 158
β-Human chorionic gonadotropin, in germ
  cell tumors, 1014, 1014t
Human herpesvirus type 6, multiple
  sclerosis from, 1449
Human immunodeficiency virus (HIV)
  in trauma, 5087
  transmission of, by allograft bone, 4617
Human immunodeficiency virus (HIV)
  infection
  in pediatric aneurysms, 3449, 3449f
  myelitis from, 4311, 4312t, 4313
  neuropathy from, 3841
  tuberculosis in, spinal, 4386–4387
  tuberculous spondylitis in, 4293–4294
Human immunodeficiency virus (HIV)
  testing, informed consent for, 409
Human leukocyte antigen (HLA) B27
  in ankylosing spondylitis, 4459
  in posterior longitudinal ligament
    ossification, 4476
Human T-cell lymphotropic virus type I
  multiple sclerosis from, 1449
  myelitis from, 4311, 4312t, 4313
Humerus
  fracture of
    radial nerve entrapment in, 3928
    shaking-impact syndrome and, 3502f
  supracondylar process of, median nerve
    entrapment by, 3924
Hunt & Hess, 242t
Hunt and Hess grade, 1509, 1509t
Hunter-Hurler syndrome, 4479
Huntington's disease, 2676–2677,
  2717–2718, 2736
  basal ganglia–thalamocortical circuit in,
    2718
  positron emission tomography of,
    2762–2764, 2763f
  substantia nigra pars compacta in, 2706f
Hyaluronate receptors, in malignant
  glioma, 763
Hyaluronic acid, in malignant glioma, 763
Hydatid disease, spinal, 4390
Hydrocephalus
  after giant arteriovenous malformation
    surgery, 2280
  after subarachnoid hemorrhage,
    1823–1824, 1823f, 1824f
  aneurysm rupture and, 1510, 1799
  classification of, 3146–3147
  historical aspects of, 3145–3153
  in achondroplasia, 3365–3366
  in Chiari malformation type II, 3350
  in choroid plexus tumors, 3613
  in Dandy-Walker syndrome, 3285–3286,
    3287f

Multiple endocrine neoplasia type 1
(MEN-1) syndrome, pituitary tumors
in, 1170
Multiple familial polyposis. *See* Turcot's
syndrome.
Multiple myeloma, 4296t, 4298
magnetic resonance imaging of, 532,
4852–4854, 4853f
skull, 1392–1393, 1393f
spinal, 1393, 1393f, 4356, 4356f, 4850,
4852–4854, 4853f
vs. plasmacytoma, 4808–4809
Multiple organ syndrome, polyneuropathy
in, 5132
Multiple sclerosis, 1449–1456
benign, 1451–1452
blood-brain barrier in, 164
clinical presentation of, 1451–1452
course of, 1451–1452
demyelinative myelitis in, 4314, 4314f
diagnosis of, 1452–1453
differential diagnosis of, 1453, 1453t,
1455
epidemiology of, 1449
genetic basis of, 1449
hyperacute, 1452
imaging of, 541, 543f, 1452–1453
immunopathogenesis of, 1449–1450
Marburg variant, 1452
pathology of, 1450–1451
primary progressive, 1451
prognosis of, 1452
relapsing-remitting, 1451
treatment of, 1454t–1455t, 1455–1456
vertigo in, 352, 2902
vs. brain tumor, 1450t
Multiple subpial transection, 2635–2641
anesthesia in, 2636
complications of, 2640, 2640t
electrocorticography in, 2636
historical aspects of, 2635
outcomes of, 2639–2640, 2639t
pathology of, 2638, 2639f
patient selection for, 2635–2636
principle of, 2635
seizure outcome after, 2578, 2640–2641
transections in, 2636, 2637f, 2638, 2638f
transector for, 2637, 2637f
Multiple system atrophy, 2703
akinetic-rigid form, 2708
cytoplasmic inclusions in, 2713–2714
neurodegeneration in, clinical subtypes
and, 2713–2714
pathogenesis of, 2714
positron emission tomography of, 2761
striatal neurons in, 2708
substantia nigra pars compacta in, 2706f
α-synuclein in, 2703
vs. Parkinson's disease, 2735
Muscimol, in intracerebral hemorrhage,
1740–1741
Muscle(s)
agonist, 2891
antagonist, 2891
asymmetry of, 3822, 3823f
biopsy of, 3963–3964
needle, 3964
open, 3964
disorders of, weakness in, 270
nociceptors of, 2921
progressive atrophy of, in lower motor
neuron degenerative disease, 4319
stretch of. *See* Stretch reflex.
synergistic, 2891

Muscle(s) (*Continued*)
testing of, in peripheral nerve disorders,
3822–3823, 3823f
ventral lumbar, 4705–4706, 4706f, 4707f
Muscle bulk, pediatric, assessment of, 3178
Muscle fiber action potential, spontaneous,
peripheral nervous system
abnormalities with, 3856, 3856t
Muscle fibers
complex repetitive discharges from, 3856
in spasticity, 2879–2880
Muscle lengthening, for cerebral palsy,
3732
Muscle relaxants, 1508
cerebrovascular effects of, in traumatic
brain injury, 5131–5132, 5132t
for failed back syndrome, 4337
for tracheal intubation, 557
in craniotomy, 5150
Muscle spindle, 2875–2876, 2876f, 3809,
3810f
Muscle strength, pediatric, assessment of,
3178–3179, 3178t
Muscle tone, pediatric, examination of,
3177–3178
Musculocutaneous nerve, entrapment of,
3933
Mutagenesis, 818
Mutism
after medulloblastoma surgery, 1038
akinetic, in frontal lobe tumors, 830
ependymoma surgery and, 3629
medulloblastoma surgery and, 1004,
3645–3646
transcallosal surgery and, 1258–1259
Myasthenia gravis
ion channels in, 225t
ocular, 323
pathology of, 3816
physical features of, 270
Myasthenic syndrome, 270
Mycobacterium tuberculosis, 1440
infectious aneurysms from, 2102
Mycoplasma pneumoniae, myelitis from,
4313
Mydriasis, pharmacologic, 322
Myelencephalon, in Chiari malformation
type II, 3352
Myelin, 86–87, 86f
central nervous system repair inhibition
by, 4168–4169
in axonal regeneration, 204
repair of, cellular transplantation in,
4164
Myelin internode, 86, 86f, 87, 88f
Myelin sheath, 3810, 3811f
Myelin-associated glycoprotein, inhibitory
activity of, 4169
Myelination, 63t, 64, 64t, 86–87, 86f
pediatric, 3462
Myelin-blocking antibodies, 4169
Myelitis
acute necrotizing, 4314
bacterial, 4312t, 4313
demyelinative, in multiple sclerosis,
4314, 4314f
epidural abscess in, 4313
fungal, 4312t, 4313
noninfectious inflammatory, 4313–4314,
4314f
parasitic, 4312t, 4313
postinfectious, 4313–4314
postvaccinal, 4313–4314
transverse, in multiple sclerosis, 1452
viral, 4311–4313, 4312t

Myelocele, spina bifida aperta with, 4316
Myelocystocele, 3224–3225, 3225f,
3280–3281, 3280f, 4316
anatomy in, 3225
epidemiology of, 3225
etiology of, 3226
history of, 3225
outcome of, 3226
pathogenesis of, 3225–3226
prenatal diagnosis of, 3226
terminal, 3215, 4267, 4268f
treatment of, 3226
Myelodysplasia, 3245
Myelography
computed tomography, of pyogenic
spinal infection, 4368, 4369f
spinal, 505–506
Myeloma globulin, in multiple myeloma,
4854
Myelomeningocele, 4256–4259, 4258f, 4259f
anatomy in, 3215–3216
Chiari malformation type II in, 3215,
3216f, 3217f, 3223–3224, 3351
chromosomal abnormalities in, 3219
differential diagnosis of, 3219
epidemiology of, 3217
etiology of, 3217–3219, 3218t
examples of, 3215, 3216f
historical aspects of, 3155, 3157f
history of, 3216
hydrocephalus in, 3216
latex allergy in, 3224
orthopedic consultation in, 3224
pathogenesis of, 3217
pediatric, 3215–3224
perinatal management of, 3220–3223,
3222f
prenatal counseling for, 3219–3220
prenatal diagnosis of, 3219
prognosis of, 3219–3220
sibling risk in, 3220
spina bifida aperta with, 4316
surgery for, 3221–3223, 3222f
complications of, 3223–3224
in neonates, 3194, 3194f
terminology for, 3215
Myelopathy
cervical, 4397
in rheumatoid arthritis, 4573
in cervical spondylosis. *See* Cervical
spondylotic myelopathy.
in perimedullary arteriovenous fistula,
2394
progressive
in conus medullaris arteriovenous
malformations, 2371f
in dural arteriovenous fistula,
2366–2367, 2367f
in intradural arteriovenous
malformations, 2370, 2370f
sensory patterns in, 272
spinal cord, radiation therapy and, 4046
Myelotomy, 3029
for spasticity, 2866t, 2870
Myerson's sign, 269
Myoblastoma, 3947t, 3948
Myocardial infarction, carotid
endarterectomy and, 1645
Myocardial ischemia
in subarachnoid hemorrhage, 1869
surgery and, 549–550
Myocardium, hypothermia effects on, 1533
Myoclonus, 2722, 2738, 2751
clinical manifestations of, 833
definition of, 2729

Myoclonus *(Continued)*
dystonia with, 2721
pediatric, assessment of, 3179–3180
segmental, 2722
Myoclonus-dystonia, 2737
Myofascial pain syndrome
in cerebral palsy, 3728
low back pain in, 4330, 4351
Myopathy
critical illness, 5131–5132, 5132f
in sarcoidosis, 1436
ion channel disorders in, 225t
weakness in, 270
Myosin light chain kinase, in cerebral
vasospasm, 1848
Myositis ossificans, 3947, 3947f, 3947t
Myotonia
ion channels in, 225t
pediatric, 3178
sodium channel, 225t
Myotonia congenita, ion channels in, 225t
Myxedema coma, treatment of, 293–294
Myxochondroma, 1365

N450K, in achondroplasia, 3362
Na-K-ATPase
in blood-brain barrier ion transport, 162
in neuronal potassium uptake, 228, 230
Nalidixic acid, pseudotumor cerebri from,
1423
Narcotics
for failed back syndrome, 4336
in craniotomy, 5150
in intracranial pressure management,
5127, 5127t
Nasal bone, in craniofacial trauma, 5262
Nasal cavity, complications in,
transsphenoidal surgery and, 569,
1182–1183
Nasoiniac line, 630–631, 631f
Nasopharynx
juvenile angiofibroma of, 1351–1359. *See
also* Angiofibroma, juvenile
nasopharyngeal.
squamous cell carcinoma of, 1398, 1399f
National Adult Reading Test, 5189
National Institutes of Health Stroke Scale,
242t, 1498, 1499t
Natriuresis, after subarachnoid
hemorrhage, 1829–1830
Natural history studies, 250–251
assessment of, 258
Nausea, 275
Neck
pain in
dorsal rhizotomy for, 3041–3042
hyperextension-hyperflexion injury
and, 4918
surgery for, 3025t
penetrating injuries to, 1670
trauma assessment of, 5088–5089
zones of, 1670, 1670f
Necrosis, 82–83
impending, 1601, 1601t
in astrocytoma, 835–836
in glioblastoma multiforme, 843f–844f,
844
in malignant phenotype, 771, 772f
radiation, in arteriovenous
malformation, 2195–2196, 2195f,
2196t
vs. apoptosis, 130–132, 131f
Necrotizing enterocolitis, after
myelomeningocele repair, 3223

Neglect, reporting obligations in, 411
Nelson's syndrome, 1199–1200
Neonates
emergency surgery on, 3193–3194, 3194t
vein of Galen malformation in, 3435,
3435f
Neoplasia, cranial destruction in, 430
Neoplastic meningitis, 1231–1234
Neovascularization, angiogenic-induced,
821–822
Nernst equation, 218, 3812
Nerve cell body, 72f, 73, 77–78
Nerve conduction, 86–87, 86f
Nerve conduction studies, 3851–3857
fundamentals of, 3851–3852, 3851f
F-wave in, 3855, 3855f
H-reflex in, 3855, 3855f
in carpal tunnel syndrome, 3857–3858
in peripheral nerve trauma, 3860, 3861
in radiculopathy, 3859
in ulnar neuropathy, 3858–3859
indications for, 3851
late responses in, 3855, 3855f
of compound muscle action potential,
3853–3855, 3854f
of sensory nerve action potential,
3852–3853, 3852f, 3853f
repetitive stimulation in, 3855–3856
Nerve fibers
myelinated, 3958–3960, 3960f
unmyelinated, 3960, 3960f
Nerve grafts, historical aspects of, 3803
Nerve growth factor, 195, 3805
after peripheral nerve injury, 3967
brain-derived, 197, 200
development and, 3975
in brain injury recovery, 5031
in central nervous system repair,
4165–4166
in distal nerve stump, 200
in inflammation, 2956
in nervous system regeneration, 4155
neurotropic function of, 4165
Nerve of Henle, 3898
Nerve of Kuntz, sectioning of, 3099f, 3100
Nerve plexus injury, 3969–3973
diagnosis of, 3970
severity of, 3970, 3971f
treatment of, 3970, 3972–3973,
3972f–3974f
Nerve roots
avulsion of, 3970, 3971f
pain in, 3821
cervical, inflammation of, 505f
disease involvement of, 271–272, 271f,
272f
in cervical laminoforaminotomy, 4416
intraoperative electrophysiologic
monitoring of, 4203–4204, 4216–4222
paresis of, after cervical laminectomy,
4425
selective injection of, 2975–2976
Nerve sheath tumor, 3941, 4296t, 4300,
4301f
benign, 3942–3946, 3943f–3945f, 3946t
surgical results for, 3945–3946, 3945f,
3946t
pediatric, 3714, 3714f
spinal cord, 4040, 4817–4818, 4818f
treatment of, 4822–4824
Nerve stump, distal
cellular responses in, 199–200
cytokines in, 200
extracellular matrix proteins in, 200
growth factors in, 200

Nerve stump *(Continued)*
neurotrophic factors in, 200
pathway specificity in, 200–201
prolonged denervation of, 201
regeneration in, 198–199
Nervous system
pattern formation in, 78, 79f
redundancy in, 3785
vicarious functioning in, 3785
Nervous system injury, functional
recovery after, 3784–3786
Neural blockade, 2970–2984
complications of, 2972
diagnostic, 2970, 2971t
fluoroscopy in, 2972–2974, 2973f, 2974f
limitations of, 2970–2972
risks of, 2972
standards for, 2972
therapeutic, 2970
training for, 2972
Neural cell transplantation, 93, 94f
Neural compression syndrome
decompressive surgery for, 4337
low back pain in, 4330–4331
reoperation for, 4339
Neural crest
fate of, 4255
formation of, 4243
Neural folds, fusion of, 4250–4251
Neural foramina, stenosis of, 515
osteophytes and, 509, 512f
Neural induction, 47
primary, 78
Neural placode, 3215, 3216f
Neural plate
bending of, 4248–4250, 4249f
shaping of, 4246, 4248, 4248f
Neural tube
formation of, 4243, 4244f
patterning of, 51, 51t
regionalization of, 50–51
segmentation of, 48, 48t, 50–51
Neural tube defect, 4256–4259, 4258f,
4259f. *See also* Myelomeningocele.
alpha fetoprotein screening for, 3219
anticonvulsants and, 3218
definition of, 3215
diabetes mellitus and, 3218–3219
folate deficiency and, 3217–3218
obesity and, 3219
open, folic acid deficiency and, 3257
risk factors for, 3218t
Neuralgia
cranial, 3018t
postherpetic, 2989t, 3842
dorsal rhizotomy for, 3041
mesencephalotomy for, 3077–3078
vs. trigeminal neuralgia, 2988
trigeminal. See Trigeminal neuralgia.
Neurapraxia
grading of, 3825–3826, 3825t
needle electromyography of, 3860–3861
nerve conduction studies of, 3860
Neuraxis, rostrocaudal and metameric
specification of, 4255–4256
Neurectomy, 3028
for trigeminal neuralgia, 3003
Neuregulins, in brain tumors, 727
Neurenteric cyst, 1226–1229, 3272–3273,
4263–4266, 4263f–4267f, 4317
at C1–2, 4813f, 4814
at craniovertebral junction, 4813f, 4814
imaging of, 535, 536f, 1227f–1228f,
1228–1229
vs. ependymal cyst, 1229

Prolactinoma, 1170
  clinical presentation of, 1185
  in pregnancy, 1188–1189
  laboratory studies for, 1185–1186
  macro-, 1185
    surgery for, 1188
  medical treatment of, 1186–1187
    in pregnancy, 1189
  micro-, 1185
    surgery for, 1187–1188
  radiation therapy for, 4036
  radiosurgery for, 4063
  surgery for, 1187–1189
    in pregnancy, 1189
    indications for, 1187, 1187t
    recurrence after, 1188
  tumor progression in, 1185
Proliferating cell nuclear antigen
  as tumor proliferation marker, 693–694
  in glioblastoma, 4097
  in meningioma, 1103, 1103f
Pronator syndrome, median nerve
    compression in, 3924–3925
Pronator teres muscle, median nerve
    entrapment at, 3924
Prone position, 597t, 600, 602–604, 602f
  complication avoidance in, 561–562
  dependent edema in, 563
  for craniotomy, 628–630, 629f
  in posterior cervical approach, 635–636
  orbital complications from, 576
Propionibacterium
  pyogenic spinal infections from, 4365
  shunt infection by, 3422–3423
Propofol, 1508
  cerebral physiology and, 551
  in craniotomy, 5149–5150
  in epilepsy surgery, 2621
  in ischemia protection, 1521
Proprioception
  pediatric, testing of, 3183–3184
  sensory nerve fibers in, 3809
Propriospinal multisynaptic ascending
    system, 2930
Proptosis, orbital tumors and, 1371
Prosencephalic vein, median, 3434
Prostaglandins
  in cerebral vasospasm, 1848–1849
  synthesis of, 2959
Prostate, transurethral resection of, for
    bladder outlet retention, 380
Prostatism, nocturia with, 365
Protease inhibitors, as angiogenesis
    antagonist, 776–777, 777t
Proteases
  in angiogenesis, 775t
  in apoptosis, 1519
  in axonal degeneration, 199
Protein
  as tumor antigens, 677
  phosphorylation of, in cell death, 127
  regulatory, in bone growth, 4614, 4614t
  synthesis of, in cell death, 132
Protein analysis, 752–753, 753f
Protein C, in cerebral venous thrombosis,
    1723
Protein kinase C system, in cerebral
    vasospasm, 1848
Protein truncation test, 753
Proteoglycans
  in axonal growth failure, 205
  in bone, 4230
  in malignant glioma, 762–763

Proton radiosurgery, 4123–4129
  evolving technology in, 4129
  historical perspective on, 4123
  physical principles of, 4123–4127,
    4124f–4126f
  technique of, 4128–4129
  treatment principles for, 4127–4128,
    4128f
  vs. linac radiosurgery, 4115–4116
Proto-oncogenes, 739
Protuberance, 29
Prourokinase, trials of, 1496
Psammoma bodies, 1101, 1101f
P-selectin, in cerebral ischemia, 140–141
Pseudallescheria boydii, infectious
    intracranial aneurysms from, 2102
Pseudarthrosis
  after scoliosis surgery, 4566
  complication avoidance in, 577
Pseudoaneurysms
  displacement artifact and, 1579f
  internal carotid artery, 1880, 1883f
  peripheral nerve involvement in, 3949
  traumatic, 2131, 5208, 5209f–5210f
    after débridement, 5237
Pseudobulbar palsy, medulloblastoma
    surgery and, 3645–3646
Pseudochondroplasia, atlantoaxial
    instability in, 3543
Pseudocoma, 293
Pseudoephedrine
  for bladder outlet incontinence, 380–381
  spontaneous intracerebral hemorrhage
    in, 1735
Pseudomeningocele
  brachial plexus injury with, 3491, 3491f
  cerebellar astrocytoma surgery and, 3659
  ependymoma surgery and, 3630
  postoperative, 564–565
  spinal surgery and, 574–576
Pseudomonas
  infectious aneurysms from, 2102
  pyogenic spinal infections from, 4365,
    4379f
Pseudoparkinsonism, arteriosclerotic,
    2716
Pseudopod, in craniopharyngioma, 3672,
    3672f
Pseudospondylolisthesis, 3580
Pseudotumor, orbital, 1376
Pseudotumor cerebri, 1419–1430
  causes of, 1419–1426
  cerebral venous drainage obstruction
    and, 1420–1422, 1424t
  clinical manifestations of, 1419,
    1420f–1423f
  complications of, 1426
  conversion from hydrocephalus to, 3400,
    3400f
  diagnosis of, 1426, 1427f, 1428
  endocrine dysfunction and, 1422, 1424t
  epidemiology of, 1419
  exogenous substances and, 1422–1425,
    1424t
  familial, 1426
  headache in, 1419
  imaging of, 1426, 1427f
  in pregnancy, 872–873
  lumbar puncture in, 1426
  metabolic dysfunction and, 1422, 1424t
  optic disk in, 1426, 1427f
  papilledema in, 1419, 1420f–1423f
  pathophysiology of, 1426
  systemic illness and, 1425–1426, 1425t

Pseudotumor cerebri (*Continued*)
  treatment of, 1429–1430
    during pregnancy, 1430
    venous hypertension and, 3398
Pseudoxanthoma elasticum, intracranial
    aneurysms in, 1773
Psuedopuberty, precocious, 1013
Psychiatric disorders
  after traumatic brain injury, 5296
  anterior capsulotomy for, 2859, 2859f
  anterior cingulotomy for, 2856–2857,
    2857f
  in epilepsy, 2573
  in failed back syndrome, 4337
  limbic leucotomy for, 2858–2859, 2858f
  neurosurgery for, 2853–2861
    anatomic basis for, 2854–2855
    approaches to, 2856–2861
    evaluation before, 2861
    historical perspective on, 2853–2854
    indications for, 2859–2860
    outcome in, 2860–2861
    patient selection in, 2855–2856
    repeat procedures in, 2860
    subcaudate tractotomy for, 2857–2858,
      2858f
Psychological disturbances
  after glomus jugulare tumor surgery,
    1308
  traumatic brain injury and, 5190–5191
  vs. multiple sclerosis, 1455
Psychological measurement, 385
Psychomotor function, after traumatic
    brain injury, 5188
Psychosocial problems, in achondroplasia,
    3363
Psychosocioeconomic syndrome, low back
    pain in, 4332
Psychosurgery, 2853
  politics of, 2660–2661
Ptc, 54t
PTCH/SMOH/SHH, 742–743
PTEN, in glioma, 716
PTEN/MMAC1/TEP1, 742
Pterion, 423–424, 423f
Ptosis, examination of, 266
Pudendal nerve, in lower urinary tract
    function, 362, 362f, 363f
Pulmonary edema
  in subarachnoid hemorrhage, 1826–1827,
    1869
  neurogenic, 1869
Pulmonary embolism, 563–564
Pulse repetition frequency, 1540
Pulvinar, thalamic, 10f, 11
Pumps, implantable
  complications of, 3140
  for intrathecal baclofen, 3749–3752,
    3749f, 3750f, 3753–3754
  for intrathecal drug infusion, 3136–3140,
    3137f–3139f
Pupil(s), 321–322, 322f, 323f
  abnormally large, 322, 322f
  abnormally small, 322, 323f
  dilation of, in brainstem lesions, 288,
    288f
  examination of, 266
  football, 288
  in bullet wounds, 5228, 5228t
  near-light dissociation of, 322
  oval, 288
  size of, 322
Pupillary defect, relative afferent, 302,
    304b

Pupillary response
  examination of, 265
  in Pediatric Coma Scale, 287–288, 288f
  pediatric, 3173
Pupillary sparing, relative, in oculomotor
    neuropathy, 321
Purkinje cell, 71, 72f
Pursuit tests, of vestibular function,
    345–346, 346f
Putamen, 7f, 12f, 2683
  arteriovenous malformation of, 2246
  fetal mesencephalic grafting in, 2836
  hemorrhage of, 1737, 1737f, 1746,
    1746f–1748f
Pyogenic infection, spinal, 4147, 4363–4382.
    See also specific infection.
  clinical presentation of, 4365–4366
  computed tomography of, 4366–4367,
    4367f
  conditions associated with, 4370–4371,
    4371f
  diagnosis of, 4366–4371, 4367f–4371f
  differential diagnosis of, 4371–4372
  epidemiology of, 4363–4364
  epidural, pain in, 4291, 4293, 4293f
  extraspinal manifestations of, 4371, 4371f
  laboratory findings in, 4366
  low back pain in, 4351–4352, 4351f,
    4352f
  magnetic resonance imaging of,
    4367–4368, 4368f, 4370f, 4379, 4380f
  medical management of, 4379, 4381
  microbiology of, 4365
    diagnostic, 4368–4369, 4370f
  myelography of, 4368, 4369f
  outcome of, 4381, 4382f
  pain in, 4290–4291, 4292f
  pathogenesis of, 4364–4365, 4365f
  pediatric, 4381–4382
  radiography of, 4366–4368, 4367f–4370f
  surgery for, 4372–4376, 4372f–4378f
  treatment of, 4372–4381, 4372f–4380f
Pyramid, 30f, 34
Pyramidal tract, in lower urinary tract
    function, 362
Pyrazinamide, for tuberculosis, 1441, 4387
Pyrexia, in extracranial head injury,
    5056–5057
Pyridostigmine, blood-brain barrier
    transport of, 14
Pyridoxine deficiency, neuropathy from,
    3844
Pyrimidines, halogenated, in malignant
    glioma radiosensitization, 4020
Pyruvate, in glucose metabolism, 1482,
    1483, 1484f

Quadrangular lobule, 30f, 31f
Quadrantanopsia, 2542f
Quadrigeminal cistern, cyst of, 3297–3298,
    3297f
Quadrigeminal plate, 36f, 3073
Quadrigeminal point, 21
Quadriplegia
  atlanto-occipital dislocation and,
    4928–4929
  midcervical, posterior fossa surgery and,
    555
  sitting position and, 615
  spastic, in cerebral palsy, 3724,
    3725–3727, 3729, 3731–3732,
    3747–3748

Quality-adjusted life-years, in epilepsy,
    2567, 2568f

R248C, in achondroplasia, 3362–3363
Rabies virus, myelitis from, 4311, 4312t
Race
  in bullet wounds, 5224t, 5225
  in intracranial hematoma, 5072
Rad, 4007
Radial glial cells, 61
Radial glial fibers
  disruption of, 63, 63f
  in neuroblast migration, 58, 59f
Radial nerve
  entrapment of, 3928–3930
    above elbow, 3929
  superficial sensory branch of,
    entrapment of, 3930
Radial tunnel syndrome, 3928
  magnetic resonance imaging of, 3882,
    3882f
Radial veins, 2381
Radiation
  absorbed dose of, 4006–4007
  biologic effects of, 4006, 4006f, 4007
  brain tumors and, 809–810
  carotid artery stenosis from, 1685–1687,
    1686f
  direct action of, 3999, 4006
  DNA interactions with, 3999
  effects of, 853–854
  high linear energy transfer beams in,
    4006, 4006f
  in spinal fusion healing, 4620
  indirect action of, 4006
  ionizing, 3999
  meningioma from, 1105, 1105f
  myelopathy from, familial spastic
    paraplegia in, 4319
  photon beam, 4007
  units of, 4007
  water interactions with, 3999
Radiation injury
  blood-brain barrier in, 166
  in arteriovenous malformation
    radiosurgery, 4082–4083
Radiation necrosis, after arteriovenous
    malformation radiation therapy,
    2195–2196, 2195f, 2196t
Radiation survival curve, radiosensitizer
    effect on, 4001, 4003f
Radiation therapy, 3989–3990, 4005–4012.
    See also Brachytherapy.
  additive quality of, 4001
  automation in, 4012
  buildup region in, 4001, 4002f
  clinical target volume in, 4011
  complications of, 4024
  Compton effect in, 4006, 4006f
  conformal, 4002–4003
  depth-dose analysis in, 4008
  depth-dose curves in, 4008, 4008f
  differential cell repair in, 4000
  dose in, 4000
  dose-volume histogram in, 4011, 4012f
  external beam, 4007–4008
  falloff region in, 4001, 4002f
  for benign skull base tumors, 4027–4030
  for brain metastases, 4015–4018
  for brain tumors, 659–660
  for malignant brain tumors, 4015–4024
  for pituitary tumors, 4033–4036
  for spinal cord tumors, 4042–4047

Radiation therapy (*Continued*)
  fractionated, 3999–4001, 4000f
  gross tumor volume in, 4011, 4011f
  heavy particle, 4008
  historical aspects of, 3989–3990
  hyperfractionation in, 4001
  intensity-modulated, 4012, 4142–4143
  interactions in, 4005–4006, 4006f
  isocenter in, 4000
  linear accelerators in, 4007–4008, 4007f,
    4008f
  multileaf collimators in, 4012
  pair production in, 4005–4006
  photoelectric effect in, 4005
  physics of, 4005
  planning target volume in, 4011
  prior, radiosurgical dose prescription
    effect of, 4054
  radiobiology in, 3999–4003
  side effects of, 4036
  simulation in, 4000, 4010, 4010f
  stereotactic. *See also* Radiosurgery.
    beam delivery systems for, 4138–4139
    fractionated, 4136, 4138, 4138f
      linacs for, 4115
    radiobiology of, 4002–4003
  target volume definitions in, 4011, 4011f
  treatment planning in, 4008–4009, 4009f
    computers in, 4010
    contouring in, 4010
    imaging in, 4009–4010, 4010f
    three-dimensional, 4010–4011, 4011f
  triangulation in, 4000
  types of, 4007–4008, 4007f, 4008f
  vs. stereotactic radiosurgery, 4012
Radical glial, 84
Radicular artery, 2381
  spinal nerve root and, 3033–3034
Radiculopathy
  cervical, 4396–4397
    surgery for, 4399–4400, 4399f, 4400f
    treatment of, 4412–4413, 4427
  diabetic, 3843
  electrodiagnostic studies of, 3859
  in spinal stenosis, 4521
  lower extremity, 4328
  lumbar, 4329
  upper extremity, signs/symptoms of,
    272t
Radiobiology, 3999–4003
Radiography
  skull, 419–422, 420f–422f
  spinal, 500–501, 500f, 501f, 4145–4146
Radioisotopes, positron-emitting, 477–479,
    478f, 478t
Radiolabeled compounds, in positron
    emission tomography, 480, 481t
Radiologic features, of central nervous
    system tumors, 835–854
Radionuclide imaging
  of pyogenic spinal infection, 4368, 4369f
  of spinal metastases, 4858
  of spinal tumors, 4836
    osteoid osteoma, 4837, 4838f
Radiosurgery, 4053–4069, 4131. *See also*
    under Stereotactic.
  adjuvant, 4053
  circular collimators in, 4139, 4139f, 4140f
  complications from, 2280
  dose planning for, 4054, 4076,
    4134–4136, 4135f–4137f
  extracranial, 4069, 4143
  for arteriovenous malformations,
    4073–4085
  for brain metastases, 4065–4068, 4066t,
    4067f, 4095, 4114